Dietary Reference Intakes (DRIs): Recommended Intakes for Individuals, Elements

Food and Nutrition Board, Institute of Medicine, National Academies

Life Stage Group	Calcium (mg/d)	Chromium (µg/d)	Copper (µg/d)	Fluoride (mg/d)	Iodine (µg/d)	Iron (mg/d)	Magnesium (mg/d)	Manganese (mg/d)	Molybdenum (µg/d)	Phosphorus (mg/d)	Selenium (µg/d)	Zinc (mg/d)
Infants												
0–6 mo	210*	0.2*	200*	0.01*	110*	0.27*	30*	0.003*	2*	100*	15*	2*
7–12 mo	270*	5.5*	220*	0.5*	130*	11	75*	0.6*	3*	275*	20*	3
Children												
1–3 y	500*	11*	340	0.7*	90	7	80	1.2*	17	460	20	3
4–8 y	800*	15*	440	1*	90	10	130	1.5*	22	500	30	5
Males												
9–13 y	1,300*	25*	700	2*	120	8	240	1.9*	34	1,250	40	8
14–18 y	1,300*	35*	890	3*	150	11	410	2.2*	43	1,250	55	11
19–30 y	1,000*	35*	900	4*	150	8	400	2.3*	45	700	55	11
31–50 y	1,000*	35*	900	4*	150	8	420	2.3*	45	700	55	11
51–70 y	1,200*	30*	900	4*	150	8	420	2.3*	45	700	55	11
>70 y	1,200*	30*	900	4*	150	8	420	2.3*	45	700	55	11
Females												
9–13 y	1,300*	21*	700	2*	120	8	240	1.6*	34	1,250	40	8
14–18 y	1,300*	24*	890	3*	150	15	360	1.6*	43	1,250	55	9
19–30 y	1,000*	25*	900	3*	150	18	310	1.8*	45	700	55	8
31–50 y	1,000*	25*	900	3*	150	18	320	1.8*	45	700	55	8
51–70 y	1,200*	20*	900	3*	150	8	320	1.8*	45	700	55	8
>70 y	1,200*	20*	900	3*	150	8	320	1.8*	45	700	55	8
Pregnancy												
≤18 y	1,300*	29*	1,000	3*	220	27	400	2.0*	50	1,250	60	12
19–30 y	1,000*	30*	1,000	3*	220	27	350	2.0*	50	700	60	11
31–50 y	1,000*	30*	1,000	3*	220	27	360	2.0*	50	700	60	11
Lactation												
≤18 y	1,300*	44*	1,300	3*	290	10	360	2.6*	50	1,250	70	13
19–30 y	1,000*	45*	1,300	3*	290	9	310	2.6*	50	700	70	12
31–50 y	1,000*	45*	1,300	3*	290	9	320	2.6*	50	700	70	12

NOTE: This table presents Recommended Dietary Allowances (RDAs) in **bold type** and Adequate Intakes (AIs) in ordinary type followed by an asterisk (*). RDAs and AIs may both be used as goals for individual intake. RDAs are set to meet the needs of almost all (97 to 98 percent) individuals in a group. For healthy breastfed infants, the AI is the mean intake. The AI for other life stage and gender groups is believed to cover all individuals in the group, but lack of data or uncertainty in the data prevent being able to specify with confidence the percentage of individuals covered by this intake.

SOURCES: Dietary Reference Intakes for Calcium, Phosphorus, Magnesium, Vitamin D, and Fluoride (1997); Dietary Reference Intakes for Thiamin, Riboflavin, Niacin, Vitamin B-6, Folate, Vitamin B-12, Pantothenic Acid, Biotin, and Choline (1998); Dietary Reference Intakes for Vitamin C, Vitamin E, Selenium, and Carotenoids (2000); and Dietary Reference Intakes for Vitamin A, Vitamin K, Arsenic, Boron, Chromium, Copper, Iodine, Iron, Manganese, Molybdenum, Nickel, Silicon, Vanadium, and Zinc (2001). These reports may be accessed via www.nap.edu.

Dietary Reference Intakes (DRIs): Recommended Intakes for Individuals, Macronutrients
Food and Nutrition Board, Institute of Medicine, National Academies

Life Stage Group	Carbohydrate (g/d)	Total Fiber (g/d)	Fat (g/d)	Linoleic Acid (g/d)	α-Linolenic Acid (g/d)	Protein[a] (g/d)
Infants						
0–6 mo	60*	ND	31*	4.4*	0.5*	9.1*
7–12 mo	95*	ND	30*	4.6*	0.5*	**13.5**
Children						
1–3 y	**130**	19*	ND[b]	7*	0.7*	**13**
4–8 y	**130**	25*	ND	10*	0.9*	**19**
Males						
9–13 y	**130**	31*	ND	12*	1.2*	**34**
14–18 y	**130**	38*	ND	16*	1.6*	**52**
19–30 y	**130**	38*	ND	17*	1.6*	**56**
31–50 y	**130**	38*	ND	17*	1.6*	**56**
51–70 y	**130**	30*	ND	14*	1.6*	**56**
>70 y	**130**	30*	ND	14*	1.6*	**56**
Females						
9–13 y	**130**	26*	ND	10*	1.0*	**34**
14–18 y	**130**	26*	ND	11*	1.1*	**46**
19–30 y	**130**	25*	ND	12*	1.1*	**46**
31–50 y	**130**	25*	ND	12*	1.1*	**46**
51–70 y	**130**	21*	ND	11*	1.1*	**46**
>70 y	**130**	21*	ND	11*	1.1*	**46**
Pregnancy						
14–18 y	**175**	28*	ND	13*	1.4*	**71**
19–30 y	**175**	28*	ND	13*	1.4*	**71**
31–50 y	**175**	28*	ND	13*	1.4*	**71**
Lactation						
14–18 y	**210**	29*	ND	13*	1.3*	**71**
19–30 y	**210**	29*	ND	13*	1.3*	**71**
31–50 y	**210**	29*	ND	13*	1.3*	**71**

NOTE: This table presents Recommended Dietary Allowances (RDAs) in **bold type** and Adequate Intakes (AIs) in ordinary type followed by an asterisk (*). RDAs and AIs may both be used as goals for individual intake. RDAs are set to meet the needs of almost all (97 to 98 percent) individuals in a group. For healthy breastfed infants, the AI is the mean intake. The AI for other life stage and gender groups is believed to cover needs of all individuals in the group, but lack of data or uncertainty in the data prevent being able to specify with confidence the percentage of individuals covered by this intake.

[a]Based on 0.8g protein/kg body weight for reference body weight.

[b]ND = not determinable at this time

SOURCES: Dietary Reference Intakes for Energy, Carbohydrate, Fiber, Fat, Fatty Acids, Cholesterol, Protein, and Amino Acids (2002). This report may be accessed via www.nap.edu.

SEVENTH EDITION

PERSPECTIVES IN

NUTRITION

Gordon M. Wardlaw
Ph.D., R.D.

Formerly Adjunct Associate Professor, Department of Human Nutrition
The Ohio State University

Jeffrey S. Hampl
Ph.D., R.D.

Associate Professor, Department of Nutrition
Arizona State University

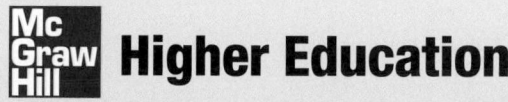

Boston Burr Ridge, IL Dubuque, IA New York San Francisco St. Louis
Bangkok Bogotá Caracas Kuala Lumpur Lisbon London Madrid Mexico City
Milan Montreal New Delhi Santiago Seoul Singapore Sydney Taipei Toronto

The McGraw·Hill Companies

 Higher Education

PERSPECTIVES IN NUTRITION, SEVENTH EDITION

Published by McGraw-Hill, a business unit of The McGraw-Hill Companies, Inc., 1221 Avenue of the Americas, New York, NY 10020. Copyright © 2007 by The McGraw-Hill Companies, Inc. All rights reserved. No part of this publication may be reproduced or distributed in any form or by any means, or stored in a database or retrieval system, without the prior written consent of The McGraw-Hill Companies, Inc., including, but not limited to, in any network or other electronic storage or transmission, or broadcast for distance learning.

Some ancillaries, including electronic and print components, may not be available to customers outside the United States.

 This book is printed on recycled, acid-free paper containing 10% postconsumer waste.

1 2 3 4 5 6 7 8 9 0 DOW/DOW 0 9 8 7 6

ISBN-13 978–0–07–282750–7
ISBN-10 0–07–282750–5

Publisher: *Colin H. Wheatley*
Senior Developmental Editor: *Lynne M. Meyers*
Marketing Manager: *Tami Petsche*
Lead Project Manager: *Peggy J. Selle*
Senior Production Supervisor: *Kara Kudronowicz*
Senior Media Project Manager: *Tammy Juran*
Media Producer: *Daniel M. Wallace*
Designer: *Rick D. Noel*
Cover Designer: *Ellen Pettengell*
(USE) Cover Image: *©Getty Images, Strawberry with Cream Splash, Lew Robertson*
Senior Photo Researcher: *John C. Leland*
Photo Research: *Mary Reeg*
Supplement Producer: *Tracy L. Konrardy*
Compositor: *Carlisle Publishing Services*
Typeface: *10/12 Galliard*
Printer: *R.R. Donnelley Willard, OH*

The credits section for this book begins on page C-1 and is considered an extension of the copyright page.

Library of Congress Cataloging-in-Publication Data

Wardlaw, Gordon M.
  Perspectives in nutrition / Gordon M. Wardlaw, Jeffrey S. Hampl.—7th ed.
    p.   cm.
  Includes bibliographical references and index.
  ISBN 978–0–07–282750–7—ISBN 0–07–282750–5 (hard copy : alk. paper)
  1. Nutrition. I. Hampl, Jeffrey S. II. Title.

QP141.W38   2007
612.3—dc22   2006009096
                                          CIP

www.mhhe.com

brief contents

contents

PART ONE   NUTRITION BASICS 1

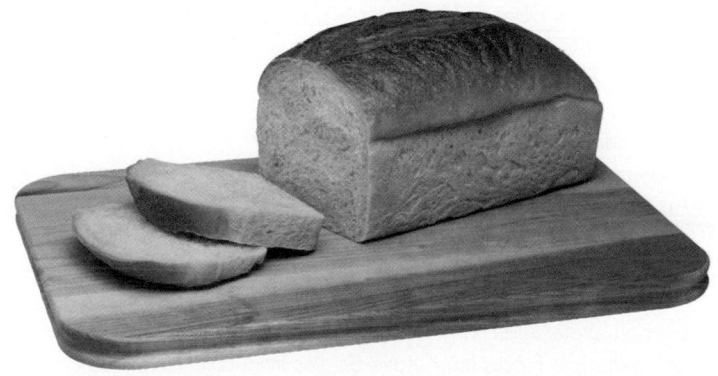

PART TWO THE ENERGY-YIELDING NUTRIENTS AND ALCOHOL 149

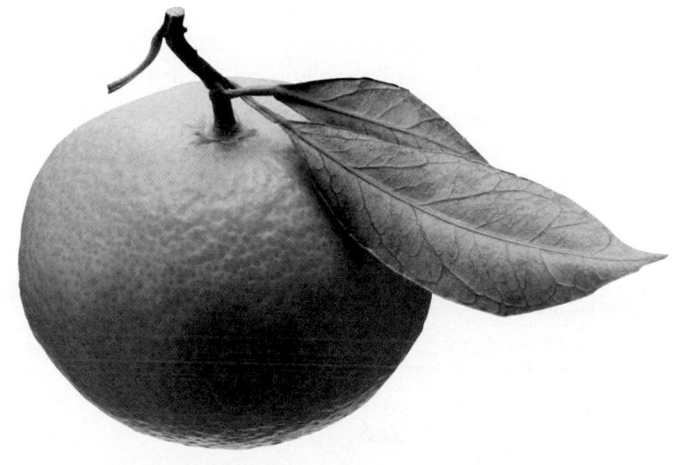

PART THREE THE VITAMINS AND MINERALS 295

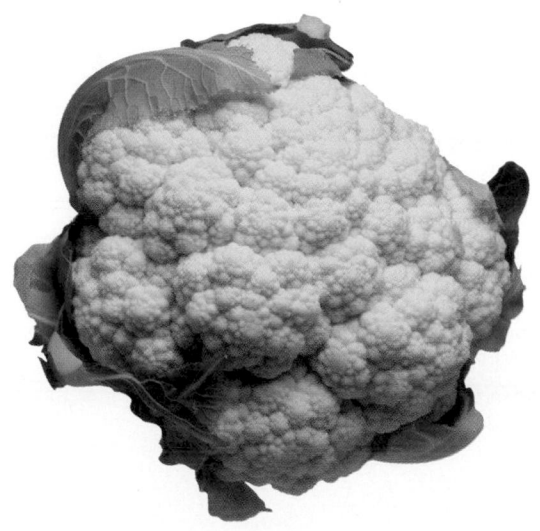

PART FOUR ENERGY BALANCE AND IMBALANCE 465

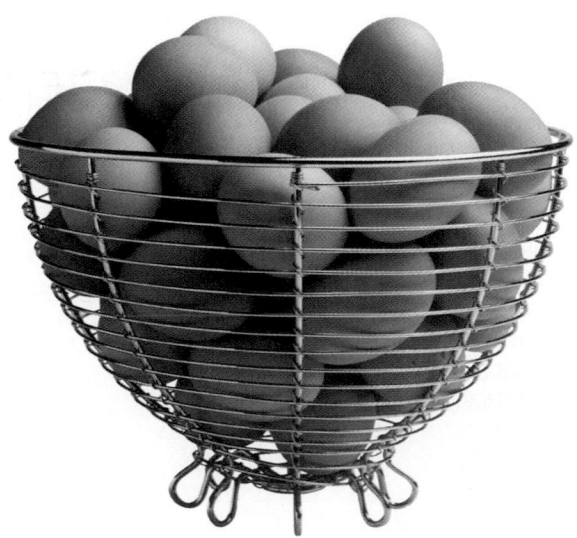

PART FIVE   NUTRITION APPLICATIONS IN THE LIFE CYCLE 581

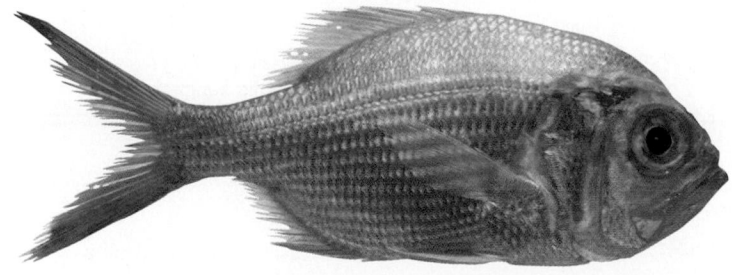

PART SIX PUTTING NUTRITION KNOWLEDGE INTO PRACTICE 689

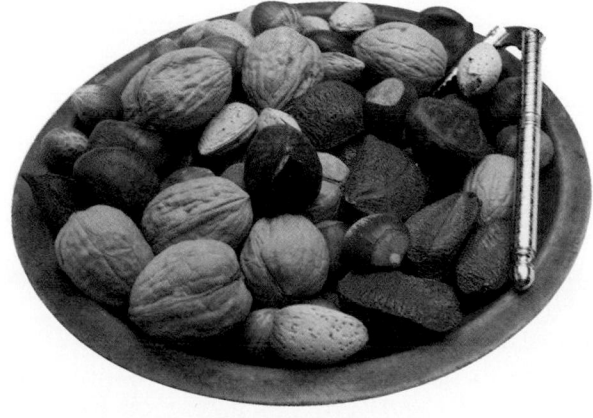

about the authors

Gordon M. Wardlaw, Ph.D., R.D., most recently taught introductory nutrition courses to students in the Department of Human Nutrition at The Ohio State University. He has recently retired from teaching, but remains active in the field. Dr. Wardlaw is the author of many articles that have appeared in prominent nutrition, biology, physiology, and biochemistry journals and was the 1985 recipient of the American Dietetic Association's Mary P. Huddleson Award. Dr. Wardlaw is a member of the American Dietetic Association, member of the American Society for Nutritional Sciences and is certified as a Specialist in Human Nutrition by the American Board of Nutrition.

Jeffrey S. Hampl, Ph.D., R.D., teaches coursework in public health nutrition in the Department of Nutrition at Arizona State University. Prior to his university appointment, Dr. Hampl worked as a nutritionist with the Special Supplemental Nutrition Program for Women, Infants, and Children (WIC) and as an outpatient dietitian in a major medical center. Dr. Hampl's research, which has been funded by the U.S. Department of Agriculture and the State of Arizona, focuses on the nutritional status of resource-constrained children and their families, and he has published articles in leading nutrition and medical journals. The winner of the 2002 Dannon Award for Excellence in Community Nutrition, Dr. Hampl is a member of the American Dietetic Association, the American Public Health Association, and the American Society for Nutritional Sciences. He is also a spokesperson for the American Dietetic Association and was the lead author for the Association's position paper on disease prevention and health promotion.

preface

TO THE INSTRUCTOR

Because you teach nutrition, you undoubtedly find it a fascinating and challenging subject. You probably also find that teaching nutrition is a challenge in and of itself. Claims and counterclaims abound regarding the need for certain dietary components. For example, one group of researchers promotes a reduction in salt intake for the general population as a means of preventing hypertension. Other researchers assert that despite excess salt intakes, most North Americans maintain normal blood pressure values. This apparent dichotomy only adds to the challenge of teaching in a rapidly changing field.

As textbook authors, we understand the importance of providing accurate, balanced, and up-to-date coverage of nutrition topics, particularly those that are controversial. To provide students with a sound introduction to the study of nutrition, we draw on as many reliable sources as possible. This seventh edition of *Perspectives in Nutrition* reflects new material from the recently published Dietary Reference Intakes by the Food and Nutrition Board, articles in major nutrition and medical journals and leading nutrition and health newsletters, and chapters in *Modern Nutrition in Health and Disease*, edited by Maurice Shils and his colleagues. We constantly scour the literature with the goal of providing clear and balanced perspectives on recent research so that you and your students can better understand and participate in the debates of current nutrition issues.

Personalized Approach to Nutrition

A prominent theme in nutrition today is *individuality*. Nutrition advice is not a one-size-fits-all proposition. For example, not all people find that saturated fat in their diet raises their blood cholesterol values above recommended standards. Individuals respond differently, often idiosyncratically, to certain nutrients. The goal of understanding how nutrients affect people as individuals is a key objective of this text.

Moreover, even at this introductory level, we do not assume that all nutrition students are alike. We incorporate opportunities, such as the Take Action activities, for students to learn more about their own health and nutrition. In this way, students can apply the knowledge they gain to improve their health. Throughout the chapters, we strive for the same objective as many of our colleagues, to educate students to become judicious consumers of both food and nutrition information. We seek to help students sort through the wealth of nutrition information and misinformation available to them. This text is designed to help them better understand and evaluate the nutrition information they encounter on cereal box labels, articles in popular magazines, nutrition- and diet-related websites, guidelines issued by government agencies, and more.

Once students have achieved a solid working knowledge of nutrition, our goal is to assist them in assessing their personal nutrition needs rather than strictly adhering to every guideline issued for an entire population. After all, a population by definition includes a scope of varying genetic and cultural backgrounds along with varying responses to diet.

As a final note, we know that students often come to this course with many preconceptions and questions about nutrition "hot topics." To address students' concerns, we have included coverage of topics that touch their lives: eating disorders, nutritional supplements, phytochemicals, vegetarianism, diets for athletes, popular (fad) diets, and complementary and alternative medical practices. (See the Chapter Highlights section of this preface for examples.) Regardless of the topic, the overall emphasis remains the same—the importance of understanding one's food choices and diet practices to best meet personal needs.

Intended Audience

We have developed this book with nutrition and science majors in mind. The chemistry, biochemistry, and physiology presented in the text assume that students have had at least some college-level science. Because this course often attracts students from a fairly broad range of majors, we have been careful to include examples and explanations that are relevant to nutrition, health education, human ecology, human performance, nursing, and other health-related majors. For students who wish to learn more or need assistance with the science involved in metabolism and body systems, additional information can be found in Appendix A, Chemistry: A Tool for Understanding Nutrition and Appendix C, Human Physiology: A Tool for Understanding Nutrition.

Key Revisions to the Seventh Edition

Creating a textbook is a dynamic process. Rather than simply updating facts and numbers with each new edition, we seek to be responsive to changing instructor and student needs. We challenge ourselves to take a fresh look at each new edition to find ways to refine and improve the book and make it a better teaching tool all around. Many of the new features in the seventh edition are a direct result of feedback we have received from instructors. Their advice on the level and presentation of science has been invaluable. We have also learned a great deal from the students in the courses we teach. Their feedback can be seen in improved illustrations and clearer discussions of difficult concepts.

Up-to-Date Nutrient Guidelines

A major component of this revision involves the continual updating of data and discussions related to the latest Dietary Reference Intakes. Chapter content has also been rewritten throughout to reflect advice provided by MyPyramid and the 2005 Dietary Guidelines for Americans.

Improved Science Coverage

Throughout the book are many dynamic new illustrations that will help students grasp important scientific concepts with greater clarity. Chapters 3 and 4 contain many new digestion and metabolism diagrams. Complex subjects such as glycolysis and the citric acid cycle have been reinterpreted with color and number sequencing to help students comprehend the steps involved in these processes.

Content Reorganization

Take Action activities are no longer specifically tied to a detailed diet analysis early in the course. Not having students create a detailed diet analysis in Chapter 2 allows you to assign a diet analysis project at any time in the course.

The Nutrition Perspective boxes at the end of the chapters have been moved into the main chapter discussion. They have been shortened and renamed Nutrition Focus to indicate the change. Some older essays have been replaced or relocated (see Contents for details).

Chapter Highlights

The following is a list of some of the key changes, updates, and enhancements that have been incorporated into the seventh edition chapters.

Chapter 1 What Nourishes You?

New Figure 1-1 on two views of macronutrients and new Figure 1-2 on the proportion of nutrients in the human body more clearly convey these important concepts.

Previous table on the benefits and risks of diet habits has been converted into Figure 1-5.

New Figure 1-6 on the scientific method now uses as an example the efficacy of the Atkins diet.

New Expert Opinion by Dr. Robert DiSilvestro discusses the use of research methods to answer the question of whether calcium intake influences weight regulation.

New Figure 1-8 shows an herbal supplement label to illustrate the FDA disclaimer on such products.

Chapter 2 The Basis of a Healthy Diet

New Expert Opinion by Dr. Barbara Rolls discusses energy density.

Figure 2-1 on nutrient density has been revised to include equal volume comparisons.

Chapter content on the MyPyramid and the 2005 Dietary Guidelines for Americans was totally rewritten to reflect the latest government advice. MyPyramid is introduced and all its components are discussed, including discretionary calories.

The 2005 Dietary Guidelines for Americans have been summarized into three major points in the chapter content. The full list of 41 guidelines is detailed in new Figure 2-8.

New Figure 2-9 represents a summary of the key information contained on a Nutrition Facts panel. This figure is part of the new Nutrition Focus feature on food labeling.

Chapter 3 Human Digestion and Absorption

Figure 3-4 has been redrawn to be a more realistic and thorough representation of the oral cavity and salivary glands.

Figure 3-5, process of swallowing; Figure 3-7, anatomy of the stomach; Figure 3-11, peristalsis; and Figure 3-13, small intestine, have all been redrawn for realism and clarity.

New Figure 3-10 illustrates the location of sphincters in the GI tract.

New Figure 3-15 shows blood circulation in the body.

New photo shows close-up of villi.

New Figure 3-18 tracks fluid intake and fluid loss in the body.

Nutrition Focus box now includes discussion and photos of gallstones, ulcers, and reflux disease damage.

Chapter 4 Metabolism

New chapter opening scenario presents a familiar situation that college students can more easily identify with.

First half of the chapter has been rewritten with the help of Dr. Eugene J. Fenster. His input simplified and clarified the challenging nature of this content.

Every figure in this chapter is either new or completely redrawn in order to help students better understand metabolism. (More detailed views of metabolic pathways can still be found in Appendix B.)

New figures more clearly show anabolism and catabolism (Figure 4-1); the stages of metabolism (Figure 4-2); end result of citric acid cycle metabolism (Figure 4-8); anaerobic metabolism (Figure 4-12); (lipolysis (Figure 4-13); beta-oxidation of fatty acids (Figure 4-14); ketosis (Figure 4-15); metabolism during feasting (Figure 4-21); and metabolism during fasting (Figure 4-22).

New Expert Opinion by Dr. Andrea Buchholtz and Dr. Dale Schoeller explores the concept of metabolic advantage for certain dietary patterns.

Chapter 5 Carbohydrates

New Expert Opinion on the health effects of fiber written by Dr. Joanne Slavin.

The latest diabetes medications and polycystic ovary syndrome are discussed in the Nutrition Focus feature on blood glucose regulation.

Tagatose is mentioned as a new alternative sweetener and is added to Figure 5-13, which shows the chemical structures of alternative sweeteners.

Recommendations for carbohydrate intake from the 2005 Dietary Guidelines for Americans are highlighted in a margin note.

Chapter 6 Lipids

Figure 6-3 on the fatty acid content of various foods has been redrawn in an easier-to-understand format. The same is true for Figure 6-8 on emulsifiers.

New Figure 6-6 on the classes of eicosanoids has been added.

Figure 6-10, fat absorption, and Figure 6-12, lipoprotein interactions, have been redrawn to include numbered sequences to assist students in navigating the steps in each process.

New Table 6-3 summarizes the roles of the various lipoproteins in the body.

New Expert Opinion by Dr. Bernhard Hennig explores the etiology of atherosclerosis.

Recommendations for fat intake from the 2005 Dietary Guidelines for Americans are featured in a margin note.

New Table 6-5 shows the *trans* fat content of common foods.

Chapter 7 Proteins

The discussion of protein turnover was moved to a more relevant position in the middle of the chapter.

Improved Figure 7-2 more clearly provides an overview of protein synthesis.

Recent findings of the ability of protein to lead to a state of satiety are mentioned.

The discussion of soy has been rewritten to reflect the generally negative results of recent intervention trials regarding soy and bone health, cholesterol-lowering ability, and treatment of menopausal symptoms.

The discussion of the evaluation of protein quality has been simplified.

Chapter 8 Alcohol

Improved Figure 8-1 more clearly demonstrates blood alcohol concentrations.

Redesigned Figure 8-3 summarizes the effects of alcohol abuse on the body.

Photo of a liver affected by cirrhosis has been added.

Recommendations for alcohol intake from the 2005 Dietary Guidelines for Americans are listed in a margin note.

Brief mention of the new medication acamprosate (Campral) has been added.

Chapter 9 The Fat-Soluble Vitamins

Figure 9-3 has been revised to better show the metabolism of vitamin A.

New Figure 9-5 demonstrates the effects of macular degeneration on vision.

Figure 9-6 now provides a clearer representation of vitamin D metabolism.

New Expert Opinion by Dr. Michael Holick on the importance of vitamin D has been added.

New Figure 9-12 summarizes the various antioxidant systems and compounds in the body.

Figure 9-13 on vitamin K metabolism has been simplified.

New Figure 9-14 explores a logical approach to supplement use.

Chapter 10 The Water-Soluble Vitamins

Homocysteine discussion has been simplified throughout the chapter. (Appendix B now contains the complete homocysteine pathway.)

Improved Figure 10-7 now shows a more realistic case of spina bifida.

Food sources of choline are featured in a margin table.

New Expert Opinion by Dr. Mark Levine and Dr. Sebastian Padayatty delves into the functions of vitamin C.

New Figure 10-11 summarizes the roles of vitamins in the body based on specific cell functions.

Chapter 11 Water and the Major Minerals

Improved Figure 11-1 provides a better visual comparison of water compartments in the body.

The osmosis discussion has been simplified and is accompanied by improved Figure 11-2.

New Figure 11-3 walks students through the steps involved in sodium flux across the cell membrane.

Water content of various foods is featured in a new margin table.

Figure 11-4 has been updated to reflect the new DRIs for water.

The hormonal regulation of blood pressure has been split into two figures to make the content easier to grasp (now Figure 11-5 and Figure 11-6).

DRIs for sodium, potassium, and chloride throughout chapter discussions have been updated.

New Expert Opinion by Dr. Marlene Most provides insights into the DASH diet.

New Figure 11-9 shows the various sites of influence on calcium balance in the body.

Latest methods for diagnosing osteoporosis and latest medications used to treat the disease are discussed.

New Figure 11-5 shows how bone density differs during a person's lifetime and why preventing severe bone loss is important.

Chapter 12 Trace Minerals

Figure 12-1 on iron metabolism has been improved.

New Table 12-2 on the factors that affect zinc absorption has been added.

Redrawn Figure 12-5 better guides students through selenium metabolism.

New photo shows mottling of teeth from excess fluoride exposure.

New Figure 12-7 summarizes the roles of minerals in the body based on specific cell functions.

The Nutrition Focus feature that looks at cancer has been moved to this chapter (previously in Chapter 10).

Chapter 13 Energy Balance and Imbalance

New statistics on the growing problem of overweight in society are added as a margin note.

Clearer discussion of basal metabolism has been provided.

Latest estimates for energy needs from MyPyramid are listed.

New Expert Opinion by Dr. Peter Havel discusses hormones and other factors that affect satiety.

Figure 13-18 has been redrawn and expanded to include the new Lap-Band procedure.

Chapter 14 Nutrition for Fitness and Sports

New Figure 14-1 highlights the benefits of physical activity.

New Figure 14-5 illustrates glycolysis.

New Figure 14-6 on metabolism during exercise has been redrawn and greatly simplified.

New Table 14-3 lists fuel use by muscles based on $VO_{2\ max.}$

New Expert Opinion by Dr. Priscilla Clarkson addresses the need for antioxidant supplementation by athletes.

New Table 14-8 shows the nutrient content of various energy bars.

Table 14-10 has been shortened to include only the major ergogenic aids commonly used today.

New Take Action box has a tool to assess physical fitness.

Chapter 15 Eating Disorders: Anorexia Nervosa, Bulimia Nervosa, Binge-Eating Disorders, and Other Conditions

New Nutrition Focus feature contains essays on the personal side of anorexia nervosa and bulimia nervosa.

Figure 15-1 summarizes the physical effects of anorexia nervosa and bulimia nervosa.

The list of medications used in the treatment of various eating disorders has been updated.

Chapter 16 Pregnancy and Breastfeeding

In Figure 16-1, a close-up of placental circulation has been added.

New Nutrition Focus feature looks at the many factors that influence pregnancy outcome.

New Expert Opinion by Dr. Lynne Bailey explains the importance of meeting folate needs before and during pregnancy.

Food plan for pregnant and lactating women has been revised to reflect the advice provided in MyPyramid.

New margin note shows the stark difference in nutrient composition between cow's milk and human milk.

Chapter 17 Nutrition from Infancy through Adolescence

Food plans for children and teenagers have been revised to reflect the advice provided in MyPyramid.

New MyPyramid for Kids has been added (Fig. 17-6).

New Expert Opinion by Dr. Carol Byrd-Bredbenner discusses social trends that are contributing to the epidemic of obesity in children today.

Chapter 18 Nutrition during Adulthood

Introductory text material has been updated to reflect the 2005 Dietary Guidelines for Americans.

New Expert Opinion by Dr. Katherine Tucker explores the importance of meeting adult nutrient needs.

New Table 18-3 provides strength training recommendations for older adults.

Chapter 19 Food and Water Safety

Figure 19-2 has been updated to reflect the latest recommendations on safe food-holding temperatures.

Statistics on mad cow disease in North America have been updated.

New discussion on the safety of our water supply, a growing concern in North America (and worldwide), has been included.

List of alternative sweeteners now includes tagatose.

Short discussion on cadmium in foods has been added.

Chapter 20 Undernutrition throughout the World

Updated content includes the pledge by industrialized nations to forgive the foreign debt of some developing countries and the devastating impact of the ongoing war in Darfur.

New Expert Opinion by Dr. Hugo Melgar-Quiñonez and Dr. Ana Claudia Zubieta discusses the effects of food insecurity worldwide.

Statistics regarding the worldwide AIDS epidemic have been updated.

New Figure 20-5 summarizes the general approaches to solving the problem of undernutrition worldwide.

Special Acknowledgments

We would like to thank Tom Hudgens for his help with this revision. Our editor, Lynne Meyers, supported and assisted us through every step of the revision and facilitated decisions that arose as we planned and produced the seventh edition. Jodi Rhomberg and Peggy Selle diligently monitored the copyediting and production tasks. All these individuals contributed key expertise to the project.

Thank You to Reviewers and Contributors

With each edition, our goal remains the same: to produce the most accurate, up-to-date, and useful textbook possible. These ambitious goals would not be achieved without the meticulous, professional assistance of colleagues who have assisted us in so many ways. Their advice and suggestions have greatly helped refine the content of this edition. We owe our sincere thanks to the following individuals:

Becky Alejandre, *American River College*
Nancy Amy, *University of California—Berkeley*
Janet B. Anderson, *Utah State University*
Kim Archer, *University of Kansas*
James Bailey, *University of Tennesee—Knoxville*
Diane Beaudry, *Shoreline Community College*
Jacqueline Berning, *University of Colorado at Colorado Springs*
Donna Beshgetoor, *San Diego State University*
Jacqueline Buell, *The Ohio State University*
Carol Byrd-Bredbenner, *Rutgers University*
Nancy L. Canolty, *University of Georgia*
Lakshmi N. Chilukrui, *University of California—San Diego*
Tina Crook, *University of Central Arkansas*
Ruth C. Davies, *Edison College*
Christine DuPraw, *San Diego Mesa College*
Eugene J. Fenster, *Longview Community College*
Cindy W. Fitch, *West Virginia University*
Betty J. Forbes, *West Virginia University*
Erin Francfort, *Idaho State University*
Leonard E. Gerber, *University of Rhode Island*
Jill Golden, *Orange Coast College*
Nanci Grayson, *University of Colorado*
Guy E. Groblewski, *University of Wisconsin—Madison*
Donna V. Handley, *University of Rhode Island*
Roschelle Heuberger, *Central Michigan University*
Beckee Hobson, *College of the Sequoias*
Kevin Huggins, *Auburn University*

Catherine Jen, *Wayne State University*
Connie Jones, *Northwestern State University of Louisiana*
Younghee Kim, *Bowling Green State University*
Allen W. Knehans, *University of Oklahoma Health Sciences Center*
Mindy Kurzer, *University of Minnesota*
Elizabeth Konz, *Lexington Community College*
Robert D. Lee, *Central Michigan University*
Linda J. Lolkus, *Indiana University Purdue University—Fort Worth*
Mary Mead, *University of California Berkeley*
Juliet Mevi-Shiflett, *Diablo Valley College*
Gaile Moe, *Seattle Pacific University*
Mohey Mowafy, *Northern Michigan University*
Kathy Munoz, *Humboldt State University*
Judy Myhand, *Louisiana State University*
Jill Patterson, *Penn State University*
Roman Paulak, *East Carolina University*
Debra Pearce, *Northern Kentucky University*
Erwina Peterson, *Yakima Valley Community College*
Nirmala V. Prabhu, *Edison College*
William R. Proulx, *State University of New York College at Oneonta*
Elizabeth Quintana, *West Virginia University*
Rebecca Roach, *University of Illinois at Urbana—Campaign*
Christian K. Roberts, *University of California—Los Angeles*
Brent J. Shriver, *Texas Tech University*
Joanne Slavin, *University of Minnesota—St. Paul*
Carole A. Sloan, *Henry Ford Community College*
Mollie Smith, *California State University—Fresno*
Bernice G. Spurlock, *Hinds Community College*
Anthony Stancampiano, *Oklahoma City Community College*
Lydia Steinman, *University of Texas at Austin*
Leeann S. Sticker, *Northwestern State University of Louisiana*
Jon Story, *Purdue University*
Robin Sytsma, *Solano Community College*
Elsie Takeguchi, *Sacramento City College*
Delores Truesdell, *Florida State University*
Jean Widdison, *Salt Lake City Community College*
Jurist Willis, *Miami-Dade Community College*

A Request to Professors Who Use This Book

As you might imagine, it is difficult to stay abreast of the vast range of nutrition science, following all the various controversies and new developments. We try our best but realize that sometimes we miss an element that deserves attention. If you find content that you question or believe warrants further consideration, feel free to contact us.

We extend our best wishes for success to you and your students.

Gordon Wardlaw Ph.D., R.D.
P.O. Box 290
Mendocino, CA 95460
E-mail: gordonmarkwardlaw@gmail.com

Jeffrey Hampl Ph.D., R.D.
Department of Nutrition
Arizona State University
7001 E. Williams Field Road
Mesa, Arizona 85212
E-mail: jeff.hampl@asu.edu

TO THE STUDENT

Cholesterol, sports drinks, food labeling, bulimia nervosa, alternative sweeteners, vegetarianism, *Salmonella* foodborne illness, and genetically engineered foods—we suspect you have heard about these topics. Which topics are important enough to be a consideration in your life or in the life of someone you know?

Americans pride themselves on their individuality. Nutritional advice should be given accordingly. For example, not all of us have high blood cholesterol and other significant risk factors for developing premature cardiovascular disease. The need to tailor dietary advice to each person's individual nature is the basic approach of this book. First, you are given a brief introduction to the study of nutrition; second, you are told how to be a knowledgeable consumer. With so much information available—both accurate and inaccurate—you should know how to make informed decisions about your nutritional well-being. Third, you are encouraged to learn the basic principles of nutrition and how to apply the concepts in this book that pertain specifically to you.

The text discusses some of the most interesting and important elements of nutrition and food consumption to help you understand both how your body works and how your food choices affect your health.

Features

Planning a New Way of Eating

Early in the text, we present many of the basic guidelines for planning a healthy diet, including a description of the USDA MyPyramid in Chapter 2. Later, in Chapter 13, we review steps involved in setting nutritional goals and designing a diet plan to attain those goals.

Understanding the World Around You

In a college environment, it is often difficult to envision how real the problem of world hunger is. Chapter 20 examines the tragedy of undernutrition and the conditions that create it. The chapter allows you to explore possible solutions that offer hope for the future of this world.

Pedagogy

The seventh edition of *Perspectives in Nutrition* incorporates some important tools to help you learn the nutrition concepts in this text. Following is a guide to those tools:

1. Each chapter begins with a Refresh Your Memory box reminding you of previous chapter content (or coursework) that will be helpful to know for understanding the current chapter. Also at the beginning of each chapter is a case scenario that allows you to apply knowledge gained from the chapter in a real-life setting. A follow-up to each case scenario is provided in the chapter at the point at which the specific content needed to answer the case scenario is covered.
2. **Chapter Objectives** help you focus your attention on key ideas in the chapter.
3. Throughout each chapter are **boldfaced key terms,** which are defined in the margin. All boldfaced terms appear with their definitions and pronunciations in the glossary at the end of the text.
4. Also throughout each chapter are **margin notes,** which further explain ideas or provide references to other chapters. Some margin notes, as well as the text itself contain URLs to nutrition-related websites.
5. The numerous **tables** throughout the text present major points.
6. The **Concept Checks,** which follow the major sections within each chapter, summarize key points. If you are having trouble understanding the material in the Concept Check, you should reread the preceding section.
7. **Critical Thinking** questions ask you to apply information as you learn it. This fosters understanding of the material.
8. **Nutrition Focus** essays within each chapter develop current topics in nutrition in greater detail.
9. Each chapter ends with a **summary,** which conveys the main ideas in the chapter, and **study questions**—both provide a review of chapter material.
10. **Annotated References** are provided to back up material presented in the chapter. If you are preparing a research paper for your class or would just like more information on specific topics, consult these sources.

11. Also at the end of each chapter are **Take Action** boxes, which relate the chapter's major concepts to your daily life. For example, you may be asked to look more carefully at your own diet, examine your family history, or apply information you've learned to friends or family.

12. A variety of supplements to this text, including dietary analysis software, are available to you. These instructional aids are designed to help you learn the major concepts developed in the text and prepare for class examinations.

13. The ARIS website www.mhhe.com/wardlawpers7 contains an online learning center with quizzes, flash cards, other activities, and web links designed to further help you learn about nutrition. This website is organized according to each chapter in the book.

A Request to Students Who Use This Book

We try our best but realize that sometimes we miss a side of an argument that deserves attention or do not make something perfectly clear. If you find content that you question or believe warrants more detail or a clearer explanation, feel free to contact us.

Gordon M. Wardlaw Ph.D., R.D.
P.O. Box 290
Mendocino, CA 95460
E-mail: gordonmarkwardlaw@gmail.com

Jeffrey S. Hampl Ph.D., R.D.
Department of Nutrition
Arizona State University
7001 E. Williams Field Road
Mesa, Arizona 85212
E-mail: jeff.hampl@asu.edu

Thoughtfully Crafted New Illustrations

The presentation of scientific concepts has been enhanced by dynamic new illustrations. Realistic renderings and careful color-coding and numbering of processes assist students in grasping difficult concepts.

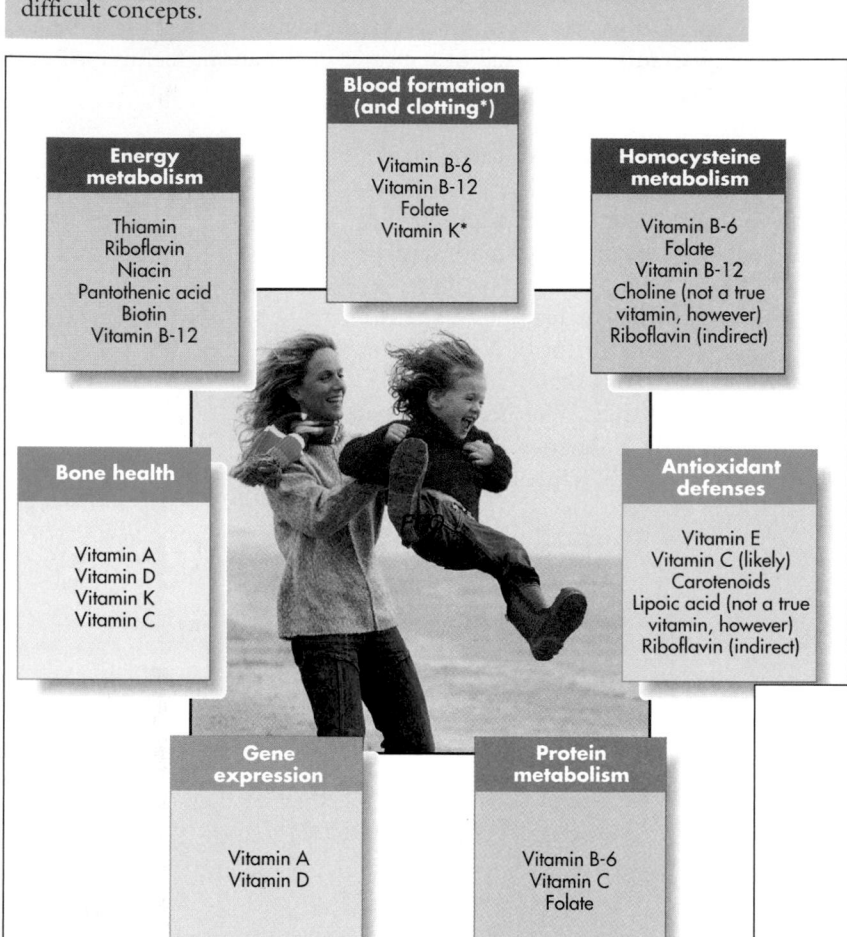

Energy metabolism

Thiamin
Riboflavin
Niacin
Pantothenic acid
Biotin
Vitamin B-12

Blood formation (and clotting*)

Vitamin B-6
Vitamin B-12
Folate
Vitamin K*

Homocysteine metabolism

Vitamin B-6
Folate
Vitamin B-12
Choline (not a true vitamin, however)
Riboflavin (indirect)

Bone health

Vitamin A
Vitamin D
Vitamin K
Vitamin C

Antioxidant defenses

Vitamin E
Vitamin C (likely)
Carotenoids
Lipoic acid (not a true vitamin, however)
Riboflavin (indirect)

Gene expression

Vitamin A
Vitamin D

Protein metabolism

Vitamin B-6
Vitamin C
Folate

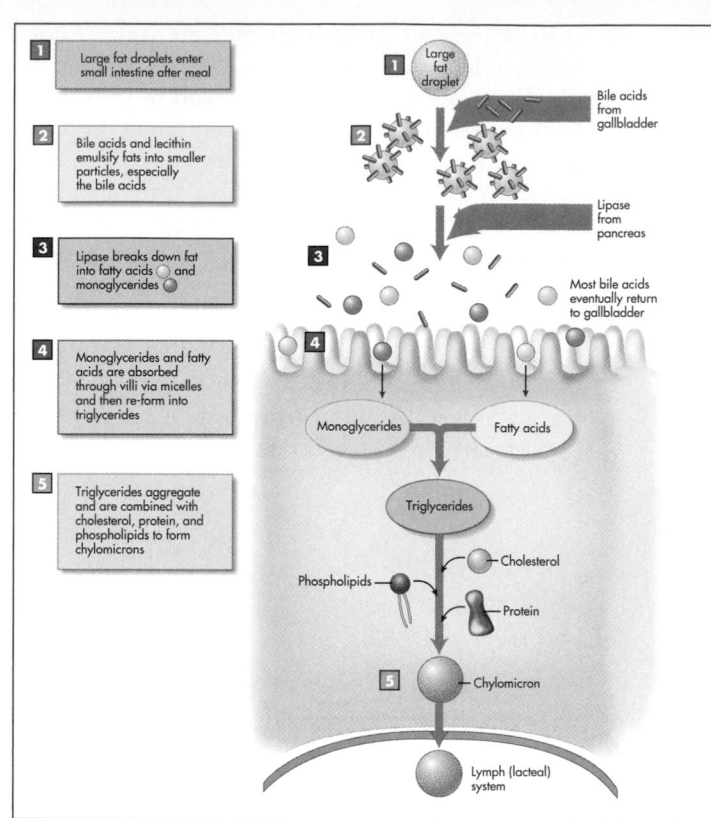

1 Large fat droplets enter small intestine after meal

2 Bile acids and lecithin emulsify fats into smaller particles, especially the bile acids

3 Lipase breaks down fat into fatty acids ◯ and monoglycerides ◉

4 Monoglycerides and fatty acids are absorbed through villi via micelles and then re-form into triglycerides

5 Triglycerides aggregate and are combined with cholesterol, protein, and phospholipids to form chylomicrons

1 Large fat droplet

Bile acids from gallbladder

Lipase from pancreas

Most bile acids eventually return to gallbladder

Monoglycerides | Fatty acids

Triglycerides

Phospholipids — Cholesterol — Protein

5 — Chylomicron

Lymph (lacteal) system

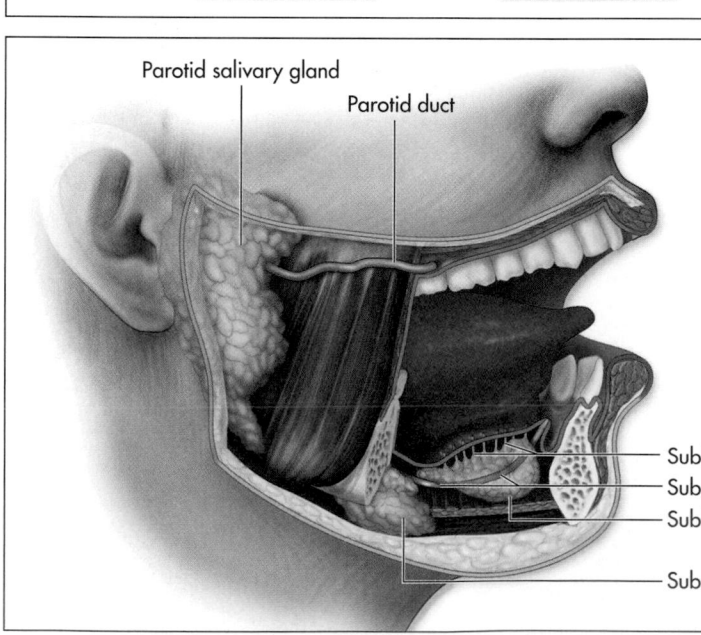

Parotid salivary gland
Parotid duct
Sublingual ducts
Submandibular duct
Sublingual salivary gland
Submandibular salivary gland

Nutrient claims, such as *"Good source,"* and health claims, such as *"Reduce the risk of osteoporosis,"* must follow legal definitions.

A Quick Guide to Nutrient Sources

% Daily Value

20% or more = *High source*
10%–19% = *Good source*
0%–5% = *Low source*

The package must include the name and address of the food manufacturer.

Ingredients are listed in descending order by weight.

Serving size is listed in household units (and grams). Pay careful attention to serving size to know how many servings you are eating; e.g., if you eat double the serving size, you must double the % Daily Values and calories.

The % Daily Values shows how a food fits into an overall 2000-kcal daily diet.

There is no % Daily Values for sugar. Limiting intake is the best advice.

% Daily Value for protein is generally not included due to expensive testing required to determine protein quality.

Only vitamin A, vitamin C, calcium, and iron are required to be listed on the label.

Nutrition Facts
Serving Size 1 Pouch (51g)
Serving Per Container 6

Amount Per Serving
Calories 250 ... Calories from Fat 70

% Daily Value*
Total Fat 7g ... 11%
Saturated Fat 2.5g ... 13%
Trans fat 1g**
Cholesterol 5mg ... 2%
Sodium 400mg ... 16%
Total Carbohydrate 38g ... 13%
Dietary Fiber <1g ... 3%
Sugars 6g
Protein 7g

Vitamin A 0% • Vitamin C 0%
Calcium 12% • Iron 8%
*Percent Daily Values are based on a 2,000 calorie diet. Your daily values may be higher or lower depending on your calorie needs:

	Calories:	2,000	2,500
Total Fat	Less than	65g	80g
Sat Fat	Less than	20g	25g
Cholest	Less than	300mg	300mg
Sodium	Less than	2,400mg	2,400mg
Total Carb		300g	375g
Fiber		25g	30g

Calories per gram:
Fat 9 • Carbohydrate 4 • Protein 4
** Intake should be as low as possible.

INGREDIENTS: ENRICHED MACARONI PRODUCT (DURUM WHEAT FLOUR, GLYCERYL MONO-STEARATE, SALT, NIACIN, FERROUS SULFATE, THIAMIN MONONITRATE [VITAMIN B1], RIBOFLAVIN [VITAMIN B2], FOLIC ACID), CHEESE SAUCE MIX (WHEY, PARTIALLY HYDROGENATED SOYBEAN OIL, MALTODEXTRIN, WHEY PROTEIN CONCENTRATE, CORN SYRUP SOLIDS, SALT, MILKFAT, SUGAR, SODIUM, NATURAL FLAVOR, CITRIC ACID, MONOSODIUM GLUTAMATE, MODIFIED FOOD STARCH, LACTIC ACID, YELLOW 5.

Dynamic Photographs

Over 100 new photographs of people in real-life situations help enliven and bring relevance to the text.

Activity
Activity is represented by the steps and the person climbing them, as a reminder of the importance of daily physical activity.

Moderation
Moderation is represented by the narrowing of each food group from bottom to top. The wider base stands for foods with little or no solid fats or added sugars. These should be selected more often. The narrower top area stands for foods containing more added sugars and solid fats. The more active you are, the more of these foods can fit into your diet.

Personalization
Personalization is shown by the person on the steps, the slogan, and the website. Find the kinds and amounts of food to eat each day at MyPyramid.gov.

Proportionality
Proportionality is shown by the different widths of the food group bands. The widths suggest how much food a person should choose from each group. The widths are just a general guide, not exact proportions. Check the website for how much is right for you.

Variety
Variety is symbolized by the 6 color bands representing the 5 food groups of the Pyramid and oils. This illustrates that foods from all groups are needed each day for good health.

Gradual Improvement
Gradual improvement is encouraged by the slogan. It suggests that individuals can benefit from taking small steps to improve their diet and lifestyle each day.

MyPyramid.gov
STEPS TO A HEALTHIER YOU

| Grains | Vegetables | Fruits | Oils | Milk | Meat & Beans |

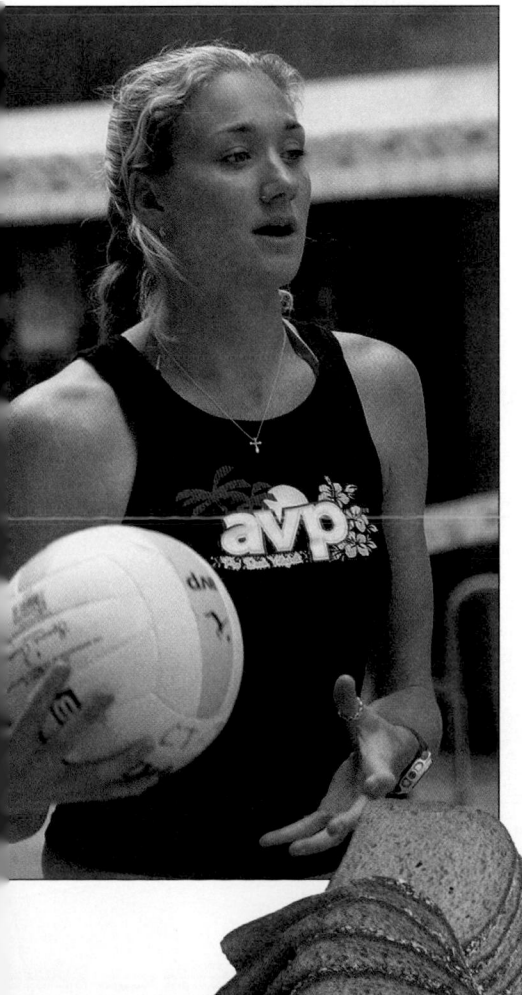

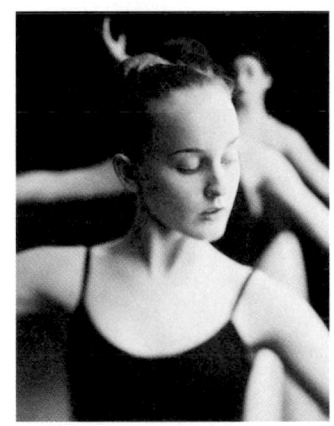

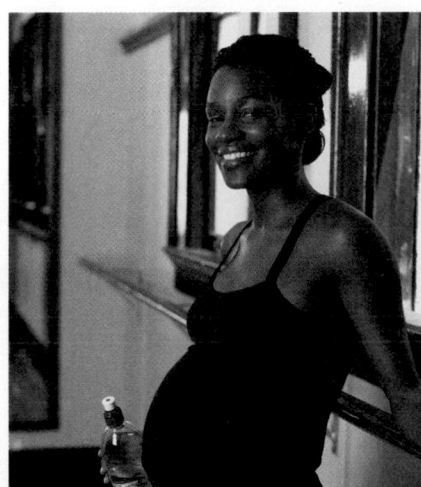

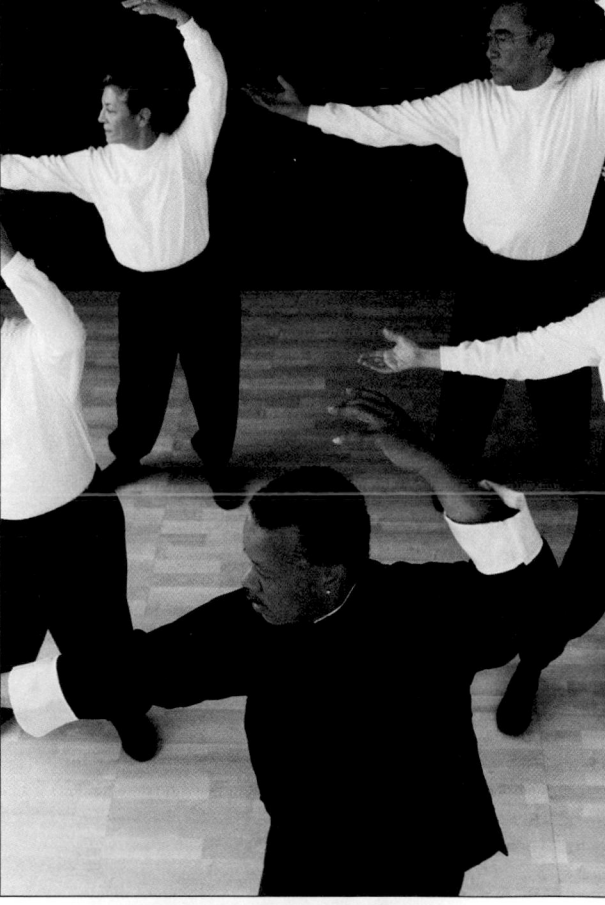

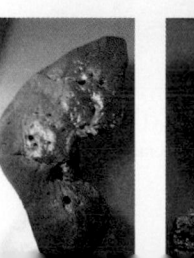

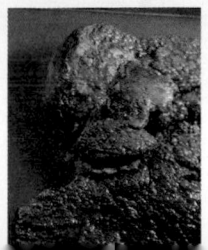

Textbook Tour

Expert Opinion

Vitamin C: Antioxidant and Pro-Ox and the Keystone of Tight Control
Mark Levine, M. D., and Sebastian J. Padayatty, M.R.C.P., Ph.D.

Is vitamin C (ascorbic acid, ascorbate) an antioxidant in humans, as popularly believed? Should vitamin C be obtained from sup... to 100-fold times th... these questions, this section presents some essential ba... tamin C physiology, biology, and chemistry.

Expert Opinion

The Importance of Energy Density in the Diet
Barbara J. Rolls, Ph.D.

With the surge in the incidence of overweight and obesity, effective dietary strategies for weight management are needed. On the surface the issue is clear-cut: simply reduce energy intake below energy expenditure. There is much debate and controversy, however, over the optimal way this goal should be achieved. Although it is unlikely that a single dietary strategy will ever fit everyone's preferences, health professionals have a responsibility to communicate to the public which strategies are considered both safe and effective.

vated body weight. My colleagues and I have shown in several studies that the effects of energy density and portion size combine to increase food intake, confirming that large portions of energy-dense foods are particularly problematic for weight management. On the other hand, large portions of foods low in energy density, such as soups and salads consumed at the start of a meal, are associated with enhanced satiety and a reduction in energy intake at the meal. Other dietary factors that have been shown to enhance satiety are increases in fiber and protein.

Designing Diets That Reduce Hunger and Enhan...

...he diet, no mat... s shifted away ...carbohydrate)

Why Focusing on Macronutrient Composition Is Not As Helpful
Both the scientific community and proponents of popular diets for weight loss have emphasized the importance of the proportions of the macronutrients in

Current Topics of Note

The latest nutrition issues reported in the media are explained in clear, scientific terms. Students learn how to read beyond the headlines to make sound nutrition judgments.

A Personalized Approach to Nutrition

The authors provide ample opportunities for students to apply nutrition concepts and guidelines to their own lives. Real-life examples and individualized activities make the material relevant and help students learn to assess the validity of nutrition claims.

II. Are You Putting the Dietary Guidelines into Practice?

As noted in this chapter, the advice provided by the 2005 Dietary Guidelines for Americans can be summariz... and a number of related activities. Fill out the following inventory to see to what extent you are following the ... Guidelines.

Food Intake

Do you:

Y N Consume a variety of nutrient-dense foods and beverages within and among th...

Choose foods that limit the intake of:
Y N Saturated fat
Y N Trans fats
Y N Cholesterol
Y N Added sugars
Y N Salt
Y N Alcohol (if used).

Emphasize in your food choices:
Y N Vegetables

CHAPTER ELEVEN — WATER AND THE MAJOR MINERAL

CHAPTER OUTLINE

Water
Water in the Body—Intracellular and Extracellular Fluid • Functions of Water • Water in Foods • Water Needs • Water-Deficiency Diseases • Water Toxicity
Minerals
Absorption, Transport, and Excretion of Minerals • Functions of Minerals • Food Sources of Minerals • North Americans at Risk for Mineral Deficiencies • Toxicity of Minerals
Sodium (Na)
Absorption, Transport, Storage, and Excretion of Sodium • Functions of Sodium • Sodium in Foods • Sodium Needs • Sodium-Deficiency Diseases • Upper Level for Sodium
Potassium (K)
Absorption, Transport, Storage, and Excretion of Pot...
Potass...

CASE SCENARIO:

Jana, a sophomore in high school, recently gave up drinking milk. She thought she could stay slim by avoiding all the calories in milk. Her mother is concerned about Jana's diet change, especially Jana's future risk of osteoporosis. Jana needs an adequate source of calcium in her diet to allow for continued bone development and maintenance of the bone mass she already has. Jana also recently started smoking, and her only physical activity is practice for the Women's Glee Club.

Jana's diet on a recent day consisted of the following items. For breakfast, she had oatmeal made with water, a banana, and a cup of fruit juice. At midmorning, she bought a snack cake from the vending machine. At lunch, she had vegetable pasta, bread with olive oil, a side salad, 1 ounce of mixed nuts, and a soft drink. For dinner, she had a hamburger along with mixed vegetables and another soft drink. As an evening snack, she had some cookies and hot tea.

FATS

- Consume less than 10 percent of energy intake from saturated fatty acids and less than 300 mg per day of cholesterol, and keep trans fatty acid consumption as low as possible.
- Keep total fat intake between 20 to 35% of energy intake, with most fats coming from sources of polyunsaturated and monounsaturated fatty acids, such as fish, nuts, and vegetable oils.
- When selecting and preparing meat, poultry, dry beans, and milk or milk products, make choices that are lean, low-fat, or fat-free.
- Limit intake of fats and oils high in saturated and/or trans fatty acids, and choose products low in such fats and oils.

Key Recommendations for Specific Population Groups
- Children and adolescents. Keep total fat intake between 30 to 35% of energy intake for children 2 to 3 years of age and between 25 to 35% of energy intake for children and adolescents 4 to 18 years of age, with most fats coming from sources of polyunsaturated and monounsaturated fatty acids, such as fish, nuts, and vegetable oils.

Latest Dietary Guidelines

Throughout the text, content has been updated to reflect MyPyramid, 2005 Dietary Guidelines for Americans, and the latest Dietary Reference Intakes.

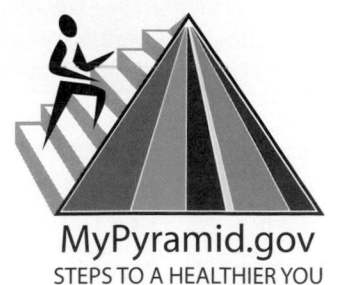

MyPyramid.gov
STEPS TO A HEALTHIER YOU

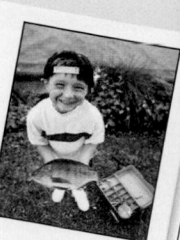

Digital Content Manager CD-ROM

If you're looking for illustrations, photographs, tables, and animations to incorporate into your lecture presentations, handouts, or quizzes, this easy-to-use CD contains hundreds of digital assets from *Perspectives in Nutrition*, 7th edition. Simply click on the chapter folder, select an image, and you're ready to import the image into the application of your choice. It's that simple!

Table 14-8 | Energy and Macronutrient Contents of Popular Energy Bars and Gels

Product	Energy (kcal)	Carbohydrates (g)	Protein (g)	Fat (g)
PowerBar Performance (chocolate)	230	45	10	2
PowerBar ProteinPlus (cookies & cream)	230	38	24	5
PowerBar PowerGel (lemon lime)	110	28	0	0
Luna Bar (cherry-covered chocolate)	180	28	10	4
Clif Bar (chocolate chip)	250	45	10	5
Clif Shot (viva vanilla)	100	24	0	0
Balance Bar (chocolate)	200	22	14	6
Balance Satisfaction (chocolate crisp)		47	12	6
Boulder Bar (chocol			10	4

Choosing energy bars is p...
be handy. Better yet, how...
a less expensive choice, ...

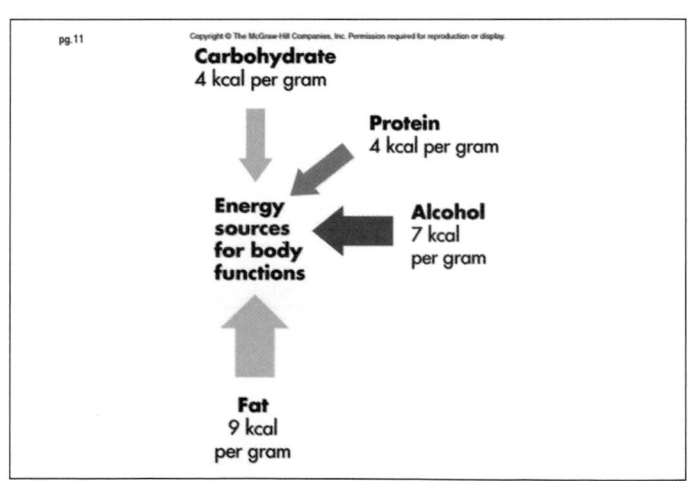

PowerPoint Lecture Outlines

A complete PowerPoint lecture outline with illustrations from the textbook is available for every chapter. Use the outline as is or modify it to match your specific course needs.

Illustrations, Photos, and Tables

Full-color digital files of the art and tables in *Perspectives in Nutrition* are logically organized and allow you to easily customize your classroom materials.

Carbohydrates

* Composed of C, H, O
* Provide a major source of fuel for the body
* Basic unit is glucose
* Simple and Complex CHO
* Energy yielding (4 kcal/gm)

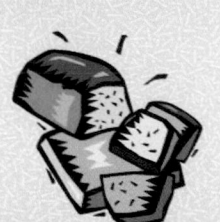

pg.11   Copyright © The McGraw-Hill Companies, Inc. Permission required for reproduction or display

Carbohydrate 4 kcal per gram

Protein 4 kcal per gram

Energy sources for body functions

Alcohol 7 kcal per gram

Fat 9 kcal per gram

Animations

Animations found on the Digital Content Manager CD-ROM allow you to harness the visual impact of processes in motion. You can import the animations into presentations or online course materials.

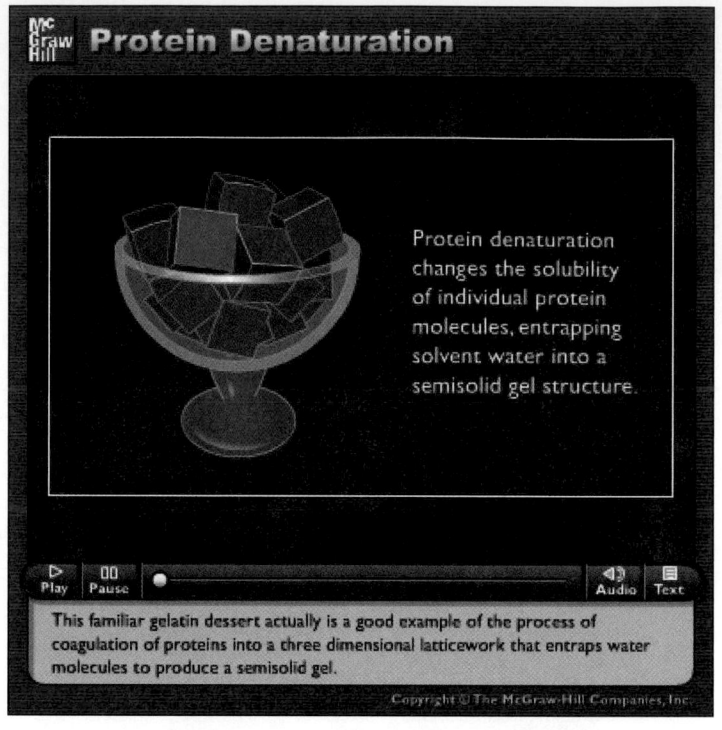

Protein Denaturation

Protein denaturation changes the solubility of individual protein molecules, entrapping solvent water into a semisolid gel structure.

This familiar gelatin dessert actually is a good example of the process of coagulation of proteins into a three dimensional latticework that entraps water molecules to produce a semisolid gel.

Copyright © The McGraw-Hill Companies, Inc.

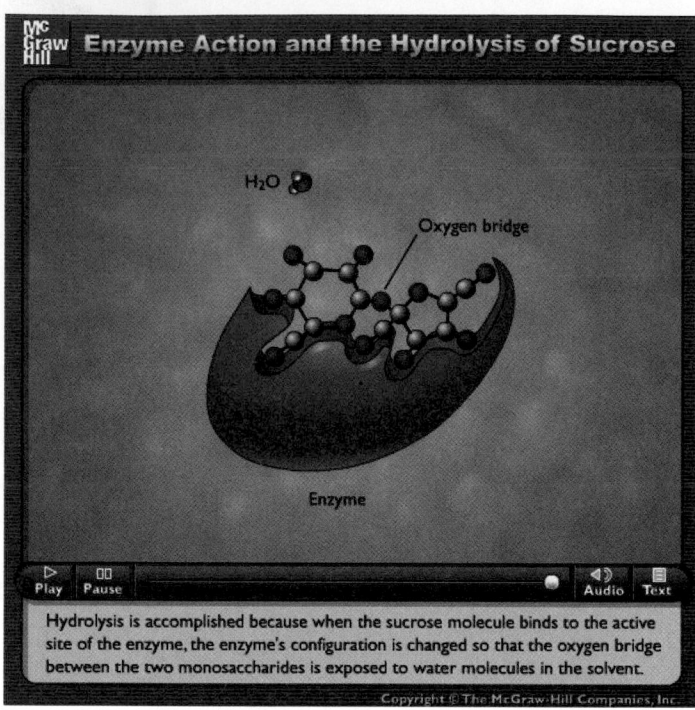

Enzyme Action and the Hydrolysis of Sucrose

H₂O

Oxygen bridge

Enzyme

Hydrolysis is accomplished because when the sucrose molecule binds to the active site of the enzyme, the enzyme's configuration is changed so that the oxygen bridge between the two monosaccharides is exposed to water molecules in the solvent.

Copyright © The McGraw-Hill Companies, Inc.

Text-Edit Art

Have you ever wished you could customize illustrations to meet your course needs? With Text-Edit Art, you can change the size, color, and labels. You can even resize or delete portions of figures.

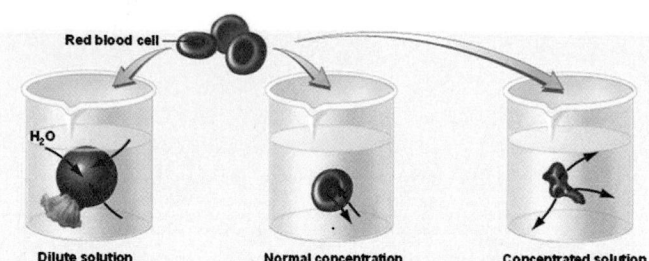

Red blood cell

H₂O

Dilute solution

Normal concentration

Concentrated solution

(a) A dilute solution with a low ion concentration results in swelling (*black arrows*) and subsequent rupture (*puff of red in the lower left part of the cell*) of a red blood cell placed into the solution.

(b) A normal concentration (a concentration of ions outside the cell equal to that inside the cell) results in a typically shaped red blood cell. Water moves into and out of the cell in equilibrium (*black arrows*), but there is no net water movement.

(c) A concentrated solution, with a high ion concentration, causes shrinkage of the red blood cell as water moves out of the cell and into the concentrated solution (*black arrows*).

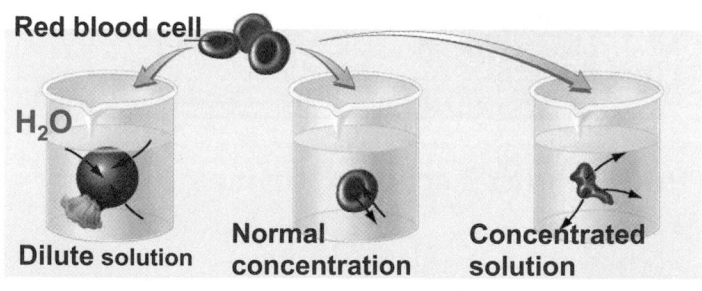

Red blood cell

H₂O

Dilute solution

Normal concentration

Concentrated solution

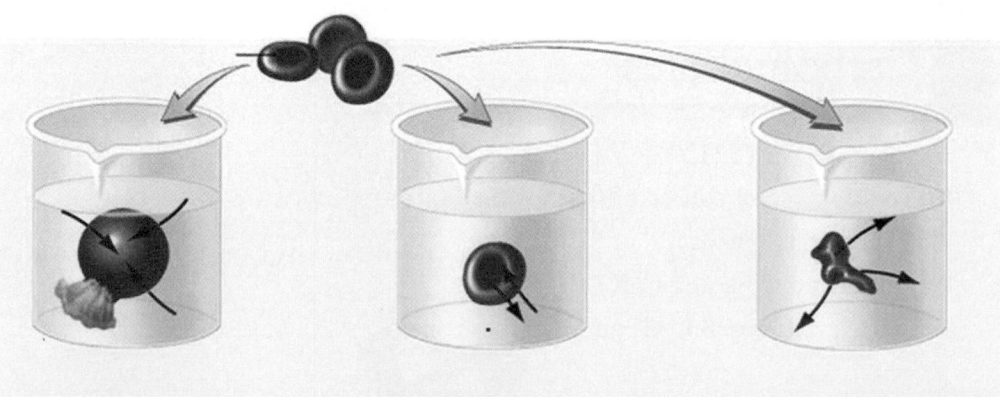

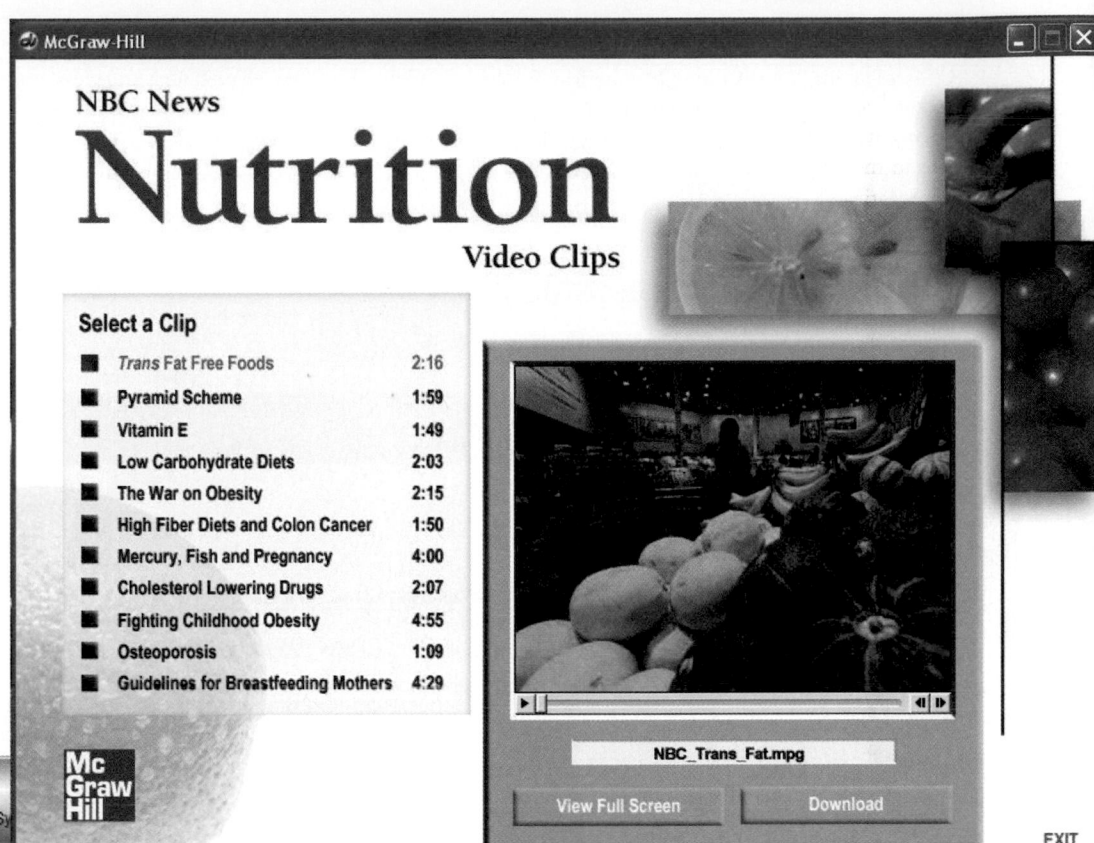

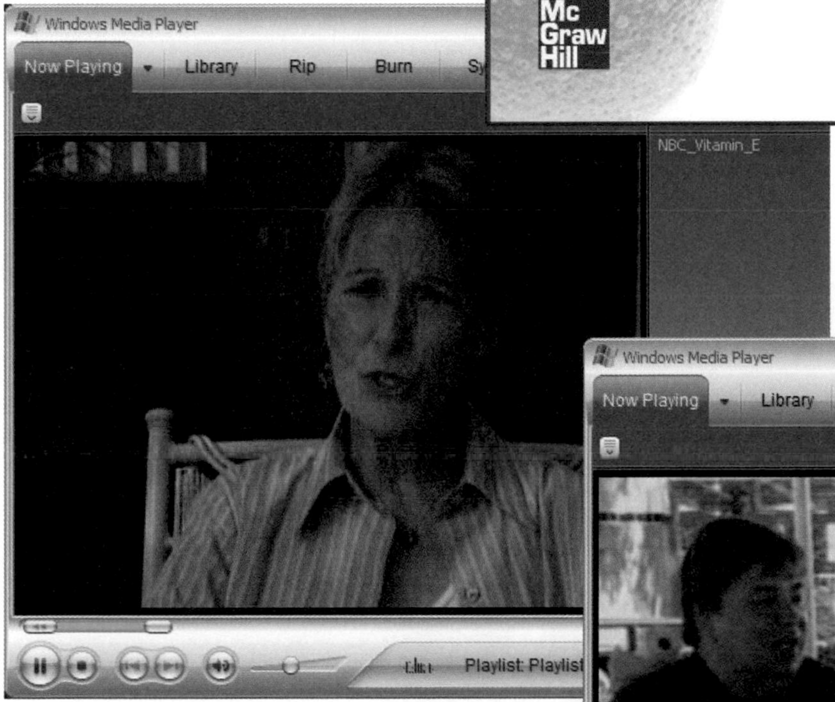

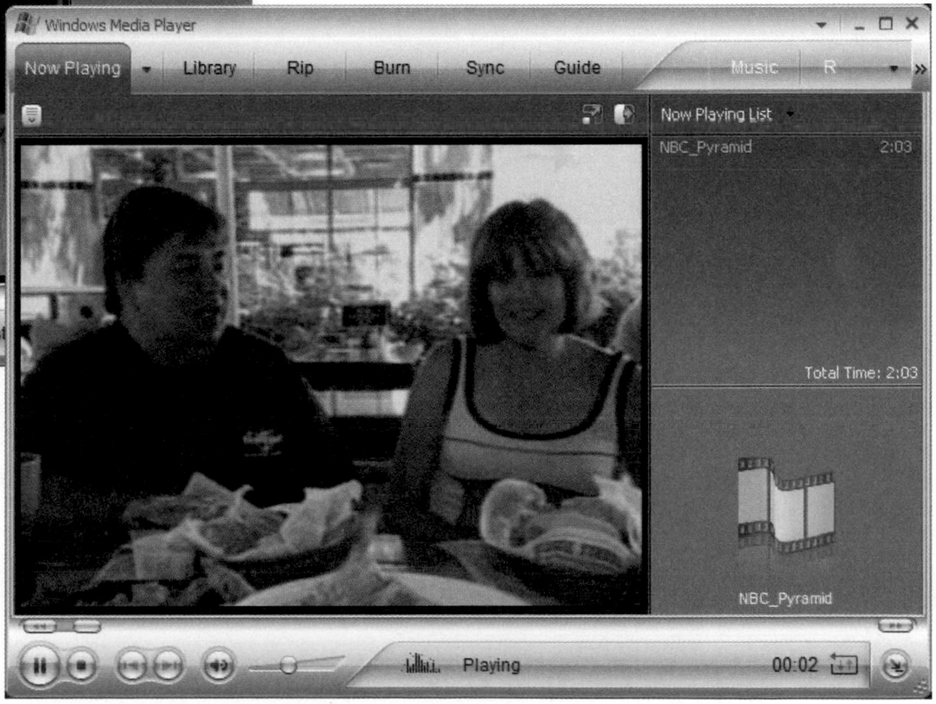

NBC News Nutrition Video Clips

Enliven your lectures with the nutrition topics that are on your students' minds. McGraw-Hill is pleased to announce that we have licensed a series of videos from NBC News. These brief clips on important nutrition issues are perfect for introducing lecture topics or class discussions. Ask your local representative about this valuable presentation CD. You and your students can also access the videos on the textbook website.

McGraw-Hill
NBC News
Nutrition
Video Clips
Select a Clip
Trans Fat Free Foods 2:16
Pyramid Scheme 1:59
Vitamin E 1:49
Low Carbohydrate Diets 2:03
The War on Obesity 2:15
High Fiber Diets and Colon Cancer 1:50
Mercury, Fish and Pregnancy 4:00
Cholesterol Lowering Drugs 2:07
Fighting Childhood Obesity 4:55
Osteoporosis 1:09
Guidelines for Breastfeeding Mothers 4:29
NBC_Trans_Fat.mpg
View Full Screen
Download
Mc Graw Hill
EXIT

Windows Media Player
Now Playing
Library
Rip
Burn
NBC_Vitamin_E
Playlist: Playlist

Windows Media Player
Now Playing
Library
Rip
Burn
Sync
Guide
Music
Now Playing List
NBC_Pyramid 2:03
Total Time: 2:03
NBC_Pyramid
Playing
00:02

ARIS

ARIS (*Assessment, Review, and Instruction System*) is an exciting, new electronic homework and course management system from McGraw-Hill. ARIS helps you and your students utilize all the resources found on the *Perspectives in Nutrition* website. Better yet, ARIS allows you to import your own content, create assignments, and post announcements. ARIS also includes an automatic grading function for quizzing and testing materials. Moreover, this dynamic McGraw-Hill tool is easily loaded into course management system such as WebCT or Blackboard. Contact your local McGraw-Hill representative for information on how you can take advantage of the power of ARIS.

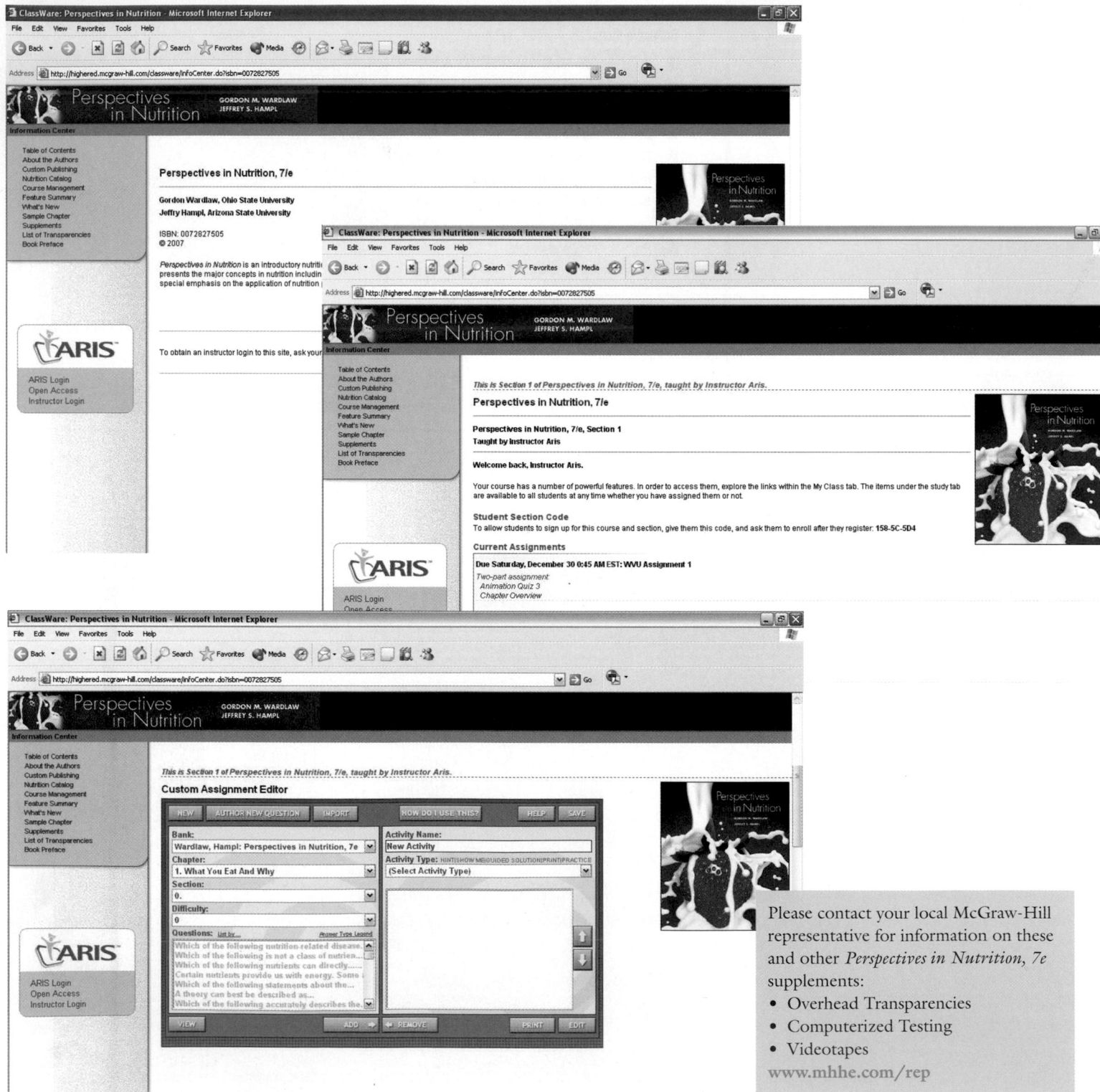

Please contact your local McGraw-Hill representative for information on these and other *Perspectives in Nutrition, 7e* supplements:
- Overhead Transparencies
- Computerized Testing
- Videotapes

www.mhhe.com/rep

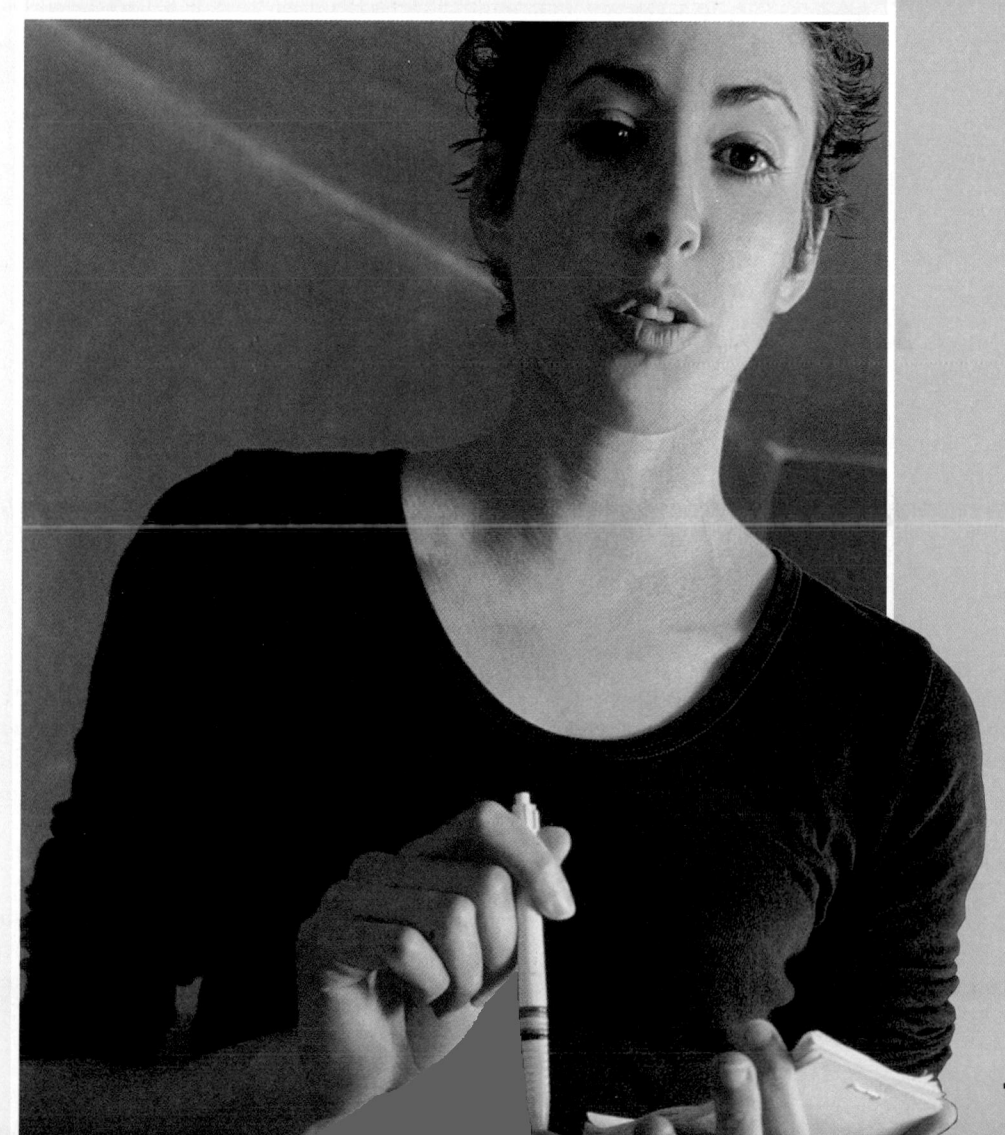

CHAPTER OUTLINE

CASE SCENARIO:

While Brenda was driving to campus last week, she heard a radio advertisement for a supplement containing a plant substance that has recently been imported from China. It supposedly gives people more energy in general, and helps people cope with the stress of daily life. This advertisement caught Brenda's attention because she has been feeling run-down lately. She is taking a full course load and has been working 30 hours a week at a local restaurant to try to make ends meet. Brenda doesn't have a lot of extra money to spare. Still, she likes to try new things, and this recent breakthrough from China sounded almost too good to be true. After searching for more information on the Internet, she discovered that the recommended dose would cost $60 per month. Because Brenda is looking for some help with her low energy level, she decides to order a one-month supply. Does this extra expense make sense to you?

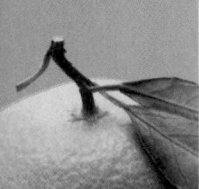

Do you need to take a balanced multivitamin and mineral supplement? Are you eating too much saturated fat, *trans* fat, and cholesterol? Is much of what you eat unsafe? Are some foods actually *junk foods*? Should you become a vegetarian? If you have asked yourself any of these questions or if you are confused about what you should eat, you are not alone. This chapter will help you sort out some of these issues as you are introduced to the science of nutrition.

As you begin this study of nutrition, keep this in mind: research over the last 40 years has shown that a healthy diet—notably one rich in fruits and vegetables—coupled with regular prolonged, vigorous exercise and strength-building exercise can both prevent and treat many age-related diseases.[3] Overall, the nutritional lifestyles of many North Americans are out of balance with their physiology.[5] And since we live longer than our ancestors did, preventing the age-related diseases that develop later in life is a more important focus today than in the past.

By optimizing dietary choices we can strive to bring the goal of a long, healthy life within reach.[15] This is the primary theme not just in this first chapter but throughout the entire book.

REFRESH YOUR MEMORY AS YOU BEGIN YOUR STUDY OF NUTRITION IN CHAPTER 1, YOU MAY WANT TO REVIEW:

* Basic concepts in chemistry in Appendix A.
* The metric system in Appendix L.

CHAPTER OBJECTIVES CHAPTER 1 IS DESIGNED TO ALLOW YOU TO:

1. Define the terms *nutrition, carbohydrates, proteins, lipids (fats), alcohol, vitamins, minerals, water, kilocalories (kcal),* and *fiber.*

2. Use the caloric values of energy-yielding nutrients to determine the total energy content (kcal) in a food or diet.

3. List the major characteristics of the North American diet and the food habits that often need to be improved.

4. Describe the various factors that affect our daily food choices.

5. List various attributes of a healthful lifestyle that are consistent with the *Healthy People 2010* goals.

6. Identify diet and lifestyle factors that contribute to the 10 leading causes of death in North America.

7. Understand the basis of the scientific method as it is used in developing hypotheses and theories in the field of nutrition.

8. Identify reliable sources of nutrition information.

9. Understand the role of genetic background in the development of nutrition-related diseases.

| Nutrition and Your Health

Bold terms in the book are defined in a glossary, which follows Chapter 20. Many bold terms are also defined in the chapter margin when first presented.

In your lifetime, you will eat about 70,000 meals and 60 tons of food. This opening chapter will take a close look at the general classes of nutrients supplied by this food, the role research plays in sorting out which food components are essential for the maintenance of health, and the powerful effect of genetic background in determining overall health.

What Actually Is Nutrition?

nutrition The science of food; the nutrients and the substances therein; their action, interaction, and balance in relation to health and disease; and the process by which the organism (i.e., body) ingests, digests, absorbs, transports, utilizes, and excretes food substances.

The American Medical Association has defined **nutrition** as "The science of food, the nutrients and the substances therein, their action, interaction, and balance in relation to health and disease, and the process by which the organism ingests, digests, absorbs, transports, utilizes, and excretes food substances."

Nutrients Come from Food

What is the difference between food and **nutrients?** Food provides both the energy and the nutrients needed to build and maintain all body cells. Many of these substances are **essential nutrients** if the body can't make them (or make enough of them) to meet needs (Note that sun exposure on the skin produces vitamin D, but some of us still need a dietary source [see Chapter 9]).[10]

For a substance to be considered essential, three characteristics are needed:

1. Its omission from the diet must lead to a decline in human biological function, such as function of the nervous system.
2. If the omitted nutrient is restored to the diet before permanent damage occurs, those aspects of human biological function hampered by its absence should regain normal function.
3. A specific biological function of the nutrient must be identified.

Why Study Nutrition?

Nutrition is one key to developing and maintaining a state of health that is optimal for you. A poor diet coupled with a sedentary lifestyle contribute to many causes of death in North America (Table 1-1).[17] These habits are known to be **risk factors** for life-threatening **chronic** diseases and deaths: **cardiovascular (heart) disease, stroke, hypertension, diabetes,** and some forms of **cancer.** (Note that Table 1-2 defines these and other key terms used in nutrition.) Not consuming enough essential nutrients in younger years also makes us more likely to suffer health consequences in later years, such as bone fractures from the disease **osteoporosis.** Iron-deficiency **anemia** is another possibility of a nutrient deficiency, especially in women and children. At the same time, taking too much of a nutrient supplement—such as vitamin A, vitamin B-6, calcium, or copper—can be harmful to organs such as bones, kidneys, and nerves. Another dietary problem, drinking too much alcohol, is associated with **cirrhosis** of the liver, some forms of cancer, accidents, and suicides.

All of these consequences of modern living are partly an "affliction of affluence." Note, however, that these diseases are often preventable. Age fast or age slowly: it is partly your choice. U.S. government scientists calculate that a poor diet and a lack of sufficient physical activity contribute to up to 350,000 fatal cases of cardiovascular disease, cancer, and diabetes each year.[17] Thus, the combination of poor diet and too little physical activity is indirectly the second leading cause of death. In addition, **obesity** is considered the second leading cause of preventable death (smoking is the first).[18]

Physical activity reflects any movement of the body caused by muscular contraction that results in the expenditure of energy. The term **exercise** in contrast is generally reserved for physical activity that is done with the intent to provide a health benefit, such as improved muscle tone or stamina.

Table 1-1 | Ten Leading Causes of Death in the United States

Rank	Cause of Death	Percent of Total Deaths
	All causes	100
1	Diseases of the heart (primarily coronary heart disease)*†‡	29
2	Cancer*† ‡	22
3	Cerebrovascular diseases (stroke)*‡ #	7
4	Chronic obstructive pulmonary diseases and allied conditions (lung diseases)‡	5
5	Accidents and adverse effects† Motor vehicle accidents All other accidents and adverse effects	4 (2) (2)
6	Diabetes*	3
7	Influenza and pneumonia	3
8	Alzheimer's disease*	2
9	Kidney disease*‡	2
10	Blood-borne infections	1

From Centers for Disease Control and Prevention, *National Vital Statistics Report,* accessed October 9, 2002. Canadian statistics are quite similar.

*Causes of death in which diet plays a part

†Causes of death in which excessive alcohol consumption plays a part

‡Causes of death in which tobacco use plays a part

#Diseases of the heart and cerebrovascular disease are included in the more global term *cardiovascular disease.*

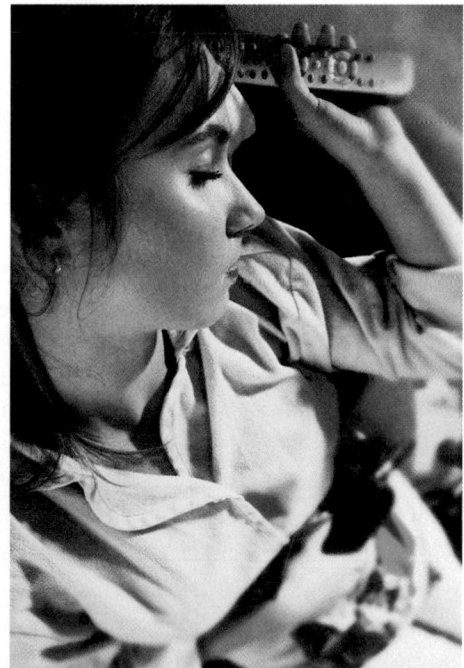

The major health problems in North America are largely caused by a poor diet, excessive energy intake, and not enough physical activity.

Table 1-2 | Glossary Terms to Aid Your Introduction to Nutrition

anemia Generally refers to a decreased oxygen-carrying capacity of the blood. This can be caused by many factors, such as iron deficiency or blood loss.

body mass index (BMI) Weight (in kilograms) divided by height (in meters) squared. A value of 25 or greater indicates a higher risk for weight-related health disorders if one is also overfat. See Table 13-3 in Chapter 13 to determine your body mass index.

cancer A condition characterized by uncontrolled growth of abnormal cells.

carbohydrate A compound containing carbon, hydrogen, and oxygen atoms; most are known as *sugars*, *starches*, and *fibers*. Supplies 4 kcal/gram.

cardiovascular (heart) disease A general term that refers to any disease of the heart and circulatory system. This disease is characterized by the deposition of fatty material in the blood vessels (hardening of the arteries), which in turn can lead to organ damage and death; also termed coronary heart disease (CHD), because the vessels of the heart are the primary sites of the disease.

cholesterol A waxy lipid found in all body cells; it has a structure containing multiple chemical rings (steroid structure). Cholesterol is found only in foods that contain animal products.

chronic Long-standing, developing over time. When referring to disease, this term indicates that the disease process, once developed, is slow and tends to remain; a good example is cardiovascular disease.

cirrhosis A loss of functioning liver cells, which are replaced by nonfunctioning connective tissue. Any substance that poisons liver cells can lead to cirrhosis. The most common cause is chronic, excessive alcohol intake.

diabetes A disease characterized by high blood glucose, resulting from either insufficient or no release of the hormone insulin by the pancreas or general inability of insulin to act on certain body cells, such as muscle cells. The two major forms are **type 1 diabetes** (requires daily insulin therapy) and **type 2 diabetes** (may or may not require insulin therapy).

essential fatty acids Fatty acids that must be supplied by the diet to maintain health. Currently only linoleic acid and alpha-linolenic acid are classified as essential ftty acids.

essential nutrient In nutritional terms, a substance that, when left out of a diet, leads to signs of poor health. The body either can't produce this nutrient or can't produce enough of it to meet its needs. Then, if added back to a diet before permanent damage occurs, the affected aspects of health are restored.

fat A general term that describes substances that dissolve in organic solvents such as benzene and ether. Fats are mostly composed of carbon and hydrogen, with relatively small amounts of oxygen and other elements.

hypertension A condition in which blood pressure remains persistently elevated. Obesity, inactivity, alcohol intake, and excess salt intake all can contribute to the problem.

kilocalorie (kcal) The heat energy needed to raise the temperature of 1000 g (1 liter) of water 1° Celsius. Also written as Calorie, with a capital C.

lipid A compound containing much carbon and hydrogen, little oxygen, and sometimes other atoms. Lipids dissolve in ether or benzene, but not in water, and include fats, oils, and **cholesterol.**

minerals Elements used in the body to promote chemical reactions and to form body structures.

nutrients Chemical substances in food that contribute to health, many of which are essential parts of a diet. Nutrients nourish us by providing energy, materials for building body parts, and factors to regulate necessary chemical processes in the body.

obesity A condition characterized by excess body fat. Typically defined in clinical settings as a **body mass index (BMI)** of 30 or above, but this cutoff is not always appropriate.

osteoporosis Decreased bone mass where no obvious disease can be found. This bone loss is related to the effects of aging, genetic background, poor diet, and hormonal changes occurring in postmenopausal women.

protein Food and body components made of amino acids; proteins contain carbon, hydrogen, oxygen, nitrogen, and sometimes other atoms, in a specific configuration. Proteins contain the form of nitrogen most easily used by the human body. Supplies 4 kcal/g.

risk factor A term used frequently when discussing diseases and the factors contributing to their development. A risk factor is an aspect of our lives—such as heredity, lifestyle choices (i.e., smoking), or nutritional habits—that may make us more likely to develop a disease.

stroke The loss of body function that results from a blood clot or other change in arteries in the brain that affects blood flow. This in turn causes the death of brain tissue. Also called a *cerebrovascular accident*.

vitamins Compounds needed in very small amounts in the diet to help regulate and support chemical reactions in the body.

water The universal solvent; chemically, H_2O. The body is composed of about 60% water. Water (fluid) needs are about 9 cups (8 fl oz each) for women and 13 cups for men per day; needs are greater if one exercises heavily (see Chapter 14).

Put together, obesity and smoking spell even more trouble for your health. And, as you will learn in Chapter 13, surgery to help treat obesity costs about $12,000 to $40,000. As always, treating health problems is much more costly than preventing them.

As you gain understanding about your nutritional habits and increase your knowledge about nutrition, you have the opportunity to dramatically reduce your risk for many common health problems.[15] For additional help, the U.S. government provides two websites that can link you to many sites providing health and nutrition information (www.healthfinder.gov and www.nutrition.gov). Three other helpful websites are www.eatright.org, www.navigator.tufts.edu, and www.webmd.com.

Interest in the Field of Nutrition Has a Long History

The science of nutrition evolved primarily from the disciplines of physiology, chemistry, and medicine.[4] Our interest in the relationship between food and the maintenance of health has a long history, beginning some 2400 years ago in Greece, during the time of Hippocrates. The Bible even contains references to the importance of certain foods, such as beans.

The science of nutrition began in the 1600s in Europe. A British physician, Sydenham, in 1674 showed that iron filings in wine can be used to treat anemia. In the 1740s, a British naval surgeon, Lind, found that the consumption of citrus fruits—lemons and limes—cures the disease **scurvy** in sailors. Between 1770 and 1794, Lavoisier and Laplace in France discovered that certain carbon-containing compounds are the source of energy for body functions. In 1816 German scientist Magendie showed that dogs fed only carbohydrate and fat lost much body protein and died within a few weeks.

By 1830, it was known that foods contain three major constituents: proteins, carbohydrates, and fats. By 1850, at least six minerals—calcium, phosphorous, sodium, potassium, chloride, and iron—had been established as essential to the diets of higher animals. Nutrition as a scientific discipline emerged as scientists realized that components in foods, some of which are present in very small amounts, contribute to health.

During the 1880s, a Japanese physician, Takaki, showed that a common disease of sailors, called **beriberi,** can be treated with evaporated milk and meat. Later research in the Dutch East Indies by both Eijkman and Grijns showed that the same disease is associated with the use of refined rice, whereas use of the whole rice grain prevented the problem. By 1901, it was assumed that refined rice lacks an essential nutrient (later called water-soluble B and then eventually found to be the vitamin thiamin), which was present in the whole-grain form.

In the 1890s, Rubner in Germany and Atwater in the United States established the energy (kcal) content of a gram of carbohydrate, fat, and protein (4, 9, 4, respectively). This research also quantified human energy output, showing that, on average, we expend about 2000 to 3000 kcal/day.

In 1906, the **amino acid** tryptophan was shown to be essential for mice by Willcock and Hopkins in Britain. By 1913, Osborne and Mendel in the United States had shown that food proteins are quite different in terms of their amino acid content.

The year 1912 was a banner year—the term *vitamine* was coined by Polish scientist Funk at this time to describe certain compounds present in very small amounts in foods that promote health. *Vita* came from the Latin for "life," and *amine* came from the term for nitrogen bonded to carbon (technically, called an amine). (The *e* was dropped from *vitamine* to form *vitamin* in the 1920s, when it was shown that some vitamins do not contain nitrogen.)

By 1915, nutrition experts knew that six minerals, four amino acids, and three vitamins—A, B (later shown to be a group of vitamins), and the anti-scurvy factor (later shown to be ascorbic acid, which we also call vitamin C)—were essential nutrients.

From the 1920s to today, nutrition research has been a key part of the intense scientific inquiry that characterized the twentieth century. **Recommended Dietary Allowances (RDAs)** for nutrients were first published in the United States in 1943 in

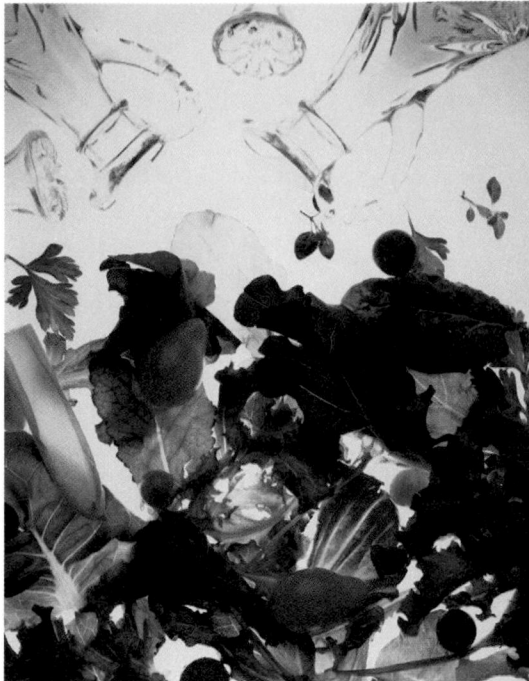

Increasing vegetable intake, such as a daily salad, is one strategy to combat development of many chronic diseases.

In the fifth century BC, Hippocrates said "Let food be your medicine and medicine be your food."

scurvy The deficiency disease that results after a few weeks to months of consuming a diet that lacks vitamin C; pinpoint hemorrhages on the skin are an early sign.

beriberi The thiamin deficiency disorder characterized by muscle weakness, loss of appetite, nerve degeneration, and sometimes edema.

amino acid The building block for proteins containing a central carbon atom with a nitrogen atom and other atoms attached.

Recommended Dietary Allowances (RDAs) Recommended intakes of nutrients that are sufficient to meet the needs of almost all individuals (97%) of similar age and gender. These are established by the Food and Nutrition Board of the National Academy of Sciences.

response to growing recognition of the poor nutritional health of many Americans. All vitamins we know of today had been characterized by 1949. The research on vitamins such as thiamin, vitamin K, vitamin C, and vitamin B-12 even led to Nobel prizes for Eijkman, Dam, Szent-Gyorgyi, and the group of researchers Minot, Murphy, and Whipple. By 1950, some 35 nutrients had been shown to be necessary to maintain human health. Today we know that the minimum diet for humans must contain about 45 essential nutrients in order to maintain health (Table 1-3).

In 1968, Dudrick in the United States was able to support the nutrient needs of dogs using only intravenous feedings of purified nutrients. Soon after, it was shown that this is also possible for humans. Thus, we had evidence that meeting the needs for nutrients known to be essential at that time sufficed to maintain health.

Over the past 40 years, interest in nutrition has grown, especially among health-conscious consumers. U.S. government policymakers stepped up their interest in nutrition after the 1969 White House conference on food, nutrition, and health, and as well increased support of federal feeding programs. Following this, more and more research, much of which was funded by the U.S. federal government, supported the role of nutrition in the maintenance of health as well as showed a link between poor nutrition (both inadequate and excessive nutrient intakes) and various health problems. To date,

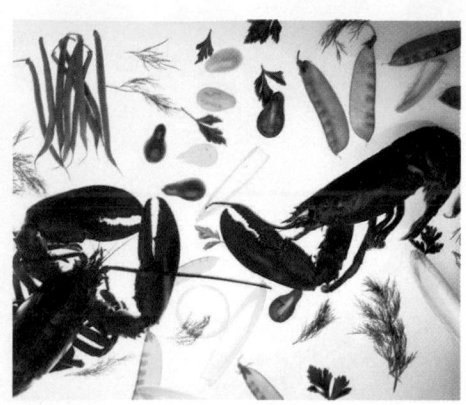

Many foods are rich sources of nutrients that we recognize today as essential for health.

glucose A six-carbon carbohydrate found in blood as well as in table sugar bound to fructose; also known as *dextrose*, it is one of the simple sugars.

Table 1-3 | Essential Nutrients in the Human Diet and Their Classes*

Energy-Yielding Nutrients		
Carbohydrate	**Fat (Lipids)†**	**Protein (Amino Acids)**
Glucose‡ (or a carbohydrate that yields glucose)	Linoleic acid (omega-6) a-Linolenic acid (omega-3)	Histidine Isoleucine Leucine Lysine Methionine Phenylalanine Threonine Tryptophan Valine

Non-Energy-Yielding Nutrients					
Vitamins		**Minerals**			
Water-Soluble	**Fat-Soluble**	**Major**	**Trace**	**Some Questionable Minerals**	**Water**
Thiamin	A	Calcium	Chromium	Arsenic	Water
Riboflavin	D§	Chloride	Copper	Boron	
Niacin	E	Magnesium	Fluoride ‖	Nickel	
Pantothenic acid	K	Phosphorus	Iodide	Silicon	
Biotin		Potassium	Iron	Vanadium	
B-6		Sodium	Manganese		
B-12		Sulfur	Molybdenum		
Folate			Selenium		
C			Zinc		

*This table includes nutrients that the current *Dietary Reference Intakes* and related publications list for humans. Some disagreement exists over the questionable minerals and certain other minerals not listed. Fiber could be added to the list of essential substances, but it is not a nutrient (see Chapter 5). Alcohol is a source of energy but is not an essential nutrient.

†The lipids listed are needed only in small amounts, about 5% of total energy needs (see Chapter 6).

‡To supply fuel for the brain and other cells as well as prevent ketosis and the muscle loss that would occur if protein were used to synthesize carbohydrate (see Chapter 5)

§Sunshine on the skin also allows the body to make vitamin D for itself (see Chapter 9).

‖Primarily for dental health (see Chapter 12)

The vitamin-like compound choline plays essential roles in the body but is not listed under the vitamin category at this time. Rough estimates of human needs for this compound recently have been set (see the inside cover of the text). Note, however, that body synthesis suffices during many stages of life (see Chapter 10 for details).

we have made much progress in the field of nutrition, but more work needs to be done, and nutrition problems still plague peoples in all parts of the world (see Chapter 20).[5]

Classes and Sources of Nutrients

To begin the study of nutrition, let's start with an overview of the various classes of nutrients. You are probably already familiar with the terms **carbohydrates, lipids** (fats and oils), **proteins, vitamins,** and **minerals** (Figure 1-1). These, plus **water,** make up the six classes of nutrients found in food (review Table 1-3).

Nutrients can then be assigned to three functional categories: (1) those that primarily provide us with energy (typically expressed in **kilocalories [kcal]**); (2) those that are important for growth and development (and later maintenance); and (3) those that act to keep body functions running smoothly. Some overlap exists among these groupings. The energy-yielding nutrients make up a major portion of most foods.[10]

Provide Energy	Promote Growth and Development	Regulate Body Processes
Most carbohydrates	Proteins	Proteins
Proteins	Lipids	Some lipids
Most lipids (fats and oils)	Some vitamins	Some vitamins
	Some minerals	Some minerals
	Water	Water

Let's now look more closely at these six classes of nutrients.

Vitamins and minerals are needed in such small amounts in the diet that they are called **micronutrients.** In contrast, because carbohydrates, proteins, lipids, and water are needed in much larger amounts, they are called **macronutrients.**

micronutrient A nutrient needed in milligram or microgram quantities in a diet.

macronutrient A nutrient needed in gram quantities in the diet.

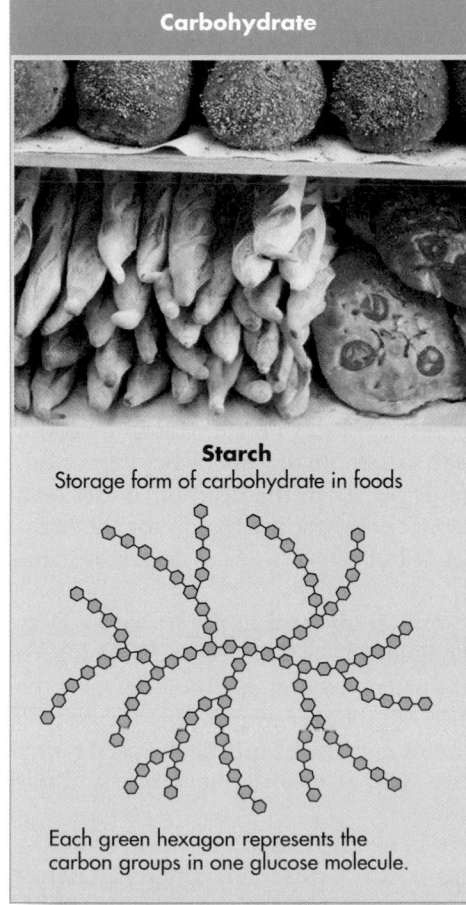

Carbohydrate

Starch
Storage form of carbohydrate in foods

Each green hexagon represents the carbon groups in one glucose molecule.

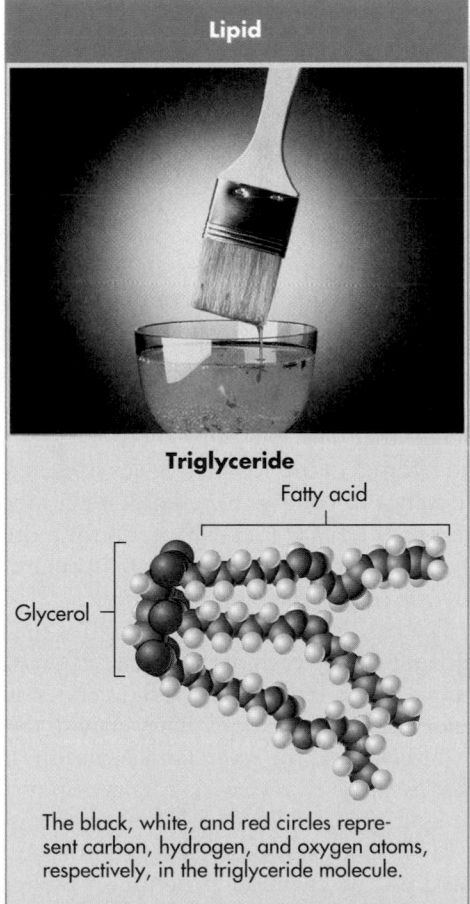

Lipid

Triglyceride

Fatty acid

Glycerol

The black, white, and red circles represent carbon, hydrogen, and oxygen atoms, respectively, in the triglyceride molecule.

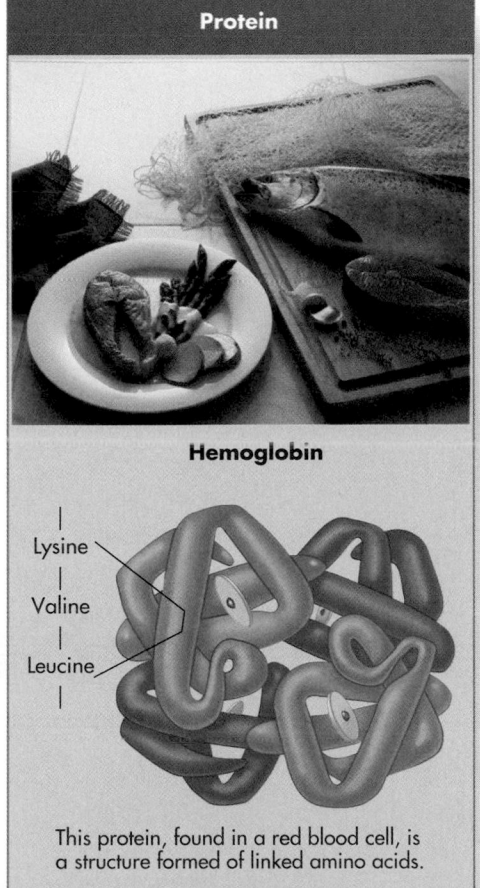

Protein

Hemoglobin

Lysine

Valine

Leucine

This protein, found in a red blood cell, is a structure formed of linked amino acids.

Figure 1-1 | Two views of carbohydrates, lipids, and proteins—chemical and dietary perspectives.

element A substance that cannot be separated into simpler substances by chemical processes. Common elements in nutrition include carbon, oxygen, hydrogen, nitrogen, calcium, phosphorus, and iron.

starch A carbohydrate made of multiple units of glucose attached together in a form the body can digest; also known as *complex carbohydrates.*

The chemistry review in Appendix A describes the shortcut notation used to draw these sugar structures. Essentially, any corner represents a carbon (unless otherwise noted), and, up to four hydrogens are present on each carbon to yield four bonds per carbon.

fiber Substances in plant foods that are not broken down by digestive processes of the stomach or small intestine. These add bulk to feces. Fiber naturally found in foods is called dietary fiber.

glycerol A three carbon alcohol used to form triglycerides.

fatty acid Major part of most lipids; composed of a chain of carbons flanked by hydrogen with an acid group

$$\begin{matrix} O \\ \| \end{matrix}$$

(—C—OH) at one end and a methyl group (—CH$_3$) at the other.

triglyceride The major form of lipid in the body and in food. It is composed of three fatty acids bonded to glycerol, an alcohol.

Carbohydrates

Carbohydrates are composed mainly of the **elements** carbon, hydrogen, and oxygen. Carbohydrates provide a major source of fuel for the body, on average 4 kcal per gram (kcal/g).[8] Small carbohydrate structures are called sugars or simple sugars. Table sugar (sucrose) is an example. It is made up of the sugars glucose and fructose. Some simple sugars, such as glucose, can chemically bond to form large storage carbohydrates, called polysaccharides or complex carbohydrates (review Figure 1-1). An example of this type of carbohydrate is the **starch** in potatoes.

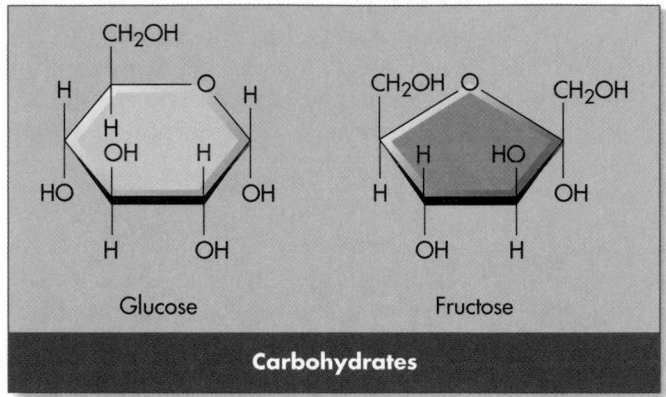

Aside from enjoying their taste, we need sugars and other carbohydrates in our diets primarily to help satisfy the energy needs of our body cells. Glucose, which the body can produce from most carbohydrates, is a major source of energy in most cells. When not enough carbohydrate is eaten to supply sufficient glucose, the body is forced to make glucose from proteins.

Digestion of some dietary starch begins in the mouth. The digestive process continues in the small intestine until starches break down into single sugar molecules (such as glucose), which are absorbed into the bloodstream using cells that line the small intestine (see Chapter 3 for more on digestion and absorption). However, the bonds between the sugar molecules in certain complex carbohydrates cannot be broken down by human digestive processes. These carbohydrates are part of what is called **fiber.** Such fiber passes through the small intestine undigested to provide bulk for feces formed in the large intestine (colon).[10] Chapter 5 focuses on carbohydrates.

Lipids

Lipids (e.g., fats, oils, and cholesterol) are composed mostly of the elements carbon and hydrogen; they contain fewer oxygen atoms than carbohydrates do. Because of this difference in composition, lipids yield more energy per gram than carbohydrates—on average, 9 kcal/g. (See Chapter 4 for more details concerning the reason for the high-energy yield of lipids.) Lipids are insoluble in water but can dissolve in certain organic solvents (e.g., ether and benzene).

The basic structure of most lipids is the three-carbon **glycerol** molecule with a **fatty acid** attached to each of the three carbons (review Figure 1-1). This form of lipid is generally called a **triglyceride.** Triglycerides are a key energy source for the body and the major form of fat in foods. They are also the major form for energy storage in the body.[10]

In this book, the more familiar term *fats* or *fats and oils* will generally be used rather than *lipids* or *triglycerides.* Fats are lipids that are solid at room temperature and oils are lipids that are liquid at room temperature.

Most lipids can be separated into two basic types—**saturated** and **unsaturated**—based on the chemical structure of their dominant fatty acids. This difference determines whether a lipid is solid or liquid at room temperature. Saturated fatty acids contain no carbon-carbon double bonds, while unsaturated fatty acids contain one or more in what is called a *cis* **configuration.** Plant oils tend to contain many unsaturated fatty acids, which makes them liquid at room temperature. Animal fats are often rich in saturated fatty acids, which makes them solid at room temperature. Almost all foods contain a variety of saturated and unsaturated fatty acids.

Lipids

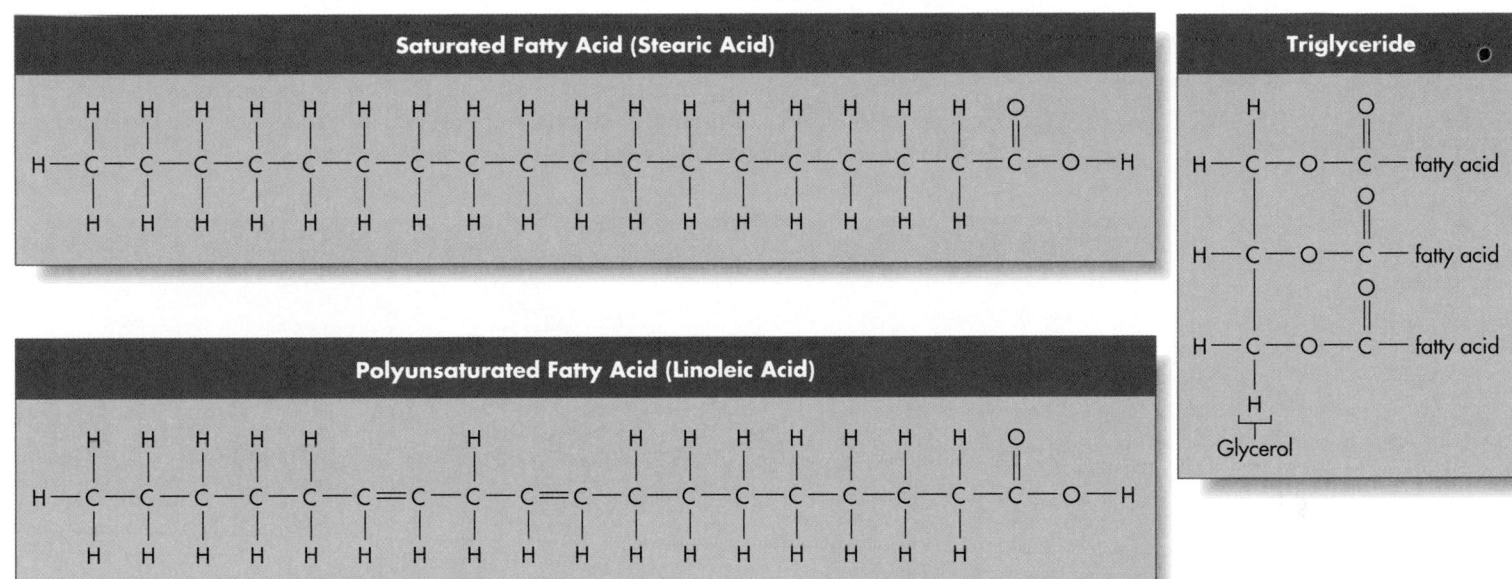

Two specific **polyunsaturated fatty acids**—linoleic acid and alpha-linolenic acid—are essential nutrients. These must come from our diets. These two fatty acids that the body can't produce, called **essential fatty acids,** perform several important functions in the body: they help regulate blood pressure and play a role in the synthesis and repair of vital cell parts. However, we need only a few tablespoons of a common vegetable oil (such as the canola or soybean oil found in supermarkets) each day to supply the essential fatty acids.[8] Adding fish in a diet at least twice a week adds to this benefit derived from the inclusion of vegetable oil. The unique unsaturated fatty acids in fish complement the healthy aspects of vegetable oil. This will be explained in greater detail in Chapter 6, which focuses on lipids.

Some foods also contain *trans* **fatty acids,** in which the unsaturated fat structure has been altered from the more typical *cis* form during food processing. These are commonly called *trans* fats and are found primarily in deep-fried foods (e.g., doughnuts and french fries), snack foods (e.g., cookies and crackers), and solid fats (e.g., stick margarine and shortening). Large amounts of *trans* fats in the diet pose certain health risks, so as with saturated fat, intake should be minimized (see Chapter 6 for details).[8] All food labels now have to list *trans* fat content (see Chapter 2 for more details concerning food labels).

Much attention has been given to eating less saturated fat in the past few years. This is because saturated fat bears a great deal of the responsibility for raising blood cholesterol. High blood cholesterol leads to clogged arteries and so can eventually lead to cardiovascular disease.

***cis* configuration** A form seen in compounds with double bonds, such as fatty acids, in which the hydrogens on both ends of the double bond lie on the same side of the plane of that bond.

polyunsaturated fatty acid A fatty acid containing two or more carbon-carbon double bonds.

trans* fatty acids** A form of an unsaturated fatty acid, usually a monosaturated one when found in food, in which the hydrogens on both carbons forming that double bond lie on opposite sides of that bond (trans* configuration).** Stick margarine, shortenings, and deep-fat fried foods in general are rich sources.

***trans* configuration** Compound in which the hydrogens lie opposite each other across a carbon-carbon double bond.

cis configuration

trans configuration

Many health-food stores market protein powders and shakes for bodybuilders and other athletes. However, the North American diet contains nearly two times the required amount of protein. Thus, these products are unnecessary.

enzyme A compound that speeds the rate of a chemical process but is not altered by the process. Almost all enzymes are proteins (some are made of nucleic acids).

Proteins

Like carbohydrates and fats, proteins are composed of the elements carbon, oxygen, and hydrogen. But unlike the other energy-yielding nutrients, all proteins also contain nitrogen. Proteins are the main structural material in the body (review Figure 1-1). For example, proteins constitute a major part of bone and muscle; they are also important components in blood, cell membranes, **enzymes,** and immune factors.[8] Furthermore, proteins can also provide energy for the body—on average, 4 kcal/g. Typically, the body uses little protein for the purpose of meeting daily energy needs. Proteins are formed by the bonding together of amino acids. Twenty common amino acids are found in food; nine of these are essential nutrients for adults, and one additional amino acid is essential for infants. Chapter 7 focuses on proteins.

Amino Acids

Alanine Valine Methionine

Vitamins

Vitamins exhibit a wide variety of chemical structures and can contain the elements carbon, hydrogen, nitrogen, oxygen, phosphorus, sulfur, and others. The main function of vitamins is to enable many **chemical reactions** to occur in the body. Some of these reactions help release the energy trapped in carbohydrates, lipids, and proteins. Remember, however, that vitamins themselves provide no usable energy for the body.[10]

chemical reaction An interaction between two chemicals that changes both participants.

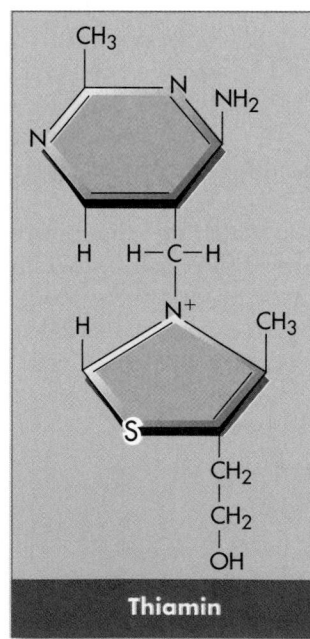

Thiamin

Vitamin C
(ascorbic acid)

The 13 vitamins are divided into two groups: four that dissolve in fat and so are **fat soluble vitamins** (vitamins A, D, E, and K) and nine that dissolve in water and so are **water soluble vitamins** (vitamin C and the B vitamins, such as thiamin). The two groups of vitamins often act quite differently. For example, cooking destroys water-soluble vitamins much more readily than it does fat-soluble vitamins. Water-soluble vitamins are also excreted from the body much more readily than are fat-soluble vitamins. Thus, the fat-soluble vitamins, especially vitamin A, are much more likely to accumulate in excessive amounts in the body, which then can cause toxicity. The vitamins are the focus of Chapters 9 and 10.

Minerals

The nutrients discussed so far are all **organic** compounds, whereas minerals are structurally very simple, **inorganic** substances, which exist as groups of one or more of the same atoms. These terms, *organic* and *inorganic*, have nothing to do with agriculture but are based on simple chemistry concepts (see Chapter 2 for a different use of the term on food labels). Inorganic substances for the most part do not contain carbon atoms.

Minerals typically function as such in the body (Na^+, K^+), or as parts of simple mineral combinations, such as bone mineral [$Ca_{10}(PO_4)_6 OH_2$]. Because of their simple structure, minerals are not destroyed during cooking. (However, they can still be lost if they leak into the water used for cooking and then discarded if that water is not consumed.) Although minerals themselves yield no energy as such for the body, they are critical players in nervous system functioning, other cellular processes, water balance, and structural (e.g., skeletal) systems.[10]

The amounts of the 16 or more essential minerals that are required in the diet for good health vary enormously. Thus, they are divided into two groups: major minerals and trace minerals, based on dietary needs. If daily needs are less than 100 mg, the mineral is put in the trace mineral class. The actual dietary requirement for some trace minerals has yet to be determined. Minerals that conduct electricity when dissolved in water are also called **electrolytes;** these include sodium, potassium, and chloride. Minerals are the focus of Chapters 11 and 12.

Water

Water is the sixth class of nutrients. Although sometimes overlooked as a nutrient, water is the macronutrient needed in the largest quantity. Water (chemically, H_2O) has numerous vital functions in the body. It acts as a **solvent** and lubricant, as a medium for transporting nutrients and waste, and as a medium for temperature regulation and chemical processes. For these reasons, and because the human body is approximately 60% water, we require about 3 liters (L)—equivalent to 3000 g or 12 cups—of a combination of water and/or beverages containing water every day.

Water is not only available from the obvious sources, but it is also the major component in some foods, such as many fruits and vegetables (e.g., lettuce, grapes, and melons). The body even makes some water as a by-product of **metabolism.**[10] Water is examined in detail in Chapter 11.

Nutrient Composition of Diets and the Human Body

The quantities of the various nutrients that people consume vary widely, and the nutrient amounts present in different foods also vary a great deal. The total daily intake of protein, fat, and carbohydrate amounts to about 500 g (about 1 lb). In contrast, the typical daily mineral intake totals about 20 g (about 4 teaspoons), and the daily vitamin intake totals less than 300 mg (1/15th of a teaspoon). Although each day we require a gram or so of some minerals, such as calcium and phosphorus, we need only a few milligrams or less of other minerals. For example, we need about 10 mg of zinc per day, which is just a few specks of the mineral.

Figure 1-2 contrasts the relative proportions of all the major classes of nutrients in a lean man and a lean woman with the proportions of both a cooked steak and french

organic Any substance that contains carbon atoms bonded to hydrogen atoms in the chemical structure.

inorganic Any substance lacking carbon atoms bonded to hydrogen atoms in the chemical structure.

electrolytes Compounds that separate into ions in water and, in turn, are able to conduct an electrical current. These include sodium, chloride, and potassium.

solvent A liquid substance that other substances dissolve in.

metabolism Chemical processes in the body that provide energy in useful forms and sustain vital activities.

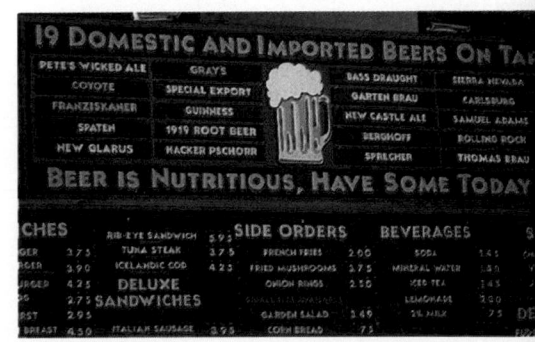

Alcoholic beverages are rich in energy, but alcohol is not an essential nutrient.

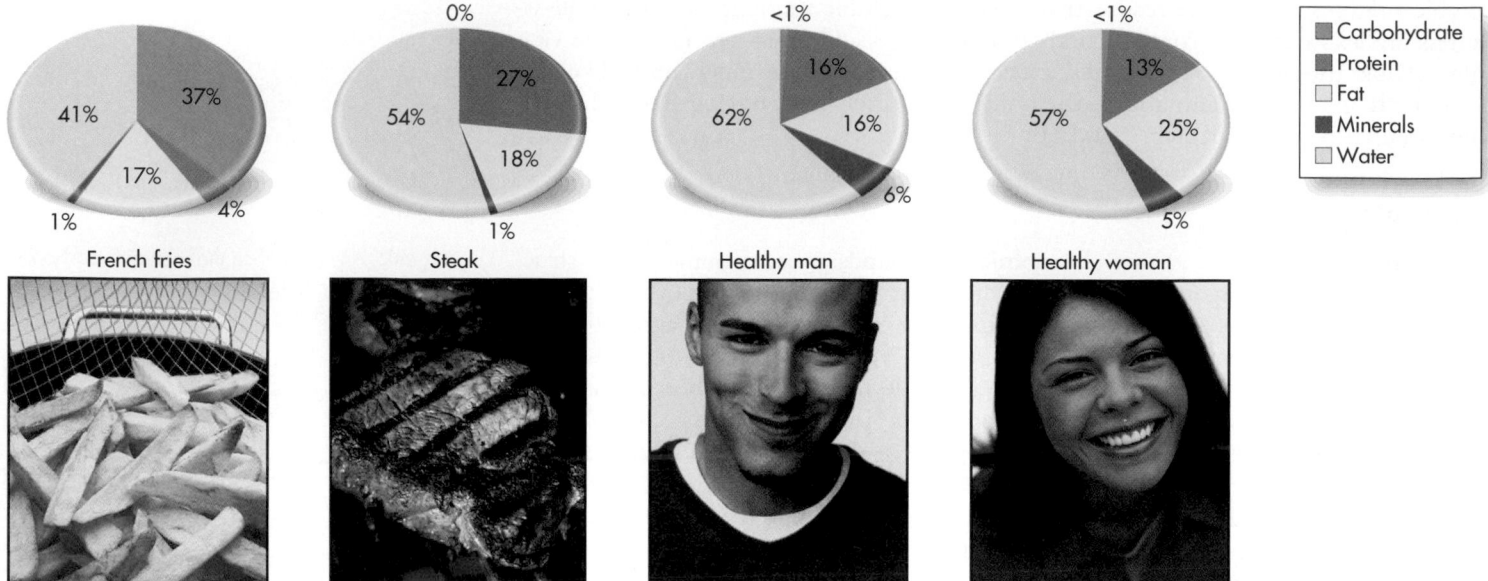

Figure 1-2 | The proportions of nutrients in the human body compared to those found in typical foods—animal or vegetable. Note that the amount of vitamins found in the body is negligible, and so is not shown.

deoxyribonucleic acid (DNA) The site of hereditary information in cells; DNA directs the synthesis of cell proteins.

genes The hereditary material on chromosomes that makes up DNA. Genes provide the blueprints for the production of cell proteins.

alcohol Ethyl alcohol or ethanol (CH_3CH_2OH).

$$H-\overset{\displaystyle H}{\underset{\displaystyle H}{C}}-\overset{\displaystyle OH}{\underset{\displaystyle H}{C}}-H$$

compound A group of different types of atoms bonded together in definite proportion (see also *molecule*). Not all chemical compounds exist as molecules. Some compounds are made up of ions attracted to each other, such as Na^+CL^- (table salt).

ion An atom with an unequal number of electrons and protons. Negative ions have more electrons than protons; positive ions have more protons than electrons.

fries. Note how the nutrient composition of the human body differs from the nutritional profiles of the foods we eat. This is because growth, development, and later maintenance of the human body are directed by the genetic material (**DNA**) inside the cell nucleus. This genetic blueprint determines how each cell uses the essential nutrients to perform body functions.[13] These nutrients can come from a variety of sources. Cells are not concerned whether available amino acids come from animal or plant sources. The carbohydrate glucose can come from sugars or starches. In sum, what you eat provides cells with basic materials to function according to the directions supplied by the **genes** housed in the cell.

Energy Sources and Uses

Humans obtain the energy needed to perform body functions and do work from carbohydrates, fats, and proteins. Foods generally provide more than one energy source.

Plant oils are one exception; these are 100% fat. **Alcohol** is also a source of energy for some of us, supplying about 7 kcal/g. It is not considered an essential nutrient, however, because it has no required function. Still, alcoholic beverages—generally also rich in carbohydrate, such as beer—contribute energy to the diet of people who drink such beverages.

The body transforms the energy trapped in carbohydrate, protein, and fat (and alcohol) into other forms of energy in order to:[10]

- Build new **compounds**
- Perform muscular movements
- Promote nerve transmissions
- Maintain **ion** balance within cells

Chapter 4 describes how that energy is released from chemical bonds and then used by body cells to support the processes just described.

You have likely noticed on food labels that the energy in food is often expressed in terms of calories. (Chapter 13 has a diagram of the instrument that can be used to measure calories in foods [bomb calorimeter].) Technically, a calorie is the amount of heat energy it takes to raise the temperature of 1 g of water 1 degree **Celsius** (1°C). Because a calorie is such a tiny measure of heat, food energy is more accurately expressed in terms of the kilocalorie (kcal), which equals 1000 calories. (If the "c" in calories is capitalized, this also signifies kilocalories.) A kcal is the amount of heat energy it takes to raise the temperature of 1000 g (1 L) of water 1°C. The term *kilo-*

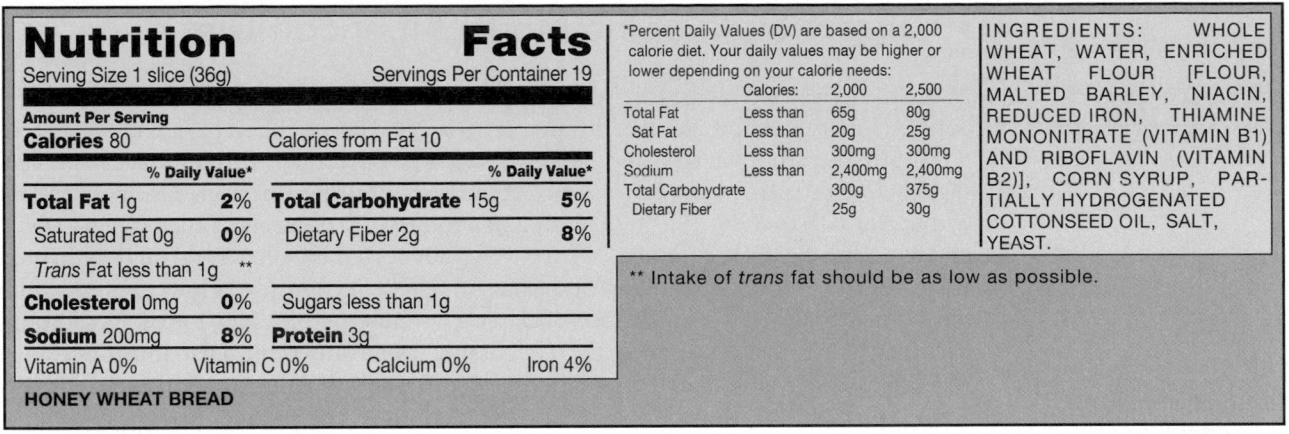

Nutrition		Facts	
Serving Size 1 slice (36g)		Servings Per Container 19	

Amount Per Serving

Calories 80		Calories from Fat 10	
	% Daily Value*		**% Daily Value***
Total Fat 1g	**2%**	**Total Carbohydrate** 15g	**5%**
Saturated Fat 0g	**0%**	Dietary Fiber 2g	**8%**
Trans Fat less than 1g	**		
Cholesterol 0mg	**0%**	Sugars less than 1g	
Sodium 200mg	**8%**	**Protein** 3g	
Vitamin A 0%	Vitamin C 0%	Calcium 0%	Iron 4%

HONEY WHEAT BREAD

*Percent Daily Values (DV) are based on a 2,000 calorie diet. Your daily values may be higher or lower depending on your calorie needs:

		Calories:	2,000	2,500
Total Fat	Less than		65g	80g
Sat Fat	Less than		20g	25g
Cholesterol	Less than		300mg	300mg
Sodium	Less than		2,400mg	2,400mg
Total Carbohydrate			300g	375g
Dietary Fiber			25g	30g

INGREDIENTS: WHOLE WHEAT, WATER, ENRICHED WHEAT FLOUR [FLOUR, MALTED BARLEY, NIACIN, REDUCED IRON, THIAMINE MONONITRATE (VITAMIN B1) AND RIBOFLAVIN (VITAMIN B2)], CORN SYRUP, PARTIALLY HYDROGENATED COTTONSEED OIL, SALT, YEAST.

** Intake of *trans* fat should be as low as possible.

Figure 1-3 | Use the nutrient values on the Nutrition Facts label to calculate the energy content of a food. Based on carbohydrate, fat, and protein content, a serving of this food (Honey Wheat Bread) contains 81 kcal ([15 × 4] + [1 × 9] + [3 × 4] = 81). The label lists 80, suggesting that the calorie value was rounded down.

calorie and its abbreviation *kcal* are used throughout this book. In everyday usage, the word *calorie* (without a capital "c") is also used loosely to mean *kilocalorie*. Any values given on food labels in calories are actually in kilocalories (Figure 1-3). A suggested intake of 2000 calories per day on a food label is really 2000 kcal.

As you have seen, carbohydrates, proteins, lipids, and alcohol provide the body with differing amounts of energy. Use the 4-9-4 rough estimates for carbohydrate, fat, and protein introduced over the last few pages to determine energy content of a food. Consider a typical deluxe hamburger sandwich:

Carbohydrate	39 grams × 4 =	156 kcal
Fat	32 grams × 9 =	288 kcal
Protein	30 grams × 4 =	120 kcal
Total		564 kcal

Note also that the 4-9-4 estimates have been adjusted for (1) **digestibility** and (2) substances not available for energy use. Such substances include waxes and some fibrous parts of plants. The energy estimates are then rounded to whole numbers.[8]

You can also use the 4-9-4 estimates to determine what portion of total energy intake is contributed by the various energy-yielding nutrients. Assume that one day you consume 290 g of carbohydrates, 60 g of fat, and 70 g of protein. This consumption yields a total of 1980 kcal ([290 × 4] + [60 × 9] + [70 × 4] = 1980). The percentage of your total energy intake derived from each nutrient can then be determined:

% of energy intake as carbohydrate = (290 × 4) ÷ 1980 = 0.59 × 100 = 59%

% of energy intake as fat = (60 × 9) ÷ 1980 = 0.27 × 100 = 27%

% of energy intake as protein = (70 × 4) ÷ 1980 = 0.14 × 100 = 14%

Check your calculations by adding the percentages together. Do they total 100?

Concept | Check

Nutrition is the study of food and nutrients—their digestion, absorption, and metabolism and their effect on health and disease. Food contains vital nutrients that are essential for good health: carbohydrates, lipids (fats and oils), proteins, vitamins, minerals, and water. Nutrients have three general functions in the body: (1) to provide materials for building and maintaining the body; (2) to act as regulators for key metabolic reactions; and (3) to participate in metabolic reactions that provide the energy necessary to sustain life. A common unit of measurement for this energy is the kilocalorie (kcal). On average, carbohydrates and protein provide 4 kcal/g of energy to the body, while lipids provide 9 kcal/g. Although not considered a nutrient, alcohol provides about 7 kcal/g. The other classes of nutrients do not supply energy but are essential for proper body functioning.

In many scientific journals, the kilojoule (kJ), rather than the kilocalorie, is used to express the energy content of food. A mass of 1 gram moving at a velocity of 1 meter/sec possesses the energy of 1 joule (J); 1000J = 1 kJ. Since heat and work are just two forms of energy, measurements expressed in terms of kilocalories (a heat measure) are interchangeable with measurements expressed in terms of kilojoules (a work measure): 1 kcal = 4.18 kJ.

digestibility The proportion of food substances eaten that can be broken down into individual nutrients in the intestinal tract for absorption into the body.

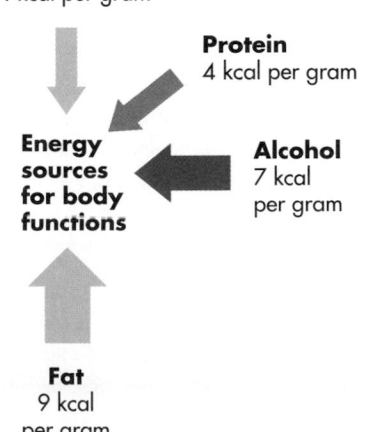

Carbohydrate
4 kcal per gram

Protein
4 kcal per gram

Energy sources for body functions

Alcohol
7 kcal per gram

Fat
9 kcal per gram

The Food and Nutrition Board also recommends limiting saturated fat, *trans* fat, and cholesterol intake when putting their diet guidelines into place.

Acceptable Macronutrient Distribution Range (AMDR) Range of intake for a specific macronutrient that is associated with a reduced risk of chronic diseases while providing for recommended intakes of essential nutrients. AMDR are set for carbohydrate, protein, and fat (various forms); each is intended to provide guidance in dietary planning.

salt Generally refers to a compound of sodium and chloride in a 40:60 ratio.

Critical | Thinking

Believing that supplements provide the nutrition her body needs, Janice regularly takes numerous supplements while paying relatively little attention to daily food choices. How would you explain to her that this practice may lead to health problems?

For suggested answers to the Critical Thinking questions in this and every chapter, see the website for this book www.mhhe.com/wardlawpers7.

▌Current State of the North American Diet

Humans derive energy mostly from carbohydrates, fats, and proteins. If we ignore alcohol, North American adults consume on average 16% of their energy intake as proteins, 50% as carbohydrates, and 33% as fats. These percentages are estimates and vary slightly from year to year and to some extent from person to person. This pattern falls within the 10% to 35%, 45% to 65%, and 20% to 35% distribution of energy intake from protein, carbohydrate, and fat, respectively, advocated by the Food and Nutrition Board of the National Academy of Sciences.[8] These recommendations apply to both the United States and Canada (see Chapter 2). These percentages for each macronutrient make up what is termed the **Acceptable Macronutrient Distribution Range (AMDR).** Note that recommendations for different distributions of energy intake among protein, carbohydrate, and fat come and go in the popular press. This will be reviewed in Chapters 5, 6, and 7.

Animal sources supply about two-thirds of protein intake for most North Americans; plant sources supply only about one-third. In many other parts of the world, it is just the opposite: plant proteins—from rice, beans, corn, and other vegetables—dominate protein intake. About half the carbohydrate in North American diets comes from simple sugars; the other half comes from starches (such as in pastas, breads, and potatoes). About 60% of dietary fat comes from animal sources and 40% from plant sources.

Assessing the Current North American Diet

Information about the North American diet comes from large surveys designed to find out what and when people eat. The U.S. government uses the National Health and Nutrition Examination Survey (NHANES) administered by the U.S. Department of Health and Human Services. In Canada, this information is gathered by Health Canada in conjunction with Agriculture and Agrifood Canada. Results from these surveys and other studies show that we eat a wide variety of foods. Many people are meeting their nutrient needs; some are not. Chapter 2 will look at this situation in more detail. For now, note that studies show that some of us should choose more foods that are rich in iron, calcium, magnesium, potassium, vitamin A, various B vitamins, vitamin C (especially smokers), vitamin D, vitamin E, zinc, and fiber.[3] Daily intake of a balanced multivitamin and mineral supplement to help meet these nutrient needs is also a strategy, but does not make up for a poor diet in all respects, such as for calcium, potassium, and fiber intake (see Chapter 9 for more on supplement use).

Routinely, experts recommend that we pay more attention to balancing energy intake with need. An excess intake of energy is usually tied to an overindulgence in sugar, fat, and alcoholic beverages.[7] African Americans and Hispanics in particular may need to pay special attention to the amount of **salt** and alcohol in their diets. This is because they have a greater chance of developing hypertension than do other ethnic groups in North America, and these substances are two of the many factors linked to elevated blood pressure. Actually, a careful look at salt and alcohol intake—along with saturated fat, *trans* fat, cholesterol, and total energy intake—is a useful and recommended task for all adults.[5]

Many North Americans would benefit from a more helpful balance of foods in their diets—greater moderation in the intake of some foods is needed, such as sugared soft drinks and fried foods, while increasing the variety of other foods, such as fruits and vegetables.[19] Few adults currently meet the "5 A Day" minimum recommendation for total servings of vegetables (≥ 3) and fruits (≥ 2).

What Influences Our Food Choices?

We eat primarily for nourishment—we have to eat to survive. But food means far more to us than that. Food symbolizes much of what we think about ourselves. Throughout our lives, we spend 13 to 15 years eating. Important reasons for the specific foods we choose are:[23]

- *Flavor, texture, and appearance.* These are the most important factors determining our food choices. Creating more flavorful foods that are both healthy and profitable is a major focus of the food industry (referred to as "better for you" products).
- *Early influences.* These expose us to various people, places, and situations and go on to influence our lifelong food choices. Many aspects of ethnic diet patterns (discussed more fully in Chapter 2) begin as we are introduced to foods as children.
- *Routines and habits.* Most of us eat from a core group of foods: about 100 basic items account for 75% of an individual's total food intake. Overall, food habits and food availability and convenience strongly influence choices.
- *Nutrition, or what we think of as "healthy foods."* North Americans who tend to make health-related food choices are often well-educated, middle-class professionals. These same people are generally health oriented, have active lifestyles, and focus on weight control.
- *Advertising.* The food industry in the United States alone spends well over $34 billion annually on advertising. Some of this advertising is helpful, such as when it promotes the importance of calcium and fiber intake. However, the food industry also advertises highly sweetened cereals, cookies, cakes, and pastries because such products can reap the greatest profits.
- *Restaurants.* Today, about half of all food dollars in North America is spent on meals outside of home. This food is often very high in energy, served in overly generous portions, and of poorer nutritional quality compared to foods made at home. However, over the past 10 years, restaurants have placed healthier items on their menus.
- *Social changes.* Many of us today have increasingly busy lives. This creates the need for convenience. Supermarkets now supply already-prepared meals, microwave entrees, and various quick-prep frozen products.
- *Economics.* Food cost is important but plays only a moderate role in food choices for many of us, because North Americans spend only about 10% of after-tax income on food (this percentage will be greater for low-income people). However, as income increases, so do meals eaten away from home.

Daily food intake is a complicated mix of innate (e.g., genetic) and social influences.[21] These factors are depicted in Figure 1-4. Chapters 13 and 15 will look at issues of food choice with specific reference to weight control and eating disorders. What influences your food intake on a daily basis? How are you the same as or different from the typical North American?

Improving Our Diets

More efforts by the general public are needed to lower saturated fat, *trans* fat, sugar, and cholesterol intakes and to improve variety in our diets, but our cultural diversity, varied cuisines, and generally high nutritional status should be points of pride for North Americans. Today we can choose from a tremendous variety of food products, the result of multifaceted cultural currents and innovation by food manufacturers.

During the past hundred years, North America has led the world in creating new food products.[20] From toaster pastries to microwave popcorn, the variety of food products in a typical supermarket is nearly limitless. Today we are eating more breakfast cereals, pizza, pasta entrees, stir-fried meats and vegetables served on rice, salads, vitamin- and mineral-fortified juices, tacos, burritos, and fajitas than ever before. Sales of whole milk are down, whereas in the same time period sales of fat-free and 1% low-fat milk have increased. Consumption of frozen vegetables, rather than canned vegetables, is also on the rise. Still, soft drinks are more popular than milk, although not as beneficial to the diet.[6]

One recent trend by food manufacturers has been to promote meal replacement bars (also called "energy" bars). These bars typically contain about 180–250 kcal, with

Scientists suspect we are born with a taste for sweets and over time acquire a taste for fat.

According to Dr. Andrew Weil, the primary danger from food is overindulgence.

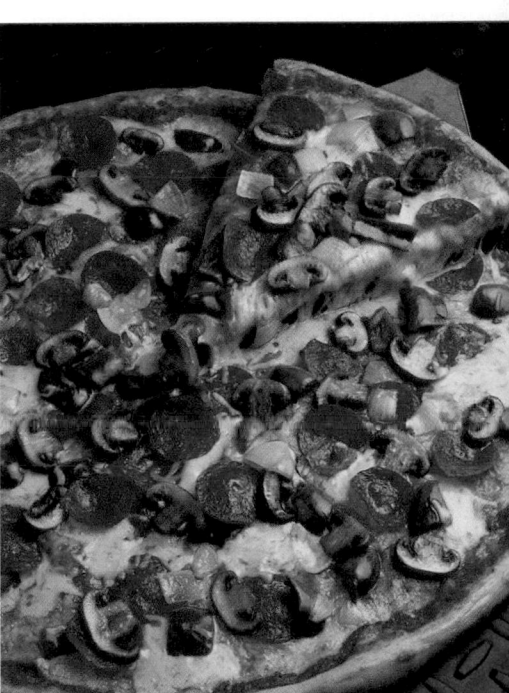

A market research firm surveyed the eating habits of people in 2000 North American households. The top meal choice was pizza, followed by ham sandwich, hot dog, peanut butter and jelly sandwich, steak, macaroni and cheese, turkey sandwich, cheese sandwich, hamburger on a bun, and spaghetti.

Figure 1-4 | Food behavior is influenced by many sources, some of which are shown. Which are important in your life?

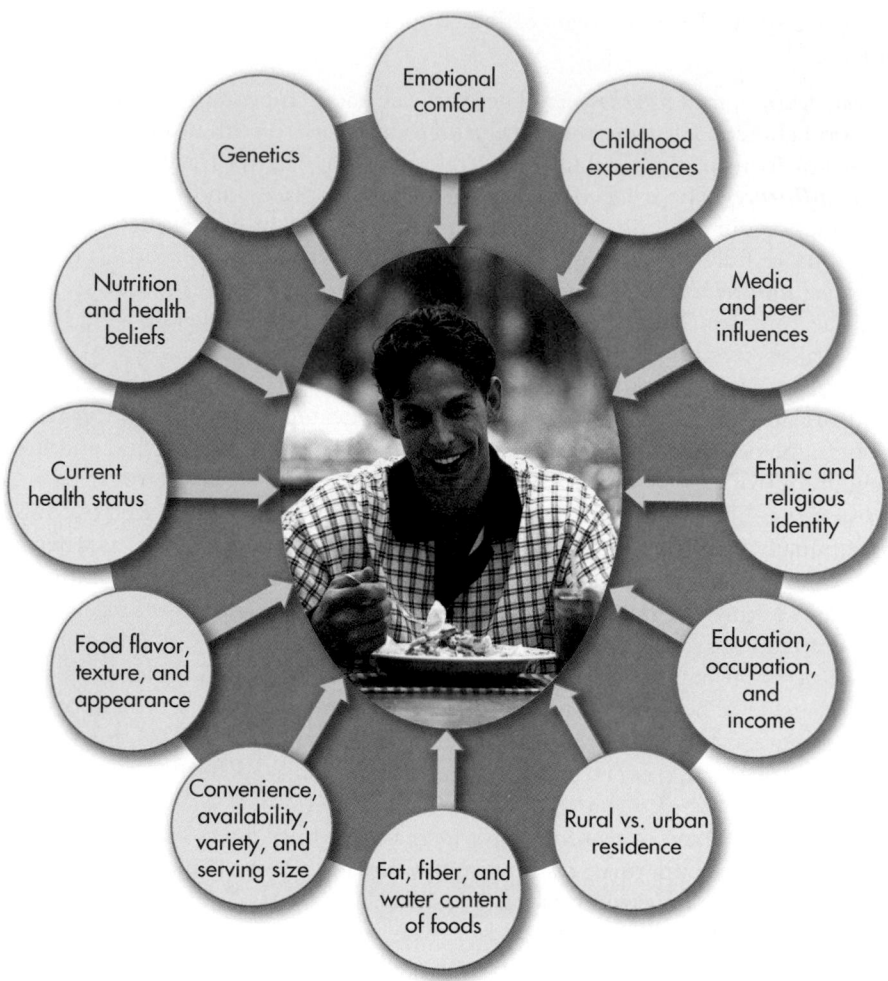

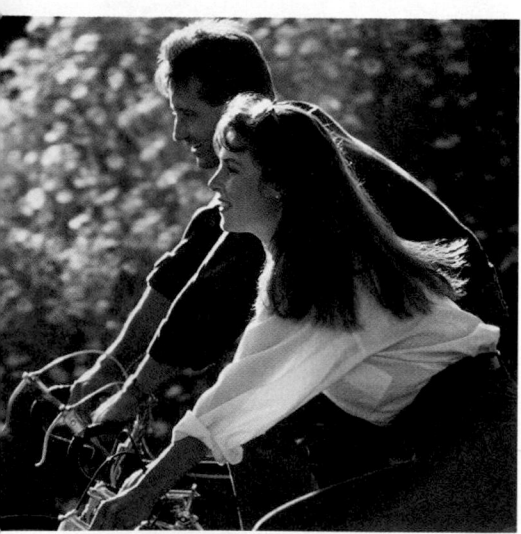

Regular physical activity complements a healthy diet; practice both each day. Whether it's all at once or in segments throughout the day, ideally incorporate 30 to 60 minutes or more of such activity into your daily routine.

a protein:carbohydrate:fat ratio typical of common diets. However, some bars replace much of the carbohydrate with protein. All of the bars are fortified with vitamins and minerals in amounts ranging from about 25 to 100% of typical human needs. Some people find that these bars provide a convenient way to consume a meal (or snack) on the run while also focusing on certain nutrients they may underconsume, such as the vitamin folate or the mineral calcium. Critics suggest these products are really just the nutritional equivalent of a low-fat yogurt and piece of fruit.

North Americans currently are living longer, and many enjoy better general health. Many also have more money and more diverse food and lifestyle choices to consider. The nutritional consequences of these trends are not fully known. Deaths from cardiovascular disease, for example, have dropped dramatically since the late 1960s, partly because of better medical care and diets. Still, if affluence leads to sedentary lifestyles and high intakes of saturated fat, *trans* fat, cholesterol, sodium, sugar, and alcohol, health problems can result.[5] For example, obesity is a growing problem in our population.[18] Because of better technology and greater choices, we can have a much better diet today than ever before—if we know what choices to make.

The goal of this book is to help you find the best path to good nutrition. Nutrition experts often say that there are no "junk" or bad foods.[1] Obviously, though, many foods and beverages available in supermarkets, such as pastries and sugar-rich soft drinks, provide fewer nutrients in comparison with energy content and, thus, contribute to less nutritious food habits.[14] One's overall diet is the proper focus in a nutritional evaluation. Chapter 2 will emphasize this point and show you how to balance your diet. As you reexamine your nutritional goals, remember that your health is largely your responsibility (Figure 1-5).

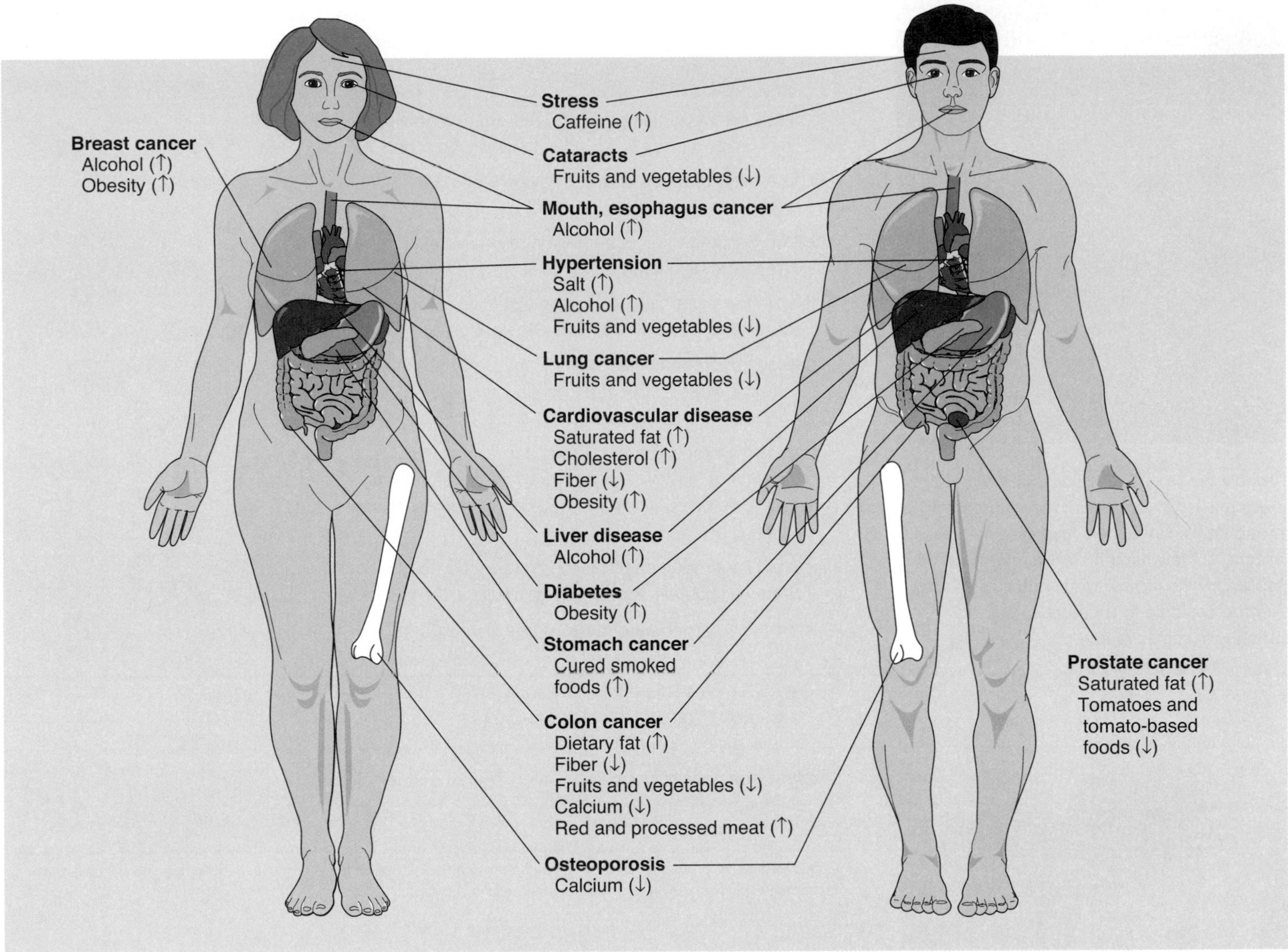

Stress
Caffeine (↑)

Cataracts
Fruits and vegetables (↓)

Mouth, esophagus cancer
Alcohol (↑)

Breast cancer
Alcohol (↑)
Obesity (↑)

Hypertension
Salt (↑)
Alcohol (↑)
Fruits and vegetables (↓)

Lung cancer
Fruits and vegetables (↓)

Cardiovascular disease
Saturated fat (↑)
Cholesterol (↑)
Fiber (↓)
Obesity (↑)

Liver disease
Alcohol (↑)

Diabetes
Obesity (↑)

Stomach cancer
Cured smoked
foods (↑)

Colon cancer
Dietary fat (↑)
Fiber (↓)
Fruits and vegetables (↓)
Calcium (↓)
Red and processed meat (↑)

Osteoporosis
Calcium (↓)

Prostate cancer
Saturated fat (↑)
Tomatoes and
tomato-based
foods (↓)

Figure 1-5 | Some possible health problems associated with poor dietary habits. An upward arrow (↑) indicates excessive intake while a downward arrow (↓) indicates low intake or deficiency. In addition to those habits listed in the figure, no illicit drug use, adequate sleep (7–8 hours), adequate water and related fluid intake, and a reduction in stress (practice better time management, relax, meditate, listen to music, have a massage, and stay physically active) provide a more complete approach to good nutrition and health. Add to this approach maintaining close relationships with others and a positive outlook on life. Finally, consultation with health-care professionals on a regular basis is important. Early diagnosis is especially useful for controlling the damaging effects of many diseases. Prevention of disease is an important investment of one's time, including during the college years.

Health Objectives for the United States for the Year 2010 Include Numerous Nutrition Objectives

Health promotion and disease prevention have been public health strategies in the United States and Canada since the late 1970s. One part of this strategy is *Healthy People 2010*, a report issued in 2000 by the U.S. Department of Health and Human Services' Public Health Service.[12] This report consists of health promotion and disease prevention objectives for the year 2010 and assigns each of the objectives to appropriate U.S. federal agencies to address. Many nutrition-related objectives are part of the overall plan (Table 1-4).

The main objectives of *Healthy People 2010* are to promote healthful lifestyles and to reduce preventable death and disability. Minority groups in particular are the focus of *Healthy People 2010* programs, because overall health status currently lags in these population groups, especially with respect to hypertension, type 2 diabetes, and obesity.

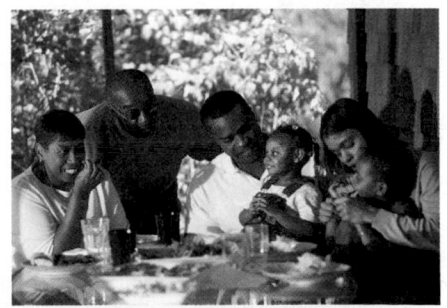

A healthy diet benefits people of all ages.

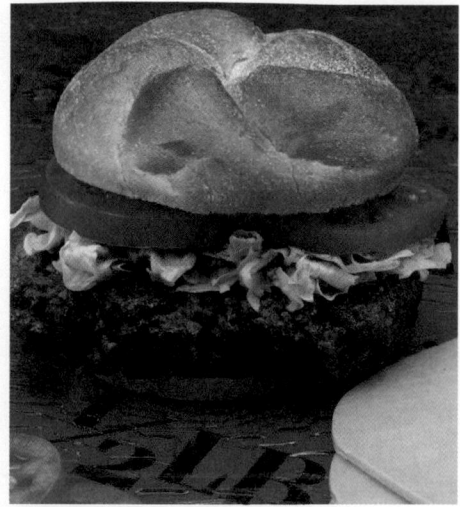

Probably the worst food-related trend in North America is large servings of foods, especially in restaurants. Consumers might see these as a bargain, but few need the extra energy supplied by the increased serving sizes. One response could be to share the oversized portion with someone else.

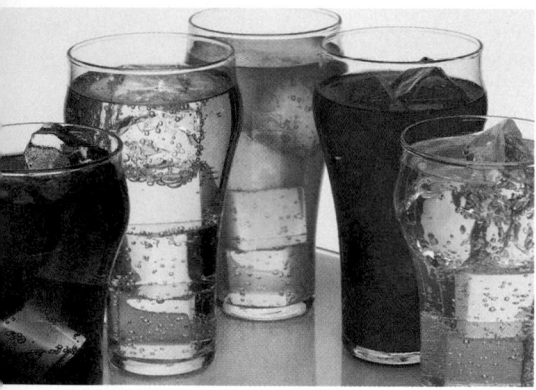

Today soft drinks are more popular than milk although not as beneficial to the diet. Soft drinks account for about 10% of the energy intake of teenagers in North America and in turn contribute to generally poor calcium intakes seen in this age group.

Table 1-4 | A Sample of Nutrition-Related Objectives from *Healthy People 2010*

	Target	Current Estimate
Increase the proportion of adults who are at a healthy weight (defined as a body mass index between 18.5 and 25).	60%	35%
Reduce the proportion of adults who are obese (body mass index of 30 or more).	15%	23%
Reduce the proportion of children and adolescents who are overweight or obese.	5%	10%
Increase the proportion of persons age 2 years and older who consume at least two daily servings of fruit.	75%	28%
Increase the proportion of persons age 2 years and older who consume at least three daily servings of vegetables, with at least one-third being dark green or deep yellow vegetables.	50%	3%
Increase the proportion of persons age 2 years and older who consume at least six daily servings of grain products, with at least three being whole grains (e.g., whole wheat bread and oatmeal).	50%	7%
Increase the proportion of persons age 2 years and older who consume less than 10% of energy intake from saturated fat.	75%	36%
Increase the proportion of persons age 2 years and older who consume 6 g or less of salt (2300 mg or less of sodium) daily.	65%	5%
Increase the proportion of persons age 2 years and older who meet dietary recommendations for calcium (see inside cover of this book).	75%	46%
Reduce iron deficiency among young children and females of childbearing age.	6%	10%

Note: Related objectives include those addressing osteoporosis, various forms of cancer, diabetes prevention and treatment, food allergies, cardiovascular disease (coronary heart disease and stroke), low birth weight, nutrition during pregnancy, breastfeeding, eating disorders, physical activity, and alcohol use (see later chapters).

Concept | Check

North Americans generally have a variety of food available to us. However, some of us could improve our diets by focusing on rich food sources of iron, calcium, vitamin A, various B vitamins, vitamin C, vitamin D, vitamin E, potassium, magnesium, zinc, and fiber. In addition, many of us should reduce our consumption of energy, sugar, saturated fat, *trans* fat, cholesterol, salt, and alcoholic beverages. These recommendations are consistent with an overall goal to attain and maintain good health. Our specific food choices depend on taste, texture, and appearance of foods; habits and routines; health knowledge and concerns; advertising; and various social trends such as increased use of restaurants.

Using Scientific Research to Determine Nutrient Needs

How do we know what we know about nutrition? How has this knowledge been gained? In a word, research. Like other sciences, the research that sets the foundation for nutrition has developed through the use of the *scientific method*, a testing procedure designed to detect and eliminate error. The first step is the observation of a natural phenomenon. Scientists then suggest possible explanations, called **hypotheses,** about its cause. Distinguishing a true cause-and-effect relationship from mere coincidence can be difficult. For instance, early in the past century, many patients in mental

hypotheses Tentative explanations by scientists to explain a phenomenon.

hospitals suffered from the disease **pellagra,** which suggested a possible relationship between mental illness and this disease. In time, it became clear that this supposed connection was simply coincidental; the real culprit was the poor diet common in mental institutions at that time (see Chapter 10 for details).

To test hypotheses and eliminate coincidental explanations, scientists perform controlled scientific **experiments.** The data gathered from these experiments may either support or refute each hypothesis. If the results of many experiments support a hypothesis, the hypothesis becomes generally accepted by scientists and can be called a **theory** (such as the theory of gravity). Very often, the results from one experiment suggest a new set of questions to be answered (Figure 1-6).

pellagra A disease characterized by inflammation of the skin, diarrhea, and eventual mental incapacity; results from an insufficient amount of the vitamin niacin in the diet.

experiments Tests made to examine the validity of a hypothesis.

theory An explanation for a phenomenon that has numerous lines of evidence to support it.

The Scientific Method

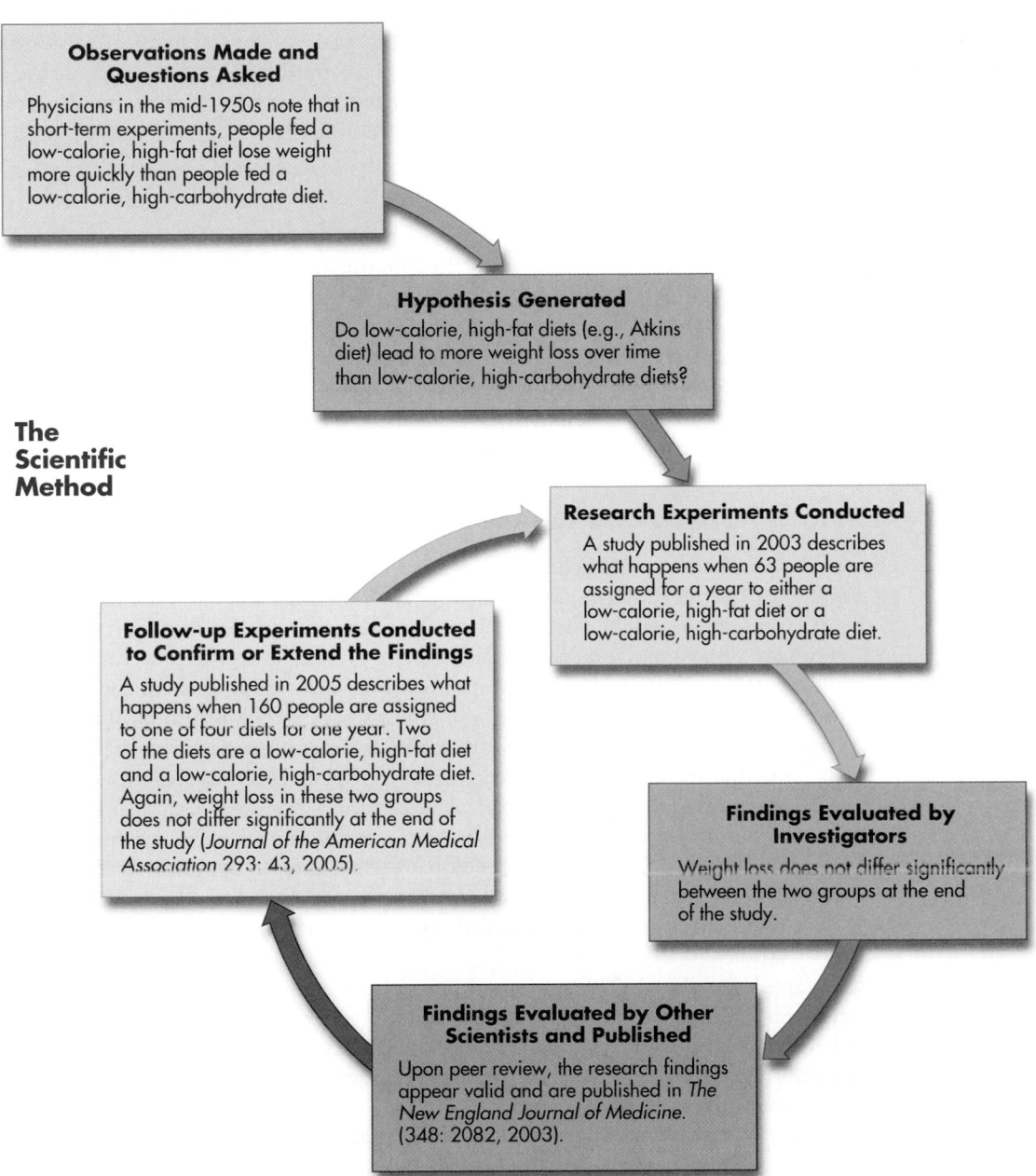

Observations Made and Questions Asked

Physicians in the mid-1950s note that in short-term experiments, people fed a low-calorie, high-fat diet lose weight more quickly than people fed a low-calorie, high-carbohydrate diet.

Hypothesis Generated

Do low-calorie, high-fat diets (e.g., Atkins diet) lead to more weight loss over time than low-calorie, high-carbohydrate diets?

Research Experiments Conducted

A study published in 2003 describes what happens when 63 people are assigned for a year to either a low-calorie, high-fat diet or a low-calorie, high-carbohydrate diet.

Follow-up Experiments Conducted to Confirm or Extend the Findings

A study published in 2005 describes what happens when 160 people are assigned to one of four diets for one year. Two of the diets are a low-calorie, high-fat diet and a low-calorie, high-carbohydrate diet. Again, weight loss in these two groups does not differ significantly at the end of the study (*Journal of the American Medical Association* 293: 43, 2005).

Findings Evaluated by Investigators

Weight loss does not differ significantly between the two groups at the end of the study.

Findings Evaluated by Other Scientists and Published

Upon peer review, the research findings appear valid and are published in *The New England Journal of Medicine.* (348: 2082, 2003).

Figure 1-6 | Implementing the scientific method using low-calorie, high-fat diets as an example. Scientists consistently follow these steps in conducting scientific research. It is important not to embrace a nutrition or other scientific concept until it has been thoroughly tested using the scientific method. Incidentally, in the final study few people on the low-calorie, high-fat diet were able to follow the guideline of <50 g of carbohydrates per day.

ulcer Erosion of the tissue lining, usually in the stomach (gastric ulcer) or the upper small intestine (duodenal ulcer). These are generally referred to as peptic ulcers.

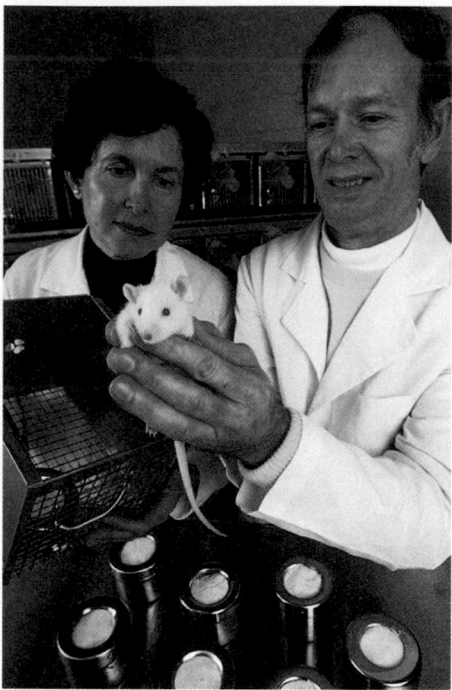

Research using laboratory animals contributes to our nutrition knowledge.

epidemiology The distribution and determinants of disease in human populations.

infectious disease Any disease caused by invasion of the body by microorganisms, such as bacteria, fungi, or viruses.

The scientific method requires a skeptical attitude. Scientists must not accept proposed hypotheses and theories until they are supported by considerable evidence, and they must reject those that fail to pass critical analysis. Likewise, students should adopt a healthy skepticism and be critical of many current ideas about nutrition.[2] Dr. Robert DiSilvestro discusses this concept further in the Expert Opinion, p. 22.

A recent example of this need for skepticism involves stomach **ulcers.** Not so many years ago, "everyone knew" that stomach ulcers were caused mostly by a stressful lifestyle and a poor diet. Then, in 1983, an Australian physician, Marshall, reported in a respected medical journal that ulcers are usually caused by a common microorganism called *Helicobacter pylori.* Furthermore, he stated that a cure is possible using antibiotics. At first, other physicians were skeptical about this finding and continued to prescribe medications such as antacids that reduce stomach acid. But as more studies were published and patients were cured of ulcers using antibiotics, the medical profession eventually accepted the findings. (He was even given the Nobel Prize for Medicine in 2005 for this discovery.) Today, ulcers are managed for the most part by medications that destroy the pathogen. We can expect that scientific discoveries will always be subject to challenge and change.

As you will see, sound scientific research requires that:

1. Questions are asked.
2. Hypotheses are generated to explain the phenomena.
3. Research is conducted (experiments).
4. Incorrect explanations are rejected.
5. The most likely explanation is used as the basis for a model.
6. Research results are subjected to review by other scientists and published in a scientific journal.
7. The results are confirmed by more experiments and studies.

Asking Questions and Generating Hypotheses

Historical events have provided clues to important relationships in nutrition science. In the fifteenth and sixteenth centuries, for example, many European sailors on the long voyages to the Americas developed the disease scurvy. The sailors ate very few fruits and vegetables, and eventually a British naval surgeon, Lind, discovered that lime juice prevented or cured scurvy. After this, sailors were given a ration of lime juice, earning them the nickname "limeys." This simple practice ensured a healthy workforce for the British navy and helped it dominate the seas worldwide. About 200 years later, scientists identified vitamin C, the nutrient present in the lime juice and other fruits and vegetables that prevents scurvy.

In a related approach to using historical observation, scientists establish nutritional hypotheses by studying the dietary and disease patterns among various populations in today's world. If one group tends to develop a certain disease but another group does not, scientists can speculate about the role diet plays in this difference. The study of diseases in populations is called **epidemiology** and ultimately forms the basis for many laboratory studies.

An example of the use of epidemiology occurred in the 1920s, in the United States, when Goldberger noticed that residents in mental institutions—but not their caretakers—suffered from pellagra. He reasoned that if pellagra were an **infectious disease,** both groups would suffer from it. Since they did not, he concluded that pellagra is caused by a dietary deficiency.

Historical and epidemiological findings can suggest hypotheses about the role of diet in various health problems. Proving the role of particular dietary components, however, requires controlled experiments. For instance, once the high incidence of pellagra in mental institutions during the 1920s was linked to poor diet, various foods were given to patients who had the disease. These experiments showed that yeast and high-protein foods could cure these patients if the disease was not in its final stage, indicating that pellagra results from a deficiency of some nutrient present in these foods. Eventually, this nutrient was found to be the B vitamin called niacin.

Laboratory Animal Experiments

When scientists cannot test their hypotheses by experiments with humans, they often use laboratory animals. Much of what we know about human nutritional needs and functions has been generated from laboratory animal experiments. Still, human experiments are the most convincing to scientists. In the 1930s, scientists showed that a pellagra-like disease seen in dogs, called *blacktongue,* is cured by nicotinic acid. Only when nicotinic acid actually cured pellagra in humans were scientists convinced that nicotinic acid (later classified as the vitamin niacin) was the critical dietary factor.

Still, the use of humans in certain types of experiments is considered unethical. Although some people argue that laboratory animal experiments are also unethical, most people believe that the careful, humane use of animals is an acceptable alternative to using human subjects. For example, most people would think it is reasonable to feed rats a low-copper diet to study the importance of this mineral in the formation of blood vessels. Almost universally, however, people would object to a similar study in infants.

The use of laboratory animal experiments to study the role of nutrition in certain human diseases depends on the availability of an **animal model**—a disease in such animals that closely mimics a particular human disease. However, most human chronic diseases do not occur in laboratory animals. If no animal model is available and human experiments are ruled out, scientific knowledge often cannot advance beyond what can be learned from epidemiological studies.

Human Experiments

Various experimental approaches are used to test research hypotheses in humans, including case-control and double-blind studies.

Case-Control Study

In a **case-control study,** scientists compare individuals who have the condition in question, such as lung cancer, with individuals who do not have the condition. Comparisons are made only between groups that are matched for other major characteristics (e.g., age, race, and gender) not being studied. You can think of such a study as a "mini" epidemiological study. This type of study may identify factors other than the disease in question, such as fruit and vegetable intake, that differ between the two groups, thus providing researchers with clues about the cause, progression, and prevention of the disease. However, without a controlled experiment, researchers cannot definitely claim cause and effect.[16]

Double-Blind Study

An important approach for more definitive testing of hypotheses is the **double-blind study,** in which a group of participants—the experimental group—follows a specific protocol (e.g., consuming a certain food or nutrient), and participants in a corresponding **control group** conform to their normal habits. People are randomly assigned to each group, such as by the flip of a coin. Scientists then observe the experimental group over time to see if there is any effect that is not found in the control group. Sometimes individuals are used as their own control: first they are observed for a period of time, and then they are treated and their responses noted.

Two features of a double-blind study help reduce the introduction of bias (prejudice), which can easily affect the outcome of an experiment. First, neither the participants nor the researchers know which individuals are in the experimental group and which are in the control group. Second, the expected effects of the experimental protocol are not disclosed to the participants or researchers until after the entire study is completed. This approach reduces the possibility that researchers may see the change they want to see in the participants to prove a certain "pet" hypothesis, even though such a change did not actually occur. This approach also reduces the chance that the

animal model Study of disease in laboratory animals that duplicates human disease. This can be used to understand more about human disease.

case-control study Studies in which individuals who have the condition in question, such as lung cancer, are compared with individuals who do not have the condition.

double-blind study An experiment in which neither the participants nor the researchers are aware of each participant's assignment (test or placebo) or the outcome of the study until it is completed. An independent third party holds the code and the data until the study has been completed.

control group Participants in an experiment who are not given the treatment being tested.

Before researchers conduct any research process using humans (or laboratory animals), they must first obtain approval from the Human Use (or Animal Use) Committee at their university or company. The committee determines if the experimental protocol is valid and assesses the risks and benefits of the potential therapy to the subject and, when appropriate, society at large. In human studies, the committee insists that a document depicting the risks and benefits of the study be developed, which the participants must receive and sign. The process is called *informed consent,* meaning the participant knows what he or she is expected to do in the research study and the associated risks.

Expert Opinion

Using Research to Answer a Question—Does Calcium Really Help with Weight Loss?

Robert DiSilvestro, Ph.D.

Obesity continues to be a major problem in many countries. The public would like a magic bullet that can safely produce major weight loss without the need for changes in diet or exercise habits. If the public can't have that, the next best alternative is something that can give a modest boost to the weight loss effects of a proper diet and exercise. One such "something" could be calcium.

Is this idea really true? We don't actually know. It could be true for some circumstances and not for others. There are also studies that don't support the story. In addition, there is more than one way to interpret those studies that do seem to support a calcium–body weight connection.

How Could Calcium Help with Weight Control?

You may think that calcium is just involved in bone health. Calcium is involved in bone health, but it may also help with weight control in at least two ways:

- Calcium binds to some of ingested fat, which stops absorption of that fat.
- As calcium intake goes up, production of a hormone made from vitamin D goes down; this hormone favors body fat production over breakdown.

Each of these mechanisms is reasonable based on how the body works and based on some research in isolated cells and experimental animals. However, the practical issue is how much these mechanisms fluctuate with typical variations in human calcium intake. In other words, calcium intake may not turn these mechanisms up or down much except at extremely low or extremely high calcium intakes. In addition, the effects of calcium intake may occur only when some other circumstances are also true (i.e., at certain levels of fat and protein intake, certain levels of exercise, etc.). If the other circumstances needed to bring about a calcium effect are rare, then most people would not obtain a body weight benefit from a high calcium intake.

There is one human study supporting the idea that calcium can have some effect on dietary fat absorption. In this short-term study, people were fed diets for one week in which calcium intake was manipulated mainly via dairy products. The high calcium intake reduced dietary fat absorption, as shown by higher fat excretion in the feces. However, the amount of energy lost this way was not enormous. It is also not known if the number would be lower, higher, or the same with different types of diets. The net energy loss in this study could be important if maintained for a long time, but it still might account for only about 9 lb loss (about 4 kg) per year.

In this short study, the higher calcium intake via dairy had no effect on two measures relevant to the other mechanism by which calcium may affect body fat use. Still, a longer time of increased calcium intake may be needed for such effects. This idea is supported by a longer study. In this study, which was a diet survey study, a measure of body fat use was proportional to calcium intake. However, it is not known if the calcium directly caused the effect or if calcium intake is really just an indicator of some other behavior.

Diet Surveys Support, But Don't Prove, a Calcium–Body Weight Connection

A number of studies have analyzed the diet patterns of different groups of people. Some of these studies find that intake of calcium and/or dairy products show some relationship to body weight. Still, when diet surveys are compared to some health parameter, it is hard to distinguish a direct relationship from a purely coincidental one. For example, a high calcium intake may cause the lower body weight, or a high calcium intake may just be indica-

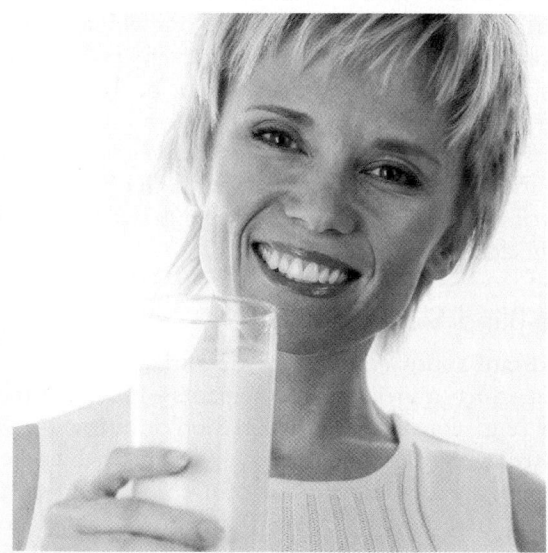

Whether calcium intake contributes to weight control is a hotly-contested research question.

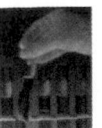

tive of health consciousness. Moreover, not all diet survey studies show a relationship between calcium intake and body weight. This finding is not surprising, because body weight is affected by numerous factors.

It has been suggested that some of the studies that do not show a calcium-weight connection may not have examined a wide enough range of calcium intakes. On the other hand, it is not clear whether the range of calcium intakes in the studies with the negative results are much different from the range in the studies with positive results.

Retrospective Analysis of Calcium Intervention Studies Is Interesting but Not Conclusive

A number of studies have been done in which calcium was given for a reason other than to study body weight. In some of these studies, body weight was measured just for general information purposes. When this data was reanalyzed, in some cases increased calcium intake looked like it might impact body weight. However, because these studies didn't control for factors such as energy intake and because the results were not totally consistent, these studies cannot be fully conclusive.

Experimental Animal Studies Are Useful But Are Not the Last Word

Work in experimental animals supports the idea that calcium intake can affect processes involved in body weight gain and in body fat accumulation. Even so, these results do not guarantee that typical calcium intake variations in people—who have many other factors affecting their body weight—will significantly impact body weight control. Also, in an unpublished study from our laboratory, in mice fed excess energy and fat, doubling calcium intake did not limit excess weight gain. However, calcium intake may impact body weight in mice with different ranges of calcium intakes or with different background diets.

Calcium Intervention–Weight Loss Studies Give Mixed Results

If calcium intake can have a distinct effect on body weight in most types of people, this effect should show up in calcium–weight loss intervention trials. In these trials, distinct amounts of calcium are given to people as supplements or dairy products, and attention is paid to other aspects of diet (i.e., energy intake). One research group has generated two papers on such studies. In each case, a high calcium intake produced a greater weight and/or fat loss than did a low calcium diet, with dairy products being more effec-

tive than calcium supplements. One criticism of these studies is that the low calcium group as well as the calcium supplement group lost less weight than would be expected from the energy restriction alone. Furthermore, the dairy group lost just the amount of weight expected from dietary energy restriction alone. Did the dairy group simply have the best compliance to the weight loss diet? It remains to be seen if the subsequent studies, which are only presented now as meeting reports, reinforce this concern.

There are three intervention studies that do not see a statistically significant weight loss effect of increased calcium intake, though one saw a small trend in that direction. One of these studies increased calcium intake via supplements, another used dairy products, and a study from our laboratory had some people take supplements or consume 1% low-fat milk. Our study, which is only published at present as a meeting report summary, included supervised exercise as part of the weight loss regimen.

One difference between the three studies that did not show an effect and the two studies from one laboratory that did is the calcium content of the low calcium diet. The two studies that report an effect of calcium each used 400 to 500 mg of dietary calcium per day in the low calcium group. In contrast, the studies showing no effect had the low calcium intake set at 700 to 800 mg per day. Perhaps calcium intake and/or body calcium functional status must be changed drastically to have an effect on weight loss. Also, because both studies with 400 to 500 mg background calcium intake come from one research group, there could be something else about the study design that distinguishes these studies from those of other groups.

So, What's the Real Story?

Based on data so far, calcium and/or dairy intake will not produce large amounts of weight losses all by itself. Also, variations in calcium intake will not affect body weight in every circumstance. What is not known is whether calcium can affect body weight in some circumstances, and what, if any, these circumstances are. If calcium intakes need to change from very low (i.e., 400 mg/day) to very high to see an effect, not many people will be helped. Although it is common for people to consume less than the recommended amounts of calcium, very few people consume only 400 mg of calcium per day. At the moment, the best advice is to follow the traditional approaches to weight loss or maintenance but to meet calcium needs in case calcium intake does help.

Dr. DiSilvestro is Professor of Human Nutrition at The Ohio State University, Columbus, Ohio. He received a Ph.D. in biochemistry from Purdue University and is well known for his work in copper and zinc metabolism. He has recently begun to study calcium as well.

placebo A fake medicine used to disguise the roles of participants in an experiment; if fake surgery is performed, it is called a *sham operation*.

Two other common types of studies are migrant and cohort. Migrant studies look at changes in health in people who move from one country to another. Cohort studies start with a healthy population and follow them, looking for the development of disease.

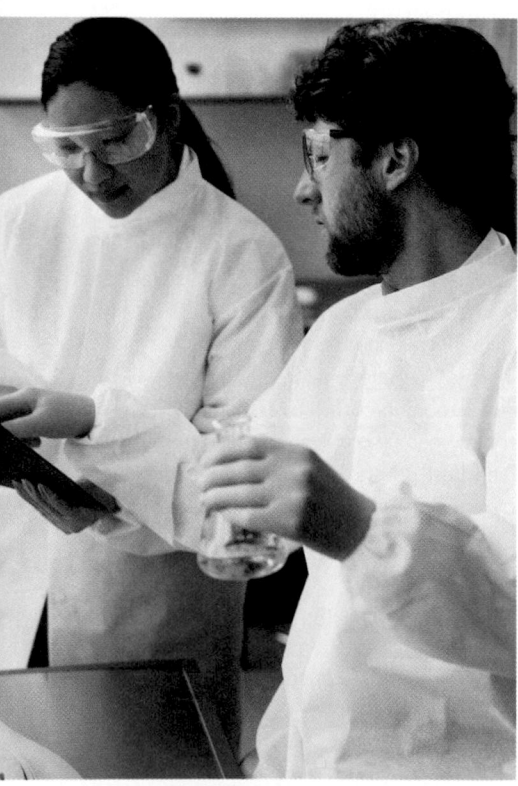

Careful research contributes to nutrition knowledge, more so than does personal experience.

persons participating begin to feel better simply because they are involved in a research study or are receiving a new treatment, a phenomenon called the *placebo effect*.

Derived from the Latin word *placebo,* meaning "I shall please," the placebo effect cannot be explained by pharmacological or other direct physical action. It may instead be linked to a simple reduction in stress and anxiety. Overall, it is critical to make allowances for the placebo effect in research studies.

In a double-blind experiment, the control group often receives a sugar pill (or other placebo treatment) to camouflage who is in which group and thereby to eliminate the bias introduced by the placebo effect. During the course of the experiment, neither the researchers nor the participants know who is getting the real treatment and who is getting a placebo. Sometimes only a single-blind protocol is possible, in which the participants (and possibly some of the researchers) are kept in the dark. Either way, now it is up to the experimental treatment—not just the practice of both groups taking a pill—to show an effect, if one is possible.

A recent example illustrates the need to test hypotheses based on epidemiological observations in double-blind studies.[16] Epidemiologists using primarily case-control studies found that smokers who regularly consumed fruits and vegetables had a lower risk for lung cancer than did smokers who ate few fruits and vegetables. Some scientists proposed that beta-carotene, a pigment present in many fruits and vegetables, could reduce the damage that tobacco smoke creates in the lungs. This hypothesis helped fuel sales of supplements of beta-carotene.

However, in double-blind studies involving heavy smokers, the risk of lung cancer was found to *be higher* for those who took beta-carotene supplements than for those who did not (note that this is not true for the small amount of beta-carotene found naturally in foods). Some investigators criticized this research, arguing that the beta-carotene was given too late in the smokers' lives to be of much use, but even these critics did not suspect that the supplement would increase cancer risk. Soon after these results were reported, the U.S. federal agency supporting two other large ongoing studies that employed beta-carotene supplements called a halt to the research, stating that these supplements are ineffective in preventing both lung cancer and cardiovascular disease.

Overall, health and nutrition advice provided by grandparents, parents, friends, and other well-meaning individuals can't be verified unless it is put to the ultimate scientific test—blinded studies.[16] Until that is done, we can't be sure that the substance or procedure in question is truly effective. When people say, "I get fewer colds now that I take vitamin C," they overlook the fact that many cold symptoms disappear quickly with no treatment; the apparent curative effect of vitamin C or any other remedy is often coincidental rather than causal to the natural healing process.

All consumers need to become more sophisticated about science, its accepted standards of evidence, and its current limitations. Failure to do so leads many to a frantic pursuit of fraudulent remedies. To ignore science is to risk learning about the dangers of various health practices primarily from being harmed by them. Medical science does not ignore novel approaches to disease prevention and cure. Anecdotes and personal experiences can be important clues leading to fruitful experimentation, but they are not credible evidence.[2]

Peer Review of Experimental Results

Once an experiment is complete, scientists summarize the findings and seek to publish the results in scientific journals. Generally, before such results are published in scientific journals, they are critically reviewed by other scientists familiar with the subject. The objective of this peer review is to ensure that only high-quality research findings are published. This is an important step because most scientific research in this country is funded by the federal government, nonprofit foundations, drug companies, and

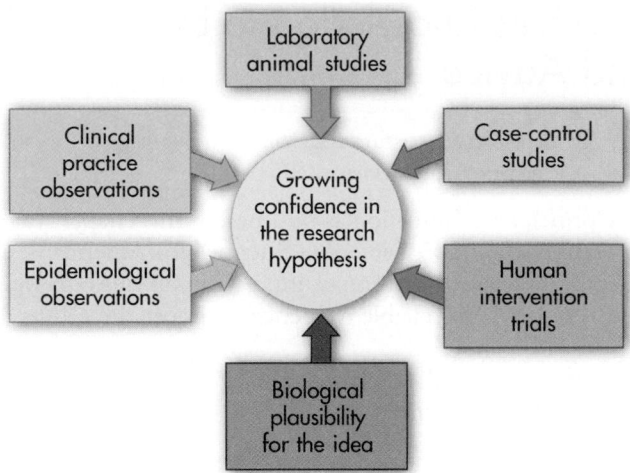

Figure 1-7 | Data from a variety of sources can come together to support a research hypothesis. For example, epidemiological studies show that type 2 diabetes is characteristically found in obese populations, when compared with leaner populations. Physicians notice in clinical practice that type 2 diabetes is much more likely in their obese patients than in their leaner patients. Case-control studies show that obese patients are much more likely to have type 2 diabetes than the leaner comparison group that is matched for other characteristics. Laboratory animal studies show that overfeeding that eventually leads to obesity often leads to the development of type 2 diabetes. Finally, human intervention trials show that weight loss can correct type 2 diabetes in many people. Laboratory researchers also show that the enlarged fat cells associated with obesity are much less responsive to the hormonal signals involved in blood glucose regulation (see Chapter 5). All these lines of data come together with biological plausibility from various laboratory studies to support the research hypothesis that obesity can lead to type 2 diabetes.

other private industries. All these funding sources can have strong expectations about the research outcomes. In theory, the scientists conducting these research studies will be fair in evaluating their results and will not be influenced by the funding agency. Peer review helps ensure that the researchers are as objective as possible. This then helps ensure that results published in **peer-reviewed journals,** such as the *American Journal of Clinical Nutrition, The New England Journal of Medicine,* and the *Journal of the American Dietetic Association,* are much more reliable than those found in popular magazines or promoted on television talk shows. Unfortunately, hyped-up press releases from reputable journals and major universities are the main sources for the information presented in the popular media, and claims are seldom scrutinized by journalists themselves for accuracy and scientific validity.

peer-reviewed journal A journal that publishes research only after two or three scientists who were not part of the study agree the study was well conducted and the results are fairly represented. Thus, the research has been approved by peers of the research team.

Follow-Up Studies

Even if an acceptable protocol has been followed and the results of a study have been accepted by the scientific community, one experiment is never enough to prove a particular hypothesis or provide a basis for nutritional recommendations. Rather, the results obtained in one laboratory must be confirmed by experiments conducted in other laboratories and possibly under varying circumstances. Only then can we really trust and use the results. The more lines of evidence available to support an idea, the more likely it is to be true (Figure 1-7). It is important to avoid rushing to accept new ideas as fact or incorporating them into your health habits until they are proved by several lines of evidence.[2]

How to Use This Knowledge to Evaluate Nutrition Claims and Advice

Based on what has been covered so far, the following suggestions should help you make healthful and logical nutrition decisions:[16]

1. Apply the basic principles of nutrition as outlined in this chapter (along with those listed in My Pyramid, the 2005 Dietary Guidelines for Americans, and related resources in Chapter 2) to any nutrition claim, including ones on websites. Do you note any inconsistencies? Do reliable references support the claims? Beware of the following:
   - Testimonials about personal experience
   - Disreputable publication sources
   - Dramatic results (rarely true)
   - Lack of evidence from supporting studies made by other scientists

2. Examine the background and scientific credentials of the individual, organizations, or publication making the nutritional claim. Usually, a reputable author is one whose educational background or present affiliation is with a nationally recognized university or medical center that offers programs or courses in the field of nutrition, medicine, or a closely allied specialty.

3. Be wary if the answer is "Yes" to any of the following questions about a health-related nutrition claim:
   - Are only advantages discussed and possible disadvantages ignored?
   - Are claims made about "curing" disease? Do they sound too good to be true?
   - Is extreme bias against the medical community or traditional medical treatments evident? Physicians as a group strive to cure diseases in their patients, using what proven techniques are available. They do not ignore reliable cures.
   - Is the claim touted as a new or secret scientific breakthrough?

4. Note the size and duration of any study cited in support of a nutrition claim. The larger it is and the longer it went on, the more dependable its findings. Also consider the type of study: epidemiology versus case-control versus double-blind. Keep in mind that "contributes to," "is linked to," or "is associated with" does not mean "causes."

5. Beware of press conferences and other hype regarding the latest findings. Much of this will not survive more detailed scientific evaluation.

6. When you meet with a nutrition professional, you should expect that he or she will do the following:
   - Ask questions about your medical history, lifestyle, and current eating habits.
   - Formulate a diet plan tailored to your needs, as opposed to simply tearing a form from a tablet that could apply to almost anyone.
   - Schedule follow-up visits to track your progress, answer any questions, and help keep you motivated.
   - Involve family members in the diet plan, when appropriate.
   - Consult directly with your physician and readily refer you back to your physician for those health problems a nutrition professional is not trained to treat.

7. Be skeptical of practitioners who prescribe **megadoses** of vitamin and mineral supplements for everyone.

8. Examine product labels carefully. Be skeptical of any product promotion not clearly stated on the label. A product is not likely to do something that is not specifically claimed on its label or package insert (legally part of the label).

This cautious approach to nutrition-related advice and products is even more important today because of sweeping changes in U.S. law passed in 1994. The Dietary Supplement Health and Education Act (DSHEA) of 1994 classified vitamins, minerals, amino acids, and herbal remedies as "foods," effectively restraining the U.S. Food and Drug Administration (FDA) from regulating them as heavily as food additives and

megadose Intake of a nutrient far beyond estimates of needs or what would be found in a balanced diet; 2 to 10 times human needs is a starting point for such a dosage.

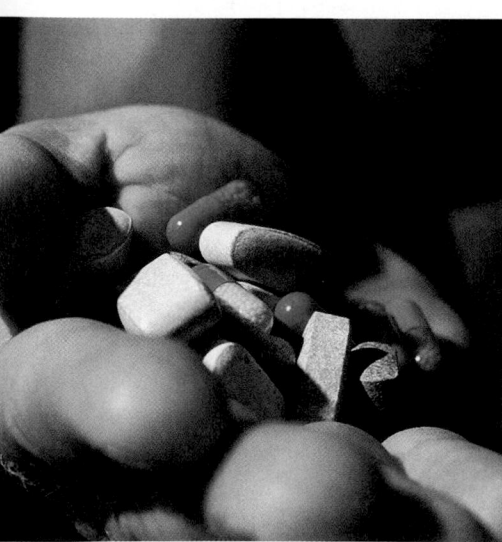

Taking numerous nutrient supplements can lead to health problems. Chapter 9 will explore the appropriate and safe use of nutrient supplements in detail.

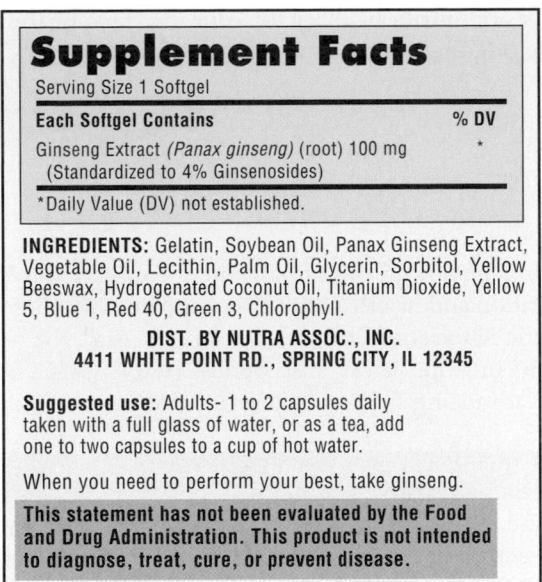

Supplement Facts
Serving Size 1 Softgel

Each Softgel Contains	% DV
Ginseng Extract *(Panax ginseng)* (root) 100 mg (Standardized to 4% Ginsenosides)	*
*Daily Value (DV) not established.	

INGREDIENTS: Gelatin, Soybean Oil, Panax Ginseng Extract, Vegetable Oil, Lecithin, Palm Oil, Glycerin, Sorbitol, Yellow Beeswax, Hydrogenated Coconut Oil, Titanium Dioxide, Yellow 5, Blue 1, Red 40, Green 3, Chlorophyll.

DIST. BY NUTRA ASSOC., INC.
4411 WHITE POINT RD., SPRING CITY, IL 12345

Suggested use: Adults- 1 to 2 capsules daily taken with a full glass of water, or as a tea, add one to two capsules to a cup of hot water.

When you need to perform your best, take ginseng.

This statement has not been evaluated by the Food and Drug Administration. This product is not intended to diagnose, treat, cure, or prevent disease.

Figure 1-8 | FDA disclaimer on a supplement label. Keep in mind that although FDA requires the highlighted statement, it does not mean the supplement has been tested or endorsed by FDA.

drugs. According to this act, rather than the manufacturer having to prove a dietary supplement is safe, FDA must prove it is unsafe before preventing its sale. In contrast, the safety of food additives and drugs must be demonstrated to FDA's satisfaction before they are marketed.

Currently, a dietary supplement (or herbal product) can be marketed in the United States without FDA approval if (1) there is a history of its use or other evidence that it is expected to be reasonably safe when used under the conditions recommended or suggested in its labeling, and (2) the product is labeled as a dietary supplement. (FDA can act if the product turns out to be dangerous, as with the recent ban on the supplement ephedra after numerous deaths.) The labels on such products are allowed to claim a benefit related to a classic nutrient-deficiency disease, describe how a nutrient affects human body structure or function (called structure/function claims; see the section on nutrition labeling in Chapter 2 for details), and claim that general well-being results from consumption of the ingredients. Examples could be "maintains bone health" or "improves blood circulation." However, the labels of products bearing such claims also must prominently display a disclaimer regarding FDA support in boldface type (Figure 1-8). Despite this warning, when consumers find these products on the shelves of supermarkets, health-food stores, and pharmacies, they may mistakenly assume FDA has carefully evaluated the products. (The effectiveness and safety of many herbal and related products is discussed in Chapter 18.)

The fact remains that many of us are willing to try untested nutrition products and believe in their miraculous effects. Popular products claim to increase muscle growth, enhance sexuality, boost energy, reduce body fat, increase strength, supply missing nutrients, increase longevity, and even improve brain function. Clearly, many nutritional products commonly found in stores are not strictly regulated in terms of effectiveness. The actual amount of product in the package and potency are also often in question. In general, national brands are more reliable with respect to these questions. Finally, few have been thoroughly evaluated by reputable scientists. So if you embark on a self-cure by means of such products, you will probably waste money and possibly risk ill health. A better approach is to consult a physician or **registered dietitian** first.[2] You can find a registered dietitian in North America by visiting www.eatright.org or www.dietitians.ca, consulting the Yellow Pages in the telephone directory, contacting the local dietetics association, or calling the dietary department of a local hospital. Make sure the person has the credentials "R.D." after his or her name ("R.D.N." is also used in Canada). This indicates the person has completed rigorous classroom and clinical training in nutrition and participates in continuing education. Appendix K also lists

The American Dietetic Association has a toll-free hotline, (800) 366-1655, that provides dietitian referrals through the Nationwide Nutrition Network and nutrition messages in English and Spanish. You can also find out more about nutrition on their website www.eatright.org. In Canada, use www.dietitians.ca.

registered dietitian (R.D.) A person who has completed a baccalaureate degree program approved by the American Dietetic Association, performed at least 900 hours of supervised professional practice, and passed a registration examination.

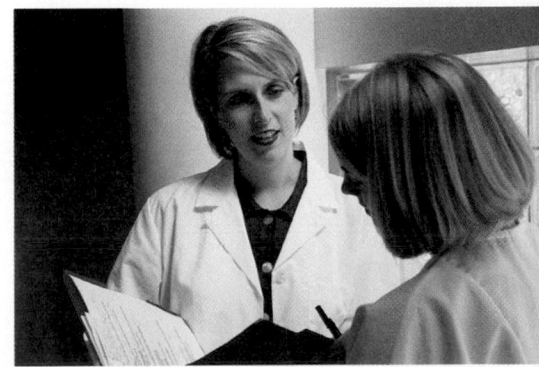

Registered dieticians are a reliable source of nutrition advice.

Recently, major nutrition organizations put together 10 red flags that they consider signals for poor nutrition advice:

1. Recommendations that promise a quick fix
2. Dire warnings of dangers from a single product or regimen
3. Claims that sound too good to be true
4. Simplistic conclusions drawn from a complex study
5. Recommendations based on a single study
6. Dramatic statements that are refuted by reputable scientific organizations
7. Lists of "good" and "bad" foods
8. Recommendations made to help sell a product
9. Recommendations based on studies published without peer review
10. Recommendations from studies that ignore differences among individuals or groups

many reputable sources of nutrition advice for your use. Finally, the following websites can help you evaluate ongoing nutrition and health claims:

www.acsh.org
www.quackwatch.com
www.ncahf.org
dietary-supplements.info.nih.gov
www.fda.gov

These sites are maintained by groups or individuals committed to providing reasoned and authoritative nutrition and health advice to consumers. Another information source is the American Dietetic Association at www.eatright.org. Also, the website for this book provides information on the latest discoveries (www.mhhe.com/wardlawpers7). Nutrition is a rapidly advancing field and there are always new findings.

Case Scenario | Follow-Up

Brenda should be cautious about taking any supplement, especially one advertised as a "recent breakthrough." As you have read, dietary supplements are not closely regulated by FDA; a general statement such as "increases energy" would be considered a structure/function claim and such product labeling does not require prior approval by FDA. Furthermore, FDA will not have evaluated either the safety or effectiveness of such a product. Even harmful dietary supplements are difficult for FDA to recall. There is also a chance that the supplement could contain little or none of the advertised ingredient. Unfortunately, Brenda will find all this out the hard way and will be out $60. Her hard-earned money would be better spent on a nutritious diet and a medical checkup at the student health center. All consumers need to be cautious about nutrition information, especially regarding dietary supplements marketed as cure-alls and breakthroughs—Let the buyer beware!

Concept | Check

The scientific method is the procedure for testing the validity of possible explanations of a phenomenon, called hypotheses. Experiments are conducted to either support or refute a specific hypothesis. Once we have much experimental information that supports a specific hypothesis, it then can be called a theory. Ideally, experiments are conducted in a blinded fashion, where the subjects and researchers (preferably both) do not find out the results of an experiment until after the experiment is completed. This reduces bias in the results and minimizes the placebo effect. All of us need to be skeptical of new ideas in the nutrition field. We should wait until many lines of experimental evidence support a concept before adopting any suggested dietary practice.

Genetics and Nutrition

The growth, development, and maintenance of cells and ultimately of the entire organism are directed by genes present in the cells. The genes contain the codes that control the expression of individual traits, such as height, eye color, and susceptibility to many diseases. An individual's genetic risk for a given disease is an important factor, although often not the only factor, in determining whether he or she develops that disease.[13]

Interest in the human genetic code and its relationship to specific diseases has exploded in recent years. The U.S. government through the Human Genome Project and a private company have each sequenced the more than 35,000 genes present on human chromosomes. These efforts have not actually sequenced the genes of just one person, but have compiled a composite genome based on the DNA contributed by a few individuals. Each gene essentially represents a recipe, noting the ingredients (specifically, amino acids) and how those ingredients should be put together. The human genome then would be the cookbook.

It is likely that soon it will be relatively easy to screen a person's DNA for genes that increase the risk for disease. Currently, a woman can pay about $2700 to be tested for a **mutation** in the BRCA1 and BRCA2 genes; these mutations greatly increase the risk for breast cancer (see a later section in this Nutrition Focus). To date, scientists have developed about 600 genetic tests. Many are for very rare diseases and fortunately often are much less expensive than the test for the BRCA genes. These genetic tests are especially valuable for families plagued by certain illnesses, but more routine testing of now-healthy people to predict future risks of cancer or other diseases is poised to grow rapidly. This field is brand new and is about to mushroom into a significant part of medical practice, as almost every medical condition has a genetic component. Most, however, are not single gene disorders but instead arise from alterations in a number of genes.

Each year new links between specific genes and diseases are reported. Decoding of the human genome could ultimately allow for tailoring of diets with respect to individual nutrient needs or the individual's response to certain diet patterns. In addition, it is thought that this greater availability of genetic information could ultimately transform the practice of medicine, allowing for the prediction

years in advance of what illnesses will likely eventually develop in a person.[10] The hope is then to replace genes that encourage diseases, such as cancer and Alzheimer's, with those that do not. Such information as well may provide opportunities for physicians in the future to diagnose disease more accurately and to prescribe individual medical therapies, instead of treating all patients with the same disease using essentially the same therapy. It is likely that many medications may be more appropriate in certain people given their genetic traits.

An exciting application of the Human Genome Project is DNA microarrays, also called gene chips. About 100,000 pieces of DNA can be loaded onto a chip the size of a fingernail. Blood can be processed and then placed on the chip and rapidly tested for altered genes. Genetic material binding to certain areas on the chip can signal a healthy form of a specific gene or alternately a form that is associated with disease. Currently, about 75 laboratories in the United States are using this technology to investigate disease risk.[9]

Nutritional Diseases with a Genetic Link

Most chronic diseases in which nutrition plays a role are also influenced by genetics. The risks of developing cardiovascular disease, hypertension, obesity, diabetes, cancer, and osteoporosis are influenced by interactions between genetic and nutritional factors. Studies of families, including those with twins and adoptees, provide strong support for the effect of genetics in these disorders. In fact, family history is considered to be one of the important risk factors in the development of many nutrition-related diseases.[22]

Cardiovascular Disease

About one in every 500 people in North America has a defective gene that greatly delays cholesterol removal from the bloodstream. As you will learn in Chapter 6, this and other genetic effects lead to an increased risk of developing cardiovascular disease at a young age. Diet changes can help these people, but medications and possibly surgery may be needed to address these problems.

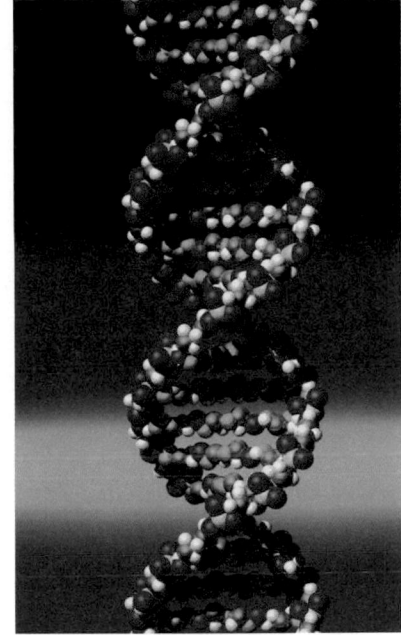

Genes are present on DNA—a double helix. The cell nucleus contains most of the DNA in the body.

mutation A change in the chemistry of a gene that is perpetuated in subsequent divisions of the cell in which it occurred; a change in the sequence of the DNA.

(continued)

Hypertension

An estimated 10 to 15% of the North American population is very sensitive to salt intake. When these salt-sensitive individuals consume too much salt, their blood pressure climbs above the desirable range. The fact that more of these people are African American than White suggests a genetic component. At present, the only way to determine whether individuals with hypertension are salt sensitive is to place them on a salt-restricted diet and see if their blood pressure falls. Note also that many cases of hypertension are unrelated to salt sensitivity and are caused by other factors (see Chapter 11).

Obesity

Most obese North Americans have at least one parent who is also obese. Findings from many human studies suggest that a variety of genes (likely 250 or more) are involved in the regulation of body weight (see Chapter 13 for more details). Little is known, however, about the specific nature of these genes in humans or how the actual changes in body metabolism (such as lower energy use in general or fat use in particular) are produced.

Still, although some individuals may be genetically predisposed to store body fat, whether they actually do so depends on how much excess energy they ultimately consume. A common concept in nutrition is that *nurture* (how people live and the environmental factors that influence them) allows *nature* (each person's genetic potential) to be expressed. Although not everyone with a genetic tendency toward obesity develops this condition, he or she does have a higher lifetime risk than individuals without a genetic predisposition to obesity.

Diabetes

Both of the two common types of diabetes—type 1 and type 2—have genetic links, as revealed by family and twin studies. Only sensitive and expensive testing can determine who is at risk. The form of diabetes involved in about 90% of all cases, type 2 diabetes, also has a strong link to obesity. A genetic tendency for type 2 diabetes is expressed once a person becomes obese but often not before, again illustrating that nurture affects nature (see Chapter 5 for more details).

Cancer

A few types of cancer (e.g., some forms of colon, prostate, and breast cancer) have a strong genetic link, and genetics may play a role in others. Still, obesity alone increases the risk of several forms of cancer. And one-third of all cancers result from smoking. Again, genetics is often not enough; environment also contributes to the risk profile (see Chapter 12 for more details).

Osteoporosis

Bone mass and resulting bone strength is similar in twins as well as in mothers and their daughters. The exact relative importance of genetic versus dietary factors is unknown, but a number of genes have been shown to contribute to a person's overall risk of low bone mass. In any case, children and adolescents need to consume sufficient calcium to build strong, dense bones, thus reducing the risk of osteoporosis in later life. Adults should continue that practice. The porous bones that are a result of osteoporosis greatly increase the risk of fractures, especially in the wrist, spine, and hip. As discussed in Chapter 11, the risk of osteoporosis in women can be greatly reduced by a combination of medical and nutritional means if therapy is started at least by midlife.

Your Genetic Profile

From this discussion, you can see that a family history of certain diseases raises your risk of developing those diseases. By recognizing your potential for developing a particular disease, you can avoid behavior that contributes to it. For example, women with a family history of breast cancer should avoid becoming obese, should minimize alcohol use, and should obtain mammograms regularly. In general, the greater number of your relatives who had a genetically transmitted disease and the closer they are related to you, the greater your risk. One way to assess your risk is to put together a family tree of illnesses and deaths by compiling a few key facts on your primary relatives: siblings, parents, aunts and uncles, and grandparents.

Figure 1-9 shows an example of a family tree (also called a genogram). High-risk conditions include two or more first-degree relatives in a family

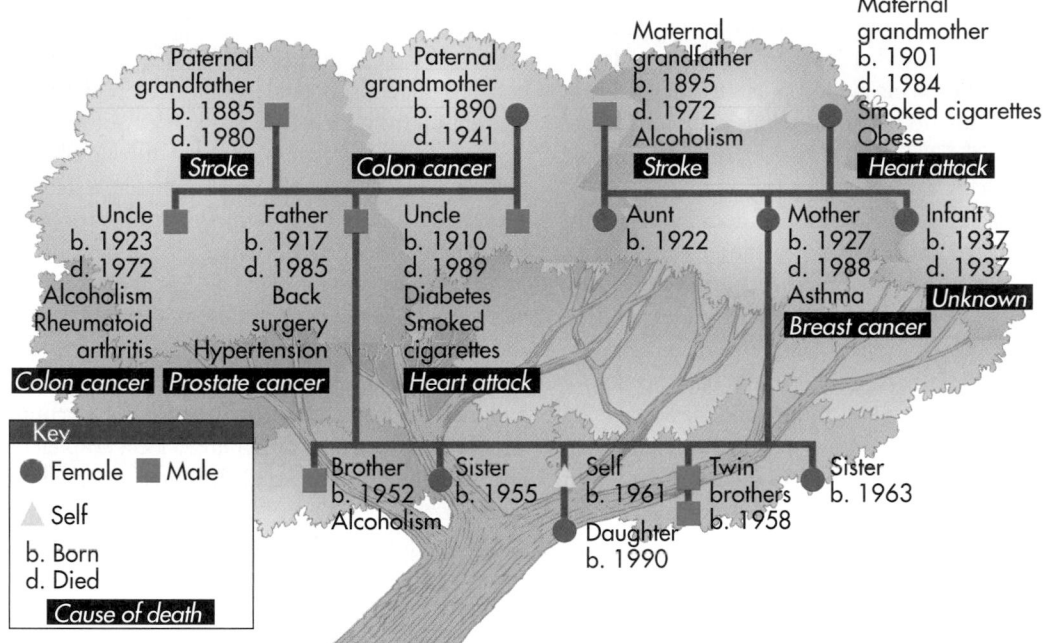

Figure 1-9 | Example of a family tree for Eugene, designated as "Self" at the trunk of the tree. The gender of each family member is identified by color (blue squares for males, orange circles for females). Dates of birth (b) and death (d) are listed below each family member. If deceased, the cause of death is highlighted using white text against a black background. In addition to causes of death, medical conditions the family members experienced are noted beneath each name. Create your own family tree of frequent diseases using the figure in the second Take Action section as a guide. Then show your family tree to your physician to get a more complete picture of what the information means for your health.

with a specific disease (first-degree relatives include one's parents, siblings, and offspring). Another sign of risk of inherited disease is development of the disease in a first-degree relative before age 50 to 60 years.[22] In the family in Figure 1-9, prostate cancer killed the man's father. Knowing this, the son should be tested regularly for prostate cancer. His sisters should consider frequent mammograms and other preventive practices because their mother died of breast cancer. Because heart attack and stroke are also common in the family, all the children should adopt a lifestyle that minimizes the risk of developing these conditions, such as a moderate animal fat and sodium intake. Colon cancer is also evident in the family, so careful screening throughout life is important.

Gene Therapy

Scientists are currently developing therapies to correct some genetic disorders. Typically, the gene of interest is inserted into a **virus,** and then this virus is injected into the target tissue. For example, a gene that stimulates blood vessel growth has been inserted into a virus, and this combination has been injected into the hearts of people with poor heart circulation. This gene therapy has led to improvement in health. In addition, a number of infants worldwide were treated for a severe immune deficiency disease with genetic therapy by putting new genes in their white blood cells. Many are alive and well today. Scientists hope that one day gene therapy applications such as these can be used to treat many diseases, especially inherited diseases. Still, much more research is needed for that to happen on a routine basis.

Genetic Testing

In recent years, scientists have developed ways of testing a person's genes for the likelihood of developing certain diseases. For cases such as Huntington's disease, a degenerative brain disorder, a positive gene test guarantees the eventual development of the disease. However, with diseases such as cancer, a positive gene test simply indicates a greater risk for developing the disease. In addition to the diseases mentioned, risk factors for birth defects, certain forms of muscular dystrophy, and a host of other diseases can be detected through genetic testing.

Check out the website www.hhs.gov/familyhistory for more information of using a family tree in health-related evaluations.

virus The smallest known type of infectious agent, many of which cause disease in humans. They do not metabolize, grow, or move by themselves. They reproduce by the aid of a living cellular host. Viruses are essentially a piece of genetic material surrounded by a coat of protein.

(continued)

phenylketonuria (PKU) A disease caused by a defect in the ability of the liver to metabolize the amino acid phenylalanine into the amino acid tyrosine. Toxic by-products of phenylalanine can then build up in the body and lead to mental retardation.

Today in the United States, newborns are routinely tested for **phenylketonuria,** an inherited metabolic disease that leads to mental retardation and other problems if appropriate treatment is not given. Infants found to have this disorder are put on a special diet, which reduces development of the disease (see Chapter 4 for details).

Because genetic background does influence disease risk, certain dietary advice is more beneficial for some people than for others. For example, people prone to osteoporosis, as mentioned earlier, need to be more aware of calcium intake. Overall, the benefits of genetic testing include the opportunity for more individualized nutrition and health advice, more informed decisions by couples attempting to have children (i.e., alternatives such as adoption or therapeutic abortion), increased surveillance for the disease, and the ability to plan appropriately for the future.[11] However, it is not possible, given the limit on resources presently allocated to medical care in North America, to identify all people at genetic risk for the major chronic diseases and other health problems. In addition, in many cases genetic susceptibility does not necessarily guarantee development of the disease. And, in almost all cases, there is no way to cure a specific gene alteration—only the health problems that result can be treated. Thus, the wisdom of genetic testing is an open question. Perhaps preventive measures and careful scrutiny for the specific genetically linked diseases using one's family tree would suffice.

Researchers also are concerned that people who are found to have genetic alterations that in-

Genetic analysis for disease susceptibility will be more common in the future as the genes that increase risk for various diseases are isolated and decoded.

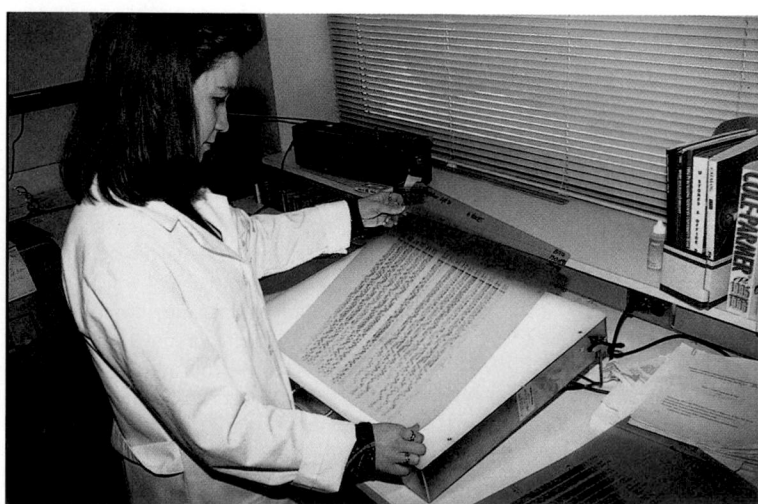

crease disease risk may face job and insurance discrimination. Testing positive could also lead to unnecessary radical treatment. As well, a seemingly hopeless diagnosis could result in depression or withdrawal from life when a cure is out of reach.[11]

Some experts recommend that anyone considering genetic testing should first undergo genetic counseling. Genetic counselors are trained to analyze family history and evaluate risk of developing or passing along an inherited disease. They can also help determine whether testing is worth the time and trouble, since genetic tests are primarily for people whose family history puts them at especially high risk of having a genetic defect. Genetic counselors can be found by contacting a local hospital or nearby university-affiliated hospital or medical school.

In the final analysis, would you rather know if you were at risk for a specific disease that a genetic test could point out? If so, ask your physician about the possibility and wisdom of testing you for the genetically linked diseases in your family tree. Also, be aware that, throughout this book, discussions will point out how you can personalize nutrition advice based on your genetic background. In this way, you can identify and avoid the "controllable" risk factors that would contribute to the development of genetically linked diseases present in your family.

The following web links will help you gather more information about genetic conditions and testing:

www.geneticalliance.org Alliance of Genetic Support Groups.

www.kumc.edu/gec/support Information on genetic conditions and rare conditions.

cancernet.nci.nih.gov/p_genetics.html Genetics information from the National Cancer Institute.

www.nhgri.nih.gov National Human Genome Research Institute (at the NIH) home page. Describes latest research findings, discusses ethical issues, and provides a talking glossary.

www.faseb.org/genetics Compilation of major genetics societies throughout the world. Information on genetics meetings, society policy statements, and so on.

vector.cshl.org Cold Spring Harbor Labs DNA Learning Center home page; includes animation of genetic techniques.

www.ncgr.org National Center for Genomic Resources home page.

Summary

1. Nutrition is the study of the food substances vital for health and the study of how the body uses these substances to promote and support growth, maintenance, and reproduction of cells. Research in the field has been especially vigorous from the past century to the present.

2. Nutrients in foods fall into six classes: (1) carbohydrates, (2) lipids (mostly fats and oils), (3) proteins, (4) vitamins, (5) minerals, and (6) water. The first three, along with alcohol, provide energy for the body to use.

3. The body transforms the energy contained in carbohydrate, protein, and fat into other forms of energy, which allow the body to function. Fat provides, on average, 9 kcal/g, whereas protein and carbohydrate each provides, on average, 4 kcal/g. Vitamins, minerals, and water do not supply energy to the body but are essential for proper body function.

4. A basic plan for health promotion and disease prevention includes eating a varied diet, performing regular physical activity, not smoking, not abusing nutrient supplements (if used), consuming adequate fluid, getting adequate sleep, limiting alcohol intake (if consumed), and limiting or coping with stress.

5. The primary focus of nutrition planning should be on food, not on dietary supplements. The focus on foods to supply nutrient needs avoids the possibility of severe nutrient imbalances.

6. Results from large nutrition surveys in the United States and Canada suggest that some of us need to concentrate on consuming foods that supply more of certain vitamins and minerals and fiber. Regular use of a balanced multivitamin and mineral supplement is another strategy to make up for some dietary shortcomings.

7. The flavor, texture, and appearance of foods primarily influence our food choices. Several other factors also help determine food habits and choices: our upbringing, various social and cultural factors, the image we want to project to others, convenience, economics, emotional state, and concerns about health.

8. The scientific method is the procedure for testing the validity of possible explanations of a phenomenon, called hypotheses. Experiments are conducted to either support or refute a specific hypothesis. Once we have much experimental information that supports a specific hypothesis, it then can be called a theory. All of us need to be skeptical of new ideas in the nutrition field, waiting until many lines of experimental evidence support a concept before adopting any suggested dietary practice.

9. Genetic background influences the risk for many health-related diseases. Examining one's family tree provides clues for an individual to such risks. Preventive measures are then important to implement, especially with respect to diet.

Study Questions

1. Name one chronic disease associated with poor nutrition habits. Now list a few corresponding risk factors.

2. Explain the concept of energy as it relates to foods. What are the fuel (energy) values used for a gram of carbohydrate, fat, protein, and alcohol?

3. Identify three ways that water is used in the body.

4. Wendy's Big Bacon Classic contains 44 g carbohydrate, 36 g fat, and 37 g protein. Calculate the percentage of energy derived from fat.

5. Describe two types of fat and explain why the differences are important in terms of overall health.

6. According to national nutrition surveys, which nutrients tend to be underconsumed by many adult North Americans? Why is this the case?

7. List four health objectives for the United States for the year 2010. How would you rate yourself in each area? Why?

8. List one food habit you should work on to improve your health. Indicate why and list three actions to take.

9. What nutrition-related disease is common in your family? What step or steps could you take at this point to minimize your risk?

10. List one nutrition claim you have heard recently that sounds too good to be true. What do you suspect is the motive of the person providing the advice?

BOOST YOUR STUDY

Check out the **Perspectives in Nutrition: Online Learning Center** www.mhhe.com/wardlawpers7 for quizzes, flash cards, activities, and web links designed to further help you learn about what nourishes you.

Annotated References

1. ADA Reports: Position of the American Dietetic Association: Total diet approach to communicating food and nutrition information. *Journal of the American Dietetic Association* 102:100, 2002.

The American Dietetic Association states that there are no good or bad foods, only good or bad diets or eating styles. No single food or type of food ensures good health, just as no single food or type of food is necessarily detrimental to health. Adults should emphasize adequacy of the total diet over time, the importance of obtaining nutrients from foods, and portion control, coupled with weight control and regular physical activity.

2. ADA Reports: Position of the American Dietetic Association: Food and nutrition misinformation. *Journal of the American Dietetic Association* 102:260, 2002.

   Much food and nutrition misinformation pervades North American society. Individuals should carefully consider the training of those who give such advice, and be assured that registered dietitians are a reliable source.

3. ADA Reports: Position of the American Dietetic Association and Dietitians of Canada: Nutrition and women's health. *Journal of the American Dietetic Association* 104:984, 2004.

   Comprehensive look at health issues related to nutrition that women often face. Widely advocated are diets rich in fruits, vegetables, and whole-grain breads and cereals, with some low-fat dairy and lean meat choices. Individual nutrients likely to be underconsumed include calcium, iron, vitamin D, vitamin E, and folate.

4. Carpenter, KJ, Harper AE: Evolution of knowledge of the essential nutrients. In Shills ME and others (eds.): *Modern nutrition in health and disease.* 10th ed. Philadelphia, PA: Lippincott: Williams & Wilkins, 2006.

   A short history of nutrition is provided in the context of the definition of an essential nutrient.

5. Cordain L and others: Origins and evolution of the Western diet: Health implications for the 21st century. *American Journal of Clinical Nutrition* 81:341, 2005.

   In recent human history the overall diet has included a great number of foods rich in refined sugars, refined flours, salt, and fatty meats. This change has resulted in a decline in diet quality for many of us in the modern world.

6. Cotton PA and others: Dietary sources of nutrients among U.S. adults, 1994 to 1996. *Journal of the American Dietetic Association* 104:921, 2004.

   The five leading energy sources for American adults are (in order): yeast bread, beef, cakes/cookies/quick breads/doughnuts, soft drinks/soda, and milk. The soft drinks/soda and cake etc. categories also have been moving up in the order compared to the 1980s. Clearly many adults need to improve their dietary choices.

7. Drewnowski, A, Levine AS: Sugar and fat— From genes to culture. *Journal of Nutrition* 133:829S, 2003.

   Added sugars and fats account for greater than 50% of energy intake in the typical North American diet. Their overconsumption is being blamed for a wide range of chronic diseases, from cardiovascular disease to obesity and diabetes. Fat and sugar seem to appeal to emotions and are the dominant object for food cravings. We need to consider this as we choose foods rich in fat and sugar.

8. Food and Nutrition Board: *Dietary reference intakes for energy, carbohydrate, fiber, fat, fatty acids, cholesterol, protein, and amino acids.* Washington DC: The National Academy Press, 2002.

   This report provides the latest guidance for macronutrient intakes. With regard to the amounts of carbohydrate, fat, and protein in a diet, this should be 45 to 65%, 20 to 35%, and 10 to 35%, respectively.

9. Friend SH, Stoughton RB: The magic of microarrays. *Scientific American,* p. 44, February 2002.

   DNA microarrays—also called gene chips—are likely to soon revolutionize medical care. Individuals will be able to have their own genetic background analyzed; this will help physicians diagnose diseases and tailor health advice. The process of using DNA microarrays is described in detail.

10. Gropper SS and others: Advanced nutrition and human metabolism. 4th ed. Belmont, CA: Thomson Wadsworth, 2005.

    Excellent source for the latest findings in nutrition science.

11. Guttmacher AF, Collins FC: Realizing the promise of genomics in biomedical research. *Journal of the American Medical Association* 294:1399, 2005.

    This article reviews the potential for using the genetic profile of a person when providing health-related advice. Genetic testing will likely have a big impact on health care in the future.

12. *Healthy People 2010* targets healthy diet and healthy weight as critical goals. *Journal of the American Dietetic Association* 100:300, 2000.

    Many of the nutrition goals included in Healthy People 2010 *are enumerated. Two key goals are to reduce obesity and inactivity in the American population.*

13. Jackson K: Pioneering the frontier of nutrigenomics. *Today's Dietitian* p. 34, November 2004.

    An exciting development in nutrition will be the ability to use a person's genetic profile to provide more precise nutrition guidance by dietitians and other clinicians. This article discusses this possibility.

14. Junk food or junky choices? *Tufts University Health & Nutrition Letter,* p. 3, September 2003.

    Some sweet or high-fat foods can be safely incorporated into an otherwise healthy diet. This healthy diet should be rich in fruits, vegetables, and whole-grain breads and cereals and should contain some low-fat and fat-free dairy choices and lean protein sources. A person's total dietary intake is what determines the quality of a diet.

15. Lubin F and others: Lifestyle and ethnicity play a role in all-cause mortality. *Journal of Nutrition* 133:1180, 2003.

    Dietary habits that reduce all-cause mortality include focusing on both high-fiber foods and those low in saturated fat and cholesterol. Positive lifestyle habits include regular physical activity and avoiding smoking and obesity.

16. Making sense of medical news. *Consumer Reports on Health,* p. 8, May 2005.

    Consumers need to be wary of health claims made in the news media, as much of this information is suspect from a scientific standpoint. The article reviews many questions that should be asked before any health-related claim is accepted and put into practice.

17. Mokdad AH and others: Actual causes of death in the United States, 2000. *Journal of the American Medical Association* 291:1238, 2004.

    Smoking is the leading cause of preventable death in the United States, with obesity a close second. A combination of a poor diet and inactive lifestyle accounts for about one-third of all deaths in the United States.

18. Olshansky SJ and others: A potential decline in life expectancy in the United States in the 21st century. *The New England Journal of Medicine* 352:1138, 2005.

    The growing problem of overweight and obesity in our society is likely to lead to more overall premature deaths. An alarming concern is that this widespread increase in body weight could result in a life expectancy of fewer years for today's children compared to their parents. Reversing this trend of greater overweight and obesity thus is crucial.

19. Paeratakul S and others: Fast-food consumption among U.S. adults and children: Dietary and nutrient intake profile. *Journal of the American Dietetic Association* 103:1332, 2003.

    Regular intake of fast food contributes a lot of fat and energy to a diet. Such foods can also crowd out more healthful foods in a diet. Regular fast-food consumers would be wise to focus on lower-fat items and greatly limit or avoid sugared soft drinks and french fries.

20. Sloan AE: What, when, and where Americans eat. *Food Technology* 57(8):48, 2003.

    The North American diet is undergoing constant change; this includes introduction of new food products as well as new types of restaurants. This article describes the 10 leading trends in regard to these and other changes.

21. Tholin S and others: Genetic and environmental influences on eating behavior: The Swedish Young Male Twins Study. *American Journal of Clinical Nutrition* 81:564, 2005.

    Genetics plays a distinct role in the development of eating habits, such as emotional eating or restrained eating. Genetics may be linked to the amount of various hormones and other physiological factors that can influence eating habits.

22. Wattendorf DJ, Hadley DW: Family history: The three-generation pedigree. *American Family Physician* 72:441, 2005.

    Reviewing family health history is a valuable tool, in assessing a person's future health risks. As discussed in the article, sharing such information with one's physician can be very important.

23. Wetter AC and others: How and why do individuals make food and physical activity choices? *Nutrition Reviews* 59(3):S11–S20, 2001.

    Health habits are influenced by a number of factors: beliefs, values, life experiences, socioeconomic status, educational attainment, interpersonal relationships, life stage, and social roles. Each decision made regarding health practices depends on input from these and other factors.

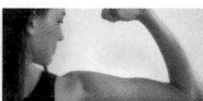

Take | Action

I. Examine Your Eating Habits More Closely.

Choose one day of the week that is typical of your eating pattern. List all foods and drinks you consume for 24 hours. In addition, write down the approximate amounts of food you ate in units, such as cups, ounces, teaspoons, and tablespoons. Check Figure 2-7 in Chapter 2 for examples of appropriate serving units for different types of foods, such as meat and vegetables.

After you record the amount of each food and drink consumed, indicate why you chose to consume the item. Use these suggested abbreviations to indicate why you picked that food or drink.

FLVR	Flavor/texture	ADV	Advertisement	PEER	Peers
CONV	Convenience	WTCL	Weight control	NUTR	Nutritive value
EMO	Emotions/comfort	HUNG	Hunger	$	Cost
AVA	Availability	FAM	Family/cultural	HLTH	Health

There can be more than one reason for choosing a particular food or drink.

Application

Now ask yourself what your most frequent reason is for eating or drinking. To what degree is health or nutritive value a reason for your food choices? Should you make these reasons higher priorities?

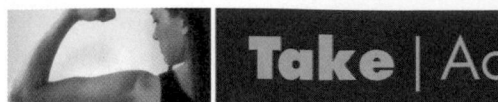

II. Create Your Family Tree for Health-Related Concerns

Adapt this diagram to your own family tree. Under each heading, list year born, year died (if applicable), major diseases that developed during the person's lifetime, and cause of death (if applicable). Figure 1-9 provides one such example.

Note that you are likely to be at risk for any diseases listed. Creating a plan for preventing such diseases when possible, especially those that developed in your family members before age 50 to 60 years, is advised. Speak with your physician about any concerns arising from this exercise.

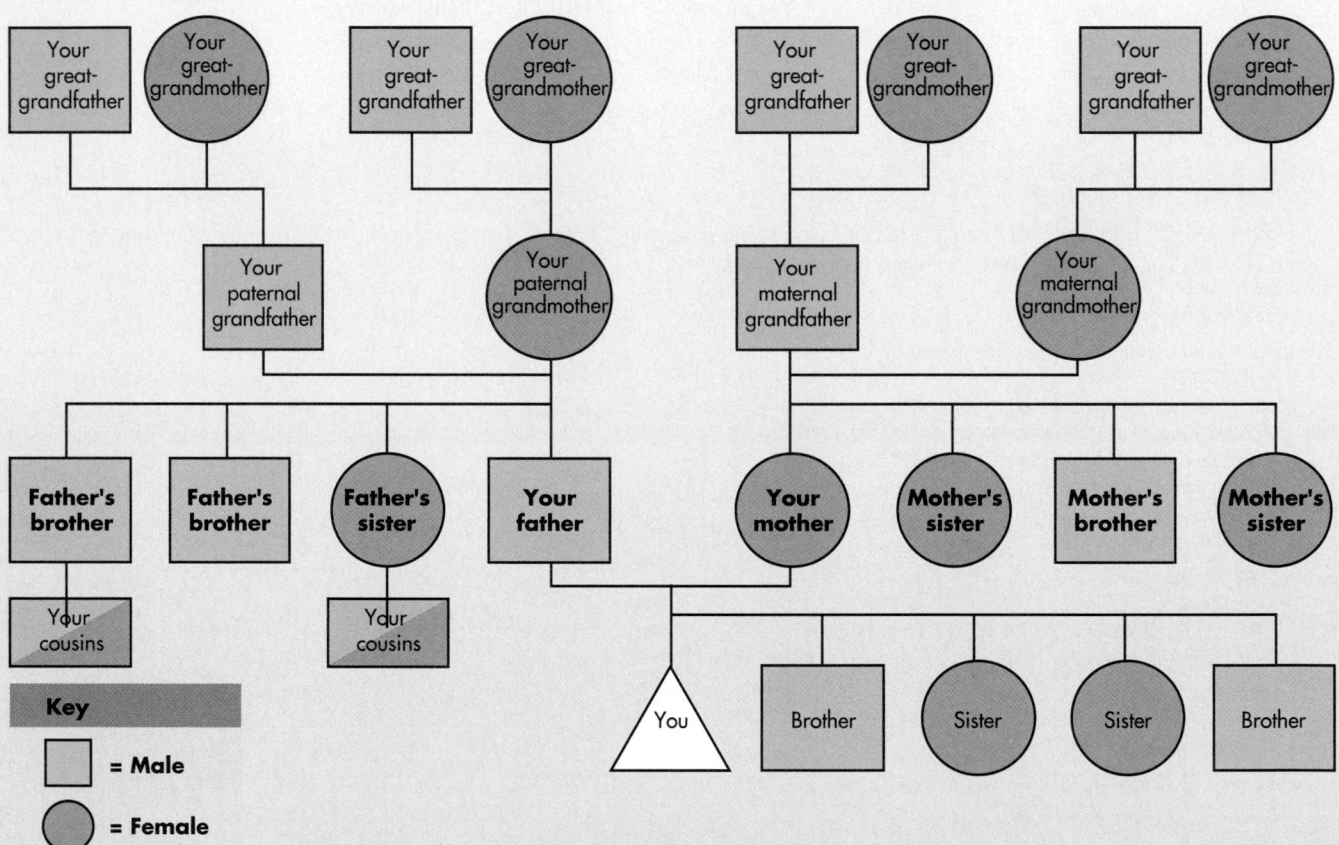

CHAPTER OUTLINE

CASE SCENARIO:

Andy is like many other college students. He grew up on a quick bowl of cereal and milk for breakfast and a hamburger, french fries, and cola for lunch, either in the school cafeteria or at a local fast-food restaurant. At dinner, he generally avoided eating any salad or vegetables, and by 9 o'clock he was deep into bags of chips and cookies. Andy has taken these habits to college. He prefers coffee for breakfast and possibly a chocolate bar. Lunch is still mainly a hamburger, french fries, and cola, but pizza and tacos now alternate more frequently than when he was in high school. One thing Andy really likes about the restaurants surrounding campus is that, for just about half a dollar more, he can *supersize* his meal. This helps him stretch his food dollar; searching out value meals for lunch and dinner now has become part of a typical day.

Can you provide some dietary advice for Andy? Start with his positive habits and then provide some constructive criticism based on what you now know.

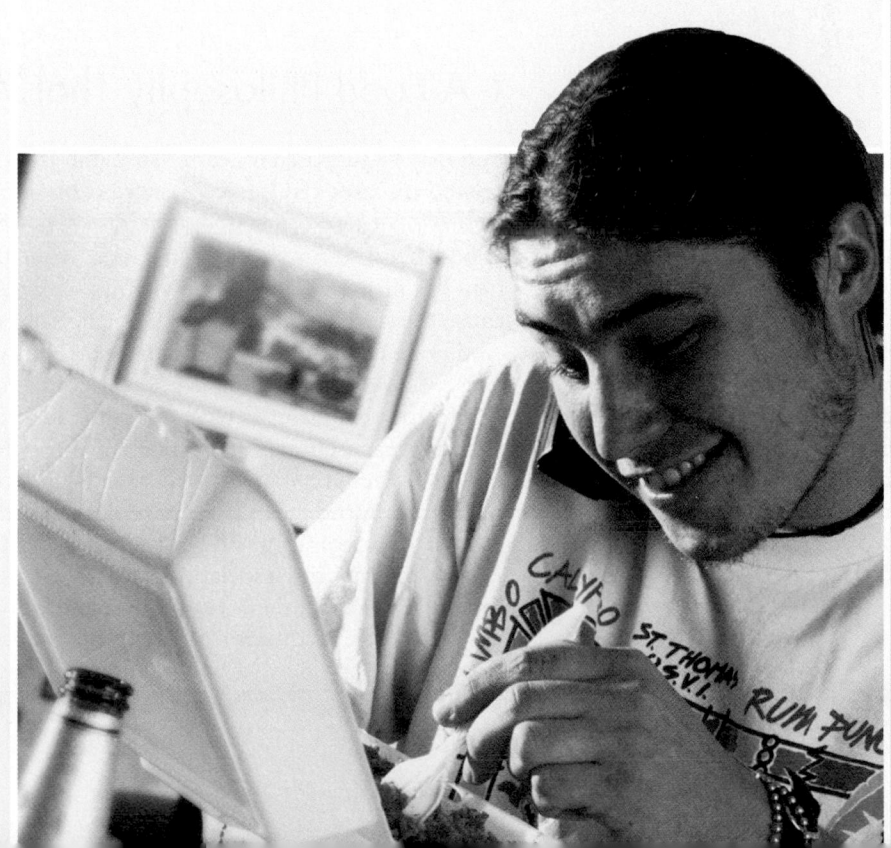

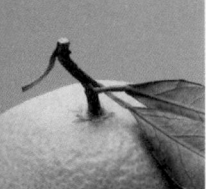

How many times have you heard wild claims about how healthful certain foods are for you? As consumers focus more and more on diet and disease, food manufacturers are asserting that their products have all sorts of health benefits. Supermarket shelves have begun to look like an 1800s medicine show. "Take fish oil capsules to avoid a heart attack." "Eat more olive oil and oat bran to lower blood cholesterol." Hearing these claims, you would think that food manufacturers have solutions to all our health problems.[8]

Advertising aside, nutrient intakes out of balance with our needs—such as excess energy, saturated fat, cholesterol, *trans* fat, salt, alcohol, and sugar—are linked to many leading causes of death in North America, including obesity, hypertension, cardiovascular disease, cancer, liver disease, and type 2 diabetes. Physical inactivity is also too common. In Chapter 2, you will explore the components of a healthy diet—a diet that will minimize your risks of developing nutrition-related diseases. The goal is to provide you with a firm understanding of basic diet-planning concepts before you study the nutrients in detail.[4]

CHAPTER OBJECTIVES CHAPTER 2 IS DESIGNED TO ALLOW YOU TO:

1. Develop a healthy eating plan based on the concepts of variety, balance, moderation, nutrient density, and energy density.

2. Outline the ABCDEs of nutrition assessment: anthropometric, biochemical, clinical, dietary, and economic.

3. Describe what the Recommended Dietary Allowances (RDAs) represent and how these relate to the other standards included in the new Dietary Reference Intakes.

4. Learn the food groupings used in the MyPyramid food guide.

5. Review the 2005 Dietary Guidelines for Americans and the diseases these guidelines are designed to prevent or minimize.

6. Describe what a nutrition label currently consists of and which health claims and label descriptors are allowed on a food package.

REFRESH YOUR MEMORY AS YOU BEGIN YOUR STUDY OF DIET PLANNING IN CHAPTER 2, YOU MAY WANT TO REVIEW:

- The terms in the margin in Chapter 1 and Table 1-2.
- The impact of the Dietary Supplement Health and Education Act (DSHEA) on certain label claims in Chapter 1.
- The impact of genetic background on the risk of developing certain chronic diseases in Chapter 1.

A Food Philosophy That Works

You may be surprised to learn that minimizing your risk of developing common nutrition-related diseases can be accomplished by doing what you've heard many times before: *consume a variety of foods balanced by a moderate intake of each food.* A variety of foods is best because no one food meets all your nutrient needs. Meat provides protein and iron but little calcium and no vitamin C. Eggs also provide protein but little calcium because the calcium is mostly in the shell. Cow's milk contains calcium, but very little iron. And none of these foods contain fiber. Thus you need a variety of foods in your diet because the required nutrients are scattered among many foods.[2]

Health professionals have recommended the same basic diet and health plan for the past 40 years: control how much you eat, focus on the major food groups, and stay physically active. Whole-grain breads and cereals, fruits, and vegetables have always been among the foods emphasized for our diet for these past 40 years.[10]

It is disappointing, however, that according to a recent survey conducted by the American Dietetic Association, two of five people in the United States believe that following a healthful diet means completely giving up foods they enjoy. To the contrary, a healthful diet requires only some simple planning and doesn't have to mean deprivation and misery. Besides, eliminating favorite foods typically doesn't work for "dieters" in the long run. The best plan consists of learning the basics of a healthful diet—a

Some people would like to live mostly on french fries. What is the nutrient content of french fries? Check the food composition table in Appendix N for the vitamin C content of french fries. How many servings would you need to eat to meet vitamin C needs (75 to 95 mg/day)?

(Answer: 4 to 5 servings)

variety and balance of foods from all food groups and moderate consumption of all foods.[10] Let's now fine-tune this advice by focusing on variety, balance, moderation, nutrient density, and energy density.

Variety Means Eating Many Different Foods

Variety in your diet means choosing a number of different foods within any given food group, rather than eating the "same old thing" day after day. Variety makes meals more interesting and helps ensure that a diet contains sufficient nutrients. For example, carrots—a rich source of a pigment that forms vitamin A in our bodies—may be your favorite vegetable; however, if you choose carrots every day as your only vegetable source, you may miss out on the vitamin folate. Other vegetables, such as broccoli and asparagus, are rich sources of this nutrient. This concept is true of all classes of foods: fruits, vegetables, grains, and so on. Different foods within each class vary somewhat in the nutrients they contain, but they generally provide similar types of nutrients.

A benefit of variety in the diet, especially within the fruit and vegetable groups, is the inclusion of a rich supply of what scientists call **phytochemicals.** These plant components are not considered essential nutrients in the diet. Still, many of these substances provide significant health benefits.[1] Considerable research attention is focused on various phytochemicals in reducing the risk for certain diseases (e.g., cancer). You can't just buy a bottle of phytochemicals—they are generally available only within whole foods. Current multivitamin and mineral supplements contain few or none of these beneficial plant chemicals.

Numerous population studies show reduced cancer risk among people who regularly consume fruits and vegetables. This is true for cancer of the gastrointestinal (GI) tract, breast, lung, and bladder. Researchers surmise that some phytochemicals present in the fruits and vegetables block the cancer process.[13] The cancer process and the specific roles of some phytochemicals in this regard are described in the Nutrition Focus in Chapter 12. For now, realize that cancer develops over many years via a multistep process. If a phytochemical blocks any one of the steps in this process, it reduces the chances that cancer will ultimately appear in the body. Some phytochemicals have also been linked to a reduced risk of cardiovascular disease. Could it be that because humans evolved on a wide variety of plant-based foods, the body developed with a need for these phytochemicals, along with the various nutrients present, to maintain optimal health?

It will likely take many years for scientists to unravel the important effects of the myriad of phytochemicals in foods, and it is unlikely that all will ever be available or effective in supplement form. For this reason, leading nutrition and medical experts suggest that a diet rich in fruits, vegetables, and whole-grain breads and cereals is the most reliable way to obtain the potential benefits of phytochemicals.[6] Table 2-1 lists some phytochemicals under study, with their common food sources. Table 2-2 provides a number of suggestions for including more phytochemicals in your diet, as does the website www.5aday.com and 5aday.nci.nih.gov.

Balance Means Not Overconsuming Any Single Type of Food

One way to balance your diet as you consume a variety of foods is to select foods from the six major food groups every day:[15]

- Grains
- Vegetables
- Fruits
- Milk
- Meat & Beans
- Oils

A dinner consisting of a bean burrito, lettuce and tomato salad with oil and vinegar dressing, a glass of milk, and an apple covers all groups.

Variety—choose different types of foods within each food group.

Balance—choose foods from all six food groups.

Moderation—control portion size so that balance and variety are possible in your diet.

phytochemical A chemical found in plants. Some phytochemicals may contribute to a reduced risk of cancer or cardiovascular disease in people who consume them regularly.

Some research suggests that increasing variety in a diet can lead to overeating. Thus, as you include a wide variety of foods in your diet, pay attention to total energy intake as well.

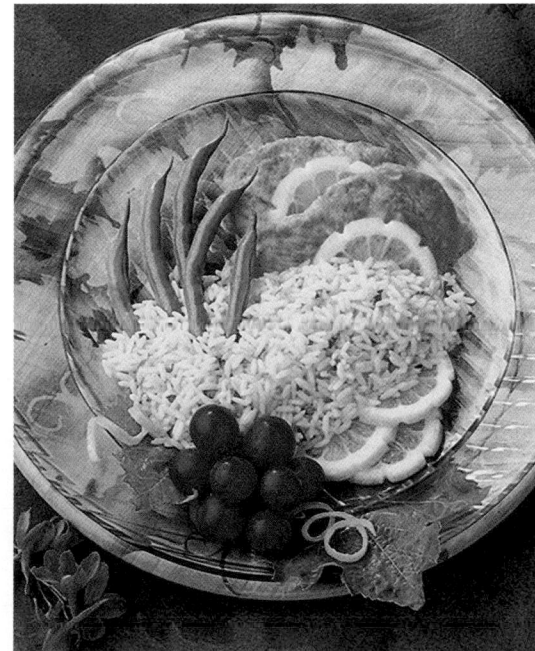

Focus on nutrient-rich foods as you strive to meet your nutrient needs. The more colorful your plate, the greater the content of nutrients and phytochemicals.

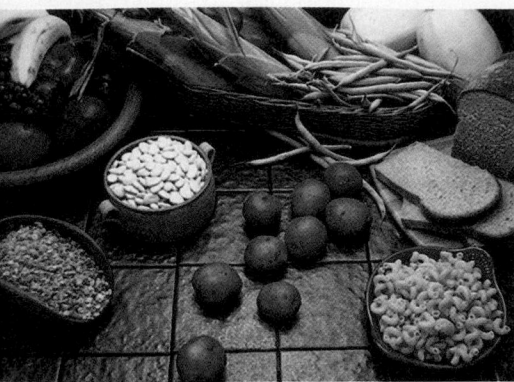

Fruits, vegetables, beans, and whole-grain breads and cereals are typically rich in phytochemicals.

Table 2-1 | Some Phytochemical Compounds under Study[6]

Phytochemical	Food Sources
Allyl sulfides/organosulfurs	Garlic, onions, leeks
Saponins	Garlic, onions, licorice, legumes
Carotenoids (e.g., lycopene)	Orange, red, yellow fruits and vegetables (egg yolks are a source as well)
Monoterpenes	Oranges, lemons, grapefruit
Capsaicin	Chili peppers
Lignans	Flaxseed, berries, whole grains
Indoles	Cruciferous vegetables (broccoli, cabbage, kale)
Isothiocyanates	Cruciferous vegetables, especially broccoli
Phytosterols	Soybeans, other legumes, cucumbers, other fruits and vegetables
Flavonoids	Citrus fruit, onions, apples, grapes, red wine, tea, chocolate, tomatoes
Isoflavones	Soybeans, other legumes
Catechins	Tea
Ellagic acid	Strawberries, raspberries, grapes, apples, bananas, nuts
Anthocyanosides	Red, blue, and purple plants (eggplant, blueberries)
Fructooligosaccharides	Onions, bananas, oranges (small amounts)
Resveratrol	Grapes, peanuts, red wine

Some related compounds under study are found in animal products, such as sphingolipids (meat and dairy products) and conjugated linoleic acid (meat and cheese). These compounds are not phytochemicals per se because they are not from plant sources, but they have been shown to have health benefits.

Foods rich in phytochemicals are now part of a family of foods referred to as **functional foods.**[6] A functional food is a food that provides health benefits beyond those supplied by the traditional nutrients it contains. Since a tomato contains the phytochemical lycopene, it can be called a functional food. You may hear this term more from the food industry in the future.

Moderation Refers Mostly to Portion Size

Although moderating portion size is a good practice, eating moderately requires planning your entire day's diet so that you don't overconsume nutrient sources. For example, if you eat something relatively high in fat, salt, and energy, such as a bacon cheeseburger, you should eat foods that are less concentrated sources of the same nutrients, such as fruits and salad greens at other meals that same day. This aids in balancing your diet. If you prefer whole milk to low-fat or fat-free milk, reduce the fat elsewhere in your meals. Try low-fat salad dressings, or use jam rather than butter or margarine on toast. Overall, strive to simply moderate serving sizes of some foods rather than eliminate these foods altogether.

Many nutrition experts agree that there are no exclusively "good" or "bad" foods. Even so, many North Americans have diets that lack the foundations of a healthy food plan—variety, balance, and moderation.[3,16] Consuming diets that are overloaded with foods high in fatty meats, fried foods, sugared soft drinks, and refined starches can result in substantial risk for nutrition-related chronic diseases.

Nutrient Density Focuses on Nutrient Content

Nutrient density has gained acceptance in recent years as an assessment of the nutritional quality of an individual food. To determine the nutrient density of a food, simply compare its vitamin or mineral content with the amount of energy it provides. A food is said to be nutrient dense if it provides a large amount of a nutrient for a relatively small amount of energy (compared with other food sources). The higher a food's nutrient density, the better it is as a nutrient source. Comparing the nutrient density of different foods is an easy way to estimate their relative nutritional quality. Generally, nutrient density is determined with respect to individual nutrients. For example, many fruits and vegetables have a high content of vitamin C compared with their modest energy content, that is, they are nutrient-dense foods for vitamin C. Moreover, as Figure 2-1 shows, fat-free milk is much more nutrient dense than is a sugared soft drink for many nutrients.

nutrient density The ratio derived by dividing a food's contribution to nutrient needs by its contribution to energy needs. When its contribution to nutrient needs exceeds its energy contribution, the food is considered to have a favorable nutrient density.

Table 2-2 | Tips for Boosting the Phytochemical Content of a Diet

- Include vegetables in main and side dishes. Add these to rice, omelets, potato salad, and pastas. Try broccoli or cauliflower florets, mushrooms, peas, carrots, corn, or peppers.

- Look for quick-fixing grain side dishes in the supermarket. Pilafs, couscous, rice mixes, and tabbouleh are just a few that you'll find.

- Choose fruit-filled cookies, such as fig bars, instead of sugar-rich cookies. Use fresh or canned fruit as a topping for puddings, hot or cold cereal, pancakes, and frozen desserts.

- Put raisins, grapes, apple chunks, pineapple, grated carrots, zucchini, or cucumber into coleslaw, chicken salad, or tuna salad.

- Be creative at the salad bar: Try fresh spinach, leaf lettuce, red cabbage, zucchini, yellow squash, cauliflower, peas, mushrooms, or red or yellow peppers.

- Pack fresh or dried fruit for snacks away from home instead of grabbing a candy bar or going hungry.

- Add slices of cucumber, zucchini, spinach, or carrot slivers to the lettuce and tomato on your sandwiches.

- Try one or two vegetarian meals per week: beans and rice or pasta; Chinese vegetable stir fry; or spaghetti and tomato sauce.

- When daily protein intake more than meets recommended amounts, reduce the meat, fish, or poultry in recipes by one-third to one-half and add more vegetables and legumes such as soy.

- Keep a bowl of fresh vegetables in the refrigerator for snacks.

- Choose fruit or vegetable juices instead of soft drinks, preferably 100% juice varieties.

- Substitute tea for coffee or soft drinks on a regular basis.

- Have a bowl of fruit on hand.

- Switch from crisphead lettuce to leaf lettuce, such as romaine.

- Use salsa as a dip for chips in place of creamy dips.

- Choose whole-grain breakfast cereals, breads, and crackers.

- Add flavor to your plate with ginger, rosemary, basil, thyme, garlic, onions, parsley, and chives in place of salt.

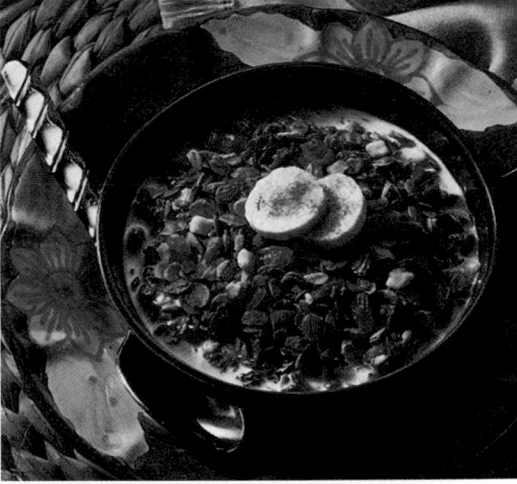

Choosing whole-grain cereals is an excellent way to increase the nutrient content of a diet. Ideally, the cereal should have at least 3 g of fiber per serving.

Critical | Thinking

Andy, described in this chapter's Case Scenario, would benefit from more variety in his diet. What are some practical tips he can use to increase his fruit and vegetable intake?

As noted previously, menu planning focuses mainly on the total diet—not on the selection of one critical food as key to an adequate diet. Nonetheless, nutrient-dense foods—such as fat-free and low-fat milk, lean meats, legumes (beans), oranges, carrots, broccoli, whole-wheat bread, and whole-grain breakfast cereals—do help balance less nutrient-dense foods—such as cookies and potato chips—which many people like to eat. The latter are often called empty-calorie foods because they tend to be high in sugar and/or fat but few other nutrients.

Eating nutrient-dense foods is especially important for people who tend not to eat a lot of food. This includes some older people and those following weight-loss diets.

Energy Density Especially Influences Energy Intake

Energy density is a concept that has captured the attention of nutrition scientists in recent years.[9] Energy density of a food is determined by comparing the energy content with the weight of food. A food that is rich in energy but weighs relatively little is considered energy dense. Examples include nuts, cookies, fried foods in general, and fat-free processed snacks such as pretzels. Foods with low energy density include fruits, vegetables, and any food that incorporates lots of water during cooking, such as oatmeal (Table 2-3). Dr. Barbara Rolls discusses energy density in detail in the Expert Opinion, p. 43.

energy density A comparison of the energy content of a food with the weight of the food. An energy-dense food is high in energy content but weighs very little (e.g., many fried foods), whereas a food low in energy density, such as an orange, weighs a lot but is low in energy content.

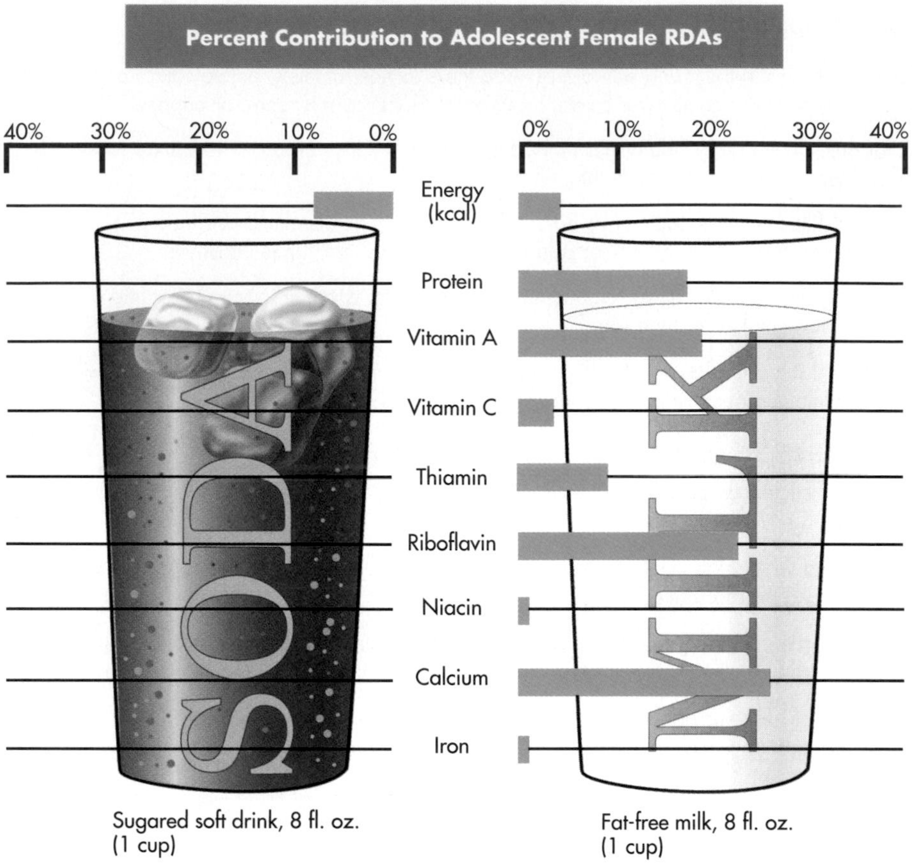

Figure 2-1 | Comparison of the nutrient density of a sugary soft drink with that of fat-free (i.e., skim) milk. Choosing a glass of fat-free milk makes a significantly greater contribution to nutrient intake than does a sugary soft drink. An easy way to determine nutrient density from this chart is to compare the lengths of the bars indicating vitamin or mineral contribution with the bar that represents energy content. For the soft drink, no nutrient surpasses energy content. Fat-free milk, in contrast, has longer nutrient bars for protein, vitamin A, the vitamins thiamin and riboflavin, and the mineral calcium. Including many nutrient-dense foods in your diet is a good way to meet nutrient needs.

Percent Contribution to Adolescent Female RDAs

40% 30% 20% 10% 0%		0% 10% 20% 30% 40%	

Energy (kcal)
Protein
Vitamin A
Vitamin C
Thiamin
Riboflavin
Niacin
Calcium
Iron

Sugared soft drink, 8 fl. oz. (1 cup)

Fat-free milk, 8 fl. oz. (1 cup)

Table 2-3 | Energy Density of Common Foods (Listed in Relative Order)

Very Low Energy Density (less than 0.6 kcal/g)	Low Energy Density (0.6 to 1.5 kcal/g)	Medium Energy Density (1.5 to 4 kcal/g)	High Energy Density (greater than 4 kcal/g)
Lettuce	Whole milk	Eggs	Graham crackers
Tomatoes	Oatmeal	Ham	Fat-free sandwich cookies
Strawberries	Cottage cheese	Pumpkin pie	Chocolate
Broccoli	Beans	Whole-wheat bread	Chocolate chip cookies
Salsa	Bananas	Bagels	Tortilla chips
Grapefruit	Broiled fish	White bread	Bacon
Fat-free milk	Fat-free yogurt	Raisins	Potato chips
Carrots	Ready-to-eat breakfast cereals with 1% low-fat milk	Cream cheese	Peanuts
Vegetable soup	Plain baked potato	Cake with frosting	Peanut butter
	Cooked rice	Pretzels	Mayonnaise
	Spaghetti noodles	Rice cakes	Butter or margarine
			Vegetable oils

Data adapted from Rolls B, Barnett RA: *Volumetrics*. New York: HarperCollins, 2000.

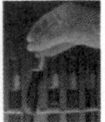

Expert Opinion

The Importance of Energy Density in the Diet
Barbara J. Rolls, Ph.D.

With the surge in the incidence of overweight and obesity, effective dietary strategies for weight management are needed. On the surface the issue is clear-cut: simply reduce energy intake below energy expenditure. There is much debate and controversy, however, over the optimal way this goal should be achieved. Although it is unlikely that a single dietary strategy will ever fit everyone's preferences, health professionals have a responsibility to communicate to the public which strategies are considered both safe and effective.

Designing Diets That Reduce Hunger and Enhance Satiety

The biggest problem in weight management is adherence to the diet, no matter what its composition. Because of this problem, the focus has shifted away from the macronutrient composition of the diet (e.g., fat vs. carbohydrate) toward dietary factors that affect hunger and satiety (the feeling of fullness and satisfaction after eating). Since weight loss is achieved through energy restriction, adherence is more likely if hunger is controlled and dieters feel satisfied.

Short-term studies show that the energy density (kcal/g) of the diet affects both the amount consumed and how satisfied people feel. Foods low in energy density provide bigger portions for a given number of calories. Water is the dietary component that has the biggest impact on the energy density of foods. Water adds weight but no calories and therefore decreases the energy density. Increasing the water content of recipes (for example, by the addition of vegetables) is associated with reduced energy intake and enhanced satiety. Whereas water decreases energy density, fat increases it because fat has 9 kcal/g, or more than twice that of carbohydrates and protein (both have 4 kcal/g). People overeat high-fat foods not only because they taste good but also because fat packs so many calories into a relatively small amount of food.

A surprising finding in recent years, both in controlled lab studies and in studies of free-living individuals, has been the demonstration that people tend to eat a consistent weight or volume of food over a day or two. Furthermore, they are relatively insensitive to calories while they are eating. A number of lab-based studies show that when offered unlimited amounts of similar dishes with different energy densities, people consume a consistent weight of food. Thus, when the food offerings contain fewer calories per gram, people consume less energy but still report feeling just as full and satisfied. If people eat foods high in energy density, they have to restrict portions to avoid excessive energy intake.

In our current "obesigenic" food environment in which we are surrounded by tasty, inexpensive, energy-dense foods in huge portions, it is difficult to avoid overeating. Indeed, a number of studies find that eating out, particularly at fast-food restaurants, is associated with increased intake and ele-

vated body weight. My colleagues and I have shown in several studies that the effects of energy density and portion size combine to increase food intake, confirming that large portions of energy-dense foods are particularly problematic for weight management. On the other hand, large portions of foods low in energy density, such as soups and salads consumed at the start of a meal, are associated with enhanced satiety and a reduction in energy intake at the meal. Other dietary factors that have been shown to enhance satiety are increases in fiber and protein.

Why Focusing on Macronutrient Composition Is Not As Helpful

Both the scientific community and proponents of popular diets for weight loss have emphasized the importance of the proportions of the macronutrients in diets for weight loss. In the 1980s and 1990s the focus was on reducing the amount of fat in the diet. Remember the proliferation of fat-free or reduced-fat products? This emphasis on fat reduction was reflected in an evidence-based report published by the National Institutes of Health in 1998 that

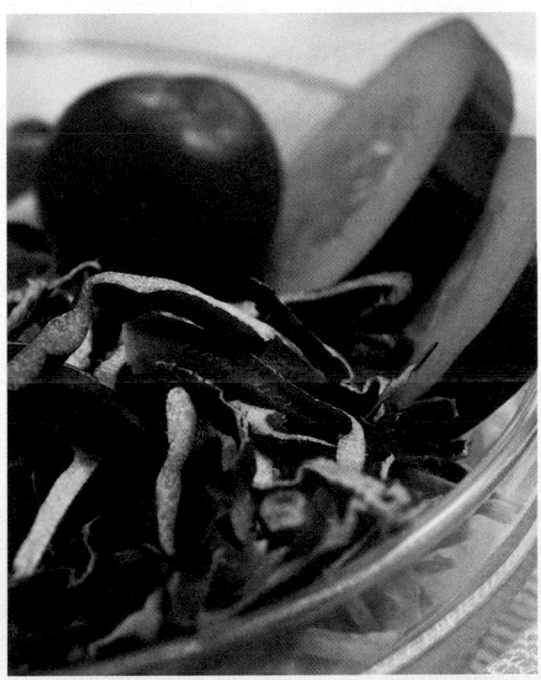

Salads are low in energy density if we limit additional calories from salad dressing, and especially minimize bacon bits, cheese, and croutons.

(continued)

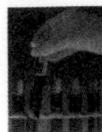

assessed the data from 48 randomized, controlled trials of weight-loss diets. The report found that on lower-fat diets (20 to 30% of calories) people lost weight, and this weight loss was associated with a reduction in energy intake. The emphasis on fat reduction in the 1998 report was related to the fact that most of the clinical trials meeting the criteria for inclusion focused on the fat content of the diet. Since then, the emphasis has shifted to restricting carbohydrates and increasing protein intake. A number of clinical trials have shown that low-carbohydrate, high-protein diets are associated with significant weight loss over 6 to 12 months. As with low-fat diets, energy intake on low-carbohydrate diets was reduced; this reduction was probably due to the restriction of food choices. The verdict is not yet in on how these alterations in the proportions of macronutrients affect health or whether adherence to such restrictive programs is possible in the long term.

It remains to be proven whether variations in the macronutrient composition of the diet can significantly affect the rate of weight loss when energy intake is held constant. There are small differences in the metabolic effects of the macronutrients, but well-controlled metabolic studies have found that these differences have only a small impact on weight loss.

Use Energy Density As a Guide to Food Choices

Using energy density as a guide to food choices not only enhances satiety but also leads consumers to foods that health professionals routinely encourage:

vegetables, fruits, whole grains, legumes, lean protein, and low-fat dairy products. Furthermore, despite the emphasis on weight loss, the key to weight management is actually prevention of weight gain; this goal will also require innovative strategies to reduce the energy density of the diet.

In summary, optimal diets for weight management should

- Provide adequate amounts of foods and nutrients from a variety of food groups
- Fit with consumer's preferences, be affordable, and be readily available
- Emphasize quality rather than quantity
- Help control hunger and promote satiety through reductions in the energy density of the diet

Dr. Barbara Rolls is Guthrie Chair of Nutrition in the Department of Nutritional Sciences at The Pennsylvania State University, University Park, Pennsylvania. She obtained a B.A. in biology from The University of Pennsylvania and a Ph.D. in physiology from The University of Cambridge, England. She is past president of both the Society for the Study of Human Ingestive Behavior and the North American Association for the Study of Obesity. She is on the editorial boards of leading journals and is the coauthor of four books, including Thirst *and* The Volumetrics Weight-Control Plan: Feel Full on Fewer Calories. *Her research interests include the controls of food and fluid intake, especially as they relate to obesity, eating disorders, and aging.*

One more dietary strategy to consider is increased meal frequency. Eating smaller, more frequent meals and snacks provides benefits to the body—such as lower blood glucose, cholesterol, and triglycerides—since body metabolism is not as overwhelmed as it is with large meals. In addition, fasting for much of a day may lead to overeating once eating resumes. As long as overall energy intake remains appropriate, spreading food throughout the day is a healthy practice. One idea is to pack a lunch and consume it throughout the day rather than all at once at noontime.

Overall, foods with lots of water and fiber provide a low-energy-density contribution to a meal and help a person feel full, whereas foods with high energy density must be eaten in greater amounts in order to contribute to fullness.[9] This is one more reason to support a diet rich in fruits, vegetables, and whole-grain breads and cereals, a pattern that also is typical of many ethnic diets throughout the world. Still, favorite foods, even if they are high in energy density, can have a place in your dietary pattern, but you will have to plan for them.[7] For example, chocolate is a very energy-dense food, but a small portion at the end of a meal can supply a satisfying finale. In addition, foods with high energy density can help people with poor appetites, such as some older people, to maintain or gain weight.

The following sections of Chapter 2 describe various states of nutritional health and provide tools and nutrient guidelines for planning healthy diets to support overall health.

Concept | Check

Basic diet-planning concepts include consuming a variety of foods, balancing a diet by consuming foods from each of the six food groups, and moderating portion size with each food choice so that the diet is not excessive in energy. Choosing nutrient-dense foods, such as fat-free milk, fruits, vegetables, and whole-grain breads and cereals, helps create a diet with many nutrients but not excessive in energy content. Many of these foods are also rich sources of phytochemicals, supplying an even greater health benefit to the diet. Consuming foods of low energy density, such as fruits and vegetables, may also help in weight control in that these foods provide satiety after a meal because of their large weight but relatively little energy content.

States of Nutritional Health

The body's nutritional health is determined by the sum of its **nutritional status** with respect to each needed nutrient. We recognize three general categories: desirable nutrition, **undernutrition,** and **overnutrition.** The common term **malnutrition** can refer to either overnutrition or undernutrition. Neither state is conducive to good health.

Desirable Nutrition

The nutritional status for a particular nutrient is optimal when body tissues have enough of the nutrient to support normal metabolic functions as well as surplus stores to be used in times of increased need.[5] A desirable nutritional state can be achieved by obtaining essential nutrients from a variety of foods.

Undernutrition

Undernutrition occurs when nutrient intake does not meet nutrient needs. Any surpluses are then put to use and health begins to decline. Many nutrients are in high demand because of the constant cycle of cell loss and later regeneration in the body, such as in the gastrointestinal tract. For this reason, certain nutrient stores are exhausted rapidly, including many of the B vitamins. Therefore, a regular intake is needed.[5] In addition, some women in North America do not consume sufficient iron to meet monthly losses and eventually deplete their iron stores. Reduced biochemical functions and ultimately clinical evidence of an iron deficiency can develop (Table 2-4).

nutritional status The nutritional health of a person as determined by anthropometric measurements (height, weight, circumferences, and so on), biochemical measurements of nutrients or their by-products in blood and urine, a clinical (physical) examination, a dietary analysis, and economic evaluation.

undernutrition Failing health that results from a long-standing dietary intake that does not meet nutritional needs.

overnutrition A state in which nutritional intake greatly exceeds the body's needs.

malnutrition Failing health that results from long-standing dietary practices that do not meet nutritional needs.

Table 2-4 | Categories of Nutritional Status with Respect to Iron*

General Condition	Condition with Respect to Iron
Overnutrition: nutrients consumed in excess of body needs (degree of toxicity varies for each nutrient)	Results in toxic damage to liver cells; may contribute to cardiovascular disease
Desirable nutrition: nutrients consumed to support body functions and stores of nutrients for times of increased need	Adequate liver stores of iron, adequate blood values for iron-related compounds
Undernutrition: nutrient intake does not meet nutrient needs; biochemical changes then take place	Many changes in body functions associated with a decline in iron status (e.g., iron-containing proteins and pigments in the blood drop below acceptable amounts [e.g., 12 ng/ml] and oxygen supply to body tissues is reduced); eventual pale complexion; fatigue upon exertion; "spooning" of the nails in a severe deficiency; poor body temperature regulation

*This general scheme can apply to all nutrients. Iron was chosen because you are likely to be familiar with this nutrient. Note that ng refers to nanograms, or 10^{-9} grams.

biochemical lesion An indication of reduced biochemical function (e.g., low concentrations of nutrient by-products or enzyme activities in the blood or urine) resulting from a nutritional deficiency.

subclinical Disease or disorder that is present but not severe enough to produce signs and symptoms that can be detected or diagnosed.

clinical lesion A sign seen on physical examination or a symptom perceived by the patient resulting from a nutritional deficiency.

A *sign* is a feature visible on examination, such as flaky skin. A *symptom* is a change in body function that is not necessarily apparent to an examiner. An example is stomach pain.

Reduced Biochemical Functions

Once nutrient stores are depleted, a continuing nutritional deficit drains body tissues further. The body can only compensate to a certain point.[5] When tissue concentrations of an essential nutrient fall sufficiently low, a **biochemical lesion** results and the body's metabolic processes eventually slow down or even stop. Diminished enzyme function often is the cause of the slowdown in biochemical function. This type of nutrient deficiency is termed **subclinical** because there are no overt signs or symptoms. At the subclinical stage for poor iron status, concentrations of hemoglobin (a red blood cell protein) in the blood are lower than considered healthy; the synthesis of hemoglobin requires iron.

Clinical Signs and Symptoms

If a biochemical deficit becomes severe, clinical signs and symptoms eventually develop and become outwardly apparent.[5] It is then possible to note **clinical lesions** in the body, perhaps in the skin, hair, nails, tongue, or eyes. In the case of an iron deficiency, the complexion may become very pale in Caucasians, and fatigue can quickly develop during even moderate activity.

Overnutrition

Prolonged consumption of more nutrients than the body needs can lead to overnutrition. In the short run, for instance a week or two, overnutrition may cause only a few symptoms, such as stomach distress from excess fiber or iron intake. But if an excess intake continues, some nutrients may increase to toxic amounts, which can lead to serious disease.[5] For example, too much vitamin A can have negative effects, particularly in children, pregnant women, and older adults.

The most common type of overnutrition in industrialized nations—excess intake of energy-yielding nutrients—often leads to obesity. In the long run, obesity can then lead to other serious diseases, such as type 2 diabetes and certain forms of cancer. Use the website shapeup.org to learn more about the importance of avoiding this form of overnutrition.

For most vitamins and minerals, the gap between desirable intake and overnutrition is wide. Even if people take a typical balanced multivitamin and mineral supplement daily, they probably won't receive a harmful amount of any nutrient. However, the gap between optimal intake and overnutrition is very narrow for vitamin A, calcium, iron, copper, and other minerals. Thus, if you take nutrient supplements, keep a close eye on your total vitamin and mineral intake both from food and from supplements to avoid toxicity. Men in general and older women should be especially cautious of supplements containing iron (see Chapter 9 for further advice on use of nutrient supplements).

▌How Can Your Nutritional State Be Measured?

To find out how nutritionally fit *you* are, a nutritional assessment—either whole or in part—needs to be performed (Table 2-5). Generally, this is performed by a physician, often with the aid of a registered dietitian.

Analyzing Background Factors

Since family history plays an important role in determining nutritional and health status, it must be carefully recorded and critically analyzed as part of a nutritional assessment. Other related background parameters include: (1) a medical history, especially for any disease states or treatments that could impede nutrient absorptive processes or ultimate use; (2) a list of medications taken; (3) a social history; (4) information about the person's level of education since poorly educated people have a greater risk for poor health; and (5) economic status to determine the ability of the person to purchase, transport, and cook food.[5]

Table 2-5 | Conducting an Evaluation of Nutritional Health

Parameters	Example
Background	Medical history (e.g., current diseases, past surgeries, current weight, weight history, and current medications) Social history (marital status, cooking facilities) Family history Education attainment Economic status
Nutritional	Anthropometric assessment: height, weight, skinfold thickness, arm muscle circumference, and other parameters Biochemical (laboratory) assessment of blood and urine: enzyme activities, concentrations of nutrients or their by-products Clinical assessment (physical examination): general appearance of skin, eyes, and tongue; rapid hair loss; sense of touch; ability to walk Dietary assessment: usual intake or record of previous days' meals

Evaluating the ABCDEs

In addition to background factors, four nutritional parameters complete the picture of nutritional status. **Anthropometric assessment** measurements of height, weight (and weight changes), skinfolds, and body circumferences provide an outline of the current state of nutrition. Measures of body composition are easy to obtain and are generally reliable. However, an in-depth examination of nutritional health is impossible without the more expensive process of **biochemical assessments.** This involves the measurement of the concentrations of nutrients and nutrient by-products in the blood, urine, and feces and of specific blood enzyme activities.[5]

For example, in Chapter 10 you will learn that the status of the vitamin thiamin in the body is measured in part by determining the activity of an enzyme called transketolase used in the breakdown of glucose. It is possible to isolate that enzyme from cells, such as red blood cells, and determine if it can process its starting products quickly enough. To test for this, cells are broken open and thiamin is added to the preparation to see if this speeds the rate of the transketolase enzyme by more than 25%. If so, we say that the red blood cells lack sufficient thiamin for the enzyme to function at maximal capacity.

During a **clinical assessment,** the health professional searches for any physical evidence of diet-related diseases (e.g., high blood pressure). Possible problem areas are assessed when the health professional takes a close look at the person's diet **(dietary assessment),** including a record of at least the previous few days' intake. Finally, the **economic assessment** (from the background analysis), which impacts the person's ability to purchase and prepare foods needed to maintain health, provides further detail to the picture. Now the true nutritional state of a person emerges.[5] Taken together, these five parameters form the ABCDEs of nutritional assessment: **a**nthropometric, **b**iochemical, **c**linical, **d**ietary, and **e**conomic (Figure 2-2).

Recognizing the Limitations of Nutritional Assessment

A long time may elapse between the initial development of poor nutritional health and the first clinical evidence of a problem. Recall that a diet high in saturated (typically solid) fat often increases blood cholesterol, but without producing any clinical evidence for years. However, when the blood vessels become sufficiently blocked by cholesterol and other materials, chest pain during physical activity or a **heart attack** may occur. Much of the current nutrition research is designed to develop better methods for early detection of nutrition-related problems such as heart attack risk.

anthropometric assessment Pertaining to the measurement of body weight and the lengths, circumferences, and thicknesses of parts of the body.

biochemical assessment An assessment focusing on biochemical functions (e.g., concentrations of nutrient by-products or enzyme activities in the blood or urine) related to a nutrient's function.

clinical assessment An assessment that focuses on a person's physical evidence of diet-related diseases, for example, general appearance of skin, eyes, and tongue; evidence of rapid hair loss; sense of touch; and ability to cough and walk.

dietary assessment An assessment that focuses on the typical food choices of the person, relying mostly on the recounting of one's usual intake or a record of one's previous days' intake.

economic assessment An assessment that focuses on the ability of the person to purchase, transport, and cook food. The person's weekly budget for food purchases is also a key factor to consider.

heart attack Rapid fall in heart function caused by reduced blood flow through the heart's blood vessels. Often part of the heart dies in the process. It is technically called a *myocardial infarction.*

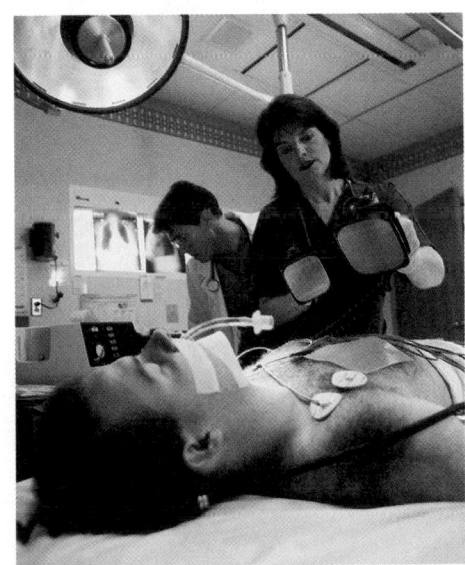

The first evidence that one's diet is out of balance with one's physiology could be a heart attack. About 25% of all heart attack victims do not survive the event.

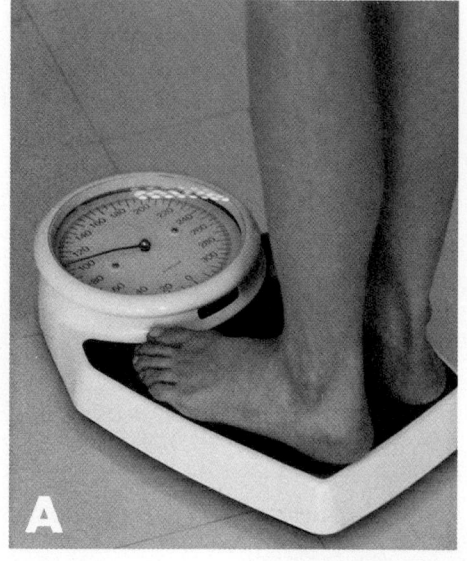

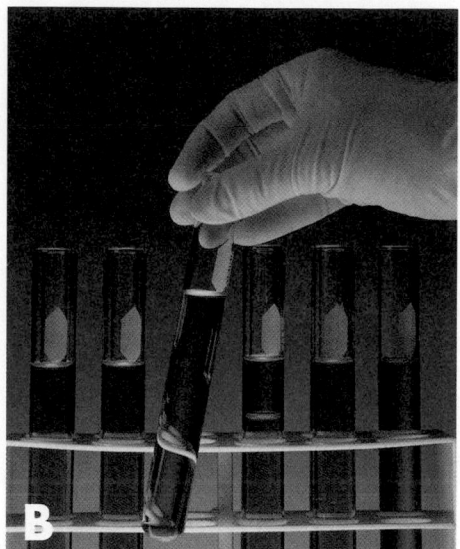

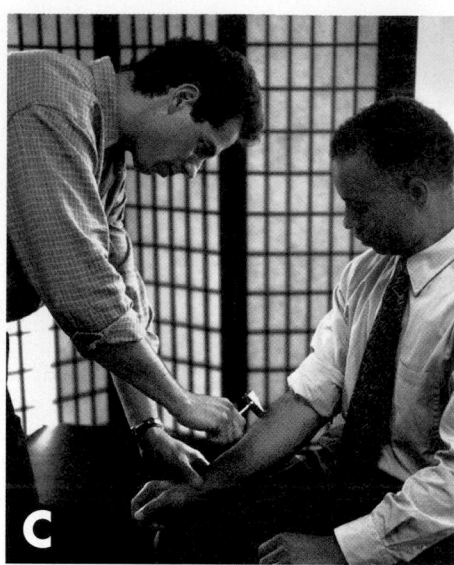

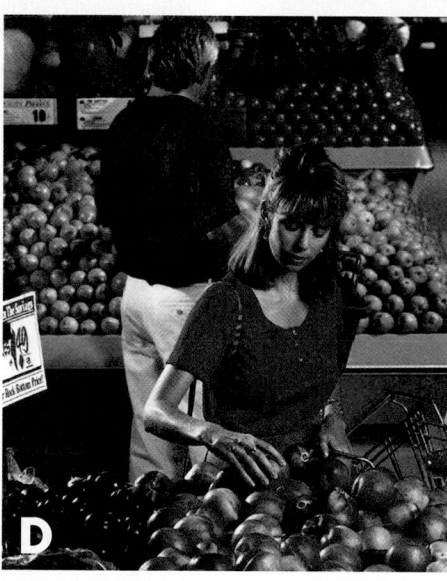

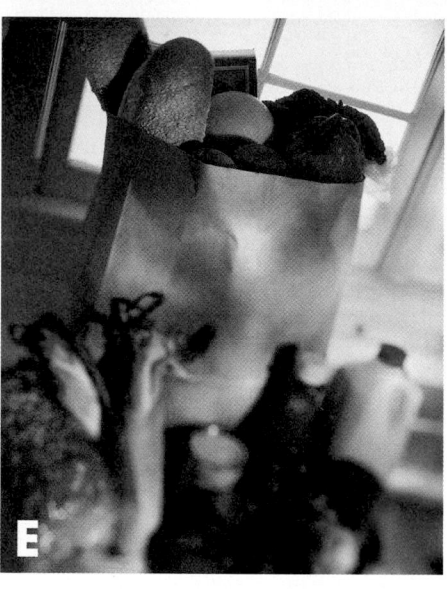

Figure 2-2 | (a) **A**nthropometric, (b) **B**iochemical, (c) **C**linical, and (d) **D**ietary information helps determine a person's nutritional status. (e) **E**conomic status adds further information, rounding out the **ABCDEs** of nutritional assessment.

Another example of a serious health condition with delayed symptoms is low bone density resulting from a calcium deficiency—a particularly relevant issue for adolescent females. Many young women consume well below the needed amount of calcium but often suffer no ill effects in their younger years. However, the bone structures of these women with low calcium intakes do not reach full potential during the years of growth, which makes osteoporosis more likely later in life.

Furthermore, clinical symptoms of nutritional deficiencies—diarrhea, an irregular walk, and facial sores—are not very specific. These may have different causes. Because it can take a long time for signs and symptoms to develop and since these also can be quite vague, it is often difficult to establish a link between an individual's current diet and nutritional state.[5]

Concern about the State of Your Nutritional Health Is Important

Figure 1-5 in Chapter 1 portrayed the close relationship between nutrition and health. The good news is that people who focus on maintaining nutritional health are apt to enjoy a long, vigorous life. For example, a recent study found that women who observe a healthy lifestyle experienced an 80% reduction in risk for heart attacks compared to women without such healthy practices.[18] Here is a list of what these healthy women did:

- Consumed a healthy diet that
  - Was varied
  - Was rich in fiber
  - Included some fish
  - Was low in animal fat and *trans* fat
- Avoided becoming overweight
- Regularly drank a small amount of alcohol
- Exercised for at least 30 minutes daily
- Did not smoke

Concept | Check

A desirable nutritional state results when the body has enough nutrients to function fully and contains stores to use in times of increased needs. When nutrient intake fails to meet body needs, undernutrition develops. Symptoms of such an inadequate nutrient intake can take months or years to develop. Overloading the body with nutrients, leading to overnutrition, is another potential problem to avoid. Nutritional state can be assessed by using anthropometric, biochemical, clinical, dietary, and economic assessments (ABCDEs).

Setting Nutrient Needs— Dietary Reference Intakes (DRIs)

Using the tools of nutrition research discussed in Chapter 1 and those of nutrition assessment just discussed in this chapter, it is possible to determine the amount of each nutrient needed by the human body. People have pursued this question for centuries. Before World War II, when many men were rejected from military service because of the effects of poor nutrition on their health, the need for official dietary recommendations was recognized. In 1941, a group of 25 scientists formed the first Food and Nutrition Board. They established dietary standards for evaluating the nutritional intakes of large populations and for planning agricultural production, first published in 1943.[20]

The framework of the latest recommendations from the Food and Nutrition Board are called **Dietary Reference Intakes (DRIs)** and have been released in stages throughout the last 10 years.[2]

Under the umbrella of the DRIs, five sets of standards have been established: Estimated Average Requirements (EARs), Recommended Dietary Allowances (RDAs), Adequate Intakes (AIs), Estimated Energy Requirements (EERs), and Tolerable Upper Intake Levels (Upper Levels, or ULs) (see the inside cover of this textbook).[20] All refer to intake averaged over a number of days, not a single day. Following is a more detailed discussion of each of these standards.

Estimated Average Requirements (EARs)

Estimated Average Requirements (EARs) are the nutrient intake that is estimated to meet the needs of 50% of the individuals in a certain age and gender group (Figure 2-3). To set an Estimated Average Requirement, the Food and Nutrition Board must be able to agree on a specific measurable functional marker to use for establishing nutrient adequacy. Such markers are typically the activity of an enzyme in the body or the ability of a cell to maintain physiological health.[20] (The specific markers used for various nutrients will be discussed in Chapters 9 through 12.) If no measurable functional marker is available, no Estimated Average Requirement can be set, such as for the mineral calcium. The Estimated Average Requirement also includes an adjustment for the amount of each nutrient that passes through the digestive tract unabsorbed. At the

A practical example using the ABCDEs for evaluating nutritional state can be illustrated in a person who chronically abuses alcohol. Upon evaluation, the physician notes:

(a) Low weight-for-height, recent 10-lb weight loss, muscle wasting in the upper body

(b) Low amounts of the vitamins thiamin and folate in the blood

(c) Psychological confusion, facial sores, and uncoordinated movement

(d) Dietary intake of little more than alcohol-fortified wine and hamburgers for the last week

(e) Currently residing in a homeless shelter; $35.00 in his wallet; unemployed

Evaluation: This person needs professional attention, including nutrient repletion.

Critical | Thinking

Tom loves to eat hamburgers, fries, and lots of pizza with double amounts of cheese. He rarely eats any vegetables and fruits but, instead, snacks on cookies and ice cream. He insists that he has no problems with his health, is rarely ill, and doesn't see how his diet could cause him any health risks. How would you explain to Tom that despite his current good health, his diet could predispose him to future health problems?

Dietary Reference Intakes (DRIs) The term used to encompass the latest nutrient recommendations made by the Food and Nutrition Board of the National Academy of Sciences. These include RDAs.

Estimated Average Requirement (EARs) An amount of nutrient intake that is estimated to meet the needs of 50% of the individuals in a specific age and gender group.

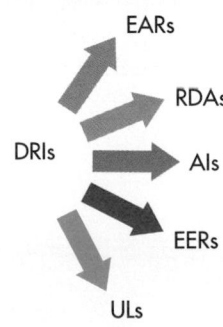

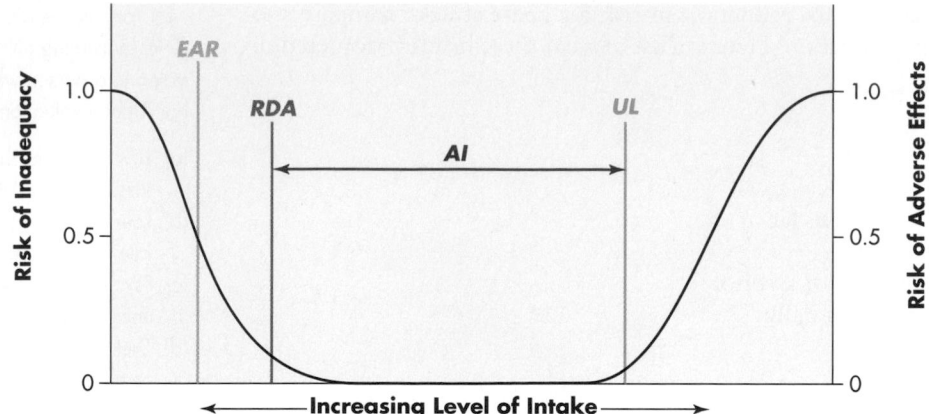

Estimated Average Requirement (EAR): A nutrient intake value that is estimated to meet the requirement of half the healthy individuals in a life stage and gender group. When set for a nutrient, an intake below the Estimated Average Requirement is likely inadequate for an individual.

Recommended Dietary Allowance (RDA): The dietary intake level that is sufficient to meet the nutrient requirement of nearly all (97% to 98%) healthy individuals in a particular life stage and gender group. When set for a nutrient, aim for this intake.

Adequate Intake (AI): A recommended intake value based on observed or experimentally determined approximations or estimates of nutrient intake by a group (or groups) of healthy people that is assumed to be adequate — used when an RDA cannot be determined. When set for a nutrient, aim for this intake.

Tolerable Upper Intake Level (Upper Level or UL): The highest level of nutrient intake that is likely to pose no risk of adverse health effects for almost all individuals in the general population. As intake increases above the Upper Level, the risk of adverse effects increases.

Figure 2-3 | Dietary Reference Intakes (DRIs). This figure shows that 50% of North Americans would have an inadequate intake by consuming the *Estimated Average Requirement (EAR)*, whereas 50% would have their needs met. Only about 2 to 3% of this group of people would have an inadequate intake if each were to meet the *Recommended Dietary Allowance (RDA)*; 97 to 98% would have their needs met. At intakes between the RDA and the *Tolerable Upper Intake Level (Upper Level or UL)*, the risk of either an inadequate diet or adverse effects from the nutrient in question is close to 0. The Upper Level is then the highest level of nutrient intake that is likely to pose no risks of adverse health effects to almost all individuals in the general population. At intakes above the Upper Level, the margin of safety to protect against adverse effects is reduced. The *Adequate Intake (AI)*, set for some nutrients instead of an RDA, lies somewhere between the Estimated Average Requirement and the Upper Level. In determining the Adequate Intake for a nutrient, it is expected that the amount exceeds the RDA for that nutrient, if an RDA were known. Thus, the Adequate Intake should cover the needs of more than 97 to 98% of individuals. The actual degree to which the Adequate Intake exceeds the RDA is likely to differ among the various nutrients and population groups. The Food and Nutrition Board states that there is no established benefit for healthy individuals if they consume nutrient intakes above the RDA or Adequate Intake.

Estimated Average Requirement, the needs of the other 50% of the population would not be met for the nutrient. Thus, the Estimated Average Requirement can only be used to evaluate the adequacy of diets of a group of people, not individuals.[20] Specific Estimated Average Requirements are listed in Appendix M.

Recommended Dietary Allowances (RDAs)

Recommended Dietary Allowances (RDAs) represent intake of a nutrient that is sufficient to meet the needs of nearly all individuals (97 to 98%) in an age and gender group (see the inside cover). RDAs are based on a multiple of the Estimated Average Requirements (generally the RDA = EAR × 1.2). Because of this relationship, an RDA can be set for a nutrient only if the Food and Nutrition Board has enough information to determine an Estimated Average Requirement. Additional consideration in setting an RDA also can be given to a nutrient's ability to prevent chronic disease rather than just prevent deficiency.[20]

Setting One RDA: Vitamin C

The amount of vitamin C needed each day to prevent scurvy is about 10 mg. However, as you will learn in Chapter 10, vitamin C has other functions as well, some of which are involved in the workings of the immune system (see Appendix C for details on the

Recommended Dietary Allowances (RDAs) Recommended intakes of nutrients that are sufficient to meet the needs of almost all individuals (97 to 98%) of similar age and gender.

immune system). Based on this relationship, the concentration of vitamin C in one component of the immune system—notably, white blood cells (specifically neutrophils)—can be used as a marker for vitamin C adequacy in an individual. The Food and Nutrition Board concluded that near-maximal saturation of white blood cells with vitamin C is, in fact, the best marker for optimal vitamin C status. It takes, on average, a daily intake of about 75 mg for men and about 60 mg for women for near-saturation of white blood cells. These average amounts then become the Estimated Average Requirement for young adult men and women.

The Estimated Average Requirement for vitamin C is multiplied by 1.2 to yield the RDA; in this case, the RDA becomes 90 mg/day for men and 75 mg/day for women. Other age groups have slightly different recommendations; smokers should add 35 mg/day to the RDA for their age and gender (see Chapter 10 for details).

Putting the RDA for Vitamin C to Use

If you total the amount of vitamin C you eat in 1 week and divide by 7, you will have your average daily vitamin C consumption. If that value is close to the RDA, you are most likely consuming enough vitamin C. Even if you eat less than the RDA, you will not likely suffer ill effects; your needs are most likely less than the RDA, which is set to include almost all individuals, some of whom probably need more vitamin C than you do. As a general rule, however, the further you stray below the RDA on a regular basis—particularly as you approach the Estimated Average Requirement—the greater your risk of a nutritional deficiency.[20] Symptoms of a vitamin C deficiency may be subtle and develop slowly. It takes a long time to detect problems such as a weakened immune system and even poor wound healing. If you suspect that your diet is not nutritious enough, don't wait for warning signs to develop. Start eating a diet that meets the RDAs set for vitamin C (and all the other nutrients listed for your age and gender), rather than risk the development of health problems from poor nutrition.

Adequate Intakes (AIs)

Nutrients for which there is not enough information to establish an Estimated Average Requirement are assigned **Adequate Intakes (AIs)** (see the inside cover). Adequate Intakes are based on estimates of the average nutrient intake that appears to maintain a defined nutritional state (e.g., bone health) in a certain population.[20] Adequate Intakes have been set for essential fatty acids, fiber, some B-vitamins, the vitamin-like compound choline, vitamin D, and some minerals such as calcium and fluoride. In addition, Adequate Intakes are set for infants under 1 year of age because experimentally studying the effects of nutrient deficiencies in infants would be unethical.

Estimated Energy Requirements (EERs)

RDAs and Adequate Intakes for nutrients are set high enough to meet the needs of almost all healthy individuals. In contrast, a different standard is used to express energy needs, called **Estimated Energy Requirements (EERs)**.[4] These refer to the average needs for various age groups and genders (see the inside cover). Unlike for most vitamins and minerals, excess energy consumed (above energy needs) is not excreted. Thus, to promote weight maintenance, a more conservative standard is used for energy needs than for nutrient needs. Overall, an Estimated Energy Requirement is only a rough estimate, because energy needs depend on energy use, and in some cases the need for growth or human milk production. For most adults, the ability to obtain and maintain a healthy weight is the best yardstick of energy balance—energy intake matching energy output.

Tolerable Upper Intake Levels (Upper Levels, or ULs)

The **Tolerable Upper Intake Levels (ULs)** is the maximum level of daily intake of a nutrient that is unlikely to cause adverse health effects in almost all people (97 to 98%) in a population (see the inside cover).[20] The number applies to chronic daily use and is

Adequate Intakes (AIs) Recommendations for nutrient intake when not enough information is available to establish an RDA. AIs are based on observed or experimentally determined estimates of the average nutrient intake that appears to maintain a defined nutritional state (e.g., bone health) in a specific population. Used when no RDA can be set.

Estimated Energy Requirements (EERs) An estimate of the amount of energy intake that will balance energy needs of an average person within specific gender, age, and other considerations.

Tolerable Upper Intake Levels (ULs) Maximum chronic daily intake of a nutrient that is unlikely to cause adverse health effects in almost all people in a population. This number applies to a chronic daily use.

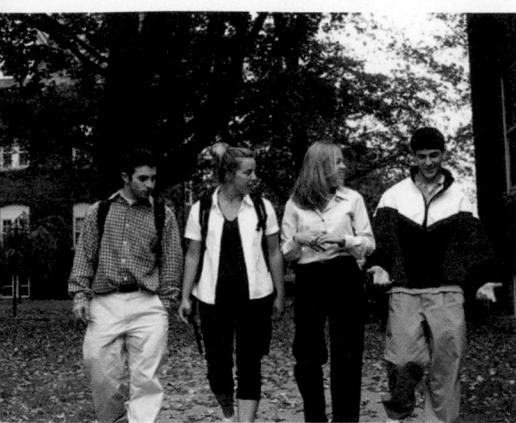

Energy needs in adulthood are based on an energy intake required to maintain weight.

The Dietary Reference Intakes apply to both the United States and Canada because scientists from both countries worked together to establish them.

set to protect even very susceptible people in the healthy general population. For vitamin C the amount is 2000 mg/day. Intakes greater than this amount can cause diarrhea and inflammation of the stomach lining.

The Upper Level is not a goal for nutrient intake but, rather, is a ceiling below which nutrient intake should remain. Still, for many of us there is a margin of safety above the UL before any adverse effects are likely to occur. Not enough information is available to set an Upper Level for all nutrients, but this does not mean that toxicity from these nutrients is impossible. Furthermore, there is no clear-cut evidence that intakes above the RDA or Adequate Intake confer any additional health benefits for most of us.

The Upper Level for most nutrients is based on the combined intake of food, water, supplements, and fortified foods. Four exceptions are the vitamin niacin and the minerals magnesium, zinc, and nickel, for which the Upper Level for each refers only to nonfood sources, such as medicines and supplements. This is because toxicity due to dietary intake of niacin, magnesium, zinc, or nickel is unlikely.[2]

Appropriate Uses of the DRIs

The DRIs are intended mainly for diet planning (Table 2-6). Specifically, a diet plan should aim to meet any RDAs set. If no RDA has been determined for a nutrient, use the Adequate Intake as a guide. Finally, the Upper Level for a nutrient should not be exceeded (Figure 2-4).[2,20] Keep in mind also that none of these dietary standards are necessarily appropriate amounts for individuals who are already undernourished or for those with diseases that require higher intakes. This concept will be covered in Chapters 9 through 12.

Concept | Check

Dietary Reference Intakes are set for specific nutrients in order to guide food intake. These standards include Recommended Dietary Allowances (RDAs), Adequate Intakes (AIs), and Tolerable Upper Intake Levels (Upper Levels, or ULs). Recommended Dietary Allowances represent the nutrient needs for healthy individuals. RDAs are established for specific age and gender categories. No one knows his or her own nutritional requirements; the best general rule is that the further you stray from nutrient standards set for your age and gender, especially below the Estimated Average Requirement (EAR), the greater your chance of having a nutritional deficiency or toxicity. Adequate Intakes are set when there is not enough information to set a more precise RDA. An Estimated Energy Requirement (EER) has also been set for various ages and genders. Intakes above Upper Levels generally should not be consumed on a long-term basis unless a physician prescribes the amount and monitors the person carefully, because toxic effects are possible.

Table 2-6 | Putting the DRIs for Nutrient Needs to Use

RDA	Recommended Dietary Allowance. Use to evaluate your current intake for a specific nutrient. The further you stray above or below this value, the greater your chances of developing nutritional problems.
AI	Adequate Intake. Use to evaluate your current intake of nutrients, but realize that an AI designation implies that further research is required before scientists can establish a more definitive number.
EER	Estimated Energy Requirement. Use to estimate your energy needs according to your height, weight, gender, age, and physical activity pattern.
UL	Upper Level. Use to evaluate the highest amount of daily nutrient intake that is unlikely to cause you adverse health effects in the long run. This number applies to chronic use and is set to protect even very susceptible people in the healthy general population. As your intake increases above the Upper Level, the potential for adverse effects generally increases.

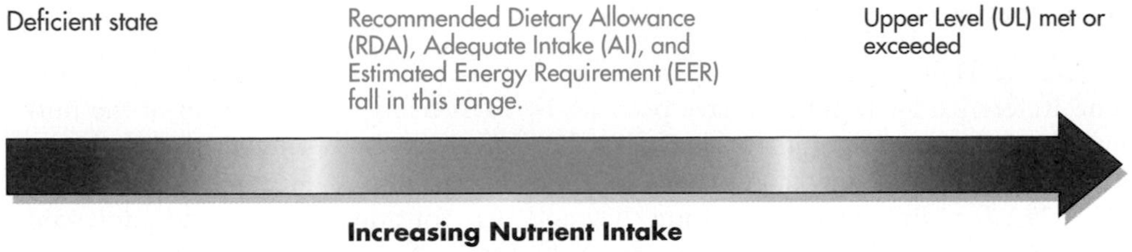

Deficient state

Recommended Dietary Allowance (RDA), Adequate Intake (AI), and Estimated Energy Requirement (EER) fall in this range.

Upper Level (UL) met or exceeded

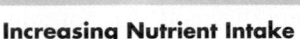

Increasing Nutrient Intake

Figure 2-4 | Think of the nutrient standards that are part of DRIs as snapshots along a line. As nutrient intake increases, the Recommended Dietary Allowance (RDA) for the nutrient, if set, is eventually met and a deficient state is no longer present. An individual's needs most likely will be met because RDAs are set high to include almost all people. Related to the RDA concept of meeting an individual's needs are the standards of Adequate Intake (AI) and the Estimated Energy Requirement (EER). These can be used to estimate an individual's needs for some nutrients and energy, respectively. Still, keep in mind that these standards do not share the same degree of accuracy as the RDA. For example, EER may have to be adjusted upward if the individual is very physically active. Finally, as nutrient intake increases above the Upper Level (UL), poor nutritional health is again likely. However, this poor health is due now to the toxic effects of a nutrient rather than to those of a deficiency.

Recall from Chapter 1 that the Food and Nutrition Board has also established Adequate Macronutrient Distribution Ranges (AMDRs) for intake of carbohydrate, protein, fat, and certain other nutrients. These recommendations complement those made as part of the DRIs (e.g., RDAs).[20]

Daily Values (DVs): The Standards Used for Food Labeling

The DRIs and accompanying nutrient standards are not used in food labeling because they are age and gender specific. We can't have different packages for men and women or for teens and adults. The US Food and Drug Administration (FDA) has developed a set of generic standards, called **Daily Values,** that are used to express the nutrient content of foods for the Nutrition Facts panel on food labels. The content of a particular nutrient is listed on labels as a percentage of the Daily Value. These percentages serve as a benchmark for evaluating the nutrient content of foods. They do not, however, represent a set of tailor-made recommendations for an adult. You will see why once the method for setting Daily Values is described.

The Daily Values are based on two sets of dietary standards. The first, **Reference Daily Intakes (RDIs),** are for vitamins and minerals. The second, **Daily Reference Values (DRVs),** are standards for protein and various dietary components that have no RDA or other established nutrient standard (e.g., total fat). These two terms—*Reference Daily Intakes* and *Daily Reference Values*—do not appear on labels. To make reading labels less confusing for consumers, the term *Daily Value* is used to represent the combination of these two sets of dietary standards, since the differences between Reference Daily Intakes and Daily Reference Values for typical consumers are inconsequential. For health professionals and nutrition experts, though, it is important to understand how nutrition label information (Reference Daily Intakes vs. Daily Reference Values) is actually derived:

Daily Values Standard nutrient-intake values developed by FDA and used as a reference for expressing nutrient content on nutrition labels. The Daily Values include two types of standards—RDIs and DRVs.

Reference Daily Intakes (RDIs) Nutrient-intake standards set by FDA based on the 1968 RDAs for various vitamins and minerals. RDIs have been set for four categories of people: infants, toddlers, people over 4 years of age, and pregnant or lactating women. Generally the highest RDA value out of all categories is used as the RDI. The RDIs constitute part of the Daily Values used in food labeling.

Daily Reference Values (DRVs) Nutrient-intake standards established for protein, carbohydrate, and some dietary components lacking an RDA or a related nutrient standard, such as total fat intake. The DRVs for sodium and potassium are constant; those for the other nutrients increase as energy intake increases. The DRVs constitute part of the Daily Values used in food labeling.

Daily Values, used on food labels, are a combination of RDI and DRV standards.

RDIs: For food labels, standards set for nutrients that have RDAs or other established nutrient standards

DRVs: For food labels, standards set for many nutrients that do not have RDAs or other established nutrient standards

Reference Daily Intakes (RDIs)

Reference Daily Intakes (RDIs) make up the majority of the Daily Values (DVs). The Reference Daily Intakes have been set by FDA using a compilation of the nutrient standards published in 1968. Essentially, Reference Daily Intakes use the highest RDA values of any age category set in 1968. For example, consider iron: In 1968, the RDA for adult men was 10 mg/day and that for adult women and adolescents was 18 mg/day. The iron Reference Daily Intake for adults is the higher value: 18 mg/day. Table 2-7 lists the Reference Daily Intakes used for various age groups.

The Reference Daily Intake values currently in use, which are based on the 1968 RDAs, are generally slightly higher than current RDAs and related nutrient standards. FDA plans to eventually revise the Reference Daily Intakes to reflect the latest nutrient standards.

Daily Reference Values (DRVs)

The Daily Values for some food constituents are based on Daily Reference Values (DRVs) rather than RDIs. Daily Reference Values cover certain dietary components that have no RDA or related nutrient standard at this time, such as saturated fatty acids and cholesterol. (Protein is the exception, because it has a DRV and also an RDA.) Overall, the Daily Reference Values for energy-yielding nutrients are based on 30% of total energy intake from fat, 60% from carbohydrate, and 10% from protein.

Using the Daily Values

Note that some of the Daily Values, such as those for saturated fat, total fat, and fiber, are related to total energy intake. By accounting for this, you can evaluate your diet even if your energy intake is more or less than the standard energy intake, 2000 kcal, used on the food label. For example, if you consume only 1600 kcal per day, the total percentage of Daily Value for each of these nutrients should add up to no more than 80% because $1600 \div 2000 = 0.8$, or 80%. If you eat 2800 kcal, your total percentage of Daily Value for each nutrient in all the foods you eat in one day can add up to 140%, because $2800 \div 2000 = 1.4$, or 140%. However, the % Daily Values for some dietary constituents, such as cholesterol and sodium, are not adjusted for differences in energy intake.

In the same way, you can calculate the amount of a certain nutrient you have left in a day by using the % Daily Value. For example, if you consume 2000 kcal per day, your total fat intake for the day should be 65 g or less. If you consume 10 g of fat at breakfast, you have 55 g, or 85%, of your Daily Value left for the rest of the day.

The Nutrition Facts panel on the label of a food product lists various components of the food as a percentage of their Daily Values (for details, see this chapter's Nutrition Focus, titled Using Food Labels in Diet Planning). Use this information on food labels to learn more about your food choices. Unfortunately most adults do not do this. To practice using this information, suppose that one serving of a macaroni and cheese product contains 15% of the Daily Value for iron. Since the Daily Value for iron is 18 mg, this product contains about 3 mg of iron per serving ($18 \times 0.15 = 2.7$ mg).

Canada also has a set of Daily Values for use on food labels (see Appendix D).

Nutrition educators often instruct patients to look only at the total amount of a nutrient (shown on the left side of the Nutrition Facts panel) rather than the % Daily Value when watching a specific nutrient. This is because the % Daily Value is not correct unless that person consumes 2000 kcal/day. For example, if a person is to limit his or her saturated fat intake to 20 g per day, the % Daily Value does not provide adequate information to assess grams of saturated fat consumed in a day.

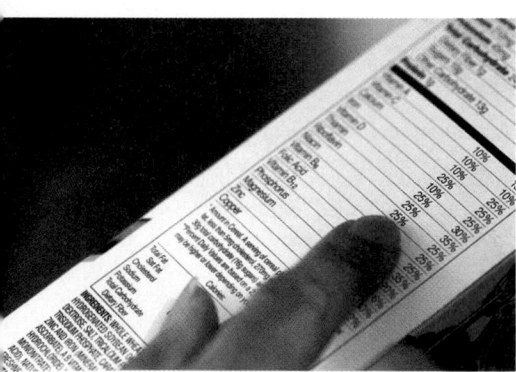

Use the Nutrition Facts label to learn more about the nutrient content of the foods you eat. Nutrient content is expressed as a percent of Daily Value. Canadian food laws and related food labels have a slightly different format (review Appendix D).

Concept | Check

Daily Values are currently used as a benchmark for representing the nutrient content of foods on nutrition labels. Nutrient content is expressed as a percentage of the Daily Value for a nutrient, which in turn is based on a Reference Daily Intake (RDI) or Daily Reference Value (DRV). The Reference Daily Intakes for vitamins and minerals constitute the majority of Daily Values and are based on the 1968 RDA standards. The Daily Reference Values have been set for some nutrients that don't have an RDA or Adequate Intake, such as fat and cholesterol. To decrease confusion, the Daily Value is the only term that appears on food labels.

Table 2-7 | Comparison of Daily Values with the Latest RDAs and Other Nutrient Standards[1]

Dietary Constituent	Unit of Measure	Current Daily Values for People over 4 Years of Age	RDA or Other Current Dietary Standard	
			Males 19 Years Old	Females 19 Years Old
Total Fat[2]	g	<65–<107	—	—
Saturated fatty acids[2]	g	<20–<36	—	—
Protein[2]	g	50–80	56	46
Cholesterol[3]	mg	<300	—	—
Carbohydrate[2]	g	300–480	130	130
Fiber	g	25–37	38	25
Vitamin A	μg Retinol activity equivalents	1000	900	700
Vitamin D	International units	400	200	200
Vitamin E	International units	30	22–33	22–33
Vitamin K	μg	80	120	90
Vitamin C	mg	60	90	75
Folate	μg	400	400	400
Thiamin	mg	1.5	1.20	1.10
Riboflavin	mg	1.7	1.30	1.10
Niacin	mg	20	16	14
Vitamin B-6	mg	2	1.30	1.30
Vitamin B-12	μg	6	2.40	2.40
Biotin	mg	0.3	0.03	0.03
Pantothenic acid	mg	10	5	5
Calcium	mg	1000	1000	1000
Phosphorus	mg	1000	700	700
Iodide	μg	150	150	150
Iron	mg	18	8	18
Magnesium	mg	400	400	310
Copper	mg	2	0.9	0.9
Zinc	mg	15	11	8
Sodium[4]	mg	<2400	1500	1500
Potassium[4]	mg	3500	4700	4700
Chloride[4]	mg	3400	2300	2300
Manganese	mg	2	2.3	1.8
Selenium	μg	70	55	55
Chromium	μg	120	35	25
Molybdenum	μg	75	45	45

Abbreviations: g = gram; mg = milligram; μg = microgram

[1]Daily Values are generally set at the highest nutrient recommendation in a specific age and gender category. Many Daily Values exceed current nutrient standards. This is in part because aspects of the Daily Values were originally developed in the early 1970s using estimates of nutrient needs published in 1968. The Daily Values have yet to be updated to reflect the current state of knowledge. Note also that the Daily Values for some nutrients (e.g., total fat, saturated fatty acids, protein, carbohydrate, and fiber) increase as energy intake increases above 2000 kcal/day.

[2]The lowest Daily Values are based on a 2000 kcal diet. All based on a caloric distribution of 30% from fat (and one-third of this total from saturated fat), 60% from carbohydrate, and 10% from protein as energy intake ranges from 2000 kcal/day to 3200 kcal/day.

[3]Based on recommendations of federal agencies

[4]The considerably higher Daily Values for sodium and chloride are there to allow for more diet flexibility, but the extra amounts are not needed to maintain health.

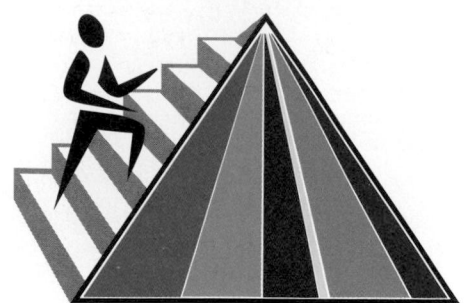

MyPyramid.gov
STEPS TO A HEALTHIER YOU

Appendix D contains the Canadian Food Guide to Healthy Eating.

▌ Recommendations for Food Choice

The following sections will describe various guidelines for planning healthy diets.

MyPyramid—A Menu-Planning Tool

Since the early twentieth century, researchers have worked to clarify the science of nutrition into practical terms, so that people with no special training could estimate whether their nutritional needs were being met. A seven food-group plan, based on foods traditionally eaten by people in North America, was one of the first formats designed by USDA. Daily food choices had to include items from each group. This plan had been simplified by the mid-1950s to a four food-group plan: a milk group, a meat group, a fruit and vegetable group, and a bread and cereal group. In 1992 this plan was illustrated using a pyramid shape.

In April 2005 USDA unveiled their latest food guide plan, MyPyramid. Entitled "Steps to a Healthier You," MyPyramid provides a more individualized approach to improving diet and lifestyle than did previous food guides. Overall, MyPyramid translates the latest nutrition advice into 12 separate pyramids based on energy needs (1000 to 3200 kcal/day).[15] Its goal is to provide advice that will help consumers live longer, better, and healthier lives. (MyPyramid replaces the Food Guide Pyramid introduced in 1992.)

The MyPyramid symbol represents the recommended proportion of foods from each food group that creates a healthy diet. Physical activity is a new element in the pyramid. To benefit from the individualized advice that is the hallmark of the plan, however, consumers need to utilize the website, MyPyramid.gov.[14]

MyPyramid, pictured in Figure 2-5, is designed to illustrate:

- *Personalization,* demonstrated at the MyPyramid website, MyPyramid.gov.
- *Gradual improvement,* encouraged by the title "Steps to a Healthier You."
- *Physical activity,* represented by the steps and the person climbing them.
- *Variety,* symbolized by the six color bands representing the five food groups and oils. Foods from all groups are needed each day for good health. Orange is used for grains, green for vegetables, red for fruits, yellow for oils, blue for milk and milk products, and purple for meat & beans.
- *Proportionality,* indicated by the different widths of the food group bands. The widths suggest how much food a person should choose from each group. The bands are wider for grains, vegetables, and fruits because these groups should form the bulk of one's diet. The narrowest band is for oils, indicating these should be eaten sparingly. All the widths are just a general guide, however, and not exact proportions. Check MyPyramid.gov for the amount that is right for you.
- *Moderation,* represented by the narrowing of each food group from bottom to top. The wider base represents foods with little or no solid fats, added sugars or caloric sweeteners, and salt. These should be selected more often to get the most nutrition from energy consumed.

An innovative aspect of MyPyramid is the interactive technology found on MyPyramid.gov. Here is a list of the programs:

MyPyramid Plan provides a quick estimate of what and how much food a person should eat from the different food groups based on age, gender, and activity level.

MyPyramid Tracker provides more detailed information on diet quality and physical activity status by comparing a day's worth of foods eaten to the guidance provided by MyPyramid. It allows the user to select from 8000 foods and 600 activities. Nutrition and physical activity messages are based on the need to maintain current weight or to lose weight.

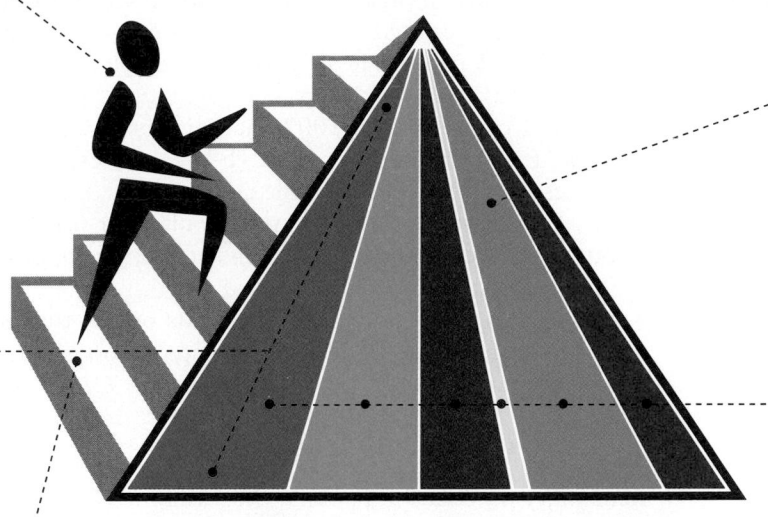

Activity
Activity is represented by the steps and the person climbing them, as a reminder of the importance of daily physical activity.

Moderation
Moderation is represented by the narrowing of each food group from bottom to top. The wider base stands for foods with little or no solid fats or added sugars. These should be selected more often. The narrower top area stands for foods containing more added sugars and solid fats. The more active you are, the more of these foods can fit into your diet.

Personalization
Personalization is shown by the person on the steps, the slogan, and the website. Find the kinds and amounts of food to eat each day at MyPyramid.gov.

Proportionality
Proportionality is shown by the different widths of the food group bands. The widths suggest how much food a person should choose from each group. The widths are just a general guide, not exact proportions. Check the website for how much is right for you.

Variety
Variety is symbolized by the 6 color bands representing the 5 food groups of the Pyramid and oils. This illustrates that foods from all groups are needed each day for good health.

Gradual Improvement
Gradual improvement is encouraged by the slogan. It suggests that individuals can benefit from taking small steps to improve their diet and lifestyle each day.

MyPyramid.gov
STEPS TO A HEALTHIER YOU

| Grains | Vegetables | Fruits | Oils | Milk | Meat & Beans |

Figure 2-5 | The anatomy of MyPyramid. USDA's new MyPyramid symbolizes a personalized approach to healthy eating and physical activity. The symbol has been designed to be simple. It has been developed to remind consumers to make healthy food choices and to be active every day.

Inside MyPyramid provides in-depth information for every food group, including recommended daily amounts in commonly used measures, like cups and ounces, with examples and everyday tips. The section also includes recommendations for choosing healthy oils, **discretionary calories,** and physical activity (refer to Table 2-8 on page 58 for a listing of discretionary calories. Basically this term refers to the energy intake allowed from food choices rich in added sugars or solid fat. For most of us, very few discretionary calories are available in daily diet planning).

Start Today provides tips and resources that include downloadable suggestions on all the food groups and physical activity and a worksheet to track one's diet.

Putting MyPyramid into Action

To put MyPyramid into action, you first need to estimate your energy needs (the website helps you with the calculation). Figure 2-6 provides a rough guide.

Once you have determined the energy allowance that is appropriate for you, you can use Table 2-9 to discover how your energy needs correspond to the recommended number of servings from each food group.

discretionary calories The amount of energy theoretically allowed in a diet after the person has met overall nutrition need. This generally small amount of energy gives individuals the flexibility to consume some foods and beverages that may contain alcohol (e.g., beer and wine), added sugars (e.g, soft drinks, candy, and desserts), or added fats that are part of moderate- or high-fat foods (e.g., many snack foods).

Table 2-8 | Discretionary Calories Allowed in a Diet

Energy Intake (kcal)	Discretionary Calories (kcal)
1000	165*
1200	171*
1400	171*
1600	132
1800	195
2000	267
2200	290
2400	362
2600	410
2800	426
3000	512
3200	648

The overall intent is to not exceed this discretionary calorie allowance—the combination of foods and beverages with alcohol, added sugars, or added fats.

*The amount of discretionary calories is higher for 1000 to 1400 kcal diets than for a 1600 kcal diet because these diets with less energy are intended for children 2 to 8 years of age. Adults typically need at least 1600 kcal.

Counting Servings

MyPyramid provides serving sizes of foods for the various food groups in household units:

- *Grains:* 1 slice of bread, 1 cup of ready-to-eat breakfast cereal, or 1/2 cup cooked rice, pasta, or cooked cereal counts as a one-ounce equivalent.
- *Vegetables:* 1 cup of raw or cooked vegetables or vegetable juice or 2 cups of raw leafy greens counts as 1 cup.
- *Fruits:* 1 cup of fruit or 100% fruit juice or 1/2 cup of dried fruit counts as 1 cup.
- *Milk:* 1 cup of milk or yogurt, 1 1/2 ounces of natural cheese, or 2 ounces of processed cheese counts as one cup.
- *Meat & Beans:* 1 ounce of meat, poultry, or fish, 1 egg, 1 tablespoon of peanut butter, 1/4 cup cooked dry beans, or 1/2 ounce of nuts or seeds counts as a one-ounce equivalent.
- *Oils:* A teaspoon of any oil from plants or fish that is liquid at room temperature counts as a serving, as do such servings of foods rich in oils (e.g., mayonnaise and soft margarine).

Planning Menus with MyPyramid

Remember the following points when using MyPyramid to plan your daily menus:

1. The guide does not apply to infants or children under 2 years of age.
2. No one food is absolutely essential to good nutrition. Each food is rich in some nutrients but deficient in at least one essential nutrient (Table 2-10).
3. No one food group provides all essential nutrients in adequate amounts. Each food group makes an important, distinctive contribution to nutritional intake.
4. Variety is the key to success of the guide and is first guaranteed by choosing foods from all the groups. Furthermore, one should consume a variety of foods within each group. (When choosing products in the milk group, be especially careful to look at saturated fat content to minimize that intake.)
5. The foods within a group may vary widely with respect to nutrients and energy content. For example, the energy content of 3 oz of baked potato is 98 kcal, whereas that of 3 oz of potato chips is 470 kcal. Compare an orange and an apple with respect to vitamin C using the food composition table in Appendix N.

Pay close attention to the stated serving size for each choice when following MyPyramid. This aids in controlling total energy intake. See Figure 2-7 for a convenient guide to estimating common household measures. Note that serving sizes listed for one serving in a MyPyramid group or on a food label are often less than is typically served in restaurants today.

	Energy Intake Range (kcal)	
Children	Sedentary ⟶	Active
2–3 years	1000 ⟶	1400
Females		
4–8 years	1200 ⟶	1800
9–13	1600 ⟶	2200
14–18	1800 ⟶	2400
19–30	2000 ⟶	2400
31–50	1800 ⟶	2200
51+	1600 ⟶	2200
Males		
4–8 years	1400 ⟶	2000
9–13	1800 ⟶	2600
14–18	2200 ⟶	3200
19–30	2400 ⟶	3000
31–50	2200 ⟶	3000
51+	2000 ⟶	2800

Sedentary means a lifestyle that includes only the light physical activity associated with typical day-to-day life.

Active means a lifestyle that includes physical activity equivalent to walking more than 3 miles per day at 3 to 4 miles per hour in addition to the light physical activity associated with typical day-to-day life.

Figure 2-6 | Estimates of energy needs provided by MyPyramid.

Table 2-9 | MyPyramid Recommendations for Daily Amounts of Foods to Consume from the Six Food Groups Based on Energy Needs

Energy Intake	1000	1200	1400	1600	1800	2000	2200	2400	2600	2800	3000	3200
Fruits	1 c	1 c	1.5 c	1.5 c	1.5 c	2 c	2 c	2 c	2 c	2.5 c	2.5 c	2.5 c
Vegetables[1,2]	1 c	1.5 c	1.5 c	2 c	2.5 c	2.5 c	3 c	3 c	3.5 c	3.5 c	4 c	4 c
Grains[3]	3 oz-eq	4 oz-eq	5 oz-eq	5 oz-eq	6 oz-eq	6 oz-eq	7 oz-eq	8 oz-eq	9 oz-eq	10 oz-eq	10 oz-eq	10 oz-eq
Meat & Beans[2]	2 oz-eq	3 oz-eq	4 oz-eq	5 oz-eq	5 oz-eq	5.5 oz-eq	6 oz-eq	6.5 oz-eq	6.5 oz-eq	7 oz-eq	7 oz-eq	7 oz-eq
Milk[4]	2 c	2 c	2 c	3 c	3 c	3 c	3 c	3 c	3 c	3 c	3 c	3 c
Oils[5]	3 tsp	4 tsp	4 tsp	5 tsp	5 tsp	6 tsp	6 tsp	7 tsp	8 tsp	8 tsp	10 tsp	11 tsp
Discretionary calorie allowance[6]	165	171	171	132	195	267	290	362	410	426	512	648

Abbreviations: c = cup or cups; oz-eq = ounces or equivalent; tsp = teaspoon

[1]Vegetables are divided into five subgroups (dark green vegetables, orange vegetables, legumes, starchy vegetables, and other vegetables). Over a week's time a variety of vegetables should be eaten, especially green and orange vegetables.

[2]Dry beans and peas can be counted *either* as vegetables (dry beans and peas subgroup) *or* in the meat & beans group. Generally, individuals who regularly eat meat, poultry, and fish would count dry beans and peas in the vegetable group. Individuals who seldom eat meat, poultry, or fish (vegetarians) would consume more dry beans and peas and count some of them in the meat & beans group until enough servings from that group are chosen for the day.

[3]At least half of these servings should be whole-grain varieties.

[4]Most of these servings should be fat-free or low fat.

[5]Limit solid fats such as butter, stick margarine, shortening, and meat fat as well as foods that contain these.

[6]Discretionary calories refers to food choices rich in added sugars or solid fat.

Table 2-10 | Nutrient Contributions of Groups in the MyPyramid Food Guide Plan

Food Category	Major Nutrient Contributions	Food Category	Major Nutrient Contributions
Milk	Calcium Phosphorus Carbohydrate Protein Riboflavin Vitamin D Magnesium Zinc	Fruits (con't)	Magnesium Potassium Fiber
Meat & Beans	Protein Thiamin Riboflavin Niacin Vitamin B-6 Folate[1] Vitamin B-12[2] Phosphorus Magnesium[1] Iron Zinc	Vegetables	Carbohydrate Vitamin A Vitamin C Folate Magnesium Potassium Fiber
		Grains	Carbohydrate Thiamin Riboflavin[3] Niacin Folate[4] Magnesium[5] Iron[3,4] Zinc[4] Fiber[5]
Fruits	Carbohydrate Vitamin A Vitamin C Folate	Oils	Fat Essential fatty acids Vitamin E

[1]Primarily in plant protein sources

[2]Only in animal foods

[3]If enriched

[4]Whole grains and some enriched/fortified products

[5]Whole grains

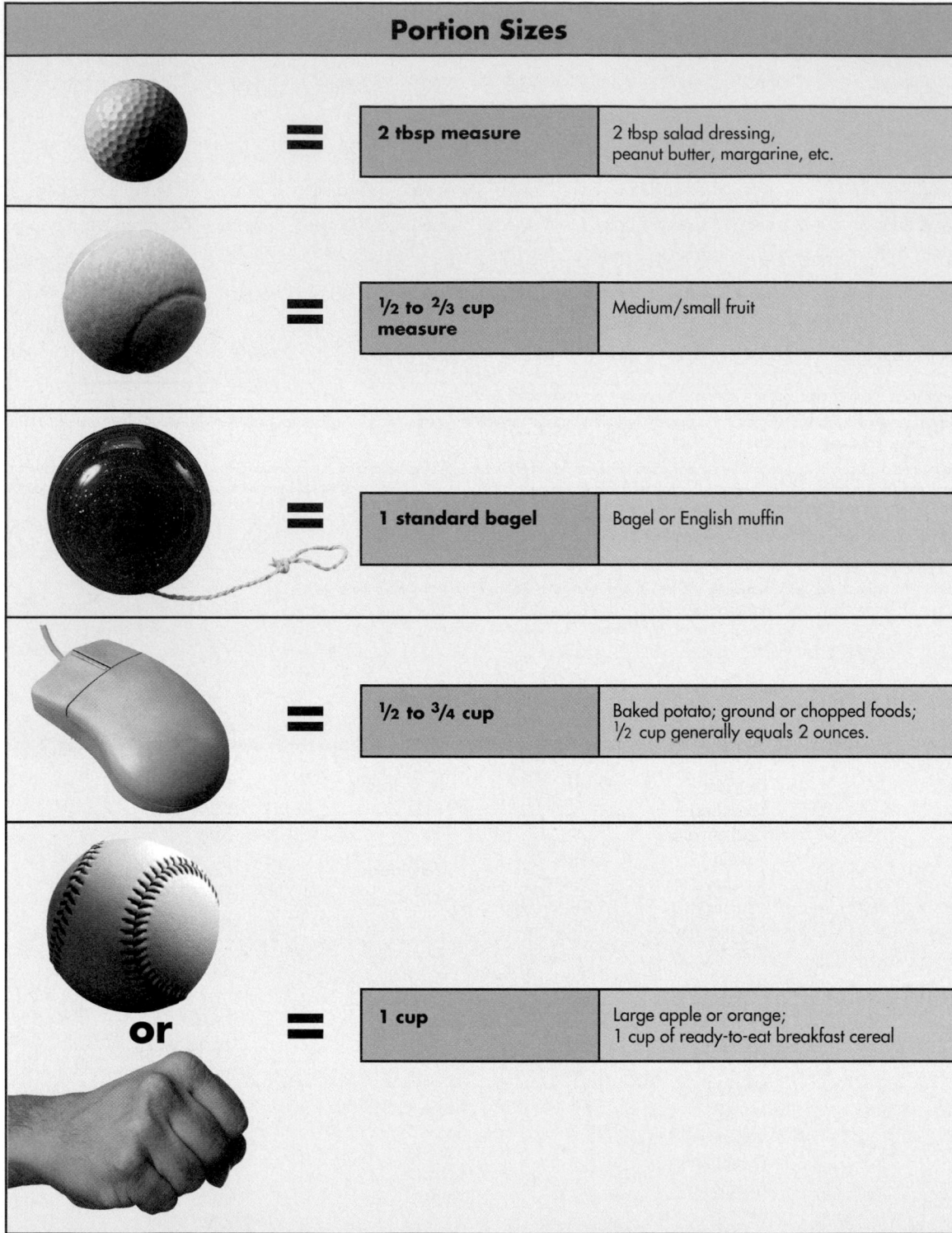

Portion Sizes		
=	**2 tbsp measure**	2 tbsp salad dressing, peanut butter, margarine, etc.
=	**½ to ⅔ cup measure**	Medium/small fruit
=	**1 standard bagel**	Bagel or English muffin
=	**½ to ¾ cup**	Baked potato; ground or chopped foods; ½ cup generally equals 2 ounces.
or =	**1 cup**	Large apple or orange; 1 cup of ready-to-eat breakfast cereal

Figure 2-7 | A golf ball, tennis ball, small yo-yo, computer mouse, baseball, and fist make convenient guides to judge MyPyramid serving sizes. Additional handy guides include:

thumb = 1 oz of cheese
4 stacked dice = 1 oz cheese
thumb tip to first joint = 1 tsp
small (individual-size) matchbox = 1 oz meat
bar of soap or deck of
   cards = 3 oz meat

palm of hand = 3 oz
1 ice cream scoop = 1/2 cup
handful = 1 or 2 oz of a
   snack food
Ping-Pong ball = 2 tbsp

Overall, MyPyramid incorporates the foundations of a healthy diet: variety, balance, and moderation. The nutritional adequacy of diets planned using this tool, however, depends on selection of a variety of foods (Table 2-11).[15] In addition, to ensure enough vitamin E, vitamin B-6, magnesium, and zinc—nutrients sometimes low in diets based on this plan—consider the following advice:

1. Choose primarily low-fat and fat-free items from the milk group. By reducing energy intake in this way, you can select more items from other food groups. If milk causes intestinal gas and bloating, emphasize yogurt and cheese. (See Chapter 5 for details on the problem of lactose maldigestion and lactose intolerance).

Table 2-11 | Putting MyPyramid into Practice

Meal	Food Group
Breakfast	
1 small orange	Fruits
3/4 cup Low-Fat Granola	Grains
with 1 cup fat-free milk	Milk
1/2 toasted, small raisin bagel	Grains
with 1 tsp soft *trans* fat-free margarine	Oils
Optional: coffee or tea	
Lunch	
Turkey sandwich	Grains
2 slices whole-wheat bread	Meat & Beans
2 oz turkey	
1 small apple	Fruits
1 oatmeal-raisin cookie (small)	Discretionary calories
Optional: diet soft drink or iced tea	
3 P.M. Study Break	
6 whole-wheat crackers	Grains
1 tbsp peanut butter	Meat & Beans
1 cup fat-free milk	Milk
Dinner	
Tossed salad	
1 cup romaine lettuce	Vegetables
1/2 cup sliced tomatoes	Vegetables
1 1/2 tbsp Italian dressing	Oils
1/2 carrot, grated	Vegetables
3 oz broiled salmon	Meat & Beans
1/2 cup rice	Grains
1/2 cup green beans	Vegetables
with 1 tsp soft *trans* fat-free margarine	Oils
Optional: coffee or tea	
Late-Night Snack	
1 cup "light" fruit yogurt	Milk
Nutrient Breakdown	
1800 kcal	
Carbohydrate	56% of kcal
Protein	18% of kcal
Fat	26% of kcal

This menu meets nutrient needs for all vitamins and minerals for an average adult.

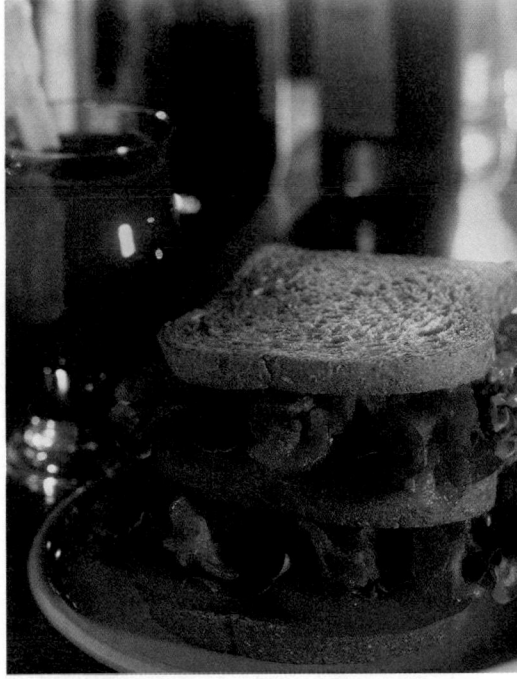

Typical restaurant portions contain numerous servings from the individual groups in MyPyramid.

What about physical activity? Walking, gardening, briskly pushing a baby stroller, climbing the stairs, playing soccer, or dancing the night away are all good examples of being physically active. For health benefits, physical activity should be moderate or vigorous and add up to at least 30 minutes on most or all days of the week. For weight loss or preventing weight gain, about 60 minutes a day may be needed. (The same goal applies to children and teenagers in general.) For maintaining prior weight loss, at least 60 to 90 minutes a day may be required.

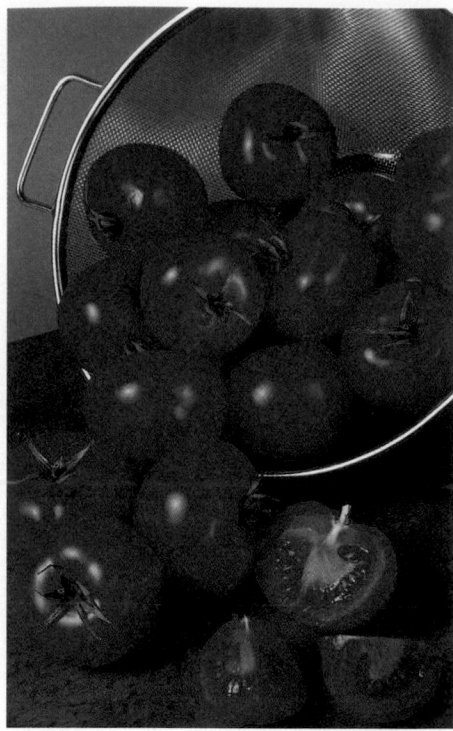

Tomatoes are a rich source of nutrients and phytochemicals.

2. Include plant foods that are good sources of protein, such as beans and nuts, at least several times a week because many are rich in vitamins (such as vitamin E), minerals (such as magnesium), and fiber.

3. For vegetables and fruits, try to include a dark green vegetable for vitamin A and a vitamin C–rich fruit, such as an orange, every day. Don't focus primarily on potatoes (e.g., french fries) for your vegetable choices. Surveys show that fewer than 5% of adults eat a full serving of a dark green vegetable on any given day. Increased consumption of these foods is important because they contribute vitamins, minerals, fiber, and phytochemicals.

4. Choose whole-grain varieties of breads, cereals, rice, and pasta because they contribute vitamin E and fiber. A plate about two-thirds covered by grains, fruits, and vegetables and one-third or less covered by protein-rich foods promotes this diet advice. A daily serving of a whole-grain, ready-to-eat breakfast cereal is an excellent choice because the vitamins (such as vitamin B-6) and minerals (such as zinc) typically added to it, along with fiber, help fill in the potential nutrient gaps just listed.

5. Include some plant oils on a daily basis, such as those in salad dressing, and eat fish at least twice a week. This supplies you with health-promoting fatty acids.

Rating Your Current Diet

Regularly comparing your daily food intake with MyPyramid recommendations for your age, gender, and degree of physical activity is a relatively simple way to evaluate your overall diet. Strive to meet the recommendations.[15] (The diets of most adults fail in this evaluation, especially with respect to servings of milk and milk products, vegetables, fruits, and whole-grain breads and cereals.[16]) If meeting the recommendations is not possible, identify the nutrients that are low in your diet based on the nutrients found in each food group (review Table 2-10). For example, if you do not consume enough servings from the milk group, your calcium intake is most likely too low. You need to then find foods you enjoy that supply calcium, such as calcium-fortified orange juice. Customizing MyPyramid to accommodate your own food habits may seem a daunting task now, but it is not difficult once you gain some additional nutrition knowledge.

Getting Going

Start putting MyPyramid into practice and use the MyTracker feature to follow your progress. Implementing even small diet and exercise changes can have positive results. Better health will likely follow as you strive to meet your nutrient needs and balance your physical activity and energy intake. In addition, follow the guidance from the *2005 Dietary Guidelines for Americans* (discussed in the next section) regarding alcohol and sodium intake and safe food preparation.

Concept | Check

MyPyramid translates the general needs for carbohydrate, protein, fat, vitamins, and minerals into the recommended number of daily servings from each of five major food groups. It is a convenient and valuable tool for planning daily menus.

Dietary Guidelines—Another Tool for Menu Planning

MyPyramid was designed to help meet nutritional needs for carbohydrate, protein, fat, vitamins, and minerals. However, most of the major chronic "killer" diseases in North America, such as cardiovascular disease, cancer, and alcoholism, are not primarily associated with deficiencies of these nutrients. Deficiency diseases such as beriberi (thiamin deficiency), scurvy (vitamin C deficiency), and pellagra (niacin deficiency) are no longer common in North America. For many North Americans, the primary dietary culprit is overconsumption of one or more of the following: total energy intake,

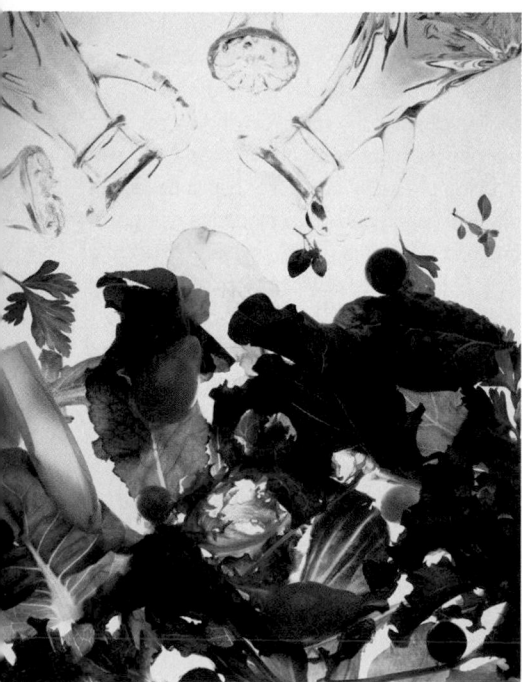

A salad with leafy green vegetables contributes many nutrients to a diet.

saturated fat, cholesterol, *trans* fat, alcohol, and sodium (salt). (Underconsumption of calcium, iron, folate and other B-vitamins, vitamin C, vitamin D, vitamin E, potassium, magnesium, and fiber is also a problem for some people.)

In response to concerns regarding these killer disease patterns, since 1980 the USDA and U.S. Department of Health and Human Services (DHHS) have published **Dietary Guidelines for Americans** (Dietary Guidelines for short) to aid diet planning. Compared to past reports, the latest *Dietary Guidelines for Americans* (2005) places stronger emphasis on monitoring one's energy intake and increasing physical activity.[11] This is because more of us are becoming overweight each year.

The report identifies 41 key recommendations, of which 23 are for the general public and 18 are for special populations. They are grouped into nine general topics:

- Adequate nutrient intake within calorie needs
- Weight management
- Physical activity
- Specific food groups to encourage
- Fats
- Carbohydrates
- Sodium and potassium
- Alcoholic beverages
- Food safety

Figure 2-8 lists the key recommendations within each general topic. The advice provided refers to people 2 years and older and will undoubtedly coincide with what you have already heard or read:[17]

- Consume a variety of nutrient-dense foods and beverages within and among the basic food groups of MyPyramid while choosing foods that limit the intake of saturated and *trans* fats, cholesterol, added sugars, salt, and alcohol (if used). Foods to emphasize are vegetables, fruits, legumes (beans), whole grains, and fat-free or low-fat milk or equivalent milk products.
- Maintain body weight in a healthy range by balancing energy intake from foods and beverages with that expended. For the latter, engage in at least 30 minutes of moderate-intensity physical activity, above usual activity, at work or home on most days of the week.

Appendix D contains nutrient guidelines for Canadians.

Dietary Guidelines for Americans General goals for nutrient intakes and diet composition set by the USDA and the U.S. Department of Health and Human Services.

ADEQUATE NUTRIENTS WITHIN ENERGY NEEDS

- Consume a variety of nutrient-dense foods and beverages within and among the basic food groups while choosing foods that limit the intake of saturated and *trans* fats, cholesterol, added sugars, salt, and alcohol.

- Meet recommended intakes within energy needs by adopting a balanced eating pattern, such as MyPyramid.

Key Recommendations for Specific Population Groups

- *People over age 50.* Consume vitamin B-12 in its crystalline form (i.e., fortified foods or supplements).

- *Women of childbearing age who may become pregnant.* Eat foods high in iron from animal products and/or consume iron-rich plant foods or iron-fortified foods with an enhancer of iron absorption, such as vitamin C–rich foods.

- *Women of childbearing age who may become pregnant and those in the first few months of pregnancy.* Consume adequate amount of the synthetic form of the B vitamin folate (i.e., folic acid) daily (from fortified foods or supplements) in addition to food forms of folate found in a varied diet.

- *Older adults, people with dark skin, and people exposed to insufficient ultraviolet band radiation (i.e., sunlight).* Consume extra vitamin D from vitamin D–fortified foods and/or supplements.

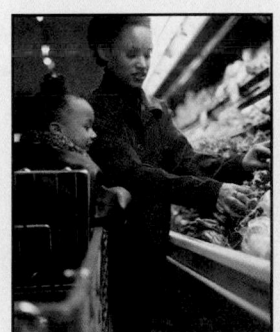

Figure 2-8 | Key recommendations within each general topic from the latest Dietary Guidelines for Americans.

continued

WEIGHT MANAGEMENT

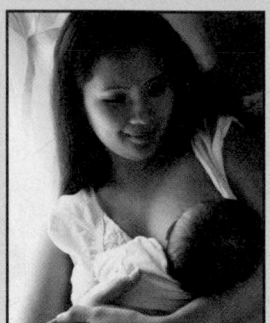

- To maintain body weight in a healthy range, balance energy intake from foods and beverages with energy expended.

- To prevent gradual weight gain over time, make small decreases in energy intake from food and beverages and increase physical activity.

Key Recommendations for Specific Population Groups

- *Those who need to lose weight.* Aim for a slow, steady weight loss by decreasing energy intake while maintaining an adequate nutrient intake and increasing physical activity.

- *Overweight children.* Reduce the rate of body weight gain while allowing for growth and development. Consult a health-care provider before placing a child on a weight-reduction diet.

- *Pregnant women.* Ensure appropriate weight gain as specified by a health-care provider.

- *Breastfeeding women.* Moderate weight reduction is safe and does not compromise weight gain of the nursing infant.

- *Overweight adults and overweight children with chronic diseases and/or on medication.* Consult a health-care provider about weight-loss strategies prior to starting a weight-reduction program to ensure appropriate management of other health conditions.

PHYSICAL ACTIVITY

- Engage in regular physical activity and reduce sedentary activities to promote health, psychological well-being, and a healthy body weight.

- To reduce the risk of chronic disease in adulthood: Engage in at least 30 minutes of moderate-intensity physical activity, above usual activity, at work or home on most days of the week.

- For most people, greater health benefits can be obtained by engaging in physical activity of more vigorous intensity or longer duration.

- To help manage body weight and prevent gradual, unhealthy body weight gain in adulthood: Engage in approximately 60 minutes of moderate- to vigorous-intensity activity on most days of the week while not exceeding energy needs.

- To sustain weight loss in adulthood: Participate in at least 60 to 90 minutes of daily moderate-intensity physical activity while not exceeding energy needs. Some people (men over 40 years of age and women over 50 years of age) may need to consult with a health-care provider before participating in this level of activity.

- Achieve physical fitness by including cardiovascular conditioning, stretching exercises for flexibility, and resistance exercises or calisthenics for muscle strength and endurance.

Key Recommendations for Specific Population Groups

- *Children and adolescents.* Engage in at least 60 minutes of physical activity on most, preferably all, days of the week.

- *Pregnant women.* In absence of medical complications, incorporate 30 minutes or more of moderate-intensity physical activity on most, if not all, days of the week. Avoid activities with a high risk of falling or abdominal trauma.

- *Breastfeeding women.* Be aware that neither acute nor regular exercise adversely affects the mother's ability to successfully breastfeed.

- *Older adults.* Participate in regular physical activity to reduce functional declines associated with aging and to achieve the other benefits of physical activity identified for all adults.

Figure 2-8 | Key recommendations within each general topic from the latest Dietary Guidelines for Americans. *(continued)*

FOOD GROUPS TO ENCOURAGE

- Consume a sufficient amount of fruits and vegetables while staying within energy needs. Two cups of fruit and 2 1/2 cups of vegetables per day are recommended for a reference 2000 kcal intake, with higher or lower amounts depending on one's energy needs.

- Choose a variety of fruits and vegetables each day. In particular, select from all five vegetable subgroups (dark green vegetables, orange vegetables, legumes, starchy vegetables, and other vegetables) several times a week.

- Consume 3 or more ounce-equivalents of whole-grain products per day, with the rest of the recommended grains coming from enriched or whole-grain products. In general, at least half the grains should come from whole grains.

- Consume 3 cups per day of fat-free or low-fat milk or equivalent milk products.

Key Recommendations for Specific Population Groups

- *Children and adolescents.* Consume whole-grain products often; at least half the grains should be whole grains. Children 2 to 8 years should consume 2 cups per day of fat-free or low-fat milk or equivalent milk products. Children 9 years of age and older should consume 3 cups per day of fat-free or low-fat milk or equivalent milk products.

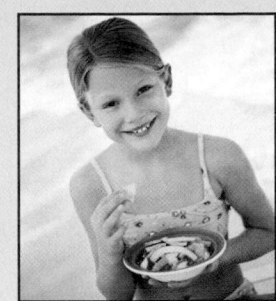

FATS

- Consume less than 10 percent of energy intake from saturated fatty acids and less than 300 mg per day of cholesterol, and keep *trans* fatty acid consumption as low as possible.

- Keep total fat intake between 20 to 35% of energy intake, with most fats coming from sources of polyunsaturated and monounsaturated fatty acids, such as fish, nuts, and vegetable oils.

- When selecting and preparing meat, poultry, dry beans, and milk or milk products, make choices that are lean, low-fat, or fat-free.

- Limit intake of fats and oils high in saturated and/or *trans* fatty acids, and choose products low in such fats and oils.

Key Recommendations for Specific Population Groups

- *Children and adolescents.* Keep total fat intake between 30 to 35% of energy intake for children 2 to 3 years of age and between 25 to 35% of energy intake for children and adolescents 4 to 18 years of age, with most fats coming from sources of polyunsaturated and monounsaturated fatty acids, such as fish, nuts, and vegetable oils.

CARBOHYDRATES

- Choose fiber-rich fruits, vegetables, and whole grains often.

- Choose and prepare foods and beverages with little added sugars or caloric sweeteners, such as amounts suggested by MyPyramid.

- Reduce the incidence of dental caries by practicing good oral hygiene and consuming sugar- and starch-containing foods and beverages less frequently.

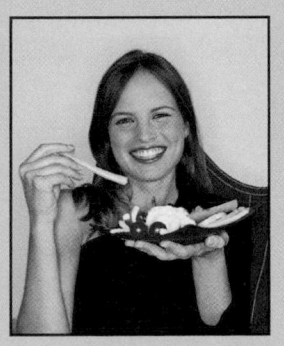

Figure 2-8 | Key recommendations within each general topic from the latest Dietary Guidelines for Americans. *(continued)*

SODIUM AND POTASSIUM

- Consume less than 2300 mg of sodium per day (approximately 1 tsp of salt).

- Choose and prepare foods with little salt. At the same time, consume potassium-rich foods, such as fruits and vegetables.

Key Recommendations for Specific Population Groups

- *Individuals with hypertension, blacks, and middle-aged and older adults.* Aim to consume no more than 1500 mg of sodium per day, and meet the potassium recommendation (4700 mg per day) with food.

ALCOHOLIC BEVERAGES

- Those who choose to drink alcoholic beverages should do so sensibly and in moderation—defined as the consumption of up to one drink per day for women and up to two drinks per day for men. (12 oz of a regular beer, 5 oz of wine or 1 1/2 oz of 80 proof distilled spirits count as a drink for purposes of explaining moderation.)

- Alcoholic beverages should not be consumed by some individuals, including those who cannot restrict their alcohol intake, women of childbearing age who may become pregnant, pregnant and lactating women, children and adolescents, individuals taking medications that can interact with alcohol, and those with specific medical conditions.

- Alcoholic beverages should be avoided by individuals engaging in activities that require attention, skill, or coordination, such as driving or operating machinery.

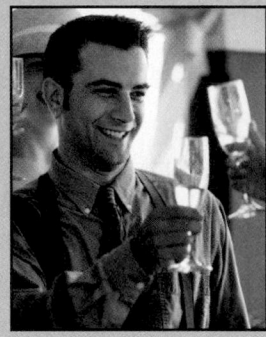

FOOD SAFETY

To avoid microbial foodborne illness:

- Clean hands, food contact surfaces, and fruits and vegetables. Meat and poultry should *not* be washed or rinsed to avoid spreading bacteria to other foods.

- Separate raw, cooked, and ready-to-eat foods while shopping, preparing, and storing foods.

- Cook foods to a safe temperature to kill microorganisms.

- Chill (refrigerate) perishable food promptly and defrost foods properly.

- Avoid raw (unpasteurized) milk or any products made from unpasteurized milk, raw or partially cooked eggs or foods containing raw eggs, or raw or undercooked meat and poultry, unpasteurized juices, and raw sprouts.

Key Recommendations for Specific Population Groups

- *Infants and young children, pregnant women, older adults, and those who are immunocompromised.* Do not eat or drink raw (unpasteurized) milk or any products made from unpasteurized milk, raw or partially cooked eggs or foods containing raw eggs, raw or undercooked meat and poultry, raw or undercooked fish or shellfish, unpasteurized juices, and raw sprouts.

- *Pregnant women, older adults, and those who are immunocompromised.* Only eat certain deli meats and frankfurters that have been reheated to steaming hot.

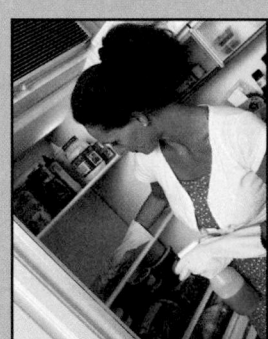

Figure 2-8 | Key recommendations within each general topic from the latest Dietary Guidelines for Americans. *(continued)*

- Practice safe food handling when preparing food. This includes cleaning hands, food contact surfaces, and fruits and vegetables before preparation, and cooking foods to a safe temperature to kill microorganisms.

A basic premise of the Dietary Guidelines is that nutrient needs should be met primarily through consuming foods.[17] Foods provide an array of nutrients and other compounds that may have beneficial effects on health. In certain cases, fortified foods and dietary supplements may be useful sources of one or more nutrients that otherwise might be consumed in less than recommended amounts. These practices are especially important for people whose typical food choices lead to a diet that cannot meet one or more nutrient recommendations, such as for vitamin E or calcium. However, dietary supplements are not a substitute for a healthful diet.

Practical Use of the Dietary Guidelines

The Dietary Guidelines are designed to meet nutrient needs while reducing the risk of obesity, hypertension, cardiovascular disease, type 2 diabetes, alcoholism, and foodborne illness.

The Dietary Guidelines are not difficult to implement (Table 2-12).[15] Despite popular misconceptions, this overall diet approach is not especially expensive. Fruits, vegetables, and low-fat and fat-free milk are no more expensive than the chips, cookies, and sugared soft drinks they should in part replace.

Note also that diet recommendations for adults have been issued by other scientific groups, such as the American Heart Association, Office of the U.S. Surgeon General, National Academy of Sciences, American Cancer Society, Canadian Ministries of Health (see Appendix D), and World Health Organization. All are consistent with the spirit of the Dietary Guidelines. These groups encourage people to modify their eating behavior in ways that are both healthful and pleasurable.

The Dietary Guidelines and You

When using the Dietary Guidelines, you should consider your own state of health. Make specific changes and see whether they are effective. Note that results are sometimes disappointing, even when you are following a diet change very closely. Some people can eat a lot of saturated fat and still keep blood cholesterol under control. Other people, unfortunately, have high blood cholesterol even if they eat a diet low in saturated fat. Differences in genetic background are a key cause, as you learned in Chapter 1. Your diet should be planned with this individuality in mind, taking into account your current health status and family history for specific diseases. However, tailoring a unique nutrition program for every North American citizen is currently unrealistic. MyPyramid and the Dietary Guidelines provide typical adults with simple advice that can be actively practiced by anyone willing to take a step toward good health.[11,15]

There is no "optimal" diet. Instead, there are numerous healthful diets. Visit the website of the International Food Information Council (ific.org). This site is a great resource for current nutrition information.

Concept | Check

Dietary Guidelines for Americans have been set by a variety of private and government organizations. These guidelines are designed to reduce the risk of developing obesity, hypertension, type 2 diabetes, cardiovascular disease, alcoholism, and foodborne illness. To do so, they recommend eating a variety of foods, which is fostered by following MyPyramid. They also recommend performing regular physical activity, aiming for a healthy weight, and moderating total fat, saturated fat, *trans* fat, salt, sugar, and alcohol intake, while focusing more on fruits, vegetables, and whole-grain products in daily menu planning. Safe food preparation and storage are also highlighted.

A brochure designed for the public based on the 2005 Dietary Guidelines for Americans is entitled "Finding Your Way to a Healthier You." It communicates the major themes of the 2005 Dietary Guidelines for Americans but uses simpler messages. The 2005 Dietary Guidelines for Americans (and the consumer brochure) are available at www.healthierus.gov/dietaryguidelines.

Advice from the American Dietetic Association suggests five basic principles with regard to diet and health.

- Be realistic, making small changes over time.
- Be adventurous, trying new foods regularly.
- Be flexible, balancing some sweet and fatty foods with physical activity.
- Be sensible, including favorite foods in smaller portions.
- Finally, be active, including physical activity in daily life.

Critical | Thinking

Shannon has grown up eating the typical American diet. Having recently read and heard many media reports about the relationship between nutrition and health, she is beginning to look critically at her diet and is considering making changes. However, she doesn't know where to begin. What advice would you give her?

The **Exchange System** is a final menu-planning tool. This tool organizes foods based on energy, protein, carbohydrate, and fat content. The result is a manageable framework for designing diets, especially for treatment of diabetes. For more information on the Exchange System see Appendixes E and F.

Table 2-12 | Recommended Diet Changes Based on the Dietary Guidelines

If You Usually Eat This,	Try This Instead	Benefit
White bread	Whole-wheat bread	• Higher nutrient density, due to less processing • More fiber
Sugary breakfast cereal	Low-sugar, high-fiber cereal with fresh fruit	• Higher nutrient density • More fiber • More phytochemicals
Cheeseburger with french fries	Hamburger and baked beans	• Less saturated fat and *trans* fat • Less cholesterol • More fiber • More phytochemicals
Potato salad	Three-bean salad	• More fiber • More phytochemicals
Doughnuts	Bran muffin or bagel with light cream cheese	• More fiber • Less fat
Regular soft drinks	Diet soft drinks	• Less energy
Boiled vegetables	Steamed or sauteed vegetables	• Higher nutrient density, due to reduced loss of water-soluble vitamins
Canned vegetables	Fresh or frozen vegetables	• Higher nutrient density, due to reduced loss of heat-sensitive vitamins • Lower in sodium
Fried meats	Broiled meats	• Less saturated fat
Fatty meats, such as ribs or bacon	Lean meats, such as ground round, chicken, or fish	• Less saturated fat
Whole milk	Low-fat or fat-free milk	• Less saturated fat • Less energy • More calcium
Ice cream	Sherbet or frozen yogurt	• Less saturated fat • Less energy
Mayonnaise or sour cream salad dressing	Oil and vinegar dressings or light creamy dressings	• Less saturated fat • Less cholesterol • Less energy
Cookies	Popcorn (air popped with minimal margarine or butter)	• Less energy and *trans* fat
Heavily salted foods	Foods flavored primarily with herbs, spices, lemon juice	• Lower in sodium
Chips	Pretzels	• Less fat

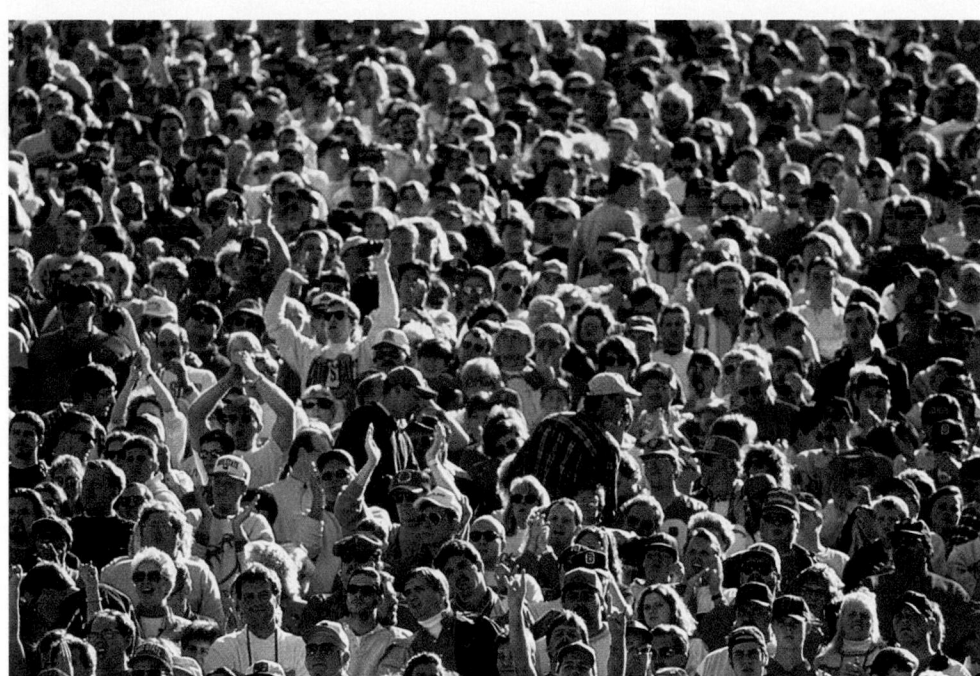

Nutrition recommendations are often made on a population-wide basis. However, in some cases, it would be more appropriate if these were made on an individual basis once a person's particular health status is known.

Case Scenario | Follow-Up

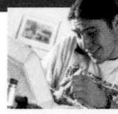 The most positive aspect of Andy's diet is that it contains adequate protein, zinc, and iron because it is rich in animal protein. On the downside, his diet is low in calcium, some B vitamins (such as folate), and vitamin C. This is because it is low in dairy products, fruits, and vegetables. It is also low in many of the phytochemical (plant-based) substances discussed at the beginning of Chapter 2. In addition, his fiber intake is low because fast-food restaurants primarily use refined grain products rather than whole-grain products. And since most super-sized options apply to foods rich in fat (french fries) and sugar (soft drinks), his diet is likely excessive in those two components.

He could alternate between tacos and bean burritos to gain the benefits of plant proteins in his diet. He could choose a low-fat granola bar instead of the candy bar for breakfast, or he could take the time to eat a bowl of whole-grain breakfast cereal with low-fat or fat-free milk to increase fiber and calcium intake. He could also order milk at least half the time at his restaurant visits and substitute diet soft drinks for the regular variety. This would help *moderate* his sugar intake. Overall, Andy could improve his intake of fruits, vegetables, and dairy products if he focused more on variety in food choice and balance among the food groups.

NUTRITION FOCUS

Using Food Labels in Diet Planning

Recall from Chapter 1 that the nutrition label uses the term *calorie* to express energy content in some cases but kilocalorie (kcal) values are actually listed.

Today, nearly all foods sold in the supermarket must be labeled with the product name, name and address of the manufacturer, amount of product in the package, and ingredients listed in descending order by weight. This food and beverage labeling is monitored in North America by government agencies such as the US Food and Drug Administration (FDA) in the United States. The listing of certain food constituents is also required—specifically, on a Nutrition Facts panel (Figure 2-9). Use this information to learn more about what you eat.

The following components must be listed: total calories (kcal), calories from fat, total fat, saturated fat, *trans* fat, cholesterol, sodium, total carbohydrate, fiber, sugars, protein, vitamin A, vitamin C, calcium, and iron. In addition to these required components, manufacturers can choose to list polyunsaturated and monounsaturated fat, potassium, and others. Listing these components is *required,* however, if a claim is made about the health benefits of the specific nutrient (see the section entitled Health Claims on Food Labels) or if the food is fortified with that nutrient.

Recall that the percentage of the Daily Value is usually given for each nutrient per serving. It is important to understand that these percentages are based on a 2000 kcal diet. Therefore, they are not as applicable to people who require considerably more or less than 2000 kcal per day with respect to fat and carbohydrate intake.

Nutrient and herbal supplement labels have a different layout that includes a "Supplement Facts" heading. Chapters 1 and 9 show examples of these labels.

Serving sizes on the Nutrition Facts panel must be consistent among similar foods. This means that all brands of ice cream, for example, must use the same serving size on their label. However, these serving sizes may differ from those of MyPyramid since those of food labels are based on typical serving sizes. In addition, food claims made on packages must follow legal definitions (Table 2-13). For example, if a product claims to be "low sodium," it must have 140 mg of sodium or less per serving.

Many manufacturers list the Daily Values set for dietary components such as fat, cholesterol, and carbohydrate on the Nutrition Facts panel. This can be useful as a reference point. As noted, they are based on 2000 kcal; if the label is large enough,

Canada has established a set of health claims for their nutrition labels (see Appendix D).

amounts based on 2500 kcal are listed as well for total fat, saturated fat, carbohydrate, and other components.

Exceptions to Food Labeling

Foods such as fresh fruits and vegetables, fish, meats, and poultry currently are not required to have Nutrition Facts labels. However, many grocers and some meat packers have voluntarily chosen to provide their customers with information about these products. Nutrition Facts labels on meat products will likely be required in the coming years. The next time you are at the grocery store, ask where you might find information on the fresh products that do not have a Nutrition Facts panel. You will likely find a poster or pamphlet near the product; often, these pamphlets contain recipes that use your favorite fruit, vegetable, or cut of meat. They may even assist you in your endeavor to improve your diet.

Because protein deficiency is not a public health concern in the United States, declaration of the % Daily Value for protein is not mandatory on foods for people over 4 years of age. If the % Daily Value is given on a label, FDA requires that the product be analyzed for protein quality. Because this procedure is expensive and time-consuming, many companies opt not to list a % Daily Value for protein rather than undergo the expense. However, labels on food for infants and children under 4 years of age must include the % Daily Value for protein, as must the labels on any food carrying a claim about protein content (see Chapter 17).

Health Claims on Food Labels

As a marketing tool directed toward the health-conscious consumer, food manufacturers like to assert that their products have all sorts of health benefits. After reviewing hundreds of comments on the proposed rule allowing health claims, FDA, which has legal oversight over most food products, has decided to permit some health claims with certain restrictions.

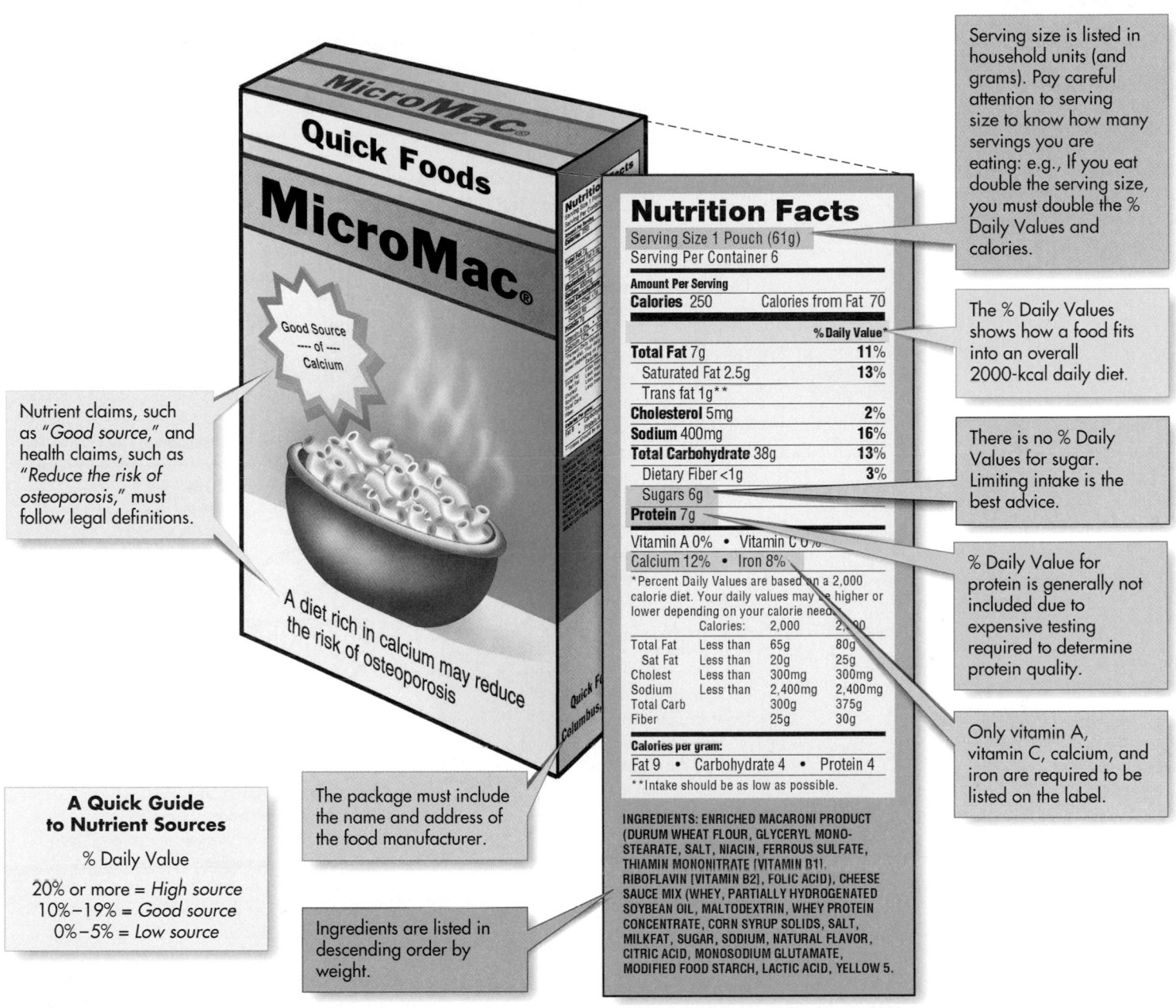

Serving size is listed in household units (and grams). Pay careful attention to serving size to know how many servings you are eating: e.g., If you eat double the serving size, you must double the % Daily Values and calories.

The % Daily Values shows how a food fits into an overall 2000-kcal daily diet.

Nutrient claims, such as "Good source," and health claims, such as "Reduce the risk of osteoporosis," must follow legal definitions.

There is no % Daily Values for sugar. Limiting intake is the best advice.

% Daily Value for protein is generally not included due to expensive testing required to determine protein quality.

Only vitamin A, vitamin C, calcium, and iron are required to be listed on the label.

A Quick Guide to Nutrient Sources

% Daily Value

20% or more = High source
10%–19% = Good source
0%–5% = Low source

The package must include the name and address of the food manufacturer.

Ingredients are listed in descending order by weight.

Nutrition Facts

Serving Size 1 Pouch (61g)
Serving Per Container 6

Amount Per Serving

Calories 250   Calories from Fat 70

	% Daily Value*
Total Fat 7g	11%
Saturated Fat 2.5g	13%
Trans fat 1g**	
Cholesterol 5mg	2%
Sodium 400mg	16%
Total Carbohydrate 38g	13%
Dietary Fiber <1g	3%
Sugars 6g	
Protein 7g	

Vitamin A 0% • Vitamin C 0%
Calcium 12% • Iron 8%

*Percent Daily Values are based on a 2,000 calorie diet. Your daily values may be higher or lower depending on your calorie needs.

		Calories: 2,000	2,500
Total Fat	Less than	65g	80g
Sat Fat	Less than	20g	25g
Cholest	Less than	300mg	300mg
Sodium	Less than	2,400mg	2,400mg
Total Carb		300g	375g
Fiber		25g	30g

Calories per gram:

Fat 9 • Carbohydrate 4 • Protein 4

**Intake should be as low as possible.

INGREDIENTS: ENRICHED MACARONI PRODUCT (DURUM WHEAT FLOUR, GLYCERYL MONO-STEARATE, SALT, NIACIN, FERROUS SULFATE, THIAMIN MONONITRATE [VITAMIN B1], RIBOFLAVIN [VITAMIN B2], FOLIC ACID), CHEESE SAUCE MIX (WHEY, PARTIALLY HYDROGENATED SOYBEAN OIL, MALTODEXTRIN, WHEY PROTEIN CONCENTRATE, CORN SYRUP SOLIDS, SALT, MILKFAT, SUGAR, SODIUM, NATURAL FLAVOR, CITRIC ACID, MONOSODIUM GLUTAMATE, MODIFIED FOOD STARCH, LACTIC ACID, YELLOW 5.)

Figure 2-9 | The Nutrition Facts panel on a current food label. This nutrition information is required on virtually all processed food products. The % Daily Value listed on the label is the percentage of the generally accepted amount of a nutrient needed daily that is present in 1 serving of the product. You can use the % Daily Values to compare your diet with current nutrition recommendations for certain diet components. Let's consider fiber. Assume that you consume 2000 kcal per day, which is the energy intake for which the % Daily Values listed on labels have been calculated. If the total % Daily Value for dietary fiber in all the foods you eat in one day adds up to 100%, your diet meets the recommendations for fiber. Food labels also contain the name and address of the food manufacturers. This allows consumers to contact the manufacturer if they desire.

Table 2-13 | Definitions for Comparative and Absolute Nutrient Claims on Food Labels

Sugar
- **Sugar free:** less than 0.5 g per serving
- **No added sugar; without added sugar; no sugar added:**
  - No sugars were added during processing or packing, including ingredients that contain sugars (for example, fruit juices, applesauce, or jam).
  - Processing does not increase the sugar content above the amount naturally present in the ingredients. (A functionally insignificant increase in sugars is acceptable for processes used for purposes other than increasing sugar content.)
  - The food that it resembles and for which it substitutes normally contains added sugars.
  - If the food doesn't meet the requirements for a low- or reduced-calorie food, the product bears a statement that the food is not low calorie or calorie reduced and directs consumers' attention to the Nutrition Facts panel for further information on sugars and calorie content.
- **Reduced sugar:** at least 25% less sugar per serving than reference food

Calories
- **Calorie free:** fewer than 5 kcal per serving
- **Low calorie:** 40 kcal or less per serving and, if the serving is 30 g or less or 2 tbsp or less, per 50 g of the food
- **Reduced or fewer calories:** at least 25% fewer kcal per serving than reference food

Fiber
- **High fiber:** 5 g or more per serving. (Foods making high-fiber claims must meet the definition for low fat, or the level of total fat must appear next to the high-fiber claim.)
- **Good source of fiber:** 2.5 to 4.9 g per serving
- **More or added fiber:** at least 2.5 g more per serving than reference food

Fat
- **Fat free:** less than 0.5 g of fat per serving
- **Saturated fat free:** less than 0.5 g per serving, and the level of *trans* fatty acids does not exceed 0.5 g per serving
- **Low fat:** 3 g or less per serving and, if the serving is 30 g or less or 2 tbsp or less, per 50 g of the food. 2% milk can no longer be labeled

low-fat, as it exceeds 3 g per serving. *Reduced fat* is the term used instead.
- **Low saturated fat:** 1 g or less per serving and not more than 15% of kcal from saturated fatty acids
- **Reduced or less fat:** at least 25% less per serving than reference food
- **Reduced or less saturated fat:** at least 25% less per serving than reference food

Cholesterol
- **Cholesterol free:** less than 2 mg of cholesterol and 2 g or less of saturated fat per serving
- **Low cholesterol:** 20 mg or less cholesterol and 2 g or less of saturated fat per serving and, if the serving is 30 g or less or 2 tbsp or less, per 50 g of the food
- **Reduced or less cholesterol:** at least 25% less cholesterol and 2 g or less of saturated fat per serving than reference food

Sodium
- **Sodium free:** less than 5 mg per serving
- **Very low sodium:** 35 mg or less per serving and, if the serving is 30 g or less or 2 tbsp or less, per 50 g of the food
- **Low sodium:** 140 mg or less per serving and, if the serving is 30 g or less or 2 tbsp or less, per 50 g of the food
- **Light in sodium:** at least 50% less per serving than reference food
- **Reduced or less sodium:** at least 25% less per serving than reference food

Other Terms
- **Fortified or enriched:** Vitamins and/or minerals have been added to the product in amounts in excess of at least 10% of that normally present in the usual product. Enriched generally refers to replacing nutrients lost in processing, whereas fortified refers to adding nutrients not originally present in the specific food.
- **Healthy:** An individual food that is low fat and low saturated fat and has no more than 360 to 480 mg of sodium or 60 mg of cholesterol per serving can be labeled "healthy" if it provides at least 10% of the Daily Value for vitamin A, vitamin C, protein, calcium, iron, or fiber.
- **Light or lite:** The descriptor *light* or *lite* can mean two things: first, that a nutritionally altered product contains one-third fewer kcal or

half the fat of reference food (if the food derives 50% or more of its kcal from fat, the reduction must be 50% of the fat) and, second, that the sodium content of a low-calorie, low-fat food has been reduced by 50%. In addition, "light in sodium" may be used for foods in which the sodium content has been reduced by at least 50%. The term *light* may still be used to describe such properties as texture and color, as long as the label explains the intent—for example, "light brown sugar" and "light and fluffy."
- **Diet:** A food may be labeled with terms such as *diet, dietetic, artificially sweetened,* or *sweetened with nonnutritive sweetener* only if the claim is not false or misleading. The food can also be labeled *low calorie* or *reduced calorie.*
- **Good source:** *Good source* means that a serving of the food contains 10 to 19% of the Daily Value for a particular nutrient. If 5% or less it is a **low source.**
- **High:** *High* means that a serving of the food contains 20% or more of the Daily Value for a particular nutrient.

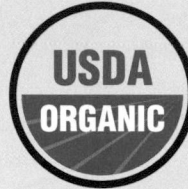

- **Organic:** Federal standards for organic foods allow claims when much of the ingredients do not use chemical fertilizers or pesticides, genetic engineering, sewage sludge, antibiotics, or irradiation in their production. At least 95% of ingredients (by weight) must meet these guidelines to be labeled "organic" on the front of the package. If the front label instead says "made with organic ingredients," only 70% of the ingredients must be organic. For livestock, the animals need to be allowed to graze outdoors and as well be fed organic feed. They also cannot be exposed to large amounts of antibiotics or growth hormones.
- **Natural:** The food must be free of food colors, synthetic flavors, or any other synthetic substance.

The following terms apply only to meat and poultry products regulated by USDA.
- **Extra lean:** less than 5 g of fat, 2 g of saturated fat, and 95 mg of cholesterol per serving (or 100 g of an individual food)
- **Lean:** less than 10 g of fat, 4.5 g of saturated fat, and 95 mg of cholesterol per serving (or 100 g of an individual food)

Many definitions are from FDA's *Dictionary of Terms,* as established in conjunction with the 1990 Nutrition Education and Labeling Act (NELA).

Currently, FDA limits the use of health messages to specific instances in which there is significant scientific agreement that a relationship exists between a nutrient, food, or food constituent and the disease.[8] The claims allowed at this time may show a link between the following:

- A diet with enough calcium and a reduced risk of osteoporosis
- A diet low in total fat and a reduced risk of some cancers
- A diet low in saturated fat and cholesterol and a reduced risk of cardiovascular disease (typically referred to as heart disease on the label)
- A diet rich in fiber—containing grain products, fruits, and vegetables and a reduced risk of some cancers
- A diet low in sodium and high in potassium and a reduced risk of hypertension and stroke
- A diet rich in fruits and vegetables and a reduced risk of some cancers
- A diet adequate in the synthetic form of the vitamin folate (i.e., folic acid) and a reduced risk of neural tube defects (a type of birth defect)
- Use of sugarless gum and a reduced risk of tooth decay, especially when compared with foods high in sugars and starches
- A diet rich in fruits, vegetables, and grain products that contain fiber and a reduced risk of cardiovascular disease. Oats (oatmeal, oat bran, and oat flour) and **psyllium** are two fiber-rich ingredients that can be singled out in reducing the risk of cardiovascular disease, as long as the statement also says the diet should also be low in saturated fat and cholesterol.
- A diet rich in whole-grain foods and other plant foods as well as low in total fat, saturated fat, and cholesterol and a reduced risk of cardiovascular disease and certain cancers
- A diet low in saturated fat and cholesterol that also includes 25 g/day of soy protein and a reduced risk of cardiovascular disease. The statement "one serving of (name of food) provides _____ g of soy protein" must also appear as part of the health claim.
- Fatty acids from oils present in fish and a reduced risk of cardiovascular disease
- Margarines containing plant stanols and sterols and a reduced risk of cardiovascular disease (see Chapter 6 for more details on plant stanols and sterols).

A "may" or "might" qualifier must be used in any statement.

In addition, before a health claim can be made for a food product, it must meet two general requirements. First, the food must be a "good source" (before any fortification) of fiber, protein, vitamin A, vitamin C, calcium, or iron. The legal definition of *good source* appears in Table 2-13. Second, a single serving of the food product cannot contain more than 13 g of fat, 4 g of saturated fat, 60 mg of cholesterol, or 480 mg of sodium. If a food exceeds any one of these requirements, no health claim can be made for it despite its other nutritional qualities. For example, even though whole milk is high in calcium, its label can't make the health claim about calcium and osteoporosis because whole milk contains 5 g of saturated fat per serving.

In addition, the product must meet criteria specific to the health claim being made. For example, a health claim regarding fat and cancer can be made only if the product contains 3 g or less of fat per serving, which is the standard for low-fat foods.

Overall, claims on foods fall into one of four categories:

- Health claims—closely regulated by FDA
- Preliminary health claims—regulated by FDA but evidence may be scant for the claim
- Nutrient claims—closely regulated by FDA (review Table 2-13)
- Structure/function claims—as discussed in Chapter 1, these are not FDA approved or necessarily valid

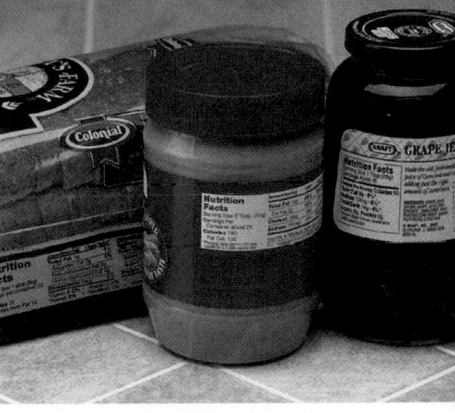

The nutrition information on the food labels on these three products can be combined to indicate nutrient intake for a peanut butter and jelly sandwich.

psyllium A type of dietary fiber found in the seeds of the plantago plant.

In December 2002, FDA created three new preliminary classes of health claims. The agency announced that it would now allow health claims for foods based on incomplete scientific evidence as long as the label qualified it with a disclaimer such as "this evidence is not conclusive."[8] These preliminary health claims haven't shown up on many foods at this time (nuts, such as walnuts, and fish have been some of the first examples). These claims also cannot be used on foods considered unhealthy (review Table 2-13 for the definition of *healthy* with regard to a food).

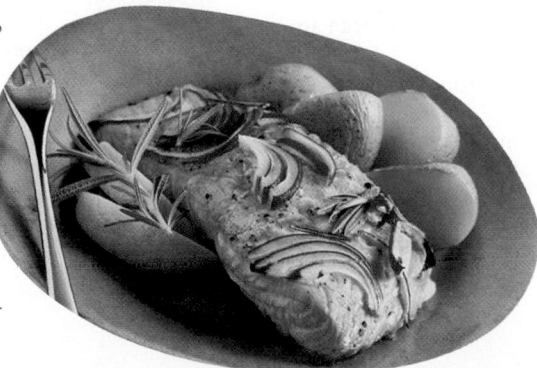

Eating fish at least twice a week contributes to overall health.

Summary

1. *Variety, balance,* and *moderation* are three watchwords of diet planning.
2. Nutrient density is a useful concept. It reflects the nutrient content of a food in relation to its energy content. Nutrient-dense foods are relatively rich in nutrients in comparison with energy content.
3. Energy density of a food is determined by comparing content with the weight of food. A food that is rich in energy but weighs relatively little, such as nuts, cookies, fried foods in general, and most snack foods (including fat-free brands), is considered energy dense. Foods with low energy density include fruits, vegetables, and any food that incorporates lots of water during cooking, such as oatmeal.
4. A person's nutritional state can be categorized as *desirable nutrition,* in which the body has adequate stores for times of increased needs; *undernutrition,* which may be present with or without clinical symptoms; and *overnutrition,* which can lead to vitamin and mineral toxicities and various chronic diseases.
5. Evaluation of nutritional state involves analyzing background factors as well as anthropometric, biochemical, clinical, dietary, and economic assessments. It is not always possible to detect nutritional inadequacies via nutrition assessment because signs and symptoms of deficiencies are often nonspecific and may not appear for many years.
6. Recommended Dietary Allowances (RDAs) are set for many nutrients. These amounts yield enough of each nutrient to meet the needs of healthy individuals within specific gender and age categories. Adequate Intakes (AIs) are used when not enough information is available to set an RDA. Estimated Energy Requirements (EERs) provide a benchmark for energy needs. Tolerable Upper Intake Levels (Upper Levels, or ULs) for nutrient intake have been set for some vitamins and minerals. All of the many dietary standards fall under the term *Dietary Reference Intakes (DRIs).* Daily Values are used as a basis for expressing the nutrient content of foods on the Nutrition Facts panel and are based for the most part on the RDAs published in 1968.
7. MyPyramid is designed to translate nutrient recommendations into a food plan that exhibits variety, balance, and moderation. The best results are obtained by using low-fat or fat-free dairy products; incorporating some vegetable proteins into the diet in addition to animal-protein foods; including citrus fruits and dark green vegetables; and emphasizing whole-grain breads and cereals.
8. Dietary Guidelines for Americans have been issued to help reduce chronic diseases. The guidelines emphasize eating a variety of foods; performing regular physical activity; maintaining or improving weight; moderating consumption of fat, *trans* fat, cholesterol, sugar, salt, and alcohol; eating plenty of whole-grain products, fruits, and vegetables; and safely preparing and storing foods, especially perishable foods.
9. Food labels are a useful tool to track your nutrient intake and learn more about the nutritional characteristics of the foods you eat. Any health claims listed must follow criteria set by FDA.

Study Questions

1. Describe the philosophy underlying the creation of MyPyramid. What dietary changes would you need to make to meet the pyramid guidelines on a regular basis?
2. Trace the progression, in terms of physical results, of a person who went from an undernourished to an overnourished state.
3. How could the nutritional status of the person at each state in question 2 be evaluated?
4. Describe the intent of the Dietary Guidelines for Americans. Point out one criticism for its general application to all North American adults.
5. Based on the discussion of the Dietary Guidelines for Americans, suggest two key dietary changes the typical North American adult should consider making.
6. How do RDAs and Adequate Intakes differ from Daily Values in intention and application?
7. How would you explain the concepts of nutrient density and energy density to a fourth-grade class?
8. Nutritionists encourage all people to read labels on food packages to learn more about what they eat. What four nutrients could easily be tracked in your diet if you read the Nutrition Facts panels regularly on food products?
9. Explain why consumers can have confidence in FDA-approved health claims on food packages.
10. Relate the importance of variety in a diet, especially with regard to fruit and vegetable choices, to the discovery of various phytochemicals in foods.

BOOST YOUR STUDY

Check out the **Perspectives in Nutrition: Online Learning Center** www.mhhe.com/wardlawpers7 for quizzes, flash cards, activities, and web links designed to further help you learn about various tools for diet planning.

Annotated References

1. ADA Reports: Position of the American Dietetic Association: Functional foods. *Journal of the American Dietetic Association*, 104:814, 2004.

   Functional foods are foods that have health-promoting properties beyond those provided by nutrient content alone. The many potential benefits of functional foods are described in the article. Still, since foods naturally contain numerous different nutrients and phytochemicals, an important focus is to consider any functional food to be a part of an otherwise healthy diet, especially one rich in fruits and vegetables.

2. Barr SI and others: Planning diets for individuals using the Dietary Reference Intakes. *Nutrition Reviews* 61:352, 2003.

   This article describes appropriate uses of the Recommended Dietary Allowances, Adequate Intakes, and Tolerable Upper Intake Levels. Dietary intakes from individuals is best evaluated with the Recommended Dietary Allowances and Adequate Intakes. Upper Levels should not be exceeded on a chronic basis.

3. DeBoer SW and others: Dietary intake of fruits, vegetables, and fat in Olmsted County, Minn. *Mayo Clinic Proceedings* 78:161, 2003.

   Most of the adults in this diet survey consumed less than the recommended amounts of fruits and vegetables and more fat than is recommended. Efforts are needed to convince adults in general to follow a healthier diet.

4. Food and Nutrition Board: *Dietary reference intakes for energy, carbohydrate, fiber, fat, fatty acids, cholesterol, protein, and amino acids.* Washington DC: National Academy Press, 2002.

   This report provides the latest guidance for macronutrient and energy intakes. Energy intake in adulthood should generally match energy output so weight maintenance is achieved.

5. Hammond KA: Dietary and clinical assessment. In Mahan LK, Escott-Stump S (eds.): *Krause's food, nutrition, and diet therapy.* 11th ed. Philadelphia: WB Saunders, 2004.

   Excellent chapter on the assessment of nutritional status. The following chapter in this textbook (Chapter 17) by T.H. Carlson compliments the discussion with a detailed look at biochemical assessment of nutritional status.

6. Hasler CM: Functional foods: Benefits, concerns, and challenges—A position paper from the American Council on Science and Health. *Journal of Nutrition* 132:3772, 2002.

   We now know that our diet and its constituents from both plant and animal sources provide more than the essential nutrients such as protein and vitamins, namely a variety of phytochemical and other components that also contribute to health. Foods rich in specific phytochemicals are often termed functional foods. This article lists a variety of phytochemicals under study as well as current approved health claims for food labels.

7. Kral TVE and others: Combined effects of energy density and portion size on energy intake in women. *American Journal of Clinical Nutrition* 79:962, 2004.

   The combination of increasing portion size and increasing energy density resulted in a greater food intake in the women in this study. The researchers suggest that both factors may be contributing to the excess energy intake seen in some adults.

8. Liebman B: Claims crazy: Which ones can you believe? *Nutrition Action HealthLetter* 30(5):1, 2003 (June).

   Consumers can rely on the accuracy of the various health claims approved by FDA. Structure/function claims and the forthcoming preliminary health claims (i.e., those that must carry a disclaimer concerning FDA approval) should be viewed cautiously.

9. Liebman B: Bigger means: Smaller waists. *Nutrition Action HealthLetter*, p. 1, June 2005.

   The article contains a discussion on energy density and practical applications to a daily diet. Highlighted is the work of Dr. Barbara Rolls, the author of this chapter's Expert Opinion.

10. Marcus JB: New age foods for disease prevention. *Today's Dietitian*, p. 24, May 2003.

    Fruits, vegetables, nuts, and whole grains are good sources of phytochemicals. Dietary guidance should be based on consuming these foods, ideally in their whole state.

11. Meadows M: Healthier eating. *FDA Consumer*, p. 10, May–June 2005.

    The latest Dietary Guidelines for Americans (2005) are reviewed. The article provides practical advice to put these guidelines into action—a task too few adults are doing well.

12. Meerschaert CM. One size does not fill all—The New Food Guidance System. *Today's Dietitian*, p. 42, August, 2005.

    This article discusses the pros and cons of the new MyPyramid plan promoted by USDA. It also reviews the various tools offered on the www.mypyramid.gov website.

13. Milner JA: Molecular targets for bioactive food components. *Journal of Nutrition* 134:2492S, 2004.

    The phytochemicals found in a healthy diet provide numerous health benefits. These affect cell metabolism at a very basic level, in turn helping to prevent diseases such as cancer.

14. Mitka M: Government unveils a new food pyramid. *Journal of the American Medical Association* 293:2581, 2005.

    Both the pros and cons of MyPyramid are raised by nutrition and medical experts. The biggest criticism is that the tool is practically useless unless a person logs on to the MyPyramid website to find out the details regarding the diet plan.

15. Rebuilding the pyramid. *Tufts University Health & Nutrition Letter*, p. 1, June 2005.

    The latest nutrition advice from MyPyramid is discussed. Applying the recommendations to everyday life is highlighted.

16. Reeves MJ, Rafferty AP: Healthy lifestyle characteristics among adults in the United States, 2000. *Archives of Internal Medicine* 165:854, 2005.

    Few adults (about 3% of those in the survey) are following all of the four keys to a healthy lifestyle. The keys are nonsmoking, healthy weight, consuming a combination of at least 5 fruit and vegetables servings per day, and performing at least 30 minutes of physical activity 5 days or more per week.

17. Revised Dietary Guidelines to help Americans live better lives. *FDA Consumer*, p. 18, March–April 2005.

    This article summarizes the latest dietary guidelines in simple terms. Colorful graphics are included to emphasize the major points.

18. Stampfer JM and others: Primary prevention of coronary heart disease in women through diet and lifestyle. *The New England Journal of Medicine* 343:16, 2000.

    Women who consume a varied diet (one rich in fiber, includes some fish, and is low in fried foods and animal fat), avoid overweight, drink small amounts of alcohol, exercise on a daily basis for about 30 minutes, and avoid smoking reduce their risk of heart attack by over 80% compared to other women.

19. Uncle Sam's diet book. *Tufts University Health & Nutrition Letter*, p. 1, March 2005.

    Implementation of the latest Dietary Guidelines for Americans is discussed. The authors suggest that even small changes that conform to this plan can provide health benefits.

20. Yates AA: Dietary Reference Intakes: Rationale and Applications. In Shils ME and others (eds.): *Modern nutrition in health and disease.* 10th ed. Philadelphia, PA: Lippincott Williams & Wilkins, 2006.

    The author provides a detailed discussion of the rationale and development of the Dietary Reference Intakes. Included is a discussion of how to implement the various standards.

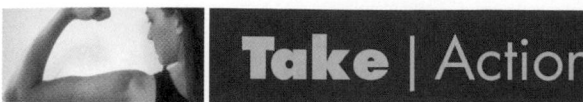

Take | Action

I. Does Your Diet Meet MyPyramid Recommendations?

Using your food-intake record from Chapter 1, place each food item in the appropriate group of the accompanying MyPyramid chart. That is, for each food item, indicate how many servings it contributes to each group based on the amount you ate (see page 58 for serving sizes). Note that many of your food choices may contribute to more than one group. For example, toast with soft margarine contributes to two categories: (1) the grains group; and (2) the oils group. After entering all the values, add the number of servings consumed in each group. Finally, compare your total in each food group with the recommended number of servings shown in Table 2-9 or obtained from the www.MyPyramid.gov website. Enter a minus sign (−) if your total falls below the recommendation or a plus sign (+) if it equals or exceeds the recommendation.

Indicate the Number of Servings from MyPyramid That Each Food Yields:

Food or Beverage	Amount Eaten	Milk	Meat & Beans	Fruits	Vegetables	Grains	Oils
Group totals							
Recommended servings							
Shortages in numbers of servings							

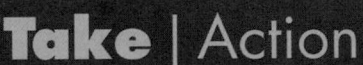 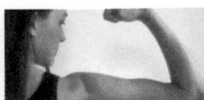

Take | Action

II. Are You Putting the Dietary Guidelines into Practice?

As noted in this chapter, the advice provided by the 2005 Dietary Guidelines for Americans can be summarized into three main points and a number of related activities. Fill out the following inventory to see to what extent you are following the basic intent of the Guidelines.

Food Intake

Do you:

Y N   Consume a variety of nutrient-dense foods and beverages within and among the basic food groups of MyPryamid?

Choose foods that limit the intake of:

Y N   Saturated fat

Y N   *Trans* fats

Y N   Cholesterol

Y N   Added sugars

Y N   Salt

Y N   Alcohol (if used).

Emphasize in your food choices:

Y N   Vegetables

Y N   Fruits

Y N   Legumes (beans)

Y N   Whole grain breads and cereals

Y N   Fat-free or low-fat milk or equivalent milk products

Body Weight

Y N   Maintain body weight in a healthy range by balancing energy intake from foods and beverages with energy expended

Y N   Engage in at least 30 minutes of moderate-intensity physical activity, above usual activity, at work or home on most days of the week.

Safe Food Handling

Y N   Clean hands, food contact surfaces, and fruits and vegetables before preparation

Y N   Cook foods to a safe temperature to kill microorganisms

Figure 2-8 points to other health practices that are part of the 2005 Dietary Guidelines for Americans, but this abbreviated list includes the major points to consider.

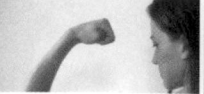

Take | Action

III. Applying the Nutrition Facts Label to Your Daily Food Choices

Imagine that you are at the supermarket looking for a quick meal before a busy evening. In the frozen food section, you find two brands of frozen cheese manicotti (see labels *a* and *b*). Which of the two brands would you choose? What information on the Nutrition Facts label contributed to this decision?

_____

_____

_____

_____

Nutrition Facts
Serving Size 1 Package (260g)
Servings Per Container 1

Amount Per Serving

Calories 390   Calories from Fat 160

	% Daily Value*
Total Fat 18g	**27**%
Saturated Fat 9g	**45**%
Trans Fat 2g	★★
Cholesterol 45mg	**14**%
Sodium 880mg	**36**%
Total Carbohydrate 38g	**13**%
Dietary Fiber 4g	**15**%
Sugars 12g	
Protein 17g	

Vitamin A 10%   •   Vitamin C 4%

Calcium 40%   •   Iron 8%

*Percent Daily Values are based on a 2,000 calorie diet. Your daily values may be higher or lower depending on your calorie needs:

	Calories:	2,000	2,500
Total Fat	Less than	65g	80g
Sat Fat	Less than	20g	25g
Cholesterol	Less than	300mg	300mg
Sodium	Less than	2,400mg	2,400mg
Total Carbohydrate		300g	375g
Dietary Fiber		25g	30g

Calories per gram:
Fat 9 • Carbohydrate 4 • Protein 4

★★Intake of *trans* fat should be as low as possible.

(a)

Nutrition Facts
Serving Size 1 Package (260g)
Servings Per Container 1

Amount Per Serving

Calories 230   Calories from Fat 35

	% Daily Value*
Total Fat 4g	**6**%
Saturated Fat 2g	**10**%
Trans Fat 1g	★★
Cholesterol 15mg	**4**%
Sodium 590mg	**24**%
Total Carbohydrate 28g	**9**%
Dietary Fiber 3g	**12**%
Sugars 10g	
Protein 19g	

Vitamin A 10%   •   Vitamin C 10%

Calcium 35%   •   Iron 4%

*Percent Daily Values are based on a 2,000 calorie diet. Your daily values may be higher or lower depending on your calorie needs:

	Calories:	2,000	2,500
Total Fat	Less than	65g	80g
Sat Fat	Less than	20g	25g
Cholesterol	Less than	300mg	300mg
Sodium	Less than	2,400mg	2,400mg
Potassium		3,500mg	3,500mg
Total Carbohydrate		300g	375g
Dietary Fiber		25g	30g

Calories per gram:
Fat 9 • Carbohydrate 4 • Protein 4

★★Intake of *trans* fat should be as low as possible.

(b)

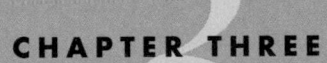

CHAPTER THREE

HUMAN DIGESTION AND ABSORPTION

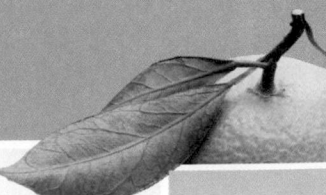

CHAPTER OUTLINE

CASE SCENARIO:

Elise is a 20-year-old college sophomore. Over the last few months, she has been experiencing regular bouts of heartburn. This usually happens after a large lunch or dinner. Occasionally she has even bent down after dinner to pick up something and had some stomach contents travel back up her esophagus and into her mouth. This especially frightened Elise, so she visited the University Health Center.

The nurse practitioner at the Center told Elise it was good she came in for a checkup. She suspects she has a disease called gastroesophageal reflux disease (GERD). She tells Elise that this can lead to serious problems if not controlled, such as a rare form of cancer. She provides Elise with a pamphlet describing GERD and schedules an appointment with a physician for further evaluation.

What type of dietary habits likely contribute to Elise's symptoms of GERD? What types of medications have been especially useful for treating this problem? Overall, how will Elise cope with this health problem, and will it ever go away?

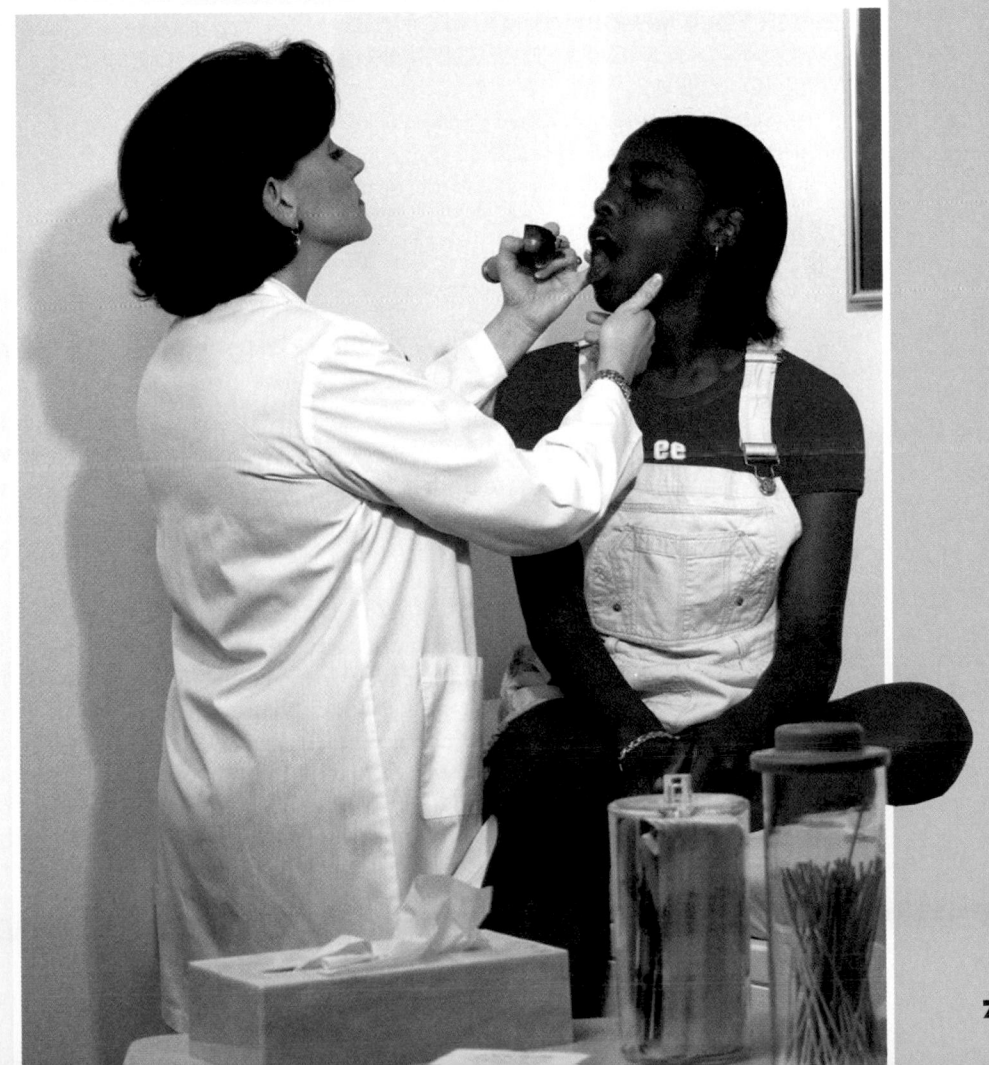

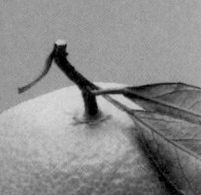

Merely eating food won't nourish you. You must first digest the food—in other words, break it down into usable forms of the essential nutrients that can be absorbed into the bloodstream. Once nutrients are taken up by the bloodstream, they can be distributed to and used by body cells.[18]

We rarely think about, let alone control, digesting and absorbing foods. Except for a few voluntary responses—such as deciding what and when to eat, how well to chew food, and when to eliminate the remains—most digestion and absorption processes control themselves. We don't consciously decide when the pancreas will secrete digestive substances into the small intestine or how quickly foodstuffs will be propelled down the intestinal tract. Various hormones and the nervous system mostly control these functions.[5] Your only awareness of these involuntary responses may be a hunger pang right before lunch or a "full" feeling after eating that last slice of pizza.

In this chapter you will examine digestion and absorption as well as some related aspects of the human physiology that support nutritional health. In the process you will become acquainted with the basic anatomy (structure) and physiology (function) of the circulatory and endocrine systems. These and other body systems control our nutritional status, and the nutrients derived from food contribute to the proper functioning of these systems.[7]

CHAPTER OBJECTIVES CHAPTER 3 IS DESIGNED TO ALLOW YOU TO:

1. Define *tissue, organ,* and *organ system.*

2. List some characteristics of the 12 organ systems and outline a role for each related to nutrition, especially the cardiovascular system, lymphatic system, endocrine system, nervous system, immune system, and urinary system.

3. Outline the overall processes of digestion and absorption, including the roles played by the organs of the gastrointestinal tract and the related accessory organs: liver, gallbladder, and pancreas.

4. Become familiar with some specific enzymes and hormones that act in digestion of the various nutrient groups.

5. Identify the major nutrition-related gastrointestinal health problems and typical approaches to treatment.

REFRESH YOUR MEMORY AS YOU BEGIN YOUR STUDY OF HUMAN DIGESTION AND ABSORPTION IN CHAPTER 3, YOU MAY WANT TO REVIEW:

- The basic chemical composition of carbohydrates, proteins, and lipids in Chapter 1.
- Cell structure and function in Appendix C.
- Physiology of the major body systems (aside from the digestive system) in Appendix C.

---

tissues Collections of cells adapted to perform a specific function.

organ A group of tissues designed to perform a specific function—for example, the heart, which contains muscle tissue, nerve tissue, and so on.

organ system A collection of organs that work together to perform an overall function.

adenosine triphosphate (ATP) The main energy currency for cells. ATP energy is used to promote ion pumping, enzyme activity, and muscle contraction.

▌The Cell Is the Basis of Human Physiology

The body is composed of trillions of cells. Each cell is a self-contained, living entity. (Review Appendix C if you are unfamiliar with the parts of a cell, such as the plasma membrane or mitochondria.) Cells of the same type join together, typically using intercellular substances, to form **tissues,** such as muscle tissue. One, two, or more tissues combine in a particular way to form more complex structures, called **organs.** All organs contribute to nutritional health, and a person's overall nutritional state determines how well each organ functions. At a still higher level of coordination, several organs can cooperate for a common purpose to form an **organ system,** such as the digestive system. Overall, the human body is an organism made up of a coordinated unit of many highly structured organ systems (Figure 3-1).[18]

Chemical reactions occur constantly in every living cell: the production of new substances is balanced by the breaking down of older ones, as exemplified by the constant formation and degradation of bone. For this turnover of substances to occur, cells require a continuous supply of energy in the form of dietary carbohydrate, protein, and/or fat. Almost all cells need oxygen to transform the energy in these nutrients to a form of energy the body can use—**adenosine triphosphate,** or **ATP** (see Chapter 4 for more on ATP). Cells also need water; building supplies, especially amino acids and

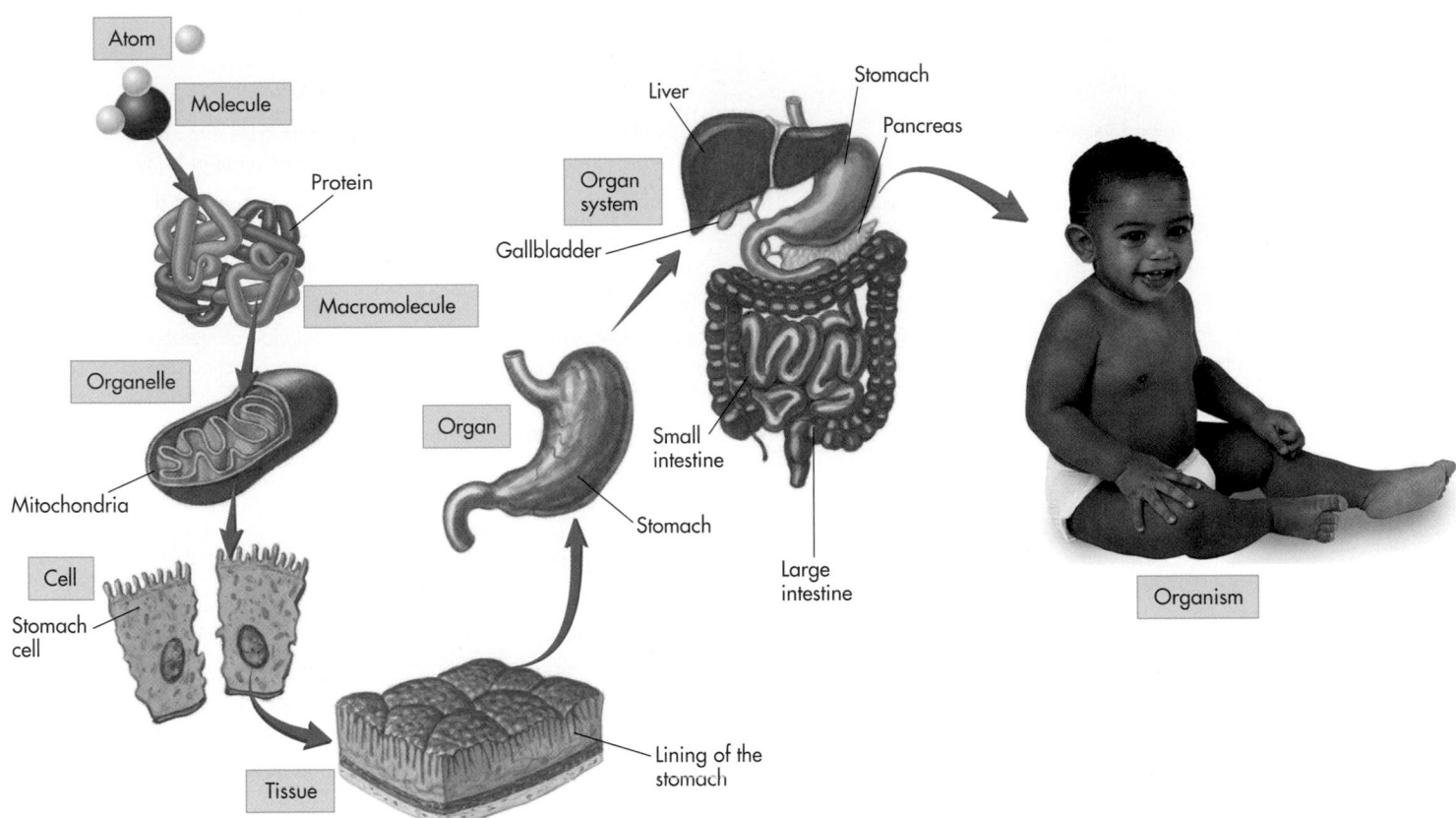

Figure 3-1 | Levels of organization of the human body. Each level is more complex than the previous level. The organ system shown is the gastrointestinal (GI) tract.

minerals; and chemical regulators, such as the vitamins. All of these substances enable the tissues, constituted from individual cells, to function properly.

Adequately supplying all nutrients to the body's cells begins with a healthful diet. To ensure optimal use of nutrients, the body's cells, tissues, organs, and organ systems also must work efficiently.[2]

Organization of the Human Body

Tissue comprises groups of similar cells working together to accomplish a specialized task. Humans are composed of four primary types of tissue: **epithelial, connective, muscle,** and **nervous.** Epithelial tissue is composed of cells that cover surfaces both outside and inside the body. These cells secrete important substances, absorb nutrients, and excrete waste. Connective tissue supports and protects the body, stores fat, and produces blood cells. Muscle tissue is designed for movement. Nervous tissue found in the brain and spinal cord is designed for communication. These four tissues form various organs and, ultimately, organ systems (review Figure 3-1).[18]

This chapter focuses on the digestive system. The nutrients we consume in food are unavailable until they have been processed by the digestive system. Using chemical and mechanical means to alter food, nutrients can be released and absorbed into the body for distribution to body tissues. Table 3-1 summarizes the components and functions of the digestive system and various other organ systems as well.

Sometimes organs within a system can serve another system. For example, the primary function of the digestive system is to convert the food we eat into absorbable nutrients. At the same time, the digestive system serves the immune system by

epithelial tissue The surface cells that line the outside of the body and all passageways within it.

connective tissue Cells and their protein products that hold different structures in the body together. Some structures are made up of connective tissue—notably, **tendons** and **cartilage.** Connective tissue also forms part of bone and the nonmuscular structures of arteries and veins.

muscle tissue A type of tissue adapted for contraction.

nervous tissue Tissue composed of highly branched, elongated cells that transport nerve impulses from one part of the body to another.

Table 3-1 | Organ Systems of the Body

System	Major Components	Functions Related to Nutrition
Cardiovascular	Heart, blood vessels, and blood	Transports nutrients, waste products, gases, and hormones throughout the body and plays a role in the immune response and the regulation of body temperature
Lymphatic	Lymph vessels, lymph nodes, and other lymph organs	Removes foreign substances from the blood and lymph, combats disease, maintains tissue fluid balance, and aids in fat absorption
Nervous	Brain, spinal cord, nerves, and sensory receptors	A major regulatory system: detects sensation, controls movements, and controls physiological and intellectual functions
Endocrine	Endocrine glands, such as the pituitary, thyroid, and adrenal glands	A major regulatory system: participates in the regulation of metabolism, reproduction, and many other functions through the production and subsequent action of hormones
Immune	White blood cells, lymph vessels and nodes, spleen, thymus gland, and other lymph tissues	Provides defense against foreign invaders
Digestive	Mouth, esophagus, stomach, intestines, and accessory structures, namely the liver, gallbladder, and pancreas	Performs the mechanical and chemical processes of digestion, absorption of nutrients, processing of nutrients (especially the liver), and elimination of wastes
Urinary	Kidneys, urinary bladder, and the ducts that carry urine	Removes waste products from the circulatory system and regulates blood acid-base balance, overall chemical balance, and water balance
Integumentary	Skin, hair, nails, and sweat glands	Protects the other organ systems, regulates temperature, prevents water loss, and produces a substance that converts to vitamin D upon sun exposure
Skeletal	Bones, associated cartilage, and joints	Protects, supports, and allows body movement, produces blood cells, and stores minerals
Muscular	Smooth, cardiac, and skeletal muscle	Produces body movement, maintains posture, and produces body heat
Respiratory	Lungs and respiratory passages	Exchanges gases (oxygen and carbon dioxide) between the blood and the air and regulates blood acid-base (pH) balance
Reproductive	Gonads, accessory structures, and genitals	Performs the processes of reproduction and influences sexual functions and behaviors

The cardiovascular and lymphatic organ systems together make up the circulatory system and so contribute to circulatory functions in the body. The endocrine and nervous organ systems contribute to the regulatory functions. The digestive, urinary, integumentary, and respiratory organ systems contribute to the excretory functions, while the muscular and skeletal organ systems contribute to storage capabilities in the body.

preventing dangerous pathogens from invading the body and causing illness. As you study nutrition, you will note the multiple roles played by many organs (Figure 3-2). Appendix C contains more details on these and other body systems.

The overriding theme of the study of human nutrition is to understand the actions of nutrients as they affect different cells, tissues, organs, and organ systems. Nutrient intake impacts each organ system, and a particular organ system uses nutrients in a particular way.[2]

The Physiology of Digestion

gastrointestinal (GI) tract Comprises the main sites in the body used in digestion and absorption of nutrients. The tract consists of the mouth, esophagus, stomach, small intestine, large intestine, rectum, and anus.

digestion The process by which large ingested molecules are mechanically and chemically broken down to produce smaller molecules that can be absorbed across the wall of the GI tract.

The **gastrointestinal (GI) tract** is a long tube stretching from the mouth to the anus (Figure 3-3). This tube, also known as the *alimentary canal*, is partitioned from the body in such a way that nutrients must pass through its walls to be absorbed into the bloodstream. Just eating a food is not enough—most nutrients must be **digested** and all nutrients must be absorbed to be of use to body cells. Certain diseases may hamper digestion and/or absorption, denying the body use of nutrients in a meal.[2] A common example is the diarrhea that accompanies many diseases.

The GI tract is a complex system that performs a variety of physiological functions: movement **(motility),** secretion, digestion, absorption, elimination, and nutrient

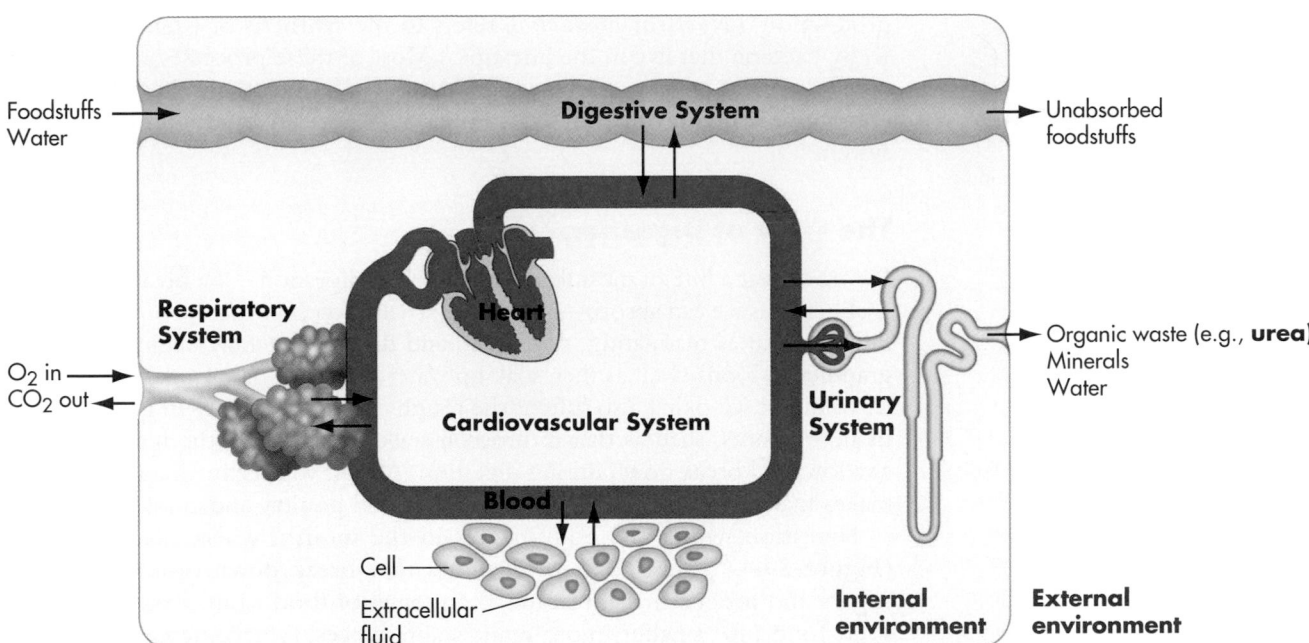

Figure 3-2 | Exchanges of nutrients occur between our external environment and the internal environment of the circulatory system via the digestive system (which includes the liver, gallbladder, and pancreas), respiratory system, and urinary system. Overall, the human body is a combination of 12 systems working together to support cell needs.

Figure 3-3 | Major organs of the gastrointestinal (GI) tract (1, 2, 3, 7, 8, and 9) and accessory organs (4, 5, and 6) used in digestion and absorption of nutrients.

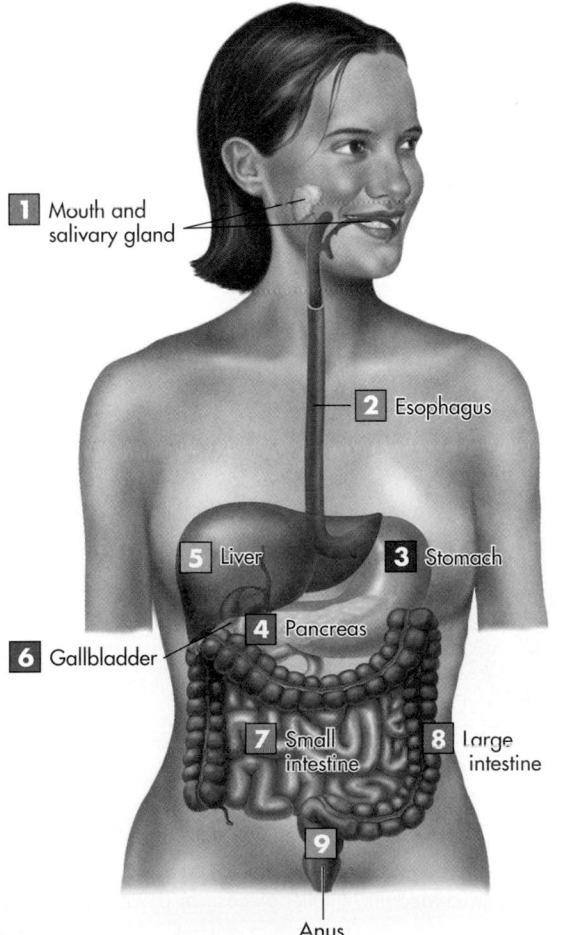

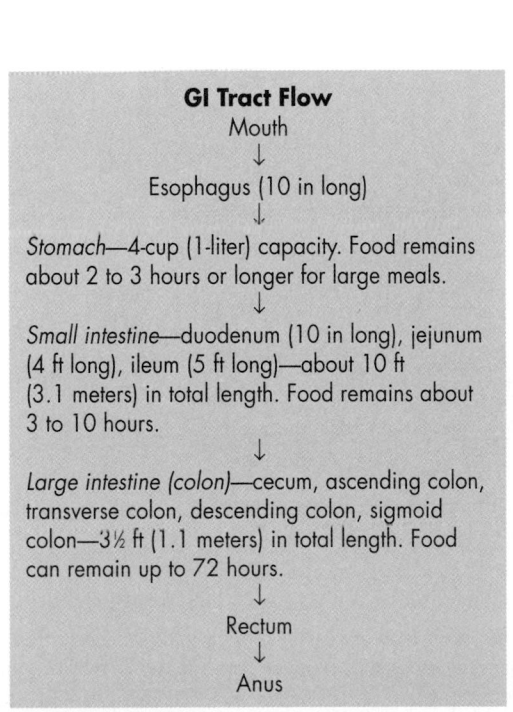

GI Tract Flow

Mouth
↓
Esophagus (10 in long)
↓
Stomach—4-cup (1-liter) capacity. Food remains about 2 to 3 hours or longer for large meals.
↓
Small intestine—duodenum (10 in long), jejunum (4 ft long), ileum (5 ft long)—about 10 ft (3.1 meters) in total length. Food remains about 3 to 10 hours.
↓
Large intestine (colon)—cecum, ascending colon, transverse colon, descending colon, sigmoid colon—3½ ft (1.1 meters) in total length. Food can remain up to 72 hours.
↓
Rectum
↓
Anus

hormone A compound with a specific site of synthesis that, when secreted into the bloodstream, controls the function of cells in its target organ or organs. Hormones can be amino acidlike (epinephrine), proteinlike (insulin), or fatlike (estrogen).

saliva A watery fluid, produced by the salivary glands in the mouth, that contains lubricants, enzymes, and other substances.

mucus A thick fluid secreted by glands throughout the body. It contains a compound that has both a carbohydrate and a protein nature. It acts as both a lubricant and a means of protection for cells.

bolus A mass of food that is swallowed.

lysozyme A set of enzyme substances produced by a variety of cells; it can destroy bacteria by rupturing cell membranes.

umami A brothy, meaty, savory flavor in some foods. Monosodium glutamate enhances this flavor when added to foods.

production. (*Nutrient production* refers to the synthesis of vitamins, such as vitamin K, by bacteria that live in the intestine.) Most of these processes are under autonomic control; that is, they are involuntary. Almost all functions involved in digestion and absorption are controlled by **hormones**, hormonelike compounds, and the nervous system.[3]

The Flow of Digestion

Before we eat a bite of most foods, the work of digestion—the breakdown of foods into usable forms we can absorb—is already partially accomplished. Cooking or other preparations, such as marinating, pounding, and dicing, generally begin the process. Starch granules in foods swell as they soak up water during cooking, making them much easier to digest. Cooking also softens the tough connective tissues in meats and the fibrous tissue of plants, such as that in broccoli stalks. As a result, the food is easier to chew, swallow, and break down during digestion. As you will see in Chapter 19, cooking also makes many foods, such as eggs, meat, fish, and poultry, much safer to eat.

Digestion within the body begins in the mouth, where glands produce **saliva** (Figure 3-4).[3] Saliva contains enzymes that break down carbohydrates to simple sugars and **mucus** that lubricates the morsel of food (Table 3-2). Chewing divides solid food into smaller, more manageable pieces, which increases the surface area exposed to the saliva. The food is now referred to as a **bolus**. Saliva also contains **lysozyme**, a set of enzymes that kill bacteria by rupturing their cell membranes. Finally, saliva bathes the teeth with fluoride and other substances that protect against decay (see Chapter 5 for details).

The tongue contains taste receptors for sweet, salt, sour, and bitter tastes.[7] The salty taste is due to sodium ions (Na^+) enhanced by chloride ions (Cl^-). The sour taste is due to the presence of hydrogen ions (H^+). Bitter and sweet tastes are generated by specific components in the food that interact with membrane receptors on the tongue. A fifth taste sensation called **umami** has been proposed.[10] This taste sensation is elicited by monosodium glutamate, a substance often added to restaurant foods to enhance flavor. Brothy, meaty, and savory are examples of umami sensations, such as for mushrooms.

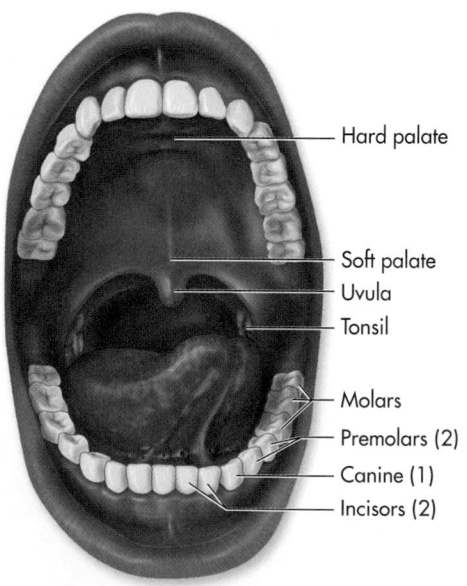

(a)

- Hard palate
- Soft palate
- Uvula
- Tonsil
- Molars
- Premolars (2)
- Canine (1)
- Incisors (2)

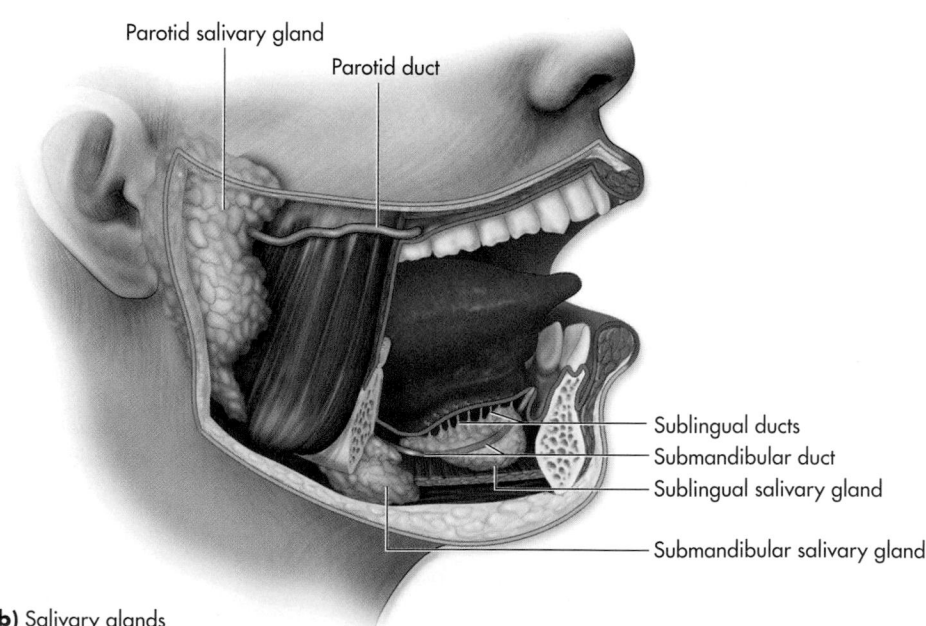

- Parotid salivary gland
- Parotid duct
- Sublingual ducts
- Submandibular duct
- Sublingual salivary gland
- Submandibular salivary gland

(b) Salivary glands

Figure 3-4 | (a) The oral cavity is the beginning of the GI tract. Incisor and canine (pointed) teeth are useful in tearing food, such as from a chicken leg. Molars (flat teeth) are used to grind food into smaller pieces. (b) The salivary glands near the oral cavity produce saliva to aid in swallowing and digesting food.

Table 3-2 | Important Secretions and Products of the Digestive Tract

Secretion	Site of Production	Purpose
Saliva	Mouth	Contributes to starch digestion, lubrication, swallowing
Mucus	Mouth, stomach, small intestine, large intestine	Protects cells, lubricates
Enzymes **(amylases, lipases, proteases)**	Mouth, stomach, small intestine, pancreas	Promote digestion of foodstuffs into particles small enough for absorption
Acid	Stomach	Promotes digestion of protein among other functions
Bile **(bile acids, cholesterol,** and **lecithins)**	Liver (stored in gallbladder)	Suspends fat in water to aid fat digestion in the small intestine
Bicarbonate	Pancreas, small intestine	Neutralizes stomach acid when it reaches the small intestine
Hormones **(gastrin, secretin, cholecystokinin, gastric-inhibitory peptide)**	Stomach, small intestine	Stimulate production and/or release of acid, enzymes, bile, and bicarbonate; help regulate peristalsis and overall GI tract flow

This sensation of flavor is then augmented by input from approximately 6 million **olfactory** cells in the nose. When we chew a food, chemicals are released that stimulate the nasal passages. Thus, it makes perfect sense that when we are sick and our noses are stuffed up and congested, even our most favorite foods will not taste as good as they normally do. Flavor is also affected by human genetic variation in both taste and olfactory sensations. The ability to detect bitter substances—such as in broccoli or cabbage—is one example. This ability is important since some bitter substances are also quite toxic.[10]

A variety of diseases and drugs, as well as the effects of aging, can alter the sense of taste. Overall, flavor is a complex combination of taste, olfaction, physical sensations from certain chemicals in foods (such as in chili peppers), and textural sensations.

The mouth and stomach are connected by the 10-inch-long esophagus. At its entrance is a valvelike flap of tissue, the **epiglottis,** that prevents food from being lodged in the trachea (windpipe).[5] When food is swallowed it lands on the epiglottis, which then covers the larynx (the opening of the trachea). Breathing automatically stops. These involuntary responses ensure that swallowed food travels only down the esophagus, aided by muscle contractions of the esophagus and by gravity (Figure 3-5). If food travels down the trachea, choking may occur (the victim will not be able to speak or breathe). A series of techniques to treat such a person is called the Heimlich Maneuver (see www.heimlichinstitute.org for details).

As food exits the esophagus, it enters the stomach. The stomach is essentially a holding tank with a capacity of about 4 cups (1 L).[5] Note that stomach size can vary, and its volume can be expanded to about 16 cups (4 L) if needed. In contrast, stomach volume can be reduced surgically as a radical treatment for obesity (more on this in Chapter 13). The stomach continues the digestive process by secreting very strong acid (hydrochloric acid [HCl]) from the **parietal cells** as well as enzymes from the **chief cells**

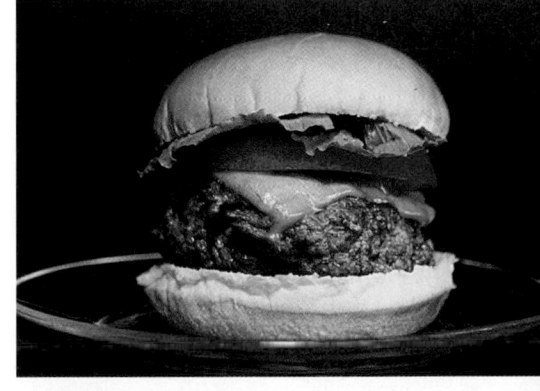

The body digests the foods presented. Despite what you may have heard or read, the order in which foods are eaten plays no role in digestion.

olfactory Sense of smell.

epiglottis Flap that folds down over the trachea during swallowing.

parietal cell Gastric gland cell that secretes hydrochloric acid and intrinsic factor.

chief cell Gastric gland cell that secretes pepsinogen, precursor of pepsin.

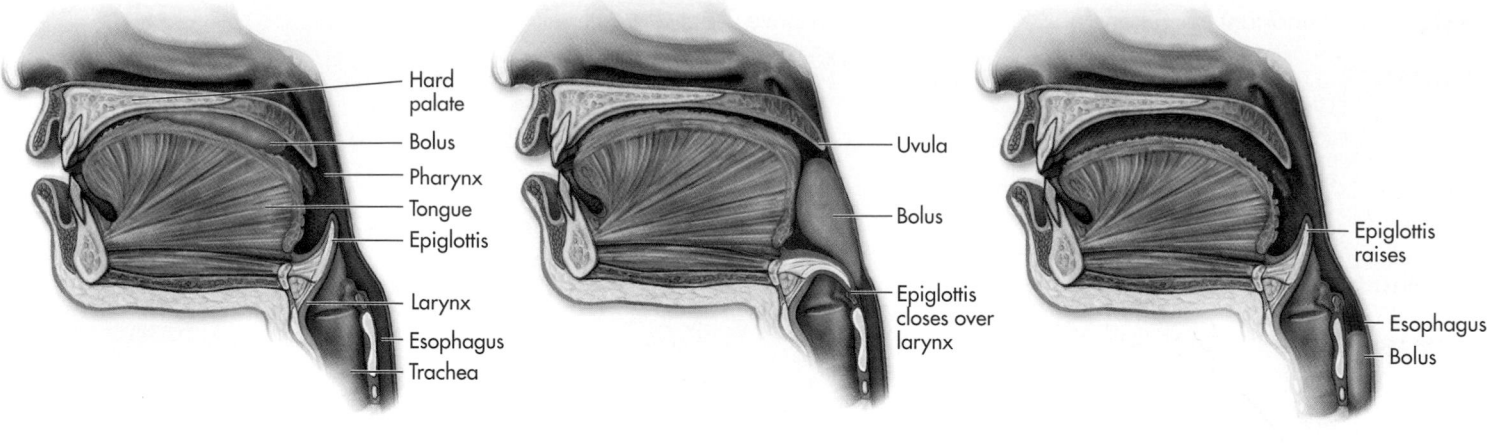

(a) Bolus of food is pushed by tongue against hard palate and then moves toward pharynx.

(b) As bolus moves into pharynx, the epiglottis closes over larynx.

(c) Esophageal muscle contractions push bolus toward stomach. The epiglottis then returns to it's normal position.

Figure 3-5 | The process of swallowing. Swallowing occurs as the food bolus is forced (a) into the pharynx from the oral cavity, (b) through the pharynx, and (c) into the esophagus on the way to the stomach. Choking occurs when the bolus becomes lodged in the trachea, blocking air to the lungs, instead of passing into the esophagus.

chyme A mixture of stomach secretions and partially digested food.

Another term to describe the stomach is *gastric.*

(Figures 3-6 and 3-7). This acid and enzymes are then slowly mixed into the food. The resulting soupy mass of food and secretions is called **chyme.** The chyme is usually ready to leave the stomach within 1 to 4 hours after food is eaten. The more solid the chyme, the longer it takes to leave the stomach.

The hydrochloric acid produced by the stomach is very important. It destroys the biological activity of ingested proteins. Otherwise protein substances such as certain plant and animal hormones in food could go on to affect human functions. For the most part bacteria and viruses in foods are also destroyed. In addition, the acid converts some inactive stomach enzymes into active forms and solubilizes dietary minerals such as calcium so they can be more easily absorbed.[9]

Figure 3-6 | The pH scale. The diagonal line indicates the proportionate concentration of hydrogen ions (H^+) to hydroxide ions (OH^-) at each pH value. Any pH value above 7 is basic, while any pH value below 7 is acidic. As pH decreases, each lower pH unit has ten times the amount of hydrogen ions than the previous unit. Therefore, only a small change in pH can have a drastic affect on a cell, and so on organ systems.

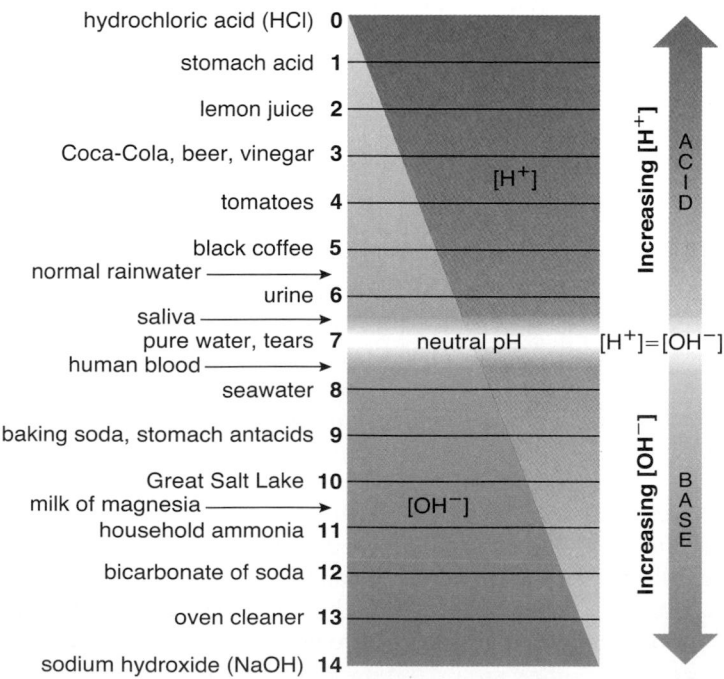

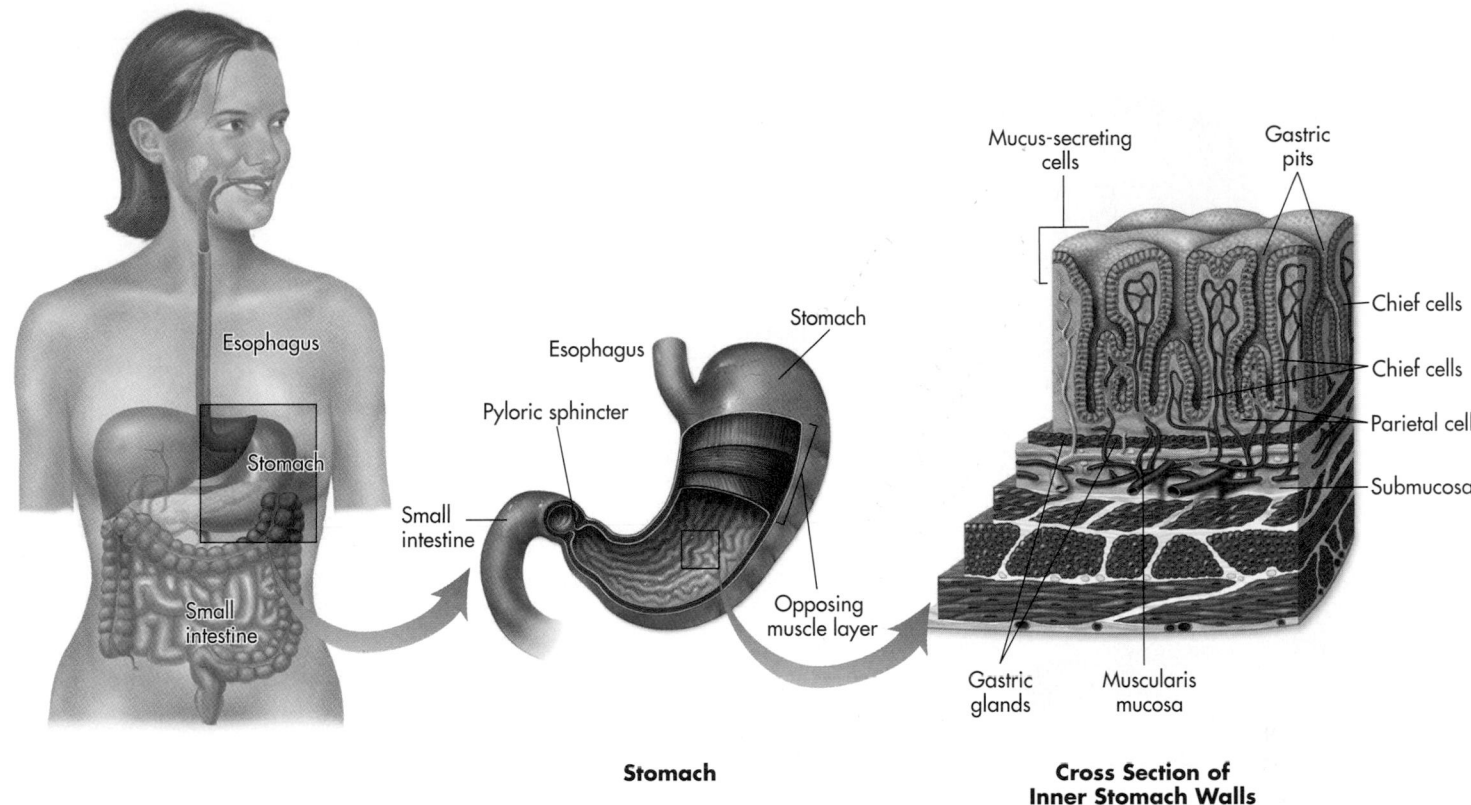

Figure 3-7 | Physiology of the stomach. Surface mucous cells produce mucus for protection from stomach acid and enzymes. Parietal cells produce the hydrochloric acid (HCl) and chief cells produce the enzymes. Mucous neck cells, scattered among the cells in the gastric pits, also produce mucus.

You might wonder how the stomach protects itself from the acid and enzymes it produces. First, the stomach has a thick layer of mucus secreted by surface mucous cells and mucous neck cells in the stomach lining. (Goblet cells perform a similar function in the intestines.) This mucus helps prevent the stomach from "digesting" itself. The production of acid and enzymes in the stomach is tied to the release of a specific hormone called gastrin. This release does not occur except when we are thinking about eating or are actually in the process of eating. Lastly, as the concentration of acid in the stomach increases, acid production tapers off, also because of hormonal control.[9]

One other important function of the stomach is the production of a substance called **intrinsic factor.** This vital material is essential for the absorption of one of the B vitamins, vitamin B-12 (see Chapter 10).[3]

The stomach empties into the small intestine, which is coiled below it in the abdomen (Figure 3-8). The small intestine is divided into three sections: the first part, the duodenum, is about 10 in. long (0.3 m); the middle segment, the jejunum, is about 4 ft long (1.3 m); and the last section, the ileum, is about 5 ft long (1.6 m).[5] The small intestine is considered small because of its narrow diameter (1 in. [2.5 cm]), not its length. Most digestion is completed in the duodenum and upper jejunum, with the help of enzymes made by intestinal cells and the pancreas. Muscular contractions in the small intestine constantly mix the food with digestive fluids, enhancing digestion. A meal remains in the small intestine about 3 to 10 hours.

The small intestine empties into the large intestine (also called the colon). This organ is about 3½ ft long (1.1 m) and is separated into five sections: cecum, ascending colon, transverse colon, descending colon, and sigmoid colon.[5] Little digestion occurs in this organ (95% of total digestion has already taken place in the small intestine). Food that reaches the large intestine is mostly indigestible. This residue remains in the large intestine for about 24 to 72 hours before elimination from the body as **feces.**

Production of mucus relies on the presence of compounds called **prostaglandins.** Heavy use of aspirin and related **NSAID** medications can cause breakdown of the stomach wall because they inhibit prostaglandin production. This in turn lessens the barrier between gastric cells and the highly acidic gastric secretions.[5]

prostaglandin (PG) One of several potent hormonelike compounds made of polyunsaturated fatty acids that produce diverse effects in the body.

NSAIDs Nonsteroidal anti-inflammatory drugs; includes aspirin, ibuprofen (Advil®), and naproxen (Aleve®).

intrinsic factor A substance present in stomach secretions that enhances vitamin B-12 absorption.

feces Substances discharged from the bowel during defecation, including undigested food residue, dead GI tract cells, mucus, bacteria, and other waste material.

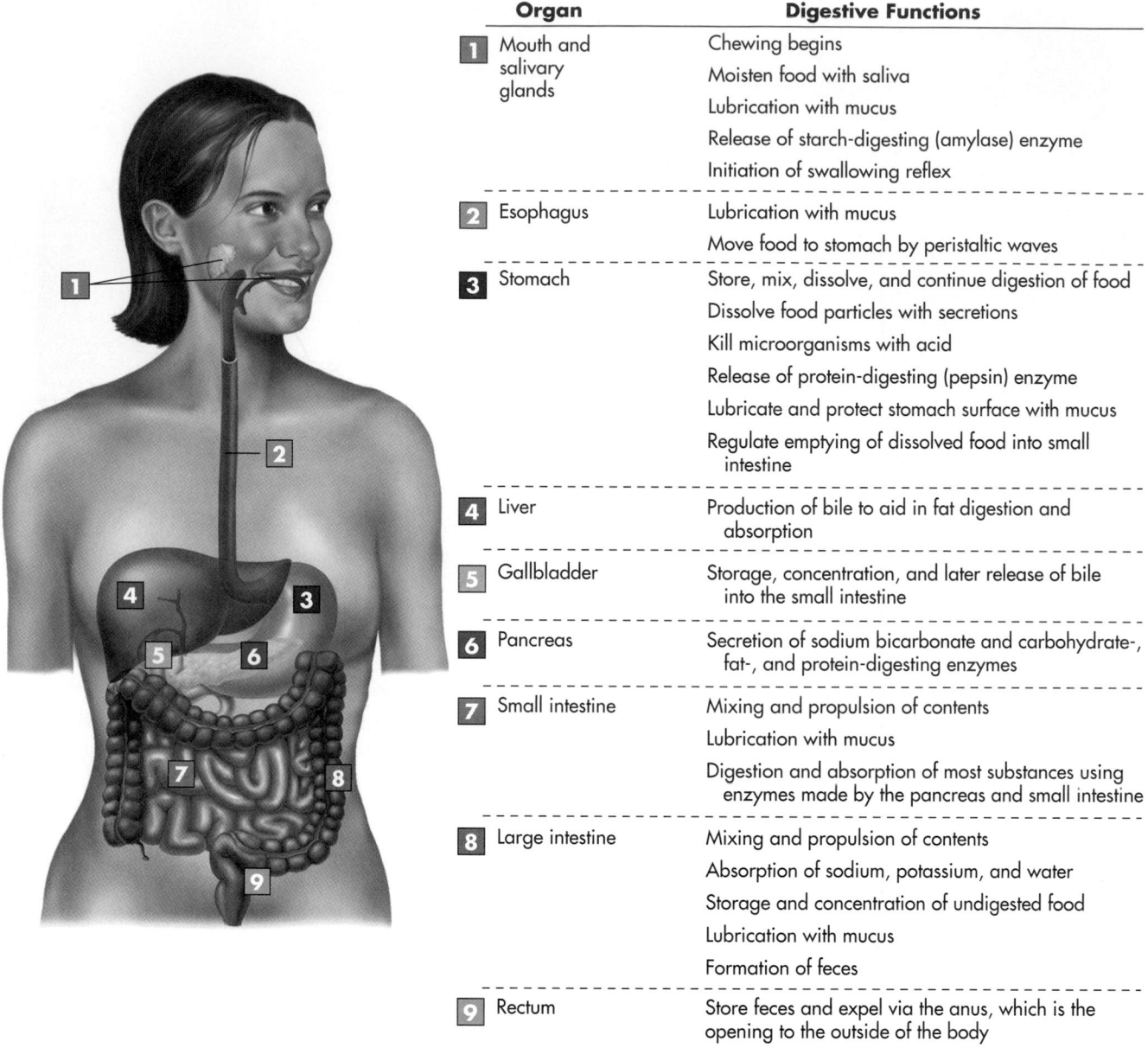

Organ	Digestive Functions
1 Mouth and salivary glands	Chewing begins
	Moisten food with saliva
	Lubrication with mucus
	Release of starch-digesting (amylase) enzyme
	Initiation of swallowing reflex
2 Esophagus	Lubrication with mucus
	Move food to stomach by peristaltic waves
3 Stomach	Store, mix, dissolve, and continue digestion of food
	Dissolve food particles with secretions
	Kill microorganisms with acid
	Release of protein-digesting (pepsin) enzyme
	Lubricate and protect stomach surface with mucus
	Regulate emptying of dissolved food into small intestine
4 Liver	Production of bile to aid in fat digestion and absorption
5 Gallbladder	Storage, concentration, and later release of bile into the small intestine
6 Pancreas	Secretion of sodium bicarbonate and carbohydrate-, fat-, and protein-digesting enzymes
7 Small intestine	Mixing and propulsion of contents
	Lubrication with mucus
	Digestion and absorption of most substances using enzymes made by the pancreas and small intestine
8 Large intestine	Mixing and propulsion of contents
	Absorption of sodium, potassium, and water
	Storage and concentration of undigested food
	Lubrication with mucus
	Formation of feces
9 Rectum	Store feces and expel via the anus, which is the opening to the outside of the body

Figure 3-8 | Physiology of the GI tract. Many organs cooperate in a regulated fashion to allow digestion and subsequent absorption of nutrients in foods.

bile A liver secretion that is stored in the gallbladder and released through the common bile duct into the duodenum. It is essential for the digestion and absorption of fat.

The terminus of the large intestine is attached to the rectum, which is connected to the anus. These final sections of the GI tract work with the large intestine to prepare the feces for elimination through the anus.[5]

The liver, pancreas, and gallbladder work with the GI tract but are not a physical part of it. They are thus called accessory organs.[18] The liver provides **bile,** which aids in fat digestion and absorption by suspending fat in water, creating many tiny fat droplets. Bile is stored in the gallbladder until needed. The bile duct leads from the gallbladder and connects with the pancreatic duct, which allows digestive enzymes and other products from the pancreas, such as sodium bicarbonate ($NaHCO_3$), to be mixed with bile before entering the duodenum for digestion. This bicarbonate neutralizes the acidic chyme as it enters the duodenum. The latter section entitled Gastrointestinal Control Valves: Sphincters discusses the role of bicarbonate in the small intestine in greater detail.

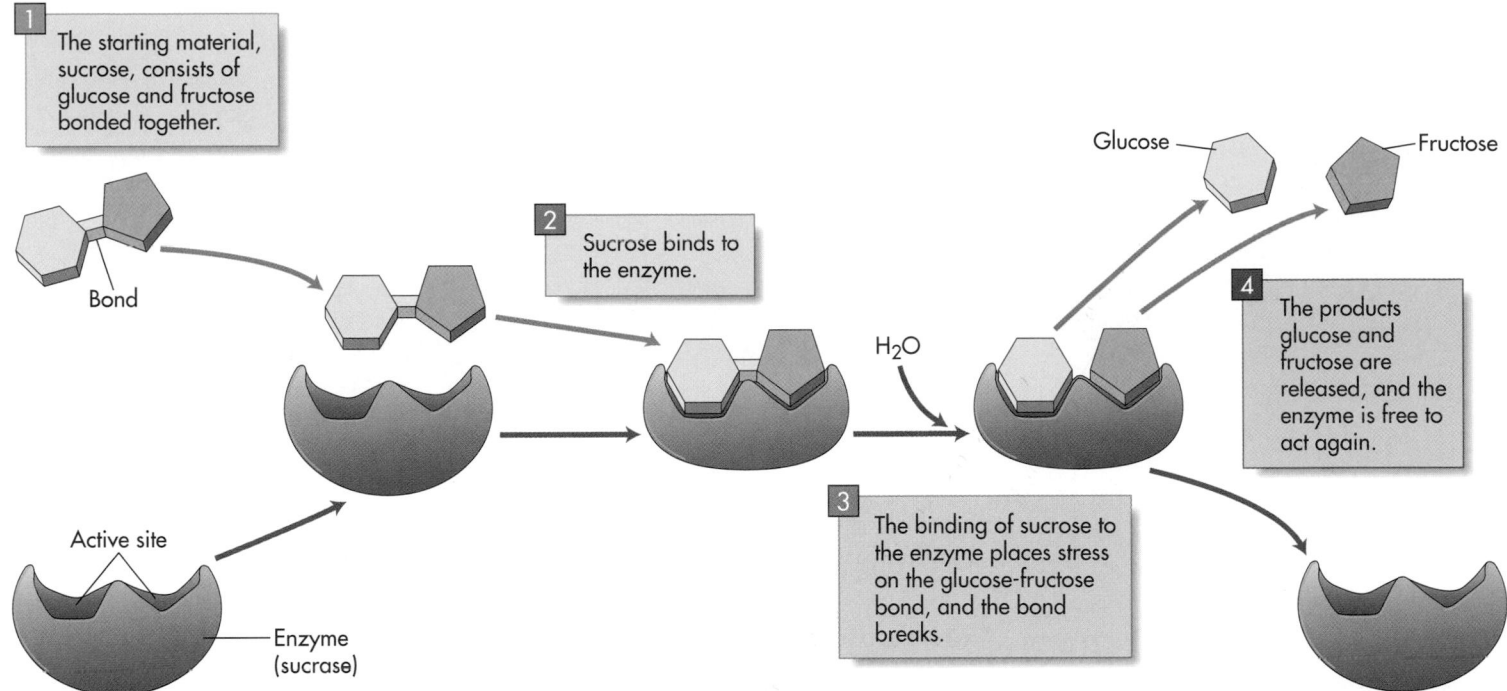

Figure 3-9 | A model of enzyme action. Enzymes increase the speed with which chemical reactions occur, but they are not altered themselves as they do so. In the reaction illustrated here, the enzyme sucrase is splitting the sugar sucrose into two simpler sugars: glucose and fructose. Only these simpler sugars are absorbed from the small intestine to enter the bloodstream. Note that sometimes energy input is needed to push the reaction along, but not in this case.

A Closer Look at Enzymes in Digestion

Enzymes speed up digestion by catalyzing chemical reactions. This catalysis brings certain molecules close together and then creates a favorable environment for the intended reaction. The enzyme lowers the amount of activation energy needed for the action to proceed (Figure 3-9). (Appendix A provides more detail on enzyme action.) Enzymes usually act only on a specific substance; for example, enzymes that recognize table sugar (sucrose) ignore milk sugar (lactose). It is also possible for some of these enzymes to digest the digestive tract itself. For this reason, nerve and hormonal mechanisms in the digestive tract control enzyme release. Enzymes are released as needed, but generally not at other times.[7]

Digestion utilizes a chemical process known as **hydrolysis,** in which water is used to split large molecules into smaller ones. The process eventually yields basic molecules, which can be absorbed through the intestinal wall.

A few digestive enzymes are made by the mouth and stomach. Most, however, are synthesized by the pancreas and small intestine (Chapters 5, 6, and 7 will review these enzymes in detail).[9] The pancreas is capable of responding to changes in nutrient intake with appropriate changes in enzyme production. Increased protein intake leads to increased protein digestive capability. This result is likely linked to the ability of the hormone **cholecystokinin (CCK)** to increase the synthesis of protein-digesting enzymes by the pancreas. Diets high in fat and low in carbohydrate lead to an increase in fat-digesting enzymes.

When either the small intestine or the pancreas is diseased, inadequate quantities of important digestive enzymes may be produced. This scarcity can result in incomplete digestion and very limited absorption.[2] In such cases, nutrients in the undigested food travel into the large intestine rather than being absorbed into the bloodstream. In the large intestine the undigested food is metabolized into acids and gases by bacteria.[2] The resultant feces appear foamy and greasy because of trapped gases and the

The naming system for enzymes is often quite simple. The first part of the enzyme name usually indicates the target; the ending is then -ase. For example, sucrase is the enzyme that digests the sugar sucrose.

hydrolysis A chemical reaction in which a compound is broken down by the addition of water. One product receives a hydrogen ion (H^+), while the other product receives a hydroxyl ion (OH^-). Hydrolytic enzymes break down compounds using water in this manner.

cholecystokinin (CCK) A hormone that stimulates enzyme release from the pancreas and bile release from the gallbladder.

Table 3-3 | Gastrointestinal Tract Hormones

Hormone	Stimulus to Secretion	Secreted by	Action
Gastrin	Food in the stomach, especially proteins, caffeine; spices; alcohol	Pyloric region of the stomach and upper duodenum	Stimulates parietal cells to produce acid, stimulates chief cells to produce enzyme that begins digestion of protein
Secretin	Acid chyme, partially digested protein	Duodenum, jejunum	Stimulates pancreas to produce bicarbonate
Cholecystokinin (CCK)	Food, especially fat and proteins in duodenum	Duodenum, jejunum	Stimulates contraction of gallbladder, secretes pancreatic digestive enzymes, inhibits stomach motility
Gastric inhibitory peptide	Protein and fat in chyme	Small intestine	Inhibits stomach motility, stimulates insulin secretion

presence of undigested fat. Intestinal malabsorption also often causes a distended abdomen because of intestinal gas.[11]

Gastrointestinal Hormones—A Key to Orchestrating Digestion

Four hormones, part of the endocrine system, primarily regulate the GI tract: gastrin, secretin, cholecystokinin, and gastric inhibitory peptide (Table 3-3).[6] The term *hormone* comes from the Greek "to stir or excite." To be a true hormone, a regulatory compound must have a specific synthesis site from which it enters the bloodstream to reach target cells. Note that hormones are not available to all cells in the body, but only act in those cells with the appropriate receptor protein. These receptors are highly specific for a certain hormone and are generally found on the cell membrane. (A few hormones can penetrate the cell membrane and bind to receptors on DNA.)

Many hormonelike compounds, such as vasoactive intestinal peptide, bombesin, substance P, and somatostatin, also control important aspects of GI function.[5] These compounds diffuse from cells or nerve endings to nearby cells. Many hormonelike compounds are found in the intestine and the brain. When a person thinks about eating or prepares to eat, the whole GI tract begins to prime itself for action. Hormonelike substances participate in this process. The cells that synthesize these hormones and hormonelike compounds are scattered throughout the GI tract.

Gastrointestinal Control Valves: Sphincters

A **sphincter** is a circular muscle arrangement (as in the anus) that acts as a valve to regulate passage or flow of material. The intestinal tract includes several sphincters, which respond to stimuli from nerves, hormones, hormonelike compounds, and pressure that builds up around them (Figure 3-10).

The flow of food through the esophagus is controlled by the upper and lower esophageal sphincters.[18] The lower esophageal sphincter (also known as the *cardiac sphincter* due to its proximity to the heart) prevents backflow (reflux) of stomach contents into the esophagus. It generally opens only in response to muscle contractions in the esophagus, which propel ingested food down to the stomach.

The lower esophageal sphincter for the most part should remain closed, as the stomach contents are highly acidic. If stomach acid comes in contact with the esophagus, it can cause a pain known as **heartburn.**

The **pyloric sphincter,** located at the junction of the stomach and first part of the small intestine (duodenum), controls the movement of the stomach contents into the small intestine. Under hormonal and nervous system control, the pyloric sphincter allows only a few milliliters (about a teaspoon) of stomach contents at a time to squirt into the small intestine. This rate allows bicarbonate ions released from the pancreas to efficiently

People who have pancreatic disease may not produce sufficient enzymes for digestion. In cystic fibrosis, excess production of mucus may block release of enzymes from the pancreas. This results in malabsorption of nutrients and associated discomfort. An affected person may be prescribed replacement enzymes, which are taken right before eating. Usually these are coated to protect against destruction by acid in the stomach.

sphincter A muscular valve that controls flow of foodstuff in the GI tract.

heartburn Pain caused by stomach acid backing up into the esophagus and irritating the tissue in that organ.

pyloric sphincter Ring of smooth muscle between the stomach and the duodenum.

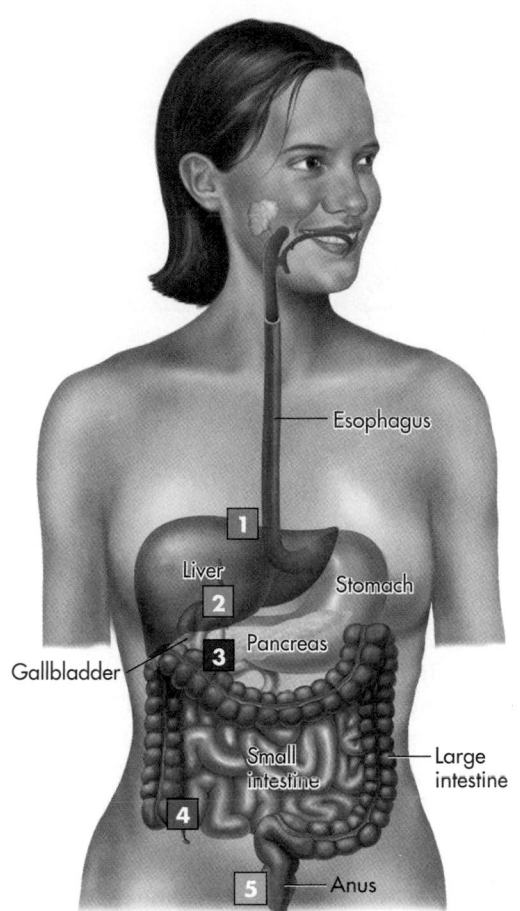

	Sphincter	Function
1	Lower esophageal sphincter	Prevent backflow (reflux) of stomach contents into the esophagus
2	Pyloric sphincter	Control the flow of stomach contents into the small intestine
3	Sphincter of Oddi	Control the flow of bile into the small intestine
4	Ileoceal sphincter	Prevent the contents of the large intestine from reentering the small intestine
5	Anal sphincters	Prevent defecation until person desires to do so

Figure 3-10 | Sphincters of the GI tract. These ringlike muscles control the flow of contents through the GI tract in response to stimuli from nerves, hormones, hormonelike compounds, and pressure that builds up around the sphincters.

neutralize the hydrogen ions coming from the stomach acid. This neutralization is critical to reduce the risk of acid erosion of the small intestine. Such erosion might produce an **ulcer.** The pyloric sphincter also prevents backflow of intestinal contents into the stomach, thereby protecting the stomach lining from bile in the intestinal contents.[18]

The **sphincter of Oddi** lies at the end of the common bile duct. When the hormone **cholecystokinin (CCK)** stimulates the gallbladder to contract during digestion, the sphincter of Oddi relaxes and allows the output of the gallbladder and much of that from the pancreas to flow from the common bile duct to the duodenum.[18]

The **ileocecal sphincter** is found at the end of the small intestine and opens in response to the presence of intestinal contents in its vicinity. Otherwise the sphincter remains closed to prevent the contents of the large intestine from backing up into the small intestine.[18] In this way bacteria from the large intestine are prevented from invading and colonizing the small intestine. The small intestine must have a relatively low concentration of bacteria because bacteria can compete for nutrients and disrupt absorption, especially for fat.

At the far end of the large intestine are two anal sphincters, one under voluntary control.[18] Once toilet-trained, a child can determine when to relax the sphincter to allow for **defecation,** and when to keep it constricted.

Gastrointestinal Muscularity: Mixing and Propulsion

Food is propelled down the GI tract by a process called **peristalsis.**[9] Watching a snake swallow its prey graphically illustrates the process. Most of the GI tract has two layers of muscles—circular and longitudinal. Peristalsis consists of a coordinated squeezing

ulcer Erosion of the tissue lining, usually in the stomach (gastric ulcer) or upper small intestine (duodenal ulcer). The general condition in either area is often termed a *peptic ulcer.*

sphincter of Oddi Ring of smooth muscle between the common bile duct and the upper part of the small intestine (duodenum). Also called the hepatopancreatic sphincter.

ileocecal sphincter Ring of smooth muscle between the ileum of the small intestine and the colon.

defecation expulsion of feces from rectum.

peristalsis A coordinated muscular contraction that propels food down the GI tract.

Figure 3-11 | Peristalsis and segmentation. A swallowed bolus is propelled through the GI tract by coordinated contraction and relaxation of the muscles of the GI wall. (a) Peristalsis is a wave of contraction that moves the bolus ahead of the wave through the GI tract toward the anus. (b) Segmentation is a back-and-forth action in the small intestine that breaks apart the bolus into increasingly smaller pieces and mixes them with digestive juices.

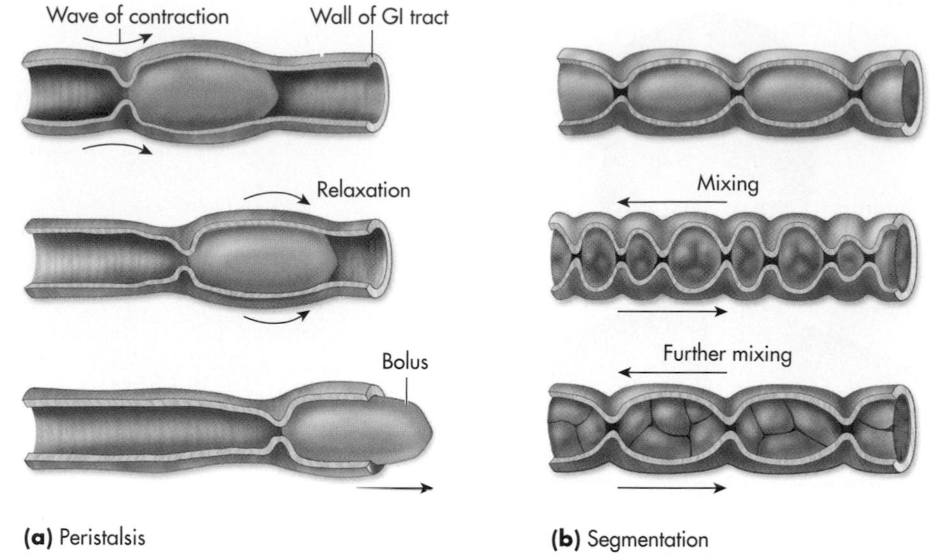

(a) Peristalsis

(b) Segmentation

and shortening of these muscles (Figure 3-11). This process begins in the esophagus in the form of two waves of muscle action closely following each other. In the stomach, peristaltic waves create a mixing and grinding action as often as three times per minute during digestion. The stomach wall is composed of three opposing muscle layers (circular, diagonal, and longitudinal), which in combination enable the stomach to contract in enough directions to fully mix food with gastric juices (review Figure 3-7).[5]

The most prominent peristalsis occurs in the small intestine, where contractions occur about every 4 to 5 seconds. The large intestine has comparatively sluggish waves of peristalsis (called haustrations). These lead to occasional **mass movements** to help eliminate the feces.

mass movement A peristaltic wave that simultaneously coordinates contraction over a large area of the large intestine. Mass movements propel material from one portion of the large intestine to another and from the large intestine into the rectum.

Concept | Check

The gastrointestinal (GI) tract includes the mouth, esophagus, stomach, small intestine, large intestine (colon), rectum, and anus. Associated with the GI tract are the salivary glands, liver, gallbladder, and pancreas. Together these organs perform the digestion and absorption needed to extract nutrients from food and deliver them to the bloodstream.

Hormones, such as gastrin and cholecystokinin (CCK), regulate digestion. Sphincters throughout the GI tract control the flow of food by blocking the passage between organs until the proper time.

In the GI tract, a coordinated muscular activity called peristalsis propels food from the esophagus to the anus. Segmentation in the intestines divides and mixes the contents, aiding digestion and absorption. Enzymes produced by cells in the mouth, stomach, pancreas, and small intestine digest the food to forms of nutrients that can be absorbed. The time from ingestion of food to the eventual elimination of the feces from the body is usually about 1 to 3 days.

When the Digestive Processes Go Awry

The fine-tuned organ system we call the digestive system can develop problems. Knowing about these common problems can help you avoid or lessen them.

Ulcers

About 25 million North Americans develop ulcers during their lifetimes. The principal causes are an acid-resistant bacterial infection *(Helicobacter pylori [H. pylori])*, the heavy use of aspirin and related NSAID medications, and disorders that cause excessive acid production in the stomach (Figure 3-12). And, after being out of favor for some years, stress is now regarded as a predisposing factor for ulcers, especially if the person is infected with *H. pylori* or has certain anxiety disorders.

As the stomach lining deteriorates in ulcer development and loses its mucus layer protection, the acid further erodes the stomach tissue. Acid can also erode the tissue lining of the first part of the small intestine. *Peptic ulcer* is the general term for both these conditions. Most ulcers in young people occur in the small intestine; in older people they occur primarily in the stomach.

The typical symptom of an ulcer is pain about 2 hours after eating. Stomach acid acting on a meal irritates the ulcer after most of the meal has moved from the site of the ulcer.

The primary risk associated with an ulcer is the possibility that it will erode entirely through the stomach or intestinal wall. The GI contents could then spill into the body cavities, causing a major infection. In addition, an ulcer may erode a blood vessel, leading to massive blood loss into the stomach or small intestine. For these reasons, it is important not to ignore the early warning signs of ulcer development.

In the past, milk and cream therapy—the so-called Sippy diet—was used to help cure ulcers. Clinicians now know that milk and cream are two of the worst foods a person with an ulcer could eat. The calcium in these foods stimulates stomach acid secretion and actually inhibits ulcer healing.

Today, a combination of approaches is used for ulcer therapy.[13] People infected with *H. pylori* are given antibiotics as well as stomach acid–blocking medications called **proton pump inhibitors** (e.g., omeprazole [Prilosec], esomeprazole [Nexium], lansoprazole [Prevacid]) and possibly bismuth to eradicate *H. pylori*. (Recall that *proton* is another term for the

Two other common GI tract disorders, lactose malabsorption/intolerance and diverticulosis, are covered in Chapter 5. Note that low-fiber diets are the common cause of the latter disorder.

proton pump inhibitor A medication that inhibits the ability of gastric cells to secrete hydrogen ions. Examples are esomeprazole (Nexium) and lansoprazole (Prevacid). Low doses of this class of medications are also available without prescription (e.g., omeprazole (Prilosec).

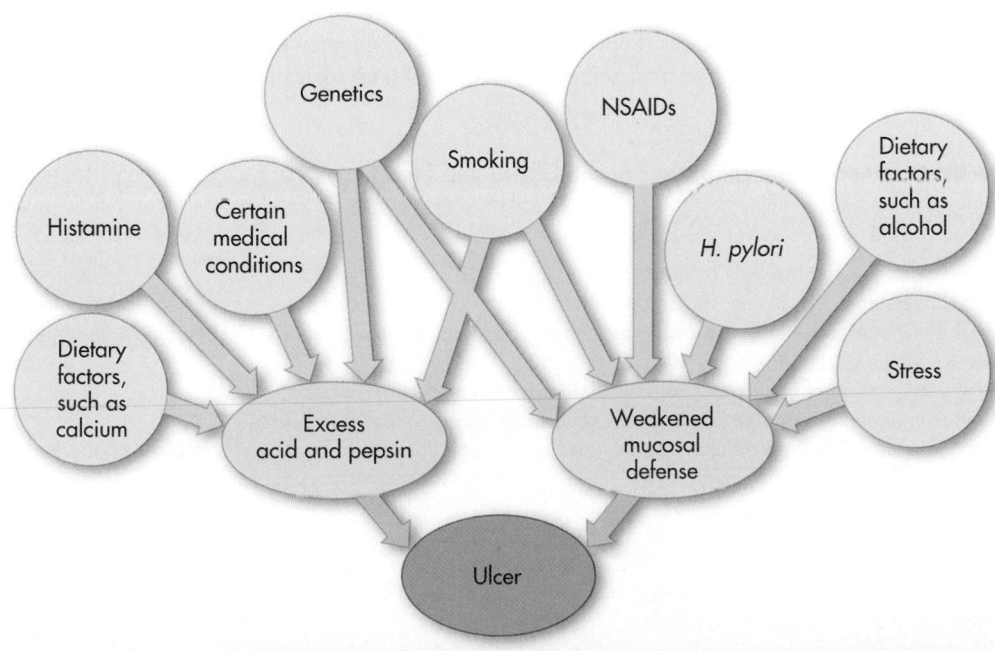

Figure 3-12 | Development of a peptic ulcer. *H. pylori* bacteria and NSAIDs (e.g., aspirin) cause ulcers by impairing mucosal defense, especially in the stomach. In the same way, smoking, genetics, and stress can impair mucosal defense, as well as cause an increase in the release of pepsin and stomach acid. All these factors can contribute to ulcers.

(continued)

H₂ blockers Medications such as cimetidine (Tagamet) that block the increase of stomach acid production caused by histamine.

histamine A breakdown product of the amino acid histidine that stimulates acid secretion by the stomach and has other effects on the body, such as contraction of smooth muscles, increased nasal secretions, relaxation of blood vessels, and constriction of airways.

Aspirin is part of the class of medications called nonsteroidal anti-inflammatory drugs (NSAIDs). Also included are ibuprofen (Motrin or Advil) and naproxen (Aleve).

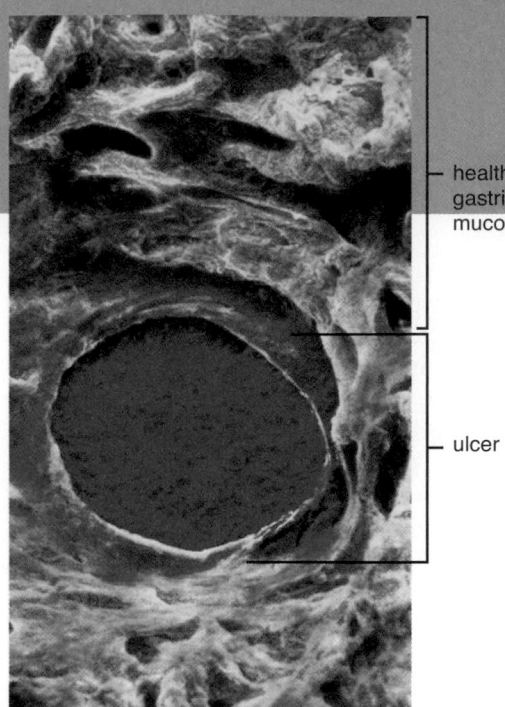

healthy gastric mucosa

ulcer

Close-up of a stomach ulcer. This needs to be treated or eventual perforation of the stomach is possible.

hydrogen ion that creates acidity.) In many cases, there is a 90% cure rate for *H. pylori* infections in the first week of this treatment. Recurrence is unlikely if the infection is cured, but an incomplete cure almost certainly leads to repeated ulcer formation.

Antacid medications may also be part of ulcer care, as is a class of medicines called **H₂ blockers.** These include cimetidine (Tagamet), ranitidine (Zantac), and famotidine (Pepcid), all of which block **histamine**-related acid secretion

in the stomach. Some of these medications are now available over the counter in nonprescription doses for cases of indigestion and heartburn (see next section). Medications that coat the ulcer, such as sucralfate (Carafate), are also commonly used.

People with ulcers should also refrain from smoking and minimize the use of aspirin and related NSAIDs. These practices reduce the mucus secreted by the stomach. A medication used to treat arthritis pain, called "Cox-2 inhibitor" (celecoxib [Celebrex]), is less likely to cause stomach ulcers and, so, has been used as a replacement for NSAIDs. It does offer some advantages over NSAIDS, but is not totally safe for some people, such as those with a history of cardiovascular disease or strokes. Overall, this combination of lifestyle therapy and medical treatment has so revolutionized ulcer therapy that dietary changes are of minor importance today. Current diet-therapy approaches recommend simply avoiding foods that increase ulcer symptoms (Table 3-4).

Note also that stomach acid is not a problem for people not prone to or currently experiencing ulcers. Because stomach acid performs important functions, antacids, despite their usual presence alongside the breath mints in a convenience store, should not be used excessively. Abuse by overingesting antacids containing magnesium (and many do) could result in magnesium toxicity.

Table 3-4 | Recommendations to Prevent Ulcers and Heartburn from Occurring or Recurring

Ulcers
1. Stop smoking if you are now a smoker.
2. Avoid large doses of aspirin, ibuprofen, and other NSAID compounds unless a physician advises otherwise. For people who must use these medications, FDA has approved an NSAID combined with a medication to reduce gastric damage.
3. Limit consumption of coffee, tea, and alcohol (especially wine), if this helps.
4. Limit consumption of pepper, chili powder, and other strong spices, if this helps.
5. Eat nutritious meals on a regular schedule; include enough fiber (see Chapter 5 for sources of fiber).
6. Chew foods well.
7. Lose weight if you are currently overweight.

Heartburn
1. Observe the recommendations for ulcer prevention.
2. Wait about 2 hours after a meal before lying down.
3. Don't overeat at mealtime. Smaller meals that are low in fat are advised.
4. Try elevating the head of the bed (6-inch blocks).

Heartburn

About half of North American adults experience occasional heartburn. This gnawing pain in the upper chest is caused by the movement of acid from the stomach into the esophagus, and so, the more serious form of this problem is called **gastroesophageal reflux disease (GERD)**.[8] Unlike the stomach, the esophagus produces very little mucus to protect it, so acid quickly erodes the lining of the esophagus, causing pain. Symptoms may also include nausea, gagging, coughing, or hoarseness. GERD is characterized by such symptoms of acid reflux two or more times per week. People who have GERD experience occasional relaxation of the lower esophageal sphincter. Typically it should be relaxed only during swallowing, but in individuals with GERD it is relaxed at other times as well.

Certain physical conditions can lead to heartburn. For example, both pregnancy and obesity result in increased production of estrogen and progesterone. These hormones relax the lower esophageal sphincter, making heartburn more likely.[15] In the latter case, adipose tissue turns certain circulating hormones into estrogen; thus, the more adipose tissue, the more estrogen is produced. The Case Scenario Follow-Up describes the therapy options for GERD and related heartburn.

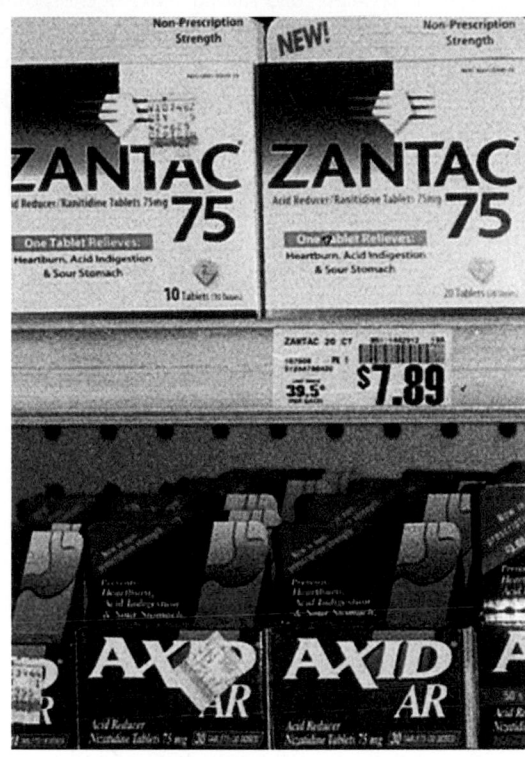

gastroesophageal reflux disease (GERD) Disease that results from stomach acid backing up into the esophagus. The acid irritates the lining of the esophagus, causing pain.

A number of over-the-counter medications are marketed for heartburn. Attention to diet and lifestyle, however, is generally a more important measure to take.

Constipation and Laxatives

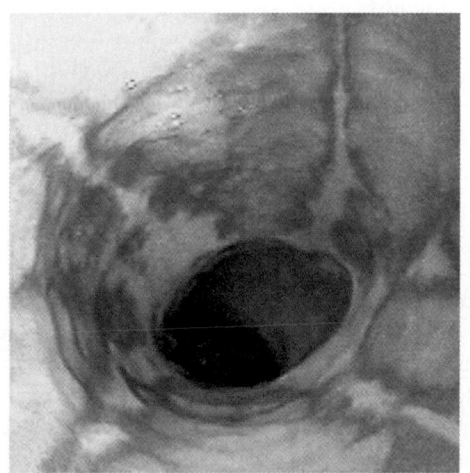

An endoscopic view of the esophagus that shows the signs of reflux esophagitis.

Constipation, which is difficult or infrequent evacuation of the bowels, is commonly reported by adults, especially older adults (the colon becomes more sluggish as we age). Slow movement of fecal material through the large intestine causes constipation. As fluid is increasingly absorbed during the extended time the feces stay in the large intestine, they become dry and hard.

Constipation can result when people regularly inhibit their normal bowel reflexes for long periods. People may ignore normal urges when it is inconvenient to interrupt occupational or social activities. Muscle spasms of an irritated large intestine can also slow the movement of feces and contribute to constipation. Medications such as antacids as well as calcium and iron supplements can also cause constipation.

constipation A condition characterized by infrequent bowel movements.

(continued)

Perhaps you have heard that taking laxatives after overeating prevents deposition of body fat from the excess energy intake. This erroneous and dangerous premise has gained popularity among followers of numerous fad diets. You may temporarily feel less full after using a laxative because laxatives hasten emptying of the large intestine and increase fluid loss. Most laxatives, however, do not speed the passage of food through the small intestine, where digestion and most nutrient absorption take place. As a result, you can't count on laxatives to prevent fat gain from excess energy intake.

laxative A medication or other substance that stimulates evacuation of the intestinal tract.

Critical | Thinking

Joci is considering going on a new diet that emphasizes eating only fruits before noon, meat at lunchtime, and starch and vegetables at dinner. In addition, the diet recommends "cleansing" the intestines with laxatives and enemas every other week. What reasons would you give Joci to steer clear of this regimen? What are some possible harmful effects that could result?

hemorrhoid A pronounced swelling in a large vein, particularly veins found in the anal region.

Eating foods with plenty of fiber, such as whole-grain breads and cereals, along with drinking more fluid to avoid dehydration, helps treat typical cases of mild constipation.[14] More serious cases require **laxative** therapy as well (see the next paragraph). Fiber stimulates peristalsis by drawing water into the large intestine and helping form a bulky, soft fecal output. Eating dried fruits also can help stimulate the bowel. In addition, people with constipation may need to develop more regular bowel habits; allowing the same time each day for a bowel movement can help train the large intestine to respond routinely. Finally, relaxation facilitates regular bowel movements, as does regular physical activity.

Laxatives can lessen more serious cases of constipation.[14] These work by irritating the intestinal nerve junctions to stimulate the peristaltic muscles, or by drawing water (by means of bulk-forming fiber) into the intestine to enlarge fecal output. The larger output stretches the peristaltic muscles, making them rebound and then constrict. Regular use of laxatives, however, should be under the supervision of a physician. Overall, for most people the bulk-forming fiber laxatives are the safest to use.

Hemorrhoids

Hemorrhoids, also called *piles,* are swollen veins of the rectum and anus. The blood vessels in this area are subject to intense pressure, especially during bowel movements. Added stress to the vessels from pregnancy, obesity, prolonged sitting, violent coughing or sneezing, or straining during bowel movements, particularly with constipation, can lead to a hemorrhoid. Hemorrhoids can develop unnoticed until a strained bowel movement precipitates symptoms, which may include pain, itching, and bleeding.

Itching, caused by moisture in the anal canal, swelling, or other irritation, is perhaps the most common symptom. Pain, if present, is usually aching and steady. Bleeding may result from a hemorrhoid and may appear in the toilet as a bright red streak in the feces. The sensation of a mass in the anal canal after a bowel movement is symptomatic of an internal hemorrhoid that protrudes through the anus.

Anyone can develop a hemorrhoid, and about half of adults over age 50 do. Pressure from prolonged sitting or exertion is often enough to bring on symptoms, although diet, lifestyle, and possibly heredity play a role. For example, a low-fiber diet can lead to hemorrhoids as a result of constipation and straining during bowel movements.[20] If you think you have a hemorrhoid, you should consult your physician. Rectal bleeding, although usually caused by hemorrhoids, may also indicate other problems, such as cancer.

A physician may suggest a variety of self-care measures for hemorrhoids. Pain can be lessened by applying warm, soft compresses or sitting in a tub of warm water for 15 to 20 minutes. Dietary recommendations are the same as those for treating mild constipation, emphasizing the need to consume adequate fiber and fluid. Over-the-counter remedies, such as Preparation H, can also offer relief of symptoms.

Irritable Bowel Syndrome

Many adults (25 million or more in the United States) have irritable bowel syndrome, a combination of cramps, gassiness, bloating, and irregular bowel function (diarrhea, constipation, or alternating episodes of both). It is more common in young women than in young men. The disease leads to about 3.5 million physician visits each year in the United States.

Symptoms associated with irritable bowel syndrome include visible abdominal distension, pain relief after a bowel movement, increased stool frequency with pain onset, looser stools with pain onset, mucus in the feces, and a feeling of incomplete elimination even after a bowel movement.[12]

The cause is thought to be altered intestinal peristalsis coupled with a decreased pain threshold for abdominal distension. In the latter case a minor amount of abdominal bloating causes pain that the average person would not sense. It is also noteworthy that up to 50% of sufferers report a history of verbal or sexual abuse.

Therapy is individualized and can include a trial of high-fiber foods and yogurt as well as elimination diets that focus on avoiding dairy products and gas-forming foods, such as legumes and certain vegetables (cabbage, beans, and broccoli) and fruits (grapes, raisins, cherries, and cantaloupe). The person should have only moderate caffeine intake or eliminate caffeine-containing foods and beverages altogether. Low-fat and more frequent, small meals may help the person since large meals can trigger contractions of the large intestine. Other strategies include a reduction in stress, psychological counseling, antidepressants, and other medications, such as diphenoxylate (Lomotil), alosetron (Lotronex), and tegaserod (Zelnorm).[12]

Referral to a registered dietitian can be beneficial, because many patients experience improvement with the elimination of specific problem foods, such as gas-forming foods. A good patient/physician relationship is also important for the treatment of irritable bowel syndrome. Although irritable bowel syndrome can be uncomfortable and upsetting, it is essentially harmless; it carries no risk for cancer or other serious digestive problems. The website www.ibsgroup.org provides further information.

Diarrhea

Diarrhea, a GI tract disease that generally lasts only a few days, is defined as increased fluidity, frequency, or amount of bowel movements compared to a person's usual pattern. Most cases of diarrhea result from infections in the intestines, with bacteria and viruses the usual offending agents. They produce substances that cause the intestinal cells to secrete fluid rather than absorb fluid. Another form of diarrhea can be caused by consumption of substances that are not readily absorbed, such as the sugar alcohol **sorbitol** found in sugarless gum (see Chapter 5).[2] When consumed in large amounts such unabsorbed substances draw excess water into the intestine, leading to diarrhea. Treatment of diarrhea generally requires drinking lots of fluid (to compensate for fluid losses); reduced intake of the poorly absorbed substance also is important if that is a cause. Prompt treatment—within 24 to 48 hours—is especially important for infants and older people, because they are more susceptible to the effects of dehydration associated with diarrhea (see Chapters 17 and 18). Diarrhea that lasts more than 7 days in adults should be investigated by a physician because it can be a symptom of more serious intestinal disease, especially if there is also blood in the feces.

sorbitol An alcohol derivative of glucose.

Gallstones

Gallstones are a major cause of illness and surgery, affecting 10 to 20% of U.S. adults. The stones themselves are pieces of solid material that develop in the gallbladder when substances in the bile—primarily cholesterol (80% of gallstones) and bile pigments (20%)—form crystal-like particles. Gallstones vary in size and may be as small as a grain of sand or as large as a golf ball.

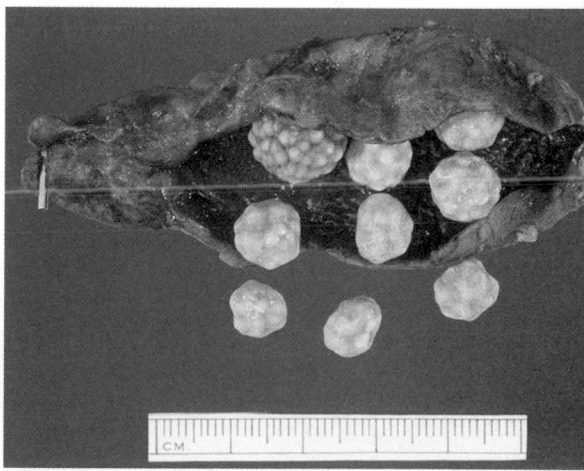

Gallbladder and gallstones seen after surgical removal from the body. Size and composition of the stones vary from one case to another.

(continued)

Gallstones are caused by a combination of factors, with excess weight being the primary modifiable factor, especially in women 20 to 60 years of age.[17] Excess body weight tends to reduce the amount of bile salts in bile, resulting in relatively more cholesterol in bile. Excess body weight also tends to reduce the ability of the gallbladder to empty properly. High blood insulin, which can develop from excess body weight, can also increase the cholesterol content of bile. Other risk factors include genetic background (e.g., Native Americans), advanced age (> 60 years for both women and men), reduced activity of the gallbladder (the gallbladder contracts less than normal), altered bile composition (too much cholesterol, too much **bilirubin,** or not enough bile salts), and diet (e.g., low-fiber diets). Excess estrogen from pregnancy, hormone replacement therapy, or birth control pills can lead to gallstones (from increased cholesterol levels in bile and decreased gallbladder movement). Gallstones also tend to develop in people who have diabetes (due to high blood insulin and triglycerides) liver cirrhosis, gallbladder infections, and various other diseases. In addition, gallstones may develop during rapid weight loss or prolonged fasting; as the liver metabolizes more body fat for energy needs, it secretes more cholesterol into the bile.

Most people with gallstones do not have symptoms; stones are usually detected during an examination for another illness. Symptoms can include intermittent pain in the right upper abdomen, pain between the shoulder blades or the right shoulder, nausea, or gas and bloating. Attacks may last from 20 to 30 minutes or as long as several hours. Once a true attack occurs, subsequent attacks are much more likely.

Sometimes gallstones may make their way out of the gallbladder and into the bile ducts. This blockage of flow can lead to fever, intermittent pain in the right upper abdomen, nausea with some vomiting, and **jaundice.** A blockage may also interfere with the flow of digestive enzymes from the pancreas into the small intestine, leading to inflammation of the pancreas.

Surgical removal of the gallbladder is the most common method for treating gallstones (500,000 surgeries per year in the United States). Nonsurgical treatments, used only in special situations, involve oral therapy with medications that dissolve gallstones. This treatment works best for small cholesterol gallstones.

Prevention of gallstones includes maintaining a healthy weight and avoiding overweight, especially for women. Avoiding rapid weight loss (> 3 lb per week), limiting intake of animal protein and focusing more on plant protein take, and following a high-fiber diet can help as well. Regular physical activity is also important. In addition, moderate caffeine and alcohol intake confers some protection.[17]

A Recap

Overall, typical medical disorders of the GI tract arise from differences in anatomical features and lifestyle habits among individuals. Because of the importance of various nutrition and lifestyle habits—such as adequate fiber and fluid intake, regular physical activity, not smoking, or not abusing NSAID medications—nutrition and lifestyle therapy is often effective in treating GI tract disorders.

The Physiology of Absorption

Most nutrient **absorption** occurs in the small intestine; the stomach and large intestine participate to a minor extent. The small intestine can ultimately absorb about 95% of the food energy it receives in the form of protein, carbohydrate, fat, and alcohol. In general, only water, a portion of alcohol intake, and a few forms of fats are absorbed to a significant extent by the stomach. Some minerals, water, and **short-chain fatty acids** (produced by bacterial action) are absorbed in the large intestine.[3]

The extent and efficiency of absorption in the small intestine are linked to its incredible surface area. The wall of the small intestine is folded, and within the folds are fingerlike projections called villi (Figure 3-13). The "fingers" trap nutrients between each

absorption The process by which nutrient molecules are absorbed by the GI tract and enter the bloodstream.

short-chain fatty acids Fatty acids that contain fewer than 6 carbon atoms.

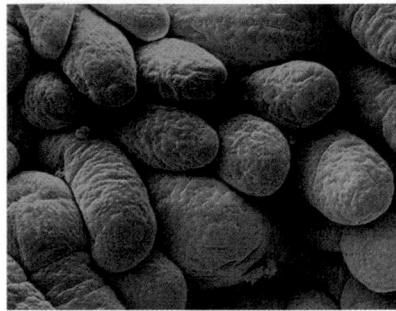

A close-up view of the intestinal villi.

Figure 3-13 | Organization of the small intestine. The small intestine has several structural levels. Because of the folds in the intestinal wall, the villi "fingers" that project into the intestine, and the brush border on each absorptive cell that makes up the villi, the surface area for absorption is up to 600 times that of a simple tube.

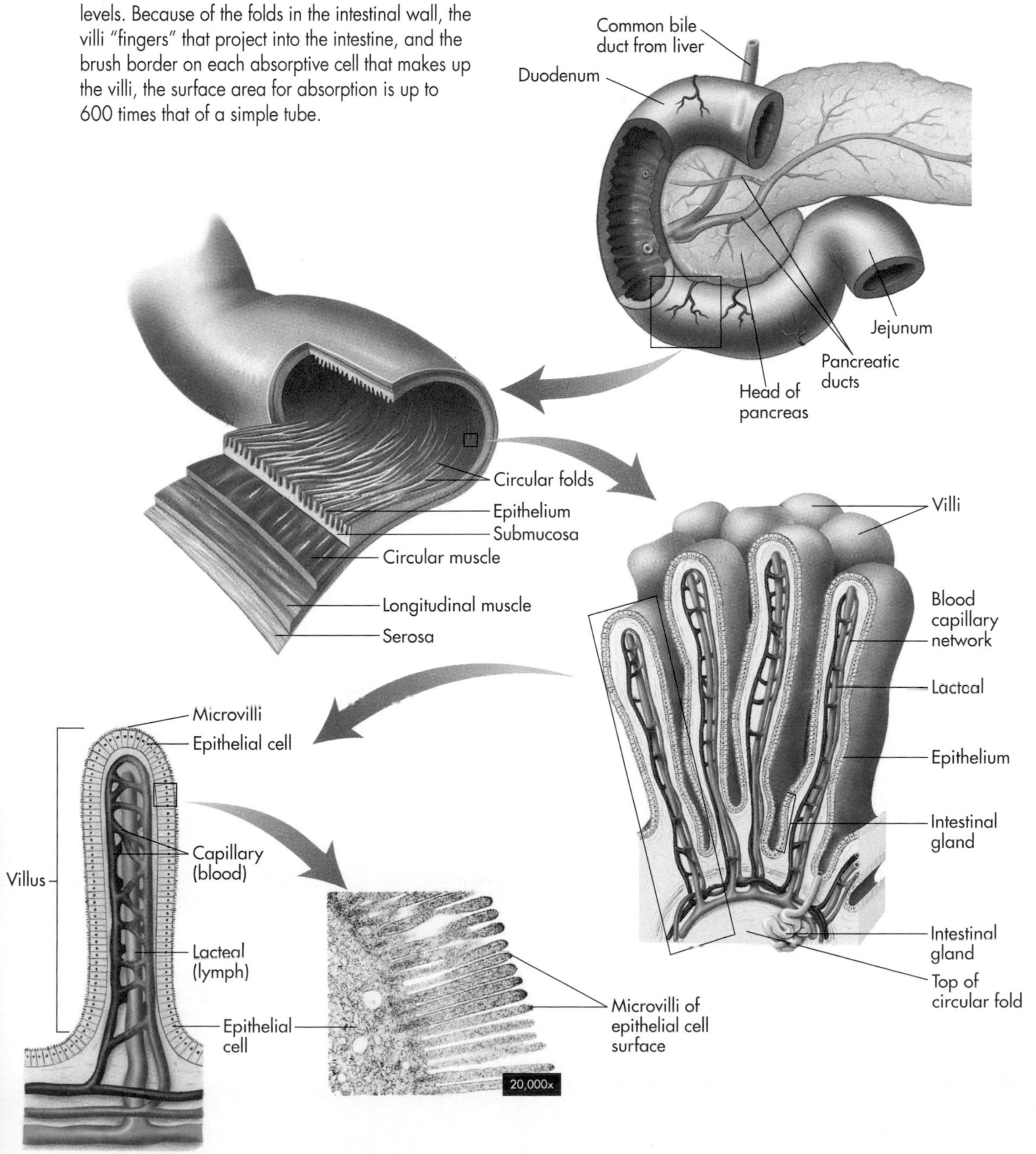

Common bile duct from liver
Duodenum
Jejunum
Pancreatic ducts
Head of pancreas

Circular folds
Epithelium
Submucosa
Circular muscle
Longitudinal muscle
Serosa

Villi
Blood capillary network
Lacteal
Epithelium
Intestinal gland
Intestinal gland
Top of circular fold

Microvilli
Epithelial cell
Villus
Capillary (blood)
Lacteal (lymph)
Epithelial cell
Microvilli of epithelial cell surface
20,000x

absorptive cells A class of cells, also called *enterocytes*, that cover the surface of the villi (fingerlike projections in the small intestine) and participate in nutrient absorption.

glycocalyx Projections of proteins on the *microvilli;* they contain enzymes to digest protein and carbohydrate.

mucosa Mucous membrane consisting of cells and supporting connective tissue. In the digestive tract there is also a layer of smooth muscle supporting the mucosa. Mucosa lines cavities that open to the outside of the body, such as the stomach and intestine, and generally contains glands that secrete mucus.

Critical | Thinking

Cancer treatments often involve the use of medications (chemotherapy) to prevent rapid cell production and growth. Cancer cells are the intended target. Diarrhea is a common side effect of chemotherapy. Why would this happen?

passive diffusion Absorption that requires permeability of the substance through the wall of the small intestine and a concentration gradient higher in the intestinal contents than in the absorptive cell.

lumen The inside of a tube, such as the inside cavity of the GI tract.

other to enhance absorption. Each villus "finger" is made up of numerous **absorptive cells** (enterocytes). Each of these cells has a brush border, made up of microvilli and covered with **glycocalyx.** Intestinal enzymes are often found on the glycocalyx. All these folds, fingers, and indentations in the small intestine increase its surface area 600 times beyond that of a simple tube.[5]

Absorptive Cells

The absorptive cells of the small intestine lie side by side with mucus-forming goblet cells as well as endocrine cells that produce hormones and hormonelike substances. All these cells form a principal part of the intestinal **mucosa.** The absorptive cells are produced in open-ended pits (called *crypts*) buried deep in the mucosa of the small intestine. They then migrate from the crypts to the tips of the villi. As the cells migrate, they mature, and their absorptive efficiency increases. By the time they reach the tips of the villi, however, they have been partially degraded by digestive enzymes and are ready to be sloughed off. Newly formed absorptive cells constantly migrate from the crypts to replace dying ones; this replacement takes approximately 2 to 5 days.[7] Since cell production requires a variety of nutrients, groups of cells undergoing constant replacement have a correspondingly enhanced need for nutrients. For this reason, the small intestine rapidly deteriorates during a nutrient deficiency or in semistarvation even though many of the old cells can be broken down and their components reused.

If a disease causes the villi to lie down, the surface area of the small intestine decreases and malabsorption results. This happens in **celiac disease** (also called *gluten-induced enteropathy*). This disease is caused by an allergic response to a protein called *gluten,* found in wheat, rye, barley, and buckwheat. To prevent attacks, any foods derived from these grains must be avoided.[1]

Types of Absorption

The wall of the small intestine absorbs nutrients through various means and processes that are illustrated in Figure 3-14:[18]

- **Passive diffusion:** When the nutrient concentration is higher in the cavity (**lumen**) of the small intestine than in the absorptive cells, the difference in nutrient concentration drives the nutrient into the absorptive cells by diffusion. Passive diffusion allows for the absorption of fats, water, and some minerals.

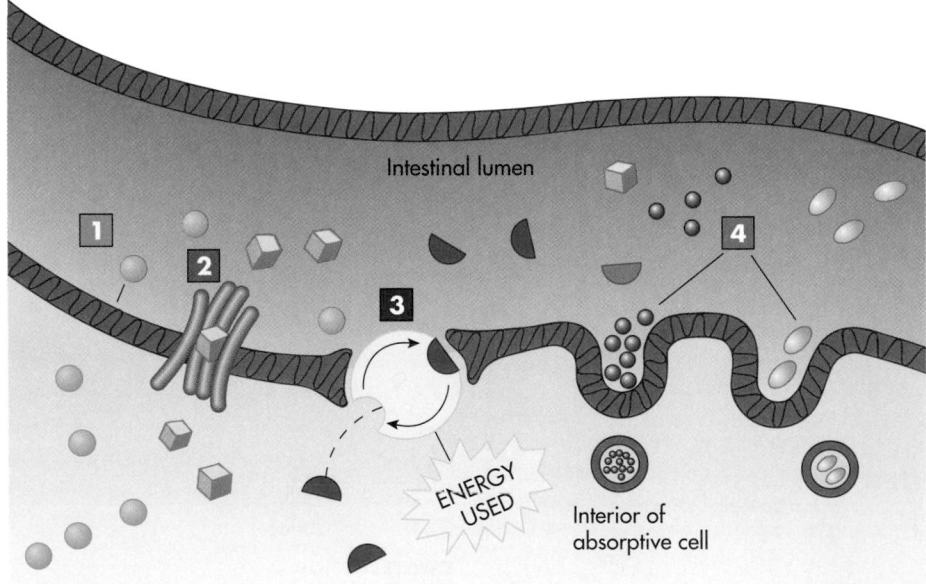

Figure 3-14 | Nutrient absorption relies on four major absorptive processes. Passive diffusion (color green) is simple diffusion of nutrients across the absorptive cell membranes. Facilitated diffusion (color blue) uses a carrier protein to move nutrients down a concentration gradient. Active absorption (color red) involves a carrier protein as well as energy to move nutrients (against a concentration gradient) into absorptive cells. Phagocytosis and pinocytosis (color orange) are forms of active transport in which the absorptive cell (yellow) membrane engulfs a nutrient to bring it into the cell.

- **Facilitated diffusion:** A difference in concentration is not enough to drive absorption of some nutrients into the absorptive cells by diffusion alone. Sometimes carrier proteins or other processes are required for absorption. Fructose is one example of a compound that makes use of facilitated diffusion.
- **Active absorption:** In addition to the need for a carrier protein, some nutrients also require energy input to move from the lumen of the small intestine into the absorptive cells. This mechanism makes it possible for cells to take up nutrients even when they are consumed in low concentrations. Some sugars, such as glucose, are actively absorbed, as are amino acids.
- **Phagocytosis and pinocytosis:** In a further means of active absorption, absorptive cells literally engulf compounds (phagocytosis) or liquids (pinocytosis). In these processes a cell membrane forms an indentation of itself so that when particles or fluids move into the indentation, the cell membrane surrounds and engulfs them. This process is especially used when a breastfeeding infant absorbs immune substances from human milk.

Portal and Lymphatic Circulation in Absorption

The villi in the intestine are drained by two different sets of vessels, portal and lymphatic (Figure 3-15). The nutrients follow one of these systems for absorption based on solubility in either (1) water or (2) organic solvents, such as chloroform and benzene. The nutrients that are soluble in water (proteins, carbohydrates, short- and **medium-chain fatty acids,** B vitamins, and vitamin C) are absorbed into the blood. Blood leaves the heart via the arteries, travels to the small intestine, and eventually ends up at the capillary beds inside the villi (review Figure 3-15).[3] The blood exits the capillary beds and collects in a large **portal vein,** which leads directly to the liver. This direct path enables the liver to process absorbed nutrients before they enter the general circulation. Blood flow used for portal absorption accounts for 30% of the heart's total output.

The **lymphatic system** also drains the villi. The lymphatic vessels carry particles that are either fat soluble (long-chain fatty acids and the fat-soluble vitamins A, D, E, and K) or too large to pass through the capillaries into the bloodstream (large proteins that escape from the bloodstream and **chylomicrons** that form after the absorption of fat).[3] Substances are squeezed through the spongelike vessels of the lymphatic system by muscular activity (see Figure C-5 in Appendix C). The lymphatic vessels from the intestine drain into the thoracic duct, which stretches from the abdomen to the neck. This duct is connected to the bloodstream via a large vein near the neck, the left subclavian vein.[5]

Enterohepatic Circulation

During meals, bile circulates through the liver to the gallbladder, through the small intestine into the portal vein, and then returns to the liver. This recycling is called **enterohepatic circulation** (Figure 3-16). Approximately 98% of the bile is recycled; only 1 to 2% is removed from the body by elimination in the feces.[3] (See Chapter 6 for a practical application of the knowledge of this process, employed by a class of blood cholesterol–lowering medications and certain brands of margarine and salad dressings.)

Concept | Check

The small intestine is the major site for absorption. Numerous folds and fingerlike projections increase the surface area to 600 times that of a simple tube. This provides a large area for nutrient absorption. Absorptive cells have a life span of 2 to 5 days, so the lining of the small intestine is constantly being renewed. These cells perform passive diffusion, promoted by a concentration gradient; facilitated diffusion, promoted by a concentration gradient plus a carrier; and active absorption, which uses energy in addition to a carrier to work against a concentration gradient. Absorptive cells also engulf compounds and liquids via

facilitated diffusion Absorption in which a carrier shuttles substances into the absorptive cell but no energy is expended. A concentration gradient higher in the intestinal contents than in the absorptive cell drives the absorption.

active absorption Absorption using a carrier and expending ATP energy. In this way the absorptive cell can absorb nutrients, such as glucose, against a concentration gradient.

endocytosis (phagocytosis/pinocytosis) Forms of active absorption in which the absorptive cell forms an indentation in its membrane, and particles (phagocytosis) or fluids (pinocytosis) entering the indentation are then engulfed by the cell.

medium-chain fatty acids A fatty acid that contains 6 to 10 carbons. Short-chain fatty acids contain fewer than 6 carbons.

portal vein A large vein leaving from the intestine and stomach that connects to the liver.

lymphatic system A system of vessels that can accept fluid surrounding cells and large particles, such as products of fat absorption. This lymph fluid eventually passes into the bloodstream via the lymphatic system.

chylomicron Lipoprotein made of dietary fats that are surrounded by a shell of cholesterol, phospholipids, and protein. Chylomicrons are formed in the absorptive cells (enterocytes) in the small intestine after fat absorption and travel through the lymphatic system to the bloodstream.

enterohepatic circulation A continual recycling of compounds between the small intestine and the liver; bile acids are one example of a recycled compound.

Critical | Thinking

The medical history of a young girl who is greatly underweight shows that she had three-quarters of her small intestine removed after she was injured in a car accident. Explain how this accounts for her underweight condition, even though her medical chart shows that she eats well.

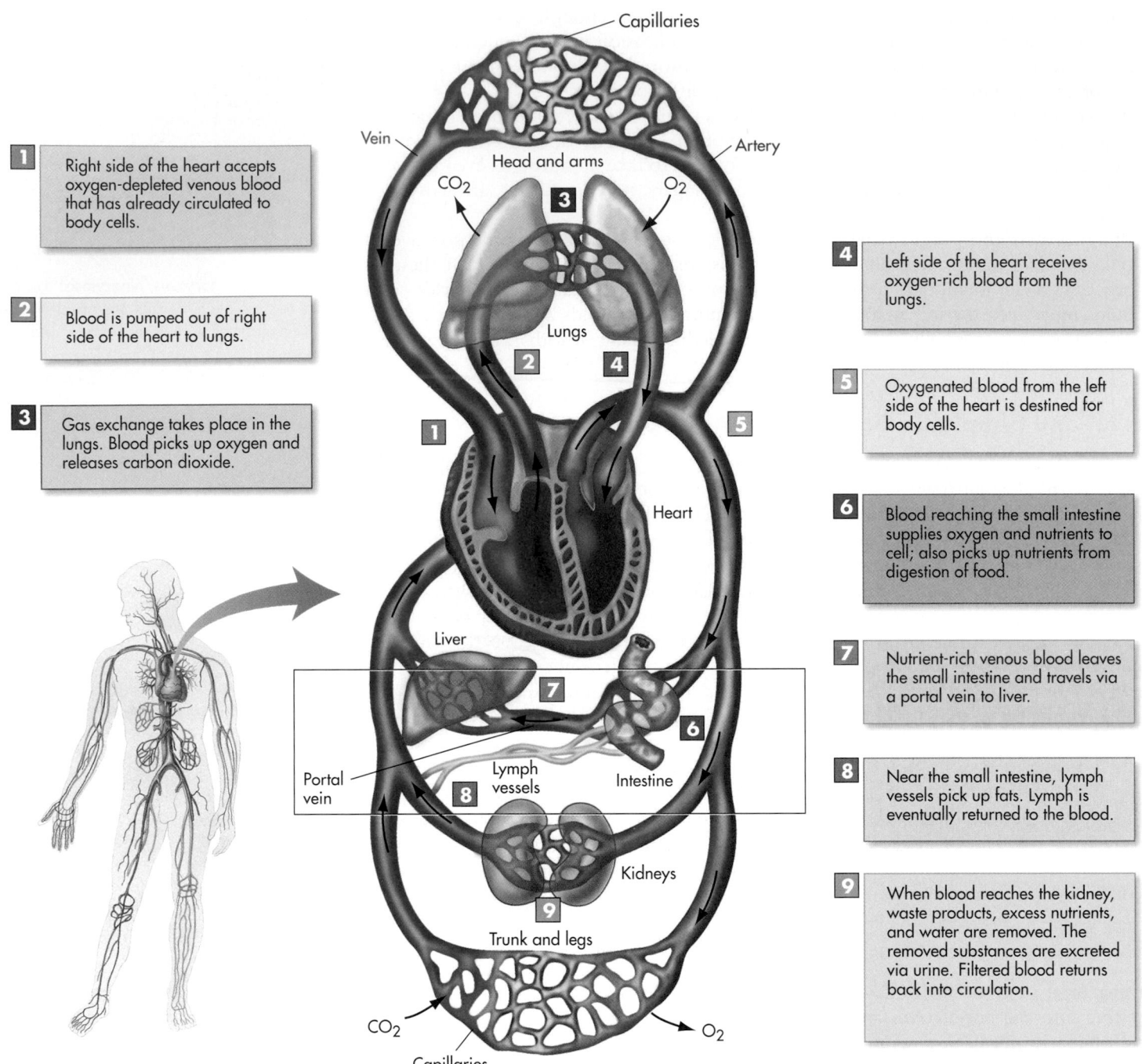

1 Right side of the heart accepts oxygen-depleted venous blood that has already circulated to body cells.

2 Blood is pumped out of right side of the heart to lungs.

3 Gas exchange takes place in the lungs. Blood picks up oxygen and releases carbon dioxide.

4 Left side of the heart receives oxygen-rich blood from the lungs.

5 Oxygenated blood from the left side of the heart is destined for body cells.

6 Blood reaching the small intestine supplies oxygen and nutrients to cell; also picks up nutrients from digestion of food.

7 Nutrient-rich venous blood leaves the small intestine and travels via a portal vein to liver.

8 Near the small intestine, lymph vessels pick up fats. Lymph is eventually returned to the blood.

9 When blood reaches the kidney, waste products, excess nutrients, and water are removed. The removed substances are excreted via urine. Filtered blood returns back into circulation.

Figure 3-15 | Blood circulation through the body. This figure shows the paths that blood takes from the heart to the lungs (1–3), back to the heart (4), and through the rest of the body (5–9). The reddish-orange color indicates blood that is richer in oxygen; blue is for blood carrying more carbon dioxide. Keep in mind that arteries and veins go to all parts of the body. Pay particular attention to sites 7 and 8. These sites are key parts of the process of nutrient absorption.

endocytosis (phagocytosis/pinocytosis). The products of absorption, if water soluble, pass into the portal vein that drains the intestine and enter the liver. The products of fat digestion mostly enter the lymphatic system and then the bloodstream. Some participants in digestion, such as bile, are reabsorbed after use in the small intestine and returned to the liver, to be sent back again to the small intestine during another round of digestion. This circulation is called *enterohepatic circulation*.

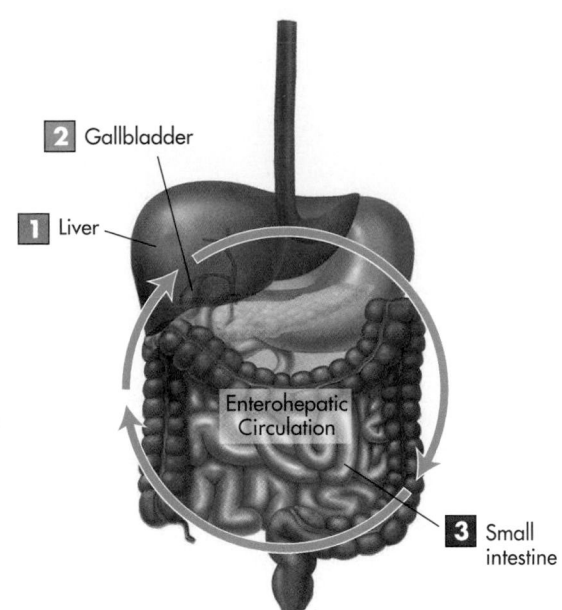

2 Gallbladder

1 Liver

Enterohepatic
Circulation

3 Small
intestine

Figure 3-16 | Enterohepatic circulation. To view this circulation, start at the liver. It secretes substances, such as bile acids, that collect in the gallbladder. The gallbladder empties these substances into the small intestine. There, some of the substances are then absorbed by the small intestine and returned to the liver through a portal vein. In this way some substances, such as bile acids, can be recycled by the liver for reuse.

Absorption Is Completed in the Large Intestine

The small intestine is responsible for about 90% of the water absorbed from the GI tract (Figure 3-17). This absorption reduces the 10 liters (L) the GI tract receives (3 L of dietary fluid plus 7 L of GI tract secretions) to about 1.5 L. The remnants of digestion that enter the large intestine are the remaining water, some minerals, and undigested food fibers and starches. Only a minor amount (5%) of carbohydrate, protein, and fat escapes absorption in the small intestine.[3]

The large intestine absorbs primarily sodium and potassium, along with some water, leaving very little water unabsorbed (Figure 3-18). This absorption occurs mostly in the first half of the large intestine. Short-chain fatty acids made from both the bacterial **fermentation** of some plant fibers and undigested starches are also absorbed in the large intestine, along with some vitamins synthesized by bacteria, such as vitamin K and biotin. Dr. Steve Hertzler discusses the latest findings on the effects of this bacterial action in the Expert Opinion on probiotics.[7,16] By the time the contents of the large intestine pass through the first two-thirds of its length, a semisolid mass is formed. This mass remains in the large intestine until peristaltic waves and mass movements push it into the rectum for elimination through the anus (Table 3-5).[5]

fermentation The metabolism, without the use of oxygen, of carbohydrates to alcohols, acids, and carbon dioxide.

Table 3-5 | A Summary of Digestion Functions, Organ by Organ

Organ	Functions
Mouth	Chewing of food Some digestion of starch
Esophagus	Passageway
Stomach	Food storage; acidity kills bacteria Some digestion of protein
Small intestine	Final digestion of all energy-yielding nutrients Absorption of nutrients
Large intestine	Absorption of water and some minerals; storage of nondigestible remains
Anus	Elimination of waste as feces
Liver	Production of bile
Gallbladder	Storage and release of bile
Pancreas	Production and release of enzymes and bicarbonate into the small intestine

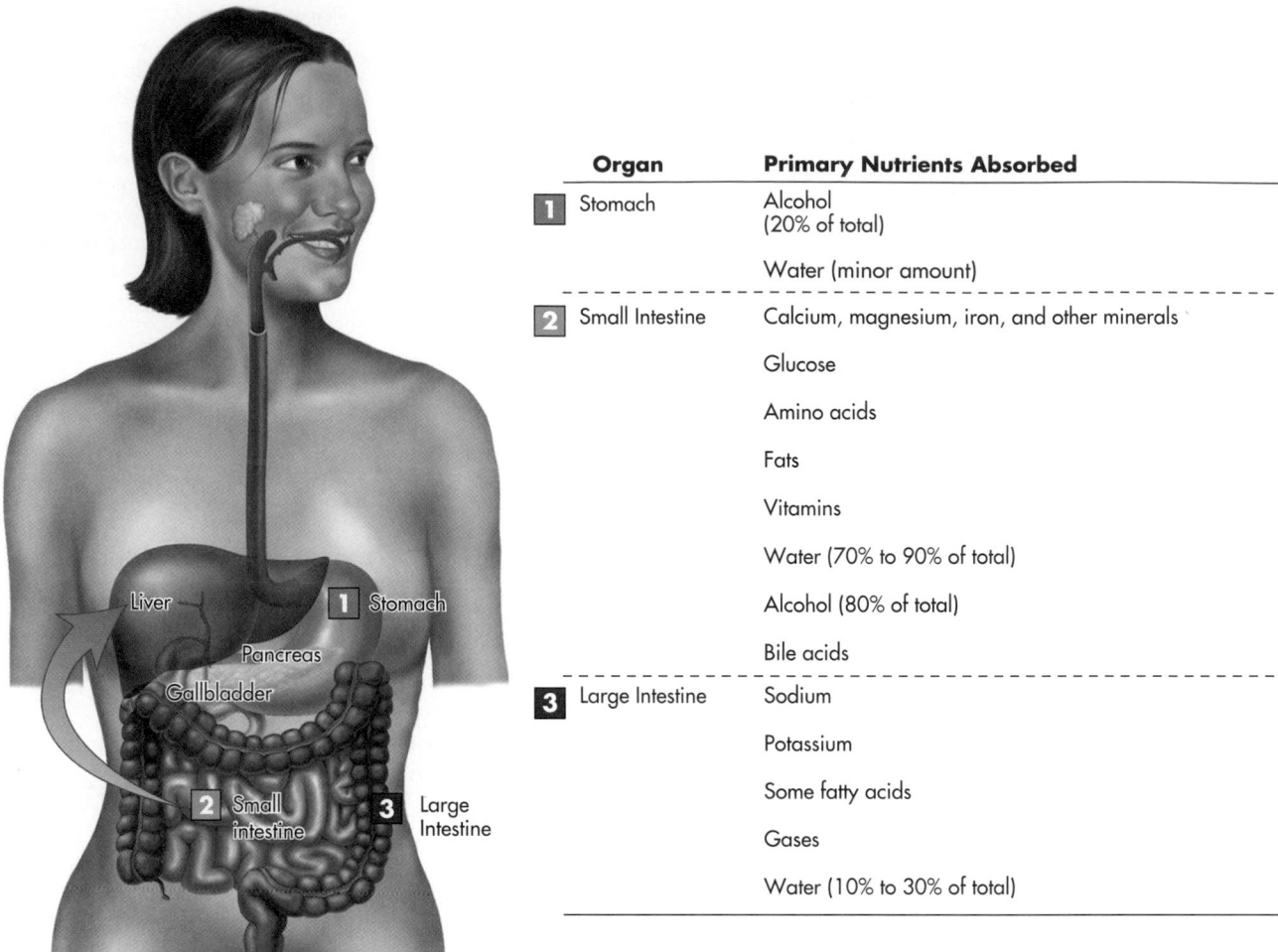

Organ	Primary Nutrients Absorbed
1 Stomach	Alcohol (20% of total)
	Water (minor amount)
2 Small Intestine	Calcium, magnesium, iron, and other minerals
	Glucose
	Amino acids
	Fats
	Vitamins
	Water (70% to 90% of total)
	Alcohol (80% of total)
	Bile acids
3 Large Intestine	Sodium
	Potassium
	Some fatty acids
	Gases
	Water (10% to 30% of total)

Figure 3-17 | Major sites of absorption along the GI tract. Note that some absorption of vitamin K and biotin takes place in the large intestine. All nutrients except most of those that are fat soluble travel through the portal vein to the liver after their absorption.

The presence of feces in the rectum powerfully stimulates defecation. This process involves muscular reflexes in the sigmoid colon and rectum as well as relaxation of the two anal sphincters (one internal and one external; only the external sphincter is under voluntary control). The feces primarily consist of indigestible plant fibers, tough connective tissue from animal foods, and bacteria from the large intestine.[7]

Storage Capabilities of the Body

Nutrient intake also directly influences nutrient absorption. For example, vitamin C in a meal increases iron absorption in the same meal because it changes iron into a more absorbable state.

The human body must maintain reserves of nutrients. Otherwise, we would need to eat continuously. Storage capacity varies for each nutrient. Most fat is stored at sites designed specifically for this—adipose tissue. Short-term storage of carbohydrate occurs in muscle and liver, and the blood maintains a small reserve of glucose and amino acids. Many vitamins and minerals are stored in the liver, while other nutrient stores are found at other sites in the body.[18]

When people do not meet their nutrient needs, some nutrients are obtained by breaking down a tissue that contains high concentrations of the nutrient. Calcium is taken from bone and protein is taken from muscle. These nutrient losses in cases of long-term deficiency harm these tissues.

Many people believe that if too much of a nutrient is obtained—for example, from a vitamin or mineral supplement—only what is needed is stored and the rest is excreted

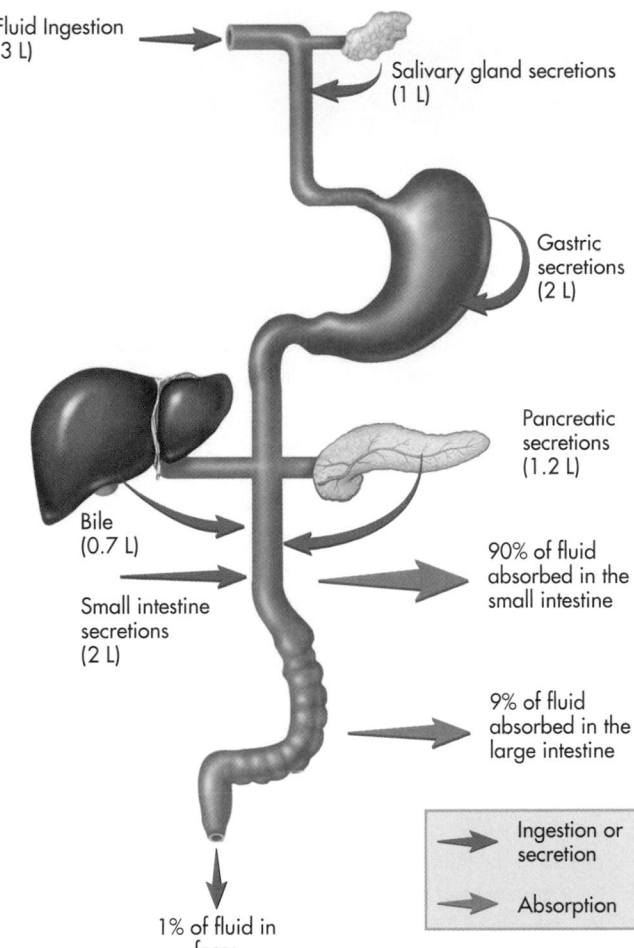

Fluid Ingestion
(3 L)

Salivary gland secretions
(1 L)

Gastric
secretions
(2 L)

Pancreatic
secretions
(1.2 L)

Bile
(0.7 L)

90% of fluid
absorbed in the
small intestine

Small intestine
secretions
(2 L)

9% of fluid
absorbed in the
large intestine

Ingestion or
secretion

Absorption

1% of fluid in
feces

Figure 3-18 | Fluid volumes in the GI tract. The body primarily relies on the small intestine to absorb the fluid that enters the GI tract from ingestion and various secretions.

by the body. This is true for many vitamins and minerals. However, large dosages of vitamin A can cause harmful side effects because it is not readily excreted. This is one reason why obtaining your nutrients primarily (or exclusively) from a balanced diet, rather than relying on supplements, is the safest means to acquire the building blocks you need to maintain good health.

This review of human anatomy and physiology from a digestion and absorption perspective sets the stage for a more detailed understanding of the nutrients. Chapters 5, 6, and 7 will build on this information.

Concept | Check

Some water and mineral absorption occurs in the large intestine. The remaining contents form the feces, which consist primarily of indigestible plant fibers, tough connective tissue from animal foods, and bacteria. Nutrients are constantly present in the blood for immediate use and are stored to a greater or lesser extent in body tissues for later use when sufficient amounts from food intake are unavailable. However, when the body suffers a nutrient deficiency caused by an inadequate diet, it breaks down vital tissues for their nutrients, which can lead to ill health. Additionally, too much of any nutrient can be detrimental. It's best to focus primarily (or exclusively) on obtaining all essential nutrients from a balanced diet.

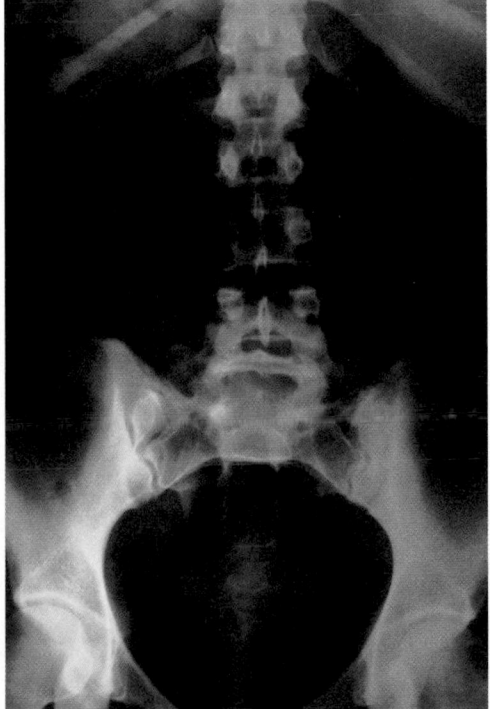

The skeletal system provides a reserve of calcium for day-to-day needs when dietary intake is inadequate. Long-term use of this reserve, however, reduces bone strength.

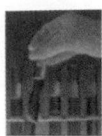

Expert Opinion

Probiotics and Human Health
Steve Hertzler, Ph.D., R.D.

The Bacteria Down Below

How much do you weigh? Have you ever stopped to think that a full 1.25 kg (almost 3 lb) of your body weight is made up of microorganisms? There are about 100 trillion microbial cells in the body, an amount that is 10 times larger than the number of human cells. The vast majority of these cells exist in the gastrointestinal tract, mainly in the colon. On a daily basis, these microbes perform many metabolic functions, some of them beneficial to our health and some that are potentially damaging. Striking an appropriate balance between a healthy and unhealthy intestinal microflora is becoming increasingly recognized as an important contributor to overall health. Probiotics are one such strategy for maintaining this balance. (A related term is prebiotics. These compounds stimulate the growth of bacteria in the colon [e.g., fructooligosaccharides]).

The sales of probiotics in the United States have increased by 19% annually for the last two years, with estimated sales of $764 million for 2005 (includes yogurts and cultured drinks). Are probiotics worth this kind of investment?

Probiotics: A Definition

Probiotics, a phrase that originated in Greek as "for life," are defined by the World Health Organization as "live microorganisms which, when administered in adequate amounts, confer a health benefit on the host." Thus, the probiotic approach involves the feeding of live bacterial cells, mainly lactic acid–producing bacteria (e.g., the *Lactobacillus* or *Bifidobacterium* genera), in foods or as dietary supplements. Numerous studies have shown that lactic acid produced by these organisms tends to inhibit the growth of less acid-tolerant organisms such as *Escherichia coli* and the genus *Clostridium* that are generally regarded as harmful.

Challenges for Probiotics in the Body

Key requirements for the successful use of probiotics are the survival of the probiotic organism as it makes its way through the gastrointestinal tract and the subsequent colonization of the organism in the gut. The hurdles that probiotic bacteria face include destruction by stomach or bile acids and competition with other bacteria in the colon. One method for overcoming this problem is the selection of probiotic bacteria that are highly resistant to stomach and bile acids and that also possess the ability to colonize the gas-trointestinal tract. This approach required meticulous laboratory testing of many bacterial strains using *in vitro* (i.e., test tube) systems that can only roughly approximate actual conditions inside the body.

Probiotics and the Gastrointestinal Tract

Despite the challenges associated with probiotic survival, the evidence for the health benefits of certain probiotics continues to accumulate, especially for conditions of the gastrointestinal tract. For example, the use of probiotics to reduce the colonization of the stomach by *Helicobacter pylori*, the main causative agent of stomach ulcers, is one promising approach. Several *Lactobacillus* strains have been shown to be inhibitory toward the growth of *H. pylori*, both in a test tube and in experimental animals (mice). However, studies in humans have shown only limited or no success of probiotics, and probiotics have never been as effective as medical treatments for eradication of this organism. Some studies suggest that it may take up to 18 weeks of probiotic administration for beneficial effects to be observed.

It appears that probiotics are particularly important for helping to maintain the integrity of the intestinal wall, which serves as a barrier to incoming disease-causing microorganisms and toxins. This benefit is likely the result of the interaction between probiotic bacteria and immune cells found in the wall of the intestine. Such an interaction can reduce inflammation, a key factor in diseases such as Crohn's disease and ulcerative colitis. There are exciting new findings that a type of *E. coli* (the Nissle 1917 strain) given daily for 1 year was just as effective as a standard medication (mesalazine) in maintaining the remission of ulcerative colitis. The specific type of *E. coli* used in this study is safe and had no greater side effects than mesalazine treatment. Further, a new study suggests that probiotics, the *Bifidobacterium infantis* 35624 strain in particular, may be effective in reducing the symptoms of irritable bowel syndrome by limiting a tendency toward inflammation.

Finally, some of the strongest evidence for probiotics relates to the prevention and treatment of several types of diarrhea, including traveler's diarrhea, relapsing *Clostridium difficile*–induced enteritis and diarrhea, rotavirus diarrhea in infants, antibiotic-associated diarrhea, and diarrhea associated with tube feedings in hospitalized patients. A meta-analysis (summary of several studies grouped together) of 9 studies showed a 61 to 66% reduction in the risk of antibiotic-associated diarrhea when probiotics were given concurrently. Probiotic organisms used

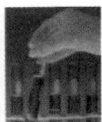

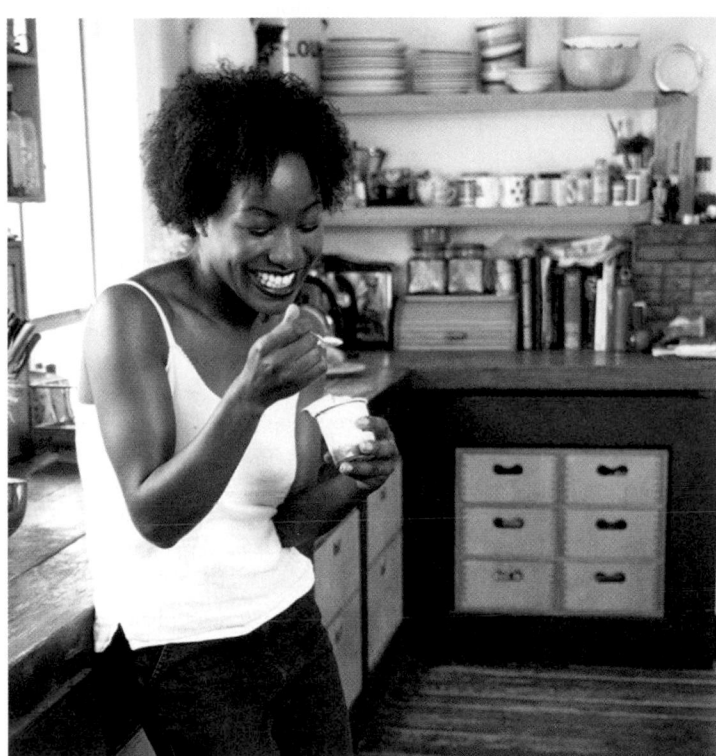

Yogurt is a convenient source of probiotic bacteria for your diet. These bacteria contribute to GI tract health.

for the prevention and treatment of diarrhea include *Lactobacillus rhamnosus* GG, *Saccharomyces boulardii*, *Enterococcus faecium* SF68, *Bifidobacterium bifidum*, and *Streptococcus thermophilus*. In addition to the prevention of diarrhea caused by pathogenic microganisms, diarrhea caused by lactose intolerance can be reduced as well. Previous studies have clearly shown that fermented dairy foods such as yogurt, which contain live cultures, can improve lactose digestion in the small intestine. My laboratory has demonstrated that kefir, a type of fermented milk that is like a drinkable yogurt, improves lactose digestion similarly to yogurt.

Probiotics and Allergy

Because of the involvement of probiotics in immune responses, there has recently been great interest in whether probiotics may lessen the chances of allergies to foods or other substances. The exposure of infants to the probiotic *Lactobacillus* GG at the time near birth reduces by 50% the number of cases of atopic eczema (skin rash due to allergy) at the age of 2 years. Further, a recent study suggests that this benefit is maintained up to the age of 4. It is unclear yet whether probiotics have an effect on respiratory allergic diseases that develop later in life. However, in this recent study, the excretion of lower levels of nitric oxide in the breath of children exposed to probiotics suggests that the placebo group may have had more underdiagnosed or subclinical respiratory allergic diseases.

Probiotics: The Advantages and Disadvantages

The research literature on probiotics has expanded greatly in recent years and covers many more conditions than have been mentioned in this feature. Probiotics may be involved in the prevention of various infections (e.g., yeast infections), may help to lower blood cholesterol and blood pressure, and may be involved to some degree in cancer prevention. In addition, probiotics are relatively inexpensive (a month's supply of *Lactobacillus* GG, sold under the brand name Culturelle, costs only about $20). So, what are the potential downsides of probiotics? First, many of the probiotic bacterial strains used in research are not available to the general public. Second, because probiotics are typically classified as dietary supplements in the United States, they are not subject to strict regulation by FDA for product quality, efficacy, and safety in the same way that pharmaceuticals are. Thus, "the buyer beware" attitude still applies to most probiotic supplements on the market. Clearly, the future for probiotics is bright, but much work needs to be done to ensure that consumers can purchase reliable and effective products.

Dr. Hertzler is currently Assistant Professor of Human Nutrition at The Ohio State University. He earned his Ph.D. in human nutrition from The University of Minnesota in 1995 and studies carbohydrate metabolism, glycemic index, lactose intolerance, and probiotics.

Summary

1. The basic structural unit of the human body is the cell. Cellular structure varies according to the type of job the cell must perform.
2. Cells join together to make up tissues; tissues unite to form organs; and organs work together as an organ system.
3. The gastrointestinal (GI) tract consists of the mouth, esophagus, stomach, small intestine, large intestine (colon), rectum, and anus. Most absorption of nutrients occurs in the small intestine.
4. The salivary glands, liver, gallbladder, and pancreas participate in digestion and absorption. Products from the last three organs enter the small intestine where enzymes and bile play important roles in digesting protein, fat, and carbohydrates.
5. The GI tract contains valves (sphincters) that control the flow of food. Muscular contractions, called *peristalsis,* propel the food down the GI tract. Segmentation contractions mechanically break down and mix the intestinal contents. Nerves, hormones, and hormonelike compounds control the activity of the sphincters and peristaltic and segmentation processes.
6. The mouth chews food to break it into smaller parts, increasing its surface area, which enhances enzyme activity. Some starch digestion occurs in the mouth. Protein digestion begins in the stomach. Carbohydrate and protein digestion are finished in the small intestine, where fat digestion begins in earnest and is completed. Some plant fibers are digested by the bacteria present in the large intestine; undigested plant fibers exit the body in the feces.
7. Digestive enzymes are secreted by the mouth, stomach, pancreas, and cells forming the wall of the small intestine. Bile needed for fat digestion is synthesized by the liver, stored in the gallbladder, and released in digestion.
8. The major absorptive sites are fingerlike projections in the small intestine called *villi.* The absorptive cells that cover the villi are replaced every 2 to 5 days. Thus the intestinal lining continually renews itself. Absorptive cells can perform passive diffusion, facilitated diffusion, and active absorption, as well as endocytosis (phagocytosis/pinocytosis), a specific type of active absorption.
9. Water-soluble compounds in the absorptive cells, such as glucose and amino acids, enter the portal vein that drains the intestine and travel to the liver. Fat-soluble compounds enter the lymphatic system, which eventually connects to the bloodstream. Some substances used in digestion, such as bile, are absorbed by the small intestine, sent back to the liver through the portal vein, and released into the small intestine again to act in further digestion of food. This recycling is called enterohepatic circulation.
10. Final water and mineral absorption, as well as absorption of products from bacterial metabolism of some plant fibers, occurs in the large intestine. Once the feces enter the rectum, the impetus for elimination is strong.
11. Limited stores of nutrients are present in the blood for immediate use and stored to a greater or lesser extent in body tissues for later use when sufficient food is unavailable. When the body suffers a nutrient deficiency it breaks down vital tissues for their nutrients, which can lead to ill health. Additionally, too much of any nutrient can be detrimental.

Study Questions

1. Identify at least one contribution to overall nutrition status provided by each of the 12 organ systems of the body.
2. Contrast passive diffusion and active absorption. Indicate the role of ATP, if any.
3. Outline the possible results on digestion and absorption of a diseased pancreas.
4. Describe why the small intestine is better suited than the other GI tract organs to carry out the absorptive process.
5. Identify the two organs that empty their contents into the small intestine. How do the digestive substances made by these organs contribute to the digestion of food?
6. Where is hydrochloric acid (HCl) secreted, and how is its production regulated? What are its roles in digestion?
7. Describe the actions of the digestive hormones.
8. Describe the actions of the digestive enzymes and explain how they function in digestion.
9. How is blood routed through the digestive system? Which nutrients enter the bloodstream directly? Which nutrients are first absorbed into the lymph?
10. The body has the ability to recycle some substances. How is this true for the digestive tract?

Annotated References

1. Against the grain: Who needs to avoid wheat? *Consumer Reports on Health*, p. 10, July 2005.

   Although a high-fiber diet leads to many health benefits, using wheat products to achieve such a goal is harmful for people with celiac disease. It is especially important that people who experience flushing, itching, hives, vomiting, or breathing difficulties within two hours of eating wheat be tested for the disease. The article discusses methods of diagnosis and treatment for celiac disease.

2. Baum C and others: Gastrointestinal disease. In Bowman BA, Russell RM (eds.): *Present knowledge in nutrition.* 8th ed. Washington, DC: ISLI Press, 2001.

   Disruption in any number of the steps in the digestive process can lead to malabsorption and in turn to protein, energy, and micronutrient deficiencies. Just as the GI tract is essential for nutrient utilization, ingested nutrients also play an active role in maintaining gastrointestinal health and function.

3. Bender DA, Mayes PA: Nutrition, digestion and absorption. In Murray RK and others (eds.): *Harper's illustrated biochemistry.* 26th ed. New York: Lange Medical Books/McGraw-Hill, 2003.

   Most foodstuffs ingested are initially unavailable to humans; they cannot be absorbed by the digestive system until broken down into smaller molecules. This chapter provides a clear step-by-step description of this digestion and subsequent absorption.

4. Devault KR: Gastroesophageal reflux: Medical and surgical options. *American Family Physician* 68:1271, 2003.

   Medications such as proton pump inhibitors are helpful in treating gastroesophageal reflux disease. The surgical treatments are much more risky, and so use must be carefully considered.

5. Ganong WF: *Review of medical physiology.* 25th ed. New York: Lange Medical Books/McGraw-Hill, 2001.

   This text is an excellent resource for learning more about digestion and absorption. Specific chapters refer to the general process of digestion and absorption as well as regulation of gastrointestinal function.

6. Granner DK: Hormones of the pancreas and gastrointestinal tract. In Murray RK and others (eds.): *Harper's biochemistry.* 25th ed. Stamford, CT: Appleton & Lange, 2000.

   The gastrointestinal tract secretes many hormones, perhaps more than any other organ system. Gastrointestinal hormones assist in all the functions of the GI tract, including the propelling of foodstuffs to sites of digestion, providing the proper environment for digestive processes, and moving digestive products across the intestinal mucosa.

7. Gropper SS and others: Advanced nutrition and human metabolism. 4th ed. Belmont, CA: Thomson Wadsworth, 2005.

   Chapter 2 of this textbook provides a detailed description of the digestive processes of the human body. Students seeking more details about digestion and absorption will find this chapter helpful.

8. Heidelbaugh JJ and others: Management of gastroesophageal reflux disease. *American Family Physician* 68:1311, 2003.

   It is important to treat recurring heartburn because it can lead to a form of esophageal cancer. Reducing the size of meals and elevating the head of the bed are two lifestyle considerations. Acid-blocking medications are very helpful; types and use of such medications are summarized in the article.

9. Klein S and others: The alimentary tract in nutrition: In Shils ME and others (eds.): *Health and disease.* 10th ed. Philadelphia, PA: Lippincott. Williams & Wilkins, 2006.

   This chapter is a review of the GI tract structure, blood supply, nervous system control, GI tract hormones, nutrient absorption, intestinal microorganisms, and immune system. The response of the GI tract to food is also explained.

10. Le Coutre J: Taste: the metabolic sense. *Food Technology* 57(8):34, 2003.

    The primary taste sensations are sweet, salt, sour, and bitter. Umami rounds out the list. Research into the use of this knowledge of taste perception to improve the taste of some foods is ongoing.

11. Liebman B: Who you gonna call? Gasbusters. *Nutrition Action Healthletter*, p. 1, May 2003.
    This article focuses on an interview with Dr. Michael Levitt, a noted expert on intestinal gas. Causes and treatment for uncomfortable cases are reviewed, such as the possible link to lactose maldigestion, sorbitol intake, and consumption of beans and various vegetables. Some people are bothered more by this gas production than others; some people experience few or no symptoms from daily gas production.

12. Mertz HR: Irritable bowel disease. *The New England Journal of Medicine* 349:2136, 2003.
    The most common symptoms of irritable bowel syndrome include a change in the appearance or frequency of stools, and abdominal pain that is relieved by defecation. Affected people should especially seek medical help if weight loss, GI tract bleeding, fever, or frequent nighttime symptoms are present. In some cases increasing fiber intake is helpful. Regular yogurt consumption may also be helpful because it can increase the concentration of beneficial types of bacteria that reside in the large intestine.

13. Meurer LN, Bower DJ: Management of Helicobactor pylori infection. *American Family Physician* 65:1327, 2002.
    Helicobactor pylori is the cause of most peptic ulcer disease and is also a risk factor for gastric cancer. Eradication of this organism is important for ulcer healing and reducing the risk of ulcer reoccurrence. Generally a two-week period of antibiotics and acid suppression is employed. Follow-up testing with analysis of breath or fecal samples is recommended for people who do not respond to therapy.

14. Muller-Lisser SA and others. Myths and misconceptions about constipation. *American Journal of Gastroenterology* 100:232, 2005.
    Increasing fiber intake and avoiding dehydration often helps in mild cases of constipation. More difficult cases require a careful physician evaluation and likely the use of laxatives and other medications. Often the latter are very helpful and are reviewed in the article.

15. Nilsson M and others: Obesity and estrogen as risk factors for gastroesophageal reflux symptoms. *Journal of the American Medical Association* 290:66, 2003.
    Obesity is a major risk factor for gastrointestinal reflux disease. Production of estrogen by adipose tissue is one likely reason for the relationship. Weight loss reverses the course of the disease and so is very beneficial to these persons.

16. Sanders ME: Probiotics: Considerations for human health. *Nutrition Reviews* 61(3):91, 2003.
    Probiotic microorganisms may play an important role in helping the body protect itself from infection, especially that which arises along the interior surfaces of the gastrointestinal tract. In North America foods currently containing probiotics are exclusively dairy products, such as yogurt, some forms of milk, some forms of cottage cheese, and a few other products.

17. Schardt D: Not everybody must get stones. *Nutrition Action Healthletter*, p. 8, November 2004.
    Excess body weight is the primary modifiable risk factor for developing gallbladder stones. Low-fiber diets are also implicated.

18. Seeley RR and others: *Anatomy and physiology.* 7th ed. Boston: McGraw-Hill, 2006.
    This text provides comprehensive coverage of the anatomy and physiology of the gastrointestinal tract as well as other related body systems.

19. Smith L: Updated ACG guidelines for diagnosis and treatment of GERD. *American Family Physician* 71:2376, 2005.
    The article outlines the diagnosis and treatment of GERD. The authors suggest that simple diet and lifestyle changes, such as avoiding high-fat meals and not lying down immediately after a meal, can help treat the disease in many cases.

20. The low-down on hemorrhoids. *UC Berkeley Wellness Letter*, p. 4, July, 2004.
    Hemorrhoids are commonly experienced by many adults. Measures to reduce such risk and as well treat the problem are discussed, such as an adequate fluid and fiber intake. Fortunately hemorrhoids rarely lead to serious health problems.

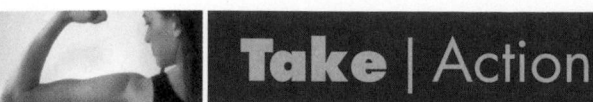

I. Are You Taking Care of Your Digestive Tract?

All of us need to think about the health of our digestive tracts. There are symptoms we need to notice as well as habits we need to practice in order to protect our GI tracts. The following assessment is designed to help you examine habits and symptoms associated with the health of your digestive tract. The Nutrition Focus in the chapter explained why these habits are important to examine. Put a *Y* in the blank to the left of the question to indicate yes and an *N* to indicate no.

_____ 1. Are you currently experiencing greater than normal stress and tension?

_____ 2. Do you have a family history of digestive tract problems (e.g., ulcers, hemorrhoids, diverticulosis, constipation, lactose intolerance)?

_____ 3. Do you experience pain in your stomach region about 2 hours after you eat?

_____ 4. Do you smoke cigarettes?

_____ 5. Do you take aspirin frequently?

_____ 6. Do you have heartburn at least once per week?

_____ 7. Do you commonly lie down after eating a large meal?

_____ 8. Do you drink alcoholic beverages more than two or three times per day?

_____ 9. Do you experience abdominal pain, bloating, and gas about 30 minutes to 2 hours after consuming milk products?

_____ 10. Do you often have to strain while having a bowel movement?

_____ 11. Do you consume less than 9 cups (women) to 13 cups (men) of a combination of water and other fluids per day?

_____ 12. Do you perform physical activity (e.g., jog, swim, walk briskly, row, stair climb) less than 30 minutes on fewer than 5 days of the week?

_____ 13. Do you eat a diet relatively low in fiber (recall that significant fiber is found in whole fruits, vegetables, legumes, nuts and seeds, whole-grain breads, and whole-grain cereals)?

_____ 14. Do you frequently have diarrhea?

_____ 15. Do you frequently use laxatives or antacids?

Interpretation

Add up the number of yes answers you gave and record the total in the blank to the right. _____

If your score is from 8 to 15, your habits and symptoms put you at risk for experiencing future digestive tract problems. Take particular note of the habits to which you answered yes. Consider trying to cooperate more with your digestive tract.

II. Investigate Over-the-Counter Medications for Treating Common GI Tract Problems

Visit your local pharmacy and check out the medications on sale for treating indigestion, heartburn, constipation, diarrhea, and hemorrhoids. Select one category and compare four brands for

1. Price/usual daily dose
2. Active ingredients
3. Warning to users
4. Advice as to when to see a physician

Write a critique of your discoveries about these products, and summarize what you would say about the safety and efficacy of these products.

METABOLISM

CHAPTER OUTLINE

CASE SCENARIO:

Ana loves to eat, and she typically eats large quantities of food at pizza parties and family gatherings. However, she doesn't want to develop a weight problem. Both her mother and father are overweight, and they both have type 2 diabetes. One of Ana's friends tells her that she can avoid both overweight and type 2 diabetes while eating as much as she wants as long as she avoids carbohydrates and eats a lot of high-fat foods. Another friend tells Ana that this is not true. Instead, she should focus on high-protein foods. Then a third friend tells Ana that she can eat as much as she wants as long as most of each meal is made up of carbohydrates that come from fruits, vegetables, and starches such as pasta.

All of Ana's friends think they know how each of these energy-yielding nutrients (fats, proteins, and carbohydrates) behaves in the body, how each of these nutrients contributes to the amount of energy she consumes, and what becomes of that food energy. The friend who tells Ana to avoid carbohydrates thinks that carbohydrates are more likely to be converted into body fat compared to the fat present in food. The friend who tells Ana to focus on eating protein thinks that the body "burns" all the energy from protein, and so proteins in the diet cannot contribute to body fat. By the end of this chapter you will know which of Ana's friends is correct.

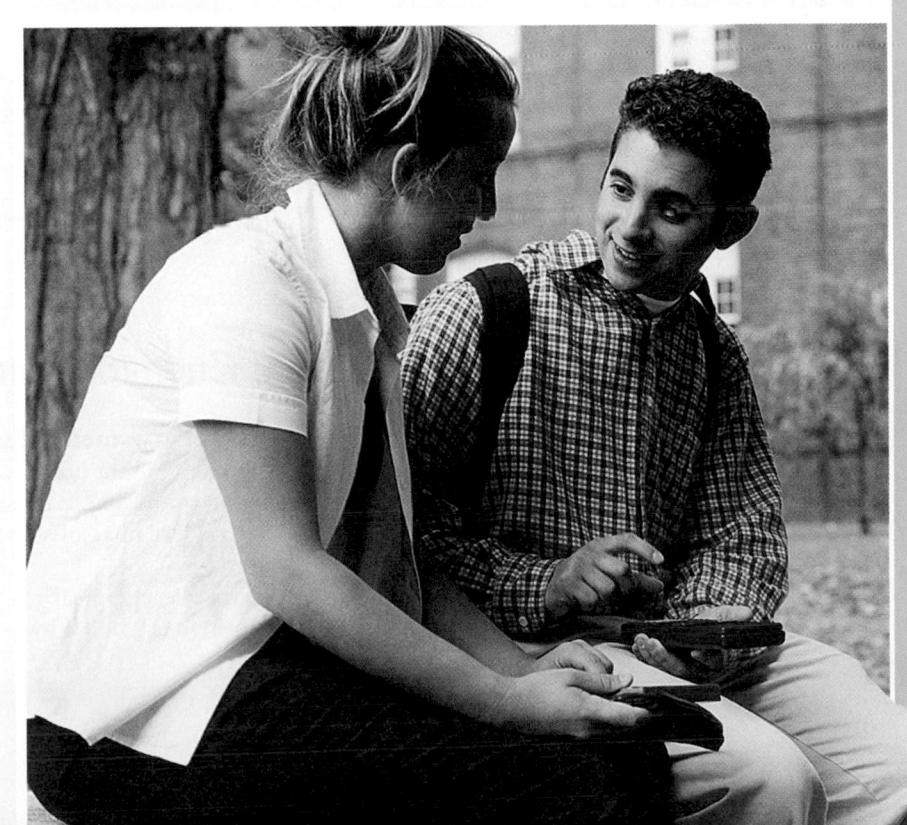

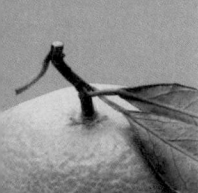

*M*etabolism refers to the entire network of chemical processes involved in maintaining life. It encompasses all the sequences of chemical reactions that occur in the body. These biochemical reactions enable us to release and use energy from foods, synthesize one substance from another, and prepare waste products for excretion.[2] Although it may seem that an overwhelming number of reactions take place within your body, all of them can be categorized as one of two classes. One class puts different molecules together, while the other class takes molecules apart. Reactions that put molecules together require energy. The source of this energy is the energy released when other molecules are broken apart.

Studying metabolism can help you comprehend a variety of nutrition concepts. Understanding metabolism clarifies how carbohydrates, proteins, fats, and alcohol are interrelated. You will see, for example, how the carbons in proteins become the carbons of glucose, and why the carbons of most fatty acids *cannot* become the carbons of glucose.

Studying metabolic pathways in the cell also sets the stage for examining the roles of vitamins and minerals. Many vitamins and minerals contribute to the enzyme activity that supports metabolic reactions in the cell.[8] Overall, the functions of both macronutrients and micronutrients will be easier to understand if you are familiar with the basic metabolic processes in the cell.

CHAPTER OBJECTIVES CHAPTER 4 IS DESIGNED TO ALLOW YOU TO:

1. Define the terms *energy metabolism, anabolism, catabolism, aerobic metabolism,* and *anaerobic metabolism.*

2. Describe aerobic and anaerobic metabolism of glucose with reference to lactate production.

3. Describe why adenosine triphosphate (ATP) is considered the energy source of the cell.

4. Outline how the energy potential of glucose, fatty acids, amino acids, and alcohol is extracted—using metabolic pathways such as glycolysis, the citric acid cycle, and the electron transport chain—and eventually deposited into ATP.

5. Describe the roles vitamins and minerals play in energy metabolism.

6. Explain the origin of CO_2 and H_2O generated by energy metabolism.

7. Describe the central role of acetyl-CoA in cell metabolism.

8. State the source of ketone bodies and their role in energy metabolism.

9. Describe the fate of energy from macronutrients during the fed state.

10. Describe the fate of energy-yielding substances in the body during the fasting state.

11. Briefly explain how metabolism is regulated.

REFRESH YOUR MEMORY AS YOU BEGIN YOUR STUDY OF METABOLISM IN CHAPTER 4, YOU MAY WANT TO REVIEW:

• Various components of the macronutrient classes—carbohydrates, proteins, and lipids—in Chapter 1.
• Basic chemistry concepts in Appendix A.
• The components of the cell and functions of various organelles in Appendix C.
• Enzyme function and regulation in Chapter 3.
• Hormone function in Chapter 3.

---

*M*etabolism = anabolism + catabolism

intermediate A chemical compound formed in one of many steps in a metabolic pathway.

*V*irtually every step in any pathway depends on an enzyme to initiate the specific chemical reaction.

Metabolism: Chemical Reactions in the Body

As noted in the chapter overview, **metabolism** refers to the entire network of chemical processes involved in maintaining life. It encompasses all the sequences of chemical reactions that occur in the body. These chemical reactions enable cells to release and use energy from foods, convert one substance into another, and prepare waste products for excretion.[2]

A progression of metabolic chemical reactions from beginning to end is called a *pathway.* Compounds formed as the pathway proceeds are called **intermediates.**

Anabolic and Catabolic Reactions

Anabolic pathways build compounds (Figure 4-1). Energy must be expended for anabolic processes to take place. For example, to make sucrose (table sugar) plants combine together the simple sugars glucose and fructose.

$$\text{ANABOLISM}$$
$$\text{glucose + fructose} \xrightarrow[\text{H}_2\text{O}]{} \text{sucrose}$$

In addition, the chemical reactions that synthesize –C–C– bonds (fatty acid synthesis),

–C–N– bonds (protein synthesis), –C–N– bonds (urea synthesis), and –C–O–
bonds[2] (triglyceride synthesis) require anabolic energy input (see Appendix A for details). The chemical elements and compounds used to form the new substances often are called *building blocks*.

Conversely, **catabolic** pathways break down compounds into small units. The sucrose molecule discussed in the anabolism example will be broken down into glucose and fructose in the GI tract during digestion.

$$\text{CATABOLISM}$$
$$\text{sucrose} \xrightarrow[\text{H}_2\text{O}]{} \text{glucose + fructose}$$

Later, the complete catabolism of this glucose and fructose results in the release of carbon dioxide (CO_2) and water (H_2O). Energy is released in the process: some is trapped for cell use and the rest is lost as heat. Recall from Chapter 1 that cells use this energy for four specific purposes: building compounds, contracting muscles, conducting nerve impulses, and pumping ions (e.g., across cell membranes).[2]

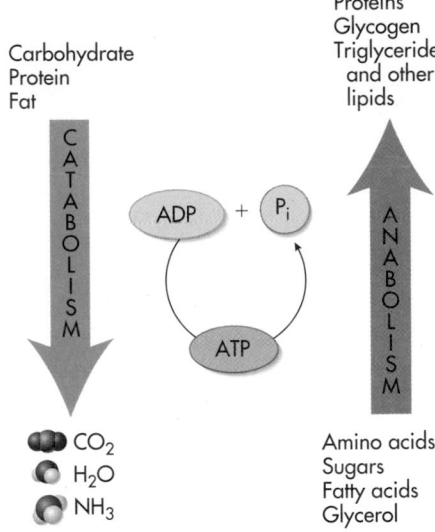

Figure 4-1 | Anabolism and Catabolism. Anabolism relies on catabolism to provide the needed energy input from ATP.

Stages of Energy Production

The production of energy for cell use occurs in three stages.[2] In the first stage, large food molecules, e.g., proteins, are broken down during digestion and absorption into smaller units, in this case amino acids. In the second stage, most of these and other smaller compounds are further degraded to the two-carbon intermediate compound **acetic acid** $\left(\text{CH}_3\text{C–OH}\right)$, the acid found in vinegar. In the third stage, acetic acid (termed acetate or an acetyl group when a hydrogen ion is missing) is degraded to carbon dioxide and water (Figure 4-2). Some of the energy released in this catabolic process drives the synthesis of **adenosine triphosphate (ATP)**. ATP is energy in a form that cells use (Figure 4-3a). Chapter 3 introduced the first stage, digestion and absorption. This chapter examines the last two stages.

Energy for the Cell

The energy that human cells use comes from chemical bonds found between the atoms in carbohydrate, fat, protein, and alcohol. This energy is originally placed there during **photosynthesis,** when plants use solar energy to make glucose and other organic (carbon-containing) compounds. The chemical reactions in photosynthesis form compounds that contain more energy than carbon dioxide and water, the building blocks used. Virtually all organisms use the sun—either directly, or indirectly as we do—as their source of energy (Figure 4-3b).[2]

The by-products of eventual human energy metabolism are carbon dioxide, water, and heat. Overall, chemical energy from ingested food that passes through body cells is eventually and irretrievably dissipated to the environment as heat.

Acids commonly lose a hydrogen ion at the pH found in human cells (pH 7.4). When that ion is lost, the name of the acid is changed by dropping the reference to acid and adding an *ate* ending. Thus, *acetic acid* become *acetate.*

adenosine triphosphate (ATP) The main energy currency for cells. ATP energy is used to promote ion pumping, enzyme activity, and muscular contraction.

photosynthesis The process by which plants use energy from the sun to produce energy-yielding compounds, such as glucose.

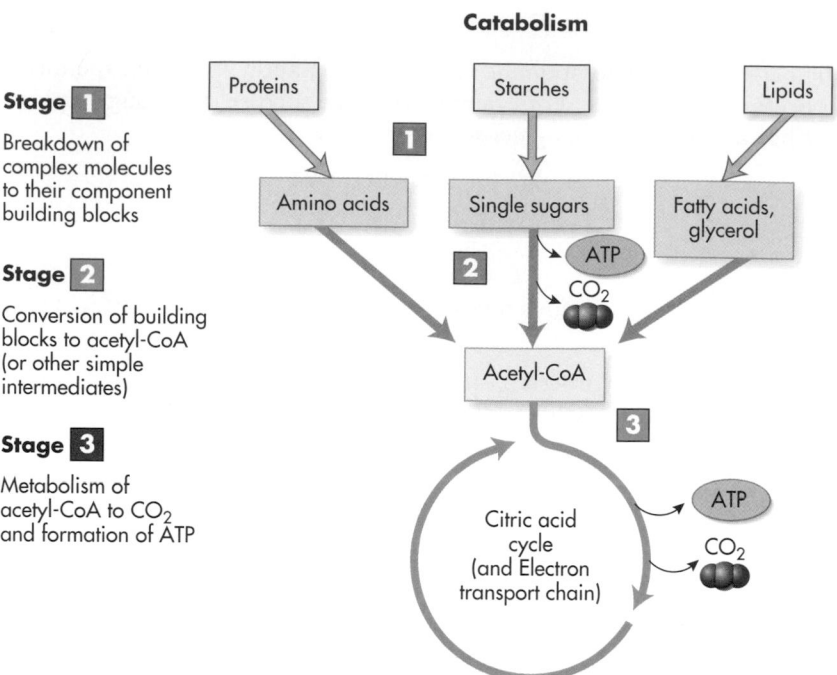

Catabolism

Stage 1

Breakdown of complex molecules to their component building blocks

Stage 2

Conversion of building blocks to acetyl-CoA (or other simple intermediates)

Stage 3

Metabolism of acetyl-CoA to CO_2 and formation of ATP

Proteins → Amino acids

Starches → Single sugars → ATP → CO_2

Lipids → Fatty acids, glycerol

Acetyl-CoA

Citric acid cycle (and Electron transport chain) → ATP → CO_2

Figure 4-2 | Three stages of catabolism (steps 1–3).

respiration The use of oxygen; in the human organism, the inhalation of oxygen and the exhalation of carbon dioxide; in cells, the oxidation (electron removal) of food molecules, to obtain energy.

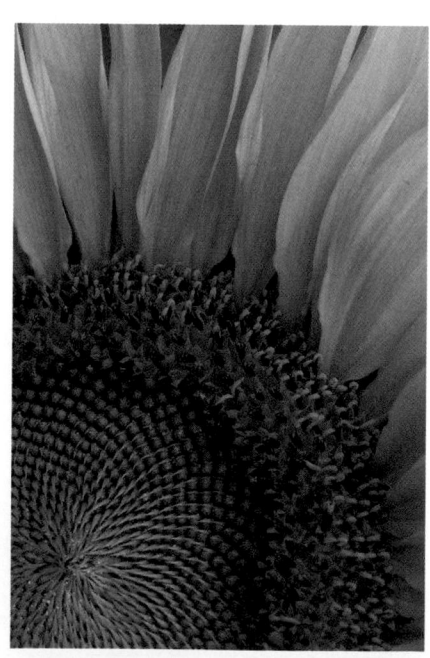

Sunflowers capture solar energy and transfer it into chemical energy in the form of protein, carbohydrate, and fat in the sunflower seeds.

Thus, in human **respiration,** the starting materials are energy-yielding compounds such as glucose, which, through an elaborate multistep process, are converted to end products such as carbon dioxide and water (e.g., $C_6H_{12}O_6 + 6\ O_2 \rightarrow \rightarrow 6\ CO_2 + 6\ H_2O$). This process results in the transfer of energy from food to cells, which in turn allows energy-requiring pathways in cells to function.[3]

Many chemical reactions in the body could not occur without the addition of outside energy supplied by food. Outside energy permits compounds, such as some forms of amino acids, to be transformed into products such as glucose. And although amino acids and glucose molecules themselves contain the energy needed for synthesis of still other compounds, these and other energy-yielding molecules provide neither the right amount of energy for a chemical reaction nor a form of energy that cells can use directly. For example, a glucose molecule contains over 100 times more energy than required to facilitate an individual chemical reaction in a cell. Thus, a cell must have a means of breaking down energy-yielding molecules to release and then convert the chemical energy trapped in them into smaller, usable energy forms.[2]

Adenosine Triphosphate (ATP) as an Energy Source

To release the energy in ATP, cells split it into adenosine diphosphate (ADP) plus P_i, a free (inorganic) phosphate group (Figure 4-4). ADP can also be split into adenosine monophosphate (AMP) plus P_i to yield energy, in a reaction muscles are capable of performing during intense exercise when ATP is in short supply (ADP + ADP → ATP + AMP). Only energy in ATP and its derivatives can be used directly by the cell.[10]

Every cell contains catabolic pathways that release energy to allow ADP to combine with P_i to form ATP. An enzyme later can break the ATP bond to release energy needed for anabolic reactions. ATP itself is very stable. It actually takes an enzyme to unlock the energy that is stored in the molecule.[10]

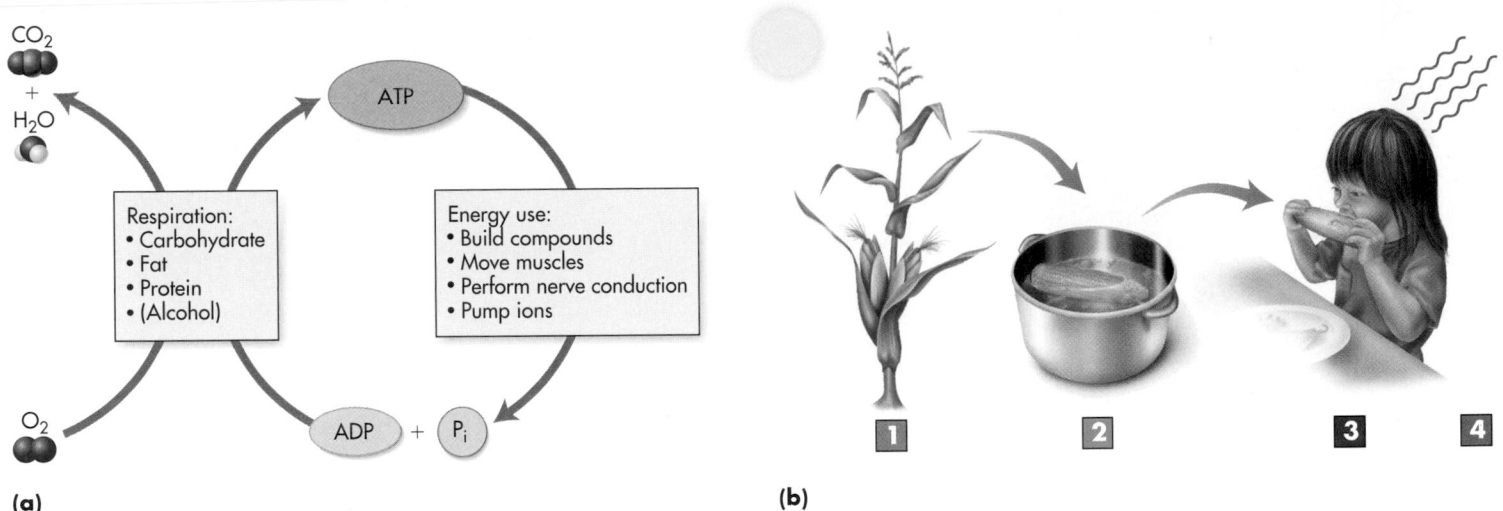

Figure 4-3 | Solar energy input and human energy output. (*a*) ATP synthesis and use. Energy from foods is used to synthesize ATP. The ATP then provides energy for the cell. (*b*) The corn plant uses solar energy to synthesize glucose from carbon dioxide and water (step *1*). We cook and eat the corn (step *2*), transferring much of the energy in the glucose from the corn to ATP energy for our cells to use (step *3*). Eventually, this energy leaves our bodies as heat (step *4*). Some energy may be stored as fat if we overeat, and a small amount is lost in urine and feces.

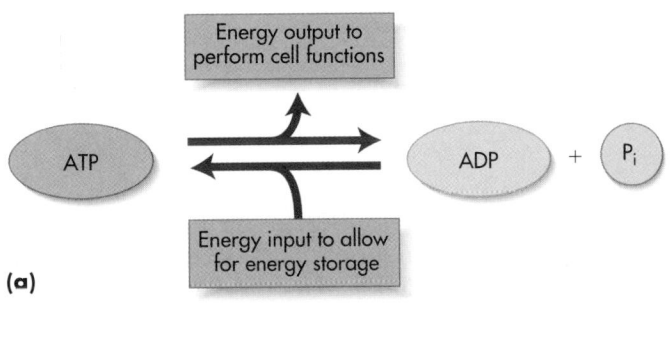

Figure 4-4 | ATP stores and yields energy. ATP is the high-energy state; ADP is the lower-energy state. (*a*) When ATP is broken down to ADP plus P_i, energy is released for cell use. When energy is trapped by ADP plus P_i, ATP can be formed. (*b*) ATP represents a storage form of energy for cell use because it contains high energy bonds. P_i is the abbreviation for an inorganic phosphate group.

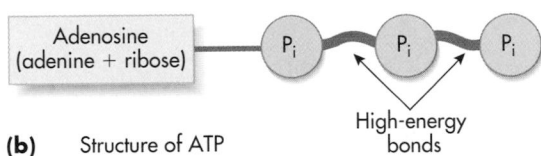

During metabolism, a cell is constantly breaking down ATP in one site while rebuilding it in another. An exhausted muscle cell has a very high concentration of ADP and a very low concentration of ATP. When this happens, muscle cell activity, such as muscle contraction, may slow down or cease altogether. A low ATP concentration then stimulates metabolic processes that produce ATP. Only by resynthesizing needed ATP can the muscle cell ready itself for future action.[10]

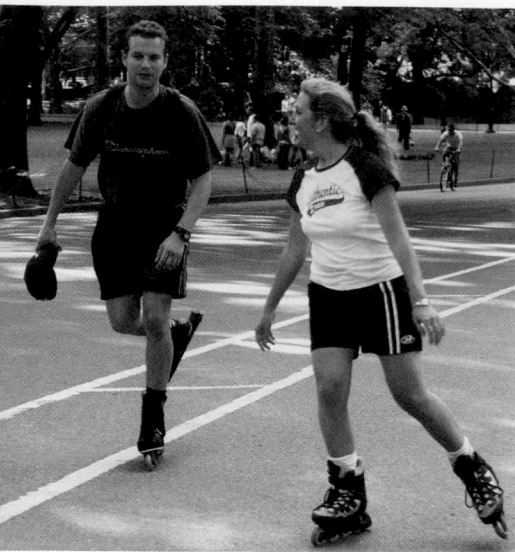

The energy used to perform physical activity is in the form of ATP.

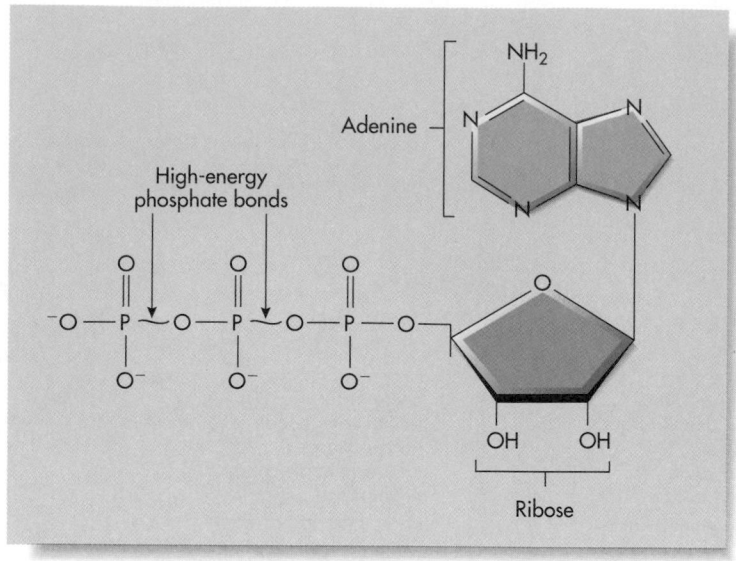

Chemical structure of adenosine triphosphate (ATP).

Oxidation-Reduction Reactions: Key Processes in Energy Metabolism

Oxidation-reduction reactions form a vital link between the energy-yielding nutrients and the formation of ATP.

A substance is *oxidized* when it loses one or more electrons.
A substance is *reduced* when it gains one or more electrons.

Electron flow governs oxidation-reduction processes. If one substance loses electrons (is oxidized), another substance must gain electrons (is reduced). The two processes go together; one cannot occur without the other.[8]

Consider the oxidation-reduction reaction involving iron:

$$Fe^{2+} \leftrightarrow Fe^{3+} + e^-$$

Here, Fe^{2+} has lost an electron (has been oxidized) ($Fe^{2+} \rightarrow Fe^{3+} + e^-$). Alternately, Fe^{3+} can gain an electron (be reduced) ($Fe^{3+} + e^- \rightarrow Fe^{2+}$). This oxidation and reduction of iron occurs during the transport of oxygen to body cells.

Oxidation-reduction reactions involving carbon-containing compounds are somewhat more difficult to visualize. A simple rule has been developed to determine oxidation-reduction reactions in these compounds. If the compound gains oxygen or loses hydrogen, it has been oxidized. If it loses oxygen or gains hydrogen, the compound has been reduced. The following process illustrates this definition.

$$CH_3-CH_3 \quad \underset{\text{reduction}}{\overset{\text{oxidation}}{\rightleftarrows}} \quad CH_3-CH_2-OH$$

ethane $\quad$ ethanol

$$CH_3-\overset{O}{\underset{\parallel}{C}}-\overset{O}{\underset{\parallel}{C}}-O^- \quad \underset{\text{reduction}}{\overset{\text{oxidation}}{\rightleftarrows}} \quad CH_3-\overset{OH}{\underset{H}{C}}-\overset{O}{\underset{\parallel}{C}}-O^-$$

pyruvate $\quad$ lactate

Now that you are familiar with oxidation and reduction reactions, you can examine the term **antioxidant.** This term is typically used to describe a compound that can donate electrons to oxidized compounds, putting them into a more reduced (stable) state. Oxidized compounds tend to be highly reactive; they seek electrons from other compounds to stabilize their chemical configuration. Dietary antioxidants such as vitamin E donate electrons to these highly reactive compounds, in turn, putting these oxidized compounds into a less reactive state (see Chapter 9 for details).

This method of determining oxidation and reduction—determining oxygen and hydrogen exchange—is used extensively in nutrition. For example, in the reaction illustrated, pyruvate (made from glucose) is reduced to form lactate by gaining two hydrogens. This happens during intense exercise (see Chapter 14). Lactate is oxidized back to pyruvate by losing two hydrogens.

Scientists generally use the terms *oxidation* and *reduction* as verbs or adjectives. When the terms are used as verbs, pyruvate is said to be *reduced* to lactate, and lactate is said to be *oxidized* to pyruvate. When the terms are used as adjectives, lactate is said to be the *reduced* form of pyruvate, while pyruvate is the *oxidized* form of lactate.

The Role of Enzymes and Vitamins in Oxidation-Reduction Reactions

Oxidation-reduction reactions in the body are controlled by enzymes. One important class of these enzymes, designated *dehydrogenases,* removes hydrogens from energy-yielding nutrients or their breakdown products. These hydrogens are eventually donated to the final acceptor, oxygen, to form water. In the process, large amounts of energy are transferred to ADP plus P_i to make ATP.[2]

Two B vitamins, niacin and riboflavin, assist dehydrogenase enzymes and, in turn, play a role in transferring the hydrogens from glucose to oxygen in the metabolic pathways of the cell.[8] Niacin functions as the **coenzyme** named **nicotinamide adenine dinucleotide (NAD).** This oxidized form can accept one hydrogen ion and two electrons to become NADH + H$^+$. (The extra hydrogen ion remains free in the cell.) In other words, the oxidized form of niacin, NAD$^+$, is reduced to form NADH + H$^+$. Note that NAD$^+$ indicates it has one less electron than in its complete configuration. By accepting two electrons and one hydrogen ion, NAD$^+$ becomes NADH + H$^+$, with no net charge on the coenzyme.

Riboflavin plays a similar role. In its oxidized form, the coenzyme form is known as **flavin adenine dinucleotide (FAD).** When it is reduced (gains two hydrogens, equivalent to two hydrogen ions and two electrons), it is known as FADH$_2$.

The reduction of oxygen (O) to form water (H$_2$O) is the ultimate driving force for life, because it is vital to the way cells synthesize ATP. Thus, oxidation-reduction reactions are a key to life.

coenzyme A compound that combines with an inactive protein, called an apoenzyme, to form a catalytically active protein, called a holoenzyme. In this manner, coenzymes aid in enzyme function.

nicotinamide adenine dinucleotide (NAD) A compound that readily accepts and donates electrons and hydrogen ions; formed from the vitamin niacin.

flavin adenine dinucleotide (FAD) A compound that readily accepts and donates electrons and hydrogen ions; formed from the vitamin riboflavin.

Concept | Check

Metabolism encompasses all the sequences of chemical reactions in the body. Anabolic processes build compounds using energy input, whereas catabolic processes break down compounds into small units, yielding energy. Adenosine triphosphate (ATP) is the form of energy used by a cell. The synthesis of ATP from ADP and P_i involves the transfer of energy from foodstuffs. This process uses oxidation-reduction reactions, in which electrons (along with hydrogen ions) are transferred from energy-yielding macronutrients eventually to oxygen. This reaction forms water and releases much energy, which can be used to produce ATP.

▌ ATP Production

This section will look at how cells convert the energy found in food to energy stored in the high-energy phosphate bonds of ATP. It will begin by examining how cells produce ATP from carbohydrates. Once you understand this process, you will turn your attention to how ATP is produced using the energy stored in fats and proteins. Along the way you will see how these energy-yielding processes are interconnected. (Cells can also produce ATP using the energy stored in alcohol; that process is discussed in Chapter 8.)

As each of the subsequent pathways is described, a good way to understand them is to diagram each step as you go. Afterward, compare your figures with those provided throughout the chapter. In addition, more detailed pathways can be found in Appendix B.

aerobic Requiring oxygen.

anaerobic Not requiring oxygen.

cytosol The water-based phase of the cytoplasm; excludes organelles such as mitochondria.

mitochondria The main sites of energy production in a cell. They also contain the pathway for oxidizing fat for fuel, among other metabolic pathways.

If oxygen is present, cellular respiration may be **aerobic.** In the absence of oxygen, **anaerobic** respiration will occur. Aerobic respiration is far more efficient than anaerobic respiration at producing ATP. As an example, starting with a single molecule of glucose, aerobic respiration will result in the net gain of 30 to 32 ATP. In contrast, anaerobic respiration is limited to a net gain of 2 ATP per glucose.

The four stages of aerobic respiration can be explained using glucose as an example (Figure 4-5):[2,11]

1. *Glycolysis.* This pathway breaks glucose down into pyruvate. This breakdown of glucose also results in the production of NADH + H$^+$. As well, energy released during glycolysis generates a net production of two molecules of ATP. Glycolysis occurs in the **cytosol** of cells.

2. *Transition reaction.* In this pathway, pyruvate is further oxidized to form an acetyl group CH$_3$–$\overset{\text{O}}{\overset{\|}{\text{C}}}$–O, which is then bonded to coenzyme A (CoA) to form acetyl-CoA. The transition reaction produces NADH + H$^+$ and releases carbon dioxide (CO$_2$) as a waste product. The transition reaction takes place within **mitochondria** of cells. Note that it is in these cellular structures that the reactions of aerobic respiration occur.

3. *Citric acid cycle.* In this pathway, the acetyl-CoA produced by the transition reaction enters into the citric acid cycle, with the end result being the production of NADH + H$^+$, FADH$_2$, ATP, and CO$_2$. The CO$_2$ is then released as a waste product. Like the transition reaction, the citric acid cycle takes place within mitochondria of cells.

4. *Electron transport chain.* The NADH + H$^+$ and FADH$_2$ produced by stages 1 through 3 of respiration enter this pathway. In the electron transport chain, NADH + H$^+$ is oxidized to NAD$^+$, and FADH$_2$ is oxidized to FAD. At the end of the electron transport chain, oxygen is combined with hydrogen ions (H$^+$) and electrons to form water. It is in the electron transport chain that the majority of the ATP is produced; keep in mind that it is an aerobic process. The electron transport chain takes place within mitochondria of cells.

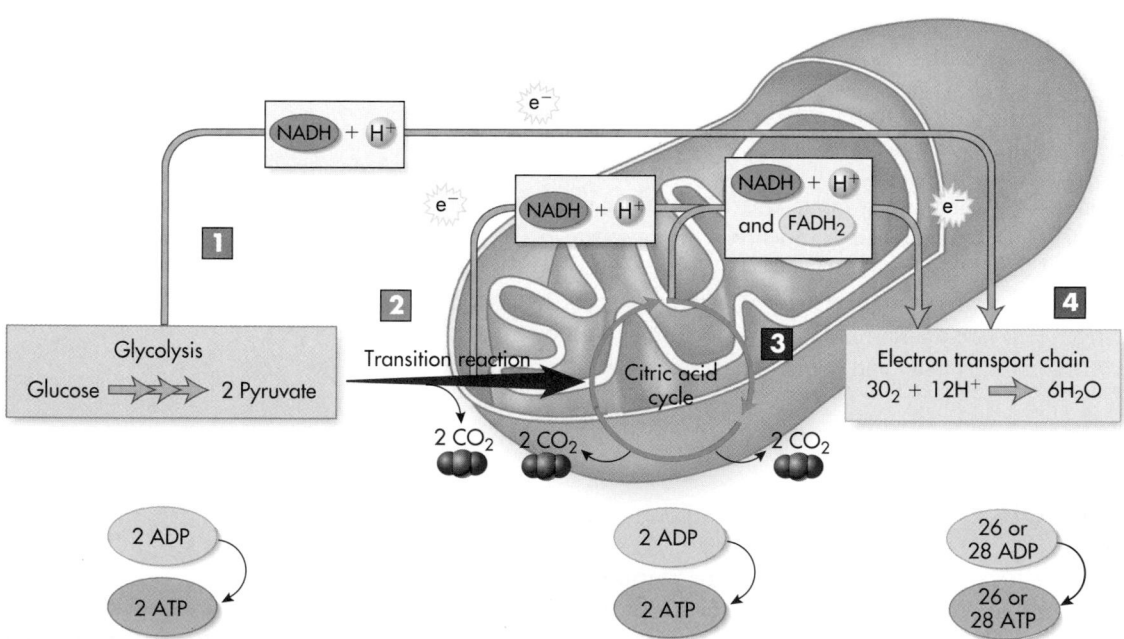

Figure 4-5 | The four phases of energy metabolism. Glycolysis in the cytoplasm produces pyruvate (step 1), which enters mitochondria if oxygen is available. The transition reaction (step 2) and the citric acid cycle that follow occur inside the mitochondria (step 3). Also, inside mitochondria, the electron transport chain receives the electrons that were removed from glucose breakdown products (step 4). The result of glucose breakdown is 30 to 32 ATP, depending on the particular cell.

Carbohydrate Metabolism

Because glucose is the main carbohydrate involved in cell metabolism, this section will track its step-by-step metabolism as an example of carbohydrate metabolism. The metabolic pathways that comprise the complete oxidation of one glucose molecule can be summarized in a single, simplified equation:

$$\underset{\substack{\text{glucose} \quad \text{oxygen}}}{C_6H_{12}O_6 + 6O_2} \quad \rightarrow \quad \underset{\substack{\text{carbon} \quad \text{water} \\ \text{dioxide}}}{6CO_2 + 6H_2O} + \text{energy}$$

oxidation

Reduction

In this equation the conversion of $C_6H_{12}O_6$ to CO_2 represents an oxidation process, whereas the conversion of O_2 to H_2O represents a reduction process.

Some of the energy that is released in this reaction is used to produce ATP, but much of the energy is simply released as heat. However, this heat should not be considered wasted energy. It is used to maintain the body temperature needed to support each cell's metabolic reactions.[2]

Glycolysis

Glycolysis literally means "breaking down glucose." The glycolysis pathway has a dual role: It degrades carbohydrates such as glucose to generate energy, and it provides building blocks for synthesizing needed cell compounds, such as glycerol for triglyceride synthesis.[11]

Before glycolysis can begin, a cell must obtain glucose. Only a few types of cells, such as liver and kidney cells, can produce their own glucose from certain amino acids, and only liver and muscle cells store glucose to a major extent. This glucose is stored as **glycogen.** Liver and muscle cells break down the glycogen to glucose (or a closely related form). Other body cells must obtain glucose from the bloodstream, so the body needs to maintain a fairly constant concentration of blood glucose to survive (see Chapter 5 for details). The product of glycolysis is two units of a three-carbon compound called *pyruvate* (Figures 4-6 and 4-7).

To begin glycolysis, a phosphate group from ATP is added to glucose, which makes the glucose more reactive (step 1). Another phosphate group from ATP is added to the newly formed glucose-phosphate compound (step 2), which then splits into two 3-carbon-phosphate compounds (step 3). These are converted through a series of steps into two molecules of the 3-carbon compound pyruvate (step 4). Thus, in glycolysis a cell starts with a 6-carbon glucose molecule and produces two molecules of the 3-carbon compound pyruvate. In the process, four hydrogens (containing a total of four electrons) are removed (step 5), and four ATP are generated (steps 6 and 7). The electrons and hydrogen ions are picked up by a carrier—in this case, NAD^+. Recall that each NAD^+ (oxidized form) accepts two electrons and one hydrogen ion, yielding $NADH + H^+$ (reduced form).[3]

The end result of glycolysis includes the synthesis of 2 $NADH + 2H^+$. There is also a net gain of two ATP. This arises because it takes two ATP to "prime" glucose for further metabolism (steps 1 and 2), but four ATP are then produced from each glucose molecule (steps 6 and 7), yielding a net gain of two ATP. These two ATP represent only about 5% of the total ATP that can be produced by the complete oxidation of one glucose molecule. Most of the energy still resides in the pyruvate molecules and the NADH + H^+ produced. (The latter must enter the electron transport chain to yield ATP.)

Glucose is not the only carbohydrate that can produce ATP by glycolysis. Other simple carbohydrate forms, such as fructose, also can be converted to intermediate compounds found in the glycolysis pathway. These compounds then follow the remaining steps in the pathway.

glycolysis The metabolic pathway that converts glucose into 2 molecules of pyruvate acid, with the net gain of 2 ATP and 2 $NADH + 2H^+$.

glycogen A carbohydrate made of multiple units of glucose with a highly branched structure; sometimes known as *animal starch*. It is the storage form of glucose in humans and is synthesized (and stored) in the liver and muscles.

Glucose

Pyruvate

Figure 4-6 | Glycolysis simplified. The process begins with one glucose ($C_6H_{12}O_6$) (step 1) and ends with two pyruvates ($C_3H_4O_3$) (step 4). Some ATP is both used (steps 1 and 2) and produced by the process (steps 6 and 7). The four electrons and two of the hydrogen ions released are captured by 2 NAD^+ (step 5). The other two hydrogen ions float free in the cytosol. Pyruvate then can undergo further metabolism in the citric acid cycle.

A new tool for understanding how we as individuals differ in the metabolic response to nutrients may lie in the ability to track the actual metabolic intermediates made to form this response, such as how we respond to exposure from different fatty acids. This approach, called *metabolomics,* should be more accurate than merely looking for differences in DNA between individuals to predict dietary responses. Reference no. 7 reviews this new tool of research.

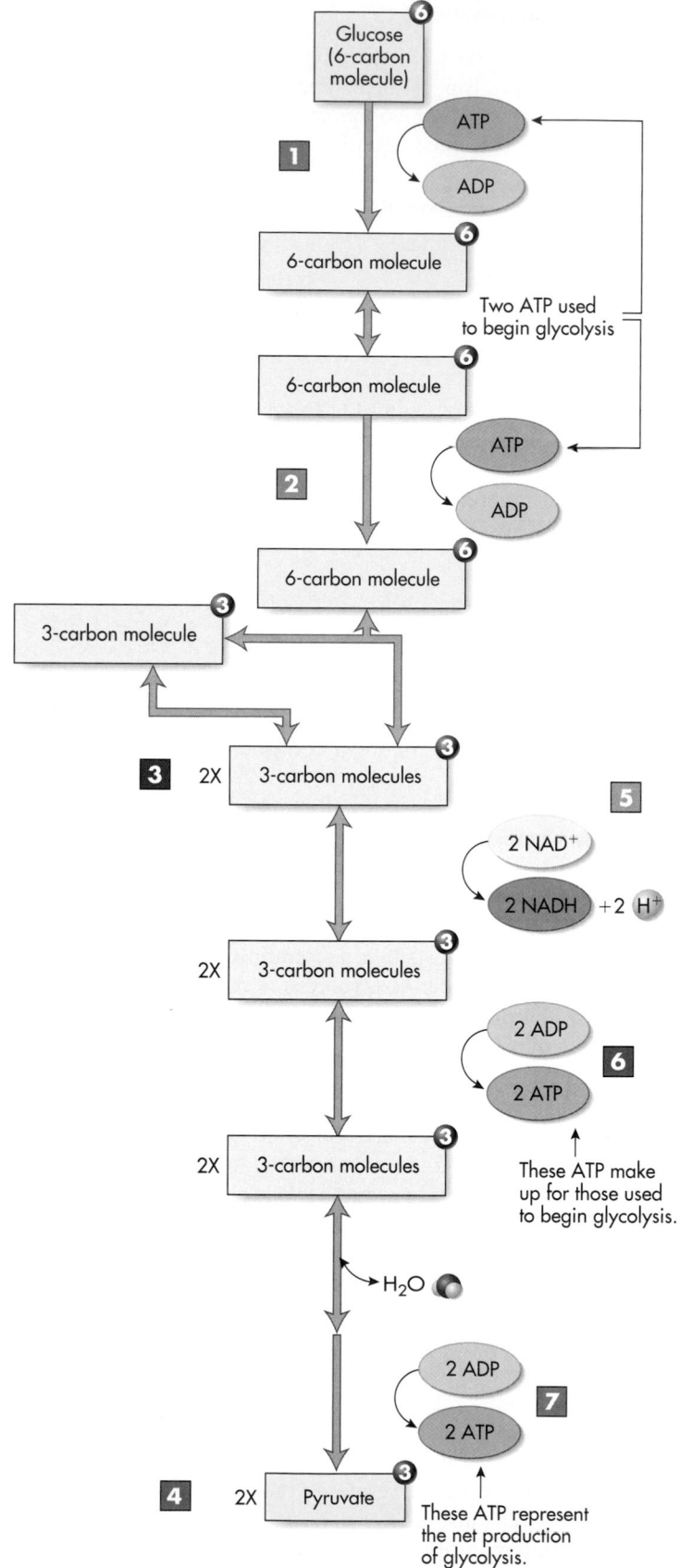

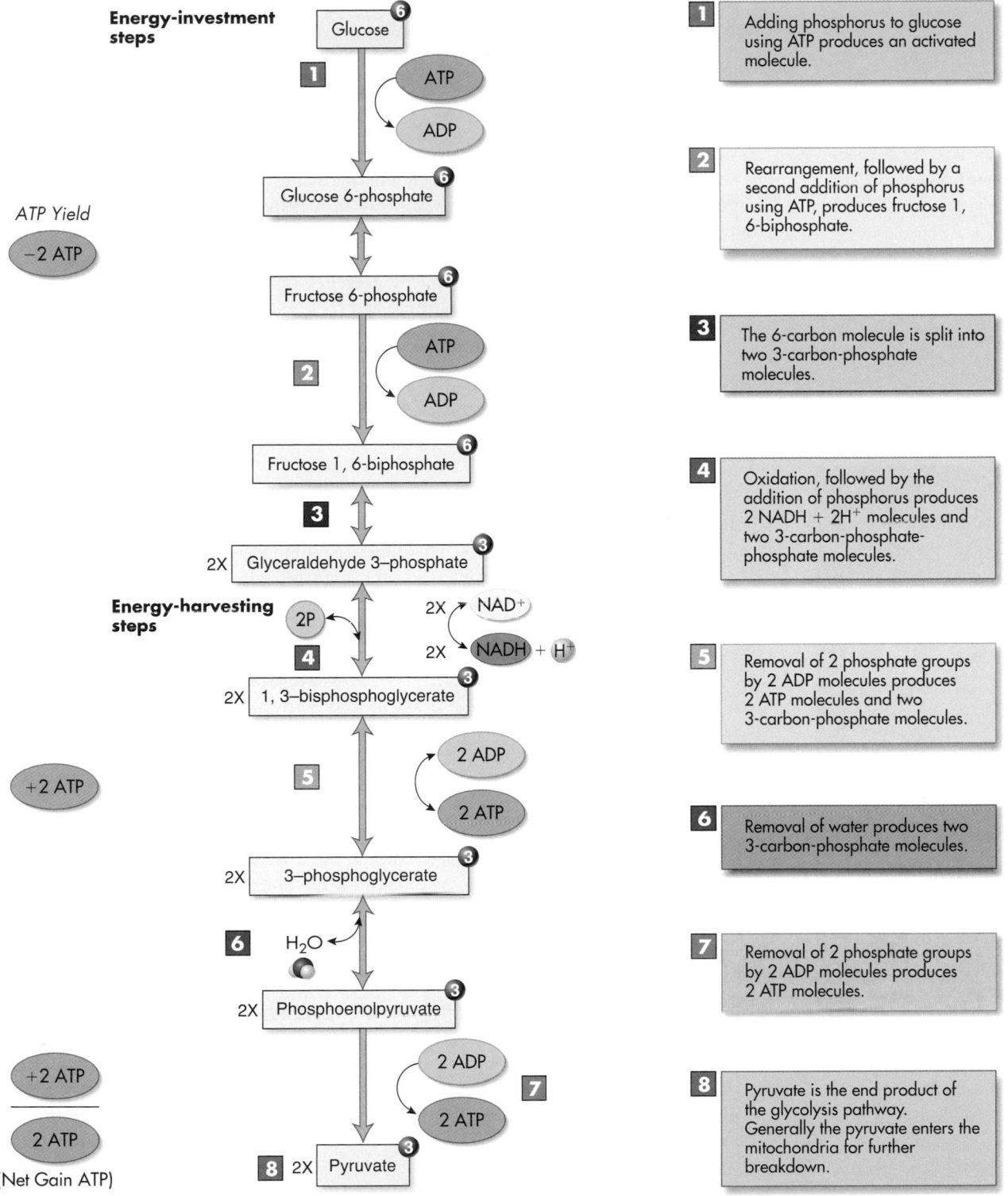

Figure 4-7 | Glycolysis, step by step. This metabolic pathway begins with glucose and ends with pyruvate. Net gain of two ATP molecules can be calculated by subtracting those used during the energy-investment steps from those produced during the energy-harvesting steps. Text in boxes to the far right explains the reactions. See Figure B-1 in Appendix B for a more detailed view of glycolysis.

The two pyruvate molecules formed at the end of glycolysis still contain much stored energy. Pyruvate passes from the cytosol into mitochondria, where the transition reaction converts pyruvate into a form that can enter the citric acid cycle.[3]

Transition Reaction

In order to enter the citric acid cycle, pyruvate must be converted to an acetyl group in a process called a transition reaction. The pyruvate is then attached to coenzyme A (CoA), forming acetyl-CoA. This overall reaction is irreversible, which has important metabolic consequences, as you will see. The conversion of pyruvate to acetyl-CoA requires the B vitamins thiamin, riboflavin, niacin, and pantothenic acid. For this reason, carbohydrate metabolism depends on the presence of these vitamins.[8]

The transition reaction oxidizes pyruvate and reduces NAD^+. It can be summarized as:

$$\text{pyruvate} + \text{CoA} + NAD^+ \rightarrow \text{acetyl-CoA} + CO_2 + NADH + H^+$$

Note that each glucose yields 2 pyruvate for the transition reaction. As with the $NADH + H^+$ produced by glycolysis, the $NADH + H^+$ produced by the transition reaction will eventually enter the electron transport chain.

> ### Concept | Check
>
> To begin glycolysis, two phosphate groups from two ATP molecules are added to glucose to make the glucose more reactive. This doubly phosphorylated glucose continues through glycolysis in the form of various intermediates (steps 1–3). Eventually one of the intermediates is split into two molecules of a 3-carbon compound. Each of these 3-carbon compounds goes through a series of chemical reactions (steps 4–7) to become the 3-carbon pyruvate. Thus, in glycolysis, glucose with 6 carbons, 12 hydrogens, and 6 oxygens ($C_6H_{12}O_6$) is converted to two molecules of pyruvate, each composed of 3 carbons, 4 hydrogens, and 3 oxygens ($C_3H_4O_3$). In the process, 4 hydrogens (containing 4 protons and 4 electrons) are removed, allowing NAD^+ to be reduced to form $NADH + H^+$. Each NAD^+ has accepted 2 electrons and 1 proton, producing NADH (the extra H^+ is an unbound proton). Also produced in this phase of glycolysis is four ATP. However, since two ATP are needed to "prime" glucose (steps 1 and 2), there is a net gain of only two ATP per glucose. Next, each pyruvate typically enters the transition reaction and is oxidized to a 2-carbon acetyl group carried by coenzyme A, and 2 NAD^+ are reduced to form 2 $NADH + 2 H^+$. CO_2 is a waste product of the reaction.

Citric Acid Cycle

The acetyl-CoA molecules produced by the transition reaction enter the citric acid cycle. The citric acid cycle is a series of chemical reactions used by cells to convert the carbons of an acetyl group to carbon dioxide while at the same time harvesting energy in order to produce ATP (Figure 4-8).[10] Each complete turn of the citric acid cycle produces $NADH + H^+$ and $FADH_2$, which, like the $NADH + H^+$ generated by glycolysis and the transition reaction, will enter the electron transport chain. The details of the citric acid cycle can be found in Figure 4-9.

How the Citric Acid Cycle Works

To begin the citric acid cycle, acetyl-CoA combines with a 4-carbon compound, oxaloacetate, to form the 6-carbon compound citrate (Figure 4-9, step 1). In the process, the corresponding CoA molecule is released and can be reused. During one complete turn of the citric acid cycle, the 6-carbon citrate molecule is metabolized back to a 4-carbon oxaloacetate molecule (steps 2–8) and 2-carbon dioxide molecules are released (steps 3 and 5). The cycle is now ready to begin again with oxaloacetate and another acetyl-CoA.

CoA is short for coenzyme A. The A stands for acetylation because CoA provides the two carbon acetyl group to start the citric acid cycle.

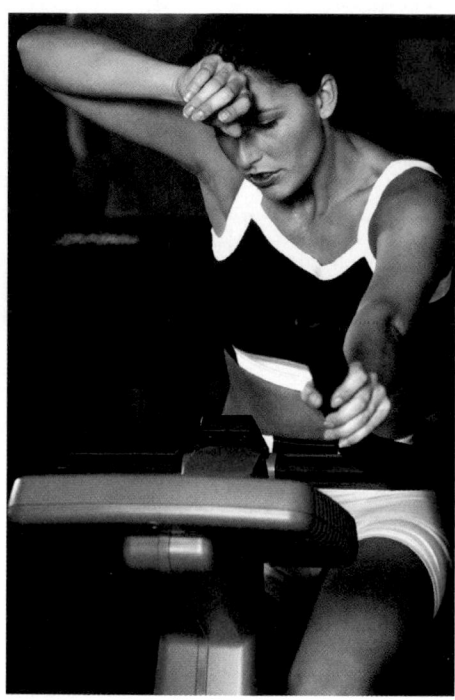

Metabolism is part of everyday life, and such activity increases when we increase physical activity.

Other names for the citric acid cycle are the tricarboxylic acid cycle (TCA cycle) and the Krebs cycle, named after Sir Hans Krebs, the scientist who first described it.

GTP from the citric acid cycle goes on to form ATP.

Overview of the Citric Acid Cycle

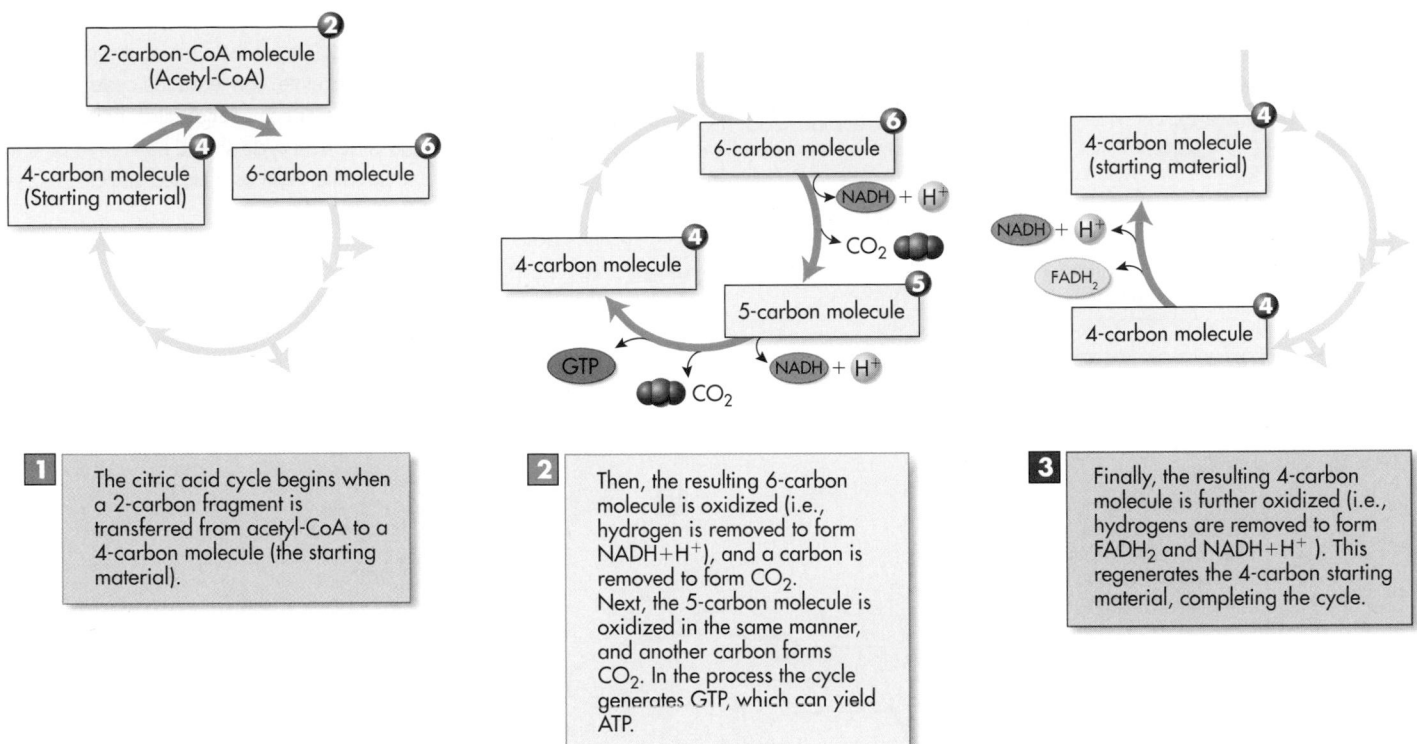

Figure 4-8 | How the citric acid cycle works.

Each complete turn of the citric acid cycle yields potential ATP in the form of guanosine triphosphate (GTP) (step 6) as well as $NADH + H^+$ (steps 2, 4, and 8) and $FADH_2$ (step 7). When reviewing this overall reaction, focus on the input of an acetyl group that was produced by the oxidation of pyruvate and on the output of GTP, $NADH + H^+$, $FADH_2$, and CO_2.

From the Citric Acid Cycle to the Electron Transport Chain

In aerobic respiration, a cell starts with a 6-carbon glucose and eventually produces 6 CO_2, 10 $NADH + H^+$, 2 $FADH_2$, and 4 ATP. It takes two turns of the citric acid cycle to process one glucose, because the glucose was split into two 3-carbon fragments as a result of glycolysis.

All the carbons in glucose are released in the form of carbon dioxide. The carbon dioxide eventually leaves the body by way of the lungs. In the process, ATP is synthesized directly by both glycolysis and the citric acid cycle, and $NADH + H^+$ and $FADH_2$ are produced.

The final pathway of aerobic respiration is the electron transport chain. Most of the ATP produced during aerobic respiration is produced by the electron transport chain. The $NADH + H^+$ and $FADH_2$ produced previously by other reactions are used to supply the energy needed for ATP synthesis in the electron transport chain. In this way, much more of the energy released from glucose metabolism is transferred to ATP (Figure 4-10).[2]

The Electron Transport Chain

Most cells perform the electron transport chain. This metabolic process, called **oxidative phosphorylation,** requires the minerals iron and copper. Iron is a component of **cytochromes** in the electron transport chain, and copper is a component of an enzyme present.

During the first steps of the **electron transport chain,** both $NADH + H^+$ and $FADH_2$ are oxidized (i.e., their hydrogens are removed; review Figure 4-9). The details of these steps

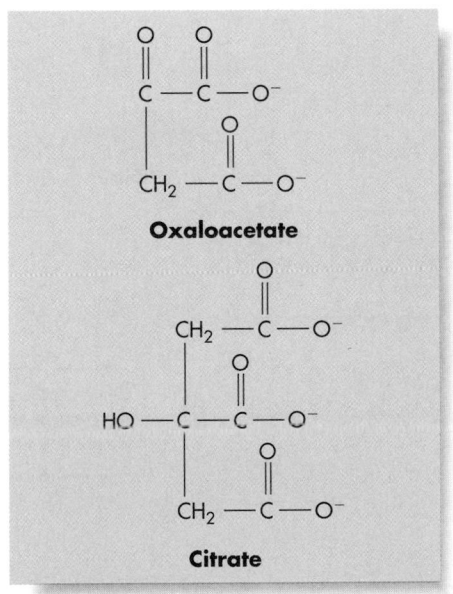

oxidative phosphorylation The process by which energy derived from the oxidation of $NADH + H^+$ and $FADH_2$ is transferred to ADP + P_i to form ATP.

cytochrome Electron-transfer compound that participates in the electron transport chain.

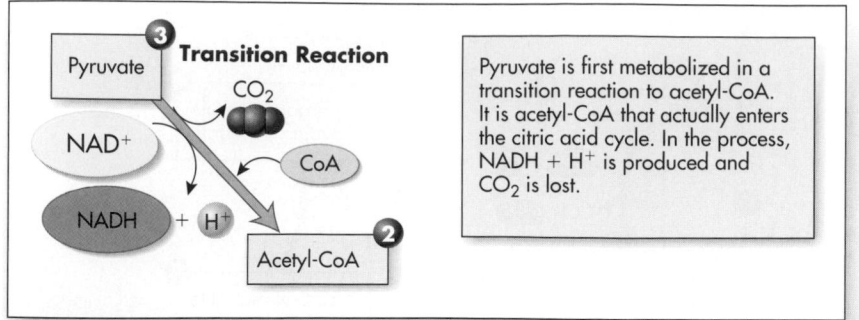

Transition Reaction

Pyruvate

CO_2

NAD^+

CoA

NADH + H^+

Acetyl-CoA

Pyruvate is first metabolized in a transition reaction to acetyl-CoA. It is acetyl-CoA that actually enters the citric acid cycle. In the process, NADH + H^+ is produced and CO_2 is lost.

Intermediates of the citric acid cycle, such as oxaloacetate, can leave the cycle and go on to form other compounds, such as glucose. Thus, the citric acid cycle should be viewed as a traffic circle rather than as a closed circle.

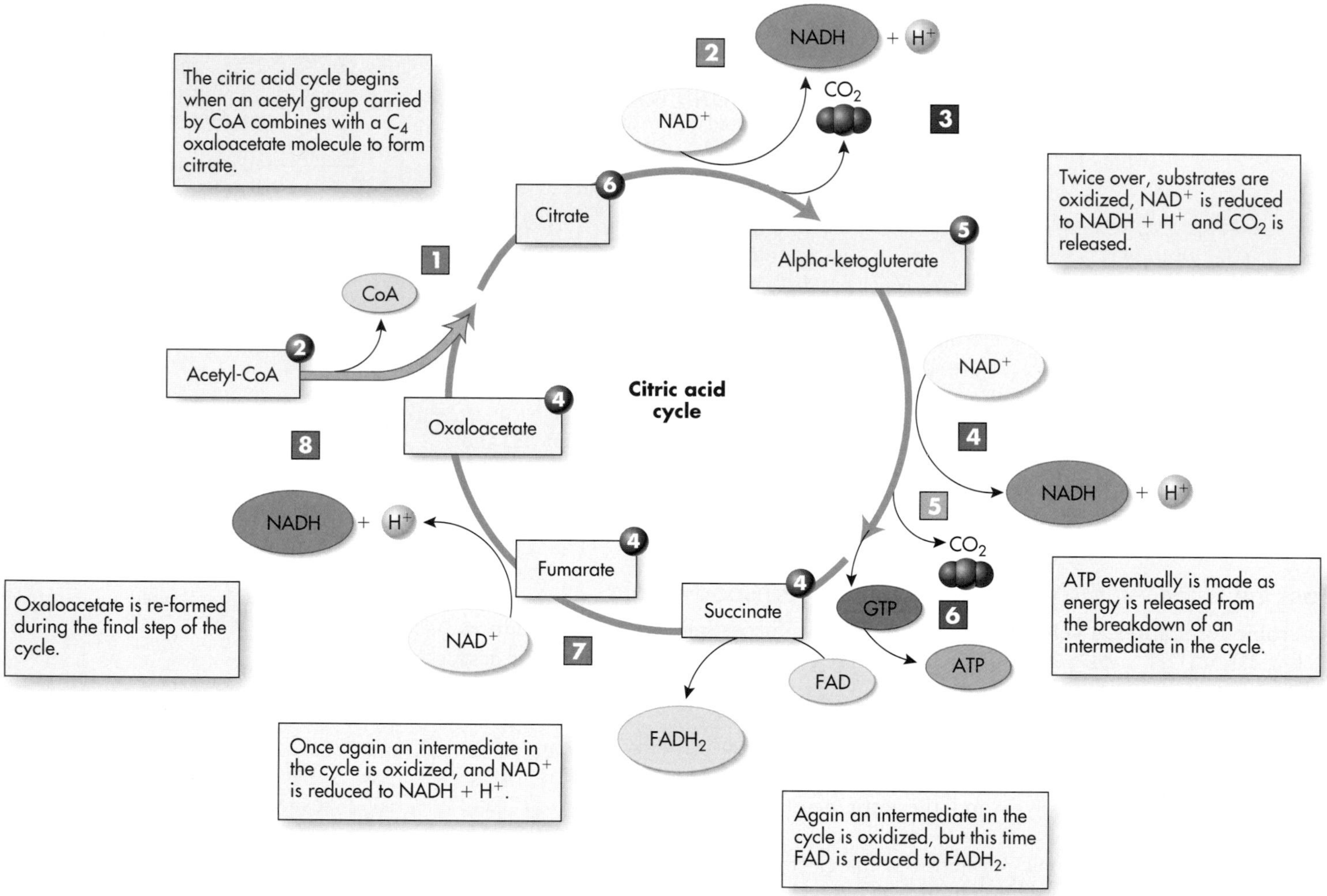

The citric acid cycle begins when an acetyl group carried by CoA combines with a C_4 oxaloacetate molecule to form citrate.

Twice over, substrates are oxidized, NAD^+ is reduced to NADH + H^+ and CO_2 is released.

NADH + H^+

NAD^+

CO_2

Citrate

Alpha-ketogluterate

CoA

Acetyl-CoA

Citric acid cycle

Oxaloacetate

NAD^+

NADH + H^+

NADH + H^+

Fumarate

Succinate

CO_2

GTP

ATP

FAD

NAD^+

$FADH_2$

ATP eventually is made as energy is released from the breakdown of an intermediate in the cycle.

Oxaloacetate is re-formed during the final step of the cycle.

Once again an intermediate in the cycle is oxidized, and NAD^+ is reduced to NADH + H^+.

Again an intermediate in the cycle is oxidized, but this time FAD is reduced to $FADH_2$.

Figure 4-9 | The transition reaction and the citric acid cycle. The net result of one turn of this cycle of reactions (steps 1–8) is the oxidation of an acetyl group to two molecules of CO_2 and the formation of three molecules of NADH + H^+ and one molecule of $FADH_2$. One GTP molecule also results, which eventually forms ATP. The citric acid cycle turns twice per glucose molecule. Note that oxygen does not participate in any of the steps in the citric acid cycle. It instead participates in the electron transport chain (described on page 123). See Figure B-2 in Appendix B for a more detailed view of the citric acid cycle.

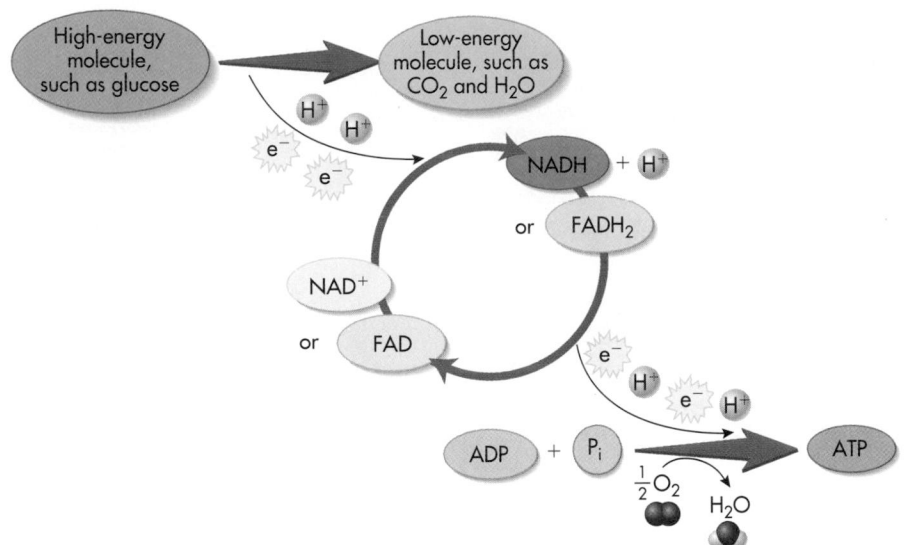

Figure 4-10 | Simplified depiction of electron transfer in energy metabolism. High-energy compounds, such as glucose, give up electrons and hydrogen ions to NAD^+ and FAD. The $NADH + H^+$ and $FADH_2$ that are formed transfer these electrons and hydrogen ions, using specialized electron carriers, to oxygen to form water (H_2O). The energy yielded by the entire process is used to generate ATP from ADP and P_i.

in the pathway are illustrated in Figure 4-11, steps 1 and 2. Pairs of electrons are then separated by coenzyme Q (CoQ) (step 3). Thus, although $NADH + H^+$ and $FADH_2$ transfer their hydrogens to the electron transport chain, the hydrogen ions (H^+), having been separated from their electrons ($H \rightarrow H^+ + e^-$), are not carried down the chain with the electrons. After the pairs of electrons have been separated, each is passed along a group of iron-containing cytochromes. At each transfer from one cytochrome to the next, some energy is given off. A portion is eventually used to generate ATP from ADP and P_i, but much is simply released as heat. At the end of the chain of cytochromes, oxygen, hydrogen ions, and electrons are united to form water: $1/2 C_2 + 2H^+ + 2e^- \rightarrow H_2O$ (step 4).[3]

The key thing to remember here is that the net result of the electron transport chain is the production of ATP and water (steps 4 and 5).

Just How Many ATP Are Produced?

Once the $NADH + H^+$ and $FADH_2$ have transferred their hydrogens to the electron transport chain, they are again in the form of NAD^+ and FAD and are ready to shuttle more hydrogens to the electron transport chain. In Figure 4-11, step 1, $NADH + H^+$ donates its chemical energy to an FAD-related compound called flavin mononucleotide (FMN). In contrast, $FADH_2$ donates its chemical energy at a latter point in the electron transport chain (Figure 4-11, step 2). This different placement of FAD and NAD^+ in the electron transport chain results in a difference in ATP production. Each $NADH + H^+$ in a mitochondrion releases enough energy to form the equivalent of 2.5 ATP, while each $FADH_2$ releases enough energy to form the equivalent of 1.5 ATP.[2]

Of all the ATP yielded by the complete oxidation of glucose, almost 90% are synthesized in the electron transport chain.

So This Is Why Oxygen Is Important

Because oxygen is essential to the processes of the electron transport chain, the electron transport chain is part of aerobic metabolism. $NADH + H^+$ and $FADH_2$ produced during the citric acid cycle can be regenerated into NAD^+ and FAD only by the eventual transfer of their electrons and hydrogen ions to oxygen, as occurs in the electron transport chain. The citric acid cycle has no ability to oxidize $NADH + H^+$ and $FADH_2$ back to NAD^+ and FAD. This is ultimately why oxygen is essential to many life forms; a final acceptor of the electrons and hydrogen ions generated from the breakdown of energy-yielding nutrients is needed. Without oxygen, most of our cells are unable to extract enough energy from energy-yielding nutrients to sustain life.[2]

electron transport chain A series of reactions using oxygen to convert $NADH + H^+$ and $FADH_2$ molecules to free NAD^+ and FAD molecules with the donation of electrons and hydrogen ions to oxygen, yielding water and ATP.

Note that a product called Coenzyme Q-10 is sold as a nutrient supplement in health food stores (the number 10 signifies that it is the form found in humans). However, when the mitochondria need coenzyme Q, they make it. Thus, to maintain overall health, people do not need to take in coenzyme Q in their diet or in the form of a supplement. (Such use may be helpful, however, in people with heart failure; see Chapter 18.)

Figure 4-11 | Organization of the electron transport chain. As electrons move from one molecular complex to the other, hydrogen ions (H⁺) are pumped from the mitochondrial matrix into the intermembrane space (steps 1–4). (Note that each mitochondrion has an inner and outer membrane.) As hydrogen ions flow down a concentration gradient from the intermembrane space into the mitochondrial matrix, ATP is synthesized by the enzyme ATP synthase (step 5). ATP leaves the mitochondrial matrix by way of a channel protein. See Figure B-3 in Appendix B for a more detailed view of the electron transport chain.

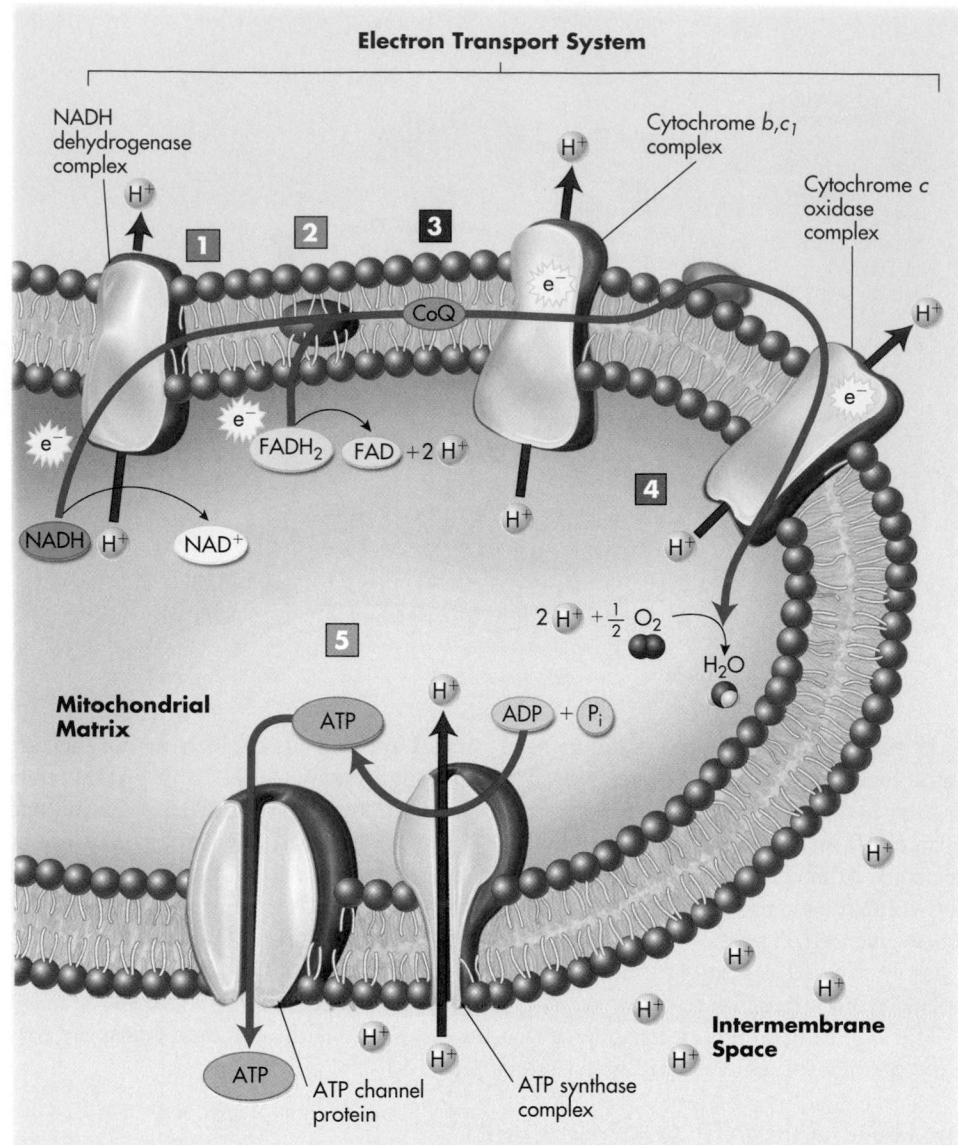

A number of defects have been described related to the metabolic processes that take place in mitochondria. A variety of medical interventions can be used to treat the muscle weakness and muscle destruction typically arising from these disorders; the use of specific nutrients and related metabolic intermediates in treatment is reviewed in reference no. 9.

Summary: The Electron Transport Chain Results in the Production of ATP and Water

The electron transport chain involves the passage of electrons along a series of electron carriers. As electrons are passed along from one carrier to the next, small amounts of energy are released. Some of this energy is ultimately used to generate ATP. NADH + H⁺ and FADH₂ supply both hydrogen ions and electrons to the electron transport chain. At the end of the electron transport chain, hydrogen ions, electrons, and oxygen combine to form water.

Concept | Check

In the citric acid cycle, a 2-carbon acetyl group in the form of acetyl-CoA combines with a 4-carbon oxaloacetate molecule to form the 6-carbon citrate molecule. Through various chemical reactions, the cycle releases two carbon dioxide molecules and eventually yields another oxaloacetate, the starting material. This new oxaloacetate can combine with another acetyl-CoA molecule to begin the process again. The NADH + H⁺ and FADH₂ produced by glycolysis, the transition reaction, and the citric acid cycle donate their electrons and hydrogen ions to the electron transport chain, yielding water and ATP and in the process regenerating NAD⁺ and FAD.

Critical | Thinking

While looking at electron microscopy slides of muscle cells, you observe various organelles. However, the large number of mitochondria you see is remarkable. Your instructor asks you to explain this observation to your classmates. How would you do so?

Expert Opinion

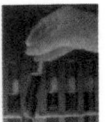

Does a Metabolic Advantage Exist for the High-Protein Diet?

Andrea C. Buchholz, Ph.D., R.D., and Dale A. Schoeller, Ph.D.

High-protein/low-carbohydrate weight-loss diets have become very popular. Despite initial skepticism by many investigators, results from a number of studies have shown that these diets do *initially* yield greater weight losses than do high-carbohydrate/low-fat diets. On average, high-protein diets result in a 12-week weight loss that is 2.5 kg greater, and in a 24-week weight loss that is 4.0 kg greater, than the weight loss on high-carbohydrate/low-fat diets. Assuming that this weight loss has the typical composition of 80% fat mass and 20% fat-free mass:

2.5 kg × 80% fat mass	× 1000 g/kg × 9.5 kcal/g fat[a]	=	19,000 kcal
2.5 kg × 20% fat-free mass	× 1000 g/kg × 1.1 kcal/g fat-free mass[b]	=	550 kcal
Total kcal represented by 2.5 kg weight loss		**=**	**19,550 kcal**
4.0 kg × 80% fat mass	× 1000 g/kg × 9.5 kcal/g fat	=	30,400 kcal
4.0 kg × 20% fat-free mass	× 1000 g/kg × 1.1 kcal/g fat-free mass	=	880 kcal
Total kcal represented by 4.0 kg weight loss		**=**	**31,280 kcal**

[a]9.5 kcal/g is the gross energy density of fat mass. It is higher than the 9 kcal/g metabolizable energy for dietary fat because there is no adjustment for incomplete absorption.

[b]1.1 kcal/g is the energy density of fat-free mass. It is calculated from the gross energy value of protein adjusted for urinary energy losses due to incomplete metabolism and the percentage of fat-free mass that is protein.

Thus, the difference in weight loss after 12 to 24 weeks of treatment reflects a 19,550 to 31,280 kcal difference in energy balance, respectively, or roughly 200 kcal/day. This finding has caused several investigators to ask whether a high-protein weight-loss diet provides a metabolic advantage to the body.

Weight loss occurs because of negative energy balance, when energy expenditure exceeds energy intake. Given that protein, fat, and carbohydrate are all used for energy metabolism but that the yield of ATP produced can vary slightly depending on the route of metabolism, it is reasonable to consider that diets differing in macronutrient distribution may influence total energy expenditure. If a particular diet were to increase total energy expenditure relative to another, then for the same energy intake, energy balance would be more negative for that diet and weight loss would likely be greater. Is it possible that individuals on a high-protein diet "burn" more energy than those on a high-carbohydrate/low-fat diet?

In controlled studies in which participants consume the same amount of energy and in which protein intake is held constant and fat is substituted for carbohydrate diet, neither total energy expenditure nor resting metabolism of those participants on a high-carbohydrate differ from those on a high-fat diet. However, increasing protein intake from 15% to 30 to 35% of total energy intake *does* increase resting metabolism and the degree to which the body must increase energy expenditure to digest, absorb, and process the macronutrients. This increase in energy use in sedentary individuals is estimated to be 41 kcal/day on a 1500 kcal/day energy intake. This amount represents only 20% of the 200 kcal/day difference in energy balance between the two diets. Thus, if there is a metabolic advantage associated with a high-protein diet, it is only a small one.

If the difference in total energy expenditure does not adequately explain the 200 kcal/day energy imbalance between a high-protein/low-carbohydrate diet and a high-carbohydrate/low-fat diet, then there must be a difference in energy intake. One important consideration in studies comparing weight-loss treatments is the accuracy of participants' energy intake data. Ideally, weight-loss studies are conducted in free-living participants. While this situation is desirable because it provides results under real-life conditions, it also means that participants are ultimately responsible for their dietary reports. Because of the well-known tendency of people to underreport their dietary intake, actual intake may be 10 to 50% greater than what is reported in diet records. Even if meals are provided to participants, noncompliance can occur and dietary intakes are likely to be higher than prescribed. Thus, researchers' knowledge of actual dietary intakes of free-living participants in weight-loss studies—regardless of macronutrient distribution—are numerically uncertain.

Even if participants accurately reported their dietary intakes, there would still remain the potential for errors in the calculation of metabolizable energy

(continued)

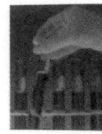

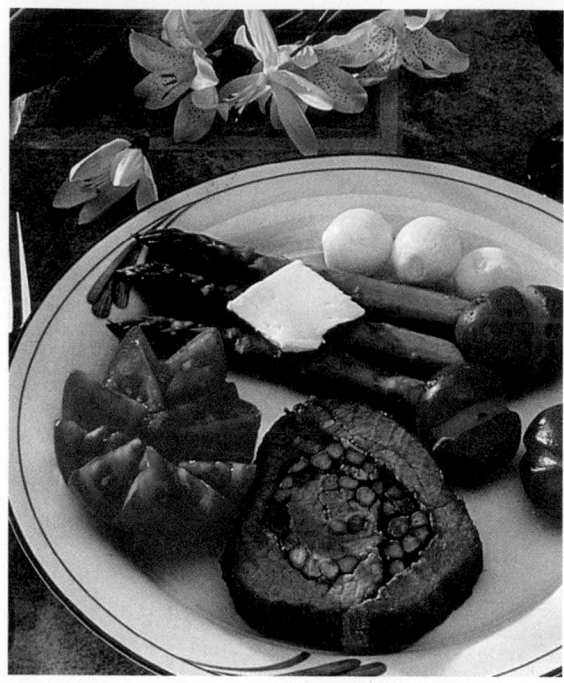

Carbohydrate, protein, fat, and alcohol all contribute chemical energy to the body.

sumed food and the chemical energy lost in feces (due to incomplete absorption) and urine (due to incomplete catabolism). The metabolizable energy values commonly used today are the general factors of 4 kcal/g for carbohydrate, 9 kcal/g for fat, and 4 kcal/g for protein described by Atwater in the early 1900s. However, Atwater clearly demonstrated that these factors were *average* values: although they can be used to calculate the metabolizable energy of a whole diet, they are in error to some degree for most single food items. This problem is due to differences in the bioavailability and chemical structure of individual macronutrients. These general factors have been found to overestimate measured metabolizable energy by 1 to 18%, particularly for high-fiber foods. This overestimation might explain some of the difference in weight loss observed on two diets differing in macronutrient distribution even if the diets are prescribed under controlled conditions. That is, while *calculated* energy intakes may be similar between two groups of participants following diets differing in macronutrient distribution, *actual* energy intakes may be lower in one group relative to the other, and thus weight loss would likely be greater. Experimental data, however, are lacking.

Greater negative energy balance, and thus weight loss, has been observed in individuals consuming a high-protein/low-carbohydrate diet than those consuming a high-carbohydrate/low-fat weight-loss diet. Experimental evidence shows that the small metabolic advantage of the high-protein diet does not adequately explain this energy imbalance. The energy imbalance must therefore be due to differences in energy intake. However, the cause is difficult to determine because of widespread underreporting of energy intakes and because of possible errors in calculated versus metabolizable energy intakes. Further research on the effects of a high-protein diet on energy intake is needed.

intake. In considering this issue, it is worthwhile to briefly review thermodynamics. The first law of thermodynamics states that energy can neither be created nor destroyed, but only transformed. Thus, the human body is constantly transforming energy—in this case, potential energy stored in C–C and C–H bonds—by oxidizing food to produce heat while using some of that energy by shuttling it to ATP for use in muscle contraction, ion pumping, and chemical synthesis. The human body, however, is not a perfect engine and cannot utilize all the potential energy available in food. This is the concept of metabolizable energy, or the difference between the gross energy of con-

Dr. Buchholz is Assistant Professor of Foods and Nutrition at the University of Guelph. She earned a Ph.D. in nutritional sciences from the University of Toronto. Dr. Schoeller is Professor of Nutritional Science at the University of Wisconsin–Madison. He earned a Ph.D. in chemistry from Indiana University. Both have research interests in energy metabolism and body composition.

Aerobic Respiration

As a result of the pathways of aerobic respiration, some of the energy in food is converted to a form of energy that cells can use rather than just being converted immediately to heat, as would have happened if you had ignited the food with a match. The ATP yield from the complete aerobic breakdown of one glucose is 30 to 32 ATP. These ATP account for about 40% of the energy found in one molecule of glucose. The remaining energy (60%) escapes as heat via all the reactions that take place in which ATP, GTP, NADH + H^+ and $FADH_2$ are not made.[2] The same 40:60 ratio applies to the energy metabolism of fatty acids and amino acids. That ratio is fairly efficient given that, for comparison, an automobile engine captures only about 10% of the chemical energy in gasoline. The human body is about four times more efficient than an automobile in extracting energy from carbon-based compounds. In the Expert Opinion, Dr. Andrea Buchholz and Dr. Dale Schoeller discuss whether diet composition influences this efficiency, as is claimed by some weight-loss diets (e.g., low carbohydrate diets).

Glycogen Metabolism

Glycogen synthesis involves adding glucose molecules to an existing glycogen molecule. Glycogen provides liver and muscle cells with a short-term storage form of glucose. Later, when glucose is needed, glycogen breakdown yields glucose as a glucose-phosphate compound, which eventually enters into glycolysis. However, there is a difference in the way the body uses the glycogen stored in liver cells and the glycogen stored in muscle cells. The glucose-phosphate compound formed when the liver breaks down glycogen can eventually be released as glucose into the bloodstream. Therefore, this glucose is available to all the cells of the body. In contrast, the glucose-phosphate compound formed when muscle cells break down glycogen is available for use only by that muscle.

Anaerobic Respiration

Some cells lack mitochondria and so are not capable of aerobic respiration. Other cells are capable of turning to anaerobic respiration when oxygen is lacking. When performed, this anaerobic respiration is not nearly as efficient as aerobic respiration, because it converts only about 5% of the energy in a molecule of glucose to energy stored in the high-energy phosphate bonds of ATP.[2]

Anaerobic Glycolysis

The anaerobic glycolysis pathway encompasses glycolysis and the conversion of pyruvate to lactate (Figure 4-12).

Anaerobic Glycolysis in Red Blood Cells

For cells, such as red blood cells, that lack mitochondria, anaerobic glycolysis is the only available method for making ATP. Such cells lack the oxygen-requiring (aerobic) pathway needed for using $NADH + H^+$ for ATP synthesis, and they also lack the ability to use this process to recycle $NADH + H^+$ back to NAD^+. Therefore, when red blood cells convert glucose to pyruvate, $NADH + H^+$ builds up in the cell. Eventually, the NAD^+ concentration falls too low to permit glycolysis to continue, because most of the NAD^+ present is in the form $NADH + H^+$.[3]

The pathway that regenerates NAD^+ anaerobically involves a reaction that combines pyruvate with $NADH + H^+$ to form lactate (review Figure 4-12). In the process, $NADH + H^+$ turns into NAD^+. The reaction that produces lactate to regenerate NAD^+ can be summarized as:

$$pyruvate + NADH + H^+ \rightarrow lactate + NAD^+$$

The lactate produced by the red blood cell is then released into the bloodstream, picked up primarily by the liver, and synthesized back into pyruvate, glucose, or some other intermediate in aerobic respiration.

Anaerobic Glycolysis in Muscle Cells

Like red blood cells, muscles that are being exercised also produce lactate when they run out of NAD^+. By regenerating NAD^+, the production of lactate allows anaerobic glycolysis to continue. Muscle cells can then make the ATP required for muscle contraction even if little oxygen is present. However, as you will find out in Chapter 14, it will become more difficult to contract those muscles as the lactate concentration builds up.

When respiring anaerobically, some microorganisms such as yeast produce ethanol, a type of alcohol, instead of lactate from glucose. Other microorganisms produce various forms of short-chain fatty acids. All this anaerobic metabolism is referred to as fermentation.

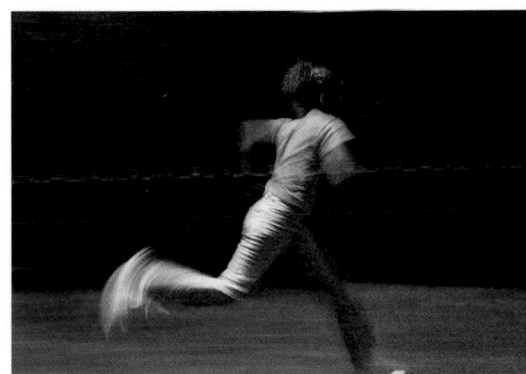

Quick bursts of activity rely on the production of lactate to help meet the ATP energy demand.

Figure 4-12 | Anaerobic glycolysis with lactate as the end product. This process "frees" NAD^+ and it returns to the glycolysis pathway to pick up more hydrogen ions and electrons.

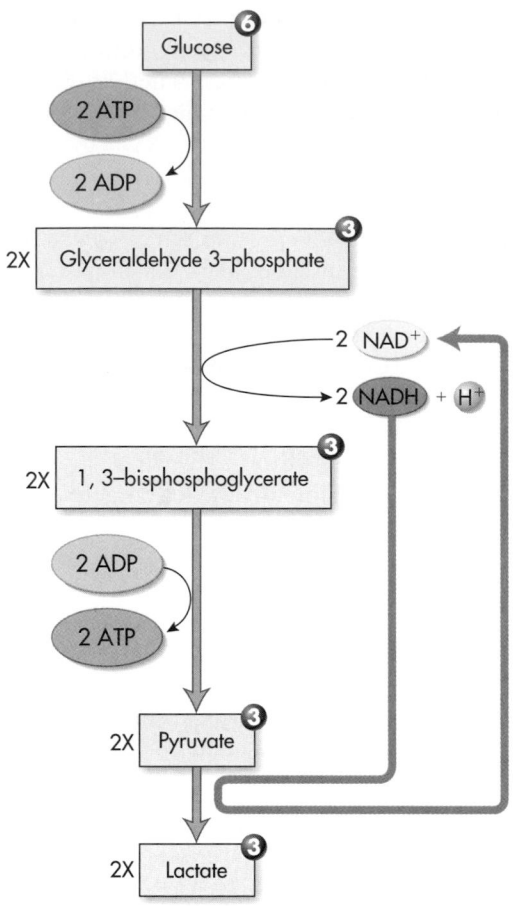

Aerobic and Anaerobic Respiration

Cells need to release energy stored in food fuels and then trap as much of this energy as possible in the form of ATP. The body cannot afford to lose all energy immediately as heat, even though some heat is necessary for maintenance of body temperature. Glycolysis (aerobic and anaerobic), the transition reaction, the citric acid cycle, and the electron transport chain accomplish many tasks in the body. Most important, however, is that they enable cells to capture some of the chemical energy in food in the form of ATP, which then acts as cellular fuel.[2]

Lipolysis: Fat Breakdown

lipolysis The breakdown of triglycerides to glycerol and fatty acids.

peroxisome Cell organelle that uses oxygen to remove hydrogens from compounds. This produces hydrogen peroxide (H_2O_2), which breaks down into O_2 and H_2O.

carnitine A compound used to shuttle fatty acids from the cytosol of the cell into mitochondria.

Lipolysis is part of a process of splitting—breaking down—triglycerides into free fatty acids and glycerol. The further breakdown of the fatty acids for energy production is called *fatty acid oxidation,* because the donation of electrons from fatty acids to oxygen is the net reaction in the energy-yielding process. This process takes place in the mitochondria and **peroxisomes** of the cell, but only mitochondria can use the energy released to form ATP.

Fatty acids are liberated from triglyceride storage in adipose cells by an enzyme called *hormone-sensitive lipase.* The activity of this enzyme is increased by the hormones glucagon, growth hormone, epinephrine, and others, and is decreased by the hormone insulin. The fatty acids are taken up from the bloodstream by cells and are shuttled from the cell cytosol into the mitochondria using a carrier called **carnitine** (Figure 4-13).[5]

Lipolysis

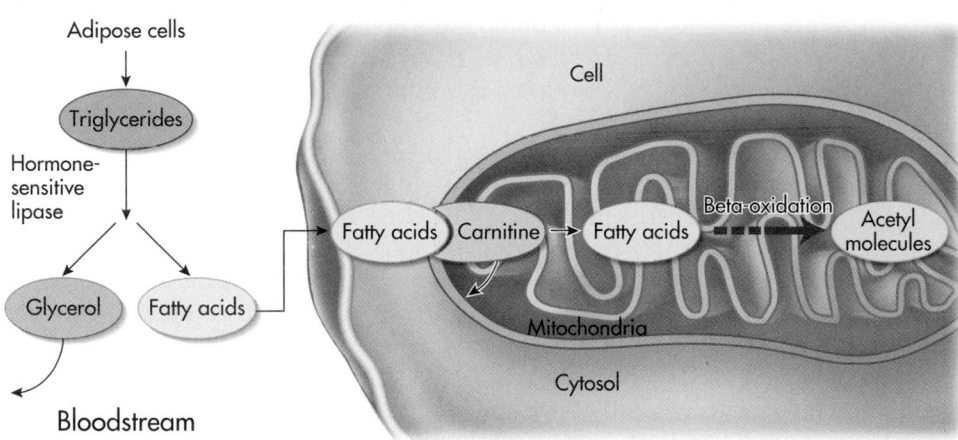

Figure 4-13 | Lipolysis. Because of the action of hormone-sensitive lipase, fatty acids are released from triglycerides in adipose cells and enter the bloodstream. (Hormones such as epinephrine increase the activity of this enzyme.) The fatty acids are taken up from the bloodstream by various cells and shuttled into the inner portion of the cell mitochondria. This shuttling utilizes carnitine. The fatty acid then undergoes beta-oxidation to yield acetate molecules, half as many as the number of carbons in the fatty acid.

Making ATP from Fatty Acids

Almost all fatty acids in nature are composed of an even number of carbons, ranging from 2 to 26. The first step in transferring the energy in such a fatty acid to ATP (fatty acid oxidation) is to cleave the carbons, two at a time, and convert the two-carbon fragments to acetyl-CoA. The process of converting a free fatty acid to multiple acetyl-CoA molecules is called **beta-oxidation,** because the second carbon on a fatty acid (counting after the acid $\left[\begin{matrix} O \\ \| \\ -C-OH \end{matrix} \right]$ end) is called the *beta carbon.*[2] This is where the reaction begins. During beta-oxidation, NADH + H$^+$ and FADH$_2$ are produced. So as with glucose, a fatty acid is eventually degraded into the 2-carbon compound acetate, in the form of acetyl-CoA. Some of the chemical energy contained in the starting compound is transferred to NADH + H$^+$ and FADH$_2$ (Figure 4-14).

The acetyl-CoA enters the citric acid cycle, and two carbon dioxides are released, just as with the acetyl-CoA produced from glucose. Thus, the breakdown product of both glucose and fatty acids, acetyl-CoA, uses a common pathway—the citric acid cycle. One big difference, however, is that a 16-carbon fatty acid yields 104 ATP, whereas the 6-carbon glucose yields only 30 to 32 ATP. That results in a ratio of about 7 ATP per carbon for fatty acids versus about 5 ATP per carbon for glucose. This difference results from the greater number of C–H bonds per carbon in a fatty acid compared to glucose. It is the oxidation of these chemical bonds that provides most of the energy to drive ATP synthesis. Note that many of the carbons in glucose are also bonded to hydroxyl groups (–OH) rather than only to hydrogen atoms, as is primarily the case with fatty acids. Thus, as a whole, the carbons of glucose exist in a more oxidized state. This is why fats yield more kcals/g than carbohydrates (9 versus 4)—fats are less oxidized (more reduced) than carbohydrates.[2]

In healthy people, cells produce the carnitine needed for synthesis, and carnitine supplements provide no benefit. In patients hospitalized with acute illnesses, however, carnitine synthesis may be inadequate for their needs. These patients may need to have carnitine added to their intravenous total parenteral nutrition solutions.

beta-oxidation The breakdown of a fatty acid into numerous acetyl-CoA molecules.

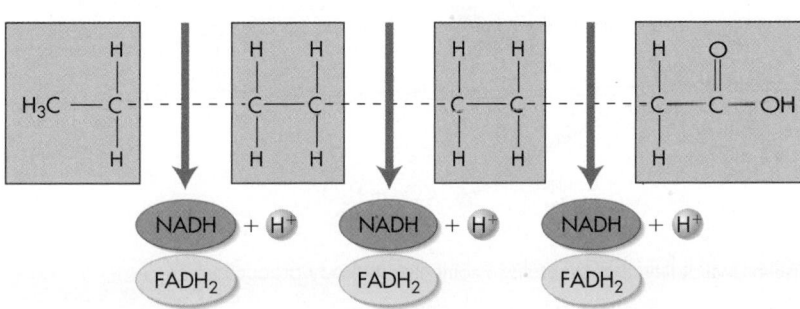

Figure 4-14 | Beta-oxidation of fatty acids. In beta-oxidation, each 2-carbon fragment (acetyl group) yields electrons and hydrogen ions to form NADH + H$^+$ and FADH$_2$ as the fragments are split off the parent fatty acid. The 2-carbon acetyl molecule then typically enters the citric acid cycle (as acetyl-CoA).

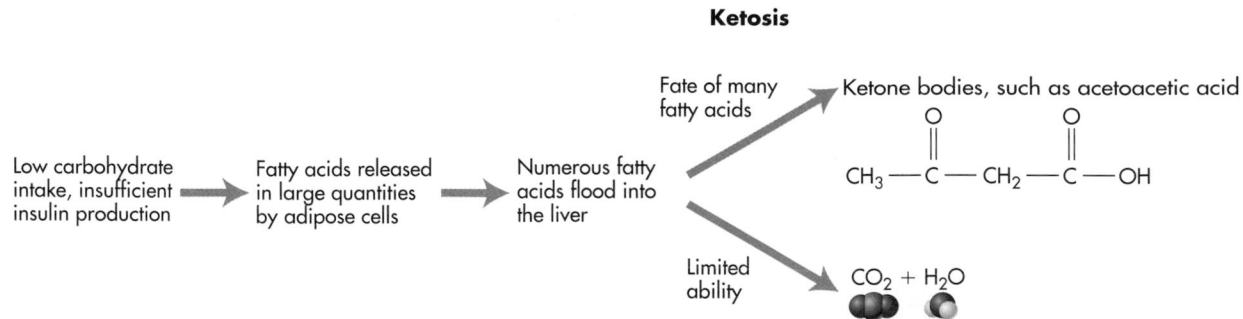

Pyruvate

Oxaloacetate

ketone bodies Incomplete breakdown products of fat, containing three or four carbons. Most contain a chemical group called a ketone, hence the name. An example is acetoacetic acid.

ketosis The condition of having a high concentration of ketone bodies and related breakdown products in the bloodstream and tissues.

No matter how many carbons a fatty acid contains, it is usually broken down into acetyl-CoA. Occasionally, a fatty acid has an odd number of carbons, so the cell forms many acetyl-CoA, plus one 3-carbon compound (propionyl-CoA). This enters the citric acid cycle directly, bypassing acetyl-CoA. It can then go on to yield NADH + H$^+$, FADH$_2$, and carbon dioxide, and even other products such as glucose.

Carbohydrate Aids Fat Metabolism

In addition to its role in energy production, the citric acid cycle provides compounds that leave the cycle and enter biosynthetic pathways. This means that even though most oxaloacetate is reused in the cycle, a minimum amount of synthesis must still be maintained because this removal from the citric acid cycle for biosynthetic reactions could slow citric acid cycle activity. One potential source of this additional oxaloacetate is pyruvate. Thus, as fatty acids create acetyl-CoA, carbohydrates such as glucose are needed to keep the concentration of pyruvate high enough to resupply oxaloacetate to the citric acid cycle. Overall, the entire pathway for fatty acid oxidation works better when carbohydrate is available.

Ketogenesis is Producing Ketone Bodies from Fatty Acids

Ketone bodies are products of incomplete fatty acid oxidation.[13] Hormonal imbalances—chiefly, inadequate insulin production to balance glucagon action in the body—allow for the development of some metabolic conditions that lead to significant production of ketone bodies called *ketosis* (Figure 4-15).

1. Fatty acids stored in adipose cells are rapidly released into the bloodstream. A fall in blood insulin is the key reason, because insulin inhibits lipolysis and, instead, favors fat storage. The bulk of the increase in fatty acids in the blood is taken up by the liver.
2. Fatty acid oxidation to acetyl-CoA predominates over fatty acid synthesis in the liver because the presence of a high amount of free fatty acids inhibits the first step in fatty acid synthesis.
3. As the liver takes up the fatty acids and degrades them to acetyl-CoA, the capacity of the citric acid cycle to process the resulting acetyl-CoA molecules decreases. This is mostly because the metabolism of fatty acids to acetyl-CoA yields many ATP, and high amounts of ATP slow citric acid cycle activity in liver cells. Essentially, there is no need to use the citric acid cycle—the main role of which is to transfer energy from fuels for use in ATP synthesis—when the cells have plenty of ATP already. Other possible contributors include lack of enough oxaloacetate or coenzyme A to allow for all the fatty acids to be oxidized in the citric acid cycle.

Ketosis

Low carbohydrate intake, insufficient insulin production → Fatty acids released in large quantities by adipose cells → Numerous fatty acids flood into the liver

Fate of many fatty acids → Ketone bodies, such as acetoacetic acid

Limited ability → CO_2 + H_2O

Figure 4-15 | Key steps in ketosis. Any condition that limits insulin availability to cells results in some ketone body production.

These metabolic changes encourage the liver cells to first form acetyl-CoA and then unite two acetyl-CoA molecules to form a 4-carbon compound. This compound is further metabolized and eventually secreted into the bloodstream as the ketone bodies acetoacetic acid and two related compounds, beta-hydroxybutyric acid and acetone.

Most ketone bodies are subsequently converted back into acetyl-CoA in other body cells, which use the ketone bodies for fuel. The acetyl-CoA is then pushed through the citric acid cycle. One of the ketone bodies formed (acetone) leaves the body via the lungs, giving the breath of a person in ketosis a characteristic, fruity smell.

Ketosis in Semistarvation or Fasting

When a person is in a state of semistarvation or fasting, carbohydrate availability falls, and so insulin production falls. This fall in blood insulin then causes fatty acids to flood into the bloodstream and eventually form ketone bodies, as just described. The heart, muscles, and some parts of the kidneys then use ketone bodies for fuel. After a few days of ketosis, the brain also begins to metabolize ketone bodies for energy.

This adaptive response is important to semistarvation or fasting. As more body cells begin to use ketone bodies for fuel, the need for glucose as a body fuel diminishes. This then reduces the need for the liver and kidneys to produce glucose from amino acids (and as well from the glycerol released from lipolysis), sparing much body protein from being used as a fuel source. The maintenance of body protein mass is a key to survival in semistarvation or fasting. Death is seen when about half of the body protein is depleted, usually coming after about 50 to 70 days of total fasting. In prolonged fasting, about half the energy needs are met by the use of ketone bodies; only 5% of energy use comes from glucose that was made from amino acids.[20]

Ketosis in Diabetes

In type 1 diabetes, little to no insulin is produced. This lack of insulin does not allow for normal carbohydrate and fat metabolism. Without sufficient insulin and the related inability to readily utilize carbohydrate, excess production of ketone bodies occurs.[18] If the concentration of ketone bodies rises too high in the blood, the excess spills into the urine, pulling the electrolytes sodium and potassium with it. Eventually, severe ion imbalances occur in the body. The blood also becomes more acidic because two of the three forms of ketone bodies contain acid groups. The resulting condition, known as *diabetic ketoacidosis (DKA)*, can induce coma or death if not treated immediately, such as with insulin, electrolytes, and fluids (see Chapter 5 for more details). Ketoacidosis usually occurs only in ketosis caused by uncontrolled type 1 diabetes; in fasting, blood concentrations of ketone bodies usually do not rise high enough to cause the problem.

▌ Lipogenesis: Building Fatty Acids

Lipogenesis is the formation of lipid. The majority of the pathways used are found in the cytosol of liver cells. Ingested protein or carbohydrate that the body does not use immediately can be converted into triglycerides and stored as such. Some of the protein can reside in amino acid pools in the body, but the amount is not significant. Most carbohydrate is stored as glycogen, but the total amount rarely exceeds 350 g in the entire body. Thus, when a lot of amino acids and/or glucose are left over in the body after a large meal containing protein and/or carbohydrate, some of the carbons can be used to synthesize fatty acids. (It is typically of minor importance in humans, however.)[17] This process requires ATP and the B-vitamins biotin, niacin, and pantothenic acid. Because ATP is used, lipogenesis is an energy-losing proposition for a liver cell.

In lipogenesis, the liver begins with carbons from glucose and the carbons from amino acids that are metabolized to acetyl-CoA. Cells in the liver bond the acetate

Critical | Thinking

The use of a very-low-carbohydrate diet to induce ketosis for weight loss is covered in Chapter 13. Why is careful physician monitoring needed if this type of diet is followed?

lipogenesis The building of fatty acids using derivatives of acetyl-CoA.

malonyl-CoA Building block in fatty acid synthesis: HO–C–CH$_2$–C–Coenzyme A

very-low-density lipoprotein (VLDL) The lipoprotein created in the liver that carries both the cholesterol and the lipids taken up from the bloodstream by the liver and those that are newly synthesized by the liver.

parts of acetyl-CoA molecules (actually in the form of **malonyl-CoA**) together in a series of steps to form a 16-carbon saturated fatty acid, palmitic acid. Insulin increases activity of a key enzyme used in the pathway (fatty acid synthase). This 16-carbon fatty acid can later be lengthened to an 18- or 20-carbon chain either in the cytosol or mitochondria.[2] Ultimately, the fatty acids are joined to a form of glycerol (produced during glycolysis from glyceraldehyde 3-phosphate) to yield a triglyceride. The triglyceride is later released to the general circulation as a **very-low-density lipoprotein,** or **VLDL** (see Chapter 6). Cells that take up fat may use it for ATP production, or it may be stored in cells (mostly adipose cells), along with other fats that originate from dietary intake.

Concept | Check

Fatty acids are degraded into numerous acetyl-CoA molecules. These molecules participate in the citric acid cycle and electron transport chain to yield carbon dioxide, water, and ATP. To synthesize fat, a cell binds numerous acetate molecules together to form a fatty acid. Three fatty acids can then be joined to glycerol to yield a triglyceride. If acetyl-CoA oxidation in liver cells is limited, such as in cases of long-term fasting, the acetyl-CoA resulting from fatty acid oxidation tends to force the production of ketone bodies. These ketone bodies enter the bloodstream and are eventually metabolized to carbon dioxide and water (after being converted back to acetyl-CoA) by various cells. In lipogenesis, carbons originally donated by acetyl-CoA are used to form fatty acids.

| Protein Metabolism

Protein metabolism begins after proteins are degraded into amino acids. To use an amino acid for fuel, cells must first split off the amino group (–NH$_2$) (see Chapter 7). These pathways often require vitamin B-6 to function. Removal of the amino group produces **carbon skeletons,** which mostly enter the citric acid cycle. Some carbon skeletons also yield acetyl-CoA or pyruvate (Figure 4-16).[3]

carbon skeleton What remains of an amino acid after the amino group has been removed.

Amino acid metabolism mostly takes place in the liver. Only branched-chain amino acids—leucine, isoleucine, and valine—are metabolized primarily at other sites—in this case, the muscles.[8] Branched-chain amino acids are added to some liquid meal replacement supplements given to hospitalized patients. Some fluid replacement formulas marketed to athletes also contain branched-chain amino acids (see Chapter 14).

The steps in protein synthesis are covered in Chapter 7.

It is important to note that some carbon skeletons enter the citric acid cycle as acetyl-CoA, whereas others form intermediates of the citric acid cycle or glycolysis. Any part of the carbon skeleton that can bypass acetyl-CoA and enter the citric acid cycle directly, or form pyruvate, can eventually become part of glucose via gluconeogenesis. Such is true for the amino acids alanine, methionine, arginine, histidine, aspartic acid, and others (review Figure 4-15).[2]

Producing Glucose from Amino Acids and Other Compounds

gluconeogenesis The production of new glucose by metabolic pathways in the cell. Amino acids derived from protein usually provide the carbons for this glucose.

The entire pathway to produce glucose from compounds such as certain amino acids—**gluconeogenesis**—is present only in liver cells and in certain kidney cells. A typical starting material for this process is oxaloacetate, which is derived primarily from the carbon skeletons of some amino acids, mostly the amino acid alanine. Pyruvate can also be converted to oxaloacetate (review Figure 4-16).

The 4-carbon oxaloacetate loses one carbon dioxide and converts to a 3-carbon compound phosphoenolpyruvate, which then reverses the path back through glycolysis to glucose. It takes two of this 3-carbon compound to produce the 6-carbon glucose. Some steps in gluconeogenesis are simply a reversal or variation of the glycolysis pathway. This entire process requires ATP as well as coenzyme forms of the B-vitamins biotin, riboflavin, niacin, and B-6.[3]

To learn more about gluconeogenesis, examine Figure 4-16, which traces the pathway in converting glutamic acid, an amino acid, to glucose. Glutamic acid first loses its amino group to form its carbon skeleton. This enters the citric acid cycle directly and is converted by stages to oxaloacetate. Oxaloacetate loses one carbon as carbon dioxide, and the 3-carbon phosphoenolpyruvate produced then moves through glycolysis to form glucose. Eventually, two glutamic acid molecules are needed to form one glucose molecule.

Gluconeogenesis from Typical Fatty Acids Is Not Possible

Why can't a typical fatty acid be turned into glucose? A fatty acid with an even number of carbons—the typical form in the body—breaks down into many acetyl-CoA molecules. The step between pyruvate and acetyl-CoA is irreversible; acetyl-CoA can never re-form into pyruvate once the carbon dioxide molecule is lost. The only option

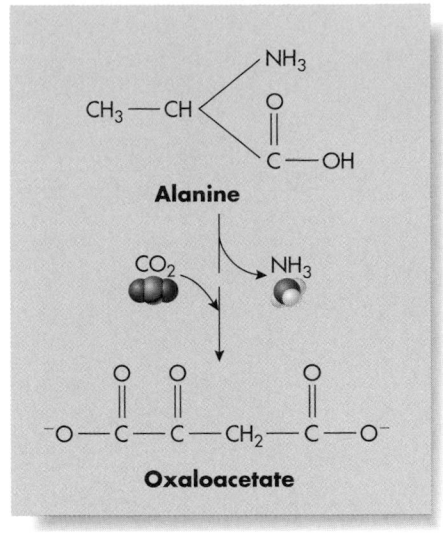

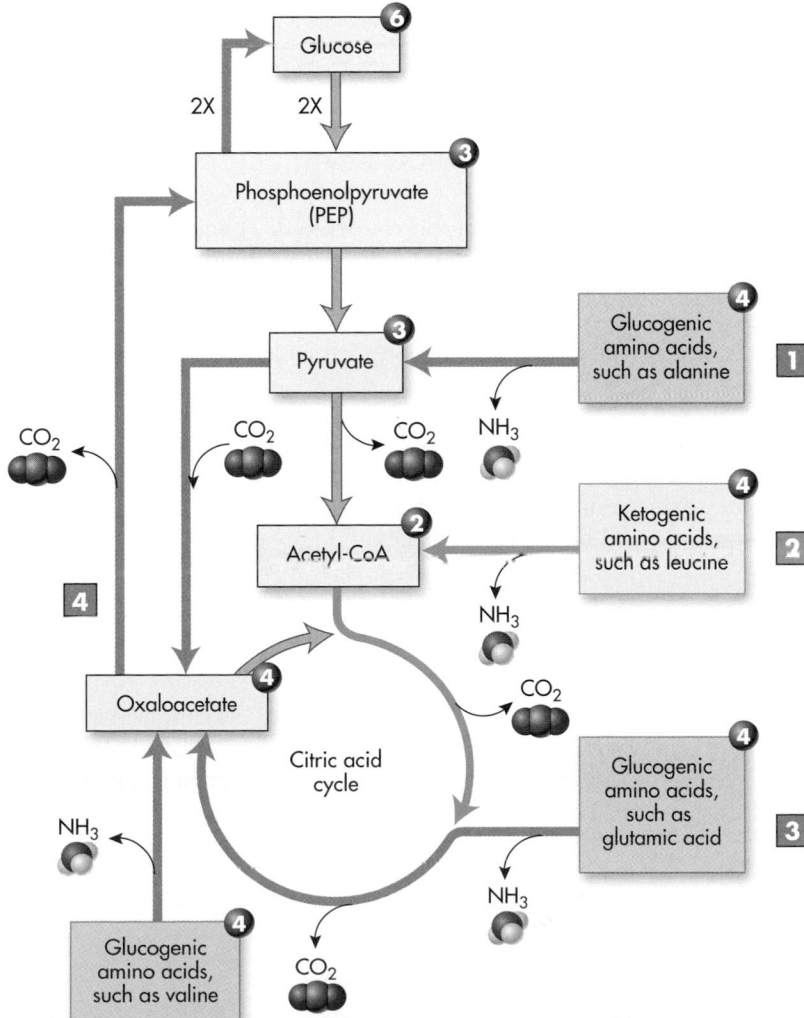

Figure 4-16 | Gluconeogenesis. Carbon skeletons of amino acids that become pyruvate (such as alanine, glycine, cysteine, serine, and threonine) (step 1) or enter directly into the citric acid cycle (such amino acids include asparagine, arginine, aspartic acid, histidine, glutamic acid, glutamine, isoleucine, methionine, proline, valine, and phenylalanine) (step 3) or are called *glucogenic amino acids* because these carbons can become the carbons of glucose. Any parts of carbon skeletons that become acetyl-CoA are called *ketogenic* because these carbons cannot become parts of glucose molecules (step 2). These include leucine and lysine, and parts of isoleucine, phenylalanine, tryptophan, and tyrosine. The deciding factor is whether part or all of the carbon skeleton of the amino acid yields a "new" oxaloacetate molecule during metabolism, two of which are needed to form glucose (step 4).

then for acetyl-CoA, besides forming fatty acids or ketones, is to combine with oxaloacetate in the citric acid cycle. However, two carbons of acetyl-CoA are added to oxaloacetate at the beginning of the citric acid cycle, and two carbons are subsequently lost as carbon dioxide when citrate converts back to the starting material, oxaloacetate. So at the end of one cycle no carbons are left to turn into glucose. Thus it is impossible to convert typical fatty acids into glucose.[3]

The only part of a triglyceride that can become glucose is the glycerol portion. Propionyl-CoA formed from the metabolism of odd-chain fatty acids can do the same. Glycerol enters into the glycolysis pathway, and propionyl-CoA can directly enter the citric acid cycle at succinyl-CoA. Propionyl-CoA can then flow through the citric acid cycle to oxaloacetate and then through the process of gluconeogenesis to convert to glucose. Glycerol can follow the gluconeogenesis pathway from glyceraldehyde 3-phosphate to glucose. Glucose yield from these compounds is insignificant, however, because the body produces little propionyl-CoA and only about 10% of the molecular weight of a triglyceride is glycerol.[2]

Recall from the earlier discussion on ketosis that if there is an insufficient amount of carbohydrate in the body to meet ongoing needs, the liver and kidneys are forced to synthesize glucose from body protein to support the energy needs of the brain and red blood cells. Liver and kidney cells primarily begin with carbon skeletons from amino acids that are able to directly enter the citric acid cycle or form pyruvate. These compounds are converted to oxaloacetate, then to a 3-carbon intermediate compound, phosphoenolpyruvate, and finally to glucose. Initially when a person fasts, the liver performs about 90% of total body gluconeogenesis. This falls to about 60% in prolonged fasting.

Disposing of Excess Amino Groups from Amino Acid Metabolism

The catabolism of amino acids yields amino groups ($-NH_2$), which then form ammonia (NH_3). The ammonia needs to be excreted because its buildup is toxic to cells. The liver prepares the amino groups for excretion in the urine using the urea cycle. During the urea cycle, two nitrogen groups—one ammonia group and one amino group—react through a series of steps with carbon dioxide molecules to form urea (H_2NCNH_2) and water. Eventually, urea is excreted in the urine (Figure 4-17).[3] In liver disease, ammonia can build up to toxic concentrations in the blood, whereas in kidney disease the toxic agent is urea. The form of nitrogen in the blood—ammonia or urea—is a diagnostic tool for detecting liver or kidney disease.

Concept | Check

Individual amino acids lose an amino group and become carbon skeletons. Many carbon skeletons can be further metabolized so that they enter either the citric acid cycle or the glycolysis pathway. The carbons can then proceed through gluconeogenesis to form new glucose. If the carbon skeleton forms acetyl-CoA, glucose production is not possible from that part of the amino acid. The amino groups go on to form part of urea, which is excreted from the body in urine.

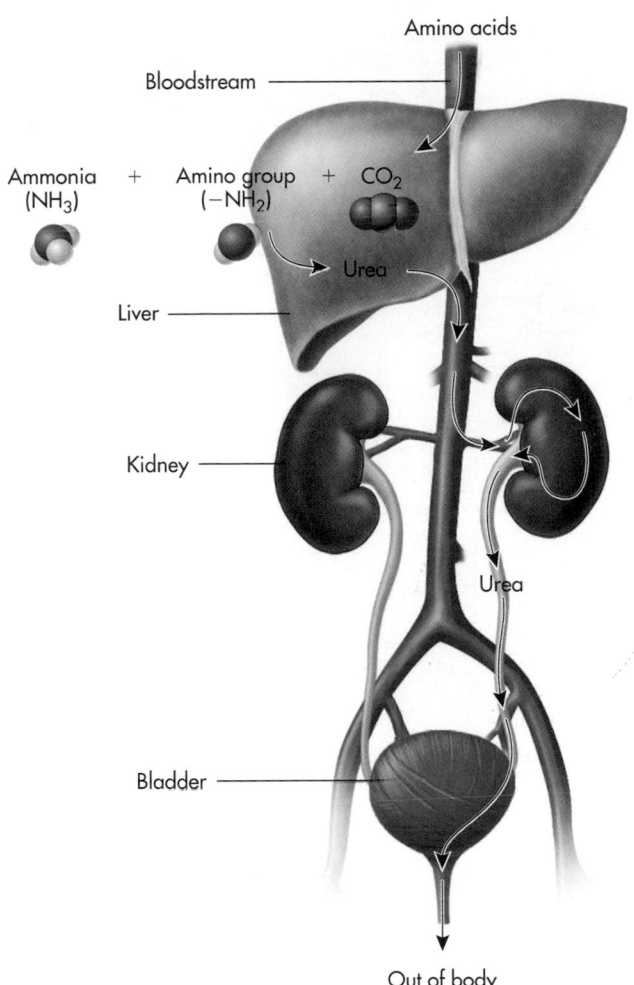

Amino acids

Bloodstream

Ammonia   +   Amino group   + CO_2
(NH_3) $(-NH_2)$

Liver

Urea

Kidney

Urea

Bladder

Out of body

Figure 4-17 | Disposal of excess amino groups. The nitrogen groups, one as ammonia and the other as an amino group, form part of urea, which is excreted in urine (H_2NCNH_2). The nitrogen groups originally came from amino acids that went through transamination reactions and ultimately deamination to yield the free nitrogen groups.

What Happens Where: A Review

Glycolysis takes place in the cytosol of a cell. The end product of glycolysis, pyruvate, enters the mitochondria, where it is further degraded in the citric acid cycle. The $NADH + H^+$ made in the cytosol during glycolysis must be shuttled into the mitochondria if the electron transport chain is to be used to convert $NADH + H^+$ back to NAD^+ and simultaneously produce ATP. The type of shuttle determines how many ATP each $NADH + H^+$ yields. Generally, 2.5 ATP are formed. One type of shuttle system results in the loss of one potential ATP, so only 1.5 ATP result.[2]

Fatty acid oxidation also occurs in the mitochondria. The product of beta-oxidation, acetyl-CoA, is metabolized by the citric acid cycle in the mitochondria. Fatty acids are synthesized primarily in the cytosol.[2]

Gluconeogenesis begins in the mitochondria with the production of oxaloacetate. Oxaloacetate eventually returns to the cytosol, where new glucose is produced. The same is true for the urea cycle; some stages occur in the cytosol and some in the mitochondria (Figure 4-18).[2]

Figure 4-18 | A bird's-eye view of cell metabolism. Note that acetyl-CoA forms a crossroads for many pathways and that the citric acid cycle can also be used to help build compounds, such as certain amino acids. Anabolic and catabolic processes may appear to share the same pathways, but generally this is true for only a few steps. Separate enzymes control anabolic and catabolic flow in a pathway. This allows the cell significant control over metabolism, since a specific set of enzymes can be activated to promote either anabolism or catabolism. If the chemical reactions in anabolism and catabolism were catalyzed by the same set of enzymes, the direction of flow of compounds through these pathways would be dictated exclusively by the concentration of the starting materials rather than by the cell's changing needs for energy or synthesis of needed compounds.

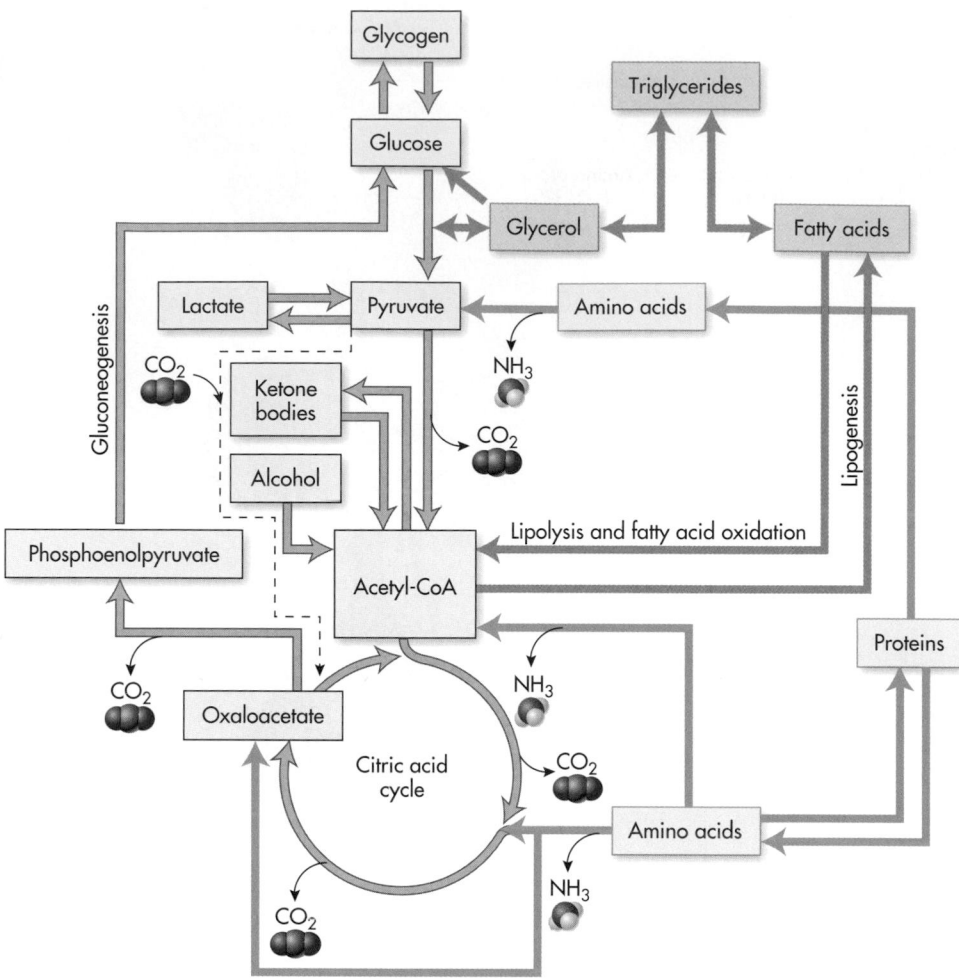

Since the electron transport chain yields most of the ATP for the cell, the mitochondria are the cell's major energy-producing organelles. Cells that need to make a lot of ATP, such as muscle cells, have thousands of mitochondria, whereas cells that need very little ATP, such as adipose cells, have fewer mitochondria.

Energy metabolism can take many forms in the body. By stringing together the glycolysis pathway and the citric acid cycle, cells can convert carbohydrates into fatty acids, convert carbohydrates into carbon skeletons for synthesis of certain amino acids, and use the energy in carbohydrates to form ATP (review Figure 4-18). These pathways can also turn carbon skeletons of some amino acids into carbon skeletons of others. Furthermore, they can convert carbon skeletons from some amino acids to glucose or have them drive ATP synthesis. Finally, fatty acids can provide energy for ATP synthesis or produce ketone bodies. The glycerol part of the triglyceride can either be converted into glucose and be used for fuel, or can contribute to ATP synthesis via participation in glycolysis, citric acid cycle, and electron transport chain metabolism (Table 4-1).

▌ Regulating Metabolism

Among the organs, the liver plays the major role in regulating metabolism: it responds to hormones and makes use of vitamins. Additional means of regulating metabolism involve enzymes, ATP concentrations, and minerals.[3]

Table 4-1 | Summary of Energy-Yielding Nutrient Metabolism

Nutrient in Diet	Contributes to Energy Needs?	Yields Glucose?	Yields Amino Acids for Body Proteins?	Yields Fat for Adipose Tissue Stores?	Energy Cost of Conversion to Adipose Tissue Stores
Carbohydrate (glucose)	Yes	Yes	Yes, can provide carbons for the carbon skeletons of certain amino acids	Yes, but not readily	High
Lipid (triglycerides)	Yes	Generally not; the glycerol present provides a minimal amount	Indirectly by adding carbons to oxaloacetate that then can form a carbon skeleton for certain amino acids from a citric acid cycle intermediate	Yes	Minimal
Protein (amino acids)	Yes, but generally not much	Yes, excess amino acids can be converted to glucose	Yes, but not readily	Yes	High

The Liver

The liver is the location of many nutrient interconversions (Figure 4-19). Most nutrients must pass first through the liver after absorption into the body. What leaves the liver is often different from what entered. Key metabolic functions of the liver include conversions between various forms of simple sugars, fat and cholesterol synthesis, production of ketone bodies, amino acid metabolism, urea production, and alcohol metabolism. Nutrient storage is an additional liver function.[8]

Enzymes

Enzymes are the key regulators of metabolic pathways; both their presence and their rate of activity are critical to chemical reactions in the body. Enzyme synthesis and rates of activity are controlled by cells and by the products of the reactions in which the enzymes participate. For example, a high-protein diet leads to increased synthesis of enzymes associated with amino acid catabolism and gluconeogenesis. Within hours of a shift to a low-protein diet, the synthesis of enzymes associated with amino acid metabolism will slow.[3]

Critical | Thinking

If you had unlimited resources to design a drug that inhibits lipogenesis, which aspect of cellular respiration would you look to affect? What unintended metabolic consequences might result from using such a drug? Reviewing Figure 4-18 might help you answer this question.

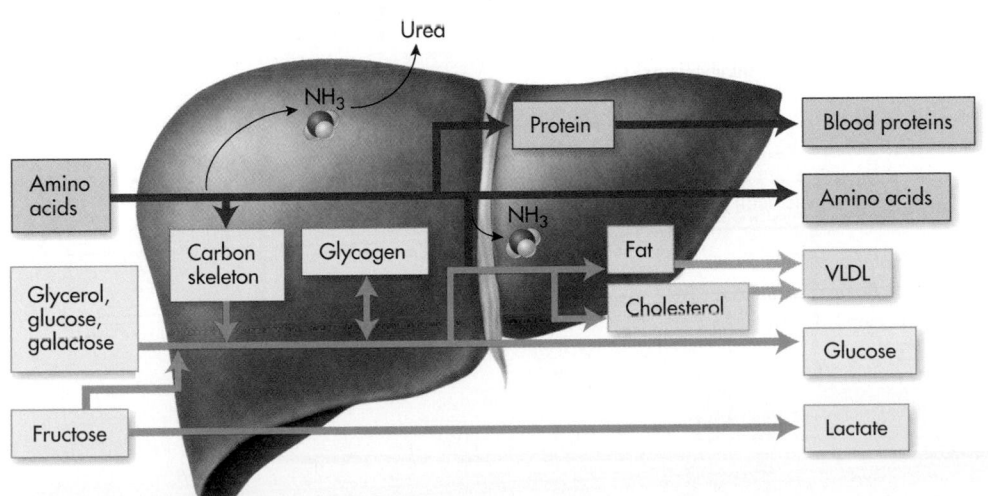

Figure 4-19 | Liver metabolism. Most nutrients must pass first through the liver after absorption into the body. What leaves the liver is often different from what entered. VLDL stands for very-low-density lipoprotein. This lipoprotein carries fat from the liver to other body cells (see Chapter 6 for details).

Hormones

Hormones, including insulin, serve as regulators of metabolic processes. Low levels of insulin in the blood promote gluconeogenesis, protein breakdown, and lipolysis. Increased blood insulin promotes the synthesis of glycogen, fat, and protein.

ATP Concentrations

ATP concentration in a cell plays a role in the regulation of metabolism. High ATP concentrations decrease energy-yielding reactions such as glycolysis and promote anabolic reactions, such as lipogenesis, that use ATP. High ADP concentrations, on the other hand, stimulate energy-yielding pathways.[12]

Vitamins and Minerals

Many vitamins and minerals participate in metabolic pathways (Figure 4-20). Most notable are the B-vitamins thiamin, riboflavin, niacin, pantothenic acid, biotin, vitamin B-6, folate, and vitamin B-12 as well as the minerals iron and copper. Because so many metabolic pathways depend on nutrient input, health problems can develop from nutrient deficiencies.[8] The roles that vitamins and minerals play in metabolism will be discussed in greater detail in Chapters 9, 10, 11, and 12.

> **Concept** | Check
>
> Glycolysis takes place in the cytosol of the cell; the transition reaction, citric acid cycle, and electron transport chain occur in mitochondria. Fatty acid oxidation occurs in mitochondria; fatty acids are synthesized mostly in the cytosol. Both urea formation and gluconeogenesis take place in both mitochondria and the cytosol. Hormone balance, enzyme activity, and the need for ATP all influence the rate at which these metabolic pathways operate. Because many metabolic pathways converge at acetyl-CoA, it is central to energy metabolism.

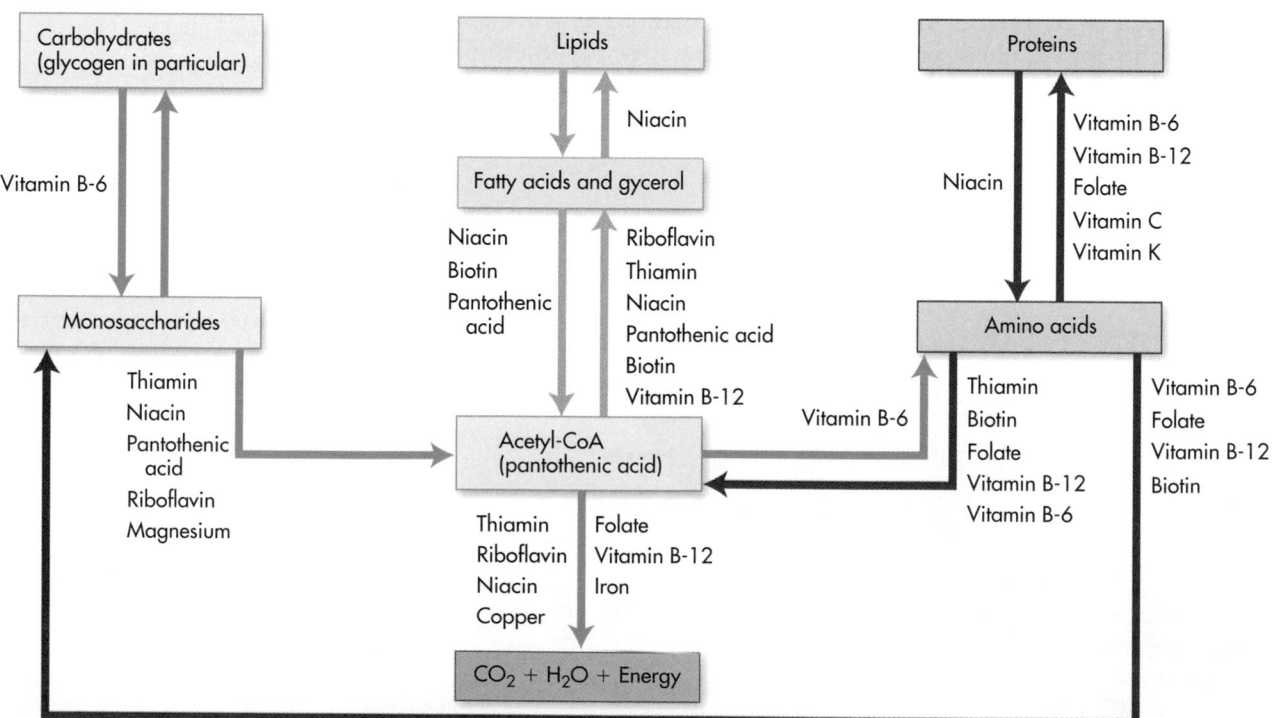

Figure 4-20 | Many vitamins and minerals participate in the metabolic pathways.

Fasting and Feasting

This chapter ends with a brief discussion of the consequences of fasting and feasting. Some of the material in this section will repeat what you have already learned, and some will serve as a preview for subsequent chapters.

Fasting

When individuals fast, their metabolic rate slows, reducing their need for energy. The decrease in metabolic rate is due to decreased food intake and organ breakdown (protein breakdown). With the resultant fall in insulin production, fasting encourages gluconeogenesis, protein breakdown, and fat breakdown with subsequent production of ketone bodies (Figure 4-21).[5,13] Loss of body protein, as it is broken down for energy, is rapid until the nervous system adapts to using ketone bodies for energy. For the first few days of a fast, protein supplies about 90% of needed glucose, with the remaining 10% coming from glycerol. (In prolonged fasting, about half the body's energy needs are met by ketone bodies; only 5% of energy use comes from glucose that was made from amino acids.)

Sodium and potassium depletion can also result as the two elements are drawn into the urine along with ketone bodies. Finally, increased blood urea levels result because of the breakdown of protein.

The maintenance of body protein mass is a key to survival in semistarvation or fasting. Death is seen when about half the body protein is depleted, usually coming after about 50 to 70 days of total fasting.

Feasting

The most obvious result of feasting is the accumulation of body fat. In addition, feasting, with the resultant increase in insulin production by the pancreas, encourages the burning of glucose for energy needs as well as the synthesis of glycogen and, to a lesser extent, protein and fat (Figure 4-22).[5,17]

Excess Carbohydrate

Any carbohydrate consumed in excess will first be used to ensure that glycogen stores are maximized. Once glycogen stores have been filled, the consumption of carbohydrate will stimulate carbohydrate catabolism. This then lessens the need for any fat

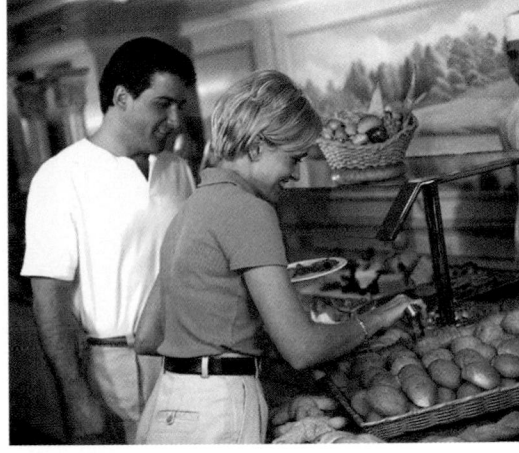

Feasting especially encourages the synthesis of glycogen and storage of fat.

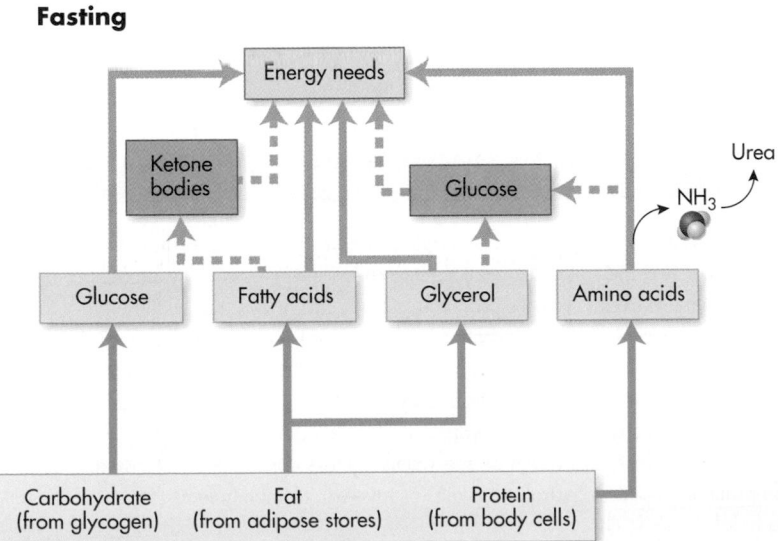

Figure 4-21 | Fasting (solid line) initially encourages use of glucose, fatty acids, and amino acids for energy needs. Prolonged fasting (dashed line), which ends up depleting glycogen stores, leads to increased production of glucose from both glycerol and certain carbon skeletons of amino acids. This supplies glucose to glucose-dependent cells, such as red blood cells. Ketone body production also increases.

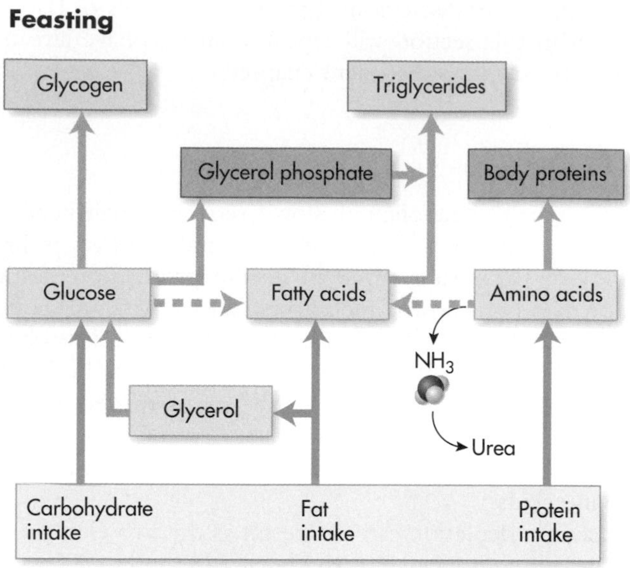

Figure 4-22 | Feasting (solid line) encourages glycogen and triglyceride synthesis and storage and allows amino acids to participate in the synthesis of body proteins. Minimal synthesis (dashed line) of fatty acids using glucose or carbon skeletons of amino acids occurs unless intake is quite excessive in comparison to overall energy needs.

Feasting

catabolism. There are two caveats to this statement. First, recall that carbohydrate consumption stimulates insulin secretion, and increased amounts of insulin in the blood have an affect on fat metabolism. Second, if excess energy is consumed, carbohydrate can be synthesized into fat and so contribute to body fat stores. However, again this pathway is not very active in humans.[17] In addition, it is energetically expensive to convert carbohydrate to body fat (review Table 4-1).

Excess Protein

Contrary to what you may have heard, increased protein/amino acid consumption does not promote muscle development. Any protein consumed in excess will first stimulate increased protein catabolism and then will contribute to fat synthesis and the accumulation of body fat.[8] However, the energy cost of converting protein into body fat is higher than it is for the conversion of dietary fat to body fat (review Table 4-1).

Excess Fat

Unlike the consumption of excess carbohydrate and protein, consumption of fat does not promote fat catabolism. Most of the fat in a meal goes immediately into storage in adipose cells.[8] Furthermore, compared to the conversion of carbohydrate and protein, relatively little energy is required to convert dietary fat into body fat. Therefore, high-fat diets promote accumulation of body fat (review Table 4-1).

Fasting encourages

Glycogen breakdown
Fat breakdown
Gluconeogenesis
Synthesis of ketone bodies

Feasting encourages

Glycogen synthesis
Protein synthesis
Fat synthesis
Urea synthesis

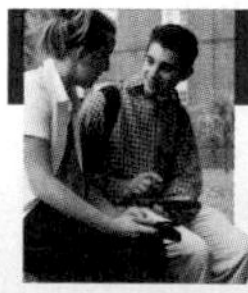

Case Scenario| Follow-Up

As you have learned in this chapter, one of Ana's friends got it wrong and the other two did not quite get it right. While it requires a large amount of energy to convert either carbohydrate or protein into body fat, it takes very little energy to convert dietary fat into body fat. In addition, a gram of fat contains more energy than a gram of either carbohydrate or protein, so if Ana eats equal amounts of carbohydrate (or protein) and fat, she will obtain more energy from the fat than from the carbohydrate (or protein). Still, Ana says she likes to eats a lot, but this does not mean that she is allowed as much carbohydrate or protein as she wants. Excess consumption of any energy-yielding nutrients—carbohydrate, protein, or fat—will ultimately lead to the accumulation of body fat.

Inborn Errors of Metabolism

Your knowledge of metabolism has a very practical application: some people have inborn errors of metabolism. This means that the person lacks a specific enzyme to perform normal metabolic functions. The metabolic pathway in which this enzyme is supposed to participate now no longer functions properly. Typically this will cause alternative metabolic products to be formed, some of which are toxic to the body.

How does a person develop an inborn error of metabolism? The person inherits defective gene coding for a specific enzyme from both parents. Both parents are likely to be carriers in that they have one healthy gene and one defective gene for the enzyme in their chromosomes. Each parent then donates the defective form of the gene to the offspring, causing the offspring to have two defective copies of the gene, and therefore little or no activity of the enzyme that the gene normally would produce. Chapter 7 will cover in detail how a gene is used to produce proteins such as enzymes. For now, realize that if a person has a defective gene, he or she will produce a defective protein based on the instructions contained in that defective gene. There is also the possibility that one or both parents may actually have the disease themselves and not simply be carriers. Generally, however, these individuals are counseled against having children, or at the very least should see a genetic counselor to assess the risk of passing the inborn error of metabolism on to their offspring.

Some characteristics of inborn errors of metabolism include the following:[19]

- They appear soon after birth. Such a disorder is suspected when otherwise physically well children develop loss of appetite, vomiting, dehydration, physical weakness, or developmental delays soon after birth. For some of these conditions, infants are screened for the potential to have a specific inborn error of metabolism, such as phenylketonuria (PKU). (Review the discussion of PKU in Chapter 1.)
- They are very specific, involving only one or a few enzymes. These enzymes usually participate in catabolic pathways (in which compounds are degraded), such as for the amino acid phenylalanine.
- No cure is possible, but typically they can be controlled. This control might include reducing intake

of the substance that must be catabolized, such as phenylalanine. Other examples of therapies in specific cases include pharmacological doses of vitamins, such as vitamin B-12, and replacement of the blocked product, such as the amino acid tyrosine in PKU (see the next section for details).[9]

Phenylketonuria

The majority of cases of PKU occur because the enzyme phenylalanine hydroxylase does not function efficiently in the liver. Because of this, phenylalanine builds up in the blood of the person with PKU. If not corrected early (within 30 days of birth), this buildup of phenylalanine leads to production of toxic phenylalanine by-products, such as phenylpyruvic acid, which then can lead to severe mental retardation.[6]

PKU occurs in about one per 10,000 births. Most carriers can be detected with a simple blood test. People of Irish descent are especially affected. Today, most infants are diagnosed within a few days of life and are started on a phenylalanine-restricted diet.[14] This diet utilizes a low-phenylalanine infant formula, which is very expensive. During infancy, nutritional needs can change on a weekly basis, so these infants are monitored continually through blood phenylalanine testing.

Phenylalanine, protein, and energy intakes must be carefully monitored.[1] The amino acid phenylalanine is an essential nutrient, which means that even someone with PKU has to obtain phenylalanine from his or her diet; however, the amount of phenylalanine consumed needs to be monitored[6] carefully to prevent toxic amounts from building up.

Starting in infancy, special formulas are available to provide nutrients for individuals with PKU. Because infants have high-protein needs, satisfying protein requirements—without also having high intakes of phenylalanine—is impossible without these specially prepared formulas. Some of these formulas provide no phenylalanine; others provide a small amount. For infants, formulas are designed to provide about 90% of protein needs and 80% of energy needs. Human milk or regular infant formula then can be used to make up the difference.[19]

Later in life, foods can be used to make up the difference, especially foods low in phenylalanine. Fruits and vegetables are naturally low in

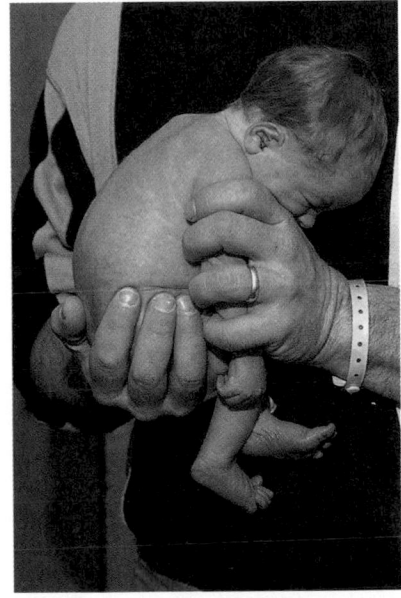

An infant who does not develop properly may have an inborn error of metabolism. A physician needs to investigate this possibility.

$$\text{Normal:} \quad \text{phenylalanine} \xrightarrow{\text{sufficient phenylalanine hydroxylase activity}} \text{tyrosine}$$

$$\text{PKU:} \quad \text{phenylalanine} \xrightarrow{\text{reduced phenylalanine hydroxylase activity}} \begin{cases} \text{phenylpyruvic acid} \\ \text{phenyllactic acid} \\ \text{other related products} \end{cases}$$

Children with PKU must be careful not to consume diet soft drinks containing aspartame, which contains phenylalanine.

galactosemia A rare genetic disease characterized by the buildup of the single sugar galactose in the bloodstream, resulting from the inability of the liver to metabolize it. If present at birth and left untreated, this disease can cause severe mental retardation and cataracts in the infant.

phenylalanine, and breads and cereals have a moderate amount. Dairy products, eggs, meats, nuts, and cheeses are very high in phenylalanine and so are not allowed on the diet. Diet soft drinks and other foods and beverages containing the alternative sweetener aspartame are also not allowed because these contain phenylalanine (see Chapter 5 for details). Older children and adults can use a formula that is very low in phenylalanine, which allows the person to consume more foods but still limits intake of phenylalanine. Overall, the majority of the person's nutrient intake throughout life will come from a special formula. Note that this formula has a very disagreeable smell and taste.

The diet is ideally followed for life. Physicians used to recommend that it was appropriate to end the diet after age 6 because brain development was complete. Later it was found, however, that diet discontinuation led to decreased intelligence and behavior problems such as aggressiveness, hyperactivity, and inattention.[19]

If a woman with PKU has abandoned the diet, she needs to return to the diet at least 6 months before becoming pregnant.[4] Otherwise the fetus—even though it does not have PKU—will be exposed to a high blood phenylalanine and related toxic products from the mother. This could result in miscarriage, or the infant could be born with a low birth weight or heart defects.

Galactosemia

In **galactosemia,** two principal specific enzyme defects lead to a reduction in the galactose metabolism to glucose (a third form is very rare). Galactose then builds up in the bloodstream, which can lead to very serious bacterial infections, mental retardation, and cataracts in the eye. An infant with galactosemia typically develops vomiting after a few days of consuming infant formula or breast milk. Both contain much galactose as part of the milk sugar lactose. This child will be switched to a soy formula. In addition, all dairy products and other lactose-containing products (butter, milk solids), organ meats, and some fruits and vegetables must be avoided. Strict label reading is also important for controlling the disease because lactose can be found in a variety of products. Note that even in well-controlled cases, slight mental retardation (such as speech delays) and cataracts are seen. Galactosemia occurs in 1 in 65,000 births.[15]

Glycogen Storage Disease

Glycogen storage disease is a group of diseases that result from the inability to metabolize glycogen to glucose in the liver. There are a number of possible enzyme defects along the pathway from glycogen to glucose. The most common forms cause poor physical growth, low blood glucose, and liver enlargement, and occur in 1 in 60,000 births. Low blood glucose results because liver glycogen breakdown is typically used to maintain blood glucose between meals (see Chapter 5 for details). People with glycogen storage disease typically have to consume frequent meals in order to regulate blood glucose. They also consume raw cornstarch between meals; this is slowly digested and so helps maintain steady blood glucose. Careful monitoring of blood glucose is very important in these people in order to know when blood glucose is too low and needs to be treated.[19]

A number of other very rare inborn errors of metabolism involve various amino acids, fatty acids, and the sugars fructose and sucrose. Typically, in large hospitals and in state health departments, physicians, nurses, and registered dietitians can help affected persons and their families with these and other inborn errors of metabolism.[19]

Summary

1. Plants capture solar energy by way of photosynthesis. Virtually all energy available to fuel the human body ultimately comes from the sun as solar energy.

2. ATP is the major form of energy used for cellular metabolism. As ATP breaks down to ADP plus P_i, energy is released from the broken bond. In humans, metabolic pathways make it possible to extract energy from C–H bonds in food and transform it into ATP; in the process, some energy is lost as heat.

3. In glycolysis, glucose is degraded into two pyruvate molecules, yielding NADH + H$^+$ (a form of potential energy) and ATP. Pyruvate can proceed through aerobic pathways to form carbon dioxide and water. Pyruvate also can react with NADH + H$^+$ in an anaerobic pathway to form lactate. Both pathways allow NADH + H$^+$ to eventually be re-formed into NAD$^+$, which is needed for glycolysis to continue.

4. Prior to entry into the citric acid cycle, pyruvate is formed into acetyl-CoA in what is called a transition reaction. One NADH + H$^+$ is produced and one carbon dioxide molecule is released.

5. Acetyl-CoA undergoes many metabolic conversions in the citric acid cycle, eventually yielding two more carbon dioxide molecules. In this way, the citric acid cycle accepts two carbons from acetyl-CoA and yields two carbons as carbon dioxide. In the process, NADH + H$^+$, FADH$_2$, and a form of energy that can yield ATP directly (GTP) are formed.

6. NADH + H$^+$ and FADH$_2$ enter the electron transport chain to yield numerous ATP molecules. Water forms as oxygen combines with the electrons and hydrogen ions (released from NADH + H$^+$ and FADH$_2$) in the electron transport chain.

7. In fatty acid oxidation, 2-carbon fragments are cleaved from a fatty acid at a time, producing multiple acetyl-CoA molecules. These enter the citric acid cycle and electron transport chain, and as did the acetyl-CoA that arose from carbohydrate breakdown, yield carbon dioxide, NADH + H$^+$, FADH$_2$ and ATP. Likewise, these NADH + H$^+$ and FADH$_2$ enter the electron transport chain to yield numerous ATP molecules and water.

8. In fat synthesis (lipogenesis), acetyl groups in effect are combined to yield a fatty acid, primarily the 16-carbon palmitic acid. These fatty acids can then react with a form of glycerol to produce a triglyceride.

9. During low carbohydrate intakes and uncontrolled diabetes, more acetyl-CoA is produced in the liver than can be metabolized to carbon dioxide and water. This excess acetyl-CoA is synthesized into ketone bodies, which flood into the bloodstream and are metabolized by other tissues, such as nervous tissue.

10. When amino acids are broken down, they lose their amino groups and become carbon skeletons. These can be metabolized to other compounds that enter the citric acid cycle, eventually yielding energy for ATP synthesis. Some carbon skeletons can be formed into oxaloacetate, an intermediate found in the citric acid cycle, which in turn can be used to form glucose. Converting the carbon skeletons of amino acids to glucose is part of a process known as gluconeogenesis.

11. Acetyl-CoA molecules, and thus fatty acids in general, cannot participate in gluconeogenesis.

12. Glycolysis takes place in the cytosol of a cell, whereas the transition reaction, the citric acid cycle, and the electron transport chain take place in the mitochondria. Fatty acid oxidation takes place in the mitochondria, and fatty acids for the most part are synthesized in the cytosol. The synthesis of urea and the pathway for gluconeogenesis both take place partly in the cytosol and partly in the mitochondria. Urea is made in the liver, while glucose is made in the liver and kidneys.

13. Acetyl CoA is pivotal in cell metabolism because carbohydrates, proteins, amino acids, fatty acids, and alcohol all can yield acetyl-CoA during their metabolism. The coordination of various metabolic pathways for food fuels allows the carbons of glucose to become the carbons of fatty acids and the carbons of some amino acids to become the carbons of glucose.

14. The vitamins thiamin, niacin, riboflavin, biotin, pantothenic acid, and vitamin B-6 and the minerals magnesium, iron, and copper play important roles in the metabolic pathways.

15. The body responds to fasting by reducing its metabolic rate. During a fast the body breaks down both amino acids and fats for energy. The loss of protein can ultimately cause death. A consequence of the breakdown of lipids is the formation of ketone bodies, which can provide energy to certain body cells, and ketosis.

16. Feasting results in the accumulation of body fat. The use of protein as an energy source will increase urea synthesis.

Study Questions

1. Many vitamins and minerals are used in energy metabolism. Identify three vitamins and/or minerals and describe their roles in ATP synthesis.

2. For what purposes do cells use ATP energy?

3. Explain how the ATP concentration is maintained in a cell. What is the key stimulus to ATP production?

4. What is the "common denominator" compound of the many pathways of energy metabolism (citric acid cycle, glycolysis, beta oxidation, etc.)? Why is it considered important in the body's chemical processes?

5. What is lactate, and how and where is it formed in the cell? Which tissues produce the most lactate? Why?

6. Trace the steps in gluconeogenesis from body protein to the formation of glucose.

7. How are fat and carbohydrate metabolism related? Use the term *ketosis*.

8. List the metabolic processes discussed throughout this chapter and their location in the cell.
9. Describe the reason most fatty acids do not turn into glucose in the body.
10. Explain how physicians can use certain aspects of protein metabolism to diagnose kidney or liver disease.

Annotated References

1. Acosta PB and others: Nutrient intakes and physical growth of children with phenylketonuria undergoing nutrition therapy. *Journal of the American Dietetic Association* 103:1167, 2003.

   It is very important for people with PKU to meet protein needs without exceeding energy needs. Exceeding protein needs somewhat might provide even more benefit in terms of growth. Use of the medical food designed for this disease is the cornerstone for meeting protein and overall nutrition needs.

2. Berg JM and others: *Biochemistry.* 5th ed. New York: WH Freeman, 2002.

   Excellent textbook covering the latest findings in metabolism. Details regarding the concepts discussed in this chapter are available. There are also detailed figures showing the various metabolic pathways.

3. Champe PC and others: *Biochemistry.* 3rd ed. Philadelphia, PA: Lippincot Williams & Wilkens, 2005.

   This textbook provides colorful and highly annotated figures that illustrate the various biochemical pathways in a cell. The text descriptions are also easy to follow, making this a very helpful book for learning more about metabolism.

4. Committee on Genetics: Maternal phenylketonuria. *Pediatrics* 107:427, 2001.

   Phenylketonuria during pregnancy is highly toxic to the growing fetus and may result in growth retardation and significant birth defects. The best outcomes of pregnancy occur when strict control of maternal phenylalanine is achieved before conception and then continued throughout the pregnancy.

5. Foster DW: The role of the carnitine system in human metabolism. *Annals of the New York Academy of Sciences* 1033:1, 2004.

   In the fed state, in terms of glucose metabolism, the liver primarily stores any available glucose as glycogen. In contrast, in the fasted state the liver produces much glucose. This article reviews the role of the carnitine system (and other biological systems) in this switch in overall metabolism.

6. Gassio R and others: Cognitive functions in classic phenylketonuria and mild hyperphenyl-alanaemia: Experience in paediatric population. *Developmental Medicine and Child Neurology* 47:443, 2005.

   Controlling blood phenylalanine concentrations in phenylketonuria is crucial for allowing for normal brain and cognitive development. Even mild increases above normal ranges in blood phenylalanine proved harmful in this study.

7. German JB and others: Metabolomics in practice: Emerging knowledge to guide future dietetic advice toward individualized health. *Journal of the American Dietetic Association* 105:1425, 2005.

   A new tool in the understanding of how we as individuals differ in the metabolic response to nutrients may lie in the ability to track the actual metabolic intermediates made to form this response, such as how we respond to exposure from different fatty acids. This approach is called metabolomics and should be more accurate than merely looking for differences in DNA between individuals to predict dietary responses. The article reviews this new tool of research.

8. Gropper SS and others: *Advanced nutrition and human metabolism.* 4th ed. Belmont CA: Thomson/Wadsworth, 2005.

   This textbook is excellent for reviewing the integration of nutrients into the various metabolic pathways. The authors also provide a helpful review of cell metabolism as a backdrop to understanding the various metabolic pathways found in the cell.

9. Marriage B and others: Nutritional cofactor treatment in mitochondrial disorders. *Journal of the American Dietetic Association* 103:1029, 2003.

   A number of defects have been described related to the metabolic processes that take place in mitochondria. A variety of medical interventions can be used to treat the muscle weakness and muscle destruction typically found in these disorders; the use of specific nutrients and related metabolic intermediates in treatment is reviewed in this context.

10. Mayes PA, Bender DA: The citric acid cycle: The catabolism of acetyl-CoA. In Murray RK and others (eds.): *Harper's biochemistry.* 26th ed. New York: Appleton & Lange Medical Books/McGraw Hill, 2003.

    The citric acid cycle is a series of reactions in the mitochondria that brings about the catabolism of acetyl-CoA, liberating hydrogen ions. Upon oxidation, these hydrogen ions lead to the release of most of the available energy of tissue fuels and eventual capture as ATP.

11. Mayes PA, Bender DA: Overview of metabolism. In Murray RK and others (eds.): *Harper's biochemistry.* 26th ed. New York: Appleton & Lange Medical Books/McGraw Hill, 2003.

    In the breakdown of carbohydrate, proteins, and fat for energy needs, all the pathways lead to the production of acetyl-CoA.

12. Mayes PA, Botham KM: Bioenergetics: The role of ATP. In Murray RK and others (eds.): *Harper's biochemistry.* 26th ed. New York: Appleton & Lange Medical Books/McGraw Hill, 2003.

    ATP is a high-energy compound because of its chemical structure. The great amount of energy released on breakdown of ATP to ADP and P_i is because of the relief of the repulsion between phosphate groups. ATP acts as the "energy currency" of the cell, transferring energy from substances of higher energy potential to those of lower energy potential.

13. Mayes PA, Botham KM: Oxidation of fatty acids: Ketogenesis. In Murray RK and others (eds.): *Harper's biochemistry.* 26th ed. New York: Appleton & Lange Medical Books/ McGraw Hill, 2003.

    Ketosis does not occur unless there is an increase in the level of circulating free fatty acids in the bloodstream. These free fatty acids are the precursors of ketone bodies made by the liver.

14. National Institutes of Health Consensus Development Panel: National Institutes of Health Consensus Development Conference Statement: Phenylketonuria: screening and management, October 16–18, 2000. *Pediatrics* 108:972, 2001.

    Genetic testing for phenylketonuria has been in place for almost 40 years and has been very successful in preventing severe mental retardation in thousands of children and adults. Metabolic control of phenylketonuria is necessary across the life span of such individuals.

15. Ridel KR and others: An updated review of the long-term neurological effects of galactosemia. *Pediatric Neurology* 33(3):153, 2005.

    Limiting galactose intake in galactosemia is critical for lessening the neurological and other organ system decline that takes place in this disorder. Still, some decline will be seen, particularly in the nervous system.

16. Saudubray JM and others: Clinical approach to inherited metabolic disorders in neonates: An overview. *Seminars in Neonatology* 7(1):3, 2002.

   There are almost 100 inborn errors of metabolism that can start in infancy; about 20 are amenable to treatment. Typically the infant is born after a normal pregnancy and delivery but soon deteriorates physically for no apparent reason and does not respond to typical medical therapy. Presenting symptoms are seizures, evidence of liver failure, various heart disorders, and hypoglycemia.

17. Timlin MT, Parks EJ: Temporal pattern of de novo lipogenesis in the postprandial state in healthy men. *American Journal of Clinical Nutrition* 81:35, 2005.

   Production of fatty acids using carbons from other macronutrients such as glucose, termed de novo lipogenesis, is seen after meals. Still, as found in this study, it is generally of minor importance with regard to the increase in blood triglycerides seen after a meal.

18. Trachtenbarg DE: Diabetic ketoacidosis. *American Family Physician* 71:1659, 2005.

   The ketosis that can develop in poorly treated type 1 diabetes is potentially very harmful to health and thus needs to be treated immediately. The article reviews such treatment, including provision of insulin and intravenous fluids.

19. Trahms CM: Medical nutrition therapy for metabolic disorders. In Mahan LK, Escott-Stump S (eds.): *Krause's food, nutrition, and diet therapy.* 11th ed. Philadelphia: WB Saunders, 2004.

   Excellent chapter on the medical nutrition therapy for inborn errors of metabolism. The chapter provides much detail on the role of nutrition in such disorders.

20. VanItallie TB, Nufert TH: Ketones: Metabolism's ugly duckling. *Nutrition Reviews* 61:327, 2003.

   This article contains a detailed discussion of ketone production and possible medical applications. Of particular interest is the historical account of the study of ketones in human metabolism.

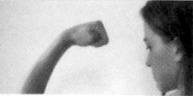

Take | Action

I. Put Your Knowledge of Metabolism into Practice

A friend is very overweight and describes to you his method of weight loss. He fasted completely for 1 week and then initiated a strict diet of 400 to 600 kcal/day under a physician's supervision. The food energy comes from a liquid formula, which he drinks for breakfast. He skips lunch and eats a small dinner of 3 ounces of protein, 1/2 cup of vegetables, 1 cup of fruit, and two starch items (a small potato, a piece of bread, etc.). He has lost approximately 25 lb in 12 weeks.

Based on your knowledge of energy metabolism, answer the following questions he poses:

1. During the fasting stage, what were the likely sources of energy for the body's cells? What metabolic processes occurred to provide glucose for red blood cells? brain? kidneys?

2. During the restrictive phase, how did the metabolic processes in the body most likely change from the fasting state?

II. Reinforce Your Knowledge of Metabolism

By this stage in your education, you have likely had a number of exposures to the topic of cell metabolism. Review your textbooks or notes from previous courses that discussed metabolism and see how the following topics were presented from the standpoint of that discipline. For example, coverage of glycolysis might have a different emphasis in a biology class than in a nutrition class.

ATP

Glycolysis

Citric acid cycle

Electron transport chain

Hormones that regulate aspects of metabolism:

Insulin

Glucagon

Enzyme activity

A general knowledge of metabolism will benefit you throughout a career in the sciences, whether in the health sciences or the biological sciences. Understanding metabolism especially will help you see how new developments in your field relate to cell function.

CARBOHYDRATES

CASE SCENARIO:

Myeshia is a 19-year-old African American female who recently read about the health benefits of calcium. She decided to increase her intake of dairy products, and to start, she drank 1 cup of 1% milk at lunch. Not long afterward, she experienced bloating, cramping, and gassiness. She suspected that the source of this pain was the milk she consumed, especially because her parents and her sister had complained of the same problem. She wanted to determine if the milk was, in fact, the cause of her gastrointestinal discomfort. So the next day she substituted a cup of yogurt for the glass of milk at lunch. Subsequently, she did not have any pain. What has Myeshia discovered? What component of milk is likely causing the problem?

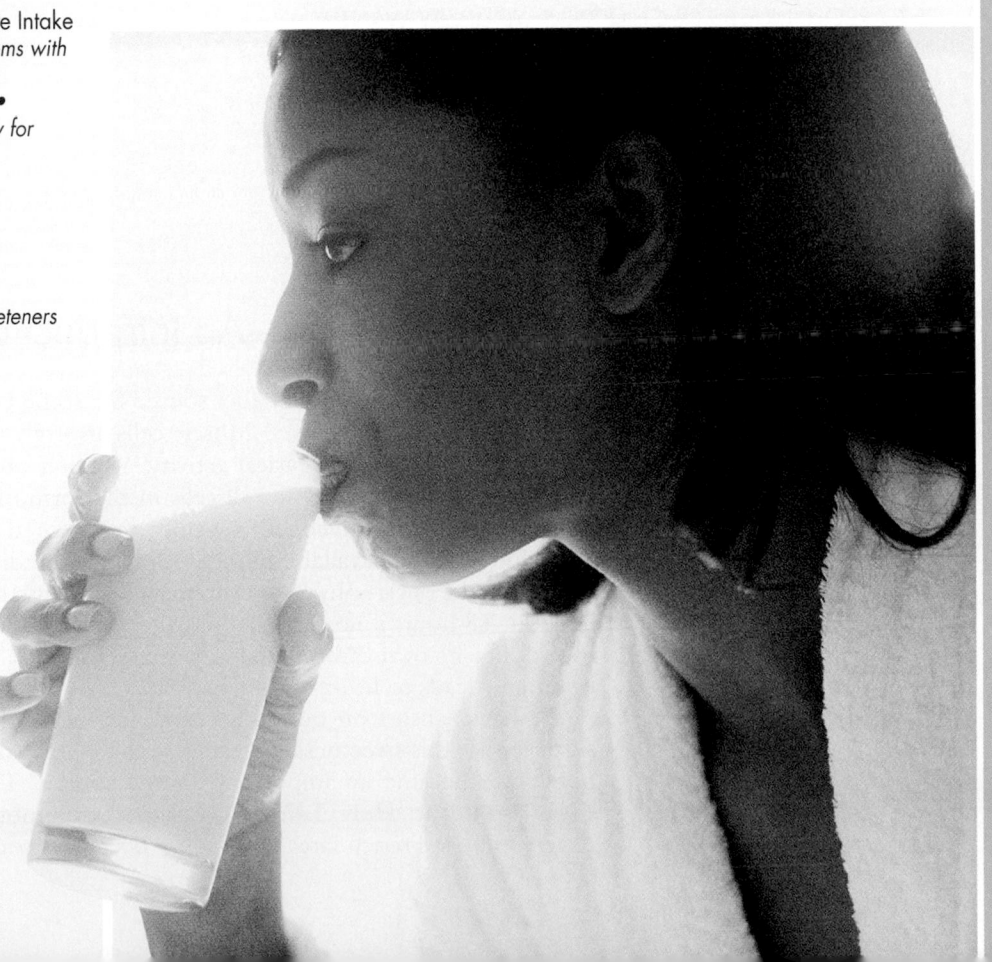

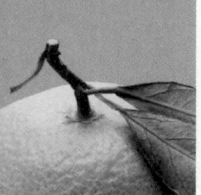

What did you eat to obtain the energy you are using right now? Chapters 5, 6, and 7 will examine this question by focusing on the main nutrients the human body uses for fuel. These energy-yielding nutrients are mainly carbohydrates (on average, 4 kcal/g) and fats and oils (on average, 9 kcal/g). Little of the other common fuel—protein (on average, 4 kcal/g)—is used for that purpose by the body.

It is likely that you have recently eaten some fruits, vegetables, dairy products, cereal, breads, and pasta. All these foods supply carbohydrates. Unfortunately, the benefits of these foods are often misunderstood.[1] As a result people think carbohydrate-rich foods are fattening—they are not. Pound for pound, carbohydrates are much less fattening than fats and oils. Furthermore, high-carbohydrate foods—especially fiber-rich foods such as fruits, vegetables, whole-grain breads and cereals, and legumes—have been promoted by many experts for the important health benefits these foods supply.[32] Some people think sugars necessarily cause hyperactivity—not so, according to well-designed scientific investigations. Almost all carbohydrate-rich foods, except pure sugars, provide essential nutrients and should generally constitute 45 to 65% of our daily energy intake.[11] Let's take a closer look at carbohydrates, including why the current trend toward carbohydrate bashing is misguided.

CHAPTER OBJECTIVES CHAPTER 5 IS DESIGNED TO ALLOW YOU TO:

1. Identify the basic structures and food sources of the major carbohydrates: monosaccharides, disaccharides, polysaccharides (e.g., starches and fiber).

2. List the functions of carbohydrate in the body and the problems that result from not eating enough carbohydrate.

3. Outline the beneficial effects of fiber on the body.

4. State the RDA for carbohydrate and various guidelines for carbohydrate intake.

5. Recognize food sources of carbohydrate.

6. List some alternative sweeteners that can be used to reduce sugar intake.

7. Describe the regulation of blood glucose and the nutrients that can become blood glucose.

8. Identify the consequences of lactose maldigestion/intolerance and diabetes, and list dietary measures to take to reduce the risk for developing, as well as managing, these health problems.

REFRESH YOUR MEMORY AS YOU BEGIN YOUR STUDY OF CARBOHYDRATES IN CHAPTER 5, YOU MAY WANT TO REVIEW:
- The health claims on food labels for various carbohydrates in Chapter 2.
- The anatomy and physiology of digestion and absorption in Chapter 3.
- The processes of glycolysis, gluconeogenesis, and ketosis in Chapter 4.

Fruits such as peaches are an excellent source of carbohydrate.

Carbohydrates—An Introduction

Carbohydrates are a primary fuel source for some cells, such as those in the nervous system and red blood cells.[14] Muscle cells also rely on a dependable supply of carbohydrate to fuel intense physical activity. Yielding on average 4 kcal/g, carbohydrates are a readily available fuel for all cells in the form of blood glucose and stored in the liver and muscles as glycogen. Carbohydrate stored in the liver can be used to maintain blood glucose availability in times when the diet does not supply enough. Still, regular intake of carbohydrate is important, because liver glycogen stores are exhausted in about 18 hours if no carbohydrate is consumed. After that point, the body is forced to produce its own carbohydrate from the amino acids in body and food protein; this eventually leads to health problems.[14]

We have sensors on our tongues that recognize sweet carbohydrates. Researchers surmise that this sweetness indicated a safe energy source to early humans, and so carbohydrate became an important energy source. The returning Crusaders brought sugar from the Holy Land to Europe. Columbus introduced sugarcane to the Americas. The French later grew sugar beets as a source of sugar.[14]

Primarily choosing the healthiest carbohydrate sources, while moderating intake of those that are less healthful, contributes to a healthy diet.[32] It is difficult to eat so little carbohydrate that body needs are not met, but it is easy to overconsume the carbohydrates that can contribute to health problems. This chapter explores this concept further as it looks at carbohydrates in detail.

Structures and Functions of Simple Carbohydrates

Most forms of carbohydrates are composed of carbon, hydrogen, and oxygen in the ratio of 1:2:1, respectively. The general formula is $(CH_2O)n$, where n represents the number of times the ratio is repeated. The chemical formula for glucose is $C_6H_{12}O_6$, or $(CH_2O)_6$.[20] The simpler forms of carbohydrates are called **sugars** and often take the form of single or double sugars, called **monosaccharides** and **disaccharides,** respectively. The more complex forms of carbohydrates are **polysaccharides,** typically either **starches** or **fibers.**

As discussed in Chapter 4, plants use carbon dioxide, water, and energy (from the sun) to produce the carbohydrates we eat. Recall from that chapter this complex process is called photosynthesis (Figure 5-1).

$$CO_2 + H_2O \rightarrow (CH_2O)n + O_2$$

Monosaccharides: Glucose, Fructose, and Galactose

The common monosaccharides (*mono* meaning "one" and *saccharide* meaning "sugar") are glucose, fructose, and galactose. Glucose is the most common monosaccharide in the body, but we eat very little of it as such. Other names for glucose are *dextrose* or *blood sugar*. In Figure 5-2, the chemical structure of glucose is shown in both its linear and ring forms. Glucose exists in the body in the ring form. Because it is a six-carbon monosaccharide, glucose is called a **hexose** (*hex* meaning "six," for six carbons; *ose* is the standard word ending for carbohydrates).[20]

Fructose is also a hexose. Unlike glucose, it can form either a five- or six-member ring (review Figure 5-2). Fructose, also called levulose, is found in

- Fruit
- Honey (about half fructose, half glucose)
- **High-fructose corn syrup,** which is used in the production of soft drinks, frozen desserts, and confections. The presence of fructose in these products makes it a common sugar in our diets. In most North American diets, fructose accounts for about 8 to 10% of total energy intake.

Fructose, after absorption by the small intestine and transport to the liver, is almost all metabolized to glucose or to intermediates in the glycolysis pathway. Some fructose is then converted to glycogen, **lactic acid,** or fat, depending on the amount consumed.

sugar A simple carbohydrate with the chemical composition $(CH_2O)n$. Most sugars form ringed structures when in solution. Generally refers to monosaccharides and disaccharides.

monosaccharide A class of simple sugars, such as glucose, which is not broken down further during digestion.

disaccharides A class of sugars formed by the chemical bonding of two monosaccharides.

polysaccharides Carbohydrates containing many glucose units, from 10 to 1000 or more.

starch A carbohydrate made of multiple units of glucose attached together in a form the body can digest; also known as *complex carbohydrate.*

fiber Substances in plant foods that are not broken down by the digestive processes that take place in the stomach or small intestine. Fibers naturally found in foods are called dietary fiber.

hexose A general term describing a carbohydrate containing six carbons.

fructose A monosaccharide with six carbons that forms a five-membered or six-membered ring with oxygen in the ring; found in fruits and honey.

lactic acid A three-carbon acid, also called lactate, that is formed during anaerobic cell metabolism; a partial breakdown product of glucose.

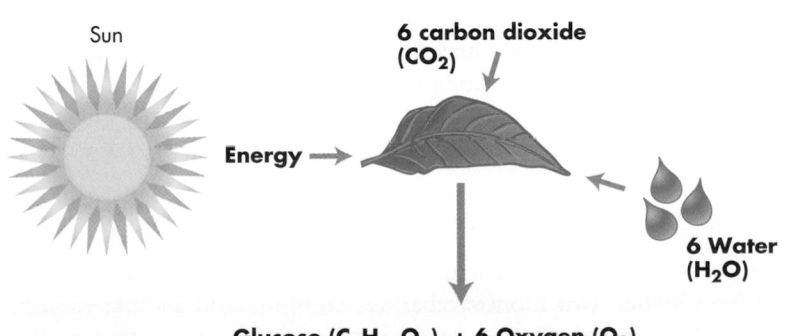

Figure 5-1 | A summary of photosynthesis. Plants use carbon dioxide, water, and energy to produce carbohydrates such as glucose. Glucose is then stored in the leaf but can also undergo further metabolism to form starch and fiber in the plant.

Figure 5-2 | Forms of the six-carbon monosaccharides—fructose, glucose, and galactose—shown in the linear form and in the ring form where each corner represents a carbon atom unless otherwise indicated. (Appendix A reviews this shortcut notation.) This ring structure is the predominant form when in solution. Only the D-isomer forms of these monosaccharides are metabolized by the body. (Appendix A also reviews the concepts of isomers.)

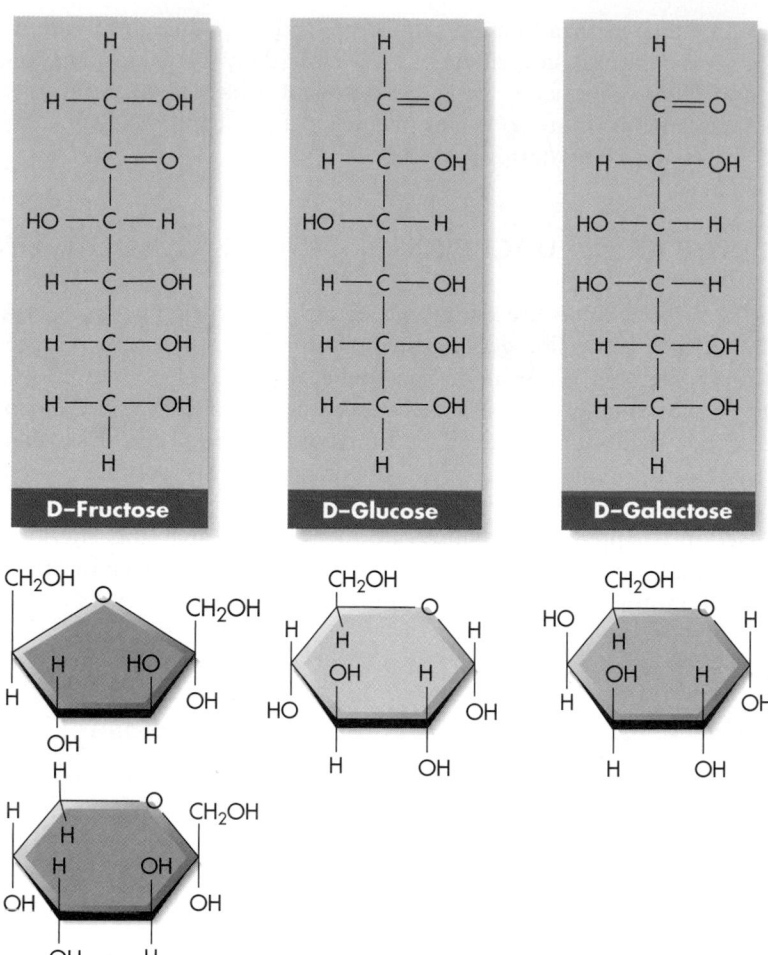

galactose A six-carbon monosaccharide; an isomer of glucose.

sorbitol An alcohol derivative of glucose that yields about 3 kcal/g but is slowly absorbed from the small intestine. It is used in some sugarless gums and dietetic foods.

condensation reaction Chemical reaction in which a bond between two molecules is formed by the elimination of a small molecule, such as water.

maltose Glucose bonded to glucose.

sucrose Fructose bonded to glucose; table sugar.

lactose A sugar composed of glucose linked to another sugar called galactose.

Synthesis of lactic acid and fat is stimulated by fructose intakes that are two or more times typical intakes.[14]

Galactose is the third major monosaccharide of nutritional importance. Comparison of the structure of this simple sugar with that of glucose shows that the two structures are almost identical, except that the hydrogen (–H) and the hydroxyl group (–OH) on carbon-4 are reversed (review Figure 5-2). Galactose is not usually found free in nature in large quantities but, rather, combines with glucose to form a disaccharide called *lactose* (found in milk and other dairy products). Once absorbed into the body, galactose is converted into glucose in the liver, which can be used to provide immediate energy or is stored as *glycogen*.[20]

Another monosaccharide found in nature is **ribose,** a five-carbon sugar (or pentose; *penta* means "five"). This is present in a cell's genetic material. Very little ribose is present in our diet; we produce this sugar from other foods we eat.[20]

Finally, a few sugar alcohols are present in foods and will be discussed later in this chapter, in the section on nutritive sweeteners in foods. Currently, the major sugar alcohol used in the manufacture of foods and beverages is **sorbitol.**[35]

Once you are familiar with the chemical forms of the sugars, it is much easier to understand how they are interrelated, combined, digested, metabolized, and synthesized.

Disaccharides: Maltose, Sucrose, and Lactose

Carbohydrates containing two sugar units are called disaccharides (*di* means "two"). These are formed when two monosaccharides combine and a water molecule is split off in what is called a **condensation reaction.** The three most common disaccharides found in nature are **maltose, sucrose,** and **lactose.** All contain glucose (Figure 5-3).[20]

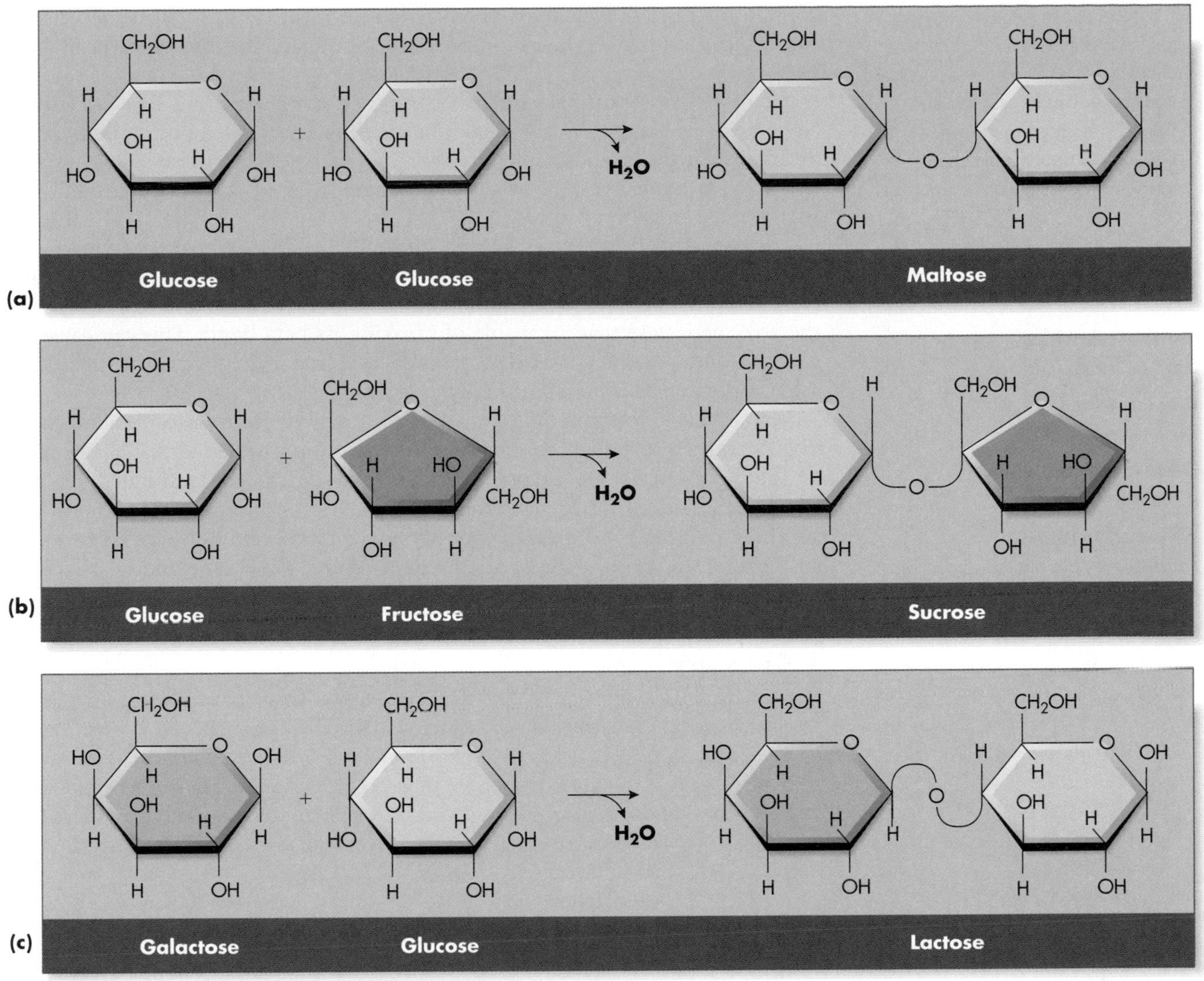

Figure 5-3 | Joining of two monosaccharides to form a disaccharide. (a) Maltose is made up of two glucose molecules and is formed in germinating grains. (b) Sucrose, or common table sugar, is made up of glucose and fructose. (c) Lactose, or milk sugar, is made up of glucose and galactose. Note that lactose contains a different type of bond (beta, or β) from that of maltose and sucrose (alpha, or α), a property that makes lactose difficult to digest for individuals who produce less of the enzyme lactase.

One carbon on each participating monosaccharide is chemically bonded together by oxygen. Two forms of this C—O—C bond exist in nature, called **alpha (α) bonds** and **beta (β) bonds,** and are depicted slightly differently. As shown in Figure 5-3, maltose and sucrose contain the alpha form, whereas lactose contains the beta form. Many carbohydrates contain long chains of glucose with the individual molecules bonded together by either alpha or beta bonds. Using what is called a **hydrolysis reaction,** humans can digest these carbohydrates, but only if the glucose molecules are linked by alpha bonds.[14] This topic will be covered later in this chapter, when fiber is discussed.

Maltose consists of two glucose molecules joined by an alpha bond. When seeds sprout, they produce enzymes that break down the polysaccharides (starch) to sugars such as maltose and glucose. These sugars provide the energy for the plant to grow. In a process called malting, the sprouting process is stopped by heat. This is the first step in the production of alcoholic beverages such as beer. In the absence of oxygen yeast converts most of the carbohydrates to ethanol (alcohol) and carbon dioxide in a process called fermentation (discussed in Chapter 4). There will be more about the production of alcohol products in Chapter 8. Few other food products and beverages

alpha (α) bond A type of chemical bond that can be digested by human intestinal enzymes; drawn as C-O-C.

beta (β) bond A type of chemical bond that cannot be broken by human intestinal enzymes during digestion when it is part of a long chain of glucose molecules (e.g., cellulose); drawn as C-O-C.

hydrolysis reaction A chemical reaction in which a bond between two molecules is broken by the inclusion of a water molecule. The water donates a hydrogen to one reactant and a hydroxyl (–OH) group to the other reactant.

A common misconception is that honey contains vitamins and minerals. You can prove to yourself that honey is no more nutritious than sucrose by consulting Appendix N. Only the sweetener molasses, a by-product of sucrose production, contains any appreciable amount of minerals. However, our consumption of molasses is very low.

Simple forms
> **Monosaccharides**
> Glucose, fructose, galactose
> **Disaccharides**
> Sucrose, lactose, maltose
> **Oligosaccharides**
> Raffinose, stachyose
> **Polysaccharides**
> Starches (amylose and amylopectin), glycogen

Complex forms
> Most fibers

raffinose An indigestible oligosaccharide made of three monosaccharides (galactose-glucose-fructose).

stachyose An indigestible oligosaccharide made of four monosaccharides (galactose galactose-glucose-fructose).

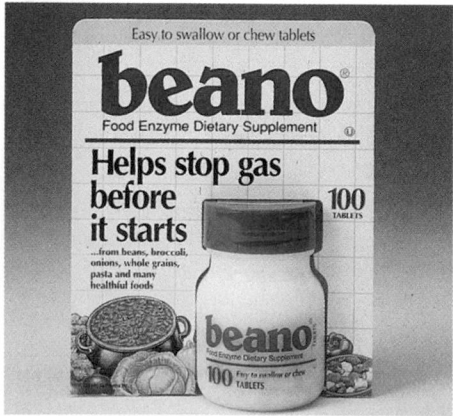

Beano can be used to reduce intestinal gas produced by bacterial metabolism of oligosaccharides in the large intestine.

contain maltose. In fact, most maltose that we ultimately digest in the small intestine is produced during the digestion of starch (see a later section on carbohydrate digestion in this chapter).

Sucrose, common table sugar, is composed of glucose and fructose linked via an alpha bond.[20] Large amounts of sucrose are found naturally only in plants, such as sugarcane, sugar beets, and maple tree sap. The sucrose from these sources may be purified to various degrees. Brown, white, and powdered sugars are common forms of sucrose sold in grocery stores.[1]

Lactose, the primary sugar in milk and milk products, consists of glucose joined to galactose by a beta bond. As discussed in a later section of this chapter, many people are unable to digest large amounts of lactose because they don't produce enough of the enzyme lactase that is capable of breaking its beta bond. This can cause intestinal gas, bloating, cramping, and discomfort as the unabsorbed lactose is metabolized into acids and gases by bacteria in the large intestine.[28]

You are likely to encounter many different words referring to monosaccharides and disaccharides or products containing these simple sugars. Note that all the terms listed in Table 5-4 later in the chapter are names for sugars either naturally present in food products or added during their manufacture. These monosaccharides and disaccharides are often referred to as *simple sugars* because they contain only one or two sugar units and, therefore, have a simple chemical structure. Food labels lump all these sugars under one category, listing them as "sugars."[1]

> ### Concept | Check
> Monosaccharides are single sugars. From a nutritional standpoint, the important monosaccharides are glucose, fructose, and galactose. Disaccharides are double sugars. The major disaccharides in the diet are sucrose (glucose bonded to fructose), maltose (glucose bonded to glucose), and lactose (glucose bonded to galactose). The disaccharides have either alpha or beta bonds. Our bodies are unable to break down most of the beta bonds. Once absorbed into the body, most carbohydrates are ultimately transformed into glucose by the liver.

Oligosaccharides: Raffinose and Stachyose

From a nutritional standpoint, oligosaccharides contain 3 to about 10 single sugar units (*oligo* means "scant"). (Chemists and biochemists, however, lump disaccharides in the oligosaccharide category as well.)[20] Two oligosaccharides of nutritional importance are **raffinose** and **stachyose,** which are found in legumes, such as kidney beans. These oligosaccharides are constructed of typical monosaccharides but are bonded together in such a way that digestive enzymes cannot break them apart. Thus, when we consume legumes, raffinose and stachyose remain undigested on reaching the large intestine. There, bacteria metabolize them, producing gas and other by-products.[14]

Many people have no trouble digesting legumes, but others experience unpleasant side effects from intestinal gas. An enzyme preparation called Beano, which prevents these side effects, can help such people if taken right before a meal. Once consumed, the enzyme preparation works in the digestive tract to break down many of the indigestible oligosaccharides in legumes (and other vegetables). Beano is made from mold, so persons sensitive to molds may react allergically and should avoid it or use with caution. For more information or free samples, contact the manufacturer (800-257-8650).

Structures and Functions of the More Complex Carbohydrates

The polysaccharides, often referred to as *complex carbohydrates*, include some that are digestible (e.g., starch) and some that are largely indigestible, such as fiber.[14]

Digestible Polysaccharides: Starch and Glycogen

Polysaccharides contain many monosaccharide units, up to 1000 or more. Most polysaccharides of nutritional importance are synthesized from glucose, such as when vegetables turn glucose into starch during maturation. This makes peas and corn sweetest when they are young. Starch, the major digestible polysaccharide in our diet, is the storage form of energy in plants. There are two types of plant starch—**amylose** and **amylopectin**—both of which are a source of energy for plants and the animals that eat plants.[20]

Both amylose and amylopectin contain many glucose units linked by alpha (digestible) bonds. The primary difference between the two types of starch is that amylose is a straight-chain polymer, whereas amylopectin is highly branched (Figure 5-4). Cooking increases the digestibility of these starches by making them more soluble in water and thus more available for attack by digestive enzymes. Amylose and amylopectin are found in potatoes, beans, breads, pasta, rice, and other starchy products, typically in a ratio of about 1:4. Amylopectin raises blood glucose much more readily than amylose, since its numerous branches provide many opportunities for digestive enzyme activity. The enzymes act only at the ends of the glucose chains. The more numerous the branches of a starch, the more sites (ends) are available for enzyme action (see the discussion of glycemic index and glycemic load in a later section of this chapter).[20]

The branches in amylopectin also allow it to form a very stable starch gel, enabling it to retain water and resist water seepage. Food manufacturers commonly use starches rich in amylopectin in sauces and gravies for frozen foods because they remain stable over a wide temperature range. Food manufacturers may also use processes to bond the starch molecules to one another, further increasing food stability. The resulting

amylose A straight-chain type of starch composed of glucose units.

amylopectin A branched-chain type of starch composed of glucose units.

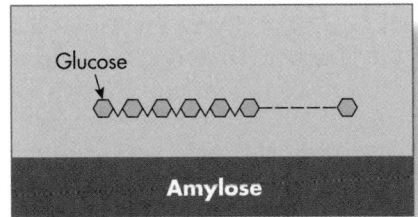

Amylose

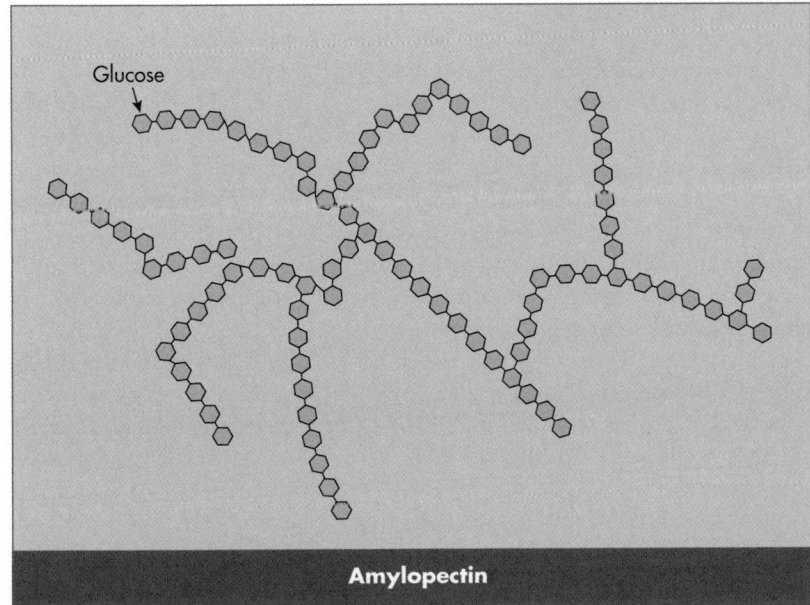

Amylopectin

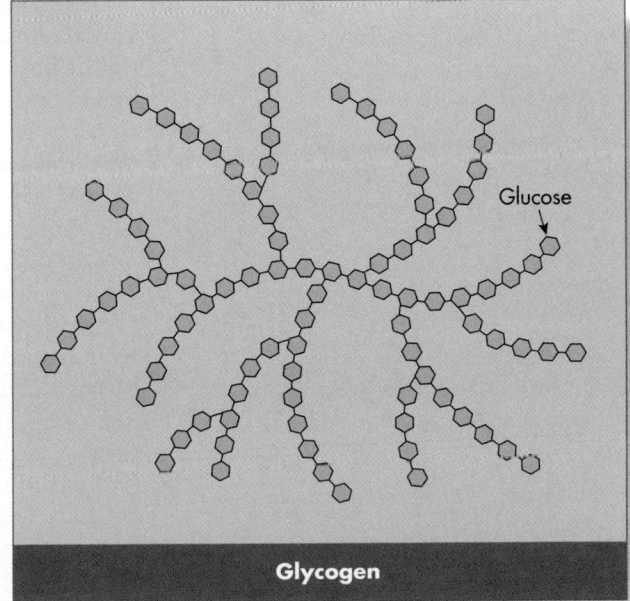

Glycogen

Figure 5-4 | Some common starches. We consume essentially no glycogen. All glycogen found in the body is made by our cells, primarily in the liver and muscles.

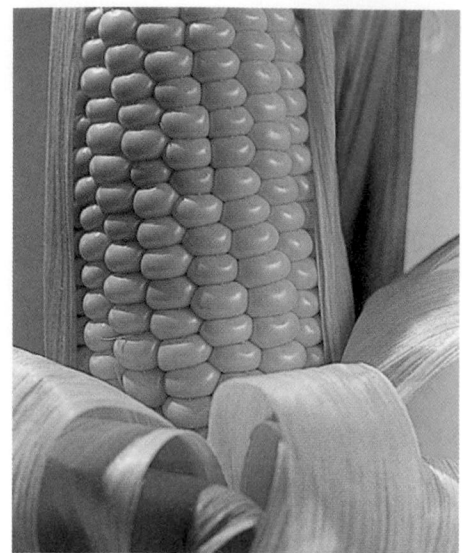

As some vegetables age, their sugars are converted to starches.

dietary fiber Fiber found in food.

functional fiber Any fiber added to foods that has shown to provide health benefits.

cellulose A straight-chain polysaccharide of glucose molecules that is undigestible because of the presence of beta bonds; part of insoluble fiber.

hemicellulose A mostly insoluble fiber containing galactose, glucose, and other monosaccharides bonded together.

pectin A soluble fiber containing chains of various monosaccharides; characteristically found between plant cell walls.

gums A soluble fiber containing chains of galactose and other monosaccharides; characteristically found in exudates from plant stems.

mucilages A soluble fiber consisting of chains of galactose and other monosaccharides; characteristically found in seaweed.

lignins An insoluble fiber made up of a multiringed alcohol (noncarbohydrate) structure.

insoluble fibers Fibers that mostly do not dissolve in water and are not generally metabolized by bacteria in the large intestine. These include cellulose, some hemicelluloses, and lignins; more formally called nonfermentable fibers.

product, called **modified food starch,** is used in baby foods, salad dressings, and instant puddings.

Glycogen, the storage form of carbohydrate in humans and other animals, is a glucose polymer with alpha bonds and numerous branches. The amount of carbohydrate in a diet greatly influences the amount of glycogen stored. The structure of glycogen is similar to that of amylopectin, but the branching patterns are more complicated (review Figure 5-4). As with amylopectin, glycogen, because it is so highly branched, is quickly broken down by enzymes in body cells in which it is stored.[20]

The liver and muscles are the major storage sites for glycogen. Because only about 120 kcal of glucose are available as such in body fluids, muscle and liver storage sites for carbohydrate energy—amounting to about 1800 kcal—are extremely important.[14] As noted in this chapter's introduction, the 400 kcal of glycogen made by the liver can be turned into blood glucose, while the 1400 kcal of glycogen made by muscle cells cannot. Still, glycogen in muscle cells supplies glucose for muscle use, especially during high-intensity and endurance exercise. (See Chapter 14 for a detailed discussion of carbohydrate use during physical activity.)

Indigestible Polysaccharides: Fibers

Folklore surrounding fiber or "roughage" has been a part of American culture since the 1800s. In the 1820s and 1830s, a minister named Sylvester Graham traveled up and down the East Coast extolling the virtues of fiber. He left us a legacy—the graham cracker. However, today's graham cracker bears little resemblance to the whole-grain product he promoted. The next wave of fiber frenzy crested in the mid-1870s with Dr. John Harvey Kellogg and his brother William of breakfast cereal fame. Dr. Kellogg became the first person to earn a million dollars from "health foods." One of his patients was Charles W. Post, who followed the Kelloggs' lead and started the Post Toasted Cornflakes Company. In 1901 alone, Post netted $1 million from his Grape-Nuts cereal and other products. As you will see, present-day scientific evidence supports this early promotion of fiber as part of a healthy diet.

The term *fiber* refers to the **dietary fiber** that is found naturally in foods as well as to other forms of fiber that may be added to foods. This second category is called **functional fiber;** any of these fibers must show beneficial effects in humans to be included in this latter category. **Total fiber** (or just the term *fiber*) is then the combination of dietary fiber and functional fiber in the food product.[11] Currently the Nutrition Facts label includes only the category dietary fiber; the label has yet to be updated to reflect the latest definition of fiber by the Food and Nutrition Board.

In terms of their chemical composition, fibers are composed primarily of the nonstarch polysaccharides **cellulose, hemicelluloses, pectins, gums,** and **mucilages.** The only noncarbohydrate components of dietary fibers are **lignins,** which include complex alcohol derivatives (Table 5-1). Almost all forms of fiber come from plants, and as a group, none are digested in the human stomach or small intestine.[14]

Cellulose is a straight-chain glucose polymer similar to amylose; however, unlike amylose, which contains alpha bonds, the glucose units in cellulose are linked by beta bonds. As noted earlier, glucose molecules joined by beta bonds are not broken down by human digestive enzymes. Thus, cellulose is not digestible by humans and is classified as a dietary fiber, not a starch. Because the long glucose chains of cellulose are linear, they can pack closely together, forming fibrous structures with great strength. Overall, cellulose, hemicelluloses, and lignins form the structural part of the plant. A cotton ball is pure cellulose. Bran fiber is rich in hemicelluloses. Since bran layers form the outer covering of all seeds, **whole grains** (i.e., those with the bran and other components left intact) are good sources of this fiber (Figure 5-5).[32] The woody fibers in broccoli are partly lignins. As a class, these undigestible dietary fibers generally do not dissolve in water and thus are called **insoluble fibers** (or nonfermentable fibers).

Pectins, gums, and mucilages are found inside and around plant cells. They help "glue" plant cells together (review Figure 5-5). These dietary fibers either dissolve or

Table 5-1 | Classification of Dietary Fibers

Type	Noncomponent(s)	Physiological Effects	Major Food Sources
Insoluble (Nonfermentable)			
Noncarbohydrate	Lignins	Increases fecal bulk	Whole grains
Carbohydrate	Cellulose Hemicelluloses	Increases fecal bulk Decreases intestinal transit time	All plants Wheat, rye, rice, vegetables
Soluble (Viscous)			
Carbohydrate	Pectins, gums, mucilages, some hemicelluloses	Delays gastric emptying; slows glucose absorption; can lower blood cholesterol	Citrus fruits, oat products (beta-glucan in particular), beans, thickeners added to foods

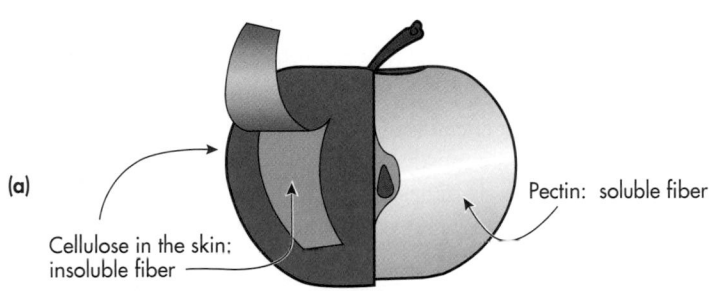

(a)

Cellulose in the skin: insoluble fiber

Pectin: soluble fiber

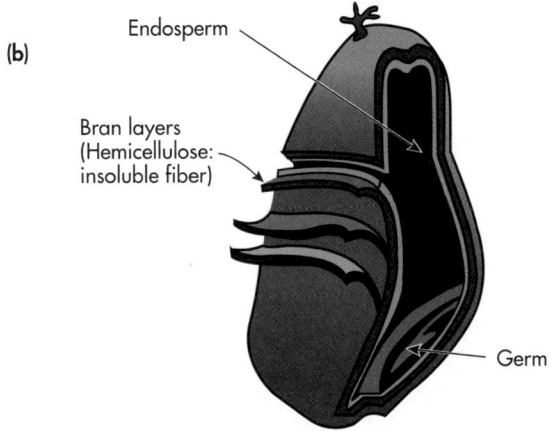

(b)

Endosperm

Bran layers (Hemicellulose: insoluble fiber)

Germ

Figure 5-5 | Various forms of fiber. (a) The skin of an apple consists of the insoluble fiber cellulose, which provides structure for the fruit. The soluble fiber pectin "glues" the fruit cells together. (b) The outside layer of a wheat kernel is made of layers of bran—insoluble fiber—making this whole grain a good source of fiber. Fruits, vegetables, whole grains, and legumes such as beans are rich in fiber.

Critical | Thinking

Celia decides to go on a diet and buys over-the-counter pills. You look at the ingredients and note that the pills contain psyllium, a word you recognize from the nutrition course you're taking. What is one possible effect of the psyllium in these diet pills?

swell when put into water and thus are called **soluble fibers** (or viscous fibers).[11] Some forms of hemicellulose also fall into this soluble-fiber category. Soluble fibers such as gum arabic, guar gum, locust bean gum, and various pectins are present in numerous food products, especially salad dressings, inexpensive ice creams, jams, and jellies. Other rich sources of soluble fibers include fruits and vegetables in general, soybean fiber, rice bran, and **psyllium** seeds (found in many commercial fiber laxatives).

One workable definition of fiber is "the foodstuffs that remain undigested as they enter the large intestine." There is really no common property that characterizes various fibers except their ability to resist digestion in the small intestine. Since some fibers—especially the soluble fibers—are fermented by bacteria in the large intestine, it is not accurate to say that fiber is just what fibers are found in the feces.[11]

Bacteria in the large intestine ferment soluble fibers into products such as short-chain fatty acids (e.g., acetic acid, butyric acid, and propionic acid) and gases, such as hydrogen (H_2) and methane (CH_4). These acids, especially butyric acid, provide fuel

soluble fibers Fibers that either dissolve or swell in water and are metabolized (fermented) by bacteria in the large intestine; these include pectins, gums, and mucilages; more formally called viscous fibers.

psyllium A mostly soluble type of dietary fiber found in the seeds of the plantago plant (native to India and Mediterranean countries).

Currently food labels use the term *soluble fiber* rather than the more formal *viscous fiber*. We will use *soluble fiber* in this and other chapters since it is still the term found on the Nutrition Facts label. It is likely that the term *soluble* will be phased out in the future and replaced with the term *viscous*.

An outmoded term used for fiber is *crude fiber*. This term arose during the early 1900s to reflect the amount of indigestible foodstuff present in animal feed. The animal feed was boiled for 1 hour in acid and for another hour in an alkaline solution. The remains of that chemical digestion was called crude fiber; it consisted mostly of cellulose and lignins. All other types of fiber were destroyed by the chemical action.

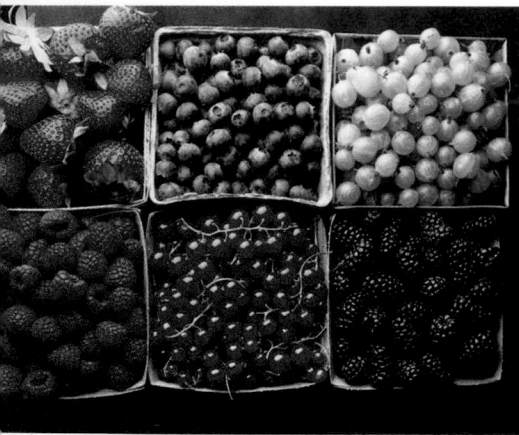

In the search for fiber sources, don't overlook berries. Just 1/2 cup contains up to 3 g of fiber. They are also rich sources of various beneficial phytochemicals.

amylase Starch-digesting enzyme from the salivary glands or pancreas.

maltase An enzyme made by absorptive cells of the small intestine; this enzyme digests maltose to two glucoses.

for the cells in the large intestine and enhance their health.[14] All these products can also be absorbed into the bloodstream. As a result of bacterial metabolism, soluble dietary fibers yield about 1.5 to 2.5 kcal/g on average, although the actual value is still in question. For this reason, high-fiber foods should not be looked at as calorie-free, though they are often lower in energy content per serving than low-fiber alternatives.

When intake of fiber is high, its metabolism by bacteria can cause methane and hydrogen to increase in the breath. This is not harmful. In addition, the body tends to adapt over time to a high-fiber intake, leading to less gaseous symptoms and adjusting to the increased pressure that develops in the large intestine.

Concept | Check

Amylose, amylopectin, and glycogen—all storage forms of glucose—are polysaccharides. Amylose and amylopectin combine in varying proportions to form food starch, such as that found in potatoes and bread. Glycogen is a storage form of glucose in humans. Liver glycogen yields a ready source of blood glucose.

Fiber is essentially the portion of ingested food that remains undigested as it enters the large intestine. Fiber components include cellulose, hemicelluloses, lignins, pectins, gums, and mucilages. There are two general classes of fiber: insoluble (nonfermentable) and soluble (viscous). Insoluble fibers are mostly made up of cellulose, hemicelluloses, and lignins. Soluble fibers are made up mostly of pectins, gums, and mucilages. Both insoluble and soluble fibers are resistant to human digestive enzymes, but bacteria in the large intestine can break down soluble fibers.

Carbohydrate Digestion and Absorption

Food preparation can be viewed as the start of carbohydrate digestion because cooking softens the tough fibrous tissue of plants, such as broccoli stalks. When starches are heated, the starch granules swell as they soak up water, making them much easier to digest. All these effects of cooking generally make these foods easier to chew, swallow, and break down during digestion.

Digestion

The enzymatic digestion of starch begins in the mouth. Saliva contains an enzyme called salivary **amylase** which mixes with the starchy products during the chewing of the food. This amylase breaks down starch into many smaller units (e.g., disaccharides, such as maltose) (Figure 5-6).[14] You can observe this conversion while chewing a saltine cracker. Prolonged chewing of the cracker causes it to taste sweeter as some starch breaks down into the sweeter sugars, such as maltose. Still, food is in the mouth for such a short amount of time that this phase of digestion is negligible. In addition, once the food moves down the esophagus and reaches the stomach, the acidic environment (pH 1–2) inactivates salivary amylase.

After the carbohydrates have reached the small intestine—where the pH of 7 or more is well-suited for further carbohydrate digestion—the pancreas releases enzymes, such as pancreatic amylase.

The original carbohydrates in a food will be present as such in the small intestine as monosaccharides (mostly any glucose and fructose present as such in food). The disaccharides will include maltose from starch breakdown, lactose mainly from dairy products, and sucrose from food. The polysaccharides in the food that were first acted on in the mouth now are digested further by pancreatic amylase. Any disaccharides are digested to their monosaccharide units once they reach the wall of the small intestine. There specialized enzymes on the absorptive cells digest each disaccharide into the monosaccharide components. The enzyme **maltase** acts on maltose to produce two

Carbohydrates

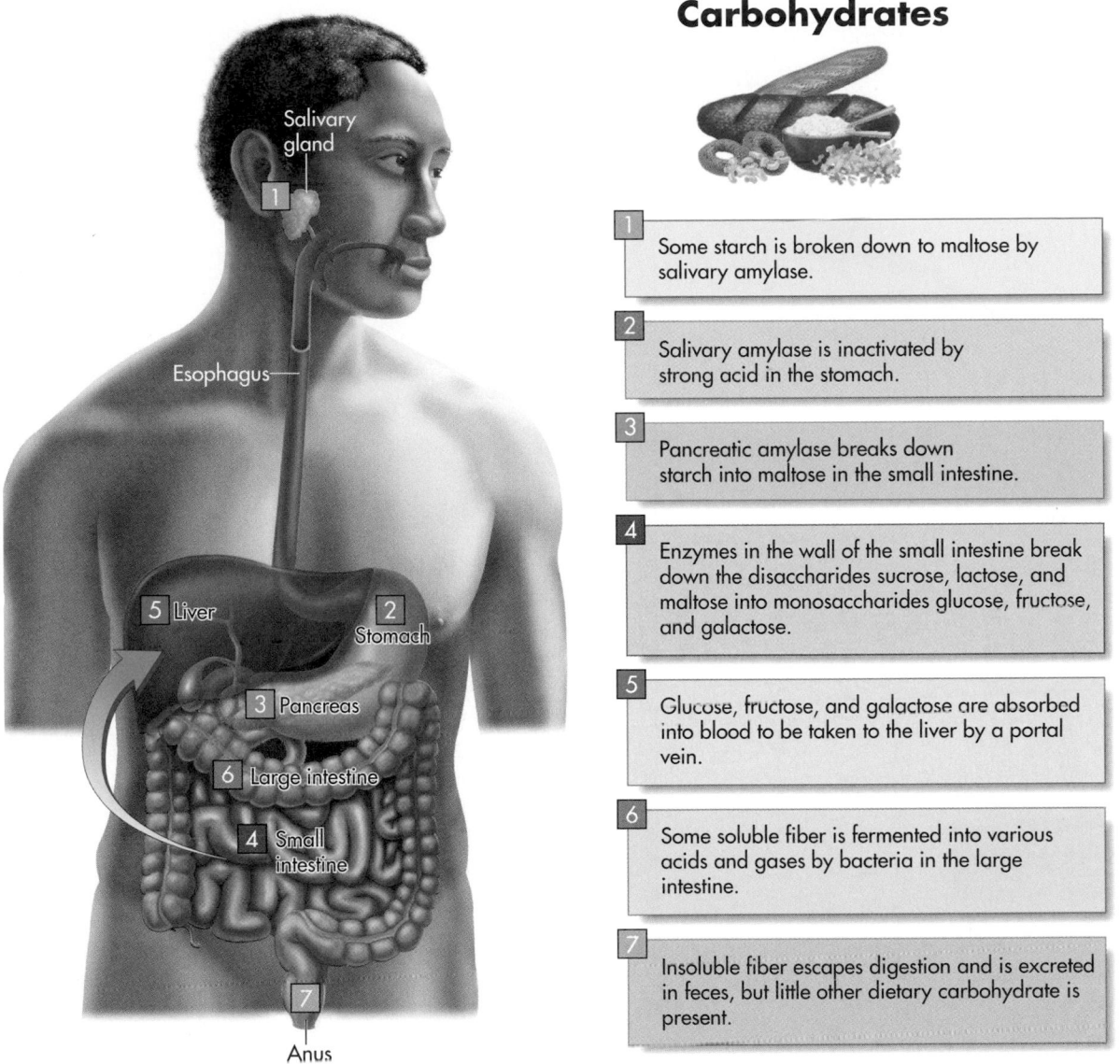

1. Some starch is broken down to maltose by salivary amylase.

2. Salivary amylase is inactivated by strong acid in the stomach.

3. Pancreatic amylase breaks down starch into maltose in the small intestine.

4. Enzymes in the wall of the small intestine break down the disaccharides sucrose, lactose, and maltose into monosaccharides glucose, fructose, and galactose.

5. Glucose, fructose, and galactose are absorbed into blood to be taken to the liver by a portal vein.

6. Some soluble fiber is fermented into various acids and gases by bacteria in the large intestine.

7. Insoluble fiber escapes digestion and is excreted in feces, but little other dietary carbohydrate is present.

Figure 5-6 | Carbohydrate digestion and absorption. Enzymes made by the mouth, pancreas, and small intestine participate in the process of digestion. Most carbohydrate digestion and absorption take place in the small intestine. Note that Chapter 3 covered the physiology of digestion and absorption in detail.

glucose molecules. **Sucrase** acts on sucrose to produce glucose and fructose. **Lactase** acts on lactose to produce glucose and galactose.[14]

When considering carbohydrate digestion, you should remember that the key digestive enzymes come from the pancreas and the cells of the intestinal wall. Intestinal diseases can interfere with the digestion of sugars such as maltose, lactose, and sucrose. Some of the carbohydrates therefore escape digestion and are not absorbed. When these unabsorbed carbohydrates eventually reach the large intestine, the bacteria there digest the sugars, producing acids and gases as by-products (review Figure 5-6). If produced in large amounts, these gases can cause abdominal discomfort. People recovering from intestinal disorders, such as diarrhea or severe foodborne illness, may need to avoid lactose for a few weeks because of temporary lactose malabsorption. A few weeks is sufficient time for the small intestine to resume producing enough lactase enzyme to allow for more complete lactose digestion (see the later section on lactose malabsorption and intolerance).[28]

sucrase An enzyme made by absorptive cells of the small intestine; this enzyme digests sucrose to glucose and fructose.

lactase An enzyme made by absorptive cells of the small intestine; this enzyme digests lactose to glucose and galactose.

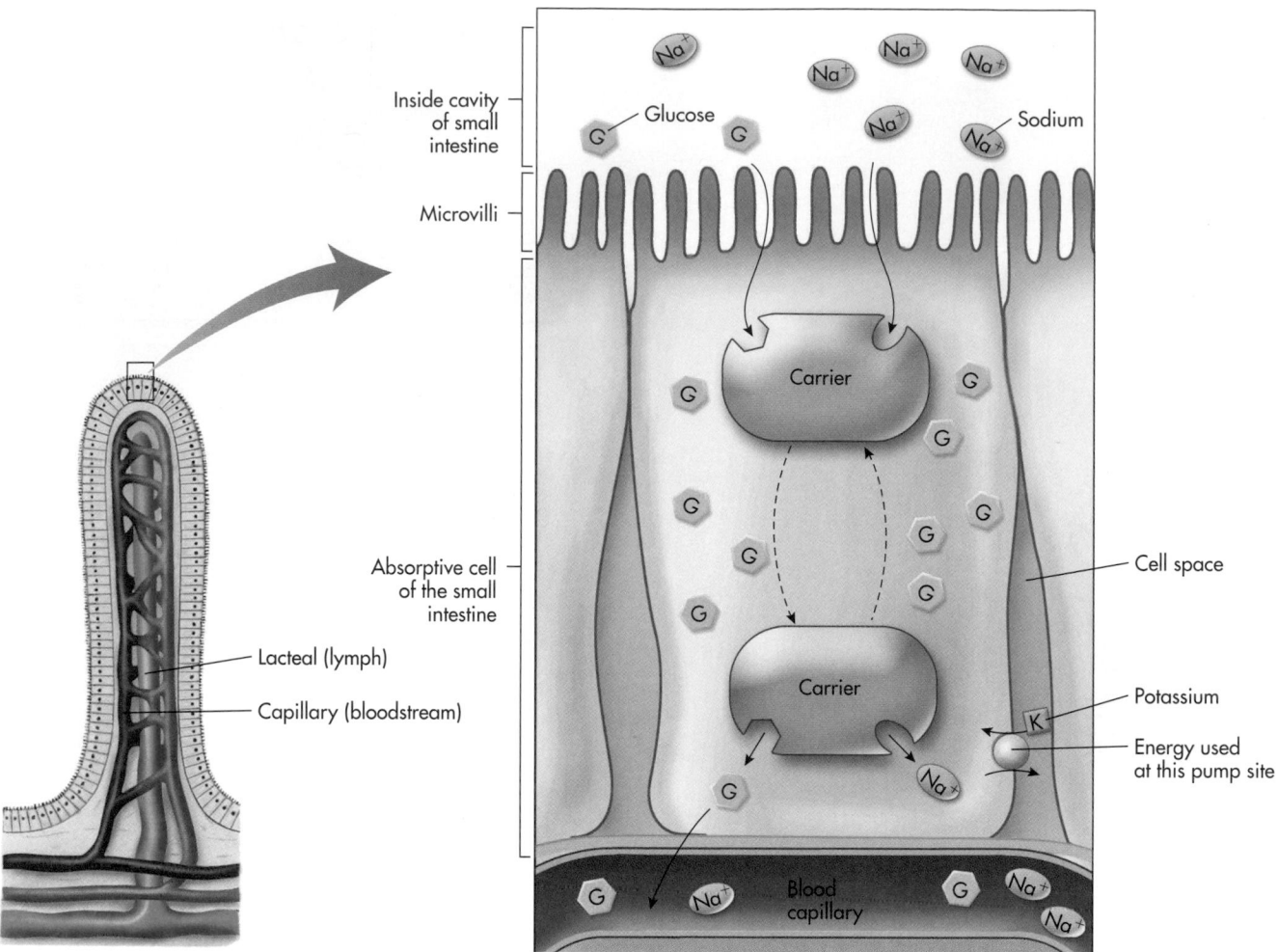

Figure 5-7 | Active absorption of glucose in the absorptive cells that make up the villi in the small intestine. Glucose and sodium pass across the absorptive cell membrane in a carrier-dependent, energy-requiring process. The energy is used for maintaining a low concentration of sodium in the cell. Once inside the absorptive cell, glucose can exit by facilitated diffusion down its concentration gradient and enter the bloodstream.

Absorption

With the exception of fructose, simple sugars found naturally in foods and those formed as by-products of earlier starch digestion in the mouth and small intestine follow an active absorption process.[14] Recall from Chapter 3 that this process requires a specific carrier and energy input in order for the substance to be taken up by the absorptive cells in the small intestine. Glucose and its close relative, galactose, undergo active absorption. They are pumped into the absorptive cells along with sodium (Figure 5-7). The ATP energy used in the process is actually needed to pump the sodium ion back out of the absorptive cell.

Fructose on the other hand is taken up by the absorptive cells via facilitated diffusion. In this case, a carrier is used, but no energy input is needed.[14] This absorptive process is slower than that seen with glucose or galactose. Thus, large doses of fructose are not readily absorbed and can contribute to diarrhea by remaining in the small intestine and attracting water via osmosis. (Chapter 11 will discuss osmosis in detail.)

Once glucose, galactose, and fructose enter the intestinal cells, glucose and galactose remain in that form, while some fructose is metabolized to glucose. All the single sugars in the absorptive cells are transported via a portal vein that is attached to the liver. The liver then exercises its metabolic options:

- transforming the monosaccharides into glucose and then releasing this glucose directly into the bloodstream for transport to organs, such as the brain, muscles, kidneys, and adipose tissues
- producing glycogen (the storage form of carbohydrate)
- producing fat

Of these three options, producing fat is the least likely, except when carbohydrate is consumed in very high amounts and energy needs are exceeded.[14]

A small portion of starch (about 10%) is called *resistant starch* because it resists digestion. The reason for the lack of digestion varies depending on the specific form of resistant starch in a food. This resistant starch travels down to the large intestine. There some of the starch is metabolized by bacteria and the resulting acids and gases are absorbed.[14] This entire process also takes place for any undigested lactose present in the large intestine. As mentioned before, scientists suspect that some of these products actually promote the health of the large intestine by providing a source of energy.

Concept | Check

Carbohydrate digestion is the process of breaking down larger carbohydrates into their absorbable components. The enzymatic digestion of starches begins in the mouth with salivary amylase. Enzymes made by the pancreas and absorptive cells of the small intestine complete the digestion of carbohydrates to single sugars in the small intestine. Primarily following an active absorption process, the single sugars (glucose and galactose)—either resulting from the digestive process or present in the meal—are then taken up by absorptive cells in the intestine. Fructose undergoes facilitated diffusion; once in the absorptive cell most is metabolized to glucose. All the monosaccharides then enter a portal vein that terminates in the liver. The liver finally exercises its metabolic options, primarily producing glucose and glycogen from the monosaccharides.

Functions of Glucose and Other Sugars in the Body

Glucose yields energy, but it has many other functions as well. The functions also apply to most carbohydrates because other sugars can generally be converted to glucose, and more complex carbohydrates (e.g., starches) are broken down to yield glucose.

Glucose is also used to synthesize the ribose and deoxyribose sugars used in RNA and DNA synthesis, respectively.

Yielding Energy

The main function of glucose is to act as a source of energy to body cells. Certain tissues, such as red blood cells and most parts of the brain, derive almost all their energy from glucose. In fact, except when the diet contains almost no carbohydrates, the brain and the rest of the **central nervous system** use mostly glucose for fuel. Glucose can also fuel muscle cells and other body cells, but many of these cells usually use fatty acids to meet energy needs.[14]

central nervous system (CNS) The brain and spinal cord portions of the nervous system.

Sparing Protein from Use as an Energy Source

Glucose is protein-sparing. That is, the amino acids that make up dietary protein can be used to make body tissues or to perform other vital processes only when carbohydrate intake provides enough glucose for body needs. This is because if you do not consume enough carbohydrate to yield that glucose, your body is forced to make it from other nutrients, such as amino acids found in muscle tissue and other organs. This process is termed **gluconeogenesis,** which means "production of new glucose"

gluconeogenesis The production of new glucose by metabolic pathways in the cell. Amino acids derived from protein usually provide the carbons for this glucose.

(review Chapter 4 for details).[14] If the process continues for weeks, these organs can become partially weakened. Generally, North Americans consume ample protein, so sparing protein is not an important role of carbohydrate in the diet. It does become important in some energy-reduced diets and in starvation. (Chapters 7 and 20 discuss specific effects of starvation.)

The life-threatening wasting of protein that occurs during long-term fasting (or starvation) has prompted companies that produce products used for rapid weight loss to include enough carbohydrate to supply 100 g/day or more. This significantly decreases protein breakdown and thus helps protect vital tissues and organs, including the heart, during rapid weight loss.

Preventing Ketosis

An adequate intake of carbohydrates—glucose, other sugars, or starch—is necessary for the complete metabolism of fats to carbon dioxide (CO_2) and water (H_2O) in the body. A low-carbohydrate intake, 50 to 100 g/day, leads to a decline in release of the hormone **insulin** into the bloodstream. This then leads to release of a large amount of fatty acids from adipose cells. The subsequent incomplete breakdown of these fatty acids in the liver then results in formation of ketone bodies—acetoacetic acid and its derivatives.[14] Chapter 4 covered in detail this condition, called ketosis.

In starvation, people do not consume enough carbohydrate, so ketone bodies soon appear in the blood. Again, this is the normal metabolic response to a fuel shortage. Over time, part of the brain and other tissues can use these ketone bodies for fuel. In fact, the use of ketone bodies by the brain and other organs, such as the heart, is an important adaptive mechanism for survival during starvation.[14] If part of the brain could not use ketone bodies, the body would be forced to produce much more glucose from protein to support the brain's energy needs. The resulting self-cannibalization would rapidly break down muscles, the heart, and other organs, severely limiting the body's ability to tolerate starvation.

In untreated type 1 diabetes, excessive production of ketone bodies can occur, partly because there is not enough insulin to allow for normal glucose metabolism. In such cases, the resulting ketosis can cause numerous complications (see the Nutrition Focus near the end of this chapter for further discussion of diabetes).[2]

▌ Functions of Fiber

Fiber adds bulk to the feces, making bowel movements easier. This is especially true for insoluble fibers. When enough fiber is consumed, the stool is large and soft because many types of plant fibers attract water. The larger size stimulates the intestinal muscles, which aids elimination. Consequently, less pressure is necessary to expel the feces.

When too little fiber is eaten, the opposite can occur: the stool may be small and hard. Constipation may result, which can force one to exert excessive pressure in the large intestine during defecation. This high pressure can force parts of the large intestine wall to pop out from between the surrounding bands of muscle, forming small pouches called **diverticula.**[9] Multiple diverticula are normally present (Figure 5-8). **Hemorrhoids** may also result from excessive straining during defecation.

Diverticula are asymptomatic in about 80% of affected people; that is, they are not noticeable. The asymptomatic form of this disease is called **diverticulosis.** If the diverticula eventually become inflamed, the condition is known as **diverticulitis.** Intake of fiber should then be reduced to limit further bacterial activity. Once the inflammation subsides, a high-fiber diet, along with regular physical activity, is advised to ease bowel movements, and reduce the risk of a future attack.[9]

Additional health benefits can accrue from eating fiber-rich foods. A diet high in fiber likely aids weight control and reduces the risk of developing obesity.[16] The bulky nature of high-fiber foods fills us up without yielding much energy. The foods also take a long time to chew. Increasing intake of foods rich in fiber is one strategy for re-

---

insulin A hormone produced by beta cells of the pancreas. Among other processes, insulin increases the synthesis of glycogen in the liver and the movement of glucose from the bloodstream into muscle and adipose cells.

The sweetness of sugars improves the taste of many foods, such as grapefruit. In addition, sugars provide certain functional properties to foods, such as texture, body, and browning capacity.

diverticula Pouches that protrude through the exterior wall of the large intestine.

hemorrhoid A pronounced swelling of a large vein, particularly veins found in the anal region.

diverticulosis The condition of having many diverticula in the large intestine.

diverticulitis An inflammation of the diverticula caused by acids produced by bacterial metabolism inside the diverticula.

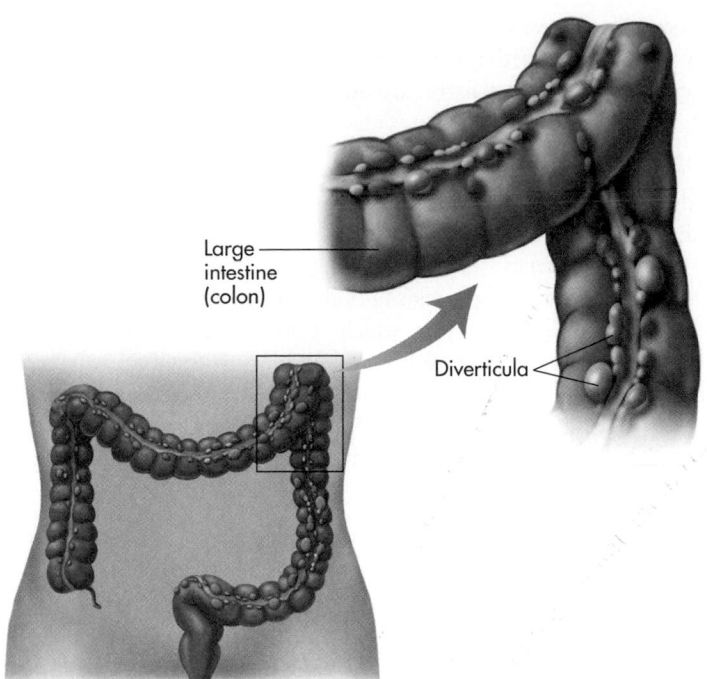

Figure 5-8 | Diverticula in the large intestine. A low-fiber diet increases the risk of developing diverticula. About one-third of people over age 45 have the disease, while two-thirds of people over 85 do.

maining satisfied after a meal (review the discussion on energy density in Chapter 2). This is yet another reason to question low-carbohydrate diet claims—where is the whole-grain fiber going to come from?

Over the past 30 years, many population studies have shown a link between increased fiber intake and a decrease in colon cancer development. However, some recent research has refuted the relationship between intake of fiber and colon cancer development, while other research has been supportive.[4,22] Currently, most of the research on colon cancer is focusing on the potential preventive effects of fruits, vegetables, whole-grain breads and cereals, and legume intakes (rather than fiber per se); regular exercise; the use of aspirin and related pain medications; and meeting vitamin D, folate, magnesium, selenium, and calcium needs. Smoking, obesity in men, excessive alcohol use, starch- and sugar-rich foods, and processed and red meat intake are under study as potential causes.[17,22] Overall, the health benefits to the colon that stem from a high-fiber diet are for the most part due to the nutrients that are commonly part of high-fiber foods, such as vitamins, minerals, phytochemicals, and in some cases essential fatty acids. Thus it is more advisable to increase fiber intake using fiber-rich foods rather than mostly relying on fiber supplements.

When consumed in large amounts, soluble fibers slow glucose absorption from the small intestine and so contribute to better blood glucose regulation. This effect can be helpful in the treatment of diabetes. In fact, adults whose main carbohydrate source is low-fiber foods are much more likely to develop diabetes than those who have high-fiber diets (see the Nutrition Focus near the end of this chapter).[24]

A high intake of soluble fiber also inhibits absorption of cholesterol and bile acids (cholesterol rich) from the small intestine, thereby somewhat reducing blood cholesterol and possibly reducing the risk of cardiovascular disease and gallstones. The short-chain fatty acids resulting from bacterial degradation of soluble fiber (e.g., proprionic acid) also probably reduce cholesterol synthesis in the liver. In addition, the slower glucose absorption that occurs with diets high in soluble fiber is linked to a decrease in insulin release. Because insulin stimulates cholesterol synthesis in the liver, this reduction in insulin may contribute to the ability of soluble fiber to lower blood cholesterol. Overall, a fiber-rich diet containing fruits, vegetables, legumes, and whole-grain breads and cereals (including whole-grain breakfast cereals) is advocated as part of a strategy

Critical | Thinking

Karla has a family history of colon cancer, and at age 20 she is curious about the lifestyle factors she can employ to prevent developing the disease. What advice would you provide her?

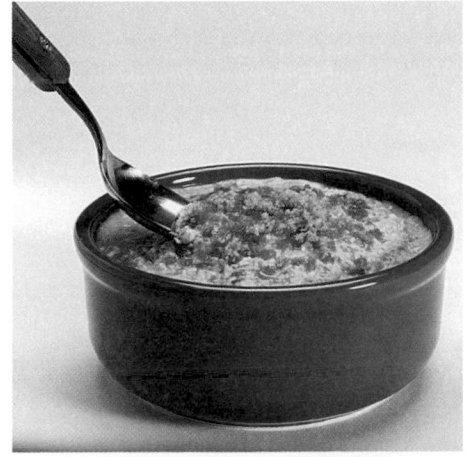

Oatmeal is a rich source of soluble fiber. FDA allows a health claim for the benefits of oatmeal to lower blood cholesterol that arise from the effects of this soluble fiber.

Recall from Chapter 2 that FDA has approved the following claim: "Diets rich in whole-grain foods and other plant foods and low in total fat, saturated fat, and cholesterol may decrease the risk for cardiovascular (heart) disease and certain cancers."

to reduce risk of cardiovascular disease (coronary heart disease and stroke).[16] This is the primary reason why criticizing carbohydrates as a group is misguided. The healthy sources of carbohydrates just listed are an important part of a diet.

Concept | Check

Carbohydrates provide glucose for the energy needs of red blood cells and parts of the brain and central nervous system. Eating too little carbohydrate forces the production of glucose (via gluconeogenesis), using carbons from amino acids. These amino acids are derived from the breakdown of proteins in body organs. An inadequate carbohydrate intake also inhibits efficient fat metabolism, which in turn can lead to ketosis.

Fiber forms a vital part of the diet by adding mass to the feces, which eases elimination. Fiber-rich foods also help in weight control and reduce the risk of developing obesity and cardiovascular disease. Soluble fiber can also be useful for controlling blood glucose in patients with diabetes and in lowering blood cholesterol. Whole grains, vegetables, legumes, and fruits are excellent sources of fiber.

Carbohydrate Needs

The RDA for carbohydrates is 130 g/day for adults.[11] This is based on the amount needed to supply adequate glucose for the brain and central nervous system, without having to rely on partial replacement of glucose by ketone bodies as an energy source. Exceeding this amount somewhat is fine; the Food and Nutrition Board recommends that carbohydrate intake should range from 45 to 65% of total energy intake.[11] North Americans consume about 180 to 330 g of carbohydrates per day. The top five carbohydrate sources for U.S. adults are white bread, soft drinks, cookies and cakes (including doughnuts), sugars/syrups/jams, and potatoes. Clearly, many of us should take a closer look at our main carbohydrate sources and strive to improve these from a nutritional standpoint.

In North America, carbohydrates supply about 50% of dietary energy intake for adults. Worldwide, however, carbohydrates account for about 70% of all energy consumed. In some countries, carbohydrates account for up to 80% of the energy consumed.

A later section entitled Health Concerns Related to Carbohydrate Intake provides a further look at a desirable amount of carbohydrate in a diet.

The Carbohydrate Continuum

Currently, other recommendations for carbohydrate intake are made in the scientific literature and popular press. Aside from the low intakes used to induce ketosis as part of a plan for quick weight loss (note that this diet is not recommended for long-term use; see Chapter 13), recommendations vary from 40% of energy intake in *The Zone* diet plans to more than 70% in the *Pritikin Program* and *Eat More, Weigh Less* plan. The Nutrition Facts panel on food labels uses 60% of energy intake as the standard for recommended carbohydrate intake. In addition, one recommendation on which almost all experts agree is that our carbohydrate intake should be based primarily on fruits, vegetables, whole-grain breads and cereals, and legumes, not mostly on refined grains and sugar.[1,32]

How Much Fiber Do We Need?

The Adequate Intake for fiber for adults is 25 g/day for women and 38 g/day for men. This is based on a goal of 14 g/1000 kcal in a diet.[11] After age 50 the Adequate Intake falls to 21 g/day and 30 g/day, respectively. The rationale for the Adequate Intake is the ability of fiber to reduce the risk of cardiovascular disease (and likely many cases of diabetes). The Daily Value used for fiber on food and supplement labels is 25 g for a 2000 kcal diet. In North America, the average intake of whole-grain breads and cereals is less than one serving per day; fiber intake averages 14 g/day for women and

Dr. Joanne Slavin discusses fiber in detail in the Expert Opinion in this chapter.

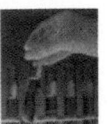

Expert Opinion

Fiber—Finally a Nutrient
Joanne L. Slavin, Ph.D., R.D.

Dietary fiber has a long and checkered past. In 300 BC, Hippocrates noted that coarse brown bread produced a lot of feces and that this was good for us. This simple fact has been rediscovered many times, including at the start of the modern cereal industry when the Kellogg brothers and C. W. Post got into the act of promoting high-fiber foods. Later, in the 1970s Dr. Denis Burkitt traveled the world showcasing pictures of large fecal specimens of rural Africans, who incidentally rarely developed Western diseases such as cardiovascular disease or colon cancer. As noted by Dr. Burkitt, having a phone in the bathroom would be of no use to the rural African because a high-fiber fecal sample is passed in much less time than it takes to make or answer a phone call.

So what is this wonder compound? Dietary fiber is essentially the polysaccharide leftover of digestion. The physiological effect of fiber in intact foods is often greater than that found with isolated fiber fractions. In epidemiologic studies, whole-grain breads and cereals, vegetables, and fruits are often more protective against diseases than fiber supplements. Thus, fiber intake may be a marker of a healthy diet rather than just a nutrient that can be isolated and added back to the diet.

In 2002, the Dietary Reference Intakes (DRIs) for the first time included fiber as a nutrient. *Dietary fiber* was defined as nondigestible carbohydrates and lignin that are intrinsic and intact in plants. Foods high in dietary fiber include whole-grain breads and cereals, legumes, vegetables, and fruits. Another class of fiber, *functional fiber,* was defined as nondigestible carbohydrates extracted from foods that have beneficial physiological effects in humans. Functional fiber is found in bulk laxatives, fortified foods, beverages, and dietary supplements. *Total fiber* was then defined as the sum of *dietary fiber* and *functional fiber.*

Soluble and Insoluble Fiber—Outmoded Terms

Previously, dietary fiber was divided into soluble and insoluble fiber in an attempt to assign physiological effects to chemical types of fiber. Oat bran and psyllium, two mostly soluble fibers, have health claims for the ability to lower blood lipids. Wheat bran and other, more insoluble fibers are linked to laxation. Yet, scientific support that soluble fibers lower blood cholesterol while insoluble fibers increase stool size is inconsistent at best. A meta-analysis (combined analysis of a number of studies) testing the effects of pectin, oat bran, guar gum, and psyllium on blood cholesterol found that 2 to 10 g/day of soluble fiber was associated with small but significant decreases in total- and LDL-cholesterol concentrations. Resistant starch and inulin, both considered soluble fibers under the new definitions do not, however, affect blood cholesterol. Thus, not all soluble fibers lower blood cholesterol, and other traits, such as viscosity of fiber, play roles.

Constipation is more likely on low-fiber intakes and risk of colon cancer is inversely related to stool weight. Still, the association of insoluble fiber with laxation also is inconsistent. Fecal weight increases 5.4 g/g of wheat bran fiber (mostly insoluble), 4.9 g/g of fruit and vegetable fiber (soluble and insoluble), 3 g/g of isolated cellulose (insoluble), and 1.3 g/g of isolated pectin (soluble). Many other fiber sources are mostly soluble but still enlarge stool weight, such as oat bran and psyllium.

Furthermore, besides food intake, other factors also affect stool size. Stress associated with exams or athletic competition can speed intestinal transit. A morning cup of coffee can contribute to a regular bowel habit. Medications, both laxatives designed to speed transit and other drugs, alter bowel function and fecal composition. There is a large variation in daily stool weight even among subjects on rigidly controlled diets of the exact same composition. A USDA study that examined the predictors of stool weight when completely controlled diets were fed to normal volunteers found that personality was a better predictor of stool weight than fiber intake. In particular, outgoing subjects were more likely to produce higher stool weights than subject who were less so.

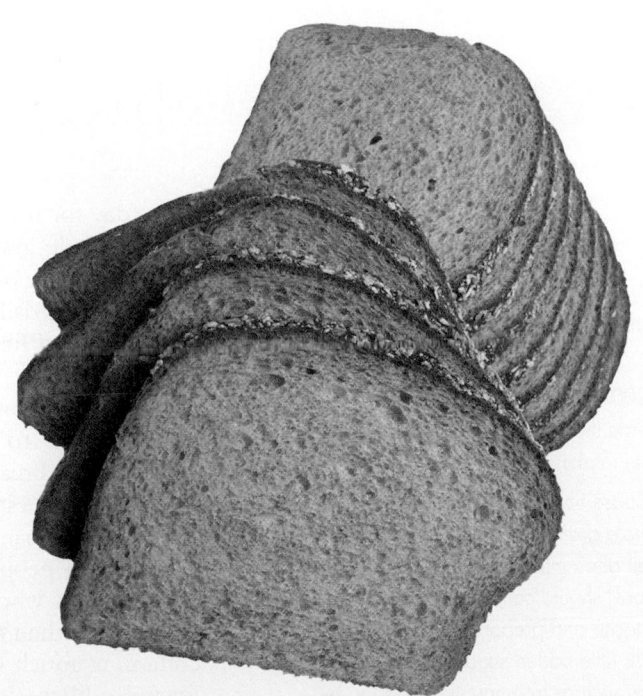

Make most of your grain choices whole grains.

Viscous and Nonfermentable Fiber— A Better Classification?

The disparities between the amounts of soluble and insoluble fiber measured chemically and the magnitude of their physiological effects led the Food and Nutrition Board to recommend that the terms *soluble* and *insoluble fibers* gradually be eliminated and be replaced by other properties, perhaps *viscosity* and *fermentability*. Measuring *dietary fiber* and *functional fiber* by the new definitions will also take new approaches. First, we must decide on the criteria for functionality. If fermentability and viscosity are accepted as important criteria, in vitro tests for these properties would need to be developed. Tests for functional properties of dietary fiber could include a reduction in blood cholesterol, improvements in bowel function, and modulation of blood glucose. Evaluation of these studies could be based on a biologically significant change. For example, does a particular functional fiber have a similar blood cholesterol–lowering effect as oat bran, or does it increase wet stool weight similar to wheat bran? Does a particular fiber control blood glucose by an acceptable amount, perhaps relative to a standard, effective fiber? Another approach would be model systems for these attributes. For example, a fecal bulking index has been described in rats. Still, no perfect system will be found to evaluate and test the physiological effects of a complex substance such as fiber.

Fiber Needs and Intakes

Average fiber intakes in the United States fall woefully short of the current Adequate Intakes set for various ages and genders. In contrast, vegetarians among us routinely consume this amount or more, and the fiber intake of Paleolithic man (the fruit and nut gatherer and wild game slayer) has been estimated at about three to four times the current recommendations.

The Future of Fiber

Some research studies support that stool size is protective against colon cancer and that fiber may be helpful for digestive diseases such as irritable bowel syndrome and diverticulosis. Many of the diseases of public health significance—obesity, cardiovascular disease, type 2 diabetes, colon cancer, and constipation—may be prevented or treated by increasing the amounts and varieties of fiber-containing foods. Promotion of such a food plan across the lifespan by health-care professionals and subsequent implementation by our population should contribute to overall better health.

Dr. Slavin is a professor in the Department of Food Science and Nutrition, University of Minnesota, St. Paul. She has conducted many human feeding studies on dietary fiber, whole grains, fruits, vegetables, soy, and flax. Besides her pursuit of the fiber research, she teaches Life Cycle Nutrition and Human Nutrition. She has published more than 100 refereed scientific articles and speaks widely on choosing carbohydrate sources wisely.

The 2005 Dietary Guidelines for Americans provide the following advice regarding carbohydrate intake:

- Choose fiber-rich fruits, vegetables, and whole grains often. (In general, at least half one's intake of grains [3 ounces or more] should come from whole grains.)
- Choose and prepare foods and beverages with little added sugars or caloric sweeteners, such as in amounts suggested by MyPyramid.
- Reduce the incidence of dental caries by practicing good oral hygiene and consuming sugar- and starch-containing foods and beverages less frequently.

19 g/day for men. This low intake is attributed to the lack of knowledge on the benefits of whole-grain foods as well as the lack of ability to recognize whole-grain products at the time of purchase. Thus, most of us should increase our fiber intake. At least three of your daily servings of grains should be whole grains. Eating a high-fiber cereal ($\geq$ 3 g of fiber per serving) for breakfast is one easy way to increase fiber intake (Figure 5-9).[18]

Table 5-2 shows a diet containing 25 or 38 g of fiber within very moderate energy intakes. Diets to meet the fiber recommendations are possible if you regularly eat whole-wheat bread, fruits, vegetables, and beans. Use the first Take Action exercise in this chapter to estimate the fiber content of your diet. What is *your* fiber score?

Note that manufacturers list enriched white (refined) flour as wheat flour on food labels. Most people think that if "wheat flour" or "wheat bread" is on the label, they are buying a whole-wheat product. Not so. If the label does not list "whole-wheat flour" first, then the product is not primarily a whole-wheat bread and thus does not contain as much fiber as it could. Careful reading of labels is important in the search for more fiber—look especially for whole grains.

Keep in mind, however, that any nutrient can lead to health problems when consumed in excess, including carbohydrate and fiber. The terms *high-carbohydrate, high-fiber,* and *low-fat* do not mean *zero calories.* Carbohydrates help moderate energy intake in comparison with fats, but high-carbohydrate foods still contribute to total energy intake, so they have to be accounted for.[1]

Nutrition Facts (Left Label)

Serving Size 1 cup (55g/2.0 oz.)
Servings Per Container 10

Amount Per Serving	Cereal	Cereal with ½ Cup Vitamins A & D Skim Milk
Calories	170	210
Calories from Fat	10	10
	% Daily Value**	
Total Fat 1.0g*	2%	2%
Sat. Fat 0g	0%	0%
Trans Fat 0g		*
Cholesterol 0mg	0%	0%
Sodium 300mg	13%	15%
Potassium 340mg	10%	16%
Total Carbohydrate 43g	14%	16%
Dietary Fiber 7g	28%	28%
Sugars 16g		
Other Carbohydrate 20g		
Protein 4g		
Vitamin A	15%	20%
Vitamin C	20%	22%
Calcium	2%	15%
Iron	65%	65%
Vitamin D	10%	25%
Thiamin	25%	30%
Riboflavin	25%	35%
Niacin	25%	25%
Vitamin B$_6$	25%	25%
Folic acid	30%	30%
Vitamin B$_{12}$	25%	35%
Phosphorus	20%	30%
Magnesium	20%	25%
Zinc	25%	25%
Copper	10%	10%

*Amount in cereal. One half cup skim milk contributes an additional 40 calories, 65mg sodium, 6g total carbohydrate (6g sugars), and 4g protein.
**Percent Daily Values are based on a 2,000 calorie diet. Your daily values may be higher or lower depending on your calorie needs:

	Calories:	2,000	2,500
Total Fat	Less than	65g	80g
Sat Fat	Less than	20g	25g
Cholesterol	Less than	300mg	300mg
Sodium	Less than	2,400mg	2,400mg
Potassium		3,500mg	3,500mg
Total Carbohydrate		300g	375g
Dietary Fiber		25g	30g

Calories per gram:
Fat 9 • Carbohydrate 4 • Protein 4

*Intake of *trans* fat should be as low as possible.

Ingredients: Wheat bran with other parts of wheat, raisins, sugar, corn syrup, salt, malt flavoring, glycerin, iron, niacinamide, zinc oxide, pyridoxine hydrochloride (vitamin B$_6$), riboflavin (vitamin B$_2$), vitamin A palmitate, thiamin hydrochloride (vitamin B$_1$), folic acid, vitamin B$_{12}$, and vitamin D.

Nutrition Facts (Right Label)

Serving Size: ¾ Cup (30g)
Servings Per Package: About 17

Amount Per Serving	1 Cup Cereal	Cereal With ½ Cup Skim Milk
Calories	170	200
Calories from Fat	0	5
	%Daily Value**	
Total Fat 0g*	0%	1%
Saturated Fat 0g	0%	1%
Trans Fat 0g		*
Cholesterol 0mg	0%	1%
Sodium 60mg	2%	4%
Potassium 80mg	2%	8%
Total Carbohydrate 35g	9%	11%
Dietary Fiber 1g	4%	4%
Sugars 20g		
Other Carbohydrate 13g		
Protein 3g		
Vitamin A	25%	30%
Vitamin C	0%	2%
Calcium	0%	15%
Iron	10%	10%
Vitamin D	10%	20%
Thiamin	25%	25%
Riboflavin	25%	35%
Niacin	25%	25%
Vitamin B$_6$	25%	25%
Folic acid	25%	25%
Vitamin B$_{12}$	25%	30%
Phosphorus	4%	15%
Magnesium	4%	8%
Zinc	10%	10%
Copper	2%	2%

*Amount in Cereal. One-half cup skim milk contributes an additional 65mg sodium, 6g total carbohydrate (6g sugars), and 4g protein.
**Percent Daily Values are based on a 2,000 calorie diet. Your daily values may be higher or lower depending on your calorie needs:

	Calories:	2,000	2,500
Total Fat	Less than	65g	80g
Sat. Fat	Less than	20g	25g
Cholesterol	Less than	300mg	300mg
Sodium	Less than	2,400mg	2,400mg
Potassium		3,500mg	3,500mg
Total Carbohydrate		300g	375g
Dietary Fiber		25g	30g

Calories per gram:
Fat 9 • Carbohydrate 4 • Protein 4

*Intake of *trans* fat should be as low as possible.

Ingredients: Wheat, Sugar, Corn Syrup, Honey, Caramel Color, Partially Hydrogenated Soybean Oil, Salt, Ferric Phosphate, Niacinamide (Niacin), Zinc Oxide, Vitamin A (Palmitate), Pyridoxine Hydrochloride (Vitamin B6), Riboflavin, Thiamin Mononitrate, Folic Acid (Folate), Vitamin B12 and Vitamin D.

Figure 5-9 | Reading the Nutrition Facts on food labels helps us choose more nutritious foods. Based on the information from these nutrition labels, which cereal is the better choice for breakfast? Consider the amount of fiber in each cereal. Do the ingredient lists give you any clues? (Note: Ingredients are always listed in descending order by weight on a label.) When choosing a breakfast cereal, it is generally wise to focus on those that are rich sources of fiber. Simple sugar content can also be used for evaluation. However, sometimes this number does not reflect added sugar but simply the addition of fruits, such as raisins, complicating the evaluation.

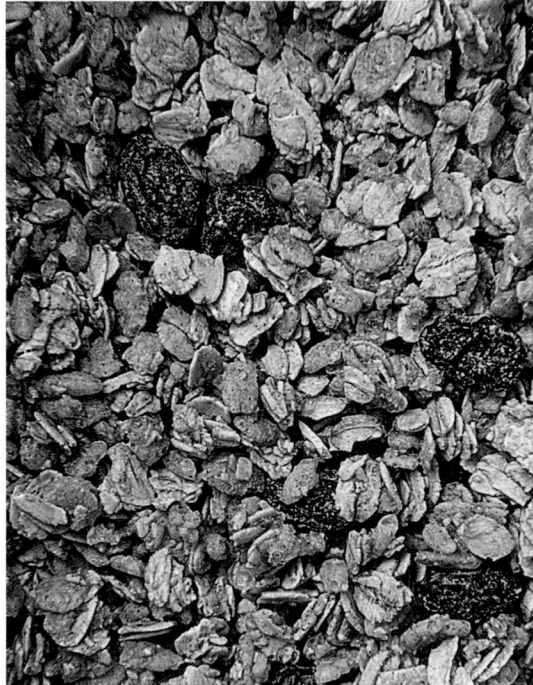

Whole-grain foods, such as granola, are excellent sources of fiber.

*H*ealthy People 2010 has the following goals related to carbohydrate intake:

- Increase the proportion of persons age 2 years and older who consume at least six daily servings of grain products, with at least three being whole grains.
- Increase the proportion of persons age 2 years and older who consume at least two daily servings of fruit.
- Increase the proportion of persons age 2 years and older who consume at least three daily servings of vegetables, with at least one-third being dark green or orange vegetables.

Concept | Check

The RDA for carbohydrate is 130 g/day. The typical North American diet provides 180 to 330 g/day. A reasonable goal is to have about half our energy intake coming from starch. Total carbohydrate intake should constitute about 60% of our energy intake, with a range of 45 to 65%. This goal should allow for the recommended intake of 25 to 38 g of fiber/day for women and men, respectively.

Table 5-2 | Sample of Menus Containing 1600 kcal and 25 g of Fiber, and 2000 kcal and 38 g of Fiber*

Menu	Serving Size	25 g Fiber		Serving Size	38 g Fiber	
		Carbohydrate Content (g)	Fiber Content (g)		Carbohydrate Content (g)	Fiber Content (g)
Breakfast						
Orange juice (with pulp)	1 cup	28	0.5	1 cup	28	0.5
Wheaties	3/4 cup	17	2	3/4 cup	17	2
2% milk	1/2 cup	6	—	1/2 cup	6	—
Whole-wheat toast	1 slice	13	2	1 slice	13	2
Margarine	1 tsp	—	—	1 tsp	—	—
Coffee		1	—	—	1	—
Lunch						
Lean ham	2 oz	—	—	2 oz	—	—
Whole-wheat bread	2 slices	26	4	2 slices	26	4
Mayonnaise	2 tsp	2	—	2 tsp	2	—
Lettuce	1/4 cup	—	0.2	1/4 cup	—	0.2
Cooked white beans	1/3 cup	15	4	1 cup	45	12
Pear (with skin)	1/2	12	2	1	25	4
1% milk	1/2 cup	6	—	1/2 cup	6	—
Snack						
Carrot (as carrot sticks)	1	8	2	1	8	2
Dinner						
Broiled chicken (no skin)	3 oz	—	—	3 oz	—	—
Baked potato (large, with skin)	1/2	15	1.5	1	30	3
Margarine	1 1/2 tsp	—	—	1 1/2 tsp	—	—
Cooked green beans	1 cup	10	4	1 cup	10	4
Margarine	1/2 tsp	—	—	1/2 tsp	—	—
1% milk	1 cup	12	—	1 cup	12	—
Apple (with peel)	1/2	16	1.8	1	32	3.7
Snack						
Raisin bagel	1	39	1.2	1	39	1.2
Total		226 g	25 g		300 g	38 g

*The overall diet pattern is based on MyPyramid. Breakdown of approximate energy content: carbohydrate, 55%; protein, 20%; fat, 25%.

Health Concerns Related to Carbohydrate Intake

Aside from the health risks related to ketosis, both excessive fiber and excessive sugar intakes can pose health problems. Too much lactose in the diet is also a problem for some people.

Problems with High-Fiber Diets

Very high intakes of fiber—for example, 60 grams per day—can pose some health risks, especially when fluid intake is low. This combination can leave the stool very hard and painful to eliminate. In more severe cases, the combination of excess fiber and insufficient fluid may contribute to blockages in the intestine, which may require surgery.

Aside from problems with the passage of materials through the GI tract, a very high fiber diet may also decrease the availability of nutrients. Certain components of fiber may bind to essential minerals, keeping them from being absorbed. For example, when fiber is consumed in large amounts, zinc and iron absorption may be hindered. In children, a very high fiber intake may reduce overall energy intake, because fiber can quickly fill a child's small stomach before food intake meets energy needs.

Problems with High-Sugar Diets

The main problem with consuming an overabundant amount of sugar is that it provides empty calories (i.e., is low in other nutrients) and increases the risk for dental decay.

Diet Quality Declines When Sugar Intake Is Excessive

Overcrowding the diet with sweet treats can leave little room for important, nutrient-dense foods, such as dairy products and vegetables. Children and teenagers are at the highest risk for overconsuming empty calories in place of nutrients that are essential for growth. Many children and teenagers are drinking an excess of sugared soft drinks and other sugar-containing beverages and much less milk than ever before. Milk contains calcium and vitamin D, both of which are essential for bone health; therefore, this exchange of soft drinks for milk can compromise bone health.

Supersizing sugar-rich beverages is also a growing problem; for example, in the 1950s a typical serving size of a soft drink was a 6½ ounce bottle, and now a 20 ounce plastic bottle is a typical serving. This one change in serving size contributes 170 extra kcal of sugars to the diet. Most convenience stores now offer cups that will hold 64 ounces of soft drinks. Filling up on sugary soft drinks in place of foods is not a healthy practice, but enjoying an occasional soft drink or limiting intake to one 12 fl. oz. serving a day is generally fine. Switching to diet soft drinks is also an easy way to spare the simple sugar calories.

The sugar found in cakes, cookies, and ice cream supplies extra energy that promotes weight gain, unless an individual is physically active. Today's low-fat and fat-free snack products usually contain lots of added sugar to produce a product with an acceptable taste. The result is to produce a high-calorie food that is equal to or greater in energy content than the high-fat food product it was designed to replace.

With regard to sugar intake, the World Health Organization suggests that sugars added to foods during processing and preparation ("added sugars") should provide no more than about 10% of total daily energy intake; an upper limit of 25% has been set by the Food and Nutrition Board. Diets that go beyond this upper limit become scarce in more healthy foods.[11]

A moderate intake of about 10% of energy intake corresponds to a maximum of approximately 50 g (or 12 tsp) of sugars per day, based on a 2000 kcal diet. Most of the sugars we eat come from foods and beverages to which sugar has been added during processing and/or manufacture. On average, North Americans eat about 82 g of added sugars daily, amounting to about 16% of energy intake. Major sources of added sugars include soft drinks, cakes, cookies, fruit punch, and dairy desserts, such as ice cream. Following the recommendation of having no more than 10% of added energy intake from "added sugars" is easier if sugary soft drinks and sweet desserts such as cakes, cookies, and ice cream (full- and reduced-fat) are consumed sparingly (Table 5-3).[1]

Excessive Sugar Intake Can Lead to Dental Caries

Sugars in the diet (and starches that are readily fermented in the mouth, such as crackers and white bread) also increase the risk of developing **dental caries**.[29] Recall that caries, also known as cavities, are formed when sugars and other carbohydrates are metabolized into acids by bacteria that live in the mouth (Figure 5-10). These acids dissolve the tooth enamel and underlying structure. Bacteria also use the sugars to make plaque, a sticky substance that both adheres acid-producing bacteria to teeth and diminishes the acid-neutralizing effect of saliva.[1]

There is a widespread notion that high-sugar intakes by children cause hyperactivity, typically part of the syndrome called *attention deficit hyperactivity disorder (ADHD)*. However, most researchers find that sucrose may actually have the opposite effect. A high-carbohydrate meal, if also low in protein and fat, has a calming effect and induces sleep; this effect may be linked to changes in the synthesis of certain neurotransmitters in the brain, such as serotonin. If there is a behavior problem, it is probably the excitement or tension in situations in which sugar-rich foods are served, such as at birthday parties and on Halloween.

An excess intake of sugared soft drinks has recently been linked to a risk for both weight gain and type 2 diabetes in adults.[25]

dental caries Erosions in the surface of a tooth caused by acids made by bacteria as they metabolize sugars.

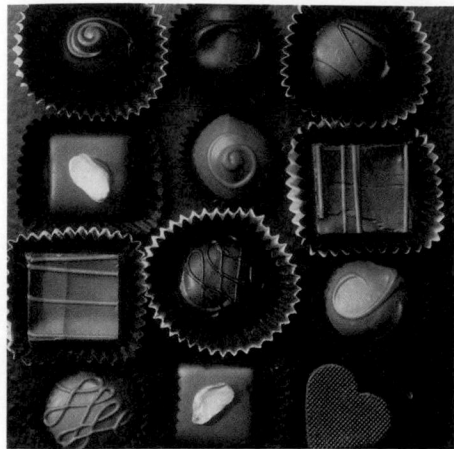

Many foods we enjoy are sweet. These should be eaten in moderation.

Table 5-3 | Suggestions for Reducing Simple-Sugar Intake

At the Supermarket

• Read ingredient labels. Identify all the added sugars in a product. Select items lower in total sugar when possible.

• Buy fresh fruits or fruits packed in water, juice, or light syrup, rather than those packed in heavy syrup.

• Buy fewer foods that are high in sugar, such as prepared baked goods, candies, sugared cereals, sweet desserts, soft drinks, and fruit-flavored punches. Substitute vanilla wafers, graham crackers, bagels, English muffins, and diet soft drinks, for example.

• Buy reduced-fat microwave popcorn to replace candy for snacks.

In the Kitchen

• Reduce the sugar in foods prepared at home. Try new low-sugar recipes or adjust your own. Start by reducing the sugar gradually until you've decreased it by one-third or more. Consider using Splenda to substitute for some sugar.

• Experiment with spices such as cinnamon, cardamom, coriander, nutmeg, ginger, and mace to enhance the flavor of foods.

• Use home-prepared items (with less sugar) instead of commercially prepared ones that are higher in sugar.

At the Table

• Use less of all sugars. This includes white and brown sugars, honey, molasses, syrups, jams, and jellies.

• Choose fewer foods high in sugar, such as prepared baked goods, candies, and sweet desserts.

• Reach for fresh fruit instead of cookies or candy for dessert or between-meal snacks.

• Add less sugar to foods—coffee, tea, cereal, and fruit. Get used to using half as much; then see if you can cut back even more.

• Cut back on the number of sugared soft drinks, punches, and fruit juices you drink. Substitute water, diet soft drinks, and whole fruits rather than fruit juice.

Modified from USDA *Home and Garden Bulletin* No. 232-5, 1986.

Figure 5-10 | Dental caries. Bacteria can collect in various areas on a tooth. Using simple sugars such as sucrose, bacteria then create acids that can dissolve tooth enamel, leading to caries. If the caries process progresses and enters the pulp cavity, damage to the nerve and resulting pain are likely. The bacteria also produce plaque whereby they adhere to the tooth surface.

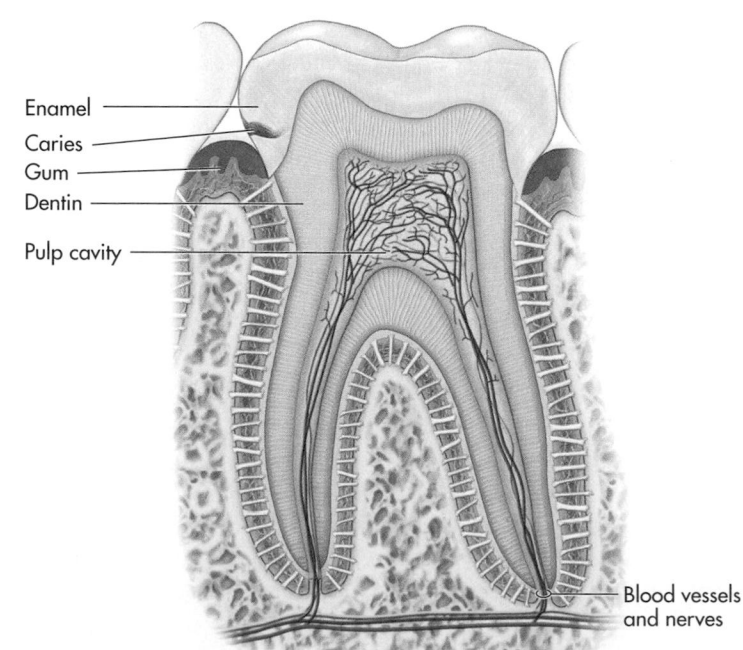

The worst offenders in terms of promoting dental caries are sticky and gummy foods high in sugars, such as caramel, because they stick to the teeth and supply the bacteria with a long-lived carbohydrate source. Although liquid sugar sources (e.g., fruit juices) are not as potent at causing dental caries as sticky and gummy foods, they still warrant consideration.[29]

Snacking regularly on sugary foods is also likely to cause caries because it gives the bacteria on the teeth a steady source of carbohydrate from which to continually make acid. Sugared gum chewed between meals is a prime example of a poor dental habit. Still, sugar-containing foods are not the only foods that promote acid production by bacteria in the mouth. As mentioned, if starch-containing foods (e.g., crackers and bread) are held in the mouth for a long time, they can be acted on by enzymes in the mouth that break down the starch to sugars; bacteria can then produce acid from these sugars. Overall, the sugar and starch content of a food and its ability to remain in the mouth largely determine its potential to cause caries.

Fluoridated water and toothpastes have contributed to fewer dental caries in North American children over the past 20 years because of fluoride's tooth-strengthening effect (see Chapter 12). Research has also indicated that certain foods—such as cheese, peanuts, and sugar-free chewing gum—can actually help reduce the amount of acid on teeth. In addition, rinsing the mouth after meals and snacks reduces the acidity in the mouth. Certainly, good nutrition, habits that do not present an overwhelming challenge to oral health (e.g., chewing sugar-free gum), and routine visits to the dentist all contribute to improved dental health.[29]

High Glycemic Index and Glycemic Load Also Deserve Consideration

Our bodies react uniquely to different sources of carbohydrates, such that a serving of a high-fiber food such as brown rice results in lower blood glucose levels compared to the same size serving of mashed potatoes. Researchers have developed two tools that are useful in predicting the blood glucose response to various foods.

The first of these tools is **glycemic index (GI),** which is a ratio of the blood glucose response to a given food compared to a standard (typically, glucose or white bread) (Table 5-4).[5] Glycemic index is influenced by starch structure, fiber content, food processing, physical structure, food temperature, and other macronutrients in the meal, such as fat. Foods with particularly high glycemic index values are potatoes, especially baking potatoes (due to higher amylopectin content compared to red potatoes), mashed potatoes (due to greater surface area exposed), short grain white rice, honey, and jelly beans. A major shortcoming of glycemic index is that the number is based on a serving of food that would provide 50 grams of carbohydrate. As you can imagine, this amount of food may not reflect the amount typically consumed.

Another way of describing how different foods affect blood glucose (and insulin) levels is **glycemic load (GL).** The glycemic load takes into account the glycemic index and the amount of carbohydrate consumed, and in doing so actually better reflects a food's effect on one's blood glucose than glycemic index alone.[5] To calculate the glycemic load of a food, the grams of carbohydrate in a serving of the food are multiplied by the glycemic index of that food, and then divided by 100 (since glycemic index is actually a percentage). For example, vanilla wafers have a glycemic index of 77, and a small serving contains 15 g of carbohydrate. This yields a glycemic load of 12.

$$(77 \times 15) \div 100 = 12$$

So even though the glycemic index of vanilla wafers is considered high, the glycemic load calculation shows that the impact of this food on blood glucose levels is fairly low (review Table 5-4).

Critical | Thinking

John and Mike are identical twins who like the same games, sports, and foods. However, John likes to chew sugar-free gum and Mike doesn't. At their last dental visit, John had no cavities, but Mike had two. Mike wants to know why John, who chews gum after eating, doesn't have cavities and he does. How would you explain this to him?

glycemic index (GI) The blood glucose response of a given food compared to a standard (typically, glucose or white bread).

glycemic load (GL) The amount of carbohydrate in a food multiplied by the glycemic index of that carbohydrate. The result is then divided by 100.

A term you might see on food labels is "net carbs." This term has no legal FDA-approved definition. It is used to describe the content of carbohydrates that increase blood glucose. Fiber and sugar alcohol content are subtracted from total carbohydrate content to yield "net carbs," because these have a negligible effect on blood glucose. Still, sugar alcohols and some fibers do yield energy.

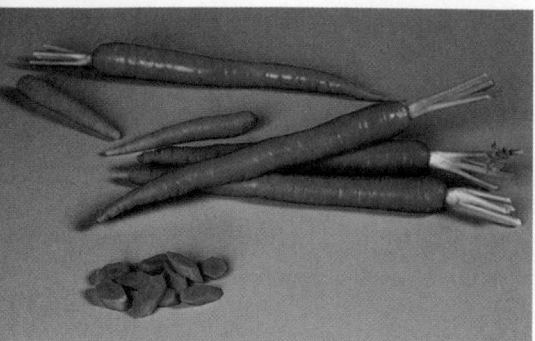

Carrots, criticized in the popular press for having a high glycemic index (which isn't even true), actually contribute a low glycemic load to a diet.

Y ou might wonder why the glycemic index and glycemic load of white bread and whole-wheat bread are similar. This is because whole-wheat flour is typically so finely ground that it is quickly digested. Thus, the effect of fiber in slowing digestion and related absorption of glucose is no longer present. Some experts suggest we focus more on minimally processed grains, such as coarsely ground whole-wheat flour and steel-cut oats, to get the full benefits of these fiber sources.

Table 5-4 | Glycemic Index (GI) and Glycemic Load (GL) of Common Foods

Reference food glucose = 100
Low GI foods—below 55
Intermediate GI foods—between 55 and 69
High GI foods—more than 70

Low GL foods—below 10
Intermediate GL foods—between 11 and 19
High GL foods—more than 20

	Serving Size (grams)	Glycemic Index (GI)*	Carbohydrate (grams)	Glycemic Load (GL)
Pastas/Grains				
Brown rice	1 cup	55	46	25
White, long grain	1 cup	56	45	25
White, short grain	1 cup	72	53	38
Spaghetti	1 cup	41	40	16
Vegetables				
Carrots, boiled	1 cup	49	16	8
Sweet corn	1 cup	55	39	21
Potato, baked	1 cup	85	57	48
New (red) potato, boiled	1 cup	62	29	18
Dairy Foods				
Milk, whole	1 cup	27	11	3
Milk, skim	1 cup	32	12	4
Yogurt, low-fat	1 cup	33	17	6
Ice cream	1 cup	61	31	19
Legumes				
Baked beans	1 cup	48	54	26
Kidney beans	1 cup	27	38	10
Lentils	1 cup	30	40	12
Navy beans	1 cup	38	54	21
Sugars				
Honey	1 tsp	73	6	4
Sucrose	1 tsp	65	5	3
Fructose	1 tsp	23	5	1
Lactose	1 tsp	46	5	2
Breads and Muffins				
Bagel	1 small	72	30	22
Whole-wheat bread	1 slice	69	13	9
White bread	1 slice	70	10	7
Croissant	1 small	67	26	17
Fruits				
Apple	1 medium	38	22	8
Banana	1 medium	55	29	16
Grapefruit	1 medium	25	32	8
Orange	1 medium	44	15	7
Beverages				
Apple juice	1 cup	40	29	12
Orange juice	1 cup	46	26	13
Gatorade	1 cup	78	15	12
Coca-Cola	1 cup	63	26	16
Snack Foods				
Potato chips	1 oz	54	15	8
Vanilla wafers	5 cookies	77	15	12
Chocolate	1 oz	49	18	9
Jelly beans	1 oz	80	26	21

*Based on a comparison to glucose

Source: Foster-Powell K and others: International table of glycemic index and glycemic load. *American Journal of Clinical Nutrition* 76:5, 2002.

Why are we concerned with the effects of various foods on blood glucose? Foods that have a high glycemic load elicit a large release of insulin from the pancreas. Chronically high insulin output leads to many harmful effects on the body: high blood triglycerides, increased fat deposition in the adipose tissue, increased tendency for blood to clot, increased fat synthesis in the liver, and a more rapid return of hunger after a meal (insulin rapidly lowers the macronutients in the blood as it stimulates their storage, signaling hunger). Over time, this increase in insulin output may actually cause the muscle cells to become resistant to the action of insulin and eventually lead to diabetes and cardiovascular disease in some people.[5]

There are many ways to address this problem of high glycemic load foods. The most important is to not overeat these foods at any one meal. This greatly minimizes their effects on blood glucose and the subsequent increase in insulin release. At each meal consider substituting at least one food that has a low glycemic load for one with a higher value, such as long grain rice or spaghetti for short grain white rice. Combining a low glycemic load food, such as an apple, kidney beans, milk, or salad with dressing, with a high glycemic load food also reduces the effect on blood glucose. In addition, maintaining a healthy body weight and performing regular physical activity further reduces the effects of a high glycemic load diet.

A focus on low glycemic load carbohydrates can help in the treatment of diabetes;[5] Chapter 14 discusses the use of foods with different glycemic load values in planning diets for athletes.

Sugars and Refined Starches and the Metabolic Syndrome

Despite the current trend to "demonize" carbohydrates, the only time a carbohydrate-rich diet may not be recommended is when a person's blood triglycerides are high, in turn contributing to the **metabolic syndrome.** (This syndrome will be covered further in Chapter 6.) Note that about 25% of North American adults have this condition. Actually, the chief culprits contributing to high blood triglycerides are not often carbohydrates as a class of nutrients but excessively large meals full of foods rich in simple sugars and refined starches but low in fiber. In addition, too little physical activity (and obesity) worsens the metabolic syndrome.[6] These practices should not form the basis of daily habits, but unfortunately, they do for many adults.

Problems with Lactose Intake, Especially for Some People

Lactose maldigestion is a normal pattern of physiology that often begins to develop after early childhood, at about ages 3 to 5 years. It can lead to symptoms of abdominal pain, gas, and diarrhea after consuming lactose, especially when eaten in large amounts. This *primary* form of lactose maldigestion is estimated to be present in about 75% of the world's population, although not all these individuals experience symptoms. (When significant symptoms develop after lactose intake, it is then called lactose intolerance.) Another form of the problem, *secondary* lactose maldigestion, is a temporary condition in which lactase production is decreased in response to an underlying disease, such as intestinal diarrhea.[28]

The symptoms of lactose maldigestion and intolerance include gas, abdominal bloating, cramps, and diarrhea. The bloating and gas are caused by bacterial fermentation of lactose in the large intestine. The diarrhea is caused by undigested lactose in the large intestine as it draws water from the circulatory system into the large intestine.

In North America, approximately 25% of adults show signs of decreased lactose digestion in the small intestine. Many lactose maldigesters are Asian Americans, African

metabolic syndrome A condition in which the person has poor blood glucose regulation, hypertension, increased blood triglycerides, and other health problems. This condition is usually accompanied by obesity, lack of physical activity, and a diet high in refined carbohydrates; also called Syndrome X.

lactose maldigestion (primary and secondary) Primary lactose maldigestion occurs when production of the enzyme lactase declines for no apparent reason. Secondary lactose maldigestion occurs when a specific cause, such as long-standing diarrhea, results in a decline in lactase production. When significant symptoms develop after lactose intake, it is then called lactose intolerance.

It is hypothesized that approximately 3000 to 5000 years ago, a genetic mutation occurred in regions that relied on milk and dairy foods as a main food source, allowing those individuals (mostly in northern Europe, pastoral tribes in Africa, and the Middle East) to retain the ability to maintain high lactase output for their entire lifetime. This was not seen in other populations in the world, and so such digestive capability was not retained in those areas of the world.

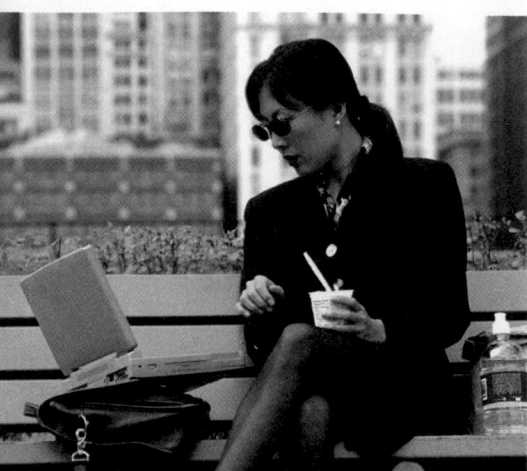

Use of yogurt helps lactose maldigesters meet calcium needs.

Americans, and Latino/Hispanic Americans, and the occurrence increases as people age. Still, many of these individuals can consume moderate amounts of lactose with minimal or no gastrointestinal discomfort because of eventual lactose breakdown by bacteria in the large intestine.[28] Thus, it is unnecessary for these people to greatly restrict their intake of lactose-containing foods, such as milk and milk products. These calcium-rich food products are important for maintaining bone health. Obtaining enough calcium and vitamin D from the diet is much easier when milk and milk products are included in a diet.

Recent studies have shown that nearly all individuals with decreased lactase production can tolerate 1/2 to 1 cup of milk with meals, and that most individuals adapt to intestinal gas production resulting from the fermentation of lactose by bacteria in the large intestine.[28] Combining lactose-containing foods with other foods also helps because certain properties of foods can have positive effects on lactose digestion. For example, fat in a meal slows digestion, leaving more time for lactase action. Hard cheese and yogurt also are more easily tolerated than milk. Much of the lactose is lost in the production of cheese, and the active bacteria cultures in yogurt digest the lactose when these bacteria are broken apart in the small intestine and release their lactase. In addition, an array of products, such as low-lactose milk and lactase pills, are available to assist lactose maldigesters when needed.

Concept | Check

North Americans eat about 82 g of sugars each day. Most of these sugars are added to foods and beverages in processing. To reduce consumption of sugars, one must reduce consumption of items with added sugars, such as some baked goods, sweetened beverages, and presweetened ready-to-eat breakfast cereals. This practice can help reduce the development of dental caries and likely improve diet quality and various other aspects of health. High-fiber diets must be accompanied by adequate fluid intakes to avoid constipation. Lactose maldigestion is a condition that results when cells of the intestine do not make sufficient lactase, the enzyme necessary to digest lactose, resulting in symptoms such as abdominal gas, pain, and diarrhea. Most people with lactose maldigestion can tolerate cheeses and yogurt as well as moderate amounts of milk. When significant symptoms develop after lactose intake, it is called lactose intolerance.

Case Scenario | Follow-Up

Myeshia suspected she had a problem with milk because when she consumed it during one meal, she developed bloating and gas. She tried to reduce these symptoms by eating yogurt, and she was successful. As you just learned, yogurt is tolerated better than milk by people with lactose maldigestion because the bacteria that are present in yogurt digest much of the lactose. Note, however, that many people with lactose maldigestion can consume moderate amounts of milk with few or no symptoms from the lactose present.

When Blood Glucose Regulation Fails

Improper regulation of blood glucose can lead to either **hyperglycemia** (high blood glucose) or **hypoglycemia** (low blood glucose). High blood glucose is most commonly associated with diabetes (technically, *diabetes mellitus*), a disease that affects about 6% of North Americans. The diagnostic criteria is based on a fasting blood glucose of 126 mg/dl or greater (dl represents 100 ml [deciliter]). Of those affected, it is estimated that about one-third to one-half of these people do not know that they have the disease. In addition, about 15% of our population shows evidence of insulin resistance but not actual diabetes (indicated by a fasting blood glucose of 100–125 mg/dl).[2] Diabetes leads to about 200,000 deaths each year in North America, and the number of new cases is climbing yearly. New recommendations promote testing fasting blood glucose in adults over age 45 every 3 years to help diagnose these missed cases. In contrast, low blood glucose is a much rarer condition.

Regulation of Blood Glucose

Under normal circumstances, blood glucose usually varies between about 70 and 99 mg/dl of blood in the fasting state, which is normally established a few hours after a meal is eaten. If blood glucose rises above 170 mg/dl, glucose begins to spill over into the urine. This leads to hunger and thirst, and eventually to weight loss. If blood glucose falls below 40 to 50 mg/dl, a person begins to feel nervous, irritable, and hungry and may develop a headache. (It is not too surprising that a headache results because the brain is fueled almost entirely by glucose.)

The liver is the main organ for controlling the amount of glucose that is eventually found in the bloodstream. Since it is the first organ to screen the sugars absorbed from the small intestine, the liver serves as a guard, helping control the amount of glucose that enters the bloodstream after a meal (review Figures 5-6).[14]

The pancreas is another important site of blood glucose control. Small amounts of insulin are released by the pancreas as soon as a person starts to eat. Once much of the dietary glucose enters the bloodstream, the pancreas releases large amounts of insulin, which affects blood glucose in a variety of ways. Insulin promotes increased glycogen synthesis and thus glucose storage in the liver as well as increased glucose uptake by muscle cells, adipose cells, and some other cells. Both of these actions of insulin lower blood glucose and help return it to the normal fasting range within a few hours after a person eats. In addition, insulin reduces gluconeogenesis by the liver.

Other hormones counteract the effects of insulin. When a person has not eaten carbohydrates for a few hours, the amount of glucose in the blood is maintained by the hormone glucagon, which is also released from the pancreas. Glucagon prompts the breakdown of glycogen in the liver, resulting in the release of glucose to the bloodstream. Glucagon also enhances gluconeogenesis. In these ways, glucagon helps restore blood glucose to normal concentrations (Figure 5-11).[14]

When a person has not eaten for a few hours, the hormones epinephrine (adrenaline) and norepinephrine also are released, but from the adrenal glands and nearby nerve endings. These hormones trigger the breakdown of glycogen in the liver; the resulting glucose is released into the bloodstream. These hormones are responsible for the "fight or flight" reaction. They are released in large amounts in response to a perceived threat, such as a car approaching head-on. The resulting rapid release of glucose into the bloodstream promotes quick mental and physical reactions. Other hormones, such as cortisol and growth hormone, also help regulate blood glucose (Table 5-5).

In essence, the actions of insulin on blood glucose are balanced by the actions of glucagon, epinephrine, norepinephrine, cortisol, and other hormones. If hormonal balance is not maintained, such as during overproduction or underproduction of insulin or glucagon, major changes in blood glucose concentrations occur.[14] This system of checks and balances for blood glucose regulation is typical of how the body maintains blood and other tissue concentrations of its key constituents within fairly narrow ranges.

Diabetes Mellitus

There are two major forms of diabetes: **type 1 diabetes** (formerly called insulin-dependent or juvenile-onset diabetes), and **type 2** (formerly called non–insulin-dependent or adult-onset) **diabetes** (Table 5-6). The change in names to type 1 and

hyperglycemia High blood glucose, above 125 mg/dl of blood on a fasting basis.

hypoglycemia Low blood glucose, below 40 to 50 mg/dl of blood.

Previously, a fasting blood glucose of 140 mg/dl was required to diagnose diabetes. Recently, though, amounts in the 120 mg/dl range have been found to cause tissue damage. For this reason, the diagnostic cutoff for diabetes using fasting blood glucose has been decreased to 126 mg/dl. The corresponding cutoff value taken 2 hours after a 75 g glucose load is 200 mg/dl.[2]

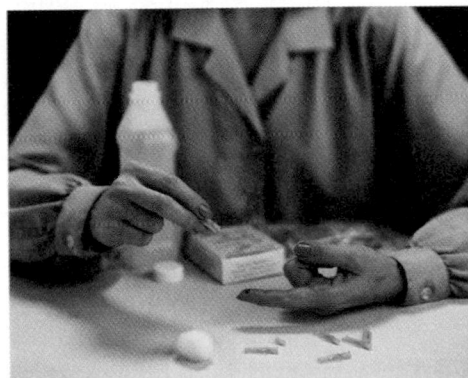

Regularly checking blood glucose is part of diabetes therapy today.

type 1 diabetes A form of diabetes in which the person is prone to ketosis and requires insulin therapy.

type 2 diabetes A form of diabetes in which ketosis is not commonly seen. Insulin therapy can be used but is often not required. This form of the disease is often associated with obesity.

Traditional symptoms of diabetes, known as the three polys, are polyuria (excessive urination), polydipsia (excessive thirst), and polyphagia (excessive hunger). No one symptom is diagnostic of diabetes. Other symptoms—such as unexplained weight loss, exhaustion, blurred vision, tingling in hands and feet, frequent infections, poor wound healing, and impotence—often accompany traditional symptoms.[2]

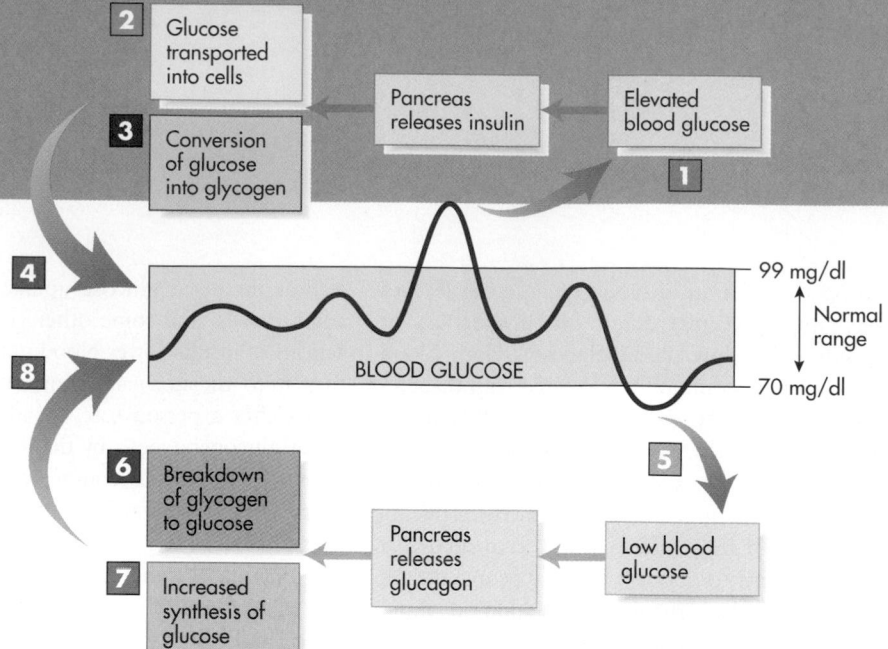

Figure 5-11 | Regulation of blood glucose. Insulin and glucagon are key factors in controlling blood glucose. When blood glucose rises above the normal range (1), insulin acts to lower it (2 and 3). Blood glucose then falls back into the normal range (4). When blood glucose falls below the normal range (5), glucagon leads to the opposite effect of insulin (6 and 7). This then restores blood glucose to the normal range (8). Other hormones, such as epinephrine, norepinephrine, cortisol, and growth hormone, also contribute to blood glucose regulation (see Table 5-5 for details). The same is true for the mineral chromium (see Chapter 12).

Table 5-5 | Role of Various Hormones in the Regulation of Blood Glucose

Hormone	Source	Target Organ or Tissue	Overall Effect on Organ or Tissue	Effect on Blood Glucose
Insulin	Pancreas	Liver, muscle, adipose tissue	Increases glucose uptake by muscles and adipose tissue, increases glycogen synthesis, suppresses gluconeogenesis	Decrease
Glucagon	Pancreas	Liver	Increases glycogen breakdown, with release of glucose by the liver; increases gluconeogenesis	Increase
Epinephrine Norepinephrine	Adrenal glands and nerve endings	Liver, muscle	Increases glycogen breakdown, with release of glucose by the liver; increases gluconeogenesis	Increase
Cortisol	Adrenal glands	Liver, muscle	Increases gluconeogenesis by the liver, decreases glucose use by muscles and other organs	Increase
Growth hormone	Adrenal glands	Liver, muscle, adipose tissue	Decreases glucose uptake by muscles, increases fat mobilization and utilization, increases glucose output by the liver	Increase

type 2 diabetes stems from the fact that many type 2 diabetics eventually must also rely on insulin injections as a part of their treatment.[2] In addition, many children today have type 2 diabetes. A third form, called gestational diabetes, occurs in some pregnant women (see Chapter 16). It is usually treated with an insulin regimen and diet, and resolves after delivery of the baby. However, pregnant women who develop gestational diabetes are at high risk for developing diabetes later in life.[2]

Type 1 Diabetes

Type 1 diabetes often begins in late childhood, around the age of 8 to 12 years, but can occur at any age. The disease runs in certain families, indicating a clear genetic link. Children usually are admitted to the hospital with abnormally high blood glucose and ketosis.[2]

The onset of type 1 diabetes is generally associated with decreased release of insulin from the pan-

Table 5-6 | Comparing and Contrasting Type 1 and Type 2 Diabetes

	Type 1 Diabetes	Type 2 Diabetes
Occurrence	5–10% of cases of diabetes	90% of cases of diabetes
Cause	Immune system attack of the pancreas	Insulin resistance
Risk Factors	Moderate genetic predisposition	Strong genetic predisposition Obesity Sedentary life style Ethnicity
Characteristics	Distinct symptoms (frequent thirst, hunger, and urination) Ketosis	Mild symptoms, especially in early phases of the disease (fatigue and nighttime urination) Generally ketosis does not occur
Cell Response to Insulin	Normal	Resistant
Treatment	Insulin* Diet Exercise Aspirin Medications to lower blood cholesterol (e.g., statins)	Diet Exercise Oral medications to lower blood glucose Insulin (in advanced cases) Aspirin Medications to lower blood cholesterol (e.g., statins)
Complications*	Cardiovascular disease Kidney disease Nerve disease Blindness	Cardiovascular disease Kidney disease Nerve damage Blindness
Monitoring	Blood glucose Urine ketones HbA1c	Blood glucose HbA1c

*In both cases maintaining a healthy blood lipid profile and normal blood pressure is vital to avoid these complications (see Chapters 6 and 11 for strategies). A new medication to lower blood glucose that can be used with insulin is pramlintide (Symlin).[37]

A common clinical method to determine a person's success in controlling blood glucose is to measure glycated (also termed glycosylated) hemoglobin (hemoglobin A1c). Over time, blood glucose attaches to (glycates) hemoglobin in red blood cells, and especially when blood glucose remains elevated. A hemoglobin A1c value of over 7% indicates poor blood glucose control. An acceptable value is 6% or less. Elevated blood glucose also leads to glycation of various proteins and fats in the body, forming what are called advanced glycation (also called glycoxidation) end products. These have been shown to be toxic to cells, especially those of immune system, circulatory system, and kidneys.[2,12]

creas. As insulin in the blood declines, blood glucose increases, especially after eating. When blood glucose exceeds the kidney's threshold, excess glucose spills over into the urine—hence the term *diabetes mellitus*, which means "flow of much urine" *(diabetes)* that is "sweet" *(mellitus)*. Figure 5-12 shows a typical glucose tolerance curve observed in a patient with this form of diabetes, following a test load of 75 g (15 teaspoons) of glucose.

An exciting finding regarding the cause of type 1 diabetes may help physicians treat this disease or even prevent its onset in the future. Most cases of type 1 diabetes begin with an immune system disorder, which causes destruction of the insulin-producing beta cells in the pancreas. Most likely, a virus or protein foreign to the body sets off the **autoimmune** destruction. In response to their destruction, the affected beta cells release other proteins, which stimulate a more furious attack. Eventually, the pancreas loses its ability to synthesize insulin, and the clinical stage of the disease begins.[2] Consequently, early treatment to stop the immune-linked destruction in children may be important. Research on this is ongoing.

Before 1921, if a person had type 1 diabetes, a high-fat, low-calorie diet was recommended. This approach was found to be the best way to control blood glucose. It was somewhat effective but resulted in poor growth in childhood and was difficult to implement. In the early part of the 1900s, a clinician could walk into a diabetes ward in a hospital and see scores of young, emaciated children. The isolation of insulin by Banting and Best in 1921 and the first use of it soon after in children opened a new door in diabetes care.

Today, type 1 diabetes is treated by insulin therapy, either with injections two to six times per day or with an insulin pump.[7] The pump dispenses insulin at a steady rate into the body, with greater amounts delivered after a meal. (Just approved is an inhaled form of insulin.) Dietary therapy includes three regular meals and one or more snacks (including one at bedtime), and a regulated ratio of carbohydrate:protein:fat to maximize insulin action and minimize swings in blood glucose.[3] If one does not eat often enough, the injected insulin can cause

autoimmune Immune reaction against normal body cells; self against self.

Figure 5-12 | Glucose tolerance test. A comparison of blood glucose concentrations in untreated diabetic and healthy (normal) persons after consuming a 75 g test load of glucose.

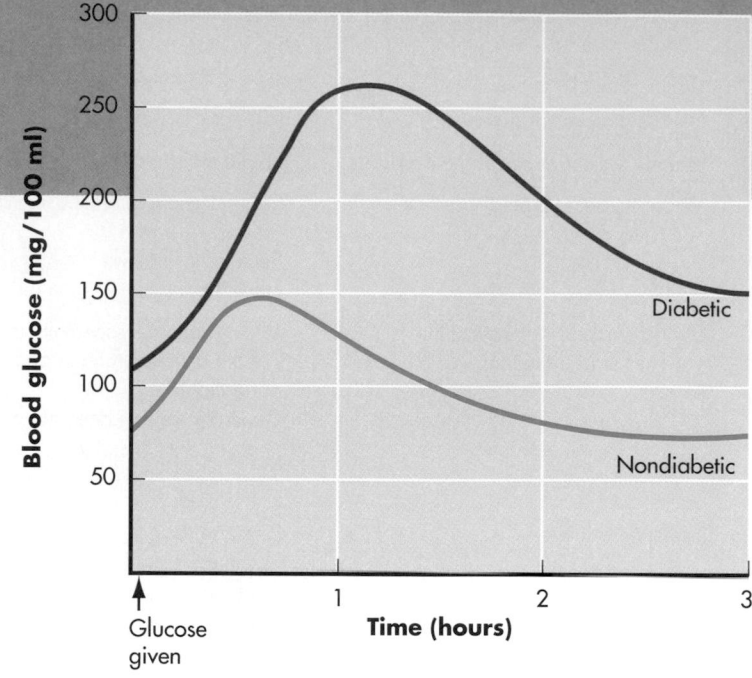

carbohydrate counting A diet method that assigns a certain number of food exchanges or carbohydrate grams to each meal and snack. Insulin is matched to carbohydrate intake (i.e., 1 unit of insulin per 10 to 15 g of carbohydrates), and carbohydrate grams can come from several combinations of exchanges.

severe hypoglycemia, because it acts on whatever glucose is available. The diet should, include ample fiber and polyunsaturated fat, supply an amount of energy in balance with energy needs, be low in animal fats, *trans* fats (e.g., stick margarine and shortenings), and cholesterol and be moderate in high glycemic load carbohydrates. Meeting magnesium needs is also helpful, as is regular coffee consumption (if desired). Both likely contribute to blood glucose regulation.[21,24]

Type 1 patients often make excellent candidates for learning the concept of **carbohydrate counting,** a method that focuses on the amount of carbohydrates in each food choice. Type 1 patients are often very familiar with the exchange system and are motivated enough to learn how to use it to count carbohydrate intake. This method results in improved blood glucose control with a wider selection of foods.[2]

Because people with diabetes (type 1 as well as type 2) are at a high risk for cardiovascular disease and related heart attacks, they should take an aspirin each day (generally 75 mg/day to 162 mg/day) if their physicians find no reason not to do so. As discussed in Chapter 6, this practice reduces the risk of heart attack. Use of medications to lower elevated blood cholesterol (e.g., "statins," discussed in Chapter 6) is also widely advocated.[19]

The hormone imbalances that occur in people with untreated type 1 diabetes lead to mobilization of body fat, which is released into liver cells. Ketosis follows because the fat is mostly converted to ketone bodies. These can rise excessively in the blood, eventually forcing ketone bodies into the urine. These pull sodium and potassium ions with them into the urine. This series of events can contribute to a chain reaction that eventually leads to dehydration, ion imbalance, coma, and even death, especially in patients with poorly controlled type 1 diabetes. Treatment includes insulin and fluids as well as sodium, potassium, and chloride.[2]

Other complications of diabetes can be degenerative conditions, such as blindness, cardiovascular disease, and kidney disease; all are caused by poor blood glucose regulation. Nerves can also deteriorate, resulting in many changes that decrease proper nerve stimulation. When this occurs in the intestinal tract, intermittent diarrhea and constipation result. Because of nerve deterioration in the arms, hands, legs, and feet, many people with diabetes lose the sensation of pain associated with injuries or infections. Not having as much pain, they often delay treatment of hand or foot problems. This delay, combined with a rich environment for bacterial growth (bacteria thrive on glucose), sets the stage for damage and death of tissues in the extremities, sometimes leading to the need for amputation of feet and legs. High blood glucose also contributes to a rapid buildup of fats in blood vessel walls, which eventually limits the blood supply to various organs such as the heart.[2]

Current research, such as the Diabetes Control and Complications Trial (DCCT), and other recent follow-up studies has shown that the development of blood vessel deterioration (e.g., cardiovascular disease and strokes) and nerve complications of diabetes can be delayed with aggressive treatment directed at keeping blood glucose within the normal range.[8,31] The therapy poses some risks of its own, such as hypoglycemia, so it must be implemented under the close supervision of a physician.

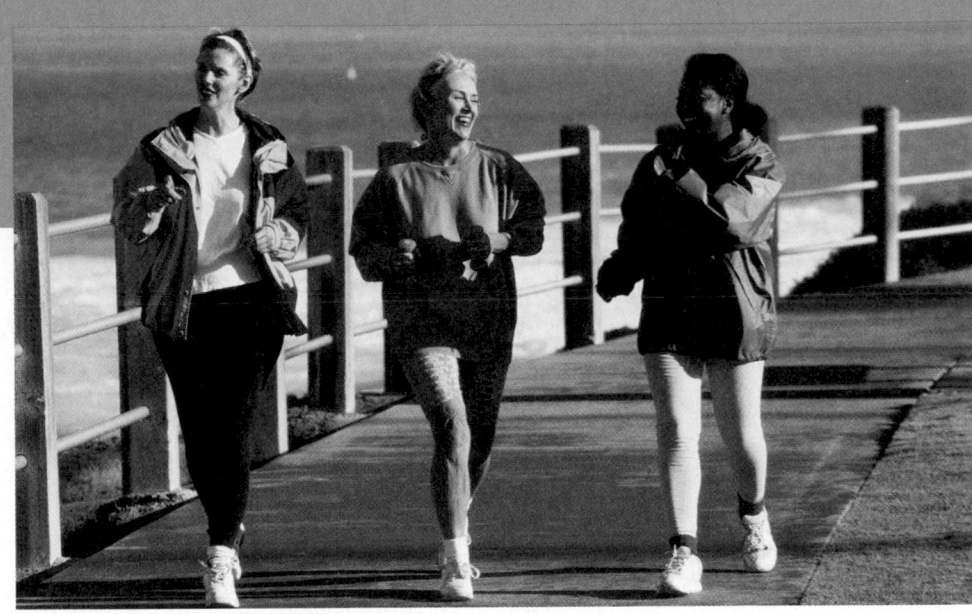

Regular exercise is a key part of a plan to prevent (and control) type 2 diabetes.

A person with diabetes generally must work closely with a physician and dietitian to make the correct alterations in diet and medications and to perform physical activity safely. Physical activity enhances glucose uptake by muscles independent of insulin action, which in turn can lower blood glucose.[15] This outcome is beneficial, but people with diabetes need to be aware of their own blood glucose response to physical activity and plan appropriately.

Type 2 Diabetes

Type 2 diabetes typically begins after age 40. This is the most common type of diabetes, accounting for about 90% of the cases diagnosed in North America. Minority populations such as Latino/ Hispanic, African Americans, Asian Americans, Native Americans, and Pacific Islanders are at particular risk.[2] As noted in this section's introduction, the number of people affected with this form of diabetes is especially on the rise, primarily because of widespread inactivity and obesity in our population. In fact, recently there has been a substantial increase in type 2 diabetes in children, due mostly to an increase in overweight in this population (coupled with limited physical activity). Type 2 diabetes is also genetically linked, so family history is a very important risk factor. However, the initial problem is not with the beta cells of the pancreas. Instead, it arises with the insulin receptors on the cell surfaces of certain body tissues, especially muscle tissue. In this case, blood glucose is not readily transferred into cells, so the patient develops hyperglycemia as a result of the glucose remaining in the bloodstream. The pancreas attempts to increase insulin output to compensate, but there is a limit to its ability to do this. Thus, rather than insufficient in-

sulin production, there is an abundance of insulin, particularly during the onset of the disease. As the disease develops, pancreatic function can fail, leading to reduced insulin output.[2] Because of the genetic link for type 2 diabetes, those who have a family history should be careful to avoid risk factors such as obesity (especially fat stores in the abdominal region); a diet rich in animal and *trans* fats, cholesterol, and high glycemic load foods; and inactivity.[3,30,34,36] Meeting needs for vitamin B-6, folate, and vitamin B-12 to control homocysteine levels in the blood is also important (see the discussion on homocysteine in Chapter 10 to learn more about homocysteine and how it is related to these vitamins).[27] Limiting red meat is also recommended, because the iron present in it has been linked to the development of type 2 diabetes. Being tested regularly for hyperglycemia is also important.[33]

Many cases of type 2 diabetes (about 80%) are associated with obesity (especially fat located in the abdominal region), but the hyperglycemia is not directly caused by the obesity. In fact, some lean people can develop type 2 diabetes. Obesity associated with oversized fat cells simply increases the risk for insulin resistance by the body, in turn increasing the risk for type 2 diabetes.[13,34]

Type 2 diabetes linked to obesity often disappears as weight is lost because the smaller adipose cells become less insulin resistant and make more of a beneficial hormone called adiponectin. This hormone aids in blood glucose regulation by increasing insulin action. Achieving a healthy weight should therefore be a primary goal of treatment, but even limited weight loss can lead to better blood glucose regulation.[13] Oral medications can also help. Some examples are medications that reduce glucose production by the liver (metformin

Polycystic ovary syndrome is another cause of type 2 diabetes in women. Excess facial and body hair, irregular menstrual periods, infertility, and obesity typically are seen in these women as well.[10]

Recently people with diabetes have been cautioned not to cook high-protein foods at high temperatures for prolonged periods of time.[12] This leads to the advanced glycation (also called gly-coxidation) end products discussed in this section forming in foods. Use of a lower power setting with a microwave oven, lower oven temperatures, and minimal use of prolonged broiling and prolonged frying are advised, as well as moderation in coffee and cola intake. (These latter two foods also are sources of advanced glycation end products.) Note that fruits, vegetables, starches, and milk are low in these substances.

For more information on diabetes, consult the following websites: www.diabetes.org and ndep.nih.gov

[Glucophage]), increase the ability of the pancreas to release insulin (glipizide [Glucotrol]), and increase the body's response to its own insulin (rosiglitazone [Avandia]). Another class of oral agents works by delaying carbohydrate digestion and glucose absorption (acarbose [Precose]). A tablet is taken with the first bite of each meal and may be combined with other therapy.[2] (Note that pregnant women cannot use these oral medications because they will affect the blood glucose of the developing fetus.) Finally, a new class of medication may be used but must be injected (exenatide [Byetta]).[37]

Sometimes it may be necessary to provide insulin injections in type 2 diabetes because nothing else is able to control blood glucose. (This eventually becomes the case in about half of all cases of type 2 diabetes.)[2] Regular physical activity also helps the muscles take up more glucose.[13] And regular meal patterns, with an emphasis on control of energy intake, consumption of low glycemic load foods, with ample fiber, is important therapy. Note that nuts fulfill the last two goals. (An almost daily [$\geq 5\times$/week] intake of nuts was even shown to reduce the risk of developing type 2 diabetes in one recent study.) Some intake of sugars is fine with meals, but again these must be substituted for other carbohydrates, not simply added to the meal plan.[2] Distributing carbohydrates throughout the day is also important, because this helps minimize the high and low swings in blood glucose concentrations. Moderate alcohol use is fine (one serving per day).[24] One recent study showed that this practice substantially reduced heart attack risk in people with type 2 diabetes. Still, diabetics must be warned that alcohol can lead to hypoglycemia and that people with type 2 diabetes must test themselves regularly for this possibility.

People with type 2 diabetes who have high blood triglycerides should moderate their carbohydrate intake and increase their intake of unsaturated fat and fiber.[30]

Although many cases of type 2 diabetes can be relieved by reducing excess fat stores,[36] many people are not able to lose weight. They remain affected with diabetes and may experience the degenerative complications seen in type 1 diabetes.[15] Ketosis, however, is not usually seen in type 2 diabetes.

Finally, medications to lower elevated blood cholesterol should be employed.[19] Meeting magnesium needs is also important.[21] Moderate use of coffee may also be helpful.

Hypoglycemia

People with diabetes who are taking insulin sometimes have hypoglycemia if they don't eat frequently enough. Hypoglycemia can also develop in nondiabetic individuals. The two common forms of nondiabetic hypoglycemia are termed *reactive* and *fasting.*[2]

Reactive hypoglycemia (also called postprandial hypoglycemia) is described as irritability, nervousness, headache, sweating, and confusion 2 to 4 hours after eating a meal, especially a meal high in simple sugars. The cause of reactive hypoglycemia is unclear, but it may be overproduction of insulin by the pancreas in response to rising blood glucose. Some researchers are unwilling even to acknowledge the existence of reactive hypoglycemia, pointing out that the symptoms are more likely tied to recent, intense exercise, psychological stress, medication use, or excess alcohol consumption. **Fasting hypoglycemia** usually is caused by pancreatic cancer, which may lead to excessive insulin secretion. In this case, blood glucose falls to low concentrations after fasting for about 8 hours to 1 day. This form of hypoglycemia is rare.

The diagnosis of hypoglycemia requires the simultaneous presence of low blood glucose and the typical hypoglycemic symptoms. Blood glucose of 40 to 50 mg/100 ml is suggestive, but just having low blood glucose after eating is not enough evidence to make the diagnosis of hypoglycemia.[2] Although many people think they have hypoglycemia, few actually do.

Healthy people may occasionally experience some hypoglycemic symptoms, such as irritability, headache, and shakiness, if they have not eaten for a prolonged period of time. Although not diagnostic of hypoglycemia, if you sometimes have symptoms of hypoglycemia, the standard nutrition therapy is one we all could follow. You need to eat regular meals, make sure you have some protein and fat in each meal, and eat low glycemic load carbohydrates with ample soluble fiber. Avoid meals or snacks that contain little more than sugar. If symptoms continue, try small protein-containing snacks between meals or fruits and juice. Fat, protein, and soluble fiber in the diet tend to moderate swings in blood glucose. Finally, moderate intakes of caffeine and alcohol.

Carbohydrates in Foods

The food components that yield the highest percentage of energy from carbohydrates are table sugar, honey, jam, jelly, fruit, and plain baked potatoes because these items are rich sources of carbohydrate. Corn flakes, rice, bread, and noodles all contain at least 75% of energy as carbohydrates. Foods with moderate amounts of carbohydrate energy are peas, broccoli, oatmeal, dry beans and other legumes, cream pies, french fries, and fat-free milk. In these foods, the carbohydrate content is diluted either by protein, as in the case of fat-free milk, or by fat, as in the case of a cream pie. Foods with essentially no carbohydrates include beef, eggs, chicken, fish, vegetable oils, butter, and margarine.

In planning a high-carbohydrate diet, you should emphasize whole grains, fruits, and vegetables.[1,32] On the other hand, you can't create a diet high in carbohydrate energy from chocolate, potato chips, and french fries because these foods contain too much fat. Overall, the percentage of energy from carbohydrate must be considered along with the total amount and type of carbohydrate in a food when planning a healthy high-carbohydrate diet.

The various substances that impart sweetness to foods fall into two broad classes: nutritive sweeteners, which can be metabolized to yield energy, and alternative sweeteners, which provide no food energy. As shown in Table 5-7, the alternative sweeteners are much sweeter on a per-gram basis than the nutritive sweeteners.[1]

Nutritive Sweeteners

Both sugars and sugar alcohols provide energy along with sweetness. Sugars are found in many different food products, whereas sugar alcohols have rather limited uses.

Sugars

All the monosaccharides (glucose, fructose, and galactose) and disaccharides (sucrose, lactose, and maltose) that were discussed earlier in this chapter are designated *nutritive sweeteners* (Table 5-8).[1] The sweetness of sucrose makes it the benchmark against which all other sweeteners are measured. Sucrose is obtained from sugarcane and sugar beet plants. Most of the sucrose and the other sugars we eat are from foods and beverages to which sugar has been added during processing and/or manufacturing. The major sources are soft drinks, candy, cakes, cookies, pies, fruit drinks, and dairy desserts, such as ice cream. The rest of the sugar in our diets is present naturally in foods, such as fruits, or comes from the sugar bowl. During food processing, the sugar content is often increased. The more processed the food, generally the higher the simple-sugar content.

A sweetener used frequently today by the food industry is high-fructose corn syrup, which is usually 55% fructose, but can range from 40 to 90% fructose. High-fructose corn syrup is made by treating cornstarch with acid and enzymes. This treatment breaks down much of the starch into glucose. Then some of the glucose is converted by enzymes into fructose. The final syrup is usually as sweet as sucrose. Its major advantage is that it is cheaper than sucrose. Also, it doesn't form crystals, and it has better freezing properties. High-fructose corn syrups are used in soft drinks, candies, jam, jelly, other fruit products, and desserts (e.g., packaged cookies).[1]

In addition to sucrose and high-fructose corn syrup, brown sugar, turbinado sugar, honey, maple syrup, and other sugars are also added to foods. Turbinado sugar is a partially refined version of raw sucrose; it has a slight molasses flavor. Brown sugar is essentially sucrose containing some molasses; either the molasses is not totally removed from the sucrose during processing or it is added back to the sucrose crystals.

Maple syrup is made by boiling down and concentrating the sap that runs during the late winter in sugar maple trees. Most pancake syrup sold in supermarkets is not actually maple syrup, which is quite expensive. Instead, it is primarily corn syrup and high-fructose corn syrup with maple flavor added.

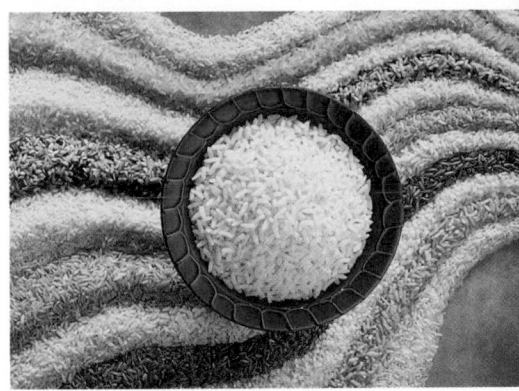

Rice is a rich source of carbohydrate.

Food Sources of Carbohydrate

Food Item	Carbohydrate (grams)	Energy from carbohydrate (%)
Baked potato (1 each)	51	91
Cola drink (12 fluid oz)	39	100
Plain M&Ms (1.5 oz)	30	58
Banana (1 each)	28	96
Cooked rice (1/2 cup)	22	90
Cooked corn (1/2 cup)	21	81
Light Yogurt (1 cup)	19	77
Kidney beans (1/2 cup)	19	72
Spaghetti noodles (1/2 cup)	19	87
Orange (1 each)	16	94
Seven-grain bread (1 slice)	12	75
Fat-free milk (1 cup)	12	56
Pineapple chunks (1/2 cup)	10	89
Cooked carrots (1/2 cup)	8	87
Peanuts (1 oz)	6	7

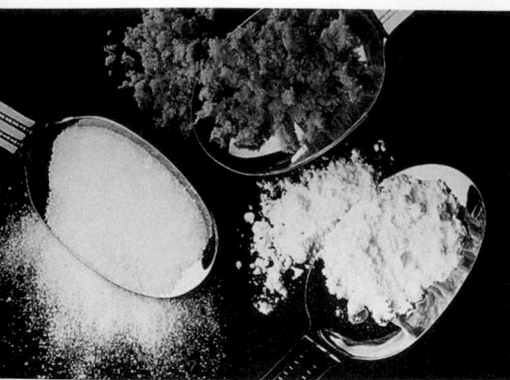

There are many forms of sugar available for purchase.

Stevia comes from a South American shrub; it is 100 to 300 times sweeter than sucrose and provides no energy. This sweetener has been used in small amounts by the Japanese since the 1970s. FDA has not approved the use of stevia in foods, but stevia can be purchased at natural- and health-food stores as a dietary supplement.[1]

Table 5-7 | The Sweetness of Sugars and Alternative Sweeteners

Type of Sweetener	Relative Sweetness* (Sucrose = 1)	Typical Sources
Sugars		
Lactose	0.2	Dairy products
Maltose	0.4	Sprouted seeds, some alcoholic beverages
Glucose	0.7	Corn syrup, honey
Sucrose	1.0	Table sugar, most sweets
Invert sugar†	1.3	Some candies, honey
Fructose	1.2–1.8	Fruit, honey, some soft drinks
Sugar Alcohols		
Sorbitol	0.6	Sugarless candies, sugarless gum
Mannitol	0.7	Sugarless candies
Xylitol	0.9	Sugarless gum
Alternative Sweeteners		
Cyclamate	30	Not currently in use in the United States, but available in Canada
Aspartame (Equal)	180 to 200	Diet soft drinks, diet fruit drinks, sugarless gum, powdered diet sweetener
Acesulfame-K (Sunette)	200	Sugarless gum, diet drink mixes, powdered diet sweeteners, puddings, gelatin desserts
Saccharin (Sweet 'n Low)	300	Diet soft drinks
Sucralose (Splenda)	600	Diet soft drinks, tabletop use, sugarless gums, jams, frozen desserts
Neotame	7000 to 13,000	Tabletop sweetener, baked goods, frozen desserts, diet soft drinks, jams and jellies
Tagatose (Naturlose)	0.9	Ready-to-eat cereals, diet soft drinks, health bars, frozen yogurt, fat-free ice cream, candies, frosting, chewing gum

From the American Dietetic Association, 1993, and other sources.

*On a per gram basis

†Sucrose broken down into glucose and fructose

Table 5-8 | Names of Sugars Used in Foods

Sugar	Honey
Sucrose	Corn syrup or sweeteners
Brown sugar	High-fructose corn syrup
Confectioner's sugar (powdered sugar)	Molasses
Turbinado sugar	Date sugar
Invert sugar	Maple syrup
Glucose	Dextrin
Sorbitol	Dextrose
Levulose	Fructose
Polydextrose	Maltose
Lactose	Caramel
Mannitol	Fruit sugar

Honey is a product of plant nectar that has been altered by bee enzymes. The enzymes break down much of the nectar's sucrose into fructose and glucose. As was noted earlier in this chapter, honey offers essentially the same nutritional value as other simple sugars—a source of energy and little else. However, honey is not safe to feed to infants because it can contain spores of the bacterium *Clostridium botulinum*. These spores can become active, leading to fatal foodborne illness. Honey does not pose the same threat to adults because the acidic environment of an adult's stomach inhibits the growth of the bacteria. An infant's stomach, however, does not produce much acid, making infants susceptible to the threat that this bacterium poses (see Chapters 17 and 19).

Sugar Alcohols

The sugar alcohol sorbitol, as well as **mannitol** and **xylitol,** are used as nutritive sweeteners.[35] Although sugar alcohols contribute energy (about 1.5–3 kcal/g), they are absorbed and metabolized to glucose more slowly than sugars. In large quantities sugar alcohols can cause diarrhea. In fact, any products whose foreseeable consumption may result in a daily ingestion of 50 g of sorbitol or mannitol must bear this labeling statement: "Excess consumption may have a laxative effect."

Sugar alcohols must be listed on labels, and if only one sugar alcohol is used in a product it must be distinguished; however, if two or more are used in one product they are grouped together under the heading "sugar alcohols." The actual energy value is calculated taking in account each sugar alcohol, so that when one reads the total energy content of a product, it includes the sugar alcohols in the overall amount.

Sorbitol and xylitol are used in sugarless gum, breath mints, and candy. These are not readily metabolized by bacteria in the mouth and thus do not promote dental caries as readily as do simple sugars such as sucrose. Recall from Chapter 2 that such a health claim can be made on these products.

Alternative Sweeteners

Often called artificial sweeteners, alternative sweeteners enable people with diabetes to enjoy the flavor of sweetness while controlling sugars in their diets; they also provide noncaloric or very-low-calorie sugar substitutes for persons trying to lose (or control) body weight. Alternative sweeteners include **saccharin, cyclamate, aspartame, neotame, sucralose, acesulfame-K,** and **tagatose** (Figure 5-13).[1] Alternative sweeteners yield little or no energy when consumed in amounts typically used in food products. All but cyclamate are currently available in the United States. Cyclamate was banned for use in the United States in 1970, although it has never been conclusively proved to cause health problems when used appropriately. Cyclamate is used in Canada as a sweetener in medicines and as a tabletop sweetener.

Saccharin

The oldest alternative sweetener, saccharin is currently approved for use in more than 90 countries. Saccharin was once thought to pose a risk of bladder cancer based on studies using laboratory animals, but today it is no longer listed as a potential cause of cancer in humans because the earlier research is now considered weak and inconclusive.[1]

Aspartame

Aspartame is in widespread use throughout the world. It has been approved for use by more than 90 countries, and its use has been endorsed by the World Health Organization, the American Medical Association, the American Diabetes Association, and the American Academy of Pediatrics Committee on Nutrition.[1] When the NutraSweet company held the patent on aspartame, it was sold as NutraSweet when added to foods and Equal when sold as a powder. Now, though, other companies manufacture aspartame.

The components of aspartame are the amino acids phenylalanine and aspartic acid, along with methanol. Recall that amino acids are the building blocks of proteins, so aspartame is more of a protein than a carbohydrate. Aspartame yields about 4 kcal/g, but it is 180 to 200 times sweeter than sucrose. Thus, only a small amount of aspartame is needed to sweeten a food or beverage, so the amount of energy added is

mannitol An alcohol derivative of fructose.

xylitol An alcohol derivative of the five-carbon monosaccharide xylose.

saccharin An alternative sweetener that yields no energy to the body; it is 300 times sweeter than sucrose.

cyclamate An alternative sweetener that yields no energy to the body; it is 30 times sweeter than sucrose.

aspartame An alternative sweetener made from two amino acids and methanol; it is 200 times sweeter than sucrose.

neotame A general-purpose nonnutritive sweetener that is approximately 7000 to 13,000 times sweeter than table sugar. It has a chemical structure similar to aspartame. Neotame is heat stable and can be used as a tabletop sweetener as well as in cooking applications. It is not broken down to its amino acid components in the body after consumption.

sucralose An alternative sweetener that has chlorines in place of some hydroxyl (–OH) groups on sucrose. It is 600 times sweeter than sucrose.

acesulfame-K An alternative sweetener that yields no energy to the body; it is 200 times sweeter than sucrose.

tagatose An isomer of fructose that is 90% as sweet as sucrose. Tagatose is poorly absorbed, so it yields only 1.5 kcal/g to the body.

INGREDIENTS: SORBITOL, GUM BASE, MANNITOL, GLYCEROL, HYDROGENATED GLUCOSE SYRUP, XYLITOL, ARTIFICIAL AND NATURAL FLAVORS, ASPARTAME, RED 40, YELLOW 6 AND BHT (TO MAINTAIN FRESHNESS). PHENYLKETONURICS: CONTAINS PHENYLALANINE.

Sugarless Gum

Sugar alcohols can be found in sugarless gum. The alternative sweetener aspartame is also used to sweeten this product. Note the warning for people with PKU that this product with aspartame contains phenylalanine.

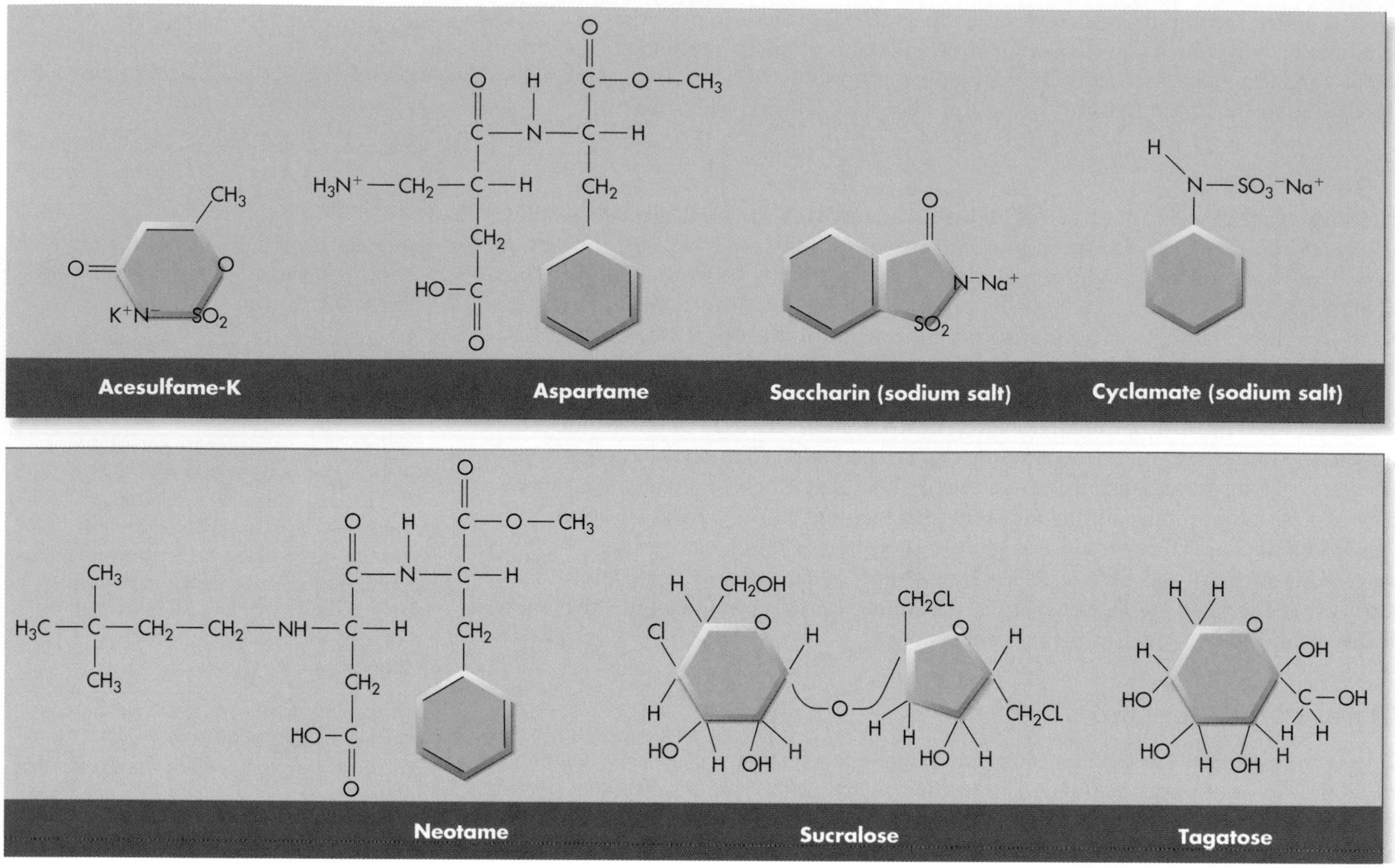

Figure 5-13 | Chemical structures of alternative sweeteners. Note that Cyclamate is available in Canada, but not in the United States.

insignificant unless the product is abused. Today aspartame is used in beverages, gelatin desserts, chewing gum, toppings and fillings in precooked bakery goods, and cookies. Aspartame does not cause tooth decay. Like other proteins, however, aspartame is damaged when heated for a long time and thus loses its sweetness if used in products that are cooked or heated.[1]

Some complaints have been filed with FDA by people claiming to have had adverse reactions to aspartame: headaches, dizziness, seizures, nausea, and other side effects. It is important for people who are sensitive to aspartame to avoid it, even though the percentage of people being affected is likely to be small. The relatively limited number of complaints about aspartame, considering its wide use in food products, means that most people can use it.

The acceptable daily intake of aspartame set by FDA is 50 mg/kg of body weight per day.[1] This is equivalent to about 14 cans of diet soft drink for an adult or about 80 packets of Equal. Aspartame appears to be safe for pregnant women and children, but some scientists suggest cautious use by these groups, especially young children, who need ample food energy to grow.

Persons with an uncommon genetic disease called phenylketonuria (PKU), which interferes with the metabolism of phenylalanine, should avoid aspartame because of its high phenylalanine content. (PKU was discussed in Chapter 4.)

Neotame

Neotame is approved by FDA for use as a general-purpose sweetener in a wide variety of food products other than meat and poultry. Neotame is a nonnutritive, high-intensity sweetener that is approximately 7000 to 13000 times sweeter than table sugar depending on its food application.[1] It has a chemical structure similar to aspartame. Neotame is heat stable and can be used as a tabletop sweetener as well as in cooking applications. Examples of uses for which it has been approved include baked goods, nonalcoholic beverages (including soft drinks), chewing gum, confections and frostings, frozen desserts, gelatins and puddings, jams and jellies, and processed fruits and fruit juices, toppings, and syrups. Neotame is safe for use by the general population, including children, pregnant and lactating women, and people with diabetes. In addition, no special labeling for people with phenylketonuria is needed because after consumption neotame is not broken down in the body to its amino acid components.

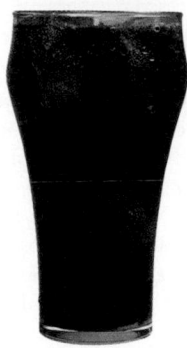

Soft drinks are typical sources of either sugars or alternative sweeteners, depending on the type of soft drink chosen.

Acesulfame-K

The alternative sweetener acesulfame-K (the K stands for potassium) is approved for use in more than 40 countries and is sold for use in the United States as Sunette. Acesulfame-K is 200 times sweeter than sucrose. It contributes no energy to the diet because it is not digested by the body, and it does not cause dental caries.[1]

Unlike aspartame, acesulfame-K can be used in baking because it does not lose its sweetness when heated. In the United States, it is currently approved for use in chewing gum, powdered drink mixes, gelatins, puddings, baked goods, tabletop sweeteners, candy, throat lozenges, yogurt, and nondairy creamers; additional uses may soon be approved. One recent trend is to combine it with aspartame in soft drinks.

Sucralose

Sucralose, sold as Splenda, is 600 times sweeter than sucrose. It is made by substituting three chlorines (Cl) for three hydroxyl groups (–OH) on sucrose.[1] FDA has approved sucralose's use as an additive to foods such as soda, gum, baked goods, syrups, gelatins, frozen dairy desserts such as ice cream, jams, and processed fruits and fruit juices and for tabletop use. Sucralose doesn't break down under high heat conditions and can be used in cooking and baking. It is also excreted as such in the feces. The little that is absorbed is excreted in the urine. Canadians had access to sucralose before its U.S. introduction.

Tagatose

Tagatose, sold as Naturlose, is an isomer of fructose and is almost as sweet as sucrose. It is poorly absorbed and so yields only 1.5 kcal/g to the body. Besides its low-energy contribution, its use does not lead to dental caries or an increase in blood glucose, and it has a prebiotic effect because it is fermented in the large intestine (review prebiotics in Chapter 3). Tagatose is approved for use in ready-to-eat cereals, diet soft drinks, health bars, frozen yogurt, fat-free ice cream, soft confectionary, hard confectionary, frosting, and chewing gum.

Concept | Check

Foods that are essentially all carbohydrate are sugars, jam, jelly, fruit, and plain baked potatoes. Grains and vegetables are also rich sources of carbohydrate. Six major alternative sweeteners are available in the United States today: saccharin, aspartame, neotame, acesulfame-K, sucralose, and tagatose. Canadians also have access to cyclamate. These alternative sweeteners can aid in the goal of reducing sugar intake.

Summary

1. The common monosaccharides are glucose, fructose, and galactose. Once these are absorbed into the small intestine and delivered to the liver, much of the fructose and galactose is converted to glucose.

2. The major disaccharides are sucrose (glucose plus fructose), maltose (glucose plus glucose), and lactose (glucose plus galactose). When digested, these yield their component monosaccharides.

3. One major group of polysaccharides consists of storage forms of glucose: starches in plants and glycogen in humans. In these polymers, the multiple glucose units are linked by alpha bonds, which can be broken by human digestive enzymes, releasing the glucose units. The main plant starches—straight-chain amylose and branched-chain amylopectin—are digested by enzymes in the mouth and small intestine. In humans, glycogen is synthesized in the liver and muscle tissue from glucose. Under the influence of hormones, liver glycogen is readily broken down to glucose, which can enter the bloodstream.

4. Fiber is composed primarily of the polysaccharides cellulose, hemicelluloses, pectins, gums, and mucilages as well as the noncarbohydrate lignins. These substances are not broken down by human digestive enzymes. However, soluble (also called viscous) fiber is fermented by bacteria in the large intestine.

5. Some starch digestion occurs in the mouth. Carbohydrate digestion is completed in the small intestine. Some plant fibers are digested by the bacteria present in the large intestine; undigested plant fibers become part of the feces. Monosaccharides in the intestinal contents mostly follow an active absorption process. They are then transported via the portal vein that leads directly to the liver.

6. Carbohydrates provide energy (on average, 4 kcal/g), protect against wasteful breakdown of body protein, and prevent ketosis. The RDA for carbohydrate is 130 g/day to meet the energy needs of the central nervous system. If carbohydrate intake is inadequate to supply the body's needs, protein is metabolized to provide glucose (gluconeogenesis) for energy needs. However, the price is loss of body protein, ketosis, and eventually a general body weakening. For this reason, very-low-carbohydrate diets are not recommended for extended periods (greater than 4 to 6 weeks).

7. Insoluble (also called nonfermentable) fiber provides bulk to the feces, thus easing bowel movements. In high doses, soluble (also called viscous) fiber can help control blood glucose in diabetic people and lower blood cholesterol.

8. Diets high in complex carbohydrates are encouraged instead of high-fat diets. A goal of about half of energy as complex carbohydrates is a good one, with about 45 to 65% of total energy intake coming from carbohydrates in general. Foods to consume are whole-grain breads and cereals, pasta, legumes, fruits, and vegetables. Many of these foods are rich in fiber.

9. Moderating sugar intake, especially between meals, reduces the risk of dental caries. Other health benefits include a reduced glycemic load for a meal or snack and an improvement in diet quality. Alternative sweeteners, such as aspartame, aid in reducing intake of sugars.

10. Table sugar, honey, jelly, fruit, and plain baked potatoes are some of the most concentrated sources of carbohydrates. Other high-carbohydrate foods, such as pie and fat-free milk, are diluted by either fat or protein. Nutritive sweeteners in food include sucrose, high-fructose corn syrup, brown sugar, and maple syrup.

11. The ability to digest large amounts of lactose often diminishes with age. People in some ethnic groups are especially affected. This condition develops early in childhood and is referred to as *lactose maldigestion*. Undigested lactose travels to the large intestine, resulting in such symptoms as abdominal gas, pain, and diarrhea. Most people with lactose maldigestion can tolerate cheese and yogurt and moderate amounts of milk.

Study Questions

1. Identify the three major disaccharides. Describe how each plays a part in the human diet.

2. How do amylose, amylopectin, and glycogen differ from one another? Why can these differences be important metabolically and in food processing?

3. What are some roles that fiber plays in the diet?

4. What are the possible effects of a diet too high in fiber (or too low in fluid relative to fiber content)?

5. Briefly describe the chemical structure, sweetness, and food uses of alternative sweeteners.

6. Why do we need carbohydrates in the diet? Briefly describe two reasons.

7. State the RDA for carbohydrate and summarize current carbohydrate intake recommendations.

8. Write a list of suggestions for a patient who has been diagnosed with lactose maldigestion. Design a 1-day sample menu that provides adequate calcium (1000 mg) for this patient.

9. How does type 1 diabetes differ from type 2 diabetes in cause and treatment?

10. What treatment is recommended for the typical form of hypoglycemia?

BOOST YOUR STUDY

Check out the **Perspectives in Nutrition: Online Learning Center** www.mhhe.com/wardlawpers7 for quizzes, flash cards, activities, and web links designed to further help you learn about carbohydrates.

Annotated References

1. ADA Reports: Position of the American Dietetic Association: Use of nutritive and non-nutritive sweeteners. *Journal of the American Dietetic Association* 104:225, 2004.

   When currently recommended diet practices are met, such as the Dietary Guidelines for Americans, use of some nutritive and nonnutritive sweeteners is acceptable. The text of the article explores in detail both classes of sweeteners, in turn supporting this overall conclusion.

2. American Diabetes Association: Standards of care in diabetes. *Diabetes Care* 28:S36, 2005.

   This article provides a comprehensive look at the treatment of diabetes. Goals for therapy and medical tools to help reach those goals are highlighted.

3. Anderson JW and others: Carbohydrate and fiber recommendations for individuals with diabetes. *Journal of the American College of Nutrition* 23(1):5, 2004.

   The carbohydrate : protein : fat ratio (in terms of energy intake) in a diabetic diet should be 55% or more : 12% to 15% : less than 30%. The diet should provide 25 to 50 grams of fiber per day, and low glycemic load foods should form the bulk of daily food choices.

4. Bingham SA and others: Dietary fibre in food and protection against colorectal cancer in the European Prospective Investigation into Cancer and Nutrition (EPIC): An observational study. *The Lancet* 36:1496, 2003.

   A diet rich in high-fiber foods is associated with a 40% reduction in colorectal cancer risk—especially in the colon—compared to a diet low in fiber. It is not known if fiber per se, or something in the high-fiber foods (e.g., phytochemicals), is the reason for the effect. Thus, one's focus should be on a diet rich in high-fiber foods, not fiber supplements.

5. Brand-Miller J: Glycemic load and chronic disease. *Nutrition Reviews* 61(5):S49, 2003.

   A diet rich in high glycemic load carbohydrates increases the risk of developing cardiovascular disease and type 2 diabetes. Such a diet may also contribute to obesity, colon cancer, and breast cancer. Following a diet rich in low glycemic load carbohydrates is on the other hand beneficial in these regards, especially if one is sedentary or obese.

6. Deen D: Metabolic syndrome: Time for action. *American Family Physician* 69(12):2875, 2004.

   The metabolic syndrome leads to many deleterious effects on the body. Weight control and regular physical activity are key parts of a plan for the prevention and treatment of the metabolic syndrome.

7. Diabetes. *Mayo Clinic Health Letter* (Suppl.) February 2004.

   Excellent summary of diabetes—from causes to treatments. Weight control, a healthy diet, and regular exercise are an important part of the latter.

8. Diabetes Control and Complications Trial/Epidemiology of Diabetes Interventions and Complications Research Study Group: Intensive diabetes treatment and cardiovascular disease in patients with type 1 diabetes. *The New England Journal of Medicine* 353:2643, 2005.

   People with diabetes who tightly control their blood glucose can reduce their risk of heart attacks and strokes by approximately 50 percent. The authors suggest that doctors encourage their patients to embrace this aggressive approach and work harder at controlling blood glucose levels.

9. Diverticular disease: The importance of getting enough fiber. *Mayo Clinic Health Letter* 23(2):1, 2005.

   Meeting your fiber needs is very important for preventing diverticular disease. To do so, eat plenty of fruits, vegetables, and whole-grain products. Regular physical activity also helps prevent the problem.

10. Ehrmann DA: Polycystic ovary syndrome. *The New England Journal of Medicine* 352:1223, 2005.

    One symptom that often accompanies polycystic ovary syndrome is hyperglycemia and related diabetes. Women at risk for this disease typically have irregular menstrual cycles, infertility, ovarian cysts, severe acne, excess facial or body hair, hypertension, obesity, type 2 diabetes, and other problems. Overproduction of male hormones and insulin resistance are at the root of these problems. This article discusses the diagnosis and treatment of the disease.

11. Food and Nutrition Board: *Dietary reference intakes for energy, carbohydrate, fiber, fat, fatty acids, cholesterol, protein, and amino acids.* Washington, DC: National Academy Press, 2002.

    This report provides the latest guidance for macronutrient intakes. With regard to carbohydrate, the RDA has been set at 130 g/day. Carbohydrate intake should range from 45 to 65% of energy intake. Sugars added to foods should constitute no more than 25% of energy intake.

12. Goldberg T and others: Advanced glycoxidation end products in commonly consumed foods. *Journal of the American Dietetic Association* 104:1287, 2004.

    Foods especially low in advanced glycoxidation end points include fruits, vegetables, starches, and milk. In contrast, meats and other high protein foods cooked or otherwise processed at high temperatures are rich sources of these compounds.

13. Hu G and others: Physical activity, body mass index, and risk of type 2 diabetes in patients with normal or impaired glucose regulation. *Archives of Internal Medicine* 164(8):892, 2004.

    Increasing physical activity can reduce the risk of developing type 2 diabetes. Weight control is also important; this weight control advice includes people who already have poor glucose control and are overweight.

14. Keim NL and others: Carbohydrates. In Shils ME and others (eds): *Modern nutrition in health and disease.* 10th ed. Philadelphia, PA: Lippincott Williams & Wilkins, 2006.

    Current review of the various dietary carbohydrates and their related metabolism. Digestion and absorption of carbohydrates is also covered.

15. Klein S and others: Weight management through lifestyle modification for the prevention and management of type 2 diabetes. *American Journal of Clinical Nutrition* 80:257, 2004.

    Overweight and obesity are important causes of type 2 diabetes. Moderate weight loss and increased physical activity can both forestall and improve poor blood glucose regulation.

16. Koh-Banerjee P and others: Changes in whole-grain, bran, and cereal fiber consumption in relation to 8-y weight gain among men. *American Journal of Clinical Nutrition* 80:1237, 2004.

    A diet rich in whole grain breads and cereals is associated with less weight gain over time compared to a diet rich in refined grains. This is especially true for foods with at least 25% whole grain content.

17. Larsson SC and others: Magnesium intake in relation to risk of colorectal cancer in women. *Journal of the American Medical Association* 293:86, 2005.

    A diet rich in magnesium is associated with a lower risk of developing colorectal cancer. The authors recommend that adults increase fruit, vegetable, bean, and whole grain intake to meet magnesium needs, as other components in these foods (e.g., various phytochemicals) also contribute to a lower risk for developing colorectal cancer.

18. Liu S and others: Is intake of breakfast cereals related to total and cause-specific mortality in men? *American Journal of Clinical Nutrition* 77:594, 2003.

    Regular intake of a whole-grain breakfast cereal reduces the risk of cardiovascular mortality and total mortality in men, while regular use of a refined grain cereal has the opposite effect. By substituting a high-fiber cereal for a low-fiber cereal, adults could experience a substantial impact on overall health.

19. Lo V and others: Statin therapy in patients with type 2 diabetes. *American Family Physician* 72:866, 2005.

   Keeping blood cholesterol in a desirable range is important for reducing cardiovascular disease risk in people with diabetes. Use of statin drugs to attain this clinical goal is widely advocated (if needed) in people with type 2 diabetes.

20. Mayes PA, Bender DA: Carbohydrates of physiological significance. In Murray RK and others (eds); *Harper's illustrated biochemistry.* 26th ed. New York, NY, Lange Medical Books/McGraw-Hill, 2005.

   Concise review of the chemical structures and related features of dietary carbohydrates. Both sugars and starches are included in the discussion.

21. Mitka M: Researchers examine effects of dietary magnesium on type 2 diabetes. *Journal of the American Medical Association* 291:1056, 2004.

   Meeting magnesium needs is important for people with diabetes. This practice likely contributes to better blood glucose regulation. Rich food sources, rather than magnesium supplements, are advocated.

22. Park Y and others: Dietary fiber intake and risk of colorectal cancer. *Journal of the American Medical Association* 2849, 2005.

   Dietary fiber intake was not shown to prevent colorectal cancer in this pooled analysis of numerous studies examining the relationship. Other dietary factors, such as meeting needs for the vitamin folate and the mineral calcium, and limiting alcohol and red meat intake, are probably more important to consider.

23. Salzman H, Lillie D: Diverticular disease: diagnosis and treatment. *American Family Physician* 72:1229, 2005.

   Meeting fiber needs helps reduce the risk of developing diverticular disease. Treatment of diverticulitis includes use of antibiotics and some dietary restrictions, as reviewed by the authors.

24. Schulze MB and others: Dietary pattern, inflammation, and incidence of type 2 diabetes in women. *American Journal of Clinical Nutrition* 82:675, 2005.

   A diet rich in sugar-sweetened soft drinks, refined grains, and processed meat was associated with a three-times greater risk of developing type 2 diabetes in this study. Protective foods included regular intake of vegetables as well as some intake of wine and coffee. This effect was especially shown in people who also maintained a healthy body weight.

25. Schulze MB and others: Sugar-sweetened beverages, weight gain, and incidence of type 2 diabetes in young and middle-aged women. *Journal of the American Medical Association* 292(8):927, 2004.

   A high consumption of sugared soft drinks is associated with weight gain and type 2 diabetes. The key factor is likely the large amounts of rapidly absorbed sugars in these products.

26. Schulze MB and others: Glycemic index, glycemic load, and dietary fiber intake and incidence of type 2 diabetes in younger and middle-aged women. *American Journal of Clinical Nutrition* 80:348, 2004.

   A diet rich in rapidly absorbed carbohydrates and low in cereal fiber is associated with an increased risk of developing type 2 diabetes. Thus the types of carbohydrates chosen for a diet are important to consider.

27. Soinio M and others: Elevated plasma homocysteine level is an independent predictor of coronary heart disease events in patients with type 2 diabetes mellitus. *Annals of Internal Medicine* 140:94, 2004.

   Elevated blood homocysteine is an independent risk factor for developing type 2 diabetes. Consuming adequate amounts of the vitamins folate, vitamin B-12, and vitamin B-6 are important in controlling blood homocysteine.

28. Swagerty D and others: Lactose intolerance. *American Family Physician* 65:1845, 2002.

   Lactose maldigestion and intolerance result from a deficiency in the lactose-digesting enzyme, lactase. This is present in up to 15% of Northern Europeans, 22% of American Whites, 70% of Indians, 80% of Blacks and Hispanics, and 100% of Native Americans and Asians. Most individuals with lactose maldigestion and intolerance can consume small amounts of dairy products without experiencing symptoms, and yogurts with live cultures tend to be especially well tolerated.

29. Sweeteners can sour your health. *Consumer Reports on Health*, p. 8, January 2005.

   Limiting simple sugars in a diet is important in order to lessen the risk of developing obesity, diabetes, and dental caries as well as increasing diet quality. Moderate use of the alternative sweeteners listed in the article helps one meet that goal.

30. Tanasescu M and others: Dietary fat and cholesterol and the risk of cardiovascular disease among women with type 2 diabetes. *American Journal of Clinical Nutrition* 79:999, 2004.

   A diet rich in cholesterol and saturated fat and low in polyunsaturated fat increases cardiovascular disease risk in persons with type 2 diabetes. The authors recommend that such people instead consume more fats rich in monounsaturated fat.

31. Tesfaye S and others: Vascular risk factors and diabetic neuropathy. *The New England Journal of Medicine* 352:341, 2005.

   Controlling blood glucose is an important part of reducing the risk of developing nerve-related disease in people with diabetes. Controlling body weight, blood triglycerides, and blood pressure are also important measures to take, as well as not smoking.

32. The whole grain story. *Tufts University Health & Nutrition Letter,* p. 4, July 2005.

   Regular whole-grain consumption may help prevent cardiovascular disease, unnecessary weight gain, and the metabolic syndrome. This is easier to do so today because many whole-grain products are now available.

33. Tirosh A and others: Normal fasting plasma glucose levels and type 2 diabetes in young men. *The New England Journal of Medicine* 353:1454, 2005.

   As fasting blood glucose increases the risk of developing type 2 diabetes also increases. Thus it is critical to have fasting blood glucose measured on a regular basis and make appropriate dietary and lifestyle adjustments to lower it when needed.

34. Wang Y and others: Comparison of abdominal adiposity and overall obesity in predicting risk of type 2 diabetes in men. *American Journal of Clinical Nutrition* 81:555, 2005.

   Obesity and excess upper body fat stores are both risk factors for developing type 2 diabetes. Avoiding both conditions is important, especially excess upper body fat distribution.

35. Warshaw HS: FAQs about polyols. *Today's Dietitian*, p. 37, April 2004.

   Polyols (e.g., sugar alcohols) yield from 0.2 to 3.0 kcal/g, so they still need to be considered when calculating the energy content of a diet. A major attribute of these products is that they do not increase the risk for dental caries.

36. Weinstein AR and others: Relationship of physical activity vs. body mass index with type 2 diabetes in women. *Journal of the American Medical Association* 292:1188, 2004.

   Both elevated body mass index and physical inactivity are independent predictors of developing diabetes. However, the association with elevated body mass index is much greater than that of physical inactivity.

37. Yaraki L: New medications for diabetes management. *Today's Dietitian*, p. 20, July 2005.

   The author reviews the latest medications available for the treatment of diabetes. These can be added to the typical medications that have been available for a number of years, such as oral hypoglycemic agents and insulin.

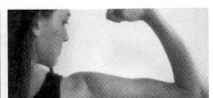

Take | Action

I. Estimate Your Fiber Intake

To roughly estimate your daily fiber consumption, determine the number of servings that you ate yesterday from each food category listed here. If you are not meeting your needs, how could you do so? Multiply the serving amount by the value listed and then add up the total amount of fiber.

Food	Servings	Grams
Vegetables		
(serving size: 1 cup raw leafy greens or 1/2 cup other vegetables)	_____ × 2	_____
Fruits		
(serving size: 1 whole fruit; 1/2 grapefruit; 1/2 cup berries or cubed fruit; 1/4 cup dried fruit)	_____ × 2.5	_____
Beans, lentils, split peas		
(serving size: 1/2 cup cooked)	_____ × 7	_____
Nuts, seeds		
(serving size: 1/4 cup; 2 tbsp peanut butter)	_____ × 2.5	_____
Whole grains		
(serving size: 1 slice whole-wheat bread 1/2 cup whole-wheat pasta, brown rice, or other whole grain; 1/2 each bran or whole-grain muffin)	_____ × 2.5	_____
Refined grains		
(serving size: 1 slice bread; 1/2 cup pasta, rice, or other processed grains; 1/2 each refined bagels or muffins)	_____ × 1	_____
Breakfast cereals		
(serving size: check package for serving size and amount of fiber per serving)	_____ × grams of fiber per serving	_____
Total Grams of Fiber =		_____

Adapted from Fiber: Strands of protection. *Consumer Reports on Health,* p. 1, August 1999.

How does your total fiber intake for yesterday compare with the general recommendation of 25 to 38 g of fiber per day for women and men, respectively? If you are not meeting your needs, how could you do so?

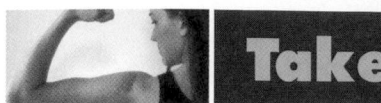

Take | Action

II. Can You Choose the Sandwich with the Most Fiber?

Assume the sandwiches on the blackboard here are available at your local deli or sandwich shop. All the sandwiches provide about 350 kcal. The fiber content ranges from about 1 gram to about 7.5 grams. Rank the sandwiches from the highest amount of fiber to the lowest amount; then check your answers at the bottom of the page.

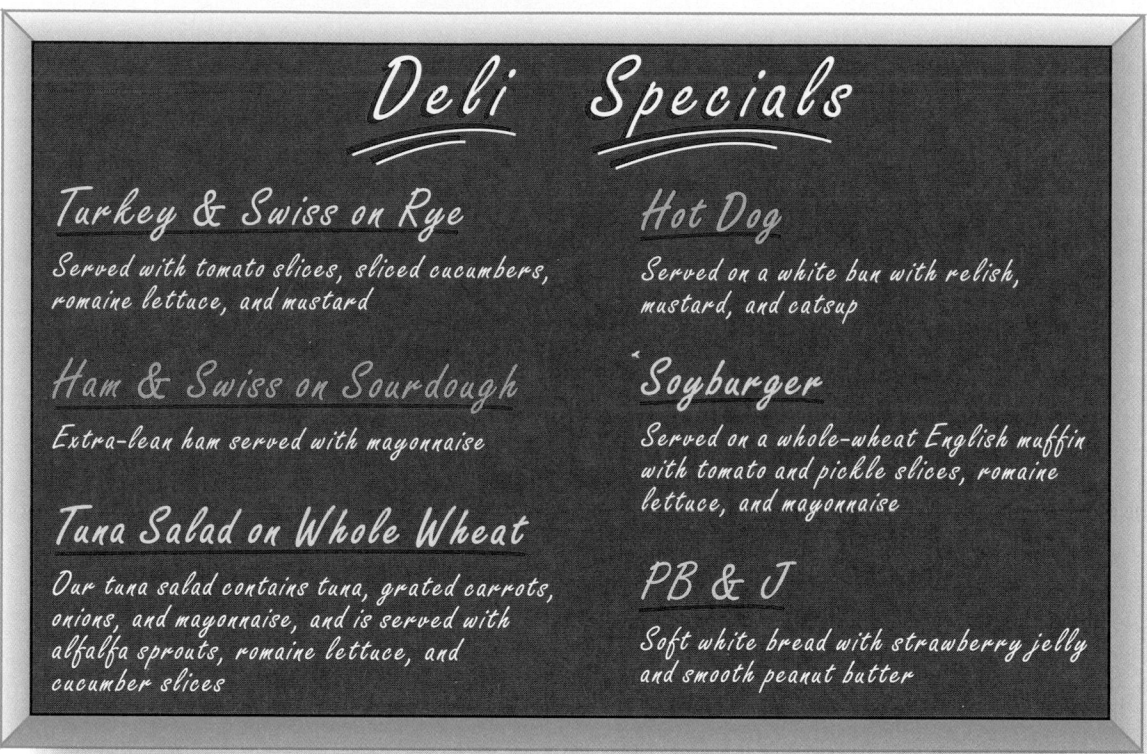

Deli Specials

Turkey & Swiss on Rye

Served with tomato slices, sliced cucumbers, romaine lettuce, and mustard

Ham & Swiss on Sourdough

Extra-lean ham served with mayonnaise

Tuna Salad on Whole Wheat

Our tuna salad contains tuna, grated carrots, onions, and mayonnaise, and is served with alfalfa sprouts, romaine lettuce, and cucumber slices

Hot Dog

Served on a white bun with relish, mustard, and catsup

Soyburger

Served on a whole-wheat English muffin with tomato and pickle slices, romaine lettuce, and mayonnaise

PB & J

Soft white bread with strawberry jelly and smooth peanut butter

Answer Key:
1. Soyburger: 7.5 g, 2. Tuna Salad on Whole Wheat: 7 g, 3. Turkey & Swiss on Rye: 4g, 4. PB&J: 3 g, 5. Ham & Swiss on Sourdough: 1.5g, 6. Hot Dog: 1 g.

LIPIDS

6

CHAPTER OUTLINE

CASE SCENARIO:

Jackie is a 21-year-old health-conscious individual in her third year of nursing school. She recently learned that a diet high in saturated fat can contribute to high blood cholesterol and that exercise is beneficial for the heart. Jackie now takes a brisk 30-minute walk each morning before going to class, and she has started to cut as much fat out of her diet as she can, replacing it mostly with carbohydrates. A typical day for Jackie begins with a bowl of Fruity Pebbles with 1 cup of skim milk and 1/2 cup of apple juice. For lunch, she might pack a turkey sandwich on white bread with lettuce, tomato, and mustard; a small package of fat-free pretzels; and a handful of reduced-fat vanilla wafers. Dinner could be a large portion of pasta with some olive oil and garlic mixed in, and a small iceberg lettuce salad with lemon juice squeezed over it. Her snacks are usually plain popcorn, baked chips, low-fat cookies, fat-free frozen yogurt, or fat-free pretzels. She drinks diet soft drinks throughout the day as her main beverage.

Do you think Jackie has found healthy ways to reduce fat in her diet? Point out some positive practices. How would you suggest that Jackie change her diet to make it more heart healthy?

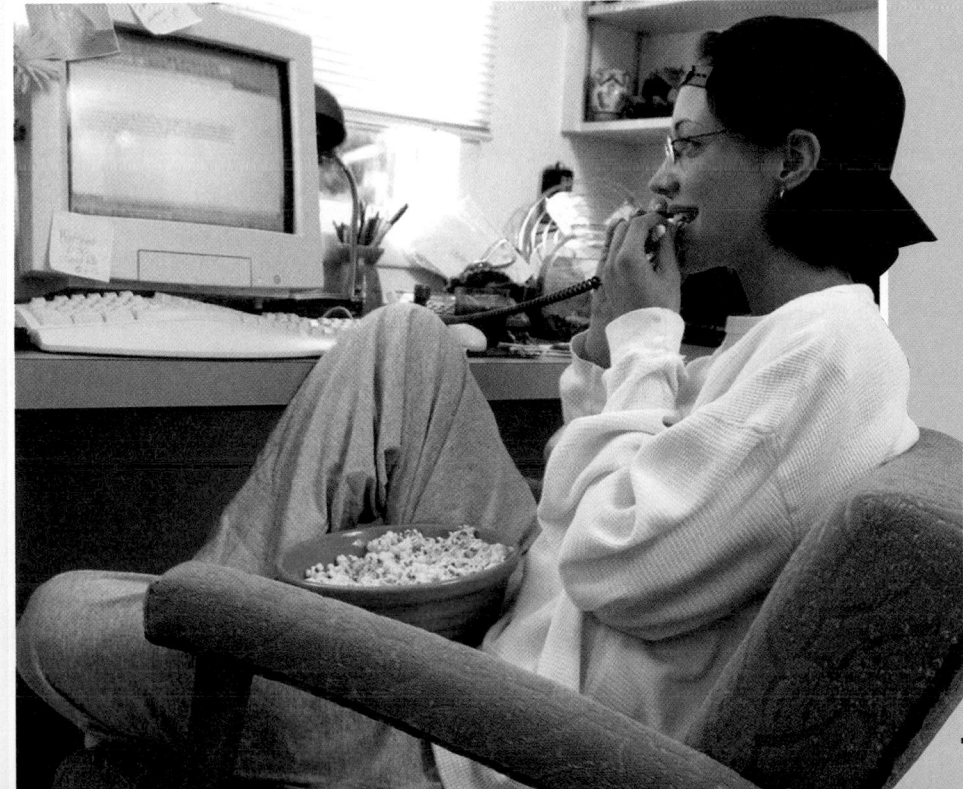

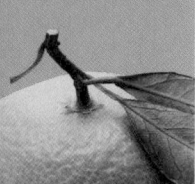

Your doctor informs you that your "triglycerides are too high." Your bill from a medical laboratory reads "Blood lipid profile—$55." A health food advertisement suggests using garlic supplements to lower blood cholesterol. Advertisers plug foods "lowest in saturated fat." All these substances—triglycerides, saturated fat, and cholesterol—are lipids, a collective term referring to fats and oils.

Lipids contain more than twice the energy per gram (on average, 9 kcal) as proteins and carbohydrates (on average, 4 kcal each). Consumption of most saturated fatty acids and *trans* fatty acids also contributes to the risk of cardiovascular disease (CVD).[7] For these reasons, some concern about lipids is warranted, but certain lipids also play vital roles both in the body and in foods. Their presence in the diet is essential to good health. In general, lipids such as those in vegetable oils should comprise 20 to 35% of our total energy intake.[7]

This chapter looks at lipids in detail—their forms, functions, metabolism, and food sources. It will also look at the link between lipid intake and the major "killer" disease in North America: cardiovascular disease, which involves the arteries of the heart (coronary heart disease) as well as other arteries in the body.

CHAPTER OBJECTIVES CHAPTER 6 IS DESIGNED TO ALLOW YOU TO:

1. List four classes of lipids (fats) and the role of each in nutritional health.
2. Distinguish between fatty acids and triglycerides.
3. Differentiate among saturated, monounsaturated, and polyunsaturated fatty acids in terms of structure and food sources.
4. Name the two essential fatty acids and explain why they are called "essential."
5. Name the classes of lipoproteins and classify them according to their functions.
6. Discuss the implications of various fats, including omega-3 fatty acids, with respect to cardiovascular disease.
7. Recognize dietary sources of *trans* fats and how they affect chronic disease risk.
8. Identify available fat replacements.
9. Characterize the symptoms of cardiovascular disease and highlight some known risk factors.

REFRESH YOUR MEMORY AS YOU BEGIN YOUR STUDY OF LIPIDS IN CHAPTER 6, YOU MAY WANT TO REVIEW:

- Legal definitions for various labeled descriptors, such as "low-fat" and "fat-free," in Chapter 2.
- The concept of energy density in Chapter 2.
- The process of digestion and absorption and gastrointestinal hormones in Chapter 3.
- The glycemic load of foods in Chapter 5.

Lipids: Common Properties and Main Types

Humans need very little fat in their diet to maintain health. In fact, daily consumption of 2 to 4 tablespoons of plant oil incorporated into foods and at least twice weekly consumption of fatty fish such as salmon or tuna meet the body's need for the essential fatty acids.[7] If fish is not consumed, the essential fatty acids in canola oil, soybean oil, flax seeds (and oils), and walnuts can contribute some of the same health benefits as those found in fish. Thus, one could follow a purely vegetarian diet containing about 10% of energy from fat and still maintain health. However, as long as saturated fat, cholesterol, and partially hydrogenated fat (technically called *trans* fat) is minimized, fat intake can be considerably higher than that 10% allotment. Recent recommendations from the Food and Nutrition Board suggest that fat intake can be as high as 35% of energy intake.[7] After learning more about lipids—fats, oils, and related compounds—in this chapter, you can decide for yourself how much fat you want to consume as well as how to track your daily intake.

Lipids are a diverse group of chemical compounds. They share one main characteristic: They do not readily dissolve in water but do so in organic solvents, such as chloroform, benzene, and ether. Think of an oil and vinegar salad dressing. The oil is not soluble in the water-based vinegar; on standing, the two separate into distinct layers, with oil on top and vinegar on the bottom.

Triglycerides are the most common type of lipid found in the body and in foods. As noted in Chapter 1, each triglyceride molecule consists of three fatty acids attached to glycerol. **Phospholipids,** and **sterols** such as cholesterol, are also classified as lipids, although their structures can be quite different from the structure of triglycerides.[20] All these lipid compounds are described in this chapter.

As explained in Chapter 1, lipids that are solid at room temperature are called *fats,* and lipids that are liquid are called *oils.* Most people use the word *fat* to refer to all lipids because they don't realize there is a difference. As already noted, however, *lipid* is a generic term that includes triglycerides and many other substances. To simplify the discussion, this chapter primarily uses the term *fat;* however, as you will see later, not all the substances called fats truly are fats. When necessary for clarity, the name of a specific lipid, such as cholesterol, will be used. This word usage is consistent with the way many people use these terms in health care settings.

Fatty Acids: The Simplest Form of Lipids

The fatty acid is common to most lipids, both those in the body and in foods. It is basically a long chain of carbons linked together and flanked by hydrogens. At one end of the molecule, designated the *alpha end,* is an acid (specifically a carboxyl [$-C-OH$])

$$\overset{O}{\overset{\|}{}}$$

group. At the other end, called the *omega* (ω) *end,* is a methyl group ($-CH_3$) (Figure 6-1*a*). In the Greek alphabet, *alpha* is the first letter and *omega* is the last.

If all the chemical bonds between the carbons are single connections and the carbons are filled with hydrogens, a fatty acid is said to be **saturated** (Figure 6-1*a*).[20] To understand this concept, picture a sponge saturated (filled) with water. In this sense, the fatty acid is saturated with hydrogen.

As noted earlier, most fats high in saturated fatty acids, such as animal fats, remain solid at room temperature. A good example is the solid fat surrounding a piece of uncooked steak at room temperature. Chicken fat, semisolid at room temperature, contains less saturated fat. In some foods, such as whole milk, saturated fats are suspended in liquid, so the solid nature of these fats at room temperature is less apparent. Any fat in milk actually consists of a combination of liquid and solid fats, as will be discussed shortly.

If a fatty acid is unsaturated, hydrogens are missing from the carbon chain—specifically, at the area of the carbon-carbon double bonds. If a fatty acid has one double bond between the carbons, it is **monounsaturated** (Figure 6-1*b*).[20] Canola and olive oils contain a high percentage of monounsaturated fatty acids. If two or more bonds between the carbons are double bonds, the fatty acid is **polyunsaturated** and thus even less saturated with hydrogens (Figure 6-1*c, d*).[20] Corn, soybean, sunflower, and safflower oils are rich in polyunsaturated fatty acids. Fats in foods are not composed of a single type or category of fatty acid. Rather, each dietary fat is a complex mixture of different fatty acids.

Saturated fatty acids are linear, allowing them to pack tightly together. In contrast, unsaturated fatty acids have a kinked shape and thus pack together only loosely (Figure 6-2). The loose organization of unsaturated fats is more easily disrupted by heat than is the more ordered organization of saturated fats. Thus, dietary fats high in unsaturated fatty acids melt at a lower temperature than fats high in saturated fatty acids (especially **long-chain** ones [12 carbons or longer]).

As mentioned in Chapter 1, monounsaturated and polyunsaturated fatty acids in their natural form usually are in the *cis* form. By definition, the hydrogens are on the same side of the carbon-carbon double bond. When oils are solidified to aid in food formulation, some hydrogens are transferred to opposite sides of the carbon-carbon double bond, creating the *trans* configuration, or a ***trans* fatty acid.** As seen in Figure 6-2, the *trans* bond allows the backbone to remain straight like a saturated fatty acid. The

phospholipid Any of a class of fat-related substances that contain phosphorus, fatty acids, and a nitrogen-containing component. The phospholipids are an essential part of every cell.

sterol A compound containing a multi-ring (steroid) structure and a hydroxyl group (–OH).

In some cases *n* is used rather than *omega* (ω). Thus, the term you see may be either n-3 or ω-3 fatty acids.

saturated fatty acid A fatty acid containing no carbon-carbon double bonds.

monounsaturated fatty acid A fatty acid containing one carbon-carbon double bond.

polyunsaturated fatty acid A fatty acid containing two or more carbon-carbon double bonds.

long-chain fatty acids Fatty acids that contain 12 or more carbons.

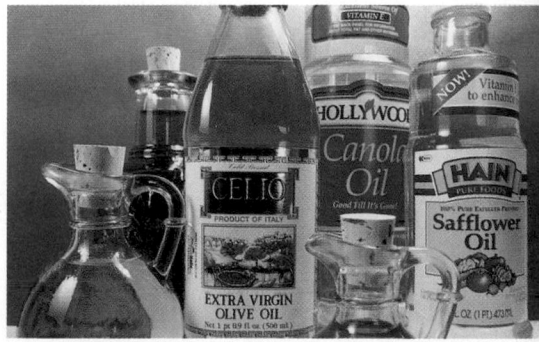

While plant oils may look similar, they can vary in specific fatty acid content. For example, safflower oil is rich in polyunsaturated fat, while olive and canola oils are rich in monounsaturated fat.

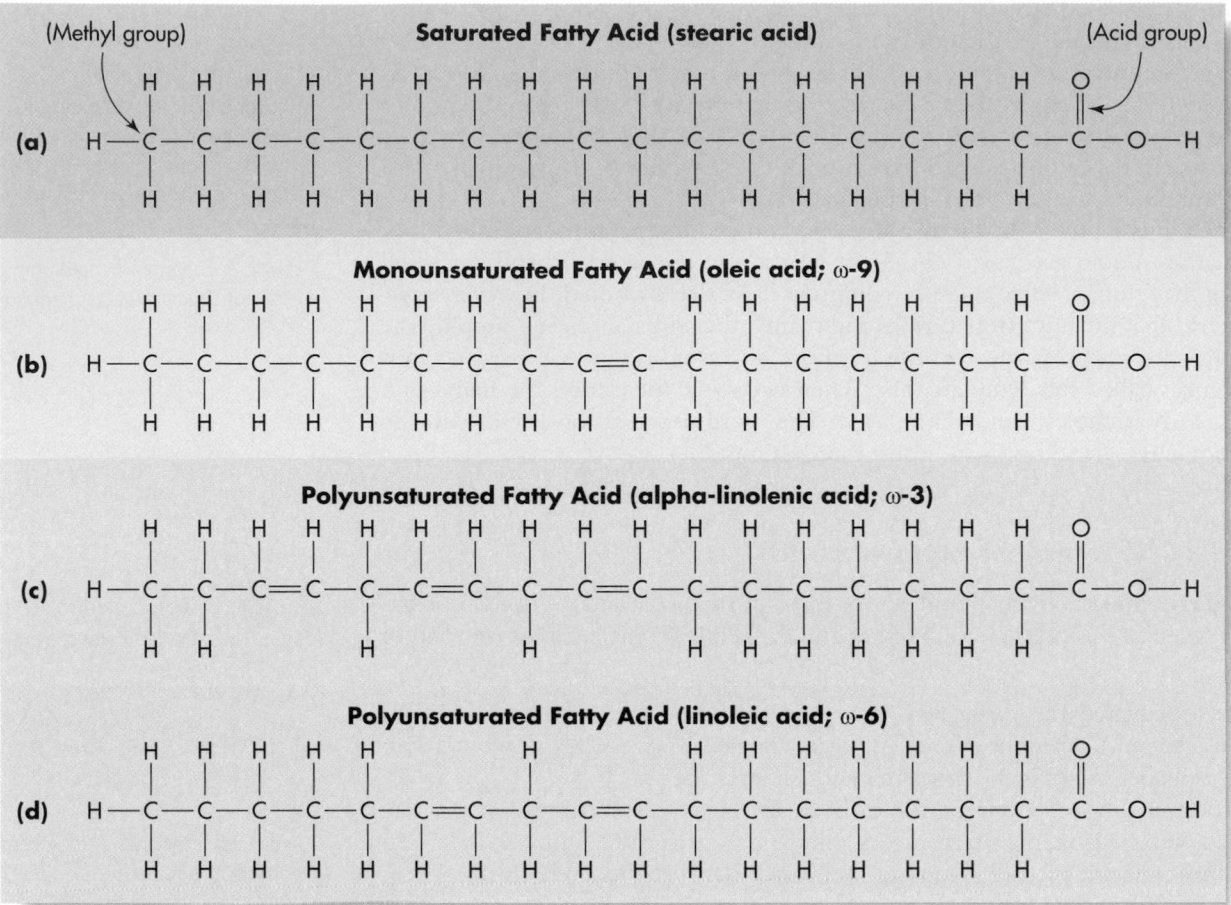

Figure 6-1 | Chemical forms of saturated, monounsaturated, and polyunsaturated fatty acids. Each of the depicted fatty acids contains 18 carbons, but they differ from each other in the number and location of double bonds. The linear shape of saturated fatty acids, as shown in (a), allows them to pack tightly together and so form a solid at room temperature. In contrast, unsaturated fatty acids have "kinks" where double bonds interrupt the carbon chain (see Figure 6-2). Thus, unsaturated fatty acids pack together only loosely and are usually liquid at room temperature.

trans fatty acid A form of an unsaturated fatty acid, usually a monounsaturated one when found in food, in which the hydrogens on both carbons forming the double bond lie on opposite sides of that bond. A *cis* fatty acid has the hydrogens lying on the same side of the carbon-carbon double bond.

medium-chain fatty acid A fatty acid that contains 6 to 10 carbons.

short-chain fatty acids Fatty acids that contain fewer than six carbon atoms.

omega-3 (ω-3) fatty acid An unsaturated fatty acid with the first double bond on the third carbon from the methyl end (–CH₃).

omega-6 (ω-6) fatty acid An unsaturated fatty acid with the first double bond on the sixth carbon from the methyl end (–CH₃).

production and health effects of *trans* fatty acids will be covered in more detail later in the chapter.

Overall, a fat or an oil is classified as saturated, monounsaturated, or polyunsaturated based on the nature of the fatty acids present in the greatest concentration (Figure 6-3).

Triglycerides that contain primarily saturated fatty acids are solid at room temperature, especially if the fatty acids have a long chain. **Medium-chain** saturated fatty acids (6 to 10 carbons long), such as those in coconut oil, produce liquid oils at room temperature. This remains true even though coconut oil consists primarily of saturated fatty acids, because the shorter chain length overrides the effect of saturation. **Short-chain** saturated fatty acids (less than 6 carbons long) also form liquid oils at room temperature. Dairy fats are sources of these short-chain fatty acids. Triglycerides containing primarily polyunsaturated or monounsaturated fatty acids are also usually liquid at room temperature. These are not affected by chain length.

Essential Fatty Acids

The actual location of the carbon-carbon double bonds in the carbon chain of a *cis* polyunsaturated fatty acid makes a big difference in how the body metabolizes it. If the first double bond starts at three carbons from the methyl (omega) end of the fatty acid, it is an **omega-3 (ω-3) fatty acid** (see Figure 6-1c). If the first double bond starts at six carbons from the methyl end of the fatty acid, it is an **omega-6 (ω-6) fatty acid** (see Figure 6-1d). Following the same scheme, an omega-9 fatty acid has the first double

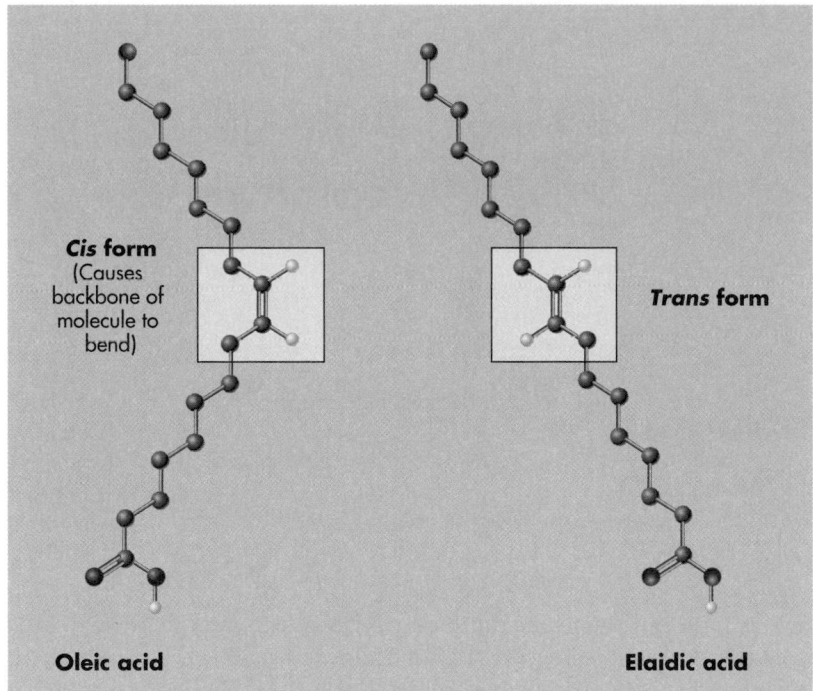

Figure 6-2 | *Cis* and *trans* isomers of fatty acids. *Cis* fatty acids are more common in foods than are *trans* fatty acids. The latter are primarily found in foods containing partially hydrogenated fats—notably, stick margarine, shortening, and deep fat-fried foods. The Food and Nutrition Board suggests limiting intake as much as possible.[7] Later in this chapter you will see why.

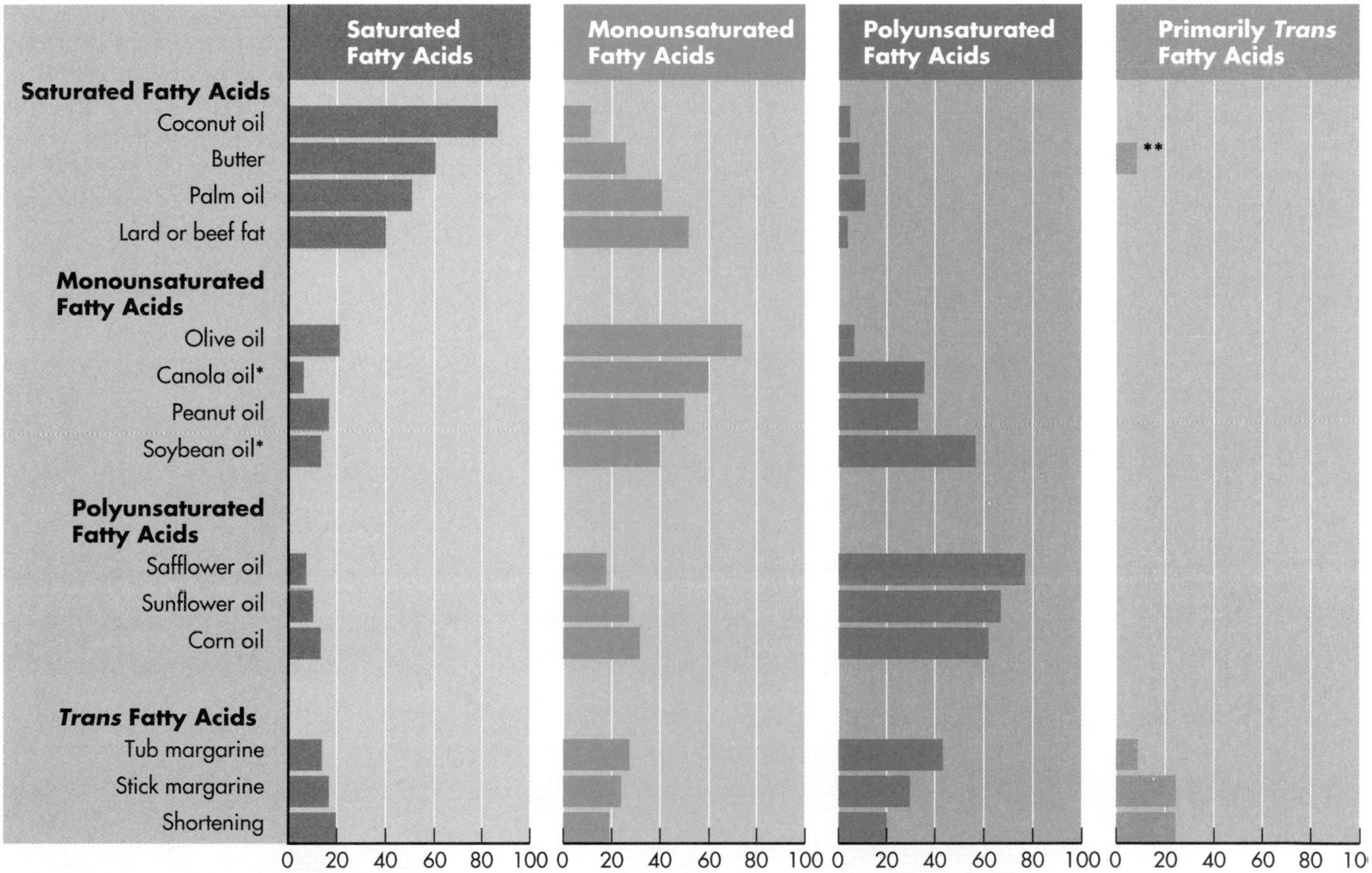

Cis form (Causes backbone of molecule to bend)

Trans form

Oleic acid

Elaidic acid

	Saturated Fatty Acids	Monounsaturated Fatty Acids	Polyunsaturated Fatty Acids	Primarily *Trans* Fatty Acids
Saturated Fatty Acids				
Coconut oil				
Butter				**
Palm oil				
Lard or beef fat				
Monounsaturated Fatty Acids				
Olive oil				
Canola oil*				
Peanut oil				
Soybean oil*				
Polyunsaturated Fatty Acids				
Safflower oil				
Sunflower oil				
Corn oil				
Trans Fatty Acids				
Tub margarine				
Stick margarine				
Shortening				

Note that fats are also typically rich in monounsaturated fatty acids (40 to 50% of total fatty acids).
*Rich source of the omega-3 fatty acid alpha-linolenic acid (7% and 12% of total fatty acid content for soybean oil and canola oil, respectively).
**The natural *trans* fatty acids in butter are not harmful and may even have health-promoting properties, such as preventing certain forms of cancer.

Figure 6-3 | Saturated, monounsaturated, polyunsaturated, and *trans* fatty acid composition of common fats and oils (expressed as % of all fatty acids in the product).

Figure 6-4 | The essential fatty acid (EFA) family. All are available from dietary sources; linoleic acid and alpha-linolenic acid are the essential fatty acids and must be consumed because body synthesis does not take place. The other fatty acids in this figure can be synthesized to some extent from the essential fatty acids.

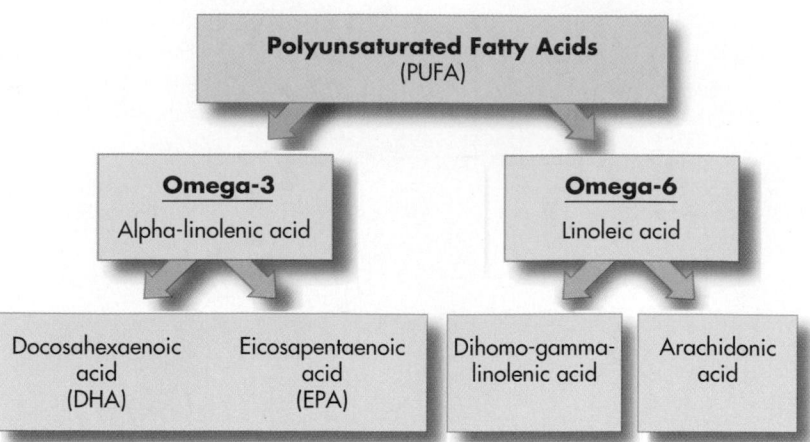

alpha-linolenic acid An essential omega-3 fatty acid with 18 carbons and three double bonds (C18:3, ω-3).

linoleic acid An essential omega-6 fatty acid with 18 carbons and two double bonds (C18:2, ω-6).

oleic acid An omega-9 fatty acid with 18 carbons and one double bond (C18:1, ω-9).

essential fatty acids Fatty acids that must be supplied by the diet to maintain health. Currently, only linoleic acid and alpha-linolenic acid are classified as essential.

eicosanoids Hormonelike compounds synthesized from polyunsaturated fatty acids, such as arachidonic acid. Within this class of compounds are prostacyclins, prostaglandins, thromboxanes, and leukotrienes.

bond starting nine carbons from the methyl end of the fatty acid. In foods, **alpha-linolenic acid** is the major omega-3 fatty acid; **linoleic acid** is the major omega-6 fatty acid; and **oleic acid** is the major omega-9 fatty acid.[20]

Because we must obtain linoleic acid (ω-6) and alpha-linolenic acid (ω-3) from foods in order to maintain health, they are called **essential fatty acids** (Figure 6-4). These omega-3 and omega-6 fatty acids form parts of vital body structures, perform important roles in immune system function and vision, help form cell membranes, and produce hormonelike compounds called **eicosanoids** (Figure 6-5*a*, *b*, *c*, and *d*).[21] This dietary necessity arises because cells in the human body can produce carbon-carbon double bonds in a fatty acid only starting at the ninth carbon numbered from the methyl end. In other words, human cells do not produce the enzyme to place double bonds between the methyl end and the ninth carbon.[20] On the other hand, omega-9 fatty acids can be synthesized in the body because the double bond falls after the ninth carbon.[20]

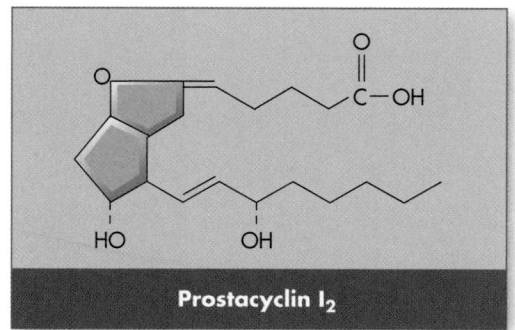

Prostacyclin I₂

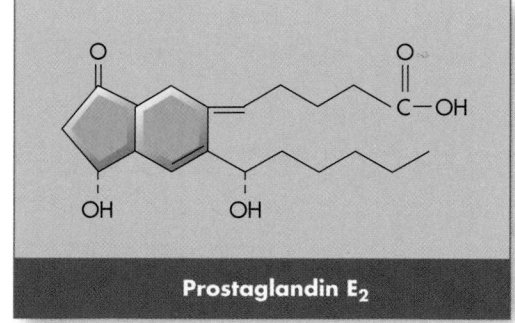

Prostaglandin E₂

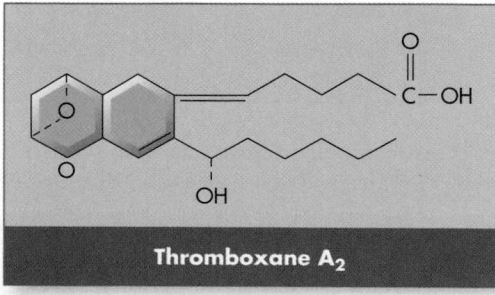

Thromboxane A₂

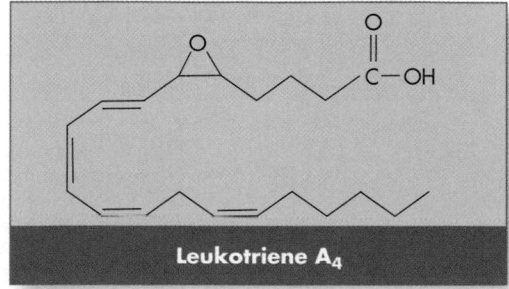

Leukotriene A₄

Figure 6-5 | The family of common eicosanoids: prostacyclins, prostaglandins, thromboxanes, and leukotrienes.

Still, we need to consume only about 2 to 4 tablespoons of plant oils each day to meet essential fatty acid needs.[7] We can easily get that much via mayonnaise, salad dressings, tub margarine, and other foods. Regular consumption of whole-grain breads and cereals and vegetables also helps supply essential fatty acids.

We also need to specifically include a regular intake of alpha-linolenic acid or one of its related omega-3 fatty acids, **eicosapentaenoic acid (EPA) and docosahexaenoic acid (DHA).** This would almost certainly require at least twice weekly consumption of broiled or baked (not deep fried, as this process increases *trans* fatty acid content) fatty fish, such as salmon, tuna, sardines, herring, mackerel, whitefish, trout, swordfish, and halibut. All are sources of omega-3 fatty acids (Table 6-1). Regular intake of canola or soybean oil or consumption of walnuts or flax seeds and flax oil also supplies a steady source of omega-3 fatty acids.[7]

A Closer Look at Metabolism and the Role of Essential Fatty Acids in the Body

Omega-3 and omega-6 fatty acids are further metabolized by cells so they can contribute to the synthesis of the biologically active eicosanoids mentioned earlier. Eicosanoids are referred to as local hormones because they act in the immediate vicinity of production and are not carried by the blood to some distant site like typical hormones. Eicosanoids are synthesized from fatty acids taken from phospholipids in the cell membrane plus free fatty acids and other sources within a cell. The eicosanoids then bind to receptors on the cell membrane surface or to adjacent cell membrane surfaces to initiate a response.[21]

Eicosanoids fall into three separate groups. One group (group 1) is derived from **dihomo-gamma-linolenic acid,** an omega-6 fatty acid with 3 double bonds. Another group (group 2) is derived from **arachidonic acid,** an omega-6 fatty acid with four double bonds. A third group (group 3) is derived from eicosapentaenoic acid, the omega-3 fatty acid with 5 double bonds discussed in the previous section.[20]

To produce the parent fatty acids for group 1 and group 2 eicosanoid synthesis, linoleic acid is lengthened to 20 carbons and undergoes desaturation, in which hydrogens are removed to yield carbon-carbon double bonds. The second reaction in this process yields the group 1 fatty acid, dihomo-gamma-linolenic acid. The last reaction produces the group 2 fatty acid, arachidonic acid (Figure 6-6).[21]

eicosapentaenoic acid (EPA) An omega-3 fatty acid with 20 carbons and five carbon-carbon double bonds (C20:5, ω-3). It is present in large amounts in fish oils and is slowly synthesized in the body from alpha-linolenic acid; it is a precursor to some eicosanoids.

docosahexaenoic acid (DHA) An omega-3 fatty acid with 22 carbons and six carbon-carbon double bonds (C22:6, ω-3). It is present in large amounts in fish oils and is slowly synthesized in the body from alpha-linolenic acid. DHA is especially present in the retina and brain.

dihomo-gamma-linolenic acid An omega-6 fatty acid with 20 carbons and three double bonds; the precursor to some eicosanoids.

arachidonic acid An omega-6 fatty acid with 20 carbon atoms and 4 carbon-carbon double bonds, a precursor to some eicosanoids.

Table 6-1 | Omega-3 Fatty Acids in Fish (grams per 3 ounce serving)

Atlantic salmon	1.8
Anchovy	1.7
Sardines	1.4
Rainbow trout	1.0
Coho salmon	0.9
Bluefish	0.8
Striped bass	0.8
Tuna, white, canned	0.7
Halibut	0.4
Catfish, channel	0.2

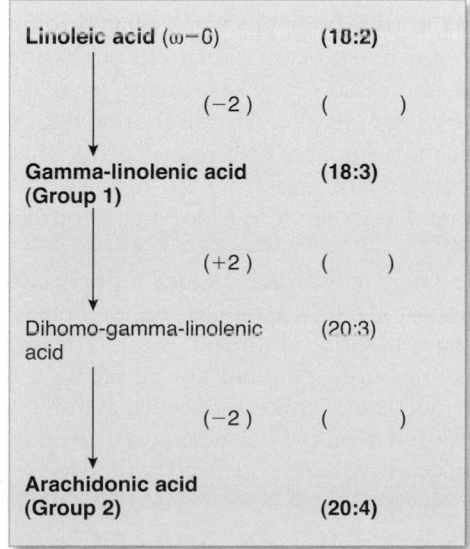

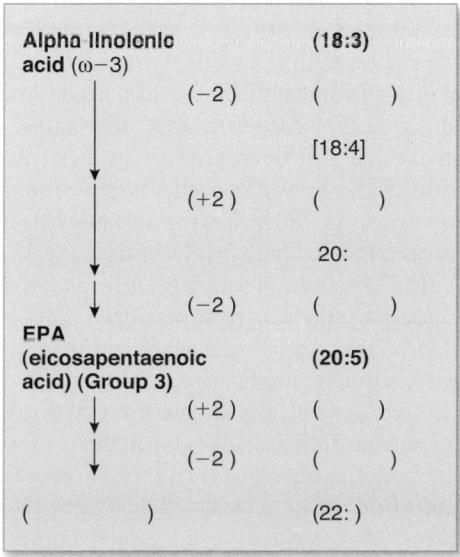

Figure 6-6 | Metabolism of omega-6 linoleic acid to arachidonic acid, and omega-3 alpha-linolenic acid to eicosapentaenoic acid and docosahexaenoic acid.

cyclooxygenase An enzyme used to synthesize prostaglandins, thromboxanes, and other eicosanoids.

lipoxygenase An enzyme used to synthesize leukotrienes and some other types of eicosanoids.

prostacyclin (PGI) Eicosanoid made by the blood vessel walls that is a potent inhibitor of blood clotting.

prostaglandin (PG) One of several potent eicosanoid compounds made of polyunsaturated fatty acids that produce diverse effects in the body.

thromboxane (TX) Eicosanoid made by blood platelets that is a stimulant of blood clotting.

leukotrienes (LT) An eicosanoid involved in inflammatory or hypersensitivity reactions, such as asthma.

endothelial cells A layer of flat cells lining the blood and lymphatic vessels and the chambers of the heart.

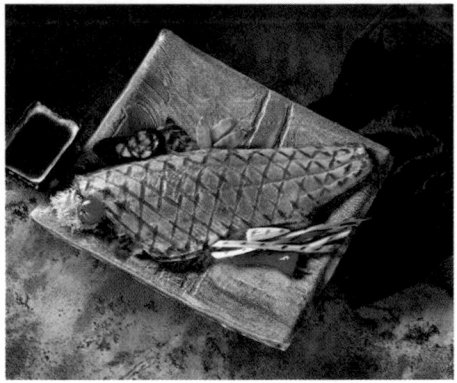

Eating fish at least two times a week is a healthy practice, because many fish are rich in omega-3 fatty acids. Especially emphasize species low in mercury, such as salmon and sardines (see Chapter 19 for details).

hemorrhagic stroke Damage to part of the brain resulting from rupture of a blood vessel and subsequent bleeding within or over the internal surface of the brain.

mega-3 fatty acids also are suspected to be helpful in managing the pain of inflammation associated with rheumatoid arthritis (by suppressing immune system responses) and may help with certain behavioral disorders and mild cases of depression.[21]

To produce the parent fatty acid for group 3 eicosanoid synthesis, alpha-linolenic acid is elongated to 20 carbons and two more carbon-carbon double bonds are added to produce eicosapantaenoic acid. (Eicosapantaenoic acid is also elongated to 22 carbons and has one more carbon-carbon double bond added to produce docosahexaenoic acid; however, this compound does not form eicosanoids.)[20]

Each of the parent fatty acids (dihomo-gamma-linolenic acid, arachadonic acid, and eicosapentaenoic acid) produces a particular set of eicosanoids. As the eicosanoids are synthesized, they take up oxygen by one of two enzyme systems: **cyclooxygenase** and **lipoxygenase,** forming distinct groups of eicosanoids. (Cyclooxygenase is the enzyme that aspirin and ibuprofen inhibit.) The eicosanoids made using cyclooxygenase (e.g., **prostacyclins, prostaglandins, thromboxanes**) or lipoxygenase (e.g., **leukotrienes**) are important and potent regulators of vital body functions such as blood pressure, labor, blood clotting, immune response, inflammation, and secretions of the stomach.[21]

A Closer Look at Omega-3 Fatty Acids

The thromboxanes derived from the cyclooxygenase pathway have a significant effect on blood clotting function. Thromboxane A is made by platelets and both stimulates blood clotting and causes blood vessels to constrict. Both are critical events when someone is bleeding profusely (hemorrhaging). (The name *thromboxane* comes from its function of forming a thrombus, or clot.) In contrast, prostacyclin I, produced by the **endothelial cells** that line blood vessel walls, is an important inhibitor of blood clotting. Thus the thromboxanes and the prostacyclins are antagonists.[21]

There is one important caveat: the balancing act between the group 2 forms (made from arachidonic acid) of thromboxane A and prostacyclin result in greater blood clotting activity than the same combination of group 3 forms (made from eicosapentaenoic acid). The thromboxane A produced from arachidonic acid is an especially powerful stimulator of blood clotting. All in all, the balance sheet is shifted toward less blood clotting in people whose diet contains some eicosapentaenoic acid to offset the effects of arachidonic acid.[21]

These eicosanoid actions were discovered many years ago in studies of Greenland Eskimos. They exhibit diminished clotting ability. Their diet is very high in fish oils containing eicosapentaenoic acid. Some studies show that people who eat fish about twice a week (total weekly intake: 8 oz [240g]) have lower risks for heart attacks than do people who rarely eat fish. In these cases, the omega-3 fatty acids in fish oil are probably acting to reduce blood clotting. As discussed in detail in the Nutrition Focus section of this chapter, blood clots are part of the heart attack process. In addition, omega-3 fatty acids can have a favorable effect on heart rhythm in some people. This effect also reduces the risk of heart attack in those people.[5]

Remember, however, that blood clotting is a normal body process. Certain groups of people, such as Eskimos in Greenland, eat so much seafood that their blood-clotting ability can be significantly impaired. An excess of omega-3 fatty acid intake can allow uncontrolled bleeding and may cause **hemorrhagic stroke.** However, the risk of stroke has not been seen in studies using moderate amounts of omega-3 fatty acids. Studies also have shown that large amounts of omega-3 fatty acids from fish (2 to 4 g/day or more; one 3 oz serving of fatty fish has about 1.6 g) can lower blood triglycerides in people with high triglyceride concentrations.[7]

In some instances, fish oil capsules can be safely substituted (under a physician's guidance) for fish consumption if a person does not like fish. However, unless a physician recommends otherwise, individuals who have bleeding disorders, who are taking anticoagulant medications, or who are anticipating surgery should not be taking fish oil capsules because of the increased risk of hemorrhagic stroke. Generally, about 1 g of omega-3 fatty acids (about three capsules) from fish oil per day is required to enjoy the benefits of reduced risk for cardiovascular disease that are associated with fish consumption twice a week. The larger doses of omega-3 fatty acids needed to reduce blood triglycerides would surely require fish oil supplements. (Note that freezing fish oil capsules before consumption will reduce the fishy aftertaste.)

Effects of a Deficiency of Essential Fatty Acids

If humans fail to consume enough essential fatty acids (linoleic acid and alpha-linolenic acid), their skin becomes flaky and itchy, and diarrhea and other symptoms such as infections often are seen. Growth and wound healing may be restricted, and anemia can develop. These signs of deficiency have been seen in people who were fed **total parenteral nutrition** solutions containing little or no fat for 2 to 3 weeks as well as in infants receiving formulas low in fat. However, because our bodies need the equivalent of only about 2 to 4 tablespoons of plant oils a day, even a low-fat diet will provide enough essential fatty acids if it follows a balanced plan, such as MyPyramid.[7]

Concept | Check

Lipids are a group of compounds that dissolve in organic solvents but do not dissolve readily in water. They include fatty acids, triglycerides, phospholipids, and sterols. Fatty acids differ from one another mainly in the number and location of the double bonds between carbons in the carbon chain. Saturated fatty acids contain no carbon-carbon double bonds; that is, they are fully saturated with hydrogens. Monounsaturated fatty acids contain one carbon-carbon double bond, and polyunsaturated fatty acids contain two or more carbon-carbon double bonds. These unsaturated fatty acids exist in a *cis* configuration in their natural state. Food processing can change this *cis* configuration to a *trans* configuration, creating a *trans* unsaturated fatty acid.

Length of the carbon chain in fatty acids affects the consistency of triglycerides at room temperature. Specifically, long-chain saturated fatty acids (greater than or equal to 12 carbons) form solid varieties at room temperature, whereas medium-chain (6 to 10 carbons) and short-chain (less than 6 carbons) saturated fatty acids form liquid varieties at room temperature, as do triglycerides composed of monounsaturated and polyunsaturated fatty acids.

If a double bond first occurs starting at the third carbon from the methyl ($-CH_3$) end of the carbon chain, the fatty acid is an omega-3 fatty acid. If a double bond first occurs starting at the sixth carbon, it is an omega-6 fatty acid. Because humans can't synthesize omega-3 and omega-6 fatty acids, which perform vital functions in the body when made into various eicosanoids, they are designated *essential fatty acids*, indicating that they must be included in the diet to maintain health. Eicosanoids made from omega-3 fatty acids reduce blood clotting and inflammation compared to those made from omega-6 fatty acids.

Triglycerides

Fats and oils in foods are mostly in the form of triglycerides. The same is true for fats found in body structures. Some fatty acids are transported in the bloodstream attached to proteins, but most fatty acids do not exist in the body as such. Instead, they form into triglycerides.[22]

Triglycerides contain a simple three-carbon alcohol, glycerol, which serves as a backbone for the three attached fatty acids. A fatty acid is attached to each of the three hydroxyl groups ($-OH$) of glycerol. Three water molecules are released in the process of bonding three fatty acids to glycerol (Figure 6-7). Note that triacylglyceride is the chemical name of the molecule, because *acyl* refers to a fatty acid that has lost its hydroxyl group, and a hydroxyl group is lost when each fatty acid attaches to glycerol.

The bonds between glycerol and each fatty acid are called *ester bonds*. The process of chemically attaching fatty acids to glycerol is called **esterification**. The release of fatty acids from glycerol is called *deesterification*.

By breaking off (deesterifying) one of the fatty acids of a triglyceride molecule, a **diglyceride** (glycerol with two attached fatty acids) is formed. The deesterification of two of the fatty acids on a triglyceride produces a **monoglyceride** (glycerol with one attached fatty acid). Free fatty acids, monoglycerides, and glycerol—but not triglycerides—can cross cell membranes because of their smaller size.[14]

The leukotrienes produced through the lipoxygenase pathway cause slow, prolonged contractions of smooth muscles in airways (and the gastrointestinal tract), especially group 2 forms (made from arachidonic acid). Medication to block leukotriene production has been developed to treat some forms of allergies and asthma.[21]

total parenteral nutrition The intravenous provision of all necessary nutrients, including the most basic forms of protein, carbohydrates, lipids, vitamins, minerals, and electrolytes. This solution is generally infused for 12 to 24 hours a day in a volume of about 2 to 3 L.

Critical | Thinking

Advertisements often claim that fats are bad. Your classmate Mike asks, "If fats are so bad for us, why do we need to have any in our diets?" How would you answer him?

esterification The process of attaching fatty acids to a glycerol molecule, creating an ester bond and releasing water. Removing a fatty acid is called deesterification; reattaching a fatty acid is called reesterification.

diglyceride A breakdown product of a triglyceride consisting of two fatty acids bonded to a glycerol backbone.

monoglyceride A breakdown product of a triglyceride consisting of one fatty acid bonded to a glycerol backbone.

Figure 6-7 | Forming a triglyceride via esterification. This process yields water as a by-product as ester bonds are formed. The *R* represents the fatty acids.

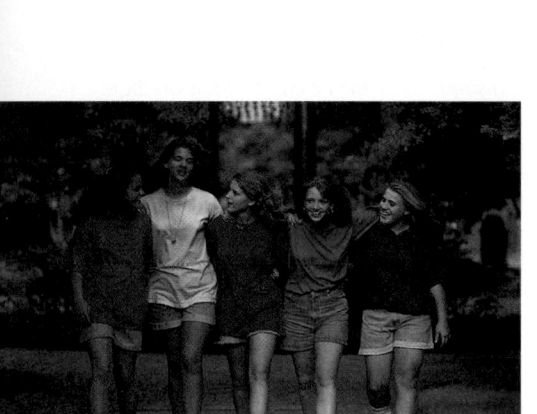

Glycerol + 3 fatty acids → Triglyceride + 3 H₂O

During digestion, enzymes in the small intestine eventually break down the triglycerides in the foods to free fatty acids and monoglycerides; only a small portion of dietary triglycerides is broken down completely to free fatty acids and glycerol.[14] After the free fatty acids, monoglycerides, and any free glycerol enter the intestinal cells, most of these components are rebuilt into new triglycerides (see the section in this chapter titled Fat Digestion and Absorption). The reattachment of fatty acids to glycerol is called *reesterification*. Every time a triglyceride enters or leaves a cell, it must also be deesterified; after entering a cell, the free fatty acids are reesterified into triglycerides. Thus, the body must continually break down and rebuild triglycerides.[22]

Roles of Triglycerides in the Body

Many key functions of fat in the body use triglycerides. Triglycerides contribute to energy storage, insulation, and transportation of fat-soluble vitamins.

Providing Energy for the Body

Triglycerides contained in the diet and stored in adipose tissue provide the fatty acids that are the main fuel for muscles while at rest and during light activity.[22] Only in endurance exercise, such as long-distance running and cycling, or in short bursts of intense activity, such as a 200-meter run, do muscles oxidize a lot of carbohydrate in addition to fatty acids supplied by triglycerides. Other body tissues also use fatty acids for energy. Overall, about half the energy used by the entire body at rest and during light activity comes from fatty acids. On a whole-body basis, the use of fatty acids in skeletal and cardiac muscle cells is balanced by the use of glucose in the nervous system and red blood cells. Recall from Chapter 4 that cells also need carbohydrate to efficiently process fatty acids for fuel.

Storing Energy for Later Use

We store energy mainly in the form of triglycerides.[22] The body's ability to store fat is essentially limitless. Its fat storage sites, adipose cells, can increase about 50 times in weight. If the amount of fat to be stored exceeds the ability of the cells to expand, the body can form new adipose cells. (This topic is discussed further in Chapter 13.)

An important advantage of using triglycerides to store energy in the body is that they are energy dense. Recall that these yield, on average, 9 kcal/g, whereas proteins and carbohydrates yield less than half that much. In addition, triglycerides are chemically very stable, so they are not likely to react with other cell constituents, making

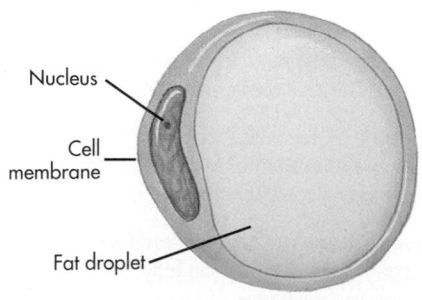

When at rest or during light activity, the body uses mostly fatty acids for fuel.

Nucleus

Cell membrane

Fat droplet

Adipose cell

them a safe form for storing energy. Finally, when we store triglycerides in adipose cells, we store little else in terms of energy-yielding compounds; adipose cells contain about 80% lipid and only 20% water and protein.[22] In contrast, imagine if we were to store energy as muscle tissue, which is about 73% water. Body weight linked to energy storage would increase dramatically.

Insulating and Protecting the Body

The insulating layer of fat just beneath the skin is made mostly of triglycerides. Fat tissue also surrounds and protects some organs—kidneys, for example—from injury. We usually don't notice the important insulating function of fat tissue because we wear clothes and add more as needed. But a layer of insulating fat is quite apparent in animals, particularly those in cold climates. Polar bears, walruses, and whales all build a thick layer of fat tissue around themselves to insulate against cold-weather environments. The extra fat also provides energy storage for times when food is scarce.

People with **anorexia nervosa** often lose 25% or more of body weight and become about as fat free as is biologically possible. In turn, they lose the insulating property of fat storage. In place of the layer of fat tissue under the skin, people with anorexia nervosa often develop downy hair, called **lanugo,** all over their body. These hairs insulate the body by standing up and trapping warm air.

Transporting Fat-Soluble Vitamins

Triglycerides and other fats in food carry fat-soluble vitamins to the small intestine and aid their absorption. If the small intestine is diseased, however, it may not be able to adequately digest and absorb fat from foods. When this happens, the unabsorbed fat carries the fat-soluble vitamins—A, D, E, and K—into the large intestine. From there, they are eliminated in the feces, and the body loses the benefits of the vitamins. If the disease doesn't resolve quickly, medical attention is necessary.

People who absorb fat poorly, such as those with the disease cystic fibrosis, are also at risk for deficiencies of fat-soluble vitamins. A similar risk accrues from taking mineral oil as a laxative at mealtimes. Because the body cannot digest or absorb mineral oil, the undigested oil carries the fat-soluble vitamins from the meal into the feces, where they are eliminated.

▌Phospholipids

Phospholipids are another class of lipid. Like triglycerides, they are built on a backbone of glycerol. However, at least one fatty acid is replaced with a compound containing phosphorus (and often other elements, such as nitrogen).[14] Many types of phospholipids exist in the body, especially in the brain. They form important parts of cell membranes. The various forms of **lecithins** are common examples of phospholipids. These are found in body cells, where they participate in fat digestion in the intestine. Peanuts contain lecithins in abundance, as do liver, wheat germ, soybeans, and egg yolks. It is not necessary to consume phospholipids, such as lecithins, in the diet because the body can synthesize them and use them when and where they are needed.

Cell membranes are composed primarily of phospholipids. A cell membrane looks much like a sea of phospholipids with protein "islands" (review Figure C-1 in Appendix C). Among their many roles, the proteins form receptors for hormones, function as enzymes, and act as transporters for nutrients. About 5 to 15% of cell membrane fatty acids is made up of arachidonic acid. This serves as a source for eicosanoid synthesis.[21] (Some cholesterol is also present in the cell membrane.)

Some phospholipids, such as lecithins, function as **emulsifiers.** These allow fat and water to mix. By breaking fat globules into small droplets, emulsifiers

Unabsorbed fatty acids also can bind minerals, such as calcium and magnesium, and draw them into the feces for elimination. This can harm mineral status (see Chapter 11).

anorexia nervosa An eating disorder involving a psychological loss or denial of appetite followed by self-starvation; related in part to a distorted body image and to various social pressures commonly associated with puberty.

lanugo Downlike hair that appears after a person has lost much body fat through semistarvation. The hair stands erect and traps air, acting as insulation for the body to compensate for the relative lack of body fat, which usually functions as insulation.

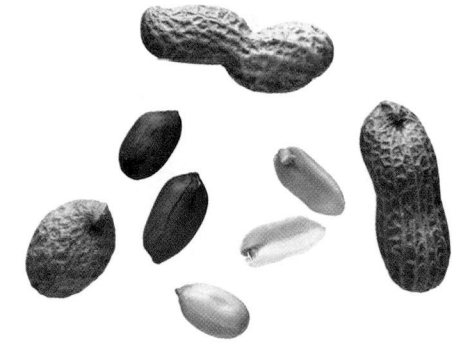

Peanuts are a source of lecithins, as are wheat germ and egg yolks.

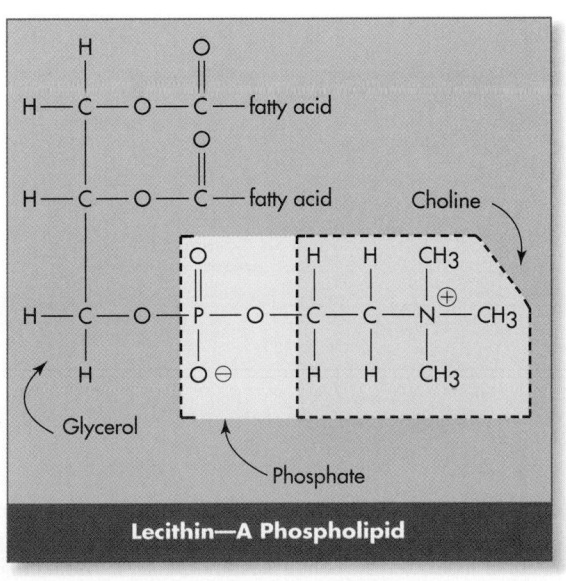

Lecithin—A Phospholipid

emulsifier A compound that can suspend fat in water by isolating individual fat droplets using a shell of water molecules or other substances to prevent the fat from coalescing.

bile acids Emulsifiers synthesized by the liver and released by the gallbladder during digestion.

micelles Water-soluble spherical structures formed by lecithin and bile acids in which the hydrophobic parts of the molecules face inward and the hydrophilic parts face outward. Lipids enclosed within micelles do not separate out into an oily layer as they normally do when mixed with water.

enable a fat to be suspended in water. Here's how the process works: The fatty acid ends of lecithins attract fat. The phosphorus and nitrogen at the other end of lecithins form an area containing positive and negative charges. This area attracts water. Because water is attracted to the charges on lecithin, this part of lecithin is called hydrophilic, which means "loving water." The parts with fatty acids are called hydrophobic, because they don't attract (they "fear") water.

When an emulsifier is mixed with oil and water in the proper proportions, it forms spherical structures in which the hydrophobic parts of the emulsifier molecules are oriented toward the interior and the hydrophilic parts toward the exterior (Figure 6-8). In this way, the emulsifier acts as a bridge between the oil and water by forming tiny oil droplets surrounded by thin shells of water.

The body's main emulsifiers are the lecithins and **bile acids,** which are produced by the liver and released into the small intestine via the gallbladder during digestion. By breaking up the fat globules, the emulsifiers create more fat surface for fat-digesting enzymes to act on. These very stable emulsified products are called **micelles** (see the section in this chapter titled Digestion).[14]

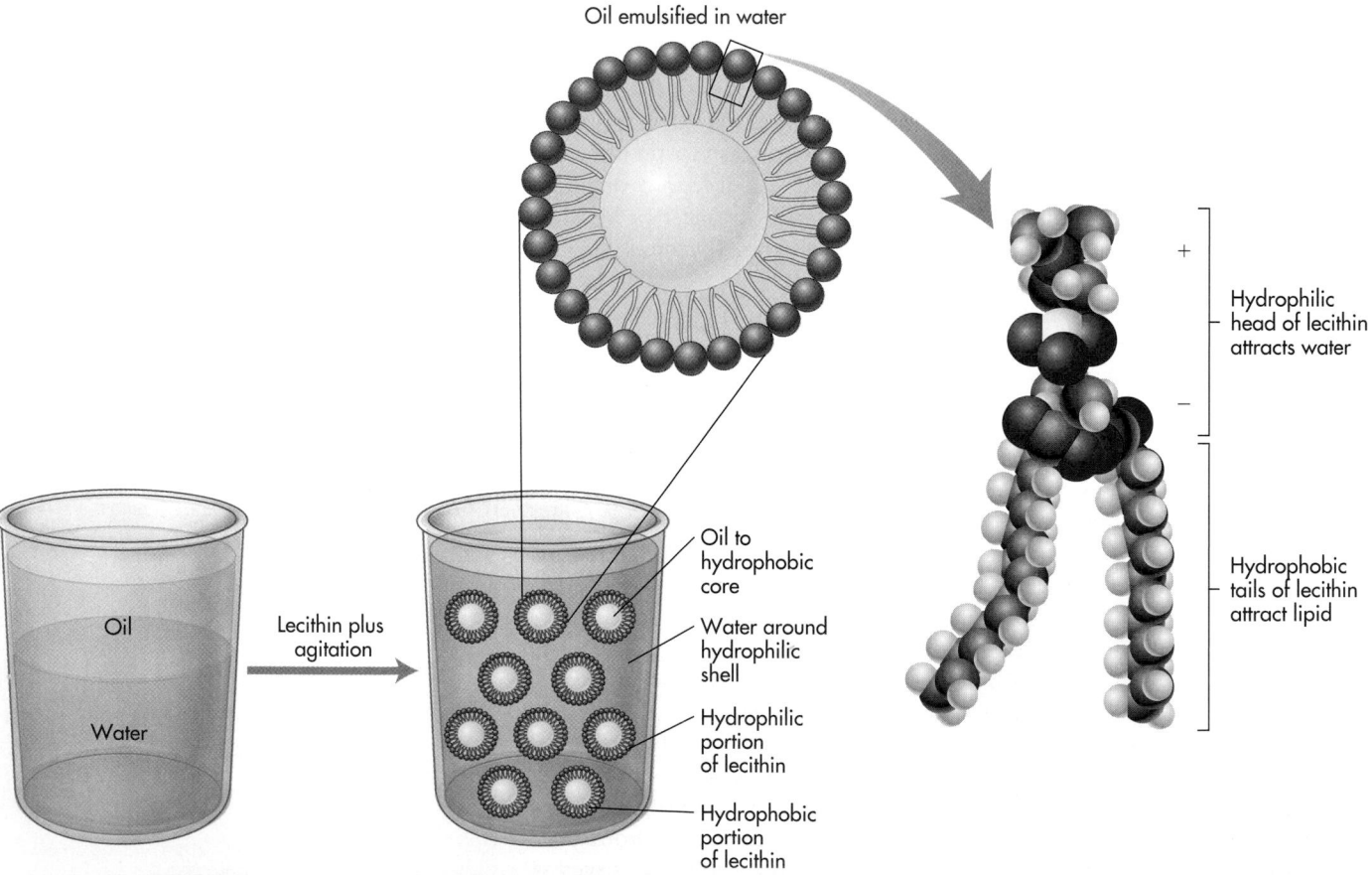

Oil emulsified in water

Oil to hydrophobic core

Water around hydrophilic shell

Hydrophilic portion of lecithin

Hydrophobic portion of lecithin

Oil

Water

Lecithin plus agitation

Hydrophilic head of lecithin attracts water

Hydrophobic tails of lecithin attract lipid

Figure 6-8 | Emulsification and emulsifiers. Emulsifiers organize oil and water into droplets of oil surrounded by water. The emulsifier molecules form a bridge between the oil and water molecules, isolating one from the other. In the droplet, oil enters the central core, while water surrounds the core. The emulsifier molecules are sandwiched between the two. Formation of such emulsions is a key step in digestion of dietary fat and is important in the manufacture of certain food products, such as mayonnaise and cakes.

Cholesterol

Testosterone

Sterols

Sterols are the last class of lipids this chapter covers. Their characteristic multiringed structure makes them different from the other lipids already discussed. Consider the sterol cholesterol. This waxy substance doesn't look like a triglyceride—it doesn't have a glycerol backbone or any fatty acids. Still, because it doesn't readily dissolve in water, it is a lipid. The main building block for the synthesis of cholesterol in the body is acetyl-CoA, a derivative of the two-carbon fatty acid **acetic acid.** (Synthesis of longer fatty acids, triglycerides, and phospholipids also makes use of acetyl-CoA.)[23]

Cholesterol forms part of some important hormones, such as the estrogens, testosterone, and a form of the active vitamin D hormone—namely, 1,25(OH$_2$) vitamin D. Cholesterol is also the precursor of bile acids, which are needed for fat digestion. Finally, cholesterol is an essential structural component of cell membranes and the particles that transport lipids in the blood, as discussed in the next section.[17] The cholesterol content of the heart, liver, kidney, and brain is quite high, reflecting its critical role in these organs.

Cholesterol is made by body cells (two-thirds of total daily body exposure) and is consumed in the diet (about one-third of total daily body exposure). Each day, our cells produce approximately 875 mg of cholesterol. Of this, about 400 mg is used to make new bile acids to replenish those lost in the feces and about 50 mg is used to make steroid hormones. With respect to diet, we consume about 180 to 325 mg of cholesterol per day from animal-derived food products, with men consuming the higher amount compared to women (Table 6-2). Of that, we absorb about 40 to 60%. There is no need to consume cholesterol per se, because body cells can make all that they need.[7]

Plants do not produce cholesterol. When companies market their bottles of vegetable oil with labels that say "cholesterol-free," they're trying to persuade uninformed consumers to buy their brand. In fact, all brands of vegetable oil are cholesterol-free. Although plants do not make cholesterol, they do make other sterols.[17] Ergosterol, for example, can form a type of vitamin D. Plants also make a sterol called sitostanol, which is now incorporated into Take Control margarine. Eating such a margarine introduces a higher-than-usual amount of sterols into the small intestine, where the plant sterols can interfere with the reabsorption of cholesterol and bile acids (which are made from cholesterol) and, hence, reduce the risk of cardiovascular disease.[18] Although studies show that sterol-rich margarine is effective in lowering blood cholesterol, the product is quite expensive.

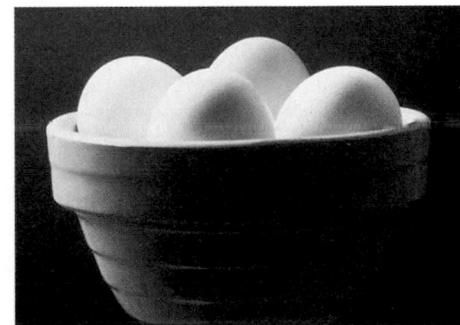

Eggs are the principal source of cholesterol in the North American diet. The Food and Nutrition Board suggests limiting intake of this and other high-cholesterol foods.

Table 6-2 | Cholesterol Content of Selected Foods in Ascending Order

Food	Amount	Cholesterol (mg)	Food	Amount	Cholesterol (mg)
Fat-free milk	1 cup	4	Oysters, salmon	3 oz	40
Mayonnaise	1 tbsp	10	Clams, halibut, tuna	3 oz	55
Butter	1 pat	11	Chicken, turkey* (white meat)	3 oz	70
Lard	1 tbsp	12	Beef,* pork	3 oz	75
Cottage cheese	1/2 cup	15	Lamb, crab	3 oz	85
Fat-reduced milk (2%)	1 cup	22	Shrimp, lobster	3 oz	110
Half-and-half	1/4 cup	23	Heart (beef)	3 oz	165
Hot dog	1	29	Egg (egg yolk)*†	1	210
Ice cream, ~ 10% fat	1/2 cup	30	Liver (beef)	3 oz	410
Cheese, cheddar*	1 oz	30	Kidney	3 oz	540
Whole milk*	1 cup	34	Brains	3 oz	2640

*Leading contributors of cholesterol to the North American diet.

†Egg whites are cholesterol-free.

Concept | Check

Triglycerides are the major form of fat in the body and in food. They are used for and stored as energy, they insulate and protect body organs, and they transport fat-soluble vitamins. Phospholipids have both hydrophilic and hydrophobic parts and so are effective emulsifiers—compounds that can suspend fat in water. Phospholipids also form parts of cell membranes and various compounds in the body. Cells produce all the phospholipids the body needs. Cholesterol, a sterol, forms part of cell membranes, some hormones, and bile acids; it is essential to the body. Cholesterol is found in animal products and is synthesized by body cells; if sufficient amounts are not ingested, the body makes what it needs.

Fat Digestion and Absorption

Given the right conditions, about 95% of fat consumed is digested and then absorbed.[14]

Digestion

Fat digestion begins in the mouth and stomach, using the enzymes lingual lipase (mostly in infancy) and gastric lipase, respectively.[14] These enzymes break down triglycerides containing short- and medium-chain fatty acids, such as those found in milk fat into free fatty acids and diglycerides. Because fat may remain in the stomach for up to 2 to 4 hours, there is an opportunity to digest some of these triglycerides and to absorb the fatty acids released through the stomach wall. The short- and medium-chain fatty acids then enter the portal vein. In contrast, long-chain fatty acids are not acted on until they reach the small intestine (Figure 6-9).

Once the fat reaches the small intestine, the hormone cholecystokinin (CCK) is released from certain intestinal cells. This hormone stimulates the release of bile from the gallbladder and lipase from the pancreas.[14] The bile contains bile acids, lecithin, and cholesterol. The lipase travels through the pancreatic duct to be mixed with bile in the common bile duct; finally, both enter together into the small intestine. In the small intestine, pancreatic lipase contributes to fat digestion by digesting (specifically hydrolyzing) the triglycerides into monoglycerides and free fatty acids. The amount of

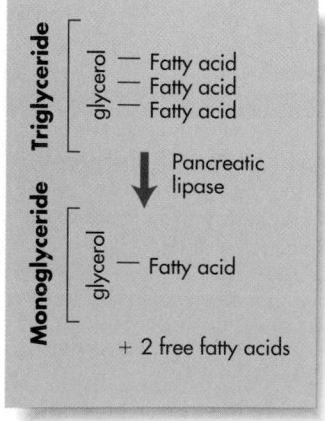

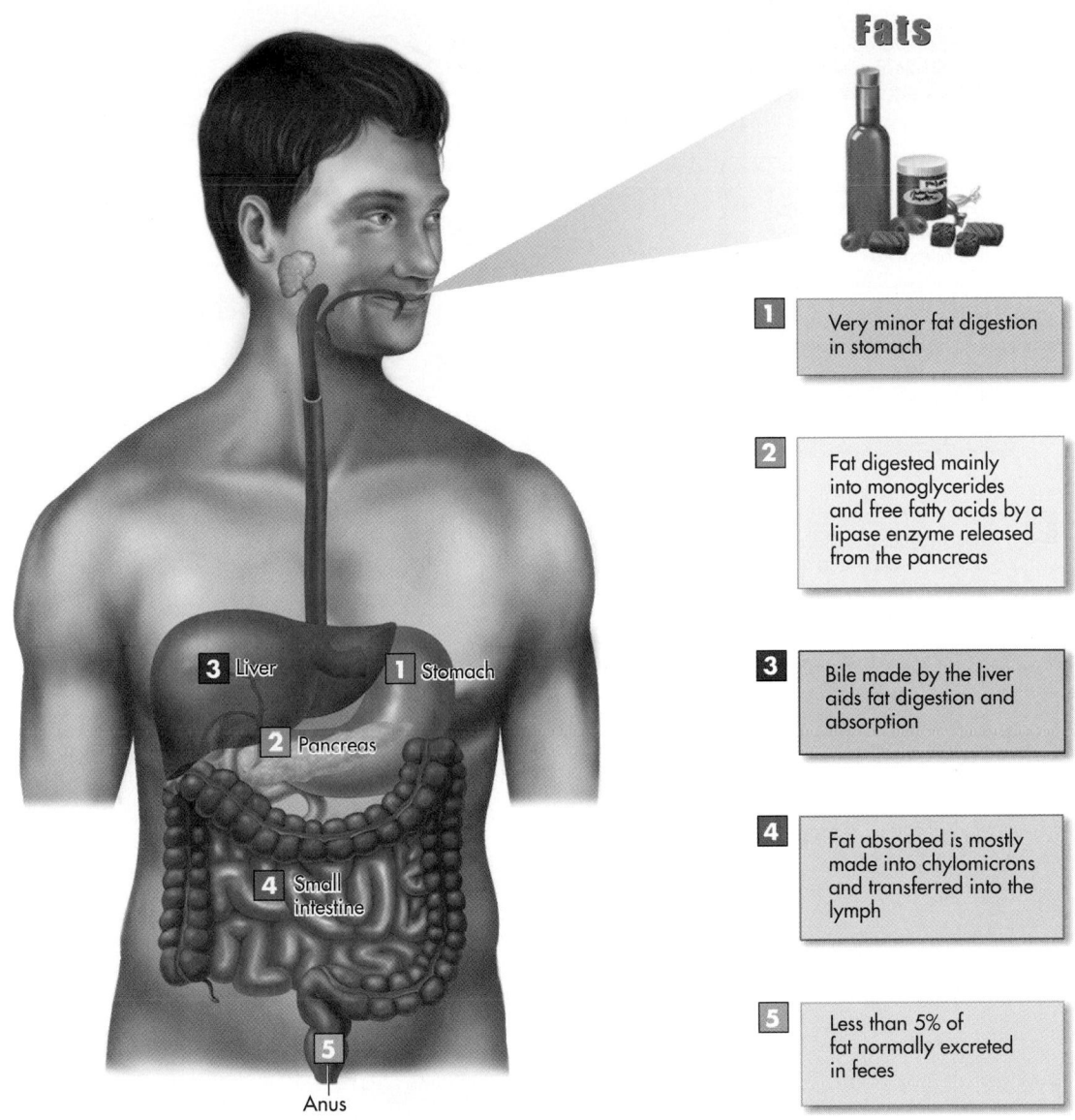

Fats

1. Very minor fat digestion in stomach

2. Fat digested mainly into monoglycerides and free fatty acids by a lipase enzyme released from the pancreas

3. Bile made by the liver aids fat digestion and absorption

4. Fat absorbed is mostly made into chylomicrons and transferred into the lymph

5. Less than 5% of fat normally excreted in feces

Figure 6-9 | A summary of fat digestion and absorption. Chapter 3 covered general aspects of this process.

pancreatic lipase released is much greater than what is needed in most circumstances to digest the fat in a meal. This "overkill" makes fat digestion very rapid and thorough in the right circumstances, which include the presence of bile acids and lecithin from the gallbladder and a protein called **colipase.** Colipase is found in pancreatic secretions, and it functions by ensuring the attachment of lipase to the lipid droplet.[14]

Because fat is hydrophobic, it needs a medium that will carry it throughout the intestinal tract. Bile acids help do this by emulsifying the fatty substances in the small intestine into micelles, as previously discussed. Emulsification improves digestion and absorption because as large fat globules are broken down into smaller ones, the total surface area for lipase action increases (Figure 6-10).[14]

With regard to phospholipid and cholesterol digestion, phospholipase enzymes from the pancreas and glandular cells in the wall of the small intestine digest phospholipids. The eventual products are glycerol, fatty acids, phosphoric acid, and remaining constituents such as choline. Cholesterol esters (cholesterol with a fatty acid attached) are broken down to cholesterol and free fatty acids.[17]

colipase A protein secreted by the pancreas that changes the shape of pancreatic lipase, facilitating its action.

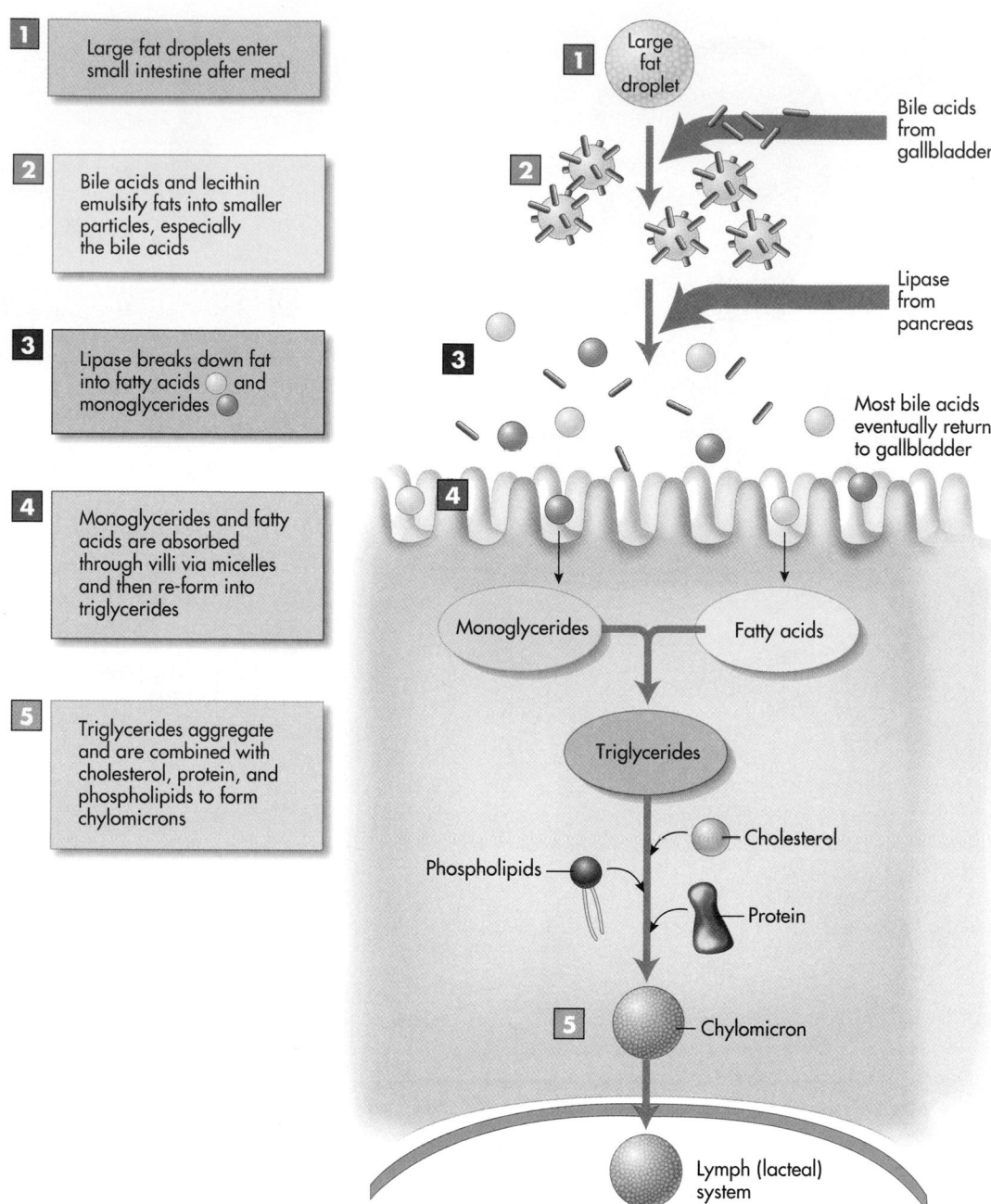

1 Large fat droplets enter small intestine after meal

2 Bile acids and lecithin emulsify fats into smaller particles, especially the bile acids

3 Lipase breaks down fat into fatty acids ◯ and monoglycerides ⬤

4 Monoglycerides and fatty acids are absorbed through villi via micelles and then re-form into triglycerides

5 Triglycerides aggregate and are combined with cholesterol, protein, and phospholipids to form chylomicrons

1 Large fat droplet

Bile acids from gallbladder

Lipase from pancreas

Most bile acids eventually return to gallbladder

Monoglycerides

Fatty acids

Triglycerides

Phospholipids

Cholesterol

Protein

5 Chylomicron

Lymph (lacteal) system

Figure 6-10 | A simplified look at absorption of triglycerides made up of long-chain fatty acids. These long-chain fatty acids, which primarily form monoglycerides and free fatty acids, are absorbed through the use of bile acids and re-formed into triglycerides in the absorptive cells. The triglycerides are then formed into chylomicrons and enter the lymphatic system. Note that short- and medium-chain fatty acids for the most part pass directly into the portal circulation (not depicted). Under normal conditions, about 95% of dietary fat is absorbed, primarily as chylomicrons. Only a small portion is found in the feces.

Absorption

The lipid content of the micelles is absorbed into the brush border of the absorptive cells lining the duodenum and jejunum. Through this process about 95% of dietary fat is absorbed.[14] The carbon chain length of fatty acids and monoglycerides absorbed then affects their fate after absorption. If a fatty acid is a short- or medium-chain variety (less than 12 carbons), it is water-soluble and probably travels out of the absorptive cell (enterocyte) and through the portal vein connected to the liver. If the fatty acid is a long-chain variety (12 or more carbons), it is first re-formed into a triglyceride molecule in the absorptive cell. After further packaging (described in the next section), it enters circulation via the lymphatic system carrying with it fat-soluble vitamins and absorbed cholesterol (review Figure 6-10).[14]

The leftover bile acids (and some of the cholesterol released in the bile) are reabsorbed in the ileum and returned to the liver (by the portal vein) to be used again in fat digestion (about 98% of bile acids are recycled; only 1 to 2% are eliminated in the feces).[14] Recall from Chapter 3 that this recycling is termed enterohepatic circulation. Using medicines that block some of this reabsorption of bile acids is one way to treat high blood cholesterol. The liver takes cholesterol from the bloodstream to form replacement bile acids. Soluble fiber in the diet can also bind to bile acids to produce the same effect.[7]

Fats Carried in the Bloodstream

The incompatibility of fat and water presents a challenge in transporting fats through the watery media of blood and lymph systems.

Carrying Dietary Fats Utilizes Chylomicrons

Once the various dietary fats are digested and absorbed into the small intestine cells, most of the by-products of digestion—glycerol, monoglycerides, and fatty acids—are re-formed into triglycerides. They are then packaged into **lipoprotein** particles—large droplets of lipid surrounded by a thin shell of phospholipid, cholesterol, and protein (Figure 6-11). The lipoprotein particles produced by intestinal cells are called **chylomicrons**.[22] The shell around a chylomicron allows the lipid it is carrying to float freely in the water-based blood. Some of the proteins present—namely, **apolipoproteins**—also help other cells identify this particle as a chylomicron.

After being assembled in intestinal cells, chylomicrons enter the lymphatic system and travel to the thoracic duct, which is located along the spinal column. This duct opens into a large vein in the neck called the subclavian vein. Chylomicrons enter the general circulation of the bloodstream at that point (see Figure C-5 in Appendix C for a view of lymphatic circulation).

Once chylomicrons enter the bloodstream, the triglycerides in the chylomicrons are broken down by **lipoprotein lipase** into fatty acids and glycerol. This enzyme is attached to the inside wall of blood vessels. Muscle cells, adipose cells, and other cells in the vicinity then absorb most of the fatty acids.[22] Cells can immediately use absorbed fatty acids for energy needs, or they can re-form them into triglycerides and store them as such. Muscle cells tend to metabolize fatty acids, whereas adipose cells tend to store them. (Table 6-3).

After a person eats a meal, the whole process of clearing chylomicrons from the blood via lipoprotein lipase activity takes about 2 to 10 hours, depending in part on fat content. After 12 to 14 hours of fasting, the chylomicrons should be totally absent from the bloodstream. People should fast for 12 to 14 hours before having certain blood tests to ensure that chylomicrons, whose presence could affect the results, have been cleared.

Transporting Lipids Mostly Made by the Body Uses Very-Low-Density Lipoproteins

The liver produces some fat and cholesterol.[22] The source of the needed carbon, hydrogen, and energy to make such substances as glycerol, fatty acids, triglycerides, and cholesterol includes the carbohydrate and protein the liver takes up from the bloodstream.

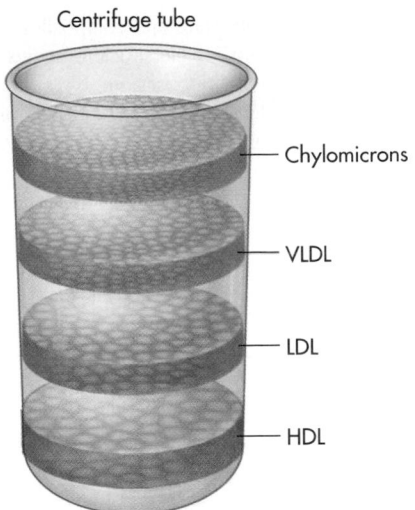

Centrifuge tube

— Chylomicrons

— VLDL

— LDL

— HDL

One way to measure the amount of chylomicrons, VLDL, LDL, and HDL particles in the bloodstream is to centrifuge the serum portion of the blood at high speed for about 24 hours in a sucrose-rich solution. The lipoproteins settle out in the centrifuge tube based on their density, with chylomicrons at the top and HDLs at the bottom.

lipoprotein A compound found in the bloodstream containing a core of lipids with a shell composed of protein, phospholipid, and cholesterol.

chylomicron Lipoprotein made of dietary fats surrounded by a shell of cholesterol, phospholipids, and protein. Chylomicrons are formed in the absorptive cells (enterocytes) of the small intestine after fat absorption and travel through the lymphatic system to the bloodstream.

apolipoprotein A protein attached to the surface of a lipoprotein or embedded in its outer shell. Apolipoproteins can help enzymes function, act as a lipid-transfer protein, or assist in the binding of a lipoprotein to a cell-surface receptor.

lipoprotein lipase An enzyme attached to the outside endothelial cells that line the capillaries in the blood vessels; it breaks down triglycerides into free fatty acids and glycerol.

Figure 6-11 | Structure and composition of lipoproteins. This lipoprotein structure allows fats to circulate in the bloodstream. Note that for each class of lipoprotein, there are various subclasses of slightly different composition, including those based on their different apolipoproteins.

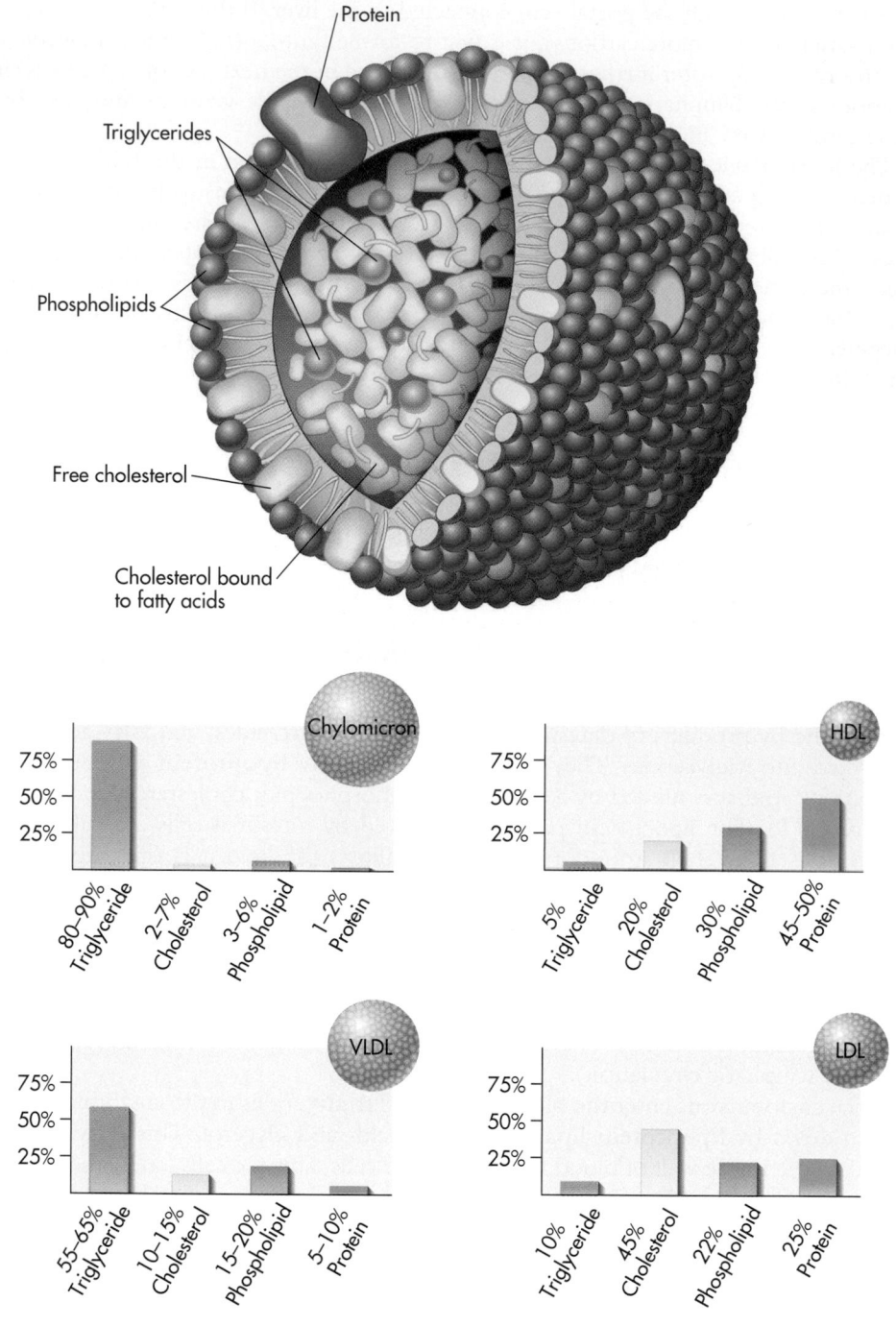

Table 6-3 | Composition and Roles of the Major Lipoproteins in the Blood

Lipoprotein	Primary Component	Key Role
Chylomicron	Triglyceride	Carries dietary fat from the small intestine to cells
VLDL	Triglyceride	Carries lipids both taken up and made by the liver to cells
LDL	Cholesterol	Carries cholesterol made by the liver and from other sources to cells
HDL	Protein	Contributes to cholesterol removal from cells and, in turn, excretion of it from the body

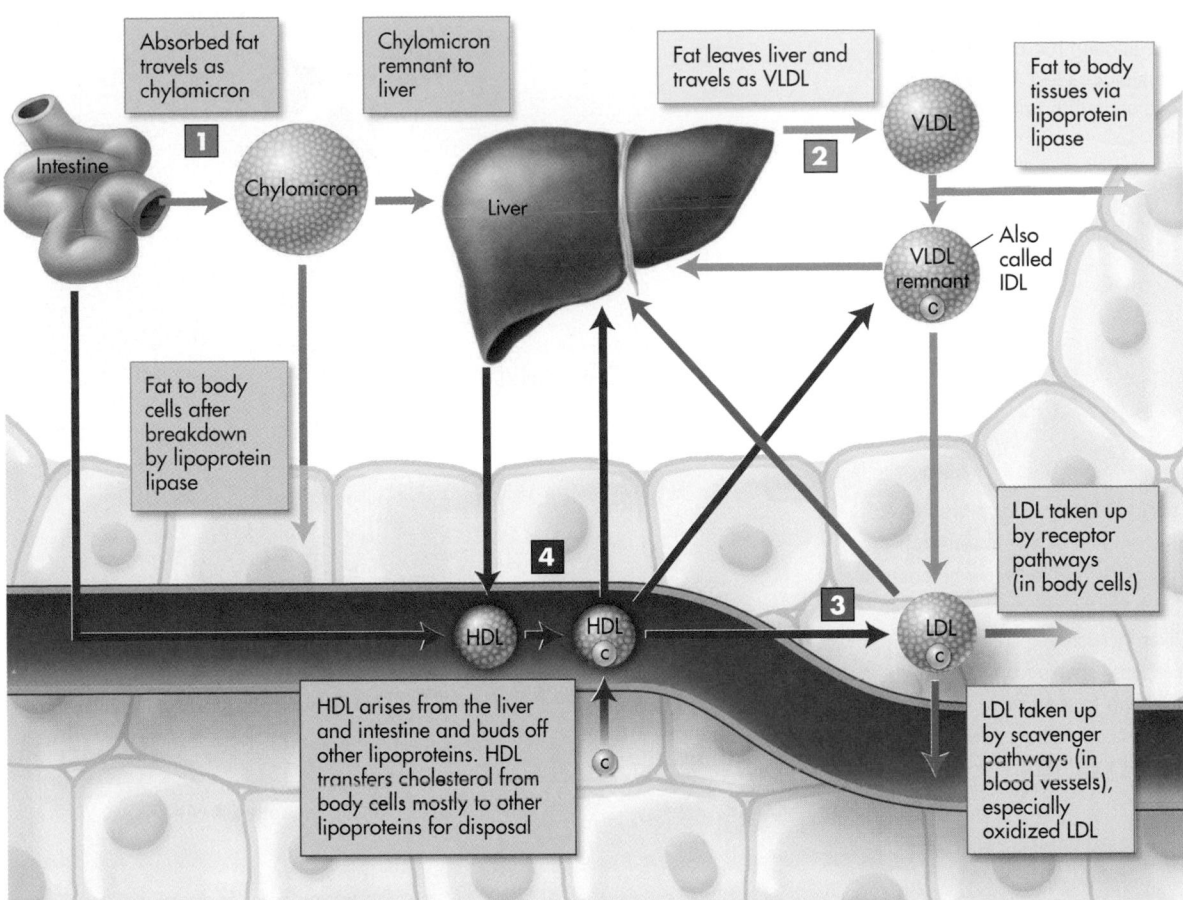

Figure 6-12 | Lipoprotein interactions. (1) Chylomicrons carry absorbed fat to body cells. (2) VLDL carries fat taken up from the bloodstream by the liver, as well as any fat made by the liver, to body cells. (3) LDL arises from VLDL and carries mostly cholesterol to cells. (4) HDL arises from body cells, mostly in the liver and intestine as well as from particles that bud off the other lipoproteins. HDL carries cholesterol from cells to other lipoproteins and to the liver for excretion.

*Intermediate Density Lipoprotein.

However, free fatty acids taken up from the bloodstream by the liver are the major source for triglyceride synthesis.[22] The liver coats the cholesterol and triglycerides that collect, including some taken up from the bloodstream, with a shell of protein and lipids. This process produces what is called a **very-low-density lipoprotein (VLDL)** fraction (Figure 6-12).

When the VLDL leaves the liver, the enzyme lipoprotein lipase on the blood vessels breaks down the triglyceride in the VLDL into fatty acids and glycerol. Again, fatty acids and glycerol are released into the bloodstream and are taken up by the body cells. Because fats are less dense than water, the VLDL becomes proportionately denser as triglyceride is released. Much of what eventually remains of the VLDL fraction becomes particles called low-density lipoprotein (LDL) fraction. LDL is composed primarily of cholesterol.[22]

LDL particles are absorbed from the bloodstream by receptors on cells, internalized, and broken down. Most LDL is taken up by receptors on liver cells.[22] Diets low in saturated fat and cholesterol encourage this process, whereas diets high in those lipids can reduce LDL uptake by the liver.[7] The cholesterol and protein parts absorbed then are transported throughout the cell. By this process, called the **receptor pathway for cholesterol uptake,** cells take up some of the building blocks necessary for cell growth and development (Figure 6-13).[14]

very-low-density lipoprotein (VLDL) The lipoprotein created in the liver that carries both the cholesterol and the lipids taken up from the bloodstream by the liver and those that are newly synthesized by the liver.

receptor pathway for cholesterol uptake A process by which LDL is bound by cell receptors and incorporated into the cell.

Figure 6-13 | Transport of LDL into cells. LDL receptors capture circulating LDL and release it inside the cell to be metabolized. Once free of their load, LDL receptors return to the cell surface to await new LDL.

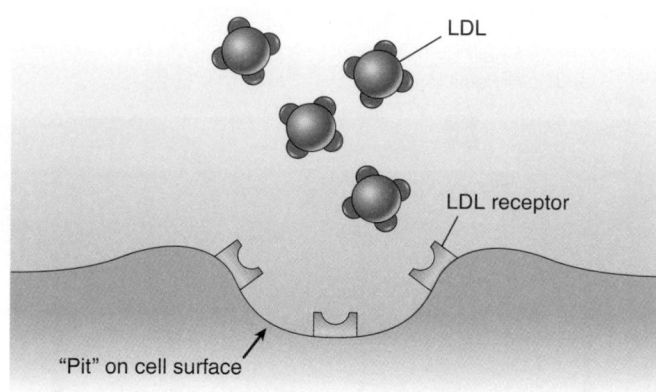

Cells have pits on the surface, which contain LDL receptors.

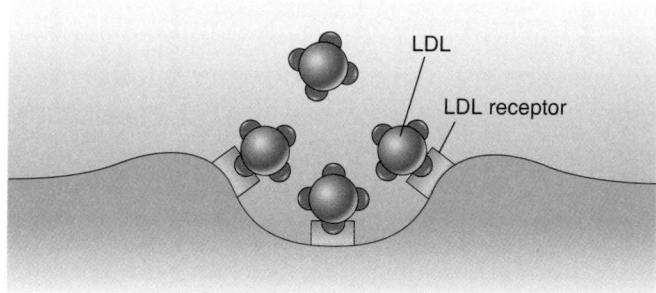

LDL binds to the LDL receptors in the pits.

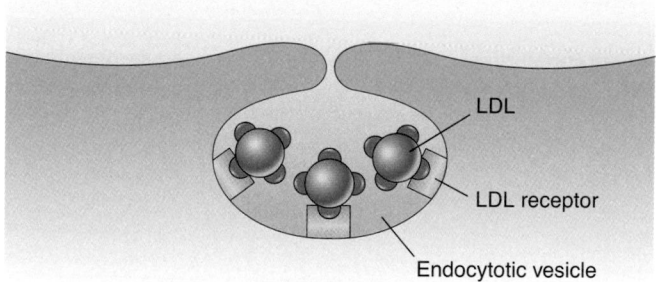

The LDL, bound to LDL receptors, is taken into the cell by endocytosis.

It appears that saturated fatty acids promote an increase in the amount of free cholesterol (not attached to fatty acids) in the liver, whereas unsaturated fatty acids do the opposite. As free cholesterol in the liver increases, it causes the liver to reduce cholesterol uptake from the bloodstream, contributing to elevated LDL in the blood. (*Trans* fatty acids are thought to act in the same ways as saturated fatty acids.)[14]

scavenger pathway for cholesterol uptake A process by which LDL is taken up by scavenger cells embedded in the blood vessels.

oxidized LDL LDL that has been damaged by free radicals. Such damage is seen both in the lipids and proteins that make up this lipoprotein.

A second process, called the **scavenger pathway for cholesterol uptake,** can also remove LDL from the circulation. This pathway is carried out by certain "scavenger" white blood cells, which leave the bloodstream and bury themselves in blood vessels. These scavenger cells detect modified LDL (e.g., **oxidized LDL**) within the vessel wall, engulf it, and then digest it. Once within the scavenger cells, the oxidized LDL generally is prevented from reentering the bloodstream.[24] Over time, cholesterol builds up in the scavenger cells, and more so when the amount of LDL in the bloodstream is excessive.

When scavenger cells have collected and deposited cholesterol for many years at a heavy pace, cholesterol builds up on the inner blood vessel walls—especially in arteries—and **plaque** develops (see Figure 6-14 in the Nutrition Focus). Diets rich in saturated fat, *trans* fat, and cholesterol encourage this process.[7] The plaque eventually mixes with connective tissue (collagen) and is then covered with a cap of smooth muscle cells and calcium. **Atherosclerosis,** also referred to as *hardening of the arteries,* develops as plaque thickens in the vessel. This thickening eventually chokes off the blood supply to organs, setting the stage for a heart attack and other problems, or it breaks apart and leads to clot formation in this or another artery. Dr. Bernhard Hennig covers this topic in more detail in the Expert Opinion in this chapter.

A final critical participant in this extensive process of fat transport is high-density lipoprotein (HDL). Its high proportion of protein makes it the heaviest (densest) lipoprotein. The liver and intestine produce most of the HDL in the blood. It roams the bloodstream, picking up cholesterol from dying cells and other sources. HDL donates the cholesterol to other lipoproteins for transport back to the liver to be excreted. Some HDL travels directly back to the liver. Another beneficial function of HDL is that it blocks oxidation of LDL.[22]

Many studies demonstrate that the amount of HDL in the bloodstream can closely predict the risk for cardiovascular disease. The risk increases with low HDL because little blood cholesterol is transported back to the liver and excreted. Women tend to have high amounts of HDL, especially before **menopause,** whereas low amounts are more common in men.

Because high amounts of HDL slow the development of cardiovascular disease, any cholesterol carried by HDL can be considered "good" cholesterol. By convention, then, cholesterol carried by LDL would be "bad" cholesterol because high amounts of LDL speed the development of cardiovascular disease. Still, LDL is only a problem when it is too high in the bloodstream; lower amounts are needed as part of routine body functions.[14]

Concept | Check

In the mouth and stomach, lingual and gastric lipase, respectively, break down short- and medium-chain triglycerides into smaller components. A minor amount is absorbed through the stomach wall. All end up in the portal vein and are transported to the liver. In the small intestine, the enzyme pancreatic lipase digests long-chain triglycerides into monoglycerides and free fatty acids. These breakdown products diffuse into the absorptive cells of the small intestine and are mostly resynthesized into triglycerides. The bloodstream carries absorbed dietary fat as chylomicrons.

Lipid synthesized by the liver is carried in the bloodstream as very-low-density lipoprotein (VLDL). Once a VLDL has most triglycerides removed by lipoprotein lipase, it eventually becomes low-density lipoprotein (LDL), which is rich in cholesterol. LDL is picked up by receptors on body cells, especially liver cells. Scavenger cells in the arteries may do the same, speeding the development of atherosclerosis. This is especially true for any LDL that has been modified (e.g., oxidized). High-density lipoprotein (HDL) picks up cholesterol from cells and transports it primarily to other lipoproteins for eventual transport back to the liver. HDL also decreases LDL oxidation, thereby reducing LDL in atherosclerotic plaque. Elevated amounts of LDL in the bloodstream is a major risk factor associated with cardiovascular disease, as is low amounts of HDL.

plaque A cholesterol-rich substance deposited in the blood vessels; it contains various white blood cells, smooth muscle cells, connective tissue (collagen), cholesterol and other lipids, and eventually calcium.

atherosclerosis Buildup of fatty material (plaque) in the arteries, including those surrounding the heart.

menopause The cessation of menses in women, usually beginning at about age 50.

Two approaches have been shown to cause regression of atherosclerosis in the body. One employs a **vegan** diet and other lifestyle changes that are part of the Dr. Dean Ornish program. The other employs aggressive LDL lowering with medications.

vegan A person who eats only plant foods.

NUTRITION FOCUS

Lipoproteins and Cardiovascular Disease

Cardiovascular disease typically involves the coronary arteries and thus is frequently termed *coronary heart disease* (CHD) or *coronary artery disease* (CAD). Because the buildup of atherosclerosis slows blood flow in the arteries, the disease is also called *ischemic heart disease* (IHD). **Ischemia** represents an obstruction of blood flow. The general term for this obstruction is **stenosis.**

ischemia Lack of blood flow due to mechanical obstruction of the blood supply, mainly from arterial narrowing.

stenosis Narrowing or stricture of a duct or canal.

myocardial infarction Death of part of the heart muscle.

cerebrovascular accident (CVA) Death of part of the brain tissue due typically to a blood clot; also termed a stroke.

Healthy People 2010 has set a goal of reducing death from coronary heart disease by 30% compared with today's incidence.

homocysteine An amino acid not used in protein synthesis, but instead arises during metabolism of the amino acid methionine. Homocysteine is likely toxic to many cells, such as those lining the blood vessels.

A heart attack can strike with the sudden force of a sledgehammer, with pain radiating up the neck or down the arm. It can sneak up at night, masquerading as indigestion, with slight pain or pressure in the chest. Many times, the symptoms are so subtle in women that it often is too late once she or the health professional realizes that a heart attack is taking (or has recently taken) place. If there is any suspicion at all that a heart attack is taking place, the person should first chew an aspirin (325 mg) thoroughly and then call 911. Aspirin helps reduce the blood clotting that precipitates a heart attack. Typical warning signs are:

- Intense, prolonged chest pain or pressure, sometimes radiating to other parts of the upper body (men and women)
- Shortness of breath (men and women)
- Sweating (men and women)
- Nausea and vomiting (especially women)
- Dizziness (especially women)
- Weakness (men and women)
- Jaw, neck, and shoulder pain (especially women)
- Irregular heartbeat (men and women)

Cardiovascular disease (CVD) is the major killer of North Americans. Each year about 500,000 people die of coronary heart disease in the United States, about 60% more than die of cancer. The figure rises to almost 1 million if strokes and other circulatory diseases are included in the global term *cardiovascular disease*. About 1.5 million people in the United States each year have a heart attack. The overall male-to-female ratio for heart disease is about 2:1. Women generally lag about 10 years behind men in developing the disease. Still, it eventually kills more women than any other disease—twice as many as cancer. And for each person in North America who dies of cardiovascular disease, 20 more (over 13 million people) have symptoms of the disease.

Development of Cardiovascular Disease

The symptoms of cardiovascular disease develop over many years and often do not become obvious until old age. Nonetheless, autopsies of adults under 20 years of age have shown that many of them had atherosclerosis in their arteries. This finding indicates that atherosclerosis buildup can begin in childhood, although it usually goes undetected for quite some time.

Coronary heart disease and strokes are associated with inadequate blood circulation in the heart and brain. Blood supplies the heart muscle and brain—and other body organs—with oxygen and nutrients. When blood flow via the coronary arteries surrounding the heart is interrupted, the heart muscle can be damaged. A heart attack, or **myocardial infarction,** may result (Figure 6-14). This may cause the heart to beat irregularly or to stop altogether. About 25% of people do not survive their first heart attack. If blood flow to parts of the brain is interrupted long enough, part of the brain dies, causing a **cerebrovascular accident (CVA),** or stroke. When a stroke causes loss of muscle control, death may occur.

More than 95% of all heart attacks are caused by blood clots that stop blood flow to the heart or brain. Continuous formation and breakdown of blood clots in blood vessels is a normal process. However, in areas where atherosclerotic plaque has built up, clots are more likely to form a blockage, diminishing or cutting off the supply of blood to the arteries that serve the heart (coronary arteries) or brain (carotid arteries). Actually, the most dangerous lesions aren't the large, advanced ones but the smaller, unstable lesions covered by a thin fibrous cap. In essence, heart attacks generally are caused not by total blockage of the coronary arteries by plaque but by disruption of a partial blockage, leading to eventual clot formation.

Atherosclerotic plaque is probably first deposited to repair injuries in a vessel lining. It develops especially at points where an artery branches into two arteries. Much stress is placed on an artery at these points from the changes in blood flow that occur at the branch point. The *athero* in *atherosclerosis* comes from the Greek and means "gruel or paste." This process of damage repair is part of the initiation phase of atherosclerosis.

The damage that starts plaque formation can be caused by smoking, diabetes, hypertension, **homocysteine** (likely, but not a major factor), and LDL itself.[4,9,25] Viral and bacterial infections are also implicated as well as ongoing blood vessel inflammation.[12] (There is a test for this ongoing inflammation

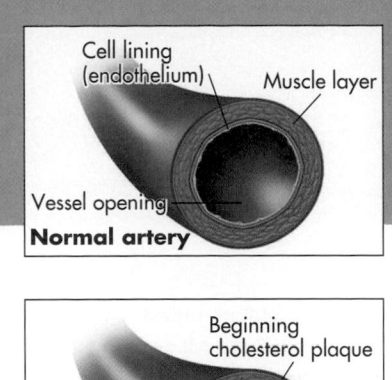

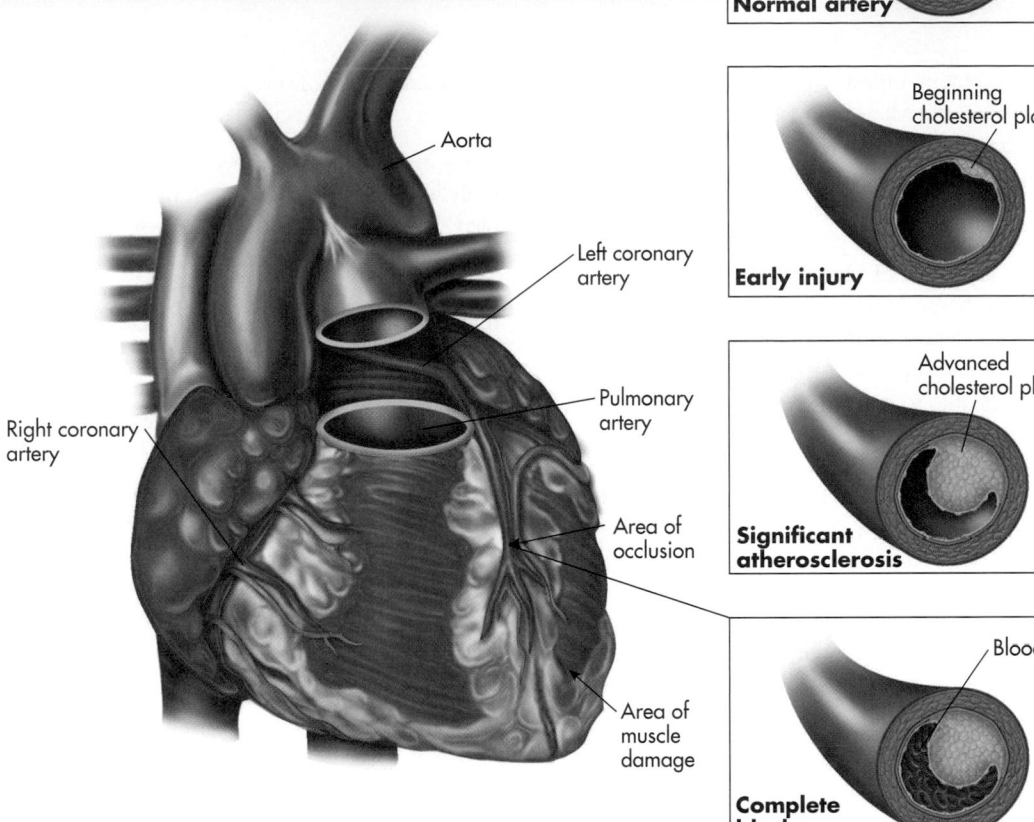

Figure 6-14 | The road to a heart attack. Injury to an artery wall begins the process. This is followed by a progressive buildup of plaque in the artery walls. The heart attack represents the terminal phase of the process. Blockage of the left coronary artery by a blood clot is evident. The heart muscle that is served by the portion of the coronary artery beyond the point of blockage lacks oxygen and nutrients and is damaged and may die. This damage can lead to a significant drop in heart function and often total heart failure.

[evidenced by elevated C-reactive protein in the blood]). Note also that these plaques can develop in arteries throughout the body, not just in the coronary arteries. This explains the use of the term *cardiovascular disease* to describe the general condition.

Some nutrients have antioxidant properties. These likely reduce LDL oxidation in the bloodstream and thus slow LDL uptake into scavenger cells, a process that was described in this chapter in the section titled Fats Carried in the Bloodstream. Fruits, vegetables, nuts, and plant oils are rich in such antioxidants (e.g., the various **carotenoids** and vitamin E). Eating fruits, vegetables, nuts, and plant oils regularly is one positive step we can take to reduce cholesterol buildup and slow the progression of cardiovascular disease.[6] Foods that are especially rich sources of antioxidants include red, black, and pinto beans; berries (blueberries, cranberries, blackberries, strawberries, etc.), fresh and dried plums (prunes); cherries; apples; pecans; and potatoes. (Coffee and tea are also sources.) Consuming

megadoses of antioxidant vitamins such as vitamin E to do the same thing is controversial. Chapter 9 will discuss this controversy in detail. Currently, the American Heart Association does not support the use of vitamin E in an effort to reduce cardiovascular disease risk.[16] Large-scale studies of people with existing cardiovascular disease have shown no benefit from megadose vitamin E therapy (200–400 mg/day; about 400–800 IU/day).[16,19] Other studies are ongoing, using people with cardiovascular disease and those with no evidence of such disease. Still, some experts suggest that megadose vitamin E use (up to 200 mg [400 IU] per day) may be helpful for *preventing* cardiovascular disease, but should be taken under a physician's guidance. This caution is because, in some cases, the megadose use of antioxidant supplements can cause harm, especially if one is taking certain anticoagulant medications or large doses of aspirin, which reduce blood clotting, because vitamin E also reduces blood clotting. On the other hand, an excessive intake of iron probably speeds LDL oxidation, making it unwise to take an

A number of large-scale trials testing the hypothesis that megadose vitamin E therapy (e.g., 600 IU every other day) can help prevent cardiovascular disease in otherwise healthy males and females are underway. The results for the females have recently been reported. This intervention generally failed to show any clear benefit. Results for the men are due by 2007.

carotenoids Plant pigments, in fruits and vegetables that range in color from yellow to orange to red.

When 28-year-old gold medalist Sergei Grinkov died suddenly of a heart attack while ice skating, researchers investigated the case and discovered a protein abnormality in his blood. This abnormal protein caused Grinkov's blood to clot more easily than normal. Grinkov was otherwise healthy, with an elevated total blood cholesterol, but normal HDL, blood triglycerides, and LDL. The main risk factor he had was that his father died of heart disease at the age of 52. It is thought that up to 25% of North Americans have this same protein abnormality and that the only sign is a family history of heart-related death under age 60. For this reason, it is wise for all adult North Americans to have a careful evaluation of cardiovascular disease risks conducted by a physician.

Most commonly, LDL-cholesterol is not actually measured in a serum sample but is calculated using the following equation: LDL-cholesterol = total cholesterol − HDL-cholesterol − (triglycerides/5). This formula cannot be used, however, if blood triglycerides are >350 mg/dl. Recently laboratories have also implemented a test that measures LDL-cholesterol directly (without the use of this formula). Refer to Table 6-4 for typical LDL-cholesterol cutoff values.

systolic blood pressure The pressure in the arterial blood vessels associated with the pumping of blood from the heart.

diastolic blood pressure The pressure in the arterial blood vessels when the heart is between beats.

iron supplement unless a physician prescribes it. People who experience iron storage disease and men in general should pay special attention to this warning (see Chapter 12).

In the next phase of the development of atherosclerosis, called the progression phase, plaque thickens as layers of cholesterol (part of LDL), connective tissue (collagen), smooth muscle, and calcium are deposited. Arteries harden and narrow as plaque builds up, making them less elastic. They are thus unable to expand to accommodate alterations in blood pressure.

Affected arteries become further damaged as blood pumps through them and pressure increases. Finally, in the terminal phase of this entire process, a clot or spasm in a plaque-clogged artery leads to a myocardial infarction.

Factors that typically bring on a heart attack in a person at risk include dehydration, acute emotional stress (such as firing an employee), strenuous physical activity when not otherwise physically fit (shoveling snow, for example), waking suddenly during the night or just getting up in the morning (linked to an abrupt increase in blood pressure and stress), and consuming high-fat meals (increases blood clotting).

Risk Factors for Cardiovascular Disease

Many of us are free of the risk factors that contribute to rapid development of atherosclerosis. If so, the advice of health experts is to simply consume a balanced diet, perform regular physical activity, have a complete fasting lipoprotein analysis performed at age 20 or beyond, and reevaluate risk factors every 5 years.[10]

People who face the highest risk for premature cardiovascular disease have genetic defects that substantially block the clearance of chylomicrons and triglycerides from the blood, reduce LDL uptake by the liver, limit synthesis of HDL, or enhance blood clotting. Other medical conditions, such as certain forms of liver and kidney disease, low concentrations of thyroid hormone, and use of certain medications to treat hypertension, can increase LDL and thus increase the risk for cardiovascular disease.

For most people, however, the most likely risk factors are:

- Total blood cholesterol over 200 mg/dl especially when it is at or over 240 mg/dl and coupled with LDL-cholesterol at or over 160 mg/dl (130 mg/dl is used for the cutoff if a person has two or more other risk factors).[10] The term *LDL-cholesterol* (and *HDL-cholesterol*) is used when expressing the serum concentration because it is the cholesterol content of these lipoproteins that is actually measured. The reference standard for expressing blood lipid concentrations also generally refers to the serum concentration. Recall that serum concentration is what remains after blood clots; blood is then centrifuged to remove all red and white blood cells and clotting factors. Although *blood cholesterol* is a common term, the value actually refers to the concentration in the serum portion of the blood.

- Smoking. The smoking factor generally negates the female advantage of later presentation of the disease and is the main cause of about 20% of cardiovascular disease deaths.[25] A combination of smoking and oral contraceptive use worsens matters even more. Smoking greatly increases the ultimate expression of a person's genetically linked risk for cardiovascular disease and even increases risk if one's blood lipids are low. Smoking also makes blood more likely to clot. Even exposure to secondhand smoke is discouraged.

- Hypertension. **Systolic blood pressure** over 140 (millimeters of mercury) and **diastolic blood pressure** over 90 indicate hypertension. More healthy blood pressure values are <120 and <80, respectively. (Treatment of hypertension is reviewed in Chapter 11.)

- Diabetes. This disease negates the female advantage. Insulin increases cholesterol synthesis in the liver, in turn increasing LDL release into the bloodstream. Recently, diabetes has even been removed from the list of risk factors, because its presence virtually guarantees development of cardiovascular disease and so puts such a person in the high-risk group even if LDL-cholesterol is not elevated.[4]

This group of four risk factors describes about 90% of the total risk for developing cardiovascular

hyperlipidemia The presence of an abnormally large amount of lipids in the circulating blood.

dyslipidemia Generally refers to a state in which various blood lipids, such as LDL or triglycerides, are markedly elevated or, in the case of HDL, very low.

metabolic syndrome A condition in which the person has poor blood glucose regulation, hypertension, increased blood triglycerides, and other health problems. This condition is usually accompanied by obesity, lack of physical activity; and a diet high in refined carbohydrates. Also called Syndrome X.

disease.[9] Still, other risk factors also need to be considered:

- HDL-cholesterol under 40 mg/dl, especially when the ratio of total cholesterol to HDL-cholesterol is 3.5:1 or less. Women often have high values for HDL-cholesterol; therefore it is important for this factor to be measured in women to establish cardiovascular disease risk. A value ≥60 mg/dl is especially protective.
- Age. Men over 45 years and women over 55 years are at greater risk.
- Family history of premature cardiovascular disease, especially before age 50.
- Obesity (especially fat accumulation in the waist). Typical adult weight gain is a chief contributor to the increase in LDL-cholesterol that is seen with aging. Obesity leads to insulin resistance in many people, creating a diabetes-like risk.[4] Obesity also increases inflammation in the body and reduces the production of the hormone adiponectin by adipose cells. High amounts of this hormone in the bloodstream contribute to a lower risk of developing a heart attack.
- Inactivity. Exercise conditions the arteries to adapt to physical stress. Regular exercise also improves insulin action in the body. The corresponding reduction in insulin output leads to a reduction in lipoprotein synthesis in the liver. Both regular aerobic exercise and resistance exercise are recommended.[8,26] A person with existing cardiovascular disease should seek physician approval before starting such a program, as should older adults (see Chapter 14).

Table 6-4 outlines some blood cholesterol profiles. If any of your blood cholesterol values fall in the category labeled "High," consult your physician because you may be at risk for cardiovascular disease. According to the National Heart, Lung, and Blood Institute, about 50% of all American adults have elevated blood cholesterol. The combined or individual risk factors of high LDL and high triglycerides are referred to as **hyperlipidemia** or **dyslipidemia.**

Researchers are currently trying to unravel and quantify still other factors that may be linked to premature cardiovascular disease. An example is the connection between inadequate intake of vitamin B-6, folate, and vitamin B-12, which can lead

Table 6-4 | Fasting Blood Cholesterol Profile (mg/dl)

LDL, Cholesterol	
<70	Therapeutic: If one has cardiovascular disease and other risk factors, such as diabetes
<100	Optimal
100–129	Near optimal/ above optimal
130–159	Borderline high
160–189	High
≥190	Very high
Total Cholesterol	
<200	Desirable
200–239	Borderline high
≥240	High
HDL, Cholesterol	
<40	Low
≥60	High
Triglycerides	
<100	Optimal
100–149	Near optimal
150–199	Borderline high
200–499	High
≥500	Very high

to increased homocysteine in the blood. Homocysteine damages the cells lining the blood vessels, in turn promoting atherosclerosis. It is probably only a minor risk factor, but likely causes some cases (see Chapter 10 for a detailed discussion of homocysteine).

The term *risk factor* is not intended to mean causality; nevertheless, the more risk factors one has, the greater the chances of ultimately developing cardiovascular disease. A good example is a person with **metabolic syndrome,** who would have abdominal obesity, high blood triglycerides, low HDL-cholesterol, hypertension, and evidence

As noted in the chapter, aspirin in small doses reduces blood clotting by reducing thromboxane A production; it is often used under a physician's guidance to treat people at risk for heart attack or stroke, especially if one has already occurred. About 80 to 160 mg/day is needed for such benefits. Individuals who may especially benefit from aspirin therapy are men over 40 if risk factors are present, men over 50 even if risk factors are not present, postmenopausal women, and people with diabetes, hypertension, or a family history of cardiovascular disease.[10]

of insulin resistance (e.g., high fasting blood glucose) and increased blood clotting. This profile raises the risk for cardiovascular disease considerably.[11] About 20 to 25% of North American adults are so affected. On a positive note, premature cardiovascular disease is rare in people who have low LDL-cholesterol, have normal blood pressure, and do not smoke or have diabetes. By minimizing these four risk factors, by following the dietary recommendations of the American Heart Association on pages 223–224 (such as limiting saturated fat, *trans* fat, and cholesterol intake) and by staying physically active, you will most likely reduce many of the other controllable risk factors listed.[8,15,25] In other words, develop and follow a total lifestyle plan. Medications may also be added to lower blood lipids, as discussed later in this chapter. Finally, if a person has a family history of cardiovascular disease but the usual risk factors aren't present, a rarer defect might be the cause. In this case, having a detailed physical examination for other potential causes is advised.

Medical Interventions for Cardiovascular Disease

Diet and lifestyle strategies to reduce cardiovascular disease risk are appropriate for both **primary prevention** (where a heart attack has not yet taken place but the person has risk factors or where clinical symptoms of cardiovascular disease are evident) and **secondary prevention** (after a heart attack has taken place). However, some people need even more aggressive therapy added to their regimen. The clearest indication for this more aggressive approach is in secondary prevention, but its use in primary prevention in cases of very abnormal blood lipoprotein patterns and diabetes also deserves consideration.

Medications are the cornerstone of this more aggressive therapy.[10] The National Cholesterol Education Program in the United States has developed a formula based on age, total blood cholesterol, HDL-cholesterol, smoking history, and blood pressure to determine who needs such medications. Check out this formula at http://hin.nhlbi.nih.gov/atpiii/calculator.asp. Currently, medications work to lower LDL-cholesterol in

one of two ways. Statins (e.g., fluvastatin [Lescol], lovastatin [Mevacor], simvistatin [Zocor]), and atorvastatin [Lipitor] reduce cholesterol synthesis in the liver. This then reduces the cholesterol content in the liver cells. The cells respond by increasing LDL receptor activity in order to pull cholesterol from the bloodstream to make up for the loss. Recall that LDL is 50% cholesterol. Statins can reduce LDL-cholesterol up to as much as 60%, depending on the drug used and the prescribed dosage. The cost of being on one of the statin drugs ranges from $1600–$13000 per year, depending on the dose needed. Use can also lead to side effects, such as muscle damage, and so requires physician supervision.[2]

A second group of medications binds bile acids in the small intestine, as does soluble fiber, and leads to their elimination, forcing the liver to synthesize new bile acids. The liver removes LDL from the blood to do this. For this reason, these drugs are called bile acid sequestrants or resins (e.g., cholestyramine [Questran] and colestipol [Colestid]). These medications taste gritty and therefore are not very popular with patients. Generally, the resins are not used alone in adults because of this unpleasant texture.

A third group of drugs can be used to lower blood triglycerides by decreasing the triglyceride production of the liver. These include gemfibrozil (Lopid) and megadoses of the vitamin nicotinic acid (extended-release form is called Niaspan). The use of nicotinic acid does result in pesky side effects (e.g., flushing), but these are typically manageable. Finally, a fourth, and relatively new class of drugs reduces cholesterol absorbtion from that found in bile in the small intestine (ezetimibe [Zetia]). Today it is very common to combine two or more medications to reach currently accepted goals for primary and secondary prevention (e.g., LDL of < 70 mg/dl for those at very high risk; review Table 6-4).[10]

It is troubling to note that, currently, many North American adults with evidence of cardiovascular disease quit risk-reducing therapy within the first year of diagnosis. Part of this problem is due to the cost and side effects of some of the medications typically used. Overall, mortality from cardiovascular disease is reduced when treatment to lower elevated LDL-cholesterol in people who

The two most common surgical treatments for coronary artery blockage are percutaneous transluminal coronary angioplasty (PTCA) and coronary artery bypass graft (CABG). PTCA involves the insertion of a balloon catheter into an artery. Once it is advanced to the area of the lesion, the balloon is expanded to crush the lesion. This method works best when only one vessel is blocked, and it may be held open with metal mesh, called a stent. CABG involves the removal and use of a saphenous vein from the leg or use of the mammary arteries. The saphenous vein or mammary artery is sewn to the main heart vessel (aorta). It is then used to bypass the blocked artery. The procedure can be performed on one or more blockages.[3]

are at high risk for such disease or who have had a heart attack is followed for a few years or more by a physician. Furthermore, new research shows that plaque even regresses in arteries when high LDL-cholesterol is treated aggressively.[10] It is suspected that these aggressive therapies to lower LDL-cholesterol stabilize the development of atherosclerotic plaque, thereby lowering the risk of rupture and reducing the chance of myocardial infarction caused by clot formation.

Other Possible Medical Therapies for Cardiovascular Disease

FDA has approved two margarines that have positive effects on blood cholesterol levels—Benecol and Take Control. As discussed in the section in this chapter titled Sterols, these margarines contain plant stanols/sterols. The plant stanols/sterols work by reducing cholesterol absorption in the small intestine and lowering its return to the liver. The liver responds by taking up more cho-

lesterol from the blood so it can continue to make bile acids. The studies done on the cholesterol-lowering effect of these margarines have found that 2 to 5 g of plant stanols/sterols per day reduces total blood cholesterol by 8 to 10% and LDL-cholesterol by 9 to 14% (similar to what is seen with some cholesterol-lowering drugs).[17,18]

Benecol is made from plant stanols that are extracted from wood pulp. This product is sold as margarine and has been added to salad dressings. Take Control is made from plant sterols that are isolated from soybeans. The recommended amount for both is about 2 to 3 g per day as part of at least two meals; this works out to about 2 tablespoons of Take Control or 1 tablespoon of Benecol per day. Use would cost about $1.00 per day, because these margarines are more expensive than regular margarines.

For people who have borderline high total blood cholesterol (between 200 and 239 mg/dl), these margarines can be helpful in avoiding future drug therapy. Recently plant stanols/sterols have also been made available in pill form and have been put in some brands of orange juice.

Another Dimension of Fat: Properties in Food

Various fats play important roles in foods. Much ingenuity must go into the production of fat-reduced products to preserve flavor and texture. In some cases, "fat-free" also means tasteless.

Fat in Food Provides Some Satiety and Flavor

Fat in foods has generally been considered to be the most **satiating** of all the macronutrients. However, this assumption has been called into question because recent studies show that protein and carbohydrate probably lead to more satiety (gram for gram). High-fat meals do provide satiety, but primarily because one consumes a lot of energy in the process. A high-fat meal is likely to be an energy-rich meal.

Fat components in foods provide important textures and carry flavors. If you've ever eaten a high-fat yellow cheese or cream cheese, you probably agree that fat melting on the tongue feels good. The fat in reduced-fat and whole milk also gives body, which fat-free milk lacks, and the most tender cuts of meat are high in fat, visible as the marbling

satiety A state in which there is no longer a desire to eat; a feeling of satisfaction.

Expert Opinion

Atherosclerosis: An Update
Bernhard Hennig, Ph.D., R.D.

Atherosclerosis: More Than High Blood Cholesterol

An extensive body of experimental as well as epidemiological evidence established a causal relationship between elevated blood cholesterol and atherosclerosis. Cholesterol-lowering medications that block cholesterol synthesis in the liver (e.g., atorvastatin [Lipitor] and other so-called statin medications) were developed to address this problem. Large clinical trials have demonstrated that statins can effectively decrease low-density lipoprotein (LDL) cholesterol and increase the activity of the LDL receptor. There is strong evidence that the reduction of LDL-cholesterol lowers the incidence of cardiovascular events in primary prevention (where a heart attack has not taken place but the person has risk factors or related clinical symptoms) and secondary prevention (after a heart attack has taken place). However, new research findings suggest that atherosclerosis is not just a passive process of lipid accumulation in blood vessels but rather is a chronic inflammatory process that results from the interactions between blood lipoproteins and cellular components derived from circulating white blood cells as well as from the endothelial cells, smooth muscle cells, and the extracellular contents of the arterial wall.

Overall Pathology of Atherosclerosis

The development of genetically modified laboratory animals has provided a powerful approach for studying individual genes and their relationship to different phases of the pathology of atherosclerosis. Strong evidence suggests that inflammatory processes mark all stages of atherosclerosis, from early endothelial cell activation to eventual rupture of the atherosclerotic plaque and clot formation. The inside lining of blood vessels is protected by the endothelium. The endothelial cells found there play an active role in physiological processes such as regulation of muscle tone, permeability of a blood vessel, and blood clotting. Activation and dysfunction of endothelial cells—for example, by oxidized LDL, infectious microorganisms, or free radicals associated with cigarette smoking—is a critical underlying cause of the initiation of the cardiovascular disease process. Endothelial cell activation, combined with an increase in the production of both inflammatory factors made by white blood cells and adhesion molecules, regulates not only the entry of white blood cells (primarily macrophages derived from circulating monocytes) into the blood vessel wall, but also a switch from anticoagulant-stimulating to coagulant-stimulating activity.

A fatty streak is formed as a result of macrophage uptake of oxidized LDL. Migrating and reproducing smooth muscle cells and platelets that are attracted to the site further augment the atherosclerotic lesion process. The continuous release of hydrolytic enzymes, inflammatory factors, and growth factors by cells within the vessel wall induces further damage, and eventually an atherosclerotic plaque with a fibrous cap forms. Eventual thinning and rupture of the fibrous cap covering the atherogenic plaque then is a stimulus to clotting events. Continued inflammation from the influx and activation of macrophages and the release of protein-digesting enzymes causes degradation of the vessel. This rupture then leads to possible hemorrhage, clot formation, and final arterial blockage.

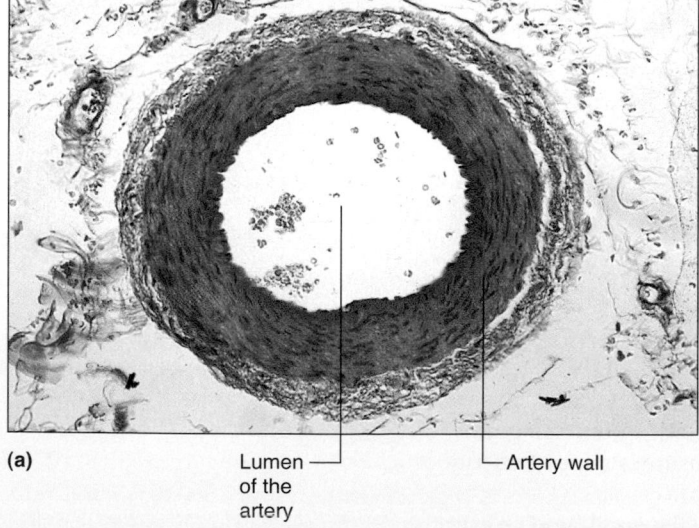

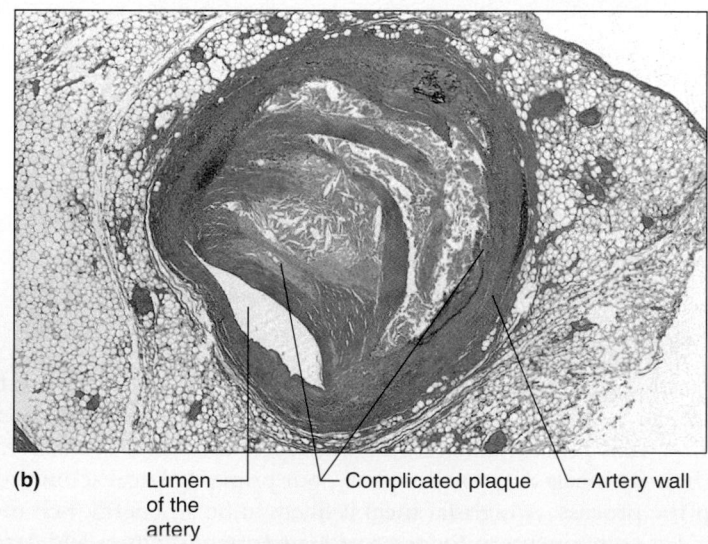

(a) Lumen of the artery — Artery wall

(b) Lumen of the artery — Complicated plaque — Artery wall

Atherosclerosis. (a) Cross section of a healthy coronary artery. (b) Cross section of a coronary artery with advanced atherosclerosis.

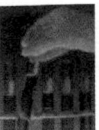

New Developments in Atherosclerosis

Oxidative stress and a low level of chronic inflammation are believed to be critical underlying factors in the pathology of atherosclerosis. A major factor in inflammatory responses is nuclear factor Kappa B (κB). This nuclear factor binds to specific sites on DNA and in turn activates associated genes. It resides in the cytosol of a cell in an inactive (bound) form. Once released (now in unbound form) through the action of oxidative stress and various inflammatory factors, it then travels to the nucleus and binds to DNA. This oxidative stress-sensitive process is critical in the regulation of inflammatory and immune system genes, cell reproduction, and cell death. Overall, as the binding of this nuclear factor to DNA increases, so does further inflammation and oxidative damage. New research suggests that blood levels of C-reactive protein (CRP) provide a predictive value for this inflammation and the degree of cardiovascular disease.

Understanding molecular aspects of production and inhibition of cyclooxygenase enzymes (COX), and especially COX-2, will help explain the involvement of the eicosanoids in the overall pathology of atherosclerosis. Many studies also are underway to understand regulatory mechanisms of nitric oxide synthesis. Nitric oxide is a signaling molecule that regulates many aspects of atherosclerosis, including oxidative stress, platelet aggregation, white blood cell adherence, smooth muscle cell reproduction, and blood pressure.

High-density lipoproteins (HDL) are important in reverse cholesterol transport by accepting cholesterol from cells throughout the body, including macrophages, and by interacting with scavenger receptors and cholesterol transporters. Of special interest are also HDL-associated enzymes called paraoxonases, which protect blood lipids from oxidation, decrease macrophage uptake of oxidized LDL, and inhibit cholesterol synthesis.

Exciting areas of recent research include the protective effects of peroxisome proliferator activated receptors. These are a family of nuclear receptors that bind specific compounds, such as unsaturated fatty acids and certain medications. This binding to DNA via this receptor then ultimately controls the activity of key genes involved in the regulation of metabolism, inflammation, and clotting. The receptors are found in blood vessels, including endothelial cells. Medications that increase activity of these receptors, such as fibrates used in treating elevated blood triglycerides (e.g., gemfibrozil [Lopid]) and glitazones used in treating diabetes (e.g., rosiglitazone [Avandia]) have been shown in some (but not all) studies to reduce inflammation in response to a variety of stimuli.

New Risk Factors and Explanations

In addition to traditional risk factors, such as age, gender, blood cholesterol, blood pressure, and smoking, more recent risk factors include high blood triglycerides (triglyceride-rich lipoprotein remnants, and free fatty acids as well), diabetes (glycemic load of the diet and insulin resistance in the person), smaller LDL particles, lipoprotein (a), angiotensin II (a factor involved in blood pressure regulation; discussed further in Chapter 11), C-reactive protein, modified (e.g., oxidized or otherwise altered) LDL, elevated blood homocysteine, and obesity. Even stress, depression, and loneliness are getting attention as important factors to consider.

Obesity, in particular increased abdominal fat or fat accumulation around organs, is an especially important risk factor for atherosclerosis that needs more attention because of its association with high blood lipids, diabetes and insulin resistance, hypertension, reduced output of the beneficial hormone adiponectin by enlarged adipose cells, and the metabolic syndrome. There also is evidence that an increase in this overall oxidative stress and inflammation in the body may be an important mechanism by which obesity increases the incidence of atherosclerosis.

Treatment Options for Atherosclerosis

Nutrition, including a healthy lifestyle and aerobic exercise, should remain the primary focus on prevention and treatment of atherosclerosis and related cardiovascular diseases. A major goal for our diets should be decreased consumption of refined foods (e.g., foods high in energy but lacking nutrients and phytochemical compounds that exhibit antioxidant and anti-inflammatory properties). Obesity and associated risk factors and a sedentary lifestyle with lack of physical activity are critical obstacles in conquering blood vessel diseases such as atherosclerosis. A diet high in whole foods; fiber and antioxidant nutrients, including micronutrients (e.g., zinc, selenium); vitamins E and C; carotenoids; and numerous polyphenols (e.g., resveratrol, quercetin) will help to control and reduce not only oxidative insults and inflammation but also high blood lipids and high blood glucose typically seen after meals. For example, polyphenolic phytochemicals stabilize the blood vessel endothelium both as antioxidants and as molecules that help regulate these cells. Furthermore, regular aerobic exercise induces protective cardiovascular adaptations by, for example, inducing genes that code for antioxidant enzymes and antiatherogenic signaling pathways (e.g., nitric oxide produced by endothelial cells). The medications mentioned in this Expert Opinion, as well as others that affect inflammatory processes and blood pressure regulation, (e.g., medications that block the action of angiotensin II) may also be a necessary part of the overall treatment approach for blood vessel diseases such as atherosclerosis. Finally, individual genetic profiling and related technologies will assist in future therapeutic approaches in health and disease.

Dr. Hennig is Professor in Nutrition and Toxicology at the University of Kentucky. He received his Ph.D. in biochemistry and nutrition from Iowa State University. After a postdoctoral appointment with the Cardiovascular Center, College of Medicine at the University of Iowa, Iowa City, Dr. Hennig joined the University of Kentucky. His research emphasis can be summarized as the utilization of tissue culture and animal models in the study of nutrition, toxicology, and atherosclerosis, with an emphasis in the role of nutrients and toxins on biochemical and molecular mechanisms of vessel endothelial cell function, injury, and protection. Dr. Hennig has published extensively and has received several national award recognitions for his research.

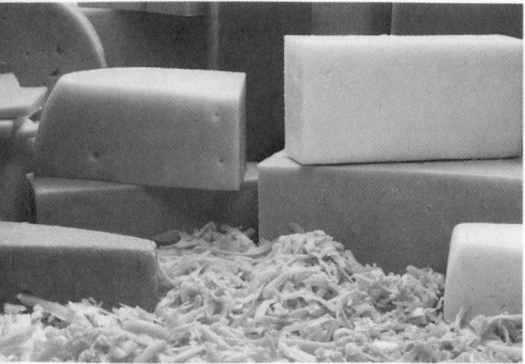

Fat is an important component of the flavor and overall appeal of cheese.

hydrogenation The addition of hydrogen to a carbon-carbon double bond, producing a single carbon-carbon bond with two hydrogens attached to each carbon. Because hydrogenation of unsaturated fatty acids in a vegetable oil increases its hardness, this process is used to convert liquid oils into more solid fats, which are used in making margarine and shortening. *Trans* fatty acids are a by-product of hydrogenation of vegetable oils.

of meat. In addition, many flavorings dissolve in fat. Heating spices in oil intensifies the flavors of an Indian curry or a Mexican dish by carrying the flavors to the sensory cells in the mouth that discriminate taste and smell. For these reasons, a person who has been following a typical North American diet will probably need some time to adjust to the taste of a lower-fat diet. For example, if one changes from drinking whole milk to 1% low-fat milk but then after a few weeks switches back to the whole milk, it will taste more like cream than milk. One has thus adjusted to the flavor of the low-fat milk and will likely now find the whole milk to be not as palatable.

Hydrogenation of Fatty Acids in Food Production Increases *Trans* Fatty Acid Content

As mentioned previously, most fats with long-chain saturated fatty acids are solid at room temperature, and those with unsaturated fatty acids are liquid at room temperature. In some kinds of food production, solid fats work better than liquid oils. In pie crust, for example, solid fats yield a flaky product, whereas crusts made with liquid oils tend to be greasy and more crumbly. If they are used to replace solid fats, oils with unsaturated fatty acids often must be made more saturated (with hydrogen), because this solidifies the vegetable oils into shortenings and margarines. Hydrogen is added by bubbling hydrogen gas under pressure into liquid vegetable oils in a process called **hydrogenation** (Figure 6-15). The fatty acids aren't fully hydrogenated to the saturated fatty acid form, because this would make the product too hard and brittle. Partial hydrogenation—leaving some monounsaturated fatty acids—creates a semisolid product.

Figure 6-15 | How liquid oils become solid fats. (*a*) Unsaturated fatty acids are present in liquid form. (*b*) Hydrogens are added (hydrogenation), changing some carbon-carbon double bonds to single bonds and producing some *trans* fatty acids. (*c*) The partially hydrogenated product is likely to be used in margarine or shortening or for deep-fat frying.

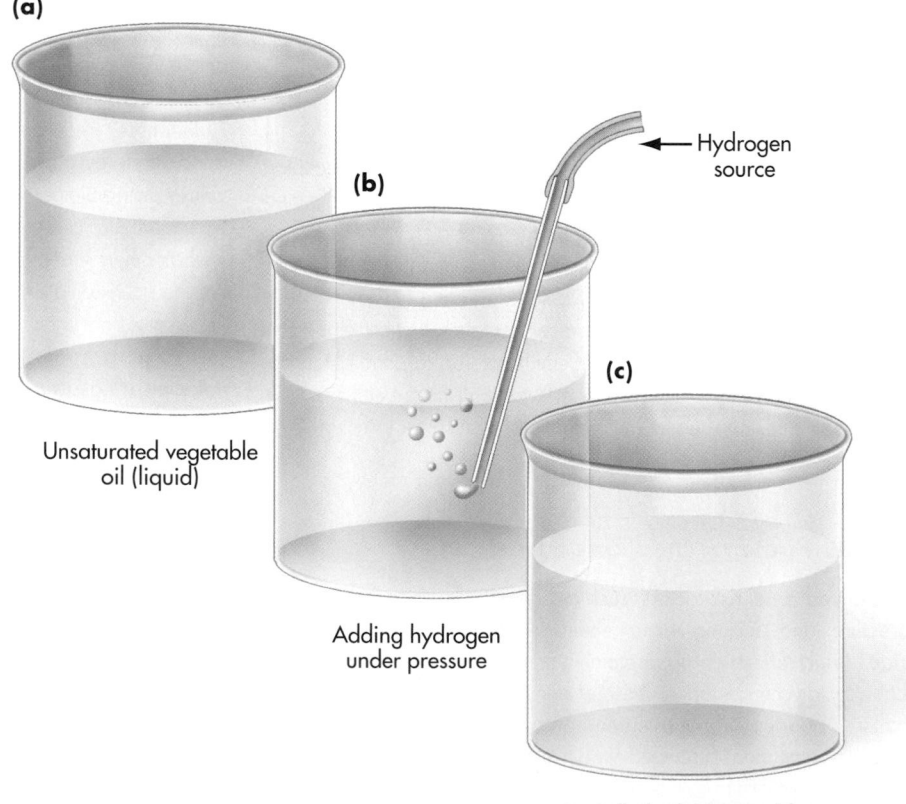

The process of hydrogenation produces *trans* fatty acids, as was described earlier in this chapter. Most natural monounsaturated and polyunsaturated fatty acids exist in the *cis* form, causing a bend in the carbon chain, whereas the straighter carbon forms of *trans* fat more closely resemble saturated fatty acids. This may be the mechanism whereby *trans* fats increase LDL. In addition, *trans* fats lower HDL and increase inflammation in the body. People with elevated LDL especially should limit intake of partially hydrogenated fat and thus *trans* fat. The average person need not be overly concerned as long as *trans* fat intake is not excessive and the diet is adequate in polyunsaturated fat. However, because *trans* fatty acids serve no particular role in maintaining body health, the latest Dietary Guidelines for Americans, the American Heart Association, and the Food and Nutrition Board each recommend minimal *trans* fat intake.[7,15]

As public pressure has persuaded manufacturers to eliminate the tropical oils rich in saturated fat (palm, palm olein, and coconut) from food processing, partially hydrogenated soybean oil—rich in *trans* fat—has become the major replacement. Currently, *trans* fat intake in North America is estimated to contribute about 3 to 4% of total energy intakes, amounting to 10g per day, on average. Table 6-5 lists typical sources.

FDA is now requiring the *trans* fat content in foods on the Nutrition Facts label. (The food labels in Canada also must list *trans* fat content.) FDA hopes to make consumers more aware of the amounts of *trans* fat in foods as well as the negative health consequences associated with their excessive consumption. North American companies are already responding to this issue by creating products that are free of *trans* fat. For example, Promise, Smart Beat, and some Fleischmann's margarines are lower in or free of *trans* fat (less than 0.5 g/serving is the labeling standard for *trans*-free) compared to typical margarines.

This addition of the *trans* fat listing on labels helps consumers at the supermarket, but when dining out, consumers are "left in the dark" as to which foods contain *trans* fat. Knowing which foods are low in *trans* fat when ordering at a restaurant is difficult because information about preparation methods and precise fat composition is rarely available. To minimize *trans* fat intake, a general guideline is to limit consumption of

You may be surprised to learn that some *trans* fatty acids occur naturally. The bacteria that live in the rumens of some animals (cows, sheep, and goats, for example) produce *trans* fatty acids that eventually appear in foods such as beef, milk, and butter. These naturally occurring *trans* fats are currently under study for possible health benefits, including prevention of cancer. About 20% of *trans* fatty acids in our diets come from this source.[17]

Table 6-5 | Total Fat, Saturated Fat, and *Trans* Fat Content of Typical Sources of *Trans* Fat (in descending order of *trans* fat)

Food Item	Serving Size	Fat (grams)	Saturated Fat (grams)	*Trans* Fat (grams)
French fried potatoes (fast-food variety)	Medium size	26.9	6.7	7.8
Doughnut	1	18.2	4.7	5.0
Cake, pound	1 slice	16.4	3.4	4.3
Shortening	1 tbsp	13.0	3.4	4.2
Potato chips	Small bag	11.2	1.9	3.2
Margarine, stick	1 tbsp	11.0	2.1	2.8
Cookies (cream-filled)	3	6.1	1.2	1.9
Margarine, tub	1 tbsp	6.7	1.2	0.6
Butter	1 tbsp	10.8	7.2	0.3
Milk, whole	1 cup	6.6	4.3	0.2
Mayonnaise (soybean oil)	1 tbsp	10.8	1.6	0

The five major sources of *trans* fat are (in order): cakes, cookies, crackers, pies, and bread; margarine; fried potatoes; potato chips, corn chips, and popcorn; and shortening used in the home.

Source: http://www.cfsan.fda.gov/~dms/qatrans2.html

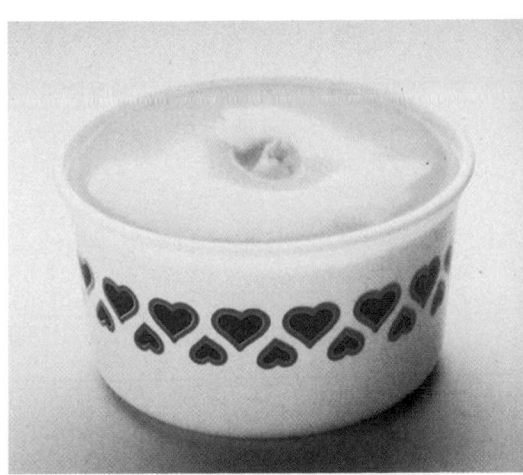

Tub margarine is much lower in *trans* fat than stick margarine or shortenings. Some newer brands of tub margarines are even free of *trans* fatty acids (< 0.5 g/serving).

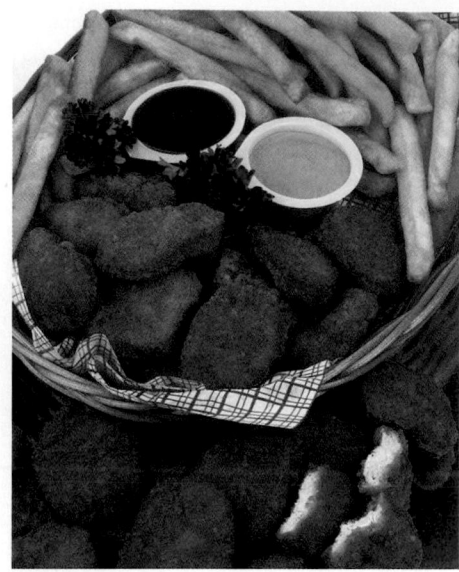

French fries and other fried foods are a common source of fat and *trans* fatty acids for many adults. For those who choose to consume these products on a regular basis a small serving size is recommended, especially if a person has elevated blood lipids.

rancid Containing products of decomposed fatty acids; they yield unpleasant flavors and odors.

BHA, BHT Butylated hydroxyanisole and butylated hydroxytoluene—two common synthetic antioxidants added to foods.

fried (especially deep-fat fried) food items, any pastries or flaky bread products (such as pie crusts, crackers, croissants, and biscuits), and cookies.

Limiting *trans* fat at home is a much easier task. Most importantly, use little or no stick margarine or shortening. Instead, substitute vegetable oils and softer tub margarines (those whose labels list vegetable oil or water as the first ingredient). Avoid deep-fat frying any food in shortening. Substitute baking, panfrying, broiling, steaming, grilling, or deep-fat frying in unhydrogenated vegetable oils. Replace nondairy creamers with reduced-fat or fat-free milk, because most nondairy creamers are rich in partially hydrogenated vegetable oils. Finally, read the ingredients on food labels, using the tips listed in this section to estimate *trans* fat content.

Fat Rancidity Limits Shelf Life of Foods

Decomposing oils emit a disagreeable odor and taste sour and stale. Stale potato chips are a good example. The double bonds in unsaturated fatty acids break down, producing rancid by-products. Ultraviolet light, oxygen, and certain procedures can break double bonds and, in turn, destroy the structure of polyunsaturated fatty acids. Saturated fats and *trans* fats can much more readily resist these effects because they contain fewer carbon-carbon double bonds.

Rancidity is not a major problem for consumers because, although eating rancid oils can cause sickness, the odor and taste generally discourage us from eating enough to become sick. However, rancidity is a problem for manufacturers because it reduces a product's shelf life. To increase shelf life, manufacturers often add partially hydrogenated plant oils to products. Foods most likely to become rancid are deep-fried foods and foods with a large amount of exposed surface (such as powdered eggs or powdered milk). The fat in fish is also very susceptible to rancidity because it is highly polyunsaturated.

Antioxidants such as vitamin E help protect foods against becoming **rancid.** Antioxidants guard against the fat breakdown caused by various agents, such as metals found as impurities in vegetable oils. The vitamin E in plant oils reduces the breakdown of double bonds in fatty acids. (The role of vitamin E is explained more fully in Chapter 9.) When food manufacturers want to prevent rancidity in polyunsaturated fats, they often add the synthetic antioxidants **BHA** and **BHT.** (Chapter 19 discusses the safety of these and other food additives.) Look for these food additives in salad dressings, cake mixes, and other products that contain fat. They can even be added to a food's paper packaging. Vitamin C may also be added for the same reason. Manufacturers also tightly seal products and use other methods to reduce oxygen levels inside packages.

Emulsifiers Improve Many Food Products

Food manufacturers add emulsifiers in the preparation of many food products, primarily to improve texture. For example, lecithins, monoglycerides and diglycerides, polysorbate 60, and other emulsifiers are added to salad dressings to keep the vegetable oil suspended in water (review Figure 6-8). Eggs added to cake batters likewise emulsify the fat with the milk. Monoglycerides and related compounds are also good emulsifiers and, for that reason, are sometimes used in cake mixes and salad dressings. Over the next few days, examine the labels of salad dressings and cake mixes, and see how many emulsifiers are listed.

Concept | Check

Fat has a variety of roles in foods, including that of contributing to flavor and texture. Fat also provides the pleasurable mouth feel of many of our favorite foods, intensifies the taste of many spices, and tenderizes many popular cuts of meat.

Hydrogenation of unsaturated fatty acids is the process of adding hydrogen to carbon-carbon double bonds to produce single bonds. This results in the creation of some *trans* fatty acids. Hydrogenation changes vegetable oil to solid fat. It is wise to monitor *trans* fat intake, because this form of fat raises LDL, lowers HDL, and increases inflammation in the body.

The carbon-carbon double bonds in polyunsaturated fatty acids are easily broken, yielding products responsible for rancidity. The presence of antioxidants, such as vitamin E in oils, naturally protects unsaturated fatty acids against oxidative destruction. Manufacturers can use hydrogenated fats and add natural or synthetic antioxidants to reduce the likelihood of rancidity.

Emulsifiers, such as lecithins, monoglycerides and diglycerides, and polysorbate 60 are added to salad dressings and other fat-rich products to keep the vegetable oils and other fats suspended in the water.

Recommendations for Fat Intake

There is no RDA for total fat intake for adults, although there is an Adequate Intake set for total fat for infants (see Chapter 17). The most specific recommendations for fat intake come from the American Heart Association (AHA).[15] Because many North Americans are at risk for developing cardiovascular disease, AHA promotes dietary and lifestyle goals aimed at reducing this risk. The AHA recommendations for the general public are presented in Table 6-6. In Table 6-7, a more detailed list of recommendations is provided for people who currently are at high risk or have cardiovascular disease.

To reduce risk for cardiovascular disease, the AHA recommends that total fat intake should not exceed 20 to 30% of total energy intake, which equates to 47 to 70 g/day for a person who consumes 2100 kcal daily. Within that fat allowance, no more than 7 to 10% of total energy intake should come from saturated fat and *trans* fat combined. These are the primary fatty acids that raise LDL. In addition, cholesterol should amount to a maximum of 200 to 300 mg/day.[7,15] Table 6-8 is an example of a diet that adheres to these guidelines. Compare these recommendations to North Americans' actual dietary intake patterns of these fats: 33% of energy from total fat, about 13% of energy from saturated fat, and 180 to 320 mg of cholesterol each day.

Both the National Cholesterol Education Program (NCEP) and the Food and Nutrition Board are in agreement with the advice of the AHA. One exception in the latest guidelines from the NCEP is that fat intake could be as high as 35% of total energy intake as long as intakes of saturated fat, cholesterol, and *trans* fat are minimized. The Food and Nutrition Board combines the AHA and NCEP recommendations, suggesting that fat provide a range of 20 to 35% of energy intake.[7] It is important to

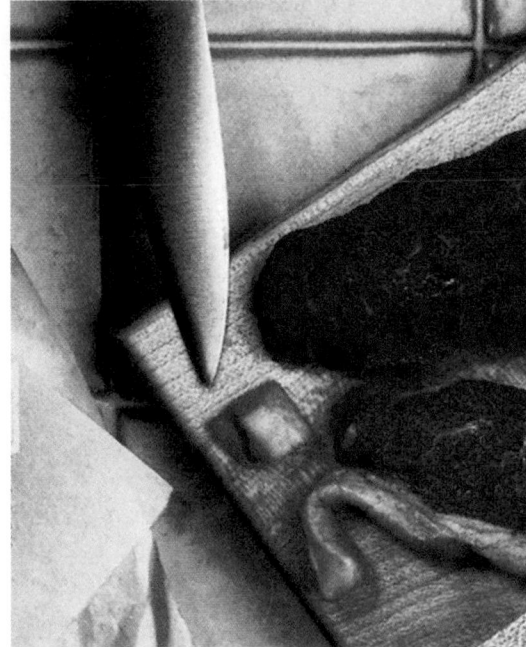

Trimming the fat from meats before cooking helps reduce your saturated fat intake. Also, limit use of meat that is highly marbled with fat (seen as streaks of fat).

Moderating alcohol and sugar intake, avoiding overeating and obesity, consuming fish on a regular basis, not smoking, and performing regular physical activity are the primary lifestyle interventions to lower blood triglycerides.[15]

One goal of *Healthy People 2010* is to increase the proportion of persons age 2 years and older who consume less than 10% of energy intake from saturated fat.

Table 6-6 | Current Dietary Guidance for the General Population (2 Years of Age and Older) from the American Heart Association

Population Goals	Major Guidelines
Overall healthy eating pattern	Include a variety of fruits, vegetables, grains, low-fat or fat-free dairy products, fish, legumes, poultry, and lean meats.
Appropriate body weight	Match energy intake to overall needs, with appropriate changes to achieve weight loss when indicated.
Desirable blood cholesterol profile	Limit foods high in saturated fat and cholesterol, and substitute unsaturated fat from vegetables, fish, legumes, and nuts.
Desirable blood pressure	Limit salt and alcohol (see Table 6-7); maintain a healthy body weight; and follow a diet with an emphasis on vegetables, fruits, and low-fat or fat-free dairy products.

Exercising for at least 45 minutes four times a week can increase HDL by about 5 mg/dl. Losing excess weight (especially around the waist) and avoiding smoking and overeating also help maintain or raise HDL, as does moderate alcohol consumption.[15]

Table 6-7 | Specific Dietary Recommendations from the American Heart Association, Especially for Those People at High Risk or Who Currently Have Cardiovascular Disease

Diet	Consume at least:
	• 5 servings of fruits and vegetables each day. Up to 9 servings per day is advised if the person has hypertension. • 6 servings of grains, including some whole grains, each day. • At least 2 (3-oz) servings of fish per week (or 1 g of a combination of omega-3 fatty acids from fish oil supplements per day). • 25 g of fiber each day, including some sources of soluble fiber.*
	Consume no more than: • 30% of energy intake from total fat or 20% if blood lipids are still too high. • 10% of energy intake as saturated fat, or 7% if blood lipids are still too high, as well as limit *trans* fat intake (included in saturated fat gram allowance). • 300 mg of cholesterol per day (on average), or 200 mg per day if blood lipids are still too high or the person has diabetes or cardiovascular disease. • 6 g of salt each day (6 g equals 2400 mg of sodium). • 2 alcoholic drinks per day for men or one drink for women or anyone age 65 and older.
	Additional advice includes: • Specifically meeting vitamin B-6, folate, vitamin B-12, and potassium needs, limiting sugar intake, and possible use of soy protein and stanol/sterol-containing margarines. Megadose vitamin E supplements are not recommended at this time, and vitamin C and beta-carotene supplements provide no benefit.
Body weight	• Maintain a **body mass index** between 18.5 and 25. Waist circumference should not exceed 40 inches (102 centimeters) in men or 35 inches (88 centimeters) in women (see Chapter 13 for details).
Physical activity	• 30 to 60 minutes of brisk activity on most, if not all, days of the week.

These specific recommendations apply to individuals 2 years of age and older. The latest guidelines from the National Cholesterol Education Program in the United States also concur with this advice for high-risk individuals, except that fat could be as high as 35% of total energy intake if saturated fat intake is 7% of energy intake or less and cholesterol intake does not exceed 200 mg/day.

*Note that the latest guidance for fiber from the Food and Nutrition Board is that men consume 38 g/day, while 25 g/day is fine for women.

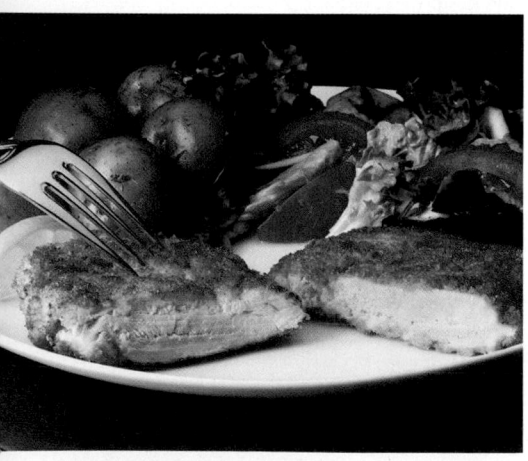

If you are looking to decrease the amount of saturated and *trans* fats in your diet, it is a good idea to opt for lower-fat substitutes for some your current high-fat food choices. How do you think this meal compares with the chicken nuggets and french fries meal on p. 222?

note that in addition to fat intake, controlling total energy intake is also significant, because weight control is a vital component of cardiovascular disease prevention.

Regarding essential fatty acids, the Food and Nutrition Board has issued recommendations for both omega-6 and omega-3 fatty acids. The amounts listed here work out to about 5% of energy intake for the total of both essential fatty acids.[7] Infants and children have lower needs (see Chapter 17). Consumption of fish at least twice a week is one step toward meeting requirements for essential fatty acids.

	Men (g/day)	Women (g/day)
Linoleic acid (omega-6)	17	12
Alpha-linolenic acid (omega-3)	1.6	1.1

The typical North American diet derives about 7% of energy from polyunsaturated fatty acids and thus meets essential fatty acid needs. An upper limit of 10% of energy intake as polyunsaturated fatty acids is often recommended, in part because the breakdown (oxidation) of those fatty acids present in lipoproteins is linked to increased cho-

Table 6-8 | Daily Menu Examples Containing 2000 kcal and 30 or 20% of Energy as Fat

30% of Energy as Fat		20% of Energy as Fat	
Food	Fat (g)	Food	Fat (g)
Breakfast			
Orange juice, 1 cup	0.5	Same	0.5
Shredded wheat, 3/4 cup	0.5	Shredded wheat, 1 cup	0.7
Toasted bagel	1.1	Same	1.1
Tub margarine, 3 teaspoons	11.4	Tub margarine, 2 teaspoons	7.6
1% low-fat milk, 1 cup	2.5	Fat-free milk, 1 cup	0.6
Lunch			
Whole-wheat bread, 2 slices	2.4	Same	2.4
Roast beef, 2 ounces	4.9	Light turkey roll, 2 ounces	0.9
Mayonnaise, 3 teaspoons	11.0	Mayonnaise, 2 teaspoons	7.3
Lettuce	—	Same	—
Tomato	—	Same	—
Oatmeal cookie, 1	3.3	Oatmeal cookie, 2	6.6
Snack			
Apple	—	Same	—
Dinner			
Chicken tenders frozen meal	18.0	Fat-free chicken tenders	—
Dinner roll, 1	2.0	Same	2.0
Margarine, 1 teaspoon	3.8	Same	3.8
Banana	0.6	Same	0.6
1% low-fat milk, 1 cup	2.5	Fat-free milk, 1 cup	0.6
Carrot sticks, 10	—	Same	
Snack			
Raisins, 2 teaspoons	—	Raisins, 1/2 cup	—
Air-popped popcorn, 3 cups	1.0	Air-popped popcorn, 6 cups	2.0
Margarine, 2 teaspoons	7.6	Same	7.6
Totals	**73.1**		**44.3**

Monitoring by a physician is important if fat is restricted to 20% of energy intake because the resulting increase in carbohydrate intake can increase blood triglycerides in some people, which is not a healthful change. Over time, however, the initial problem of high blood triglycerides on a low-fat diet may self-correct, as has been shown in people following a vegan diet for a year or more. Their blood triglycerides increased initially on the diet but, within a year, fell to normal values as long as they emphasized carbohydrate sources high in fiber, controlled (or improved) body weight, and followed a regular exercise program.

lesterol deposition in the arteries. Depression of immune function is also suspected to be caused by an excessive intake of polyunsaturated fatty acids.[7]

Major sources of fat in the typical North American diet include animal flesh, whole milk, pastries, cheese, margarine, and mayonnaise. In contrast, the major sources of fat in the Mediterranean diet include liberal amounts of olive oil and the fat found in the small amounts of animal flesh and dairy products in the diet. The main sources of fat in a vegan diet plan are a scant amount of vegetable oil used in cooking and the small amounts found in various plant foods.

In summary, the general consensus among nutrition experts suggests that limitation of saturated fat, cholesterol, and *trans* fat intake should be the primary focus and that the diet needs to contain some omega-3 and omega-6 fatty acids (Table 6-9). Furthermore, if fat intake exceeds 30% of total energy intake, the extra fat should come from monounsaturated fat.[7]

Most people probably have no idea how much of the energy content of their diets comes from fat. Using the information on food labels and recording and analyzing daily food intake allows you to track your fat intake.

Fats in Food

Table 6-9 provides an example of the amount of fat in foods in a day's menu. The foods richest in fat are salad oils, butter, margarine, and mayonnaise. All contain close to 100% of energy as fat (Table 6-10). In fat-reduced margarines, water replaces some

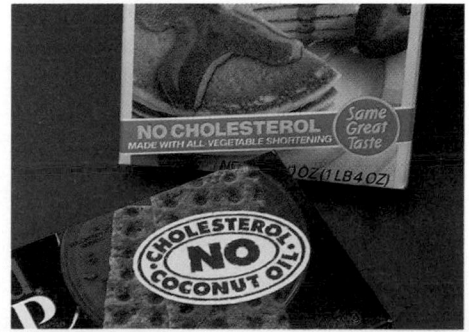

Manufacturers now offer a variety of low cholesterol foods.

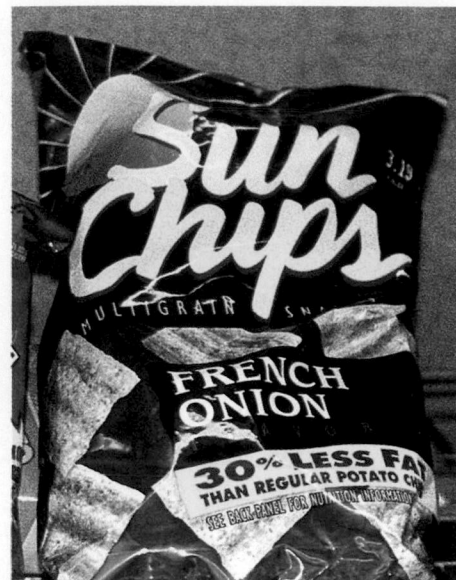

Many manufacturers offer products that are lower in fat than the traditional product. Even though these products are lower in fat, portion size and the total calories supplied still must be considered.

T he advice to consume 20 to 30% of energy as fat does not apply to infants and toddlers below the age of 2 years. These youngsters are forming new tissue that requires fat, especially in the brain, so their intake of fat and cholesterol should not be greatly restricted.[7]

C holesterol is found only in the animal foods we eat (review Table 6-2). An egg yolk contains about 210 mg of cholesterol. This is our main dietary source of cholesterol, along with meats and whole milk. Some plants contain related sterols, but none we typically eat contains cholesterol.[17]

Table 6-9 | Tips for Avoiding Too Much Fat, Saturated Fat, Cholesterol, and *Trans* Fat

	Eat Less of These Foods	Eat More of These Foods
Grains, cereals, rice, and pasta	• Pasta dishes with cheese or cream sauces • Croissants • Pie crust	• Whole-grain breads • Whole-grain pasta • Brown rice
Vegetables	• French fries • Vegetables cooked in butter, cheese, or cream sauces	• Fresh, frozen, baked, or steamed vegetables
Fruit	• Fruit pies	• Fresh, frozen, or canned fruits
Milk, yogurt, and cheese	• Whole milk • High-fat cheese	• Fat-free and reduced-fat milk • Reduced-fat/part-skim cheese
Meats, poultry, fish, dry beans, eggs, and nuts	• Bacon • Sausage • Organ meats (e.g., liver) • Egg yolks	• Fish • Skinless poultry • Lean cuts of meat (with fat trimmed away) • Soy products • Egg whites/egg substitutes
Fats, oils, and sweets	• Butter and stick margarine • Cheesecake • Pastries • Doughnuts • Ice cream • Potato chips	• Angel food cake • Fig bars • Animal or graham crackers • Air-popped popcorn • Low-fat frozen desserts (e.g., yogurt, sherbet, ice milk) • Canola oil or olive oil • Tub or liquid margarine (in small amounts)

of the fat. Typical margarines are 80% fat by weight (11 g/tbsp). Some fat-reduced margarines are as low as 30% fat by weight (4 g/tbsp). The extra water added to these margarines can cause texture and volume changes when used in recipes.[1] Cookbooks can provide guidance for appropriate use of these products by suggesting alterations in recipes to compensate.

Walnuts, bologna, avocados, and bacon have about 80% of energy as fat. Peanut butter and cheddar cheese have about 75%. Marbled steak and hamburgers (ground chuck) have about 60%, and chocolate bars, ice cream, doughnuts, and whole milk have about 50% of energy as fat. Eggs, pumpkin pie, and cupcakes have 35%, as do lean cuts of meat, such as top round (and ground round) and sirloin. Bread contains about 15%. Cornflakes, sugar, and nonfat milk have essentially no fat. Careful label reading is necessary to determine the true fat content of food—these are only rough guidelines.

Animal fats, which contain about 40 to 60% of total fat as saturated fatty acids, are the chief contributors of saturated fatty acids to the North American diet. Saturated fatty acids with 12, 14, and 16 carbons (lauric acid, myristic acid, and palmitic acid, respectively) are the primary contributors to elevated LDL. Of these, the 14-carbon myristic acid is mainly responsible for elevating LDL.[7] Dairy fats are rich sources of myristic acid. The 16-carbon palmitic acid also increases LDL, primarily when there is more than 200 to 300 mg of cholesterol in the diet and LDL is already elevated. The saturated fatty acids with 12, 14, or 16 carbons generally constitute about 25 to 50%

Table 6-10 | Food Sources of Fat

Food Item	Fat (g)	Energy from Fat (%)
T-bone steak (3 oz)	17	66%
Mixed nuts (1 oz)	16	78%
Canola oil (1 tbsp)	14	100%
Hamburger with bun (1 each)	12	39%
Margarine (1 tbsp)	12	100%
Avocado (1/2 cup)	11	86%
Cheddar cheese (1 oz)	10	74%
Whole milk (1 cup)	8	49%
Chicken breast with skin (3 oz)	7	36%
Whole milk yogurt (8 oz)	7	28%
Snack crackers (1 oz)	7	45%
Baked beans (1/2 cup)	7	31%
M&M chocolate candies (1 oz)	6	39%
Flax seeds (1 tbsp)	3	62%
Fig Newton cookies (2 each)	3	23%

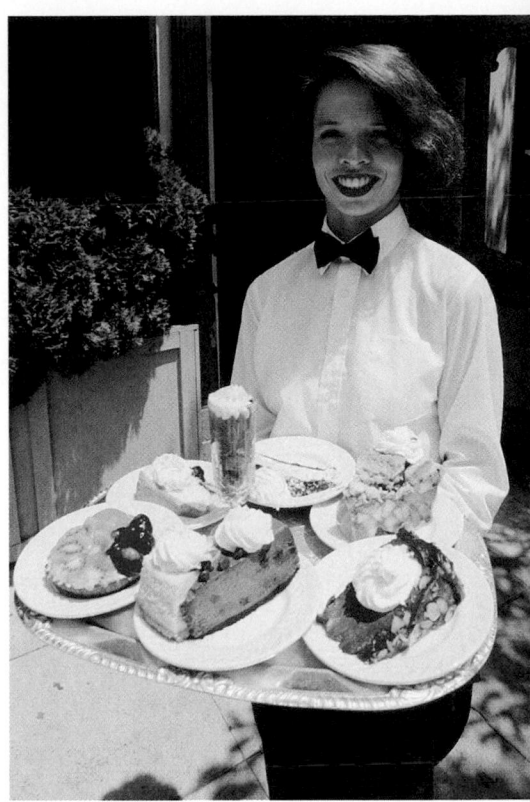

The North American diet contains many high-fat foods—including candy, cookies, and desserts. Portion control is the key to enjoying these foods while still controlling energy intake.

of the total fat in animal foods. In general, dairy fats and meat are rich in the fatty acids that raise LDL. In some plant oils, these saturated fatty acids also make up a notable percentage of the total fat—for example, cottonseed oil (27%) and coconut oil (89%).

Plant oils contain mostly unsaturated fatty acids, ranging from 73 to 94% of total fat. Canola oil, olive oil, and peanut oil contain moderate to high amounts of total fat as monounsaturated fatty acids (49 to 77%). Some animal fats are also good sources of monounsaturated fatty acids (30 to 47%) (review Figure 6-3). Corn, cottonseed, sunflower, soybean, and safflower oils contain mostly polyunsaturated fatty acids (54 to 77%) in terms of total fat. These plant oils supply the majority of the linoleic acid and alpha-linolenic acid in the North American food supply. Note that plant oils vary in their content of polyunsaturated fatty acids. Oils that are similar in appearance still may vary significantly in fatty acid composition.

Fat Replacement Strategies Are Available

Currently, five types of fat replacements are available to food manufacturers. Addition of these substances during manufacturing yields products that, to varying degrees, satisfy consumers' desire for reduced-fat products that are still tasty.[1]

Water, Starch Derivatives, and Fibers

The first and simplest fat replacement is water. The addition of water yields a product, such as diet margarine, with less fat per serving than the normal product. Starch derivatives that bind water form a second type of fat replacement. The resulting gel replaces some of the mouth feel lost by the removal of fat. Z trim is one example. It is made from the hulls or bran of various plants, including oats, peas, soybeans, rice, corn, and wheat. Other starch derivatives commonly used by food manufacturers include the fiber cellulose, Maltrin, Stellar, and Oatrim. These substances are used in a variety of foods, including luncheon meats, salad dressings, frozen desserts, table spreads, dips, baked goods, and candies. Most starch derivatives yield some energy, but at least half the amount that is in fat. Note that these starch derivatives cannot be used in fried foods.[1]

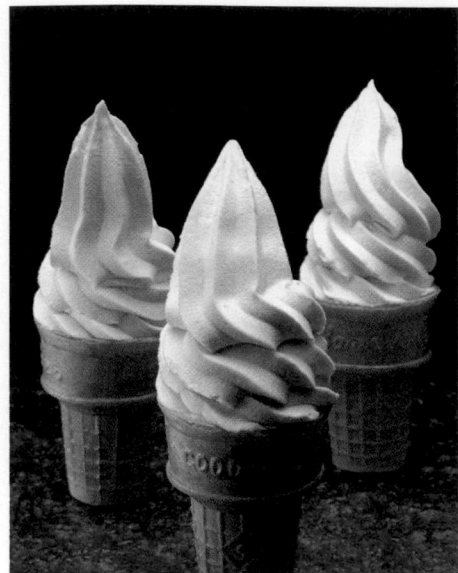

Fat replacements such as gum fiber are typically seen in soft serve ice cream.

So far, fat replacements have had little impact on our diets, partly because the currently approved forms either are not very versatile or have not been used extensively by manufacturers. The public, in fact, has shown very little interest in the use of fat replacers such as olestra. In addition, fat replacements are not practical to use in the foods that contribute the greatest quantity of fat to our diets—beef, cheese, whole and reduced-fat milk, and pastries.[1]

Canada has not approved the use of olestra in food products; the United States is the only country that permits the use of this fat substitute in foods.[1]

Gum fiber extracted from plants can also be used to replace fat. This thickens a product and replaces some of the body that fat provides. Diet salad dressings and fat-reduced ice cream have gums added for this reason.

Protein-Derived Fat Replacements

Still another type of fat replacement on the market consists of proteins that have been treated to produce microscopic, mistlike protein globules. Both egg and milk proteins can be used. When these substances replace fat in a food product, they feel like fat in the mouth, although the product does not contain any fatty acids. One example is Dairy-Lo, which is used in milk and other dairy products, baked goods, frostings, salad dressings, and mayonnaise-type products. Such fat replacements yield some energy— but only about 1 to 2 kcal/g. They have this low-energy value for two reasons: proteins contain only 4 kcal/g, and the products have a high water content.[1]

Engineered Fats and Related Products

The last form of fat replacement is engineered fat. This type of product is synthesized in the laboratory from various food constituents. Olestra (Olean) is a good example. It is made by chemically bonding fatty acids to sucrose (table sugar). The resulting product cannot be digested by either the human digestive enzymes or bacteria that live in the intestinal tract. Therefore, olestra is not absorbed and so provides no energy for the body.

Olestra can replace much of the fat in salad dressing and cakes and was the first fat replacement that could be used in fried foods. Olestra was approved by FDA in 1996 for use in fried snack foods, such as potato chips.[1]

The major problem associated with the use of olestra is that it binds the fat-soluble vitamins A, D, E, and K, thus reducing their absorption. To compensate, the manufacturer adds these vitamins to food products containing olestra. Other suspected problems, such as GI tract discomfort, have not been supported by careful research. Thus, warnings about use of olestra and GI tract disturbances, which used to be required on labels for olestra-containing foods, are no longer mandatory.

Food manufacturers are working on other types of engineered fats that either wholly or partially escape absorption by the body. One example is salatrim, which is marketed under the name Benefat and yields only about 5 kcal/g. It is composed of some saturated fatty acids that are poorly absorbed by the body. This product has been used in reduced-fat chocolate.

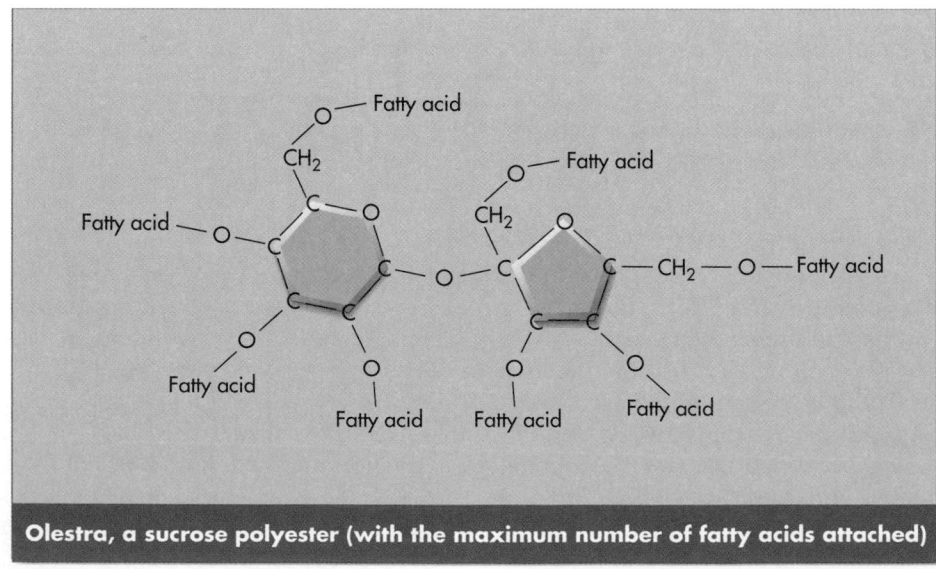

Olestra, a sucrose polyester (with the maximum number of fatty acids attached)

Fat Is Hidden In Some Foods

Some fat discussed so far is obvious: butter on bread, mayonnaise in potato salad, and marbling in raw meat. Fat is harder to detect in other foods that also contribute significant amounts of fat to our diets. Fat is hidden in whole milk, pastries, cookies, cake, cheese, hot dogs, crackers, french fries, and ice cream. When we try to cut down on fat intake, hidden fats need to be considered along with the more obvious sources.

A place to begin searching for hidden fat is on the Nutrition Facts labels of foods you buy. Some signals from the ingredient list that can alert you to the presence of fat are animal fats, such as bacon, beef, ham, lamb, pork, chicken, and turkey fats; lard; vegetable oils; nuts; dairy fats, such as butter and cream; egg and egg-yolk solids; and partially hydrogenated shortening or vegetable oil. Conveniently, the label lists ingredients by order of weight in the product. If fat is one of the first ingredients listed, you are probably looking at a high-fat product. Use food labels to learn more about the fat content of the foods you eat (Figure 6-16).

Table 2-14 in Chapter 2 listed the definitions for various fat descriptors on food labels, such as "low-fat," "fat-free," and "reduced-fat." Recall that "low-fat" indicates, in most cases, that a product contains no more than 3 g of fat per serving. Products that are marketed as "fat-free" must have less than 1/2 g of fat per serving. A claim of "reduced-fat" means the product has at least 25% less fat than is usually found in that food. When there is no Nutrition Facts label to inspect, controlling portion size is a good way to control fat intake.

Whether or not to choose a fat-rich food should depend on how much fat you have eaten or will eat for that particular day. If you plan to eat high-fat foods at your evening meal, you could reduce your fat intake at a previous meal in order to balance overall fat intake for the day.

Wise Use of Reduced-Fat Foods Is Important

In recent years, manufacturers have introduced reduced-fat versions of numerous food products. The fat content of these alternatives ranges from 0% in fat-free Fig Newtons to about 75% of the original fat content in other products. However, the total energy content of most fat-reduced products is not substantially lower than that of their conventional versions. Generally, when fat is removed from a product, something must be added—commonly, sugars—in its place. It is very difficult to reduce both the fat and sugar contents of a product at the same time. For this reason, many reduced-fat products (e.g.,

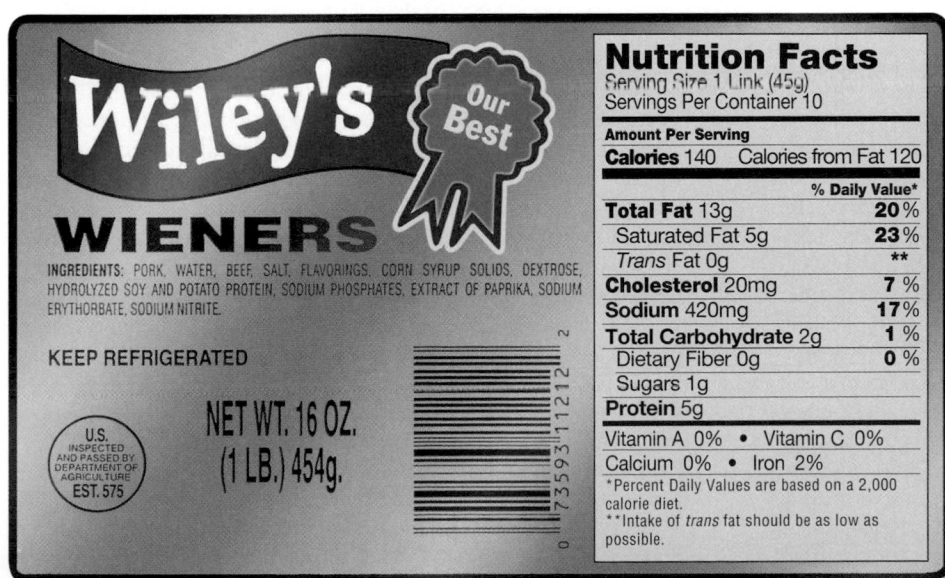

Figure 6-16 | Reading labels helps locate hidden fat. Who would think that wieners (hot dogs) can contain about 85% of energy content as fat? Looking at the hot dog itself does not suggest that almost all its energy content comes from fat, but the label shows otherwise. Do the math: $(13 \text{ g} \times 9 \text{ kcal/g})/140 \text{ kcal} = 0.84$, or 84%.

When many North Americans think of a low-fat diet, they include reduced-fat versions of pastries, cookies, and cakes. When health professionals refer to a low-fat diet, they often have a very different plan in mind: one that focuses primarily on fruits, vegetables, and whole-grain breads and cereals.[6,13]

cakes and cookies) are still very energy dense. Use the Nutrition Facts label to guide the portion size you choose.[1]

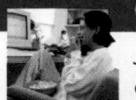

Case Scenario | Follow-Up

Jackie's approach to lowering blood cholesterol does not incorporate the best choices; she has excluded a great deal of fat in her diet by merely replacing it with refined carbohydrates. To make a shift to a more heart-healthy diet, Jackie would need to include at least two fruit and three vegetable servings a day along with more whole-grain products (such as whole-wheat bread and a breakfast cereal that has at least 3 g of fiber per serving). Lowering fat as drastically as she has is not really necessary, especially for a 21-year-old female who is physically active. Jackie could allow a more liberal amount of fat in her diet by including more monounsaturated fats (canola oil and olive oil as well as fats found in nuts and avocados). These do not increase blood cholesterol. In addition to allowing more liberal fat intake from monounsaturated oils and including more fruits, vegetables, and whole-grain breads and cereals, Jackie would benefit from including good sources of omega-3 fatty acids (fatty fish, flaxseeds, walnuts, or soybean and canola oil). One option is to use a canola oil-and-vinegar dressing on her salad rather than lemon juice.

Critical | Thinking

Allison has decided to start eating a low-fat diet. She has mentioned to you that all she needs to do is add less butter, oil, or margarine to her foods and she will dramatically lower her fat intake. How can you explain to Allison that she needs to be aware of the hidden fats in her diet as well?

Concept | Check

There is no RDA for total fat intake. We need about 5% of total energy intake from plant oils to meet the Adequate Intakes set for essential fatty acids. Eating fish at least twice a week is also advised to supply omega-3 fatty acids. Many health-related agencies recommend a diet containing no more than 35% of energy intake as fat, with limited amounts of saturated fat, cholesterol, and *trans* fatty acids. The current North American diet contains about 33% of energy content as fat, with about 13% of energy content as saturated fat and about 3% as *trans* fatty acids. Fat-dense foods—those with more than 60% of total energy as fat—include plant oils, butter, margarine, mayonnaise, walnuts, bacon, avocados, peanut butter, cheddar cheese, steak, and hamburger. Of the foods we typically eat, cholesterol is found naturally only in those of animal origin, with eggs being a primary source. Fat is often hidden in foods such as whole milk, pastries, cookies, cake, cheese, hot dogs, crackers, french fries, ice cream, and fast food. Fat free doesn't mean calorie free; moderation in the use of fat-reduced products is still important.

Summary

1. Compared with carbohydrates and proteins, lipids are a group of relatively oxygen-poor compounds that dissolve in organic solvents, such as chloroform, benzene, and ether. Saturated fatty acids contain no carbon-carbon double bonds. Monounsaturated fatty acids contain one carbon-carbon double bond. *Trans* fatty acids also typically contain one carbon-carbon double bond, but it is in a *trans* rather than *cis* configuration. Polyunsaturated fatty acids contain two or more carbon-carbon double bonds in the carbon chain.

2. In omega-3 polyunsaturated fatty acids, the first of the carbon-carbon double bonds is located three carbons from the methyl end of the carbon chain. In omega-6 polyunsaturated fatty acids, the first carbon-carbon double bond counting from the methyl end occurs at the sixth carbon. Both omega-3 and omega-6 fatty acids are essential fatty acids; these must be included in the diet to maintain health. Body cells can synthesize hormone compounds called eicosanoids from both omega-3 and omega-6 fatty acids. Eicosanoids made from omega-3 fatty acids reduce blood clotting and inflammation more so than eicosanoids made from omega-6 fatty acids.

3. Triglycerides are formed from a glycerol backbone with three fatty acids. Triglycerides rich in long-chain saturated fatty acids tend to be solid at room temperature, whereas those rich in polyunsaturated fatty acids are liquid at room temperature. Triglyceride is the major form of fat in both food and the body. It allows for efficient energy storage, protects certain organs, transports fat-soluble vitamins, and helps insulate the body.

4. Phospholipids are derivatives of triglycerides. Phospholipids are important parts of cell membranes, and some act as efficient emulsifiers.

5. Cholesterol forms vital biological compounds, such as hormones, components of cell membranes, and bile acids. Cells in the body make cholesterol whether we eat it or not. It is not a necessary part of an adult's diet.

6. Fat digestion takes place primarily in the small intestine. Lipase enzyme released from the pancreas digests the long-chain triglycerides into smaller breakdown products—namely, monoglycerides (glycerol backbones with single fatty acids attached) and fatty acids. The breakdown products are then taken up by the absorp-

tive cells of the small intestine. These products are mostly remade into triglycerides and combined with cholesterol, protein, and other substances to yield a chylomicron. Chylomicrons enter the lymphatic system, in turn passing into the bloodstream.

7. Lipids are carried in the bloodstream by various lipoproteins, which are particles consisting of a central triglyceride core encased in a shell of protein, cholesterol, and phospholipid. Chylomicrons are released from intestinal cells and carry lipids arising from dietary intake. Very-low-density lipoprotein (VLDL) and low-density lipoprotein (LDL) carry lipids both taken up and synthesized in the liver. High-density lipoprotein (HDL) picks up cholesterol from cells and acts in allowing transport of it back to the liver.

8. In the blood, elevated amounts of LDL and low amounts of HDL are strong predictors of the risk for cardiovascular disease.

9. Fat adds flavor and texture to foods and provides some satiety after meals. Some phospholipids are used in foods as emulsifiers, which suspend fat in water. When fatty acids break down, food becomes rancid, resulting in a foul odor and unpleasant flavor.

10. Hydrogenation is the process of converting carbon-carbon double bonds into single bonds by adding hydrogen at the point of un-

saturation. Hydrogenation of fatty acids in vegetable oils changes the oils to solid fats and helps reduce rancidity, which results from the breakdown of fatty acids. Hydrogenation also increases the *trans* fatty acid content. High amounts of *trans* fatty acids in the diet are discouraged, because they increase LDL and reduce HDL.

11. There is no RDA for total fat intake. We need about 5% of total energy intake from plant oils to obtain the needed essential fatty acids based on the Adequate Intake for these nutrients. Fish is a rich source of omega-3 fatty acids and should be consumed at least twice a week.

12. Many health agencies and scientific groups suggest a fat intake of no more than 30 to 35% of energy intake. If fat intake exceeds 30% of total energy intake, the diet should emphasize monounsaturated fat. The typical North American diet contains about 33% of total energy as fat.

13. Fat-reduced products aid in the goal of reducing fat intake, but they still must be eaten in moderate amounts to maintain control of total energy intake.

Study Questions

1. Describe the chemical structures of saturated and polyunsaturated fatty acids and their different effects in both food and the human body.

2. Relate the need for omega-3 fatty acids in the diet to the recommendation to consume fish twice a week.

3. Describe the structures, origins, and roles of the four major blood lipoproteins.

4. What are the recommendations of health-care professionals regarding fat intake? What do these recommendations mean in terms of actual food choices?

5. What are two important attributes of fat in food? How are these different from the general functions of lipids in the human body?

6. Describe the significance of and possible uses for reduced-fat foods.

7. Does a person's cholesterol intake tell the whole story with respect to cardiovascular disease risk?

8. List the four main risk factors for the development of cardiovascular disease.

9. What three lifestyle factors decrease the risk of cardiovascular disease development?

10. When are medications most needed in cardiovascular disease therapy, and how in general do the various classes of medications operate to reduce risk?

BOOST YOUR STUDY

Refer to *Perspectives in Nutrition: Online Learning Center* www.mhhe.com/wardlawpers7 for quizzes, flash cards, activities, and web links designed to further help you learn about dietary lipids.

Annotated References

1. ADA Reports: Position of the American Dietetic Association: Fat replacers. *Journal of the American Dietetic Association* 105:266, 2005.
   The majority of fat replacers, when used in moderation by adults, can be safe and useful adjuncts to lowering the fat content of foods and may play a role in decreasing total dietary energy and fat intake.

2. Cholesterol: How low should you go? *Consumer Reports on Health*, p. 8, March 2004.
   Good review of the diet and medication regimens used to lower blood cholesterol. Despite the power of medications to lower blood cholesterol, lifestyle changes are also needed to get the full effect of the medications.

3. Coronary bypass: *Mayo Clinic Health Letter* 22(4):1, 2004.
   Complete description of coronary bypass surgery is provided.

4. Coulston AM and Peragallo-Ditto KV: Insulin resistance syndrome: A potent culprit in cardiovascular disease. *Journal of the American Dietetic Association* 104(2): 176, 2004.
   Insulin resistance as evidenced by mild increases in fasting blood glucose leads to many deleterious effects on the body. Weight loss (when needed) along with regular physical activity and a diet rich in whole grains, fruits, vegetables, and low-fat dairy products helps treat the condition.

5. Covington MB: Omega-3 fatty acids. *American Family Physician* 70(1):133, 2004.
   Omega-3 fatty acids can reduce the risk of sudden cardiac death in people with cardiovascular disease. These fatty acids also have anti-inflammatory effects.

6. Djousse L and others: Fruit and vegetable consumption and LDL cholesterol. *American Journal of Clinical Nutrition* 79:213, 2004.
   Regular fruit and vegetable intake can reduce LDL cholesterol. It is important to put these recommendations into practice.

7. Food and Nutrition Board: *Dietary reference intakes for energy, carbohydrate, fiber, fat, fatty acids, cholesterol, protein, and amino acids.* Washington

DC: The National Academy Press, 2002.

This report provides the latest guidance for macronutrient intakes. With regard to fat intake, Adequate Intakes were set for omega-6 and omega-3 fatty acids. Intake of total fat can range from 20 to 35% of total energy intake. Intake of saturated fat, cholesterol, and trans fat should be minimal because these dietary constituents are not essential nutrients and are associated with increasing risk for cardiovascular disease.

8. Ford ES and others: Sedentary behavior, physical activity, and the metabolic syndrome among U.S. adults. *Obesity Research* 13(3):608, 2005.

Sedentary behavior is an important potential determinant of the presence of metabolic syndrome. An increase in physical activity could in contrast result in substantial decreases in the prevalence of metabolic syndrome.

9. Greenland P and others: Major risk factors as antecedents of fatal and nonfatal coronary heart disease events. *Journal of the American Medical Association* 290:891, 2003.

Cardiovascular disease deaths predominate in people with four major factors: elevated total cholesterol, elevated blood pressure, cigarette smoking, and diabetes. Presence of one or more of these risk factors predicted such deaths in almost 90% of all cases, emphasizing the importance of considering all these major risk factors.

10. Grundy SM and others: Implications of recent clinical trials for the National Cholesterol Education Program Adult Treatment Panel III Guidelines. *Circulation* 110:227, 2004.

This report outlines the goals for LDL cholesterol for people at various risk classifications for developing cardiovascular disease. The newest guideline is to lower LDL cholesterol to less than 70 mg/dl for those at high risk for or who have cardiovascular disease.

11. Grundy SM and others: Diagnosis and management of the metabolic syndrome. *Circulation* 112:2735, 2005.

The constellation of metabolic risk factors known as metabolic syndrome is strongly associated with type 2 diabetes mellitus or the risk for this condition. These metabolic risk factors consist of atherogenic dyslipidemia (elevated triglycerides and apolipoprotein B, small LDL particles, and low HDL-cholesterol concentrations), elevated blood pressure, elevated plasma glucose, a prothrombotic state, and a proinflammatory state. The most important of these underlying risk factors are abdominal obesity and insulin resistance.

12. Hansson GK: Inflammation, atherosclerosis, and coronary artery disease. *New England Journal of Medicine* 352:1685, 2005.

This article contains an excellent review of the role of inflammation in causing cardiovascular disease.

13. Jensen MK and others: Intakes of whole grains, bran, and germ and the risk of coronary heart disease in men. *American Journal of Clinical Nutrition* 80:1492, 2004.

This study supports the reported beneficial association of whole-grain intake with coronary heart disease and suggests that the bran component of whole grains could be a key factor in this relation.

14. Jones JH, Kubow S: Lipids, sterols, and their metabolites. In Shils ME and others (eds): *Modern nutrition in health and disease.* 10th ed. Philadelphia, PA: Lippincott Williams & Wilkins, 2006.

Current review of the various dietary lipids and their related metabolism. Digestion and absorption of these lipids is also covered.

15. Krauss RM and others: AHA Dietary Guidelines: Revision 2000: A statement for healthcare professionals from the Nutrition Committee of the American Heart Association. *Circulation* 102:2284, 2000.

This report contains the latest advice for the public regarding diet and cardiovascular disease from the American Heart Association. The revised guidelines place an increased emphasis on the need for weight control and a heart-healthy diet.

16. Kris-Etherton PM and others: Antioxidant vitamin supplements and cardiovascular disease. *Circulation* 110:637, 2004.

There is no scientific data to clearly justify the use of antioxidant supplements such as vitamin E for the prevention of cardiovascular disease. It is much more important to focus on a healthy diet, regular physical activity, and control of blood pressure.

17. Kritchevsky D: Cholesterol and other dietary sterols. In Shils ME and others (eds): *Modern nutrition in health and disease.* 10th ed. Philadelphia, PA: Lippincott Williams & Wilkins, 2006.

Current review of the role of cholesterol in health and disease, including the various factors that influence its production in the body.

18. Lau VWY and others: Plant sterols are efficacious in lowering plasma LDL and non-HDL cholesterol in hypercholesterolemic type 2 diabetic and nondiabetic persons. *American Journal of Clinical Nutrition* 81: 1351, 2005.

The risk of developing cardiovascular disease is twofold to sevenfold higher in type 2 diabetics than in nondiabetic persons, and this study shows that plant sterol consumption decreases the risk of cardiovascular disease in this population.

19. Lonn E and others: Effects of long-term vitamin E supplementation on cardiovascular events and cancer: A randomized controlled trial. *Journal of the American Medical Association* 293:1338, 2005.

No significant differences were noted between the vitamin E supplementation group and the control group in the incidence of cancer or deaths related to cancer in this study.

20. Mayes PA, Botham KM: Lipids of physiological significance. In Murray RK and others (eds); *Harper's illustrated biochemistry.* 26th ed. New York, NY, Lange Medical Books/McGraw-Hill, 2003.

Concise review of the chemical structures and related features of dietary lipids.

21. Mayes PA, Botham KM: Metabolism of unsaturated fatty acids and eicosanoids significance. In Murray RK and others (eds); *Harper's illustrated biochemistry.* 26th ed. New York, NY, Lange Medical Books/McGraw-Hill, 2003.

Overview of the metabolism of fatty acids, with a special focus on eicosanoids.

22. Mayes PA, Botham KM: Lipid storage and transport. In Murray RK and others (eds); *Harper's illustrated biochemistry.* 26th ed. New York, NY, Lange Medical Books/McGraw-Hill, 2003.

Detailed depiction of the pathways used in lipoprotein metabolism in the body.

23. Mayes PA, Botham KM: Cholesterol synthesis, transport, and excretion. In Murray RK and others (eds); *Harper's illustrated biochemistry.* 26th ed. New York, NY, Lange Medical Books/McGraw-Hill, 2003.

Overview of the metabolism of cholesterol, as well as a review of its specific contribution to various forms of elevated blood lipids seen in humans.

24. Meisinger C and others: Plasma oxidized low-density lipoprotein, a strong predictor for acute coronary heart disease events in apparently healthy, middle-aged men from the general population. *Circulation* 112:651, 2005.

Elevated concentrations of oxidized low-density lipoprotein are predictive of future coronary heart disease events in apparently healthy men.

25. Millen BE and others: Dietary patterns, smoking, and subclinical heart disease in women. *Journal of the American Dietetic Association* 104:208, 2004.

A public health priority for women is to promote healthy lifestyle behaviors, especially healthy eating and the avoidance of smoking.

26. Thompson PD and others: Exercise and physical activity in the prevention and treatment of atherosclerotic cardiovascular disease. *Circulation* 107:3109, 2003.

Habitual physical activity prevents the development of cardiovascular disease and reduces symptoms in patients with established cardiovascular disease.

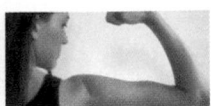

Take | Action

I. Are You Eating a Diet That Includes Many Saturated Fat and *Trans* Fatty Acid Sources?

Instructions: In each row of the following list, circle your typical food selection from either column A or B.

Column A		Column B
Bacon and eggs	or	Ready-to-eat whole-grain breakfast cereal
Doughnut or sweet roll	or	Whole-wheat roll, bagel, or bread
Breakfast sausage	or	Fruit
Whole milk	or	Reduced-fat, low-fat, or fat-free milk
Cheeseburger	or	Turkey sandwich, no cheese
French fries	or	Plain baked potato with salsa
Ground chuck	or	Ground round
Soup with cream base	or	Soup with broth base
Macaroni and cheese	or	Macaroni with marinara sauce
Cream/fruit pie	or	Graham crackers
Cream-filled cookies	or	Granola bar
Ice cream	or	Frozen yogurt, sherbet, or reduced-fat ice cream
Butter or stick margarine	or	Vegetable oils or soft margarine in a tub

Interpretation

The foods listed in column A tend to be high in saturated fat, *trans* fatty acids, cholesterol, and total fat. Those in column B generally are low in these dietary components. If you want to help reduce your risk of cardiovascular disease, choose more foods from column B and fewer from column A.

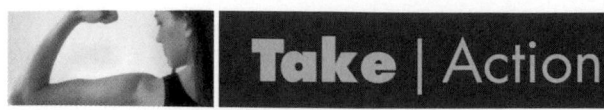
Take | Action

II. Applying the Nutrition Facts Label to Your Daily Food Choices

Imagine that you are at the supermarket looking for a quick snack to help you keep your energy up during afternoons. In the snack section, you settle on two choices (see labels a and b). Which of the two brands would you choose? What information on the Nutrition Facts labels contributed to your decision?

Nutrition Facts

Serving Size: 2 bars (42g)
Servings Per Container: 6

Amount Per Serving	**2 bars**	
Calories 180	Calories from Fat 50	

		% Daily Value*
Total Fat 6g		**9**%
Saturated Fat 0.5g		**3**%
Trans fat 0g		**
Cholesterol 0mg		**0**%
Sodium 160mg		**7**%
Total Carbohydrates 29g		**10**%
Dietary Fiber 2g		**8**%
Sugars 11g		
Protein 4g		

Iron	6%

Not a significant source of Vitamin A, Vitamin C, and calcium.

** Intake of *trans* fat should be as low as possible.

* Daily values are based on a 2,000 calorie diet. Your daily values may be higher or lower depending on your calorie needs:

** Intake should be as low as possible.	Calories	2,000	2,500
Total Fat	Less than	65g	80g
Saturated Fat	Less than	20g	25g
Cholesterol	Less than	300mg	300mg
Sodium	Less than	2,400mg	2,400mg
Total Carbohydrates		300g	375g
Dietary Fiber		25g	30g

INGREDIENTS: WHOLE GRAIN ROLLED OATS, SUGAR, CANOLA OIL, CRISP RICE WITH SOY PROTEIN (RICE FLOUR, SOY PROTEIN CONCENTRATE, SUGAR, MALT, SALT), HONEY, BROWN SUGAR SYRUP, HIGH FRUCTOSE CORN SYRUP, SALT, SOY LECITHIN, BAKING SODA, NATURAL FLAVOR, PEANUT FLOUR, ALMOND FLOUR, HAZELNUT FLOUR, WALNUT FLOUR, PECAN FLOUR.

(a)

Nutrition Facts

Serving Size: 2 cookies (38g)
Servings Per Container: about 12

Amount Per Serving	
Calories 180	Calories from Fat 70

		% Daily Value*
Total Fat 7g		**11**%
Saturated Fat 2g		**10**%
Trans fat 2g		**
Cholesterol 0mg		**0**%
Sodium 100mg		**4**%
Total Carbohydrate 26g		**9**%
Dietary Fiber 1g		**4**%
Sugars 12g		
Protein 2g		

Vitamin A 0%	•	Vitamin C 0%	
Calcium 0%	•	Iron	2%

** Intake of *trans* fat should be as low as possible.

* Daily values are based on a 2,000 calorie diet. Your daily values may be higher or lower depending on your calorie needs:

** Intake should be as low as possible.	Calories	2,000	2,500
Total Fat	Less than	65g	80g
Saturated Fat	Less than	20g	25g
Cholesterol	Less than	300mg	300mg
Sodium	Less than	2,400mg	2,400mg
Total Carbohydrates		300g	375g
Dietary Fiber		25g	30g

Calories per gram: • Fat 9 • Carbohydrate 4
• Protein 4

INGREDIENTS: ENRICHED FLOUR (WHEAT FLOUR, NIACIN, REDUCED IRON, THIAMINE MONONITRATE, RIBOFLAVIN, FOLIC ACID), SUGAR, VEGETABLE OIL SHORTENING (PARTIALLY HYDROGENATED SOYBEAN, COCONUT, COTTONSEED, CORN AND/OR SAFFLOWER AND/OR CANOLA OIL), CORN SYRUP, HIGH FRUCTOSE CORN SYRUP, WHEY (A MILK INGREDIENT), CORN STARCH, SALT, SKIM MILK, LEAVENING (BAKING SODA, AMMONIUM BICARBONATE), ARTIFICIAL FLAVOR, SOYBEAN LECITHIN, COLOR (CONTAINING FD&C YELLOW #5 LAKE).

(b)

CASE SCENARIO:

Shannon is a freshman in college. She lives in a campus residence hall and teaches aerobics in the afternoon. She eats two or three meals a day at the residence hall cafeteria and snacks between meals. Shannon and her roommate both decided to become vegetarians because they recently read on the Internet an article describing the health benefits of a vegetarian diet. Yesterday her vegetarian diet consisted of a danish pastry for breakfast and a tomato-rice dish (no meat) with pretzels and a diet soft drink for lunch. In the afternoon, after her aerobics class, she had two cookies. At dinnertime, she had a vegetarian sub sandwich with two glasses of fruit punch. In the evening, she had a bowl of popcorn.

What is missing from Shannon's current diet plan? Which foods should be emphasized on a vegetarian diet? How could she improve her new diet to meet her nutritional needs?

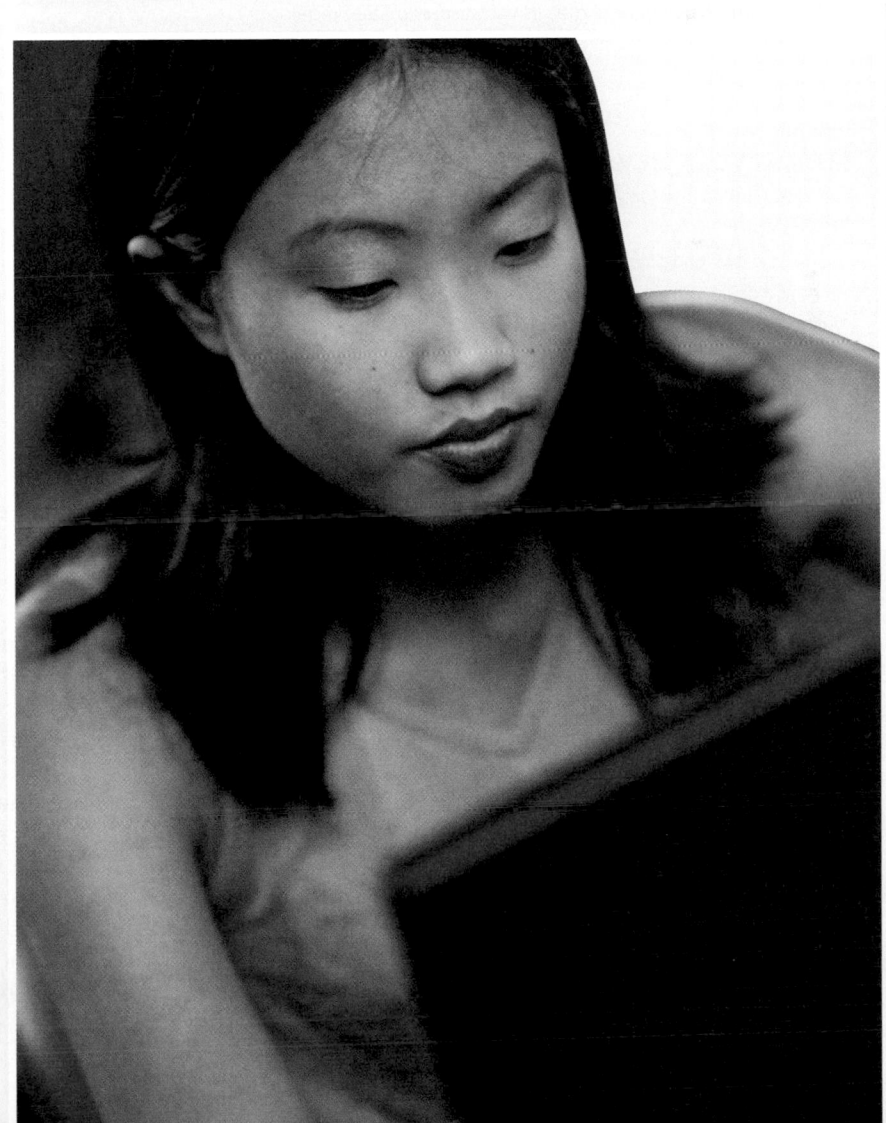

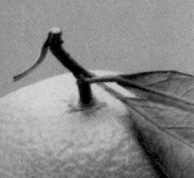

Consuming enough protein is vital for maintaining health.[10] Proteins form important structures in the body, make up a key part of the blood, help regulate many body functions, and can fuel body cells.[18] This term *protein* comes from the Greek word *protos*, which means "to come first." In the developing world, such a primary focus on protein in diet planning is important because diets in those areas of the world can be deficient in protein. In contrast, diets in industrialized countries are generally rich in protein, and therefore a specific focus on eating enough protein for the most part is not needed.

High-protein diets have come and gone over the past 30 years. Recently, these have become very popular as weight-loss diets, with some containing about 35% of energy as protein.[16] This figure falls within the latest advice for protein intake from the Food and Nutrition Board (10 to 35% of energy intake), so in general these diets are appropriate if otherwise nutritionally sound (e.g., they follow MyPyramid).[10] Still, as discussed in Chapter 13, these types of weight-loss diets are hardly a magic bullet for weight loss.

This chapter takes a close look at protein, including the benefits of plant proteins in a diet. It will also examine vegetarian diets: their benefits, and their risks if not properly planned.

CHAPTER OBJECTIVES CHAPTER 7 IS DESIGNED TO ALLOW YOU TO:

1. Describe how amino acids make up proteins.
2. Distinguish between essential and nonessential amino acids.
3. Explain why adequate amounts of each of the essential amino acids are required for protein synthesis.
4. List the primary functions of protein in the body.
5. List the factors that influence protein needs, and calculate the RDA for protein for an adult when a healthy weight is given.
6. Describe what is meant by positive nitrogen balance, negative nitrogen balance, and nitrogen equilibrium in terms of protein status in the body.
7. Distinguish between high-quality and lower-quality proteins and the sources of each, and describe how two lower-quality proteins can be complementary for each other and so provide enough of all the essential amino acids for a diet.
8. Outline two methods used to measure protein quality of foods, including assessment of biological value.
9. Describe how protein-energy malnutrition can eventually lead to disease in the body.
10. Develop vegetarian diet plans that meet the body's nutrient needs.

REFRESH YOUR MEMORY AS YOU BEGIN YOUR STUDY OF PROTEINS IN CHAPTER 7, YOU MAY WANT TO REVIEW:
- The anatomy and physiology of digestion and absorption in Chapter 3.
- Amino acid use in energy metabolism in Chapter 4.
- The processes of gluconeogenesis and ketosis in Chapter 4.
- The disease phenylketonuria (PKU) in the Nutrition Focus in Chapter 4.
- The immune system in Appendix C.

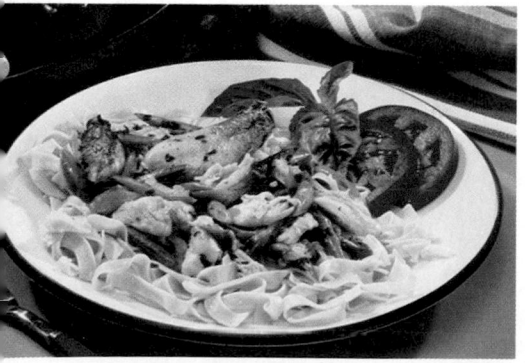

Small amounts of animal protein in a meal easily add up to meet daily protein needs.

▌Proteins—Vital to Life

Thousands of substances in the body are made of proteins. Aside from water, proteins form the major part of lean body tissue, totaling about 17% of body weight.[18] Much of this lean body mass is made up of muscle tissue. Amino acids—the building blocks for proteins—contain a special form of nitrogen: essentially, nitrogen bonded to carbon. Plants combine nitrogen from the soil with carbon and other elements to form amino acids. They then bond these amino acids together to make proteins. We get the nitrogen we need by consuming dietary proteins. Proteins are thus very important because they supply nitrogen in a form we can readily use—namely, amino acids. Directly using simpler forms of nitrogen is, for the most part, impossible for humans.

Proteins are crucial to the regulation and maintenance of the body. Body functions such as blood clotting, fluid balance, hormone and enzyme production, visual processes, and cell repair require specific proteins. The body makes proteins in many configurations and sizes so that they can serve these greatly varied functions.[18] All these proteins use the amino acids in the protein-containing foods we eat, plus some arising from cell synthesis. Proteins also can be broken down to supply energy for the body—on average, 4 kcal/g.[10]

If you fail to consume an adequate amount of protein for weeks at a time, many metabolic processes slow down. This is because the body does not have enough amino acids available to build the proteins it needs. For example, the immune system no longer functions efficiently when it lacks key proteins, thereby increasing the risk of infections, disease, and eventually death.[18]

Amino Acids

Amino acids contain carbon, hydrogen, oxygen, and nitrogen, and some contain sulfur. Body proteins are made using the 20 common amino acids, each with different metabolic destinies in the body (e.g., some can be made into glucose or hormones) and varying composition.[18] Each amino acid is composed of a central carbon bonded to four groups. The first three of these groups are a nitrogen group ($-NH_2$), called an amino group (or amine group), an acid group ($-\overset{\overset{O}{\|}}{C}-OH$), and a hydrogen ($-H$). The fourth group, often signified by R, completes the amino acid. In the margin is the basic model of an amino acid and structures of two amino acids, glycine and alanine. The chemical structures of the rest of the amino acids are shown in Appendix A.

Amino Acid Form and Function

The form that the R portion of the amino acid takes determines the type name of the amino acid. If R is a hydrogen, the amino acid is glycine; if R is a methyl group ($-CH_3$), the amino acid is alanine; and so on. Some amino acids have chemically similar R portions. These related amino acids form special classes, such as acidic amino acids, basic amino acids, or branched-chain amino acids. This distinction with regard to classes of amino acids has important practical implications. For instance, branched-chain amino acids are used for fuel by the muscles, especially during injury and other related forms of trauma.[18] Liquid formulas used to feed hospitalized patients may be enriched with branched-chain amino acids in order to provide ample amounts. The same holds true for some fluid replacement drinks marketed to athletes (see Chapter 14).

The body needs to use 20 common forms of amino acids to function. Although they are all important, 11 of these amino acids are considered **nonessential** (also called *dispensable*)—it isn't necessary to consume them because our bodies make them using other amino acids we consume (Table 7-1). The nine amino acids the body cannot make are known as **essential** (also called *indispensable*)—they must be obtained from foods. This is because body cells cannot make the needed carbon backbone (also called carbon skeleton) of the amino acid, cannot put a nitrogen group on the needed carbon backbone, or just cannot do the whole process fast enough to meet body needs.[10]

Two amino acids—cysteine and tyrosine—are synthesized in the body from methionine and phenylalanine, respectively. Both methionine and phenylalanine are essential amino acids. Cysteine and tyrosine must be made from their essential amino acid counterparts unless they are consumed in the diet. If cysteine and tyrosine are consumed, the body can synthesize protein from them directly. Thus, consumption of cysteine and tyrosine then frees the essential amino acids methionine and phenylalanine to contribute directly to protein synthesis. Therefore, cysteine and tyrosine are classed as **semiessential** (also called *conditionally dispensable*) amino acids. In some scenarios, such as infancy or adults with traumatic injury, other amino acids are also considered semiessential (review Table 7-1).[10]

Both nonessential and essential amino acids are present in foods that contain protein. If you don't consume enough food to yield a sufficient supply of essential amino acids, your body first struggles to conserve what essential amino acids it can. However,

"Generic" amino acid

Glycine

L-alanine

The L isomer, rather than a D isomer, is the form of amino acid used by the body for protein synthesis.

nonessential amino acids Amino acids that can be synthesized by a healthy body in sufficient amounts; there are 11 nonessential amino acids. These are also called *dispensable amino acids.*

essential amino acids Amino acids that cannot be synthesized by humans in sufficient amounts or at all and therefore must be included in the diet; there are 9 essential amino acids. These are also called *indispensable amino acids.*

semiessential amino acids Amino acids that, when consumed, spare the need to use an essential amino acid for their synthesis. Tyrosine in the diet, for example, spares the need to use phenylalanine for tyrosine synthesis. These are also called *conditionally essential amino acids.*

Because two cysteine molecules can bind to form a new amino acid called cystine, the number of nonessential amino acids is sometimes listed as 12. If this form of cysteine is not counted as a unique form, then there are 11 nonessential amino acids. The discussion in this chapter does not count cystine and thus uses the figure of 20 amino acids in foods: 9 essential and 11 nonessential.

Table 7-1 | Classification of Amino Acids

Essential Amino Acids	Nonessential Amino Acids
Histidine	Alanine
Isoleucine*	Arginine[†]
Leucine*	Asparagine
Lysine	Aspartic acid
Methionine	Cysteine[†]
Phenylalanine	(Cystine)
Threonine	Glutamic acid
Tryptophan	Glutamine[†]
Valine*	Glycine[†]
	Proline[†]
	Serine
	Tyrosine[†]

*A branched-chain amino acid

[†]These amino acids are also classed as semiessential.

eventually your body progressively slows production of new proteins until at some point you will break down protein faster than you can make it. When this happens, health deteriorates. Therefore, the two main functions of proteins in our diets are (1) to provide the nine essential amino acids needed by our bodies and (2) to provide either the nonessential amino acids our bodies use, or nitrogen from an amino acid that in turn can be used to make the nonessential amino acids.[10]

Transamination and Deamination

A common metabolic process for synthesizing nonessential amino acids is called **transamination.** This process requires vitamin B-6. Figure 7-1 illustrates transamination: pyruvic acid (this is not an amino acid) accepts the amino group ($-NH_2$) from the amino acid glutamic acid and becomes the amino acid alanine.[10]

Some amino acids, such as glutamic acid, can simply lose their amino group without transferring it to another carbon skeleton. This process is called **deamination.** The amino group, in the form of ammonia, is incorporated into **urea** in the liver. The urea is then transferred through the bloodstream to the kidneys and is mostly excreted in the urine. Once an amino acid breaks down to its amino-free carbon skeleton, the carbon skeleton can be used for fuel or synthesized into other compounds, such as glucose (review Chapter 4).[10]

Essential and Nonessential Amino Acids in Perspective

Eating a balanced diet can supply us with both the essential and nonessential amino acid building blocks needed to maintain good health. This section takes a more detailed look at this concept of essential amino acids, especially in relation to nonessential amino acids.

Physiological Aspects

The disease phenylketonuria (PKU) illustrates the importance of one essential amino acid. Recall from Chapter 4 that a person with PKU has a limited ability to metabolize the essential amino acid phenylalanine. Normally, the body uses an enzyme to convert

transamination The transfer of an amino group from an amino acid to a carbon skeleton to form a new amino acid.

deamination The removal of an amino group from an amino acid.

urea Nitrogenous waste product of protein metabolism; The major source of nitrogen in the urine; chemically $NH_2-\overset{O}{\overset{\|}{C}}-NH_2$.

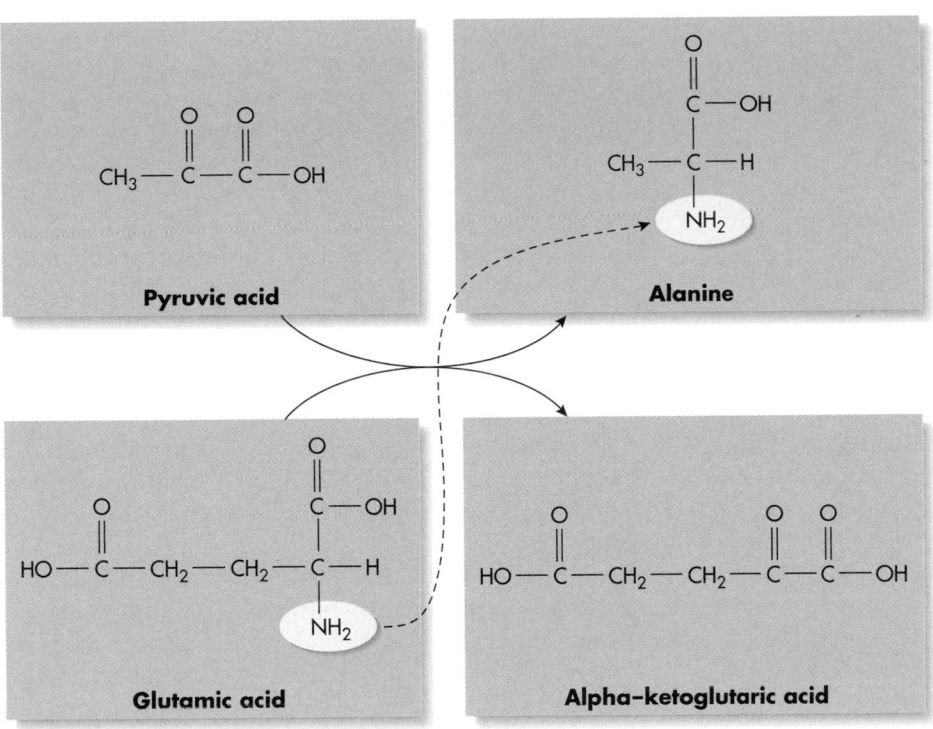

Figure 7-1 | Transamination. This pathway allows cells to synthesize nonessential amino acids. In this example, pyruvic acid gains an amino group to form the amino acid alanine.

By looking only at the bottom half of the reaction, deamination is seen when glutamic acid loses its amino group, but there is not a transfer of the amino group to a carbon skeleton.

much of our dietary phenylalanine intake into the nonessential amino acid tyrosine by adding a hydroxyl group (–OH).

In PKU-diagnosed persons, this enzyme activity may be grossly or mildly insufficient in processing phenylalanine to tyrosine. When the enzymes cannot synthesize enough tyrosine, both amino acids must be derived from foods. The key point here is that now tyrosine becomes *essential* in terms of dietary needs because the body can't produce enough of it.[10]

Dietary Considerations—Protein Quality

Animal and plant proteins can differ greatly in their proportions of essential and nonessential amino acids. Animal proteins contain ample amounts of all nine essential amino acids. (Gelatin—made from the animal protein collagen—is an exception because it loses one essential amino acid during processing and is low in other essential amino acids.) With the exception of soy protein, plant proteins don't match our need for essential amino acids as precisely as animal proteins. Many plant proteins, especially those found in grains, are low in one or more of the nine essential amino acids.[14]

As you might expect, human tissue composition resembles animal tissue more than it does plant tissue. These similarities enable us to use proteins from any single animal source more efficiently to support growth and maintenance than we do those from any single plant source. For this reason, animal proteins, except gelatin, are considered **high-quality** (also called **complete**) **proteins**—they contain all nine essential amino acids we need in sufficient amounts. Individual plant sources of proteins, except for soybeans, are considered **lower-quality** (also called **incomplete**) **proteins** when compared to high-quality proteins because they are either quite low in or missing one or more of the nine essential amino acids. This arises because their amino acid patterns are quite different from ours. Thus, a single plant protein, such as corn, cannot support body growth and maintenance if consumed alone. To obtain a sufficient amount of the nine essential amino acids, a variety of plant proteins needs to be consumed, because each plant protein lacks adequate amounts of one or more of the essential amino acids.[14]

Critical | Thinking

Rina is 7 months pregnant and has read about various tests that her baby will undergo when he or she is born. How can you explain to Rina the purpose and significance of one of those tests, the one that screens for PKU?

high-quality (complete) proteins Dietary proteins that contain ample amounts of all nine essential amino acids.

lower-quality (incomplete) proteins Dietary proteins that are low in or lack one or more essential amino acids.

limiting amino acid The essential amino acid in the lowest concentration in a food or diet relative to body needs.

complementary proteins Two food protein sources that make up for each other's inadequate supply of specific essential amino acids; together they yield a sufficient amount of all nine and so provide high-quality (complete) protein for the diet.

This chapter has a section titled "Evaluation of Protein Quality," which describes methods to measure protein quality. As you might guess, the result depends on how closely the essential amino acid pattern in a food resembles that found in human tissue.

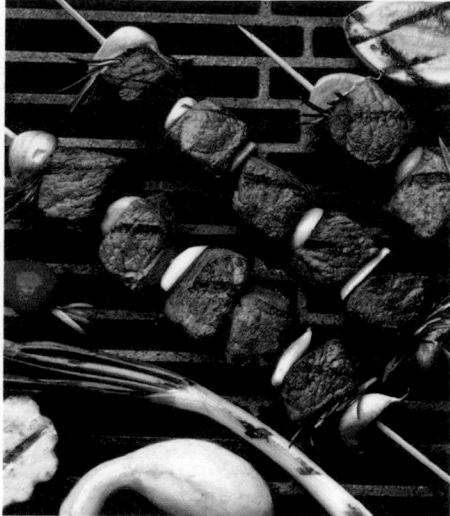

When combined with vegetables, high-protein foods such as meats also help balance the amino acid content of the diet.

When only lower-quality protein foods are consumed, enough of the nine essential amino acids needed for protein synthesis may not be obtained. Therefore, except for soy protein, a greater amount of this type of protein is needed to meet the needs of protein synthesis. Moreover, once any of the nine essential amino acids in the plant protein is used up, further protein synthesis becomes impossible. The remaining amino acids are used for energy or converted to carbohydrate or fat and stored as such. Because the depletion of just one of the essential amino acids prevents protein synthesis, the process illustrates the *all-or-none principle:* either all nine essential amino acids are available or none can be used. The remaining amino acids would then be used for energy or converted to carbohydrate or fat. The essential amino acid in smallest supply in a food or diet in relation to body needs becomes the limiting factor (called the **limiting amino acid**) because it limits the amount of protein the body can synthesize.[18]

For example, assume the letters of the alphabet represent the 20 or so different amino acids we consume. If *A* represents an essential amino acid, we need four of these letters to spell the hypothetical protein *ALABAMA.* If the body had an *L,* a *B,* and an *M,* but only three *A*s, the "synthesis" of *ALABAMA* would not be possible. *A* would then be seen as the limiting amino acid.

When two or more dietary proteins are combined to compensate for deficiencies in essential amino acid content in each protein, the proteins are called **complementary proteins** (Table 7-2). Mixed diets generally provide high-quality protein because a complementary protein pattern results. Therefore, healthy adults should have little concern about balancing foods to yield the proteins needed to obtain enough of all nine essential amino acids. Even on plant-based diets, complementing proteins need not be consumed at the same meal by adults. Meeting amino acid needs over the course of a day is a reasonable goal because there is a ready supply of amino acids from those present in body cells and in the blood (see Figure 7-8 on page 249).[18] In addition, adults need only about 11% of their total protein requirement to be supplied by essential amino acids. (The estimated needs for essential amino acids for infants and preschool children are about 40% of total protein intake.) Typical diets supply an average of 50% of protein as essential amino acids.

Critical | Thinking

Leon, a vegetarian, has heard of the "all-or-none principle" of protein synthesis but doesn't understand how this rule applies to protein synthesis in the body. He asks you, "How important is this nutritional concept for diet planning?" How would you answer his question?

Concept | Check

The human body uses 20 different amino acids from protein-containing foods. Because a healthy body can synthesize 11 of the amino acids, it is not necessary to obtain all amino acids from foods—only 9 of these must be obtained from the diet and are therefore termed *essential amino acids.* Foods that contain all nine essential amino acids in about the proportions we need are considered high-quality (complete) protein foods. Those low in one or more essential amino acids are lower-quality (incomplete) protein foods. When different lower-quality protein foods are eaten together, the total intake of amino acids generally makes up for shortcomings of each individual food to yield a high-quality protein meal.

polypeptide Fifty to 2000 or more amino acids bonded together.

peptide bond A chemical bond formed to link amino acids in a protein.

Proteins—Amino Acids Bonded Together

One way of classifying proteins is based on the number of amino acids present. Two amino acids chemically bonded together form a dipeptide, and three amino acids form a tripeptide. An oligopeptide has more than 3 but fewer than 50 amino acids. A **polypeptide** has 50 or more amino acids. Most proteins in foods contain polypeptide chains.[10] However, specialized liquid meal replacement supplements used in hospitals often contain various small peptides because these show enhanced absorption compared with larger polypeptides (see the section in this chapter titled Protein Digestion and Absorption).

Table 7-2 | Limiting Amino Acids in Plant Sources of Protein

Food	Limiting Amino Acids	Good Plant Sources of the Limiting Amino Acids*	Traditional Food Combinations in Which the Proteins Complement Each Other
Beans and most other legumes	Methionine Tryptophan	Wheat germ, seeds, peanuts, dry roasted soybeans Seeds, peanuts, dry roasted soybeans, wheat germ	Hummus and whole-wheat flatbread
Tree nuts and seeds	Methionine Lysine	Wheat germ, peanuts, dry roasted soybeans Wheat germ; whole-grain bread; cornmeal; dark rye bread; soybeans, and other legumes	Whole-wheat bread and cashew butter Roasted soybeans with almonds
Grains (wheat, rice, oats)	Lysine	Wheat germ; whole-grain bread; cornmeal; dark rye bread; soybeans, and other legumes	Rice with beans
Vegetables	Methionine Lysine	Wheat germ, seeds, peanuts, dry roasted soybeans Wheat germ; whole-grain bread; dark rye bread; cornmeal; soybeans, and other legumes	Green beans and sunflower seeds Beans in vegetable soup

Source: *USDA National Nutrient Database for Standard Reference, Release 18*. Agricultural Research Service, Nutrient Data.

Note: As you might suspect from the information in this table, the amino acids most likely to be low in a diet are lysine, methionine, threonine, and tryptophan. If a diet is low in an amino acid, nutrition experts recommend finding a good food source to supply it. Finding the right combinations of amino acids, such as a dish of rice and beans, is recommended. Forget about amino acid supplements—they can lead to problems, such as decreased absorption of other, similar amino acids. Amino acid supplements also have a disagreeable odor and flavor and are much more expensive than food protein.

*Animal products in the diet serve the same purpose, such as when rice is consumed with fish.

Amino acids are joined by a strong, covalent (e.g., electron-sharing) **peptide bond.** An amino group ($-NH_2$) reacts with a carboxyl group ($-\overset{\overset{O}{\|}}{C}-OH$), and a water molecule is split off in an enzyme-catalyzed reaction. The body can synthesize many different proteins by joining the 20 types of common amino acids with such peptide bonds.

Protein Synthesis

Since the human genome was deciphered in 2000, interest in human genetics and the role it plays in disease has increased. This topic was discussed in Chapter 1. What wasn't covered in detail in that chapter is how cells use the genome to make body proteins.

This discussion begins with the composition of DNA, present in the nucleus of the cell. Recall from Chapter 1 that DNA is a double-stranded molecule in a helical form. Each strand of DNA is composed of four nucleotides: adenine (A), guanine (G), cytosine (C), and thymine (T). Each of the nucleotides is complementary to (binds to) another nucleotide; A and T are complementary, as are C and G. Soon you will see why that is important.

DNA contains coded instructions for protein synthesis consisting of a sequence of three nucleotides per unit of instruction (e.g., which specific amino acid is to be placed in a protein and in which order).[10] These nucleotide units (e.g., GAG) are called codons and each DNA codon represents a specific amino acid. For example, the codon CTC represents the amino acid glutamic acid. Some amino acids have only one possible

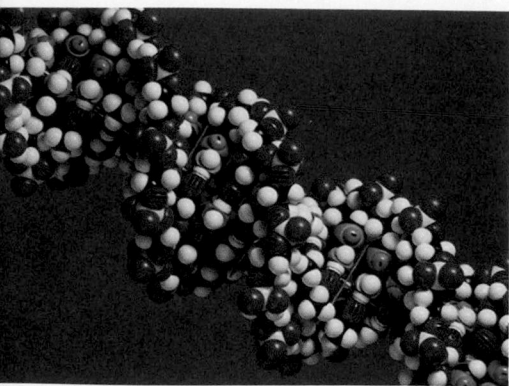

Genes are present on DNA—a double-stranded helix. The cell nucleus contains most of the DNA in the body.

DNA transcription Process of forming messenger RNA (mRNA) from a portion of DNA.

mRNA translation Synthesis of polypeptide chains at the ribosome according to information contained in strands of messenger RNA (mRNA).

A Synopsis of the Steps in Protein Synthesis Part of DNA code (gene) is transcribed to mRNA in the nucleus.

↓

mRNA leaves the nucleus and travels to cytosol.

↓

Ribosomes in the cytosol and rough endoplasmic reticulum read the mRNA code and translate that into directions for a specific order of amino acids in a polypeptide chain.

↓

To produce the polypeptide, tRNA brings the appropriate amino acid to the ribosome as dictated by the mRNA code. The amino acid is added to the existing amino acid chain, which begins with the amino acid methionine.

↓

When synthesis of the polypeptide is complete, it is released from the ribosome.

↓

Often the polypeptide will undergo further cell metabolism in order to function as a specific body protein once it folds into its active form.

codon, whereas others have as many as six. The amino acid glutamic acid actually has two codons: CTC and CTT. Having the correct codons in the DNA is critical for producing the correct protein, since the order of the codons in the DNA indicates the order of the specific amino acids needed to synthesize a particular protein.[18] This is important, because mistakes in the order or types of amino acids in a protein can result in profound health consequences (see the discussion of sickle-cell disease in the next section of this chapter).

Protein synthesis in a cell takes place in the cytosol, not in the nucleus. Thus, the DNA code used for synthesis of a specific protein must be transferred from the nucleus to the cytosol to allow for such synthesis. This transfer is the job of messenger RNA (mRNA). To produce mRNA, the DNA in the nucleus unwinds from its supercoiled state. Enzymes read the code on the DNA and transcribe that code into a complementary single-stranded mRNA molecule, called the primary transcript (Figure 7-2). This is the **DNA transcription** phase of protein synthesis. The segment that is read is the gene. In this process, A becomes uracil (U), C becomes G, T becomes A, and G becomes C. You might wonder why A did not become T, considering that A and T are complementary. It turns out that mRNA uses uracil (U) instead of thymine (T) in its code. Thus, the DNA code ACTGAT yields an mRNA of UGACUA. The actual DNA codons are ACT and GAT:

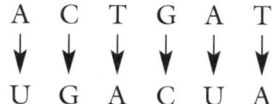

The primary transcript mRNA undergoes processing in the nucleus to remove any parts of the DNA code that do not code for protein synthesis, called introns (these actually make up much of the DNA). (The portions of the DNA that code for protein synthesis are called exons.) Some additional processing then takes place, and the final (mature) mRNA transcript is ready to leave the nucleus.

The mRNA travels to the ribosomes in the cytosol, present on the rough endoplasmic reticulum. The ribosomes read the codons on the mRNA and translate those instructions in order to produce a specific protein. This is the **mRNA translation** phase of protein synthesis. Amino acids are added one at a time to the polypeptide chain as directed by the instructions on the mRNA. Energy input from ATP is needed to add each amino acid to the growing polypeptide chain, making protein synthesis very "costly" to the body in terms of energy use. Many ribosomes can combine to simultaneously translate a large mRNA.

Protein synthesis begins at a specific starting point on the mRNA, indicated by AUG. It then continues until a specific ending (stop) codon is reached, such as UAA, UAG, or UGA.

One key participant in protein synthesis in the cytosol is transfer RNA (tRNA). These units bring amino acids to the ribosomes as needed during protein synthesis (review Figure 7-2). The tRNA carriers have a complementary code to the mRNA—such that, if an arginine were needed during synthesis, the AGA on the mRNA would correspond to UCU on the transfer RNA. Numerous tRNA carriers are present during protein synthesis to continually supply the ribosomes with needed amino acids.

Once synthesis of the polypeptide is completed, indicated by the ending codon, it is released from the ribosome, as is the mRNA. The polypeptide now twists and folds into a very complex three-dimensional structure (see the following section on protein organization for details).[18] Some polypeptides, such as the hormone insulin, also undergo further metabolism in the cell before they are functional. Generally, if synthesis of a particular protein needs to be increased in a cell, more mRNA for that protein is made.

The important message in this discussion is the relationship between DNA and the proteins eventually produced by a cell. If the DNA contains errors, an incorrect mRNA will be produced. The ribosomes will then read this incorrect message and produce an incorrect polypeptide chain. As discussed in Chapter 1, ultimately we may be able to

(a)

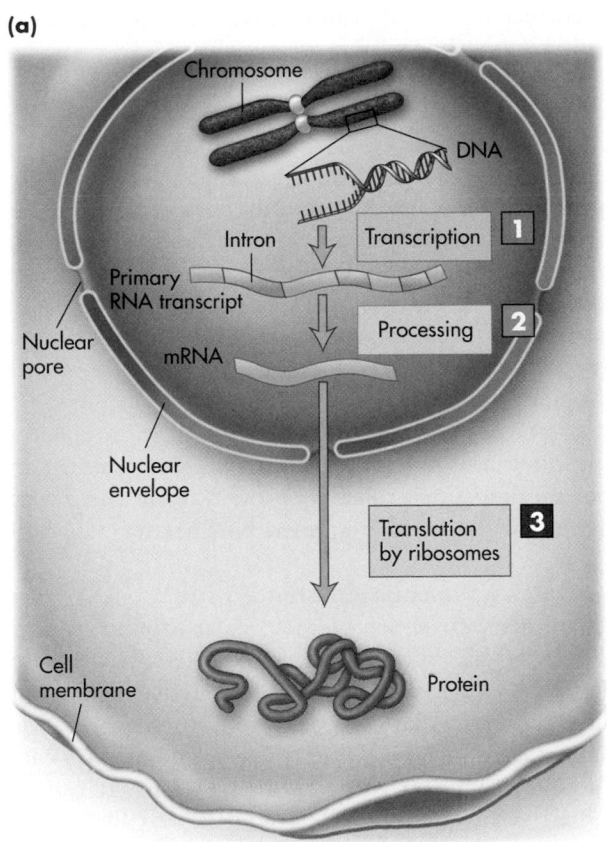

Figure 7-2 | Protein synthesis (simplified). (a) DNA present in the nucleus of the cell is composed of four nucleotides: adenine (A), guanine (G), cytosine (C), and thymine (T) (1). The DNA code is read, three nucleotides at a time, with each specific unit being called a codon. Each DNA codon represents a specific amino acid. The DNA unwinds from its supercoiled state and the code embedded in the order of the nucleotides is transcribed into a complementary messenger RNA (mRNA; labeled as the primary RNA transcript) (2). The mRNA is processed in the nucleus and then is ready to leave the nucleus. The mRNA travels to the cytosol, where the ribosomes then read the codons on the mRNA and translate those instructions in order to produce a specific protein (3). (b) Protein synthesis at the ribosomes begins at a specific starting point, indicated by AUG (4). Protein synthesis then continues by adding one amino acid at a time to the growing polypeptide chain until a specific ending (stop) codon is reached, such as UAA, UAG, or UGA (5). Transfer RNA (tRNA) units bring amino acids to the ribosomes as needed during protein synthesis (6). The tRNA carriers have a complementary code to the mRNA—such that, if an arginine were needed during synthesis, the AGA on the mRNA would correspond to UCU on the tRNA. Numerous tRNA carriers are present during protein synthesis to continually supply the ribosomes with needed amino acids. ATP is used to supply the energy needed to activate tRNA in order to form each new peptide bond. The polypeptide is then released from the ribosome when it encounters the ending (stop) codon (7). Appendix A contains the abbreviations used for the amino acids in this figure, such as "met" for "methionine."

(b)

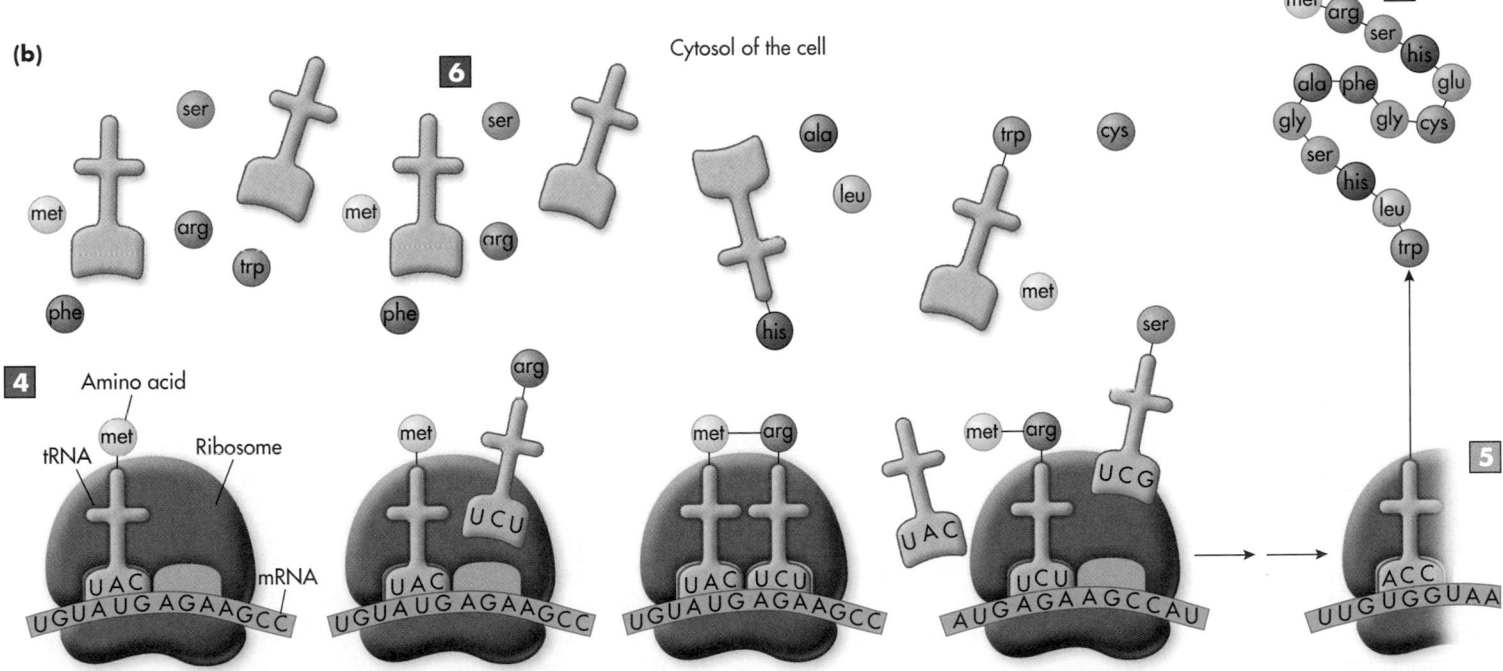

The initiation complex forms when the ribosomal subunits and the first tRNA molecule lock into a strand of mRNA at the start codon (AUG).

A tRNA carrying the amino acid specified second in the mRNA sequence plugs into the complex.

A peptide bond forms between the adjacent amino acids.

As the first tRNA detaches from the mRNA template, the second moves over, trailing its small amino acid chain. A third tRNA sits down at the vacated site, which is now situated over the next codon in the sequence.

Polypeptide released when the ribosome eventually encounters the ending (stop) codon, which in this example is UAA.

correct gene defects such that the correct DNA code can be placed in the nucleus so that the correct protein can be made by the ribosomes.

Protein Organization

The sequential order of the amino acids in the polypeptide chain, called *primary structure*, determines a protein's shape. The key point is that only correctly positioned amino acids can interact and fold properly to form the intended shape for the protein and, in turn, allow for the chemical attractions to form between amino acids near each other that are needed to stabilize the structure, such as hydrogen bonds (see Appendix A for details). This is part of what is called *secondary structure*. The resulting unique three-dimensional conformation, called *tertiary structure*, dictates the function of each protein. If a protein lacks the appropriate configuration, it cannot function.[10]

In some cases, two or more separate polypeptide units interact to form an even larger new protein form, termed a *quaternary structure* (Figure 7-3). This level of organization becomes significant when it is important to have a protein active only at certain times. A protein may be active when the units are joined but inactive when the units are separate.

Sickle-cell disease (also called **sickle-cell anemia**) illustrates what happens when amino acids are out of order in the primary structure of a particular protein. African Americans (about 3 cases per 1000 births) are especially prone to this genetic disease. It originates from a mutation in the DNA sequence and results in defective production of the protein chains of hemoglobin, a protein that carries oxygen in red blood cells. In two of its four protein chains, an error in the amino acid order occurs, one on each chain. This error produces a profound change in hemoglobin structure: It can no longer form the shape needed to carry oxygen efficiently inside the red blood cell. Instead of forming normal doughnut-shaped disks, the red blood cells collapse into crescent (or sickle) shapes (Figure 7-4). Health deteriorates, and eventually episodes of severe bone and joint pain, abdominal pain, headache, convulsions, and paralysis may occur because the sickled cells clump in the capillary beds, hampering blood flow to the target tissue. Treatment for this disease includes blood transfusions, medications (e.g., hydroxyurea) to increase red blood cell synthesis, and bone marrow transplants.

Denaturation of Proteins

Exposure to acid or alkaline substances, heat, or agitation can alter a protein's structure, leaving it in a **denatured** state (Figure 7-5). The protein can no longer perform its function. For example, once the bacteria in yogurt have synthesized enough acid

Sulfur-containing amino acids stabilize many compounds, such as the hormone insulin. Sulfur atoms can bond together (—S—S—), creating a bridge between two protein strands or two parts of the same strand. This stabilizes the structure of the molecule and is also part of what is called *secondary structure*.

sickle-cell disease (sickle-cell anemia) An illness that results from a malformation of the red blood cell because of an incorrect primary structure in part of its hemoglobin protein chains. The disease can lead to episodes of severe bone and joint pain, abdominal pain, headache, convulsions, paralysis, and even death.

denaturation Alteration of a protein's three-dimensional structure, usually because of treatment by heat, enzymes, acid or alkaline solutions, or agitation.

Figure 7-3 | Levels of protein structure. Four different levels of structure are found in proteins. The primary structure of a protein is the linear sequence of amino acids in the polypeptide chain. Secondary structure consists of areas in the polypeptide chain that have a specific shape stabilized by hydrogen and other bonds. The total three-dimensional shape of entire proteins is called tertiary structure. Some proteins also show quaternary structure where two or more protein units join together to form a larger protein, such as hemoglobin depicted in the figure.

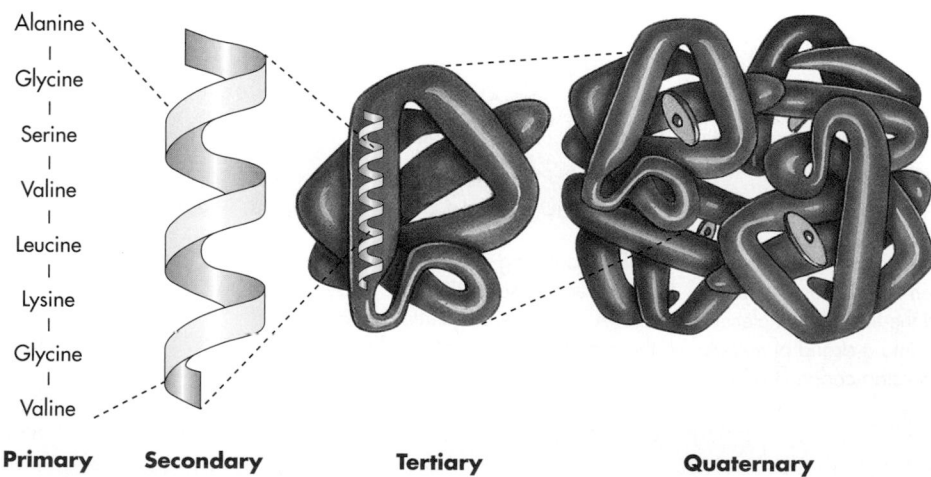

Alanine
|
Glycine
|
Serine
|
Valine
|
Leucine
|
Lysine
|
Glycine
|
Valine

Primary   **Secondary**   **Tertiary**   **Quaternary**

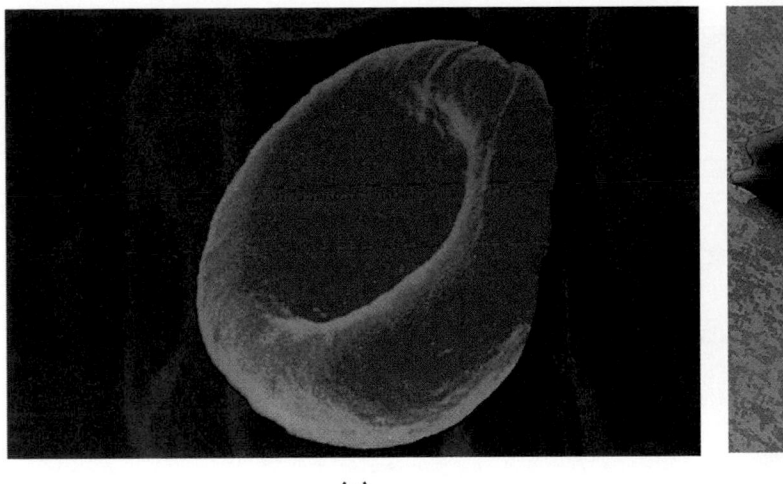

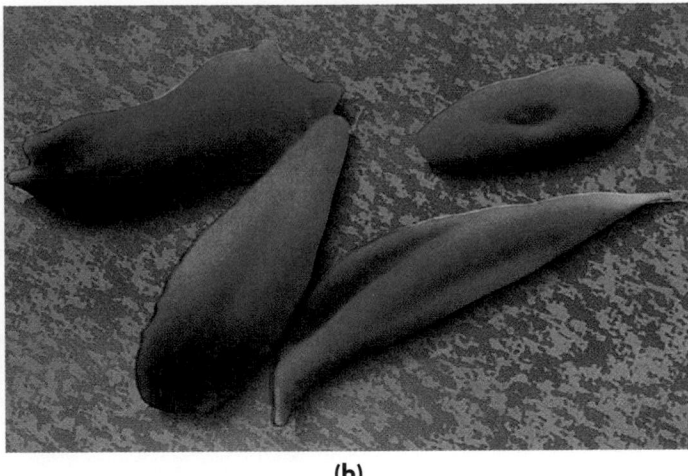

(a)

(b)

Figure 7-4 | An example of the consequences of errors in DNA coding of proteins. *(a)* Normal red blood cell; *(b)* red blood cells from a person with sickle-cell disease: note their abnormal crescent (sicklelike) shape.

and enzymes to denature some of the milk protein, the product solidifies irreversibly. Note that this or any denaturation does not affect the primary structure.

Unraveling a protein's shape often destroys its normal functioning such that it loses its biological activity. That characteristic is useful for some body processes, such as digestion.[18] The secretion of hydrochloric acid in the stomach denatures some bacterial protein, plant hormones, many active enzymes, and other forms of proteins in foods. The heat produced during cooking likewise denatures proteins. Both processes make foods in general safer to eat. Digestion is also enhanced because the unraveling increases exposure of the food to digestive enzymes. Denaturing proteins in some foods can also reduce their tendencies to cause allergic reactions.

Recall that we need proteins in the diet to supply essential amino acids—not the active proteins themselves. We dismantle dietary proteins and use their amino acid building blocks to assemble the proteins we need.

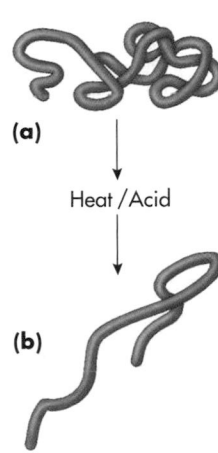

(a)

Heat /Acid

(b)

Figure 7-5 | Denaturation. *(a)* Protein showing a typical coiled state. *(b)* Protein is now partly uncoiled, exhibiting a denatured state. This uncoiling typically reduces or eliminates biological activity.

Concept | Check

Amino acids are linked together in specific sequences to form distinct proteins. DNA provides the directions for synthesizing these new proteins. Specifically, DNA directs the order of the amino acids on the protein. The amino acid order within a protein determines its ultimate shape and function. Destroying the shape of a protein denatures it. Acid conditions present during the body's digestive processes, heat, and other factors can denature proteins, causing them to lose their biological activity.

▌ Protein Digestion and Absorption

As in carbohydrate digestion, the first step in protein digestion takes place in the cooking of food. Cooking unfolds (denatures) proteins and softens tough connective tissue in meat. Cooking also makes many protein-rich foods easier to chew, swallow, and break down during later digestion and absorption.

Digestion

The enzymatic digestion of protein begins in the stomach.[10] Once proteins are denatured by stomach acid, **pepsin,** a major enzyme for digesting proteins, goes to work (Figure 7-6). Stomach acid unravels the proteins, which allows pepsin to attack the

pepsin A protein-digesting enzyme produced by the stomach.

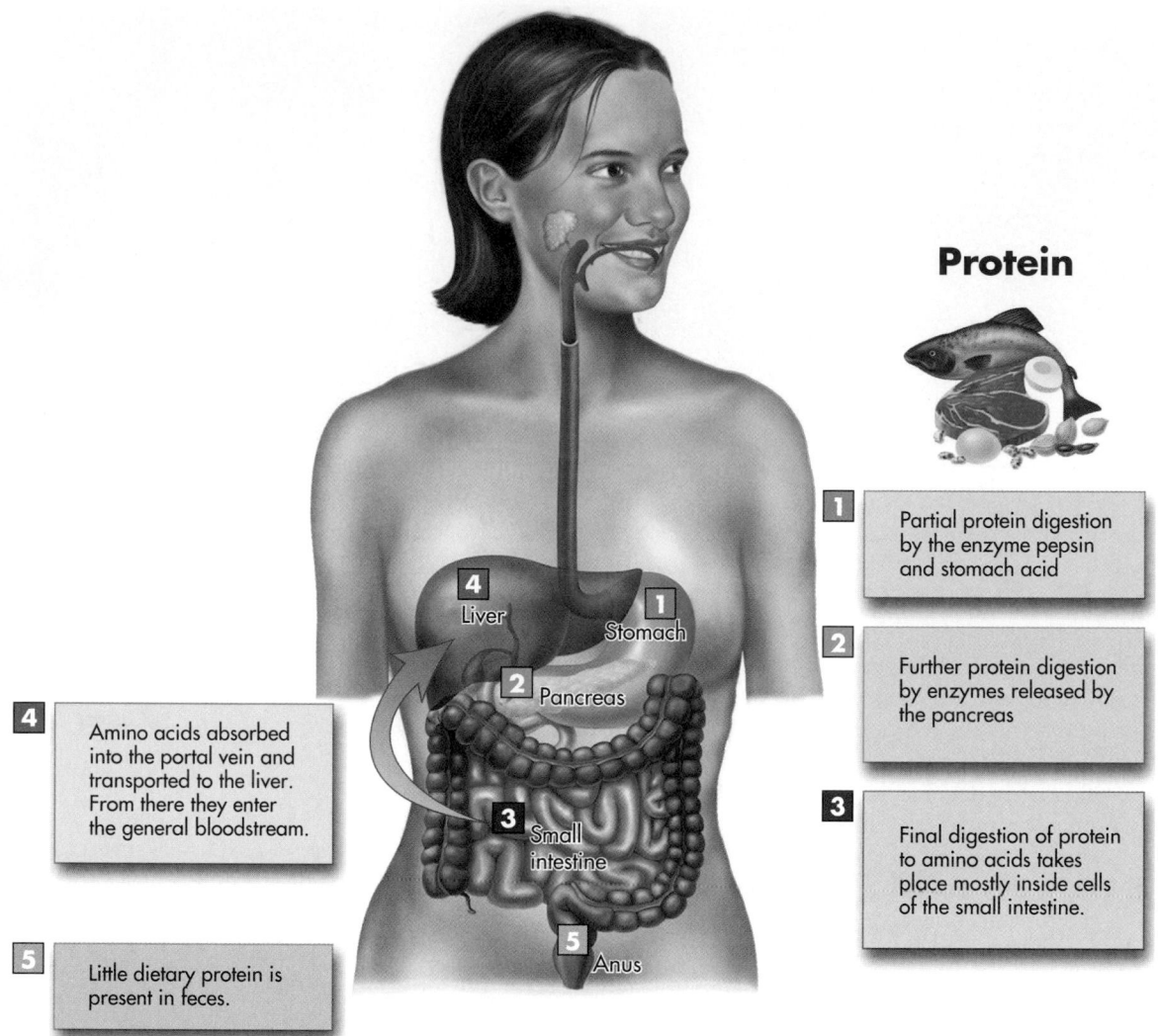

Protein

1 Partial protein digestion by the enzyme pepsin and stomach acid

2 Further protein digestion by enzymes released by the pancreas

3 Final digestion of protein to amino acids takes place mostly inside cells of the small intestine.

4 Amino acids absorbed into the portal vein and transported to the liver. From there they enter the general bloodstream.

5 Little dietary protein is present in feces.

4 Liver

1 Stomach

2 Pancreas

3 Small intestine

5 Anus

Figure 7-6 | A summary of protein digestion and absorption. Enzymatic protein digestion begins in the stomach and ends in the absorptive cells of the small intestine, where the last peptides are broken down into single amino acids. Stomach acid and enzymes contribute to protein digestion. Absorption from the intestinal lumen into the absorptive cells requires energy input.

zymogen An inactive form of an enzyme that requires the removal of a minor part of the chemical structure for it to work. The zymogen is converted into an active enzyme at the appropriate time, such as when released into the stomach or small intestine.

gastrin A hormone that stimulates enzyme and acid secretion by the stomach.

polypeptide chains and break them down into shorter chains of amino acids. Pepsin does not completely separate proteins into amino acids because it can break only a few of the many peptide bonds found in these large molecules. The reaction that takes place is a hydrolysis reaction, because water is used to break down the bond (see Appendix A).

Pepsinogen, the inactive form of pepsin (called a **zymogen**), is produced by the chief cells of the stomach. In proximity are acid-forming cells (parietal cells) and mucus-forming cells in the stomach (review Figure 3-7). If pepsin were not stored as an inactive enzyme, it would digest the stomach glands while waiting to be secreted from the pits. Once pepsinogen enters the stomach's acidic environment (pH between 1 and 2), part of the molecule is split off, forming the active enzyme pepsin.

The release of pepsin is controlled by the hormone **gastrin** (review Table 3-3). Thinking about food or chewing food stimulates gastrin-producing cells in the terminus of the stomach to release the hormone. Gastrin also strongly stimulates the stomach's parietal cells to produce acid.

The partially digested proteins move with the rest of the nutrients and other substances in a meal (chyme) from the stomach into the duodenum, the first part of the small intestine. Once in the small intestine, the polypeptide units (and any fats accompanying them) trigger the release of the hormone cholecystokinin (CCK) from the walls of the small intestine. CCK, in turn, travels through the bloodstream to its target organs, the pancreas and gallbladder. Its arrival causes the pancreas to release the protein-splitting enzymes **trypsin**, chymotrypsin, and carboxypeptidase, which are released into the small intestine in their zymogen forms and then activated by digestive secretions. Together, these digestive enzymes further divide the polypeptides into short peptides and amino acids. Eventually, digestion of all peptides into amino acids occurs using other enzymes secreted into the intestinal lumen by glands located in the wall of the small intestine as well as enzymes present inside the absorptive cells of the small intestine.[10]

trypsin A protein-digesting enzyme secreted by the pancreas to act in the small intestine.

Absorption

The small peptides and amino acids in the lumen of the small intestine are actively absorbed into the cells of the small intestine (Figure 7-7).[18] Eleven or so different transport mechanisms in the intestinal tract have been described. The absorbed small peptides,

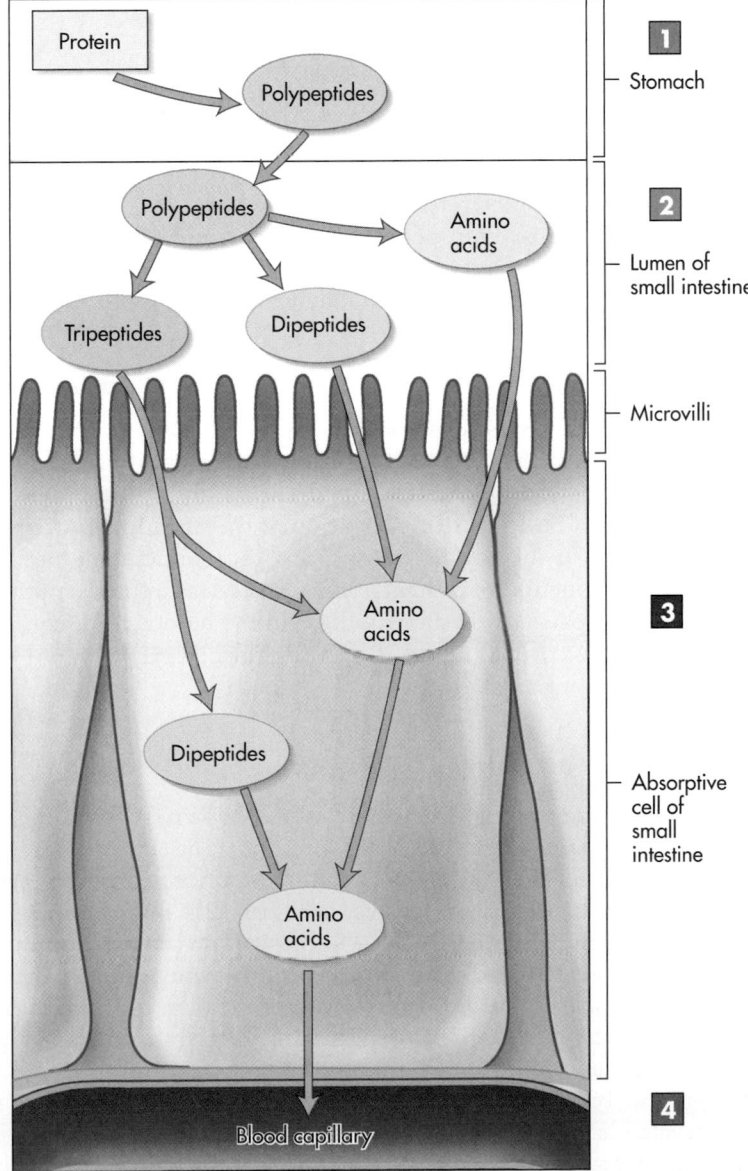

Figure 7-7 | Protein digestion takes place in the stomach (1) lumen of the small intestine (2) and the absorptive cells of the small intestine (3). Then, in a sodium-dependent, energy-requiring process (active absorption), all of the end products of protein digestion are absorbed at the microvilli surface. Any remaining peptides are broken down to amino acids within the absorptive cell. These free amino acids are released into the bloodstream (4). The enzymes used come from the stomach, pancreas, and absorptive and glandular cells that line the small intestine.

then, are eventually broken down to individual amino acids inside the intestinal cells. The amino acids travel via the portal vein that drains the intestinal tract and connects to the liver. There the amino acids are combined into protein, converted to nonessential amino acids, carbohydrate or fat, used for energy needs, or released into the bloodstream. Of these options, conversion to fat is the least likely.

Except during infancy, it is uncommon for intact proteins to be absorbed from the digestive tract. In the period of infancy (up to 4 to 5 months of age), the gastrointestinal tract is somewhat permeable to small proteins, so some whole proteins can be absorbed. Because proteins from some foods (e.g., cow's milk and egg whites) may predispose an infant to food allergies, pediatricians and registered dietitians recommend waiting until an infant is at least 6 to 12 months of age before introducing commonly allergenic foods (see Chapter 17 for details).

Concept | Check

Enzymatic protein digestion begins in the stomach. In the small intestine, protein breakdown products formed in the stomach separate into dipeptides and tripeptides and finally into amino acids as these further breakdown products enter the absorptive cells of the small intestine. The amino acids then travel via the portal vein that connects to the liver.

Functions of Proteins

Proteins function in many crucial ways in human metabolism and in the formation of body structures (Figure 7-8). We rely on foods to supply the amino acids needed to form these proteins. Note, however, that only when we also eat enough carbohydrate and fat can food proteins be used most efficiently. If we don't consume enough energy to meet energy needs, some amino acids from proteins are broken down to produce energy, rendering them unavailable to build body proteins.

Producing Vital Body Structures

Every cell contains protein. Muscle tissue, connective tissue, mucus, blood-clotting factors, transport proteins in the bloodstream, lipoproteins, enzymes, immune bodies, some hormones, visual pigments, and the support structure inside bones are mainly made of protein.[18] Half of body protein is made up of the structural proteins collagen, actin, and myosin as well as the oxygen-transporting protein hemoglobin. This structural role is the primary function of protein in the body. Measurements of the amounts of certain body proteins, particularly some of those in the blood, are used as indicators of health or disease. Excess protein in the diet doesn't necessarily enhance the synthesis of body components, but eating too little can impede it.

Protein Turnover—Adapting to Changing Conditions

protein turnover The process by which a cell breaks down existing proteins and then synthesizes new proteins. Thus the cell can adapt to changing conditions: it will have the necessary proteins as the need for them arises.

slough To shed or cast off.

Most vital body proteins are in a constant state of breakdown, rebuilding, and repair, especially in the bone marrow and the small intestine. This process, called **protein turnover**, allows cells to adapt to changing circumstances.[10] For example, when we eat more protein than necessary for health, the liver needs to make more enzymes to process the waste product from the resulting amino acid metabolism—namely ammonia—into urea. The amino acids needed to make the enzymes can come from the diet and from amino acids released from the breakdown of other proteins in cells. For example, the GI tract lining is constantly **sloughed** off. The digestive tract treats sloughed cells just like food particles and absorbs the amino acids released during their digestion. In fact, most protein breakdown products—amino acids—released throughout the body can be recycled and are added to the pool of amino acids available for future protein synthesis. Overall, protein turnover is a process by which a cell can respond

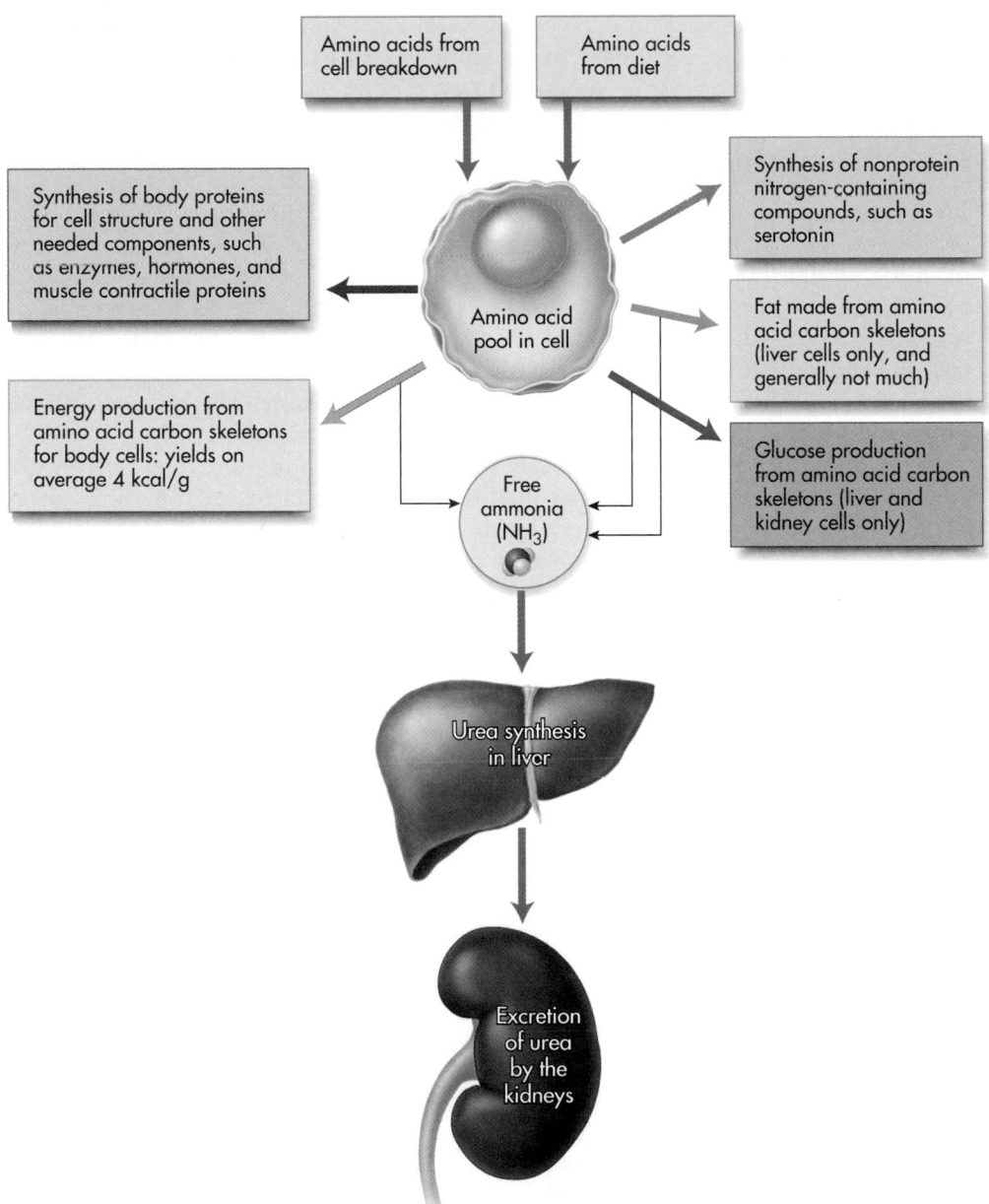

Figure 7-8 | Amino acid metabolism. The amino acid **pool** in a cell can be used to supply amino acids to form body proteins, as well as to form a variety of other possible products—such as fat and glucose—from amino acid **carbon skeletons.** The urea that results is a waste product made from the nitrogen-containing ammonia (NH_3) released during amino acid breakdown. It is excreted in the urine.

Within the figure:

- Amino acids from cell breakdown
- Amino acids from diet
- Synthesis of body proteins for cell structure and other needed components, such as enzymes, hormones, and muscle contractile proteins
- Amino acid pool in cell
- Synthesis of nonprotein nitrogen-containing compounds, such as serotonin
- Fat made from amino acid carbon skeletons (liver cells only, and generally not much)
- Energy production from amino acid carbon skeletons for body cells: yields on average 4 kcal/g
- Free ammonia (NH_3)
- Glucose production from amino acid carbon skeletons (liver and kidney cells only)
- Urea synthesis in liver
- Excretion of urea by the kidneys

pool The amount of a nutrient found within the body that can be easily mobilized when needed.

carbon skeleton What remains of an amino acid after the amino group has been removed.

to its changing environment and produce needed proteins while reducing the quantity of proteins not currently needed.

During any day, an adult makes and degrades about 250 to 300 g of protein, and many of the amino acids are recycled. By comparing 250 to 300 g with the 65 to 100 g or more of protein typically consumed by adults, you can see the importance of recycling amino acids in the body when possible.[10]

Hormones that increase protein synthesis are insulin and growth hormone. In contrast, the hormone cortisol increases protein breakdown.

A practical example of the concept of protein turnover occurs in untreated **acquired immunodeficiency syndrome (AIDS),** as seen in the developing world (see Chapter 20). Rates of protein synthesis are similar in healthy people and those with untreated or untreatable cases of AIDS, but the rates of protein degradation are much higher because of the effects of the disease. Over time, these higher rates result in much protein wasting in people with AIDS.

Critical | Thinking

Samantha's mother's blood concentration of urea is high. From a health status point of view, what might this indicate?

acquired immunodeficiency syndrome (AIDS) A disorder in which a virus (human immunodeficiency virus [HIV]) infects specific types of immune system cells. This leaves the person with reduced immune function and, in turn, defenseless against numerous infectious agents.

If a person's diet is deficient in protein for a long period of time, the rebuilding and repairing process slows. Eventually, skeletal muscles, heart, liver, blood proteins, and other organs decrease in size or volume. Only the brain resists protein breakdown.

Maintaining Fluid Balance

Blood proteins—albumins and globulins—maintain body fluid balance. Normal blood pressure in the arteries forces blood into capillary beds. The blood fluid then moves from the **capillary beds** into the spaces between nearby cells (**extracellular spaces**) to provide nutrients to those cells (Figure 7-9). Proteins in the bloodstream such as albumin are too large, however, to move out of the capillary beds into the tissues. The presence of these proteins in the capillary beds attracts the proper amount of fluid back to the blood, partially counteracting the force of blood pressure. This is especially true in the areas of the capillary beds right next to their venous connections.

With inadequate protein consumption, the concentration of proteins eventually decreases in the bloodstream. Excessive fluid then builds up in the surrounding tissues because the counteracting force produced by the smaller amount of blood proteins is too weak to pull enough of the fluid back from the tissues into the bloodstream. As fluids accumulate in the tissues, the tissues swell, causing clinical **edema**.[18] Because edema sometimes can be a sign of serious medical problems, the cause must be identified. An important step in diagnosing the cause is to measure the concentration of blood proteins, although many other medical problems also cause edema.

Contributing to Acid-Base Balance

Proteins help regulate the acid-base balance in the blood. Proteins located in cell membranes pump chemical ions in and out of cells. The ion concentrations that result from the pumping action, among other factors, keeps the blood slightly alkaline. **Buffers**— compounds that maintain acid-base conditions within a narrow range—are another

capillary bed Minute vessels one cell thick that create a junction between arterial and venous circulation. Gas and nutrient exchange occurs here between body cells and the blood.

extracellular space The space outside cells.

edema The buildup of excess fluid in extracellular spaces.

Figure C-5 in Appendix C provides a detailed view of a capillary bed.

buffers Compounds that cause a solution to resist changes in acid-base balance.

Figure 7-9 | Blood proteins in relation to fluid balance. (a) Blood proteins are important for maintaining the body's fluid balance, since they draw fluid back into the capillary bed. (b) Without sufficient protein in the bloodstream, edema develops because the counteracting force to blood pressure provided by blood proteins declines.

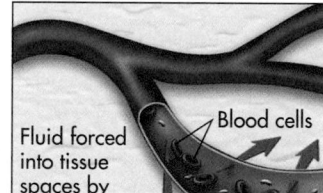
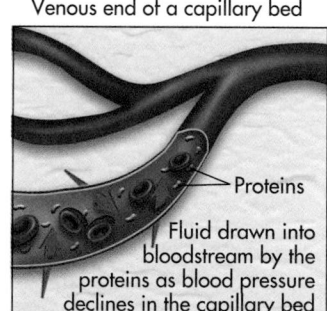
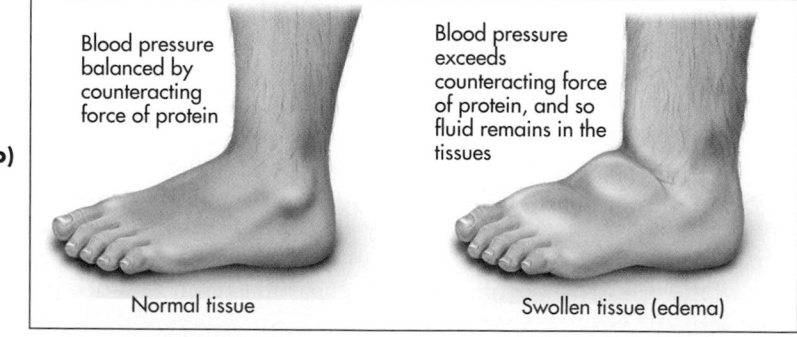

Arterial end of a capillary bed

Venous end of a capillary bed

(a) Fluid forced into tissue spaces by blood pressure generated by pumping action of heart

Blood cells

Proteins

Fluid drawn into bloodstream by the proteins as blood pressure declines in the capillary bed

(b) Blood pressure balanced by counteracting force of protein

Blood pressure exceeds counteracting force of protein, and so fluid remains in the tissues

Normal tissue

Swollen tissue (edema)

means of regulating acid-base balance in the blood. Some blood proteins are especially good buffers for the body. Hemoglobin is extremely important in maintaining normal blood pH.[10]

Forming Hormones and Enzymes

Amino acids are required for the synthesis of most hormones—our internal body messengers. Some hormones, such as the thyroid hormones, are made from only one amino acid, tyrosine. Insulin, on the other hand, is composed of 51 amino acids. These and other hormones classified as proteins perform important regulatory functions in the body, such as controlling the metabolic rate and amount of glucose taken up from the bloodstream. Almost all enzymes are also proteins or have a protein component.[18]

Contributing to Immune Function

Proteins are a key component of the cells used by the immune system, such as leukocytes and lymphocytes. Also, the antibodies produced by one type of immune cell (β-lymphocytes) are proteins.[18] These antibodies can bind to foreign proteins in the body, an important step in removing invaders from the body. Without sufficient dietary protein, the immune system lacks the materials needed to function properly. Thus, immune incompetence—**anergy**—and a protein-deficient diet often appear together. Anergy can turn measles into a fatal disease for a malnourished child. It also can encourage unusual infections, such as widespread yeast *(Candida)* growth in the mouth and throat of a hospitalized adult.[10]

Forming Glucose

In Chapter 5 you learned that the body must maintain a fairly constant concentration of blood glucose to supply energy for red blood cells and nervous tissue, such as the brain. At rest, the brain uses about 19% of the body's energy requirements, and it gets most of that energy from glucose. If you don't consume enough carbohydrate to supply the glucose, your liver (and kidneys, to a lesser extent) will be forced to make glucose from amino acids present in body tissues (review Figure 7-8). Recall from Chapter 4 that this process is called gluconeogenesis (review Figure 4-16).[10]

Making some glucose from amino acids is normal. For example, when you skip breakfast and haven't eaten since 7 P.M. the preceding evening, glucose must be manufactured. In an extreme situation, however, such as starvation, the conversion of amino acids into glucose wastes much muscle tissue and can lead to **cachexia.**

Providing Energy

Proteins supply very little energy for a weight-stable person. Two exceptions are prolonged exercise (see Chapter 14 for information about the use of amino acids for energy during exercise) and energy restriction, such as with a low-calorie diet. In these cases the carbon skeletons of amino acids are metabolized for energy.

Still, under most conditions, cells use primarily fats and carbohydrates for energy. Although proteins and carbohydrates contain the same amount of usable energy—on average, 4 kcal/g—proteins are a very costly source of energy, considering the amount of metabolism and processing the liver and kidneys must perform to use this energy source.[10]

Contributing to Satiety

Compared to the other macronutrients, proteins provide the highest feeling of **satiety** after a meal. Thus, including some protein with each meal helps control overall food intake. Many experts warn against skimping on protein when trying to reduce energy intake to lose weight. Meeting protein needs is still important and exceeding needs

Neurotransmitters, released by nerve endings, are often derivatives of amino acids. This is true for dopamine (synthesized from the amino acid tyrosine), norepinephrine (synthesized from the amino acid tyrosine), and serotonin (synthesized from the amino acid tryptophan).[10]

anergy Lack of an immune response to foreign compounds entering the body.

The vitamin niacin can be made from the amino acid tryptophan, illustrating another role of proteins.

cachexia Widespread wasting of the body due to undernutrition.

satiety A state in which there is no longer a desire to eat; a feeling of satisfaction.

Too little protein in the diet also contributes to poor bone health. This effect has been shown in older people who do not eat enough protein. For anyone following a balanced diet, this is not a concern.[8]

somewhat may provide an additional benefit when dieting to lose weight (see Chapter 13 for details).[16]

Concept | Check

Vital body structures—such as muscle, connective tissue, blood transport proteins, enzymes, hormones, buffers, and immune factors—are mainly proteins. The breakdown of existing proteins and synthesis of new proteins takes place on a minute-by-minute basis, amounting to a turnover of about 250 to 300 g a day for the entire human body. Proteins can also provide fuel for the body and can be used for glucose production.

Protein Needs

How much protein (actually, amino acids) do we need to eat each day? People who aren't growing need to eat only enough protein to match daily losses as evidenced by protein breakdown products in the urine and protein lost as such from feces, skin, hair, nails, and so on. In short, people need to balance protein intake with protein losses, producing a state of equilibrium.[10]

When a body is growing or recovering from an illness, it needs extra protein to supply the raw materials required to build new tissues. To achieve this, a person must eat more protein daily than he or she loses. In addition, the hormones insulin, growth hormone, and testosterone all stimulate this building of new tissue. Merely eating more protein does not produce additional body tissue unless the right hormonal conditions associated with the growing years or pregnancy exist. Resistance exercise (weight training) also enhances protein synthesis.

For healthy people, the amount of dietary protein needed to compensate for all evidence of protein losses can be determined by increasing protein intake until it just equals such losses. (Energy needs must be met so that amino acids are not diverted for energy use.)

To determine this balance between protein gain and loss by the body, researchers actually track nitrogen intake and loss (Figure 7-10).[10] It is much easier to quantify nitrogen intake and loss. Nitrogen makes up, on average, 16% of the weight of an amino acid, so nitrogen intake or output divided by 0.16 yields a rough estimate of protein intake or output. One can also multiply by the reciprocal of 0.16, which is 6.25:

$$\text{nitrogen (g)} \times 6.25 = \text{protein (g)}$$

To measure nitrogen balance, first a person's protein intake is monitored: this measurement includes protein that comes in the form of fluids and foods. The grams of protein consumed is divided by 6.25 to yield the approximate grams of nitrogen (N) consumed. This value is then compared with the amount of nitrogen lost from the body. Urine output for the same 24-hour period is collected and analyzed for urea nitrogen content. This value is then put into one of various formulas available to estimate total nitrogen loss from the body. Because most of the nitrogen lost from the body is in the form of urea, this approach is fairly accurate. The other factors in a specific formula account for nitrogen loss in the urine that is not in the form of urea (e.g., $0.2 \times$ urinary urea N) as well as nitrogen loss from all other body sources, such as hair, skin, feces, and other nonurine sources (e.g., 2 g).

$$\text{nitrogen balance} = \frac{\text{protein intake}}{6.25 \text{ g}} - \text{g urinary urea N} - (0.2 \times \text{urinary urea N}) - 2 \text{ g}$$

For example, suppose a person consumes 70 g of protein in a 24-hour period; during that time he excreted 7 g of nitrogen as urea. His state of nitrogen balance is 0.8, based on the following calculation:

$$\text{nitrogen balance} = \frac{70}{6.25} - 7 - (0.2 \times 7) - 2$$

$$= 0.8$$

(a)

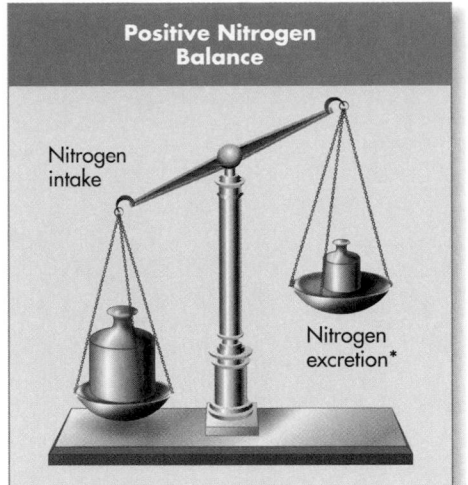

Situations in which nitrogen balance is positive:

Growth
Pregnancy
Recovery stage after illness/injury
Athletic training**
Increased secretion of certain hormones, such as insulin, growth hormone, and testosterone

(b)

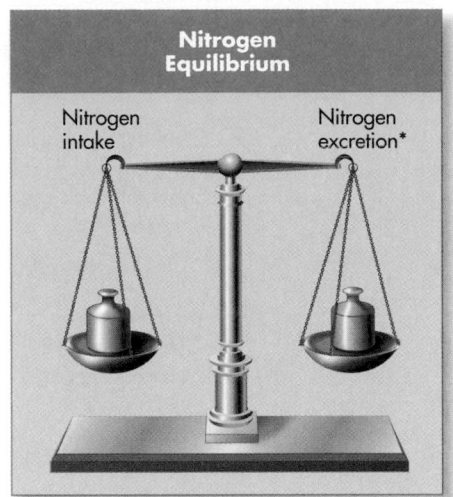

Situations in which nitrogen balance is in equilibrium:

Healthy adult meeting nutrient needs, notably protein and energy needs

(c)

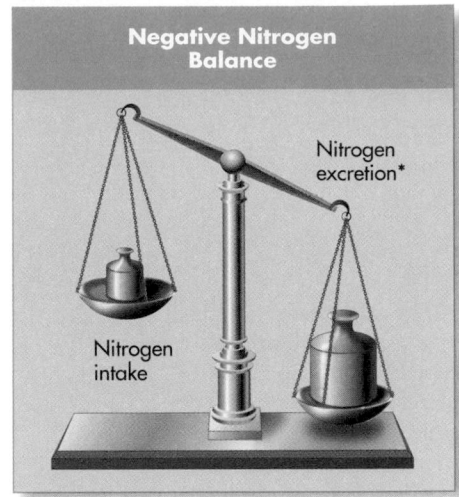

Situations in which nitrogen balance is negative:

Inadequate intake of protein (fasting, intestinal tract diseases)
Inadequate energy intake
Conditions such as fevers, burns, and infections
Bed rest (for several days)
Deficiency of essential amino acids (e.g., poor-quality protein consumed)
Increased protein loss (as in some forms of kidney disease)
Increased secretion of certain hormones, such as thyroid hormone and cortisol

---

*Based on losses of urea and other nitrogen-containing compounds in the urine as well as protein itself lost from feces, skin, hair, nails, and other minor routes.
**Only when additional lean body mass is being gained. Nevertheless, the athlete is probably already eating enough protein to support this extra protein synthesis; protein supplements are not needed.

Figure 7-10 | Nitrogen balance in practical terms. Determining this balance requires measuring nitrogen intake and loss.

Because this number is positive, the person is in a slightly positive nitrogen balance and thus in a positive protein balance. Through measurement error, however, he could also simply be in equilibrium.

Today the best estimate for the amount of protein required for nearly all adults to maintain protein equilibrium is 0.8 g of protein per kilogram (kg) of healthy body weight (the concept of healthy weight is discussed in Chapter 13). This 0.8 g/kg is the RDA for protein. Healthy weight is used as a baseline because excess fat storage doesn't contribute much to protein needs. This RDA works out to about 56 g of protein daily for a 70-kg (154-lb) man and about 46 g of protein daily for a 57-kg (125-lb) woman.[10]

Convert weight from pounds to kg:

$$\frac{154 \text{ pounds}}{2.2 \text{ pounds/kg}} = 70 \text{ kg}$$

$$\frac{125 \text{ pounds}}{2.2 \text{ pounds/kg}} = 57 \text{ kg}$$

Calculate RDA:

$$70 \text{ kg} \times \frac{0.8 \text{ g protein}}{\text{kg body weight}} = 56 \text{ g}$$

$$57 \text{ kg} \times \frac{0.8 \text{ g protein}}{\text{kg body weight}} = 46 \text{ g}$$

Pregnant and lactating women and infants and children under 19 years of age have different RDAs for protein (see Chapters 16 and 17).

The RDA for protein translates into about 8 to 10% of total energy intake.[10] The National Cholesterol Education Program in the United States recommends up to 15% of total energy intake to provide more flexibility in diet planning, in turn allowing for the variety of protein-rich foods North Americans typically consume. This amount also generally provides enough protein for the active athlete.

Table 7-3 | The Protein Contents of a 1600 kcal Diet and a 2400 kcal Diet*

1600 kcal Diet	Protein (Grams)	2400 kcal Diet	Protein (Grams)
Breakfast			
1% low-fat milk, 1 cup	8	2% reduced-fat milk, 1 cup	8
Cheerios, 1 cup	2	Cheerios, 1 cup	2
Orange	1	Eggs, soft cooked, 2	12
		Orange	1
Lunch			
Whole-wheat bread, 2 slices	5	Whole-wheat bread, 2 slices	5
Chicken breast, 2 oz	17	Chicken breast, 2 oz	17
Mayonnaise, 1 tsp	—	Provolone cheese, 2 oz	15
Tomato slices, 2	—	Tomato slices, 2	—
Carrot sticks, 1 cup	1	Mayonnaise, 1 tsp	—
Oatmeal-raisin cookie, 1	2	Oatmeal-raisin cookies, 2	4
Fig, 1 large	0.5	Figs, 2	1
Diet soft drink	—	Diet soft drink	—
Dinner			
Mixed green salad, 1 cup	—	Mixed green salad, 1 cup	—
Italian dressing, 2 tsp	—	Italian dressing, 2 tsp	—
Beef tenderloin, 3 oz	21	Beef tenderloin, 4 oz	28
Spinach pasta, 1 cup, with garlic butter, 1 tsp	7	Spinach pasta, 1 cup, with garlic butter, 1 tsp	7
Zucchini, 1/2 cup, sauteed in oil, 1 tsp	0.5	Zucchini, 1/2 cup, sauteed in oil, 1 tsp	0.5
1% low-fat milk, 1 cup	8	Carrot sticks, 1/2 cup	0.5
		2% reduced-fat milk, 1 cup	8
Snack		**Snack**	
Bagel, toasted, 1/2 of a 3 1/2" bagel	4	Bagel, toasted, 1/2 of 3 1/2" bagel	4
Jam, 2 tsp	—	Jam, 2 tsp	—
Fruited yogurt, 1 cup	<u>10</u>	Fruited yogurt, 1 cup	<u>10</u>
TOTAL	87		123

*This table illustrates how little energy needs to be consumed while still meeting the RDA for protein. It also shows how much protein we eat when we consume typical energy intakes.

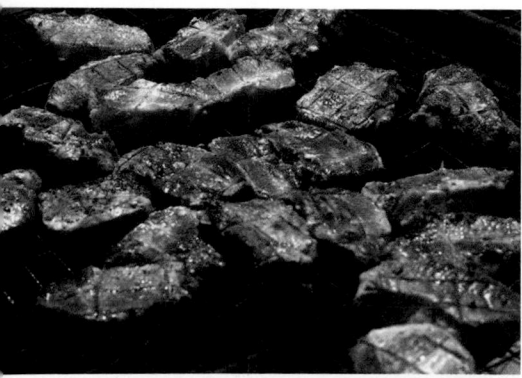

Animal protein foods are typically our main sources of protein in North America.

Approximate protein needs are listed in the inside cover of this textbook. It is easy to consume the amount of protein currently suggested each day to meet body needs (Table 7-3). North American men typically consume about 100 g of protein daily, whereas women typically consume 65 g daily.[10]

Most of us consume much more protein than RDA amounts because we like many high-protein foods and can afford to buy them. Excess protein eaten cannot be stored as such, so the carbon skeletons are put to use for other purposes or metabolized for energy needs (review Figure 7-8). Note also that mental stress, physical labor, and routine weekend sports activities do not require an increase in the protein RDA.[10]

To support the training needs of endurance and highly trained athletes, protein consumption may need to exceed the RDA. The Food and Nutrition Board does not support an increased need, but some experts suggest that an intake of 1.2–1.7 g/kg of protein per day may be needed (see Chapter 14). However, studies supporting these high intakes are few. Many North Americans also already consume that much protein, especially men. The Food and Nutrition Board also suggests that protein intake not exceed 35% of energy intake.[10] Athletes can calculate this amount and use it as an upper limit for protein intake. In addition, athletes do not need individual amino acid supplements. These are a needless expense. All of us, athletes included, can meet our protein needs using basic foods (see Chapter 14 for details).

Does Eating a High-Protein Diet Harm You?

You may wonder about the potential harm of protein intakes greatly in excess of the RDA. If diets high in protein rely mostly on animal sources for protein, they may be simultaneously low in plant sources and therefore low in fiber, some vitamins (e.g., folate), some minerals (e.g., magnesium), and phytochemicals. Additionally, high-protein foods from animals are often rich in saturated fat and cholesterol and thus do not follow the recommendations of the Dietary Guidelines for Americans or the Food and Nutrition Board in terms of reducing the risk for cardiovascular disease.[10]

Some, but not all, studies show that high-protein diets can increase calcium losses in urine. This effect when seen, however, is very minimal. For people with adequate calcium intakes, little concern about this relationship is warranted.

Excessive intake of red meat, especially processed forms, is linked to colon cancer.[6] There are several possible explanations for this connection. The curing agents used to process meats such as hot dogs, ham, and salami may cause cancer. Substances that form during cooking of red meat at high temperatures (heterocyclic amines) may also cause cancer (for a discussion of heterocyclic amines, see the Nutrition Focus section in Chapter 12). The excessive fat or low fiber contents of diets rich in red meat in general may also be a contributing factor. Because of these concerns, some nutrition experts suggest we focus more on poultry, fish, nuts, legumes, and seeds to meet protein needs. In addition, any red and other types of meat should be trimmed of all visible fat before grilling.

Some researchers have expressed concern that a high protein intake may overburden the kidneys by forcing them to excrete the extra nitrogen as urea.[9] Additionally, animal proteins may contribute to kidney stone formation in susceptible people.[5] To prevent these problems, there is some support for not exceeding protein needs. For instance, for people in the early stages of kidney disease, low-protein diets somewhat slow the decline in kidney function. Because preserving kidney function is especially important for people with diabetes and early signs of kidney disease, these people are advised against consuming a high-protein diet. For people without diabetes or kidney disease, the risk of suffering kidney failure is minimal.

The amino acids most likely to cause toxicity when consumed in large amounts are methionine, cysteine, and histidine.[12] The potential for amino acid imbalance and toxicity is too great to recommend that any be taken individually as supplements. As emphasized earlier, the body is designed to handle whole proteins as a dietary source of amino acids. When individual amino acid supplements are taken, they can overwhelm the absorptive mechanism in the small intestine, triggering amino acid imbalances in the body. These imbalances occur because groups of chemically similar amino acids compete for absorption sites in the absorptive cells. An excess of one can hamper other amino acids from being absorbed. Overall, every amino acid taken in excess can be harmful. We should stick to whole foods as sources for amino acids.

Protein in Foods

Based on the typical foods we eat in North America, about 70% of protein comes from animal sources. The most nutrient-dense source of protein is water-packed tuna, which has 87% of its energy as protein. Other good sources are meat, poultry, fish, milk and some milk products, beans, and nuts. Worldwide, 35% of protein comes from animal sources. In Africa and East Asia, only about 20% of the protein eaten comes from animal sources.

The Value of Plant Protein

Plant sources of proteins deserve more attention and use from North Americans. Many plant foods—in proportion to the amount of energy they supply—provide not only much protein but also ample magnesium and fiber (especially soluble fiber), along with

High-protein diets increase urine output, in turn posing a risk for dehydration. This is a special concern for athletes (see Chapter 14).

Infants' diets must be limited in protein because their kidneys have difficulty excreting large amounts of urea and minerals, which remain after protein metabolism. Thus, regular cow's milk must not be used for feeding young infants—it is too high in protein and other nutrients (see Chapter 17 for details).

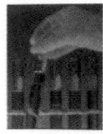

Expert Opinion

A New Appreciation for the *Nut* in Nutrition
Penny M. Kris-Etherton, Ph.D., R.D.

A marked shift has taken place in our thinking about the role of nuts in a healthy diet thanks to a substantive and growing body of scientific evidence demonstrating the health benefits of nut consumption in a number of disease states. The story began with benefits being shown for nut consumption and coronary disease; it has expanded to benefits for other diseases. Data from four large epidemiologic studies have convincingly shown that frequent consumption of nuts (1 oz of nuts consumed five times/week) is associated with a decreased risk of coronary heart disease morbidity and/or mortality in the range of approximately 30 to 50% in many different population groups. Frequent nut consumption (1 oz of nuts consumed ≥ five times/week) has been shown to decrease risk of type 2 diabetes in women by 27%, and consumption of peanut butter five times or more per week reduces risk by 21%. Similarly, comparable nut consumption decreases risk of gallbladder stones in women by 25%. In addition, there is intriguing evidence that nuts can help regulate body weight; the available evidence shows that frequent nut consumption is not associated with a higher body mass index or tendency to gain weight.

What the Specific Research Studies Show

The Adventist Health Study, a landmark prospective epidemiologic study conducted with 34,198 Seventh-Day Adventists in California, was the first study to report a protective effect of nuts on cardiovascular disease. Individuals who ate nuts ≥ 5 times/week experienced a 51% reduction in risk of having a myocardial infarction. Those who ate nuts 1 to 4 times/week had a 22% reduced risk compared with a group who ate nuts < 1 time/week.

Since this pioneering study, other epidemiologic studies have reported cardioprotective effects of nut consumption. These studies include the Iowa Women's Health Study, Nurses' Health Study, and Physicians' Health Study. In the Iowa Women's Health Study, which followed 34,500 postmenopausal women for five years, coronary mortality was inversely associated with nut consumption. Women who consumed nuts > 1 time/week had a 40% reduction in cardiovascular disease risk compared with women who ate nuts less frequently. In the Nurses' Health Study, which involved 86,016 women,

frequent nut consumption (> 5 oz/week) was associated with a 35% reduction in cardiovascular disease risk. The magnitude of risk reduction was similar for both fatal coronary heart disease and nonfatal myocardial infarction. The Physicians' Health Study, conducted with 21,454 male participants, reported that those who consumed nuts 2 or more times/week had reduced risks of sudden cardiac death (by 47%) and of total cardiovascular disease death (by 30%). Collectively, this epidemiologic evidence is compelling and has established a dose-response relationship between nut consumption and reduced cardiovascular disease risk. Moreover, subsequent analyses conducted with these databases have shown that the protective effect of nut consumption is consistent among many different population subgroups including men and women (as noted), younger and older subjects, those with or without hypertension, and subjects who vary in weight, smoking status, and physical activity level.

The emerging evidence from the Nurses' Health Study that demonstrates beneficial associations with nut consumption and decreased risk of diabetes and gallbladder stones is exciting because it has expanded the health benefits of nut consumption to other diseases. Both epidemiologic and controlled clinical trials consistently show either a lower body weight or no weight gain when nuts are included in the diet. This weight result may contribute to the beneficial association of nut consumption on diabetes and gallbladder disease. Nuts may well exert beneficial effects on other diseases linked to overweight/obesity.

Put Nuts into Focus

Researchers have conducted numerous controlled clinical studies with different nuts as well as peanuts (which are a legume). These studies differed in design and dietary control. Some studies were specifically designed to evaluate the effects of nuts on blood lipids and lipoproteins. Other studies used nuts and other fat sources to achieve a fatty acid profile of an experimental diet that was evaluated. The studies in general evaluated diets that were low in saturated fat and cholesterol because nuts were used to replace food sources of saturated fat. Both moderate-fat and low-fat diets were studied. Across di-

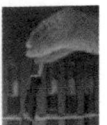

etary fat levels, experimental diets containing nuts reduced total cholesterol and low-density lipoprotein (LDL) cholesterol concentrations by about 4 to 16% and 9 to 20%, respectively. In addition, the diets that contained nuts did not reduce high-density lipoprotein (HDL) cholesterol, nor did they increase blood triglyceride levels as did the comparative low-fat, high-carbohydrate control diets. It is evident that the decrease in total and LDL cholesterol levels with the nut diets reflects the decrease in saturated fat and increase in unsaturated fat. In addition, the effects of the nut test diets on HDL cholesterol and triglycerides could be explained by their higher total fat content.

A key question is whether the effects of nuts on blood lipids are solely due to their fat and fatty acid profile, or whether there are other bioactive compounds in nuts that contribute to the blood lipid and lipoprotein responses noted. Nonetheless, it is clear that when nuts replace food sources of saturated fat, total cholesterol and LDL cholesterol are reduced, resulting in a decreased risk of cardiovascular disease. The American Heart Association Dietary Guidelines (2000) advise that to attain a desirable blood cholesterol profile, one should limit foods high in saturated fat and cholesterol and substitute unsaturated fat from vegetables, fish, legumes, and nuts. Thus, this dietary recommendation acknowledges the health benefits of unsaturated fats and recognizes nuts and legumes as important food sources of unsaturated fats.

Peanut and Tree Nut Allergies

Food allergy occurs in 6 to 8% of children 4 years of age or younger and in 4% of adults. Eight foods account for 90% of all food-related allergies; peanuts and tree nuts are two of these foods. (The other foods are milk, egg, fish, shellfish, soy, and wheat). The allergic reactions can range from a mild intolerance to a fatal allergy due to anaphylaxis. Current guidelines advise that children < 3 years of age should not eat peanuts or tree nuts. In addition, peanuts and/or tree nuts should be avoided by older children and adults with nut and peanut allergies.

Nuts as a Source of Nutrition

Nuts are a powerhouse of nutrients including unsaturated fats (both monounsaturated and polyunsaturated), plant protein, fiber, vitamin E, folic acid, vitamin B-6, niacin, magnesium, copper, zinc, and potassium, all of which can contribute to heart health. In addition, a wide range of bioactive compounds such as ellagic acid, flavonoids, phenolic compounds (including the polyphenol resveratrol), and isoflavones are present in nuts and could play a role in heart health. Mechanisms of action of these bioactive compounds that could account for the cardioprotective effects of nuts include decreased LDL oxidative susceptibility, decreased platelet aggregation, increased synthesis of cardioprotective eicosanoids, and enhanced antioxidant status. In addition, the omega-3 fatty acid (alpha-linolenic acid) in nuts may protect against sudden death and secondary coronary events. Nuts also are a source of plant sterols, which inhibit cholesterol absorption. Thus, there are multiple mechanisms by which nuts can protect against heart disease.

One ounce of nuts (an amount that fits in the palm of a hand) provides about 160 to 180 calories. Thus, nuts and legumes must be incorporated in the diet to ensure that calorie control is maintained. This can be done by substituting nuts for other fats. For example, season vegetables with nuts in place of butter or margarine; use nuts on salads with less salad dressing; use nut butters rather than dairy butter, margarine, or cream cheese. Eat a sandwich with peanut butter rather than lunch meat. Finally, nuts can be enjoyed as a healthy snack as well as a savory snack. So now, with a new appreciation for the *nut* in *nutrition*, enjoy nuts in moderation for good nutrition and heart health!

Dr. Kris-Etherton is Distinguished Professor of Nutrition in the Department of Nutritional Sciences at Pennsylvania State University. Her research focuses on different interventions, which include the use of nuts, to reduce cardiovascular disease risk.

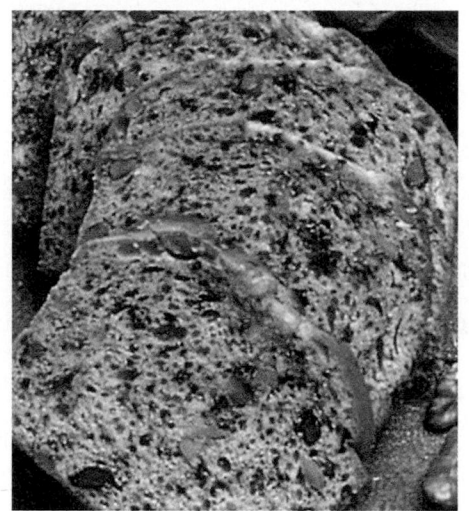

Incorporating nuts into your diet can be as simple as adding walnuts to banana bread.

ecall from Chapter 4 that consumption of beans can lead to intestinal gas because our bodies lack the enzymes to break down certain carbohydrates that beans contain. An over-the-counter preparation called Beano can greatly lessen symptoms if taken right before the meal. It is also helpful to soak dry beans in water, which leaches the indigestible carbohydrates into the water so they can be disposed. However, intestinal gas is not harmful. In fact, fermentation products of indigestible carbohydrates promote the health of your colon (review Chapter 3 for more information on probiotics and prebiotics).

Food Sources of Protein

Food Item and Amount	Protein (g)	Energy from protein (%)
Canned tuna, 3 oz	21.6	87
Broiled chicken, 3 oz	21.3	40
Beef chuck, 3 oz	15.3	30
Yogurt, 1 cup	10.6	35
Kidney beans, 1/2 cup	8.1	29
1% low-fat milk, 1 cup	8.0	31
Peanuts, 1 oz	7.3	18
Cheddar cheese, 1 oz	7.0	25
Egg, 1	5.5	32
Cooked corn, 1/2 cup	2.7	12
Seven-grain bread, 1 slice	2.6	16
White rice, 1/2 cup	2.1	8
Pasta, 1 oz	1.2	16
Banana, 1	1.2	4

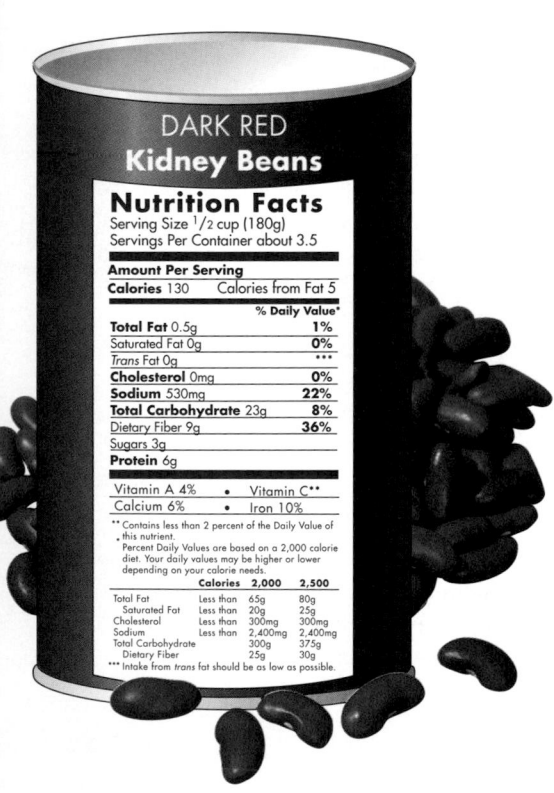

Figure 7-11 | Legumes are rich sources of protein. One-half cup meets about 10% of protein needs, but contributes only about 5% of energy needs.

other benefits, such as ample vitamin E, folate, iron, zinc, copper, and numerous phytochemicals.[15] The plant proteins we eat also contain no cholesterol and little saturated fat, unless these are added during processing. Regular use of plant proteins makes a valuable addition to a diet because these supply a variety of other nutrients.[1] Nuts are receiving much attention today.[17] Dr. Penny M. Kris-Etherton discusses why in the Expert Opinion.

Legumes are a plant family with pods that contain a single row of seeds: garden and black-eyed peas; green, black, red, great northern, lima, kidney, pinto, and garbanzo beans; lentils; peanuts; and soybeans. Dried varieties of the mature seeds—what we know as beans—also make an impressive contribution to the protein, vitamin, mineral, and fiber content of a meal. Regularly consuming these legume protein sources can add substantial amounts of nutrients to a diet (Figure 7-11).

As a way to add more plant proteins in general to your diet, consider these suggestions:

- At your next cookout, try a veggie burger instead of a hamburger. These are available in the frozen foods section of the grocery store and come in a variety of delicious flavors. Many restaurants have added veggie burgers to their menus.
- Sprinkle sunflower seeds or chopped almonds on top of your salad to add taste and texture.
- Mix chopped walnuts into the batter of banana bread, muffins, or pancakes to boost your intake of monounsaturated fats.
- Eat soy nuts (oil-roasted soybeans) as a snack when you're on the go.
- Spread some peanut butter on your bagel instead of butter or cream cheese.
- Instead of having beef or chicken tacos for dinner, heat up a can of beans (any variety; drained) in your skillet with one-half of a packet of taco seasoning and chopped tomatoes. Use this as a filling in a tortilla shell.
- Consider using soy milk, especially if you have lactose maldigestion or lactose intolerance. Look for varieties that are fortified with calcium.

A Closer Look at Soy Protein

Plant proteins from soy in particular have recently received much publicity for their supposed ability to combat a host of medical problems, including cardiovascular disease, cancer, osteoporosis, and menopausal symptoms. In 1999, it was given an FDA-approved health claim for lowering blood cholesterol. This claim is limited to foods high in soy protein, and the recommended daily intake is 25 g of such protein to acquire the benefits. Soy products were then touted as "wonder foods" and sales rose steadily. More recent studies, however, have failed to confirm much of soy's original promise; scientists are reevaluating many of the initial claims.[17] This recent saga of soy is a reminder that there are no "wonder foods." Soybeans, like most legumes, are rich in protein and phytochemicals, and can be part of a healthy, varied diet. To replace the beef patty in your hamburger with a soy patty is one to reduce your intake of cholesterol and saturated fat. Little more can be said for this form of plant protein.

Concept | Check

The Recommended Dietary Allowance (RDA) for adults is 0.8 g of protein per kg of healthy body weight. This is approximately 56 g of protein daily for a 70-kg (154-lb) person. The average North American man consumes about 100 g of protein daily, and a woman consumes about 65 g. Thus, typically we eat more than enough protein to meet our needs. Diets high in protein can compromise kidney health in people with diabetes and those with kidney disease. Diets rich in animal protein sources are generally high in saturated fat and cholesterol and likely increase risk of kidney stones, colon cancer, and cardiovascular disease.

Most protein in the North American diet comes from meat. Plant protein sources contain a wide variety of nutrients and should play an important role in one's diet.

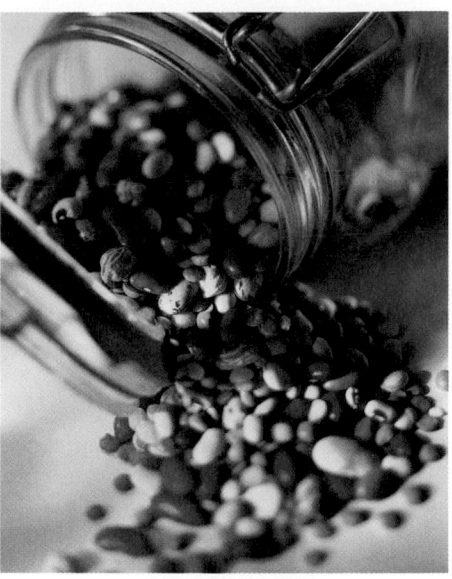

Beans are rich sources of plant proteins and add much nutritional value to a diet.

Evaluation of Protein Quality

A final consideration with regard to proteins in foods is protein quality, which is the ability of a food protein to support body growth and maintenance. Methods exist to both measure and estimate protein quality. Each has its uses and limitations. Keep in mind, also, that the concept of protein quality applies only under conditions in which the amount of protein consumed is equal to or less than the amount of protein required to meet the need for essential amino acids. When protein intake exceeds this amount, efficiency of protein use declines regardless of the balance of amino acids present. This occurs even with the highest-quality proteins because, after the need for essential amino acids has been met, the remaining essential and nonessential amino acids cannot be stored on a long-term basis and will primarily be degraded and used as a source of energy.

Biological Value

The **biological value (BV)** of a protein is a measure of how efficiently food protein, once absorbed from the GI tract, can be turned into body tissues. If a food possesses enough of all nine essential amino acids, it should allow a person to efficiently incorporate the food protein into body proteins. The biological value of a food, then, depends on how closely its amino acid pattern reflects the amino acid pattern in body tissues. The better the match, the more completely food protein turns into body protein.[18] We measure protein retention by measuring nitrogen retention in the body. Both humans and laboratory animals are used to generate data for determining biological value of food proteins.

If the amino acid pattern in a food is quite unlike tissue amino acid patterns, many amino acids in the food will not become body protein. They simply become "leftovers." Their nitrogen groups are removed and excreted in the urine as urea (review Figure 7-8). Because not much of the nitrogen is retained, the ratio of retained nitrogen to absorbed nitrogen, and the consequent biological value, is low.

$$BV = \frac{g \text{ nitrogen retained}}{g \text{ nitrogen absorbed}} \times 100$$

The concept of biological value has clinical importance whenever protein intake must be limited. This is because we want what little protein that is consumed to be used efficiently by the body. For example, protein intake during liver disease and kidney disease may need to be controlled in order to lessen the effects of the disease. In these cases, most of the protein consumed should come from high biological value sources, such as eggs, milk, and meat.

The **protein efficiency ratio (PER)** is another means of measuring a food's protein quality. FDA uses this method rather than the PDCAAS to set standards for the labeling of foods intended for infants. The PER compares the amount of weight (in grams) gained by a growing rat to the grams of protein the rat consumed during 10 days or more of eating a standard amount of protein (9.09% of its energy intake) from a single protein source. The PER of a food reflects its biological value, since both tests basically measure protein retention by body tissues. Plant proteins, because of their incomplete nature, generally yield low PER values, whereas the values for animal proteins are higher, often above 2.0.[18]

$$PER = \frac{g \text{ weight gain}}{g \text{ protein consumed}}$$

$$Chemical\ score = \frac{actual\ mg\ of\ each\ essential\ amino\ acid\ per\ g\ of\ protein}{Required\ mg\ needs\ of\ that\ essential\ amino\ acid\ per\ g\ of\ protein}$$

PDCAAS = Chemical score × digestibility

Egg-white protein has a biological value of 100, the highest biological value of any single food protein. In other words, essentially all nitrogen that is absorbed from egg protein can be retained. Milk and meat proteins also have high biological values. This makes sense because humans and other animals have similar tissue amino acid compositions. Plant amino acid patterns differ greatly from those of humans. For example, corn has only a moderate biological value of 70; it is high enough to support body maintenance, but not growth. Peanuts consumed as the only source of protein show a low biological value of about 40.

Chemical Score and Related Protein Digestibility Corrected Amino Acid Score (PDCAAS)

Protein quality of a food can be estimated by its chemical score. To calculate a food's **chemical score,** the amount of each essential amino acid provided by a gram of the food's protein is divided by an "ideal" amount for that essential amino acid per gram of food protein. The "ideal" protein pattern is based on the minimal amount (in milligrams) of each of the nine essential amino acids that is needed per gram of food protein. The lowest amino acid ratio calculated for any essential amino acid is the chemical score. Scores vary from 0 to 1.0.[18]

To then calculate the **Protein Digestibility Corrected Amino Acid Score (PDCAAS),** the most widely used measure of protein quality, the chemical score of a protein is multiplied by the digestibility of the protein (generally, 0.9 to 1.0). For example, the chemical score for wheat is 0.47. The PDCAAS for wheat is then estimated at 0.47 × 0.90, which equals about 0.40. The maximum value for PDCAAS is 1.0, which is the value of milk, eggs, and soy protein. A protein totally lacking any of the nine essential amino acids has a PDCAAS of 0, since its chemical score is 0.[10]

For nutrition labeling purposes, protein content when listed as % Daily Value is reduced if the PDCAAS is less than 1. For example, if the protein content of 1/2 cup of spaghetti noodles is 3 g, only 1.2 g will be counted when calculating % Daily Value, since the PDCAAS of wheat is 0.40 (3 g × 0.40 = 1.2). Other PDCAAS values are egg white, 1.0; soy protein, 0.92 to 0.99; beef, 0.92; and black beans, 0.53. Currently the Nutrition Facts panel rarely contains the % Daily Value for protein because the manufacturers do not want to spend the money needed to determine the PDCAAS.

Concept | Check

Protein quality refers to the ability of a protein to contribute to protein needs. Using any of the methods available for testing, individual foods with ample amounts of all nine essential amino acids show high protein quality.

Vegetarian Diets

Vegetarianism has evolved over the centuries from a necessity into an option. Historically, vegetarianism was linked with specific philosophies and religions or with science. In the sixth century B.C., Pythagoras advocated a meatless diet for its physical health, ecological, religious, and philosophical benefits.[14]

Today, about 1 in 40 adults in the United States (and about 1 in 25 adults in Canada) is a vegetarian. This rise in interest has encouraged the development of new food products such as soy-based sloppy joes, chili, tacos, burgers, and more. In addition, cookbooks that feature the use of a variety of fruits, vegetables, and seasonings are enhancing food selection for vegetarians of all degrees.

Vegetarianism is popular among college students.[14] Fifteen percent of college students in one survey said they select vegetarian options at lunch or dinner on any given day. In response, dining services offer vegetarian options at every meal, the most common being pastas with meatless sauce and pizza. Many teenagers are also turning to vegetarianism. A survey by the National Restaurant Association found that 20% of its customers want a vegetarian option when they eat out. Many customers cite health and taste as reasons for choosing vegetarian fare.

As nutrition science has grown, new information has enabled the design of nutritionally adequate vegetarian diets. It is important for vegetarians to take advantage of this information because a diet of only plants has the potential to promote various nutrient deficiencies and substantial growth retardation in infants and children.[1] People who choose a vegetarian diet can meet their nutritional needs by following a few basic rules and knowledgeably planning their diets (Table 7-4).[14]

Studies show that death rates from some chronic diseases, such as certain forms of cardiovascular disease, hypertension, many forms of cancer, type 2 diabetes, and obesity, are lower for vegetarians than for nonvegetarians.[4,11,13,14,16,18,19,21,22] Healthful lifestyles (not smoking, abstaining from alcohol and drugs, and engaging in regular physical activity) and social class bias probably partially account for these findings.

Table 7-4 | Food Group Plan for Lactovegetarians and Vegans That Also Follows MyPyramid

Group[a]	Servings		Key Nutrients Supplied
	Lactovegetarian[b]	Vegan[c]	
Grains[d]	6–11	8–11	Protein, thiamin, niacin, folate, vitamin E, zinc, magnesium, iron, and fiber
Beans and other legumes	2–3	3	Protein, vitamin B-6, zinc, magnesium, and fiber
Nuts, seeds	2–3	3	Protein, vitamin E, and magnesium
Vegetables	3–5 (include one dark green or leafy variety daily)	4–6 (include one dark green or leafy variety daily)	Vitamin A, vitamin C, and folate
Fruits	2–4	4	Vitamin A, vitamin C, and folate
Milk	3	—	Protein, riboflavin, vitamin D, vitamin B-12, and calcium

[a]Base serving size on those listed for MyPyramid (see Chapter 2). This plan yields about 1600 to 1800 kcal. Increase the number of servings, or add other foods to meet higher energy needs.

[b]Contains about 75 grams of protein in 1650 kcal.

[c]A calcium-fortified food, such as orange juice or soy milk, is needed unless a calcium supplement is used. In addition, use of a supplement source of vitamin B-12 or foods fortified with vitamin B-12 is a must. Overall, fortified soy milk makes a valuable contribution to a vegan diet. This plan contains about 79 grams of protein in 1800 kcal.

[d]One serving of vitamin- and mineral-enriched ready-to-eat breakfast cereal is recommended. Alternately, a balanced multivitamin and mineral supplement can be used to meet possible nutrient gaps.

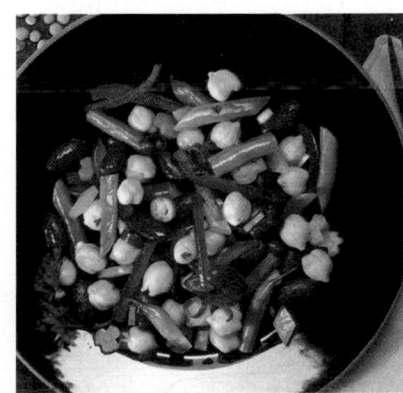

Amino acids in vegetables are best used when a combination of vegetable protein sources is consumed. Table 7-2, earlier in this chapter, lists traditional dishes in which vegetable proteins combine to provide high-quality (complete) protein in the meal.

Why Do People Become Vegetarians?

People choose vegetarianism for a variety of reasons. Some believe that killing animals for food is unethical. Hindus and Trappist monks eat vegetarian meals as a practice of their religion. In the United States, many Seventh-Day Adventists base their practice of vegetarianism on biblical texts and believe it is a more healthful way to live.

People might choose vegetarianism after realizing that animals are not efficient protein factories. Animals actually use much of the protein they eat just to maintain themselves rather than to synthesize new muscle tissue. Note that 40% of the world's grain production is used to raise meat-producing animals. Animals that humans eat sometimes eat grasses that humans cannot digest. Many, however, also eat grains that humans can eat.

People might also practice vegetarianism because it encourages a high intake of complex carbohydrates; vitamins A, E, and C; carotenoids; magnesium; and fiber while it limits saturated fat and cholesterol intake.[15] This produces a diet closely resembling that suggested in the 2005 Dietary Guidelines for Americans, covered in Chapter 2.

Food Planning for Vegetarians

There are a variety of vegetarian styles.[14] **Vegans** eat only plant foods (and as well may not use animal products for other purposes, such as leather shoes or feather pillows). **Fruitarians** primarily eat fruits, nuts, honey, and vegetable oils. This plan is not recommended because it can lead to nutrient deficiencies such as vitamin B-12 and calcium in people of all ages. **Lactovegetarians** modify vegetarianism a bit—they include dairy products and plant foods. **Lactoovovegetarians** modify the diet even further and eat dairy products and eggs as well as plant foods. Including these animal products makes food planning easier because these foods are rich in some nutrients that are missing or present in low amounts in plants (e.g., the vitamin B-12 and calcium just mentioned).[2,23] The more variety in one's diet, the easier it is to meet nutritional needs. Thus, the practice of eating no animal sources of food significantly separates the vegans and fruitarians from all other semivegetarian styles.

Most people who call themselves vegetarians consume at least some dairy products and eggs. A food-group plan has been developed for lactovegetarians and vegans (review Table 7-4). This plan includes servings of nuts, grains, legumes, and seeds to help meet protein needs. There is also a vegetable group, a fruit group, and a milk group.[14]

A vegan diet requires even more knowledge and creative planning to yield high-quality protein and other key nutrients without animal products. Earlier in this chapter, you learned about complementing proteins, whereby the essential amino acids deficient in one protein source are supplied by those of another consumed at the same meal or the next. Recall that many legumes are deficient in the essential amino acid methionine, while cereals are limited in lysine. Eating a combination of legumes and cereals, such as beans and rice, will supply the body with adequate amounts of all essential amino acids. Variety is an especially important characteristic of a nutritious vegan diet.

Low intakes of certain micronutrients can also be a problem for the vegan. At the forefront of nutritional concerns are riboflavin, vitamins D and B-12, iron, zinc, and calcium.[14]

A major source of both riboflavin and vitamin D in the typical North American diet is milk, which is omitted from the vegan diet. However, riboflavin can be obtained from green leafy vegetables, whole-grain breads and cereals, yeast, and legumes—components of most vegan diets. Alternate sources of vitamin D include fortified foods (e.g., margarine) and dietary supplements as well as regular sun exposure (see Chapter 9).

Vitamin B-12 occurs naturally only in animal foods. Plants can contain soil or microbial contaminants that provide trace amounts of vitamin B-12, but these are negligible sources of the vitamin. Because the body can store vitamin B-12 for about 4 years, it may take a long time after removal of animal foods from the diet for a deficiency to surface. If dietary B-12 inadequacy persists, deficiency can

---

hapter 6 noted that a vegan diet coupled with regular exercise and other lifestyle changes can lead to a reversal of atherosclerotic plaque in the coronary arteries.

vegan A person who eats only plant foods.

fruitarian A person who eats primarily fruits, nuts, honey, and vegetable oils.

lactovegetarian A person who consumes plant products and dairy products.

lactoovovegetarian A person who consumes plant products, dairy products, and eggs.

lead to a form of anemia, nerve damage, and mental dysfunction. These dire consequences of deficiency have been noted in the infants of vegetarian mothers whose breast milk was low in vitamin B-12.[23] Chronically low vitamin B-12 consumption may also result in excess blood concentration of homocysteine, which is likely a risk factor for cardiovascular disease. To prevent a vitamin B-12 deficiency, vegans must find a reliable source of vitamin B-12, such as fortified soy milk, ready-to-eat breakfast cereals, and special yeast grown in media rich in vitamin B-12. Use of a balanced vitamin and mineral supplement containing vitamin B-12 is another option.

For iron, vegans can consume whole-grain breads and cereals, dried fruits and nuts, and legumes.[14] Note that the iron in these foods is not absorbed as well as iron in animal foods, but a good source of vitamin C taken with these foods helps somewhat with iron absorption. Thus, a recommended strategy is to consume vitamin C with every meal that contains iron-rich plant foods. Cooking in iron pots and skillets can also add iron to the diet (see Chapter 12).

Vegans can find zinc in whole-grain breads and cereals, nuts, and legumes, but phytic acid and other substances in these foods limit zinc absorption. Grains are most nutritious when consumed as breads, because the leavening (rising of the bread dough) reduces the influence of phytic acid.[14]

Calcium-fortified foods are the vegan's best option for obtaining calcium. These include fortified soy milk, fortified orange juice, calcium-rich tofu (check the label), and certain ready-to-eat breakfast cereals, breads, and snacks. Green leafy vegetables and nuts also contain calcium, but the mineral is either not well absorbed or not very plentiful from these sources. Calcium supplements are another option (see Chapter 11). Special diet planning is required, because even a typical multivitamin and mineral supplement will not supply enough calcium to meet the body's needs.[3]

Special Concerns for Infants and Children

The populations at highest risk for nutrient deficiencies as a result of improperly planned vegetarian diets are infants and children, who are notoriously picky eaters in the first place.[14] With the use of complementary proteins and good sources of problem nutrients discussed in this section, the energy, protein, vitamin, and mineral needs of vegetarian and vegan infants and children can be met. The most common nutritional concerns for infants and children following vegetarian and vegan diets are deficiencies of iron, vitamin B-12, vitamin D, and calcium.

Vegetarian and vegan diets tend to be high in bulky, high-fiber, low-calorie foods that cause fullness. While this side effect can be a welcome advantage for adults, children have a small stomach volume and relatively high nutrient needs compared to their size and therefore may feel full before their energy needs are met. For this reason, the fiber content of a child's diet may need to be decreased by replacing high-fiber sources with some refined grain products, fruit juices, and peeled fruit. Other concentrated sources of energy for vegetarian and vegan children include fortified soy milk, nuts, dried fruits, avocados, and cookies made with vegetable oils or tub margarine.

Overall, vegetarian and vegan diets can be appropriate during infancy and childhood, but these diets must be implemented with knowledge and, ideally, professional guidance.[1] An especially informative website on vegetarianism in general is www.ivu.org, supported by the International Vegetarian Union. See also www.vrg.org and www.vegetariannutrition.net.

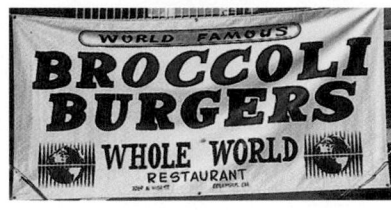

Vegetarian adaptations of traditional foods are a growing trend in our society.

M eeting omega-3 fatty acid needs also becomes an issue for vegetarians who do not eat fish. Regular use of canola oil, soybean oil, flax seeds, or walnuts is then advised to obtain alpha-linolenic acid, the omega-3 fatty acid. Seaweed and microalgae are also possible sources of omega-3 fatty acids.[7]

Case Scenario | Follow-Up

Shannon's dietary intake for this day, although lactovegetarian, is not as healthy as it could be because it does not come close to following the recommendations provided in this chapter's Nutrition Focus. Many components of a healthy vegetarian diet—whole grains, nuts, soy products, beans, two to four servings of fruit, and three to five servings of vegetables per day—are missing. With so few fruits and vegetables, her diet is also low in the many phytochemicals that are under study for numerous health benefits. It is apparent that Shannon has not yet learned to implement the concept of complementary proteins, so the quality of protein in her diet is low. Unless she makes a more informed effort at diet planning, Shannon will not reap the health benefits she had hoped for when she chose to follow a vegetarian diet.

protein-energy malnutrition (PEM) A condition resulting from regularly consuming insufficient amounts of energy and protein. The deficiency eventually results in body wasting, primarily of lean tissue, and an increased susceptibility to infections.

marasmus A disease that results from consuming a grossly insufficient amount of protein and energy; one of the diseases classed as protein-energy malnutrition. Victims have little or no fat stores, little muscle mass, and poor strength. Death from infections is common.

kwashiorkor A disease occurring primarily in young children who have an existing disease and who consume a marginal amount of energy and considerably insufficient protein in relation to needs. The child generally suffers from infections and exhibits edema, poor growth, weakness, and an increased susceptibility to further illness.

Protein-Energy Malnutrition

Rarely an isolated condition, protein deficiency usually accompanies a deficiency of dietary energy and other nutrients resulting from insufficient food intake. In developing areas of the world, people often have diets low in energy and also in protein. This state of undernutrition stunts the growth of children and makes them more susceptible to disease throughout life. (Note that undernutrition is a main focus of Chapter 20.) People who consume too little protein and food energy eventually develop **protein-energy malnutrition (PEM),** also referred to as *protein-calorie malnutrition (PCM).*[18] In its milder form, it is difficult to tell if a person with PEM is consuming too little energy or protein, or both. But if the nutrient deficiency—especially for energy—is quite severe, a deficiency disease called **marasmus** can result. When an inadequate intake of nutrients, including protein, is combined with an already existing disease (such as infection), a form of malnutrition called **kwashiorkor** can develop. Both conditions are seen primarily in children, but may also develop in adults. These two conditions form the tip of the iceberg with respect to states of undernutrition, and symptoms of these two conditions can even be present in the same person (Figure 7-12).

Kwashiorkor

Kwashiorkor is a word from Ghana that means "the disease that the first child gets when the new child comes." From birth, an infant in developing areas of the world is usually breastfed. Often by the time the child reaches 1 to 1.5 years of age, the mother is pregnant or has already given birth again, and breastfeeding is no longer possible for the first child. This child's diet then abruptly changes from nutritious human milk to starchy roots and gruels. These foods have low protein densities compared with total energy. Additionally, the foods are usually full of plant fibers, which are often bulky,

Figure 7-12 | Schema for classifying undernutrition in children. The presence of subcutaneous fat (directly underneath the skin) is a diagnostic key for distinguishing kwashiorkor from marasmus.

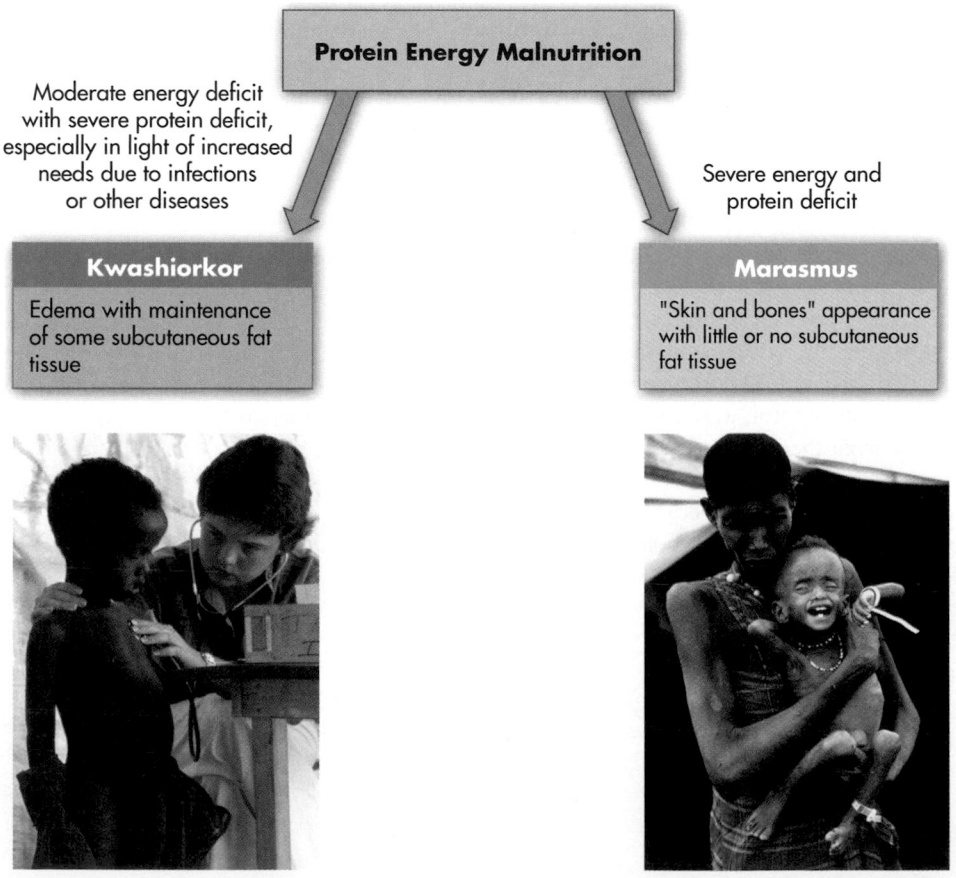

making it difficult for the child to consume enough to meet energy needs. The child typically also has infections and parasites, which acutely raise energy and protein needs, or could be exposed to toxins found in moldy grains. Overall, energy needs of these children are just barely met, at best, and their protein needs are not met, especially in view of the increased amount needed to combat infections. Usually, many vitamin and mineral needs are also far from being fulfilled. Famine victims face similar problems.

The major symptoms of kwashiorkor are apathy, diarrhea, listlessness, failure to grow and gain weight, various infections, and withdrawal from the environment. These symptoms complicate other diseases present. For example, a condition such as measles, a disease that normally makes a healthy child ill for only a week or so, can become severely debilitating and even fatal. Further signs and symptoms of the disease are changes in hair color, potassium deficiency, flaky skin, fatty infiltration in the liver, reduced muscle mass, and massive edema in the abdomen and legs. The presence of edema in a child who has some subcutaneous fat still present is the hallmark of kwashiorkor (review Figure 7-12). In addition, these children seldom move. If you pick them up, they don't cry. When you hold them, you feel the plumpness of edema, not muscle and fat tissue.

Many symptoms of kwashiorkor can be explained based on what we know about proteins. Proteins play important roles in fluid balance, lipoprotein transport, immune function, and production of tissues such as skin and hair. We should not expect children with an insufficient protein intake to grow and mature normally and they don't.

If children with kwashiorkor are helped in time—if infections are treated and a diet ample in protein, energy, and other essential nutrients is provided—the disease process reverses. They begin to grow again and may even show no signs of their previous condition, except perhaps shortness of stature. Unfortunately, by the time many of these children reach a hospital or care center, they already have severe infections. In spite of the best care, they still die. Or if they survive, they return home only to become ill again.

Marasmus

Marasmus typically occurs as an infant slowly starves to death. It is caused by diets containing minimal amounts of energy as well as too little protein and other nutrients. As previously noted, this condition is also commonly referred to as *protein-energy malnutrition,* especially when experienced by older children and adults. The word *marasmus* means "to waste away." Victims have a "skin and bones" appearance, with little or no subcutaneous fat (review Figure 7-12).

Marasmus commonly develops in infants who either are not breastfed or have stopped breastfeeding in the early months. Often the weaning formula used is improperly prepared because of unsafe water and because the parents cannot afford sufficient infant formula for the child's needs. The latter problem may lead the parents to dilute the formula to provide more feedings, not realizing that this provides only more water for the infant.

Marasmus in infants commonly occurs in the large cities of poverty-stricken countries. When people are poor and sanitation is lacking, bottle-feeding often leads to marasmus. In the cities, bottle-feeding is often necessary because the infant must be cared for by others when the mother is working or away from home. An infant with marasmus requires large amounts of energy and protein—like a preterm infant—and unless the child receives them, full recovery from the disease may never occur. The majority of brain growth occurs between conception and the child's first birthday. In fact, the brain grows fastest at the time of birth. If the diet does not support brain growth during the first months of life, the brain may not grow to its full adult size. This reduced or retarded brain growth may lead to diminished intellectual function. Both kwashiorkor and marasmus plague infants and children; mortality rates in developing countries are often 10 to 20 times higher than in the United States.

Kwashiorkor and Marasmus Malnutrition in the Hospital

Kwashiorkor can result when a hospitalized patient is fed primarily glucose intravenously for many days, such as when a slow recovery from surgery prevents normal food consumption. Or a person may feel too sick to eat, in spite of the increased nutrient needs caused by his or her disease. Intravenous glucose feeding can meet energy needs to some extent but provides no protein. As a result, the person develops edema, and often the immune function is diminished, leaving the patient at great risk for infections.

Studies have demonstrated that a hospital patient with a low body weight, low blood albumin, and a low white blood cell (especially lymphocyte) count faces a risk of complications and death that is four to six times greater than that of a patient with normal values for those three factors. In response, nutrition support teams have been formed in hospitals. One of their missions is to ensure that patients receive enough oral or balanced intravenous total parenteral nutrition support to meet their needs for energy, protein, carbohydrate, and other nutrients.

Marasmus occurs in a hospitalized patient who simply does not receive enough energy and other nutrients. This can be caused by anorexia nervosa, cancer, HIV/AIDS, and some intestinal disorders. The person either does not eat enough food or does not absorb enough nutrients from the intestinal tract to meet nutritional needs. Muscle, vital organ tissue, and fat stores waste away, and the person eventually looks like "skin and bones." Skinfold measurements of the arm can be used as an indication of marasmus. (Chapter 13 reviews this technique.) However, appearance alone is often enough to indicate the disease. Death from starvation or heart failure can result. A hospitalized person may also have mixed kwashiorkor-marasmus. This is characterized by edema in a person with greatly diminished fat stores.

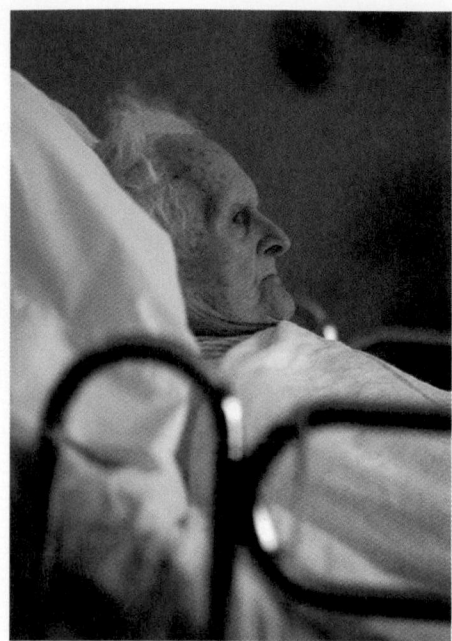

Some hospitalized patients are at risk of protein-energy malnutrition. This includes older adults recovering from surgery.

Concept | Check

Most undernutrition consists of mild deficits in energy, protein, and often other nutrients. If a person needs more nutrients because of disease and infection but does not consume enough energy and protein, a condition known as kwashiorkor can develop. The person suffers from edema and weakness. Children around age 2 are especially susceptible to kwashiorkor, particularly if they already have other diseases. Famine situations in which only starchy root products are available to eat contribute to this problem. Marasmus is a condition wherein people—infants, especially—starve to death. Symptoms include muscle wasting, absence of fat stores, and weakness. Both an adequate diet and the treatment of concurrent diseases must be promoted to regain and then maintain nutritional health. This also is true in an adult suffering from anorexia nervosa, cancer, or HIV/AIDS. The symptoms of marasmus, especially, are seen in these situations.

Summary

1. Amino acids, the building blocks of proteins, contain a very usable form of nitrogen for humans. Of the 20 common amino acids found in food, nine must be consumed as food (essential) and the rest can be synthesized by the body (nonessential).

2. High-quality, also called complete, protein foods contain ample amounts of all nine essential amino acids. Furthermore, foods derived from animal sources provide high-quality, or complete, protein. Lower-quality, or incomplete, protein foods lack sufficient amounts of one or more essential amino acids. This is typical of plant foods, especially cereal grains. Different types of plant foods eaten together often complement each other's amino acid deficits, thereby providing high-quality protein in the diet.

3. Individual amino acids are linked together to form proteins. The sequential order of amino acids determines the protein's ultimate shape and function. This order is directed by DNA in the cell nucleus. Diseases such as sickle-cell anemia can occur if the amino acids are incorrect on a polypeptide chain. When the three-dimensional shape of the protein is unfolded—denatured—by treatment with heat, acid or alkaline solutions, or other processes, the protein also loses its biological activity.

4. Protein digestion begins in the stomach, dividing the proteins into breakdown products containing shorter polypeptide chains of amino acids. In the small intestine, these polypeptide chains eventually separate into mostly dipeptides and amino acids. These are

absorbed by the enterocytes and are broken down into amino acids. The free amino acids then travel via the portal vein that connects to the liver.

5. Important body components—such as muscles, connective tissue, transport proteins in the bloodstream, visual pigments, enzymes, some hormones, and immune bodies—are made of proteins. These proteins are in a state of constant turnover. Proteins also provide carbon skeletons which can be used to synthesize glucose when necessary.

6. The protein RDA for adults is 0.8 g per kg of healthy body weight. For a typical 70-kg (154-lb) person, this corresponds to 56 g of protein daily; for a 57-kg (125-lb) person, this corresponds to 46 g/day. The North American diet generally supplies plenty of protein: men typically consume about 100 g of protein daily, and women consume about 65 g. These usual protein intakes are also of sufficient quality to support body functions.

7. Almost all animal products are rich sources of protein. The high quality of these proteins means that they can be easily converted into body proteins. Plant foods generally contain less than 20% of their energy content as protein; however, legumes are an excellent source of high-quality protein if eaten with grains or animal products.

8. Protein quality can be measured by determining the extent to which the body can retain the nitrogen contained in the amino acids absorbed; this is called biological value. In addition, the balance of essential amino acids in a food can be compared with an ideal pattern. The comparison with the ideal pattern is referred to as the chemical score. When multiplied by the degree of digestibility, the chemical score yields the Protein Digestibility Corrected Amino Acid Score (PDCAAS).

9. Undernutrition can lead to protein-energy malnutrition in the form of kwashiorkor or marasmus. Kwashiorkor results primarily from an inadequate energy and protein intake in comparison with body needs, which often increase with concurrent disease and infection. Kwashiorkor often occurs when a child is weaned from human milk and fed mostly starchy gruels. Marasmus results from extreme starvation—a negligible intake of both protein and energy. Marasmus commonly occurs during famine, especially in infants. Variations of these diseases appear in some hospitalized North Americans.

Study Questions

1. Discuss the relative importance of essential and nonessential amino acids in the diet. Why is it important for essential amino acids lost from the body to be replaced in the diet?

2. Explain the process for synthesizing nonessential amino acids. What is the chemical reaction called when an amino acid loses its amino group without transferring it to another carbon skeleton?

3. What is a limiting amino acid? Explain why this concept is a concern in a vegetarian diet. How can a vegetarian compensate for limiting amino acids in specific foods?

4. Briefly describe the organization of proteins (e.g., primary structure, etc.). How can this organization be altered or damaged? What might be a result of damaged protein organization?

5. Describe four functions of proteins. Provide an example of how the structure of a protein relates to its function.

6. How are DNA and protein synthesis related?

7. What would be one health benefit of preventing protein-energy malnutrition in children?

8. What characteristics of plant proteins could improve the North American diet? What foods would you include to provide a diet that has ample protein from both plant and animal sources but is moderate in fat?

9. Outline the major differences between kwashiorkor and marasmus.

10. What are the possible long-term effects of an inadequate intake of dietary protein among children between the ages of 6 months and 4 years?

BOOST YOUR STUDY

Check out the **Perspectives in Nutrition: Online Learning Center** www.mhhe.com/wardlawpers7 for quizzes, flash cards, activities, and web links designed to further help you learn about proteins.

Annotated References

1. ADA Reports: Position of the American Dietetic Association and Dietitians of Canada: Vegetarian diets. *Journal of the American Dietetic Association* 103:748, 2003.

   It is the position of the American Dietetic Association and Dietitians of Canada that appropriately planned vegetarian diets are healthful and nutritionally adequate and provide health benefits in the prevention and treatment of certain diseases. In some cases, however, use of fortified foods or a multivitamin and mineral supplement may be needed to meet recommendations for individual nutrients.

2. Antony AC: Vegetarianism and vitamin B-12 (cobalamin) deficiency. *American Journal of Clinical Nutrition* 78:3, 2003.

   It is vital that a vegetarian focus on meeting vitamin B-12 needs. Use of vitamin B-12-fortified foods or a vitamin and mineral supplement are two options.

3. Aronson D: Vegetarian nutrition. *Today's Dietitian*, p. 3, March 2005.

   A vegetarian diet can result in possible nutrient deficiencies. This article reviews plant food sources, such as rich sources of calcium, to counteract these risks.

4. Berkow SE, Barnard ND: Blood pressure regulation and vegetarian diets. *Nutrition Reviews* 63:1, 2005.

   Vegetarian diets are associated with lower blood pressure in humans. It is likely that the fruit, vegetables, legumes, and nuts in such a diet lead to this health benefit.

5. Borghid, L and others: Comparison of two diets for the prevention of recurrent stones in idiopathic hypercalciuria. *The New England Journal of Medicine* 346:77, 2002.

   In men with a history of calcium oxalate stones and exhibiting increased calcium in the urine, restricted intakes of animal protein and salt, combined with normal calcium intakes, provided protection against recurrence of such stones.

6. Chao A and others: Meat consumption and colorectal cancer. *Journal of the American Medical Association* 293:172, 2005.

Diets rich in red meat, especially processed meat, increase the risk of colon cancer. Protein from poultry and fish, in contrast, does not pose the same risk.

7. Davis BC, Kris-Etherton PM: Achieving optimal essential fatty acid status in vegetarians: Current knowledge and practical implications. *American Journal of Clinical Nutrition* 78(suppl): 640S, 2003.

Most of the fat in a vegetarian diet should come from nuts, seeds, olives, avocados, soy foods, and monounsaturated-rich oils, such as canola oil, olive oil, and nut oils. This practice provides a sufficient amount of essential fatty acids. Seaweed and microalgae are two possible sources for vegans of the very-long-chain omega-3 fatty acids found in fish.

8. Dawson-Hughes B: Interaction of dietary calcium and protein in bone health in humans. *Journal of Nutrition* 133:852S, 2003.

It is important to meet calcium needs to offset any possible protein-related calcium loss in the urine. In this way the combination of meeting protein and calcium needs can be beneficial to bone health.

9. Eating a high protein diet may accelerate kidney problems. *Today's Dietitian*, p. 26, April 2004.

High-protein diets may accelerate kidney disease in people who show evidence of the disease. Note that the National Kidney Foundation suggests one in nine North American adults show evidence of at least mild kidney disease.

10. Food and Nutrition Board: *Dietary reference intakes for energy, carbohydrate, fiber, fat, fatty acids, cholesterol, protein, and amino acids.* Washington DC: The National Academy Press, 2002.

This report provides the latest guidance for macronutrient intakes. With regard to protein intake, the RDA has been set at 0.8 g/kg per day. Protein intake can range from 10 to 35% of energy intake. The 10% allotment approximates the RDA, based on typical energy intakes.

11. Gardner CD and others: The effect of a plant-based diet on plasma lipids in hypercholesterolemic adults. *Annals on Internal Medicine* 142:725, 2005.

Adding plant proteins to a diet already low in saturated fat and cholesterol provides additional benefits regarding the lowering of blood cholesterol. The authors emphasize the importance of including fruits, vegetables, legumes, and whole grains in a diet.

12. Garlick PJ: The nature of human hazards associated with excessive intakes of amino acids. *Journal of Nutrition* 134:1633S, 2004.

The most toxic amino acids are methionine, cysteine, and histidine. Possible health risks from excessive intakes of other amino acids are also reviewed. These risks are seen with amino acid supplements, not whole food sources.

13. Hu F: Plant-based foods and prevention of cardiovascular disease: An overview. *American Journal of Clinical Nutrition* 78(suppl): 544S, 2003.

Plant-based diets provide numerous factors that reduce cardiovascular disease risk, such as unsaturated fats, phytochemicals, and fiber. The whole-grain breads and cereals, fruits, and vegetables in such a diet are the primary source of these factors. If desired, some lean/low-fat animal products can be added to round out a plant-based diet without decreasing its benefits.

14. Johnston PA, Sabate J: Nutritional implications of vegetarian diets. In Shils ME and others (eds): *Modern nutrition in health and disease.* 10th ed. Philadelphia, PA: Lippincott Williams & Wilkins, 2006

Current review of the nutritional advantages and possible nutritional problems arising from following various types of vegetarian diets. The authors emphasize the many benefits of including plant proteins in a diet plan.

15. Leitzmann C: Vegetarian diets: What are the advantages? *Forum of Nutrition* 57:147, 2005.

The benefits of a vegetarian diet are a lower intake of saturated fat, cholesterol, and animal protein as well as a higher intake of complex carbohydrates, fiber, magnesium, folate, vitamin C, vitamin E, carotenoids, and other phytochemicals. Well-balanced vegetarian diets are appropriate for all stages of the life cycle. The article provides evidence to support these statements and reviews other possible health benefits.

16. Lejeune MP and others: Additional protein intake limits weight regain after weight loss in humans. *British Journal of Nutrition* 93:281, 2005.

Adding 30 g of protein per day to their usual diets helped people in this study limit weight regain after weight loss. The diet of the experimental group included 18% of energy intake as protein compared to 15% in the control group. This protein intake in the experimental group would not be considered excessive given the upper limit of 35% of energy intake set by the Food and Nutrition Board.

17. Magic soybeans? Testing the promise of soy protein. *Tufts University Health & Nutrition Letter* p. 4, December 2005.

Replacing animal proteins in a diet with some soy protein helps reduce saturated fat intake, which is beneficial to health. Other purported health benefits of soy proteins themselves, such as lowering blood cholesterol, have not been supported by recent studies.

18. Matthews DE: Proteins and amino acids. In Shils ME and others (eds): *Modern nutrition in health and disease.* 10th ed. Philadelphia, PA: Lippincott Williams & Wilkins, 2006.

Detailed examination of what is known about proteins in general. This includes a review of methods to determine the protein quality of individual food proteins.

19. Newby PK: Risk of overweight and obesity among semivegetarian, lactovegetarian, and vegan women. *American Journal of Clinical Nutrition* 81:1267, 2005.

Semivegetarian women in this study were less likely to be overweight and obese compared to omnivorous women. Consuming more plant foods rich in protein and less animal protein may help individuals control their weight.

20. Nuts are on a roll. *UC Berkeley Wellness Letter*, p. 1, May 2003.

Nuts are a rich source of many nutrients and fiber but also are very energy-dense. Thus it is best to substitute nuts for other protein sources, especially those rich in saturated fat.

21. Sabate J: The contribution of vegetarian diets to human health. *Forums of Nutrition* 56: 218, 2005.

Components of a healthy vegetarian diet include a variety of vegetables, fruits, whole-grain cereals, legumes, and nuts. Such a diet contributes to overall health and increased longevity when these foods are emphasized.

22. "Vegging out" for better health? *HealthNews*, p. 8, November 2003.

Well-balanced plant-based diets can lead to numerous health benefits. One benefit may be a longer life.

23. Weiss R and others: Severe vitamin B-12 deficiency in an infant associated with a maternal deficiency and a strict vegetarian diet. *Journal of Pediatric Hematology and Oncology* 26:270, 2004.

A pregnant woman must meet vitamin B-12 needs when following a vegetarian diet. This article describes what happens when a pregnant woman deficient in vitamin B-12 goes on to breastfeed her infant, notably, development of severe anemia and nerve degeneration in the infant.

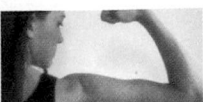

Take | Action

I. Protein and the Vegetarian

Alana is excited about all the health benefits that might accompany a vegetarian diet. However, she is concerned that she will not consume enough protein to meet her needs. She is also concerned about possible vitamin and mineral deficiencies. Use NutritionCalc Plus or Appendix N to calculate her protein intake and see if her concerns are valid.

	Protein (g)
Breakfast	
Calcium fortified orange juice, 1 cup	
Soy milk, 1 cup	
Fortified bran flakes, 1 cup	
Banana, medium	
Snack	
Calcium-enriched granola bar	
Lunch	
GardenBurger, 4 oz	
Whole-wheat bun	
Mustard, 1 tbsp	
Soy cheese, 1 oz	
Apple, medium	
Green leaf lettuce, 1 1/2 cups	
Peanuts, 1 oz	
Sunflower seeds, 1/4 cup	
Tomato slices, 2	
Mushrooms, 3	
Vinaigrette salad dressing, 2 tbsp	
Iced tea	
Dinner	
Kidney beans, 1/2 cup	
Brown rice, 3/4 cup	
Fortified margarine, 2 tbsp	
Mixed vegetables, 1/4 cup	
Hot tea	
Dessert	
Strawberries, 1/2 cup	
Angel food cake, 1 small slice	
Soy milk, 1/2 cup	
TOTAL PROTEIN (g) _____	

Alana's diet contained 2150 kcal, with _____ g (you fill in) of protein (Is this plenty for her?), 360 g of carbohydrate, 57 g of total dietary fat (only 9 g of which came from saturated fat), and 50 g of fiber. Her vitamin and mineral intake with respect to those of concern to vegetarians—vitamin B-12, vitamin D, calcium, iron, and zinc—met her needs.

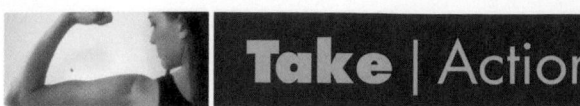

Take | Action

II. Meeting Protein Needs When Dieting to Lose Weight

Your father has been gaining weight for the last 30 years and now has developed hypertension and type 2 diabetes as a result. His physician recommends that he lose some weight by following an 1800 kcal diet. You know that it will be important for your father to meet protein needs as he tries to lose weight. Design a 1-day diet for him that contains about 20% of energy intake as protein. Table 7-3 will provide some help. Will this diet meet his protein RDA? Does the diet look like a plan you could also follow?

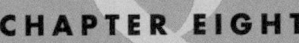

ALCOHOL

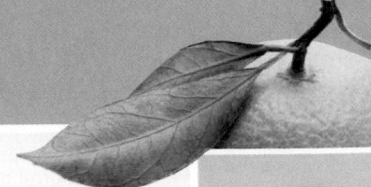

CHAPTER OUTLINE

CASE SCENARIO:

Alyssa and her boyfriend Todd are college juniors. Todd was a very serious student in high school and achieved excellent grades, but as a college student he has begun binge drinking. His grades have fallen sharply and he is becoming socially isolated. He was even arrested once for drunk driving.

Last night, Todd had eight beers and three shots of whiskey at an off-campus party he attended with Alyssa. Unfortunately, everyone who knows Todd says he tends to get angry and says things he doesn't mean when he drinks too much. He often becomes cruel and destructive to those he cares for and respects. He also has been involved in several fights.

As the party began to die down, Alyssa tried to get Todd to leave. He responded rudely and forcefully grabbed her arm. She became frightened with his aggressive behavior and left without him.

The next morning, Alyssa noticed a large bruise on her arm where Todd had grabbed her. She decided to e-mail Todd to express her anxiety about the events from the night before and his alcohol abuse. She did not want to see everything he had worked so hard for be ruined by alcohol.

What should Alyssa say in the e-mail? What long-term problems associated with such alcohol abuse should she mention? Where could Alyssa suggest that Todd go to get help with his drinking problem?

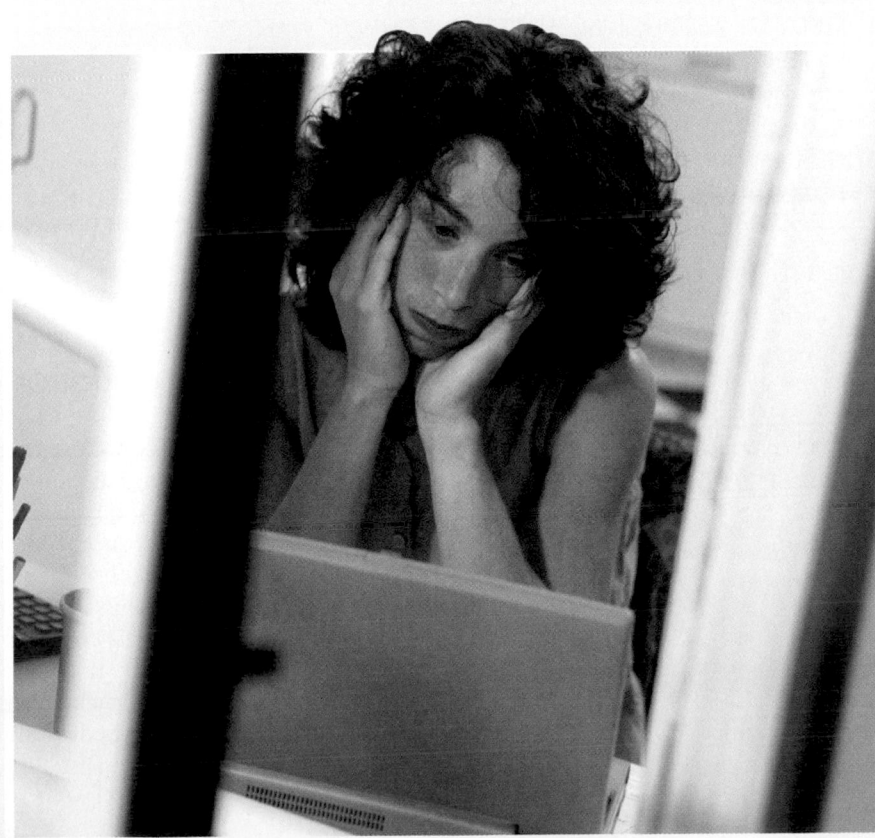

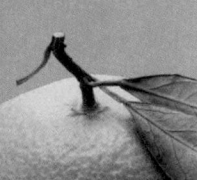

Alcohol use is an issue requiring careful attention by health professionals, law enforcement officials, the courts, elected officials, the entertainment industry, university professors, parents, students, and businesspeople engaged in the production and distribution of alcoholic beverages. Although not an essential nutrient, alcohol is a source of energy for about half of all adults, constituting about 3% of total energy intake in the North American diet when averaged across the population. Moderate consumption of alcohol by a person of legal age is an acceptable practice and has some health benefits.[10] But when consumed to excess, alcohol leads to many unfortunate consequences. It is by far the most commonly abused drug, and alcohol use can cause automobile and boating accidents; destroy families and friendships; and spur deadly behaviors such as suicide, rape, and violence. Alcohol abuse is in fact the third leading cause of preventable death in adults (behind smoking and obesity).[3]

About 55% of adults in North America drink alcohol. Nearly 4% of adults are currently classified as having alcoholism. Many current drinkers are under the legal age of 21. From teenage years through later years in life, excess alcohol intake has damaging effects on one's nutritional status and overall health.[13,18] Alcohol abuse is also a major problem in Canada.

The American Medical Association defines alcoholism as an illness characterized by significant impairment directly related to persistent and excessive use of alcohol. Impairment can involve physiological and social dysfunction, and for psychological, social, and genetic reasons some people are more vulnerable to this disorder than others.[14] Because alcohol abuse touches many lives, this chapter examines this substance in detail.

CHAPTER OBJECTIVES CHAPTER 8 IS DESIGNED TO ALLOW YOU TO:

1. Describe the process of alcohol metabolism.
2. Describe some benefits of moderate alcohol consumption and define "moderate drinking."
3. List some nutrients that are most likely to be deficient in the diet of a person who abuses alcohol.
4. Explain how alcohol abuse damages body organs, such as the liver, heart, brain, and kidneys.
5. Identify body organs most likely to develop cancer because of alcohol abuse.
6. Outline the methods used to diagnose alcohol abuse.
7. List the typical strategies used in treating alcoholism, including the typical medications employed.
8. Describe binge drinking and its risks.

REFRESH YOUR MEMORY AS YOU BEGIN YOUR STUDY OF ALCOHOL IN CHAPTER 8, YOU MAY WANT TO REVIEW:

● The role of the GI tract, liver, and pancreas in digestion and absorption in Chapter 3.
● Oxidation and reduction reactions in Chapter 4.
● Glycolysis, the citric acid cycle, and electron transport chain in Chapter 4.
● The term fermentation defined in Chapter 3 and the actual chemical reactions in Chapter 4.
● Forms of carbohydrates in Chapter 5.
● Protein-energy malnutrition in Chapter 7.

Alcohol—An Introduction

alcohol abuse Alcohol consumption that results in severe physical, psychological, or social problems.

ethanol Chemical term for the form of alcohol found in alcoholic beverages.

Given the wide spectrum of alcohol use and **alcohol abuse**—often starting in teenage and college years—knowledge of alcohol consumption and its relationship to overall health is essential to the study of nutrition. Alcohol, chemically known as **ethanol,** has played many roles throughout history. Alcohol contributes energy to the diet (about 7 kcal/g) (Table 8-1).[13] It is also used socially because it takes away inhibitions. In addition, alcoholic beverages are thirst quenchers when used as safe alternatives to polluted water (such as when water is contaminated with certain microorganisms).

Alcohol requires no digestion. It is absorbed rapidly from the GI tract by simple diffusion—no specific transport mechanisms are required for alcohol to enter a cell—so it is the most efficiently absorbed of all energy sources. Different parts of the GI

Table 8-1 | Energy, Carbohydrate, and Alcohol Content of Alcoholic Beverages*

Beverage	Amount (fluid oz)	Alcohol (g)	Carbohydrates (g)	Energy (kcal)
Beer				
Regular	12	13	13	146
Light	12	11	5	99
Distilled Spirits				
Gin, rum, vodka, bourbon, whiskey (80 proof)	1.5	14	—	96
Brandy, cognac	1.5	14	—	96
Wine				
Red	5	14	2	102
White	5	14	1	100
Dessert, sweet	5	23	17	225
Rosé	5	14	2	100
Mixed Drinks				
Manhattan	3	26	3	191
Martini	3	27	—	189
Bourbon and soda	3	11	—	78
Whiskey sour	3	14	13	144

*There is little to no fat or protein contribution to energy content.
Source: USDA.

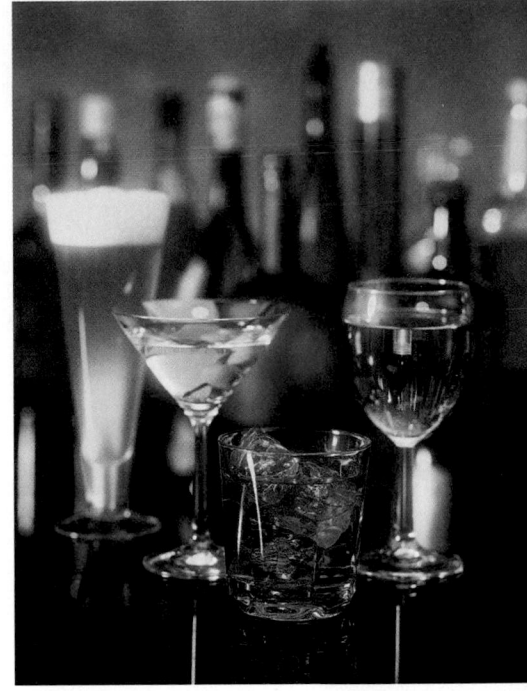

The following servings of each type of alcoholic beverage provide the same amount of alcohol (about 15 g): wine—5 oz, hard liquor—1.5 oz, beer or wine cooler—12 oz. In determining a safe level of intake, it is important to observe these serving sizes.

tract absorb alcohol at different rates. The upper parts of the small intestine absorb alcohol fastest, depending on how quickly the stomach empties, which in turn depends on the kinds of foods consumed along with the alcohol.[8] Alcohol then goes on to act on various organs, but has no cellular receptors per se, unlike other compounds that affect the body such as insulin and some fat-soluble vitamins.[13]

How Alcoholic Beverages Are Produced

Any number of natural foods can be fermented. Recall from Chapter 3 that fermentation represents the breakdown of carbohydrates without the use of oxygen. Alcohol, carbon dioxide (CO_2), and various acids are by-products. Production temperatures and composition of the food itself determine the characteristics of the final product. High-carbohydrate foods especially encourage the growth of yeast, the microorganism responsible for alcohol production. Brewer's yeast is one source of the enzyme that is necessary to make alcohol production possible.

During glycolysis, glucose is first converted to pyruvate. Yeast cells then ferment pyruvate to alcohol and carbon dioxide in a simple, two-step process. In the first step, the 3-carbon pyruvate is converted to the 2-carbon acetaldehyde in an irreversible reaction with the release of CO_2. In the second step, another enzyme donates a pair of hydrogen ions and electrons to acetaldehyde to form ethanol. This enzyme uses the B-vitamin niacin in the form of the coenzyme NADH + H$^+$ (review Chapter 4 for details). Ethanol and CO_2 are the end products of the process.

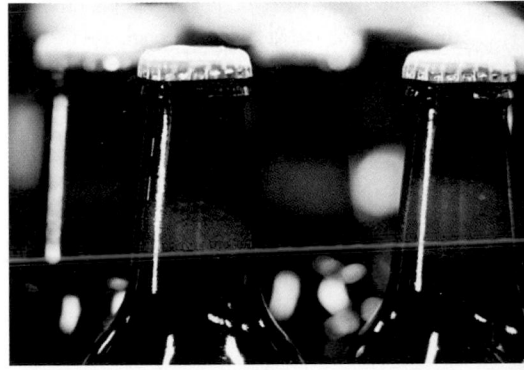

Beer is a source of alcohol and carbohydrates.

1. Glucose $\longrightarrow$ Pyruvate $\longrightarrow$ $\begin{array}{c} CO_2 \\ \text{Acetaldehyde} \end{array}$

NADH + H$^+$ NAD$^+$

2. Acetaldehyde $\longrightarrow$ Ethanol

$$\begin{array}{c} H \\ | \\ H-C-OH \\ | \\ CH_3 \\ \text{Ethanol} \end{array} \qquad \begin{array}{c} H \\ | \\ C=O \\ | \\ CH_3 \\ \text{Acetaldehyde} \end{array}$$

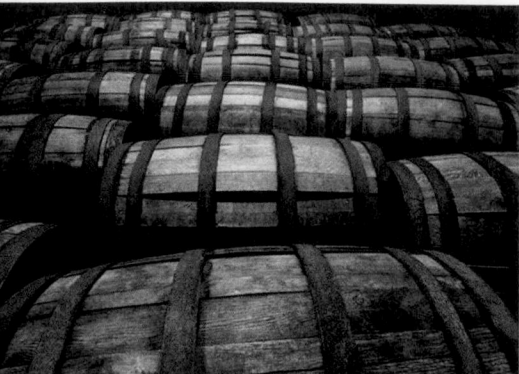

Wine is a historic beverage. It has been produced and consumed for more than 10,000 years.

distillation A physical method used to separate liquids based on their boiling points.

Alcohol proof represents twice the volume of alcohol in percentage terms in the product. Thus 80 proof vodka is 40% alcohol.

alcohol dehydrogenase An enzyme used in alcohol (ethanol) metabolism; the major enzyme used in the liver when alcohol is in low concentration.

The overall reaction is

$$C_6H_{12}O_6 + 2\ ADP + 2\ P_i \longrightarrow 2\ C_2H_5OH + 2\ CO_2 + 2\ ATP + 2\ H_2O$$

Glucose   Ethanol

Thus, under anaerobic conditions, one glucose molecule is fermented by yeast to two ethanol, two carbon dioxide, and two water molecules. The 2 ATP that result are used by the yeast for energy.

The carbohydrate must be a simple sugar, such as maltose or glucose, in order for the yeast to use it as food. If the carbohydrate is a starch, such as that found in cereal grains, it must be broken down to simpler forms, or "malted." During malting, the cereal grain seeds are allowed to sprout to produce the enzymes that break down the starches to simple sugars. The sprouting is then stopped by heating, and yeast cells and water are added to the malt. The yeast grows using the sugars for energy. When the oxygen in the vat (the mixture of water, yeast, and malt) is used up, the yeast ferments the remaining sugar to produce alcohol and carbon dioxide. After fermentation has ceased, the product is finished in a variety of ways. In some cases, the alcohol itself is recovered from the product.

Beer is made from malted cereal grain, such as barley; it is flavored with hops and brewed by slow fermentation. The carbon dioxide released is collected and used to carbonate the beer, thus producing the desirable fizz associated with a quality beverage.

Wine is the fermented juice of grapes. Climate, geographic region, and variety of grape determine the character of the wine. After fermentation, wines are often aged in barrels to decrease the acidity and remove undesirable impurities.

Distilled spirits are made from the **distillation** of the alcohol after fermentation. The difference between the boiling point of water and the boiling point of alcohol allows these two liquids to be separated by distillation and the alcohol to be recovered. Any number of fruits, vegetables, and grains can be fermented and the resulting mash distilled.

Alcohol Metabolism

After a person drinks an alcoholic beverage, his or her blood concentration of alcohol rises rapidly. Alcohol is readily absorbed into the blood from different segments of the GI tract by simple diffusion. You've probably been warned, with good reason, not to drink alcohol on an empty stomach. Alcohol absorption depends partly on the rate of stomach emptying. Food slows the stomach's emptying rate and stimulates secretions, such as hydrochloric acid, which dilute the alcohol and slow its absorption into the bloodstream.[8]

Alcohol is readily distributed into all the fluid compartments within the body because alcohol is found wherever water is distributed in the body. Alcohol moves easily through the cell membranes; however, as it does, it damages proteins in the membranes.[13]

Most of alcohol's damaging effects are seen in the liver because this is the first organ that is exposed to alcohol after absorption. The liver is also the chief site for alcohol metabolism. Although cells of the GI tract are in contact with alcohol, they are constantly being replaced because of their naturally short life span. Thus, they are not subject to the same degree of damage as liver cells, which have a much longer life span.[8]

Metabolism of alcohol is dependent on numerous factors, such as gender, race, size, physical condition, what is eaten, the alcohol content of the beverage, and even how much sleep one has had. The ability to produce the enzyme **alcohol dehydrogenase** is the key to alcohol metabolism, because it acts on about 90% of the alcohol consumed.[13] Women absorb and metabolize alcohol differently than men do. A woman cannot metabolize much alcohol in the cells that line her stomach because of low activity of alcohol dehydrogenase. Men metabolize about 30% of the alcohol ingested in this manner, but women metabolize only 10%. Women also have less body water in which to dilute the alcohol than do men (the same is also true for older men and older women). So, when a young man and a woman of similar size drink equal amounts of alcohol, a larger proportion of the alcohol reaches and remains in the woman's bloodstream. This explains why women develop alcohol-related ailments, such as **cirrhosis** of the liver, more rapidly than do men with the same alcohol-consumption habits.[2]

Most of the remaining alcohol consumed is then metabolized in the liver in the same way (by alcohol dehydrogenase) to carbon dioxide and water. Only a small percentage of alcohol intake is excreted unmetabolized through the lungs, urine, and sweat.[13] (Because the alcohol content of exhaled air maintains a constant relationship to the blood alcohol concentration in the lungs, it is used as the basis of the breathalyzer test.) As one continues to drink, one's blood alcohol concentration (BAC) continues to rise (Figure 8-1). A social drinker who weighs 150 pounds and has normal liver function metabolizes about 5 to 7 g of alcohol per hour. This is about one half of a beer or one fourth of an ordinary-sized drink. When the rate of alcohol consumption exceeds the liver's metabolic capacity, blood alcohol rises and symptoms of intoxication appear as the brain begins to be exposed to alcohol (Table 8-2).[19]

Because alcohol cannot be stored in the body, it has absolute priority in metabolism as a fuel source, taking precedence over other energy stores such as fat. When needed, the liver also has two other pathways to metabolize alcohol. Each—along with alcohol dehydrogenase—produces acetaldehyde. The other pathways are the **microsomal ethanol oxidizing system (MEOS)** and that utilizes the enzyme **catalase.** These other two pathways are also active in other cells in the body.[13]

cirrhosis A loss of functioning liver cells, which are replaced by nonfunctioning connective tissue. Any substance that poisons liver cells can lead to cirrhosis. The most common cause is a chronic, excessive alcohol intake. Exposure to certain industrial chemicals can also lead to cirrhosis.

microsomal ethanol oxidizing system (MEOS) An alternative pathway for alcohol metabolism when alcohol is in high concentration in the liver; uses rather than yields energy for the body, in contrast to alcohol dehydrogenase activity.

catalase pathway An alternative enzyme pathway to alcohol metabolism; alcohol is broken down in conjunction with the breakdown of hydrogen peroxide (H_2O_2) by this enzyme.

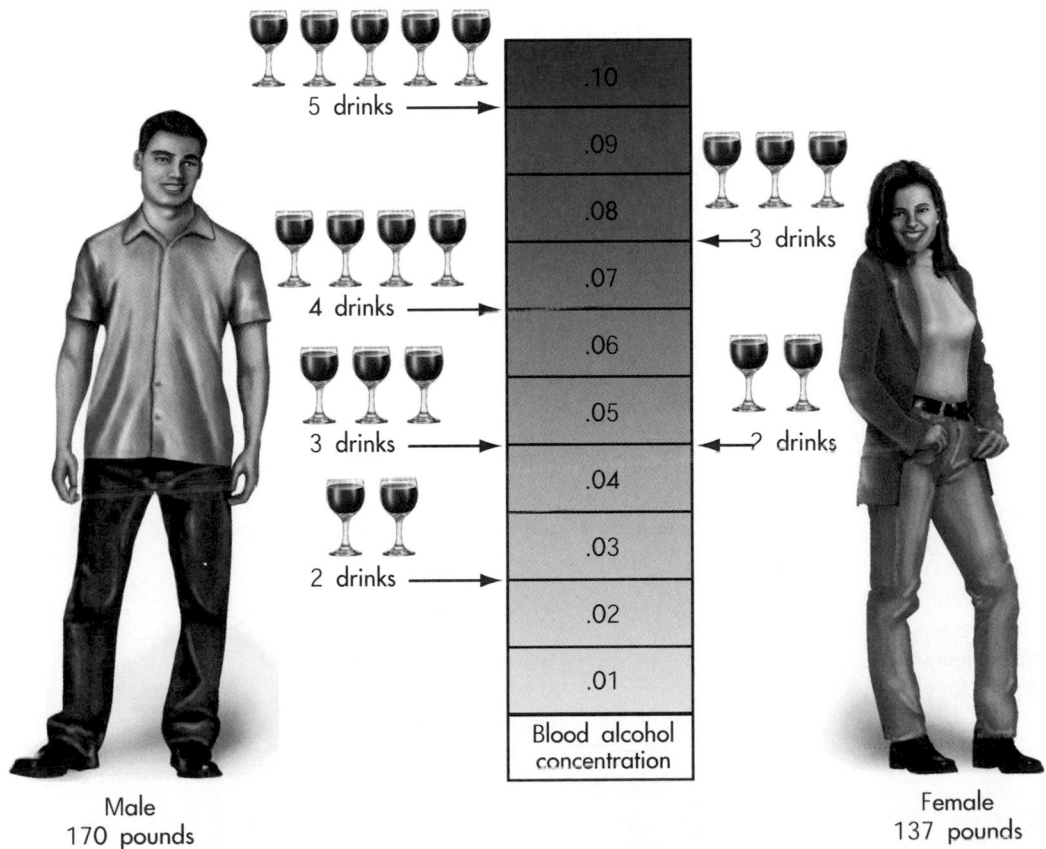

Figure 8-1 | Approximate relationship between alcohol consumption and blood alcohol concentration (BAC; units are % or mg of alcohol per 100 ml of blood). Note that effects can vary among people and whether food is also consumed. A BAC of 0.02 begins to impair driving. One is legally intoxicated at a BAC of 0.08 in the United States and throughout Canada. Recall that the following servings of each type of alcoholic beverage provide the same amount of alcohol (about 15 g): wine—5 oz, hard liquor—1.5 oz, beer or wine cooler—12 oz.

Table 8-2 | Blood Alcohol Concentration and Symptoms

Concentration*	Sporadic Drinker	Chronic Drinker	Hours for Alcohol to Be Metabolized
50 (party high) (0.05%)	Congenial euphoria; decreased tension; noticeable impairment (e.g., in driving)	No observable effect	2–3
75 (0.075%)	Gregarious	Often no effect	3–4
80–100 (0.08–0.1%)	Uncoordinated; 0.08% is legally drunk (as in drunk driving) in the United States and Canada	Minimal signs	4–6
125–150 (0.125–0.15%)	Unrestrained behavior; episodic uncontrolled behavior	Pleasurable euphoria or beginning of uncoordination	6–10
200–250 (0.2–0.25%)	Alertness lost; lethargic	Effort is required to maintain emotional and motor control	10–24
300–350 (0.3–0.35%)	Stupor to coma	Drowsy and slow	12–24
>500 (>0.5%)	Some will die	Coma	>24

*Milligrams of alcohol per 100 milliliters of blood (mg/dl).

Modified from Wyngaarder JB, Smith LH: *Cecil Textbook of Medicine,* fourth edition, Philadelphia, 1988, WB Saunders. Used with permission.

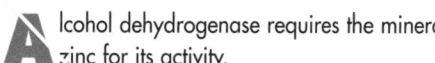 lcohol dehydrogenase requires the mineral zinc for its activity.

Alcohol Dehydrogenase Pathway

During the first step, alcohol at a low to moderate quantity is converted to acetaldehyde by the action of alcohol dehydrogenase and the coenzyme NAD^+. NAD^+ picks up two hydrogen ions and two electrons from the alcohol to form $NADH + H^+$ and produces the intermediate acetaldehyde (Figure 8-2).

$$\text{Ethanol} \xrightarrow{\quad NAD^+ \quad\quad NADH + H^+ \quad} \text{Acetaldehyde}$$

Distinctly different forms of alcohol dehydrogenase are found in the liver and the stomach. Each varies in its rate of alcohol metabolism.

The acetaldehyde formed is then converted to acetyl-CoA, again yielding $NADH + H^+$ with the aid of aldehyde dehydrogenase and coenzyme A.

$$\text{Acetaldehyde} \xrightarrow{\quad NAD^+ \quad\quad NADH + H^+ \quad} \text{Acetic acid} \xrightarrow{\quad \text{Coenzyme A} \quad} \text{Acetyl-CoA}$$

Figure 8-2 | Alcohol metabolism. At low alcohol intake, the alcohol dehydrogenase pathway in the cytoplasm is used. At high alcohol intake, the microsomal ethanol oxidizing system (MEOS) in the cytoplasm also is used. The MEOS uses rather than yields energy and accounts in general for about 10% of alcohol metabolism.

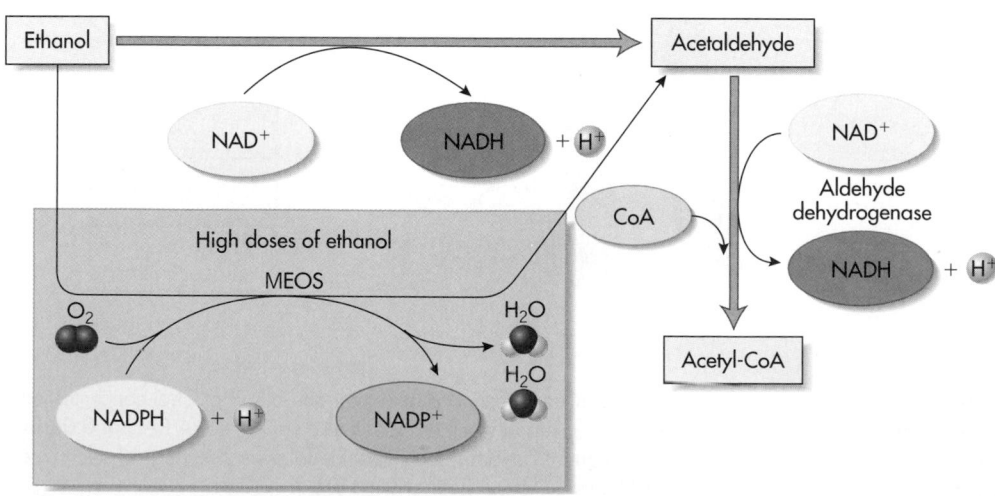

For any acetyl-CoA that enters the citric acid cycle, the NADH + H$^+$, FADH$_2$, and GTP molecules produced can then be used to synthesize ATP via the electron transport chain (review Chapter 4).

Structurally, ethanol with its hydroxyl group (–OH) resembles a carbohydrate. However, because ethanol is converted directly into acetyl-CoA, alcohol carbons cannot support glucose production. Thus, alcohol is metabolized more like a fatty acid than a carbohydrate and is considered fat in metabolic terms.[8] The related increase in NADH + H$^+$ also promotes fatty acid synthesis and reduces fatty acid use in the liver, with accumulation of body fat, especially in the abdominal region of the body.[9]

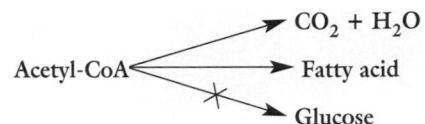

Metabolic fates of acetyl-CoA.

Microsomal Ethanol Oxidizing System (MEOS)

When a person drinks moderate to excessive amounts of alcohol, the enzyme alcohol dehydrogenase cannot keep up with the demand to metabolize all the alcohol into acetaldehyde. For this and other reasons, another enzyme system exists to metabolize alcohol. This system is called the microsomal ethanol oxidizing system (MEOS).

The liver (and other body cells as well) uses the MEOS to metabolize drugs and other substances foreign to the body. When the liver is overwhelmed with excess amounts of alcohol, it treats the excess as a foreign substance and activates the MEOS. This system uses oxygen—another niacin coenzyme (NADP$^+$)—and produces water and acetaldehyde. Once the MEOS is active, alcohol tolerance increases because the rate of alcohol metabolism increases.[13]

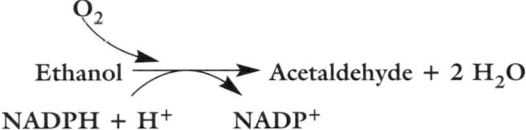

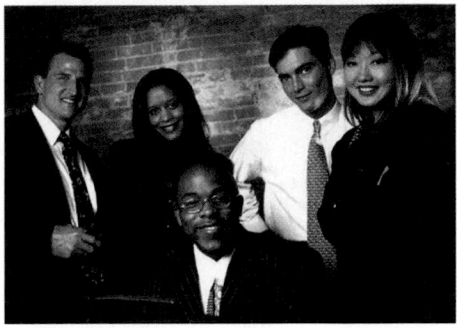

Compared with whites, some Asians and Native Americans make little of the active form of aldehyde dehydrogenase, and so are more likely to suffer from hangovers.

There are two interesting aspects of the body's reliance on MEOS. First, rather than forming the niacin-containing coenzyme NADH + H$^+$, as with alcohol dehydrogenase, the MEOS uses the niacin-containing coenzyme NADPH + H$^+$, a compound analogous to NADH + H$^+$. Rather than *yielding* "potential" ATP molecules from the first step in alcohol metabolism, by using NADPH + H$^+$ the MEOS *uses* "potential" ATP energy in the form of NADPH + H$^+$. NADPH + H$^+$ is converted to NADP$^+$. This partly explains why alcoholics do not gain as much weight as might be expected from the amount of alcohol-derived energy they consume.[13] The liver inefficiently uses excessive amounts of alcohol because it requires energy for the initial step in metabolism. A person with alcoholism wastes some energy by inducing this alternate metabolic pathway. Liver damage from alcohol, which causes other metabolic pathways to be hampered, also is implicated in the reduced energy yield associated with high alcohol consumption. In addition, alcohol slightly increases the metabolic rate of the body.

Use of the MEOS also increases the potential for a drug overdose. While the MEOS is metabolizing alcohol, the liver's capacity for metabolizing other drugs, such as many sedatives (barbiturates), is reduced, since both pathways compete for the same enzymes. If large amounts of alcohol and sedatives are consumed simultaneously, the alcohol gets preferential treatment. Because the liver is not able to metabolize the sedatives as fast as usual, the user may lapse into a coma and even die. Alcohol itself is toxic in high quantities. Mixed with sedatives, it creates an extremely lethal combination.[19]

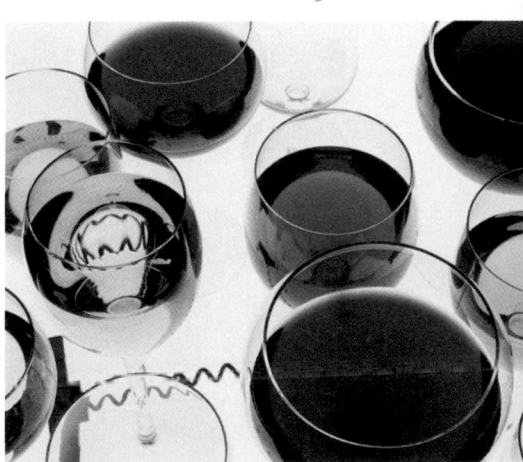

Of all the alcohol sources, red wine is often singled out as the best choice because of the added bonus of the many phytochemicals (e.g., resveretrol) present. These leach out from the grape skins as the red wine is made. Dark beer contains some phytochemicals, but a lower amount.

Catalase Pathway

The catalase enzyme found in the liver and other cells contributes to a minor pathway for metabolizing alcohol. It is located in the peroxisomes, a cell organelle.[13]

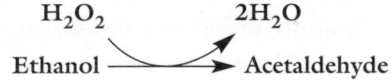

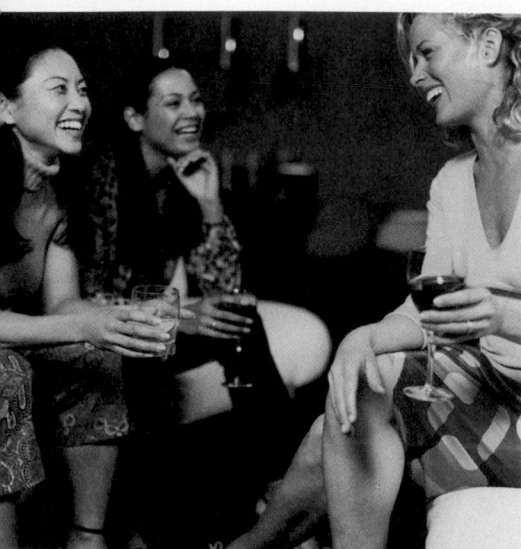

Much of alcohol's popularity is due to the pleasurable and social aspects associated with its use.

ischemic stroke A stroke caused by the absence of blood flow to a part of the brain.

Benefits of Moderate Alcohol Use

The benefits of alcohol use are linked to specific intakes of about one drink a day for men and slightly less than one for women. The type of alcoholic drink consumed does not significantly affect the benefit. Note that beer ranges considerably in its alcohol content, with malt liquor being higher in alcohol than most other forms of beer.

The benefits of moderate alcohol consumption begin with the many pleasurable and social aspects of its use. People enjoy meeting a friend over a beer or settling down to a glass of wine in the evening with dinner. These behaviors are not considered excessive as long as they are practiced by people of legal drinking age, remain under control, and cause no obvious harm. Other benefits include reduced risk of developing cardiovascular disease and cardiovascular disease–related deaths, such as from coronary heart disease. This benefit applies, however, only to middle-aged and older adults at risk for the disease who consume moderate amounts of alcohol, and not to younger adults.[1] **Ischemic stroke** risk also is decreased in light-to-moderate drinkers as opposed to those who abstain from alcoholic beverages.[16] Other potential health benefits are listed in Table 8-3.

Many of the benefits of moderate alcohol use are effective only in the short term, such as on an almost daily basis. More intermittent users and previous consumers of alcohol no longer experience the benefits of alcohol when consumption ceases.

Concept | Check

Alcohol is not an essential nutrient. It requires no digestion, and alcohol metabolism takes precedence over metabolism of the other energy-yielding nutrients. Alcohol is metabolized in the liver and other tissues. Metabolism mostly depends on the enzyme alcohol dehydrogenase. A number of individual factors, such as gender, race, and body composition, determine how a person reacts to alcohol. The microsomal ethanol oxidizing system (MEOS) is used whenever the liver detects more alcohol than can be processed by the alcohol dehydrogenase enzymes. Once the MEOS is active, alcohol tolerance increases because alcohol is being metabolized more rapidly.

The benefits of alcohol use are realized with moderate consumption. Under the correct circumstances, alcohol can be pleasurable, add to social occasions, and decrease the risk of coronary heart disease–related deaths and ischemic stroke. Mortality risk is somewhat greater in people who abstain from alcohol, and the risk appears to be decreased in men consuming up to two drinks per day. Furthermore, the protective dose of alcohol is somewhat less in women.

Health Problems from Alcohol Abuse

Despite the benefits of regular, moderate alcohol use, the risks of abuse are more numerous and harmful. Alcoholism, in and of itself, is the third leading cause of preventable death in North America.[3] In fact, excessive consumption of alcohol contributes significantly to 5 of the 10 leading causes of death in North America—heart failure, certain forms of cancer, cirrhosis of the liver, motor vehicle and other accidents, and suicides (review Table 8-3). Tobacco, often used simultaneously, interacts with alcohol in a way that reinforces its effects and causes esophageal and oral cancer. In addition, excessive alcohol drinking increases the risk of heart rhythm disturbances, hypertension, hemorrhagic stroke, osteoporosis, brain damage, colorectal and breast cancer, inflammation of the stomach lining, suppression of the immune system (and, thus, an increased risk of infections), sleep disturbances, impotence, hypoglycemia, and high blood triglycerides.[1,2,4,7,13,18] Figure 8-3 illustrates many of these risks. As mentioned before, alcohol ingestion also reduces use of fat by liver cells and promotes a positive energy balance, thus contributing to risk for obesity, especially abdominal obesity.[9] Finally, by reducing the action of antidiuretic hormone, alcohol increases urination

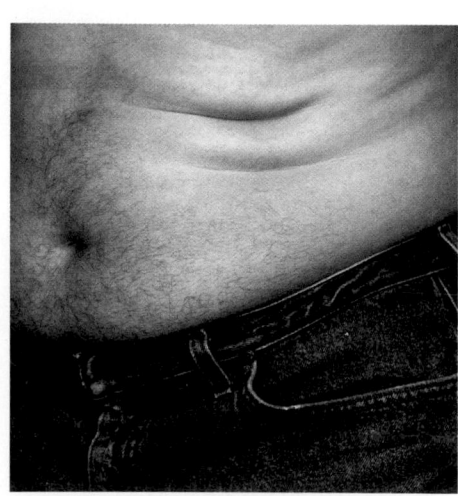

Excessive alcohol intake, notably binge drinking, encourages fat deposition, especially in the abdominal region.

Table 8-3 | A Summary of Benefits and Risks of Alcohol Use[4, 7,11,13,17,20,24]

	Benefits	Risks
Coronary heart disease	Decreased risk of death in those at high risk for coronary heart disease–related death, primarily by increasing HDL-cholesterol in some people, decreasing blood clotting, and relaxing blood vessels	Heart rhythm disturbances, heart muscle damage, increased blood triglycerides and homocysteine, and increased blood clotting
Hypertension and stroke	Mild decrease in blood pressure; fewer ischemic strokes in people with normal blood pressure; reduced death in people with hypertension	Increased blood pressure (hypertension); more ischemic and hemorrhagic strokes
Peripheral vascular disease	Decreased risk due to reduced blood clotting	No risk
Blood glucose regulation and type 2 diabetes	Some increase in insulin sensitivity and a decreased risk of death from cardiovascular disease	Hypoglycemia, reduced insulin sensitivity, and damage to pancreas (site of insulin production)
Bone and joint health	Some increase in bone mineral content in women, linked to increased estrogen output	Loss of active bone-forming cells and eventual osteoporosis (many nutrient deficiencies also contribute to the problem); increased risk of gout
Brain function	Enhanced brain function and decreased risk of dementia by increasing blood circulation in the brain	Brain tissue damage and decreased memory, especially in the teenage and young adult years
Skeletal muscle health	No benefit	Skeletal muscle damage
Cancer	No benefit	Increased risk of oral, esophageal, stomach, liver, lung, colorectal, and breast cancer, to name a few (especially if the person's diet is deficient in the vitamin folate); breast cancer risk is elevated even more if a woman is on estrogen replacement therapy (e.g., for menopausal symptoms)
Liver function	No benefit	Fat infiltration and eventual cirrhosis, especially if a person is also infected with hepatitis C; iron toxicity
GI tract disease	Decreased risk of certain bacterial infections in the stomach	Inflammation of the stomach (and pancreas); absorptive cell damage leading to malabsorption of nutrients
Immune system function	No benefit	Reduced function and increased infections
Nervous system function	No benefit	Loss of nerve sensation and nervous system control of muscles
Sleep disturbances	Some relaxation	Fragmented sleep patterns and snoring; worsens sleep apnea
Impotence and decreased libido	No benefit	Contributes to the problem in both men and women
Drug overdose	No benefit	Contributes to the problem, especially with sedatives
Obesity	No benefit	Increased abdominal fat deposition, contributes to positive energy balance
Nutrient intake	May supply some B vitamins and iron	Leads to numerous nutrient deficiencies: protein, vitamins, and minerals
Fetal health	No benefit	Variety of toxic effects on the fetus when alcohol is consumed by pregnant women (see Chapter 16)
Socialization and relaxation	Provides some benefit to socialization and leads to relaxation by increasing **serotonin** and **dopamine** neurotransmitter activity	Contributes to violent behavior and agitation
Traffic deaths and other violent deaths	No benefit (and likely even an increase in traffic accidents)	Contributes to both traffic death and violent death; note that the cost of a conviction for drunk driving is about $8000–$10,000 when the figure includes increased automobile insurance premiums.

The risks from alcohol abuse begin at intake of more than two to three drinks per day for men and one to two drinks per day for both women and adults over age 65.[21] Binge drinking (more than four drinks in a row for women and more than five drinks for men) can be especially harmful (see the Nutrition Focus in this chapter). The Swiss chemist Paracelsus (1493–1541) made the observation that "the dose determines the poison." This is especially true for alcohol, because alcohol abuse typically reduces a person's life expectancy by 15 years.)

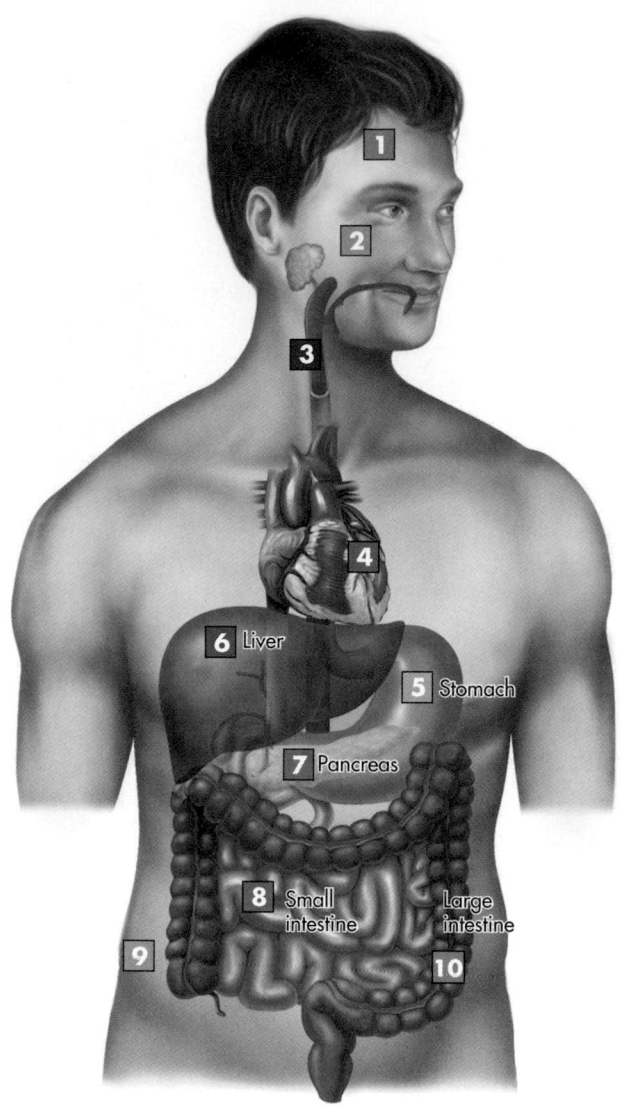

1	Impaired brain function and resulting brain damage
2	Vasodilation and resulting flushing of the skin
3	Cancer of the esophagus
4	Heart muscle damage and resulting heart failure
5	Irritation of the stomach lining and stomach cancer
6	Fatty infiltration of the liver and ultimate liver failure
7	Impaired pancreatic function and related hypoglycemia and pancreatic cancer
8	Malabsorption of nutrients in the small intestine
9	Abdominal fat deposition and fluid accumulation
10	Cancer of the colon and rectum

Figure 8-3 | Some effects of alcohol abuse on the body. Virtually every organ system is affected by alcohol. The mind-altering effects of alcohol begin soon after it enters the bloodstream. Within minutes, alcohol inhibits nerve cells in the brain. As a drug, alcohol eventually produces a **narcotic** effect on the body.[8] As Shakespeare wrote in Macbeth: "It provides the desire but takes away the performance." The heart muscle strains to cope with alcohol's depressive action. If drinking continues, rising blood alcohol causes impaired speech, vision, balance, and judgment. With an extremely high blood alcohol content, respiratory failure is possible. Over time, alcohol abuse increases the risk of liver and pancreas failure and certain forms of heart damage and cancer, among other disorders. Table 8-3 summarized all the negative effects of excessive alcohol use on physical health.

narcotic An agent that reduces sensations and consciousness.

If a person were to use beer as a nutrient source, he or she would need to consume daily:

• 40 to 55 bottles (12-oz) to meet protein needs
• 65 bottles for thiamin needs
• 6 bottles for niacin needs

and the risk for dehydration. Death from alcohol abuse usually results from respiratory failure or inhalation of vomit (the latter if the blood alcohol concentration is lower).

As a nutrient source, alcohol has little nutritional value, and thus, nutrient deficiencies are also a common result of alcoholism.[12] The protein and vitamin content is extremely low, except in beer, where it is marginal. Iron content varies from drink to drink, with red wine ranking especially high in iron. Excess use of some alcoholic beverages can even lead to iron toxicity, as well as toxicity from lead or cobalt.

Alcoholism produces many micronutrient deficiencies. These arise mostly because of poor nutrient intakes, but fat malabsorption linked to poor pancreatic function and increased urinary losses are also important in some cases.[13] On the other hand, micronutrient toxicity is also of concern, particularly with vitamin A and iron. In both cases, damage to the GI tract and liver enhance the potential for toxicity from these nutrients.[13] Dr. Charles Halsted discusses these problems in detail in the Expert Opinion. The immediate aim in nutritional treatment of alcoholism is eliminating alcohol intake. Then attention turns to replenishing nutrient stores, generally with nutrient supplements.

A Closer Look at Cirrhosis

Long-term alcohol use causes fatty liver, inflammation of the liver (alcoholic hepatitis), and eventually cirrhosis.[5] Cirrhosis is a chronic and usually relentlessly progressive disease characterized by fatty infiltration of the liver. Fatty liver occurs in response to increased synthesis of fat and decreased utilization of fat for energy needs by the liver. Eventually, the enlarged fat deposits choke off the blood supply, depriving the liver cells of oxygen and nutrients. Liver cells can accumulate so much fat that they burst and die and are replaced by connective (scar) tissue. This scarring process is called *cirrhosis*. When too many liver cells die, the liver dies, and the alcoholic patient dies. In North America, most cases of cirrhosis are caused by alcohol consumption. Cirrhosis develops in about 10 to 15% of cases of alcoholism and affects about 2 million people in the United States alone.[15] It is the second leading cause of the need for liver transplants. In addition to the amount and duration of alcohol consumption, genetic factors and individual differences determine one's risk for the disease, such as obesity, exposure to hepatotoxins (e.g., acetaminophen [Tylenol]), and infections with hepatitis C.[15] (Note that about 4 million people in the United States are infected with the virus that causes hepatitis C.) Once a person has cirrhosis, there is a 50% chance of death within 4 years, a far worse prognosis than many forms of cancer. Most of the deaths from alcoholic cirrhosis occur in people between the ages of 40 and 65 years. The actual death rate in the United States is 8.8 per 100,000 people. In 2001, 35,000 Americans died of cirrhosis.[15]

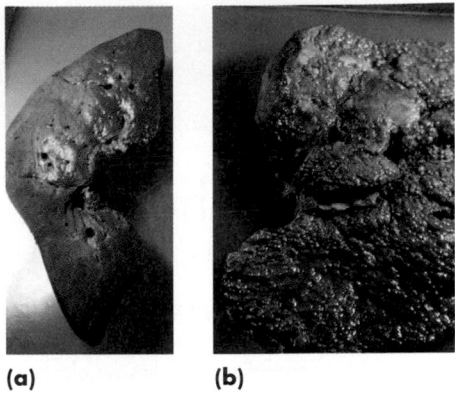

(a)   **(b)**

(*a*) Healthy liver; (*b*) liver with cirrhosis.

ascites Fluid produced by the liver, accumulating in the abdomen, that is a sign of liver failure associated with cirrhosis.

Why Does Alcohol Abuse Typically Lead to Cirrhosis?

A number of possible mechanisms underlie the liver damage from alcohol abuse. In chronic alcoholism, acetaldehyde concentration increases in the liver and is thought to be the underlying cause of the toxic effects of alcohol. Another cause of liver damage is the production of free radicals from alcohol metabolism. These highly reactive molecules destroy cell membranes and DNA and lead to chronic inflammation.[13]

No specific amount of alcohol consumption guarantees cirrhosis. Cirrhosis is commonly associated with a 10-year or longer consumption of approximately 80 g of alcohol (the equivalent of 7 beers) per day. Some evidence suggests that damage is caused by a dose as low as 40 g/day for men (3 beers) and 20 g/day for women (1 1/2 beers). Early stages of alcoholic liver injury are reversible, but moderate to advanced stages usually are not. If a person is terminally ill, a liver transplant is necessary for survival.[15]

A nutritious diet helps prevent some complications associated with alcoholism, but usually alcoholism brings about serious destruction of vital tissues regardless of the quality of the food consumed. Laboratory animal studies show clearly that even when a nutritious diet is consumed, alcohol abuse can lead to cirrhosis. Still, nutrient deficiencies compound the problem of cirrhosis because it makes the liver more vulnerable to toxic substances such as free radicals by depleting supplies of antioxidants, such as vitamin E. If present in adequate amounts, this vitamin can reduce free radical damage to the liver. A folate deficiency also compounds the damage.[13]

The overt signs of liver failure associated with cirrhosis are jaundice (the whites of the eyes and the skin turn yellow), **ascites,** and significant enlargement of the veins in the neck.[15]

Critical | Thinking

What risks and diseases could correlate with the combination of smoking and excessive alcohol use?

Concept | Check

Excessive alcohol use can result in an array of medical problems. It increases the risk of developing hypertension, certain forms of strokes and heart damage, birth defects, inflammation of the pancreas, damage to the brain, and malnutrition, to name a few.

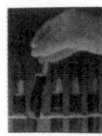

Expert Opinion

Alcohol and Nutrition
Charles H. Halsted, M.D.

Nutritional problems are common among alcoholics. Alcohol abuse can interfere with nutrient intake if alcohol replaces some or all of the food in the diet. When an individual relies on alcohol for the majority of his or her energy needs, protein-energy malnutrition can result. The symptoms of this protein-energy malnutrition are similar to those seen in children with marasmus (see Chapter 7). In addition to potential protein and energy deficiencies, deficiencies of a variety of other nutrients are possible, particularly certain vitamins and minerals.

Water-Soluble Vitamins

Excessive alcohol intake can lead to deficiencies in the water-soluble vitamins thiamin, niacin, vitamin B-6, vitamin B-12, folate, and vitamin C (see Chapter 10 for more details on these effects). Thiamin deficiency can be caused by decreased intake or decreased absorption of thiamin. The typical symptoms include **polyneuropathy** and nervous system problems. Often patients with extreme thiamin deficiency are admitted to the hospital and must be given thiamin injections to recover from this medical emergency, which, if untreated, can result in irreversible paralysis of ocular muscles, neuropathy with loss of sensation in lower extremities, loss of balance with abnormal gait, and memory loss. In patients with decreased thiamin stores, administration of large amounts of intravenous glucose can accelerate the symptoms of thiamin deficiency.

The metabolism of alcohol requires large quantities of niacin as NAD^+ and $NADP^+$, thus limiting the amount of niacin available for other metabolic activities in the body. If alcoholics consume a diet low in niacin and consume insufficient protein, they are at risk for niacin deficiency and the corresponding classic deficiency disease, pellagra.

Acetaldehyde, the primary metabolite of alcohol, can interfere with vitamin B-6 metabolism. Acetaldehyde displaces B-6 from its binding protein, re-

sulting in increased vitamin B-6 urinary excretion. If the alcoholic consumes a diet with inadequate amounts of vitamin B-6, he or she is at risk for developing **sideroblastic anemia** and peripheral neuropathy.

Excessive alcohol intake can also impair the absorption of vitamin B-12 as a result of decreased release of the digestive enzyme trypsin by the pancreas. Trypsin is needed to release vitamin B-12 from the R-protein so that it can then be bound by intrinsic factor and be absorbed by the body (see Chapter 10).

Insufficient intake of folate by an individual who abuses alcohol can be especially problematic. Folate deficiency may lead to a decreased number of absorptive cells in the small intestine, which then can result in decreased absorption of many other nutrients. **Megaloblastic anemia** is not uncommon in folate-depleted patients who consume excess alcohol.

Vitamin C deficiency can ultimately lead to the development of scurvy. When more than 30% of total energy intake comes from alcohol, vitamin C intake is usually less than the RDA. Daily supplementation may be required for weeks or months to restore blood and urinary vitamin C concentrations back to normal ranges.

Fat-Soluble Vitamins

Excessive alcohol intake can also result in deficiencies in the fat-soluble vitamins A, D, E, and K (see Chapter 9 for more details on these effects). Vitamin A deficiency may be caused by a deficient diet, by increased metabolism and biliary excretion, or by an inability of the liver to produce the vitamin A (retinol)-binding protein that delivers the vitamin to all parts of the body. Vitamin A stores in individuals with alcoholism are diminished regardless of whether dietary vitamin A intake is low, adequate, or high. Vitamin A concentrations are especially low in individuals with alcoholic cirrhosis. Chronic alcohol consumption is thought to induce metabolic systems in the liver that

---

polyneuropathy A disease process involving a number of peripheral nerves.

sideroblastic anemia A form of anemia characterized by red blood cells containing an internal ring of iron granules. This anemia may respond to vitamin B-6 treatment.

megaloblastic anemia A form of anemia characterized by large, nucleated, immature red blood cells that result from the inability of precursor cells to divide normally.

Guidance Regarding Alcohol Use

The U.S. Surgeon General's office, the National Academy of Science, and the USDA/DHHS do not specifically recommend drinking alcohol, but do not specifically discourage its use. The text of the *2005 Dietary Guidelines for Americans* (discussed in Chapter 2) does mention alcohol intake. It contains these statements:

- Those who choose to drink alcoholic beverages should do so sensibly and in moderation—defined as the consumption of up to one drink per day for women and adults age 65 and older, and up to two drinks per day for men. The definition is not intended, however, as an average over several days, but rather as the amount consumed on a single day.

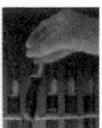

hasten the degradation of vitamin A. In addition, a pancreas damaged by alcohol releases a smaller amount of the enzymes needed to digest fat than a healthy pancreas, that, together with decreased bile secretion in alcoholic liver disease, results in decreased capacity to solubilize fat-soluble vitamins and reduced vitamin A absorption. Finally, alcohol can interact with beta-carotene, a precursor of vitamin A, ultimately reducing the amount of beta-carotene converted to vitamin A. Many alcoholics have trouble seeing in the dark (night blindness) because of this alcohol-induced vitamin A deficiency.

Vitamin D deficiency can result from inadequate dietary intake of the vitamin and/or lack of exposure to sunlight. A pancreas damaged by alcohol releases fewer fat-digesting enzymes, resulting in decreased fat absorption and consequently, decreased vitamin D absorption. A liver damaged by alcohol is compromised in its ability to convert vitamin D to the biologically active hormone form. Vitamin D deficiency can also result in reduced calcium absorption and increased parathyroid hormone secretion, both of which can lead to the development of osteoporosis.

Deficiencies in vitamins E and K also occur in individuals who have alcohol-damaged pancreases.

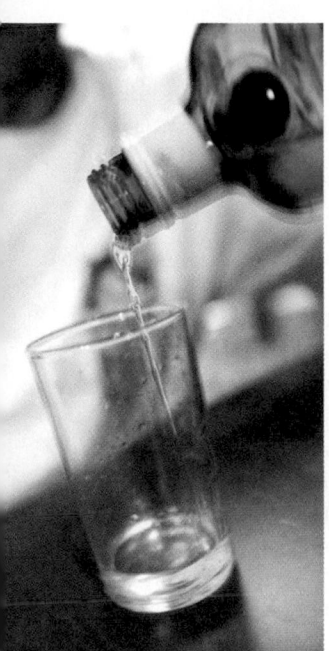

Alcoholism is a common cause of micronutrient malnutrition in North America.

Here again, the damaged pancreas is less able to release necessary digestive enzymes, leading to impaired digestion and absorption of fat and fat-soluble nutrients. Individuals with alcoholic liver disease are less able to synthesize vitamin K-dependent clotting factors, while individuals with vitamin E deficiency can develop peripheral neuropathy and tunnel vision.

Minerals

Individuals who abuse alcohol can also develop problems with magnesium, zinc, and iron metabolism (see Chapters 11 and 12 for more details on these effects). Severe alcohol abuse can result in magnesium deficiency by increasing urinary excretion of this mineral. Alcoholics can develop low blood concentrations of magnesium, which can result in **tetany,** characterized by muscle twitches, cramps, carpopedal spasms, and seizures. In addition, impairment of the central nervous system can also result. Magnesium deficiency is partly responsible for the hallucinations experienced by people withdrawing from alcohol intoxication.

Alcoholics can develop zinc deficiency as a result of decreased zinc absorption as well as increased urinary excretion. The consequences of alcoholism combined with zinc deficiency include changes in taste and smell, loss of appetite, trouble seeing at night, and impaired wound healing.

Both iron deficiency and iron overload are possible in alcoholics. Excessive alcohol consumption can damage the gastrointestinal tract and cause GI bleeding. This bleeding can eventually result in an iron deficiency. In contrast, alcohol can also increase the uptake and storage of iron in the liver, which can hasten the development of cirrhosis.

Clinicians need to be aware of the nutrition-related problems that can occur in alcoholism. Nutrient repletion is an important aspect of the treatment plan for alcoholic patients.

Dr. Halsted is Professor of Internal Medicine and Nutrition in the Division of Endocrinology, Clinical Nutrition and Vascular Metabolism at the University of California–Davis School of Medicine. Dr. Halsted is editor of the American Journal of Clinical Nutrition *and has published widely on the effects of alcohol on nutritional health.*

- Alcoholic beverages should not be consumed by some individuals, including those who cannot restrict their alcohol intake, women of childbearing age who may become pregnant, pregnant and lactating women, children and adolescents, individuals taking medications that can interact with alcohol, and those with specific medical conditions.
- Alcoholic beverages should be avoided by individuals engaging in activities that require attention, skill, or coordination, such as driving or operating machinery.

There is no recommendation for a nondrinker to start consuming alcohol for health benefits, but people of legal age who are not prone to abuse alcohol should know there's nothing wrong with moderate drinking. In fact, many studies have shown that light-to-moderate alcohol consumption has some health benefits.[10]

Healthy People 2010 set an important goal regarding alcohol use: reduce by 25% the proportion of adults who exceed the guidelines for appropriate alcohol use (currently, 73% of those who consume alcohol).

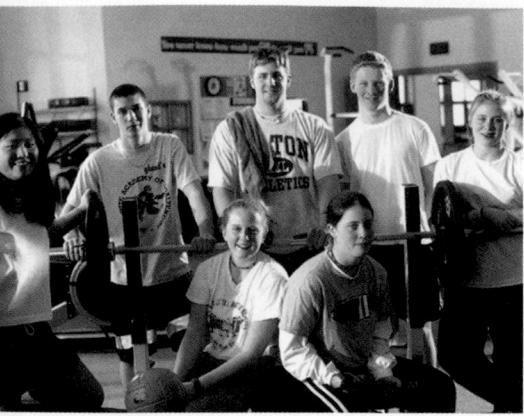

Young people benefit most from a healthy diet and exercise to decrease future risk of cardiovascular disease. There is no related benefit at this age for alcohol use.

alcohol dependence Repeated alcohol-related difficulties, such as a person's inability to control use, spending a great deal of time associated with alcohol use, continued use of alcohol despite physical or psychological consequences, persistent desire or unsuccessful efforts to cut down or control alcohol use, increased physical tolerance to alcohol's effects, and withdrawal symptoms.

Ability to "hold one's liquor" compared to the average person is a strong indicator of genetic risk.

Currently, about 32% of all North American adults have three drinks or less each week, about 22% have two drinks or less a day, and only about 11% have more than two drinks a day.

Alcohol Dependency and Abuse

Many factors determine a person's chances of developing **alcohol dependence.** Studies have shown links tying gender, genetics, ethnicity, parental influence, nurture, and depression. For some people, alcohol can be addictive and dangerous, and can eventually lead to **alcohol abuse.** Such alcohol abuse leads to 100,000 deaths in the United States each year.[18]

Genetic Influences

About 40 to 50% of a person's risk for alcoholism comes from genetic factors, although the gene or genes have not been identified.[14] The genetic influence on alcohol dependency and abuse has been shown by a number of studies, including twin and adoption research. Twins and first-degree relatives share a tendency toward alcohol addiction. Children of alcoholics have a fourfold-increased risk of developing alcoholism, even when adopted by a family with no history of alcoholism. This finding suggests that individuals with a family history of alcoholism need to be especially alert for evidence of the early signs of alcohol dependence.

Children with a family history of alcoholism should be warned of the dangers of drinking by the age of 10. At this age, they are old enough to understand the consequences of alcoholism but are not yet under the strong influence of their peers. Children as young as 10 may begin experimenting with alcohol to feel grown up, to fit in and belong to a group, to relax and feel good, to take risks and rebel against authority, or simply to satisfy curiosity. When alcoholic beverages are available in the home, it is easy for a child to sample a variety of drinks and to share them with friends.

Tolerance to alcohol may be genetic. A person tolerant to alcohol requires greater amounts of alcohol to produce the desired effect. Still, any one of us can become addicted if we drink long enough and consume ever-increasing quantities of alcohol. The lifetime risk of developing alcohol dependence is about 10 to 15% for men and 5 to 8% for women.[15]

The Effect of Gender

Gender plays a key role in alcohol metabolism, dependency, and surprisingly, treatment. The male:female ratio of alcohol dependency is 4:1, but there is evidence that women delay seeking treatment for alcohol abuse. As previously noted, the recommended limit for alcohol use is also different for men and women, because women's bodies have more fat and less muscle tissue and body water than do men's.[8] Alcohol can be diluted by water-holding muscle tissue, but not by adipose tissue. As also mentioned before, women cannot metabolize alcohol as quickly as men so it remains in their blood longer. Higher blood alcohol concentrations make women more susceptible to alcoholic liver disease, heart muscle damage, cancer, and brain injury.[2]

Ethnicity and Alcohol Abuse

Many ethnic distinctions play an important role in the probability of alcohol dependency and abuse. Compared with Caucasians, Asians and Native Americans are very susceptible to the damaging effects of alcohol for reasons discussed earlier (e.g., less aldehyde dehydrogenase activity in the liver). The major cause of death among Native Americans is motor vehicle accidents and unintentional injuries related to alcohol use. Other alcohol-related mortality statistics confronting Native Americans are suicide, homicide, domestic abuse, and fetal alcohol syndrome. African American alcoholics are at greater risk than other racial groups for tuberculosis, hepatitis C, HIV/AIDS, and other infectious diseases. Hispanic Americans are at particular risk for cirrhosis-related death.

Other Conditions

Depression and alcohol abuse often go hand in hand. Researchers have discovered that the risk for heavy drinking is higher among women with a history of depression than among women with no such history.[18] This finding holds up even when other factors that increase the risk of heavy drinking are accounted for, such as age, family history of drinking, and personality disorder. The more symptoms of depression women report, the more likely they are to drink heavily. There may be several reasons for this association. One reason is self-medication to relieve the symptoms of depression, possibly by increasing **serotonin** and **dopamine** activity in the brain. Research has shown that, although alcohol may alleviate depression in the short term, it tends to increase depression over time. A second reason is that women who are more depressed may not pay attention to their drinking and may not be concerned about the effects it can have on their health and behavior.[2]

The majority of suicides and interfamily homicides are alcohol-related. Clinicians need to be careful when dealing with depressed alcoholic patients to determine the psychological reasons for their drinking and how these behaviors might cause the death of the alcoholic or a family member. Alcohol consumption appears to be associated with youth suicide. The younger the drinker, the more likely he or she is to commit suicide.[22]

Alcohol dependence is the most common psychiatric disorder, affecting 13% of the North American population. Overall, about $185 billion is spent annually in the United States in terms of lost productivity, premature deaths, direct treatment expenses, and legal fees associated with alcoholism in the United States alone. A liver transplant costs about $150,000 and is needed in cases of excessive alcohol use. On the positive side, a typical counseling program costs only about $5000 to treat a person who is abusing alcohol.[15]

How Is Alcoholism Diagnosed?

Alcoholism is often considered a two-phase problem. Initially, it begins as problem drinking. This includes the repetitive use of alcohol, often to alleviate anxiety or solve other emotional problems. Alcohol addiction, the second phase, is defined as a true addiction following the repeated use of alcohol.

The diagnosis of alcoholism is based on a list of major criteria. Alcoholics may exhibit some or all of the following factors:[18]

- Physiologic dependence on alcohol with evidence of withdrawal symptoms when intake is interrupted
- Tolerance to the effects of alcohol, prompting greater alcohol intake to achieve the desired effect
- Evidence of alcohol-associated illnesses such as alcoholic liver disease or irreversible brain damage exhibited by memory loss, inability to concentrate, and decline in intellectual functions
- Continued drinking in defiance of strong medical and social contraindications and disruptions in normal life
- Depression and blackouts as well as impairment in social and occupational functioning

Other signs of alcoholism include the basic alcohol stigmas: alcohol odor on the breath, flushed face and reddened skin (the latter due to breakage of small blood vessels, which allows blood to seep under the skin), and nervous system disorders, such as tremors.[8] Unexplained work absences, frequent accidents, and falls or injuries of vague origin may all lead a clinician to consider the possibility of alcoholism. Laboratory tests are also helpful. These tests include measures of impaired liver

serotonin A neurotransmitter synthesized from the amino acid tryptophan that affects mood (sense of calmness), behavior, appetite, and induces sleep.

dopamine A type of neurotransmitter in the central nervous system that leads to feelings of euphoria, among other functions; it is also used to form norepinephrine, another neurotransmitter molecule.

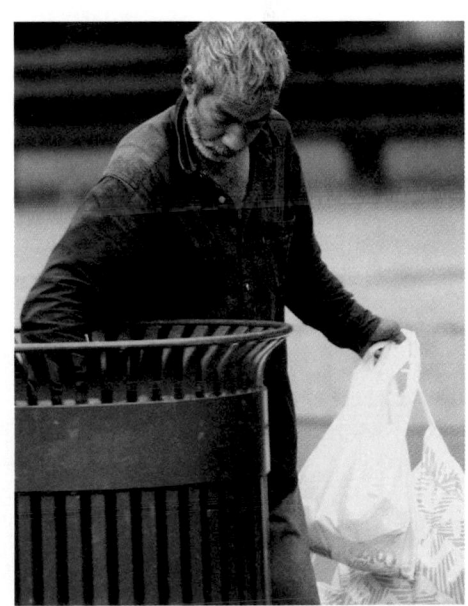

Because of a higher incidence of alcohol addiction among the homeless, many homeless individuals suffer from a wide range of alcohol-related health problems.

Alcoholics who stop drinking may substitute for their alcohol by increasing their intake of caffeine, nicotine, and simple sugars. This increase can lead to a worsening of overall nutritional status. Because heavy drinkers have poor nutrient intakes to begin with and because alcohol in itself creates so many nutritional problems, such a shift in intake has the potential to cause lifelong health consequences and so should be addressed.

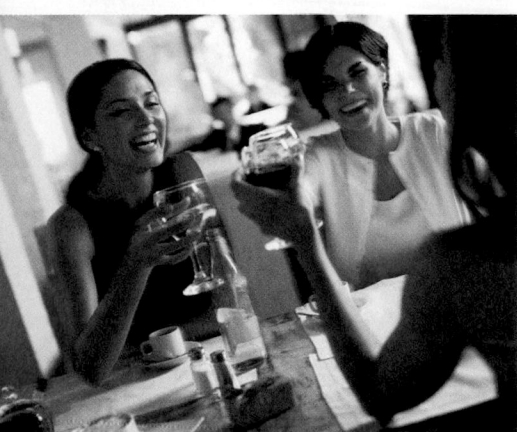

Compared to men, women more readily develop alcohol-related health problems.

Another common screening tool is the Michigan Alcohol Screening Test (MAST). It contains 22 questions. Briefer versions are also available.[23] Check out these and still other screening tools at the National Institute on Alcohol Abuse and Alcoholism website: http://www.niaaa.nih.gov/publications/niaaa-guide.

function, enlarged red blood cell size (to check for a deficiency of the B vitamin folate), and triglyceride and uric acid concentrations in the blood.[13]

Do You Have a Problem with Alcohol?

Asking a person about the quantity and frequency of alcohol consumption is an important means of detecting abuse and dependence. The CAGE questionnaire is commonly used in routine health care.[23]

C: Have you ever felt you ought to *cut* down on drinking?

A: Have people *annoyed* you by criticizing your drinking?

G: Have you ever felt bad or *guilty* about your drinking?

E: Have you ever had a drink first thing in the morning to steady your nerves or get rid of a hangover (*eye-opener*)?

More than one positive response to the CAGE questionnaire suggests an alcohol problem. Another key point to probe is tolerance: Does it take more to make you inebriated than it did in the past?

Other questions to ask along with the CAGE questionnaire are:

1. Have you had memory lapses or blackouts due to drinking?
2. Do you continue to drink even though you have health problems caused by alcohol?
3. Do you get withdrawal symptoms, such as headaches, chills, shakes, and a strong craving for alcohol and, as a result, drink more to get rid of these symptoms?
4. Do you take part in high-risk behaviors, such as having unsafe sex in a nonmonogamous relationship or driving a car or boat when under the influence of alcohol?
5. Has drinking caused trouble at home, at work, or in relationships with others?
6. Do you have to drink alcohol for any of the following reasons?
   a. To get through the day or unwind at the end of the day
   b. To cope with stressful life events
   c. To escape from ongoing problems

Answering yes to any of these questions should prompt the respondent to consult a family physician or a certified counselor for help.[18]

▌Treatment of Alcoholism

Once a diagnosis of alcohol abuse or dependence is established, one should seek the guidance of a physician to arrange appropriate treatment and counseling for the person and family. An important goal of counseling is to identify ways to compensate for the loss of pleasure from drinking. This helps the drinker confront the immediate problem of how to stop drinking. Total abstinence must be the ultimate objective. For alcoholics, there is no such thing as controlled drinking. A problem drinker cannot return safely to social drinking.[19]

The person should enter an Alcoholics Anonymous (AA) 12-step program (Al-Anon for the spouse) or another reputable therapy program for people with alcoholism.[18] One can check with a local mental health treatment center to find programs available in the community or call 800-245-4656. Substance Abuse and Mental Health Services can be reached at 800-729-6686 or www.health.org, for alcohol and drug information. In addition, one may visit the Alcoholics Anonymous web page at www.alcoholics-anonymous.org, www.al-anon.alateen.org or contact AA at:

AA World Services, Inc.
P.O. Box 459
New York, NY 10163
212-870-3400

Binge Drinking

College students are drinking more heavily and more frequently than ever before. Excessive alcohol consumption is an even bigger problem than illicit drug use on college campuses today (Table 8-4). Many college students consider drinking alcohol to be a "rite of passage" into adulthood. The largest drinking population in North America consists of young, Caucasian college students. Bars near campus typically promote heavy drinking. Alcohol producers frequently target college students with advertising and other marketing efforts. Adding to the overall problem is the fact that approximately half of all college students are not yet of legal drinking age. In fact, the annual overall cost related to underage alcohol use is estimated at more than $58 billion. This figure includes costs associated with violent crime, traffic accidents, treatment, and alcohol poisonings.[22]

Binge drinking—having four or more drinks in a row for women, or five or more for men—is common among college students. Only a minority of drinking by this group is done so in moderation,

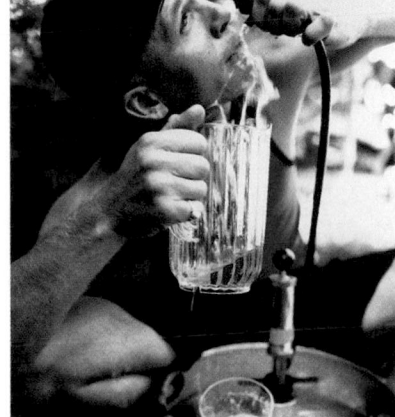

Although many young adults do not recognize the true impact of binge drinking habits, it is inherently risky in terms of their nutritional health, overall health, and safety.

Table 8-4 | Sobering Statistics on the Impact of Binge Drinking on College Campuses

Death: 1400 college students between the ages of 18 and 24 die each year from alcohol-related unintentional injuries, including motor vehicle crashes.

Injury: 500,000 students between the ages of 18 and 24 are unintentionally injured each year under the influence of alcohol.

Assault: More than 600,000 students between the ages of 18 and 24 are assaulted each year by another student who has been drinking.

Sexual abuse: More than 70,000 students between the ages of 18 and 24 are victims of alcohol-related sexual assault or date rape each year.

Unsafe sex: Each year about 400,000 students between the ages of 18 and 24 have unprotected sex and more than 100,000 students between the ages of 18 and 24 have been too intoxicated to know if they consented to having sex.

Academic problems: About 25% of college students report academic consequences of their drinking, including missing class, falling behind, doing poorly on exams or papers, and receiving lower grades overall.

Health problems/Suicide attempts: More than 150,000 students develop an alcohol-related health problem and between 1.2 and 1.5% of students indicate that they tried to commit suicide within the past year because of drinking or drug use.

Drunk driving: 2.1 million students between the ages of 18 and 24 drive under the influence of alcohol each year.

Vandalism: About 11% of college student drinkers report that they have damaged property while under the influence of alcohol.

Property damage: More than 25% of administrators from schools with relatively low drinking levels and more than 50% from schools with high drinking levels say their campuses have a "moderate" or "major" problem with alcohol-related property damage.

Police involvement: About 5% of 4-year college students are involved with the police or campus security as a result of their drinking, and an estimated 110,000 students between the ages of 18 and 24 are arrested for an alcohol-related violation such as public drunkenness or driving under the influences.

Alcohol abuse and dependence: 31% of college students met criteria for a diagnosis of alcohol abuse and 6% for a diagnosis of alcohol dependence in the past 12 months, according to questionnaire-based self-reports about their drinking.

The consequences of excessive and underage drinking affect virtually all college campuses, college communities, and college students whether they choose to drink or not.

Source: www.collegedrinkingprevention.gov/facts/snapshot.aspx

Healthy People 2010 includes an important goal regarding binge drinking: Reduce by at least one-half the number of high school and college students engaging in binge drinking (currently estimated at 32 and 40%, respectively).

Critical | Thinking

Imagine you are president of a university where there is a tradition of the "fourth-year fifth," a long-standing practice of seniors to consume a fifth of liquor during the semester prior to graduation. Every weekend between 3 and 10 students arrive in the local emergency room with alcohol poisoning or alcohol-related injuries, and there are several alcohol-related deaths each year. As the head of this institution, how do you and the Board of Trustees tackle this problem?

and the main reported purpose of drinking is "to get drunk." About 50% of college students engage in binge drinking. **Acute alcohol intoxication,** which can result from such rapid consumption of a large quantity of alcohol, is a major cause of suicide and hazing deaths related to binge drinking.

Binge drinking has a variety of contraindications. It can lead to unplanned sexual activity, injury to oneself or others, and even death. Death due to alcohol misuse can result, for example, from inhalation of vomit. In other cases, the body systems slowly shut down because of alcohol's overpowering depressant effect (Table 8-5). Other injuries can occur, resulting in paralysis or other lifelong medical problems. For example, in 2000, a student at the University of Michigan rapidly drank 20 shots to celebrate his 21st birthday and died shortly afterward, with a blood alcohol concentration of 0.39 percent. A student at Old Dominion University choked to death on his own vomit during a pledge-week drinking binge. A student on the diving team at Ohio State University became so intoxicated that he dove headfirst while diving into a mudpile at a party. He survived but is paralyzed from the neck down. Two female students in Colorado died of alcohol poisoning in 2004. Other students have drowned while intoxicated despite knowing how to swim.

Problems associated with binge drinking can affect all aspects of life. Regular binge drinking can lead to academic failure, because binge drinkers are more likely to miss class than are students who are light drinkers or abstainers. Property damage, as a result of vandalism and accidents, can be another consequence of binge drinking.[6] Students who live around binge drinkers experience more unwanted sexual advances, assaults, and insults/humiliations. Despite the array of negative outcomes, binge drinkers often do not think they have a problem, because their behavior has become so acceptable on college campuses.

According to U.S. law in all 50 states, an individual must be 21 years old to drink. In Canada, the legal age is 18 or 19, depending on the province. However, alcohol use often begins in adolescence. For example, 31% of twelfth-graders in the United States reported frequent drinking during 1999, and about 11% of all alcohol is consumed by youths under age 21. Influences on premature alcohol use are often seen in conjunction with athletics, if older, highly visible role models advertise products or are seen consuming alcohol. Peer pressure at school and on sports teams can cause many adolescents to drink. Dangerous habits become deadly when young adults choose to drive drunk or ride with friends who are intoxicated. Drinking habits created in youth may continue and worsen over time. Education and prevention strategies should focus on behavioral and psychosocial consequences because athletic performance typically does not suffer initially.

Overall, it is important that binge drinkers be aware that these habits can cause lifelong problems, especially when drinking becomes habitual.[6]

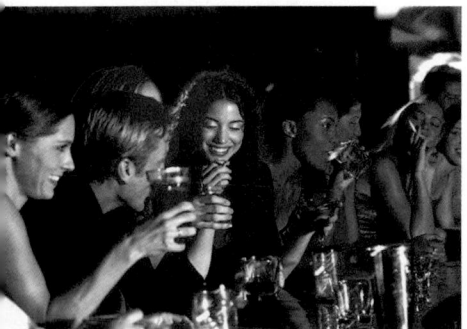

Alcohol use often begins in young adulthood and is carried into later years.

Table 8-5 | Signs and Symptoms of Alcohol Poisoning

Being aware of the warning signs and dangers of alcohol poisoning is important. It could help save the life of someone you love. The warning signs and symptoms include the following:
• Semiconsciousness or unconsciousness
• Slow respiration of eight or fewer breaths per minute or lapses between breaths of more than 8 seconds
• Cold, clammy, pale, or bluish skin
• Strong odor of alcohol, which usually accompanies these symptoms

Note: Although these are obvious warning signs of alcohol poisoning, the list is certainly not all-inclusive.

According to AA's literature, "AA is a fellowship of men and women who share their experience, strength, and hope with each other that they may solve their common problem and help others recover from alcoholism." As an informal society chartered in 1935, Alcoholics Anonymous includes more than 2 million recovered alcoholics. The only requirement for membership is the desire to stop drinking. There are no rules, regulations, dues, or fees. In addition, the group is not a political or formal organization.

It is helpful for the spouse to join the treatment program as well. AA has two types of meetings—open and closed. Alcoholics and their families and friends are invited to the open meetings, whereas the closed meetings are reserved for alcoholics only.

Current research does not support the generally negative public opinion about the prognosis for alcoholism. In most job-related alcoholism treatment programs, wherein workers are socially stable and—because of the risk to jobs and pensions—well motivated, recovery rates reach 60% or more.[19] This remarkably high cure rate is probably accounted for by early detection. Once a person moves from problem drinking to an advanced stage of alcoholism, success of treatment seldom exceed 50%. Early identification and intervention remain the most important steps in the treatment of alcoholism. Success is usually proportional to participation in AA, other social agencies' programs, and religious counseling. About 2 years of treatment should be expected.

Three medications are available to treat alcoholism.[18,25] The medication naltrexone (ReVia) blocks the craving for alcohol and the pleasure of intoxication (Figure 8-4). Disulfiram (Antabuse) causes physical reactions, such as vomiting, when drinking alcohol. It does so by blocking acetaldehyde metabolism. Acamprosate (Campral) is thought to act on neurotransmitter pathways in the brain related to alcohol abuse, decreasing the desire to drink. Detoxification drugs are also important in treating alcoholism, as is using some form of psychotherapy.

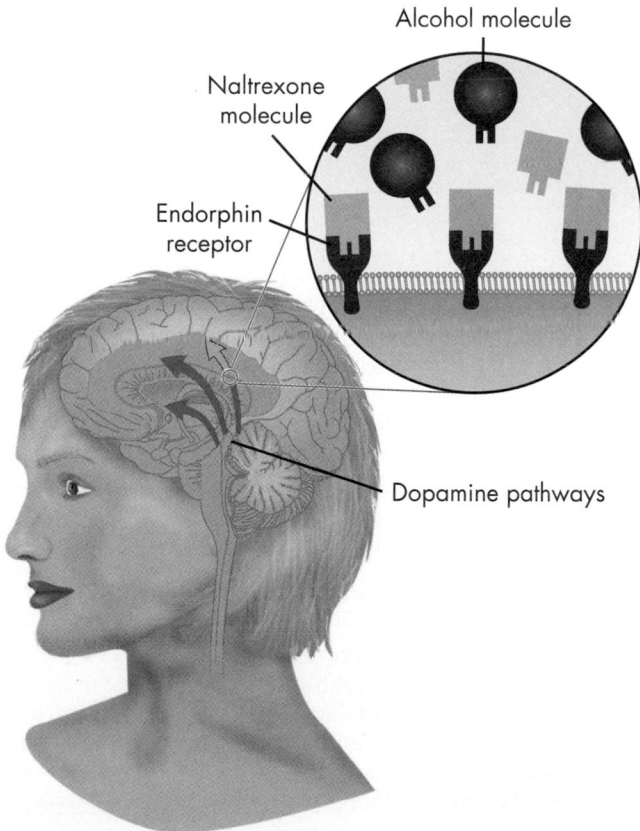

Figure 8-4 | The euphoria that arises from alcohol use involves alcohol binding to specific receptors in the brain. It is likely that this binding, in turn, causes a release of the neurotransmitter dopamine. The increase in dopamine in the brain is thought to cause the characteristic high associated with alcohol use. Naltrexone (ReVia) works by blocking alcohol's ability to bind to brain receptors. This, then, reduces dopamine release and blocks the pleasant feelings elicited by alcohol use.

To learn more about alcoholism, visit these websites:

www.niaaa.nih.gov

www.asam.org

www.mentalhelp.net/selfhelp

www.nlm.nih.gov/medlineplus/
alcoholconsumption.html

www.findtreatment.samhsa.gov

http://www.nacoa.org

Concept | Check

Treatment of alcoholism often includes the use of medicine, counseling, and social support. The clinicians involved must treat the entire person. Alcoholics Anonymous and other support groups are very helpful. Naltrexone can be prescribed to decrease alcohol intakes, as can acamprosate. Another option is disulfiram, which produces an ill feeling when the patient consumes both the medicine and alcohol. With all the treatments for alcoholism, it is important to find the one that works best for the individual with alcoholism.

Case Scenario | Follow-Up

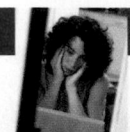

Alcohol is a central nervous system depressant and narcotic that affects both respiration and heart rate. In large quantities, alcohol can depress both systems to the point of terminating respiration and cardiac function. Obviously, this is fatal. Alcohol abuse is a common problem, and continued alcohol abuse can lead to dependence problems, although alcohol abuse and dependence are different.

As a close friend, Alyssa has a responsibility to hold Todd accountable for his actions. Sometimes it is difficult to realize that one has a drinking problem, although it may be obvious to others. Alyssa should talk privately to Todd when he is sober and calm about the most recent incident. It is important to deal with situations such as these very carefully, because the problem drinker will probably respond defensively. She could explain how his drinking is causing problems for both of them, she could tell him about the harmful consequences of his drinking, and she could refuse to go with him to any alcohol-related events, but she must be prepared to carry out her refusal. This is especially important for her because she does not want to risk further physical harm from Todd. Alyssa could talk with a counselor, who may help her learn ways to approach Todd effectively. Offering to go with Todd to a treatment program or an AA meeting and get help is one idea. There is strength in numbers, so other members of Todd's family or close friends also should be enlisted to help, under the guidance of a therapist trained in treating alcoholics.

Summary

1. Alcohol use is a complex issue because it involves psychological, social, economic, health, legal, and family issues.

2. Alcohol is metabolized in the liver and other tissues. Metabolism depends on the enzyme alcohol dehydrogenase. A number of factors, such as gender, race, and body composition, determine how a person reacts to alcohol.

3. The body uses the microsomal ethanol oxidizing system (MEOS) whenever the liver detects more alcohol than can be processed by the alcohol dehydrogenase enzymes. Once the MEOS is active, alcohol tolerance increases because alcohol is being metabolized more rapidly.

4. The benefits of alcohol use are associated with low-to-moderate alcohol consumption. These benefits include the pleasurable and social aspects of alcohol use, a reduction in various forms of cardiovascular disease-related deaths, increase in insulin sensitivity, and protection against some harmful stomach bacteria.

5. Alcohol use also creates many health risks. Excessive consumption of alcohol contributes significantly to 5 of the 10 leading causes of

death in North America. Alcohol increases the risk of developing certain forms of heart damage, inflammation of the pancreas, GI tract damage, vitamin and mineral deficiencies, cirrhosis of the liver, certain forms of cancer, hypertension, and hemorrhagic stroke—to name a few.

6. If alcohol is consumed, it should be consumed in moderation with meals. Women are advised to drink no more than one drink per day, as are adults 65 years and older; men are advised to limit intake to two drinks a day.

7. Gender, genetics, ethnic background, and ongoing depression all play a role in a person's chances of becoming alcohol dependent.

8. Early detection of alcoholism is key to successful treatment and a reduction of health-care costs. The CAGE questionnaire can help a person determine whether he or she has an alcohol problem.

9. Many methods are available to treat alcoholism. Alcoholics Anonymous and the medication ReVia are among the typical approaches.

Study Questions

1. Where in the body does most of the metabolism of alcohol take place? What is a by-product of alcohol metabolism?
2. Why does it take a woman longer than a man to metabolize alcohol?
3. List two potential health benefits of alcohol use.
4. List four problems associated with alcohol abuse.
5. Which two nutrient deficiencies are common in alcoholism? Why?
6. Define the term *one drink*. How much alcohol use is considered to be moderate for men? for women?
7. Why can some ethnic groups hold their liquor better than others can?
8. Name four criteria that might indicate that someone has a problem with alcohol. What is this group of criteria checklist called?
9. Describe a method used in treating alcoholism. What are the benefits and drawbacks?
10. What is binge drinking? Within which segment of the population is this activity increasing in popularity?

BOOST YOUR STUDY

Check out the **Perspectives in Nutrition: Online Learning Center** www.mhhe.com/wardlawpers7 for quizzes, flash cards, activities, and web links designed to further help you learn about issues surrounding alcohol use and abuse.

Annotated References

1. Alcohol and health: The pros and cons. *Mayo Clinic Health Letter*, p. 4, November 2003.

    The pros and cons of alcohol use are reviewed. Although there are health benefits from alcohol use, moderation is a key theme, and there is no recommendation to start drinking merely to gain the health benefits.

2. Alcohol—an important women's health issue. *Alcohol Alert* 62:1, 2004.

    When a woman drinks alcohol, the alcohol in her bloodstream typically reaches a higher amount than in a man even if the two are drinking the same amount of alcohol. This is because women have less body water than men. As a result, women are very susceptible to alcohol-related organ damage.

3. Alcohol-attributable deaths and years of potential life lost. *Journal of the American Medical Association* 292:2831, 2004.

    Excessive alcohol consumption is the third leading cause of preventable death in the United States. These deaths include liver cirrhosis, various cancers, unintentional injuries, and violence.

4. Alcohol's damaging effects on the brain. *Alcohol Alert* 63:1, 2004.

    Alcohol can produce detectable impairments in memory after only a few drinks. As the amount of alcohol increases, so does the degree of impairment.

5. Alcoholic liver disease. *Alcohol Alert* 64:1, 2005.

    Alcoholic liver disease includes three conditions: fatty liver, alcoholic hepatitis, and cirrhosis. The fatty liver stage is reversible when alcohol intake stops, but the other stages are not. Thus, even when stopping drinking, alcoholics will still suffer the effects of these latter two stages.

6. Brewer RD, Swahn MH: Binge drinking and violence. *Journal of the American Medical Associatioan* 294:616, 2005.

    Binge drinking is strongly associated with violence. This is an important reason to discourage binge drinking.

7. Cho E and others: Alcohol intake and colorectal cancer: A pooled analysis of 8 cohort studies. *Annals of Internal Medicine* 140:603, 2004.

    Drinking more than two drinks a day appears to increase the risk for colorectal cancer. This finding is true for men and women and is true for the various alcoholic beverages typically consumed.

8. Clairmont MA: Alcohol dependence & abuse. *Today's Dietitian* p. 14, September 2005.

    Alcohol abuse can lead to a number of nutrient deficiencies and other health problems. Drinking alcohol without concomitant food intake is especially risky as food slows alcohol absorption and thus reduces some of its negative social and health effects.

9. Dorn JM and others: Alcohol drinking patterns differentially affect central adiposity as measured by abdominal height in women and men. *Journal of Nutrition* 133:2665, 2003.

    Alcohol use increases the risk for abdominal fat deposition. Binge drinking especially was found to be a risk factor.

10. Klatsky AL: Drink to your health? *Scientific American*, p. 75, February 2003.

    Moderate alcohol use provides some health benefits, but alcohol abuse poses many health risks. In light of current knowledge, a person with an established moderate drinking pattern should generally not be advised to abstain from alcohol. However, nondrinkers should not be advised to start drinking for health reasons.

11. Leevy CM, Moroianu SA: Nutritional aspects of liver disease. *Clinics in Liver Disease* 9(1):67, 2005.

    Nutritional deficiencies are part of the cause of liver disease related to alcohol use. Still, avoidance of alcohol is needed to stop the progressive nature of alcohol-related liver disease.

12. Lieber CS: Relationships between nutrition, alcohol use, and liver disease. *Alcohol Research and Health* 7(3):220, 2003.

    Many alcoholics become malnourished because they consume too few nutrients and because of the potential of alcohol itself to reduce nutrient absorption.

13. Lieber CS: Nutrition in liver disorders and the role of alcohol. In Shils ME and others (eds): *Modern nutrition in health and disease.* 10th ed. Philadelphia, PA: Lippincott Williams & Wilkins, 2006.

    Detailed examination of alcohol metabolism and its related role in nutrition-related health disorders.

14. Liu I-Chao and others: Genetic and environmental contributions to the development of alcohol dependence in male twins. *Archives of General Psychiatry* 61:897, 2004.

    Genetic influence accounted for about 50% of the risk of alcohol dependence in this study. The effect was even seen after accounting for other psychiatric disorders, but was closer to 40%.

15. Mailliard MR, Sorrell MF: Alcoholic liver disease. In Kasper DL and others (eds.): *Harrison's Principles of Internal Medicine.* New York: McGraw-Hill, 2004.

    Alcohol is a powerful toxin to the cells of the liver and leads to liver cirrhosis in about 10% to 20% of cases of alcoholism. Women are much more susceptible to this disease than men, and so should be especially cautious about alcohol intake.

16. Mukamal KJ and others: Alcohol and risk for ischemic stroke in men: The role of drinking pattern and usual beverages. *Annals of Internal Medicine* 142:11, 2005.

Intake of more than two drinks a day increases the risk of ischemic stroke. In contrast, lesser amounts of alcohol, specifically red wine, is associated with a reduced risk of ischemic stroke.

17. Renaud S and others: Moderate wine drinkers have lower hypertension-related mortality: A prospective cohort study in French men. *American Journal of Clinical Nutrition* 80:621, 2004.

    A moderate intake of wine is associated with a lower risk of mortality from all causes in persons with hypertension. This result was seen with wine drinking, but because the study was done in France, an effect for other forms of alcoholic beverages consumed by other cultures cannot be ruled out.

18. Saitz R: Unhealthy alcohol use. *The New England Journal of Medicine* 352:596, 2005.

    This article presents a case study of a man who is abusing alcohol. Both diagnosis and treatment of alcoholism are reviewed in the process.

19. Schuckit MC: Alcohol and alcoholism. In Kasper DL and others (eds.): *Harrison's Principles of Internal Medicine*. New York: McGraw-Hill, 2004.

    Excellent review of alcoholism is presented. This chapter was used to verify much of the content of Chapter 8.

20. Stampfer MJ and others: Effects of moderate alcohol consumption on cognitive function in women. *The New England Journal of Medicine* 352:245, 2005.

    Up to one drink per day may increase cognitive function in women. An intake of more than that is not protective and even has the opposite effect.

21. Strandberg AY and others: Alcohol consumption, 29-yr total mortality, and quality of life in men in old age. *American Journal of Clinical Nutrition* 80:1366, 2004.

    Greater than three drinks per day worsened the quality of life of older men in this study. Lower intakes were not harmful but also were not found to be helpful in this group of men.

22. Underage drinking. *Alcohol Alert* 59:1 (April), 2003.

    Underage drinking may lead to a host of health problems, including traffic accidents and suicide. Early intervention to curb underage drinking is essential to prevent these and other health problems.

23. US Preventive Services Task Force: Screening and behavioral counseling interventions in primary care to reduce alcohol misuse: Recommendation statement. *American Family Physician* 70:353, 2004.

    The US Preventive Services Task Force recommends screening and behavioral counseling to reduce alcohol misuse. The CAGE questionnaire is one tool that can be used for screening purposes. Other tools are also presented.

24. Wannamethee SG and others: Alcohol drinking patterns and risk of type 2 diabetes mellitus among younger women. *Archives of Internal Medicine* 163:1329, 2003.

    Light to moderate alcohol consumption may be associated with a lower risk of type 2 diabetes among women. Intakes in excess of this amount are not more protective, however, and actually increased such risk.

25. Williams SH: Medications for treating alcohol dependence. *American Family Physician* 72:1775, 2005.

    Concise review of the medications available to treat alcohol dependence. Naltrexone and acamprosate are the most useful of the currently available medications.

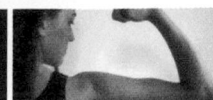

Take | Action

I. Could You or Someone You Know Have a Problem with Alcoholism?

Problem drinking often has its seeds in the teen years. Significant health consequences of this practice typically arise in adulthood. Alcohol abuse is a prominent contributor to 5 of the 10 leading causes of death in North America. The social consequences of alcohol dependency include divorce, unemployment, and poverty. The following questionnaire was developed by the National Council on Alcoholism. With this assessment, you can determine whether you or someone you know might need help.

	Yes	No
1. Do you occasionally drink heavily after disappointment, after a quarrel, or when someone gives you a hard time?		
2. When you have trouble or feel under pressure, do you drink more heavily than usual?		
3. Have you ever noticed that you're able to handle liquor better than you did when you first started drinking?		
4. Do you ever wake up the morning after you've been drinking and discover that you can't remember part of the evening before, even though your friends tell you that you didn't pass out?		
5. When drinking with other people, do you try to have a few extra drinks when others won't know it?		
6. Are there certain occasions when you feel uncomfortable if alcohol isn't available?		
7. Have you recently noticed that when you begin drinking, you're in more of a hurry to get the first drink than you used to be?		
8. Do you sometimes feel a little guilty about your drinking?		
9. Are you secretly irritated when your family or friends discuss your drinking?		
10. Have you recently noticed an increase in the frequency of memory blackouts?		
11. Do you often find that you wish to continue drinking after your friends say they've had enough?		
12. Do you usually have a reason for the occasions when you drink heavily?		
13. When you're sober, do you often regret things you have done or said while drinking?		
14. Have you tried switching brands or following different plans to control your drinking?		
15. Have you often failed to keep promises you've made to yourself about controlling or stopping your drinking?		
16. Have you ever tried to control your drinking by changing jobs or moving to a new location?		
17. Do you try to avoid family or close friends while you're drinking?		
18. Are you having an increasing number of financial and work problems?		
19. Do more people seem to be treating you unfairly without good reason?		
20. Do you eat very little or irregularly when you're drinking?		

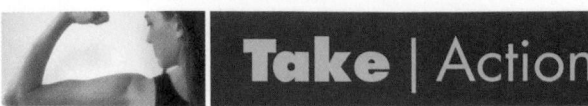

	Yes	No
21. Do you sometimes have the "shakes" in the morning and find that it helps to have a little drink?	_____	_____
22. Have you recently noticed that you can drink more than you once did?	_____	_____
23. Do you sometimes stay drunk for several days at a time?	_____	_____
24. Do you sometimes feel very depressed and wonder whether life is worth living?	_____	_____
25. Sometimes after periods of drinking do you see or hear things that aren't there?	_____	_____
26. Do you get terribly frightened after you have been drinking heavily?	_____	_____

Interpretation

These are all symptoms that may indicate alcoholism. "Yes" answers to several of the questions indicate the following stages of alcoholism:

Questions 1–8:	Potential drinking problem
Questions 9–21:	Drinking problem likely
Questions 22–26:	Definite drinking problem

It is vital that people assess themselves honestly. If you or someone you know demonstrates some or a number of these symptoms, it is important to seek help. If there is even a question in your mind, go talk to a professional about it.

II. Investigate the Energy Cost of Alcohol Use

On an upcoming weekend (Friday night through Sunday night), have a few friends keep a careful log of their alcoholic beverage intake. Include males and females. Then use Table 8-1 or your nutrient analysis software to calculate the amount of energy provided by alcoholic beverages over that time period. Assuming that an active man needs about 2800 kcal/day and an active woman needs about 2200 kcal/day, is the amount of energy provided by alcoholic beverages large (e.g., 25% or more of needs) or small (e.g., 10% or less of needs) in comparison?

THE FAT-SOLUBLE VITAMINS

CHAPTER OUTLINE

CASE SCENARIO:

Kristen works nights at a local package distribution center to make some extra money. The combination of taking a full course load at college and working nights has created a lot of stress for her. Kristen's many commitments also make it important that she not become ill. On a recent coffee break at her job, a coworker suggested she take *Nutramega* supplements to help prevent colds, flu, and other illnesses. The product's label suggests that *Nutramega* helps prevent such problems, especially those associated with the changing of seasons. The label recommends taking two to three tablets every 3 hours at the first sign of feeling ill, and two to three tablets daily for health maintenance. Kristen looks at the Supplement Facts label on the bottle and finds that each tablet contains (as a percentage of the Daily Value): 33% for vitamin A (three-quarters of which is preformed vitamin A), 700% for vitamin C, 50% for zinc, and 10% for selenium. A month's supply also costs about $50.

Should Kristen use this product? Are there health risks associated with this product, especially considering the dosage recommended on the label?

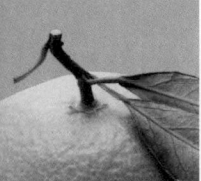

When it comes to vitamins, we often hear, "If a little is good, then more must be better." Some people believe that consuming vitamins far in excess of their needs provides them with extra energy, protection from disease, and prolonged youth. About 40% of adults in the United States take vitamin and/or mineral supplements on a regular basis, some at unsafe levels.[1] They are spending about $17 billion annually on supplements. The health-related value of this practice is hotly debated.[7,14]

Our total vitamin needs to prevent deficiency are actually quite small. In general, humans require a total of about 1 oz (28 g) of vitamins for every 150 lbs. (70 kg) of food consumed. Vitamins are found in plants and animals. Plants synthesize all the vitamins they need. Animals vary in their ability to synthesize vitamins. For example, guinea pigs and humans are two of the very few organisms that are unable to make their own supply of vitamin C.[9]

These vital nutrients are divided into two groups: the fat-soluble vitamins and the water-soluble vitamins. This chapter focuses on the functions and sources of the fat-soluble vitamins and human needs for them. (Chapter 10 reviews the water-soluble vitamins.) This chapter also explores the current controversy over vitamin and mineral supplement use.

CHAPTER OBJECTIVES CHAPTER 9 IS DESIGNED TO ALLOW YOU TO:

1. Define the term *vitamin* and list three characteristics of vitamins as a group.
2. Classify the vitamins according to whether they are fat-soluble or water-soluble.
3. List the major functions and deficiency symptoms for each fat-soluble vitamin.
4. State the conditions in which deficiencies of fat-soluble vitamins are likely to occur.
5. List three important food sources for each fat-soluble vitamin.
6. Describe toxicity symptoms from excess consumption of certain fat-soluble vitamins.
7. Evaluate the use of vitamin and mineral supplements with respect to their potential benefits and hazards to the body.

REFRESH YOUR MEMORY AS YOU STUDY CHAPTER 9 ON FAT-SOLUBLE VITAMINS, YOU MAY WANT TO REVIEW:

- Implications of the Dietary Supplement Health and Education Act (DSHEA) in Chapter 1.
- The gastrointestinal system for the digestion and absorption of fat-soluble nutrients in Chapter 3.
- Oxidation and reduction reactions in Chapter 4.
- The digestion and absorption of dietary lipids and the formation of lipoproteins in Chapter 6.
- Protein synthesis in Chapter 7.

Vitamins: Vital Dietary Components

vitamin Compound needed in very small amounts in the diet to help regulate and support chemical reactions and processes in the body.

fat-soluble vitamins Vitamins that dissolve in fat and such substances as ether and benzene but not readily in water. These vitamins are A, D, E, and K.

water-soluble vitamins Vitamins that dissolve in water. These vitamins are the B vitamins and vitamin C.

By definition, **vitamins** are essential, organic (e.g., containing carbon bonded to hydrogen) substances needed in small amounts in the diet for the normal function, growth, and maintenance of body tissues. Although vitamins themselves provide no energy to the body, some can facilitate energy-yielding chemical reactions. Vitamins A, D, E, and K dissolve in organic solvents, such as ether and benzene, and are referred to as **fat-soluble vitamins.** The B-vitamins and vitamin C, in contrast, dissolve in water and are the **water-soluble vitamins.**

Vitamins are generally indispensable in human diets because they can't be synthesized in sufficient quantities to meet individual need, or synthesis is curtailed by environmental factors, or they can't be synthesized at all. Vitamins such as niacin and vitamin D can be synthesized by the body under certain conditions, and vitamin K and biotin are synthesized to some extent by bacteria in the intestinal tract.[8,10]

To be classified as a vitamin, the compound must be organic and must meet the criteria to be an essential nutrient: (1) the body is unable to synthesize enough of the compound to maintain health; and (2) absence of the compound from the diet for a defined period of time produces deficiency symptoms that, if caught in time, are quickly cured when the substance is resupplied. A substance does not qualify as a vitamin merely because the body can't make it. Evidence must suggest that health declines when the substance is not consumed.[8,9,10]

In addition to their use in correcting deficiency diseases, a few vitamins have also proved useful as pharmacological agents in treating a limited number of nondeficiency diseases. These medical applications often require the administration of **megadoses,** well above the typical human needs for the vitamin. For example, as noted in Chapter 6, megadoses of a form of niacin can be used as part of blood cholesterol-lowering treatment for appropriately selected individuals. Another example is the use of vitamin D **analogs** for psoriasis. Nevertheless, at this time any claimed benefits for the use of vitamin supplements, especially intakes in excess of the Upper Level (if set) should be viewed critically because many unproved claims are continually being made.[8,9,10]

Both plant and animal foods supply vitamins in the human diet. Whether isolated from foods or synthesized in the laboratory, vitamins are the same chemical compounds and generally work equally well in the body. Contrary to claims in the health-food literature, "natural" vitamins isolated from foods are for the most part no more healthful than those synthesized in a laboratory, but there are exceptions. Vitamin E is about twice as potent in its natural form compared to its synthetic form.[9] On the other hand, folic acid, the synthetic form of the vitamin added to grain products, is 1.7 times more potent than the natural form, folate.[1] Some vitamins exist in several related forms that differ in chemical or physical properties. These forms exist both in nature and in synthesized vitamin supplements. It is important to have enough of the specific vitamin forms that the body can use; the various forms will be identified throughout this chapter and Chapter 10.

Historical Perspective on the Vitamins

Long before any vitamins had been identified, certain foods were known to cure illnesses brought on by what we now recognize to be vitamin deficiencies. The ancient Egyptians, for example, treated night blindness with topical applications of juice extracted from liver, a rich source of vitamin A. As you'll see, vitamin A plays a critical role in vision.[10] During the fifteenth and sixteenth centuries, British sailing ships did not carry sufficient amounts of fresh fruits and vegetables with them for long sea voyages. This resulted in a tremendous loss of life. In one expedition, 1000 men set out from England for the Pacific, but only 145 returned. The rest had died from the disease known as scurvy. Scientists eventually discovered that citrus fruits cured scurvy; after lemons and limes were included as a routine part of British sailors' rations, cases of scurvy declined greatly. We now know that this disease, marked by weakness, blood vessel rupture, and poor immune function, results from a deficiency of vitamin C.[9]

As scientists began to identify various vitamins, related deficiencies, such as scurvy, were dramatically cured. For the most part, as the vitamins were discovered, they were named alphabetically: A, B, C, D, and E. Later, some substances originally classified as vitamins were found not to be essential for humans and were dropped from the list, such as vitamin P. Other vitamins thought at first to have a single chemical form turned out to exist in many forms, so "vitamin B" now comprises eight separate entities.

It took some time to uncover the true nature of the various vitamins. For example, when scientists realized that both protein foods and nicotinic acid (a form of the vitamin niacin) can cure pellagra, they eventually went on to discover that the amino acid tryptophan can be synthesized into niacin. Finally, as mentioned, it was determined that some vitamins (such as biotin and vitamins D and K) can be synthesized by the body or bacteria present in the intestinal tract.[8,10]

We can be relatively confident that all vitamins needed by humans have been discovered. The ability of total parenteral nutrition (TPN) to support human life for years

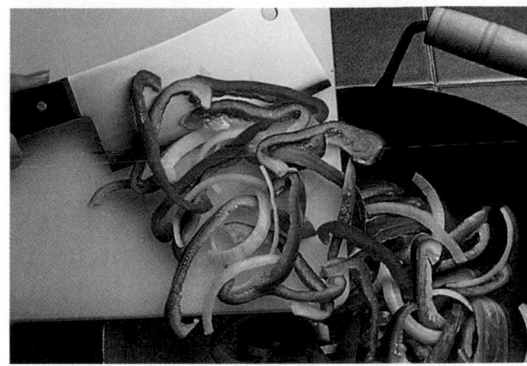

Vegetables are rich sources of many vitamins.

megadose Intake of a nutrient beyond estimates of needs to prevent a deficiency, or what would be found in a balanced diet; 2 to 10 times human needs is a starting point for such a dosage.

analog A chemical compound that differs slightly from another naturally occurring compound. Analogs generally contain extra or altered chemical groups and may have similar or opposite metabolic effects compared with the native compound; also spelled analogue.

E vidence suggests that health declines when choline, a substance the body makes, is not included in a diet during some life stages, such as growth spurts. Thus, choline has an Adequate Intake (AI) set for it and may one day be added to the list of known vitamins. Choline is discussed in more detail in Chapter 10.

strongly supports this view. With TPN, the patient receives intravenously a carefully formulated preparation containing all necessary nutrients. The gastrointestinal tract is completely bypassed, because no food or beverages are consumed. People who receive protein, carbohydrate, fat, and all known vitamins and essential minerals in this manner may continue not only to live but also to build body tissue, have a baby, heal wounds, and combat existing diseases.

Storage of Vitamins in the Body

Except for vitamin K, the fat-soluble vitamins are not readily excreted from the body.[8,9,10] In contrast, most water-soluble vitamins are generally lost from the body quite rapidly, partly because the water in cells dissolves these vitamins and flushes them out of the body via the kidneys. Two exceptions are vitamin B-12 and vitamin B-6, which are stored much more readily than the other water-soluble vitamins. Because of the limited storage of many vitamins, they should be consumed in the diet daily, although an occasional lapse in the intake of even water-soluble vitamins generally causes no harm. An average person, for example, must consume no vitamin C for 20 to 40 days before developing the first signs and symptoms of a related deficiency.[9] The signs and symptoms of a vitamin deficiency occur only when that vitamin is lacking in the diet and body stores are essentially exhausted.

Vitamin Toxicity

Although a toxic effect from an excessive intake of any vitamin is theoretically possible, toxicity of the fat-soluble vitamin A is the most likely to occur.[10] Vitamin D can also cause toxic effects, especially in infants.[8] These vitamins are unlikely to cause toxic effects unless taken in supplement (pill) form. However, vitamin A can cause toxicity with long-term intake beginning at just 2 to 4 times human needs, especially in older adults and pregnant women.[10]

Because daily use of a balanced multivitamin and mineral supplement usually supplies less than 2 times the Daily Values of the components, this practice is unlikely to cause toxic effects in adults. But consuming many vitamin pills can cause problems. See the Nutrition Focus at the end of this chapter to explore whether you should take a multivitamin and mineral supplement and, if so, how to do it safely.

Malabsorption of Vitamins

Vitamins consumed in foods must be absorbed efficiently from the intestine to meet body needs. If absorption of a vitamin is defective, a person must consume larger amounts of it to avoid deficiency symptoms. As discussed in the following section, fat malabsorption resulting from various GI tract and pancreatic diseases is associated with poor absorption of the fat-soluble vitamins.[8,9,10] Alcohol abuse and certain intestinal diseases also can lead to malabsorption of some B-vitamins (e.g., thiamin and folate), as covered in detail in Chapter 10.

> ### Concept | Check
>
> In general, the fat-soluble vitamins—A, D, E, and K—are less readily excreted than are the water-soluble B vitamins and vitamin C. Regular consumption of foods rich in both water-soluble and fat-soluble vitamins is important for health. However, the occasional inadequate consumption of any one vitamin is of little health concern, because even water-soluble vitamins persist in the body to some extent. For example, when a person ingests a vitamin-free diet, the first deficiency signs (due to lack of thiamin) will not appear for about 10 days. When taken in supplement form, the fat-soluble vitamin A poses the greatest risk of toxicity. For the most part, there is little risk of toxicity when vitamins are obtained from foods.

Critical | Thinking

Many vitamin supplements supply nutrients in amounts that exceed the Daily Values listed on the label. Miguel believes that "more is better." How can you explain to him that the supplement he is about to start taking is "worse," because it contains amounts that exceed the Daily Values by 10 times for many nutrients, including vitamin A?

The Fat-Soluble Vitamins

The discussion of the individual fat-soluble vitamins—A, D, E, and K—begins by look-ing at how they are absorbed.

Absorption of the Fat-Soluble Vitamins

You can see from the chemical structures at the beginning of each vitamin section that these vitamins are lipidlike molecules. Because these vitamins are absorbed along with dietary fat, adequate absorption of the fat-soluble vitamins depends on efficient fat ab-sorption. This, in turn, depends on fat digestion, the utilization of bile salts and pan-creatic lipase in the small intestine, and adequate absorptive capacity from a healthy intestinal wall (Figure 9-1). Under these conditions, about 40 to 90% of the fat-soluble

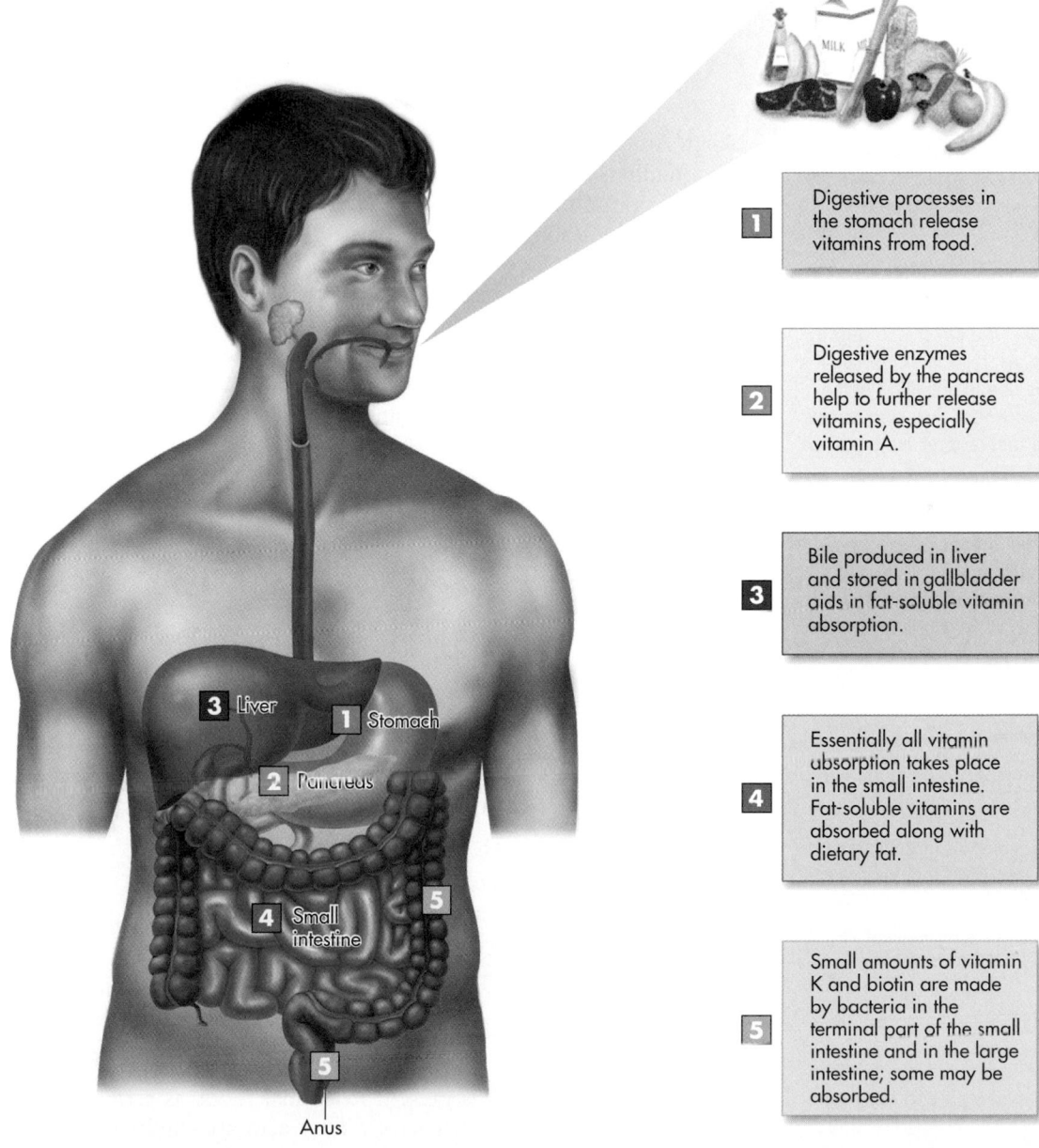

1 Digestive processes in the stomach release vitamins from food.

2 Digestive enzymes released by the pancreas help to further release vitamins, especially vitamin A.

3 Bile produced in liver and stored in gallbladder aids in fat-soluble vitamin absorption.

4 Essentially all vitamin absorption takes place in the small intestine. Fat-soluble vitamins are absorbed along with dietary fat.

5 Small amounts of vitamin K and biotin are made by bacteria in the terminal part of the small intestine and in the large intestine; some may be absorbed.

Figure 9-1 | An overview of the digestion and absorption of vitamins. Key participants in the process include bile, pancreatic enzymes, intestinal enzymes, and a healthy small intestine absorptive surface. Adequate fat digestion and absorption are critical for the ultimate absorption of fat-soluble vitamins. Carotenoids are absorbed mainly in the small intestine in conjunction with dietary fat.

eople with **cystic fibrosis, celiac disease, Crohn's disease,** or any other disease that hampers fat absorption absorb fat-soluble vitamins poorly. Some medications, such as the weight-loss drug orlistat (Xenical) discussed in Chapter 13, also interfere with fat absorption. Unabsorbed fat carries these vitamins to the large intestine, where they are incorporated into the feces and excreted. People with such conditions are especially susceptible to vitamin E and vitamin K deficiencies. A multivitamin and mineral supplement, taken under a physician's guidance, is part of the treatment for preventing the nutrient deficiencies associated with fat malabsorption. Extra vitamin E may be recommended for people with cystic fibrosis.

cystic fibrosis A disease that often leads to overproduction of mucus. Mucus can block the pancreatic duct, in turn decreasing enzyme output.

celiac disease An immunological or allergic reaction to the protein gluten in certain grains, such as wheat and rye. The effect is to destroy the intestinal enterocytes, resulting in a much reduced surface area due to flattening of the villi. The elimination of wheat, rye, and certain other grains from the diet restores the intestinal surface.

Crohn's disease An inflammatory disease of the gastrointestinal tract, but generally more pronounced in the terminal ileum. A family history is a major risk factor. The disease limits the absorptive capacity of the small intestine.

retinoids Collective term for the biologically active forms of vitamin A including retinol, retinal, and retinoic acid.

provitamin Substance that can be made into a vitamin.

carotenoids Pigment materials in fruits and vegetables that range in color from yellow to orange to red.

ee Appendix A to review *cis* and *trans* isomers.

he retinyl ester retinyl palmitate is a common form of vitamin A added to foods.

vitamins consumed are absorbed when they are taken in typical amounts. Absorption efficiency generally falls when intakes greatly exceed human needs.[8,9,10]

Distribution of the Fat-Soluble Vitamins

Once absorbed, fat-soluble vitamins are packaged and delivered to target cells throughout the body in a manner similar to that used for dietary fats—namely, by way of chylomicrons and other blood lipoproteins.[8,9,10] This process is needed because the vitamins are not water-soluble. Recall also from Chapter 6 that, as a chylomicron circulates in the bloodstream, much of its triglyceride content is removed by body cells. What remains—the remnant—is taken up by the liver. This remnant contains the fat-soluble vitamins absorbed from the diet. The liver can then "repackage" fat-soluble vitamins with new blood proteins for transport in the blood, or they can be stored in the liver for future use.

❙ Vitamin A

North Americans have little risk of developing a severe deficiency of vitamin A because this vitamin is abundant in our food supply.[10] But vitamin A deficiency constitutes one of the major public health problems in developing countries. Worldwide, vitamin A deficiency is the leading cause of nonaccidental blindness. Children from impoverished nations in Africa, Asia, and South America are especially susceptible because their inadequate intake and diminished stores of vitamin A fail to meet the increased needs associated with rapid growth. In the world's most destitute nations, hundreds of thousands of children become blind each year because they lack vitamin A.

Vitamin A refers to the preformed **retinoids,** plus the **provitamin A carotenoids** that can form retinoids.[10] Vitamin A is a ring structure with a fatty acid tail. As preformed vitamin A, it exists in three forms: retinol (an alcohol), retinal (an aldehyde), and retinoic acid. The tail terminates in one of these three chemical groups.

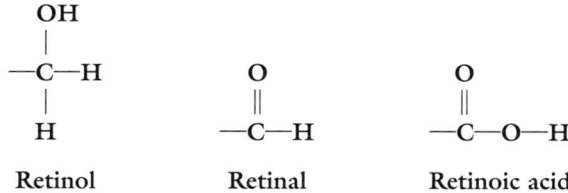

To some extent these forms can be interconverted (Figure 9-2).

The tail of the vitamin A molecule can vary from *cis* to *trans* configuration. This orientation influences the function of the specific retinoid (see the section titled Functions of Vitamin A).

Cis   *Trans*

Preformed vitamin A is present in animal foods as retinol, the alcohol form, and retinyl ester-compounds that have a fatty acid attached to retinol. The retinyl esters don't exhibit vitamin A activity but are broken down to retinol and the attached fatty acid in the intestinal tract.[10]

Provitamin A carotenoids also can be enzymatically split to form retinal within the intestinal cells or liver cells.[9] Some is also made into retinoic acid. The provitamin A

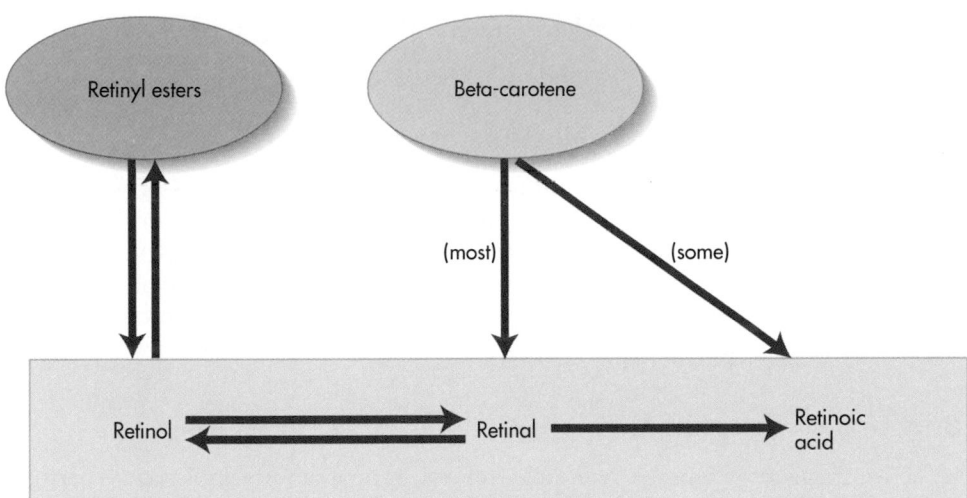

Figure 9-2 | Interconversions of beta-carotene and the various retinoids. Notice that synthesis of retinoic acid is a "dead end" in metabolic terms.

carotenoids are alpha-carotene, beta-carotene, and beta-cryptoxanthin. (The yellow-orange pigment in fruits and vegetables is due to provitamin A beta-carotene.) Other carotenoids in nature, such as lycopene, do not have vitamin A activity in humans.[9]

Absorption, Transport, Storage, and Excretion of Vitamin A

In the small intestine, retinyl esters are broken down, leaving free retinol. This process requires bile to make the retinyl esters soluble and also to activate the enzymes used, such as pancreatic lipase.

Up to 90% of retinol is absorbed into the cells of the small intestine. After absorption, a fatty acid is then attached to retinol to form a new retinyl ester. These retinyl esters are packaged into chylomicrons, along with other lipids, before entering the lymph. The chylomicrons deliver vitamin A to tissues for storage or to be used. Over 90% of the body's vitamin A storage can be found in the liver, but retinoids also are found in adipose tissue cells, kidneys, bone marrow, testicles, and eyes. Normally, the liver stores enough vitamin A to last for several months, so some time will pass before the signs and symptoms of vitamin A deficiency arise.[10]

Carotenoids are absorbed intact; this causes their absorption rate to be much lower than that of retinol. After being absorbed in the small intestine, carotenoids can be cleaved to yield retinal, which is then formed into retinol. This retinol can then have a fatty acid attached to it to become a retinyl ester and enter the lymph as part of a chylomicron. Carotenoids also can enter the bloodstream directly; however, the mechanisms that allow this to happen aren't well understood.[9]

When vitamin A as a retinoid is released from the liver into general circulation, it is bound to a protein called retinol-binding protein, produced mainly by the liver. In the bloodstream, retinol-binding protein is then bound to another protein called transthyretin (commonly known as prealbumin).[10] In contrast, when carotenoids are released from the liver, they are carried by the lipoprotein VLDL.[9]

Vitamin A is not readily excreted by the body; only some is lost in the urine. Kidney disease and aging in general increases the risk of vitamin A toxicity as this urinary route of excretion is compromised.[10]

Cellular Retinoid-Binding Proteins

Retinoids are bound to specific retinoid-binding proteins within cells that take up retinoids. There is a family of cellular retinoid-binding proteins; these hold retinoids and direct them to functional sites within the cell. Nearly all cells contain one or more

During protein-energy malnutrition, synthesis of retinol-binding protein and transthyretin (prealbumin) is reduced by the lack of sufficient availability of amino acids and energy. These proteins are used as clinical indicators of protein synthesis in a person because decreased concentrations in the blood suggest inadequate protein and energy intake.

Use of some synthetic retinoids has been shown to lead to a remission in various forms of cancer. The mechanism is probably through the fundamental role of retinoids in cell differentiation.

RXR, RAR The abbreviations for retinoid X receptor and retinoic acid receptor. These two subfamilies of retinoid receptors in the nucleus interact with retinoic acid and bind with specific sites on DNA, allowing for gene expression.

gene expression The activation of a specific site on DNA, which results in either the activation or the inhibition of the gene.

cell differentiation The process of transforming an unspecialized cell into a specialized cell.

of these binding proteins.[10] Besides transport, these binding proteins also protect retinoids from breakdown.

Retinoid Receptors in the Nucleus

One way the retinoids influence health is to bind to two main families of retinoid receptors in the cell nucleus (called **RAR** and **RXR**). Once these receptors within the cell nucleus bind forms of retinoic acid, the complex then binds to DNA. This binding regulates the formation of mRNA and the subsequent production of body proteins (and body processes) known as **gene expression.** This gene expression can go on to direct **cell differentiation** (Figure 9-3).[10]

Functions of Vitamin A

The active forms of vitamin A retinoids—retinol, retinal, and retinoic acid—perform three basic functions. These biochemical or physiologic actions are vision, the growth and development of many types of tissues, and immunity.[10]

Vision

Vitamin A (as retinal) is needed in the retina of the eye to turn visual light into nerve signals to the brain (Figure 9-4). In addition, vitamin A (as retinoic acid) is needed to maintain normal differentiation of the cells that make up the various structural components of the eye, such as the cornea and rod cells.[10]

The sensory elements of the retina consist of specialized cells known as rods and cones. Rods are responsible for the visual processes that occur in dim light, translating

Figure 9-3 | The mechanism of the action of vitamin A (as retinoic acid) on the target cell. (1) Vitamin A is carried by retinol-binding protein and transthyretin in the blood. (2) Upon release vitamin A enters the target cell, and (3) binds to cellular retinoid-binding protein. (4) Once released from this protein, vitamin A then enters the nucleus and binds to its nuclear-retinoid receptors (RAR and RXR). (5) This complex then binds to DNA, activating gene transcription. (6) The resulting messenger RNA (mRNA) has the code for the protein that (7) ultimately produces the cellular responses (see Chapter 7 for details on protein synthesis using mRNA). Nearly all cells have at least one member of the RAR and RXR families of vitamin A–binding proteins. It is interesting that vitamin D in its active hormone form acts in a similar way. However, the retinoic acid receptor (RAR) portion is replaced by the vitamin D receptor (VDR).

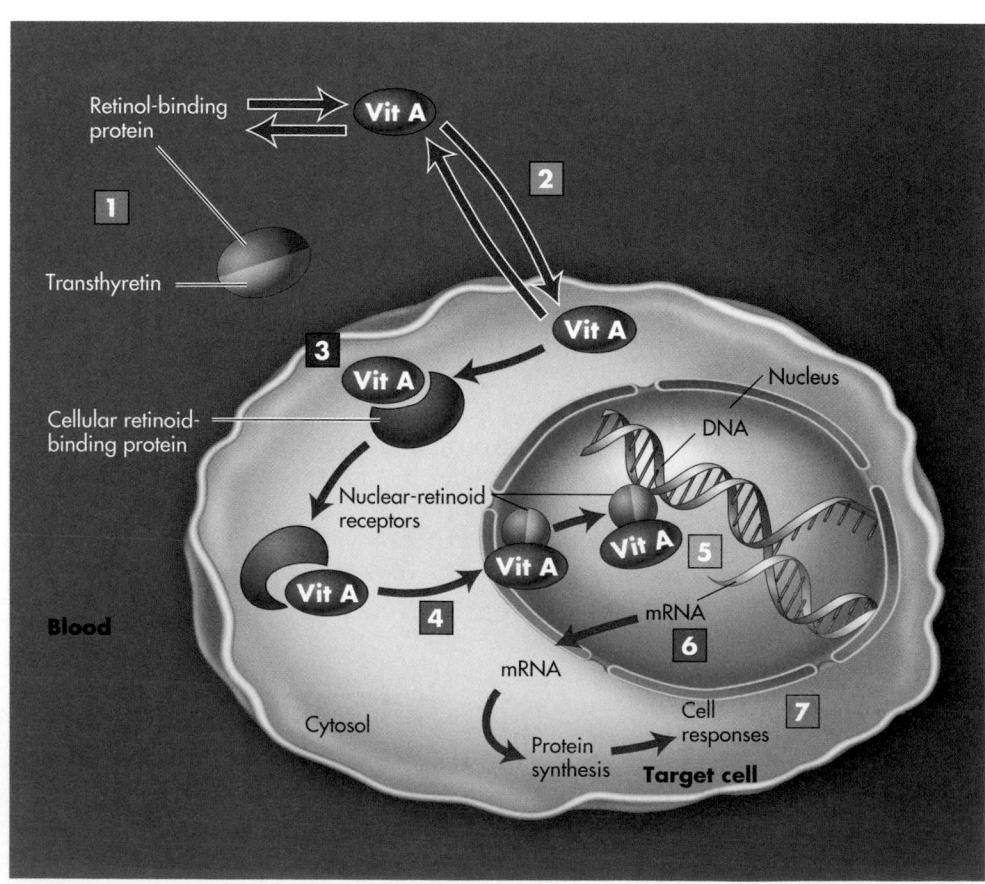

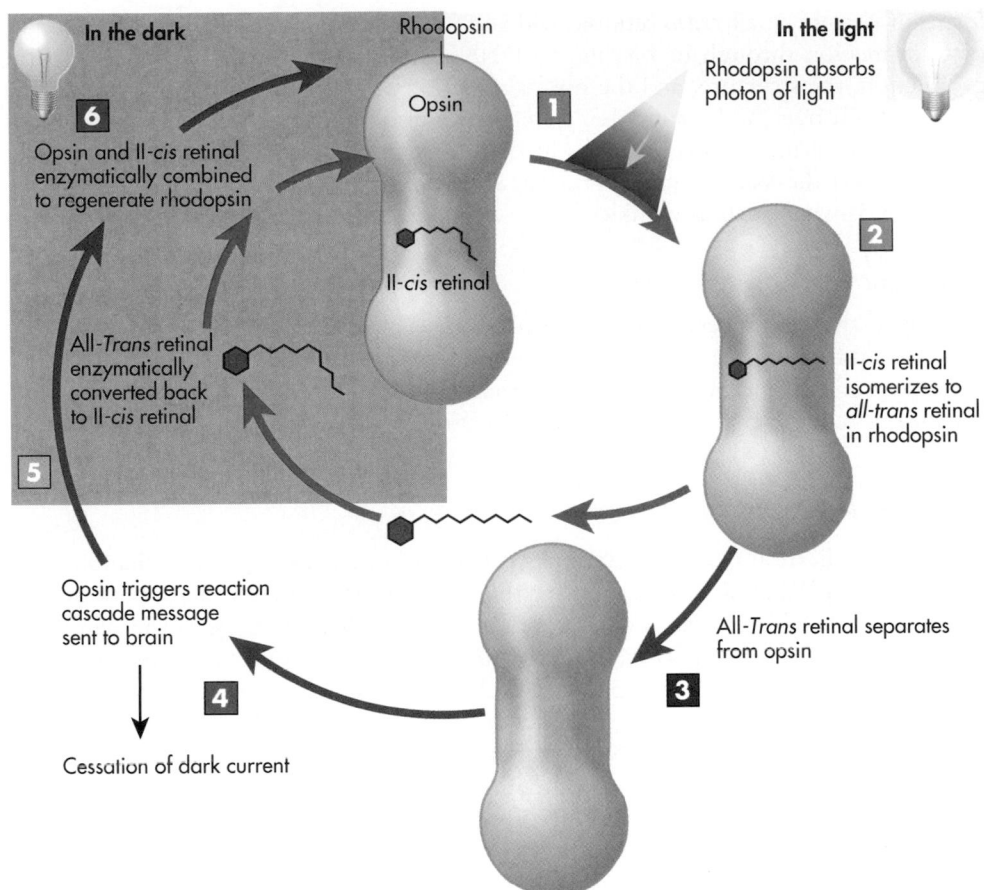

Figure 9-4 | The bleaching and regeneration of rhodopsin (1–6). The yellow background indicates the bleaching events that occur in the light; the gray background indicates the regenerative events that can occur in either light or dark conditions. Note that 11-*cis* retinal has a kink in the molecule, but all-*trans* retinal is a straight chain. As shown in Chapter 6, this change in configuration is typical when lipidlike molecules convert from *cis* to *trans* shapes.

objects into black-and-white images and detecting motion. Cones are responsible for the visual processes occurring under bright light, translating objects into color images.

In the rods, 11-*cis*-retinal binds to a protein called opsin to form the visual pigment **rhodopsin.** The absorption of a **photon** of light catalyzes a change in the shape of 11-*cis*-retinal to all-*trans* retinal, causing opsin to separate from all-*trans* retinal.[10] This isomerization event leads to a cascade of biochemical events, which trigger a change in ion permeability of the photoreceptor cells. This, in turn, initiates a signal to the nerve cells that communicate with the brain's visual center. Actually, thousands of rod cells containing millions of molecules of rhodopsin are triggered simultaneously.

In order to keep the visual processes functioning, the 11-*cis*-retinal in the rod cells must be regenerated in the pigment-containing cells in the eye. All-*trans* retinal is eventually converted back to 11-*cis*-retinal. This slow process can take several minutes. The 11-*cis*-retinal then moves back to the photoreceptor site, where it recombines with opsin and is ready for another cycle.

The release of 11-*cis*-retinal from opsin is a **bleaching process.** During exposure to bright light, the rods' rhodopsin is completely activated and cannot respond to more light until it returns to its resting state. Enzymes regenerate the initial form of rhodopsin so that it can respond to light again. When there is a limited amount of rhodopsin in the rod cells, it is difficult to adapt to seeing in dim light (night blindness).

Not all retinal is reused, so there is a pool of retinyl esters in the eye to keep a supply of vitamin A on hand. Should the pool of vitamin A be low, the process of **dark adaptation** is slowed down, and a condition known as **night blindness** develops.[10]

Growth and Differentiation of Cells

Various cells in the retina, cornea, and **epithelium** of the eye depend on retinoic acid for maintaining structural integrity. Vitamin A is delivered to these cells by tears. Vitamin A then acts in its role in gene expression and ultimate cell differentiation. Two

rhodopsin A photoreceptor in rod cells composed of 11-*cis*-retinal and opsin.

photon A unit of light intensity at the retina having the brightness of one candle.

bleaching process The process by which light depletes the rhodopsin concentration in the eye. This fall in rhodopsin concentration allows the eye to become adapted to bright light.

dark adaptation The process by which the rhodopsin concentration in the eye increases in dark conditions, allowing improved vision in the dark.

night blindness A vitamin A deficiency condition in which the retina in the eye cannot adjust to low amounts of light.

epithelium The covering of internal and external surfaces of the body, including the lining of vessels and other small cavities. It consists of epithelial cells joined by a small amount of cementing material.

Most forms of cancer arise from cells that are influenced by vitamin A. Coupled with its ability to aid immune system activity, vitamin A may be a valuable tool in the fight against cancer. This is especially true for skin, lung, bladder, and breast cancers. Still, because of the potential for toxicity, unsupervised use of megadose vitamin A supplements to reduce cancer risk is not advised.

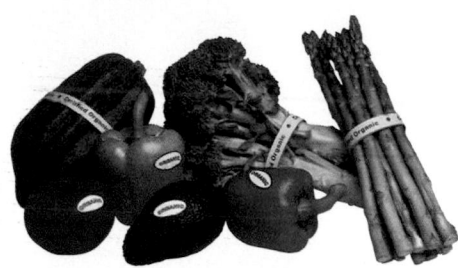

Many vegetables, such as asparagus and broccoli, are rich in provitamin A carotenoids.

forms of vitamin A, all-*trans* retinoic acid and 9-*cis*-retinoic acid, regulate finely tuned gene expression through its binding to DNA. Retinoic acid is also necessary for the production, the structure, and the normal function of epithelial cells in the lungs, trachea, skin, GI tract, and many other systems. It is also important for the formation and maintenance of mucus-forming cells in these organs.[10] Because of its effect on cells that make up the skin, forms of retinoic acid (e.g., tretinoin [Retin-A]) are used to treat skin damage, such as wrinkles. It has a modest effect.

Immunity

As early as the 1920s, researchers recognized that vitamin A (mostly as retinoic acid) is important for immune system functions, and a vitamin A deficiency is associated with decreased resistance to infections.[10] The severity of some infections, such as measles and diarrhea, is reduced by vitamin A supplementation in people who show a deficiency.

Vitamin A Analogs for Acne

The acne medication tretinoin (Retin-A) is made of one analog form of vitamin A. It is used as a topical treatment (applied to the skin) for acne. It appears to work by irritating the skin, which leads to open pores and a generalized peeling of the skin layer. It also can block the deleterious effects that skin bacteria have on acne lesions. Another derivative of vitamin A, 13-*cis* retinoic acid (Accutane), is an oral drug used to treat serious acne. It acts in part to regulate development of cells in the skin (the gene expression role discussed earlier). Note that taking high doses of vitamin A itself would not be safe.[10] Even Accutane, a less potentially toxic form, can induce toxic symptoms as well as birth defects in the offspring of women using it during pregnancy. A pregnancy test is required before Accutane is prescribed to women.

Possible Carotenoid Functions

Carotenoids may play a role in preventing cardiovascular disease in persons at high risk, possibly linked to carotenoids' antioxidant capability.[17] Until definitive studies are complete, many scientists recommend that we consume a total of at least 5 servings of a combination of fruits and vegetables per day as part of an overall effort to reduce the risk of cardiovascular disease.

Carotenoids by themselves also may help prevent cancer, acting again as antioxidants. Population studies show that regular consumption of foods rich in carotenoids decreases the risk of lung and oral cancers. The dietary carotenoid lycopene (the red pigment found in tomatoes, watermelon, and several other fruits) protects against cancer of the **prostate gland.** The proposed biological role of lycopene again may be that of an antioxidant. Because of this link to prostate cancer, some food companies (e.g., Campbell Soup Company) are even marketing their products as important sources of lycopene. The carotenoid lycopene also may decrease skin cancer risk.

In contrast to the potential benefits from carotenoids in foods, recall from Chapter 1 that recent studies from the United States and Finland failed to show a reduction in lung cancer in male smokers and nonsmokers who were given supplements of the carotenoid beta-carotene for 5 or more years. In fact, beta-carotene use in male smokers increased the number of lung cancer cases compared with the control groups. No comparable studies have been done with women. Although further research continues, most researchers are now convinced that beta-carotene supplementation offers no protection against cancer. Thus overwhelming advice is to rely on food sources of this or any other carotenoids.

Age-related **macular degeneration** (Figure 9-5) is a leading cause of legal blindness among North American adults over the age of 65. The disease is associated with changes in the macular area of the eye, which provides the most detailed vision. Age, smoking, and genetics are risk factors. The macula contains the carotenoids lutein and

prostate gland A solid, chestnut-shaped organ surrounding the first part of the urinary tract in the male. The prostate gland secretes substances into the semen.

macular degeneration A painless condition leading to disruption of the central part of the retina (in the eye) and, in turn, blurred vision.

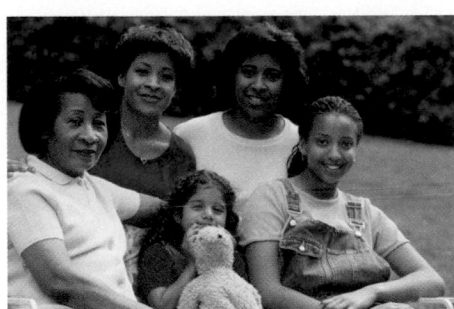

Normal vision

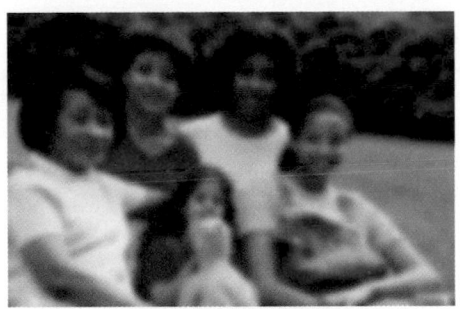

The same scene as viewed by a person with macular degeneration

Figure 9-5 | Further research is needed to better understand the relationship between macular degeneration and carotenoids. While supplementing one's diet with specific carotenoids has not yet been shown to reduce the risk of macular degeneration, research has shown that smokers are at three times greater risk than nonsmokers to develop this disease.

zeaxanthin in high enough concentrations to impart a yellow color. In some studies, the higher the total number of carotenoids (beta-carotene, lutein, and zeaxanthin) consumed in the diet, the lower was the risk for age-related macular degeneration. These carotenoids may also decrease the risk of cataracts in the eyes.[18] Although these hypotheses are interesting, the risk for these eye disorders may be reduced by a general consumption of fruits and vegetables high in carotenoids rather than the intake of these specific carotenoids. Note that multivitamin and mineral supplements formulated for older adults (e.g., Centrum Silver) are being marketed as a source of lutein.

Vitamin A in Foods

Retinoids (preformed vitamin A) are found in liver, fish, fish oils, fortified milk, and eggs. Margarine is fortified with vitamin A, as are fat-free, low-fat, and fat-reduced milks. Provitamin A carotenoids are mainly found in dark green and yellow-orange vegetables and some fruits. Carrots, spinach and other greens, winter squash, sweet potatoes, broccoli, romaine lettuce, mangoes, cantaloupe, peaches, and apricots are examples of such sources. About 70% of the vitamin A in the typical North American diet comes from animal (preformed vitamin A) sources, whereas provitamin A predominates in the diet among poor people in other parts of the world.

Beta-carotene accounts for some of the orange color of carrots. In vegetables such as broccoli, this yellow-orange color is masked by the dark-green pigment chlorophyll. Still, green vegetables contain provitamin A. Consuming a varied diet rich in green vegetables and carrots will provide enough vitamin A to meet needs.

Retinol Activity Equivalent (RAE)

At one time, the amounts of most nutrients in foods were expressed in **international units (IUs),** a crude measure of vitamin activity. Today we can directly measure very small quantities of nutrients more precisely; consequently, milligrams (1/1000 of a gram) and micrograms (1/1,000,000 of a gram) have generally replaced international units as customary units of measure, although vitamin supplements may still display the older IU values.

For vitamin A, the current unit of measurement is the retinol activity equivalent (RAE), which is basically 1 μg of retinol. In this system, 12 μg of beta-carotene yield 1 μg of vitamin A activity, and 24 μg of the other two provitamin A carotenoids (alpha-carotene and beta-cryptoxanthin) yield 1 μg of vitamin A activity.[10]

The total RAE value for a food is calculated by adding the actual weight of retinol and the adjusted equivalent weights of provitamin A carotenoids present in the food. For example, a diet that contains 500 μg retinol, 1800 μg beta-carotene and 2,400 μg alpha-carotene supplies 750 μg RAE (500 + (1800 ÷ 12) + (2400 ÷ 24) = 750 μg RAE).

Calculating Retinol Activity Equivalents

Table 9-1 is a tool for converting amounts of vitamin A and carotenes expressed in one unit of measure into another unit of measure.

Food Sources of Vitamin A

Food Item and Amount	Vitamin A (μg RAE)*
Cooked beef liver, 1 oz	3042
Sweet potato, 1/2 cup	958
Spinach, 2/3 cup	494
Mango, 1	402
Baby carrots, 5	375
Acorn squash, 2/3 cup	244
Cooked kale, 1/2 cup	206
Fat-free milk, 1 cup	150
Broccoli, 1 cup	138
Apricot, 3	137
Cheddar cheese, 1 oz	78
Romaine lettuce, 1 cup	72
Margarine, 1 pat	50
Scallions, 1 tbsp	32
Peach, 1	26

RDA for adult men, 900 μg RAE; adult women, 700 μg RAE

*Retinol activity equivalents

international unit (IU) A crude measure of vitamin activity, often based on the growth rate of animals. Today these units often have been replaced by precise measurements of actual quantities in milligrams or micrograms.

Table 9-1 | Conversion Values for Retinol Activity Equivalents

1 retinol activity equivalent (RAE)	1 IU vitamin A activity
= 1 µg of all-*trans*-retinol	= 0.3 µg of all-*trans*-retinol
= 12 µg of dietary all-*trans*-beta-carotene	= 3.6 µg of dietary all-*trans*-beta-carotene
= 24 µg of other dietary provitamin A carotenoids	= 7.2 µg of other dietary provitamin A carotenoids

The retinal equivalent (RE) is an older unit for vitamin A. This RE assumed that there was a greater contribution to vitamin A needs from carotenoids than we assume today. Food composition tables and nutrient databases may contain this older RE standard. It will take some time to update these resources.

To compare the older RE (or IU) standards to current RAE recommendations, assume that for any preformed vitamin A in a food or added to food, 1 RE (or 3.3 IU) = 1 RAE. There is no easy way to convert RE or IU units to RAE units for foods that naturally contain provitamin A carotenoids, such as carrots, spinach, and apricots. A general rule of thumb is to divide the older values for foods containing carotenoids by 2, and then do the conversion from RE or IU to RAE as shown in Table 9-1. There is also no easy way to do this calculation for food containing a mixture of preformed vitamin A and carotenoids. We will just have to wait for all the food tables to be updated. Generally speaking, any values listed for such foods provide less vitamin A than the RE or IU values suggest.

Measuring vitamin A in the blood is one way to assess a person's status. This measure is insensitive, however, because concentrations do not fall until vitamin A stores in the liver are very low.

Vitamin A Needs

The RDA for vitamin A is 900 µg Retinol Activity Equivalents (RAE) per day for adult men and 700 µg RAE per day for adult women. At this intake, adequate body stores of vitamin A are maintained, which is the basis for setting the RDA.[10] Average intakes for adult men and women in North America meet the RDA. Most adults have liver reserves of vitamin A that are three to five times greater than needed to provide good health. At present, there is no separate RDA for beta-carotene or any of the other provitamin A carotenoids.[9]

Vitamin A-Deficiency Diseases

Deficient vitamin A status may be seen in preschool children who do not eat enough vegetables. The urban poor, older adults, and people with alcoholism or liver disease (which limits vitamin A storage) can also show diminished vitamin A status, especially with respect to stores. Finally, children and adults with severe fat-malabsorption syndromes, such as celiac disease, chronic diarrhea, pancreatic insufficiency, Crohn's disease, cystic fibrosis, HIV, and AIDS, may also experience vitamin A deficiency. Such a deficiency can have widespread effects on the body.[10]

When the retinol in the blood is insufficient to replace the retinal lost during the visual cycle, the rod cells in the eye recover from flashes of light more slowly. The resulting night blindness is a common early symptom of vitamin A deficiency, as discussed earlier. As well, without enough retinoic acid, mucus-forming cells deteriorate and are no longer able to synthesize mucus, the essential lubricant used throughout the body. The eye, especially the cornea, is adversely affected by the loss of mucus, which keeps the eye surface moist and washes away dirt and other particles that settle on the eye. Deterioration of the eye results from bacterial invasion because retinoic acid plays an important role in resistance to infection. Conjunctival xerosis (abnormal dryness of the **conjunctiva** of the eye) and Bitot's spots (drying out of the eye and appearance of hardened epithelial cells) appears as vitamin A deficiency worsens. The corneal ulceration and keratomalacia (softening of the cornea) result in scarring (Figure 9-6). The ultimate

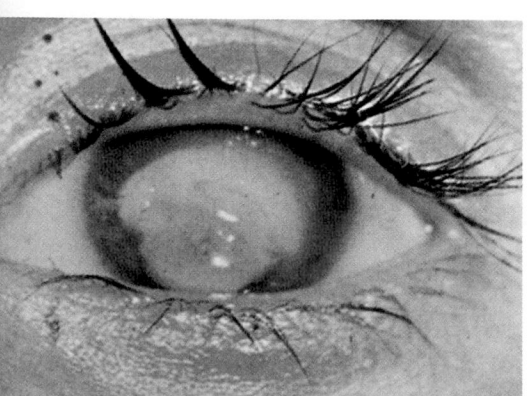

Figure 9-6 | Vitamin A deficiency can eventually lead to blindness. Note the severe effects on this eye. This problem is commonly seen today in Southeast Asia. In contrast, the leading causes of blindness in North America are accidents in children and diabetes in adults.

scarring may be barely detectable, or it could lead to loss of sight. This sequence of changes in the eye—collectively known as **xerophthalmia**—causes irreversible blindness in millions of people worldwide.

Vitamin A deficiency also produces skin changes referred to as **follicular hyperkeratosis.** Keratin, the normal component of the outer layers of skin, protects the inner layers and reduces water loss through the skin. During severe vitamin A deficiency, keratinized cells, which are normally present only in the outer layers, replace the normal epithelial cells in the underlying skin layers. Hair follicles become plugged with keratin, giving a bumpy appearance and rough texture to the skin, and the skin becomes very dry.

In areas of the world where vitamin A deficiency exists, poor growth follows. If liver vitamin A stores are established after an infant is weaned, they can supply retinol for several months or even longer. Vitamin A deficiency in children occurs most often during the postweaning period. Giving supplements of 15,000 to 60,000 μg to young children at risk may protect them for up to 6 months. Finding a suitable food to improve intake is a must for a long-term solution to vitamin A deficiency. Also, insufficient fat in the diet of these children inhibits the absorption of what little vitamin A there is in the diet.

Upper Level for Vitamin A

Signs and symptoms of toxicity from excessive vitamin A—called **hypervitaminosis A**—can appear with long-term supplement use at 2 to 4 times the RDA for preformed vitamin A, especially in pregnant women and older adults in general (Figure 9-7).[10,20] Correspondingly, the Upper Level is set at 3000 μg/day of retinol, about 4 times what the typical adult needs.[10] (This amount is based on the presence of birth defects occurring during pregnancy and liver toxicity in general with chronic intakes above this amount.)

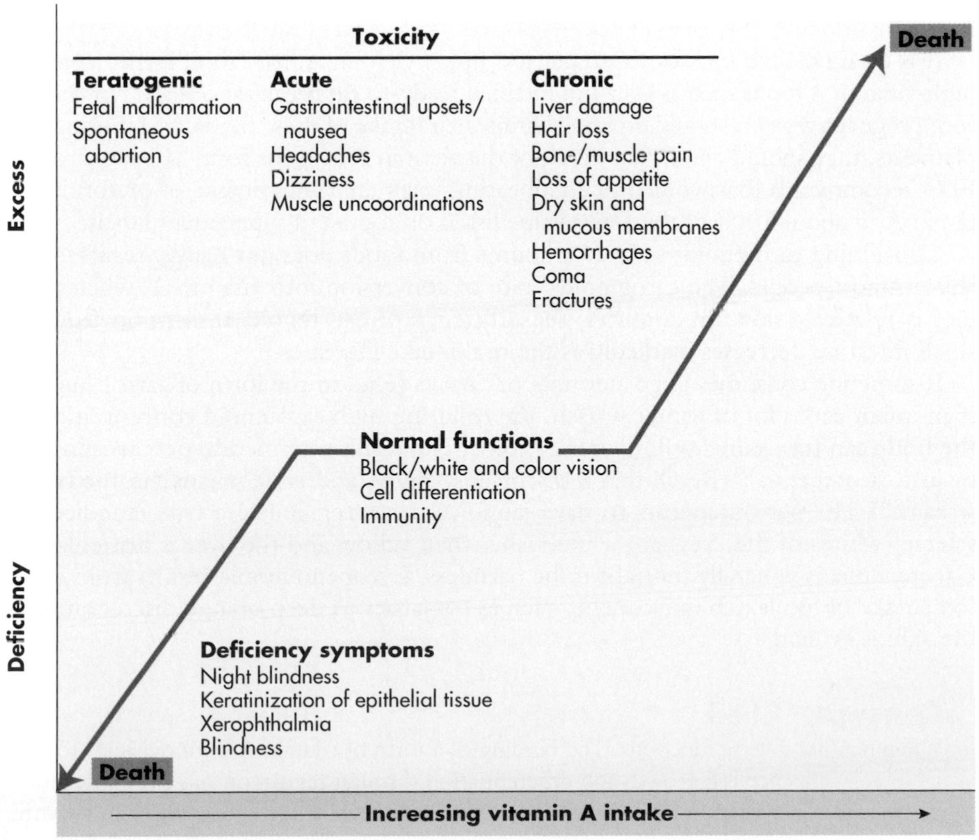

conjunctiva The mucous membrane covering the anterior surface of the eyeball and the posterior surface of the eyelids.

xerophthalmia A condition marked by dryness of the cornea and eye membranes that results from vitamin A deficiency and can lead to blindness. The specific cause is a lack of mucus production by the eye, which then leaves it more vulnerable to surface dirt and bacterial infections.

follicular hyperkeratosis A condition in which keratin, a protein, accumulates around hair follicles.

Figure 9-7 | Consuming the right amount of vitamin A is critical to overall health. A very low (deficient) or a very high (toxic) vitamin A intake (as retinoids) can produce damaging signs and symptoms and even lead to death. The severity of effects and the intake range vary among individuals.

teratogenic Tending to produce physical defects in a developing fetus (literally, "monster forming").

P eople in developing countries typically pose an exception to the rule that moderately large doses of vitamin A can cause toxicity. Because of their minimal storage of vitamin A, these people can tolerate intermittent large doses of the vitamin.

hypercarotenemia Elevated amounts of carotenoids in the bloodstream, usually caused by consuming a diet high in carrots or squash or by taking beta-carotene supplements.

Three kinds of vitamin A toxicity exist: acute, chronic, and **teratogenic.** Acute toxicity is caused by the ingestion of one very large dose of vitamin A or several large doses taken over several days (about 100 times the RDA). The effects of acute toxicity are largely GI tract upset, headache, blurred vision, and poor muscle coordination. Once the dosing is stopped, these signs disappear. Extraordinarily large doses, about 12 g (13,000 times the RDA), however, can be fatal.

In chronic toxicity, infants and adults show a wide range of signs and symptoms: bone and muscle pain, loss of appetite, various skin disorders, headache, dry skin, hair loss, liver damage, double vision, hemorrhage, vomiting, hip fractures, and coma.

Vitamin A also is particularly harmful in early pregnancy, a time when many women do not know that they are pregnant. Hypervitaminosis A may cause a spontaneous abortion or birth defects.[20]

Toxicity of vitamin A probably causes instability in retinoid-sensitive membranes and the inappropriate expression of certain genes. The treatment is simply to discontinue the supplement. Effects then decrease over the next few weeks to a month as blood concentrations fall to within a normal range. Permanent damage to the liver, bones, and eyes as well as recurrent joint and muscle pain, however, can occur with chronic ingestion of excessive amounts of the vitamin.

The most serious and tragic effects of hypervitaminosis A are teratogenic—most notably, the birth defects just mentioned. Vitamin A and its related analog forms, all-*trans*-retinoic acid (topical tretinoin [e.g., Retin-A]) and 13-*cis*-retinoic acid (oral isotretinoin, or Accutane), have been subjects of concern for years. These vitamin A analog medications are used to treat various skin disorders, such as acne and psoriasis. Accutane causes spontaneous abortion and birth defects in laboratory animals. The risk is significant for pregnant women taking large doses of vitamin A analogs. Their offspring show congenital malformations of the head, probably because neural crest cells, which are important in the development of the head and brain, are known to be very sensitive to excess amounts of vitamin A. As mentioned before, women of childbearing age need to take oral contraceptives immediately before, during, and for some time after taking these medications to prevent pregnancies that could result in such fetal malformations.

It is even possible for women to get too much vitamin A from food if they consume high-vitamin A foods such as liver and fortified ready-to eat breakfast cereals. For this reason, pregnant women should especially limit their intake of these foods, and if using supplements, they should check that much of the vitamin A is in the form of beta-carotene. FDA recommends that women of childbearing years limit their intake of preformed vitamin A to about 100% of the Daily Value listed on food and supplement labels.

Consuming carotenoids in large amounts from foods does not readily result in toxicity in most people. The carotenoids' rate of conversion into vitamin A, when possible, is relatively slow. In addition, the efficiency of carotenoid absorption from the small intestine decreases markedly as the oral intake increases.[8]

If someone consumes large amounts of carrots (e.g., in the form of carrot juice) or if an infant eats a lot of winter squash, the resulting high carotenoid concentrations in the body can turn skin a yellow-orange color. The result is termed **hypercarotenemia,** or just carotenemia.[8] (Recall that *hyper* means "high" and *emia* means "in the bloodstream.") The person appears to have jaundice; however, unlike a true jaundice, the sclerae (whites of the eyes) are white rather than yellow and the liver is not enlarged. Carotenemia is generally thought to be harmless. Lycopenodermia results from excessive intake of foods rich in lycopene, such as tomatoes. A deep orange discoloration of the skin is evident.

Concept | Check

Vitamin A has diverse functions. The binding of a form of vitamin A (retinoic acid) to DNA can influence cell growth and differentiation through regulation of gene expression. Vitamin A is important for maintaining vision and epithelial tissues, reproduction, growth, and ensuring proper function of the immune system. Vitamin A in the diet comes in two forms: retinoids (preformed vitamin A) and certain carotenoids (provitamin A). A diet that meets the RDA for vitamin A and contains plenty of carotenoid-containing fruits and vegetables is considered sound nutrition. Major food sources of vitamin A include liver, carrots, eggs, tomatoes, milk, and many vegetables. North Americans most at risk for poor vitamin A status are preschool children and alcoholics. Large doses of retinoids can be toxic, even at chronic dosages only about 2 to 4 times the RDA, especially during early pregnancy and one's older years.

Vitamin D

The status of vitamin D as a vitamin is ambiguous because, in the presence of sunlight, skin cells are capable of synthesizing a sufficient supply of the vitamin from a derivative of cholesterol. Because a dietary source is not required in this case, the vitamin is more correctly classified as a "conditional" vitamin, or **prohormone** (e.g., a precursor of an active hormone). Vitamin D achieves vitamin status because the diseases **rickets** and **osteomalacia** can be prevented and, to some extent, treated by the consumption of vitamin D-rich foods.[8]

For North Americans in general, sun exposure provides 80 to 100% of our vitamin D needs.[8] The amount of sun exposure needed by individuals to produce vitamin D (specifically vitamin D_3) depends on their skin color, age, time of day, season, and location. Experts recommend that people should expose their hands, face, and arms at least two to three times a week for 25% of the time it takes to turn one's skin pink (e.g., 5 to 10 minutes) to make enough vitamin D. Person with dark skin would need additional exposure, about 3 to 5 times the amount just recommended (or maybe even

prohormone Precursor of a hormone.

rickets A disease characterized by inadequate mineralization of the bones caused by poor calcium deposition during growth. This deficiency disease arises in infants and children with poor vitamin D status.

osteomalacia The weakening of the bones that occurs in adults as a result of poor bone mineralization linked to inadequate vitamin D status.

Humans produce vitamin D_3 (cholecalciferol), whereas supplements and fortified foods may contain vitamin D_2 (ergocalciferol). This latter compound has vitamin D activity in humans, but not as much as compared to vitamin D_3.

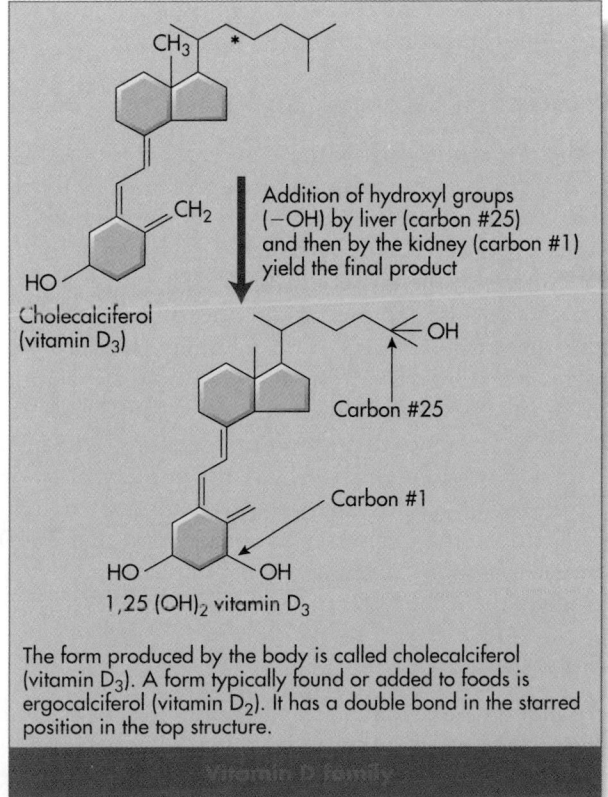

Addition of hydroxyl groups (—OH) by liver (carbon #25) and then by the kidney (carbon #1) yield the final product

Cholecalciferol (vitamin D_3)

Carbon #25

Carbon #1

1,25 $(OH)_2$ vitamin D_3

The form produced by the body is called cholecalciferol (vitamin D_3). A form typically found or added to foods is ergocalciferol (vitamin D_2). It has a double bond in the starred position in the top structure.

Vitamin D family

Aging decreases production of vitamin D_3 in the skin by about 70% when one reaches the age of 70. Older people are advised to get some sun exposure, especially during early morning and late afternoon. In this way they will receive the benefit of vitamin D_3 synthesis without also significantly increasing their risk of skin cancer.

previtamin D_3 The precursor of one form of vitamin D, produced as a result of sunlight opening a ring on 7-dehydrocholesterol in the skin.

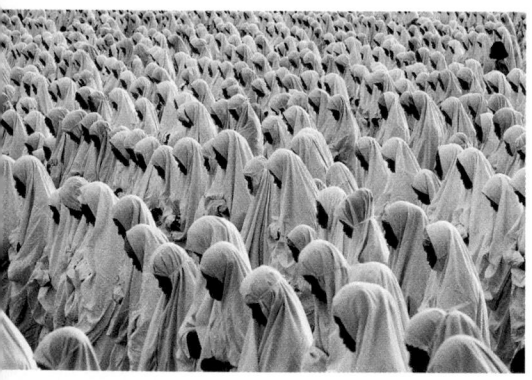

People who remain almost fully covered during the day, such as for religious reasons, produce little vitamin D_3.

more). The large amount of melanin pigment in dark-skinned people is a potent natural sunscreen. Sun exposure is effective for vitamin D synthesis only if sunscreen over SPF 8 is not used and if exposure takes place between about 8 A.M. and 4 P.M. Even this exposure is not effective at all in the winter in northern climates (e.g., above a line connecting Los Angeles, Calif., to Atlanta, Ga.). Some people may be able to use the vitamin D that was stored from summer months in their adipose cells, but most people in northern climates should find alternate vitamin D sources in the winter months.[5] Overall, anyone who does not receive enough sunshine to synthesize an adequate amount of vitamin D (the most reliable source) should seek a dietary source of the vitamin, but obtaining some sun exposure is still important.[8]

Vitamin D_3 Formation in the Skin

Synthesis of vitamin D_3 begins with provitamin D_3 (7-dehydrocholesterol), a precursor of cholesterol synthesis located in the skin. During exposure to sunlight, one ring on the molecule breaks open creating **previtamin D_3.** Over the next few hours, previtamin D_3 undergoes a chemical transformation aided by body heat, forming the more stable vitamin D_3. This change allows vitamin D_3 to enter the bloodstream, bound to a protein. It is now on its way to becoming a hormone.[6]

In Boston, Massachusetts (42° N), production of previtamin D_3 in the skin is adequate to meet needs from March through October. From November through February, the UV light is too low on the horizon to produce previtamin D_3. In Los Angeles (34° N), production of previtamin D_3 occurs throughout the year. Prolonged exposure doesn't increase the production of vitamin D_3 beyond needs, because any excess is rapidly degraded.[6]

Absorption of Vitamin D_2 from Food

Following the consumption of vitamin D_2-containing foods, about 80% of vitamin D_2 is incorporated into micelles in the small intestine and then absorbed and transported to the liver by chylomicrons through the lymphatic system. Patients with chronic fat-malabsorption syndromes (e.g., cystic fibrosis, Crohn's disease, and celiac disease) have trouble absorbing vitamin D_2 and may develop a deficiency.[8]

Metabolism, Transport, Storage, and Excretion of Vitamin D

When vitamin D (either D_3 synthesized in the skin or D_2 consumed from food or supplements) enters general circulation, it is bound to a protein. The formation of the hormone form of vitamin D from its precursor occurs in the liver and kidneys (Figure 9-8). In the liver, the vitamin is hydroxylated on carbon 25, converting it to 25-OH vitamin D. This inactive form circulates in the blood for weeks. The next stop is the kidney, the principal (but not exclusive) site for the production of $1,25(OH)_2$ vitamin D, also known as calcitriol or the hormone form of the vitamin. This form is active for about 1 day. People with chronic kidney failure have very low concentrations of circulating $1,25(OH)_2$ vitamin D, and they are routinely treated with it.[6]

Once vitamin D enters general circulation, it can be stored in adipose cells for later use or converted to 25-OH vitamin D in the liver. When there is a shortage of calcium in the blood, the parathyroid glands increase production of parathyroid hormone (PTH). Parathyroid hormone then increases the production of $1,25(OH)_2$ vitamin D in the kidney. Eventual excretion of vitamin D takes place mostly via the bile, with small amounts leaving via the urine.[8]

Functions of Vitamin D

Vitamin D has hormone functions that affect the body's use of calcium and phosphorus (Figure 9-9). The effects on calcium can have two somewhat opposite impacts on bone. On the one hand, vitamin D hormonal actions (as $1,25(OH)_2$ vitamin D) increase intestinal absorption of calcium from foods (review Figure 9-3 for the general

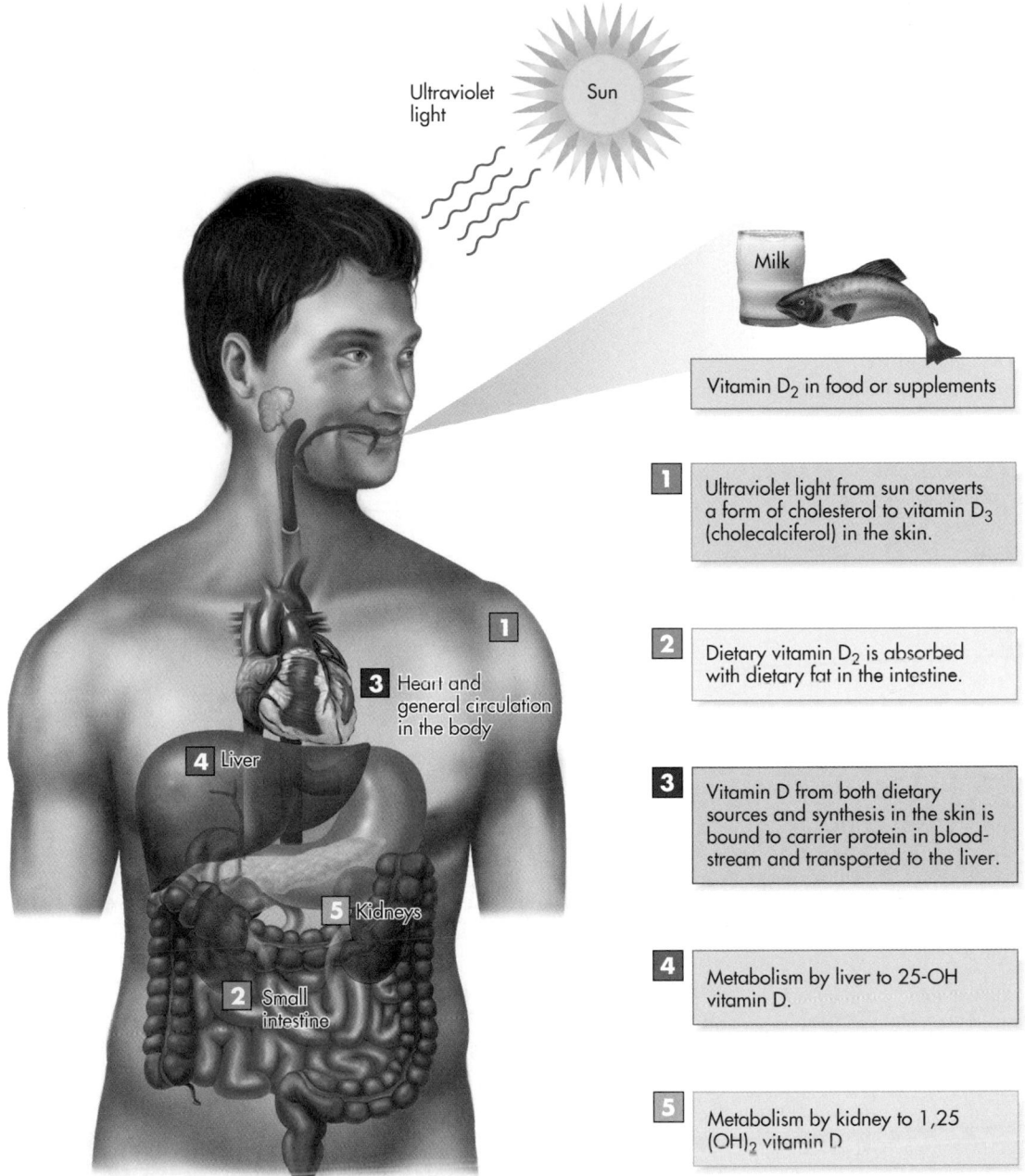

Milk

Vitamin D_2 in food or supplements

1 Ultraviolet light from sun converts a form of cholesterol to vitamin D_3 (cholecalciferol) in the skin.

2 Dietary vitamin D_2 is absorbed with dietary fat in the intestine.

3 Vitamin D from both dietary sources and synthesis in the skin is bound to carrier protein in blood-stream and transported to the liver.

4 Metabolism by liver to 25-OH vitamin D.

5 Metabolism by kidney to 1,25 $(OH)_2$ vitamin D

Sun

Ultraviolet light

3 Heart and general circulation in the body

4 Liver

5 Kidneys

2 Small intestine

Figure 9-8 | The many facets of vitamin D metabolism. Whether synthesized in the skin or obtained from dietary sources, vitamin D ultimately functions as a hormone: $1,25(OH)_2$ vitamin D.

mechanism of vitamin D action). This makes calcium available for body cells as well for incorporation into bone when there is more calcium in the blood than is needed for the other basic life functions of calcium.[6] On the other hand, vitamin D hormonal actions can release calcium from bone into the blood, working with parathyroid hormone. The latter action occurs to the greatest extent when blood calcium levels start to fall. This fall is reversed by vitamin D hormone-induced release of calcium from the bone. Although this action, if it occurs too much and too long, can weaken the bones, there is a benefit to it. Calcium is needed for many basic life functions, including heartbeat (see Chapter 11). If the bones did not supply calcium for these functions, a person could quickly have

Figure 9-9 | The active vitamin D hormone—1,25(OH)$_2$ vitamin D—and parathyroid hormone interact to control blood calcium concentration. Low blood calcium is a trigger for many hormonal responses. (1) Parathyroid hormone and 1,25(OH)$_2$ vitamin D mobilize calcium from the bone. (2) Parathyroid hormone also reduces calcium excretion by the kidneys and stimulates synthesis of 1,25(OH)$_2$ vitamin D by that organ. (3) 1,25(OH)$_2$ vitamin D by itself stimulates intestinal calcium absorption. All these responses raise blood calcium. Conversely, when calcium in the blood becomes too high, the hormone **calcitonin** responds by promoting calcium deposition in the bone (see Figure 11-10 in Chapter 11). (4) Normal amounts of calcium in the blood are needed to support nerve function, muscle action, bone health, and other functions.

calcitonin A thyroid gland hormone that inhibits bone resorption.

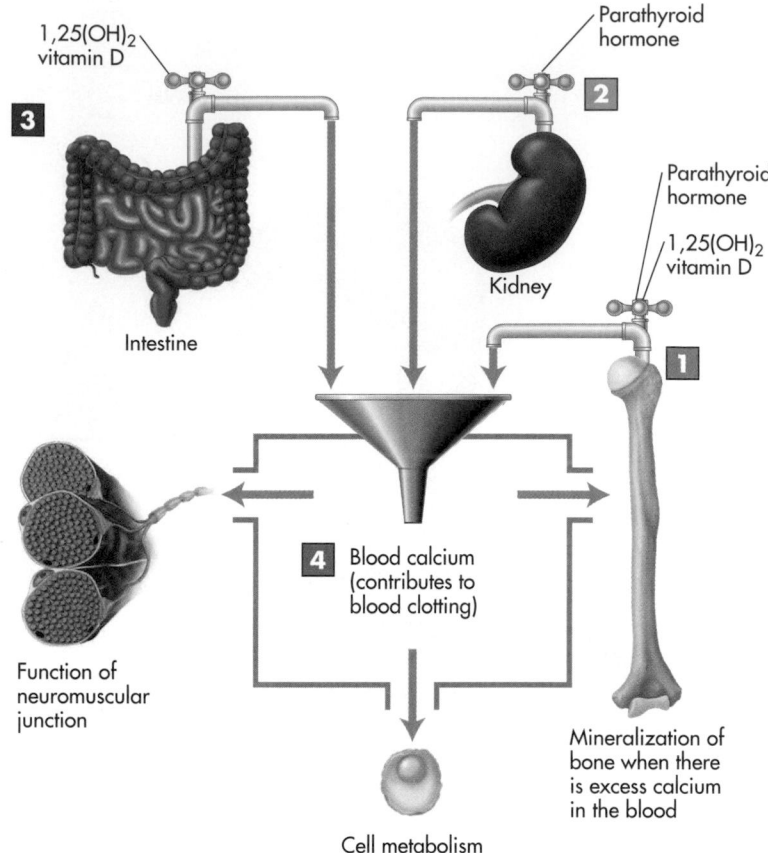

neuromuscular junction A chemical synapse between a motor neuron and a muscle fiber.

serious, even fatal, health consequences. Thus, vitamin D preserves these important functions of calcium even if dietary calcium intakes are not optimal.[6]

Vitamin D hormonal actions also help calcium with some of this mineral's regulatory functions. A prime example is providing enough calcium to maintain the function of the **neuromuscular junction** (see Chapter 11). In addition, vitamin D hormonal actions affect the body's use of phosphorus, which again partners with calcium to form calcium phosphate, the main component of bone structure.[6]

Human epidermal cells have receptors for 1,25(OH)$_2$ vitamin D in the nucleus. Activated receptors then affect the differentiation of skin cells. At present, 20 different cell types in the human body are known to be sensitive to the hormonal effects of vitamin D.[6] Its ability to affect muscle cells has been linked to a decreased risk of falling and decreased gum disease in older adults. Vitamin D is also capable of influencing differentiation in some cancer cells, such as skin, bone, and breast cancer cells. Indeed, adequate vitamin D status has been linked to a reduced risk of developing breast, ovarian, colon, and prostate cancer. Vitamin D may also contribute to lower blood pressure. Dr. Michael Holick further discusses the potential benefits of adequate vitamin D status in the Expert Opinion.

Vitamin D in Foods

Because some people may not receive enough sun exposure to generate sufficient vitamin D for the body's needs, they need to pay attention to dietary sources. Actually, few foods contain appreciable amounts of vitamin D.[8]

Good food sources of vitamin D are fatty fish (e.g., sardines and salmon), fortified milk, and some fortified breakfast cereals. In North America, milk is generally fortified with 10 µg (400 IU) per quart. Although eggs, butter, liver, and a few brands of margarine contain some vitamin D, large servings must be eaten to obtain an appreciable amount of the vitamin; thus, these foods are not considered significant sources.

Vitamin D Needs

The Food and Nutrition Board has set an Adequate Intake for vitamin D (see Chapter 2 for details about Adequate Intakes and how these standards differ from RDAs). A more precise RDA could not be set because the amount of vitamin D produced by sunlight is too variable between individuals. The Adequate Intake for vitamin D is 5 μg/day (200 IU/day) for people under age 51 and increases to 10 μg/day (400 IU/day) for people between 51 and 70 and 15 μg/day (600 IU/day) for older adults.[8] A number of experts suggest that older adults, especially those age 70 and over, who have limited sun exposure, receive about 20 to 25 μg (800 to 1000 IU) from a combination of vitamin D–fortified foods and a multivitamin and mineral supplement, with an individual supplement of vitamin D added if needed.[2,5] Providing 1250 mg (50,000 IU) once a month is another strategy. Young, light-skinned people can produce enough vitamin D from casual sun exposure on just the face and hands. The marker used to determine the Adequate Intake for young adults is the concentration of 25-OH vitamin D in the blood, the precursor to the active form of the vitamin. For older persons, indices of bone maintenance are also used.[8]

Infants are born with a supply of vitamin D. Still, the American Academy of Pediatrics recommends that breastfed infants be given a vitamin D supplement of 5 μg/day (200 IU per day) until they are weaned to infant formula and are consuming at least 500 ml of it. Note that infant formulas are fortified with vitamin D.

Vitamin D-Deficiency Diseases

Without adequate calcium and phosphorus in the blood available for deposition in the bone, the skeleton fails to mineralize properly and bones weaken and bow under pressure. When these effects occur in the growing bones of a child, the disease is called rickets (Figure 9-10). Signs of rickets include enlarged head, joints, and rib cage; a deformed pelvis; and bowed legs. In North America today, rickets is most commonly associated with fat malabsorption, such as is seen in children with cystic fibrosis, but an increase in cases has been seen related to a decrease in milk consumption and the use of clothing that, for religious or social reasons, limits skin exposure to the sun.[8,11]

Rickets in adults is called osteomalacia, which means "soft bones." It is characterized by poor calcification of newly synthesized bone. It can cause fractures in the hip, spine, and other bones. (Do not confuse this with the disease osteoporosis, which will be discussed in Chapter 11.) Osteomalacia is most likely to occur in people with kidney, stomach, gallbladder, or intestinal disease (especially when most of the intestine has been removed) and in those with cirrhosis of the liver.[8] These diseases affect both vitamin D metabolism and calcium absorption. Combinations of sun exposure and treatment with vitamin D or 1,25(OH)$_2$ vitamin D can be used to treat osteomalacia.

Studies suggest that older people and other individuals who stay indoors most of the day and ingest little or no vitamin D are at risk for developing a vitamin D deficiency. This concern is particularly important for older

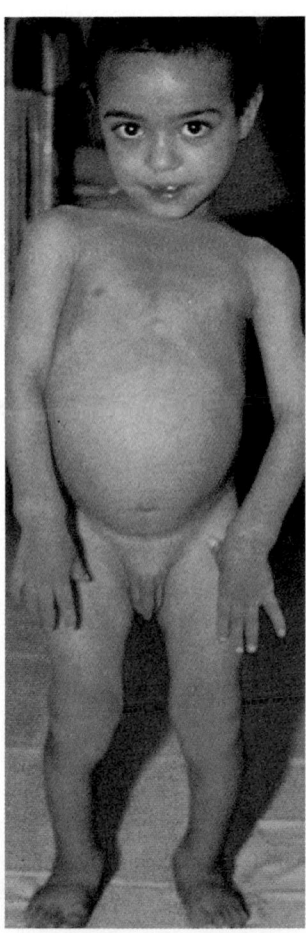

Figure 9-10 | The bowed legs of rickets, a vitamin D–deficiency disease.

Food Sources of Vitamin D		
Food Item and Amount	Vitamin D (μg)	Vitamin D (IU)
Baked herring, 3 oz	44.4	1775
Smoked eel, 1 oz	25.5	1020
Cod liver oil, 1 tbsp	11.3	453
Baked salmon, 3 oz	6.0	238
Sardines, 1 oz	3.4	136
Canned tuna, 3 oz	3.4	136
1% milk, 1 cup	2.5	99
Fat-free milk, 1 cup	2.5	98
Soft margarine, 1 tsp	1.5	60
Italian pork sausage, 3 oz	1.1	44
Soy milk, 1 cup	1.0	40
Raisin Bran cereal, 3/4 cup	1.0	38
Baked bluefish, 3 oz	0.9	34
Special K cereal, 3/4 cup	0.8	30
Cooked egg yolk, 1	0.6	25
Adequate Intake for adults, until age 50 5 μg (200 IU)		

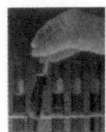

Expert Opinion

Miracle Vitamin D: Importance for Bone Health and Prevention of Common Cancers, Autoimmune Diseases, and other Disorders

Michael F. Holick, Ph.D., M.D.

Adequate vitamin D nutrition is associated with the prevention of rickets in children; therefore, little thought has been given to the consequences of vitamin D deficiency in adults. However, it is now becoming clear that vitamin D plays an important role in maintaining bone health from birth until death. Of equal importance is that vitamin D has a multitude of other biologic functions in the body that may be important for the prevention of common cancers, hypertension, and type 1 diabetes as well as a host of other common maladies that afflict older adults.

Vitamin D Sources: Exposure to Sunlight and Dietary Intakes

It is not appreciated that most of our vitamin D requirement, that is, 80 to 100%, comes from our exposure to sunlight. The body has a huge capacity to produce vitamin D_3. A person in a bathing suit exposed to sunlight or ultraviolet B radiation for an amount that would cause a light pinkness to the skin (1 minimal erythemal dose; 1 MED) will raise the blood levels of vitamin D_3 to the same degree as if the individual took between 10,000 and 25,000 IU of vitamin D_2. Anything that alters the amount of ultraviolet B radiation that penetrates into the skin will have a dramatic influence on the skin production of vitamin D_3. Increase in skin pigmentation, use of sunscreens, increase in latitude, increase in the Zenith angle of the sun due to seasonal changes, and aging all dramatically influence the skin production of vitamin D_3. The topical application of a sunscreen with an SPF of 8 will reduce it by 97.5%.

Unlike most fat-soluble and water-soluble vitamins that are plentiful i healthy diet, very few foods naturally contain vitamin D. Consumption of fish, such as salmon or mackerel, three to four times a week, or ingestio cod liver oil on a daily basis, are two natural sources. Some foods, such milk and some breads and cereals, are fortified with vitamin D. However, vitamin D content in milk in the past has been found to be highly varic and, in some cases, absent.

Vitamin D Deficiency: How Common Is It?

Vitamin D deficiency is extremely common in the U.S. adult population. M than 50% of free-living and institutionalized older adults have been repo to be vitamin D deficient. It has been assumed that young and middle-a adults are not at risk for vitamin D deficiency. However, the lifestyle of young and middle-aged adults is such that they are constantly working doors and when outdoors they wear a sunscreen because of their conc of sun exposure and risk of skin cancer. A study in Boston reported that of medical students and residents aged 18 to 29 years were vitamin D cient at the end of the winter. The NHANES III study reported that 41° African American women of childbearing age (15 to 49 years) were fc to be vitamin D deficient at the end of the winter.

Chronic vitamin D deficiency has subtle and insidious consequences for bone health and overall health and well-being for all adults and in partic older adults. Vitamin D deficiency can precipitate and exacerbate osteopo

The best way to assess a person's vitamin D status is to determine the concentration of 25-OH vitamin D in the blood.

people who live in northern climates or reside in nursing homes. Not only do these people experience little sun exposure, they also can have reduced $1,25(OH)_2$ vitamin D production from kidney resistance, which decreases conversion to the active form of the hormone.

A person with a low circulating concentration of 25-OH vitamin D should take 20 to 25 μg (800–1000 IU) of vitamin D each day until the concentration reaches the midnormal range.[2,5] People who are likely to fall into this category are dark-skinned people, older people (especially those with osteoporosis), and people with malabsorption syndromes, liver failure, and kidney disease or failure. After blood concentrations are normal, 10 μg (400 IU/day) from a multivitamin and mineral supplement should be sufficient for most people.[8] Some sun exposure would also be helpful.

Some humans show resistance to the action of certain vitamins, including vitamin D. Resistance to vitamin D can be caused either by a lack of $1,25(OH)_2$ vitamin D

because of the accompanying increase in release of parathyroid hormone. Vitamin D deficiency also causes osteomalacia, which is often associated with muscle pain, muscle weakness, bone pain, and increased risk of fracture.

Vitamin D: More Than Just Bone Health

Vitamin D is biologically inert and is metabolized in the liver to its major circulating form 25-hydroxyvitamin D [25(OH) D]. 25(OH) D is converted in the kidney to 1,25-dihydroxyvitamin D [$1,25(OH)_2$ D], which is responsible for regulating intestinal calcium absorption and stimulating bone cell synthesis. Vitamin D receptors (VDR) are present in the DNA of most tissues and immune cells in the body. $1,25(OH)_2$ D is one of the most potent inhibitors of cellular growth. In addition, $1,25(OH)_2$ D alters both activated T and B lymphocyte function. VDR is present in the kidney, and recently it was demonstrated that $1,25(OH)_2$ D down—regulates the renin/angiotension system involved in blood pressure regulation (more on this system in Chapter 11).

It is now recognized that the kidney is not the sole source for the production of $1,25(OH)_2$ D. Many other organ systems, including colon, prostate, breast, and skin have the enzymatic machinery to produce $1,25(OH)_2$ D locally. This may be the explanation for why chronic vitamin D deficiency, often associated with living at higher latitudes, is associated with increased risk of dying from colon, prostate, breast, and ovarian cancer. Exposure to ultraviolet B radiation is effective in treating moderate hypertension. In animal models $1,25(OH)_2$ D treatment was effective in preventing multiple sclerosis–like disease and type 1 diabetes. The recent observation that vitamin D supplementation of children resulted in a decreased risk of type 1 diabetes by 80% is noteworthy.

Overall, there is a great need to increase our awareness of vitamin D nutritional status and its health implications. The only method to determine vitamin D status is to measure circulating concentrations of 25(OH) D. Recently, the National Academy of Sciences has recommended that vitamin D intakes be increased for older adults to 600 IU/day. However, in the absence of exposure to any sunlight, this amount is probably inadequate. It is now estimated that in this case 1000 IU of vitamin D a day would be required to satisfy the body's needs and maintain circulating concentrations of 25(OH) D of at least 20 nanograms/ml, which is thought to be important to maximize bone health and cellular health.

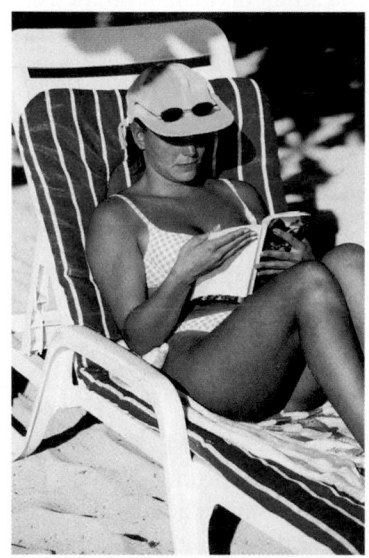

Solar radiation on the skin provides about 80 to 100% of the vitamin D humans use. This is also the most reliable way to maintain vitamin D status. Dietary vitamin D is also effective, but less so.

Dr. Holick is Professor of Medicine, Physiology, and Biophysics; Director of the General Clinical Research Center; and Director of the Bone Health Care Clinic and the Heliotherapy, Light and Skin Research Center at Boston University Medical Center. After completing a postgraduate degree in biochemistry, a medical degree, and a research postdoctoral fellowship at the University of Wisconsin–Madison, Dr. Holick completed a residency in medicine at the Massachusetts General Hospital in Boston. He has made numerous contributions to the field of the biochemistry, physiology, metabolism, and photobiology of vitamin D for human nutrition. These observations provide new insights into the role of sunlight and vitamin D nutrition in prevention of osteoporosis, some common cancers, type 1 diabetes, and other disorders. Dr. Holick has been the recipient of numerous awards and honors for more than three decades.

synthesis in the kidney or by an inability of $1,25(OH)_2$ vitamin D to bind to its receptors in the nucleus throughout the body. In both cases, the treatment is a large dose of $1,25(OH)_2$ vitamin D. This treatment works well in the first case but is not as successful in the second.

Pharmacologic Use of Vitamin D Analogs

Normal keratinocytes (skin-producing cells) require 28 to 44 days to move from the basal cell layer of the skin to the surface of the epidermis. Among patients with psoriasis, the movement takes only 4 days, which results in a scaly and embarrassing dermatitis. Today, vitamin D analogs applied to the skin are used as a safe, effective treatment of psoriasis.

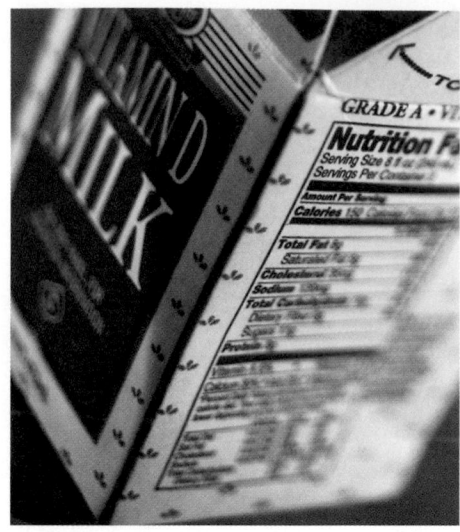

Milk is usually fortified with vitamin D as well as vitamin A.

North Americans are spending more than $1 billion on vitamin E supplements each year.

Upper Level for Vitamin D

The Upper Level for vitamin D is 50 µg/day (2000 IU/day). Too much vitamin D taken regularly can create problems, especially in some infants and young children.[8] For adults, intakes somewhat above the Upper Level appear to be safe. The Upper Level is based on the risk of overabsorption of calcium and eventual calcium deposits in the kidneys and other organs. The person also suffers the typical symptoms of high blood calcium: weakness, loss of appetite, diarrhea, vomiting, mental confusion, and increased urine output. Calcium deposits in organs cause metabolic disturbances and cell death. However, vitamin D toxicity does not result from tanning in the sun too long because the body regulates the amount made in the skin.

Concept | Check

Vitamin D is a vitamin only for people who fail to produce enough from exposure to sunlight. Most people can synthesize adequate vitamin D by the action of sunlight on the skin. Older people and breastfed infants are at risk of a vitamin D deficiency. Vitamin D is activated by the liver and kidneys to form the hormone 1,25(OH)$_2$ vitamin D. This hormone increases calcium absorption in the intestine and works with other hormones to maintain proper blood calcium concentrations and calcium metabolism in bones and other organs in the body. The hormone 1,25(OH)$_2$ vitamin D is also an important regulator of cell differentiation in many tissues of the body. Fish oils and fortified milk are good food sources of vitamin D. An excess of vitamin D can be quite toxic, especially during infancy. Sun exposure poses no risk of vitamin D toxicity.

Vitamin E

Vitamin E is the major fat-soluble antioxidant found in cells. A vitamin E deficiency in laboratory animals can result in muscular dystrophy, inability to produce viable offspring, and impotence. The link between vitamin E deficiency and inability to reproduce in rats, first noted in 1922, gave vitamin E its chemical name tocopherol (*toco* means "related to childbirth"). Overt vitamin E deficiency in humans is not common, though it does occur in a few situations.[9] Most of the interest in vitamin E is not from the deficiency standpoint, but more in terms of an optimal intake for promoting health. This area is still controversial; ongoing research may provide more insight.

Natural and Synthetic Vitamin E

It is important to take a close look at vitamin E chemistry in order to understand not only the units used to express vitamin E activity but also food and supplement labels and issues regarding potential vitamin E toxicity. As you can see in the figure on the next page, vitamin E has a long carbon tail. In this tail, the three carbon atoms with a star can exist in two different spatial orientations, designated R and S (see Appendix A to learn more about R and S stereoisomers). Such a compound with R and S possibilities at three different sites yields eight different isomers ($2^3 = 8$). Only vitamin E isomers that have the R configuration at the first starred site are active in the body; the S form leads to an unwanted "kink" in the tail of the vitamin E molecule. All the vitamin E found naturally in foods has R at that first starred carbon atom and is therefore considered active. (Actually it is R in all 3 positions, and is therefore RRR vitamin E.) Synthetic vitamin E will only have R on the first starred carbon atom in half of the isomers present, while the others will have the S configuration. Thus, only about half of the vitamin E in synthetic formulations is active in the body.[9]

When you look at food or supplement labels, however, you will not see R and S designations concerning the type of vitamin E in the product. Instead, you will see "d" and "l." These designations are another way of describing isomers, but they have been

Alpha-tocopherol

The carbon chain attached to the ringed structure exists in many possible isomer forms. The specific carbons that have isomer forms (termed R and S) are starred.

Vitamin E

inappropriately assigned to vitamin E. The d and l isomers are only appropriate when just one carbon atom in a compound has different orientations, and you know that vitamin E has three carbon atoms that have different orientations. Food and supplement labels, however, still use this older terminology because researchers did not understand much about vitamin E chemistry until recent years, and the label terminology has not been updated. From a practical standpoint, if you see d next to vitamin E on a label, all of that vitamin E will be active in the body. If you see dl on a label, only about half of that vitamin E will be active in the body.

What we call vitamin E is actually a family of eight naturally occurring compounds—four **tocopherols** (alpha, beta, gamma, delta) and four **tocotrienols** (alpha, beta, gamma, delta)—with widely varying degrees of biological activity. The most active form of the vitamin is the so-called "d" isomer of alpha-tocopherol (again, actually RRR).[9] This is the form found in nature and in varying amounts in vitamin supplements. However, recent research shows that other forms, such as gamma-tocopherol, may also be important to the body.[9]

Absorption, Transport, Storage, and Excretion of Vitamin E

The degree of absorption of vitamin E depends on the total absorption of dietary fat. Like the other fat-soluble nutrients, vitamin E must be incorporated into micelles within the lumen of the small intestine, which in turn is dependent on bile and pancreatic enzymes. Once taken up by the absorptive cells, vitamin E is incorporated into chylomicrons for transport by the lymph and eventually the bloodstream to tissues and the liver.[9] The precise degree of absorption is not known.

The chylomicron remnants release the vitamin E to the liver, which can then deliver the vitamin to the lipoproteins VLDL and HDL. Vitamin E can be stored in the liver and in adipose tissues and skeletal muscle. Eventually, vitamin E positions itself in cell membranes, where it is associated with phospholipids.[9]

Excretion of vitamin E is via the bile and urine. Because of the limited absorption of vitamin E from the intestinal tract, there is a significant amount in the feces.[9]

Functions of Vitamin E

Besides functioning as a lipid-soluble antioxidant, vitamin E also can affect a number of other body processes, such as platelet aggregation, but it is not yet known if these effects are directly related to antioxidant actions. As an antioxidant, vitamin E functions as a chain-breaking molecule that prevents the propagation of chain reactions caused by **free radicals.**[9]

Free radicals are reactive species with unpaired electrons that start oxidant chain reactions that then create **oxidative stress.** Strictly speaking, an oxidant-related reaction is any reaction in which electrons are donated to another molecule. This definition

tocopherols A group of four structurally similar compounds that have vitamin E activity. The RRR ("d") isomer of alpha-tocopherol is the most active form.

tocotrienols A group of four compounds with the same basic chemical structure as the tocopherols but containing slightly altered side chains. They exhibit much less vitamin E activity than the corresponding tocopherols.

free radical The short-lived form of a compound that has an unpaired electron, causing it to seek an electron from another compound. Free radicals are strong oxidizing agents and can be very destructive to electron-dense cell components, such as the DNA and cell membranes.

oxidative stress The damage to lipids, proteins, and DNA produced by excessive production of free radicals.

Figure 9-11 | Fat-soluble vitamin E can insert itself into cell membranes, where it helps stop free radical chain reactions. If not interrupted, these reactions cause extensive oxidative damage to cells and ultimately cell death.

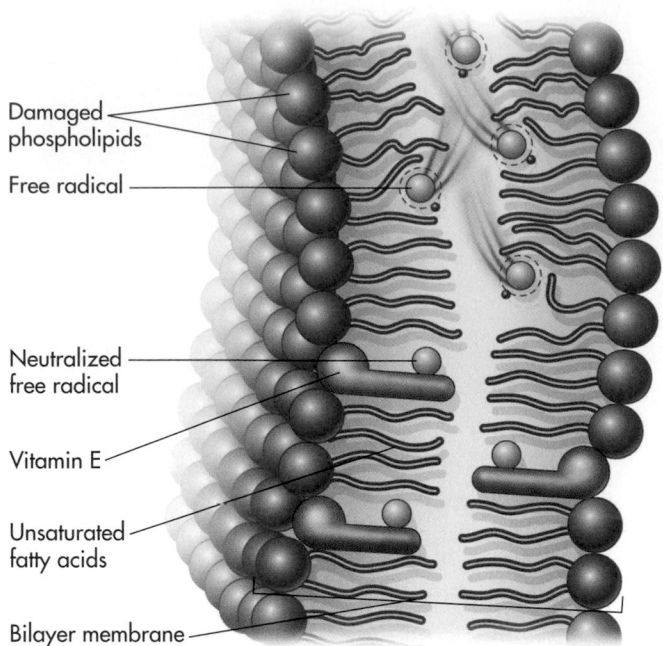

Damaged phospholipids

Free radical

Neutralized free radical

Vitamin E

Unsaturated fatty acids

Bilayer membrane

peroxyl radical A peroxide compound containing a free radical; designated R–O–O˙.

reactive oxygen species (ROS) Several oxygen derivatives produced during the formation of ATP. Formed constantly in the human body and shown to kill bacteria and inactivate proteins, they are implicated in a number of diseases and inflammatory processes.

redox agents Chemicals that can readily undergo both oxidation (loss of an electron) and reduction (gain of an electron).

includes reactions that are part of aerobic respiration. However, when the term *oxidative stress* is used, these reactions involve free radicals and produce damage to biological molecules (Figure 9-11). The health consequences of oxidative stress have been publicized extensively in regard to cardiovascular disease, cancer, skin aging, and arthritis, but oxidative stress also compromises immune function and may have many other less obvious effects.

An antioxidant is any agent that can in some manner work against the damage of oxidative stress. This can happen in a variety of ways. Vitamin E works mainly as a chain-breaking antioxidant in lipid environments.[9] A free radical reacts with an unsaturated fatty acid in a phospholipid located in a cell membrane or lipoprotein, which can start a series of reactions that includes breaking fatty acids apart and creating one type of free radical, a lipid **peroxyl radical.** The lipid peroxyl radical is symbolized by the term R–O–O˙, where R is a carbon-hydrogen chain broken off a fatty acid and the dot is an unpaired electron. This compound is also termed a **reactive oxygen species (ROS),** because it is a free radical that contains an oxygen radical. This lipid peroxyl radical then reacts with a new unsaturated fatty acid, which creates a new lipid peroxyl radical. This radical continues the chain reaction until two radicals meet and neutralize each other. By that time, however, many fatty acids have been broken apart.

Vitamin E reacts with the lipid peroxyl radical and stops the chain reaction. Thus, we use the term *chain-breaking antioxidant* ($R˙ + O_2 \rightarrow R–O–O˙$ and then $R–O–O˙$ + vitamin E-OH $\rightarrow$ R–O–O–H + vitamin E–O˙). In effect, the cell traded a very reactive free radical for a much less reactive vitamin E radical. This chain-breaking reaction is important both to protect cells from dying and limit LDL oxidation, a contributor to atherosclerosis.

A vitamin E molecule is "used up" during its chain-breaking action. However, there is some evidence that vitamin C may be able to regenerate some vitamin E to allow it to function again. This works well in vitro (in a test tube), but we don't know yet how well it works in the human body, especially since vitamin C tends to be located in watery environments while vitamin E tends to stay with lipids.[9]

Antioxidants vs. Redox Agents

Because an antioxidant protects other compounds by becoming oxidized itself, in a chemical sense antioxidants are more properly termed **redox agents.** In other words, they can readily undergo both oxidation (loss of an electron), and later reduction (regaining an electron). Nevertheless, *antioxidant* is still the most common term, even in the scientific literature.

Also keep in mind that free radicals are not all bad. As part of the immune system's arsenal against invading pathogens, white blood cells (leukocytes) generate free radicals to destroy the agents that cause infections. Also, free radicals stimulate normal cell growth and division. Overall, exposure to free radicals is part of life and for the most part essential, but the body must be able to regulate this exposure and avoid the undesirable effects, a task assigned to antioxidants.[9]

Other Antioxidant Systems in the Body

In addition to vitamin E, the body has various other mechanisms for protecting itself from oxidant damage (Figure 9-12). The body also contains numerous antioxidant enzymes such as **glutathione peroxidase, catalase,** and **superoxide dismutase.**[9]

Glutathione peroxidase catalyzes the breakdown of hydrogen peroxides (H–O–O–H) and lipid peroxides (R–O–O–H). These compounds are not radicals, but they can easily become radicals. Glutathione peroxidase eliminates peroxides before this happens. Consequently the need for vitamin E decreases because fewer free radicals will be formed. Glutathione peroxidase thus aids vitamin E in reducing oxidative damage to cells. The activity of glutathione peroxidase depends on the mineral selenium (the functional part of this enzyme) and the vitamin riboflavin. (Thioredoxin is another selenium-dependent antioxidant enzyme [see Chapter 12 for details].) An adequate dietary intake of selenium reduces the need for vitamin E, whereas an inadequate intake of selenium increases the need. The enzyme catalase performs a function similar to that of glutathione peroxidase but has a different cell location (peroxisomes).

Another important defense system in cells, the family of enzymes known as superoxide dismutase, eliminate one particular free radical called superoxide. Two of the superoxide dismutase enzymes contain copper and zinc. One is located in the cell cytosol and the other is found outside of cells. Intake of the essential nutrient copper can affect the activities of these two superoxide dismutase enzymes, but zinc intake seems to have major effects only on the enzyme that is found outside the cells. The third superoxide dismutase enzyme is found in the mitochondria and requires the mineral manganese for function.

In addition to vitamin E and antioxidant enzymes, there are still other antioxidants. Phytochemicals (such as many carotenoids) can neutralize free radicals and possibly prevent certain radicals from forming.[9]

Oxidizing agents that cells encounter include highly reactive oxygen species such as singlet oxygen ($^1O_2$), hydrogen peroxide (H_2O_2), hydroxyl radical ($^\bullet OH$), superoxide ($O_2^{\bullet -}$), ozone (O_3) and nitrogen-oxygen combinations that are typical of air pollutants ($NO^\bullet$).

glutathione peroxidase A selenium-containing enzyme that can destroy peroxides. It acts in conjunction with vitamin E to reduce free radical damage to cells.

catalase An enzyme that breaks down hydrogen peroxide to water.

superoxide dismutase Enzymes containing manganese, copper, or zinc that destroy superoxide.

Four metabolic compounds—bilirubin, uric acid, lipoic acid, and ubiquinone (coenzyme Q-10)—also are thought to provide antioxidant protection.

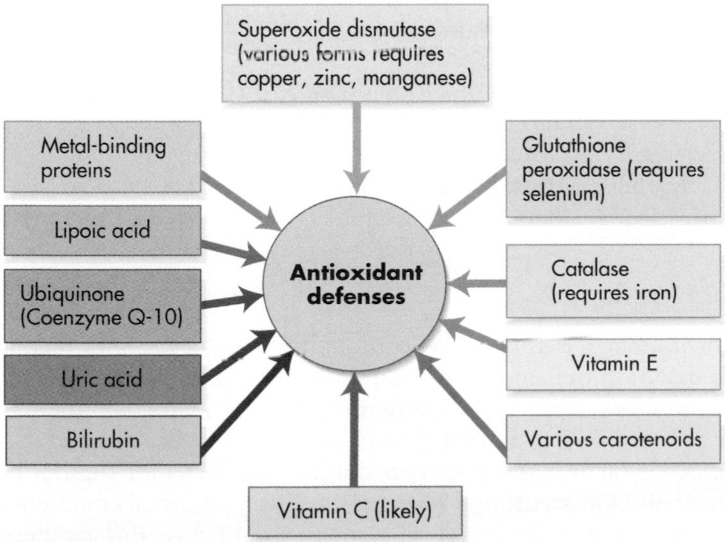

Figure 9-12 | The body does not rely solely on vitamin E for antioxidant protection. Such protection is a team effort that utilizes a number of nutrients, metabolites, and enzyme systems.

Proteins in the blood also bind metals—this limits the ability of metals to catalyze free radical production. Systems also exist in cells to repair molecules that have been oxidatively damaged, such as DNA.

Food Sources of Vitamin E

Food Item and Amount	Vitamin E (mg)	Vitamin E (IU)
Sunflower oil, 2 tbsp	16.3	24.3
Dry-roasted sunflower seeds, 1 oz	14.3	21.2
Dry-roasted almonds, 1 oz	7.5	11.1
Safflower oil, 1 tbsp	5.9	8.7
Canola oil, 2 tbsp	5.7	8.5
Wheat germ, 1/4 cup	5.2	7.7
Almonds, 1 oz	4.5	6.8
Oil-roasted sunflower seeds, 1 tbsp	3.4	5.0
Italian dressing, 2 tbsp	3.1	4.5
Mayonnaise, 1 tbsp	3.0	4.5
Avocado, 1	2.7	4.0
Chunky peanut butter, 2 tbsp	2.4	3.6
Mango, 1	2.3	3.5
Peanuts, 1 oz	2.1	3.1
Cooked asparagus, 1 cup	2.1	3.1
RDA for adults, 15 mg		

hemolysis The destruction of red blood cells, caused by the breakdown of the red blood cell membrane. This causes the cell contents to leak into the fluid portion (plasma) of the blood.

Because there are limits to how much of any one antioxidant compound can accumulate in any one cell, it may be advantageous to consume a variety of antioxidant phytochemicals along with vitamin E and vitamin C. Furthermore, some phytochemicals may be better at protecting against certain free radicals than others. For example, carotenoids may be especially good at dealing with singlet oxygen, which is not a radical itself but can initiate oxidant stress. The bottom line is that antioxidant protection is a team effort involving a number of nutrients.

This discussion raises the question of the relative role of vitamin E in oxidant protection in the body. It is unknown whether taking vitamin E supplements confers any additional protection against cardiovascular disease and cancer than that achieved by improving one's diet, performing regular physical activity, not smoking, and controlling (or improving) body weight.

All major long-term trials using megadose vitamin E therapy have failed to show any benefit in reducing heart attacks or cardiovascular disease-related death in people who have the disease. These studies have included thousands of people and had durations of approximately 5 to 7 years. As noted in Chapter 6, these results have caused most experts and some leading cardiologists to discount the benefit of megadose vitamin E therapy in high-risk people. There is even a risk of heart failure among people with diabetes or existing cardiovascular disease who take megadoses of vitamin E.

Currently, the major hope is that megadose vitamin E therapy (50 to 200 mg/day [100 to 400 IU/day]) in healthy people will *prevent* future development of cardiovascular disease. A large trial using men is currently testing this hypothesis, and results will be available by 2007. The dose used is 600 IU of natural vitamin E taken every other day (recall from Chapter 6 that results of the similar trial in women showed no clear benefit in reducing cardiovascular disease-related deaths, except in a subset of older women who showed a somewhat lower risk for sudden cardiac death[13]). At this time the American Heart Association states that it is premature to recommend vitamin E supplements to the general populations, based on current knowledge. This conclusion is in agreement with the latest report on vitamin E by the Food and Nutrition Board.[9] In addition, FDA recently denied the request of the supplement industry to make a health claim that vitamin E supplements reduce the risk of cardiovascular disease.

Vitamin E in Foods

Good food sources of vitamin E are plant oils (e.g., corn, soybean, safflower, sunflower, cottonseed, and wheat germ oil), wheat germ, asparagus, and peanuts. Products made from the plant oils—margarine, shortenings, and salad dressing—are also good sources. Finfish and shellfish add vitamin E to the diet. In addition, grain meals such as oatmeal, nuts (e.g., almonds), and seeds (e.g., sunflower seeds) are other good sources. In milling whole grains, most of the vitamin E is lost and not restored. Animal fats have practically no vitamin E.

The actual vitamin E content of a food depends on harvesting, processing, storage, and cooking because vitamin E is highly susceptible to destruction by oxygen, metals, light, and deep-fat frying. In any case, a varied diet supplies the vitamin E needed for good health. Synthetic antioxidants, such as BHA and BHT, also add to the cellular protection provided by vitamin E (see Chapter 19 for more on BHA and BHT).

Vitamin E Needs

The RDA for vitamin E is 15 mg/day of alpha-tocopherol for both men and women. The RDA is based on the amount of vitamin E needed to prevent breakdown of red blood cell membranes, a process called **hemolysis.** The 15 mg allotment is equivalent to 22 IU of a natural source and 33 IU of a synthetic source.[9]

Adults consume on average about two-thirds of the RDA for vitamin E each day.[15] Daily intake of nuts and seeds, or a ready-to-eat breakfast cereal containing vitamin E, or use of a multivitamin and mineral supplement would close this gap between typical vitamin E intakes and needs.

To convert from the older IU system, 1 IU equals about 0.45 mg, based on the synthetic (dl isomer) form of vitamin E found in most supplements. If vitamin E is from a natural source (d isomer), 1 IU equals 0.67 mg, because the natural form of vitamin E is more potent than the synthetic form.[9] Thus the 200 mg/day maximum recommendation made by some experts actually represents 300 IU (d isomer) (200/0.67 = 300) to 450 IU (dl isomer) (200/0.45 = 450). Incidentally, 200 mg/day is thought to supply the maximum amount of vitamin E that can be retained by the body over time.[9] The Daily Value used on food and supplement labels for vitamin E is 30 IU.

Vitamin E-Deficiency Diseases

Smokers are especially likely to develop a vitamin E deficiency and related oxidative damage in the body.[4] (Smoking readily destroys vitamin E in the lungs, but there is no easy way to test for this problem in clinical practice.) But studies have shown that even using megadoses of vitamin E is ineffective in preventing this damage. Others at considerable risk of a vitamin E deficiency include adults on very low-fat diets or those with fat malabsorption. **Preterm** infants are particularly susceptible to the hemolysis of red blood cells, first because they are born with limited tissue stores of vitamin E and are inefficient in absorbing vitamin E from the intestinal tract. Second, the rapid growth of preterm infants exhausts what little vitamin E stores exist. To prevent hemolytic anemia, special formulas and supplements for preterm infants are prescribed to prevent vitamin E-related disorders of preterm births.

Vitamin E deficiency occurs also as a result of a genetic abnormality in lipoprotein synthesis, because lipoproteins distribute vitamin E throughout the body. In these cases, the primary vitamin E deficiency symptom is nervous system damage. Immune function is also reduced.[9]

Upper Level for Vitamin E

The Upper Level for vitamin E is 1000 mg/day of supplemental alpha-tocopherol. Excessive amounts of vitamin E can interfere with vitamin K's role in the clotting mechanism, leading to **hemorrhage.**[3,9] The risk of insufficient blood clotting is especially high if vitamin E is taken in conjunction with anticoagulant medications (e.g., Coumadin or heavy aspirin use). In international units, the Upper Level is 1500 IU for vitamin E isolated from natural sources (d isomer; 1000/0.67 = 1500) and 1100 IU for synthetic vitamin E (dl isomer; 1000/0.45/2 = 1100). The lower IU value for the synthetic form reflects the greater number of forms present in the synthetic product, only half or less of which contribute to vitamin E activity in cells, but are still absorbed and reduce blood clotting.[9] This Upper Level is set for a healthy population. Again, individuals who are vitamin K deficient or who are taking anticoagulants or heavy doses of aspirin are especially at risk for hemorrhage from megadose vitamin E use.

There is additional concern that taking large amounts of alpha-tocopherol might decrease gamma-tocopherol activity in the body. Gamma-tocopherol is a potentially beneficial form of vitamin E (It may reduce prostate cancer risk in men). To compensate, some experts recommend that any vitamin E supplement should contain a mixture of natural (RRR) tocopherols (e.g., mixed tocopherols). This form is more expensive, however, than natural or synthetic alpha-tocopherol alone.

Concept | Check

Enzymes and other body mechanisms scavenge and minimize the formation of free radicals and other oxidative compounds, but they are not 100% effective. Hence, diet-derived antioxidants may be critical in diminishing cumulative oxidative damage and helping us to stay healthy. Vitamin E is one such nutrient that functions primarily as an antioxidant. By providing electrons to free radicals, vitamin E helps prevent oxidative damage, especially of cell membranes. The best sources of vitamin E are plant oils. When more plant oils are

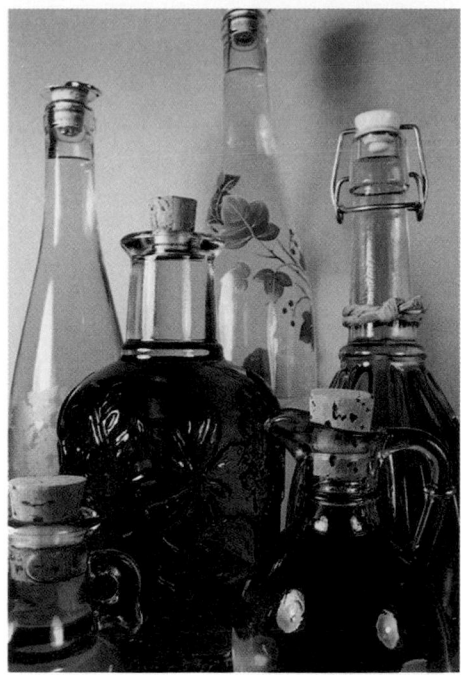

Plant oils are rich sources of vitamin E.

preterm An infant born before 37 weeks of gestation; such an infant is also referred to as premature.

hemorrhage An escape of blood from blood vessels.

One way to assess the vitamin E status of a person is to incubate a sample of his or her red blood cells with peroxide for 3 hours and then measure the extent of red blood cell destruction. A newer method uses the same procedure but measures the amount of a breakdown product of polyunsaturated fatty acids. These tests can be used in addition to measuring vitamin E in the blood.

consumed, more vitamin E is needed to protect the double bonds found in plant oils from oxidation. However, the vitamin E content in plant oils is usually high. Because of their poor vitamin E status, preterm infants are particularly susceptible to oxidative breakdown of their red blood cell membranes (hemolysis). Among adults, people who smoke or experience long-term fat malabsorption run the biggest risk of vitamin E deficiency. At present, there is controversy about whether taking large amounts of vitamin E in supplement form over a long period of time provides any special health benefits; research is ongoing. Megadose use of vitamin E reduces blood clotting, possibly leading to a hemorrhage.

Vitamin K

Vitamin K is essential for blood clotting. A Danish researcher first noted the relationship between vitamin K and blood clotting and named the fat-soluble vitamin "K" after *koagulation*, the Danish spelling for *coagulation*.

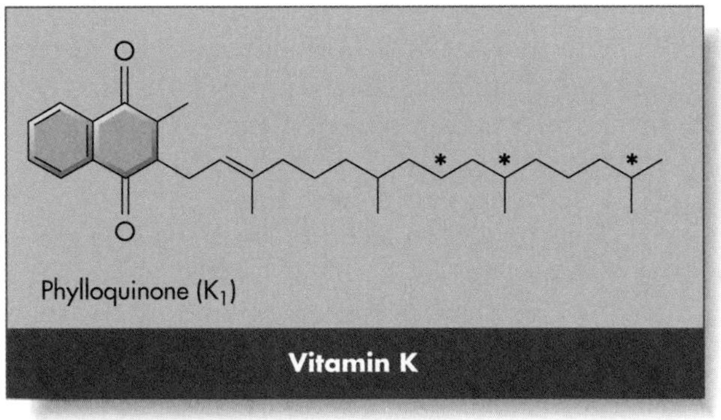

Phylloquinone (K_1)

Vitamin K

Vitamin K as phylloquinone. Menaquinones have a carbon-carbon double bond at the starred positions.

phylloquinone A form of vitamin K that comes from plants; also called vitamin K_1.

menaquinone A form of vitamin K found in fish oils and meats. It is also made by bacteria in the human intestine.

prothrombin One of the numerous proteins that participate in the formation of blood clots. Conversion of its precursor protein to the active blood-clotting factor in the liver requires vitamin K.

osteocalcin A protein produced in bone that is thought to bind calcium; the synthesis of osteocalcin is aided by vitamin K.

The family of compounds known as vitamin K includes **phylloquinone** (vitamin K_1) from plants and a family of **menaquinones** (vitamin K_2) found in fish oils and meats. The menaquinones are also synthesized by bacteria in the human intestine.[10]

Absorption, Transport, Storage, and Excretion of Vitamin K

It appears that up to 80% of dietary vitamin K as phylloquinone and menaquinone is taken up by cells that line the small intestine and is incorporated into chylomicrons. The process requires bile and pancreatic enzymes. The menaquinones synthesized by bacteria in the colon are absorbed, but the amount absorbed likely provides only 10% of the vitamin K we need. Some vitamin K is stored in the liver and some is incorporated in the lipoproteins VLDL, LDL, and HDL for transport throughout the body. Mineral oil and other nonabsorbable lipids interfere with vitamin K absorption, so their use close to meals should be discouraged. Most vitamin K excretion occurs via the bile, with a small amount of excretion via the urine.[10]

Functions of Vitamin K

Vitamin K is needed for the synthesis of seven blood-clotting factors by the liver (Figure 9-13). Vitamin K is required for the conversion of some precursor proteins to the active clotting factors. In these reactions, carbon dioxide (CO_2) is added to a glutamic acid in the precursor protein, yielding the active factor containing the unique amino acid gamma-carboxyglutamic acid. Proteins that have undergone this conversion are called Gla proteins, where "Gla" stands for gamma-carboxyglutamic acid. One

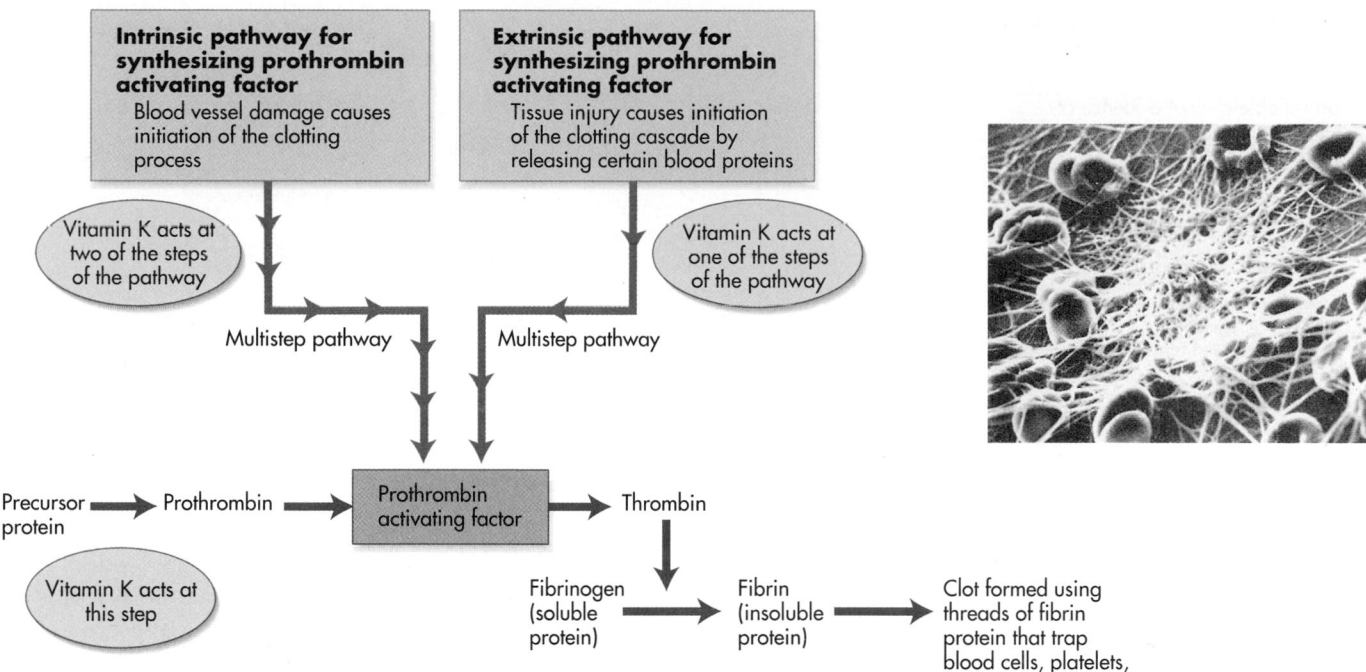

Figure 9-13 | Vitamin K metabolism. Forming a blood clot requires the participation of vitamin K in both the intrinsic and extrinsic blood-clotting pathways. Note that although the two pathways are activated by different events, there is some overlap in the pathways, but for simplicity we have not shown that. Vitamin K specifically imparts calcium-binding capacity to the proteins in these pathways, as in the conversion of a precursor protein to prothrombin, an active clotting factor.

example of this process is the conversion of a precursor protein to **prothrombin,** a participant in both pathways of the blood-clotting cascade. All these vitamin K–dependent clotting proteins depend on calcium interaction with gamma-carboxyglutamic acid to participate in the clotting reaction.[10]

In the body, vitamin K is converted to an inactive form once it has acted. It must then be reactivated for its biological action to persist. The body reactivates vitamin K readily. However, drugs such as warfarin, which strongly inhibit this reactivation process, act as powerful anticoagulants. People taking warfarin to lessen blood clotting should not consume vitamin K supplements and should have a consistent vitamin K intake.

Vitamin K also participates in the conversion of protein-bound glutamic acid residues to gamma-carboxyglutamic acid residues and the synthesis of two bone Gla proteins. The first protein is **osteocalcin,** secreted by bone-building cells. The second bone protein, called matrix Gla protein, is found in the protein matrix of bone. Low concentrations of circulating vitamin K have been associated with low bone mineral density.[12] It may be that inadequate intake of vitamin K increases the risk of hip fracture in women.[10] Finally, vitamin K may also participate in various blood vessel functions.

Dietary Sources of Vitamin K

Good food sources of vitamin K are liver, green leafy vegetables (e.g., kale, turnip greens, salad greens, cabbage, and spinach), broccoli, peas, and green beans. One reason to consume a diet rich in green vegetables is to obtain sufficient vitamin K. Other sources are vegetable oils, such as soy and canola. Vitamin K also is quite resistant to cooking losses.

Vitamin K Needs

For adult women the Adequate Intake for vitamin K is 90 μg/day, and for adult men the amount is 120 μg/day. These Adequate Intakes are based on the amount adults usually consume.[10] The Daily Value used on food and supplement labels for vitamin K is 80 μg. Average consumption is 60 to 200 μg/day, with men showing higher intakes.

Food Sources of Vitamin K	
Food Item and Amount	Vitamin K (μg)
Cooked kale, 1/2 cup	530
Cooked turnip greens, 1 cup	520
Cooked spinach, 1 cup	480
Cooked brussels sprouts, 1/2 cup	150
Raw Spinach, 1 cup	144
Cooked asparagus 1 cup	144
Cooked broccoli, 1/2 cup	110
Looseleaf lettuce, 1 cup	97
Cooked green beans, 1/2 cup	49
Raw cabbage, 1 cup	42
Sauerkraut, 1/2 cup	30
Green peas, 1/2 cup	26
Soybean oil, 1 tbsp	25
Cooked cauliflower, 1 cup	20
Canola oil, 1 tbsp	17
Adequate Intake for adult men, 120 μg; for adult women, 90 μg	

The most reliable clinical evidence of vitamin K deficiency is an increase in clotting time, which is a measure of how quickly prothrombin in the blood can form a clot. The actual vitamin K and prothrombin concentration in the blood can also be measured.

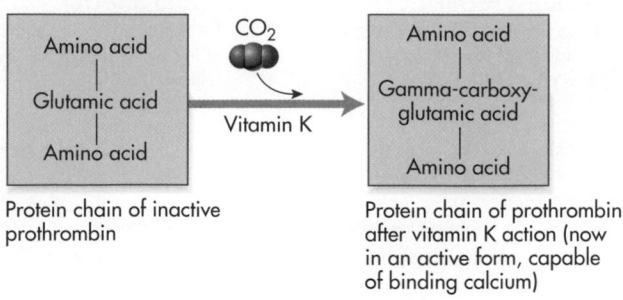

Protein chain of inactive prothrombin

Protein chain of prothrombin after vitamin K action (now in an active form, capable of binding calcium)

Vitamin K-Deficiency Diseases

A deficiency of vitamin K most likely occurs when a person takes certain types of antibiotics that disrupt vitamin K metabolism or has impaired fat absorption.[10]

Vitamin K deficiency also can occur in newborns. Their vitamin K stores are typically low at birth. Infants are at risk of defective blood clotting and eventual hemorrhage because of a lack of vitamin K. To prevent this possible vitamin K deficiency, physicians in North America routinely provide vitamin K by injections within 6 hours of delivery. Finally, some older people may be at risk of deficiency because of scant green vegetable intake.

Laboratory animal studies have shown that excessive amounts of vitamin A and vitamin E are known to antagonize the actions of vitamin K.[3,10] Vitamin A is thought to interfere with the absorption of vitamin K from the intestine. Large doses of vitamin E can lead to a decrease in vitamin K–dependent clotting factors and increased bleeding tendency. In either case, megadose supplements of these vitamins may pose a risk to vitamin K status, as noted in this chapter's discussions of upper levels for these vitamins.

The fat-soluble vitamins are reviewed in Table 9-2.

Most vitamin K consumed in a day disappears from the body in the next few days. Thus, no Upper Level for vitamin K has been set.

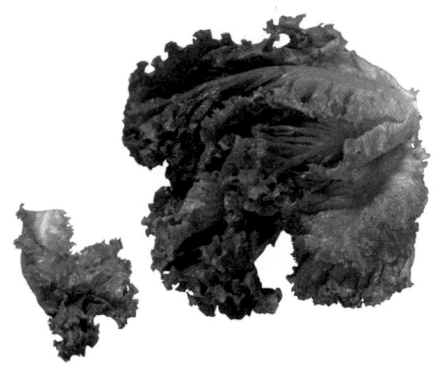

A salad containing dark greens (or other green vegetables) each day provides abundant vitamin K for a diet.

Critical | Thinking

Tim was diagnosed as having blood clots in his leg and has been using anticoagulant medications for 2 months. On examination, the doctor is surprised to find that the clots he expected to have dissolved are still there. What is a possible nutritional explanation for this finding?

Concept | Check

Vitamin K is important for blood clotting because it stimulates the conversion of precursor proteins to active clotting factors, such as prothrombin. This conversion involves the addition of carbon dioxide to glutamic acid in the precursor protein, yielding gamma-carboxyglutamic acid, which in turn can bind calcium. About 10% of the vitamin K we absorb every day comes from bacterial synthesis in the intestines, but most comes from the diet. The amount in the diet alone generally meets our needs. Thus, except for newborns and possibly some older people, a deficiency of vitamin K is unlikely, even though it is readily excreted from the body.

Table 9-2 | A Summary of the Fat-Soluble Vitamins: Their Functions, Deficiency Conditions, and Food Sources

Major Vitamin	Functions	Deficiency Symptoms	People at Risk	Sources	RDA or Adequate Intake	Toxicity Symptoms*
Vitamin A Preformed retinoids and provitamin A carotenoids	Vision in dim light and color vision, cell differentiation and growth, immunity	Poor growth, night blindness, blindness, dry skin, xerophthalmia	Rare in United States but common in preschool children living in poverty in developing countries, alcoholics	**Preformed vitamin A (retinoids):** liver, fortified milk, fish liver oils **Provitamin A (carotenoids):** red, orange, dark green, and yellow vegetables; orange fruits	700–900 μg RAE	Headache, vomiting, double vision, hair loss, dry mucous membranes, bone and joint pain, fractures, liver damage, hemorrhage, coma, teratogenic effects: spontaneous abortions, birth defects. Upper Level is 3000 μg of preformed vitamin A (10,000 IU), based on the risk of birth defects and liver toxicity.
Vitamin D Cholecalciferol D_3 Ergocalciferol D_2	Maintenance of intracellular and extracellular calcium concentrations	Rickets in children, osteomalacia in older adults	Dark-skinned individuals, older adults, breastfed infants	Vitamin D–fortified milk, fish oils	5–10 μg (200–400 IU) 15 μg > 70 yrs (600 IU)	Calcification of soft tissues, growth restriction, excess calcium excretion via the kidney. Upper Level is 50 μg (2000 IU), based on the risk of elevated blood calcium.
Vitamin E Tocopherols Tocotrienols	Antioxidant, prevention of propagation of free radicals	Hemolysis of red blood cells, degeneration of sensory neurons	Patients with fat-malabsorption syndromes, smokers (overt deficiency is rare)	Plant oils, seeds, nuts, products made from oils	15 mg alpha-tocopherol for men and women (22 IU natural form, 33 IU synthetic form)	Inhibition of vitamin K metabolism. Upper Level is 1000 mg (1100 IU synthetic form, 1500 IU natural form), based on the risk of hemorrhage.
Vitamin K Phylloquinone Menaquinone	Synthesis of blood-clotting factors and bone proteins	Hemorrhage, fractures	Those taking antibiotics for a long period of time, older adults with scant green vegetable intake	Green vegetables, liver, synthesis by intestinal microorganisms, some calcium supplements	90–120 μg	No Upper Level has been set.

*For vitamins D and E, toxicity is seen only with supplement use; foods pose no threat.

NUTRITION FOCUS

Nutrient Supplements: Who Needs Them and Why?

Because recent research on a variety of nutrient supplements has revealed a lack of product quality, the USP (United States Pharmacopeia) designation is being extended to an increasing number of nutrient supplements. The USP standards designate strength, quality, purity, packaging, labeling, speed of dissolution, and acceptable length of storage of ingredients for drugs. The purpose of applying them to vitamin and mineral supplements is to establish professionally accepted standards for these products. Consumers who buy nutrient supplements should look for a USP label when comparing similar products, such as calcium supplements. If no USP label is present, the next best approach is to purchase nationally advertised brands. Most brand name nutrient supplements aren't labeled USP because the manufacturers prefer to guarantee the products via their brand names.

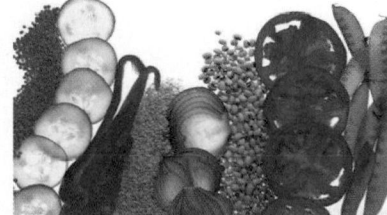

Focus first on foods that meet nutrient needs.

The term *multivitamin and mineral supplement* has been mentioned many times so far in this textbook. Often, these and other supplements are marketed as cures for anything and everything. This cure-all approach is promoted by the supplement industry and countless health-food stores, pharmacies, and supermarkets. Should you take a supplement? This decision is up to you. Currently, opinions vary even among knowledgeable scientists regarding the wisdom and safety of supplement use.[1,7,14,19]

According to the Dietary Supplement Health and Education Act of 1994 (discussed in Chapter 1), a supplement in the United States is a product intended to supplement the diet that bears or contains one or more of the following ingredients:

- A vitamin
- A mineral
- An herb or another botanical
- An amino acid
- A dietary substance to supplement the diet, which could be an extract or a combination of the first four ingredients in this list

The definition is very broad and covers a wide variety of nutritional substances. The use of dietary supplements is a common practice among North Americans and generates about $17 billion annually for the industry in the United States alone.[1] Recall also from Chapter 1 that unless FDA has evidence that a supplement is inherently dangerous or marketed with an illegal claim, it will not regulate such products closely. (The vitamin folate is an exception.) Currently, FDA has limited resources to police supplement manufacturers, and it has to act against these manufacturers one at a time. Thus, we cannot rely on FDA to protect us from vitamin and mineral supplement overuse and misuse. We bear that responsibility ourselves, coupled with professional advice from a physician or registered dietitian.[1]

Currently, the supplement manufacturers can make broad claims about their products under the "structure or function" provision of the law. The manufacturers and their products, however, cannot claim to prevent, treat, or cure a disease. Because menopause in women and aging are not diseases per se, products alleging to treat symptoms of these conditions can be marketed without FDA approval.[1] For example, a product that claims to treat hot flashes arising during menopause can be sold without any evidence to prove that the product actually works, but a product that claims to decrease the risk of cardiovascular disease by reducing blood cholesterol must have results from scientific studies that justify the claim.

Why do people take supplements? Reasons that are frequently given include the following:

- To reduce susceptibility to health problems (e.g., colds)
- To prevent heart attacks
- To prevent cancer
- To reduce stress
- To increase "energy"

Recently the U.S. Preventive Services Task Force noted there is insufficient evidence to support the recommendation of use of a multivitamin and mineral supplement by the general population. They did not discourage the practice, however.[19] Two nutrition experts from Tufts University (Dr. Alice Lichtenstein and Dr. Robert Russel) found after a careful review of the scientific literature that nutrient supplements provided no health advantage to the average adult, but noted in some cases such use is appropriate (see the next section in this feature for specific examples).[14] On the other hand, over the last few years some reputable nutrition and medical scientists have recommended supplementation of specific nutrients for most (or all) adults.[7]

The rationale for widespread use is primarily because many North Americans have been unwilling to change their food habits, such as eating ample fruits, vegetables, and whole grains. This gap can leave diets low in the vitamin folate. Adequate folate status when a woman becomes pregnant helps reduce the risk of certain birth defects (400 μg/day of synthetic folic acid is recommended). Folate also limits homocysteine in the blood, a likely risk factor for cardiovascular disease that can affect all of us. In addition, the committee appointed by the Food and Nutrition Board that sets current nutrient standards for vitamin B-12 suggested that adults over age 50 consume vitamin B-12 in a synthetic form, such as that added to ready-to-eat breakfast cereals or present in supplements. Synthetic vitamin B-12 is more easily absorbed than that found in food; this helps compensate for the fall in vitamin B-12 absorption often seen in older adults.

Recently two articles in the *Journal of the American Medical Association* also supported the use of a daily balanced multivitamin and mineral supplement.[7] Still, these and other experts, whether they support use of a multivitamin and mineral supplement or not, emphasize that many of the health-promoting effects of foods cannot be found in a bottle. Recall the discussions of phytochemicals in Chapter 2 and the benefits of fiber in Chapter 5. Supplements may contain few or no phytochemicals and typically contain no fiber. Multivitamin and mineral supplements also contain little calcium in order to keep the pill size small, and the forms of magnesium, zinc, and copper used in many supplements (oxides) are not as well absorbed as forms found in foods.

Overall, supplement use cannot fix a poor diet in all respects. Uninformed megadose supplement use also can lead to harm—currently, most nutrient toxicity is a result of supplement use.[11] Thus, you are advised to first take a good look at your dietary habits and then improve them, as outlined in Chapter 2 (see also Figure 9-14). Then you should find out which nutrient gaps remain and identify food sources that can help. Such a source could be

ready-to-eat breakfast cereals to increase vitamin E, folic acid, and vitamin B-6 intake and to provide highly absorbable forms of vitamin B-12. Calcium-fortified orange juice could be used to increase calcium intake. Milk and yogurt intake could be increased to provide more vitamin D and calcium. You need to be careful with highly fortified foods, however, because eating these products may provide the appropriate amount of nutrients in 1 serving, but eating more than 1 serving can lead to an excessive intake of some nutrients, such as vitamin A, iron, and synthetic folic acid.

If you wish to use a supplement, discuss your decision with a physician or registered dietitian, because some supplements can interfere with certain medicines.[1,14] For example, vitamin B-6 can offset the action of L dopa (used in treating Parkinson's disease), high intakes of vitamin K or vitamin E alter the action of anticlotting medications, large doses of vitamin C can interfere with certain cancer therapy regimens, excessive zinc intake can inhibit copper absorption, and large amounts of folate can mask signs and symptoms of a vitamin B-12 deficiency. Remember, you *can* get too much of a good thing.[1]

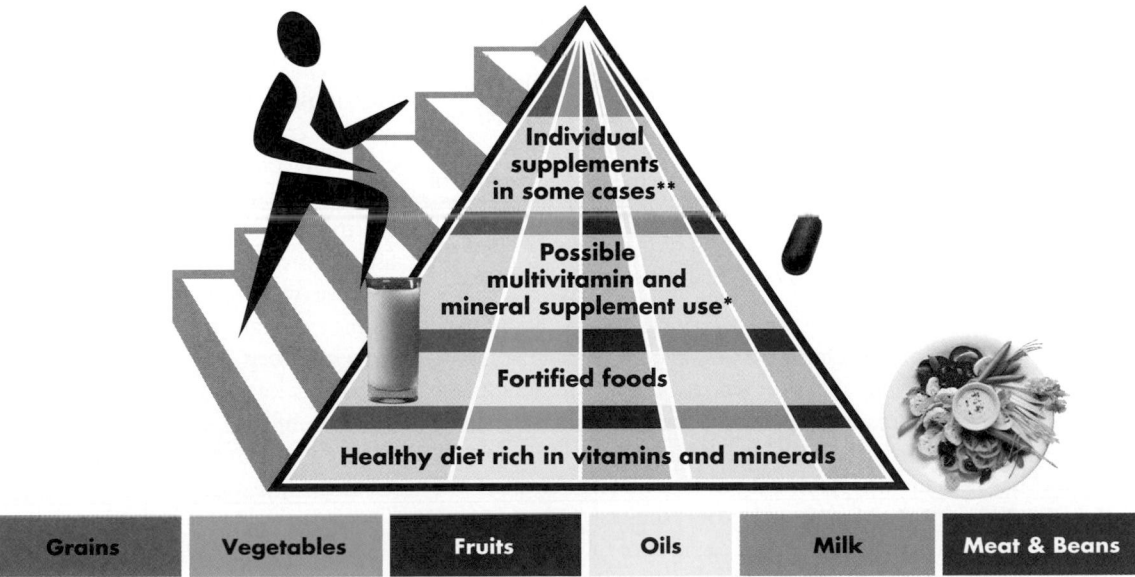

Figure 9-14 | Supplement savvy—A MyPyramid approach to the use of nutrient supplementation. Emphasizing the bottom portion of the pyramid is always the best option. Extra benefits include fiber, numerous phytochemicals, and omega-3 fatty acids.
*Men in general and older women should use iron-free formulas
**Iron and calcium supplements for younger women are two possible examples.

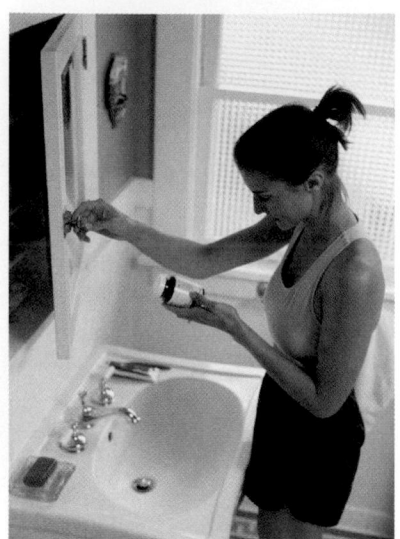

Long-term intake of just two times the Daily Value for some fat-soluble vitamins—particularly preformed vitamin A (retinoids)—can cause toxic effects. Know what you are taking if you use supplements.

As you might guess, generally the most healthy people in our population take supplements. Ironically, these are the people who least likely need to take supplements.[16]

People Most Likely to Need Supplements

Various medical and health-related organizations suggest that the following vitamin and mineral supplements can be important for certain groups of healthy people:[1,14,19]

- Women of childbearing age may need extra synthetic folic acid if their dietary patterns do not supply the recommended amount (400 μg/day).
- Women with excessive bleeding during menstruation may need extra iron.
- Women who are pregnant or breastfeeding may need extra iron, folate, and calcium.
- People with very low energy intakes (less than about 1200 kcal per day) may need a range of vitamins and minerals. This is true of some women and many older people.
- Strict vegans may need extra calcium, iron, zinc, and vitamin B-12.
- Newborns need a single dose of vitamin K, as directed by a physician.
- Some older infants may need fluoride supplements, as directed by a dentist.
- People with limited milk intake and sunlight exposure may need extra vitamin D. This includes breastfed infants and many older people.
- People with lactose maldigestion or intolerance, and those with allergies to dairy products, may need extra calcium.
- Adults over age 50 may need a synthetic source of vitamin B-12.
- People on very low fat diets or diets low in plant oils and nuts may need some extra vitamin E.

Individuals with certain medical conditions (e.g., vitamin-resistant diseases or long-standing fat malabsorption) and those who use certain medications also may require supplementation with specific vitamins and minerals. Children who are picky eaters may require supplementation as well (see Chapter 17). Finally, smokers and alcohol abusers may benefit from supplementation, but cessation of these two activities is far more beneficial than any supplementation.[4]

Which Supplement Should You Choose?

If you decide to take a multivitamin and mineral supplement, which one should you choose? As a start, choose a nationally recognized brand (from a supermarket or pharmacy) that contains about 100% of the Daily Values for the nutrients present. A multivitamin and mineral supplement should also generally be taken with or just after meals to maximize absorption. Make sure also that intake from the total of this supplement, any other supplements used, and highly fortified foods such as ready-to-eat breakfast cereals provide no more than the Upper Level for each vitamin and mineral. (See the inside cover of this textbook for Upper Levels.) This instruction is especially important with regard to preformed vitamin A (retinol) intake. Two exceptions to this upper limit cutoff are (1) both men and older women should make sure any product used is low in iron or iron-free to avoid possible iron overload (see Chapter 12 for details), and (2) somewhat exceeding the Upper Level for vitamin D is likely a safe practice for adults. Read the labels carefully to be sure of what you are taking (Figure 9-15).

Another consideration in choosing a supplement is avoiding superfluous ingredients, such as para-aminobenzoic acid (PABA), hesperidin complex, inositol, bee pollen, and lecithins. These compounds are not needed in our diets. They are especially common in expensive supplements sold in health-food stores and by mail. In addition, use of l-tryptophan and high doses of beta-carotene or fish oils is discouraged.

Five websites to help you evaluate ongoing claims and evaluate safety of supplements are:
www.acsh.org
www.quackwatch.com
www.ncahf.org
dietary-supplements.info.nih.gov
www.eatright.org
The sites are maintained by groups or individuals committed to providing reasoned and authoritative nutrition and health advice to consumers.

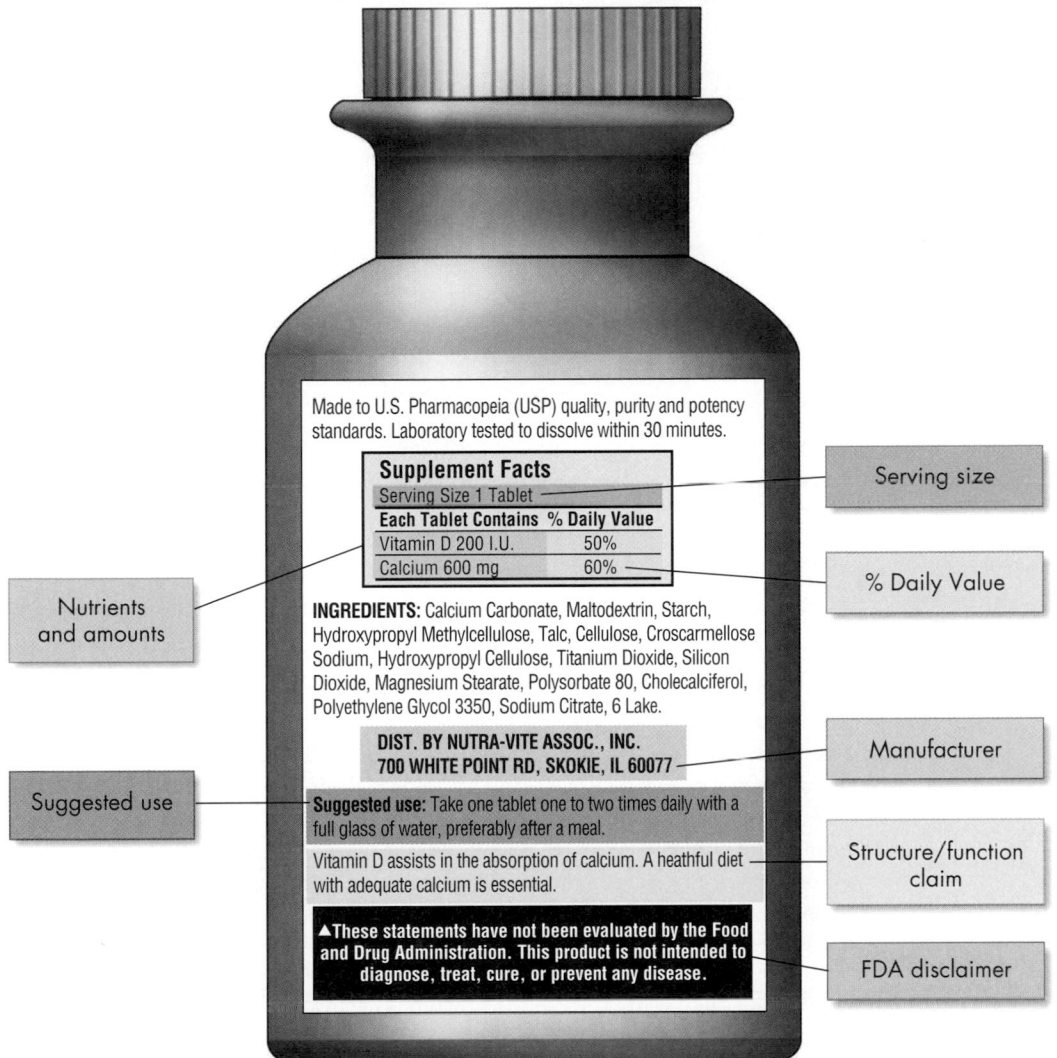

Made to U.S. Pharmacopeia (USP) quality, purity and potency standards. Laboratory tested to dissolve within 30 minutes.

Serving size

Supplement Facts

Serving Size 1 Tablet

Each Tablet Contains	% Daily Value
Vitamin D 200 I.U.	50%
Calcium 600 mg	60%

% Daily Value

Nutrients and amounts

INGREDIENTS: Calcium Carbonate, Maltodextrin, Starch, Hydroxypropyl Methylcellulose, Talc, Cellulose, Croscarmellose Sodium, Hydroxypropyl Cellulose, Titanium Dioxide, Silicon Dioxide, Magnesium Stearate, Polysorbate 80, Cholecalciferol, Polyethylene Glycol 3350, Sodium Citrate, 6 Lake.

DIST. BY NUTRA-VITE ASSOC., INC. 700 WHITE POINT RD, SKOKIE, IL 60077

Manufacturer

Suggested use

Suggested use: Take one tablet one to two times daily with a full glass of water, preferably after a meal.

Vitamin D assists in the absorption of calcium. A heathful diet with adequate calcium is essential.

Structure/function claim

▲These statements have not been evaluated by the Food and Drug Administration. This product is not intended to diagnose, treat, cure, or prevent any disease.

FDA disclaimer

Figure 9-15 | Nutrient supplements display a nutrition label that is different from that of foods. This Supplement Facts label must list the ingredient(s), amount(s) per serving, serving size, suggested use, and % Daily Value if one has been established. Note that this label also includes structure/function claims. Thus, it also must include the FDA warning that these claims have not been evaluated by the agency.

Use of *Nutramega* poses some health risks for Kristen. Taking 2 to 3 tablets every 3 hours would mean taking at least 16 tablets per day. This alone would provide an intake of vitamin A, vitamin C, and zinc well in excess of the Upper Levels for these nutrients. Intake of preformed vitamin A would be 1.3 times the Upper Level, intake of vitamin C would be 3.4 times the Upper Level, and intake of zinc would be 3 times the Upper Level. Intake of selenium, however, falls well below the Upper Level set for that nutrient. This is how the math works out:

Vitamin A

33% (0.33) times the Daily Value of 1000 μg RAE equals 330 μg RAE per tablet. Sixteen tablets would yield 5280 μg RAE. The Upper Level is 3000 μg RAE for preformed vitamin A. Because 75% of the vitamin A is preformed vitamin A, this yields 3960 μg RAE of preformed vitamin A (5280 × 0.75 = 3960), or 1.3 times the Upper Level (3960/3000 = 1.3).

Vitamin C

700% (7) times the Daily Value of 60 mg equals 420 mg per tablet. Sixteen tablets would yield 6720 mg. The Upper Level is 2000 mg. This would then yield 3.4 times the Upper Level (6720/2000 = 3.4).

Zinc

50% (0.5) times the Daily Value of 15 milligrams equals 7.5 mg per tablet. Sixteen tablets would yield 120 mg. The Upper Level is 40 mg. This would then yield 3 times the Upper Level (120/40 = 3).

Selenium

10% (0.1) times the Daily Value of 70 μg equals 7 μg per tablet. Sixteen tablets would yield 112 μg. This is less than the Upper Level of 400 μg.

The maintenance dose of two to three tablets per day poses no risk per se, but *Nutramega* is very expensive compared to the cost of the typical multivitamin and mineral supplement (a 1-month supply would cost about $2 compared to about $15 for *Nutramega*). Overall, Kristen is smart to be concerned about meeting her nutrient needs, but the stress she is under does not increase nutrient needs. A healthy diet, as shown in Table 2-11 in Chapter 2, should be her primary focus. Taking a balanced multivitamin and mineral supplement is also a reasonable practice. Actually, however, it is most important for Kristen to get adequate sleep; this health habit will best help her through her current schedule.

Summary

1. Vitamins are essential, organic compounds needed for important metabolic reactions in the body. They are not a source of energy. Instead, they promote many energy-yielding and other reactions in the body, thereby aiding in the growth, development, and maintenance of various body tissues. Vitamins A, D, E, and K are fat-soluble, whereas the B-vitamins and vitamin C are water-soluble. Fat-soluble vitamins are excreted less readily from the body and are less susceptible to cooking loss than are water-soluble vitamins.

2. Some fat-soluble vitamins pose a potential threat for toxicity, especially vitamin A. The water-soluble vitamins niacin, vitamin B-6, and vitamin C can also induce toxic signs and symptoms, but only at doses much higher than their RDAs.

3. Fat-soluble vitamins are absorbed along with dietary fat. They travel by way of the lymphatic system into general circulation, carried by chylomicrons. In disease states in which fat digestion is limited, fat-soluble vitamin status may be compromised, especially with vitamins A, E, and K.

4. Vitamin A consists of a family of retinoid compounds: retinal, retinol, and retinoic acid. A plant derivative known as beta-carotene, along with two other carotenoids, yields vitamin A after metabolism by the intestine or liver. Vitamin A contributes to the maintenance of vision, the proper development of cells (especially mucus-forming cells), and immune function. Vitamin A is found in foods of animal origin, such as liver, fish oils, and fortified milk. Carotenoids are obtained from plants and are especially plentiful in dark green and orange vegetables and in some fruits.

5. North Americans at risk for poor vitamin A status are people exhibiting limited fat absorption and alcoholics. Vitamin A can be quite toxic when taken at doses 2 to 4 times or more the RDA, but only with preformed vitamin A (retinoids). Use is especially dangerous during pregnancy because it can lead to fetal malformations.

6. For most people, vitamin D is more correctly viewed as a hormone rather than a vitamin because sufficient amounts of it can be produced by the body. Provitamin D_3 is synthesized in the skin from a derivative of cholesterol in a process that depends on ultraviolet light. With adequate sun exposure, no dietary intake of vitamin D is needed. The provitamin, whether produced in the skin or obtained from the diet, is metabolized in the liver and kidneys to yield $1,25(OH)_2$ vitamin D (or calcitriol), the active hormonal form of vitamin D. $1,25(OH)_2$ vitamin D is important for calcium absorption from the intestine, and with other hormones, it helps regulate bone metabolism. Vitamin D is found in fish oils and fortified milk.

7. Vitamin E functions as a chain-breaking antioxidant. By donating electrons to electron-seeking compounds (oxidizing agents), it neutralizes their action. One group of electron-seeking compounds, known as free radicals, can cause widespread destruction, both to cell membranes and to DNA. Vitamin E is one of several components in the body's defense system against such oxidizing agents. Vitamin E is plentiful in plant oils and food products that contain these oils. Overt vitamin E deficiency is rare; marginal status is usually associated with problems in fat absorption and smoking. To date, the use of megadose supplements of vitamin E by healthy adults to limit cardiovascular disease risk (and certain other health problems) is still a research question. Use in high-risk people has been proven ineffective in major clinical trials. Toxicity from megadose therapy involves inhibition of vitamin K activity and, correspondingly, an increased risk of hemorrhage.

8. Vitamin K contributes to the body's blood-clotting ability by facilitating the conversion of precursor proteins to active clotting factors, such as prothrombin, which promotes blood coagulation. Vitamin K also plays a role in bone metabolism. About 10% of the vitamin K absorbed each day likely comes from bacterial synthesis in the intestine; most comes from foods, primarily green leafy vegetables and vegetable oils. Vitamin K is readily excreted from the body, but the usual daily intake from diet alone meets one's needs.

9. Taking a multivitamin and mineral supplement to help meet nutrient needs is recommended by some experts, while other experts suggest that only some people need to take supplements. Taking many nutrient supplements can lead to nutrient-related toxicity, so any such use should be carefully considered. The clearest evidence for good nutrition is a diet rich in fruits and vegetables and whole-grain breads and cereals, not a primary reliance on supplements.

Study Questions

1. Describe two forms of vitamin A that are available in common foods.
2. Explain how retinal functions in vision.
3. Describe how retinoic acid participates in protein synthesis.
4. What factors determine whether a person needs a dietary source of vitamin D or can rely on self-synthesis?
5. Describe how vitamin D, parathyroid hormone, and calcitonin regulate the concentration of calcium in the blood.
6. Define a free radical and explain how vitamin E controls free radical damage.
7. List several important dietary sources for each of the fat-soluble vitamins. Identify the Adequate Intake or RDA and the Upper Level for each of the fat-soluble vitamins.
8. Identify the two primary functions of vitamin K in the body.
9. What properties of vitamin A make it a greater risk for toxicity than vitamin K?
10. Identify the North Americans most at risk for fat-soluble vitamin deficiencies.

BOOST YOUR STUDY

Check out the **Perspectives in Nutrition: Online Learning Center** www.mhhe.com/wardlawpers7 for quizzes, flash cards, activities, and web links designed to further help you learn about the fat-soluble vitamins.

Annotated References

1. ADA Reports: Position of the American Dietetic Association: Fortification and nutritional supplements. *Journal of the American Dietetic Association* 105:1300, 2005.

   The best nutritional strategy for promoting optimal health and reducing the risk of chronic disease is to wisely choose a wide variety of foods. Additional vitamins and minerals from fortified foods and/or supplements can help some people meet their nutritional needs as set by science-based nutrition standards (e.g., the Dietary Reference Intakes).

2. Bischoff-Ferrari HA and others: Fracture prevention with vitamin D supplementation. *Journal of the American Medical Association* 293:2257, 2005.

   Providing about 800 IU/day of vitamin D to older adults reduced the risk of hip fracture in this study. It appears that 400 IU/day is not sufficient to provide the same benefit.

3. Booth SL and others: Effect of vitamin E supplementation on vitamin K status in adults with normal coagulation status. *American Journal of Clinical Nutrition* 80:143, 2004.

   Supplementation with high doses of vitamin E decreased the synthesis of prothrombin, a vitamin K–dependent protein. Further research is required to elucidate the importance of the inhibitory effect that vitamin E has on vitamin K status.

4. Bruno RS and others: Alpha-tocopherol disappearance is faster in cigarette smokers and is inversely related to their ascorbic acid status. *American Journal of Clinical Nutrition* 81:95, 2005.

   Greater rates of alpha-tocopherol disappearance in smokers appear to be related to increased oxidative stress and by lower blood vitamin C (ascorbic acid) concentrations. Thus, smokers have an increased requirement for both alpha-tocopherol and ascorbic acid.

5. Dawson-Hughes B: Racial/ethnic considerations in making recommendations for vitamin D for adult and elderly men and women. *American Journal of Clinical Nutrition* 80(suppl):1763S, 2004.

   In the winter months, broad-based vitamin D supplementation to 1000 IU/day may be needed to attain adequate vitamin D status in adults. This recommendation would especially benefit black adults.

6. DeLuca HF: Overview of general physiologic features and functions of Vitamin D. *American Journal of Clinical Nutrition* 80:1689S, 2004.

   Vitamin D₃ is a prohormone produced in skin through ultraviolet irradiation of 7-dehydrocholesterol. It is biologically inert and must be metabolized in the liver, then in the kidney, before function. The hormonal form of vitamin D₃ acts through a receptor on the cell nucleus to carry out its many functions, including calcium absorption, phosphate absorption, calcium mobilization in bone, and calcium reabsorption in the kidney. Vitamin D also has several non-calcium-related functions in the body. This overview provides a brief description of the physiologic, endocrinologic, and molecular characteristics of vitamin D.

7. Fairfield K, Fletcher R: Vitamins for chronic disease prevention in adults: Scientific review and clinical applications. *Journal of the American Medical Association* 287:3116, 2002, and 287:3127, 2002.

   While vitamin deficiency diseases are no longer common in North America, many physicians are suggesting that marginal intakes of many vitamins and minerals by some North Americans may increase the risk of developing some chronic diseases, including cancer and cardiovascular disease. To help ensure optimal intakes of most of the vitamins and minerals, the authors recommend that adult North Americans consume a daily multivitamin and mineral supplement.

8. Food and Nutrition Board, Institute of Medicine: *Dietary Reference Intakes for calcium, phosphorus, magnesium, vitamin D, and fluoride.* Washington, DC: National Academy Press, 1997.

   The RDAs and related standards for vitamin D and some minerals are discussed in detail. A major change in setting these new (and all other) estimates of human needs is the use of a specific biological marker or estimate of current intakes that shows adequacy.

9. Food and Nutrition Board, Institute of Medicine: *Dietary Reference Intakes for vitamin C, vitamin E, selenium, and carotenoids.* Washington, DC: National Academy Press, 2000.

   The functions of antioxidant nutrients, how RDA and related standards were determined, and deficiency and toxicity symptoms are explained. This is the definitive report by the panel of experts on nutrient needs for dietary antioxidants.

10. Food and Nutrition Board, Institute of Medicine: *Dietary Reference Intakes for vitamin A, vitamin K, arsenic, boron, chromium, copper, iodine, iron, manganese, molybdenum, nickel, silicon, and zinc.* Washington, DC: National Academy Press, 2001.

    Recommendations for vitamin A and vitamin K intake are listed. The rationale used to set the RDA or Adequate Intake and Upper Level for these nutrients is discussed in detail.

11. Hatun S and others: Subclinical vitamin D deficiency is increased in adolescent girls who wear concealing clothing. *Journal of Nutrition* 135:218, 2005.

    Vitamin D deficiency is an important problem in Turkish adolescent girls, especially those who follow a religious dress code in which the body remains essentially covered. Vitamin D supplementation appears to be necessary for these adolescent girls.

12. Kalkwarf HJ and others: Vitamin K, bone turnover, and bone mass in girls. *American Journal of Clinical Nutrition* 80:1075, 2004.

    Better vitamin K status is associated with decreased bone turnover in healthy girls consuming a typical U.S. diet. Randomized trials are needed to further understand the potential benefits of vitamin K on bone acquisition in growing children.

13. Lee I and others: Vitamin E in the primary prevention of cardiovascular disease and cancer: The women's health study: A randomized controlled trial. *Journal of the American Medical Association* 294:56, 2005.

    The data from this large trial indicated that 600 IU of natural-source vitamin E taken every other day provided no overall benefit for major cardiovascular events or cancer. These data do not support recommending vitamin E supplementation for cardiovascular disease or cancer prevention among healthy women, but more research is warranted, because a decrease in sudden cardiac death was seen in a subset of older women in this study.

14. Lichtenstein AH, Russell RM: Essential nutrients: Food or supplements? Where should the emphasis be? *Journal of the American Medical Association* 294:351, 2005.

    There is insufficient evidence to justify a shift in public health policy from one that emphasizes a food-based diet to fulfill nutrient requirements and promote optimal health to one that emphasizes dietary supplementation. Targeted nutrient supplementation is appropriate in some cases, however, as reviewed by these authors.

15. Maras JE and others: Intake of a-Tocopherol is limited among U.S. adults. *Journal of the American Dietetic Association* 104:567, 2004.

    Vitamin E consumption in the United States does not generally meet the current RDA. Greater use of nuts, seeds, whole-grain breads and cereals, and vitamin E–rich plant oils is advocated to close the gap between intakes and needs.

16. McNaughton SA and others: Supplement use is associated with health status and health-related behaviors in the 1946 British birth cohort. *Journal of Nutrition* 135:1782, 2005.

    The healthiest individuals in this large group of people studied were the ones most likely to be taking supplements. This finding suggests that the people who actually benefit the least from the practice of taking supplements are the very people who are taking the supplements.

17. Osganian SK and others: Dietary carotenoids and the risk of coronary artery disease. *American Journal of Clinical Nutrition* 77:1390, 2003.

    Regular intake of foods rich in carotenoids is associated with a reduction in the risk of coronary artery disease. The authors conclude that greater consumption of fruits and vegetables in general remains an important public health policy recommendation.

18. Ribaya-Mercado JD, Blumberg JB: Lutein and zeaxanthin and their potential roles in disease prevention. *Journal of the American College of Nutrition* 23:6:567S, 2004.

    Lutein and zeaxanthin are carotenoids found particularly in dark-green leafy vegetables and in egg yolks. They are widely distributed in tissues and are the principal carotenoids in the eye lens and macular region of the retina. Epidemiologic studies indicating an inverse relationship between lutein and zeaxanthin intake and status and both cataract and age-related macular degeneration suggest that these compounds can play a protective role in the eye. Some studies show that lutein and zeaxanthin may also help reduce the risk of breast cancer, lung cancer, heart disease, and stroke.

19. U.S. Preventive Services Task Force: Routine vitamin supplementation to prevent cancer and cardiovascular disease: Recommendations and rationale. *Annals of Internal Medicine* 139:51, 2003.

    The health benefits of nutrient supplementation remain uncertain, whereas much evidence supports a diet high in fruit, vegetables, and legumes. Currently the clearest use of supplements is that of folic acid for the prevention of neural tube defects that develop during pregnancy. Other potential benefits of supplementation, such as a lowering of blood homocysteine, need to be established by further studies.

20. Vitamin A: "Magic bullet" that can backfire. *Tufts University Health and Nutrition Letter,* p. 4, February 2005.

    Vitamin A and its derivatives (e.g., beta-carotene) are micronutrients crucial to growth, immune function, reproductive processes, and cell physiology. While it is well-known that very high doses of vitamin A are toxic, it now appears that even moderately high doses can increase chances of birth defects, of liver disease, and possibly of hip fractures in postmenopausal women. In the United States, the only people for whom vitamin A supplements are warranted are those who have chronic GI tract diseases that lead to difficulty in absorbing nutrients.

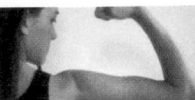

I. Preservation of Vitamins in Foods

Substantial amounts of vitamins in foods can be lost from the time a fruit or vegetable is picked until it is eaten. Heat, light, exposure to the air, cooking in water, and alkalinity are all factors that can destroy vitamins. The sooner a food is eaten after harvest, the less chance there is of nutrient loss. The following list provides some tips to aid in preserving the vitamins in food. How many of these suggestions do you employ on a regular basis?

What to Do	Why
■ Keep fruits and vegetables cool.	Enzymes in food begin to degrade vitamins once the fruit or vegetable is picked. Chilling reduces this process. Refrigerate fresh produce (except for potatoes, tomatoes, onions, and bananas) until consumed.
■ Refrigerate foods in moisture-proof, air-tight containers.	Nutrients keep best at temperatures near freezing, at high humidity, and away from air.
■ Trim, peel, and cut fruits and vegetables minimally—just enough to remove rotten or inedible parts.	Oxygen breaks down vitamins faster when more surface is exposed. Outer leaves of lettuce and other greens have more vitamins and minerals than the inner, tender leaves or stems. Potato skins and apple skins have more vitamins and minerals than the inner parts.
■ Microwave, steam, or use a pan or wok with very small amounts of fat and a tight-fitting lid to cook vegetables.	More nutrients are retained when there is less contact with water and shorter cooking time. Whenever possible, cook fruits or vegetables in their skins.
■ Minimize reheating food.	Prolonged reheating reduces vitamin content.
■ Avoid adding fats to vegetables during cooking if you plan to discard the liquid.	Fat-soluble vitamins will be lost in discarded fat. If you want to add fats to vegetables, do so after they are fully cooked and drained.
■ Avoid adding baking soda to vegetables to enhance the green color.	Alkalinity destroys much vitamin D, thiamin, and other vitamins.
■ Use frozen rather than canned fruits and vegetables.	Freezing helps retain vitamin content much better than canning. In fact, frozen vegetables are often as nutrient-rich as fresh-picked ones.
■ Store canned foods in a cool place and use them wisely.	Canned foods vary in the amount of nutrients lost, largely because of differences in storage time and temperatures. To obtain maximal nutritive value from canned goods, serve any liquid packed with the food whenever possible.

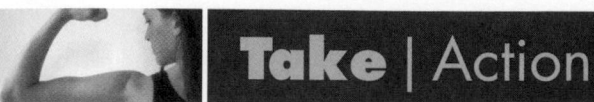

Take | Action

II. A Closer Look at Supplement Use

With the current popularity of vitamin and mineral supplements, it is more important than ever to understand how to evaluate a supplement. Study the label of a supplement you use, or one readily available from a friend or the supermarket. Then answer the following questions.

1. What is the recommended dosage of this supplement?

_____

_____

_____

2. Based on the recommended dosage, are there any individual vitamins for which the intake would be greater than 100% of the Daily Value? List these vitamins.

_____

_____

_____

3. Are any suggested intakes above the Upper Level for the nutrient?

_____

_____

_____

4. Are there any superfluous ingredients, such as herbs or flavors, in the supplement? You can often determine these by looking for ingredients that do not have a percent of Daily Value.

_____

_____

_____

5. Does at least 50% of the vitamin A in the product come from beta-carotene or other provitamin A carotenoids (to reduce risk of preformed vitamin A toxicity)?

_____

_____

_____

6. Are there any warnings on the label as to populations who should not consume this product?

_____

_____

_____

7. Are there any other signs that tip you off that this product may not be safe?

_____

_____

_____

THE WATER-SOLUBLE VITAMINS

CASE SCENARIO:

Suzanne and Ted are planning to have their first child. Ted (who completed one university-level nutrition course) has been trying to persuade Suzanne to eat a folic acid–rich breakfast cereal or take a multivitamin-mineral supplement every morning. Ted is concerned because Suzanne's sister gave birth to a child with spina bifida last year. Suzanne doesn't like to be hassled about her eating habits but admits her diet is "awful." Breakfast is usually a sweet pastry and coffee, lunch is whatever snack is available from a vending machine, and dinner is frequently eaten at a fast-food restaurant. She consumes no more than one or two servings of fruits and vegetables per day.

Is Ted correct in his concern? How concerned should Suzanne be, especially given her current diet?

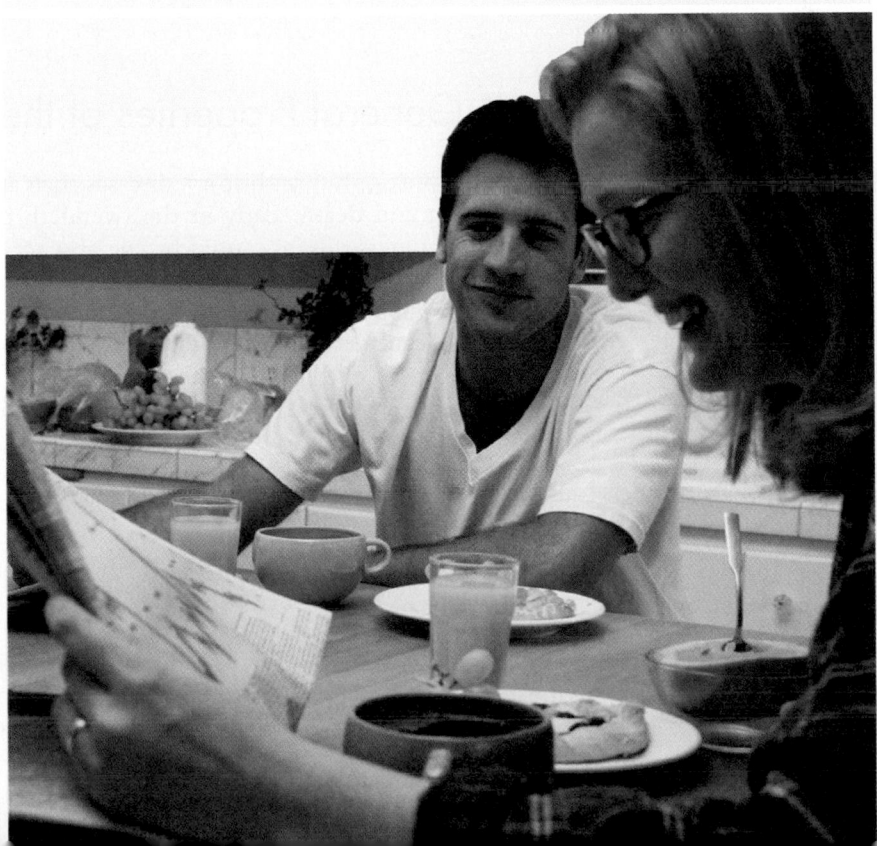

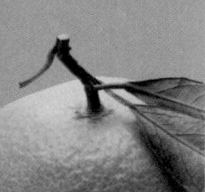

As defined in Chapter 9, vitamins are essential organic substances needed in very small amounts to support the metabolism, growth, and maintenance of cells. The water-soluble vitamins discussed in this chapter include eight B-vitamins, vitamin C, and a newcomer to the list of important nutrients, a dietary component called choline. The B-vitamins form coenzymes—organic compounds that enable certain enzymes to function. As a group, the B-vitamins are necessary for energy metabolism, transforming nutrients into characteristic cell structures and creating various proteins, lipids, and carbohydrates.[11] Vitamin C participates in a wide variety of metabolic processes, although not in the form of a coenzyme.[12] Choline is needed to form lecithin and other compounds.[29]

The Nutrition Focus briefly describes some vitamin-like compounds. People may require these compounds in their diets under atypical circumstances. These compounds, however, currently are not classified as true vitamins both because a healthy person does not require a dietary source of them and because no specific deficiency disease results when they are absent from the diet.[8]

CHAPTER OBJECTIVES CHAPTER 10 IS DESIGNED TO ALLOW YOU TO:

1. Identify the water-soluble vitamins.
2. List the major functions and deficiency symptoms for each water-soluble vitamin.
3. List three important food sources for each water-soluble vitamin.
4. Describe toxicity symptoms from excess consumption of certain water-soluble vitamins.
5. Distinguish between vitamins and nonvitamins, such as inositol and taurine.

REFRESH YOUR MEMORY AS YOU BEGIN YOUR STUDY OF THE WATER-SOLUBLE VITAMINS, YOU WILL WANT TO REVIEW:

- The gastrointestinal system for the digestion and absorption of nutrients in Chapter 3.
- Energy metabolism, especially glycolysis, the citric acid cycle, and the electron transport chain in Chapter 4.
- Oxidation-reduction reactions in Chapter 4.
- The metabolism of carbohydrates in Chapter 4.
- Amino acid metabolism and the link between DNA and protein synthesis in Chapter 7.

General Properties of the Water-Soluble Vitamins

For most of human history, diseases such as scurvy and pellagra caused enormous suffering and death. Early in the twentieth century, scientists began to recognize that these illnesses were caused by the absence of certain vital substances from the diet—now called the B-vitamins and vitamin C.[11,12] The scientists discovered that restoring these vitamins to the diet dramatically reversed these deficiency diseases if done before significant deterioration of the body took place.

The second vitamin to be discovered was designated vitamin B, according to the letter convention discussed in Chapter 9. This water-soluble substance, which can cure **beriberi,** was initially thought to be a single chemical compound. When subsequent research showed that this substance actually consists of several compounds, they were named the B-vitamins, and numbers were added to the letter B to distinguish them. Of the eight B-vitamins, only two are still commonly referred to by letter and number: vitamin B-6 and vitamin B-12. The others now are usually referred to by the following names: thiamin (previously B-1), riboflavin (previously B-2), niacin (previously B-3), pantothenic acid, biotin, and folate. The older designations, however, are sometimes used on vitamin supplement labels.

All B-vitamins function as **coenzymes.**[11] This classification falls under the general term **cofactor,** which also includes inorganic ions. Cofactors as a class are necessary for

beriberi The thiamin-deficiency disorder characterized by muscle weakness, loss of appetite, nerve degeneration, and sometimes edema.

coenzyme A compound that combines with an inactive protein, called an apoenzyme, to form a catalytically active protein, called a holoenzyme. In this manner, coenzymes aid in enzyme function.

cofactor An organic or inorganic substance that binds to a specific region on an enzyme and is necessary for the enzyme's activity.

certain enzymatic reactions to take place. Coenzymes specifically are molecules consisting of a vitamin, such as a B-vitamin, plus other chemical units. The body can make the other units and put the coenzyme together, but cannot make the B-vitamin. Because coenzymes fall under the cofactor designation, they also work with certain body enzymes to allow chemical reactions in a cell to proceed (Figure 10-1). All the eight B-vitamins participate in energy metabolism; some also have other roles in the chemical reactions that take place within cells.[11] Although vitamin C does not function as a coenzyme, it plays a role in the synthesis of several important compounds.[19]

The B-vitamins are present in foods in their coenzyme forms bound to specific proteins. After ingestion, the bound vitamin coenzymes are released as part of the general digestive processes that occur in the stomach and small intestine. The free vitamins are then absorbed in the small intestine.

Typically, about 50 to 90% of the B-vitamins in the diet are absorbed.[11] Once inside cells, the coenzyme forms of the vitamins are resynthesized. Health-food stores sell the coenzyme forms of some vitamins, although they have no specific benefits to the consumer, because vitamins are not absorbed in this form.

Because they are water soluble, most of the B-vitamins and vitamin C are more easily excreted from the body than are the fat-soluble vitamins.[8] Moreover, some of the water-soluble vitamins are readily destroyed during cooking because of heat or alkalinity; all are subject to leaching into the cooking water. Retention of the B-vitamins and vitamin C is greatest in foods that are prepared by steaming, stir-frying, microwaving, or simmering in minimal moisture (review the first Take Action in Chapter 9).

B-Vitamin and Vitamin C Status of North Americans

The nutritional status of most North Americans with respect to the B-vitamins and vitamin C is generally good. Our typical diets contain ample and varied natural sources of these vitamins.[11,12] In addition, many common foods are enriched or fortified with one or more of the water-soluble vitamins. (Table 2-14 in Chapter 2 reviewed the proper use of the terms *enriched* and *fortified*.) In some developing countries, however, deficiencies of the water-soluble vitamins are more common, and the resulting deficiency diseases pose significant public health problems. (A detailed discussion of nutritional deficiencies worldwide is presented in Chapter 20.)

Despite the generally good B-vitamin and vitamin C status of North Americans, marginal deficiencies of the water-soluble vitamins may occur, especially in smokers and older adults.[11,12] Another group that is susceptible to B-vitamin deficiencies is alcoholics. The extremely unbalanced diets of some people with alcoholism, in combination with alcohol-induced alteration of vitamin absorption and metabolism, create a significant risk.[11] (Chapter 8 covered this topic in detail.) The long-term effects of marginal deficiencies are as yet unknown, but increased risk of cardiovascular disease, cancer, and cataracts of the eye is suspected. However, in the short run, marginal deficiency in most people likely leads only to fatigue or other bothersome and unspecific signs and symptoms.[11,12]

Enrichment and Fortification of Foods with B-Vitamins

In the milling of grains, the seeds are crushed and the germ, bran, and husk layers are removed. This process leaves just the starch-containing endosperm, which is used to make flour, bread, and cereal products. Because the discarded fractions are rich in many nutrients, this time-honored milling process leads to loss of vitamins and minerals.

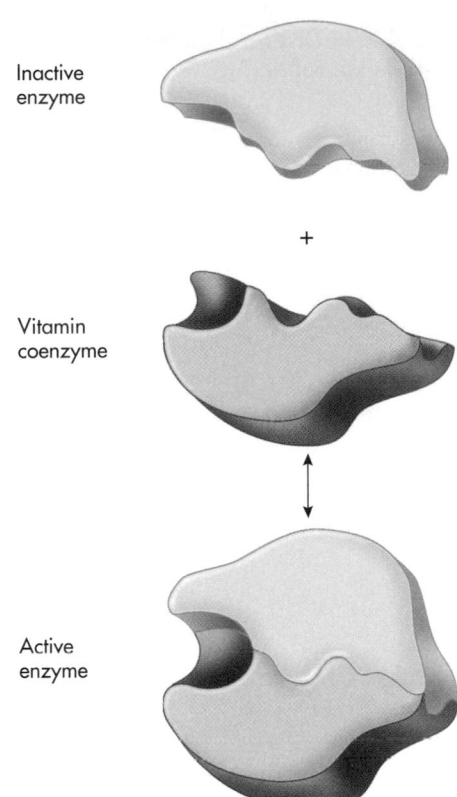

Inactive enzyme

Vitamin coenzyme

Active enzyme

Figure 10-1 | The enzyme-coenzyme interaction. The B-vitamins form coenzymes, which are compounds that enable specific enzymes to function.

Because of their role in energy metabolism, needs for many B vitamins increase somewhat as energy expenditure increases. Still, this is not a major concern because this increase in energy expenditure usually results in a corresponding increase in food intake, which contributes more B vitamins to a diet.

The Whole-Grain Advantage (whole vs. refined)

Bread:		
vitamin E	↑	17%
vitamin B-6	↑	60%
potassium	↑	92%
magnesium	↑	70%
fiber	↑	66%
Rice:		
vitamin E	↑	800%
vitamin B-6	↑	93%
potassium	↑	280%
magnesium	↑	450%
fiber	↑	550%

To counteract this nutrient loss, for many years bread and cereal products made from milled grains have been enriched with four B-vitamins—thiamin, riboflavin, niacin, and folic acid—and with the mineral iron. This enrichment program has helped protect North Americans from the common deficiency diseases associated with a dietary lack of the added nutrients.[11] This practice, however, still leaves the products with less vitamin B-6, vitamin E, magnesium, and zinc (and fiber) than that present in the whole grains. Nutrition experts therefore advocate the regular consumption of whole-grain products, such as whole-wheat bread, rather than enriched grain products.

Another reason not to depend too much on enriched foods for vitamins is that whole grains, as well as fruits and vegetables, contain many phytochemicals. Phytochemicals are not vitamins, nor even absolutely essential nutrients. However, they may still be helpful to good health (e.g., they may decrease the risk of certain diseases, such as cataracts in the eyes[7]). Recall that phytochemicals were mentioned in Chapter 2, where a list of examples of phytochemical compounds was given.

Thiamin

Thiamin consists of a central carbon to which is attached a six-member nitrogen-containing ring and a five-member sulfur-containing ring. The name comes from *thio*, meaning "sulfur," and *amine*, referring to the nitrogen groups in the molecule. In modern spelling, the *e* is dropped from the word. Its coenzyme form, thiamin pyrophosphate (TPP), participates chiefly in carbohydrate metabolism.[4]

The chemical bond between each ring and the central carbon in thiamin is easily broken by prolonged exposure to heat (overcooked foods), thus destroying the functions of the vitamin. This destruction also occurs if food is cooked in alkaline solutions (pH > 8.0). Sometimes baking soda is added to the water in which fresh green beans are cooked to retain their bright green color; this practice is not recommended.

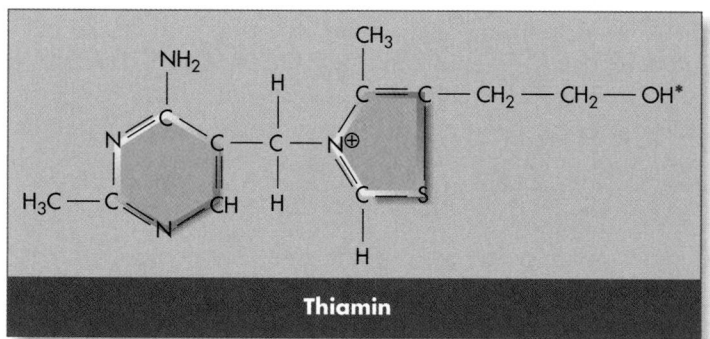

Thiamin

Thiamin has two phosphate groups added here (red asterisk) to form the coenzyme thiamin pyrophosphate (TPP).

Absorption, Transport, Storage, and Excretion of Thiamin

Thiamin is absorbed mainly in the small intestine by a sodium-dependent active absorption process. It is transported in the blood as such or in its coenzyme form by red blood cells. Storage is poor; only a small reserve is found in muscles and the liver. Any excess intake is promptly excreted in the urine.[4]

decarboxylation The action of removing one molecule of carbon dioxide from a compound.

transketolase An enzyme whose functional component is TPP (thiamin pyrophosphate); it converts glucose to various other sugars.

Functions of Thiamin

Thiamin pyrophosphate (TPP) functions in the metabolism of carbohydrates and of branched-chain amino acids (leucine, isoleucine, and valine) (Figure 10-2). It specifically participates in removal of carbon dioxide (**decarboxylation**) from these various compounds and in the action of the enzyme **transketolase**.[4] Transketolase is the enzyme

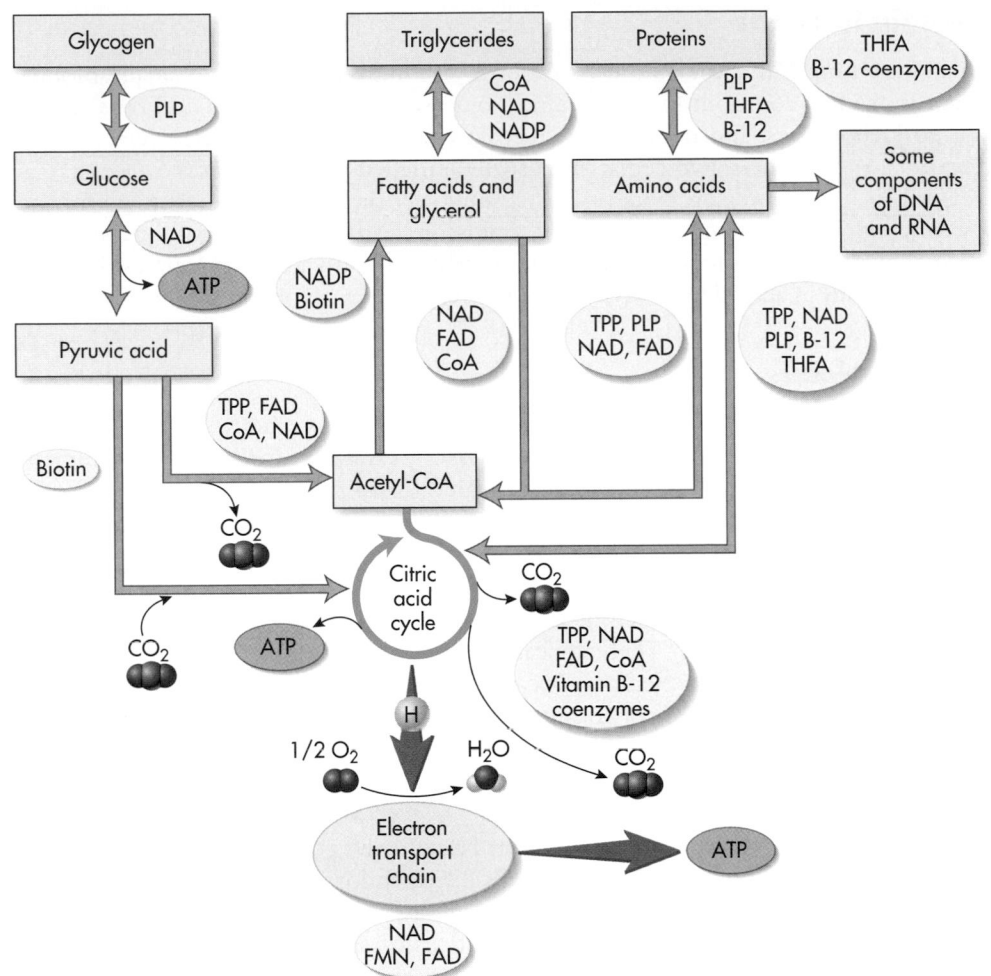

Figure 10-2 | Many metabolic pathways, including those involved in energy metabolism, use coenzyme forms of the B-vitamins: thiamin as thiamin pyrophosphate TPP; riboflavin as flavin adenine dinucleotide (FAD) and flavin mononucleotide (FMN); niacin as nicotinamide adenine dinucleotide (NAD) and nicotinamide adenine dinucleotide phosphate (NADP); pantothenic acid as coenzyme A; vitamin B-6 as pyridoxal phosphate (PLP); and folate as tetrahydrofolic acid (THFA). Vitamin B-12 exists in two coenzyme forms. Biotin exists as a cofactor. Other, minor pathways associated with energy metabolism also exist but are not depicted in this figure.

responsible for the formation of the five-carbon sugar components of RNA and DNA from the six-carbon glucose using a series of reactions called the pentose phosphate pathway.

The conversion of pyruvate to acetyl-CoA is an example of the action of thiamin; this conversion is the critical transition reaction in the aerobic metabolism of glucose.

$$\text{Glucose} \longrightarrow \text{Pyruvate} \xrightarrow[\begin{array}{c}\text{Thiamin as TPP}\\ \text{CoA} \quad \text{NAD}^+ \quad \text{NADH + H}^+\\ \downarrow\\ \text{CO}_2\end{array}]{} \text{Acetyl-CoA} \longrightarrow \text{Citric acid cycle}$$

In the citric acid cycle, TPP in a similar fashion converts the intermediate compound alpha-ketoglutarate to succinyl CoA.

$$\text{Alpha-ketoglutarate} \xrightarrow[\begin{array}{c}\text{Thiamin as TPP}\\ \text{CoA} \quad \text{NAD}^+ \quad \text{NADH + H}^+\\ \downarrow\\ \text{CO}_2\end{array}]{} \text{Succinyl-CoA}$$

TPP also plays a role in nerve function. It may aid in the synthesis of neurotransmitters and participate in the conduction of nerve impulses.

In November 1996, the United States began to experience a shortage of multivitamins for total parenteral nutrition feedings. Patients who did not receive adequate thiamin for more than 7 days developed lactic acidosis, because pyruvate could not be converted to acetyl-CoA. Instead, the pyruvate was turned into lactate.

Food Sources of Thiamin	
Food Item and Amount	*Thiamin (mg)*
Brewer's yeast, 2 tbsp	2.4
Canned lean ham, 3 oz	0.9
Pork chops, 4 oz	0.6
Wheat germ, 1/4 cup	0.5
Canadian bacon, 2 oz	0.5
Acorn squash, 1 cup	0.4
Soy milk, 1 cup	0.4
Flour tortilla, 1	0.4
Ham lunch meat, 2 pieces	0.3
Watermelon, 1 slice	0.2
Fresh orange juice, 1 cup	0.2
Cooked green peas, 1/2 cup	0.2
Baked beans, 1/2 cup	0.2
Navy beans, 1/2 cup	0.2
Corn, 1/2 cup	0.2
RDA for adult men, 1.2 mg; adult women, 1.1 mg	

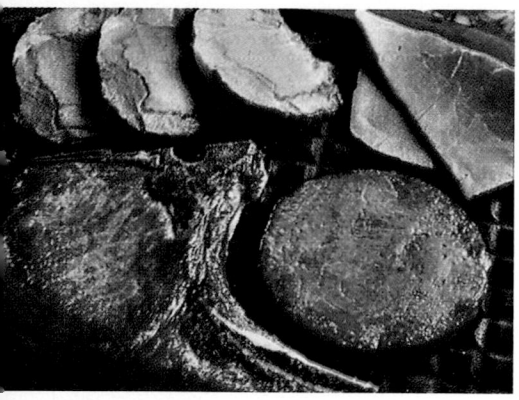

Pork is a good source of thiamin.

peripheral neuropathy Impaired sensory, motor, and reflex functions affecting arms and legs and causing calf muscle tenderness and difficulty in rising from a squatting position.

When physicians see a person suffering from unexplained delirium in the emergency room, they must consider whether it may be caused by a thiamin deficiency related to alcoholism. The treatment is an injection of thiamin. Dietary supplementation will not suffice because thiamin is absorbed slowly, especially in a person with alcoholism.

Thiamin in Foods

Thiamin is found in a wide variety of foods, although generally in a small amount. Major individual contributors of thiamin to our diets are white bread and rolls, crackers, pork, hot dogs, luncheon meats, ready-to-eat cereals, and orange juice. White bread, bakery products, and cereals are usually enriched with thiamin.

Foods rich in thiamin are pork products, sunflower seeds, legumes, wheat germ, and watermelon. Whole grains and enriched grains, green beans, asparagus, organ meats (such as liver), peanuts and other seeds, and mushrooms also are good sources. Eating a variety of foods in accord with MyPyramid is a reliable way to obtain sufficient thiamin.

Thiamin Needs

The RDA for thiamin for adult men and women is approximately 1.2 mg/day and 1.1 mg/day, respectively (refer to the inside cover of this text for vitamin recommendations for other age groups).[11] The Daily Value for thiamin used on food and supplement labels is 1.5 mg. Providing for sufficient activity of transketolase in red blood cells is used to set the RDA.

The average daily intake for thiamin in the United States for young men is close to 2 mg per day. For young women, it is approximately 1.2 mg/day. Canadian studies show a slightly lower intake. There appear to be no adverse effects with excess intake of thiamin from food or supplements because it is readily excreted in the urine. Thus, no Upper Level is established for this nutrient.[11]

Thiamin-Deficiency Diseases

The classic thiamin-deficiency disease beriberi has afflicted polished rice–eating populations for centuries. If little besides polished rice is eaten for weeks at a time, the disease develops. Because thiamin is so important to energy metabolism and because all cells need energy, it might seem that a thiamin deficiency should affect every organ and organ system.[4] However, three parts of the body are especially vulnerable to a deficiency of thiamin, as well as other B-vitamins involved in energy metabolism. One part is the nervous system because nerve cells use a lot of energy compared to most cells. In addition, the skin and GI tract are very sensitive to deficiencies of thiamin or other B-vitamins involved in energy metabolism. The reason is that skin and GI tract cells are replaced frequently, which requires much energy input. As symptoms are listed for B-vitamin deficiencies, notice how many can involve the nervous system, GI tract, or skin.

Beriberi

In Sinhalese, the language spoken by the inhabitants of Sri Lanka, the word *beriberi* means "I can't, I can't." Thiamin-deficient individuals are very weak and poorly coordinated because of impaired function of the cardiovascular, muscular, nervous, and gastrointestinal systems.

The clinical signs of thiamin deficiency include anorexia, weight loss, apathy, loss of short-term memory, confusion, GI tract distress, irritability, **peripheral neuropathy,** and muscle weakness.[4] There are two distinct types of beriberi: wet and dry. In wet beriberi, in addition to peripheral neuropathy, edema occurs along with an enlarged heart and congestive heart failure. In dry beriberi extreme muscle wasting occurs in addition to peripheral neuropathy. Some of the clinical signs of beriberi can be observed after only 7 days on a thiamin-free diet.

Wernicke-Korsakoff Syndrome

The thiamin-deficiency disease found primarily in North America is among people with heavy alcohol consumption and is called Wernicke-Korsakoff syndrome. Alcoholics have a three-pronged problem related to thiamin. Alcohol diminishes thiamin absorption, alcohol increases thiamin excretion, and alcoholics consume such a poor quality diet that there may be little, if any, thiamin in the foods and beverages consumed. Because the vitamin is not readily stored, the symptoms can occur rapidly. Changes in vision (e.g., double vision, crossed eyes, and rapid eye movements) **ataxia,** a staggering gait; and deranged mental functions characterize it. The disorientation, listlessness, memory loss, and other symptoms, including alcohol withdrawal, are due to lesions in the brain.

ataxia An inability to coordinate muscle activity during voluntary movement; incoordination.

▌ Riboflavin

Riboflavin contains three linked six-membered rings, with a sugar alcohol attached to the middle ring. The name comes from its yellow color (*flavin* means "yellow" in Latin). Riboflavin is a component of two coenzymes that play key roles in energy metabolism: flavin mononucleotide (FMN) and flavin adenine dinucleotide (FAD).[23]

Absorption, Transport, Storage, and Excretion of Riboflavin

In the stomach, HCl releases riboflavin from its bound forms. Absorption is primarily via active transport or facilitated diffusion in the small intestine. In the blood, riboflavin is transported by protein carriers. Riboflavin is converted to its coenzyme forms, FMN and FAD, in most tissues, but mainly in the small intestine, liver, heart, and kidney. A small amount of riboflavin is stored in the liver, kidneys, and heart. Any excess intake is excreted in the urine.[23] For people who take excessive amounts in supplement form, riboflavin imparts a bright yellow color to the urine.

Functions of Riboflavin

Riboflavin coenzymes have oxidation-reduction (redox) reaction functions.[23] These coenzymes either take electrons from a substrate or give electrons to a substrate. In the first case, the riboflavin coenzyme undergoes reduction (gains electrons) and the substrate undergoes oxidation (loses electrons). In other cases, the sequence is reversed (the riboflavin is oxidized and the substrate is reduced). Unlike some redox reactions, riboflavin does not exchange isolated electrons, but rather exchanges hydrogen atoms.

Riboflavin coenzymes are involved in many enzyme reactions, a number of which are critical to energy metabolism. For example, the enzyme succinate dehydrogenase is a FAD-containing enzyme that accepts hydrogens from succinate to form fumarate during the citric acid cycle. The hydrogens are then passed on to the electron transport chain.

$$\text{Succinate} \xrightarrow{\quad \text{FAD} \quad \text{FADH}_2 \quad} \text{Fumarate}$$

Another FAD-containing enzyme participates in the breakdown of fatty acids (beta oxidation) to acetyl-CoA, the entry compound for the citric acid cycle. And another riboflavin-containing coenzyme, FMN, shuttles hydrogen atoms into the electron transport chain. Still other FAD-containing enzymes help form the vitamin B-6 coenzyme, synthesize the amino acid tryptophan into the B-vitamin niacin, and participate in folate metabolism (and in this way participate indirectly in homocysteine metabolism). Metabolism of the oxidized form of glutathione (abbreviated GS; this binds to another GS to form GS-SG) to the reduced form (2 GSH) is dependent on the FAD-requiring enzyme glutathione reductase. Recall from Chapter 9 that this process is part of the cell's antioxidant defense system.

$$\text{GSSG} \xrightarrow{\quad \text{FADH}_2 \quad \text{FAD} \quad} \text{2GH}$$

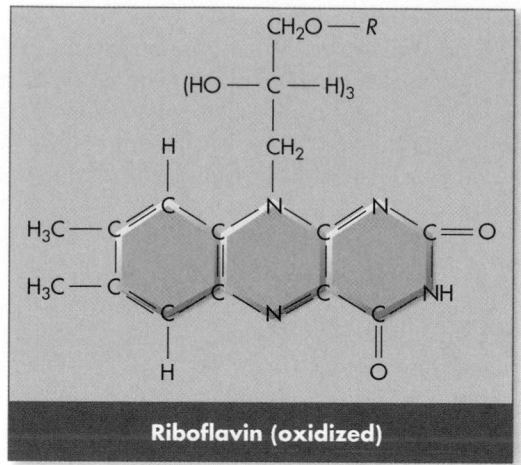

For riboflavin, the italicized *R* denotes H in the free vitamin; phosphate in FMN; and an adenine dinucleotide in FAD. In the reduced form of riboflavin, the hydrogens are shown in red in this figure.

Food Sources of Riboflavin	
Food Item and Amount	*Riboflavin (mg)*
Multigrain Cheerios, 3/4 cup	1.3
Fried beef liver, 1 oz	1.2
Steamed oysters, 10	1.1
Plain yogurt, 1 cup	0.5
Brewer's yeast, 2 tbsp	0.5
Raw mushrooms, 5	0.5
Braunschweiger sausage, 1 oz	0.4
Cooked spinach, 1 cup	0.4
1% milk, 1 cup	0.4
Buttermilk, 1 cup	0.4
Boiled egg, 1	0.3
Sirloin steak, 3 oz	0.3
Feta cheese, 1 oz	0.2
Tortilla, 1	0.2
Lean ham, 3 oz	0.2
RDA for adult men, 1.3 mg; adult women, 1.1 mg	

Riboflavin in Foods

One-quarter of the riboflavin in our diets comes from milk products. The rest of our riboflavin intake typically comes from enriched white bread, rolls, and crackers as well as from eggs and meat. Foods rich in riboflavin are liver, mushrooms, spinach and other green leafy vegetables, broccoli, asparagus, low-fat and fat-free milk, and cottage cheese.

Exposure to light (ultraviolet radiation) causes riboflavin to break down rapidly. To prevent this light-induced breakdown, paper and plastic cartons—not glass—should be used in packaging riboflavin-rich foods such as milk, milk products, and cereals.

Riboflavin Needs

The RDA for riboflavin is 1.1 to 1.3 mg/day for adults. The most commonly used method for assessing riboflavin status involves the maintenance of normal erythrocyte (red blood cell) glutathione reductase activity and urinary riboflavin excretion. These tests were used to establish the RDA.[11] The Daily Value for riboflavin used on food and supplement labels is 1.7 mg. North Americans have an intake of approximately 2.1 mg/day for men and 1.5 mg/day for women. There appear to be no adverse effects from consuming large amounts of riboflavin because of its limited absorption and rapid excretion via the urine, and so no Upper Level has been set.[11]

Riboflavin-Deficiency Diseases

The signs and symptoms associated with a pure riboflavin deficiency (technically called **ariboflavinosis**) include inflammation of the tongue (glossitis), cracking of tissue around the corners of the mouth (cheilosis), seborrheic dermatitis (a disease of the sebaceous glands of the skin), inflammation of the mouth (stomatitis) and throat, various eye and nervous system disorders, and confusion and headaches (Figure 10-3).[23] At present, little is known about the possible consequences of a marginal riboflavin deficiency. One possibility is that people may become tired more quickly during physical activity, although evidence for this is not conclusive.

The first evidence of a severe deficiency is inflammation of the mouth and tongue. The complete picture of a deficiency develops after approximately 2 months on a riboflavin-deficient diet (consuming one-fourth of the RDA). Diseases such as cancer, certain forms of cardiovascular disease, and diabetes also are known to precipitate or worsen a riboflavin deficiency. However, a deficiency disease associated with an isolated lack of dietary riboflavin is rarely seen in otherwise healthy people. And because riboflavin functions along with other B-vitamins (e.g., vitamin B-6, niacin, thiamin, and folate) in numerous metabolic pathways, some symptoms ascribed to riboflavin deficiency are actually caused by the failure of metabolic pathways associated with a lack of other nutrients. As already noted, an assortment of B-vitamins, such as riboflavin, thiamin, and niacin, is often found in the same foods.[11]

Alcoholics risk a riboflavin deficiency because they often eat a very nutrient-deficient diet. Long-term use of phenobarbital may also compromise riboflavin status because this drug produces metabolic changes in the liver that increase the breakdown of the vitamin. Marginal intakes may also be seen in people who do not consume milk or milk products. All such people would be wise to search for another, plentiful dietary source of riboflavin, such as enriched breads or ready-to-eat breakfast cereals.

> **ariboflavinosis** A condition resulting from a lack of riboflavin. The *a* means "without," and the *osis* stands for "a condition of."

Niacin

The B-vitamin niacin actually exists in two forms—nicotinic acid (niacin) and nicotinamide (niacinamide). In the body, both forms of the vitamin perform the functions associated with niacin. The two coenzyme forms of niacin are nicotinamide adenine dinucleotide (NAD^+) and nicotinamide adenine dinucleotide phosphate ($NADP^+$). Both forms participate in numerous chemical reactions in the body.[3]

Absorption, Transport, Storage, and Excretion of Niacin

Nicotinic acid and nicotinamide are readily absorbed from the stomach and the intestine by active transport and passive diffusion, so that almost all niacin consumed is absorbed. Niacin is transported from the liver to all tissues, where it is converted to its coenzyme forms, NAD^+ and $NADP^+$, which function in either oxidized or reduced forms. Niacin coenzymes are stored in the liver. Any excess niacin intake is excreted as a variety of metabolic products in the urine.[3]

Functions of Niacin

Like the coenzyme forms of riboflavin, the coenzyme forms of niacin, NAD^+ and $NADP^+$, are active participants in oxidation-reduction reactions.[3] The niacin coenzymes function in at least 200 reactions in cellular metabolic pathways, especially those used to produce ATP. NAD^+ participates in catabolic reactions, acting as an electron and hydrogen ion acceptor in glycolysis (e.g., the conversion of glucose to pyruvate) and the citric acid cycle. Under anaerobic conditions, the resulting reduced form, $NADH + H^+$, is used in converting pyruvate to lactate, thereby regenerating NAD^+.

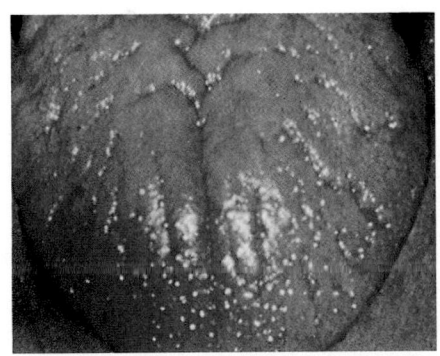

Figure 10-3 | A painful, inflamed tongue (glossitis) can signal a deficiency of riboflavin, niacin, vitamin B-6, folate, or vitamin B-12. Often more than one deficiency is the cause. Because other medical conditions can also cause glossitis, further evaluation is needed before a nutrient deficiency can be diagnosed.

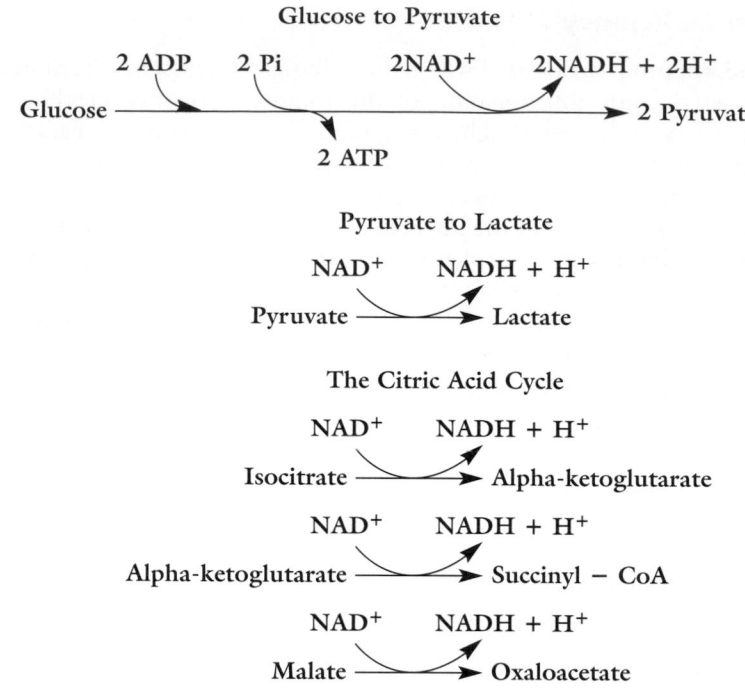

Under aerobic conditions, NADH + H$^+$ also donates an electron and hydrogen to other acceptor molecules in the electron-transport chain.

The enzyme alcohol dehydrogenase also uses NAD to convert alcohol to acetaldehyde (review Chapter 8).

Each of the reactions shown here starts with an oxidized form of a niacin coenzyme. However, synthetic pathways in the cell—those that make new compounds—use a reduced form of the niacin coenzyme, specifically NADPH + H$^+$. This coenzyme is important in the biochemical pathway for fatty-acid synthesis. Cells that synthesize a lot of fatty acids (e.g., those in the liver and female mammary glands) have higher concentrations of NADPH + H$^+$ than do cells not involved in fatty-acid synthesis (e.g., muscle cells).

Niacin in Foods

Niacin can be found in foods as the vitamin itself or as the amino acid tryptophan, which can be synthesized into niacin by the body. About 25% of the preformed niacin in North American diets comes from poultry and mixed dishes that include meat, fish, and poultry. Another 11% comes from enriched bread and bread products.

If a person is on a high-tryptophan intake, much of the tryptophan is available for synthesis of niacin, because tryptophan needs for protein synthesis are met (each 60 mg yields 1 mg of niacin). The overall number of milligrams of niacin supplied by dietary protein can be estimated by dividing dietary protein intake (in grams) by 6.[11] For example, if one consumes 90 g of protein, the body will synthesize about 15 mg of niacin. In this way we synthesize much of our need for niacin. Note that this synthesis requires input from riboflavin and vitamin B-6.

Rich sources of niacin are mushrooms, wheat bran, tuna (as well as other fish), chicken, turkey, asparagus, and peanuts. Animal proteins (except gelatin) are especially rich in tryptophan. Unlike some other water-soluble vitamins, niacin is very heat stable, and little is lost in cooking.

Food Sources of Niacin	
Food Item and Amount	Niacin (mg)
Tuna, 3 oz	11.3
Roasted chicken, 3 oz	10.1
Peanuts, 1/2 cup	9.9
Baked salmon, 3 oz	8.6
Turkey lunch meat, 3 oz	5.4
Ground beef, 3 oz	5.0
Raw mushrooms, 5	4.7
Lean steak, 4 oz	4.5
Chunky peanut butter, 2 tbsp	4.4
Fried beef liver, 1 oz	4.1
Raisin Nut Bran cereal, 3/4 cup	3.8
Tortilla, 1	2.6
Baked cod, 3 oz	2.1
Potato, 1	2.1
Broiled halibut, 3 oz	1.6
RDA for adult men, 16 mg NE; adult women, 14 mg NE	

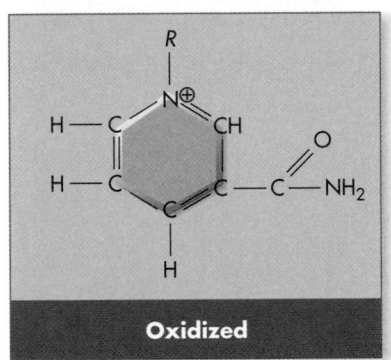

Nicotinic acid

Oxidized

Coenzyme
forms using
nicotinamide

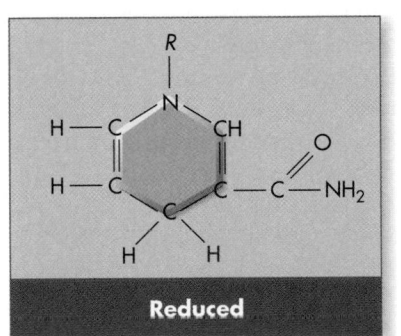

Reduced

The two coenzyme forms of niacin, NAD and NADP, contain
nicotinamide linked to adenine dinucleotide or adenine
dinucleotide phosphate, indicated by the italicized *R*. Both
coenzymes undergo oxidation and reduction by loss or
addition of an electron and a hydrogen (red in this figure).

Because food composition tables list only preformed niacin, they can underestimate the total niacin supplied by protein foods. For example, although eggs and milk lack niacin, they contain abundant tryptophan and thus indirectly contribute substantial amounts of niacin.

Populations that eat corn as a staple food are prone to a niacin deficiency called pellagra. You might therefore be surprised to learn that the niacin content of corn is similar to that of rice and considerably higher than that of most other vegetables. However, the niacin in corn is marginally absorbed because it is tightly bound by a protein. Soaking corn in an alkaline solution such as lime water (calcium hydroxide dissolved in water) releases bound niacin, rendering it more usable by the body. Look for evidence of this form of processing on the label when you buy corn-meal products such as tortillas. Because this practice was common among native peoples of Mexico and Central and South America, they did not suffer from a niacin deficiency. Early Spanish explorers of the New World took corn—a crop native to the Americas—back to Europe, but they were unaware of the importance of soaking corn in lime water.

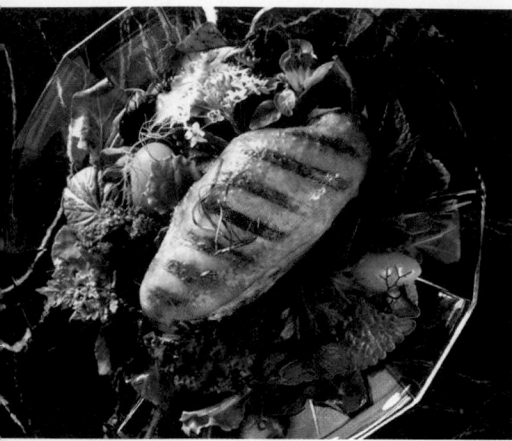

Chicken is a good source of niacin. The tryptophan present can also be metabolized to niacin.

Thus, as the use of corn as a staple spread in Europe, niacin deficiencies became widespread during the 1700s. In contrast, Spanish settlers in Latin America learned from the native populations to soak corn meal in lime water before using it in cooking. The Hispanic populations descended from these settlers continued this practice and rarely suffered from niacin deficiencies, whereas other North Americans who used untreated corn as a staple food often did.

Niacin Needs

For adult men the RDA for niacin is 16 mg/day, and for adult women it is 14 mg/day. The RDA for niacin is expressed as niacin equivalents (NE) to account for niacin received preformed from the diet as well as that synthesized from tryptophan. The primary criterion used to establish the RDA for niacin is the urinary excretion of a niacin metabolite, N-methyl nicotinamide.[11] The Daily Value for niacin used on food and supplement labels is 20 mg.

About the only population groups to exhibit a niacin deficiency in North America today are people with rare disorders of tryptophan metabolism (e.g., Hartnup's disease), alcoholics, and people with diseases that greatly impair food intake.

Niacin-Deficiency Diseases

The first official record of the niacin-deficiency disease pellagra was made by Spanish physician Casal in 1735. It was named *mal de la rosa*, or "red sickness." The typical red rash appears in areas exposed to sunlight, especially around the neck, which is today called "Casal's necklace." Later the disease was renamed *pellagra* (from Italian *pelle*, meaning "skin," and *agra*, meaning "rough").

Because almost every metabolic pathway uses either NAD^+ or $NADP^+$, it is not surprising that a niacin deficiency causes widespread damage in the body. The effects of pellagra are known as the three *D*s—dementia, diarrhea, and dermatitis (Figure 10-4). If the disease is not successfully treated, death (the fourth *D*) follows.[3] Clinical evidence of pellagra develops 50 to 60 days after instituting a niacin-deficient diet. Early symptoms include diminished appetite, weight loss, and weakness.

Pellagra is the only dietary deficiency disease ever to reach epidemic proportions in the United States. During the early 1900s, cases of pellagra increased dramatically in the southeastern region of the country, where corn—a poor source of naturally available niacin and the amino acid tryptophan—was being increasingly used as a primary component of the diet. More than 10,000 Americans died of pellagra in 1915. From the end of World War I until the end of World War II, an estimated 200,000 Americans suffered from the disease. Many people had such severe dementia that they were forced to live out their lives in mental institutions. One reason that pellagra remained a problem in the southeastern United States for so long was the misimpression that it was an infectious disease. This assumption was disproved by Dr. Joseph Goldberger, a public health specialist. He and some colleagues exposed themselves in a variety of ways to biological samples from pellagra patients to demonstrate that the disease was not infectious in nature. Goldberger also induced and cured pellagra in a prison population using dietary interventions.

The introduction of niacin-enriched grains in 1941 and improved intake of dietary protein resulting from post-wartime prosperity eventually led to the disappearance of pellagra in the United States. Pellagra is still found today throughout Southeast Asia and Africa among populations whose diets lack sufficient protein and niacin.

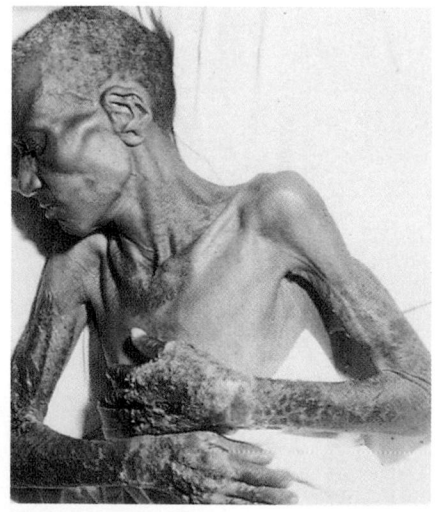

Figure 10-4 | The dermatitis of pellagra. Dermatitis on both sides of the body (bilateral) is a typical symptom of pellagra. Sun exposure worsens the condition.

Pharmacologic Use of Niacin and Upper Level for Niacin

Consuming 1.5 to 2 g of nicotinic acid per day—about 75 to 100 times the RDA—can decrease LDL-cholesterol and increase HDL-cholesterol.[3] When combined with diet, exercise, and other cholesterol-lowering drugs, megadoses of niacin can slow and even reverse the progression of atherosclerosis. Niacin prescribed for high LDL-cholesterol must have a time-release coating. Otherwise, such megadose therapy may have adverse effects, including flushing of the skin (the initial adverse effect), itching, GI tract upsets (such as nausea and vomiting), and liver damage. These effects (GI tract disturbances and liver damage) have been observed at doses of 1.5 g nicotinic acid per day. Some people experience symptoms at dosages as low as 50 mg/day. Even with the time-release coating, megadose use must be supervised by a physician because of the potential for side effects. The use of various other medications can lessen the side effects. For example, premedication with aspirin reduces the flushing reactions.

The flushing seen with excess niacin intake was considered the most appropriate effect on which to base the Upper Level. For adults, this amount is 35 mg/day of supplemental niacin and/or that from fortified foods, the point at which this symptom may begin. Note that niacin naturally found in food is not counted.[11]

Critical | Thinking

Both the vitamin niacin and protein-rich foods can cure pellagra. Why are both effective?

Concept | Check

The B-vitamins thiamin, niacin, and riboflavin function in various biochemical pathways used for the metabolism of glucose, amino acids, and fatty acids. Enriched grains are adequate sources of all three vitamins. Otherwise, pork is an excellent source of thiamin; milk is an excellent source of riboflavin; and protein foods in general are excellent sources of niacin. Deficiencies of all three vitamins can occur with alcoholism; of the three, a thiamin deficiency is the most likely. The specific deficiency symptoms typically occur in the brain and nervous system, skin, and GI tract. Cells in these tissues are very metabolically active, and those in the skin and GI tract are also constantly being replaced. Only niacin leads to toxic effects when consumed in high doses.

Pantothenic Acid

Pantothenic acid is part of coenzyme A (CoA), which plays a pivotal role in energy metabolism. This coenzyme is formed when the vitamin combines with a derivative ADP and part of the amino acid cysteine. Cysteine provides the sulfur atom, which is the functional end of the coenzyme.[27]

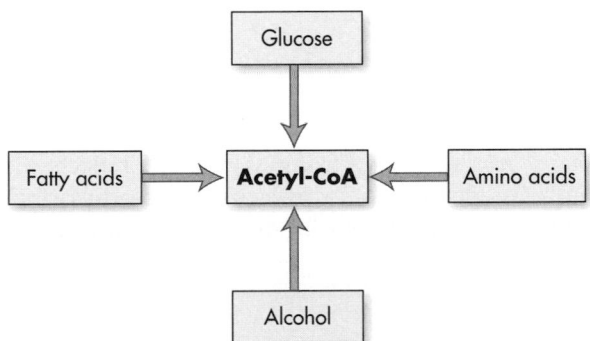

Absorption, Transport, Storage, and Excretion of Pantothenic Acid

The pantothenic acid portion of any coenzyme A in the diet is released during digestion in the small intestine. It is then absorbed as such or as a slight derivitive. Storage is minimal and is as the coenzyme form, such as is found in the liver. Excretion of pantothenic acid is via the urine.[27]

Functions of Pantothenic Acid

Coenzyme A is essential for the formation of ATP from the breakdown of carbohydrate, protein, alcohol, and fat.[27] The formation of acetyl-CoA from the two-carbon acetate that arises from their metabolism allows the acetate to enter the citric acid cycle. In another series of reactions, acetyl-CoA combines with carbon dioxide to begin the synthesis of fatty acids:

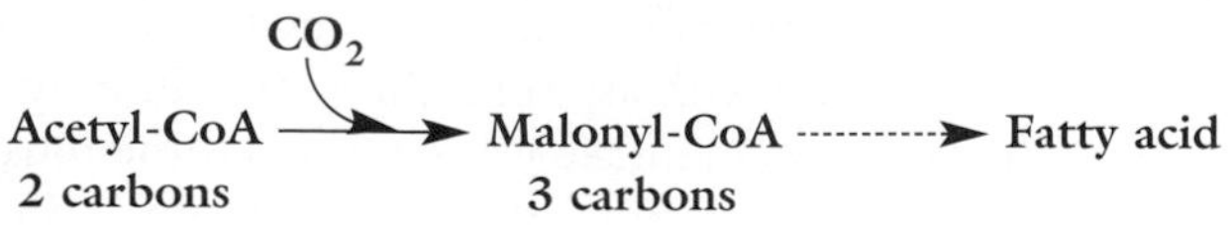

$$\text{Acetyl-CoA} \xrightarrow{\text{CO}_2} \text{Malonyl-CoA} \dashrightarrow \text{Fatty acid}$$
$$\text{2 carbons} \qquad\qquad \text{3 carbons}$$

Pantothenic acid also forms part of a compound called the *acyl carrier protein*. This protein attaches to fatty acids and shuttles them through the metabolic pathway designed to increase their chain length. Finally, pantothenic acid as coenzyme A also donates fatty acids to proteins in a process that can determine their location and function within a cell.

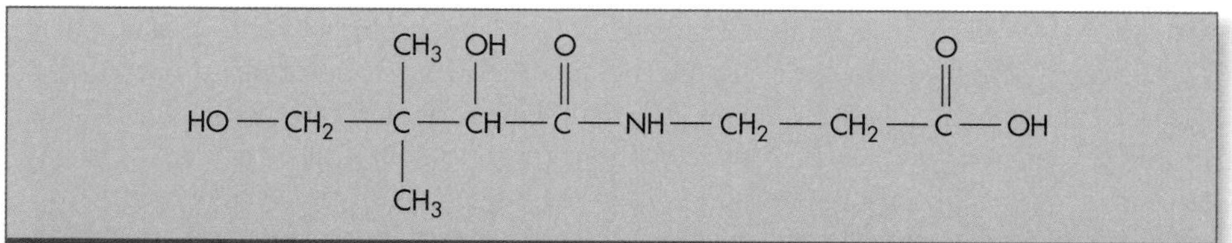

Pantothenic acid

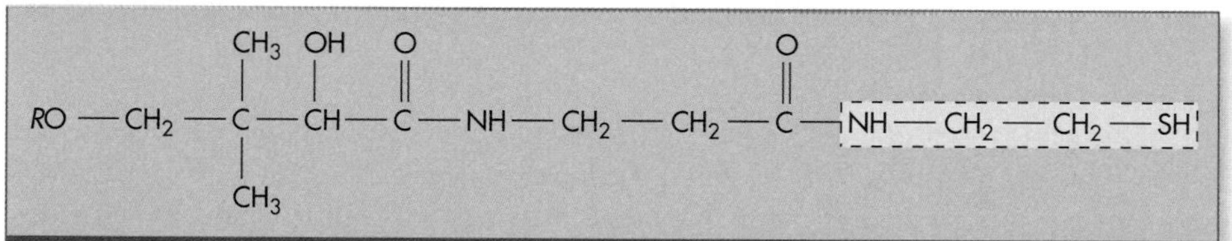

Coenzyme A (CoA)

Pantothenic acid is converted to coenzyme A by combining with a part of the amino acid cysteine (box) and with a derivative of adenosine diphosphate (ADP), represented by the italicized *R*.

Pantothenic Acid in Foods

The Greek word *pantothen*, meaning "from every side," reflects the ample supply of pantothenic acid in foods. Common sources include meat, milk, and many vegetables. Rich sources of pantothenic acid are mushrooms, liver, peanuts, eggs, yeast, broccoli, and milk.

Pantothenic Acid Needs

For adults, the Adequate Intake set for pantothenic acid is 5 mg/day. (Recall that an Adequate Intake is an acceptable intake established by the Food and Nutrition Board for some nutrients for which insufficient data are available to set an RDA.) Adults generally consume the Adequate Intake or more. The primary criterion used to estimate an Adequate Intake for pantothenic acid is the amount needed to replace urinary excretion.[11] The Daily Value for pantothenic acid used on food and supplement labels is 10 mg.

Dietary Sources of Pantothenic Acid

Food Item and Amount	Pantothenic Acid (mg)
Total corn flakes cereal, 3/4 cup	11.8
Power bar, 1	10.0
Luna bar, 1	9.9
Sunflower seeds, 1/4 cup	2.3
Fried beef liver, 1 oz	1.7
Raw mushrooms, 5	1.7
Plain yogurt, 1 cup	1.5
Acorn squash, 1 cup	1.2
Peanuts, 1/2 cup	1.0
1% milk, 1 cup	0.9
Roasted chicken breast, 3 oz	0.8
Broccoli, 1 cup	0.8
Baked potato, 1	0.7
Legumes, 1/2 cup	0.7
Cooked egg yolk, 1	0.6
Adequate Intake for adults, 5 mg	

Pantothenic Acid-Deficiency Diseases

A deficiency of pantothenic acid might occur in cases of alcoholism in which a very nutrient deficient diet is consumed. However, the effects would probably be hidden among deficiencies of thiamin, riboflavin, vitamin B-6, and folate, so the pantothenic acid deficiency might go unrecognized. When a deficiency was experimentally induced in humans, symptoms of headache, fatigue, impaired muscle coordination, and GI tract disturbances were seen. There is no known toxicity for pantothenic acid, and so no Upper Limit is set.[11]

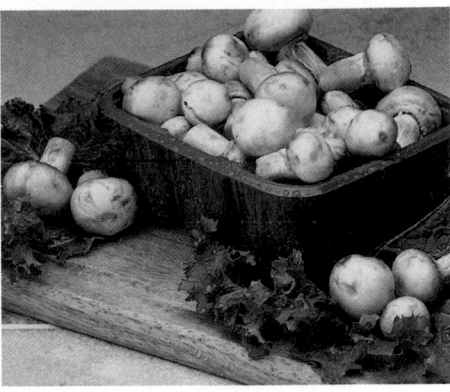

Mushrooms are a good source of pantothenic acid.

Biotin

Biotin participates in reactions in which carbon dioxide is added to a compound.

Absorption, Transport, Storage, and Excretion of Biotin

Biotin is commonly found in two forms in foods: the free vitamin and the protein-bound coenzyme form, called biocytin. In the formation of biocytin, biotin forms a bond with the amino acid lysine in a protein. Biotin is absorbed from the small intestine, whereas the biocytin form is not absorbed until the enzyme biotinidase, which is present in the small intestine, cleaves the bond linking biotin to a protein, releasing the free vitamin. Biotinidase also is involved in recycling biotin after biocytin is released from breakdown of biotin-dependent enzymes. Biotin is stored in small amounts in the muscles, liver, and brain. Biotin excretion is mostly via the urine (via bile is another route).[24]

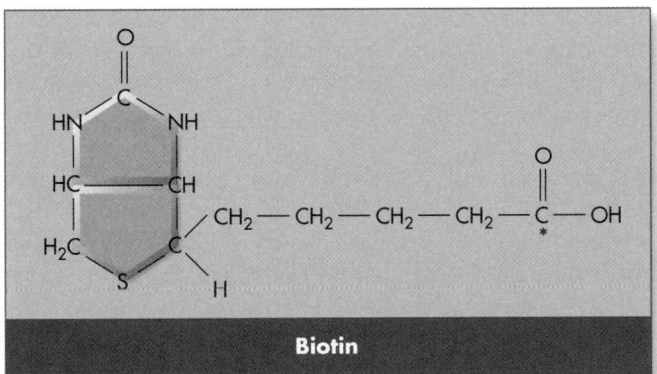

Biotin

The vitamin biotin attaches to a protein by formation of a bond between its carboxyl group (red asterisk) and lysine in a protein, yielding the bound cofactor form called biocytin.

About 1 in 60,000 infants is born with a genetic defect that leaves the infant with very low amounts of the enzyme biotinidase. Because the infant cannot readily break down biocytin arising from dietary intake and body metabolism to the free form, a biotin deficiency is likely to develop. The infant is treated with 100 μg of biotin, which is about three times typical biotin needs.

Functions of Biotin

Biotin functions as an essential cofactor for five carboxylase enzymes that add carbon dioxide to various compounds.[24] Four of the five enzymes are involved in energy and amino acid metabolism, and the other is involved in making certain fatty acids. The specific function of the first two is related to fatty acid synthesis, namely adding carbon dioxide to acetyl-CoA to form malonyl-CoA (review the previous section on pantothenic acid for the specific reaction). This reaction is the first step in the elongation of the carbon chain to form a fatty acid.

Food Sources of Biotin

Food Item and Amount	Biotin (μg)
Smooth peanut butter, 2 tbsp	30.1
Cooked lamb liver, 1 oz	11.6
Boiled egg, 1	9.3
Cooked egg yolk, 1	8.1
Low-fat yogurt, 1 cup	7.4
Wheat germ, 1/4 cup	7.2
Roasted peanuts, 5	6.5
Wheat bran, 1/4 cup	6.4
Skim milk, 1 cup	4.9
Salmon, 3 oz	4.3
Egg noodles, 1 cup	4.0
Swiss cheese, 2 oz	2.2
Cheddar cheese, 2 oz	1.7
Raw cauliflower, 1 cup	1.5
American cheese, 2 oz	1.4
Adequate Intake for adults, 30 μg	

avidin A protein found in raw egg whites that can bind biotin and inhibit its absorption; cooking destroys avidin.

A third enzyme adds carbon dioxide to the 3-carbon pyruvate to yield the 4-carbon oxaloacetate, an intermediate in the citric acid cycle. This reaction replenishes lost oxaloacetate and so helps keep the citric acid cycle functioning. In the liver and kidney, oxaloacetate also can be converted to glucose when glucose supplies are running low; this conversion is an initial step in gluconeogenesis.

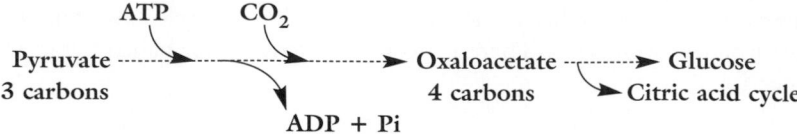

If biotin were missing, the citric acid cycle could not run effectively, and the result would be a buildup of lactate, the anaerobic by-product of glycolysis. This condition would also be accompanied by a decrease in aerobic metabolism.

A fourth biotin-dependent enzyme contributes to the breakdown of the amino acid leucine for energy needs, and a fifth does the same for the amino acids threonine, methionine, and isoleucine. Clearly, biotin is required for the metabolism of carbohydrates, amino acids, and fatty acids.

Sources of Biotin: Food and Microbial Synthesis

Biotin content of food has been determined for only a small number of foods, so foods containing biotin are not included in most food composition tables. Biotin is widely distributed in food but concentration varies considerably. Sources include whole grains, eggs, nuts, and legumes.

It is likely that the intestinal synthesis of biotin by bacteria supplies at least part of our needs, as evidenced by the rather rare incidence of biotin deficiency. In fact, we excrete more biotin than we consume. However, questions remain about the actual bioavailability of the biotin synthesized by the intestinal bacteria, because this production takes place mostly in the large intestine, whereas biotin is most efficiently absorbed from the small intestine.

A protein called **avidin** in raw egg whites binds biotin and inhibits its absorption. (Note that cooking denatures avidin in such a way that it can no longer bind biotin.) Feeding many raw egg whites to animals leads to the classic "egg-white injury" deficiency disease. An occasional raw egg would not cause this problem because it would take a regular daily consumption of 12 to 24 raw eggs to produce a biotin deficiency. Biotin deficiency resulting from consuming raw eggs has been reported, however, in people with alcoholism who eat as few as three raw eggs a day. These people also probably exist on very deficient diets.

Biotin Needs

The Adequate Intake for biotin for adults of 30 μg/day is extrapolated from the intake seen in exclusively breastfed infants. The results of such an extrapolation likely overestimate the amount needed for adults because adults require biotin only for maintenance, not for growth.[11] Diets of adults generally meet the Adequate Intake. The Daily Value for biotin used on food and supplement labels is 300 μg, 10 times our current estimate of needs. There is no Upper Level for biotin.[11]

Biotin-Deficiency Diseases

If undetected, a lack of biotinidase activity leads to a severe biotin deficiency in infants. Signs and symptoms may appear within a few months of life, beginning with a skin rash and hair loss. Other signs and symptoms include convulsions, other neurological disorders, and impaired growth. Most other well-documented cases of biotin deficiency have occurred with total parenteral nutrition when the biotin was omitted from the formula. Overall, a biotin deficiency is rare.[24]

I Vitamin B-6

Vitamin B-6 is actually a family of three compounds: pyridoxal, pyridoxine, and pyridoxamine. All three forms can be phosphorylated to the active vitamin B-6 coenzymes, the primary one being pyridoxal phosphate (PLP). The coenzymes participate in numerous metabolic reactions. The generic name for the vitamin is B-6, or pyridoxine.[20]

Absorption, Transport, Storage, and Excretion of Vitamin B-6

Both the coenzyme and free forms of vitamin B-6 can be absorbed by passive means. Vitamin B-6 as such is transported to the liver via the portal blood, where ultimately the three forms of the vitamin are phosphorylated. From the liver the phosphorylated forms (mainly PLP) are released to general circulation bound to a blood protein (albumin) for transport. The main storage of vitamin B-6 in the body takes place in muscle tissue. Excess vitamin B-6 is generally excreted in the urine.[20]

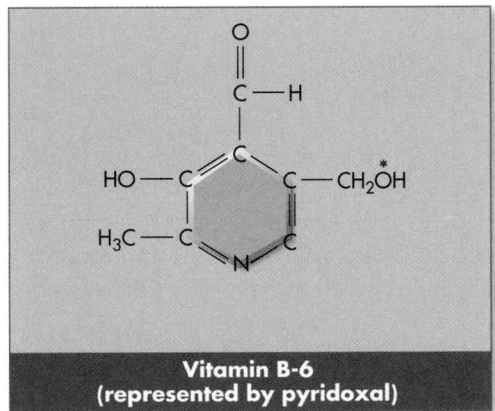

**Vitamin B-6
(represented by pyridoxal)**

Pyridoxal, one form of vitamin B-6, is converted to an active coenzyme—pyridoxal phosphate (PLP)—by the addition of a phosphate group to the hydroxyl group, indicated in this figure by the red asterisk.

Functions of Vitamin B-6

Vitamin B-6 as PLP plays a coenzyme role in more than 100 enzymatic reactions, almost all of which involve nitrogen-containing compounds.

Amino Acid Metabolism

A major role of PLP is to participate in amino acid metabolism. For example, PLP participates in reactions to form nonessential amino acids via transamination. (If we didn't have the services of PLP, every amino acid would be essential because it would have to be supplied by the diet.) PLP acts to loosen the bond between the nitrogen group ($-NH_2$) and the central carbon on the amino acid, allowing it to be removed (Figure 10-5).[20]

PLP is responsible for the interconversion of D- and L-amino acids—it acts as a **racemase.** Recall from Chapter 7 that humans only use the L form of amino acids for protein synthesis. PLP is also involved in the conversion of homocysteine to cysteine, which occurs during methionine (an amino acid) metabolism.

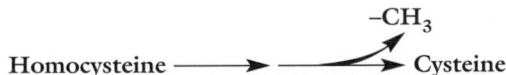

Vitamin B-6 participates in both steps of the reaction. The methyl ($-CH_3$) group is accepted by a larger molecule (the amino acid serine; see Appendix B for details).

Homocysteine is receiving much attention today, especially regarding development of brain disorders, bone disorders, and cardiovascular disease.[14,15,16,17,25,28] Meeting B vitamin needs (riboflavin, vitamin B-6, folate, and vitamin B-12) and choline needs allows for metabolism of homocysteine to nutrients, such as the amino acids methionine and cysteine. This keeps homocysteine low in the blood and so protects the body from its potentially toxic consequences.

racemase A group of enzymes that catalyzes reactions involving structural rearrangement of a molecule (e.g., conversion of D-alanine isomer to L-alanine isomer).

Figure 10-5 | An example of a transaminase enzyme pathway that utilizes vitamin B-6. This pathway allows cells to synthesize nonessential amino acids. In this example, pyruvic acid gains an amino group from glutamic acid to form the amino acid alanine.

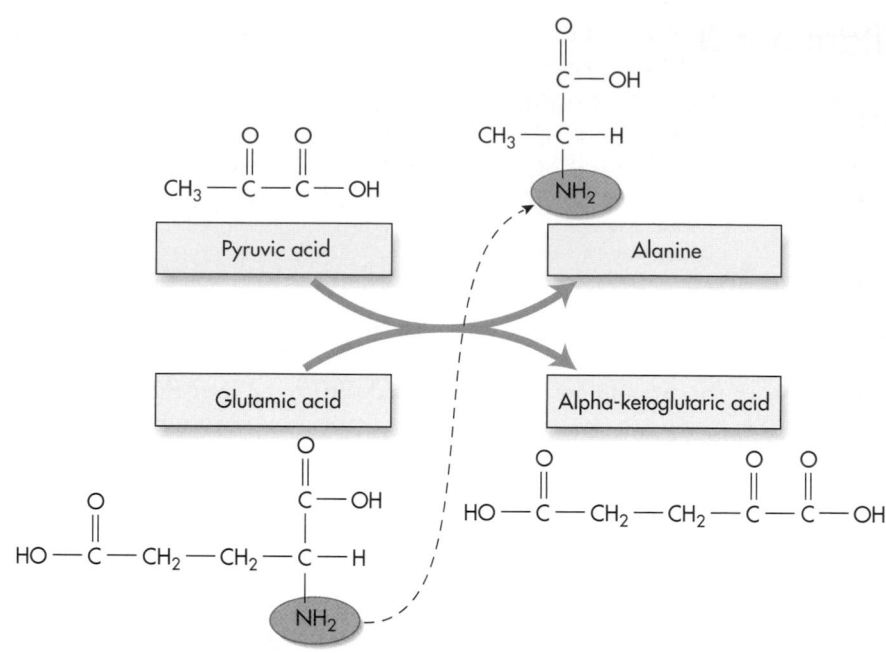

In the early 1950s, some infants were accidentally fed a commercial formula in which vitamin B-6 had been destroyed by oversterilization. The infants developed abnormal electroencephalogram (EEG) readings and experienced convulsions. The reason was probably associated with a lack of neurotransmitter synthesis in the brain. The situation was successfully treated with vitamin B-6.

Food Sources of Vitamin B-6	
Food Item and Amount	*Vitamin B-6 (mg)*
Baked salmon, 3 oz	0.8
Baked potato, 1 medium	0.7
Banana, 1	0.7
Avocado, 1	0.6
Brewer's yeast, 2 tbsp	0.5
Roasted chicken breast, 3 oz	0.5
Acorn squash, 1 cup	0.5
Special K cereal, 3/4 cup	0.5
Whole wheat bread, 1 slice	0.5
Fried beef liver, 1 oz	0.4
Roasted turkey lunch meat, 3 oz	0.4
Sirloin steak, 3 oz	0.4
Lean ham, 3 oz	0.4
Watermelon, 1 slice	0.3
Sunflower seeds, 1/4 cup	0.3
Cooked spinach, 1/2 cup	0.2
RDA for adults, 1.3 mg	

Heme Synthesis

In the red blood cell, PLP catalyzes a step in the synthesis of heme. Heme is a nitrogen-containing ring. It is inserted into certain proteins to hold iron in place. The best known of these proteins is hemoglobin, which uses the iron to transport oxygen in the blood.[20]

Carbohydrate Metabolism

PLP is part of the enzyme that releases glucose from glycogen during glycogen breakdown. Therefore, vitamin B-6 helps maintain blood glucose concentrations. This action is an exception to the rule that vitamin B-6 works with nitrogen-containing compounds. The chemistry of PLP with this glycogen breakdown enzyme differs from the typical chemistry of PLP with enzymes.[20]

Neurotransmitter Synthesis

Not only are amino acids used to build proteins, but they are also used to make nonprotein nitrogen compounds. Many of these compounds are neurotransmitters, which are important for brain function. PLP plays in the synthesis of the neurotransmitters serotonin from tryptophan, dopamine (DOPA) and norepinephrine from tyrosine, histamine from histadine, and gamma-aminobutyric acid (GABA) from glutamic acid.[20]

Vitamin Formation

PLP participates in the conversion of the amino acid tryptophan to the B-vitamin niacin.[20]

Immune Function and Lipid Metabolism

PLP affects immune function and lipid metabolism, probably via its roles in amino acid metabolism, hormone production, and possibly other functions.[20]

Vitamin B-6 in Foods

Vitamin B-6 is stored in the muscle tissues of animals, and thus meat, fish, and poultry are some of the best sources of this vitamin. Although vitamin B-6 in animal foods is often more readily absorbed than that in plant foods, whole grains also are good sources of vitamin B-6. However, vitamin B-6 is lost during the refining of grains, and it is not one of the vitamins added during enrichment. Most fruits and vegetables are not good vitamin B-6 sources, but there are some exceptions: carrots, potatoes, spinach, bananas, and avocados. Other sources of vitamin B-6 include peanut butter, garbanzo beans, and ready-to-eat breakfast cereals.

Vitamin B-6 is not stable under heat or alkaline conditions. Heat processing and other destructive processing technologies can reduce the vitamin B-6 content of a food by 10 to 50%.

Vitamin B-6 Needs

The adult RDA for vitamin B-6 is 1.3 to 1.7 mg/day. The RDA is based on the amount needed to maintain adequate PLP in the blood.[11] The Daily Value used on food and supplement labels is 2 mg. Average daily consumption of vitamin B-6 for adult men and women is somewhat above the RDA.

Vitamin B-6-Deficiency Diseases

The symptoms of vitamin B-6 deficiency include seborrheic dermatitis, **microcytic hypochromic anemia** (and occasionally a sideroblastic anemia, as described in Chapter 8), convulsions, depression, and confusion.[20] The anemia reflects a decline in heme synthesis due to an inadequate amount of PLP; the accumulation of abnormal metabolites of tryptophan in the brain or a lack of neurotransmitters may cause the convulsions. Because vitamin B-6 is essential for the formation of a type of white blood cell, a deficiency is associated with diminished immune function. These deficiencies are rare, but there are some documented occurrences, sometimes due to alcoholism or to a genetic condition that causes an anemia that can often be reversed by increased vitamin B-6 intake. When alcohol is metabolized in the body, an intermediate, acetaldehyde, is produced. Acetaldehyde decreases the formation of PLP by cells and perhaps competes with PLP for protein-binding sites.

A number of medications—especially L-DOPA, used to treat Parkinson's disease, and isoniazid, a common antituberculosis medication—reduce blood concentrations of PLP. Patients taking these medications should be advised to obtain extra vitamin B-6 under a physician's guidance. Finally, some adults have been found to exhibit signs of a mild deficiency, such as reduced immune function, a high concentration of homocysteine in the blood, and coronary artery disease.[11,14]

Pharmacologic Use of Vitamin B-6 and Upper Level for Vitamin B-6

Carpal tunnel syndrome, a nerve disorder in the wrist, has been treated with large daily doses of vitamin B-6. Results have been inconsistent, leading experts to caution about any use of megadoses of vitamin B-6 for such a purpose.

Studies of vitamin B-6 and **premenstrual syndrome (PMS)** indicate that the evidence is so shaky that it is not possible to make a definitive recommendation for taking vitamin B-6. Because there are no laboratory tests for PMS and the cause of symptoms has not yet been elucidated, well-controlled trials are needed to clarify the possible benefits and side effects of vitamin B-6 in the treatment of PMS. Some physicians, however, advise doses of 50 to 100 mg/day as a possible part of therapy. Such large doses may also help treat nausea that develops during pregnancy (see Chapter 16).

The Upper Level for adults is set at 100 mg of vitamin B-6 per day, based on development of nerve damage.[11] Intakes of 2 to 6 g of vitamin B-6 per day for 2 or more months especially can lead to irreversible nerve damage, as can long-term intakes of greater than 200 mg/day.[20] Body builders and women attempting to treat themselves for PMS have developed symptoms such as walking difficulties and hand and foot numbness. Some nerve damage in individual sensory neurons is probably reversible, but damage to ganglia (where many nerve fibers converge) is probably permanent.

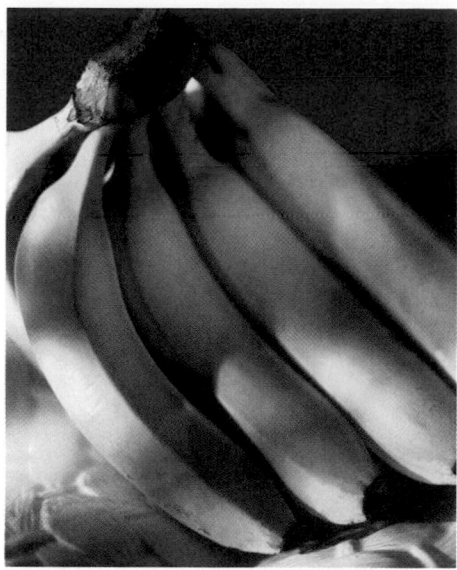

Bananas are a good plant source of vitamin B-6.

microcytic hypochromic anemia An anemia characterized by small, pale red blood cells that lack sufficient hemoglobin and thus have reduced oxygen-carrying ability. It is often also caused by an iron deficiency.

premenstrual syndrome (PMS) A disorder found in some women a few days before a menstrual period begins. It is characterized by depression, anxiety, headache, bloating, and mood swings. Severe cases are currently termed premenstrual dysphoric disorder (PDD).

Concept | Check

Pantothenic acid and biotin both participate in metabolism of carbohydrate, protein, and fat. A deficiency of either vitamin is unlikely because pantothenic acid is found in a wide variety of foods and our need for biotin is partially met by synthesis from intestinal bacteria. Vitamin B-6 is important for protein metabolism, neurotransmitter synthesis, and other key metabolic functions. Headache, anemia, nausea, and vomiting can result from a vitamin B-6 deficiency. Animal protein sources and plant foods such as potatoes, spinach, and bananas are good sources of vitamin B-6. Doses of vitamin B-6 in excess of approximately 1500 times the RDA for a few months or 150 times the RDA for long-term use can cause nerve destruction.

Folate

The word *folate* derives from the Latin word for leaf *(folium)* because dark green, leafy vegetables are among the best sources of this vitamin. It was once thought that a folate-deficient diet was virtually impossible to produce unless the diet was grossly deficient in many nutrients. Today, this attitude has changed as dietary folate intake has become a major issue of interest because of its many roles in metabolism.

Folate and vitamin B-12 produce a number of identical deficiency signs and symptoms when omitted from the diet. These two water-soluble vitamins share a close relationship because a vitamin B-12 coenzyme is needed to recycle a folate coenzyme for repeated function.[11]

What we call folate today was known earlier as either folic acid or folacin. Today, the term *folate* is a generic name for the vitamin and also refers to the various forms of the vitamin found naturally in foods. Folic acid refers specifically to the form of the vitamin found in supplements and fortified foods.

Folate consists of three parts: pteridine, para-aminobenzoic acid (PABA), and one or more molecules of the amino acid glutamic acid (glutamate). If only one glutamate molecule is present, it is designated folic acid (folate monoglutamate). In food, about 90% of the folate molecules have three or more glutamates attached and are known as polyglutamates.[26]

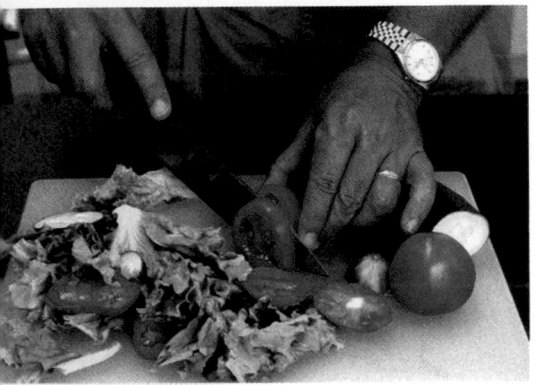

Leafy green vegetables are good sources of folate.

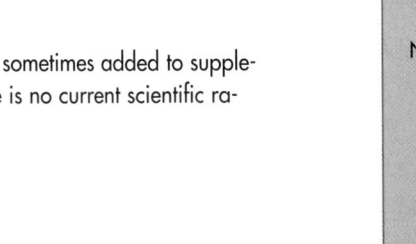

PABA by itself is sometimes added to supplements, but there is no current scientific rationale for this.

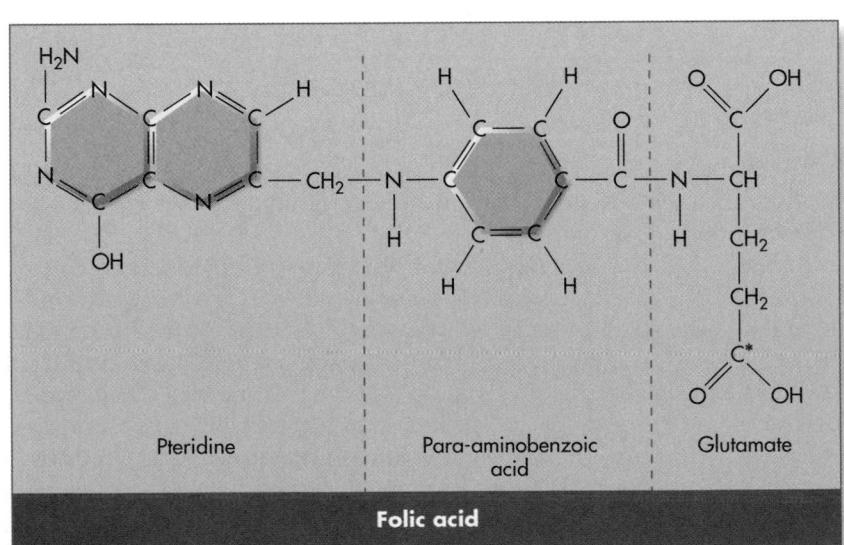

Pteridine   Para-aminobenzoic acid   Glutamate

Folic acid

Folic acid, also called folate monoglutamate, is the form absorbed in the intestine. Most of the folate naturally found in foods, however, contains additional glutamate molecules linked to the carboxyl group, indicated in this figure by the red asterisk. (These additional glutamates need to be removed before absorption.)

Absorption, Transport, Storage, and Excretion of Folate

To be absorbed, folate polyglutamates must be broken down (hydrolyzed) to the monoglutamate form in the GI tract. Enzymes, folate **conjugases,** located in the absorptive cells, allow for the removal of the excess glutamates. The monoglutamate form is then actively transported across the intestinal wall. Very large doses of folic acid from supplements are also absorbed by passive diffusion. When synthetic folic acid is consumed as a supplement and without food, it is nearly 100% bioavailable. Consumed with food, as in fortified cereal grains, absorption is slightly reduced.[11]

The portal blood draining the small intestine delivers the monoglutamate form of folate to the liver, where it is changed back to the polyglutamate form once in a cell. (This change allows folate to be trapped in a cell.) Folate is then either stored in the liver or released into the blood or bile. Most of the urinary excretion of folate exits as metabolic products. Biologically active folate is also excreted into the bile and is reabsorbed by enterohepatic circulation. Alcohol interferes with this process, which is one reason alcoholics often become folate deficient.

conjugase Enzyme systems in the intestine that enhance folate absorption; they remove glutamate molecules from polyglutamate forms of folate.

Functions of Folate

In cells, all forms of folate are readily converted to the basic coenzyme form, that transfers a single-carbon group called tetrahydrofolic acid (THFA). There are actually five active coenzyme forms of THFA. These forms participate in metabolic reactions by accepting and donating the single-carbon groups listed in the margin.

THFA transfers the following single-carbon groups: methyl ($-CH_3$), formyl ($-CH=O$), methylene ($-CH_2-$), and metheynyl ($-CH=$)

Metabolic Reactions

Transfer of these single-carbon units is needed for the synthesis of DNA and the metabolism of various amino acids and their derivatives. A crucial reaction requiring THFA is the transfer of a one-carbon methylene group ($-CH_2-$) to uridylate, forming thymidylate, an essential component of DNA and thus cell replication:

$$\text{THFA}(-CH_2-) \longrightarrow \text{THFA (free)}$$
$$\text{uridylate} \dashrightarrow \text{thymidylate} \dashrightarrow \text{DNA}$$

THFA is also needed for the synthesis of adenine and guanine of DNA, so DNA synthesis and repair may decline as a result of a folate shortage.

Because THFA is needed for DNA synthesis, folate deficiency may be induced during a common form of cancer therapy. One example is the cancer drug methotrexate. It inhibits a key aspect of folate metabolism. When methotrexate is taken in high doses, it reduces DNA synthesis throughout the body by interfering with folate metabolism. This reduction in DNA synthesis can halt the growth of cancer cells, but it also affects other rapidly proliferating cells, such as intestinal cells and red blood cells. Therefore, the typical side effects of methotrexate therapy are the same as for a folate deficiency (e.g., anemia and diarrhea). Methotrexate acting as a folate antagonist is also used to treat rheumatoid arthritis, psoriasis, asthma, alcoholic cirrhosis, and inflammatory bowel disease. When people are given methotrexate, they need to follow a high-folate diet and/or take folic acid supplements to reduce the toxic side effects of the drug. High supplemental doses generally have little or no influence on methotrexate's effectiveness.

Another key function of folate is the formation of neurotransmitters in the brain.[5] Meeting folate needs can improve the depressed state seen in some cases of mental illness.

Although folate deficiency can be induced to treat cancer, folate deficiency may also cause concern with regard to cancer. Because folate aids in the transfer of methyl groups for DNA synthesis, even mild folate deficiency may contribute to abnormal DNA integrity, which in turn affects certain cancer-protecting genes. A daily intake of 400 μg (the RDA) is thought to be chemo-preventive.

About 10% of the North American population has a defect in one aspect of folate metabolism. They may need up to twice the RDA to compensate for the reduced activity on an enzyme that converts folate to a related coenzyme form.[5] Currently, testing for this defect is not routine in medical practice, but one day it may be.

Other Functions

THFA is important in amino acid metabolism, especially the interconversions of amino acids.[5] It accepts one-carbon groups from various amino acids and is responsible for the glycine to serine reaction, (this reaction is the main methyl group source for THFA), the histidine to glutamic acid reaction, and one of the pathways in the homocysteine to methionine reaction.

Food Sources of Folate

Food Item and Amount	Folate (μg)
Asparagus, 1 cup	263
Cooked spinach, 1 cup	262
Cooked lentils, 1/2 cup	179
Black-eyed peas, 1/2 cup	179
Romaine lettuce, 1 1/2 cups	114
Great Grains cereal, 3/4 cup	114
Tortilla, 1	89
Cooked turnips, 1/2 cup	85
Cooked broccoli, 1 cup	78
Sunflower seeds, 1/4 cup	76
Fresh orange juice, 1 cup	75
Cooked beets, 1/2 cup	68
Kidney beans, 1/2 cup	65
Fried beef liver, 1 oz	62
Brewer's yeast, 1 tbsp	60
RDA for adults, 400 μg	

The use of dietary folate equivalents (DFEs) instead of the actual amount of folate in a food has some important implications. Typically, many foods will be richer in folate than the Nutrition Facts label suggests because folate content is due primarily to synthetic folic acid added to the foods, such as in enriched grains and ready-to-eat breakfast cereals. This addition contributes substantially to the DFE calculation. Another implication is that food composition tables (such as the one in the back of this book) and nutrition analysis software programs also underestimate the true folate contribution of a diet compared to folate needs because these have not been updated to DFE units.

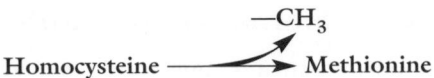

Folate participates in this reaction (and needs vitamin B-12 input to do so; see Appendix B for details).

Folate may also help maintain normal blood pressure and reduce the risk of developing colon cancer.[13,22]

Folate in Foods

The biological availability of folate varies with the source of the vitamin. The best sources, from the standpoint of amount and availability, are liver, fortified ready-to-eat breakfast cereals and other grain products, legumes, and dark green, leafy vegetables in general. Other, less rich sources of folate include eggs, dried beans, and oranges.

Food processing and preparation can destroy 50 to 90% of the folate in food. Folate is extremely susceptible to destruction by heat, oxidation, and ultraviolet light. (Vitamin C in foods helps protect folate from oxidative destruction.) It is important to eat fresh fruits and lightly cooked (or raw) vegetables on a regular basis to gain the full benefits of their folate contents.

Folate Needs and Dietary Folate Equivalents

The RDA for folate for adults is 400 μg/day, as is the Daily Value used on food and supplement labels. This quantity is based on the amount needed to maintain red blood cell folate, control blood homocysteine, and maintain normal blood folate concentrations. Also considered was the intake necessary to prevent neural tube defects for women capable of becoming pregnant (see the next section on folate deficiency).[11]

Dietary folate equivalents (DFEs) are the units used to express folate needs for all stages of life except childbearing years. (As you will learn in the next section, women of child-bearing age should meet such recommendations with synthetic folic acid.) These DFE units reflect the differences in absorption of food folate and synthetic folic acid.

To estimate the amount of DFE requires some calculations. First, determine how much of a day's food intake comes from food folate and how much comes from synthetic folic acid added to foods. When in doubt, assume all folate in a diet is derived from food in that form, except that coming from ready-to-eat breakfast cereals and refined grain products. Also include in this second category any folic acid consumed as part of dietary supplements. To calculate the DFE for the diet, multiply total synthetic folic acid intake by 1.7 and add that value to the total food folate intake.[11] The following is an example. The Daily Value for a serving of ready-to-eat breakfast cereal consumed is listed on the label as 50%, so the amount of folic acid is 200 μg per serving (Daily Value of 400 μg × 0.50). Because this folate is synthetic folic acid, the 200 μg is multiplied by 1.7, yielding 340 μg DFE. Assume the diet also contains 300 μg of food folate. To obtain the total DFE intake for the day, add the 300 μg to the 340 μg, which equals 640 μg DFE, more than enough for a man or older woman.

Folate-Deficiency Diseases

Folate deficiency can result from a low intake; inadequate absorption, which often is associated with alcoholism; increased need, most commonly occurring in pregnancy; compromised utilization, typically associated with vitamin B-12 deficiency; use of certain chemotherapy medications; and excessive excretion, linked to long-standing diarrhea.

Megaloblastic Anemia

A deficiency of folate first affects cell types that are actively synthesizing DNA; such cells have a short life span and rapid turnover rate.[5] Thus, one of the major folate-deficiency signs is changes in the early phases of red blood cell synthesis, because these cells turn over every 120 days. Without folate, the precursor cells in the bone marrow cannot divide normally to become mature red blood cells because they cannot form new DNA. The cells grow larger because there is continuous formation of RNA, leading to increased synthesis of protein and other cell components to make new cells. Hemoglobin synthesis also intensifies. However, when it is time for the cells to divide, they lack sufficient DNA for normal division. The cells thus remain in a large, immature form in the bone marrow, known as **megaloblasts** (Figure 10-6).

Unlike normal, mature red blood cells, megaloblasts retain their nuclei. Most of these cells do not make it out of the bone marrow. Any of these cells that do enter the bloodstream are called **macrocytes.** Their presence results in a form of anemia called **megaloblastic (or macrocytic) anemia.**

Large, immature cells also appear along the entire length of the GI tract during chronic folate deficiency.[5] This occurs because these cells are replaced very frequently, which means that DNA for the new cells has to be produced rapidly. In a folate deficiency, cell division in the GI tract is impaired. This change contributes to decreased absorptive capacity of the GI tract and a persistent diarrhea. White blood cell synthesis also is disrupted by a folate deficiency because these cells are made in rapid bursts during immune challenges (e.g., infections). Thus, immune function can be diminished during a folate deficiency. This effect likely can occur with milder folate deficiency than is needed to produce anemia.

megaloblast A large, nucleated, immature red blood cell in the bone marrow that results from the inability of a precursor cell to divide when it normally should.

macrocyte Literally "large cell," such as a large red blood cell.

megaloblastic anemia A form of anemia characterized by large, nucleated, immature red blood cells that result from the inability of a precursor cell to divide normally.

macrocytic anemia Anemia characterized by the presence of abnormally large red blood cells in the bloodstream.

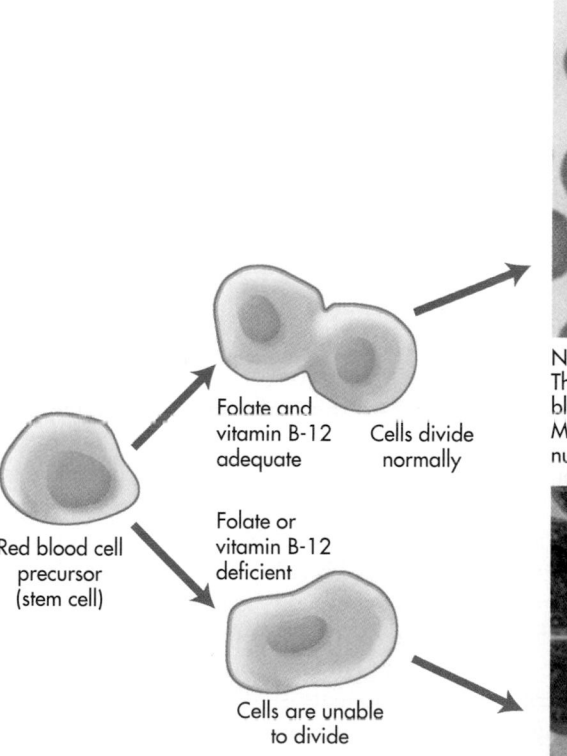
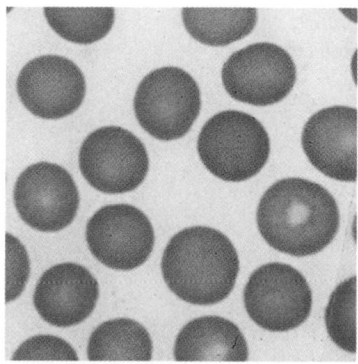

Normal blood cells in the bloodstream. The size, shape, and color of the red blood cells show that they are normal. Mature red blood cells have lost their nuclei.

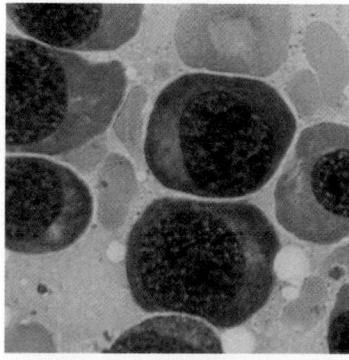

Megaloblastic blood cells seen here in the bone marrow are arrested at an immature stage of development. They still have their nuclei and are slightly larger than normal red blood cells.

Figure 10-6 | Megaloblastic anemia occurs when blood cells are unable to divide, leaving large, immature red blood cells. Either a folate or vitamin B-12 deficiency may cause this condition. Measurements of blood concentrations of both vitamins are taken to help determine the cause of the anemia.

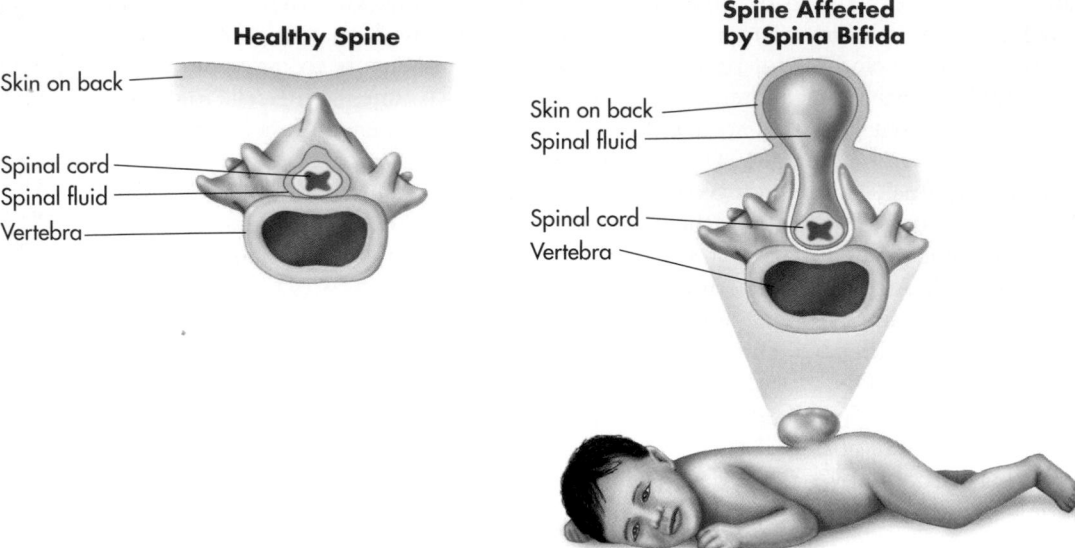

Healthy Spine

Skin on back
Spinal cord
Spinal fluid
Vertebra

Spine Affected by Spina Bifida

Skin on back
Spinal fluid
Spinal cord
Vertebra

Figure 10-7 | Neural tube defects result from a developmental failure affecting the spinal cord or brain in the embryo. Very early in fetal development, a ridge of neural-like tissue forms along the back of the embryo. As the fetus develops, this material differentiates into the spinal cord and body nerves at the lower end and into the brain at the upper end. At the same time, the bones that make up the back gradually surround the spinal cord on all sides. If any part of this sequence goes awry, many defects can appear. The worst is total lack of a brain (anencephaly). Much more common is spina bifida, in which the backbones do not form a complete ring to protect the spinal cord. Deficient folate status in the mother during the beginning of pregnancy increases the risk of neural tube defects, as does a genetic predisposition.

Women who have had a child with a neural tube defect are advised to consume 4 mg/day of folic acid beginning at least one month before any future pregnancy. This must be done under strict physician supervision. For further information about neural tube defects, see the website www.sbaa.org.

neural tube defect A defect in the formation of the neural tube occurring during early fetal development. This type of defect results in various nervous system disorders, such as spina bifida. A very severe form is anencephaly. Folate deficiency in the pregnant woman increases the risk that the fetus will develop this disorder.

Neural Tube Defects

A maternal deficiency of folate and a genetic predisposition have been linked to the development of **neural tube defects** in the fetus (Figure 10-7). These defects include spina bifida (spinal cord or spinal fluid bulge through the back) and anencephaly (absence of a brain). Approximately 2000 infants are born so affected annually in the United States. Victims of spina bifida may exhibit paralysis, incontinence, hydrocephalus, and learning disabilities. Children born with anencephaly die shortly after birth. Adequate folate nutriture is crucial for all women of childbearing years, because neural tube closure begins 21 days after conception and is completed by day 28, a time when many women are not even aware that they are pregnant. Perhaps as many as 70% of these defects could be avoided by adequate folate status before conception.[2] All research has been done with synthetic folic acid supplementation, and it appears that even women with varied diets may not consume adequate synthetic folic acid to prevent neural tube defects (400 μg/day) unless specific attention to synthetic folic acid sources, such as many ready-to-eat breakfast cereals, is given. Most grain products are now enriched or fortified with folic acid.

Because the metabolism and functions of folate and B-12 are linked, regular consumption of large amounts of folate can mask (e.g., prevent the appearance of) the primary early warning sign of vitamin B-12 deficiency—enlarged red blood cells.[11] To prevent such masking of vitamin B-12 deficiency, it is the goal of FDA to increase the synthetic folic acid intake of women of childbearing years through grain enrichment without producing excessive intake by other groups (> 1 mg/day of folic acid). This enrichment currently supplies adults in the United States with about 200 μg/day of synthetic folic acid.

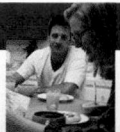

Case Scenario | Follow-Up

Suzanne and Ted should remember that spina bifida is caused by a failure of the spinal cord to close during the first 28 days of pregnancy, a time when neither Ted nor Suzanne will realize that Suzanne is pregnant. The B-vitamin folate must be available at the time of conception to prevent spina bifida and other birth defects. The fact that a close relative of Suzanne's has already produced a child with this birth defect should be a warning sign. Suzanne and Ted would be wise to seek the advice of a registered dietician to ensure that Suzanne's prepregnancy diet provides enough synthetic folic acid.

Steps in Folate Deficiency

1. Decrease in blood folate concentration
2. Decrease in red cell folate
3. Defective DNA synthesis
4. Change in structure of certain white blood cells
5. Increase in blood concentration of homocysteine (and methylmalonic acid)
6. Megaloblastic changes in bone marrow and other rapidly dividing cells
7. Increase in the size of circulating red blood cells
8. Megaloblastic (macrocytic) anemia

Other Folate Deficiency States

Folate deficiencies sometimes appear in pregnant women. They need extra folate to meet an increased rate of cell division and thus of DNA synthesis in their own bodies and in the developing fetus (600 μg DFE/day).[11] Today, prenatal care often includes prenatal multivitamin and mineral supplements fortified with folate to compensate for the extra needs associated with pregnancy.

Young women in general also often show low blood folate values. It is important for them to seek good sources of synthetic folic acid that they enjoy eating and then to eat those foods regularly, such as ready-to-eat cereals. The use of a balanced multivitamin and mineral supplement is another option. Older adults are also at risk for folate deficiency. Finally, persons suffering from alcohol abuse or taking certain prescription drugs need to recognize that they may develop a folate deficiency.

Upper Level for Folate

The Upper Level for synthetic folic acid is 1000 μg (1 mg), based on its ability to mask a vitamin B-12 deficiency when synthetic folic acid is given in high doses.[11] (However, the Upper Level does not apply to folate in foods because absorption is limited.) In response to this problem, FDA limits the amount of folic acid in nonprescription vitamin supplements for nonpregnant individuals to 400 μg when no statement of age is listed on the supplement label. When age-related doses are listed, there can be no more than 100 μg for infants, 300 μg for children, and 400 μg for adults. Prenatal supplements sold over the counter can contain 800 μg.

▌Vitamin B-12

What we call vitamin B-12 includes the free vitamin cyanocobalamin and two active coenzymes—methylcobalamin and 5-deoxyadenosylcobalamin. This vitamin has a complex structure containing the mineral cobalt.[6]

All vitamin B-12 compounds are synthesized exclusively by bacteria, fungi, and algae. Animals such as cows and sheep obtain vitamin B-12 either from bacterial synthesis in the multiple compartments of their stomachs (rumen) or from the soil they ingest while eating and grazing. The only reliable source of the vitamin for humans is animal foods. Plants do not synthesize vitamin B-12. There is minor contamination of vegetable products by bacteria and soil, but it is not a reliable source. The process of fermentation also contributes a small amount of vitamin B-12 to a food.

Vitamin B-12 (cyanocobalamin)

The cyanocobalamin form of vitamin B-12 is converted to the active coenzyme forms by replacement of the cyano group (red) with another group, such as a methyl group or a hydroxyl group.

R-protein A protein produced by the salivary glands that enhances absorption of vitamin B-12, possibly by protecting the vitamin during its passage through the stomach.

intrinsic factor A substance present in gastric juice that enhances vitamin B-12 absorption.

Absorption, Transport, Storage, and Excretion of Vitamin B-12

Absorption of vitamin B-12 is very complex. In the stomach, vitamin B-12 in food is released from proteins by the action of HCl and pepsin in gastric juice. The free B-12 binds to a protein, designated **R-protein,** that originates in the salivary glands in the mouth and is swallowed along with the food. The R-protein/vitamin B-12 complex travels to the small intestine, where it encounters pancreatic protease enzymes (e.g., trypsin), which release the vitamin. Awaiting the free B-12 is **intrinsic factor,** a proteinlike compound produced by the parietal cells in the stomach. The resulting intrinsic factor/vitamin B-12 complex travels to the terminal portion of the small intestine, the ileum, where it attaches to special receptor cells on the brush border. Several hours later, cells within the ileum absorb vitamin B-12 and transfer it to a specific blood transport protein, transcobalamin II. This vitamin-protein complex enters the portal vein that drains the small intestine and is taken up by the liver and eventually the bone marrow and red blood cells (Figure 10-8).[6]

It is assumed that 50% of dietary vitamin B-12 is absorbed by healthy adults with normal GI tract function. Vitamin B-12 is continually secreted into the bile, and most of it is reabsorbed by enterohepatic circulation. Failure in any of the links found in the absorptive process reduces absorption to 2% or less of dietary vitamin B-12.

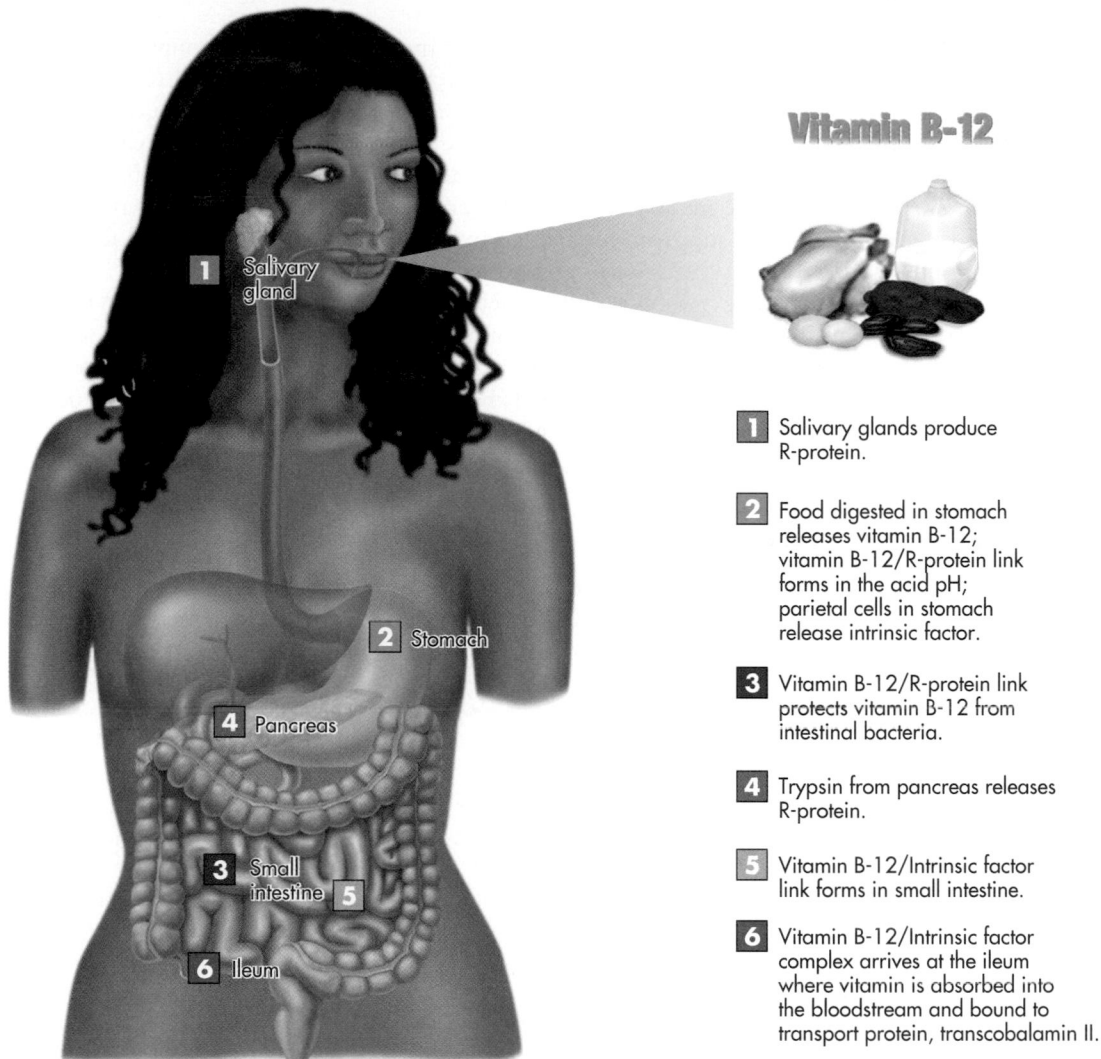

1. Salivary glands produce R-protein.

2. Food digested in stomach releases vitamin B-12; vitamin B-12/R-protein link forms in the acid pH; parietal cells in stomach release intrinsic factor.

3. Vitamin B-12/R-protein link protects vitamin B-12 from intestinal bacteria.

4. Trypsin from pancreas releases R-protein.

5. Vitamin B-12/Intrinsic factor link forms in small intestine.

6. Vitamin B-12/Intrinsic factor complex arrives at the ileum where vitamin is absorbed into the bloodstream and bound to transport protein, transcobalamin II.

Figure 10-8 | Absorption of vitamin B-12. Many factors and sites in the gastrointestinal tract participate. Defects arising in the stomach or small intestine can interfere with vitamin B-12 absorption, in turn causing pernicious anemia.

Absorption of vitamin B-12 can be disrupted by numerous defects, including the following:[1,11,26]

- Absence or defective synthesis of R-protein, pancreatic proteases, or intrinsic factor
- Defective binding of the intrinsic factor/vitamin B-12 complex to receptor cells in the ileum
- Absence (or surgical removal) of much or all of the ileum and stomach
- Bacterial overgrowth of the small intestine
- Tapeworm infestation
- Use of certain anti-ulcer medications that significantly reduce acid production by the parietal cells (e.g., omeprazole [Prilosec])
- Chronic malabsorption syndromes, as can be seen in AIDS

About 50 to 90% of the body's total supply of vitamin B-12 is stored in the liver (about 2 to 4 mg). In the body, little vitamin B-12 is excreted—just the small amount that escapes enterohepatic circulation of the bile.

mutase An enzyme that rearranges the functional groups on a molecule.

Functions of Vitamin B-12

Vitamin B-12 is associated with coenzymes that move one-carbon groups.[6] An example of an enzyme that uses a vitamin B-12 coenzyme is methylmalonyl CoA **mutase.** This enzyme requires vitamin B-12 to convert methylmalonyl CoA to succinyl CoA, an intermediate in the citric acid cycle. This reaction allows fatty acids with an odd number of carbons (most, but not all, fatty acids have an even number) to be oxidized for energy. The enzyme methionine synthase requires a vitamin B-12 coenzyme for the transfer of a methyl group from methyltetrahydrofolate to homocysteine to form methionine and tetrahydrofolate, as shown on page 356 and in Appendix B.

Vitamin B-12 coenzymes also end up helping recycle folate coenzymes. When folate coenzymes function, their chemical composition changes as various single-carbon groups are added. In a variety of chemical reactions, vitamin B-12 is needed to turn the folate coenzyme back into the original chemical structure that can resume function (e.g., free of the added single-carbon group). Vitamin B-12 also plays some roles in the nervous system, some of which are not fully understood.[11]

Vitamin B-12 in Foods

Sources of vitamin B-12 include animal products such as meat, poultry, seafood, and eggs. Especially rich sources of vitamin B-12 (μg/kcal) are organ meats (especially liver, kidneys, and heart). Another source of vitamin B-12 is dairy products.

Vitamin B-12 Needs

The RDA of vitamin B-12 for adults is 2.4 μg/day. It is based on maintaining enough vitamin B-12 in the body to adequately synthesize red blood cells.[11] The Daily Value used on food and supplement labels is 6 μg. On average, adult men consume 3 times the RDA and women consume 2 times the RDA. This high intake provides the average meat-eating person with 2 to 3 years' storage of vitamin B-12 in the liver. For men and women 51 years and older, the RDA is also 2.4 μg of vitamin B-12 per day, but this population group is advised to select foods fortified with vitamin B-12 (e.g., ready-to-eat breakfast cereals) and/or to take a supplemental form. Absorption of foodborne vitamin B-12 is hampered by the typical fall in gastric acid output seen in aging, called **achlorhydria,** but the vitamin B-12 that is added to foods or supplements is not.[1]

No adverse effects have been observed with excess vitamin B-12 intake from food or from supplements, so there is no Upper Level for this vitamin.[11]

Vitamin B-12-Deficiency Diseases

Researchers in mid-nineteenth-century England noted a form of anemia that causes death within 2 to 5 years of initial diagnosis. They called this disease **pernicious anemia** (*pernicious* literally means "leading to death").[6] We now know that this anemia is caused by a genetic problem in the production of intrinsic factor that is needed for vitamin B-12 absorption. Clinically, this disease looks like a folate-deficiency anemia, because a vitamin B-12 deficiency impairs folate function. For patients with either a folate or vitamin B-12 deficiency, many megaloblasts (macrocytes) are seen in the blood. As in folate deficiency, the cause of the anemia is an interference with normal synthesis of DNA.

A vitamin B-12 deficiency also produces nerve degeneration, which can be fatal. The neurological complications produce sensory disturbances in the legs, such as tingling and numbness (collectively referred to as **paresthesia**).[21] These unpleasant sensations often are worse in the lower legs. Walking is difficult and "position sense" is seriously affected. Many mental problems exist as well, such as loss of concentration and memory, disorientation, and dementia. As the condition worsens, bowel and bladder control is lost. Visual disturbances are common. There also are numerous GI tract problems, from a sore tongue to constipation.

Food Sources of Vitamin B-12

Food Item and Amount	Vitamin B-12 (μg)
Fried beef liver, 1 oz	31.7
Baked clams, 1 oz	15.7
Boiled oysters, 2	14.4
Brewer's yeast, 2 tbsp	3.0
Lobster, 3 oz	2.7
Pot roast, 3 oz	2.5
Plain yogurt, 1 cup	1.4
Corn Flakes cereal, 3/4 cup	1.1
Shrimp, 3 oz	1.0
1% milk, 1 cup	0.9
Soy milk, 1 cup	0.8
Boiled egg, 1	0.6
Lean ham, 3 oz	0.6
Beef hot dog, 1	0.5
Ham lunch meat, 2 oz	0.4
RDA for adults, 2.4 μg	

achlorhydria A decrease in stomach acid primarily due to age-associated loss of acid-producing gastric cells.

pernicious anemia The anemia that results from the inability to absorb sufficient vitamin B-12; it is associated with nerve degeneration, which can result in eventual paralysis and death.

paresthesia An abnormal spontaneous sensation such as of burning, prickling, and numbness.

Infants who are breastfed by vegetarian or vegan mothers can develop vitamin B-12 deficiency, accompanied by anemia and long-term neurological problems such as diminished brain growth, degeneration of the spinal cord, and poor intellectual development. The problems may have their origins during pregnancy if the mother is deficient in vitamin B-12.

Adult vegetarians can also become vitamin B-12 deficient, though if an adult becomes a vegetarian, vitamin B-12 stores in the liver can delay a severe deficiency for a long time (even years). Vegetarians have several options for obtaining vitamin B-12. If they are not vegans, they can obtain vitamin B-12 from dairy products. Eggs also contain some vitamin B-12. In addition, vegetarians can take a supplement that contains vitamin B-12 or eat food products fortified with vitamin B-12 (review Chapter 7 for further details).

People with malabsorption syndromes of any kind have an increased need for vitamin B-12. These situations include people who have had their stomach either bypassed or removed, people who have had their ileum removed, and patients with Crohn's disease or any disease involving the ileum. People who are HIV-positive with chronic diarrhea may develop vitamin B-12 deficiencies. Several other medical conditions, such as reduced secretions of the pancreas (chronic pancreatic disease) and bacterial infections of the intestinal tract, require extra vitamin B-12 because of decreased bioavailability of the vitamin from food.[6]

Older people may often have problems with absorbing vitamin B-12 due to reduced stomach production of gastric acid, which frees vitamin B-12 from food proteins. This decrease can lower vitamin B-12 absorption to the extent that it creates a marginal vitamin B-12 deficiency.[1] This deficiency is not severe enough to produce anemia, but it can cause neurological problems and elevated blood homocysteine. This degree of impaired vitamin B-12 absorption can usually be overcome by a moderate increase of oral vitamin B-12 intake via fortified foods or supplements.

Three types of therapy are possible for patients diagnosed with a major defect in vitamin B-12 absorption: monthly injections of vitamin B-12 to bypass the GI tract, use of a vitamin B-12 nasal gel (nasal absorption does not require the intrinsic factor), or weekly ingestion of vitamin B-12 supplements in megadoses (300 times the RDA), which allow absorption by passive diffusion. Most cases of vitamin B-12 deficiency among otherwise healthy people in North America result from a defect in vitamin B-12 absorption rather than from inadequate intake.[6]

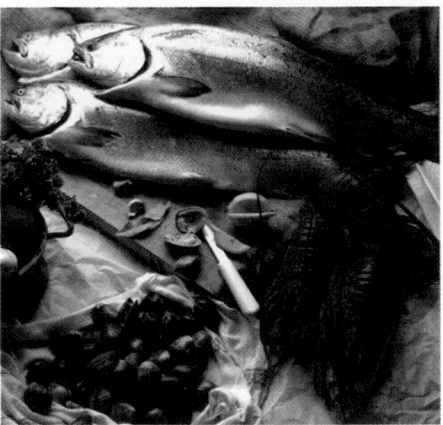

Fish, seafood, and related products are good sources of vitamin B-12.

In the 1920s, researchers found that a vitamin B-12 deficiency can be cured by consumption of massive amounts of liver or concentrated water extracts of liver. In this case, the deficiency was caused by an absorption defect. If enough of the vitamin is ingested, it can be absorbed by simple diffusion, thereby overcoming the defective R-protein/intrinsic factor system.

Concept | Check

Folate is needed for cell division because it is essential for DNA synthesis. A folate deficiency results in macrocytic anemia as well as diarrhea, inflammation of the tongue, and poor growth—all signs of inadequate cell division. Folate is found in fresh vegetables and organ meats. Folate deficiency is most commonly found in pregnant women, when needs are elevated, and in alcoholics, because alcohol interferes with absorption of folate. Vitamin B-12 is necessary for folate metabolism. Without dietary vitamin B-12, folate deficiency symptoms, such as macrocytic anemia, develop. In addition, vitamin B-12 is necessary for maintaining the nervous system; paralysis can develop from a vitamin B-12 deficiency. Vitamin B-12 is found only in animal foods; meat eaters generally have a 3- to 5-year supply stored in the liver. However, vitamin B-12 absorption may decline in older persons and is generally corrected by monthly injections of the vitamin.

Choline

For many years, choline was often included in supplements as a supposed B-vitamin. However, most nutrition experts claimed that choline was not a vitamin at all because the body makes enough of it to meet its needs. Recent research has contradicted some

Choline

of this attitude. Apparently in some cases, the body's production of choline is not sufficient to cover requirements.[29] Choline still is not considered a B-vitamin. Choline does not have a coenzyme function, and the amount of choline in the body is much greater than the amount of a typical B-vitamin.

Absorption, Transport, Storage, and Excretion of Choline

Choline is absorbed from the small intestine by way of transport proteins. Choline is taken up rapidly by the liver from the portal vein that drains the small intestine. All tissues contain some stores of choline. Some choline is excreted in the urine, but most of the excess is converted to a related donor of single-carbon groups **(betaine)**.[29]

betaine A product of choline metabolism and a methyl (CH₃) donor in methionine metabolism.

Functions of Choline

Choline functions as a precursor for acetylcholine, a neurotransmitter associated with attention, learning and memory, muscle control, and many other functions. Choline is a component of phospholipids, such as phosphatidylcholine (lecithin), a major component of the cell membrane and blood lipoproteins. Liver export of VLDL is also associated with the action of choline. The methyl (—CH₃) group of choline can be used to form methionine from homocysteine.[29]

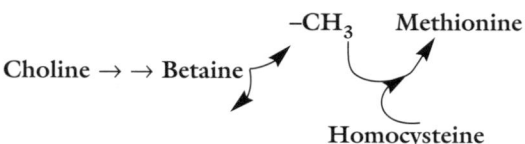

Choline in Foods

Choline is widely distributed in foods, mostly in the form of phosphatidylcholine in membranes. Milk, liver, eggs, and peanuts are rich sources. Lecithins often are added to food during processing, so this is yet another source. So much choline is available in ordinary foods that a dietary deficiency is unlikely.[10]

Choline Needs

The Adequate Intake for choline for adult men is 550 mg/day; for adult women it is 425 mg/day. These amounts are based on the intake of choline required to maintain liver function as assessed by measuring an enzyme (alanine aminotransferase) concentration in the blood.[11]

Few data exist to assess whether a dietary supply is needed at all life stages. Although Adequate Intakes are set for choline, it may be that the choline requirement can be met by body synthesis at some or all stages of life. We also consume ample choline from food, at least 700 to 1000 mg/day, so there is no need to supplement a diet with this nutrient.[10]

Choline-Deficiency Diseases

When humans were fed choline-deficient total parenteral nutrition solutions, they developed fatty livers and liver damage. Based on these observations, plus laboratory animal studies, choline has been deemed essential, at least in some life stages and health conditions.[29]

Upper Level for Choline

The Upper Level for adults is 3.5 g/day, based on development of a fishy body odor (arising from a breakdown product) and low blood pressure. Very high doses of choline have also been associated with vomiting, salivation, sweating, and GI tract effects.[11]

Food Sources of Choline

Food Item and Amount	Choline (mg)
Egg, 1	126
Cod, 3 oz	70
Chicken, 3 oz	56
Nonfat milk, 1 cup	37
Beef, 3 oz	36
Yogurt, 1 cup	31
Wheat germ, 2 tbsp	21
Peanut butter, 2 tbsp	20
Cottage cheese, 1/2 cup	20
Orange, 1	12
Broccoli, 1/2 cup	7
Squash, 1/2 cup	7
Whole-wheat bread, 1 slice	7
Apple, 1	7
Romaine lettuce, 4 leaves	6
White bread, 1 slice	3
Adequate Intake for adult men, 550 mg; adult women, 425 mg	

▌Vitamin C

Vitamin C, also known as ascorbic acid, is involved in many processes in the human body, primarily as an electron donor.[19] Ascorbic acid is needed by all other life forms, but all plants and most animals make ascorbic acid. So ascorbic acid is a vitamin only for humans, plus a few other animals: nonhuman primates, guinea pigs, a few birds, fruit bats, and some fish.

The term *vitamin C* actually refers not only to ascorbic acid but also to its oxidized form dehydroascorbic acid. Both forms are found in the foods we eat.

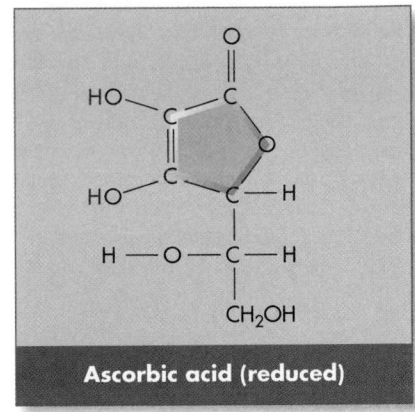

Ascorbic acid (reduced)

Absorption, Transport, Storage, and Excretion of Vitamin C

Absorption of vitamin C occurs in the small intestine by means of active transport (for ascorbic acid) and by facilitated diffusion (for dehydroascorbic acid). Efficiency of the absorptive mechanism decreases as intake increases. About 70 to 90% of vitamin C is absorbed at daily intakes between 30 and 200 mg, whereas absorption efficiency declines substantially with doses exceeding that amount. Excretion by the kidneys increases as dietary intake increases.[19]

The amount of vitamin C varies widely by tissue. High concentrations are found in the pituitary and adrenal glands, white blood cells, eyes, and brain. The lowest concentrations are in the blood and saliva. The total amount of vitamin C in the body varies over a wide range.

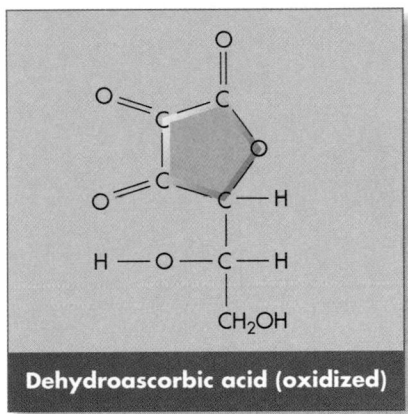

Dehydroascorbic acid (oxidized)

Ascorbic acid Vitamin C undergoes reversible oxidation and reduction by loss or addition of two hydrogens (red).

Functions of Vitamin C

Vitamin C performs a variety of important cell functions. It does so primarily by acting as a nonspecific electron donor (**reducing agent**).[19] As mentioned in conjunction with riboflavin and niacin functions, a reducing agent is a substance that donates electrons and, in turn, becomes oxidized (loses electrons). Ascorbic acid donates electrons as part of hydrogen atoms; however, unlike the coenzyme function of riboflavin or niacin, ascorbic acid donates hydrogens in a way that the electrons of the atom go to different molecules than the rest of the hydrogen. For example, vitamin C can donate electrons to metal ions, such as iron and copper. In the oxidized state, ferric iron (Fe^{3+}) can be reduced to ferrous iron (Fe^{2+}), and the cupric ion (Cu^{2+}) to the cuprous ion (Cu^+). The metals receive the electrons while the rest of the hydrogen goes elsewhere (e.g., as H^+).

Some vitamin C actions are associated with enzymes, while others are not. Even when enzymes are involved, vitamin C is not considered a coenzyme in the same way B-vitamins are because the chemistry is different. For example, a riboflavin coenzyme can modify a compound, whereas a vitamin C may act on a metal in an enzyme.

reducing agent A compound capable of donating electrons (also hydrogen ions) to another compound.

Collagen Synthesis

Collagen is the fibrous protein that gives strength to **connective tissue.** Collagen fibers are critical to the structure of bone and blood vessels, and they are essential in wound healing.

A collagen molecule is like a three-stranded rope. It consists of three-polypeptide chains wound together to form a triple helix. To get the three strands in the right shape to form the triple helix, which gives a ropelike structure, vitamin C is needed. In particular, vitamin C helps change the structure of two amino acids, lysine and proline in collagen (Figure 10-9). These are converted to hydroxylysine and hydroxyproline. The role of vitamin C in the formation of these unusual amino acids is to interact with the enzymes involved in making the conversions. These enzymes use iron as part of the catalytic process. In this process, the iron is converted from Fe^{2+} to Fe^{3+}. For the enzymes to continue functioning, the iron must be recycled to Fe^{2+}. Vitamin C, as a reducing agent, can provide electrons for this purpose.[19]

collagen The major protein of the material that holds together the various structures of the body.

connective tissue Cells and their protein products that hold different structures of the body together. Tendons and cartilage are composed largely of connective tissue. Connective tissue also forms part of bone and the nonmuscular structures of arteries and veins.

Figure 10-9. | Vitamin C is needed for the addition of hydroxyl groups (–OH) to the amino acid proline in collagen molecules (1–2). Collagen is unique among body proteins because it contains large amounts of the amino acid hydroxyproline, which is necessary for the formation of stable collagen fibers (3). Without sufficient vitamin C available to perform this task, only weak connective tissue is formed (4).

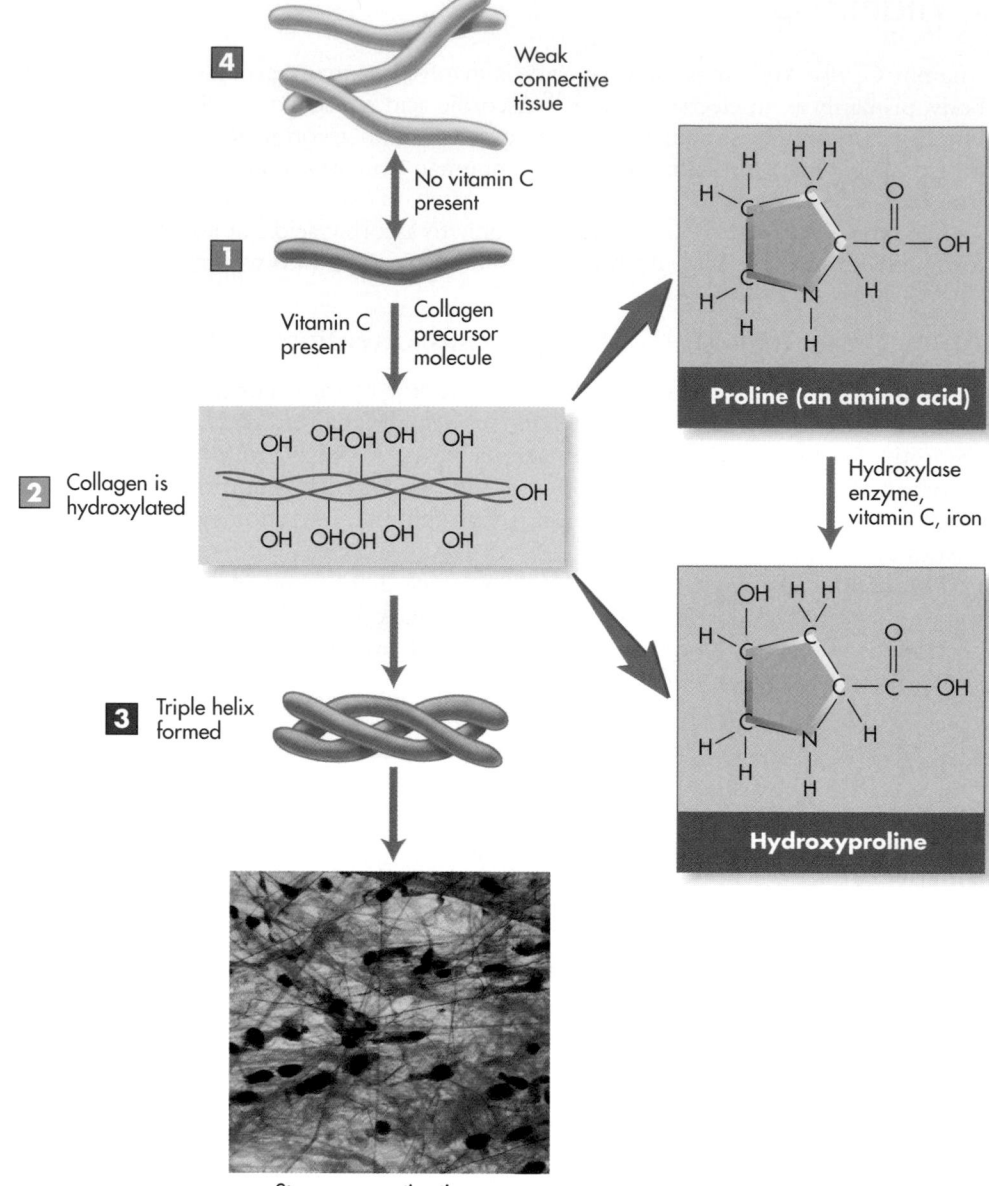

4 Weak connective tissue

No vitamin C present

1

Vitamin C present | Collagen precursor molecule

2 Collagen is hydroxylated

3 Triple helix formed

Strong connective tissue.

Proline (an amino acid)

Hydroxylase enzyme, vitamin C, iron

Hydroxyproline

Antioxidant Activity

In vitro (in a test tube), vitamin C can be an antioxidant by donating electrons to free radicals. Recall that a free radical has an unpaired electron. A vitamin C molecule can donate electrons to free radicals so that they become stable. Researchers have proposed that vitamin C in the body's water-based fluids (e.g., blood) acts just like vitamin E does in lipid-rich environments. It has also been suggested that vitamin C can recycle vitamin E and make it function more effectively.

Although these vitamin C antioxidant actions work well in a test tube, do they work the same in humans? Despite what you may have read to the contrary, we don't actually know if vitamin C plays major or minor antioxidant roles in humans.[19] Research in this area is ongoing. So far, some data suggest that vitamin C does have some important in vivo antioxidant effects. However, not all the results have been that positive. In fact, some research suggested that vitamin C can increase oxidative stress, such as in people with diabetes.[18] Dr. Mark Levine and Dr. Sebastian J. Padayatty discuss this role of vitamin C in more detail in the Expert Opinion.

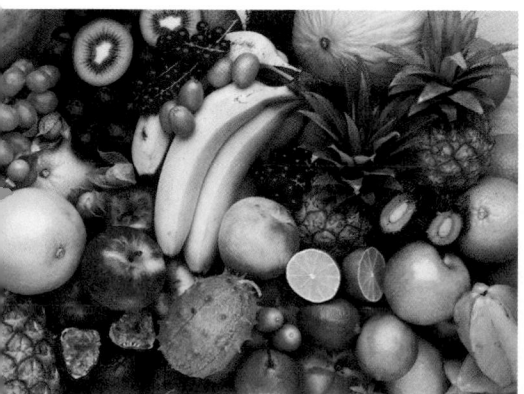

Orange, limes, lemons, and kiwi fruit are all rich sources of vitamin C.

Vitamin C is present in high concentrations in the eye, possibly to protect against photolytically generated free radicals.[19] It is also present in high concentrations in white blood cells (e.g., neutrophils), possibly for protection against the free radicals produced during immune functions.

Iron Absorption

Vitamin C added to meals modestly facilitates the intestinal absorption of nonheme iron (iron that is not in hemoglobin) because of the conversion of iron in the GI tract to ferrous iron (Fe^{2+}). Vitamin C also counters the action of certain food components that inhibit iron absorption.[12]

Synthesis of Other Vital Compounds

Carnitine is a transport compound that moves fatty acids from the cytoplasm into the mitochondria for energy production. Vitamin C participates in two separate steps in carnitine biosynthesis. The biosynthesis of the hormones and neurotransmitters norepinephrine and epinephrine depends on vitamin C as an electron donor. The conversion of the essential amino acid tryptophan to the neurotransmitter serotonin requires vitamin C. Vitamin C is necessary for the biosynthesis of thyroxine (the thyroid hormone) and many other nervous system components. Vitamin C is also involved in the biosynthesis of corticosteroids and aldosterone, the conversion of cholesterol to bile acids, and tyrosine (an amino acid) metabolism.[12]

Immune Function

White blood cells, part of the immune defenses of the body, contain the highest vitamin C concentration of all body constituents. A high concentration of vitamin C in white blood cells may provide protection against the oxidative damage associated with cellular respiration.[19] Free radicals generated during phagocytosis and **neutrophil activation,** though intended to kill bacteria or damaged tissue, can also damage the body's own immune cells. Vitamin C may reduce this self-destruction by this vitamin's antioxidant actions. Vitamin C may also have other roles in immune function. Note, however, that supplemental vitamin C beyond body needs may not necessarily improve immune function.

Vitamin C in Foods

All fruits and vegetables contain some vitamin C, but certain fruits and vegetables provide much more than others. Citrus fruits, potatoes, and green vegetables in general are good sources of vitamin C. Animal products and grains are generally not good sources. An intake of 5 servings/day of combined fruits and vegetables provides ample vitamin C. The major contributors of vitamin C to North American diets are oranges and orange juice, grapefruit and grapefruit juice, tomatoes and tomato juice, fortified fruit drinks, tangerines, and potatoes. Vitamin C is easily lost in processing and cooking. Juices are good foods to fortify with vitamin C because their acidity reduces vitamin C destruction. Vitamin C is very unstable when in contact with heat, iron, copper, and oxygen.

Vitamin C Needs

The RDA for vitamin C for adult men is 90 mg/day; for adult women it is 75 mg/day. Most of us consume this much and more. The RDA is based on near maximal vitamin C concentrations in neutrophils (a white blood cell) with minimal urinary excretion. Because smoking causes oxidative stress, the needs of smokers increases by 35 mg/day.[12] Smokers have a higher turnover of vitamin C, probably because of its antioxidant activity. Vitamin C needs are also increased by oral contraceptive use (for reasons that are

Critical | Thinking

Carlos just returned from a local mall and is excited because he saw an advertisement claiming that vitamin C will cure just about everything from colds to heart disease. How would you explain to him vitamin C's main functions in the human body?

neutrophil activation A type of white blood cell being prepared for immune response.

Food Sources of Vitamin C

Food Item and Amount	Vitamin C (mg)
Orange, 1	98
Cooked brussels sprouts, 1 cup	97
Strawberries, 1 cup	94
Grapefruit juice, 1 cup	80
Red peppers, 1/4 cup	71
Kiwi fruit, 1	57
Green pepper rings, 5	45
Tomato juice, 1 cup	45
Cooked broccoli, 1/2 cup	33
Kale, 1/2 cup	27
Raw cauliflower, 1/2 cup	23
Sweet potato, 1	17
Baked potato, 1 medium	16
Pineapple chunks, 1/2 cup	12
Cooked spinach, 1/2 cup	9
RDA for adult men, 90 mg; adult women, 75 mg	

not clear). Vitamin C needs can be increased by burns or surgery that removes a lot of tissue. Such injuries require much collagen production to replace the lost tissue. However, the medical literature does not agree on how much extra vitamin C is needed. The Daily Value for vitamin C on food and supplement labels is 60 mg.

Vitamin C-Deficiency Diseases

A deficiency of vitamin C prevents the normal synthesis of collagen, thus causing widespread and significant changes in connective tissues throughout the body. The first signs and symptoms of scurvy, the deficiency disease, appear after about 20 to 40 days on a vitamin C–free diet and include fatigue and pinpoint hemorrhages around hair follicles on the back of the arms and legs (Figure 10-10). These hemorrhages are the most characteristic sign of scurvy. In addition, there is bleeding in the gums and joints, a classic sign of connective tissue failure. Other effects of scurvy include impaired wound healing, bone pain, fractures, and diarrhea. Psychological problems, such as depression, are common in advanced scurvy.[19]

Worldwide, scurvy is associated with poverty. It is especially common in infants who are fed boiled milk (all forms of milk are poor sources of vitamin C) and are not provided with a good food source of vitamin C or a supplement.

In North America, vitamin C deficiency is most likely to occur in alcoholics and those addicted to other drugs, because such people often consume a nutrient-poor diet. Anyone who eats very few fruits and vegetables is also susceptible to vitamin C deficiency. Men in general are more at risk of vitamin C deficiency compared with women because they are more apt to eat poorly. Finally, people exposed to cigarette smoke generally have lower vitamin C status than nonsmokers.

Vitamin C Intake above the RDA

Some popular authors and speakers advocate consumption of vitamin C at amounts higher than the RDA. Surprisingly, there is not much research comparing different vitamin C intakes. Note that if vitamin C intake is above about 100 mg/day, much of the additional vitamin C is excreted in the urine. Some research also indicates that 200 mg/day is the most a person would need to maximize the health benefits of vitamin C intake. Choosing several vitamin C–rich foods each day can boost intakes to 200 mg/day.[19]

One aspect of high vitamin C intake that has drawn a lot of attention is its possible use for prevention or treatment of the common cold. This use is not focused on correcting vitamin C deficiency. Although such an intake may help with cold severity, probably by improving immune function, most of the attention has been on a high vitamin C intake by people with no deficiency. At these doses, the vitamin C could exert multiple actions, including actions that do not occur at more typical vitamin C intakes. The notion that high doses of vitamin C are useful for preventing and treating colds, and perhaps some other maladies, has gained a lot of attention. Many of the studies on this topic have concluded that high dose vitamin C use (up to about 1000 mg/day) may have small effects on cold severity (not incidence) in some people.[9]

Upper Level for Vitamin C

The Upper Level for vitamin C is 2 g/day. Regularly consuming more than that may cause stomach inflammation and diarrhea.[12] Other purported toxicity symptoms from vitamin C have been discounted in healthy people, but as noted earlier a recent study showed an increase in cardiovascular disease deaths in older women with diabetes who consumed megadose amounts.[18]

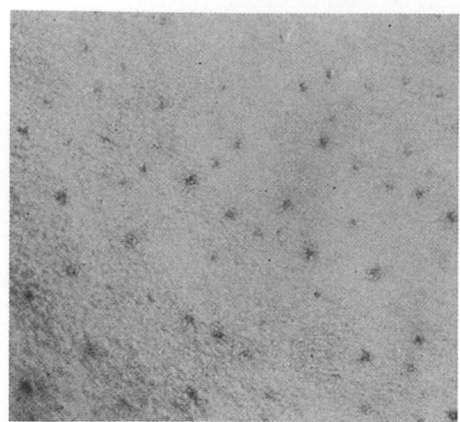

Figure 10-10 | Pinpoint hemorrhages of the skin—an early symptom of scurvy. The spots on the skin are caused by slight bleeding into hair follicles. The person also will often show inadequate wound healing—all signs of defective collagen synthesis.

Although the development of scurvy in an otherwise healthy child is rare, it is possible. A 5-year-old boy developed scurvy after eating nothing but Pop-Tarts, cheese pizza, biscuits, and water for 5 months. The boy, who was growing and maturing normally, started to limp; his gums became swollen; and small, purple spots began to appear on his skin. His baffled doctors finally diagnosed the boy as having scurvy and gave him vitamin C, and his condition began to improve within a week.

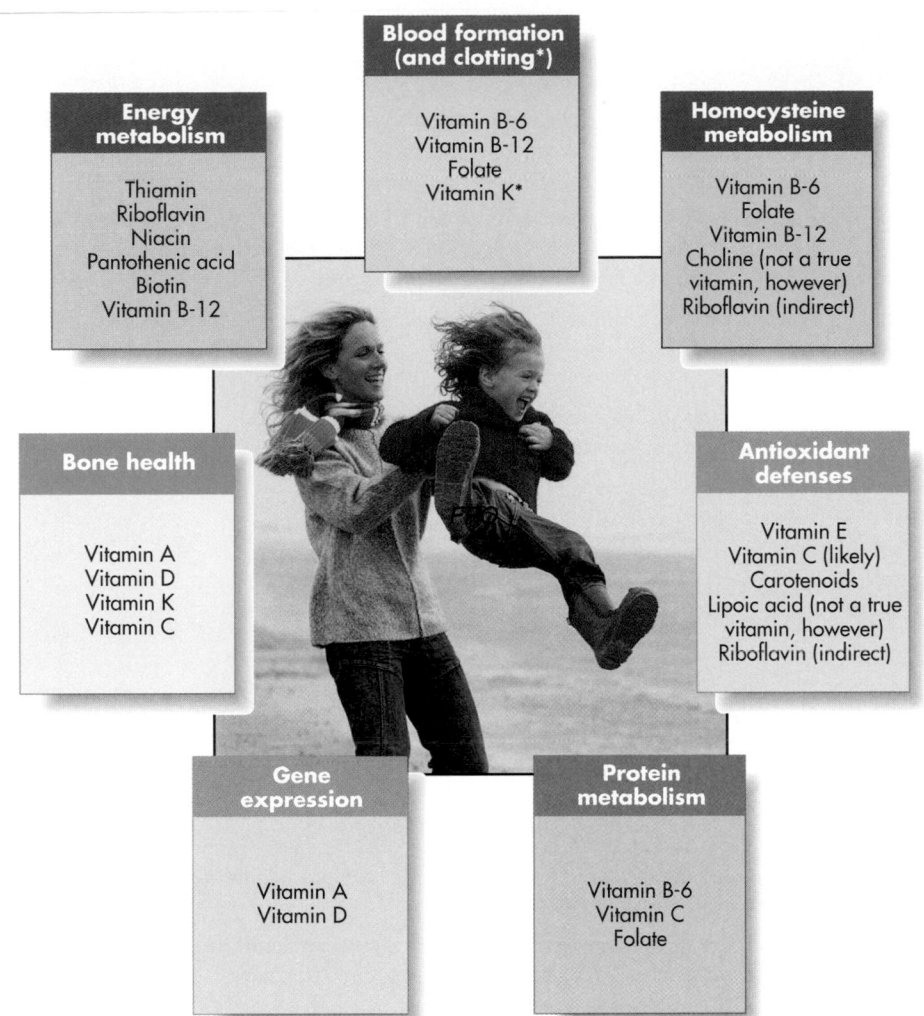

Energy metabolism

Thiamin
Riboflavin
Niacin
Pantothenic acid
Biotin
Vitamin B-12

Blood formation (and clotting*)

Vitamin B-6
Vitamin B-12
Folate
Vitamin K*

Homocysteine metabolism

Vitamin B-6
Folate
Vitamin B-12
Choline (not a true vitamin, however)
Riboflavin (indirect)

Bone health

Vitamin A
Vitamin D
Vitamin K
Vitamin C

Antioxidant defenses

Vitamin E
Vitamin C (likely)
Carotenoids
Lipoic acid (not a true vitamin, however)
Riboflavin (indirect)

Gene expression

Vitamin A
Vitamin D

Protein metabolism

Vitamin B-6
Vitamin C
Folate

Figure 10-11 | Vitamins and related nutrients (e.g., choline) work together to maintain health.

Table 10-1 summarizes much of what is known about the B-vitamins, choline, and vitamin C.

Figure 10-11 Summarizes the various roles of vitamins in the body. This figure underscores the importance of vitamin nutriture in maintaining overall health.

Concept | Check

Only guinea pigs, monkeys, some birds and fish, and humans need dietary vitamin C. It is used mainly in the synthesis of collagen, a major connective tissue protein. A vitamin C deficiency causes scurvy, which is marked by many changes in the skin and gums, such as small hemorrhages, because of reduced collagen synthesis. Vitamin C also modestly improves iron absorption and is involved in the synthesis of certain hormones and neurotransmitters. Citrus fruits, green peppers, cauliflower, broccoli, and strawberries are good sources of vitamin C. Fresh or lightly cooked foods are the best sources, because loss of vitamin C in cooking can be high. At intakes greater than about 2 g/day, vitamin C can lead to diarrhea and other GI tract problems.

People who want to experiment with large doses of vitamin C should alert their physician. High doses of vitamin C can change reactions to medical tests for diabetes (urine) or blood in the feces. Vitamin C can interact with the testing procedures because much of a high dose of vitamin C will not be absorbed, or if absorbed, will be rapidly excreted. Physicians may misdiagnose conditions when large doses of vitamin C are consumed without their knowledge.

Table 10-1 | A Summary of Water-Soluble Vitamins

Vitamin	Major Functions	Deficiency Symptoms	People Most at Risk
Thiamin	Coenzyme in energy release	Beriberi: anorexia, weight loss, weakness, peripheral neuropathy; Wernicke-Korsakoff syndrome	Alcoholics and people living in poverty
Riboflavin	Coenzyme in numerous oxidation-reduction reactions, including those of energy release	Ariboflavinosis: inflammation of mouth and tongue, cracks at corner of mouth	People taking certain medications if no dairy products are consumed
Niacin	Coenzyme in numerous oxidation-reduction reactions in energy metabolism, synthesis and breakdown of fatty acids	Pellagra: diarrhea, dermatitis, dementia (death)	Alcoholics and people living in poverty where corn is the dominant food
Pantothenic acid	Coenzyme in energy metabolism and fatty-acid synthesis	Weakness, fatigue, impaired muscle function, GI tract disturbances	None
Biotin	Cofactor for five carboxylases that participate in fatty acid, amino acid, and energy metabolism	Dermatitis, conjunctivitis, hair loss, nervous system abnormalities	Alcoholics
Vitamin B-6 (pyridoxine)	Coenzymes in amino acid metabolism, heme synthesis, lipid metabolism; homocysteine metabolism	Dermatitis, anemia, convulsion, depression, confusion	Alcoholics
Folate	Coenzyme in DNA synthesis, homocysteine metabolism	Megaloblastic (macrocytic) anemia, birth defects	Alcoholics, pregnant women, people on certain medications
Vitamin B-12 (cobalamin)	Coenzymes affecting folate metabolism, homocysteine metabolism	Megaloblastic (macrocytic) anemia, paresthesia, pernicious anemia	Older adults, vegans, HIV-positive patients, patients with malabsorption syndromes
Vitamin C (ascorbic acid)	Collagen synthesis, some antioxidant capability, hormone and neurotransmitter synthesis	Scurvy: poor wound healing, pinpoint hemorrhages, bleeding gums	Alcoholics, individuals who eat few fruits and vegetables
Choline	Precursor for acetylcholine and phospholipids; homocysteine metabolism	No natural deficiency	None

Table 10-1 | A Summary of Water-Soluble Vitamins (continued)

Dietary Sources	RDA or Adequate Intake	Toxicity*
Pork and pork products, enriched and whole-grain cereals, nuts and seeds	Men: 1.2 mg/day; women: 1.1 mg/day	None recognized
Milk, mushrooms, spinach, liver, enriched grains	Men: 1.3 mg/day; women: 1.1 mg/day	None recognized
Meat, poultry, fish, enriched and whole-grain breads and cereals; also from tryptophan conversion to niacin	Men: 16 mg NE/day; women: 14 mg NE/day	Flushing of skin; Upper Level for adults is 35 mg/day from supplements, based on flushing of skin
Widely distributed in foods	Adequate Intake for adults: 5 mg/day	None recognized
Widely distributed in foods	Adequate Intake for adults: 30 μg/day	Unknown
Animal protein foods, spinach, potatoes, bananas, salmon, sunflower seeds	Adults 19–50: 1.3 mg/day; men over 50: 1.4 mg/day; women over 50: 1.3 mg/day	None from food but excess intake from supplements causes neuropathy, skin lesions; Upper Level is 100 mg/day, based on nerve destruction
Green vegetables, liver, enriched cereal products, legumes, oranges	400 μg/day of dietary folate equivalents (Note: dietary folate equivalents are not used for women in childbearing years; actual μg folic acid is used.)	None; Upper Level for adults set at 1000 μg/day for synthetic folic acid, exclusive of food folate, based on masking vitamin B-12 deficiency
Animal foods and fortified ready-to-eat breakfast cereals	Adults 19–50: 2.4 μg/day; adults 51 and older: same, but use of fortified foods or supplements to meet needs is recommended	None recognized
Citrus fruits, strawberries, broccoli, greens	Men: 90 mg/day; women: 75 mg/day; + 35 mg/day for smokers	Diarrhea and other GI tract problems; Upper Level is 2 g/day, based on development of diarrhea
Widely distributed in foods, plus self-synthesis	Adequate Intake for men: 550 mg/day; women: 425 mg/day	Upper Level is 3.5 g/day, based on development of fishy body odor and reduced blood pressure

*Toxicity arises only from supplement use.

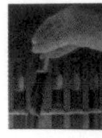

Expert Opinion

Vitamin C: Antioxidant and Pro-Oxidant Functions and the Keystone of Tight Control

Mark Levine, M. D., and Sebastian J. Padayatty, M.R.C.P., Ph.D.

Is vitamin C (ascorbic acid, ascorbate) an antioxidant in humans, as popularly believed? Should vitamin C be obtained from supplements? To answer these questions, this section presents some essential background in basic vitamin C physiology, biology, and chemistry.

The Physiology of Tight Control of Vitamin C

Researchers know now that the physiology of healthy humans is responsible for tight control of vitamin C concentrations in blood and tissues and that tight control is a function of dose. This knowledge comes from depletion-repletion studies in young healthy men and women on vitamin C–free diets. These subjects were first depleted of vitamin C and then repleted and allowed enough time to attain a steady blood concentration for each of 7 escalating doses, from 30 mg to 2500 mg daily. Between doses of 30 and 100 mg, a very steep increase occurred in fasting blood concentrations. However, the effect ceased beyond 200 mg, and fasting concentrations changed little as the vitamin C dose rose higher. Circulating white blood cells and platelets—which also provide an estimate for body tissues in general—also accumulated vitamin C in these studies, but 10-fold

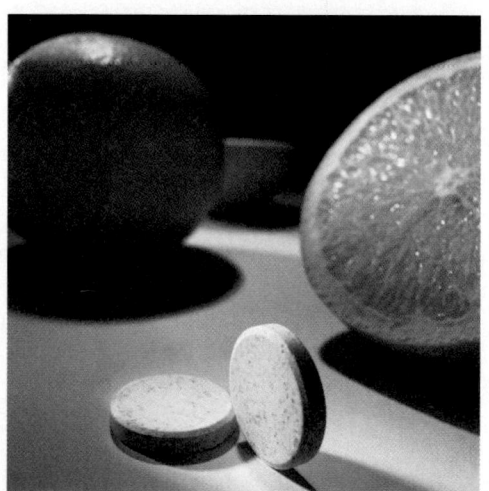

Oranges are a rich source of vitamin C. The many phytochemicals provided are an additional benefit, and something not found in vitamin C supplements.

to 100-fold times that seen in blood. As a result, cells attained their plateau internal concentrations at even lower doses than that seen in the blood.

Gate-Keeper Mechanisms for Regulating Vitamin C Concentrations

These studies indicate that blood and tissue concentrations of vitamin C are tightly controlled in relation to dose. Three gate-keeper mechanisms are responsible for this control: absorption limitations, saturable tissue transporters, and excretion by the kidneys, including both filtration and reabsorption.

For oral doses of 15 and 30 mg, bioavailability for vitamin C is about 90%, but it decreases to less than 50% for a dose of 1250 mg/day. These data show that as doses rise, the percent of the dose absorbed falls, so that intestinal absorption is one gatekeeper of tight control.

A second gate-keeper is tissue transport. With the exception of red blood cells, vitamin C is accumulated into all cells many-fold against its concentration gradient. Most tissue transport uses sodium-dependent vitamin C transporters, and these proteins transport vitamin C as such. (In specialized cases, oxidant-producing cells may transport oxidized ascorbic acid [dehydroascorbic acid] via some glucose transporters, followed by immediate intracellular transformation to the ascorbic acid form.) And as already noted, cells attain their plateau internal concentrations at even lower doses than that seen in the blood.

The third mechanism of tight control is the kidney. At doses of less than 60 mg daily, no vitamin C appears in the urine, whereas at a dose of 2500 mg/day, all absorbed vitamin C is excreted in the urine. The kidney first freely filters vitamin C and then reabsorbs it from the filtrate before ultimate excretion until the sodium-dependent transporter saturates. Once saturation occurs, excess vitamin C is excreted in urine. Overall, the kidney is a key gatekeeper of tight control.

Reducing Agent? Antioxidant? Pro-Oxidant?

For all its known functions, ascorbic acid has one action: to donate two electrons, most likely sequentially. Therefore, as a chemical electron donor, vitamin C is a reducing agent, which is usually synonymous with the term *antioxidant*.

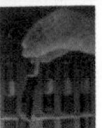

Is vitamin C an antioxidant in vivo? This is an open question. Using in vitro systems, vitamin C is definitely able to chemically reduce oxidants and to do so better than most other compounds. In vivo, however, the evidence that vitamin C is an antioxidant by itself is either lacking or not compelling. There are a number of reasons for this conclusion.

Fruits and vegetables are the primary food sources for vitamin C, and 200 to 300 mg is usually found in 5 to 9 varied servings of fruits and vegetables. Consumption of these foods is associated with health benefits and decreased disease risk for some cancers and cardiovascular diseases. However, it is unknown whether benefit is due to the vitamin itself; to vitamin C plus other fruit and vegetable components; to fruit and vegetable components independent of vitamin C; to displacement of other harmful foods by fruits and vegetables; or to other lifestyle practices of people who consume fruits and vegetables.

Vitamin C supplements have been given to subjects who have diseases believed to be associated with increased oxidant stress, such as diabetes. In most cases, supplements have not made a difference in disease progression or outcome. However, these results may be due to properties of vitamin C physiology in humans: tight control. At the beginning of this section we described the steep dose-concentration relationship for vitamin C doses below 100 mg daily. If the subjects who were enrolled in studies of ascorbic acid and oxidant stress were initially above the steep portion of the dose-concentration curve before they were given supplements, the supplements would make little difference to resulting concentrations and thus to outcome. To properly address whether vitamin C supplements affect diseases associated with oxidant stress, the subjects must, at study enrollment, have low enough initial vitamin C concentrations for supplements to substantially increase them. Although undertaking such a study is not impossible, it is certainly not easy. Thus, it remains possible that vitamin C is a functional antioxidant in vivo but that investigators have not been able to conduct the proper study to test for this.

Based on its chemistry, it is likely that vitamin C has antioxidant functions; whether there is clinical relevance to these functions is the real issue. If antioxidant functions are essential as protective mechanisms, it is predictable that redundant antioxidant protection systems exist in vivo and that vitamin C concentrations are in excess of antioxidant need. Unfortunately, it may be possible to learn whether there is a functional antioxidant role specifically for vitamin C only when its concentrations are extremely low and such function is lost. Such low concentrations may not have relevance to the healthy population, although there could be relevance to subjects whose vitamin C concentrations might fall precipitously, as for those who are critically ill. An analogous example of excess concentration in relation to need for vitamin C can be seen for collagen synthesis and scurvy. Vitamin C is essential for several steps in collagen biosynthesis. However, only with advanced deficiency (scurvy) is this need clinically apparent, suggesting that vitamin C is greatly in excess of its needed concentration for this function and that excess may be a cushion against deficiency.

Ironically, emerging evidence indicates that ascorbic acid only in pharmacologic, not physiologic, concentrations may have pro-oxidant, not antioxidant, functions. Tight control of blood concentrations normally present in humans, and the gatekeeper functions responsible, can be bypassed transiently by intravenous administration of ascorbate as a drug. In comparison to maximal oral dosing, intravenous dosing can produce blood concentrations as much as 50-fold higher until these concentrations are cleared by the kidney after several hours. Ascorbate concentrations produced by intravenous dosing might result in hydrogen peroxide concentrations forming in the extravascular space but not in blood, with ascorbic acid acting as a pro-drug for hydrogen peroxide formation. Intravenous ascorbate with resulting hydrogen peroxide formation and consequent pro-oxidant actions may have unexpected and exciting therapeutic possibilities in cancer and infection, but this work is only in its infancy.

Regardless of potential antioxidant function, vitamin C should be obtained not from supplements but from fruits and vegetables, and 5 to 9 servings should be consumed each day to meet vitamin C needs. This advice has the strongest support based on current knowledge of vitamin C.

Dr. Levine received his undergraduate degree from Brandeis University and his medical training from Harvard Medical School and the Johns Hopkins Hospital. Dr. Levine is a physician-scientist at NIDDK and currently Section Chief of Molecular and Clinical Nutrition and Senior Staff Physician. Dr. Levine is the author of more than 190 scientific journal articles, chapters, books, and abstracts. He is recognized internationally for his comprehensive biochemical and clinical work on vitamin C.

Dr. Padayatty received his medical degree from St. John's Medical College, Bangalore, India. He trained in General Internal Medicine and Endocrinology in England and the United States and received his Ph.D. from the University of Leeds, England. He is a Clinical Researcher and Staff Clinician at the National Institute of Diabetes and Digestive and Kidney Diseases, National Institutes of Health.

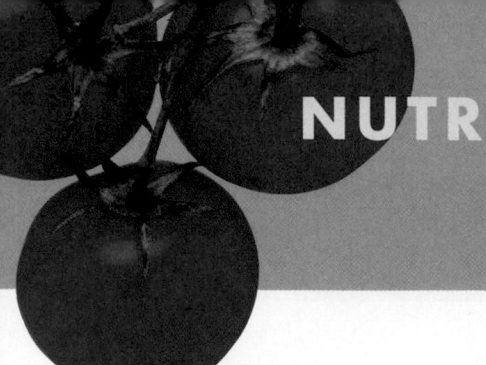

The various vitamin-like compounds discussed in this Nutrition Focus—carnitine, inositol, taurine, and lipoic acid—are necessary to maintain normal metabolism in the body. They all can be synthesized by the body, but their biosynthesis often occurs at the expense of other nutrients, such as essential amino acids. The need for these compounds often increases during times of rapid tissue growth, as in the preterm infant.[8]

Deficiencies of these vitamin-like compounds do not exist in the average healthy adult. But more research is needed to clarify whether deficiencies might arise in certain disease states and whether the compounds should be included in infant formulas and total parenteral nutrition solutions. Currently, manufacturers often add these vitamin-like compounds to infant formulas.

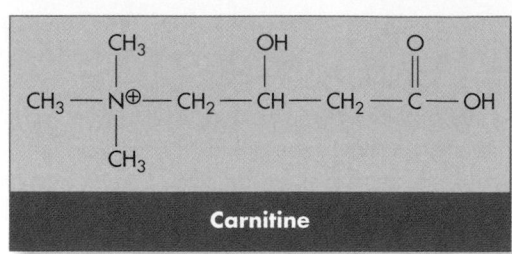

Carnitine

Carnitine

Carnitine is a relatively simple compound that can be synthesized in the liver from the amino acids lysine and methionine. Human needs for carnitine are met from both animal foods and biosynthesis.[8] Adults and children who are severely malnourished or on total parenteral nutrition can have lower-than-normal concentrations of carnitine in their blood. An inadequate supply of protein (e.g., a lack of the amino acids needed for making carnitine) leads to abnormal fatty-acid metabolism. There is speculation that people with cirrhosis may need carnitine from the diet to offset inadequate liver production.

Within the cell, carnitine transports fatty acids from the cytosol into the mitochondria, where the fatty acids are then metabolized for energy. Carnitine also aids the mitochondria in removing excess organic acids, products of metabolic pathways.

Meat and dairy products are the main sources of carnitine. We consume about 100 to 300 mg/day. Vegetarian diets are very low in carnitine because it is almost absent from plant foods. However, vegetarians show normal blood concentrations of carnitine. Consequently, it is doubtful that carnitine is necessary in the diets of healthy people. It may be considered a conditionally essential nutrient in times of recovery from disease, serious trauma, kidney dialysis, or preterm birth.

In addition, carnitine has displayed pharmaceutical usefulness in the removal of compounds that can build to toxic amounts in people with inborn errors of metabolism. Dosages approximately 10 times typical dietary intakes have also been shown to improve the condition of persons with progressive muscle disease and heart muscle deterioration. There have been some sales of carnitine supplements to promote weight loss or as an exercise aid; however, the research on these uses is still very limited.

Inositol

Of the nine possible isomers of inositol, only one—called myo-inositol—has nutritional implications for humans. The structure of inositol is related to that of glucose, from which it is synthesized in the body.

Much of the inositol in body cells occurs in phosphorylated forms, such as inositol triphosphate (IP_3), which is found free in the cell cytosol.[8] Inositol is also incorporated into the phospholipids located in cell membranes. These inositol phospholipids are important precursors of the eicosanoids,

Inositol in supplement form is promoted as treatment for insomnia. There are a variety of causes for sleep disorders, but probably none are linked to an inositol deficiency.

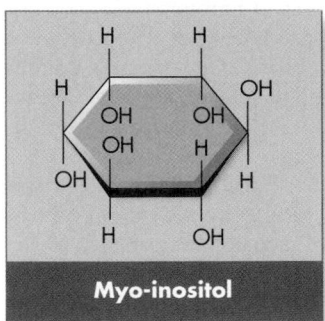

Myo-inositol

which have numerous hormonelike actions (review Chapter 6). Under certain conditions (e.g., the binding of hormones), enzymes in the cell membrane act on the inositol phospholipids, releasing IP_3. This compound, in turn, mobilizes calcium ions (Ca^{2+}) from stores within cells.

Both free inositol and inositol phospholipids are present in animal foods. Some plant foods (e.g., wheat bran) also contain inositol, mostly as part of phytic acid, a compound that binds minerals. The average North American diet provides about 1 g of inositol per day, and another 4 g/day or more are synthesized in the kidneys.

The metabolism of inositol is altered by several medical conditions. The hyperglycemia associated with diabetes inhibits inositol transport. Abnormal inositol metabolism is also noted in multiple sclerosis, kidney failure, and certain cancers. Overall, it appears that inositol is an essential nutrient only in certain medical conditions.

Taurine

Taurine is synthesized from the sulfur-containing amino acids methionine and cysteine. It is abundant in muscle, platelets, and nerve tissue. It is also attached to bile acids. Although its mechanism of action is not well understood, taurine is involved in many vital functions. It is associated with photoreceptor activity in the eye, antioxidant activity in white blood cells, the protection of pulmonary tissue from oxidation, central nervous system function, platelet aggregation, cardiac contraction, insulin action, and cell differentiation and growth.[8]

Taurine is found only in animal foods. North Americans consume about 40 to 400 mg/day. No clear cases of taurine deficiencies have been diagnosed in vegans, even though it is not found in plants, suggesting that synthesis by the body meets needs. Thus, it appears that healthy people need not worry about consuming taurine.

Taurine supplementation may be of benefit to children with cystic fibrosis. Some of these children experience increased growth when treated with taurine, perhaps because of increased fat absorption from the action of taurine as part of bile. Preterm infants supplemented with taurine may also exhibit improved fat absorption.

Lipoic Acid

Lipoic acid is used in reactions in which a carbon dioxide molecule is lost from a substrate, as when pyruvate is converted into acetyl-CoA. Lipoic acid also works with several antioxidants in the body.[8]

Even though lipoic acid serves such beneficial functions in the body, it is unnecessary to obtain it from outside sources. Rich dietary sources are meats, liver, and yeast.

One website states that many individuals are deficient in L-taurine. Because taurine is found in the central nervous system, the website claims, it controls epileptic seizures, motor tics, and facial twitches. It is also promoted as preventing cataracts and certain forms of cardiovascular disease. Scientific evidence for these claims is lacking.

$$HO-\underset{\underset{O}{\parallel}}{\overset{\overset{O}{\parallel}}{S}}-CH_2-NH_2$$

Taurine

Some supplement manufacturers claim that the body is unable to manufacture sufficient lipoic acid. They also claim that a deficiency of lipoic acid prevents antioxidants from working properly together. Research has yet to confirm such claims.

$$CH_2-CH_2-CH-CH_2-CH_2-CH_2-CH_2-\overset{\overset{O}{\parallel}}{C}-OH$$
$$\underset{S}{|}\qquad\qquad\underset{S}{|}$$

Lipoic acid

Summary

1. The B vitamins function as coenzymes. Deficiency symptoms typically show up in the skin, GI tract, brain, and nervous system.

2. Thiamin in its functional form as TPP serves as a coenzyme in energy release. Typically the only North American population that could be deficient in thiamin are alcoholics. Pork, pork products, and enriched grains are reliable sources of thiamin.

3. Riboflavin in functional form, FAD and FMN, participates in a wide variety of oxidation-reduction reactions including those in numerous metabolic pathways that produce energy. A specific riboflavin deficiency is unlikely but could accompany other B-vitamin deficiencies. Dairy products and enriched grains are good dietary sources.

4. Niacin as NAD and NADP are coenzymes. NAD is important in oxidation-reduction reactions including reactions that yield energy. A deficiency of the vitamin produces the disease pellagra. Alcoholism can lead to a deficiency. Food sources of niacin are enriched cereal grains and protein foods. The body is able to synthesize the vitamin from the amino acid tryptophan. Megadoses of niacin produce a variety of toxic symptoms.

5. Among its functions, pantothenic acid in coenzyme form (CoA) shuttles two carbon fragments from the metabolism of glucose, amino acids, fatty acids, and alcohol into the citric acid cycle during energy metabolism. A deficiency of pantothenic acid is unlikely, because it is widely distributed in foods.

6. Biotin functions as a cofactor in five enzymes that add carbon dioxide to a substance. Biotin is widely distributed in foods. No deficiency exists in healthy people. Intestinal bacteria also synthesize biotin.

7. Vitamin B-6 in coenzyme form (PLP) participates in amino acid metabolism, especially the synthesis of nonessential amino acids. It is essential in the synthesis of heme in hemoglobin, the formation of certain neurotransmitters, and the metabolism of homocysteine. Anemia, convulsions, and decreased immune response are symptoms of a deficiency. Animal protein foods, a few fruits and vegetables, and whole-grain cereals are good sources of this vitamin.

Toxic effects from excess consumption include nerve damage.

8. Folate in its many coenzyme forms (tetrahydrofolic acid) accepts one-carbon groups from various donors and donates one-carbon groups. The most notable function performed by folate is in DNA synthesis. It also participates in homocysteine metabolism. A dietary lack of the vitamin produces megaloblastic anemia and increases the risk of spina bifida. Deficiency is common among alcoholics. Folate is found in green vegetables, legumes, liver, and fortified cereal grains. Folate is destroyed by high cooking temperatures.

9. Vitamin B-12 in coenzyme form transfers one-carbon groups. Because of its interaction with folate, a deficiency of vitamin B-12 results in the same type of megaloblastic anemia as well as excess homocysteine in the blood. Defective absorption of vitamin B-12 is the cause of the deficiency disease pernicious anemia. In such cases, injection of the vitamin or another pharmacologic approach is necessary. Vitamin B-12 is found in animal foods but not in plant foods. Vegans need to look for foods fortified with the vitamin or take it as part of a multivitamin and mineral supplement.

10. Choline is a dietary component that is available from a wide variety of foods and is synthesized in the body. No natural deficiency of choline has been reported.

11. Vitamin C functions as an electron donor in many processes, including the synthesis of collagen, a protein in connective tissue. A deficiency of vitamin C causes the disease scurvy. Fresh fruits and vegetables are reliable sources of this vitamin. Like folate, vitamin C is destroyed by heat. Among North Americans, alcoholics, smokers, and individuals who don't eat many fruits or vegetables are most likely to develop a deficiency.

12. Carnitine, inositol, taurine, and lipoic acid, while participating in many important biochemical reactions in the body, are not true vitamins because they can be synthesized in the body from readily available precursors. In some medical circumstances, dietary intake may be needed to augment cellular production.

Study Questions

1. Define and explain the term *coenzyme*.

2. Which vitamins can be synthesized in the body, and how are they synthesized?

3. Explain why individual B-vitamin deficiencies are rare in North America. Which B-vitamins are added to cereal grains as part of the enrichment program?

4. Homocysteine is of some health concern today. Why?

5. Define Upper Level and explain why certain vitamins have this designation.

6. Some vitamins have an Adequate Intake designation rather than an RDA. Why?

7. Draw a map of the energy-transformation pathways in the cell and identify the biochemical reactions where B-vitamins participate in energy metabolism (Hint: review Figure 10-2).

8. Name the vitamins that have been used as pharmacologic agents, and identify the medical conditions for which they are used as therapy.

9. Draw MyPyramid and place the various B-vitamins and vitamin C into the food groups in which they are most likely to be found.

10. Suppose you read in the newspaper or hear on TV news that a "new" vitamin has been discovered. What criteria will have to be met in order for this substance to be a true vitamin?

Annotated References

1. Andres E and others: Food-cobalamin malabsorption in elderly patients: Clinical manifestations and treatments. *American Journal of Medicine* 118:1154, 2005.

   About 15% of older adults show defective vitamin B-12 absorption. This condition especially affects absorption of the vitamin B-12 found naturally in foods. Consumption of crystalline vitamin B-12 in contrast is not so affected and was found to be a useful form of therapy for the older adults in this study.

2. Bailey LB and others: Folic acid supplements and fortification affect the risk for neural tube defects, vascular disease, and cancer. Evolving science. *Journal of Nutrition* 133:1961s, 2003.

   Adequate folic acid status before and during pregnancy reduces the risk of neural tube defects by about 70%. The ability of folic acid to reduce the risk of cancer and cardiovascular disease are interesting scientific theories that need more research before clear recommendations can be made.

3. Bourgeois C and others: Niacin. In Shils ME and others (eds): *Modern nutrition in health and disease.* 10th ed. Philadelphia, PA: Lippincott Williams & Wilkins, 2006.

   Current review of niacin metabolism. Digestion and absorption and related issues such as pharmacologic use are also covered.

4. Butterworth RF : Thiamin. In Shils ME and others (eds): *Modern nutrition in health and disease.* 10th ed. Philadelphia, PA: Lippincott Williams & Wilkins, 2006.

   Current review of thiamin metabolism. Digestion and absorption and related issues such as thiamin deficiencies seen in alcoholism are also covered.

5. Carmel R: Folate. In Shils ME and others (eds): *Modern nutrition in health and disease.* 10th ed. Philadelphia, PA: Lippincott Williams & Wilkins, 2006.

   Current review folate metabolism. Digestion and absorption and related issues such as genetic causes of folate deficiencies are also covered.

6. Carmel R: Colbalamin (Vitamin B12). In Shils ME and others (eds): *Modern nutrition in health and disease.* 10th ed. Philadelphia, PA: Lippincott Williams & Wilkins, 2006.

   Current review of vitamin B-12 metabolism. Digestion and absorption and related issues such as how to properly diagnose a vitamin B-12 deficiency are also covered.

7. Christen WG and others: Fruit and vegetable intake and the risk of cataract in women. *American Journal of Clinical Nutrition* 81:1417, 2005.

   The possible beneficial effects of fruit and vegetables on the risk of many chronic diseases, including cataract, have a strong biological basis and warrant the continued recommendation to increase total intakes of fruit and vegetables.

8. Combs GF: Vitamins. In Mahan LK, Escott-Stump S (eds.): *Krause's food, nutrition, and diet therapy.* 11th ed. Philadelphia: WB Saunders, 2004.

   Excellent chapter on vitamins in general. The many vitamin-like compounds are also reviewed.

9. Douglas RM and others: Vitamin C for preventing and treating the common cold. *Cochrane Database Systematic Reviews* 18(4): CD000980, 2004.

   After a careful review of the scientific literature, megadose vitamin C therapy was found to have no effect on preventing the common cold for the average person but may decrease severity and length of such an infection to a small degree. The possible benefit is seen primarily in people experiencing periods of extreme physical exercise or very cold climactic conditions.

10. Fischer LM and others: Ad libitum choline intake in healthy individuals meets or exceeds the proposed Adequate Intake level. *Journal of Nutrition* 135:826, 2005.

    Using new and recently published data on choline levels in a large number of common foods, the authors report that healthy men and women consumed amounts of choline that were at or slightly higher than the current Adequate Intake level, but some individual subjects, especially women, consumed slightly less. Therefore the current Adequate Intake level for choline seems to be a good approximation of the actual intake of this nutrient.

11. Food and Nutrition Board, Institute of Medicine: *Dietary Reference Intakes for thiamin, riboflavin, niacin, vitamin B-6, folate, vitamin B-12, pantothenic acid, biotin, and choline.* Washington, DC: National Academy Press, 1998.

    This report explains how nutrient recommendations were established for the B vitamins and choline, with specific reference to RDA and related standards. The functions of each of the B vitamins and choline are also explained.

12. Food and Nutrition Board, Institute of Medicine: *Dietary Reference Intakes for vitamin C, vitamin E, selenium, and carotenoids.* Washington, DC: National Academy Press, 2000.

    The functions of antioxidant nutrients, how RDA and related standards were determined, and deficiency and toxicity symptoms are explained. This is the definitive report by the panel of experts on nutrient needs for dietary antioxidants.

13. Forman JP and others: Folate intake and the risk of incident hypertension among U.S. women. *Journal of the American Medical Association* 293:320, 2005.

    Meeting folate needs was associated with a decreased risk of incident hypertension, particularly in younger women.

14. Friso S and others: Low plasma vitamin B-6 concentrations and modulation of coronary artery disease risk. *American Journal of Clinical Nutrition* 79:992, 2004.

    Low plasma concentrations of the active metabolite of vitamin B-6 are independently associated with increased risk for coronary artery disease and are inversely related to major markers of inflammation.

15. Herrmann M and others: Relation between homocysteine and biochemical bone turnover markers and bone mineral density in peri- and post-menopausal women. *Clinical Chemistry and Laboratory Methods* 43:1118, 2005.

    Elevated blood homocysteine was a modest risk factor for having low bone density in this study. It is thus important for older adults to meet their needs for vitamin B-6, folate, and vitamin B-12 (notably in the crystalline form) in order to protect bone health.

16. Homocysteine Lowering Trialists' Collaboration: Dose-dependent effects of folic acid on blood concentrations of homocysteine: A meta-analysis of the randomized trials. *American Journal of Clinical Nutrition* 82:806, 2005.

    Consuming 400 μg/day of folic acid contributes to healthy blood values for homocysteine. Increasing folic acid intake to 800 μg/day provided a slightly greater effect. The authors caution that it is important to also meet vitamin B-12 needs when consuming such doses of folic acid.

17. Kuo HK and others: The role of homocysteine in multistage age-related problems: A systematic review. *Journal of Gerontological and Biological Sciences and Medicine* 60:1190, 2005.

    There is growing evidence of an association between elevated blood homocysteine and numerous health problems associated with aging, including cardiovascular disease, stroke, declining mental function, and bone loss. The proposed mechanism is the tendency for homocysteine to damage blood vessels and nerves and to inhibit the cross-linking of collagen that is important for bone synthesis (and resynthesis).

18. Lee D-H and others: Does supplemental vitamin C increase cardiovascular disease risk in women with diabetes? *American Journal of Clinical Nutrition* 80:1194, 2004.

    Vitamin C can also be a pro-oxidant and can glycate proteins. High vitamin C intake from supplements is associated with an increased risk of cardiovascular disease mortality in post menopausal diabetic women.

19. Levine M and others: Vitamin C. In Shils ME and others (eds): *Modern nutrition in health and disease.* 10th ed. Philadelphia, PA: Lippincott Williams & Wilkins, 2006.

    Current review of vitamin C metabolism, including both known and proposed roles in the body. Digestion and absorption are also covered.

20. Mackey AD and others: Vitamin B6. In Shils ME and others (eds): Modern nutrition in health and disease. 10th ed. Philadelphia , PA: Lippincott Williams & Wilkins, 2006.

    Current review of vitamin B-6 metabolism. Digestion and absorption and related issues such as the risks associated with pharmacologic use are also covered.

21. Marks PW, Zukerberg LR: Case 30-2004: A 37-year-old woman with paresthesias of the arms and legs. *The New England Journal of Medicine* 351(13):1333, 2004.

    A case of pernicious anemia with autoimmune gastritis and B-12 deficiency is successfully treated with parenteral treatments of vitamin B-12.

22. Martinez MA and others: Folate and colorectal neoplasia: Relation between plasma and dietary markers of folate and adenoma recurrence. *American Journal of Clinical Nutrition* 79:691, 2004.

    Adequate folate nutriture is associated with a lower risk of colon cancer. Intakes of about 600 μg/day showed the greatest effect. A healthy diet can easily provide this amount of folate.

23. McCormick DB: Riboflavin. In Shils ME and others (eds): *Modern nutrition in health and disease.* 10th ed. Philadelphia, PA: Lippincott Williams & Wilkins, 2006.

    Current review of riboflavin metabolism. Digestion and absorption are also covered.

24. Mock DM: Biotin. In Shils ME and others (eds): *Modern nutrition in health and disease.* 10th ed. Philadelphia, PA: Lippincott Williams & Wilkins, 2006.

    Current review of biotin metabolism. Digestion and absorption and related issues such as biotinidase deficiencies are also covered.

25. Ravaglia G and others: Homocysteine and folate as risk factors for dementia and Alzheimer disease. *American Journal of Clinical Nutrition* 82:638, 2005.

    In this study of 816 older adults, elevated blood homocysteine was associated with almost a doubling of the risk of developing Alzheimer's disease. Low concentrations of folate in the bloodstream were especially predictive of high blood homocysteine in this study, and therefore low concentrations of folate need to be avoided in older people.

26. Stover PJ: Physiology of folate and vitamin B-12 in health and disease. *Nutrition Reviews* 62(6):S3, 2004.

    This paper reviews the functions of folate and B-12, highlighting the risks of overconsumption and underconsumption.

27. Trumbo TR: Pantothenic acid. In Shils ME and others (eds): *Modern nutrition in health and disease.* 10th ed. Philadelphia, PA: Lippincott Williams & Wilkins, 2006.

    Current review of pantothenic acid metabolism. Digestion and absorption are also covered.

28. Tucker KL and others: High homocysteine and low B vitamins predict cognitive decline in aging men: The Veterans Affairs Normative Aging Study. *American Journal of Clinical Nutrition* 82:627, 2005.

    Elevated blood homocysteine concentrations predicted cognitive decline in the men in this study. Thus it is important for aging adults to meet B vitamin needs in order to maintain cognitive health.

29. Zeisel SH, Niculescu MD: Choline and phosphotidalcholine. In Shils ME and others (eds): *Modern nutrition in health and disease.* 10th ed. Philadelphia, PA: Lippincott Williams & Wilkins, 2006.

    Current review of choline metabolism. Digestion and absorption and the effects of a deficiency when induced in humans are also covered.

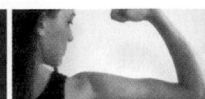

Take | Action

I. Spotting Fraudulent Claims on the Internet

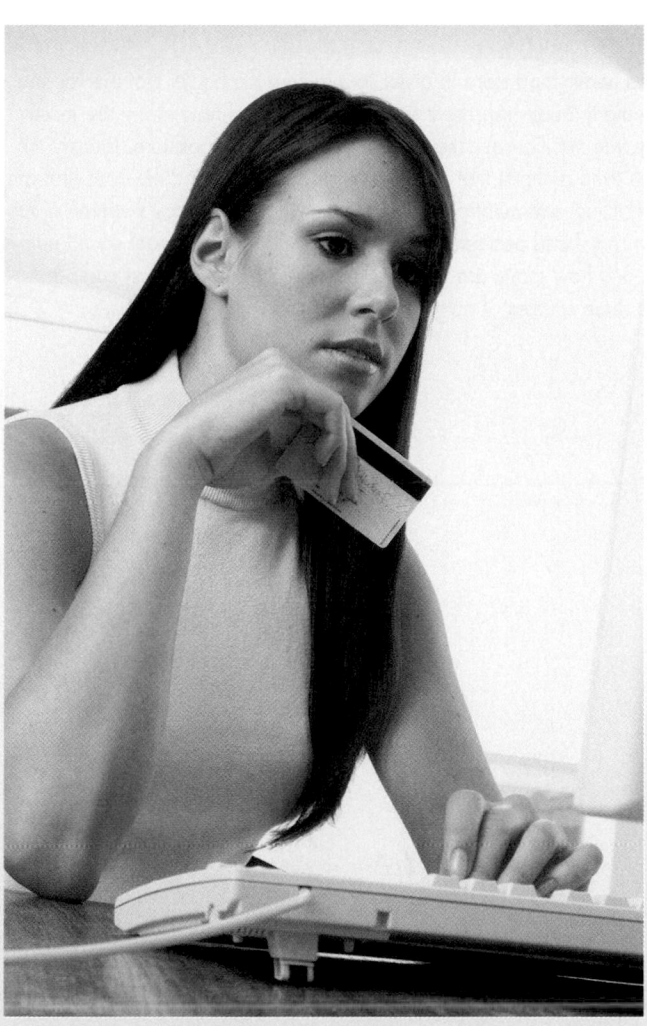

Search for vitamins and vitamin-like substances that are sold over the Internet. Then write a report concerning any claims made on behalf of these products that you consider fraudulent or misleading. Are the websites really selling vitamins, or are they actually a cover for selling something else? Compare the price of the vitamins from these sites with the price you would pay at the local supermarket or drugstore. Do any of these sites display any disclaimers or warnings about the products?

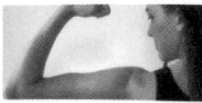

Take | Action

II. Spotting Fraudulent Claims in Popular Books for Sale at Health-Food Stores and Bookstores

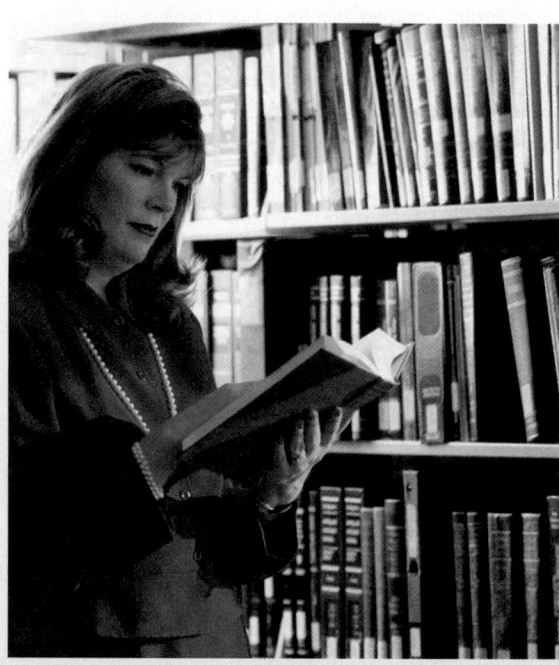

Visit a health-food store in order to examine the books that are for sale. How many books represent sound nutrition, and how many are mostly filled with nutrition quackery? Visit your campus bookstore. Identify the books (and authors) that represent sound nutrition and the ones that are mostly filled with nutrition quackery. Consult last Sunday's edition of the *New York Times* best-seller list. How many books represent sound nutrition, and how many are nutrition quackery? Write a report comparing these three sources of nutrition information.

WATER AND THE MAJOR MINERALS

CHAPTER OUTLINE

CASE SCENARIO:

Jana, a sophomore in high school, recently gave up drinking milk. She thought she could stay slim by avoiding all the calories in milk. Her mother is concerned about Jana's diet change, especially Jana's future risk of osteoporosis. Jana needs an adequate source of calcium in her diet to allow for continued bone development and maintenance of the bone mass she already has. Jana also recently started smoking, and her only physical activity is practice for the Women's Glee Club.

Jana's diet on a recent day consisted of the following items. For breakfast, she had oatmeal made with water, a banana, and a cup of fruit juice. At midmorning, she bought a snack cake from the vending machine. At lunch, she had vegetable pasta, bread with olive oil, a side salad, 1 ounce of mixed nuts, and a soft drink. For dinner, she had a hamburger along with mixed vegetables and another soft drink. As an evening snack, she had some cookies and hot tea.

What factors place Jana at risk for osteoporosis in the future? What changes to her current diet could reduce that risk?

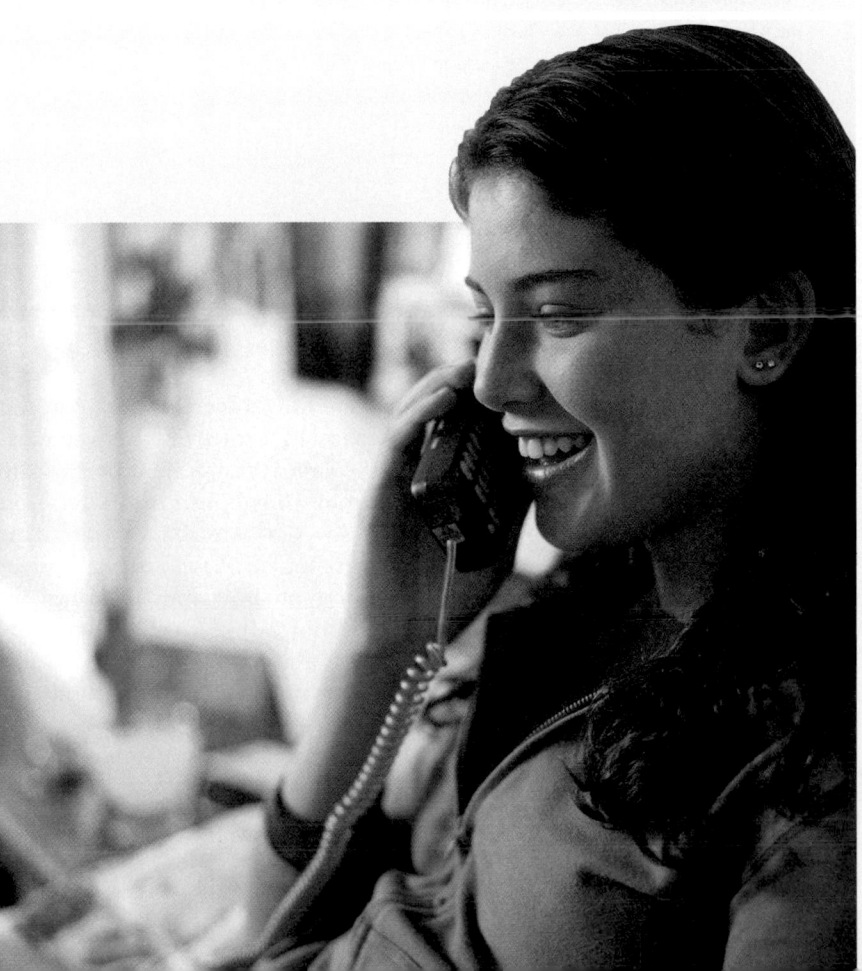

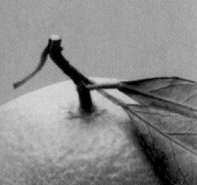

Water—the most versatile medium for a variety of chemical reactions—constitutes the major portion of human body weight. Without water, biological processes necessary to life would cease in a matter of days. We operate on about 3 to 4 liters (3 to 4 quarts) of water daily and must replenish it regularly because the body does not store water per se.[6] We recognize this constant demand for water as thirst.[2] Many nutrients, including minerals, exist in the body dissolved in water.[21] Because the functioning of minerals is related to the characteristics of water, water and its roles in the body are explored first in this chapter.

Many minerals, like water, are vital to health. They are key participants in body metabolism, muscle movement, body growth, and water balance, among other wide-ranging processes.[5,6] Some of the minerals found in our bodies—for example, vanadium and boron—may not be necessary to sustain human life. Nevertheless, we know that some mineral deficiencies can cause severe health problems.[5,6] For this reason, the study of minerals is critical to understanding human nutrition. This chapter focuses on the major minerals, such as calcium and magnesium; Chapter 12 focuses on the trace minerals, such as iron and zinc.

CHAPTER OBJECTIVES CHAPTER 11 IS DESIGNED TO ALLOW YOU TO:

1. Classify the minerals as major or trace minerals.

2. List conditions of the body, dietary factors, and other pertinent relationships that influence the absorption, retention, and availability of specific major minerals.

3. List and briefly explain the functions of water in the body as well as typical sources of intakes and losses.

4. Discuss how body water balance is maintained by the mechanisms of thirst, absorption, and hormonal regulation.

5. List key functions of the major minerals.

6. Identify possible deficiency and toxicity symptoms associated with the major minerals.

7. List at least two food sources for each major mineral.

8. Describe the processes involving minerals that aid in maintaining bone health as well as controlling blood pressure.

REFRESH YOUR MEMORY AS YOU BEGIN YOUR STUDY OF WATER AND THE MAJOR MINERALS IN CHAPTER 11, YOU MAY WANT TO REVIEW:

• MyPyramid and the 2005 Dietary Guidelines in Chapter 2.
• The functions of vitamin D and vitamin K related to calcium and bone health in Chapter 9.
• The role of vitamin C in collagen synthesis in Chapter 10.
• Intracellular and extracellular fluid compartments in Appendix C.
• The muscular and skeletal systems in Appendix C.

| Water

To appreciate how minerals operate in the body, it helps to understand the nature and general chemical properties of water as well as specific nutrient-related functions. Water is the largest component of the human body, making up 50 to 70% of the body's weight (about 10 gallons, or 40 liters). Lean muscle tissue contains about 73% water. Adipose tissue is about 20% water.[21] Thus, as fat content increases (and the percentage of lean tissue decreases) in the body, total body water decreases toward 50%.

Depending on how much fat has been stored, an adult can survive for about 8 weeks without eating food but only several days without drinking water. In a desert environment, a person wouldn't survive for more than one day without water. This difference in survival time between food and water occurs not because water is more important than carbohydrate, fat, protein, vitamins, or minerals but, rather, because the body has no storage site for water.

Water can dissolve most substances, and in doing so, it enables minerals and other chemicals to undergo biological reactions in the body (see Appendix A for details).

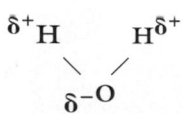

At a molecular level, water is highly polar, because the positive charges tend to be located near the hydrogens and the negative charges near the oxygen.

$$\delta^+ H \quad\quad H^{\delta^+}$$
$$\delta^- O$$

δ denotes partial charge

Water in the Body—Intracellular and Extracellular Fluid

Water flows in and out of body cells through cell membranes. Water inside cells forms part of the **intracellular fluid**—fluid within the cells. When water is outside cells or in the bloodstream, it is part of the **extracellular fluid**—fluid outside cells (Figure 11-1).[21] Extracellular fluid is further divided into **interstitial fluid**—water between cells—and **intravascular fluid**—water in the bloodstream and lymph. Interstitial fluid forms a transport link between tissue cells and the blood.

Because cell membranes are permeable to water, water shifts freely in and out of cells. For example, if blood volume decreases, water can move from the areas inside and around cells to the bloodstream to increase blood volume.

The body controls the amount of water in each compartment mainly by controlling the **electrolyte** concentrations in each compartment.[21] In solution, electrolytes such as sodium, chloride, and potassium dissociate into charged particles called ions. Water is attracted to these electrolytes and other ions. By controlling the movements of ions in and out of the cellular compartments, the body maintains the appropriate amount of water in each compartment. Where ions go, water follows (Figure 11-2).

Osmosis

Much of the movement of body water results from water's tendency to move across a semipermeable membrane so as to equalize the total particle concentration in the compartments on each side of the membrane. A semipermeable membrane is one through which water, but not particles, can pass. In the body, the particles are primarily electrolytes,

intracellular fluid Fluid contained within a cell represents about two-thirds of all body fluid.

extracellular fluid Fluid present outside the cells; it includes intravascular and interstitial fluids; represents about one-third of all body fluid.

interstitial fluid Fluid between cells.

intravascular fluid Fluid within the bloodstream (that is, in the arteries, veins, capillaries, and lymph vessels); represents about 25% of all body fluids.

electrolytes Compounds that separate into ions in water and, in turn, are able to conduct an electrical current. These include sodium, chloride, and potassium.

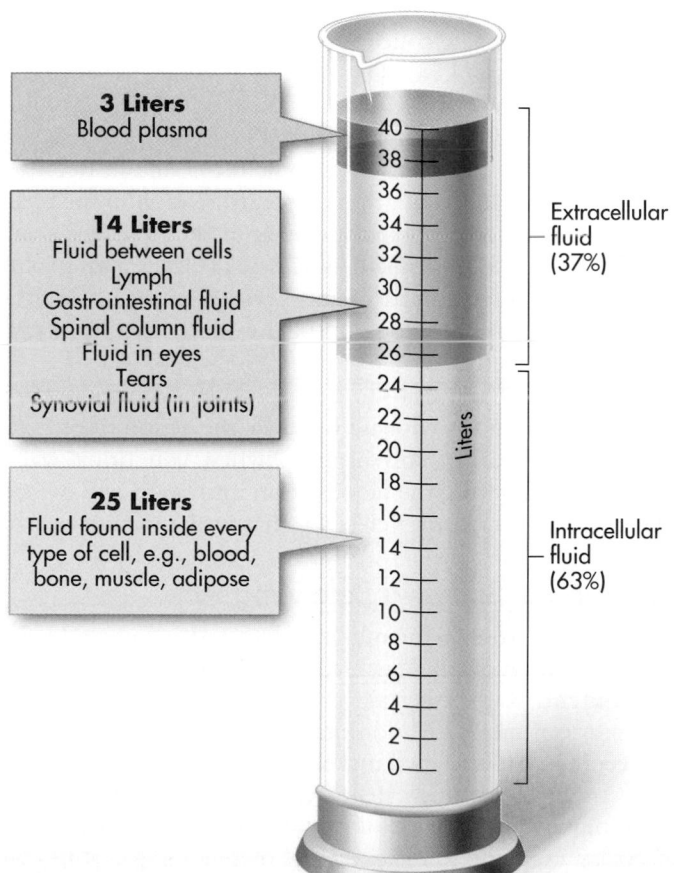

Figure 11-1 | Fluid compartments in the body. Total fluid volume is about 40 liters (about 10 gallons).

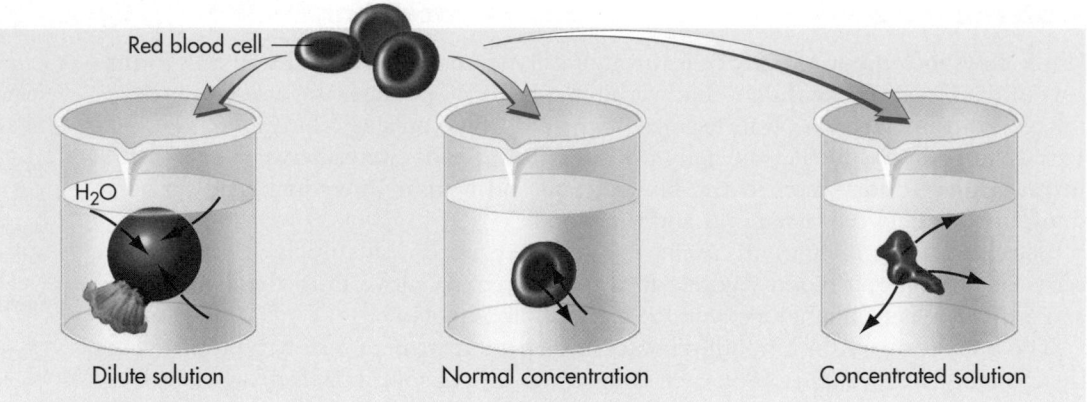

(a) A dilute solution with a low ion concentration results in swelling (*black arrows*) and subsequent rupture (*puff of red in the lower left part of the cell*) of a red blood cell placed into the solution.

(b) A normal concentration (a concentration of ions outside the cell equal to that inside the cell) results in a typically shaped red blood cell. Water moves into and out of the cell in equilibrium (*black arrows*), but there is no net water movement.

(c) A solution with a high ion concentration causes shrinkage of the red blood cell as water moves out of the cell and into the concentrated solution (*black arrows*).

Figure 11-2 | Red blood cells affected by various ion concentrations. Osmosis causes fluid to shift in and out of the red blood cells depending on the ion concentration in each flask.

osmosis The passage of a solvent (water) through a semipermeable membrane from a less concentrated compartment to a more concentrated compartment.

osmolality A measure of the total concentration of a solution; the number of particles of solute per kg of solvent.

The term **osmotic pressure** refers to the amount of force needed to prevent dilution of the compartment containing the higher particle concentration.

and the membranes are cell membranes. This passage of water (or other solvent), called **osmosis,** results in the movement of water from a less concentrated to a more concentrated solution.[21] The specific concentration is expressed as **osmolality,** representing the number of particles per kg of solvent.

Figure 11-2 illustrates how osmosis works. When particles in a solution are less concentrated than those in a closed compartment bounded by a semipermeable membrane, the compartment will be forced to become more dilute. Because particles can't pass easily across the membrane, water moves by diffusion from the relatively dilute solution to the more concentrated compartment until their particle concentrations become identical. The opposite movement would take place if the solution was more concentrated than the enclosed compartment (review Figure 11-2). Besides this effect on red blood cells, examples of osmosis are sugar pulling fluid from strawberries and a salty salad dressing wilting lettuce.

Adding water—instead of particles—to a compartment dilutes its particle concentration, so the compartment tends to donate water by the action of osmosis to more concentrated compartments nearby. This happens when you drink water. Some water absorbed by the body moves from the bloodstream into body cells, which in turn equalizes the particle concentration in the cells with that in the various nearby body sites.

Water and Ions in the Body—a Balancing Act

The movement of water across the membrane, depicted in Figure 11-3, occurs by simple diffusion. Little of this movement actually occurs across cell membranes because of their high lipid content. Rather, certain proteins in cell membranes act as channels through which water can move. In addition, cell membranes possess an extremely sophisticated gatekeeping system, which makes them selectively permeable to many electrolytes as well as other compounds.[21] For example, a specific protein located in the cell membrane can pump potassium ions into and sodium ions out of a cell. Energy is used by this sodium-potassium pump to move each of these ions against its concentration gradient. Cells use such mechanisms in addition to osmotic processes to maintain their intracellular water volume and electrolyte concentrations within quite narrow ranges.

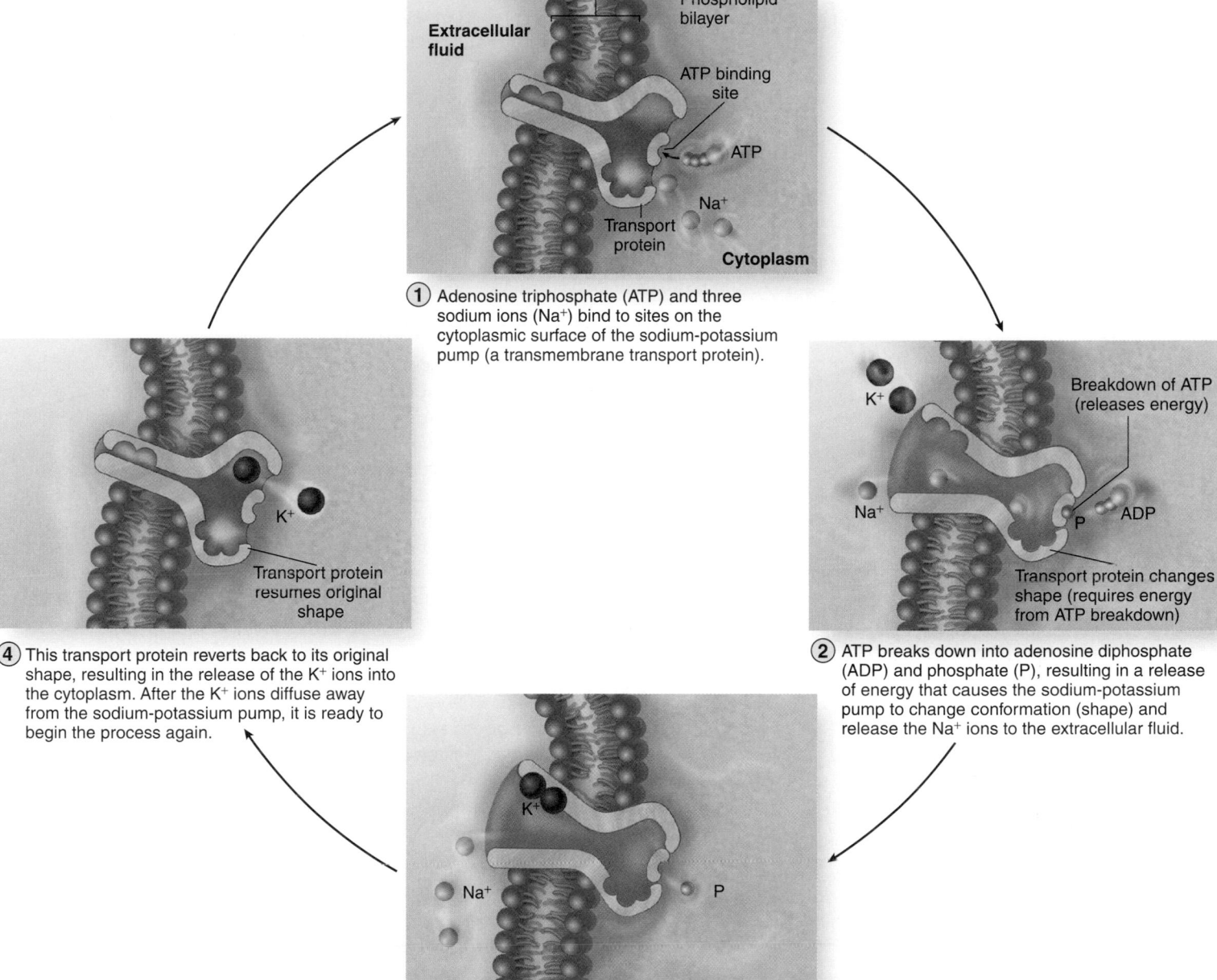

① Adenosine triphosphate (ATP) and three sodium ions (Na⁺) bind to sites on the cytoplasmic surface of the sodium-potassium pump (a transmembrane transport protein).

② ATP breaks down into adenosine diphosphate (ADP) and phosphate (P), resulting in a release of energy that causes the sodium-potassium pump to change conformation (shape) and release the Na⁺ ions to the extracellular fluid.

③ As the three Na⁺ ions diffuse away from the sodium-potassium pump into the extracellular fluid, two K⁺ ions from the extracellular fluid bind to sites on the extracellular surface of the sodium-potassium pump. At the same time, the phosphate produced earlier by ATP hydrolysis is released into the cytoplasm.

④ This transport protein reverts back to its original shape, resulting in the release of the K⁺ ions into the cytoplasm. After the K⁺ ions diffuse away from the sodium-potassium pump, it is ready to begin the process again.

Figure 11-3 | Sodium-Potassium Pump. A sodium-potassium pump has a transmembrane transport protein that uses energy to transport Na⁺ and K⁺ ions through the membrane from a region of low concentration to a region of high concentration. This continuous, active transport process can be broken down into four steps.

Positive ions (cations), such as sodium and potassium, pair with negative ions (anions), such as chloride and phosphate. Intracellular water volume depends primarily on the intracellular potassium and phosphate concentration. Extracellular water volume depends primarily on the extracellular sodium and chloride concentration.[21]

Besides balancing the ion concentrations between the inside and outside of cells, body cells must also balance ion charges. If a negative ion enters a cell, either a positive ion must also enter or another negative electrolyte must leave.[21]

Functions of Water

Because of its unique chemical and physical characteristics, water plays several key roles in metabolic processes. Water functions in several ways in the body's chemical reactions: because it is polar, it serves as a solvent for many chemical compounds; it provides a medium in which many chemical reactions occur; and it actively participates as a reactant or becomes a product in some reactions, such as in protein digestion. It also is the transport medium of the body.[6]

Water Contributes to Temperature Regulation

Water changes temperature slowly because it has a great ability to hold heat. Water has this high heat capacity (**specific heat**) because water molecules are strongly attracted to each other. In contrast, the molecules in fat are not strongly attracted to each other, and so fats exhibit lower specific heat values than water.

As the amount of heat energy contained within the body increases, water in the surrounding tissues absorbs any excess heat energy. The body then secretes fluids in the form of perspiration, which evaporates through skin pores. To evaporate water, heat energy is required, so as perspiration evaporates, heat energy is taken from the skin, cooling it in the process. This process is the main way in which the body cools itself.[6] Each quart (liter) of perspiration evaporated represents approximately 600 kcal of energy lost from the skin and surrounding tissues. Note that for this reason fever increases one's need for energy (and fluid).

Recall from Chapter 4 that about 60% of the chemical energy in food is turned directly into body heat. Only about 40% is converted to ATP energy, and almost all of that energy eventually leaves the body in the form of heat. If this heat could not be dissipated, the body temperature would rise too high and prevent enzyme systems from functioning efficiently.

However, to cool efficiently, perspiration must be allowed to evaporate. If it simply rolls off the skin or soaks into clothing, perspiration doesn't cool us much. Evaporation of perspiration occurs readily when humidity is low. This is why we feel more comfortable in hot, dry climates than in hot, humid climates.

Water Helps Remove Waste Products

Water is an important vehicle for ridding the body of waste products. Most unwanted substances in the body are water-soluble and can leave the body via the urine.[6] In addition, liver metabolism converts some fat-soluble compounds such as some fat-soluble medications and potential cancer causing substances, into water-soluble compounds. In this way they, too, can be excreted in the urine.

A major body waste product is urea. Recall from Chapter 4 that this by-product of protein metabolism contains nitrogen. The more protein we eat in excess of needs, the more nitrogen we excrete—in the form of urea—in the urine. Likewise, the more sodium we consume, the more sodium we excrete in the urine. Overall, the amount of urine a person needs to produce is determined primarily by excess protein and sodium chloride (salt) intake. By limiting excess protein and salt intakes, it is possible to limit urine output—a useful practice, for example, in space flights. This type of diet is also used to treat some kidney diseases in which the ability to produce urine output is hampered.

A typical urine volume is about 1 liter (1 quart) per day, depending mostly on the intake of fluid, protein, and sodium.[6] A somewhat greater urine output than that is fine, but less—especially less than 500 ml (2 cups)—forces the kidneys to form a very concentrated urine. The heavy ion concentration increases the risk of kidney stone formation in susceptible people, especially among men. Kidney stones are simply minerals and other substances that have precipitated out of the urine and accumulated in kidney tissues.

specific heat The amount of heat required to raise the temperature of any substance 1°C compared with the heat required to raise the temperature of the same volume of water 1°C. Water has a high specific heat, meaning that a relatively large amount of heat is required to raise its temperature; therefore, it tends to resist large temperature fluctuations.

The simplest way to determine if water intake is adequate is to observe the color of one's urine. Urine should be clear or pale yellow and have little odor, whereas concentrated urine is very dark yellow in color and has a strong odor.[4]

Other Functions of Water

Water is incompressible, so it helps form the lubricants found in knees and other joints of the body. It is the basis for saliva, bile, and **amniotic fluid.** Amniotic fluid acts as an important shock absorber surrounding the growing fetus. Electrolyte concentrations vary in each fluid compartment to accommodate specific needs, such as maintenance of a specific range in pH.[21]

Water in Foods

Water can be found in abundance in fruits and vegetables. Foods that are highest in water content include fruits and vegetables as well as milk and other beverages, such as beer. Other sources that fall between 75 and 50% water are potatoes, chicken, and steak. The foods that are less than 35% water include jam, honey, crackers, and various fats in general (Table 11-1).

Water Needs

The Adequate Intake set for total water intake per day is 3.7 liters (15 cups) for adult men and 2.7 liters (11 cups) for adult women. This amount is based primarily on typical total water in takes from a combination of fluids and foods. Fluid alone per day corresponds to about 3 liters (13 cups) for men and about 2.2 liters (9 cups) for women.[6] (The Adequate Intake does not indicate, however, that only water per se must be used to meet fluid needs.) At minimum, adults need 1 to 3 liters per day of fluid to replace daily water losses.

We consume water in various liquids, such as fruit juice, coffee, tea, soft drinks, and water itself. Note that coffee, tea, and soft drinks often contain caffeine, which increases urine output. However, the fluid consumed from these beverages is not completely lost in urine, so these fluids still help to meet water needs. Foods also supply water (Table 11-2). Water as a by-product of metabolism provides approximately 250 to 350 ml (1 to 1 1/2 cups) of additional water.

Much of the water we need is used to produce urine (500 to 1000 ml/or more). The rest compensates for typical water losses through the lungs (250 to 350 ml), feces (100 to 200 ml), and skin (450 to 1900 ml for normal perspiration)[6] (Figure 11-4). We are not normally aware of these **insensible water losses,** as opposed to losses we more easily notice, called **sensible water losses.** Urine output and heavy perspiration fall into this latter category. These numbers are also just estimates: altitude, caffeine intake, alcohol intake, and humidity can affect these individual losses. When we consider the large amount of water used to facilitate GI tract function, the loss of only 100 to 200 ml of water a day through the feces is remarkable. About 8000 ml of water enters the GI tract daily via secretions from the mouth, stomach, intestine, pancreas, and other organs. The diet supplies an additional 30 to 50% or more. The small intestine reabsorbs most of this water, while the large intestine takes up a lesser—but still important—amount. The kidneys also conserve water, reabsorbing about 97% of the water filtered from waste products.

Water-Deficiency Diseases

If you don't drink enough water, your body eventually lets you know by signaling thirst. This thirst mechanism is not always reliable, however, especially during athletic practices and events, in infancy, during illness, and in one's older years.[6] For this reason, athletes should weigh themselves before and after training sessions to determine their rate of water loss and thus their water needs. Replacing at least 75% of this weight loss is advised, especially as weight loss approaches 2%. About 2 1/2 to 3 cups (about 3/4 liter) of water are recommended per pound (about half a kilogram) of weight loss (see Chapter 14 for details on fluid use in athletics). Sick children—especially those with fever, vomiting, diarrhea, and increased perspiration—and older persons often need to be reminded to drink plenty of fluids. As Chapter 17 discusses in further detail, infants can easily become dehydrated.

amniotic fluid The fluid contained in a sac within the uterus. This surrounds and protects the fetus during its development.

Table 11-1 | Water Content (by Weight) of Various Foods

Food	Water %
Tomato	95
Lettuce	95
Beer	90
Milk	89
Orange	87
Apple	86
Potato	75
Banana	75
Chicken	64
Steak	50
Bread, whole-wheat	38
Jam	28
Honey	20
Butter	16
Crackers, saltine	4
Shortening	0

insensible water losses Water losses not readily perceived, such as water lost with each breath.

sensible water losses Water losses readily perceived, such as urine output and heavy perspiration.

Long airplane flights are another situation that demands extra fluid intake: a traveler can lose about 6 cups (1.5 liters) of water during a 3-hour flight. The dehumidified air in an airplane is so dry that it induces excessive insensible perspiration.

Table 11-2 | Water Content of a Typical Day's Food Intake*

Meal	Fluid Oz
Breakfast	
1 cup orange juice	7.2
1/2 cup fat-free milk	3.6
1/2 cup strawberries	2.7
1 cup Cheerios	0.4
Midmorning Snack	
1 cup water	8.0
1 banana	3.0
Lunch	
2 oz water-packed tuna	2.2
2 slices whole-wheat bread	0.9
1 large tomato	5.0
8 oz low-fat yogurt	6.8
1 cup water	8.0
1 kiwi fruit	2.6
Midafternoon Snack	
1 cup apple juice	8.0
4 small cookies	—
Dinner	
2 oz baked skinless chicken	1.3
2 cups romaine lettuce	4.0
2 oz sliced red peppers	1.8
1 slice bread	1.0
1 baked potato	3.5
1 cup fat-free milk	7.0
1 tbsp oil-and-vinegar dressing	0.0
1 cup of tea	8.0
Evening Snack	
12 fl oz diet soft drink	12.0
4 saltine crackers	—
Total	97 fluid ounces (12 cups)

*Adequate for a woman. A man should add 3 more cups of fluid.

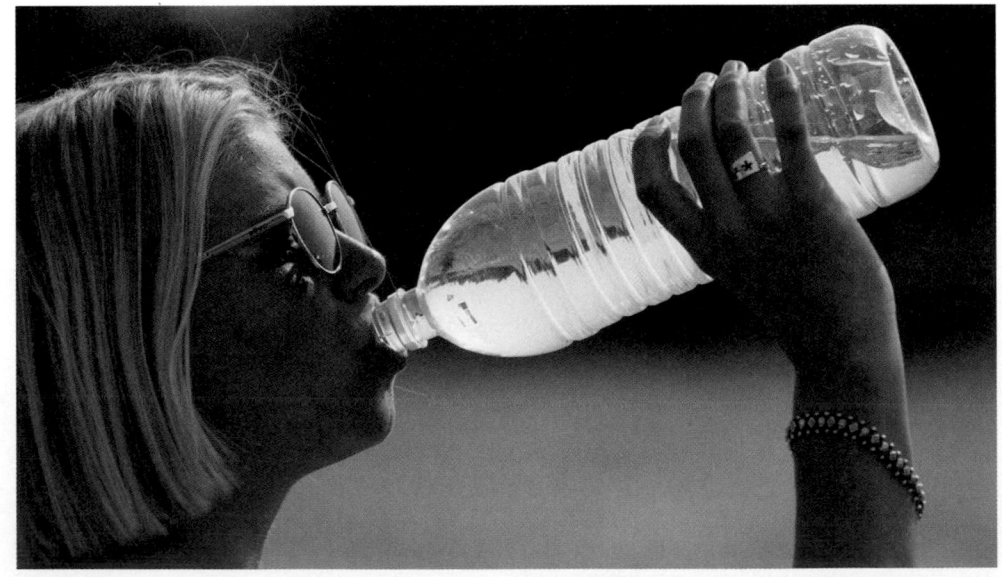

Regular intake of fluid is essential to replace daily fluid losses. A recent trend in North America is to carry water and other fluids with us.

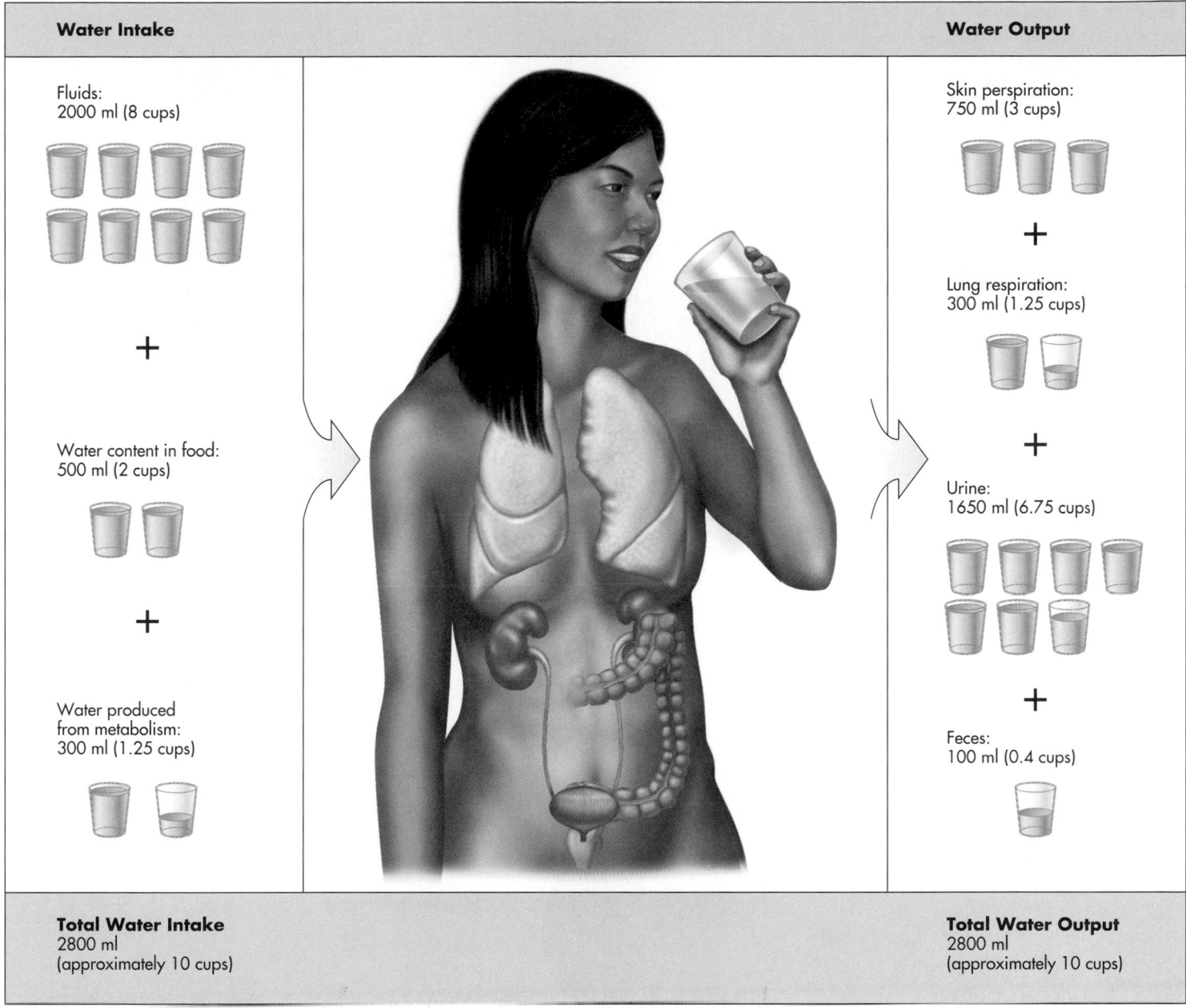

Water Intake	Water Output
Fluids: 2000 ml (8 cups)	Skin perspiration: 750 ml (3 cups)
+	+
Water content in food: 500 ml (2 cups)	Lung respiration: 300 ml (1.25 cups)
+	+
Water produced from metabolism: 300 ml (1.25 cups)	Urine: 1650 ml (6.75 cups)
	+
	Feces: 100 ml (0.4 cups)
Total Water Intake 2800 ml (approximately 10 cups)	**Total Water Output** 2800 ml (approximately 10 cups)

Figure 11-4 | Estimate of water balance—intake versus output—in a woman. We primarily maintain our volume of body fluids by adjusting water output to intake. As you can see, most water comes from the liquids we consume. Some comes from the moisture in more solid foods, and the remainder is manufactured during metabolism. Water output includes losses from the lungs, urine, skin, and feces.

What If the Thirst Message Is Ignored?

Once the body registers an increase in blood concentration, it increases fluid conservation. The pituitary gland releases **antidiuretic hormone** to force the kidneys to conserve water (Figure 11-5).[21] The kidneys respond by reducing urine flow. At the same time, as fluid volume decreases in the bloodstream, blood pressure falls. This fall initiates a sequence of events beginning in the kidneys. Signaled by highly sensitive pressure receptors, the kidneys release an enzyme called **renin** (Figure 11-6). Renin, in turn, activates a circulating blood protein originally produced in the liver called angiotensinogen to form angiotensin I. Angiotensin I is converted to **angiotensin II,** which, among other effects, causes blood vessels to constrict and triggers the adrenal

antidiuretic hormone A hormone secreted by the pituitary gland that acts on the kidneys to cause a decrease in water excretion. It is also called arginine vasopressin.

renin An enzyme formed in the kidneys and released in response to low blood pressure; it acts on a blood protein called angiotensinogen to produce angiotensin I.

angiotensin II A compound produced from angiotensin I that increases blood vessel constriction and triggers production of the hormone aldosterone.

Figure 11-5 | Antidiuretic hormone is released in response to an increased concentration of blood (1). This hormone acts on the kidney to increase water retention (2); therefore blood volume and in turn blood pressure are restored to normal values.

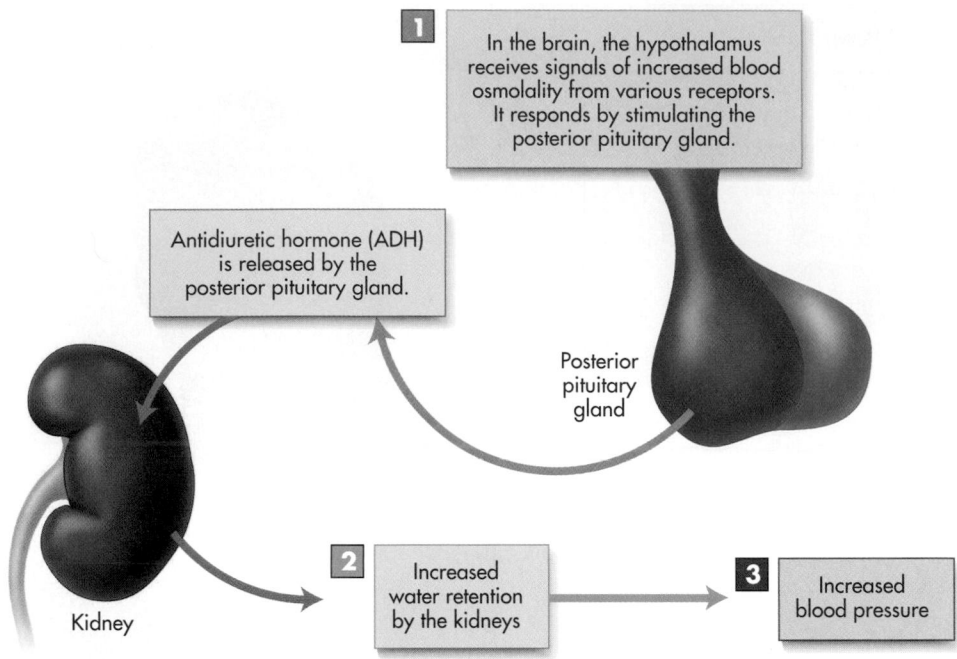

1 In the brain, the hypothalamus receives signals of increased blood osmolality from various receptors. It responds by stimulating the posterior pituitary gland.

Antidiuretic hormone (ADH) is released by the posterior pituitary gland.

Posterior pituitary gland

Kidney

2 Increased water retention by the kidneys

3 Increased blood pressure

Alcohol inhibits the action of antidiuretic hormone. One reason people feel so weak the day after heavy drinking is that they are very dehydrated. Even though they may have consumed a lot of liquid in their drinks, they have lost even more liquid because alcohol has inhibited antidiuretic hormone. Caffeine also does the same, and so produces a diuretric effect on the body.

Figure 11-6 | The renin-angiotensin system is one regulator of blood pressure. A decrease in blood pressure (1) starts the cascade of reactions (2–7) that act to restore blood pressure back into the normal range. This system functions with antidiuretic hormone to control blood pressure. Number (5) is listed twice since angiotensin II acts at both the adrenal gland and blood vessels to help regulate blood pressure.

*The angiotensin-converting enzyme (ACE) inhibitors used to treat hypertension and other disorders act at this site (see the Nutrition Focus for details). A new class of antihypertensive medications goes a step further to block the binding of angiotensin II to receptors in the body (e.g., in blood vessels). These are called angiotensin II receptor blockers (ARBs).

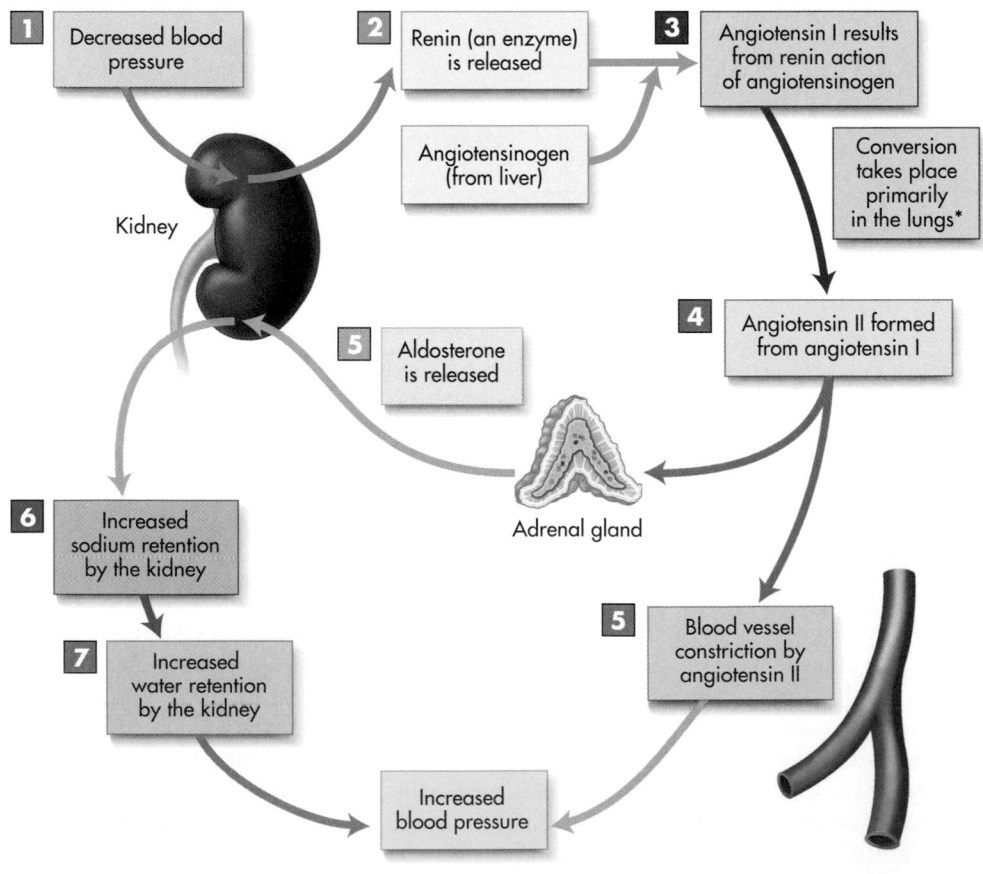

1 Decreased blood pressure

2 Renin (an enzyme) is released

Angiotensinogen (from liver)

3 Angiotensin I results from renin action of angiotensinogen

Conversion takes place primarily in the lungs*

Kidney

5 Aldosterone is released

4 Angiotensin II formed from angiotensin I

Adrenal gland

6 Increased sodium retention by the kidney

7 Increased water retention by the kidney

5 Blood vessel constriction by angiotensin II

Increased blood pressure

glands to release the hormone **aldosterone.** This hormone, in turn, signals the kidneys to retain more sodium and chloride, and therefore more water. Remember that water always follows electrolytes. Thus, low blood pressure, through this roundabout measure using the kidneys, causes increased water conservation in the body.

However, despite these mechanisms to conserve water, fluid continues to be lost via the insensible routes—feces, skin, and lungs. Those losses must be replaced. In addition, there is a limit to how concentrated urine can become. Eventually, if fluid is not consumed, the body becomes dehydrated and suffers ill effects.[6]

A Closer Look at Dehydration

By the time a person loses 1 to 2% of body weight in fluids, he or she will be thirsty. This loss of body weight contributes to fatigue as well as impaired physiological and performance responses. At a 4% loss of body weight, muscles lose significant strength and endurance. By the time body weight is reduced by 10 to 12%, heat tolerance is decreased and weakness results. At a 20% reduction, coma and death may soon follow (Figure 11-7).[6]

Water Toxicity

Too much water—whatever amount the kidneys are unable to excrete—can also lead to serious side effects, such as headache, blurred vision, cramps, convulsions, and ultimately death. Water intoxication is most likely to occur if water intake is not accompanied by sufficient electrolytes. However, an excessive amount would have to approach many quarts (liters) each day.[6]

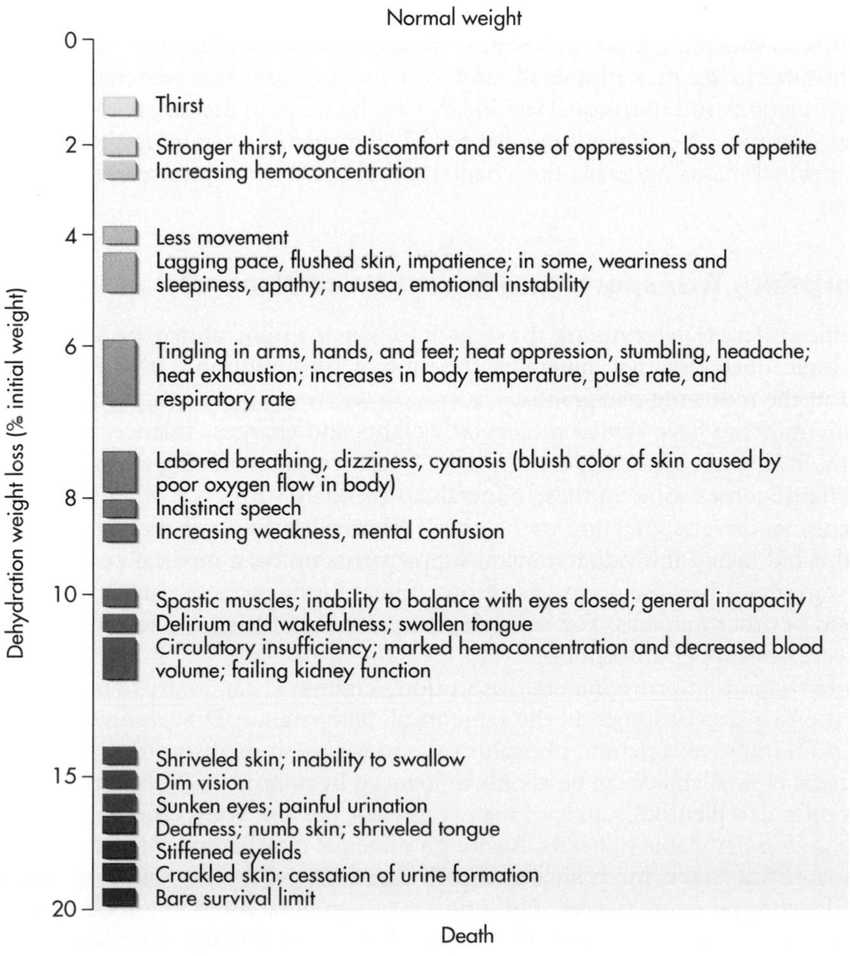

aldosterone A hormone produced in the adrenal glands that acts on the kidneys, causing them to retain sodium and, therefore, water.

Critical | Thinking

Stacy has been working in the yard with her brother Tom. They have been busy mowing the lawn and pulling weeds since noon. Tom tells Stacy that he is feeling weak and has a headache. Stacy is concerned that her brother might be somewhat dehydrated. How can his symptoms be explained? How could Tom's risk of dehydration have been decreased?

Figure 11-7 | The effects of dehydration range from thirst to death, depending on the extent of body weight loss.

Normal weight

Dehydration weight loss (% initial weight)	
0	Thirst
2	Stronger thirst, vague discomfort and sense of oppression, loss of appetite
	Increasing hemoconcentration
4	Less movement
	Lagging pace, flushed skin, impatience; in some, weariness and sleepiness, apathy; nausea, emotional instability
6	Tingling in arms, hands, and feet; heat oppression, stumbling, headache; heat exhaustion; increases in body temperature, pulse rate, and respiratory rate
8	Labored breathing, dizziness, cyanosis (bluish color of skin caused by poor oxygen flow in body)
	Indistinct speech
	Increasing weakness, mental confusion
10	Spastic muscles; inability to balance with eyes closed; general incapacity
	Delirium and wakefulness; swollen tongue
	Circulatory insufficiency; marked hemoconcentration and decreased blood volume; failing kidney function
15	Shriveled skin; inability to swallow
	Dim vision
	Sunken eyes; painful urination
	Deafness; numb skin; shriveled tongue
	Stiffened eyelids
	Crackled skin; cessation of urine formation
20	Bare survival limit

Death

As bottled water becomes more and more popular, the industry now generates more than $3 billion per year. In 1996, FDA instituted definitions for the various types of bottled water on the market; FDA also tests products for microbial and chemical content. For a list of manufacturers that meet federal guidelines, contact the International Bottled Water Association at 1-800-928-3711 or www.nsf.org. Some experts recommend that children not be given bottled water exclusively, because many brands do not contain an adequate fluoride supply to protect against dental caries. For adults, bottled water is typically an unnecessary expense, because it is often very similar to tap water. Chapter 19 reviews issues surrounding the safety of our water supply in North America, such as possible bacterial and lead contamination.

Very few people are at risk of drinking too much water, but problems do accompany some disease states and mental disorders.[6] In addition, it is also possible for some athletes to drink too much water. Endurance athletes (especially poorly trained individuals and those competing in cold conditions) may not sweat as much as they might have predicted. Thus, their water losses are not very high. They must then monitor their water intake to avoid an eventual fall in blood sodium, which is not desirable. Drinking less fluid so as not to gain weight during the activity can help prevent this problem (see Chapter 14 for details).

Concept | Check

Because our bodies cannot store water, we can survive only a few days without it. Water dissolves substances, serves as a medium for chemical reactions and as a lubricant, and aids in temperature regulation. Water accounts for 50 to 70% of body weight and distributes itself throughout the body among lean and other tissues (in both intracellular and extracellular fluids) and in urine and other body fluids. The Adequate Intake for total water intake is 2.7 liters (11 cups) for women and 3.7 liters (15 cups) for men. Thirst is the body's first sign of dehydration. If this thirst mechanism is faulty, as it may be during illness or vigorous exercise, hormonal mechanisms also help conserve water by reducing urine output. Excess fluid intake can be hazardous to a person's health.

▌ Minerals

Minerals are divided into major minerals and trace minerals, depending on the amount we need per day. Generally speaking, if we require 100 mg (1/50 of a teaspoon) or more per day of a mineral, it is considered a **major mineral,** or **macromineral;** otherwise, it is considered a **trace mineral,** or **micromineral.** Using these criteria, calcium and phosphorus are major minerals, and iron and zinc are trace minerals.

The functions and nutritional significance of the major minerals are discussed in this chapter, and the trace minerals in Chapter 12. But, before examining the properties of the individual major minerals, this chapter considers some topics relevant to all these minerals.

Absorption, Transport, and Excretion of Minerals

A significant factor determining the degree to which a mineral may be absorbed is the physiological need for that mineral at the time of consumption. Other factors are discussed in the following paragraphs.

Many minerals have similar molecular weights and charges (valences). Magnesium, calcium, iron, and copper can exist in the 2^+ valence state. Having similar size and the same charge causes some of these minerals to compete with each other for absorption mechanisms, thereby affecting each other's **bioavailability** and metabolism.[5] People should avoid taking individual mineral supplements unless a medical condition specifically warrants it because an excess of one mineral influences the absorption and metabolism of other minerals. For example, the presence of a large amount of zinc in the diet decreases copper absorption.

Some vitamins improve mineral absorption. Vitamin C can improve iron absorption when the two are consumed in the same meal. The vitamin D hormone (1,25 $(OH)_2$ vitamin D) improves calcium, phosphorus, and magnesium absorption.[5]

Mineral bioavailability can be greatly influenced by nonmineral substances in the diet. Foods offer us a plentiful supply of many minerals, but the body varies in its capacity to absorb and use available minerals. Although minerals may be present in foods, they are not bioavailable unless the body can absorb them. The ability to absorb minerals from a diet depends on many factors. The amount of a mineral listed in a food composition table does not necessarily reflect the amount that can be actually absorbed.

major mineral A mineral vital to health that is required in the diet in amounts greater than 100 mg/day; also called a macromineral.

trace mineral A mineral vital to health that is required in the diet in amounts less than 100 mg/day; also called a micromineral.

bioavailability The degree to which the amount of an ingested nutrient is absorbed and is available to the body.

Components of fiber, especially **phytic acid (phytate)** in wheat grain fiber, can limit the absorption of some minerals by chemically binding to them and preventing these from being released during digestion. As noted in Chapter 5, an intake greatly above the recommendation of 25 to 38 g/day of fiber can cause problems with mineral status of the body. However, if grains are leavened with yeast, as they are in bread, enzymes produced by the yeast can break some of the chemical bonds between phytic acid and minerals. This breakdown in some cases reduces the effect of phytates on mineral absorption. The zinc deficiencies found among some Middle Eastern populations are attributed partly to their consumption of unleavened breads, resulting in low bioavailability of dietary zinc. This issue is discussed in detail in Chapter 12.

Oxalic acid (oxalate) is another substance in plants that binds minerals and makes them less available to the body. Spinach, for example, contains plenty of calcium, but only about 5% of it can be absorbed because of the vegetable's high concentration of oxalic acid. On average, about 25% of dietary calcium is absorbed by adults, such as from milk and milk products.[5]

Once absorbed, minerals travel in the blood either in a free form or bound to proteins. For example, calcium ions can be found in the blood as such, as well as bound to the blood protein albumin. Many of the trace minerals have specific binding proteins, which transport them in the bloodstream. Trace minerals in their free form are often highly reactive and, so, would be toxic if not so bound. Many trace minerals also are bound by specific cellular proteins once taken up by cells.

Mineral excretion takes place primarily through the urine. When kidney function fails, mineral intake must be controlled in order to avoid mineral toxicity, such as with phosphorus and magnesium.[5] Some minerals, such as copper, are discharged through the bile into the intestinal tract and then excreted through the feces.

Functions of Minerals

The metabolic roles of minerals and the amounts of them in the body vary considerably (Figure 11-8). Some minerals, such as copper and selenium, function as cofactors, enabling enzymes to carry out a chemical reaction. (Recall this term was defined in

phytic acid (phytate) A constituent of plant fibers that binds positive ions to its multiple phosphate groups.

oxalic acid (oxalate) An organic acid found in spinach, rhubarb, and other leafy green vegetables that can depress the absorption of certain minerals present in the food, such as calcium.

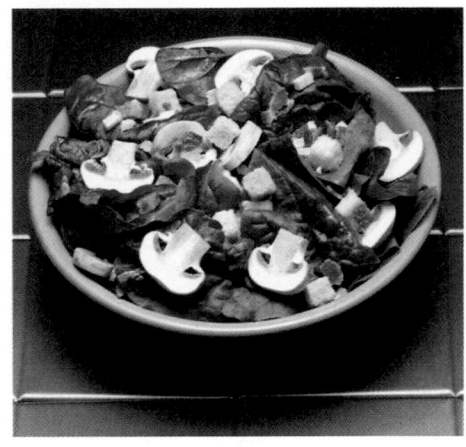

Spinach is often touted as a rich source of calcium, but little of the calcium present is bioavailable, that is, available to the body.

Figure 11-8 | Approximate amounts of various minerals present in the average human body. Other trace minerals of nutritional importance not listed include chromium, fluoride, molybdenum, selenium, and zinc.

Major minerals | Some trace minerals

Mineral	Grams in human body
Calcium	1200
Phosphorus	650
Potassium	200
Sulfur	180
Sodium	100
Chloride	100
Magnesium	30
Iron	10
Manganese	0.16
Copper	0.12
Iodide	0.03

Minerals

Chapter 9.) Minerals also are components of many body compounds. For example, iron is a component of hemoglobin in red blood cells. Sodium, potassium, and calcium aid in the transmission of nerve impulses throughout the body.[21] Body growth and development also depend on certain minerals, such as calcium and phosphorus.[19] Water balance requires sodium, potassium, calcium, and phosphorus. At all levels—cellular, tissue, organ, and whole body—minerals clearly play important roles in maintaining body functions.

Food Sources of Minerals

Minerals in the average North American's diet come from both plant and animal sources. For some minerals, animal sources are the food sources with the highest amounts and best bioavailability. For example, dairy products are rich sources of bioavailable calcium, while meat and related foods are rich sources of bioavailable iron and zinc. On the other hand, magnesium and manganese are more plentiful in plant-based foods than animal food products.

Generally the more refined a plant food—as in the case of white flour—the lower its mineral content. With regard to minerals, the enrichment process for grains adds only iron. The selenium, zinc, copper, and other minerals lost when grains are refined are not replaced. This is just one more reason to consume whole grains on a regular basis.

North Americans at Risk for Mineral Deficiencies

Typically, the major mineral at risk for being deficient in adult diets is calcium. Currently, most North Americans do not meet the recommended intake for calcium. For trace minerals, iron and zinc are most likely to be deficient in diets; these minerals are discussed in Chapter 12.

Toxicity of Minerals

Excess mineral intake can lead to toxic results, especially with the trace minerals, such as iron and copper. This potential for toxicity is yet another reason to consider carefully the use of mineral supplements. Many trace minerals are quite toxic at doses not much above typical needs, which is approximated by the Daily Value on the food or supplement label. Thus, doses of mineral supplements should be examined carefully, especially if intake will exceed the Upper Level. Such intakes should be taken only under a physician's supervision because toxicity and nutrient interactions are possible (see the inside cover of this text for Upper Levels for minerals).

The potential for toxicity is not the only reason to carefully consider the use of mineral supplements. Harmful interactions with other nutrients are possible. Also, contamination of mineral supplements—with lead, for example—is a very real possibility. Use of brands approved by United States Pharmacopeia (USP) lessens this risk. In summary, even with the best intentions, people may harm themselves using mineral supplements.

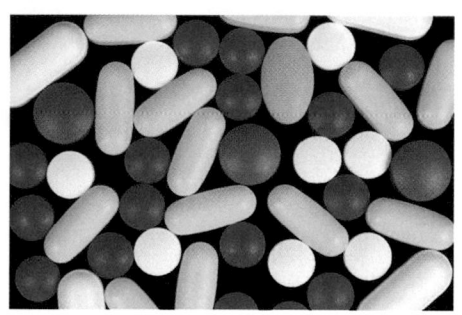

Some mineral supplements pose a high risk for toxicity. Generally, mineral intake from a supplement should not exceed 100% of the Daily Value unless otherwise specified by a physician.

Concept | Check

Minerals are vital for many body processes. Their bioavailability depends on many factors, including interactions with fiber, vitamins, and other minerals. Both animal and plant sources help us meet our mineral needs. Taking large amounts of an individual mineral supplement can greatly diminish the absorption and metabolism of other minerals. In addition, some minerals are potentially toxic at intakes not much in excess of human needs. These are two good reasons to consider carefully any use of mineral supplements that exceed the Daily Value on the label, especially if the intake is in excess of any Upper Level on a long-term basis.

Sodium (Na)

Many health professionals recommend that North Americans limit intake of sodium.[1,8,13,20] Salt contributes almost all the sodium to our diets. Salt is 40% sodium and 60% chloride. North Americans typically consume more sodium than is needed. Still, as reviewed in the Nutrition Focus in this chapter, salt intake is not the major cause of hypertension in North America (obesity and inactivity are more important).[1,15,18]

Absorption, Transport, Storage, and Excretion of Sodium

The human body absorbs almost all sodium consumed because sodium is easily absorbed from the GI tract. The body maintains a large amount of sodium in the bloodstream for use when needed. Excretion of sodium is via the kidneys into the urine.[21]

Functions of Sodium

Sodium is the major positive ion (cation) in extracellular fluid and a key factor in retaining body fluids. Sodium balance is regulated by the hormone aldosterone. Sodium also helps regulate the fluid balance of the body both within and outside the cells.[21]

As both sodium and potassium shift across the cell membrane, they create an electrical potential charge that allows muscles to contract and nerve impulses to be conducted. Sodium also participates in the absorption of other nutrients (e.g., glucose and amino acids) in the small intestine.

Sodium in Foods

About 80% of the sodium we consume is added during food manufacturing and food preparation at restaurants (Table 11-3). Sodium added in cooking and at the table provides about 10% of our intakes, and sodium naturally present in foods provides the rest,

The earliest reference to salt is in The Book of Job written about 300 B.C. At one time, it was the custom to rub salt on newborn babies as a symbol of purity and to ensure their good health. Salt was once so scarce that it was used as money. Caesar's soldiers received part of their pay in common salt. This part of their pay was known as their "salarium," and from this custom came today's word "salary." The expression "not worth his salt" meant that a man did not earn his wages.

Many commercially prepared condiments, sauces, and seasonings are high in sodium. Examples include onion, celery, and garlic seasonings; sea salt; baking powder; salad dressings; pickles; soy, steak, barbecue, chili, and Worcestershire sauces; meat tenderizer; baking soda; salt pork; brine; catsup; mustard; bouillon; monosodium glutamate (MSG); and relish.

Table 11-3 | Increase in Sodium Content of Foods during Processing*

Food Category	Sodium (mg)
Dairy Products	
Fruited yogurt, 3/4 cup	107
2% milk, 1 1/2 cups	182
Cheddar cheese, 1 3/4 oz	307
American cheese food, 2 oz	548
Meats	
Beef roast, 1 oz	17
Beef jerky, 2/3 oz	540
Pork loin, 1 oz	22
Bacon, 2 pieces	202
Ham, 1 1/2 oz	564
Vegetables	
Fresh peas, 1 cup	5
Frozen peas, 1 cup	139
Frozen peas in cheese sauce, 2/3 cup	205
Canned peas, 1 cup	372
Grain Products	
Flour, 1/3 cup	1
Bread, 2 slices	286
Saltine crackers, 12	486

*All examples in a particular group contain the same amount of food energy.

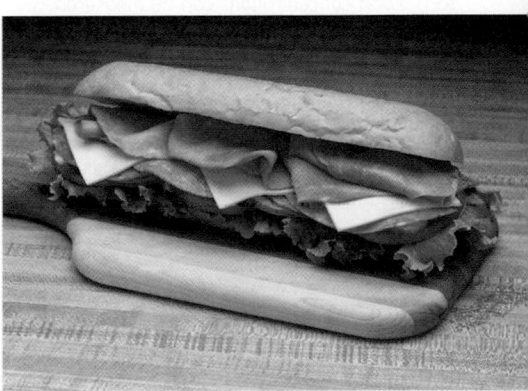

Cured meats are very high in sodium.

Food Sources of Sodium

Food Item and Amount	Sodium Content (mg)
Pepperoni pizza, 2 slices	2045
Sliced ham, 1 oz	1215
Chicken noodle soup, canned, 1 cup	1106
V8 vegetable juice, 8 oz	620
Macaroni salad, 1/2 cup	561
Hard pretzels, 1 oz	486
Hamburger with bun, 1	474
Green beans, canned, 1/2 cup	390
Saltine crackers, 6	234
Cheddar cheese, 1 oz	176
Peanut butter, 2 tbsp	156
Fat-free milk, 1 cup	127
7-grain bread, 1 slice	126
Animal crackers, 1 oz	112
Grape juice, 1 cup	10
Adequate Intake for young adults, 1500 mg	
Adequate Intake for older adults, 1200 to 1300 mg	

To assess the sodium, potassium, chloride, magnesium, or phosphorus status of a person, blood concentrations can be measured. Other methods, which are often more sensitive, when appropriate, will be noted in this chapter.

again about 10%. Almost all unprocessed foods naturally contain a little sodium; the higher amount found in milk (about 120 mg/cup) is one exception.

The more processed and restaurant food we consume, generally the higher our sodium intake is. Conversely, the more home cooking we do, the more sodium control we have.[6] Major contributors of sodium in the adult diet are white bread and rolls, hot dogs and lunch meats, cheese, soups, and foods with tomato sauce, partly because these foods are eaten so often. Foods that are especially high in sodium include salted snack foods, french fries and potato chips, and sauces and gravies.

If we ate only unprocessed foods and added no salt, we would consume about 500 mg of sodium per day.[6] Comparing 500 mg of sodium from unprocessed food with the 2300 to 4700 mg or more typically eaten by adults, it is clear that food processing and cooking contribute most of our dietary sodium. As discussed in Chapter 2, nutrition labels list a food's sodium content. When dietary sodium must be severely restricted, attention to food labels is of utmost importance. Under FDA food and supplement labeling rules, the Daily Value for sodium is 2400 mg (2.4 g). In addition, various descriptive terms, such as *sodium-free, salt-free,* and *low-sodium,* may appear elsewhere on labels (review Table 2-14 in Chapter 2). When sodium must be severely restricted in a diet, even contributions from tap water (especially from softened water, which contains more sodium), as well as medicines that contain sodium, must be considered.

Sodium Needs

The Adequate Intake set for sodium for adults under age 51 is 1500 mg/day. (See the inside cover for references to mineral needs for various age groups.) Note that 1500 mg/day is a generous amount. We really need only about 200 mg/day to maintain physiological functions. Additional sodium was added to the Adequate Intake to allow for a more varied diet in which not all foods need to be low in sodium.[6]

Should you choose to consume less sodium, you can eventually adapt to a low-sodium diet, but many typical food choices will need to be eliminated (see the first Take Action at the end of this chapter). At first, foods will taste quite flat, but eventually you will perceive more flavor as the tongue's salt receptors become more sensitive to the natural salt content of foods. By slowly reducing dietary salt and substituting garlic, oregano, other herbs, spices, and lemon juice, you can eventually become accustomed to a diet containing less sodium. Many new cookbooks offer tested recipes for flavorful low-sodium foods. Except when baking breads with yeast, omitting salt from food preparation can still yield many excellent products.

Sodium-Deficiency Diseases

Only when weight loss from perspiration exceeds about 2% of total body weight (or about 5 to 6 lb) should sodium losses be of concern.[21] Even then, merely salting foods is sufficient to restore body sodium for most people. Endurance athletes, however, may need to consume sports drinks during competition to avoid depletion of sodium (see Chapter 14). Although perspiration tastes salty on the skin, sodium is not highly concentrated in perspiration. Rather, water evaporating from the skin just leaves sodium behind. (Perspiration contains about two-thirds the sodium concentration found in blood.) Sodium depletion also can occur because of diarrhea or vomiting, especially in infants. There are special electrolyte drinks for use in such cases to replace sodium (see Chapter 17).

Upper Level for Sodium

The Upper Level for sodium for adults is 2300 mg/day (2.3g). Intakes exceeding this amount typically increase blood pressure.[6] About 95% of North American adults have sodium intakes that exceed the Upper Level. A sodium intake > 2 g/day also increases calcium loss in the urine, a problem for people who consume much salt and little calcium (and too little potassium).[3] Another health area in which salt may be a problem is kidney stone formation. A high salt intake may contribute to stone formation in certain people, linked to increased calcium excretion. A very high sodium intake overall, can be toxic, especially when the kidneys cannot excrete the excess in the urine. Sodium is especially toxic when a high intake is accompanied by a lack of water.[6]

Concept | Check

Sodium is the major positive ion in the extracellular fluid. It is important for maintaining fluid balance and conducting nerve impulses. Sodium depletion is unlikely, because the typical North American's diet has abundant sources of sodium and most of it gets absorbed. Compared to dining out or buying commercially prepared foods, preparation of foods in the home allows greater control over sodium intake. The Adequate Intake for sodium for adults is 1500 mg/day. The average adult consumes 2300 to 4700 mg or more daily. Some adults are especially sensitive to sodium. In these people, hypertension can develop as a result of high-sodium diets. Nutrition experts currently suggest that for young adults, sodium intake should be about 1500 mg (1.5 g), and should not exceed 2300 mg (2.3 g) on a regular basis. Sodium in the North American diet is provided predominantly through processed and restaurant foods.

Critical | Thinking

Mrs. Massa has recently seen and heard a lot about the amount of salt in foods. She has been surprised by the number of articles that advise the public to decrease the amount of salt in their food. If sodium is such a bad thing, Mrs. Massa wonders, why do you need to have any at all? How would you explain to her this need for some sodium?

▌Potassium (K)

Like sodium, potassium is a primary electrolyte in body fluids. Unlike sodium, potassium is associated with lower, rather than higher, blood pressure values.

Absorption, Transport, Storage, and Excretion of Potassium

The body absorbs about 90% of the potassium consumed. Most of this potassium ends up inside body cells, while some is found in the bloodstream. As with sodium, potassium balance is achieved primarily through kidney excretion or retention.[21]

Functions of Potassium

Potassium performs many of the same functions as sodium, such as fluid balance and nerve-impulse transmission. It also influences the contractility of smooth, skeletal, and cardiac muscle.[25] Potassium is the major cation inside the cell. Intracellular fluids contain 95% of the potassium in the body.[21]

Potassium in Foods

Unlike sodium, potassium is not generally added to foods. Overall, fresh fruits and vegetables are good sources of potassium. Milk, whole grains, dried beans, and meats are also sources. Major contributors of potassium to the adult diet include milk, potatoes, coffee, tomatoes, and orange juice.

Potassium Needs

The Adequate Intake for potassium for adults is 4700 mg (4.7 g) per day.[6] The Daily Value used on food and supplement labels is 3500 mg. Typically, North Americans consume on average 2000 to 3000 mg/day. Thus many of us need to increase our potassium intakes, preferably by increasing intake of fruits, vegetables, whole-grain breads and cereals, and low-fat and fat-free milk and milk products.[6] Information about a food's potassium content is required on the Nutrition Facts panel only if the food contains added potassium as a nutrient or if claims about this nutrient appear on the label. In all other cases, information is voluntary.

▌he DASH (Dietary Approaches to Stop Hypertension) study showed that when people ate 8 to 10 servings of fruits, vegetables, and nuts each day (along with low-fat dairy products)—all sources of potassium—their blood pressure went down. This trend was especially true for people who had hypertension (see the Expert Opinion by Dr. Marlene Most).

Food Sources of Potassium

Food Item and Amount	Potassium (mg)
Kidney beans, 1 cup	715
Winter squash, 3/4 cup	670
Plain yogurt, 1 cup	570
Orange juice, 1 cup	495
Cantaloupe, 1 cup	495
Lima beans, 1/2 cup	480
Banana, 1 medium	470
Zucchini, 1 cup	450
Soybeans, 1/2 cup	440
Artichoke, 1 medium	425
Tomato juice, 3/4 cup	400
Pinto beans, 1/2 cup	400
Baked potato, 1 small	385
Buttermilk, 1 cup	370
Sirloin steak, 3 oz	345
Adequate Intake for adults, 4700 mg	

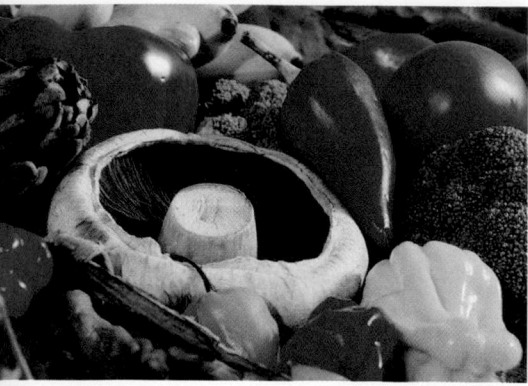

Vegetables are a rich source of potassium, as are fruits.

Potassium-Deficiency Diseases

Low blood potassium is a life-threatening problem. Symptoms often include a loss of appetite, muscle cramps, confusion, constipation, and increased urinary calcium excretion. Eventually, the heart beats irregularly, decreasing its capacity to pump blood.[21]

Some diuretics used to treat hypertension deplete potassium from the body. People who take potassium-wasting diuretics need to monitor their potassium intakes carefully. A recent study showed an increase in risk of stroke in people on these medications who did not consume enough potassium. For these people, high-potassium foods—such as fruits, fruit juices, and vegetables—are good additions to the diet, and if recommended by a physician, so are potassium chloride supplements.

A continual deficient food intake, as may be the case in alcoholism, can result in a severe potassium deficiency. This deficiency also can be evident in people with anorexia nervosa and bulimia nervosa, who have poor eating habits and whose bodies can be depleted of potassium because of vomiting (see Chapter 15). People on very low energy diets are also at risk, as are athletes who exercise heavily. As covered in Chapters 13 and 14, all these people should compensate for potentially low body potassium by consuming potassium-rich foods.

Use of potassium in supplement form to treat a deficiency or poor intake is harmless if the kidneys function normally. Thus no Upper Level has been set.[6] However, taken in excessive amounts, potassium supplements can cause GI tract upset. When the kidneys function poorly, potassium readily builds up in the blood. This buildup inhibits heart function, causing slowed heartbeat. If untreated, this condition can be fatal, because the heart eventually stops beating. Consequently, in cases of reduced kidney function, close control of potassium intake is critical.[21]

Chloride (Cl)

Chlorine is an element, but humans need the chloride ion (Cl^-).

Absorption, Transport, Storage, and Excretion of Chloride

Chloride is almost completely absorbed in the small intestine and colon. Much chloride is found in the bloodstream (associated with sodium). Like excretion of sodium and potassium, excretion of chloride occurs mainly through the kidneys.[21]

Functions of Chloride

Chloride serves as an important negative ion in the extracellular fluid. Chloride's negative charge balances the positive charges of sodium ions and in turn contributes to maintenance of electrolyte balance.[21] Chloride contributes to the function of the nervous system. Chloride also is a component of the hydrochloric acid produced in the stomach, and is used during immune responses when white blood cells attack foreign cells. Finally, chloride aids in the transport of carbon dioxide from cells to the lungs as well as the disposal of carbon dioxide by way of exhaled air.

Chloride is likely part of the blood pressure–raising property of sodium chloride (salt).

Chloride in Foods

Seaweed, olives, rye, lettuce, a few fruits, and some vegetables are naturally good sources of chloride. Chlorinated water is also a source. However, we consume most chloride as salt added to foods. Once we know a food's salt content, we can easily predict its chloride content; recall that salt is 60% chloride. Naturally occurring sodium or chloride won't significantly affect the prediction.

Chloride Needs

The Adequate Intake for chloride for adults is 2300 mg. This amount is based on the 40:60 ratio of sodium to chloride in salt (1500 mgs of sodium in a diet is accompanied by 2300 mg of chloride).[6] The Daily Value used on food and supplement labels is 3400 mg. An average daily consumption of 9 g of salt yields 5.4 g (5400 mg) of chloride.

Chloride-Deficiency Diseases

A chloride deficiency is generally unlikely because our dietary sodium chloride (salt) intake is so high. Frequent and lengthy bouts of vomiting—if coupled with a nutrient-poor diet—can cause a deficiency because stomach secretions contain much chloride.[21]

Upper Level for Chloride

As just noted, the average adult typically consumes much more than this amount. The Upper Level for chloride is 3.6 g/day. This amount is based on the amount of chloride that accompanies the Upper Level for sodium (2300 mg/day).[6] Dietary chloride has been implicated in the blood pressure–raising ability of sodium chloride.[15] Still, as one lowers sodium intake as part of hypertension therapy, chloride intake automatically falls as well.

Concept | Check

Potassium performs functions similar to those of sodium, except that it is the main positive ion (cation) found inside, not outside, cells. Potassium is vital to fluid balance and nerve transmission. A potassium deficiency—caused by an inadequate intake of potassium, persistent vomiting, or use of some diuretics—can lead to loss of appetite, muscle cramps, confusion, and heartbeat irregularities. Fruits and vegetables are generally good sources of potassium. Potassium intake can be toxic if a person's kidneys do not function properly. Chloride is the major negative ion (anion) of extracellular fluid. Chloride also functions in digestion as part of hydrochloric acid and in immune and nervous system responses. Deficiencies of chloride are highly unlikely because we eat so much salt.

NUTRITION FOCUS

Minerals and Hypertension

Symptoms of Stroke

Individuals experiencing any of the following symptoms of stroke should seek immediate treatment because physicians can administer drugs that can reduce the extent of the damage caused by most strokes (i.e., ischemic strokes). Currently about 700,000 North Americans suffer strokes each year.

- Sudden disturbances in sight, speech, and steadiness
- Sudden sleepiness or severe headache
- Sudden temporary blindness in one eye or other visual effects
- Sudden numbness, weakness, or paralysis of an arm, a leg, or an entire side of the body
- Sudden difficulty with speech or the ability to swallow
- Coma or convulsions

Regular, moderate physical activity contributes to better blood pressure control.

More than 50 million North American adults have hypertension, as does one out of two adults over age 65. Blood pressure is expressed by two numbers. The higher number represents systolic blood pressure, which is the pressure in the arteries when the heart actively pumps blood. The second value is for diastolic blood pressure, which is the artery pressure when the heart is relaxed. Optimal systolic blood pressure is less than 120 mm of mercury (mm Hg). Optimal diastolic blood pressure is less than 80 mm Hg. Elevated systolic and diastolic pressure shows a strong relationship to various diseases (especially strokes and other cardiovascular diseases).[2,11]

For adults, hypertension is defined as sustained systolic pressure exceeding 140 mm Hg or diastolic blood pressure exceeding 90 mm Hg (Table 11-4). Most cases of hypertension (about 95% of cases) have no clear-cut cause and are described as primary, or essential, in nature (e.g., essential hypertension). Kidney disease, sleep-disordered breathing (sleep apnea), and other causes often lead to the other 5% of cases, known as secondary hypertension. African Americans are more likely than Caucasians to develop hypertension and to do so earlier in life. As a result, they also suffer more from hypertension-related diseases and, so, are particularly advised to have their blood pressure checked regularly and to have any evidence of hypertension treated aggressively.

Unless blood pressure is measured periodically, the development of hypertension can be easily overlooked. Thus, hypertension is described as a silent disorder because it usually does not cause symptoms. A physician usually does not treat hypertension with medication until the diastolic blood pressure measures at least 90 mm Hg and/or the systolic blood pressure reaches 140 mm Hg on three or more occasions.[2]

Why Control Blood Pressure?

Blood pressure needs to be controlled mainly to prevent cardiovascular disease, kidney disease, strokes and related declines in brain function, poor blood circulation in the legs, problems with vision, and sudden death. All these conditions are much more likely to be found in individuals with hypertension than in people with normal blood pressure. Smoking and elevated blood lipoproteins (LDL and VLDL) further increase disease risk. Individuals with hypertension need to be diagnosed and treated as soon as possible, because the condition generally progresses to a more serious stage over time and even resists therapy if it persists for years.[2]

Causes of Hypertension

Blood pressure usually increases as a person ages. Some increase is caused by atherosclerosis. As plaque builds up in the arteries, the arteries become less flexible and cannot expand. When vessels remain rigid, blood pressure remains high. Eventually, the plaque begins to choke off the blood supply to the kidneys, decreasing their ability to control blood volume and, in turn, blood pressure.[2]

The enzyme renin, which is secreted by the kidneys and some hormonelike compounds affect blood pressure. Medications are available to reduce their effect on the renin-angiotensin system.[2,21]

Obesity is often associated with high blood pressure, especially among women. In fact, overweight people have six times greater risk of having hypertension than do lean people. Overall, obesity is considered the primary lifestyle factor related to hypertension.[1] The increase in fat mass increases the need for blood circulation. The extra miles of associated blood vessels increases work by the heart and increases blood pressure. Elevated blood insulin concentration associated with insulin-resistant

Table 11-4 | Latest Classification of Blood Pressure for Adults Age 18 Years and Older in Millimeters of Mercury (mm Hg)

Category	Systolic		Diastolic
Normal	< 120	and	< 80
Prehypertension	120–139	or	80–89
Hypertension			
Stage 1	140–159	or	90–99
Stage 2	≥ 160	or	≥ 100

adipose cells is another reason for this link to obesity. Insulin increases sodium retention in the body and accelerates atherosclerosis. Additionally, an estimated 65% of people with diabetes also have hypertension.

A weight loss of as little as 10 to 15 pounds often can decrease the need for hypertension drugs, which by themselves may cause headache, impotence, reduced exercise tolerance, persistent cough, and other side effects. The sleep apnea linked to hypertension also typically improves with weight loss.

Inactivity is considered the second leading lifestyle factor related to hypertension.[1] If an obese person can engage in regular physical activity (at least five days per week for a total of 60 minutes) and lose weight, blood pressure often returns to normal.

Excess alcohol intake is responsible for about 10% of all cases of hypertension, especially in middle-aged males and among[1] African Americans in general. It is considered the third leading lifestyle factor related to hypertension. Hypertension caused by excessive alcohol intake is usually reversible. A sensible intake for people with hypertension is two or fewer drinks per day for men and one or no drinks per day for women and older adults. (These are the same recommendations given to healthy adults.) As discussed in Chapter 8, some studies suggest that such a moderate alcohol intake reduces the risk of ischemic stroke. These data, however, should not be used to encourage alcohol use in nonconsumers.

Salt and Blood Pressure

Excess salt intake tends to increase blood pressure, particularly among African Americans, older persons, obese persons, and people in general who are susceptible to developing a problem regulating sodium concentration in the body. This last group is termed "sodium (or salt) sensitive" because they are not good at excreting excess salt via the kidney. This excess salt retention then has a tendency to increase blood pressure.[1,15] It is not clear whether the sodium ion or the chloride ion is most responsible for the effect. Still, as reviewed in this chapter,

if one reduces sodium intake, chloride intake naturally falls; the opposite is also true. For the most part, when nutrition recommendations suggest consuming less sodium, they are in essence saying "consume less salt." Because only some North Americans are susceptible to increases in blood pressure from salt intake, salt intake is only the fourth leading lifestyle factor related to hypertension. Thus, it is unfortunate that salt intake receives the major portion of public attention with regard to hypertension; obesity, inactivity, and alcohol abuse should be given much more attention, especially for people who are not sodium sensitive.[1,18] About half the people with hypertension are not sodium sensitive. However, many people with hypertension do not know whether they are sodium sensitive, and testing for this sensitivity takes a lot of time and is not routinely done.

Other Nutrients and Blood Pressure

Recent studies show that a diet rich in calcium, potassium, and magnesium (and low in sodium) may lead to a decrease in blood pressure, especially among African Americans.[1] The response is similar to that seen with typical antihypertensive medications. Dr. Marlene Most discusses this dietary approach to lowering blood pressure in detail in the Expert Opinion. Other studies also show a reduction in stroke risk among people who consume a diet rich in fruits, vegetables, and vitamin C (recall that fruits and vegetables are rich sources of potassium).[11] Overall, a diet rich in low-fat and fat-free dairy products, fruits, vegetables, whole grains, and some nuts can substantially reduce blood pressure and stroke risk for many people.[1,15]

Prevention of Hypertension

Many of the risk factors for hypertension and stroke are controllable, and appropriate lifestyle changes can reduce a person's risk (Table 11-5). Experts typically recommend that people with hypertension in the Prehypertension and Stage 1 categories attempt to lower blood pressure through

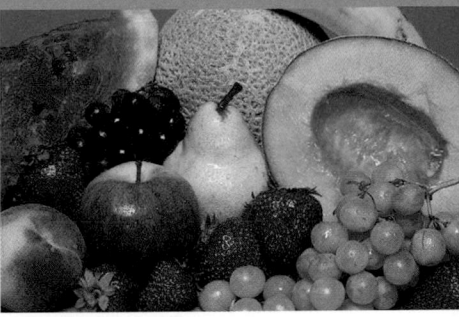

Regular intake of fruits and vegetables has been linked to a decreased risk of both hypertension and stroke.

Preliminary studies show a link between bone lead concentrations and increased risk of hypertension. More information is needed, but it is suspected that even small amounts of lead stored over decades may damage the kidneys and eventually result in hypertension. This is just one of the deleterious effects of lead exposure (see Chapter 19 for more information on lead).

The exact mechanism whereby sodium increases blood pressure is not clear. Studies suggest that a genetically influenced ability determines the ease at which the body can excrete sodium. In salt-sensitive individuals, the kidneys require an elevated blood pressure to excrete sodium from the body. Salt-sensitive individuals retain more sodium, which then leads to fluid retention. Ultimately, the fluid retention leads to increased blood volume and, in turn, the increased blood pressure needed to maintain sodium excretion.[15]

Table 11-5 | A Nutritional and Related Lifestyle Plan to Minimize Hypertension and Stroke Risk*[1,11,20,25]

1. Follow MyPyramid. A person could even consider going beyond this plan to include more fruit, vegetables, and some nuts, especially if one has hypertension.
2. Make sure to meet nutrient recommendations for calcium, potassium, and magnesium listed in this chapter.
3. Attain and maintain a healthy body weight.
4. Incorporate regular physical activity (at least five times per week for a total of 60 minutes).
5. Consume alcoholic beverages in moderation, if at all (two drinks per day maximum for men and one drink per day maximum for women and older adults).
6. Consume moderate amounts of sodium (salt) and see if any changes in blood pressure occur. The Upper Level is a reasonable starting point (2300 mg sodium or 6 g salt [1¼ tsp]) per day. One might even try to lower intake to 1500 mg/day, the Adequate Intake set for sodium.
7. Don't smoke.
8. Maintain blood lipoproteins in the normal range (see Chapter 6).
9. Moderate caffeine intake.
10. Find ways to reduce psychological stress.

*In addition, make sure to have blood pressure measured on a regular basis (i.e., yearly physical checkups).

diet and lifestyle changes before resorting to blood pressure medications. Such a focus on diet and lifestyle is important because many people discontinue their blood pressure medications because of expense and side effects.

Medications to Treat Hypertension

Potassium-wasting diuretics, such as thiazides (chlorothiazide [Diuril]), are commonly used for drug therapy to treat hypertension. People need to monitor their potassium intakes carefully while taking these drugs. Other typical medications to treat hypertension include angiotensin-converting enzyme (ACE) inhibitors (captopril [Capoten], angiotensin II receptor blockers (candesartan [Atacand]), beta-blockers (atenolol [Tenormin]), and calcium channel blockers (amlodipine [Norvasc]). A combination of two or more drugs is commonly used. The beta-blockers act to slow heart rate and cause some vasodilation, whereas the calcium channel blockers and ACE-related medications lead to general vasodilation.[2]

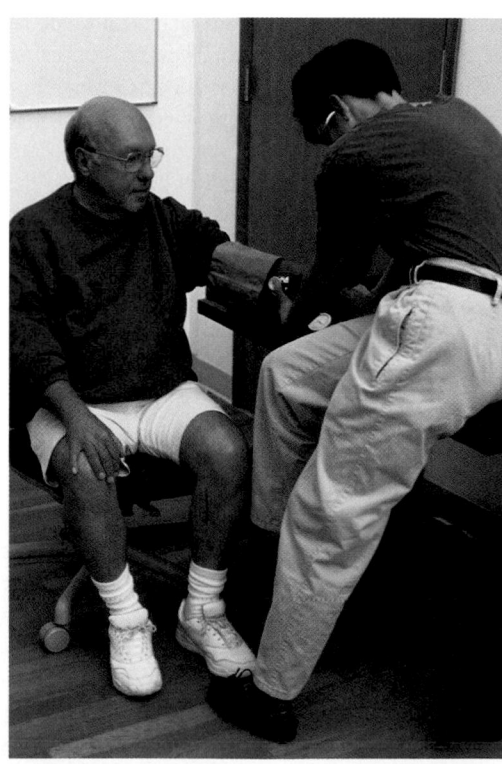

Older adults are particularly at risk of hypertension.

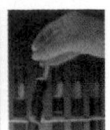

Expert Opinion

A Close Look at the DASH Diet
Marlene Most, Ph.D., R.D., F.A.D.A.

As individuals are becoming more aware of the relationship between diet and their health, they are searching for dietary means to improve health by diminishing disease risk factors. We know, for example, that a diet low in saturated fat will improve blood lipid levels, a major risk factor for cardiovascular health. Similarly, we know that some changes in diet will lower blood pressure and in turn minimize the risk of developing hypertension. These changes include reducing body weight (if overweight or obese), lowering alcohol intake, and minimizing sodium intake. Other dietary factors, such as potassium, magnesium, calcium, protein, and fiber intake, also are implicated in having a beneficial effect on blood pressure. The scientific evidence for these individual factors, however, is inconsistent or inconclusive.

Why Develop the DASH Diet?

It is plausible that the effects on blood pressure from individual nutrients are small and cannot be seen in research studies. Because many of the studies have examined the individual nutrients in supplement form rather than in foods, synergistic effects were then considered as well as the possible importance of a combination of nutrients in foods that may be needed to reduce blood pressure. Thus, the National Heart, Lung, and Blood Institute decided in 1992 to fund a study with the goal of examining dietary patterns and blood pressure. The highly successful Dietary Approaches to Stop Hypertension (DASH) diet was the end result.

What Actually Is the DASH Diet?

The DASH diet is characterized as low in fat and sodium and rich in fruits, vegetables, and low-fat dairy products. Here is the actual breakdown:

Per day	Per week
6–8 servings of grains and grain products	4–5 servings of nuts, seeds, or legumes
4–5 servings of fruit	5 servings of sweets and added sugars
4–5 servings of vegetables	
2–3 servings of low-fat or fat-free dairy products	
2 or less servings of meats, poultry, and fish	
2–3 servings of fats/oils	

Participants who consumed the DASH diet showed substantial reductions in blood pressure, especially those who had hypertension. The magnitude of the effect on blood pressure was similar to that observed with single antihypertensive drug therapy. Additionally, the diet was particularly effective for African Americans. Most impressively, the reduction in blood pressure took place rather quickly, occurring within two weeks of the dietary intervention.

Although the goal of the DASH study was to find a dietary pattern to benefit blood pressure, certain nutrients were targeted in the diet's design. These nutrients specifically included magnesium, potassium, and calcium. The diet was also designed to be low in total fat and saturated fat and moderately high in protein and dietary fiber. Sodium reduction was added in a subsequent study—3300 mg/day, 2400 mg/day, and 1500 mg/day groups. This intervention further lowered blood pressure as sodium intake declined (called DASH-Sodium).

How Do Magnesium, Potassium, Calcium, and Fiber Affect Blood Pressure?

Clinical and epidemiological studies had examined the relationship between blood pressure and magnesium consumption. Some results have shown an inverse relationship and a clear effect of magnesium. It had been shown that magnesium has a direct effect on reducing the contractile activity of smooth muscle, such as that surrounding blood vessels, which offers a plausible mechanism for magnesium's contribution to the regulation of blood pressure. On the other hand, failures of many magnesium supplementation intervention trials had been reported. Initial magnesium status appears to be important. Significant effects tend to be seen in persons in whom magnesium intake or availability initially was compromised.

Evidence from clinical studies of dietary or supplemental calcium were suggestive, but not conclusive, in the role for this mineral in modulating blood pressure. Benefits were found in persons who had low calcium intakes or metabolic conditions in which calcium availability is affected, such as pregnancy. Epidemiological studies also have provided support for higher calcium intakes and lowered blood pressure.

Potassium had the most definitive role of any micronutrient in the control of blood pressure. Potassium intake or urinary potassium is inversely associated with blood pressure. Epidemiological and intervention data have provided support for both phytosterols. Their roles in disease risk reduction are now becoming recognized, as they provide health benefits much beyond the nutrients present in the foods. It is possible that the bioactive compounds found in the DASH diet played a role in the blood pressure changes observed in the studies: For example, a probable contributing mechanism for blood pressure regulation may be through blood vessel relaxation and

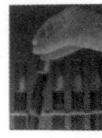

improved potassium intake from foods and supplements in people with normal blood pressure values and mild hypertension.

High-fiber diets significantly reduce blood pressure in persons with hypertension. Yet in people with normal blood pressure values, fiber supplementation only modestly reduces blood pressure or has no effect. Positive studies of fiber intake generally utilized vegetarian diets or involved the manipulation of fiber content along with other nutrients. Although suggestive, the literature did not unequivocally support a role for fiber alone in the control of blood pressure.

How Does the DASH Diet Benefit One's Total Diet?

The failure of many nutrient-specific interventions to have significant blood pressure effects may have been due to the fact that several aspects of the diet must be changed together. The most compelling data for this assertion come from studies of vegetarian diets—these diets are strongly associated with reduced blood pressure when compared to nonvegetarian diets. Vegetarian diets tend to be lower in total fat and higher in fiber, magnesium, and potassium. It had been difficult to tease out which nutrients were responsible for the lower blood pressures in vegetarians, suggesting the need for including all factors. With this in mind, the combination of nutrients in the DASH dietary pattern led to its success in blood pressure regulation.

While certain nutrient targets were achieved in the DASH diet, its focus on fruits, vegetables, and whole grains also contributed many other compounds to the diet. These foods are abundant in phytochemicals, including polyphenols, carotenoids, and endothelial cell function from the antioxidant properties of the polyphenols present in the DASH diet. The actual protective mechanisms remain to be determined, and more information will surely become available about the impact of phytochemicals in the processes sur-

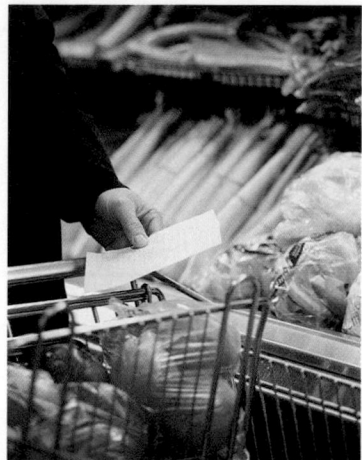

Opting for the fruits, vegetables, and low-fat foods recommended by the DASH diet represents a sound approach to nutrition for most people regardless of hypertension risk.

rounding blood pressure regulation. Consequently, the health benefits of the DASH diet may extend beyond blood pressure reduction. Look to the grocery aisles, rather than the supplement aisles in a pharmacy, for the benefits of the DASH diet. Never has the recommendation for a diet rich in low-fat and fat-free dairy products, fruits, vegetables, nuts, and whole-grain breads and cereals been so clear.

Dr. Most is Associate Professor of Research at the Pennington Biomedical Research Center in Baton Rouge, Louisiana. She is a registered dietitian and a charter fellow of the American Dietetic Association. She received her Ph.D. in Veterinary Medical Sciences, Physiology, from Louisiana State University and her M.S. and B.S. in Food Science and Nutrition from Colorado State University. Dr. Most has been principal investigator for feeding studies that examined cardiovascular benefits of various modified diets and was instrumental in the Dietary Approaches to Stop Hypertension (DASH) studies funded by the National Heart, Lung, and Blood Institute, NIH. Dr. Most has conducted NIH-funded training workshops for delivering research diets and is the author of several manuscripts and book chapters that describe controlled feeding study methodologies.

Calcium (Ca)

All cells need calcium, but more than 99% of the calcium in the body is used as a structural component of bones and teeth. This calcium represents 40% of all the minerals present in the body and equals about 2.5 lb (1200 g). As calcium circulates in the bloodstream, it supplies the calcium needs of body cells.[5]

Absorption, Transport, Storage, and Excretion of Calcium

Unlike sodium, potassium, and chloride, the amount of calcium in the body greatly depends on the amount absorbed from the diet (Figure 11-9).

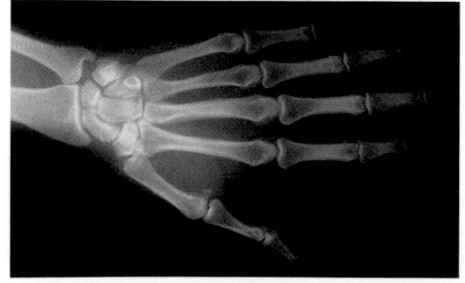

Ninety-nine percent of calcium in the body is in bones.

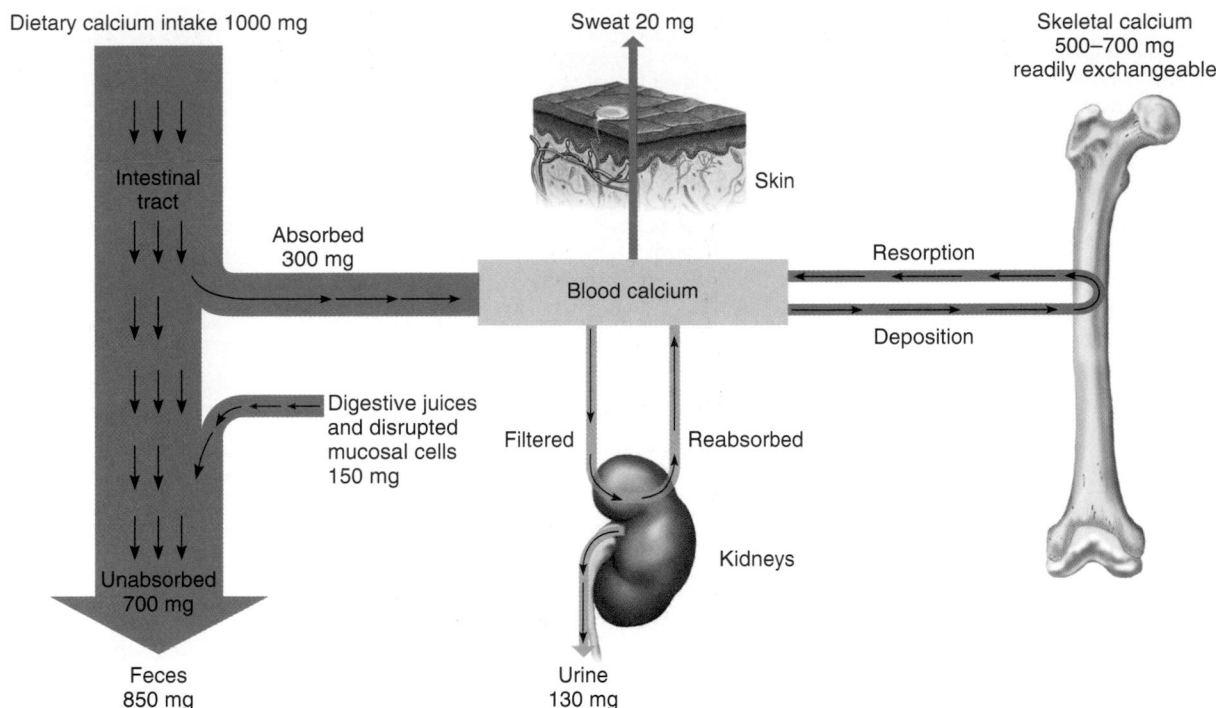

Figure 11-9 | Calcium balance in an adult. On an intake of 1000 mg, only about 300 mg are absorbed by the body, with the remaining 700 mg being excreted in the feces. To maintain calcium balance, 300 mg are excreted by a combination of the kidneys (130 mg), skin (20 mg), and secretions and cell loss into the feces (150 mg).

Absorption

Calcium absorption occurs primarily in the upper part of the small intestine because calcium requires a pH below 6 to stay in solution in an ionic state (Ca^{2+}). As the acidic stomach contents reach the small intestine, they are partially neutralized by bicarbonate released from the pancreas but are still slightly acidic, which provides a suitable environment for calcium absorption. In addition, calcium absorption within the upper small intestine depends on the active vitamin D hormone ($1,25\ (OH)_2$ vitamin D). Because the intestinal contents become more alkaline as they pass down the GI tract, calcium absorption decreases at the terminal end of the small intestine and colon, although some still occurs via passive diffusion.

Humans absorb about 25% of the calcium in the foods eaten.[5] However, when the body needs extra calcium—such as during infancy and pregnancy—absorption might reach as high as 60%. Young people tend to absorb calcium better than do older people, especially those older than 70. Postmenopausal women generally absorb the least calcium.

Other factors that enhance absorption of calcium include parathyroid hormone; dietary glucose and lactose; and normal intestinal motility (flow).

Factors limiting calcium absorption include large amounts of phytic acid in fiber; excessive amounts of dietary phosphorus; polyphenols (tannins) in tea; a vitamin D deficiency; and diarrhea.[5]

Transport, Storage, and Excretion

Each cell has a crucial need for calcium, which is supplied from the bloodstream. This need is probably the reason humans have such excellent hormonal systems to control calcium homeostasis in the body (Figure 11-10). Normal blood calcium can be maintained despite an inadequate calcium intake, because much is stored in bones.[28] (The bones, however, pay the price.) This situation makes blood calcium a poor measure of calcium status.

The tooth consists of a hard, yellowish tissue called dentin, which is covered with enamel in the crown and cementum in the root. When dentin and cementum are damaged, they can repair themselves. Damaged enamel cannot be naturally repaired because enamel is a secretion produced before the tooth erupts, and it does not have a blood supply like the other two tissues. To repair broken or damaged enamel requires the skills of a dentist. In contrast, bone is well supplied with blood vessels, so a fracture can be repaired (healed) by the body given time.

Figure 11-10 | Regulation of blood parathyroid hormone (PTH) and calcitonin are key factors in controlling blood calcium. When blood calcium rises too high (1), the thyroid gland releases calcitonin (2). This hormone restores blood calcium to the normal range (2–5). When blood calcium falls too low (6), the parathyroid gland releases parathyroid hormone (7). This hormone restores blood calcium to the normal range (7–11). On a day-to-day basis, parathyroid hormone is the most important regulator. Recall from Figure 9-9 that the actions of parathyroid hormone also involve the active vitamin D hormone (1,25 (OH)$_2$ vitamin D) in various ways.

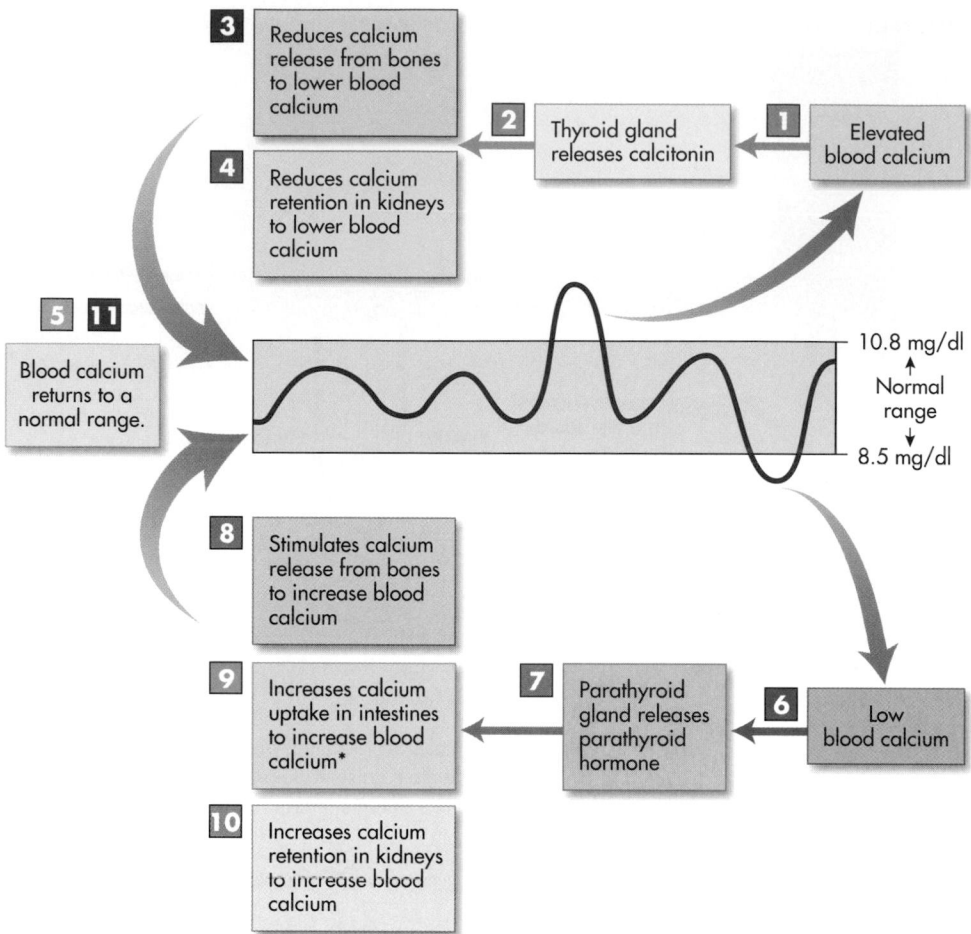

* Indirectly by increasing 1,25 (OH)$_2$ vitamin D synthesis by the kidneys

As discussed in Chapter 9, when blood calcium falls, the parathyroid gland releases parathyroid hormone. This hormone, working with 1,25 (OH)$_2$ vitamin D, increases the kidneys' retrieval of calcium before it is excreted in the urine. Parathyroid hormone also helps increase calcium absorption indirectly by increasing the synthesis of 1,25 (OH)$_2$ vitamin D. In addition, parathyroid hormone, often working in conjunction with 1,25 (OH)$_2$ vitamin D, causes increased calcium release from bones. In all these ways, then, parathyroid hormone increases blood calcium.

When blood calcium is too high, the release of parathyroid hormone falls. Then calcium loss from the kidneys increases. Synthesis of 1,25 (OH)$_2$ vitamin D also decreases; thus, calcium absorption decreases. In addition, the thyroid gland secretes the hormone calcitonin, which decreases calcium loss from bones. All these metabolic changes cause blood calcium to remain within the normal range.[28]

Other routes for calcium excretion are the skin, as well as the feces losses that result from intestinal secretions into the intestinal lumen.[5]

Functions of Calcium

Forming and maintaining bones are calcium's major roles in the body.

Bone Development and Maintenance

Despite its "dead" appearance, bone is very active metabolically. Bone contains two types of cells—**osteoblasts** and **osteoclasts**—which are integral to maintaining bones.[9] Osteoblasts secrete a collagen protein matrix that forms the support structure of bone.

osteoblasts Cells in bone that secrete mineral and bone matrix.

osteoclasts Bone cells that arise originally from a type of white blood cell. Osteoclasts secrete substances that lead to bone erosion. This erosion can set the stage for subsequent bone mineralization.

They mature to osteocytes and then secrete bone mineral, which causes bone mineralization. This mineral matures and eventually approaches the composition of $Ca_{10}(PO_4)_6OH_2$, called hydroxyapatite.[5] In contrast, osteoclasts continually break down bone in areas where bone is not needed. Osteoclast activity is stimulated by parathyroid hormone, often in conjunction with $1,25\ (OH)_2$ vitamin D. These bone cells are very active when a diet is deficient in calcium; their action releases calcium from the bone so it can enter the blood. Remember, a supply of calcium is vital to all cells, not just to bone cells.

Bone turnover (**bone remodeling**) represents a cycle of bone breakdown by osteoclasts, followed by bone rebuilding by osteoblasts. In this way, bone is re-formed when necessary to respond to the physical demands placed on it. Before new bone can be built, the old bone in that area must be partially broken down.[9]

During human growth, total osteoblast activity exceeds osteoclast activity, so we make more bone than we break down, with more bone being built in areas put under high stress. A right-handed tennis player, for example, builds more bone in that arm than in the left arm. In older years, osteoclast activity generally becomes more dominant. Most bone is built from infancy through the late adolescent years. Small increases in **bone mass** continue between 20 and 30 years of age. Genes control up to 80% of the variation in the peak bone mass ultimately built.[9]

Bone loss begins in mid-adulthood and increases significantly at menopause in women. By age 65 to 70, the rate of bone loss falls to about the same rate as before menopause. In men, bone loss is slow and steady from around age 30. Overall, this bone loss in both genders progresses without signs or symptoms. During their lifetimes, about one-third to one-half of all women go on to experience fractures associated with low bone mass, especially women who live beyond age 75.[3] In addition, some women have much more bone than others. They probably built more bone when they were young, so they are able to endure greater bone loss without experiencing fractures. In sum, many factors are associated with such a higher bone mass (Table 11-6).

Even more factors, however, are associated with low bone mass: slim figure; family history of hip fracture or osteoporosis; reduced vitamin D receptor activity in the intestine; irregular menstruation; premature menopause; use of certain medications (such as corticosteroids); excess dietary protein and caffeine (which increase calcium loss in the urine) if sufficient calcium is not consumed; and prolonged bed rest.[3]

Visual observation of the cross sections of a bone reveals two primary bone structural types in the body: **cortical** (also called compact) bone and **trabecular** (also called cancellous or spongy) bone.[9] These two bone types in turn interact within each bone to form quite an engineering marvel of strength (Figure 11-11). The entire outer surface of all bones is composed of cortical bone, which is very dense. The shafts of long bones, such as those of the arm, are almost entirely cortical bone. Trabecular bone is found in the ends of the long bones, inside the spinal vertebrae, and inside the flat bones of the pelvis. Trabecular bone forms an internal scaffolding network for a bone. It supports the outer cortical shell of the bone, especially in heavily stressed areas such as joints.

Bone strength especially depends on a person's bone mineral density (bone mass/bone width). The more densely packed the calcium-rich bone crystals are, the stronger the bone structures. Another important element of bone strength is the trabecular bone support network inside a bone.[9]

Blood Clotting

Calcium ions participate in several reactions in the cascade that leads to the formation of fibrin, the main protein component of a blood clot (review Figure 9-13 in Chapter 9).

Transmission of Nerve Impulses to Target Cells

When a nerve impulse reaches its target site—such as a muscle, other nerve cells, or a gland—the impulse is transmitted across the junction between the nerve and its target cells, called a **synapse**.[28] In many nerves, the arrival of the impulse at the target

---

bone remodeling A process by which bone is first resorbed by osteoclasts and then re-formed by osteoblasts. This process allows the body to form bone where needed, such as in areas of high mechanical stress.

bone mass The total mineral substance (such as calcium or phosphorus) in a cross section of bone, generally expressed as grams per centimeter of length.

cortical bone Dense, compact bone that constitutes the outer surface and shafts of bone; also called compact bone. Cortical bone makes up 75 to 80% of total bone mass.

trabecular bone The spongy, inner matrix of bone found primarily in the spine, pelvis, and ends of bones; also called cancellous bone. Trabecular bone makes up 20 to 25% of total bone mass.

synapse The space between the end of one nerve cell and the beginning of another nerve cell.

Table 11-6 | Diet and Lifestyle Factors Associated with Bone Status[3,10,17,19,25]

Positive Diet and Lifestyle Factors	Call to Action
Adequate diet containing a sufficient amount of protein, calcium, phosphorus, magnesium, potassium, vitamin A, vitamin B-6, folate, vitamin B-12, vitamin C, vitamin D, vitamin K, zinc, copper, fluoride, and manganese (and boron?)*	• Follow MyPyramid with special emphasis on adequate amounts of fruits, vegetables, and low-fat and fat-free milk products. • Consider use of fortified foods (or supplements) to make up for specific nutrient shortfalls, such as vitamin D, folate, and calcium.
Healthy body weight	• Be aware that low body weight (slender figure) increases the risk for low bone mass.
Normal menses	• During childbearing years, seek medical advice if menses cease (such as in cases of anorexia nervosa or extreme athletic training). • Women at menopause and beyond should consider use of current medical therapies to reduce bone loss linked to the fall in estrogen output.
Weight-bearing physical activity	• Perform weight-bearing activity because it contributes to bone maintenance, whereas bed rest and a sedentary lifestyle lead to bone loss. Strength training is especially helpful to bone maintenance.
Genetic background (family history and Black race)	• The ability to absorb calcium and regulate bone metabolism are influenced by one's genetic background.
Negative Diet and Lifestyle Factors	**Call to Action**
Excessive intake of protein, phosphorus, sodium, caffeine, wheat bran, and alcohol	• Moderate intake of these dietary constituents is recommended. Problems primarily arise if adequate calcium is not consumed. • Excessive soft drink consumption is especially discouraged.
Smoking	• Because smoking lowers estrogen output in women, smoking cessation is advised.
Use of certain medications, such as **corticosteroids**	• Corticosteroid medications lead to bone loss, so medical therapy to counteract the bone loss should be instituted if use is long term.
Celiac disease	• Malabsorption of nutrients due to this intestinal disease leads to poor bone maintenance.

*Vitamin B-6, folate, and vitamin B-12 are listed because elevated blood homocysteine is a risk factor for low bone density.

corticosteroid A steroid hormone produced by the adrenal gland, an example of which is cortisol.

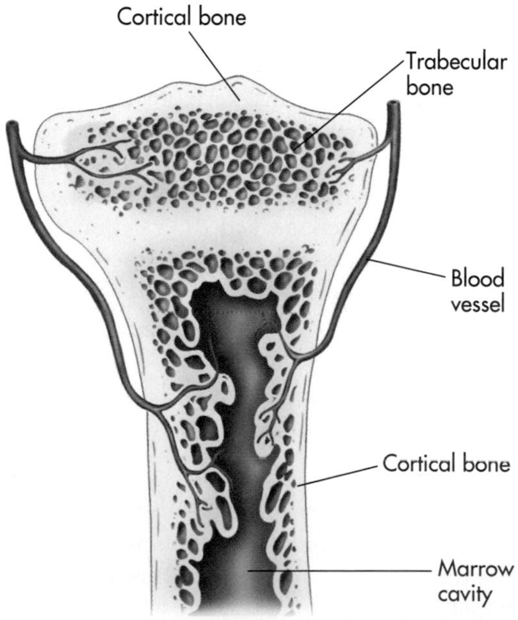

Figure 11-11 | Cortical and trabecular bone. Cortical bone forms the shafts of bones and the outer mineral covering. Trabecular bone supports the outer shell of cortical bone in various bones of the body, as in the bone pictured.

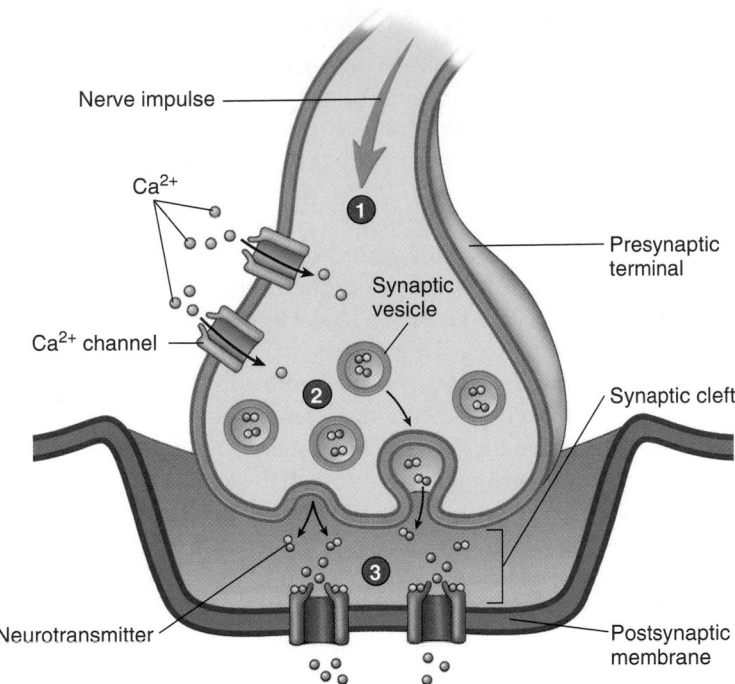

Nerve impulse

Ca²⁺

Ca²⁺ channel

Presynaptic terminal

Synaptic vesicle

Synaptic cleft

Neurotransmitter

Postsynaptic membrane

Figure 11-12 | The release of a neurotransmitter. Nerve impulses, by opening Ca²⁺ channels (1), stimulate the fusion of synaptic vesicles containing neurotransmitters with the cell membrane of the nerve terminals (2). This leads to exocytosis and the release of a neurotransmitter (3). The neurotransmitters will bind to and stimulate the postsynaptic membrane of nearby cells.

site stimulates an influx of calcium ions into the nerve from the extracellular medium. The rise in intracellular calcium ions then triggers the release of neurotransmitters from synaptic vesicles, which are responsible for storing the neurotransmitter until needed. The released neurotransmitter then carries the impulse across the synapse to the target cells (Figure 11-12).

In an entirely different process, nerve impulses develop spontaneously if insufficient calcium is available, leading to what is called hypocalcemic **tetany.** This condition is characterized by muscle spasms, because the muscles receive continual nerve stimulation. Inadequate parathyroid hormone release or action is the typical cause of **hypocalcemia.**[28]

tetany A body condition marked by sharp contraction of muscles and failure to relax afterward; usually caused by abnormal calcium metabolism.

hypocalcemia Low blood calcium, typically arising from inadequate parathyroid hormone release or action.

Muscle Contraction

The critical role of calcium in muscle contraction is most easily understood in the context of skeletal muscles, but other types of muscles use calcium in a similar fashion. When a skeletal muscle is stimulated by a nerve impulse from the brain, calcium ions are released from intracellular stores within the muscle cells. The resulting increase in the concentration of calcium ions in a muscle cell is one factor, along with ATP, that permits the contractile proteins to slide along each other.[28] This movement leads to muscle contraction. Then, to allow for subsequent relaxation, the calcium ions are returned to intracellular stores, and the contractile proteins slide apart (see Figure C-4 in Appendix C).

Cell Metabolism

Calcium ions help regulate metabolism in the cell by participating in the **calmodulin** system. When calcium enters a cell (often because of hormone action) and binds to the protein calmodulin, the resulting protein-calcium complex can regulate the activity of various enzymes, including one that breaks down glycogen to many units of glucose 1-phosphate (Figure 11-13).[28]

calmodulin A cell protein that binds calcium ions. The resulting calmodulin—Ca²⁺ complex influences the activity of some enzymes in the cell.

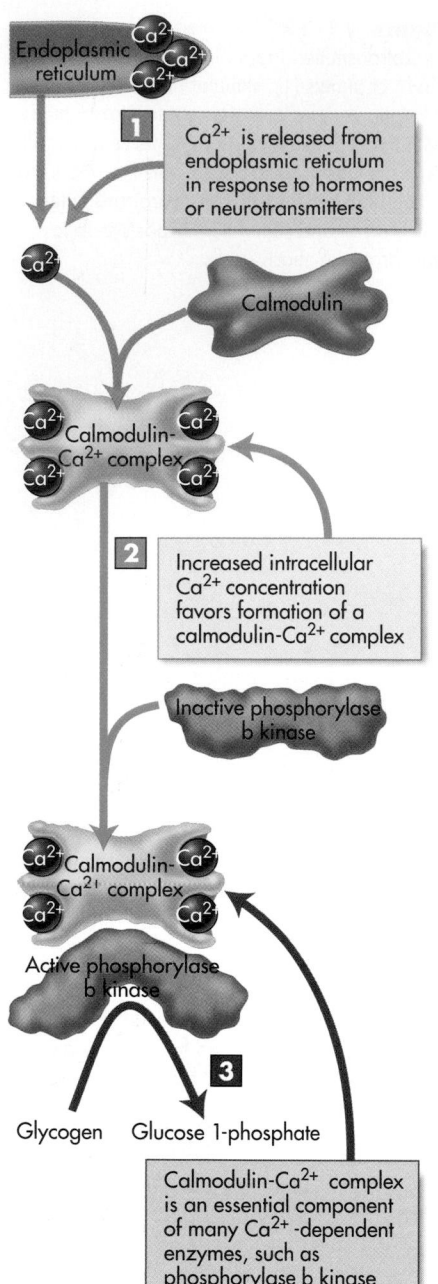

1. Ca²⁺ is released from endoplasmic reticulum in response to hormones or neurotransmitters

Endoplasmic reticulum

Calmodulin

Calmodulin-Ca²⁺ complex

2. Increased intracellular Ca²⁺ concentration favors formation of a calmodulin-Ca²⁺ complex

Inactive phosphorylase b kinase

Calmodulin-Ca²⁺ complex

Active phosphorylase b kinase

3. Calmodulin-Ca²⁺ complex is an essential component of many Ca²⁺-dependent enzymes, such as phosphorylase b kinase

Glycogen   Glucose 1-phosphate

Figure 11-13 | Calmodulin mediates many of the effects of intracellular calcium—in this case (1–3), the regulation of the breakdown of glycogen to many units of glucose 1-phosphate. Note that a kinase is an enzyme that adds a phosphorus group to another molecule.

Some calcium supplements are poorly digested because they do not readily dissolve. To test for solubility, put a supplement in 6 oz of cider vinegar. Stir every 5 minutes. It should dissolve within 30 minutes.

Other Possible Health Benefits of Calcium

Researchers have been examining links between calcium intake and risks for a wide array of diseases. An adequate calcium intake can reduce the risk of colon cancer, especially in people who consume a high-fat diet. A decreased risk of some forms of kidney stones and reduced lead absorption are other possible benefits when calcium is part of a meal. Calcium intakes of 800 to 1200 mg/day may also decrease blood pressure, compared with intakes of 400 mg/day or less. As covered in Chapter 6, calcium intakes of 1200 mg/day in combination with a low-fat, low-cholesterol diet can help people with elevated LDL improve their blood lipid profiles.

A link between a low calcium intake and overweight/obesity is also under study. Although the true benefit in this regard is not clear, an adequate calcium intake (compared to a very low intake [e.g., 400 mg/day]), coupled with a low energy intake, may promote even more weight loss than the low energy diet alone. Focusing on dairy sources of calcium is recommended because other components of dairy foods, such as some of the specific dairy proteins present, contribute to this potential weight-loss benefit.

For women, an adequate calcium intake might also reduce the risk of premenstrual syndrome and high blood pressure that can develop during pregnancy. Overall, the benefits of a diet providing adequate calcium extend beyond bone health.[5]

Calcium in Foods

Dairy products, such as milk and cheese, provide about 70% of the calcium in North American diets. The exception is cottage cheese, because most calcium is lost during production. White bread, rolls, crackers, and other foods made with milk products are secondary contributors. Leafy greens (such as spinach), broccoli, sardines, and canned salmon are also sources. However, much of the calcium in some leafy green vegetables, notably spinach, is not absorbed because of the presence of oxalic acid. This effect is not as significant, however, in kale, collard, turnip, and mustard greens. The calcium-fortified versions of orange juice, cranberry juice, and other beverages as well as calcium-fortified cottage cheese, yogurt, breakfast cereals, breakfast bars, bread, chocolate candies, and snacks also provide much calcium. Another source of calcium is soybean curd (tofu), if it is made with calcium carbonate (check the label). Note that it is the bones present in canned fish, such as salmon and sardines, that supply the calcium. Information about calcium is mandatory on food labels.

Calcium Supplements

Calcium supplements can be used by people who do not like milk or who cannot incorporate enough calcium-containing foods into their diets. Calcium carbonate, the form found in calcium-based antacid tablets, is the most common supplement used. People should take this supplement with or just after meals in doses of about 500 mg so that stomach acid produced during digestion can aid with absorption of this mineral. On the other hand, a supplement containing calcium citrate, which is acidic itself, can be taken between or with meals, or at bedtime.[28]

Here is how to determine the calcium content of typical supplements based on the percent of calcium per unit of weight and form of calcium, as listed on the supplement label.

- Calcium carbonate: 40%
- Calcium phosphate (tribasic): 38%
- Calcium citrate: 21%
- Calcium lactate: 13%
- Calcium gluconate: 9%

To calculate the amount of calcium in a supplement, simply multiply the weight of the capsule by the percentage just listed. For example, if one tablet of calcium citrate weighs 500 mg, it contains 105 mg of calcium.

$$500 \text{ mg} \times 0.21 = 105 \text{ mg}$$

With calcium supplements, interactions with other minerals are a valid concern. Perhaps most importantly, there is some evidence that calcium supplements may decrease zinc absorption. Therefore, calcium supplements should not be taken with meals rich in zinc. An effect of calcium supplementation on iron and magnesium absorption is possible; however, this effect appears to be small over the long term. To be safe, people using a calcium supplement on a regular basis should notify their physician of the practice.

Some calcium supplements contain lead. Chapter 19 points out that lead produces an array of deleterious effects on the body. Currently, FDA has no standards for lead content in food supplements. It is especially important to avoid supplements made from bonemeal, the worst offender when it comes to lead. Tablet or liquid calcium supplements with the USP seal of approval are less likely than others to contain high concentrations of contaminants. Typically, taking 1000 mg of calcium daily in divided doses of 500 mg each in the form of calcium carbonate or calcium citrate is safe.

Calcium Needs

The Adequate Intake set for calcium for adults ranges from 1000 to 1200 mg/day. For adolescents between the ages of 9 and 18, the Adequate Intake is set higher, at 1300 mg. The Adequate Intake for adults is based on the amount of calcium needed each day to offset calcium losses in urine, feces, and other routes.[5] The Adequate Intake for young people includes an additional amount to allow for increases in bone mass during growth and development. The Daily Value for calcium used on food and supplement labels is 1000 mg.

In North America, average calcium intakes range from approximately 600 to 800 mg/day for women and 800 to 1000 mg/day for men. About 25% of women consume only about 300 mg/day. Thus, dietary intakes of calcium by many women, especially young women, are well below the Adequate Intake amount, whereas intakes by most men are roughly equivalent to it. It is important for vegans to focus on eating good plant sources of calcium as well as on the total amount of calcium ingested.

Calcium-Deficiency Diseases

The most common calcium-related deficiency disease is osteoporosis, but calcium is not the only nutrient needed to maintain bone health (review Table 11-6).[10] To prevent low blood calcium, the body withdraws calcium from bone. This action preserves indispensable functions of calcium, such as those that keep the heart and muscles working. There is also some evidence that a low calcium intake may increase blood pressure and the risk of certain cancers, such as colon cancer, by affecting cell turnover. Some recent research is indicating that low calcium intake is also associated with low bone mass development in growing children.[3]

Although it is assumed that calcium intake is a factor in most cases of bone loss, the exact contribution of calcium intake versus other factors is hard to quantify. Bone loss is not due to a calcium deficiency in the same way that scurvy is due to a vitamin C deficiency. In the latter case, low vitamin C intake is typically the only factor, whereas multiple factors likely contribute to most cases of bone loss. It is difficult to pinpoint the extent to which various factors contribute to bone health, because bone-related disease can take decades to develop. Studies have to look back at what happened over a long period of time or look forward to what could happen.

Failure to maintain adequate bone mass in the body throughout life first leads to a state of **osteopenia.** Osteopenia can be caused by the vitamin D deficiency disease osteomalacia, the use of certain medications, cancer, and other conditions. The diagnosis of osteoporosis generally is made when the bone loss becomes marked and/or a fracture occurs and there is no obvious medically related cause (Figure 11-14).[3] Typically both cortical and trabecular portions of the bone are affected, particularly the trabecular portion. People who develop more bone by early adulthood can sustain

Food Sources of Calcium

Food Item and Amount	Calcium (mg)
Plain yogurt, 1 cup	450
Parmesan cheese, 1 oz	390
Fortified orange juice, 1 cup	350
Romano cheese, 1 oz	300
1% milk, 1 cup	300
Buttermilk, 1 cup	285
Swiss cheese, 1 oz	275
Spinach, 1 cup	250
Salmon (with bones), 3 oz	210
Cheddar cheese, 1 oz	200
Total Raisin Bran cereal, 3/4 cup	180
Sardines (with bones), 2 oz	170
Chocolate pudding, 1/2 cup	160
Tofu, 1/2 cup	140
Adequate Intake for adults, 1000 mg;	
Adequate Intake for adults over 50, 1200 mg	

Critical | Thinking

Manuela is a vegan. She stopped eating meat and dairy products when she was 12 years old and is now in her mid-twenties. She wants to start a family but is concerned about whether she can obtain enough calcium from her diet to ensure her baby's health. How can she consume enough calcium to meet her own and her baby's needs?

osteopenia Decreased bone mass caused by cancer, hyperthyroidism, or other reasons.

To estimate your calcium intake, use the rule of 300s. Give yourself 300 mg for calcium provided by a typical diet of moderate energy intake. Add to that another 300 mg for every 8 oz of milk or yogurt or 1.5 ounces of cheese you consume. If you eat a lot of tofu, almonds, or sardines or drink calcium-fortified beverages, use the second Take Action or food composition tables to obtain a more accurate estimate of your calcium intake.

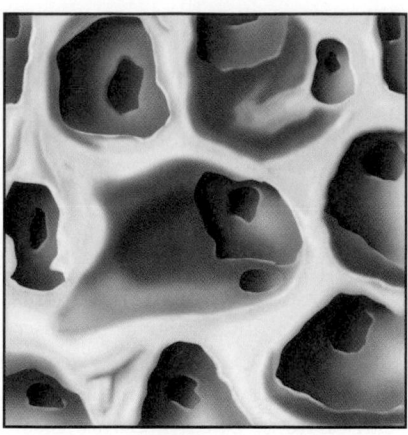
Normal trabecular bone

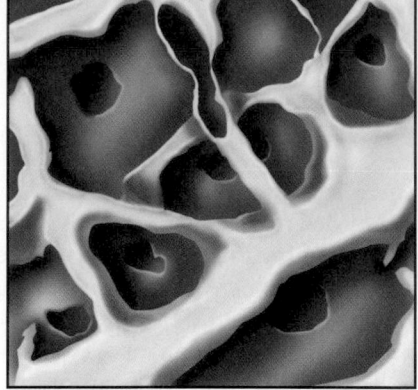
Osteoporotic trabecular bone

Figure 11-14 | Normal and osteoporotic trabecular bone. Note in the picture on the right how there is much less trabecular bone. It is especially critical for the horizontal trabeculae to extend continuously—without breaks—between the areas of vertical trabeculae. Any break in either the horizontal or more vertical trabecular beams weakens the support system of a bone and increases the risk for bone fracture. And, once these beams are broken, there is currently no way to rebuild them. This is why it is so important to limit bone loss as people age.

greater age-related bone loss with less fracture risk than those who have built less bone. Thus, osteoporosis is considered to be a pediatric disease with geriatric consequences (Figure 11-15).

Osteoporosis currently leads to approximately 2 million fractures per year, resulting in over $16 billion in direct health-care costs.[16] Many older women in North America show low values for bone mass and are therefore at risk for these fractures.

Diagnosis of Osteoporosis

Dual energy X-ray absorptiometry (DEXA) bone scan Method to measure bone density that uses small amounts of X-ray radiation. The ability of a bone to block the path of the radiation is used as a measure of bone density at that bone site.

A simple and very accurate test to identify osteoporosis is **dual energy X-ray absorptiometry (DEXA) bone scan**.[22] A DEXA scan measures bone mass and bone density in the spine, hip, and total body using a small amount of X-ray radiation. For this test, a person lies down on his or her back on a padded table while a movable imaging arm glides over the length of the body (see Figure 13-12 in Chapter 13). The procedure usually takes about 10 to 20 minutes. The ability of a bone to block the path of radiation is used as a measure of bone mass and bone density at that bone site. A very low dose of radiation is used for the DEXA—about one-tenth of the exposure from a chest X-ray.

From the DEXA measurement of bone density, a statistical analysis called a T score is generated, which compares the observed bone density to that of a person at peak bone density. T scores may be interpreted as follows:

0 to −1	Normal
−1 to −2.4	Osteopenia
−2.5 or lower	Osteoporosis

Peripheral DEXA and ultrasound are additional ways to measure the bone density of one part of the body, such as the wrist or heel. Even though peripheral methods are faster than DEXA, they are not as accurate because the density of one part of the body may not reflect the density of other areas susceptible to fractures, such as the spine.

Osteoporosis Prevention and Treatment

As women mature, different strategies for preventing osteoporosis are needed, based on the risk factors present.[3,23] Young women should meet calcium, vitamin D, and other nutrient needs and should see a physician with any sign of irregular menstrua-

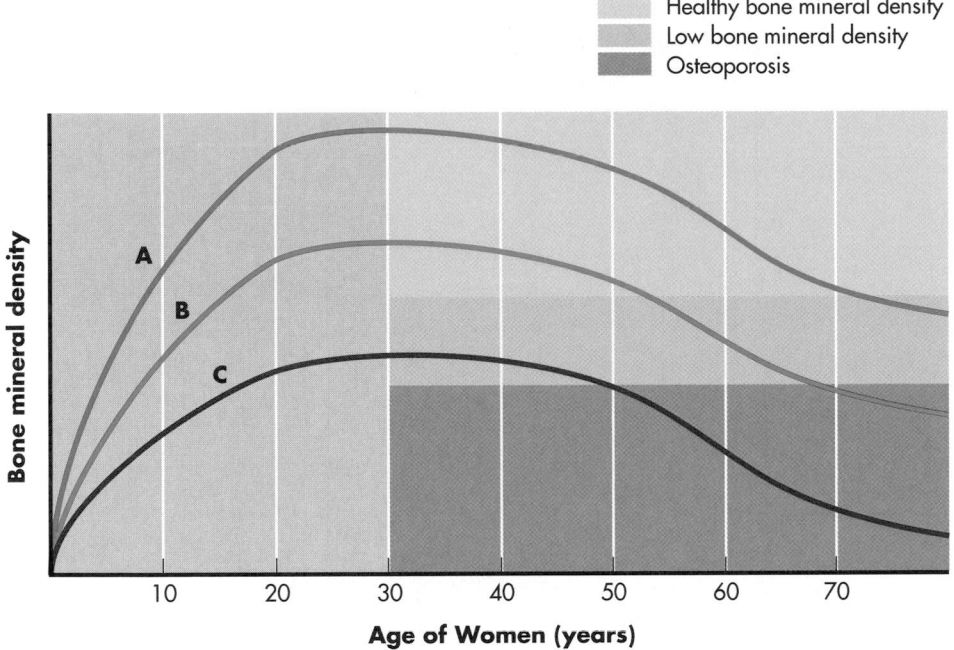

Figure 11-15 legend:
- Healthy bone mineral density
- Low bone mineral density
- Osteoporosis

Bone mineral density (y-axis)

A
B
C

Age of Women (years)
10   20   30   40   50   60   70

Figure 11-15 | The relationship between peak bone mass and the ultimate risk of developing osteoporosis and related bone fractures. Woman A developed a high peak bone mass by age 30. Her bone loss was slow and steady between ages 30 and 50 and sped up somewhat after age 50 because of the effects of menopause. Still, by age 75 the woman had a healthy bone mineral density value and did not show evidence of osteoporosis. Woman B developed an average peak bone mass and experienced the same rate of bone loss as woman A. By age 65, woman B had low bone mineral density and evidence of osteoporosis. She was now at risk of related fractures. Woman C achieved a low peak bone mass, and by following the typical pattern for bone loss, she already showed evidence of low bone mineral density and osteoporosis at age 50. Given the low calcium intakes that are common among young women today, line C is a sobering reality. Ideally, by following a diet and lifestyle pattern that contributes to maximal bone mineral density, more women will follow line A and in turn significantly reduce their risk of developing osteoporosis.

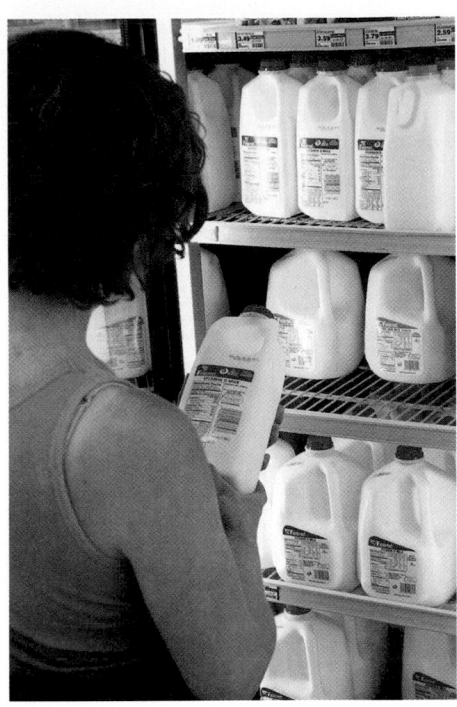

Milk is a rich as well as convenient source of calcium.

tion. In young women, regular menstruation is a main contributor to bone maintenance, as evidenced by low bone mass in some nonmenstruating female athletes and other women with irregular menstruation (e.g., those with anorexia nervosa). An active lifestyle that includes weight-bearing physical activity is also important (to build and maintain muscle mass).[12] Greater muscle mass linked to physical activity is associated with greater bone mass, because muscle keeps tension on bone.[3] Still, physical activity cannot prevent the bone loss associated with irregular menstruation. Thus, female athletes with irregular menstruation should be closely monitored by a physician.

Smoking and excessive alcohol intake decrease bone mass at any age. Smoking lowers the estrogen concentration in the blood in women, increasing bone loss. Alcohol is toxic to bone cells, and alcoholism is probably a major undiagnosed and unrecognized cause of osteoporosis. Moderation in phosphorus, caffeine, sodium, and protein intake is also advised. Excessive intakes are especially problematic when insufficient calcium is consumed.[3]

At menopause, women should discuss approved osteoporosis-related therapies with a physician. They also need to accurately track their height. A decrease of more than 1 1/2 inches from premenopausal values is a sign that significant bone loss is taking place (Figure 11-16). Currently, five medical therapies can be used to slow bone loss at menopause in women. Some can even be used in men who develop low bone mass. The approved drugs are estrogen (various forms are available); **bisphosphonates** (alendronate [Fosamax], risedronate [Actonel], and ibandronate [Boniva]); selective estrogen receptor modulators (SERMs) (raloxifene [Evista]); calcitonin (nasal form is

bisphosphonates Compounds primarily composed of carbon and phosphorus that bind to bone mineral and in turn reduce bone breakdown.

Figure 11-16 | A loss of height and a distorted body shape are common signs of osteoporosis. Monitor your adult height changes to detect early osteoporosis. All women 65 years and older should be screened for this disease. Medicare covers the cost of the needed DEXA scan. Younger women are advised to have the same test at menopause if they have associated risk factors or if the results of the screening would help them decide what treatment plan is appropriate at menopause.

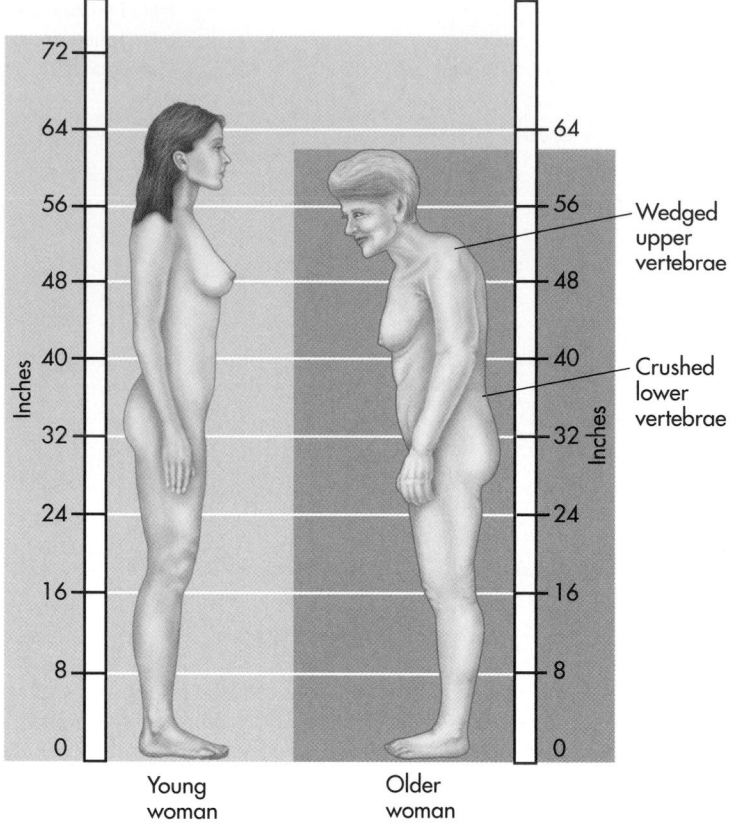

Young woman

Older woman

Wedged upper vertebrae

Crushed lower vertebrae

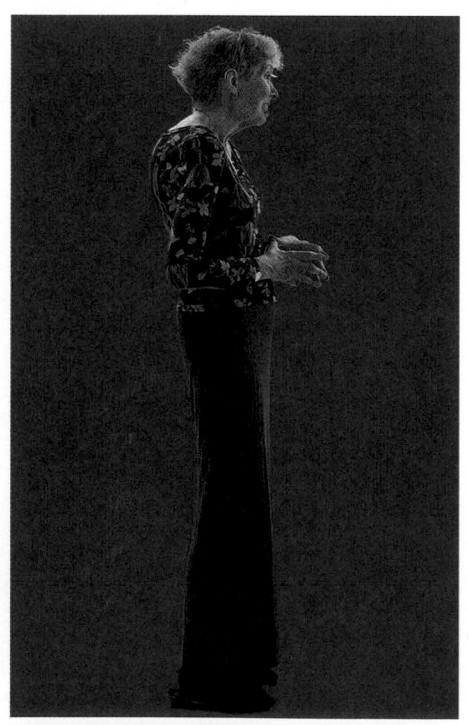

Women with osteoporosis typically develop abnormal curvature of the upper spine. This results from fractures of the weakened vertebrae. Osteoporosis can lead to both physical and emotional pain.

Miacalcin); and a form of parathyroid hormone called teriparatide (Forteo). Estrogen and SERMs blunt bone turnover by binding to receptors on bone; bisphosphonates blunt bone resorption by binding to bone mineral; calcitonin inhibits osteoclast activity and, so, bone resorption; and teriparatide stimulates new bone growth.[3,23]

All these medications have side effects, so use needs to be tailored to a person's current health status. The latest thinking is that estrogen replacement is most useful for treating menopausal symptoms such as hot flashes, whereas the bisphosphonates are most useful for preventing bone loss.[3,23,26] The recent trend to use bisphosphonates as the major form of medical therapy for osteoporosis rather than estrogen replacement stems from the observation that greater than 5 years of estrogen use increases the risk for breast and some other forms of cancer, such as in the ovaries. If a woman at menopause begins estrogen therapy to relieve related menopausal symptoms, experts suggest she should consider switching to another form of osteoporosis therapy as soon as possible.[27]

Older men and women need to stay physically active—including doing some weight-bearing and resistance activities—and they should at least meet the Adequate Intakes for calcium and vitamin D set for their particular age. This combination of physical activity and calcium and vitamin D intakes is most likely to limit bone loss in some areas of the body, such as the hip.[12,28] Still, this form of therapy does not replace the need for medical therapy in high-risk individuals. Older people also need to minimize the risk for falls, especially by limiting their use of medications and alcohol, which might disturb coordination, and they should take corrective measures if visual function is impaired. (Hip protective garments are also available to reduce hip fracture risk.)

Upper Level for Calcium

The Upper Level for calcium is 2500 mg/day, based on the risk of developing kidney stones.[5] Normally, the small intestine prevents excess calcium from being absorbed. However, if this level of control breaks down, the calcium concentration in the blood may rise and lead to calcification of the kidneys and other organs, irritability, headache, kidney failure, kidney stones in some people, and decreased absorption of other minerals. Ordinarily, calcium in food and usual doses of calcium supplements do not pose a health threat because it is present in relatively modest amounts.

Case Scenario | Follow-Up

Jana is increasing her chances of developing osteoporosis later in life because of her current high-risk lifestyle. Factors contributing to her potential risk include a poor dietary intake of calcium. Jana needs to find some reliable sources of calcium. These could include calcium-fortified juices, calcium-fortified bread and snack bars, and calcium-fortified chewable chocolate candies. Tofu (made with calcium) is another potential source, as is calcium-fortified soy milk. Meeting the Adequate Intake of 1000 mg/day for her age would not be that hard if she were to make a conscious effort to use these calcium-rich foods and/or incorporate other rich sources (which include calcium supplements). She also should rethink her rationale for avoiding milk. Fat-free milk is very low in energy content and provides much calcium. Dairy products such as milk do not lead to weight gain per se.

Concept | Check

About 99% of calcium in the body is found in the bones. Calcium requires a slightly acid pH and the vitamin D hormone for efficient absorption. Factors that reduce calcium absorption include large amounts of fiber, decreased estrogen production, and a great excess of phosphorus in the diet. Blood calcium is regulated primarily by hormones and does not closely reflect daily intake. Aside from its critical role in bone, calcium also functions in blood clotting, muscle contraction, nerve-impulse transmission, and cell metabolism. A person can decrease risk for osteoporosis by consuming adequate calcium and vitamin D; engaging in weight-bearing exercise; considering bisphosphonates or other medications that decrease bone loss (postmenopausal female); and moderating sodium, alcohol, and caffeine intake. Dairy products are rich food sources of calcium. Certain calcium-fortified foods, such as some beverages, are rich sources as well. Supplemental forms, such as calcium carbonate, are well absorbed by most people. Megadose supplementation can result in the development of kidney stones and other health problems among some people.

Phosphorus (P)

Efficient absorption plus the wide availability in food makes phosphorus a much less important major mineral than calcium in diet planning.

Absorption, Transport, Storage, and Excretion of Phosphorus

The body absorbs phosphorus quite efficiently, up to about 70% of dietary intake in adults, by passive diffusion in the GI tract. The active vitamin D hormone $1,25\,(OH)_2$ vitamin D also enhances phosphorus absorption. As pointed out in the next section, much phosphorus is stored in bones. Excretion of phosphorus is achieved by the kidneys. The degree of excretion is the primary mechanism by which blood phosphorus is regulated.[14] This mechanism differs from that of calcium, in which changes in absorption are a more significant factor.

Functions of Phosphorus

Approximately 80% is found in bones and teeth as calcium phosphate. The remainder of phosphate is found in every cell in the body and in the extracellular fluid as PO_4^{2-}. Phosphorus is a component of many enzyme systems, adenosine triphosphate (ATP),

To find out more about osteoporosis, check out the website of the National Osteoporosis Foundation (www.nof.org) or call 800-464-6700. Another helpful website is that of the National Dairy Council (www.nationaldairycouncil.org).

No form of natural calcium, such as coral calcium, is superior to typical supplement forms. People making such claims of superiority have even been prosecuted by the U.S. Federal Trade Commission for false advertising.

People who have experienced extreme weight loss and long-standing poor nutrient intake are at risk of low blood phosphorus and a related condition called refeeding syndrome. If these individuals are aggressively refed, such as in a hospital or in a famine relief setting (in the developing world), much of the small amount of phosphorus in the bloodstream will shift into cells in order to participate in essential metabolic pathways. This shift can cause blood phosphorus to be so low that respiratory failure and other critical health conditions may result. To avoid this problem, clinicians generally check blood phosphorus before feeding such a person to correct a phosphorus deficiency if present. Under such circumstances, people then are gradually refed and blood phosphorus is monitored to make sure it remains within a normal range.[14]

Food Sources of Phosphorus

Food Item and Amount	Phosphorus (mg)
Plain yogurt, 1 cup	350
Swiss cheese, 2 oz	345
Almonds, 1/2 cup	340
Sunflower seeds, 1 oz	330
1% milk, 1 cup	235
Cheddar cheese, 1.5 oz	220
Salmon, 3 oz	220
Sirloin steak, 3 oz	210
Raisin Bran cereal, 1 cup	215
Egg, 2 hard-boiled	200
Chicken breast, 3 oz	180
Roasted turkey, 3 oz	180
Pot roast, 3 oz	170
Lean ham, 3 oz	165
American cheese, 1 slice	155
RDA for adults, 700 mg	

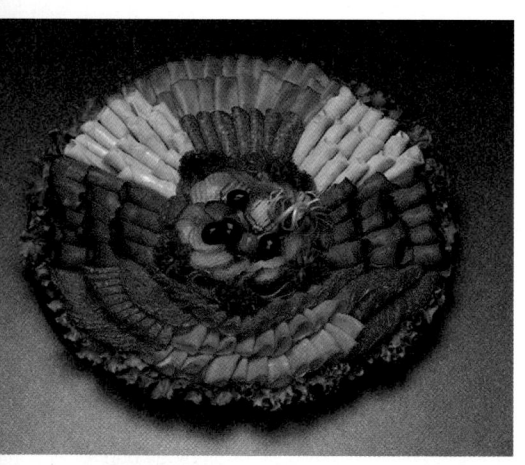

Meats are rich in phosphorus.

DNA and RNA, and the phospholipids in cell membranes. It also participates in acid-base balance.[21]

Phosphorus in Foods

Milk, cheese, yogurt, bakery products, and meat provide most of the phosphorus in the adult diet. Cereals, bran, eggs, nuts, and fish are also sources. About 20 to 30% of dietary phosphorus comes from food additives, especially in baked goods, cheeses, processed meats, and many soft drinks (about 75 mg per 12-oz [1/3 liter] serving of soft drinks).

Phosphorus Needs

The RDA is 700 mg/day. Phosphorus needs are based on the amount that maintains an adequate blood concentration.[5] Adults consume about 1000 to 1600 mg or more of phosphorus per day. Thus, a phosphorus deficiency is unlikely in healthy adults, especially because it is so efficiently absorbed. The Daily Value for phosphorus used on food and supplement labels is 1000 mg.

Phosphorus-Deficiency Diseases

A chronic deficiency of phosphorus can contribute to bone loss, decreased growth, and poor tooth development. Symptoms of rickets may occur in phosphorus-deficient children. Furthermore, symptoms of a deficiency include anorexia, weight loss, weakness, irritability, stiff joints, and bone pain. Marginal phosphorus status can be found in preterm infants, alcoholics, older people on nutrient-poor diets, people experiencing long-term bouts of diarrhea and weight loss, and people who daily use aluminum-containing antacids, which in the small intestine bind phosphorus.[14]

Upper Level for Phosphorus

The Upper Level for phosphorus in adulthood is 3 to 4 g/day, based on the risk of developing impaired kidney function.[5] High blood concentrations of phosphorus can cause calcium-phosphorus precipitates to form in body tissues as well as contribute to bone loss by inducing the release of parathyroid hormone (review Chapter 9).

A chronic imbalance in the calcium-to-phosphorus ratio in the diet, resulting from a high phosphorus intake coupled with a low calcium intake, can also contribute to bone loss.[3] This situation most likely arises when calcium needs are not met, as can occur when adolescents and adults regularly substitute soft drinks for milk or otherwise underconsume calcium.[28]

Magnesium (Mg)

Magnesium, like calcium, is a divalent cation. Because magnesium is found in chlorophyll, green leafy vegetables are rich sources.

Absorption, Transport, Storage, and Excretion of Magnesium

We normally absorb about 40 to 60% of the magnesium in our diets, but absorption efficiency can increase up to about 80% if intakes are low. Both passive and active absorption in the small intestine is used. The active vitamin D hormone 1,25 (OH)$_2$ vitamin D enhances magnesium absorption to a limited extent. Some magnesium is stored in bones; a small amount is stored in other tissues, such as muscles. The kidneys primarily regulate blood concentrations of magnesium and are able to reduce magnesium loss into the urine when blood magnesium is low.[24]

Functions of Magnesium

Magnesium has a vital role in a varying range of biochemical and physiological processes. More than 300 enzymes that utilize ATP require magnesium. Magnesium ions bind to ATP to form active ATP. One of the magnesium-dependent enzyme systems pumps sodium out of cells and potassium into cells. This process seems especially sensitive to magnesium deficiency. Magnesium also contributes to DNA and RNA synthesis. Its role in calcium metabolism contributes to bone structure. Magnesium is also important for nerve and heart function as well as insulin release from the pancreas and ultimate insulin action on cells. Other possible benefits of magnesium include decreasing blood pressure by dilation of arteries and preventing heart rhythm abnormalities.[24] Because of its ability to lower blood pressure, magnesium is used to treat hypertension that arises during pregnancy (see Chapter 16).

Magnesium in Foods

The richest sources of magnesium are plant products, such as whole grains, broccoli, squash, green leafy vegetables, beans, nuts, seeds, and chocolate. Animal products, such as milk and meats, supply some magnesium, although less than the foods just listed. Another source of magnesium is hard tap water, which contains a high mineral content (hard water also contains calcium). About 45% of dietary magnesium comes from vegetables, fruits, grains, and nuts, whereas about 30% comes from milk, meat, and eggs. Refined foods generally are low in magnesium.

Magnesium Needs

The RDA for magnesium is 400 mg/day for men 19 to 30 years of age and 310 mg/day for women 19 to 30 years of age. Magnesium needs increase slightly (an additional 10 mg/day) beyond this age for adult men and women. Magnesium needs are based on a daily intake that equals daily losses.[5] The Daily Value for magnesium used on food and supplement labels is 400 mg.

Adult men consume an average of 325 mg/day, whereas women consume closer to 225 mg/day. Women particularly should find some good food sources of magnesium that they like and eat them regularly.[7] Note that the form of magnesium in multivitamins and mineral supplements (magnesium oxide) is not well absorbed but can contribute to meeting magnesium needs.

Magnesium-Deficiency Diseases

Animals deficient in magnesium become very irritable and, with severe deficiency, eventually suffer convulsions and often die. In humans a magnesium deficiency causes an irregular heartbeat, sometimes accompanied by weakness, muscle spasms, disorientation, nausea and vomiting, and seizures. These symptoms may be related to abnormal nerve cell function due to impairment of sodium and potassium pumping. A fall in blood calcium is also seen in magnesium deficiency as well as resistance to 1,25 $(OH)_2$ vitamin D. It is possible that a chronically deficient intake of magnesium then may increase the risk of osteoporosis. Note that a magnesium deficiency develops very slowly because our bodies store it readily.[24]

Food Sources of Magnesium

Food Item and Amount	Magnesium (mg)
Spinach, 1 cup	157
Squash, 1 cup	105
Wheat germ, 1/4 cup	90
Raisin Bran cereal, 1 cup	90
Navy beans, 1/2 cup	54
Peanut butter, 2 tbsp	51
Black-eyed peas, 1/2 cup	46
Plain yogurt, 1 cup	43
Kidney beans, 1/2 cup	43
Sunflower seeds, 1/4 cup	41
Broccoli, 1 cup	37
Banana, 1 medium	34
1% milk, 1 cup	34
Watermelon, 1 slice	32
Oatmeal, 1/2 cup	28
Whole-wheat bread, 1 slice	25
RDA for adult men 400 mg RDA for adult women 310 mg	

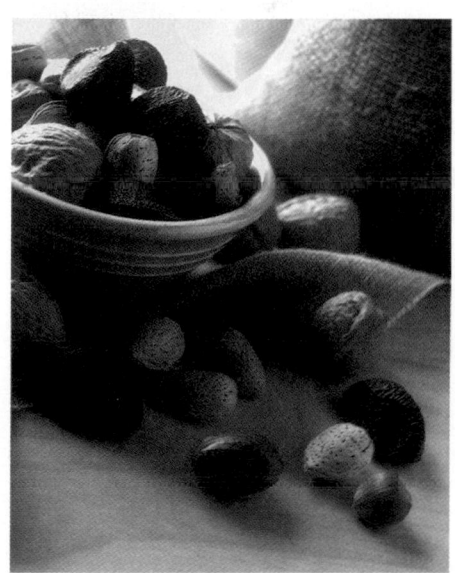

Nuts are a rich source of magnesium.

Poor magnesium status is especially found among users of certain diuretics, which increase magnesium excretion in the urine. In addition, heavy perspiration for weeks in hot climates and bouts of long-standing diarrhea or vomiting cause significant magnesium loss. Alcoholism also increases the risk of a deficiency because dietary intake may be poor and because alcohol increases magnesium excretion in the urine. The disorientation and weakness associated with alcoholism closely resemble the behavior of people with low blood magnesium. People with diabetes and some other health problems may have higher magnesium needs, which makes them vulnerable to marginal magnesium deficiency.

Upper Level for Magnesium

The Upper Level of 350 mg/day for magnesium only refers to supplement and other nonfood sources only, such as certain laxatives and antacids (e.g., Milk of Magnesia). Intakes above this amount from these sources can lead to diarrhea.[5] Toxicity also can be seen in kidney failure because the kidneys primarily regulate blood magnesium. In this case, high blood magnesium leads to weakness, nausea, slowed breathing, eventual malaise, coma, and death. Older people in general are at particular risk of magnesium toxicity, because kidney function may be compromised.

▎ Sulfur (S)

The minerals discussed so far function in the body primarily in the form of charged ions. In contrast, much of the sulfur in the body occurs in nonionic forms as an integral component of organic compounds, such as the vitamins biotin and thiamin. Because the amino acids methionine and cysteine both contain sulfur, it also is present in proteins. Disulfide bridges form when the sulfur atoms in two cysteine residues bind to each other; these bridges stabilize the structure of many protein molecules (review Chapter 7). For example, this stabilization is necessary for the formation of collagen, the protein found in connective tissue, and for keratin, which is found in nails, skin, and hair. Ionic forms of sulfur, such as sulfate (SO_4^{2-}), participate in the acid-base balance in the body, are present in many substances found in the extracellular fluid, and play an important role in some drug-detoxifying pathways in the body.[6]

We actually do not need to consume sulfur as such in our diets because proteins supply the sulfur we need. Sulfur compounds are also used to preserve foods (see Chapter 19).

Table 11-7 provides a summary of the major minerals.

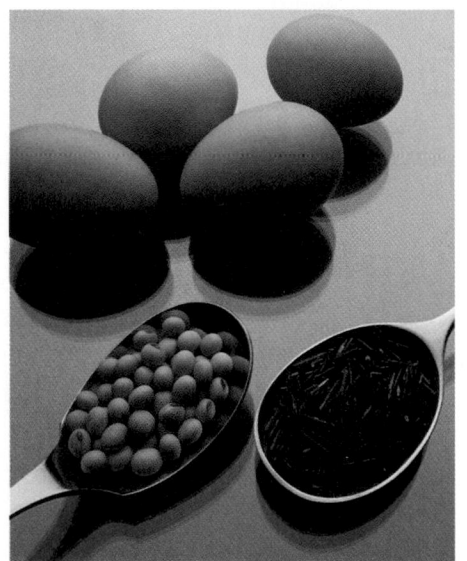

Protein-rich foods supply sulfur in the diet.

Concept | Check

Magnesium is a mineral found mostly in plant foods. It is important for nerve and heart function and as an activator of many enzymes. Whole grains (bran portion), vegetables, nuts, seeds, milk, and meats are good food sources. Sulfur is incorporated into certain vitamins and amino acids. Its ability to bond with other sulfur atoms enables it to stabilize protein structure.

Table 11-7 | A Summary of the Major Minerals

Mineral	Major Functions	RDA or Adequate Intake	Dietary Sources	Deficiency Symptoms	Toxicity Symptoms
Sodium	• Major positive ion of the extracellular fluid • Aids nerve impulse transmission • Water balance	*Age 19–50 years:* 1500 mg *Ages 51–70 years:* 1300 mg *Age 71 years or more* 1200 mg	• Table salt • Processed foods • Condiments • Sauces • Soups • Chips	• Muscle cramps	• Contributes to hypertension in susceptible individuals • Increases calcium loss in urine • Upper Level is 2300 mg
Potassium	• Major positive ion of intracellular fluid • Aids nerve impulse transmission • Water balance	4700 mg	• Spinach • Squash • Bananas • Orange juice • Milk and milk products • Meat • Legumes • Whole grains	• Irregular heartbeat • Loss of appetite • Muscle cramps	• Slowing of the heartbeat, as is seen in kidney failure
Chloride	• Major negative ion of extracellular fluid • Participates in acid production in stomach • Aids nerve impulse transmission • Water balance	2300 mg	• Table salt • Some vegetables • Processed foods	• Convulsions in infants	• Linked to hypertension in susceptible people when combined with sodium • Upper Level is 3600 mg
Calcium	• Bone and tooth structure • Blood clotting • Aids in nerve impulse transmission • Muscle contractions • Other cell functions	*Age greater than 18 years:* 1000–1200 mg *Age 9–18 years:* 1300 mg	• Milk and milk products • Canned fish • Leafy vegetables • Tofu • Fortified orange juice (and other fortified foods)	• Increased risk of osteoporosis	• May cause kidney stones and other problems in susceptible people. • Upper Level is 2500 mg
Phosphorus	• Major ion of intracellular fluid • Bone and tooth strength • Part of various metabolic compounds • Acid/base balance	*Age greater than 18 years:* 700 mg *Age 9–18 years:* 1250 mg	• Milk and milk products • Processed foods • Fish • Soft drinks • Bakery products • Meats	• Possibility of poor bone maintenance	• Impairs bone health in people with kidney failure • Poor bone mineralization if calcium intakes are low • Upper Level is 3–4 g
Magnesium	• Bone formation • Aids enzyme function • Aids nerve and heart function	*Men:* 400–420 mg *Women:* 310–320 mg	• Wheat bran • Green vegetables • Nuts • Chocolate • Legumes	• Weakness • Muscle pain • Poor heart function	• Causes diarrhea and weakness in people with kidney failure • Upper Level of 350 mg, but refers to nonfood sources (e.g., supplements) only
Sulfur	• Part of vitamins and amino acids • Aids in drug detoxification • Acid/base balance	None	• Protein foods	• None observed	• None likely

Summary

1. Water constitutes 50 to 70% of the human body. Its unique chemical properties enable it to dissolve substances as well as serve as a medium for chemical reactions, temperature regulation, and lubrication. Water also helps regulate the acid-base balance in the body. For adults, daily fluid needs as such are estimated at 9 cups (women) to 13 cups (men).

2. Many minerals are vital for sustaining life. For humans, animal products are the most bioavailable sources of most minerals. Supplements of minerals exceeding the Daily Value, and especially the Upper Level, should be taken only under a physician's supervision because toxicity and nutrient interactions are possible.

3. Sodium, the major positive ion (cation) found outside cells, is vital in fluid balance and nerve impulse transmission. The North American diet provides abundant sodium through processed foods and table salt.

4. Potassium, the major positive ion (cation) found inside cells, has functions similar to those of sodium. Milk, fruits, and vegetables are good sources. Chloride is the major negative ion (anion) found outside cells. It is important in digestion as part of gastric hydrochloric acid and in immune and nerve functions. Table salt supplies most of the chloride in our diets.

5. Calcium forms a vital part of bone structure and is very important in blood clotting, muscle contraction, nerve transmission, and cell metabolism. Calcium absorption is enhanced by stomach acid and the active vitamin D hormone. Milk and milk products are rich calcium sources. Women are particularly at risk for not meeting calcium needs. They are also typically at risk of developing osteoporosis as they age. Numerous lifestyle and medical options help reduce this risk.

6. Phosphorus aids function of some enzymes and forms part of key metabolic compounds, cell membranes, and bone. It is efficiently absorbed, and deficiencies are rare. Typical food sources are dairy products, bakery products, and meats.

7. Magnesium, a mineral found mostly in plants, is important for nerve and heart function and as an activator for many enzymes. Whole grains (bran portion), vegetables, nuts, seeds, milk, and meats are typical food sources. Sulfur is incorporated into certain vitamins and amino acids. Its ability to bond with other sulfur atoms enables it to stabilize protein structure.

Study Questions

1. Approximately how much water does a person need each day to stay healthy? Identify at least two situations that increase the need for water. Then list three sources of water in the average person's diet.

2. Why are most minerals present in higher concentrations in animal foods than in plant foods?

3. How is water eliminated from the body? What physiological forces regulate this output?

4. What is the main physiological difference between teeth and bones?

5. Identify four factors that influence the bioavailability of minerals from food.

6. What is the relationship between sodium and water balance, and how is that relationship monitored as well as maintained in the body?

7. Within what physiological system do sodium, potassium, and calcium interact? What are the individual roles of these minerals in this system?

8. What might you tell a 12-year-old child about the importance of consuming sufficient calcium?

9. In terms of total amounts in the body, calcium and phosphorus are the first and second most abundant minerals, respectively. Name two ways in which phosphorus and calcium are alike and two ways in which they differ.

10. Describe the relationship between magnesium and the function/health of the heart.

BOOST YOUR STUDY

Check out the **Perspectives in Nutrition: Online Learning Center** www.mhhe.com/wardlawpers7 for quizzes, flash cards, activities, and web links designed to further help you learn about water and the major minerals.

Annotated References

1. Appel LJ and others: Dietary approaches to prevent an treat hypertension: A scientific statement from the American Heart association. *Hypertension* 47:296, 2006.
   Latest advice from the American Heart Association on diet and hypertension. Key preventive factors are to avoid overweight and inactivity, and moderate alcohol and salt intake.

2. Chobanian AV and others: The seventh report of the joint national committee on the prevention, detection, evaluation, and treatment of high blood pressure. *Journal of the American Medical Association* 289:2560, 2003.
   This article is a comprehensive look at the various lifestyle and medical interventions to prevent and treat hypertension. Key lifestyle factors emphasized are weight reduction, regular, physical activity, reduction in salt intake, moderation in alcohol use, and following a healthy diet, such as the DASH diet.

3. Dawson-Hughes B: Osteoporsis. In Shils ME and others (eds): *Modern nutrition in health and disease.* 10th ed. Philadelphia, PA: Lippincott Williams & Wilkins, 2006.
   Current review of osteoporosis diagnosis and treatment, as well as current medical therapies for the disorder.

4. Fiske H: Measuring water's benefits and optimal intake recommendations. *Today's Dietitian,* p. 22, January 2003.
   One way to make sure we stay well hydrated is to always have no more than a pale yellow urine. For many of us hydration is not a challenge be-

cause our thirst mechanisms encourage us to drink fluid when needed. All fluids count, even those with caffeine and alcohol (but not quite as much as water itself).

5. Food and Nutrition Board, Institute of Medicine: *Dietary Reference Intakes for calcium, phosphorus, magnesium, vitamin D, and fluoride.* Washington, DC: National Academy Press, 1997.

   Dietary standards for many major minerals are discussed. The rationale used to set RDA or Adequate Intakes and Upper Levels for these nutrients is discussed in detail.

6. Food and Nutrition Board, Institute of Medicine: *Dietary Reference Intakes for water, potassium, sodium, chloride, and sulfate.* Washington, DC: National Academy Press, 2004.

   Dietary standards for water, potassium, sodium, and chloride are discussed. The rationale used to derive the Adequate Intakes, as well as the Upper Levels, are presented along with information on function, intake, and deficiency.

7. Ford ES, Mokad AH: Dietary magnesium intake in a national sample of U.S. adults. *Journal of Nutrition* 133:2879, 2003.

   Many adults currently do not meet their magnesium needs on a regular basis, particularly women who do not take a multivitamin and mineral supplement and African-Americans in general. Green vegetables, nuts, seeds, dried beans, whole grains, dairy products, and meats are good magnesium sources for a diet.

8. Havas S and others: Reducing the public health burden from elevated blood pressure levels in the United States by lowering intake of dietary sodium. *American Journal of Public Health* 94:19, 2004.

   The American public consumes far more sodium than is needed. Most of this sodium is added as salt by food manufacturers and restaurants.

9. Heaney RP: Bone biology in health and disease. In Shils ME and others (eds): *Modern nutrition in health and disease.* 10th ed. Philadelphia, PA: Lippincott Williams & Wilkins, 2006.

   Current review of bone biology in health and disease. Dietary factors such as various vitamins and minerals that affect bone health are also covered.

10. Hoolihan L: Beyond calcium. *Nutrition Today* 39(2):69, 2004.

    Meeting one's needs for calcium using dairy products may provide health benefits beyond those attributed to the calcium content alone. Incorporating milk and milk products into a diet is a good habit to develop.

11. How to prevent strokes. *Consumer Reports on Health* 16(9):1, 2004.

    This article provides detailed review of the health risks posed by strokes as well as a look at current treatments. Preventive measures include not smoking, meeting nutrient needs, reducing stress, and controlling diabetes if present.

12. Kemmler W and others: Benefits of 2 years of intense exercise on bone density, physical fit-ness, and blood lipids in early postmenopausal osteopenic women: Results of the Erlangen Fitness Osteoporosis Prevention Study (EFOPS). *Archives of Internal Medicine* 164:1084, 2004.

    A general-purpose exercise program has a positive impact on women who are in the early years of menopause. Such a program can also improve strength and endurance, reduce back pain, and improve lipid levels.

13. Khaw K-T and others: Blood pressure and urinary sodium in men and women: The Norfolk Cohort of the European Prospective Investigation into Cancer (EPIC-Norfolk). *American Journal of Clinical Nutrition* 80:1397, 2004.

    Within the usual range found in a free-living population, higher amounts of urinary sodium, an indicator of dietary sodium intake, are associated with increases in blood pressure of clinical and public health relevance. The findings reinforce recommendations to lower average sodium intakes in the general population.

14. Knochel JP: Phosphorus. In Shils ME and others (eds): *Modern nutrition in health and disease.* 10th ed. Philadelphia, PA: Lippincott Williams & Wilkins, 2006.

    Current review of phosphorus metabolism. Digestion and absorption and related issues such as clinical states that pose a risk for a deficiency use are also covered.

15. Kotchen TA, Kotchen JM: Nutrition, diet and hypertension. In Shils ME and others (eds): *Modern nutrition in health and disease.* 10th ed. Philadelphia, PA: Lippincott Williams & Wilkins, 2006.

    Current review of nutrition, diet and hypertension, including a detailed discussion of the ways in which salt intake contributes to the problem.

16. Kuehn BM: Better osteoporosis management a priority: Impact predicted to soar with aging population. *Journal of the American Medical Association* 293(20):2453, 2005.

    More than 2 million individuals in the United States will experience osteoporosis-related fractures this year, resulting in estimated medical costs of more than $16.9 billion. By 2025, the number of fractures and the associated costs are expected to rise by 48%. Despite this daunting challenge, the arsenal of tools to identify, prevent, or treat osteoporosis has grown considerably over the past 10 years. Proper diet and exercise throughout life are recognized as the most effective measures to maintain bone health.

17. Liebman B: Breaking up: Strong bones need more than calcium. *Nutrition Action Health Letter* 32(3):3, 2005.

    Good, basic overview of latest research for preventing bone loss and maintaining bone health. The article includes specific recommendations for daily exercise and for intakes of calcium, vitamin A, vitamin D, vitamin K, protein, and potassium and for fruits and vegetables in general.

18. Mitka M: Dash of dissent on salt intake advice. *Journal of the American Medical Association* 291:1686, 2004.

    Low-sodium diets especially help some people control blood pressure, but some experts contend that recommending such a diet to all adults does not have strong scientific support. There is no compelling evidence to show that low-sodium diets harm adults in general, which has led other experts to recommend routine adoption of a low-sodium diet.

19. Nieves JW: Osteoporosis: The role of micronutrients. *American Journal of Clinical Nutrition* 81:1232S, 2005.

    The effects of calcium and vitamin D on bone cannot be considered in isolation from the other components of the diet. The other micronutrients needed for optimizing bone health include magnesium, potassium, vitamin C, and vitamin K. These needs can be met with a healthy diet that is high in fruits and vegetables (≥ 5 servings per day).

20. Nowson CA: Blood pressure response to dietary modifications in free-living individuals. *Journal of Nutrition* 134:2322, 2004.

    A population-wide reduction in dietary sodium, specifically by reducing the sodium content of staple food items, together with an increase in potassium intake (through increased fruit, vegetable, and whole-grain cereal intake), would contribute to the maintenance of optimal blood pressures in the population.

21. Oh MS, Uribarri J: Electrolytes, water, and acid-base balance. In Shils ME and others (eds): *Modern nutrition in health and disease.* 10th ed. Philadelphia, PA: Lippincott Williams & Wilkins, 2006.

    Current review of water and electrolyte metabolism, and the effects of both deficiency and toxicity states for water and various electrolytes.

22. Raisz LG: Screening for osteoporosis. *The New England Journal of Medicine* 353:164, 2005.

    Measurement of bone mineral density at the lumbar spine and proximal femur by dual-energy X-ray absorptiometry bone scans is a reliable and safe way to assess the risk of fracture in postmenopausal women. However, many other factors influence fracture risk, such as genetic background and race, and should be considered in making recommendations regarding bone densitometry and therapy.

23. Rosen CJ: Postmenopausal osteoporosis. *The New England Journal of Medicine* 353:595, 2005.

    A review of the diagnosis and treatment of osteoporosis, including current medications. The author recommends biphosphonates as the most appropriate medication and also recommends meeting calcium and vitamin D needs.

24. Rude RK, Shils ME: Magnesium. In Shils ME and others (eds): *Modern nutrition in health and disease.* 10th ed. Philadelphia, PA: Lippincott Williams & Wilkins, 2006.

Current review of magnesium metabolism. Digestion and absorption and related issues such as numerous clinical examples where a deficiency might develop are also covered.

25. Schardt D: Potassium: Bones, stones, and strokes on the line. *Nutrition Action Health Letter,* p. 8, December 2004.

   Potassium is the seventh most plentiful mineral on earth, but it is much too scarce in the American diet. Consuming more potassium would help protect us against high blood pressure, strokes, kidney stones, and bone loss.

26. Stronger bones without the hype. *Consumer Reports on Health* 16(5):1, 2004.

   The article provides detailed answers to typical questions about bone health. A review of the approved osteoporosis medications is also provided.

27. U.S. Preventive Services Task Force Recommendation Statement: Hormone therapy for the prevention of chronic conditions in postmenopausal women. *American Family Physician* 72(2):311, 2005.

   The USPSTF recommends against routine use of combined estrogen and progestin for the prevention of chronic conditions in postmenopausal women. Any such use should be short term, such as for treating the initial symptoms of menopause. The American College of Obstetrics and Gynecology, the American Heart Association, the North American Menopause Society, and the Canadian Task Force on Preventive Health Care make similar recommendations.

28. Weaver CM, Heaney RP: Calcium. In Shils ME and others (eds): *Modern nutrition in health and disease.* 10th ed. Philadelphia, PA: Lippincott Williams & Wilkins, 2006.

   Current review of calcium metabolism. Digestion and absorption are also covered.

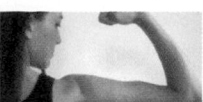

Take | Action

I. How High Is Your Sodium Intake?

Complete this questionnaire to evaluate your sodium habits with respect to typically rich sources.

How Often Do You . . .	Rarely	Occasionally	Often	Regularly (Daily)
1. Eat cured or processed meats, such as ham, bacon, sausage, frankfurters, and other luncheon meats?	☐	☐	☐	☐
2. Choose canned or frozen vegetables with sauce?	☐	☐	☐	☐
3. Use commercially prepared meals, main dishes, or canned or dehydrated soups?	☐	☐	☐	☐
4. Eat cheese, especially processed cheese?	☐	☐	☐	☐
5. Eat salted nuts, popcorn, pretzels, corn chips, or potato chips?	☐	☐	☐	☐
6. Add salt to cooking water for vegetables, rice, or pasta?	☐	☐	☐	☐
7. Add salt, seasoning mixes, salad dressings, or condiments—such as soy sauce, steak sauce, catsup, and mustard—to foods during preparation or at the table?	☐	☐	☐	☐
8. Salt your food before tasting it?	☐	☐	☐	☐
9. Ignore labels for sodium content when buying foods?	☐	☐	☐	☐
10. When dining out, choose foods with sauces or foods that are obviously salty?	☐	☐	☐	☐

The more checks you put in the "often" or "regularly" columns, the higher your dietary sodium intake is. However, not all the habits in the table contribute the same amount of sodium. For example, many natural cheeses such as cheddar are relatively moderate in sodium, whereas processed cheeses and cottage cheese are much higher. To moderate sodium intake, choose lower-sodium foods from each food group more often and balance high-sodium food choices with low-sodium ones.

Adapted from *USDA Home and Garden Bulletin* No. 232–6, April 1986.

II. Working for Denser Bones

Osteoporosis and related low bone mass affect many adults in North America, especially older women. In fact, one-third of all women experience fractures because of this disease, amounting to about 2 million bone fractures per year.

Osteoporosis is a disease you can do something about. Some risk factors can't be changed, but others, such as a poor calcium intake, can. Is this true for you? To find out, complete this tool for estimating your current calcium intake. For all the following foods, write the number of servings you eat in a day. Total the number of servings in each category and then multiply the total number of servings by the amount of calcium for each category. Finally, add the total amount for each food category to estimate your calcium intake for that day.

Does your intake meet your AI set for calcium?

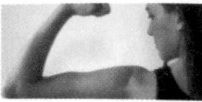

Take | Action

Food	Serving Size	Number of Servings	Calcium (mg)	Total Calcium (mg)
Plain low-fat yogurt	1 cup	_____		
Fat-free dry milk powder	1/2 cup	_____		
	Total servings	_____	× 400	= _____ mg
Canned sardines (with bones)	3 ounces	_____		
Fruit-flavored yogurt	1 cup	_____		
Milk: fat-free, reduced-fat, whole, chocolate, buttermilk	1 cup	_____		
Calcium-fortified soy milk (e.g., Silk)	1 cup	_____		
Parmesan cheese (grated)	1/4 cup	_____		
Swiss cheese	1 ounce	_____		
	Total servings	_____	× 300	= _____ mg
Cheese (all other hard cheese)	1 ounce	_____		
Pancakes	3	_____		
	Total servings	_____	× 200	= _____ mg
Canned pink salmon	3 ounces	_____		
Tofu (processed with calcium)	4 ounces	_____		
	Total servings	_____	× 150	= _____ mg
Collards or turnip greens, cooked	1/2 cup	_____		
Ice cream or ice milk	1/2 cup	_____		
Almonds	1 ounce	_____		
	Total servings	_____	× 75	= _____ mg
Chard, cooked	1/2 cup	_____		
Cottage cheese	1/2 cup	_____		
Corn tortilla	1 medium	_____		
Orange	1 medium	_____		
	Total servings	_____	× 50	= _____ mg
Kidney, lima, or navy beans, cooked	1/2 cup	_____		
Broccoli	1/2 cup	_____		
Carrot, raw	1 medium	_____		
Dates or raisins	1/4 cup	_____		
Egg	1 large	_____		
Whole-wheat bread	1 slice	_____		
Peanut butter	2 tablespoons	_____		
	Total servings	_____	× 25	= _____ mg
Calcium-fortified orange juice	6 ounces	_____		
Calcium-fortified snack bars	1 each	_____		
Calcium-fortified breakfast bars	1/2 bar	_____		
	Total servings	_____	× 200	= _____ mg
Calcium-fortified chocolate candies	1 each	_____		
Calcium supplements*	1 each	_____	× 500	= _____ mg
		Total calcium intake	=	_____ mg

Other calcium sources to consider include many breakfast cereals (100 to 250 mg per cup), and some vitamin/mineral supplements (200 to 500 mg or more per tablet).

*Amount varies, so check the label for the amount in a specific product and then adjust the calculation as needed.
Reprinted with permission from *Topics in Clinical Nutrition*, "Putting Calcium into Perspective for Your Clients," G. Wardlaw and N. Weese; 11:1, p. 29. © 1995 Aspen Publishers, Inc.

CHAPTER OUTLINE

CASE SCENARIO:

At a recent family reunion, Gina learned that an aunt was currently undergoing treatment for colon cancer. Her grandmother also explained that two other family members had died of the disease before Gina was born. After the reunion Gina decided to learn more about colon cancer and how her family history of the disease could affect her. Gina's research uncovered that 150,000 Americans are diagnosed with colon cancer each year and that her family history increased her chances of developing the disease. While searching online she came across a site that recommended 200 µg/day of the trace mineral selenium as a way to prevent the disease. She then went to her local supermarket and found that 100 selenium tablets containing 200 µg each only cost $7.50 a bottle. Gina figured this supplement was cheap "insurance" against developing the disease and so began taking 200 µg of selenium a day. Is Gina's practice harmful? Should we all follow her example? Are there other nutritional practices she should consider to help protect her from developing colon cancer?

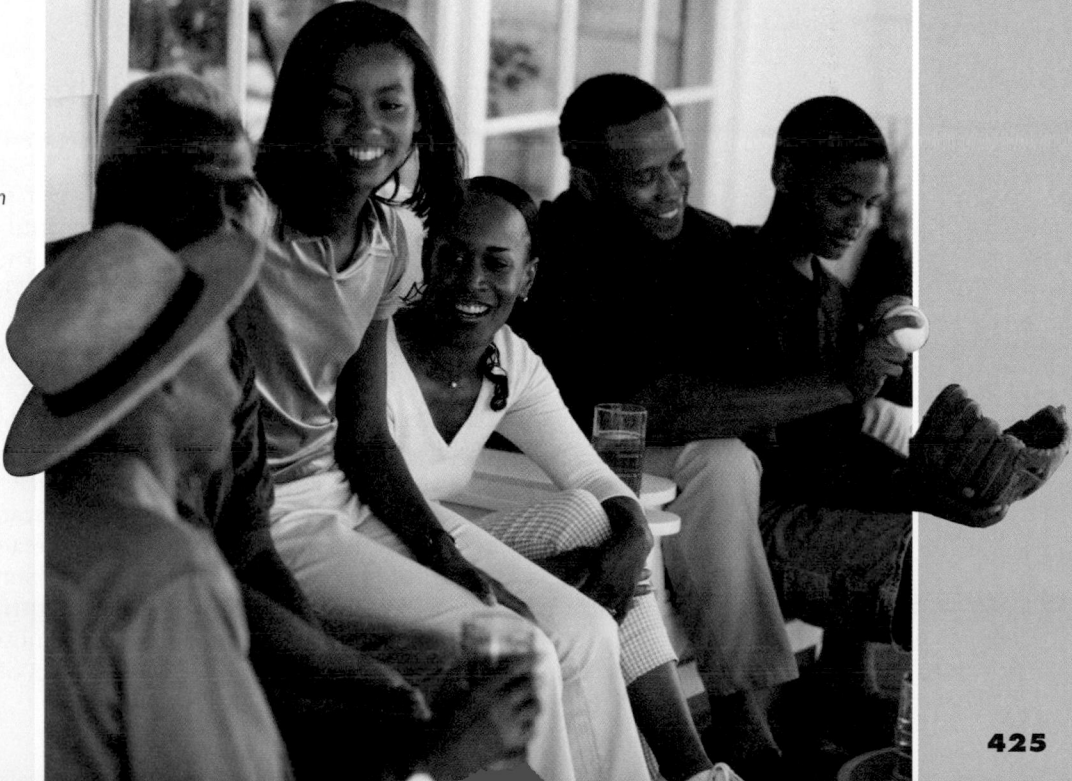

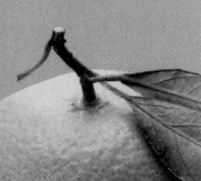

Trace minerals make up less than 1% of all minerals in the body, but their functions are absolutely essential for life.[9,10,11] A trace mineral is defined as a mineral for which our daily nutritional need is less than 100 mg. Grouping them together this way, however, is too simplistic because the functions, mechanisms of absorption, transport in the body, and metabolism of the various trace minerals vary considerably. For example, the body carefully regulates the absorption and transport of iron and copper but not selenium and iodide. This difference makes these latter trace minerals potentially toxic at intakes not much above our needs. The trace minerals are also very interactive; the abundance of one mineral in the diet and in the body can affect the absorption and metabolism of several other minerals.[10]

Information about trace minerals is one of the most rapidly expanding areas of nutrition science. With the exception of iron and iodide, the importance of trace minerals to humans has been recognized only within the last 50 years. This chapter will examine some of these new findings as well as the role played by various nutrients in cancer development and prevention.

CHAPTER OBJECTIVES CHAPTER 12 IS DESIGNED TO ALLOW YOU TO:

1. List conditions of the body, dietary factors, and other pertinent influences that determine the absorption, retention, and availability of specific trace minerals.

2. List key functions of the trace minerals.

3. Identify possible deficiency and toxicity symptoms associated with the trace minerals.

4. List at least two food sources for each trace mineral.

REFRESH YOUR MEMORY AS YOU BEGIN YOUR STUDY OF TRACE MINERALS IN CHAPTER 12, YOU MAY WANT TO REVIEW:

- Digestion and absorption processes in Chapter 3.
- The process of oxidation and reduction and the electron transport chain in Chapter 4.
- Vitamins in Chapters 9 and 10.
- Calcium in Chapter 11.
- Chemistry terms such as *valence* and *free radicals* in Appendix A.
- Respiration, the muscular and skeletal systems, cell structure and function, immunity, and the endocrine system in Appendix C.

▌ Trace Minerals—An Introduction

The terms *trace mineral* and *micromineral* are somewhat imprecise because several definitions of these terms have evolved over time. Originally the terms were used to describe minerals that were not easily quantified by existing analytical methods, but today we have precise techniques for determining the concentration of very small amounts of minerals in tissues and in foods. Thus, the definition used in this textbook relates to "a daily nutritional need of less than 100 mg." Trace minerals are dietary essentials in that they have specified biological functions and a dietary deficiency produces physiological or structural abnormalities.[9,10,11]

Discovering the importance of these trace minerals to humans has a fairly recent history, although the use of dietary iron to treat the effects of blood loss can be traced back to ancient civilizations. In 1961, scientists linked dwarfism among villagers in the Middle East to a zinc deficiency. Other researchers later recognized that an obscure form of heart deterioration in an isolated area of China was linked to a selenium deficiency. In the United States, deficiencies of some trace minerals were first observed in the late 1960s to early 1970s when these nutrients were omitted in the preparation of synthetic formulas used for total parenteral nutrition. This "accident" also led to proof that some trace minerals were essential parts of a human diet.

❚ Research on Trace Minerals

Not only are trace minerals needed in much smaller amounts than the major minerals, but the actual need for some trace minerals is also still debatable. Table 1-3 in Chapter 1 listed nine essential trace minerals but some other possible entries also were listed. Demonstrating the essential nature of this latter group of nutrients is hampered by difficulty in measuring the small amounts needed by the body and by not knowing all the functions in the body that may be associated with the trace mineral. Before presenting each trace mineral, this chapter looks at why research in this area is so complex.

Difficulties in Studying Trace Minerals

Rigorous protocols often are required to produce a trace mineral deficiency in animals. (All animal research referred to in this discussion was conducted with farm and/or laboratory animals.) The animals may need to be raised in ultraclean environments and have their diets carefully formulated from individual essential nutrients to ensure that no trace mineral contamination occurs. Stainless steel and plastic cages may also be needed so that the animals do not obtain any trace minerals, such as zinc, from chewing on the cages. Trace minerals must sometimes even be filtered from the air, and the water must be as free of trace minerals as possible. In addition, glassware used for chemical analysis may need to be rinsed repeatedly in acid to eliminate trace mineral contamination; sometimes only plastic bottles are appropriate.

Despite the difficulties encountered in experimentally producing most trace mineral deficiencies in laboratory animals, overt human deficiencies still do occur. In addition, some evidence suggests that marginal dietary intakes of certain trace minerals (e.g., iron, zinc, copper, and chromium) also occur, leading to mild, undetected deficiencies in humans.[9,10,11] The lack of precise tests to pinpoint these deficiencies is one reason there is concern but not hard evidence. Most of these tests involve blood samples. However, for many trace minerals, the blood tests most commonly used aren't sensitive measures of small changes in trace mineral status. Moreover, the values for many of these blood tests are influenced by factors not related to the trace mineral status, such as ongoing infections.

A good example of these various difficulties is the trace mineral copper. A copper deficiency is often assessed by the amount of copper, or the protein that contains most of the copper (called **ceruloplasmin**) in the blood.[16] However, based on work with laboratory rats, these values don't fall as readily during a mild copper deficiency as do some other copper-related parameters in various tissues. In addition, both laboratory animal and human studies have shown that copper or ceruloplasmin readings in the blood are affected by factors such as inflammation, pregnancy, fluctuating estrogen levels, and oral contraceptive use. For reasons like this, diagnosing marginal trace mineral deficiencies can be seen as an art that only a few researchers can reliably perform.

Another reason why marginal trace mineral deficiencies often go undetected is that the effects may be subtle and may involve interactions with other factors. For example, a marginal trace mineral deficiency might produce a change in cardiovascular disease risk factors or immune function. However, these changes are not obvious to the person affected. Even the person's physician might not recognize that these effects involve trace minerals because many other factors are involved in cardiovascular or immune function. Therefore, it is important that research with trace minerals continues. Meanwhile, you would do well to eat a balanced diet and pay attention to situations that may cause low trace mineral intakes or lead to high trace mineral needs. Many of these situations are discussed in this chapter.

Trace Mineral Needs

The primary method used to set trace mineral nutrient needs is the balance study. This is the same basic technique that is used for nitrogen balance studies (review Chapter 7). Researchers try to determine the lowest trace mineral intake that compensates for all

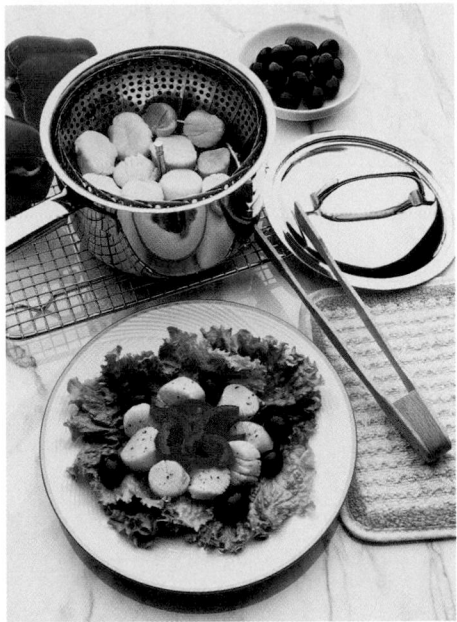

Seafood, such as scallops, is a good source of many trace minerals.

Research on trace minerals in humans still has a long way to go because our current understanding of trace mineral metabolism relies heavily on the knowledge gained from studies with farm and laboratory animals.

ceruloplasmin A blue copper-containing protein in the blood that can remove an electron from Fe^{2+} (the ferrous form) to yield Fe^{3+} (the ferric form). The Fe^{3+} form of iron can then bind with iron transport and storage proteins, such as transferrin.

The difficulty in measuring trace mineral nutrition in humans makes setting specific human needs problematic. Some trace minerals have only an Adequate Intake (AI), not a more precise RDA.

trace mineral losses from urine, feces, hair, skin, perspiration, menses, and so on. These studies are very expensive to perform. In addition, a balance study tells only the amount of dietary intake needed to maintain a specific pool of the trace mineral in the body, but this pool does not necessarily represent the amount needed to maintain all body functions or ensure good health.

Another complication is that trace minerals interact with each other. For example, an overabundance of iron in the digestive tract can interfere with the absorption of other minerals, such as zinc. Thus, to set human dietary needs for zinc, nutrition scientists must estimate the amount of iron that will be consumed to predict how much zinc the body will actually absorb.[10] Overall, quite a lot of scientific judgment must go into setting appropriate intakes for trace minerals.

Sources of Trace Minerals

Trace minerals are found in both plant and animal foods. However, the bioavailability of trace minerals is an important issue to consider, especially when planning diets. Even if a food is high in a particular trace mineral, it will not supply much to the body unless the trace mineral is absorbed well. Many factors found in foods inhibit trace mineral absorption. Mineral absorption from some sources can amount to only 1 to 6% of the total present, with the lowest percentages typically seen in plant sources.

By eating a variety of foods, you can obtain nutrients from plants grown in a variety of soils and, thus, maximize your chances of consuming adequate amounts of trace minerals. In addition, for most trace minerals, it is best to consume as many minimally processed foods as possible; generally, the more refined a food, the lower its content of trace minerals. For example, during the refining of whole wheat into white flour, much of the trace mineral content of iron, selenium, zinc, and copper is lost. The enrichment of white flour restores iron but not the other trace minerals.

Iron (Fe)

Iron is found in every living cell; total body content is about 5 g (about 1 tsp). The importance of iron for the maintenance of health has been recognized for centuries. In 4000 B.C., the Persian physician Melampus gave iron supplements to sailors to compensate for the iron lost from bleeding during battles. Today, iron deficiency and related cases of anemia are common worldwide, affecting an estimated 1 billion or more people in developing and developed countries. In most developing nations, about two-thirds of all children and women of childbearing age experience iron deficiency.[18]

Absorption, Transport, Storage, and Excretion of Iron

The body uses a variety of mechanisms to absorb iron and distribute it in the body. These various mechanisms maximize iron function and minimize iron toxicity. Although this system doesn't work perfectly if body iron is very low or very high, it still works well most of the time. The body's handling of iron is affected by a number of factors, but the most influential factor is body iron stores. If stores are low, the small intestine becomes more efficient at iron absorption. Diet composition also plays a major role. These and other factors that affect iron absorption are summarized in Table 12-1.

Iron occurs in foods in various forms. In meat, fish, and poultry, some of the iron is present as **hemoglobin** and **myoglobin,** which collectively are called **heme iron.** The rest of the iron present in these foods, as well as all the iron in vegetables, grains, and supplements, is **nonheme iron.** Heme iron is absorbed more readily than nonheme iron (generally 30% versus 2 to 10%, respectively).[10] This is one reason meat products are an efficient way to obtain iron from foods. The amount of iron in meat is also higher than the amount naturally occurring in plant foods. (This discussion, however, does not discount the value of iron in plant foods. Those sources still help

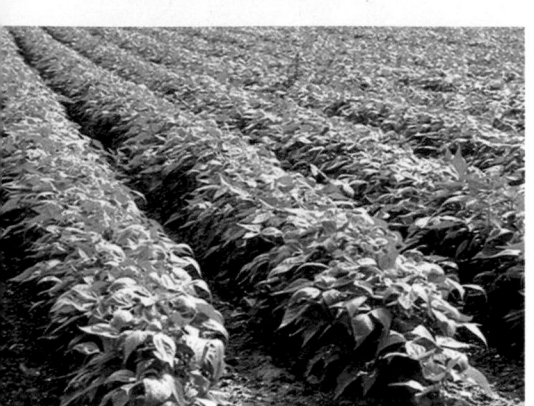

The trace mineral content of plant foods depends on the soil in which they were grown.

hemoglobin The iron-containing protein in red blood cells that transports oxygen to the body tissues and some carbon dioxide away from the tissues. It is also responsible for the red color of blood.

myoglobin The iron-containing protein that controls the rate of diffusion of oxygen (O_2) from red blood cells to muscle cells.

heme iron Iron provided from animal tissues primarily as a component of hemoglobin and myoglobin. Approximately 40% of the iron in meat is heme iron; it is readily absorbed.

nonheme iron Iron provided from plant sources and elemental iron components of animal tissues. Nonheme iron is less efficiently absorbed than heme iron, and absorption is also more closely dependent on body needs.

Table 12-1 | Factors That Affect Iron Absorption

Increase Absorption	Decrease Absorption
Gastric acid	Phytic acid (in fiber)
Heme iron in food	Oxalic acid in leafy vegetables
High body demand for red blood cells (blood loss, high altitude, physical training, pregnancy)	Polyphenols in tea, coffee, red wine, and other foods
	Full body stores of iron
Low body stores of iron	Excessive intakes of other minerals (Zn, Mn)*
Meat protein factor (MPF)	Reduced gastric acid output
Vitamin C intakes	Calcium-containing supplements and antacids (small effect in the long run)

*Especially when taken as supplements

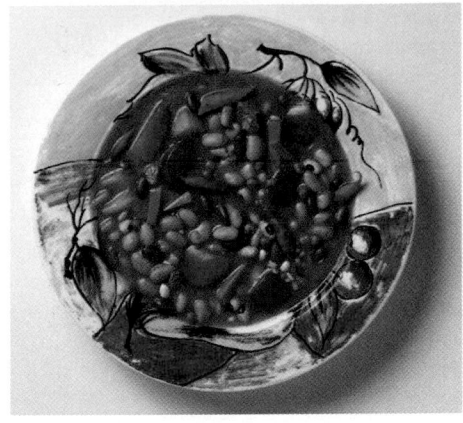

Minimally-processed foods should be the focus for your daily intake of trace minerals.

meet iron needs.) Another reason that meat is advantageous is that it helps us absorb the nonheme iron from other foods, although the exact mechanisms aren't well understood. A meat protein factor (MPF) may explain part of this effect.

Organic acids, such as vitamin C, in the foods we eat also increase nonheme iron absorption by adding an electron to Fe^{3+} (the ferric form), yielding Fe^{2+} (the ferrous form). Vitamin C then forms a complex, called a **chelate,** with Fe^{2+}, thereby enhancing absorption. For vegetarians or people who limit intake of animal flesh, combining vitamin C–rich foods with plant foods containing iron is a useful strategy.

Ferrous iron (Fe^{2+}) is absorbed better than ferric iron (Fe^{3+}) because it crosses the mucous layer of the small intestine more readily to reach the brush border of intestinal absorptive cells. There, Fe^{2+} must then have an electron removed, oxidizing it to Fe^{3+}, before it enters the absorptive cells. At the cell membrane of the brush border, Fe^{3+} binds to a receptor protein, called a membrane iron-binding protein, which finally transfers iron into the absorptive cell.

Although no iron absorption occurs in the stomach, gastric acid plays an important role in nonheme iron absorption by promoting the conversion of Fe^{3+} to Fe^{2+} and by solubilizing the iron. The decreased production of gastric acid experienced by many older people can lower both their iron absorption and ultimately their body stores of iron. Once acted on by acid in the stomach, absorption of the iron then occurs primarily in the small intestine.

Heme iron follows a different absorptive process. It is likely absorbed directly into the absorptive cells after the globin (protein) fraction has been removed. Once inside the absorptive cells, the iron is released from the heme portion.

Several dietary factors interfere with our ability to absorb iron. Phytic acid and other factors in grain fibers and oxalic acid in vegetables can all bind iron, reducing its absorption. For this reason, spinach is not a good iron source despite containing relatively high amounts of iron for a plant food. Polyphenols, such as tannins found in tea and related substances found in coffee, also reduce iron absorption.[10] People trying to rebuild iron stores are advised to reduce coffee and tea consumption, particularly at meal times. Finally, several studies have shown that calcium interferes with dietary iron absorption, but the effect is mild at best. Still, experts on calcium and iron interactions recommend that individuals with high iron requirements avoid taking calcium supplements at meals that contain most of the dietary iron. They could also consider taking calcium supplements between meals or at bedtime to avoid this potential interaction.

Because iron is essential but high intakes can be quite toxic, the body has an elaborate system to try to place iron where it belongs and inhibit iron toxicity (a few highlights of this iron processing are noted in Figure 12-1). First, cells of the small intestine make an iron-binding protein called **ferritin** in proportion to body iron stores. If

chelates Complexes formed between metal ions and substances with polar groups, such as proteins. The polar groups form two or more attachments with the metal ions, forming a ringed structure. The metal ion is then firmly bound and sequestered.

Critical | Thinking

Annie, Tom's friend, is taking a nutrition class at her university. She suggested that he consume some extra vitamin C–rich foods every day. Tom is confused by this advice, because his doctor told him that to help treat his low blood iron, Tom should increase the amount of iron in his diet but not the amount of vitamin C. How can Annie explain her recommendation to him?

ferritin A protein compound that serves as the storage form of iron in the blood and tissues.

Figure 12-1 | Iron absorption and distribution. Iron binds with a protein called apoferritin to form ferritin when stored in cells (1). If the intestinal absorptive cells are sloughed before iron is absorbed from them, the iron is not absorbed into the blood (2). This allows the body to control the absorption of iron. The mechanism for resisting absorption of excess iron, primarily that in the nonheme form, is termed a mucosal block. Iron that enters the bloodstream binds to transferrin (3) and is then distributed to various cells in the body (4). Some iron is also recycled for further use in the body.(5)

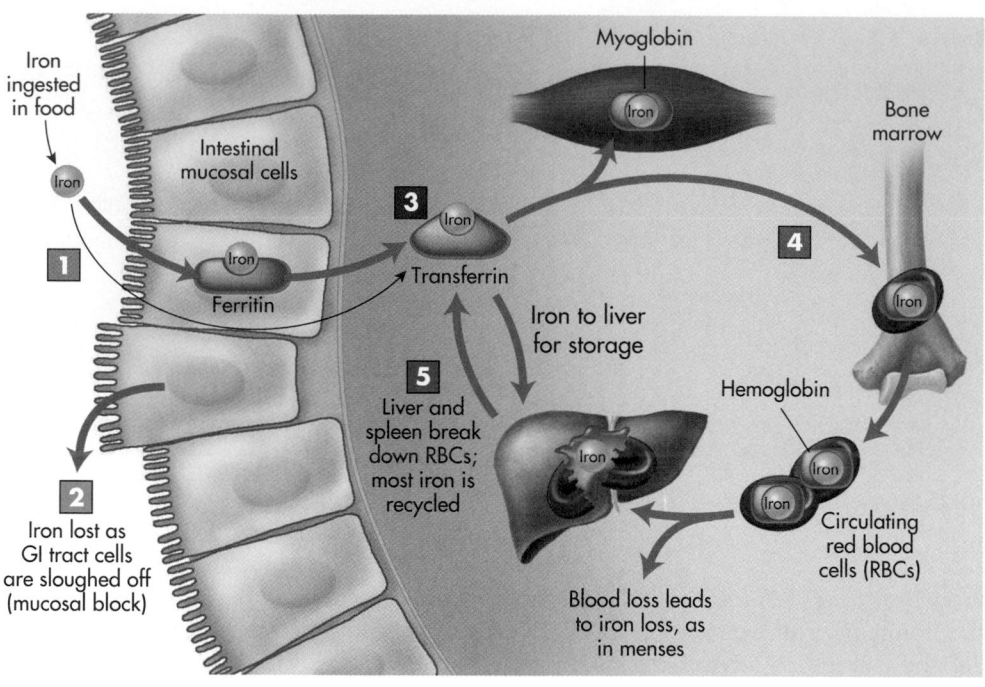

The copper-containing blood protein ceruloplasmin removes an electron from Fe^{2+}, yielding Fe^{3+}, the form bound by transferrin. Thus, copper metabolism and iron metabolism are closely linked.

transferrin A protein that transports iron in the blood.

hemosiderin An insoluble iron-protein compound in the liver. Hemosiderin stores iron when the amount of iron in the body exceeds the storage capacity of ferritin.

stores are low, little ferritin is made. This condition elevates iron absorption because ferritin is a barrier to iron reaching the bloodstream. If iron stores are high, much ferritin is made, which binds iron as it enters these intestinal cells. Much of this iron is kept from ever entering the bloodstream because after just a few days, intestinal cells are sloughed off. Any iron bound to ferritin goes back to the intestinal lumen with the cells. The process is termed a mucosal block, because this process is in effect blocking iron absorption.[10] This response of ferritin to an increase in iron stores can be fairly rapid.

After iron is absorbed from the small intestine, it can be stored in the liver. Like in the intestine, ferritin is the primary iron-binder in the liver. Iron can be transported out of the liver to other body sites using a step that involves a copper enzyme mentioned in the section that described the difficulties in studying trace minerals (ceruloplasmin). In the blood, iron is carried to these sites via a transport protein called **transferrin.** This protein then binds to receptors on cells, which take up the whole transferrin protein by a process called endocytosis, described in Chapter 3. The transferrin then finds its way to a cell organelle called the lysosome where acid releases the iron from transferrin. The released iron can then become part of various iron-containing molecules, such as certain enzymes, hemoglobin (if a red blood cell is being made), myoglobin (a protein that traps oxygen in tissues), and ferritin (which stores iron and helps prevent toxicity). In states of iron overload, another protein, called **hemosiderin,** is made to bind up much of the excess iron. This protein also helps reduce iron toxicity, but it does not prevent it. Overall, the main defense against iron toxicity is ferritin in the small intestine. If a lot of iron manages to get by this defense, then the other mechanisms become an important consideration.

Much of the iron in the body is inserted into hemoglobin, which transports oxygen in red blood cells (Figure 12-2). The iron in hemoglobin is what actually binds the oxygen. These red blood cells do eventually die, but most of the iron from hemoglobin is conserved by the body. The same is true for iron used for other purposes. Nonetheless, some iron is lost each day via the GI tract, urine, and skin. Women who are menstruating also lose iron as part of that blood loss.[10]

Functions of Iron

Iron plays an important role in many parts of the body, including immune function, cognitive development, temperature regulation, energy metabolism, and work performance.[18]

Iron is a component of two proteins that are involved in the transport and metabolism of oxygen. In hemoglobin, iron is the oxygen carrier of the blood, which transports oxygen from the lungs to all tissues and assists in the transport of some carbon dioxide back to the lungs for expiration. When the oxygen-carrying capacity of the blood begins to decline, the kidneys produce the hormone **erythropoietin,** which targets the bone marrow to produce more red blood cells.

As part of myoglobin, iron provides oxygen to skeletal and heart muscle cells. Within the mitochondria, the electron transport chain uses iron as a component of cytochromes that carry electrons from $NADH + H^+$ and $FADH_2$ to molecular oxygen. The first step in the citric acid cycle, the conversion of citrate to isocitrate, requires an iron-containing enzyme. The limitation of these three processes in iron deficiency helps explain why this condition readily leads to fatigue upon physical exertion. Iron found in enzymes in the endoplasmic reticulum contributes to many processes, such as alcohol metabolism, drug detoxification, and carcinogen excretion, especially in the liver.

Iron in peroxidase enzymes helps break down toxic oxygen species, such as hydrogen peroxide (H_2O_2). Peroxidase enzymes are found in white blood cells and platelets (clotting factors in the blood). Iron also functions as a cofactor for some other enzymes, including those involved in the synthesis of collagen, various neurotransmitters (e.g., dopamine, epinephrine, norepinephrine, and serotonin), and eicosanoids.

When iron functions in cytochromes of the electron transport chain and in iron-requiring enzymes; it can exist stably in two different valences (2^+ and 3^+). Within cytochromes and enzymes, iron will switch between these two valences, which catalyzes the movement of electrons either along the electron transport chain or as part of an enzyme reaction. This feature of iron is very useful when the iron is confined within these systems, but this ability to readily change valences also makes iron very toxic if the iron roams free. In the latter case, iron can catalyze destructive reactions, including the formation of free radicals.

As a red blood cell matures, its nucleus is expelled along with its DNA. Such a cell cannot replace itself. The red blood cell goes on to have a life span of about 120 days.

erythropoietin A hormone secreted mostly by the kidneys that enhances red blood cell synthesis and stimulates red blood cell release from bone marrow.

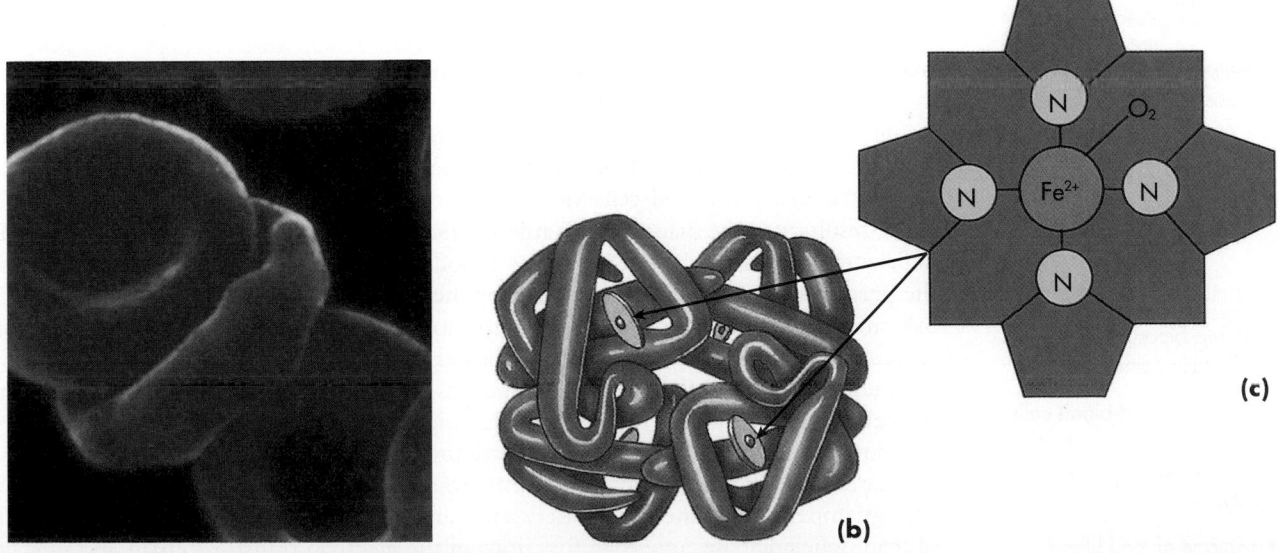

Figure 12-2 | (a) Red blood cells. (b) Most iron in the body is present in the hemoglobin molecules of the red blood cells. (c) Iron gives hemoglobin the ability to carry oxygen.

Food Sources of Iron

Food Item and Amount, with Bioavailability (in parentheses)	Iron (mg)
Oat bran cereal, 1 cup	15.0 (low)
Baked clams, 3 oz	14.0 (high)
Spinach, 1 cup	6.4 (low)
Kidney beans, 1 cup	5.3 (low)
Pot roast, 4 oz	3.9 (high)
Sirloin steak, 4 oz	3.8 (high)
Fried beef liver, 2 oz	3.6 (high)
Shrimp, 3 oz	2.7 (high)
Braunschweiger sausage, 1 piece	2.7 (high)
Flour tortilla, 1	2.4 (low)
Garbanzo beans, 1/2 cup	2.4 (low)
Navy beans, 1/2 cup	2.3 (low)
Baked potato, 1	1.7 (low)
Artichoke, 1	1.6 (low)
Whole-wheat bread, 1 slice	1.0 (low)

RDA for adult men, 8 mg;
RDA for adult women, 18 mg

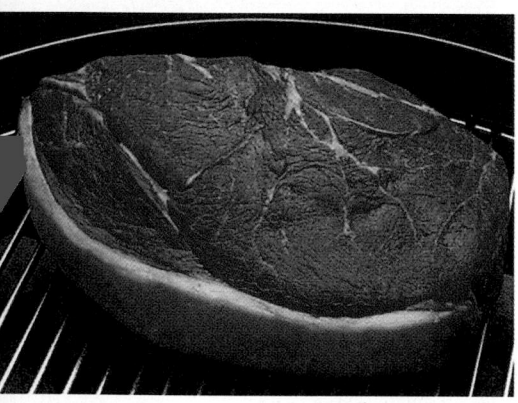

Red meat is a major source of iron in the North American diet. As noted in Chapter 7, a moderate serving about two times a week or less is a typical recommendation for red meat intake.

microcytic Describing red blood cells that are smaller than normal; literally, "small cell."

hypochromic Describing pale red blood cells lacking sufficient hemoglobin as a result of iron deficiency. Hypochromic cells have a reduced oxygen-carrying ability.

hematocrit The percentage of total blood volume occupied by red blood cells.

Iron in Foods

Because much of the iron in animal foods is heme iron, the most bioavailable form, meats are the richest sources of iron. The major iron sources in North American diets are animal foods, such as beef steaks, roasts, and hamburger. The next greatest sources are bakery products, including white breads, rolls, and crackers. Most of the iron in these products is elemental forms of iron added to refined flour as part of the enrichment process. For some cereal products, iron is added in higher amounts than used for enrichment, which makes the product a fortified product. About 5% of the iron added to grain products is absorbed. Overall, the North American diet contains about 5 to 7 mg of iron per 1000 kcal.[10] The bioavailability of the iron present in a meal depends on its form and the presence or absence of factors that influence absorption. The body's need for iron then ultimately determines how much iron actually is absorbed in the small intestine.[18]

A common cause of iron deficiency anemia in children is an overreliance on milk, a very poor source of iron, and too little meat in their diets. In the United States, a major contributor to decreasing rates of iron deficiency anemia in preschool children has been the use of iron-fortified formulas and cereals in the Special Supplemental Nutrition Program for Women, Infants, and Children (WIC program) (see Chapters 16 and 20).

Another source of iron is cooking utensils. When acidic foods, such as tomato sauce, are cooked in iron cookware, some iron from the pan is taken up by the food. Vegetarians can especially benefit from this interaction. The replacement of iron cookware with stainless steel and aluminum cookware in recent times likely has decreased the amount of iron in the diet.

Iron Needs

Because a major source of iron loss can be due to menstrual blood loss, the iron RDA varies greatly with age and gender. For adult women, the RDA is 18 mg/day, while it is 8 mg/day for adult men. The RDA for teenage girls, 15 mg/day, is slightly lower than that for adult women. The RDA for teenage boys, 11 mg/day, is slightly higher than that for adult men because of the need to support more lean tissue growth during the teenage years. All these values are based on the need to balance iron intake with iron losses. It is also assumed that 18% of dietary iron will be absorbed.[10] The Daily Value for iron used on food and supplement labels is 18 mg. The average daily intake for North American women is 12 mg, whereas among men it is about 17 mg.

Iron-Deficiency Diseases

Iron deficiency is the most common trace mineral deficiency in North America. In severe iron deficiency, there is not enough iron to produce all the hemoglobin needed, which results in iron deficiency anemia. Anemia represents any impairment in transporting oxygen in the blood; iron deficiency anemia is the most common form of anemia. When this anemia occurs, red blood cells viewed under a microscope appear small and show less color, resulting in the diagnosis of a **microcytic, hypochromic** anemia (Figure 12-3). Iron deficiency anemia can be detected by a blood measurement called **hematocrit,** which is the percent of blood volume occupied by the red blood cells. A value below 34 to 37% indicates iron deficiency anemia. An even more accurate measure is blood hemoglobin. A value less than 10 to 11 g/dl also indicates iron deficiency anemia.[18]

Anemia in any form impairs energy because aerobic respiration cannot occur without oxygen. Obvious signs of anemia include fatigue upon exertion and difficulties in mental concentration. However, aerobic respiration is also important to many unseen body processes, including those that contribute to organ system development during growth. Energy impairments due to iron deficiency anemia are also made worse by other effects of iron deficiency. Because iron functions in the electron transport chain and in the citric acid cycle, impairments in those functions impair aerobic respiration. In addition to effects on energy metabolism, iron deficiency also compromises immune function.

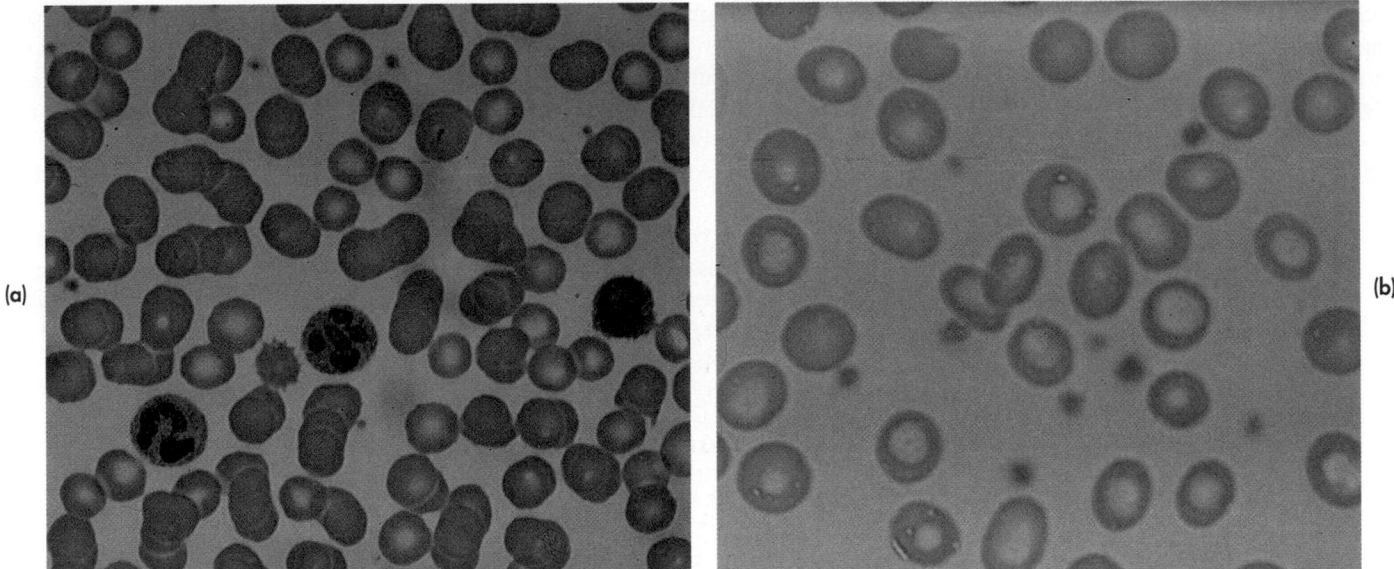

(a)

(b)

Figure 12-3 | Iron deficiency anemia. (a) Normal cells—both cell size and color are normal. (b) Iron-deficient cells—both cell size and color are decreased. The loss of color stems from the lower amount of the pigment hemoglobin. The stages of iron depletion in the body progress from (1) low ferritin in the blood to (2) low transferrin saturation in the blood to (3) microcytic hypochromic anemia.

It is very important to note that some people can have a marginal iron deficiency that does not produce anemia.[18] In this state, aerobic respiration is still impaired to some extent. However, this impairment occurs not because of anemia, but rather because of iron's other roles in aerobic respiration. In addition, immune function can be impaired. Because marginal deficiency does not involve anemia, a hemoglobin or hematocrit measurement will not detect marginal iron deficiency. For this reason, if a physician or a registered dietitian is seeing a client who shows signs of fatigue upon exertion and concentration problems, a hemoglobin or hematocrit measurement cannot be the sole means of ruling out an iron concern. Fortunately, unlike for marginal deficiencies of some other trace minerals, many clinical laboratories can perform other tests for iron status. The most common method used has been serum ferritin, but another blood measure, such as a rise in transferrin receptors in the blood, may soon become more widely used.

Many different groups are at risk for iron deficiency. In fact, it may be simpler to say who tends not to be at risk than list everyone at risk.[18] One group that tends not to be at high risk are adult males who consume meat regularly. On the other hand, young adult women, as well as teenage girls, are often at risk for iron deficiency due to blood iron losses and lower than average meat consumption.[19] Women with heavy menstrual blood losses are especially prone to iron deficiency. Pregnant women don't have to contend with menstrual blood losses, but iron is still a concern. During pregnancy, much of the body's iron is used to expand the blood supply and for other physical changes. As a person ages, iron can become a problem for both genders because food intake often declines. In addition, body iron absorption and distribution can become less efficient. At the opposite end of the age spectrum, just after birth, preterm infants (born before 37 weeks after conception) can have iron problems. During the first six months to one year of age, iron stores present at birth should be able to meet much of the infant's needs. Because these iron stores are built mostly during the last weeks of pregnancy, a preterm birth cuts short the time to build iron stores.

Two other groups of people prone to iron deficiency are children who are picky eaters (these children typically avoid iron-rich foods) and vegetarians. The latter group has a challenge to get enough iron because, as noted earlier, meat provides relatively well-absorbed dietary heme iron, plus meat promotes iron absorption from other

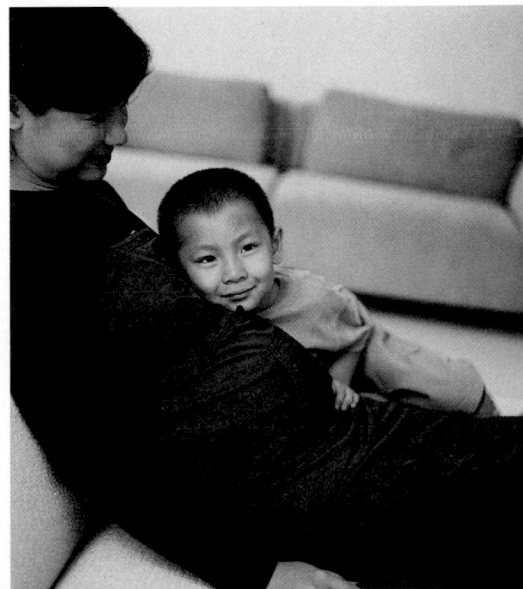

Pregnancy greatly increases iron needs, as does growth in childhood.

Consumption of dirt and similar nonfood substances may lead to iron deficiency anemia because these substances can bind much of the iron in the GI tract. The practice of eating nonfood items, termed *pica*, is discussed in Chapter 16. Blood loss caused by intestinal or bloodborne parasite infections is another common cause of anemia around the world.

hemochromatosis A disorder of iron metabolism characterized by increased absorption of iron, saturation of iron-binding proteins, and deposition of hemosiderin in the liver tissue.

Testing is available to determine the presence of the genes that are responsible for hemochromatosis. The cost is usually about $150.

Chapter 9 noted that if men, in general, and older women take a multivitamin and mineral supplement, it should be low in iron or iron-free because of their increased risk for iron toxicity.

Hemosiderosis is the storage of excess iron in the form of hemosiderin. This form of excess iron is not associated with the organ damage of hemochromatosis, because excess iron is stored in areas of normal storage. In hemochromatosis, the iron accumulates in body organs outside normal areas, such as in the liver and heart, and causes organ deterioration.

foods. Moreover, the high oxalic acid content of many vegetarian diets can further depress iron absorption. On the other hand, vegetarian diets usually are rich in vitamin C. Vegetarians should consume vitamin C–rich foods simultaneously with the few nonanimal foods that contain appreciable amounts of iron. Use of an iron-fortified ready-to-eat breakfast cereal can be useful for vegetarians, even though this iron is not as well absorbed as heme iron. Another option is a multivitamin and mineral supplement that contains iron.

Finally, the donation of 1 pint (0.5 L) of blood represents a loss of 200 to 250 mg of iron. It generally takes several months to replace this iron. Most healthy people can donate blood two to four times a year without harmful consequences; generally, women need a longer interval between donations to rebuild their iron stores. As a precaution, blood banks first screen potential donors' blood for evidence of anemia.

Upper Level for Iron

Although iron deficiency is a major public health concern, iron also poses a risk for toxicity. The Upper Level for iron is 45 mg/day. Higher amounts can lead to stomach irritation.[10] Iron's ability to alternate between two valences (2^+ vs. 3^+) is functional when confined to cytochromes and enzymes, but is toxic when not. One reason for the toxicity is that changes in iron valences can catalyze the formation of free radicals. Two prominent causes of significant iron toxicity are the genetic condition **hemochromatosis** and repeated blood transfusions. The iron absorption section in this chapter described the mucosal block that protects the body from oral iron. In hemochromatosis this mucosal block works less efficiently.[12] The iron introduced into the body through repeated blood transfusions also bypasses the protective system and can result in dangerously high iron stores in the body.[10]

Because of the body's protective system, it is generally not easy to produce severe toxicity due to oral iron consumption. One exception to this general rule involves the susceptibility of children to iron toxicity. Children are more vulnerable to oral iron poisoning than adults because their protective system cannot respond as rapidly as an adult's. The prime source of iron overload in children is the consumption of excess chewable iron-containing supplements. FDA has recently ruled that all iron supplements must carry a warning about toxicity, and those with 30 mg of iron or more per tablet must be individually wrapped.

Treatment of iron toxicity depends on the situation. For hemochromatosis, a normal treatment is periodic blood removal (the same removal process as when blood is donated to blood banks). Another approach that is used in some situations is administration of a drug that binds iron in the bloodstream and enhances its excretion. More can be found on iron overload in the accompanying Expert Opinion by Dr. Barbara Bowman and Dr. Giuseppina Imperatore. Finally, besides overt toxicity, there is some (but conflicting) evidence that mild iron toxicity contributes to health problems such as cardiovascular disease and arthritis.

Concept | Check

Iron absorption depends mostly on its form and the body's need for it. Absorption is hindered by a mucosal block, but excess iron intake can override the system, leading to toxicity. Iron absorption increases in the presence of vitamin C and decreases in the presence of large amounts of oxalates and some components of grains, such as phytic acid. Iron is most important in synthesizing hemoglobin and myoglobin, in supporting immune function, and in energy metabolism. Iron deficiency can cause a form of anemia. It is particularly important for women of child-bearing age to consume adequate iron, primarily to replace that lost in menstrual blood. Sources include red meat, pork, liver, enriched grains and cereals, and oysters. Iron toxicity usually results from a genetic disorder called hemochromatosis. This disease causes the overabsorption and accumulation of iron, which can result in severe liver and heart damage.

Zinc (Zn)

Although zinc has been recognized as an essential nutrient in animals since the early 1900s, zinc deficiency was first recognized in humans in the early 1960s in Egypt and Iran. The deficiency was determined to be the cause of growth restriction and inadequate sexual development in humans.[13] Curiously, the dietary zinc content was not that low. The key factor was that the customary diet contained almost exclusively unleavened bread and little animal protein. Unleavened bread is very high in phytic acid and other factors that decrease zinc bioavailability. Yeast fermentation in the preparation of bread dough reduces the effect of phytic acid by tenfold. In addition, parasite infestation and the practice of eating dirt also contributed to these cases of severe zinc deficiency observed in humans.

In North America, zinc deficiencies were first observed in the early 1970s in hospitalized patients receiving total parenteral nutrition. Originally, zinc was not added to the intravenous solutions, but the protein source in the solutions was based on milk protein or blood fibrin, which contain zinc. When the solutions were later changed to include mostly isolated amino acids as the protein source, zinc-deficiency symptoms quickly developed. The isolated amino acids source of protein is very low in zinc.

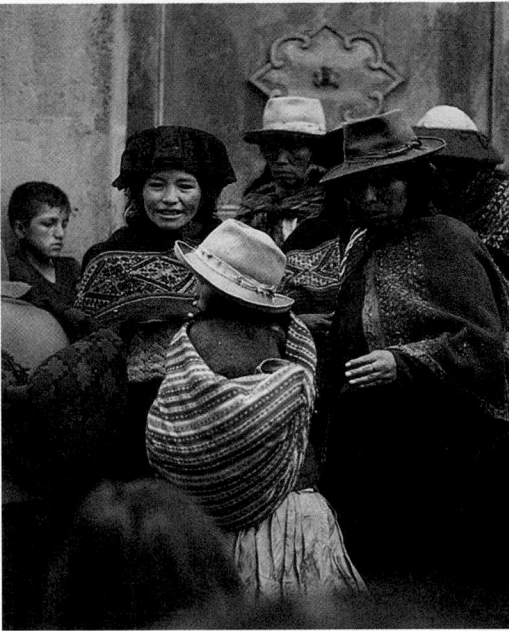

Minimal intakes of energy, protein, and zinc limit the growth of people worldwide.

Absorption, Transport, Storage, and Excretion of Zinc

Zinc is absorbed throughout the small intestine. Factors that affect the absorption of zinc include the body's need for zinc (especially important) and the composition of the meal in which zinc is consumed. These factors are summarized in Table 12-2. The absorption and transport of zinc utilizes a two-step process. The first step is the uptake or membrane binding at the mucosal surface. The second step is the transport of zinc across the mucosal cell and the release into the bloodstream, but the process is not completely understood. After entering the blood, zinc binds to blood proteins, such as albumin, for transport to the liver. The liver releases zinc into general circulation bound to proteins, such as globulins.[10] There is no storage site per se for zinc in the body. Zinc status is primarily maintained during low intakes by conserving (e.g., recycling) what zinc is available.[13]

When zinc is absorbed into intestinal cells, it induces the synthesis of **metallothionein,** a protein that binds zinc in much the same way that ferritin binds iron. Homeostatic regulation of zinc absorption may partly be due to the synthesis of metallothionein, because it hinders the movement of zinc from intestinal cells. If zinc is not transferred to the blood from the intestinal cells within their short lifetime, it is sloughed off along with the cell and excreted. Thus, a mucosal block works against the overabsorption of zinc and iron, but much more so in the case of iron. Large doses of zinc override the mucosal block. Luckily for overconsumers, zinc is also readily excreted via the pancreas into the intestinal tract and then leaves the body by way of the feces. It is also excreted in small amounts in urine and sweat.

Like iron absorption, zinc absorption is influenced by the types of food ingested. Absorption is more likely when animal protein sources are consumed, when the body's zinc needs are elevated, or when small amounts are consumed.[10,13]

metallothionein A protein that binds and regulates the release of zinc and copper in intestinal and liver cells.

Table 12-2 | Factors That Affect Zinc Absorption

Increase Absorption	Decrease Absorption
Moderate zinc intake	Phytic acid and calcium supplements
Body deficiency	Excessive zinc intake
Animal protein	Oxide form in supplements

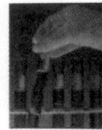

Iron Overload: Too Much of a Good Thing
Barbara A. Bowman, Ph.D., and Giuseppina Imperatore, M.D., Ph.D.

Nutritionists consider iron to be the gold standard of micronutrients, because we know more about the dietary intake, metabolism, and nutritional requirements of iron than any other trace element. Despite this extensive knowledge and the array of sophisticated techniques for evaluating iron nutrition, however, more than 1 billion people suffer from iron deficiency, which is the most prevalent micronutrient deficiency in the world.

Iron deficiency is also a significant health problem in the United States, especially in young children and women of childbearing age, particularly pregnant women. Iron deficiency is a special concern for women and children because one of its major consequences is anemia. Anemia, defined as a low concentration of hemoglobin in blood, leads to decreased work capacity in adults, developmental delays and behavioral disturbances in children, increased susceptibility to infection, and increased mortality in both children and adults. In the United States, about 3.3 million women of childbearing age and 240,000 children age 1 to 2 years have iron deficiency anemia, the most severe form of iron deficiency.

Iron overload lies at the opposite end of the spectrum of iron status. If untreated, iron overload disease, like iron deficiency, can lead to illness and even death. This section examines iron overload in more detail.

Etiology of Iron Overload

What causes iron overload? The major cause of iron overload in the United States is hereditary hemochromatosis, a genetic condition that affects about one person out of every 200 to 500 in the United States. Iron overload can also occur in chronic liver disease due to alcohol abuse, viral infections, and chronic anemias requiring frequent blood transfusions (e.g., thalassemia). The specific genetic lesion in hereditary hemochromatosis was identified in 1996, and two

major mutations have been identified. The fundamental defect involves the regulation of iron absorption. In hereditary hemochromatosis, iron absorption is excessive, and iron absorption is not reduced when iron status is normal. The human body does not have a mechanism for eliminating excess iron. Therefore, after many years of absorbing too much iron, excessive amounts of iron can accumulate in the body, leading to iron overload and tissue injury. If undetected and untreated for many years, iron levels can build up in the liver, heart, pancreas, joints, and pituitary gland and can eventually lead to liver disease, heart disease, diabetes, arthritis, and hypopituitarism with hypogonadism. People at a late stage of iron overload may have skin that turns bronze or gray. The diseases caused by iron overload usually appear by age 40 to 60, although some people are affected earlier and others never become ill. With early detection and treatment, organ damage can be prevented. However, without lifelong treatment, organ damage may be permanent and life-threatening.

Up to 1 million Americans, mostly people of European descent, have the mutation for hemochromatosis. However, far fewer actually develop iron overload. Some people have the mutation but never get iron overload, probably because clinical expression of iron overload depends on additional factors, including the severity of the metabolic defect, the amount and type of iron in the diet, other dietary factors that enhance or inhibit iron absorption, environmental factors, and blood loss (menstruation, for example).

Diagnosis and Treatment of Iron Overload

Early detection and lifelong treatment can prevent the complications of hemochromatosis. The major approach to diagnosis is a series of blood tests to measure the amount of iron in the blood, such as the extent to which transferrin is saturated with iron and the amount of ferritin in the blood. The same

---

Critical | Thinking

Zinc lozenges have received much attention as a treatment for the common cold. You tell a classmate that you do not feel that the evidence is convincing enough to recommend this practice to the general public. Your friend would like to know what it would take to convince you that zinc is a reasonable treatment for the common cold.

Functions of Zinc

It is hard to name a body process or body structure that isn't affected either directly or indirectly by zinc. Some zinc functions involve enzymes in which zinc is either part of the catalytic reaction or it stabilizes the enzyme structure. The exact number of known zinc-dependent enzymes depends on classification (i.e., two similar enzymes can be called two different enzymes or a single enzyme with different forms). Suffice it to say that over 50 (and as many as 200 or more) enzymes need zinc to function. These functions contribute to DNA and RNA synthesis, alcohol metabolism, protein metabolism and related growth and development of the body, antioxidant defenses (see the functions of copper for details), immune function, and acid/base balance in the body.[13] In addition to enzyme-related functions, zinc also stabilizes the structures of cell membrane proteins, certain hormones, and gene transcription factors (called zinc fingers). The cell membrane function has very broad effects because cell membrane stability influences the membrane receptors, which control actions in cells.

blood tests are used during treatment to monitor the amount of iron in the body and the response to treatment. Genetic testing is also being studied. However, not everyone with the mutation develops iron overload. Because of concern about the need for privacy and possible discrimination in employment and insurance, genetic screening for hereditary hemochromatosis is not recommended. People who have been diagnosed with hereditary hemochromatosis should tell their family members and urge them to get tested, too.

Treatment of iron overload is straightforward, safe, and effective. After they have been diagnosed, people with iron overload have blood removed regularly, usually a unit or pint of blood, to remove the excess iron that has accumulated. The procedure, which is called phlebotomy, is exactly the same as when blood is donated. The frequency of phlebotomy depends on how much iron has built up. When iron overload is first diagnosed, phlebotomy may be needed every week or two. When accumulated iron has been reduced to a safe amount, phlebotomy may be needed only a few times a year, but it must be continued. Health-care providers use blood testing to determine when phlebotomy treatment is needed.

People with hemochromatosis must be sure to follow their doctor's advice and get tested regularly to prevent complications from developing. For most, periodic phlebotomy will be needed for the rest of their lives. It is also important for people with hemochromatosis to avoid alcohol and raw shellfish, which can damage the liver. Dietary supplements that contain iron must not be used, and foods highly fortified with iron should be avoided. The same advice may be given as well for vitamin C supplements. Foods containing heme iron pose more of a risk than foods with nonheme iron be-

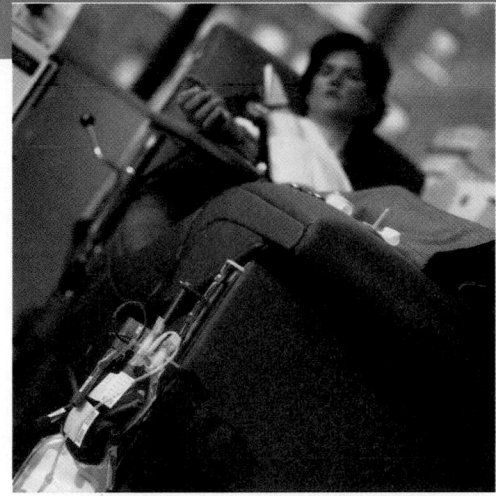

Regular donation of blood is the main intervention for treating iron overload in the body.

cause heme iron is more readily absorbed. Most people with hereditary hemochromatosis are not aware that they have a predisposition to accumulating excessive amounts of iron. If such a person were to decide to use iron supplements to increase his or her energy or to combat fatigue, for example, iron accumulation and tissue damage could be accelerated and enhanced, increasing the risk of chronic disease. For this reason, iron supplements should not be used indiscriminately but should be used only when iron deficiency has been diagnosed by a health professional and iron therapy is prescribed.

As you can see, with iron more than perhaps any other nutrient, it is critical to meet daily requirements for the proper nutrient intake—not too little, not too much, but just the right amount. Different individuals have different needs. People who don't consume enough iron to meet their needs can develop iron deficiency and eventually anemia. On the other hand, for some people, consuming too much iron every day can lead to serious illness, including death. Hereditary hemochromatosis is one of the first examples of how a gene interacts with nutrition (iron intake) to affect risk of disease. As the public and health professionals become more aware of hereditary hemochromatosis, iron overload can be detected earlier, treated more effectively, and ultimately prevented.

Drs. Imperatore and Bowman are epidemiologists at the Centers for Disease Control and Prevention in Atlanta, Ga. Dr. Imperatore is a genetic epidemiologist and Dr. Bowman is Chief of the Chronic Disease Nutrition Branch. Both are especially interested in the disease hemochromatosis.

Zinc in Foods

In general, protein-rich diets are also rich in zinc. North Americans get about 70% of their dietary zinc from animal foods. Lean meats—especially beef, other red meats, and shellfish—are among the best zinc sources. Plant sources of zinc, such as nuts, beans, and whole grains, can also deliver substantial amounts of zinc to body cells. Zinc is not part of the enrichment process so refined flours are not a good source.

Zinc Needs

The RDA for zinc of 11 mg/day for adult males and 8 mg/day for adult females is based on replacing daily losses via feces, skin, and urine. The RDA assumes that 40% of dietary zinc will be absorbed.[10] The Daily Value used on food and supplement labels for zinc is 15 mg. Average adult intakes in North America are 9 to 13 mg/day, with men showing the higher value.[19]

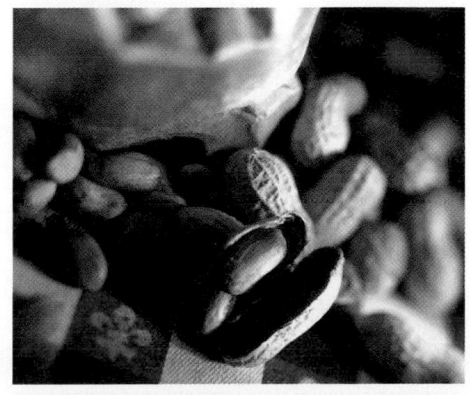

Peanuts are a plant source of zinc.

Food Sources of Zinc

Food Item and Amount	Zinc (mg)
Steamed oysters, 6	49.9
Sirloin steak, 4 oz	7.4
Peanuts, 1 cup	4.8
Pot roast, 3 oz	4.6
Special K cereal, 1 cup	3.8
Wheat germ, 1/4 cup	3.5
Lamb chops, 3 oz	2.7
Black-eyed peas, 1 cup	2.2
Plain yogurt, 1 cup	2.2
Lean ham, 3 oz	1.9
Swiss cheese, 1.5 oz	1.7
Ricotta cheese, 1/2 cup	1.7
Sunflower seeds, 1 oz	1.5
Cheddar cheese, 1.5 oz	1.3
Enriched white rice, 1/2 cup	1.1
RDA for adult men, 11 mg; RDA for adult women, 8 mg	

acrodermatitis enteropathica A rare inherited childhood disorder that results in the inability to absorb adequate amounts of zinc from the diet. Symptoms include skin lesions, hair loss, and diarrhea. If untreated, the condition can result in death during infancy or early childhood. Management of this condition is with zinc supplements.

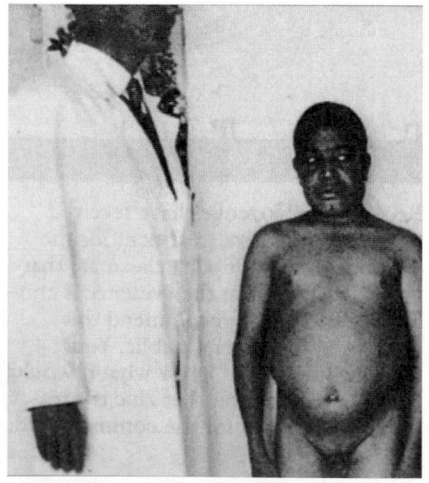

Figure 12-4 | An example of zinc deficiency. An Egyptian farm boy, age 16 years and 49 inches tall, with dwarfism and inadequate sexual development associated with a zinc deficiency.

One key issue in understanding zinc needs is body adaptation via conservation to different intakes, as mentioned in the opening section. Some research suggests that people change their zinc absorption and excretion rates to allow them to tolerate lower intakes than what is seen among people who eat relatively high amounts of zinc.[13]

Zinc-Deficiency Diseases

In a zinc deficiency, not all zinc functions decrease at the same rates. Some are impaired even in mild zinc deficiency, whereas others do not show a major impairment unless the deficiency becomes severe.[13] Cell membrane functions may be the most sensitive change to a mild zinc deficiency. Still other zinc-requiring functions manage to use zinc so effectively that they operate fairly well even in a pronounced zinc deficiency. Thus, the symptoms of zinc deficiency depend a lot on its severity. The symptoms seem also to depend on what else is taking place in the body at the same time, such that some zinc functions are affected mainly when a zinc deficiency is combined with certain other factors (e.g., the presence of another disease or a period of rapid growth).

Linking poor health with zinc deficiency can be challenging because zinc affects so many molecular processes and functions, either directly or indirectly. For example, a severe zinc deficiency can affect bone growth. There are many possible reasons for this effect on bone, including a number of zinc-dependent enzymes and hormones.

As noted at the beginning of the zinc section, severe deficiency in humans was first reported in areas of the Middle East. Symptoms included severely stunted growth, poor taste sensitivity, and impaired sexual maturation in the males (Figure 12-4).

In certain parts of the world, where poverty limits food choices, the effects of zinc deficiency can be clearly seen in children. Symptoms include severe, even fatal diarrhea, poor growth, impaired vitamin A function, and high risk of pneumonia (presumably due to impaired immune function). In these same parts of the world, zinc deficiency in pregnant women may contribute to increased infant mortality and birth defects.[13]

Besides dietary causes of severe zinc deficiency, this state can also be produced by a genetic condition in which zinc absorption is impaired. This disease, **acrodermatitis enteropathica,** is recognizable by a skin condition that develops in infancy. The condition can be treated with supplemental zinc. Preterm infants can also show signs of zinc deficiency for the same general reason described for iron and preterm infants.

Marginal zinc deficiency may occur in many people, though there are still many questions to be answered. The classic example of documented marginal zinc deficiency involves a study of a group of children in the Denver, Colorado, area. The study reported that marginal zinc deficiency was responsible for impaired growth in a number of children. Other groups that may be prone to marginal zinc deficiencies are Crohn's disease patients, people on kidney dialysis, diabetic individuals, older adults, sickle-cell anemia patients, alcoholics, and children with Down's syndrome. Vegetarians may also be vulnerable to marginal zinc status. However, there is some evidence that vegetarians adapt to low intake by reducing zinc excretion while increasing zinc absorption.[13]

Upper Level for Zinc

The Upper Level set for zinc is 40 mg/day, based on the ability of zinc to interfere with copper status as measured by a fall in the activity of copper-containing enzymes.[10] Zinc supplements at approximately 5 to 20 times the RDA can reduce HDL-cholesterol, perhaps by interfering with copper absorption. Again, this finding shows why mineral supplements should not be consumed in excess of the Upper Level on a chronic basis unless under close scrutiny of a physician. This caution includes use of zinc lozenges to treat cold symptoms for more than a week or so. (Note that these lozenges have a minor effect, if any, on cold symptoms.) Zinc intakes over 100 mg/day also result in diarrhea, cramps, nausea, vomiting, and depressed immune system function, especially if intake exceeds 2 g/day.

▌Copper (Cu)

Like iron, copper can catalyze certain reactions by alternating between two valences (Cu^+ and Cu^{2+}). Also as with iron, this property is very useful when copper is contained within enzymes or other proteins, but dangerous when not. Thus, specific chaperone proteins are used to distribute copper around the body. Copper enzymes perform a number of different functions and are quite impaired by severe copper deficiency.[16] In addition, some research suggests that moderate copper deficiency may impair copper function enough to have subtle, but important, long-term effects on health.

Absorption, Transport, Storage, and Excretion of Copper

Copper is absorbed mostly in the small intestine, with a percent absorption that can vary widely (12 to 70%).[10] The factors affecting copper absorption have not been studied as well as the factors affecting iron or zinc. However, one major factor in copper absorption can be zinc supplementation. High-dose zinc supplementation can impair copper absorption to the point of causing a severe copper deficiency. This impairment probably involves some competition between copper and zinc for a common intestinal receptor.

After intestinal absorption, copper moves rapidly into the liver and kidney, the main sites of storage. Following this initial distribution, copper transport is very controlled. Copper moves from the liver to other tissues tightly bound to the protein ceruloplasmin, which also has an enzyme function (see the functions section). Ceruloplasmin then releases copper to cells via a specific receptor. Excess copper is excreted primarily in the bile. In a genetic disorder called Wilson's disease, this excretion is impaired, which can produce copper toxicity (see the section on Upper Level for copper).

Functions of Copper

Copper functions in enzymes as a catalyst that alternates between two different valences.[16] One of these enzymes, ceruloplasmin (and possibly some other copper enzymes) are needed to transport iron from the liver to various functional sites, including where iron is inserted into hemoglobin. Ceruloplasmin may also have an antioxidant function by inhibiting iron-catalyzed formation of free radicals. An even better characterized antioxidant function for copper is its role in two of the three members of a family of enzymes known as **superoxide dismutase** (also called SOD). This family of enzymes eliminates one particular free radical known as superoxide (O_2^-). Copper is needed for function of the SOD enzyme found in the cytosol of cells (partners with zinc) and for another SOD enzyme found outside of cells (again partners with zinc). (A third SOD enzyme is found in mitochondria, but it contains only manganese.)

Copper is also part of a number of other enzymes.[16] One of these enzymes is cytochrome C oxidase, which catalyzes the last step of the electron transport chain. In this step of the chain, oxygen enters and water leaves. Another copper enzyme forms norepinephrine, which is important both as a hormone and a neurotransmitter. Still another copper enzyme, lysyl oxidase, is very important in connective tissue formation. Lysyl oxidase cross-links the strands within two structural proteins that give tensile strength to connective tissues. Connective tissue comprises a large portion of structures such as blood vessels, lungs, skin, and the protein portion of bone. The two structural proteins that are cross-linked by lysyl oxidase are elastin and collagen. The latter is the same protein whose structure is affected by vitamin C (review Chapter 10). Vitamin C is needed to put collagen in the right shape for the three individual strands to curl around each other. Lysyl oxidase completes the process by cross-linking the strands together.

One study has shown that megadose zinc supplements (80 mg/day of zinc oxide) reduces the progression of macular degeneration by 25% in people who had a moderate case of the disease. The zinc supplements worked even better when provided in combination with 400 IU of vitamin E, 500 mg of vitamin C, and 15 mg of beta-carotene. (Copper oxide [2 mg] was also included because zinc decreases copper absorption.) Although the study had some flaws, some experts suggest that adults who have evidence of moderate macular degeneration talk to their physicians and eye-care specialists about the possibility of following such a protocol.[2]

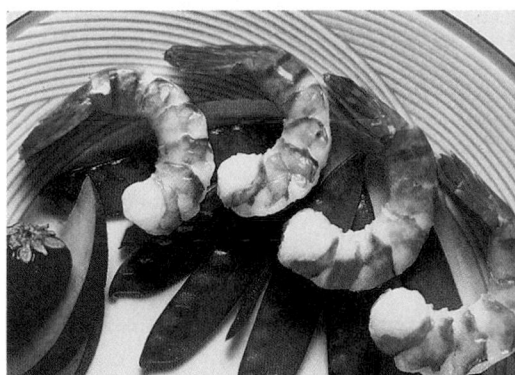

Seafood is a good source of copper.

superoxide dismutase An enzyme that can quench (deactivate) a superoxide negative free radical (O_2^-). This can contain the trace minerals copper, zinc, and manganese.

Copper is also essential to optimal immune function, though the exact reasons are still unclear. Possibly, copper antioxidant functions help protect immune cells, which are often under a lot of oxidative stress.

Food Sources of Copper

Food Item and Amount	Copper (μg)
Fried beef liver, 3 oz	3800
Power bar, 1	700
Walnuts, 1/2 cup	600
Kidney beans, 1 cup	500
Lobster, 3 oz	400
Molasses, 3 tbsp	300
Sunflower seeds, 2 tbsp	300
Shrimp, 3 oz	300
Raisin Bran cereal, 1 cup	300
Great Grains cereal, 1 cup	300
Semi-sweet chocolate, 1 oz	210
Black-eyed peas, 1/2 cup cooked	200
Wheat germ 1/4 cup	200
Milk chocolate, 1 oz	110
Whole-wheat bread, 1 slice	80
RDA for adults, 900 μg	

An inherited copper-related disease called Wilson's disease results in the accumulation of copper in the liver, brain, kidneys, and cornea of the eye. People with this disease can't incorporate copper into ceruloplasmin and also have a decreased ability to excrete copper in the bile. Some of the wide range of symptoms include liver, nervous system, and psychiatric disorders as well as kidney abnormalities. If caught early in life, treatment with agents that bind copper, such as penicillamine, or use of high dosages of zinc to block copper absorption, can prevent tissue damage and reduce the mental degeneration commonly seen in Wilson's disease.

Copper in Foods

Good food sources of copper include liver, shellfish, nuts, seeds, soy products, avocadoes, and dark chocolate. Legumes, whole-grain products, and often tap water are also important sources. Meat is a marginal source of copper. Nonetheless, the copper present can contribute at least part of one's copper needs. In addition, meat may promote copper absorption from other foods, just as it does with iron. Cow's milk is not a good copper source. Unlike some trace minerals, copper is not typically added to ready-to-eat breakfast cereals in high amounts because cereal fats can be oxidized by the copper complexes most often used for food fortification.

Copper Needs

The adult RDA for copper is 900 μg/day for adults, based on the need for normal activity of copper-containing enzymes (e.g., SOD) and proteins (e.g., ceruloplasmin) in the body.[10] The Daily Value on food and supplement labels for copper is 2 mg. The average adult intake in North America is about 1 to 1.6 mg/day. Women generally consume the smaller amount.

Copper-Deficiency Diseases

The most common cause of severe copper deficiency is high-dose zinc supplementation, which inhibits copper absorption. Prominent symptoms include iron deficiency-like anemia and a low count for one type of white blood cells.[16] Some medical situations, such as recovery from burns or kidney dialysis, may also lead to a copper deficiency. Preterm infants are also prone to copper deficiency during the first few days of life and then again during the catch-up growth period of the first year. The reason for this deficiency is the same as that noted for iron and zinc.

For a number of years, copper researchers have been interested in marginal copper deficiency. Two concerns have spurred this interest. First, many health problems, especially those involving inflammation, such as rheumatoid arthritis, may raise copper needs. Second, the types of symptoms observed in experimental animals with copper deficiency (sometimes with just a marginal deficiency) resemble common human health problems (elevated blood cholesterol, suboptimal immune function, and poor resistance to oxidative stress). Future research will likely determine how much we should be concerned about marginal copper deficiency.

Upper Level for Copper

The Upper Level for copper is 10 mg/day, based on the risk of liver damage.[10] Generally, copper toxicity in humans is not very common because intakes are usually not very high and because our bodies can regulate copper storage through excretion via the bile. At single supplemental doses of 10 to 15 mg, though, copper provided in aqueous forms tends to cause vomiting.

Concept | Check

As with iron absorption, zinc absorption is partly regulated by a mucosal block. Animal protein sources, increased body needs, and small intakes lead to increased zinc absorption. Zinc functions as a cofactor for many enzymes and is important for growth and development and for immune function. Beef, seafood, and whole grains are rich food sources of zinc. Copper functions mainly as part of enzymes and other compounds involved in iron metabolism, cross-linking of collagen, and neurotransmitter synthesis. A copper deficiency can result in a form of anemia and impaired immune function. Food sources of copper are liver, seafood, legumes, nuts, and whole grains.

▌ Selenium (Se)

Selenium deficiency and toxicity have occurred in livestock in areas where the soil is very low or very high in selenium, respectively. The same is true in humans, though the number of documented cases is fewer in humans. Selenium functions in certain enzymes and has drawn interest for its roles in antioxidant defense and thyroid hormone production as well as possible applications in cancer prevention.

Absorption, Transport, Storage, and Excretion of Selenium

Selenium enters the body in many ionic forms. Most selenium in foods is bound to derivatives of the amino acids methionine and cysteine. Because these substances are readily absorbed, the bioavailability of selenium is considerably higher than that of iron and zinc. About 50 to 100% of dietary selenium intake is absorbed, and it is not affected by one's selenium status. Because no physiological mechanism appears to control selenium absorption, selenium has a definite potential for toxicity.[11]

Not much is known about the transport of selenium. What is known is that selenium is made available for use when the particular amino acid it is bound to is catabolized. The selenium can then be incorporated into macromolecules, transported to various organs, or excreted. Homeostasis of selenium in the body is achieved through excretion, mainly via the urine and feces. Urinary excretion of selenium increases as dietary intake increases. Selenium is stored primarily bound to the amino acid methionine and as part of glutathione peroxide enzyme. Both are found throughout the body.

Functions of Selenium

Selenium is incorporated into certain enzymes as part of an amino acid known as selenocysteine (i.e., selenium bound to the amino acid cysteine).[3] Normally, the amino acid cysteine contains sulfur, but in selenocysteine, the sulfur is replaced by selenium. The best understood enzymatic function of selenium occurs as part of two enzymes, each named glutathione peroxidase (one is inside cells, whereas the other is outside cells including in the blood). Glutathione peroxidase is part of the body's antioxidant defense network described in the vitamin E section of Chapter 9. Some of this network is shown in Figure 12-5. Glutathione peroxidase eliminates peroxides, including hydrogen peroxide. These peroxides occur in the body as a by-product of certain body reactions and can also arise in other ways. Peroxide accumulation is a concern because peroxides can easily form free radicals. Another antioxidant system that uses selenium is the newly described **thioredoxin** family of enzymes.[3]

Selenium also functions in an enzyme that is part of the process that makes thyroid hormones. Thyroid hormones are very important in stimulating energy input to various body processes needed for growth or maintenance. A few other proteins in the body have been found to contain selenium, but their function is not yet known.

Selenium in Foods

Animal products are good sources of selenium, though some are better than others. Grain products and nuts are also good sources. Whole-grain products generally have more selenium than those made with white flour, though the latter can also provide selenium. The exact amount of selenium in grain products depends on the selenium content of the soil in which the grains are grown. For example, in the United States, pasta tends to be high in selenium because the durum wheat that is used tends to come from high-selenium soils in the Dakotas.

You have now seen that the absence of many nutrients from the diet can lead to anemia:

- Vitamin E deficiency can lead to hemolytic anemia (see Chapter 9).
- Vitamin K deficiency, especially coupled with use of certain antibiotics, can lead to blood loss and thus to hemorrhagic anemia (see Chapter 9).
- Vitamin B-6 deficiency can lead to microcytic anemia and sideroblastic anemia (see Chapter 10).
- Folate deficiency can lead to megaloblastic anemia (see Chapter 10).
- Vitamin B-12 malabsorption can lead to megaloblastic anemia (see Chapter 10).
- An iron deficiency can lead to microcytic hypochromic anemia.
- A copper deficiency can lead, although rarely, to iron deficiency anemia because copper aids in iron metabolism.

Some interesting research has suggested that a moderately high-dose supplement of selenium (i.e., 200 µg/day) may lower the risk of certain cancers, such as in the prostate gland. (A current trial using 200 µg/day, with mega-dose vitamin E supplementation [400 mg/day] as well, is testing that hypothesis in older men with enlarged prostate glands.)

thioredoxin A family of three selenium-dependent enzymes that have an antioxidant role and other roles in the body.

Critical | Thinking

Tammy read an article about antioxidants and their role in preventing free radical damage to cells. When Tammy went to the drugstore to take a closer look at such supplements, she saw that selenium was one of the antioxidants in the supplements. Why does selenium deserve consideration as an antioxidant?

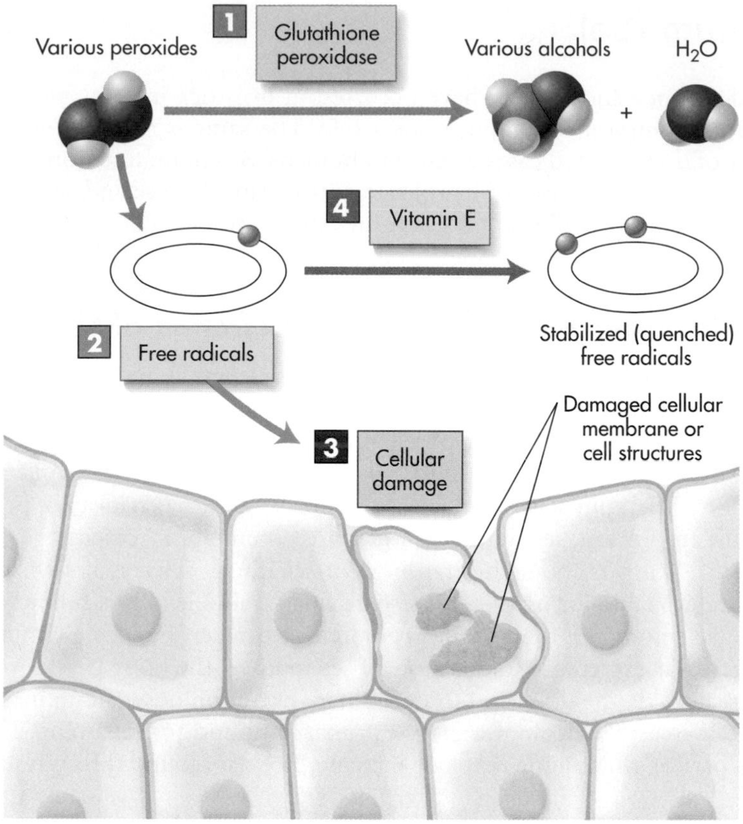

Figure 12-5 | Selenium is part of the glutathione peroxidase system (1), which breaks down peroxides, such as H_2O_2 to water (H_2O), before they can form free radicals (2) and lead to cell damage (3). This breakdown of peroxides in turn, spares some people of the need for vitamin E, which is a major free radical scavenger (4).

Food Sources of Selenium	
Food Item and Amount	*Selenium (μg)*
Tuna, 3 oz	68
Lean ham, 3 oz	42
Clams, 3 oz	41
Salmon, 3 oz	40
Egg noodles, 1 cup	35
Sirloin steak, 3 oz	28
Chicken breast, 3 oz	20
Special K cereal, 1 cup	17
Oat bran cereal, 1 cup	14
Whole-wheat bread, 1 slice	10
Cooked oatmeal, 1/2 cup	10
White bread, 1 slice	9
Raisin Bran cereal, 1 cup	4
RDA for adults, 55 μg	

Selenium Needs

The RDA for selenium is 55 μg/day for adult men and women,[11] based on the amount of selenium needed to maximize glutathione peroxidase activity in blood. In North America average intakes are about 105 μg/day from food. The Daily Value used on food and supplement labels for selenium is 70 μg.

Selenium-Deficiency Diseases

The signs and symptoms of a selenium deficiency in animals and humans include muscle pain, muscle wasting, and cardiomyopathy, which is a form of heart muscle damage.[3] These same signs and symptoms are noted when there is insufficient selenium in total parenteral nutrition solutions. Farm animals in areas with low soil concentrations of selenium (e.g., New Zealand and Finland) and humans in some areas of China develop characteristic heart muscle disorders associated with an inadequate selenium intake.

Keshan disease, a deficiency state that results in varying degrees of heart deterioration in children, is associated with inadequate selenium intake. Viral infections also seem to play a role in the disease. This disease was first observed in the Keshan province of China but since has been found elsewhere, including Finland and New Zealand. Regardless of geography, Keshan disease occurs when the soil is almost devoid of selenium. Note that although selenium is protective against development of the disease, selenium cannot correct the heart disorders once they have occurred. A selenium deficiency can also result in an accumulation of fatty acid peroxides in the heart, leading to an increased risk of blood clot formation. Additional studies have associated low blood selenium with both the incidence of myocardial infarctions and an increased death rate from cardiovascular disease. Studies have also reported a relationship between kidney disease and depressed selenium status. Further studies will be identifying the effects of supplementation and its application in the prevention of certain chronic diseases.

Upper Level for Selenium

The Upper Level is 400 μg/day for adults, based on overt signs of selenium toxicity, such as hair loss and high blood concentrations.[11] Daily intakes as low as 1 to 3 mg can cause toxicity symptoms if taken for many months. These signs and symptoms, besides hair loss, include a garlicky odor of the breath, nausea, diarrhea, fatigue, and changes in fingernails and toenails. Rashes and cirrhosis of the liver may also develop.

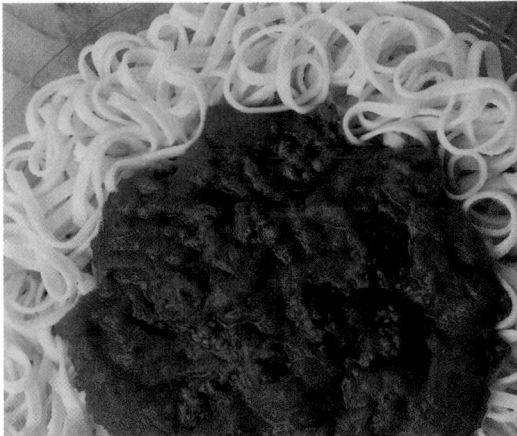

Pasta made from North American wheat is generally a good source of selenium, as is any meat in the accompanying sauce.

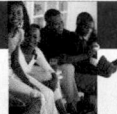
Case Scenario | Follow-Up

Gina's supplement dose of 200 μg/day, plus a typical dietary intake of 105 μg/day is below the Upper Level of 400 μg/day. Therefore, her practice is probably safe. Whether it will be helpful in reducing colon cancer risk awaits further research. Thus, widespread use of such a high dose of selenium is not currently recommended.

▌ Iodide (I)

Iodine (I_2), present in food as iodide (I^-) and other nonelemental forms, was linked to the presence of **goiter,** an enlarged thyroid gland, during World War I. Men drafted from areas such as the Great Lakes region of the United States had a much higher rate of goiter than men from some other areas of the country. The soil in these areas is very low in iodide. During the 1920s, researchers in Ohio found that goiter could be prevented in children by feeding them low doses of iodide for an extended period. Following the lead of the Swiss, American companies began adding iodide to table salt. Use of iodized salt is the major method for correcting iodide deficiencies.

goiter An enlargement of the thyroid gland that can be caused by a lack of iodide in the diet.

Absorption, Transport, Storage, and Excretion of Iodide

Iodide is efficiently absorbed along the gastrointestinal tract in its inorganic form, the most common form of dietary iodine.[10] Iodide is also easily absorbed in other forms, such as the iodate (IO_3^-) form that is added to bread. After iodide is absorbed into the bloodstream, it is transported as free ions and bound to proteins, including thyroid-binding globulin and albumin. The transported iodide is then distributed throughout the body's extracellular compartments.

About three-quarters of the iodide found in the adult human body is located in the thyroid gland. The thyroid gland actively accumulates and traps iodide from the bloodstream to support thyroid hormone synthesis. The thyroid hormones thyroxine (T_4) and triiodothyronine (T_3) are synthesized from the amino acid tyrosine and iodide. If a person's iodide intake is too low, the thyroid gland enlarges as it attempts to take up more iodide from the blood.

▌ odine (I_2), which is quite poisonous, can be used in a water solution as a topical anti-infective agent. The iodide ion (I^-) is the form of this trace mineral that is an essential nutrient. The term *iodine* is sometimes used in nutrition instead of iodide; however, to avoid confusion with this poisonous form, the term *iodide* will be used exclusively in this textbook.

Structure of thyroxine (T_4). Note that triiodothyronine (T_3) lacks one iodide (I), indicated in this figure with a red asterisk.

Food Sources of Iodide

Food Item and Amount	Iodide (μg)
Table salt, 1/2 tsp	195
Plain yogurt, 1 cup	87
Buttermilk, 1 cup	60
1% milk, 1 cup	59
Luna bar, 1	38
Soy protein bar, 1	38
Egg, 1 large	35
1% cottage cheese, 1/2 cup	28
Mozzarella cheese, 1 oz	10
RDA for adults, 150 μg	

goitrogens Substances in food and water that interfere with thyroid gland metabolism and thus may cause goiter if consumed in large amounts.

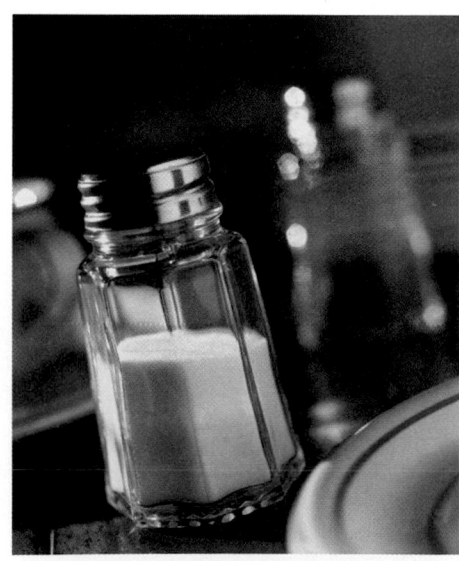

A small amount of iodized salt in one's diet helps meet iodide needs.

The kidneys are the principal route for iodide excretion. The amount of iodide found in urine is an adequate measurement of the status of iodide intake, along with current blood concentration of iodide.

Functions of Iodide

The major function of iodide is the synthesis of the thyroid hormone thyroxine (T_4).[10] Almost all organs in the body are targets for T_4, but T_4 is actually considered a pre-hormone. Within the target cell, T_4 is converted to T_3, the active form of the hormone. T_3 controls the rate of cell metabolism.

T_3 binds to DNA receptors and stimulates mRNA and protein synthesis in a way similar to that of vitamin A and vitamin D (review Figure 9-3). This action is especially important for development of the central nervous system. During periods of rapid growth (the first 6 months in utero), T_3 is crucial for normal brain development. Under normal circumstances, T_3 also increases glucose utilization and protein synthesis.

Iodide in Foods

Saltwater fish, seafood, iodized salt, molasses, and some plants contain various forms of iodide, especially the leaves of plants grown near the sea. Sea salt found in health-food stores, however, is not a good source because the iodide is lost during processing. A half teaspoon (about 2 g) of iodide-fortified salt supplies the adult RDA for iodide. The actual amount of fortification in the United States is 76 μg of iodide per gram of salt. This fortification is voluntary, however, so check the label. (In Canada such fortification is mandatory.)

The bioavailability of iodide in the diet is associated with the consumption of **goitrogens,** which are found in raw vegetables such as turnips, cabbage, brussels sprouts, cauliflower, broccoli, rutabagas, and cassava as well as other plants and even water. Goitrogens inhibit iodide metabolism by the thyroid gland and, in turn, inhibit thyroid hormone synthesis. However, goitrogens are not that important in developed countries because they are destroyed by cooking, and the foods they are found in do not play a central role in our eating patterns. They are, however, important to consider in less-developed parts of the world.

Iodide Needs

The RDA for iodide for adults is 150 μg/day.[10] This amount of iodide is needed to maintain adequate iodide uptake and turnover by the thyroid gland. The Daily Value used on food and supplement labels for iodide is also 150 μg/day. Most North Americans consume much more iodide than the RDA. Consumption is estimated to be about 190 to 300 μg/day (not including the iodide contributed by the use of iodized salt at the table), with men consuming the higher amounts.

Such intakes are typical because iodide is used as a sterilizing agent in dairies and restaurants, as a dough conditioner in bakeries, in food colorants, and in iodized salt.

Iodide-Deficiency Diseases

Some areas of Europe, such as northern Italy, have very low iodide concentrations in the soil but have yet to adopt the practice of fortifying salt with iodide. People in these areas, especially women, still suffer from goiter, as do people in areas of Latin America, the Indian subcontinent, Southeast Asia, and Africa. About 2 billion people worldwide are at risk of iodide deficiency, and nearly 700 million of these people have suffered the widespread effects of such a deficiency. Eradication of iodide deficiency is a goal of many health-related organizations worldwide.[20]

In an iodide deficiency, insufficient T_4 is produced. An adaptive response causes continual growth of the thyroid gland, eventually producing a goiter. A fall in metabolic rate and an increase in blood cholesterol are two other symptoms of thyroid hormone deficiency.[10]

Simple goiter is a painless condition, but if uncorrected it can lead to pressure on the trachea (windpipe), which may cause difficulty in breathing. In addition, other serious metabolic problems can result from low T_4 levels. Treatment with iodide can result in a slow reduction in the size of the thyroid gland, although surgical removal of part of the gland may be required in severe cases.

An iodide-deficient diet poses a major threat to pregnant women and the fetus, especially during the latter two-thirds of pregnancy. Some of the harmful documented effects include stillbirth, low birth weight, increased infant mortality, goiter, impaired mental function, and restricted development. Increasing the mother's intake of iodide prior to the fourth month of pregnancy, but preferably sooner, can prevent these abnormalities. Iodide deficiency is the major preventable cause of mental retardation worldwide.[20] The World Health Organization estimates that at least 50 million people in the world suffer from varying degrees of preventable brain damage due to the effects of iodide deficiency on fetal brain development. The resulting restriction of body growth and mental development is referred to as **cretinism.** Cretinism was common in certain areas of the United States before the program to fortify salt with iodide. Today, cretinism still appears in parts of Europe, Africa, Latin America, and Asia (Figure 12-6). Some of these areas are attempting to decrease iodide deficiency by providing iodinated vegetable oil orally or by injection in addition to the fortification of salt with iodide.

cretinism The stunting of body growth and mental development during fetal and later development that results from inadequate maternal intake of iodide during pregnancy.

Upper Level for Iodide

When very high amounts of iodide are consumed, thyroid hormone synthesis is inhibited, as in a deficiency. The Upper Level of 1.1 mg/day is based on such an effect. This effect can appear in people who eat a lot of seaweed, which is rich in iodide.

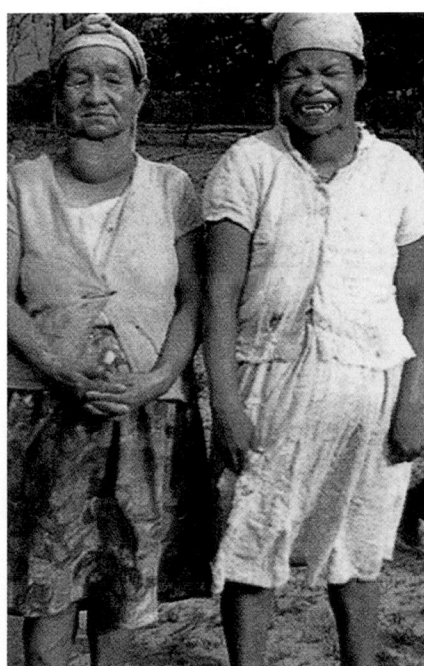
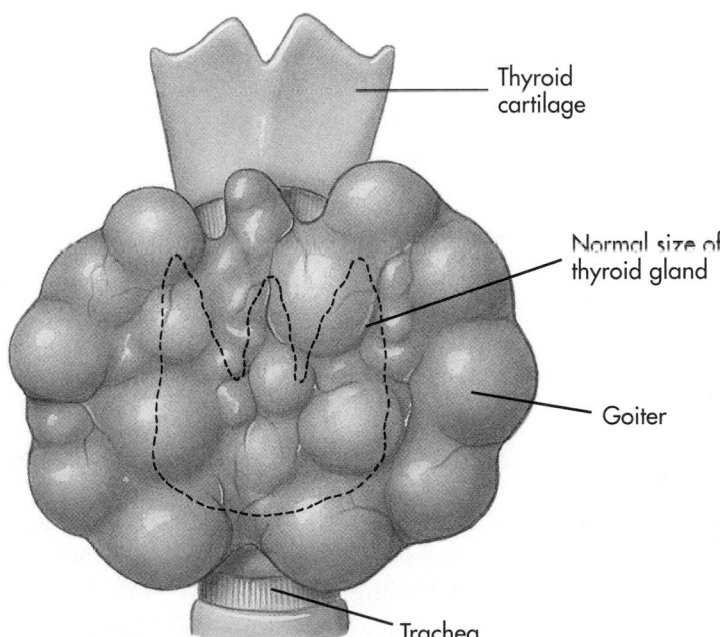

Figure 12-6 | Goiter and cretinism in Bolivia. The mother on the left is goitrous but otherwise normal. The daughter is goitrous, mentally retarded, deaf, and mute. Both mother and daughter exhibit characteristics typical of iodide deficiency.

Illustration by William Ober.

L ike chlorine, fluorine (F₂) is a poisonous gas. The fluoride ion (F⁻) is the form of this trace mineral that contributes to human health.

mottling The discoloration or marking of the surfaces of teeth from exposure to excessive amounts of fluoride (also called enamel fluorosis).

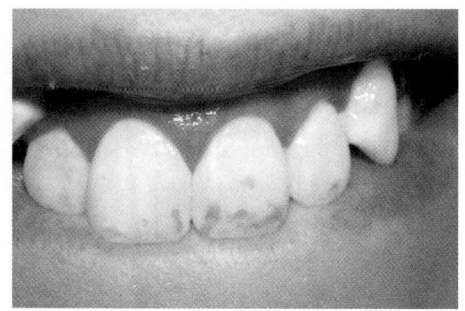

Example of mottling in a tooth caused by overexposure to fluoride.

fluorapatite A fluoride-containing, acid-resistant crystalline substance that is produced during bone and tooth development. Its presence in teeth helps prevent dental caries.

Fluoride (F)

Fluoride may not be an essential nutrient per se because all basic body functions may proceed without it. However, fluoride does have some health-promoting attributes. Dentists in the early 1900s noticed a lower incidence of dental caries in the southwestern United States, where the water naturally contained high concentrations of fluoride. Many people in these areas had small spots on the teeth, called **mottling** (or enamel fluorosis), due to deposits of fluoride. Although discolored, these mottled teeth were virtually free of dental caries. After experiments showed that fluoride in the water does indeed decrease the rate of dental caries, the controlled fluoridation of water in parts of the United States began in 1945 (review Chapter 5 concerning the development of dental caries).

People who have grown up drinking fluoridated water generally have 40 to 60% fewer dental caries than people who did not drink fluoridated water as children. Dentists can provide fluoride treatments and schools can provide fluoride tablets, but it is much less expensive and more reliable to simply add fluoride to the community's drinking water. However, not all public or private water sources contain enough fluoride. When in doubt, contact your local water plant or have the water in your home analyzed for fluoride content. If the water doesn't contain the recommended amount—1 part per million parts of water (1 ppm, or 1 mg/L)—talk to your dentist about the best means for obtaining sufficient fluoride. And although the most important clinical aspect of fluoride is its benefits in the prevention of dental caries, fluoride has also been shown to protect against the demineralization of other calcified tissues.[1]

Absorption, Transport, Storage, and Excretion of Fluoride

The absorption of fluoride occurs very rapidly. A significant proportion of dietary fluoride is absorbed in the stomach. Absorption continues to take place throughout the GI tract by passive diffusion. Overall, about 80 to 90% is absorbed. Fluoride is then transported throughout the body via the bloodstream in the ionic form.[9]

Calcified tissue deposition and renal excretion are the two major mechanisms by which fluoride is removed from circulation. An estimated 50% of the fluoride absorbed each day is deposited in the bones and teeth. The amount of fluoride deposited depends on the stage of development of the bone, with the developing stages being the most significant. The major path for the excretion of fluoride from the body occurs via the urine.

Functions of Fluoride

Although an essential function has not been described for fluoride, it is still recognized as a trace mineral with the beneficial property of protecting against the demineralization of calcified tissues.[9] The action of fluoride on the erupted teeth of children and adults is due to its effects on the metabolism of bacteria in dental plaque. It also works to reduce dental caries by

- Reducing the acid solubility of enamel by forming **fluorapatite** crystals rather than the typical hydroxyapatite crystals
- Promoting the remineralization of enamel lesions
- Increasing the deposition of minerals that restrict the development of caries
- Reducing the net rate of transport of minerals from the enamel surface

Fluoride present in bones is constantly released into the blood, and more so if the bone fluoride content is high. This blood fluoride combines with daily fluoride exposure from fluoridated water (if available) and toothpaste (if used). Blood fluoride then contributes to fluoride in the saliva, which in turn bathes the teeth to provide daily fluoride protection. Overall, lifelong fluoride exposure on a daily basis is the most beneficial way to receive the dental caries–preventive function of fluoride.

Fluoride in Foods

In North America, the major source of dietary fluoride is drinking water (but not bottled water). Typical fluoridated water contains about 0.2 mg/cup. Tea, seafood (especially marine fish that are consumed with their bones), and seaweed are among the richest dietary sources of fluoride. Estimating fluoride content in food can be difficult because water sources can vary in amount. Toothpaste, mouth rinses, and fluoride treatments performed by dentists are other sources of fluoride.

Fluoride Needs

The Adequate Intake for fluoride is 3.1 mg/day for women and 3.8 mg/day for men.[9] For infants up to 6 months of age, the Adequate Intake is 0.01 mg/day and increases to 0.5 mg/day through age 1. For children and adolescents, the fluoride Adequate Intake ranges from 0.7 to 3.2 mg/day. This range of intake provides the benefits of resistance to dental caries without causing mottling of the teeth, which is the basis for setting the Adequate Intake.

Upper Level for Fluoride

The Upper Level set for children over 9 years of age and adults is 10 mg/day, based on the risk of **skeletal fluorosis.**[9] A fluoride intake greater than 6 mg/day is a concern in childhood because this amount can mottle and weaken teeth during their developmental stage. Children who swallow large amounts of fluoridated toothpaste as part of daily tooth care are at greatest risk. Limiting the amount used to "pea" size is the best way to prevent this problem.

Concept | Check

Selenium is important for the activity of glutathione peroxidase, an enzyme that reduces the concentration of peroxides, thus lessening the free radical load in the body. In this way, selenium spares some of the need for vitamin E. A deficiency results in muscle and heart disorders. Organ meats, eggs, fish, and grains are good selenium sources; however, the selenium content in grains depends on the selenium concentration in the soil. A high selenium intake is potentially toxic. Iodide is vital in the synthesis of thyroid hormones. A prolonged insufficient intake will cause the thyroid gland to enlarge, resulting in goiter. Insufficient intake in pregnancy can lead to mental retardation in the offspring. The use of iodized salt has virtually eliminated this condition in North America. Fluoride incorporated into teeth during development makes them resistant to acid and bacterial attack, in turn reducing development of dental caries. Regular fluoride exposure also aids in the remineralization of teeth once decay begins. Most of us receive adequate amounts of fluoride from that added to drinking water and toothpaste. A high fluoride intake during tooth development can lead to spotted, or mottled, teeth.

▌ Chromium (Cr)

The importance of chromium in human diets has been recognized only in the past 40 years. Although not much is understood about this mineral, many studies suggest that chromium plays an important role in maintaining proper carbohydrate and lipid metabolism, which may help alleviate type 2 diabetes for some individuals.

Absorption, Transport, Storage, and Excretion of Chromium

Only about 0.5 to 2% of chromium from food is absorbed. However, the bioavailability of chromium in humans is difficult to assess because the concentrations in human tissues are very low. Chromium is transported in the bloodstream primarily by the

Because of its ability to increase bone mass, high doses of fluoride (>20 mg/day) are being used experimentally in adults to treat severe osteoporosis, especially that seen in the spine. Fluoride can stimulate osteoblasts (bone-forming cells) to increase the production of proteins that ultimately undergo rapid mineralization to form new bone. Such high fluoride dosages can cause significant side effects, such as stomach upset and bone pain. Ongoing research is attempting to establish an effective dose and duration of treatment.

Note that high fluoride intake in adults does not cause mottling of teeth.

skeletal fluorosis A condition caused by a greatly excessive fluoride intake, characterized by weakened skeletal structure.

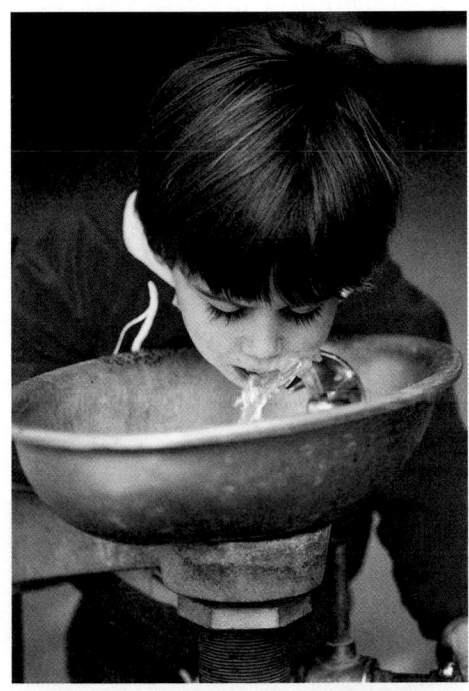

Fluoridated water is responsible for much of the decrease in dental caries throughout North America in recent years.

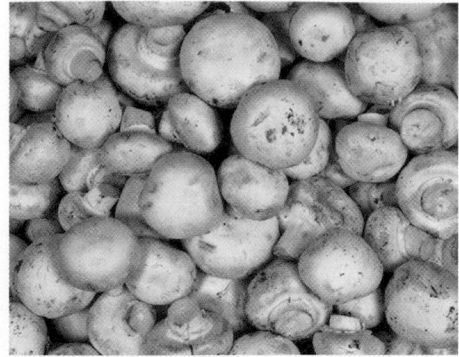

Mushrooms are a good source of chromium.

Chromium supplements have been touted to help with weight loss and exercise-induced increases in muscle mass, linked to its effect on insulin function. Most research, however, does not support this assertion. In addition, any benefit would be negligible compared to regular aerobic physical activity and some strength training.

Chromium in foods (Cr^{3+}) has not shown any toxicity, so no Upper Level has been set. Chromium toxicity has been reported in people exposed to chromium in industrial settings (specifically Cr^{6+}). Chromium poisoning damages the lungs and causes allergic responses in the skin. In addition, the most popular form of chromium in dietary supplements, chromium picolinate, appears to be absorbed in a fashion different from dietary chromium and can lead to the production of harmful free radicals.

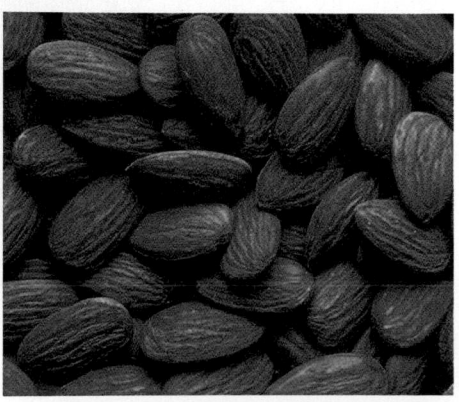

Nuts are a good source of manganese.

iron-binding protein transferrin, and it appears to be a bone-seeking trace mineral. Chromium accumulates as well in the spleen, liver, and kidneys. The excretion of chromium occurs via the feces.[10]

Functions of Chromium

The most studied function of chromium is the maintenance of glucose uptake into cells, but the actual mechanism is still under debate. One proposal is that chromium's ability to enhance insulin action occurs when a chromium-binding protein binds to insulin receptors on the cell membrane and then boosts receptor activity.[10]

Chromium in Foods

Information regarding the chromium content of various foods is scant, and most food composition tables do not include values for this trace mineral. Processed meats, organ meats (liver), whole-grain products, egg yolks, mushrooms, broccoli, nuts, some legumes (such as dried beans), and beer are the most reliable sources. Yeast is also a source. Generally speaking, whole grains and cereals contain higher concentrations of chromium than do fruits and vegetables. The amount of chromium in foods is closely tied to the local soil content of chromium. To provide yourself with an adequate chromium intake, regularly choose whole grains in preference to refined grains.

Chromium Needs

The Adequate Intake for chromium is 35 μg/day for men and 25 μg/day for women,[10] based on the amount typically found in well-balanced diets. The average dietary intake for adults in North America generally meets the Adequate Intake standards. The Daily Value used on food and supplement labels for chromium is 120 μg.

Chromium-Deficiency Diseases

A chromium deficiency is characterized by impaired glucose tolerance and elevated blood cholesterol and triglycerides. The mechanism by which chromium influences cholesterol metabolism is not known but may involve enzymes that control cholesterol synthesis. Chromium deficiency appears in people maintained on total parenteral nutrition not supplemented with chromium as well as in children suffering from undernutrition.[10] In addition, some adults may become chromium-deficient as they age, and this deficiency may contribute to the increased risk for the development of type 2 diabetes. A recent study observed that when yeast chromium was fed to older persons, there was improvement in glucose tolerance. Because sensitive measures of chromium status are not available, marginal chromium deficiencies may go undetected.

Manganese (Mn)

It is easy to confuse the mineral manganese (Mn) with magnesium (Mg). Their names are similar, and in a few metabolic pathways they can substitute for each other. Both these minerals form bridges between ATP or ADP and enzymes. In some cases, these enzymes can use either magnesium or manganese, but in many other cases, magnesium seems to be the preferred mineral. On the other hand, some enzymes prefer manganese, including an enzyme involved in glucose production and a family of enzymes that put together protein-carbohydrate complexes in the protein portion of bone. Besides bridge-forming activities, manganese is an actual part of some enzymes, much like copper, zinc, and iron. Manganese-containing enzymes include mitochondrial superoxide dismutase. Manganese enzymes also participate in the urea cycle and in carbohydrate metabolism.[10]

Based on balance studies of intakes and losses, an Adequate Intake for manganese is set at 2.3 mg/day for men and 1.8 mg/day for women.[10] It has been generally assumed that almost everyone consumes plenty of manganese, but a few studies have raised the possibility that this assumption may not always be true. Unfortunately, very little manganese research has been done in humans. The Daily Value used for manganese on food and supplement labels is 2 mg.

Foods that contain the most manganese include nuts, legumes, tea, and whole grains, but little is known about how well manganese is absorbed from various foods. Animal products generally contribute little manganese to the diet.

A concern has been raised for manganese toxicity due to some high-dose supplements. The Upper Level for manganese is 11 mg/day based on the development of nerve damage.[10]

Molybdenum (Mo)

Molybdenum is notable for its interactions with iron and copper. In particular, high intakes of molybdenum inhibit copper absorption.

Several enzymes—including **xanthine dehydrogenase** and a related form, xanthine oxidase—require molybdenum. The oxidase form of the enzyme is produced from the dehydrogenase form during tissue injury. No molybdenum deficiency has been observed in people consuming a normal diet, although deficiency signs and symptoms have appeared in people on total parenteral nutrition.[10] These symptoms include increased heart and respiration rates, night blindness, mental confusion, edema, weakness, and coma.

Good food sources of molybdenum include milk and milk products, beans, liver, whole grains, and nuts. The RDA for molybdenum is 45 μg/day for adults,[10] based on the amount needed to balance daily losses. The Daily Value used on food and supplement labels for molybdenum is 75 μg. Typical North American intakes are 75 to 110 μg/day, with the higher intakes seen in men. When laboratory animals consume high dosages of molybdenum, they develop evidence of toxicity, including anemia, weight loss, and decreased growth. The Upper Level of 2 mg/day is based on decreased growth and reproduction in laboratory animals.[10]

Table 12-3 reviews the minerals discussed so far in this chapter. Figure 12-7 summarizes the roles of major minerals and trace minerals in the body.

xanthine dehydrogenase An enzyme containing molybdenum and iron that functions in the formation of uric acid and the mobilization of iron from liver ferritin stores.

Ultratrace Minerals

Many elements of the periodic table occur in microgram/gram amounts in body tissues (Table 12-4).[8] Ultimately, some may be elevated to the status of essential nutrients, but at this time elements such as aluminum, cadmium, bromine, germanium, lead, rubidium, and tin have not been shown to have any beneficial effects in humans. In fact, lead is a danger to young children, as evidenced by toxicity to those children living in older homes contaminated with peeling lead-based paint (see Chapter 19 for more details on lead).

What follows is a discussion of five ultratrace minerals that may have a role in human nutrition. Because these minerals have not yet been determined to be essential trace minerals, no RDAs or Adequate Intakes have been set. However, because these ultratrace minerals, like all minerals, can be toxic, in some cases an Upper Level has been established.

Boron (B)

Boron has long been known as an important growth factor for plants. In humans, boron may be involved in the metabolism of steroid (cholesterol-containing) hormones, such as the active vitamin D hormone and the estrogens.[8] There appears to be

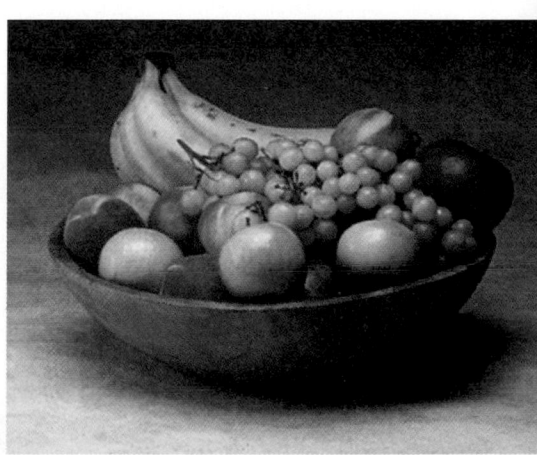

Fruits are a source of boron.

Table 12-3 | A Summary of Key Trace Minerals

Mineral	Major Functions	Deficiency Symptoms	People Most at Risk	RDA or Adequate Intake	Good Dietary Sources	Results of Toxicity
Iron	Functional component of hemoglobin and other key compounds used in respiration; immune function; cognitive development	Fatigue upon exertion; small, pale red blood cells; low blood hemoglobin values; poor immune function	Infants, preschool children, women in childbearing years	Men: 8 mg Women: 18 mg	Meats, seafood, enriched breads, fortified cereals, molasses	Gastrointestinal upset; toxicity especially seen when children consume many iron pills; toxicity also seen in people with hemochromatosis; Upper Level is 45 mg/day, based on gastric irritation
Zinc	Required for many enzymes such as those that participate in antioxidant protection; stabilizes cell membranes and other body molecules	Skin rash, diarrhea, decreased appetite and sense of taste, hair loss, poor growth and development	Vegetarians, elderly people, people with alcoholism, malnourished populations	Men: 11 mg Women: 8 mg	Seafoods, meats, whole grains	Supplement use can reduce copper absorption; can cause diarrhea, cramps, depressed immune function; Upper Level is 40 mg/day, based on interaction with copper
Copper	Aids in iron metabolism; works in antioxidant enzymes and those involved in connective tissue metabolism and hormone synthesis	Anemia, low white blood cell count, poor growth	Overzealous supplementation of zinc	900 μg	Liver, cocoa, beans, nuts, whole grains, shellfish	Excessive supplement use can cause vomiting; nervous system and liver disorders; Upper Level is 8–10 mg/day, based on liver damage
Selenium	Part of an antioxidant system	Muscle pain, muscle weakness, form of heart disease	Known only in areas of the world with low selenium content in the soil	55 μg	Meats, eggs, fish, seafoods, whole grains	Excessive supplement use can cause nausea, vomiting, hair loss, weakness, liver disease; Upper Level is 400 mg/day, based on hair loss
Iodide	Component of thyroid hormones	Goiter; mental retardation, poor growth in infancy when mother is iodide deficient during pregnancy	Major problem in most parts of the world	150 μg	Iodized salt, white bread, saltwater fish, dairy products	Inhibition of function of the thyroid gland; Upper Level is 1.1 mg/day, based on decreased T_4 synthesis
Fluoride	Increases resistance of tooth enamel to dental caries	Although not a true deficiency symptom, dental caries is a risk	Areas where water is not fluoridated	Men: 3.8 mg Women: 3.1 mg	Fluoridated water, toothpaste, dental treatments, tea, seaweed	Stomach upset; mottling (staining) of teeth during development, bone deterioration; Upper Level is 10 mg/day, based on bone problems
Chromium	Enhances insulin action	High blood glucose after eating	People on intravenous nutrition, perhaps elderly people with type 2 diabetes	25–35 μg	Egg yolks, whole grains, pork, nuts, mushrooms	Caused by industrial contamination, not dietary excess; no Upper Level set
Manganese	Cofactor of some enzymes, such as those involved in carbohydrate metabolism and antioxidant protection	None in humans	Unknown	1.8–2.3 mg	Nuts, oats, beans, tea	Nervous system disorders; Upper Level is 11 mg/day, based on nerve damage
Molybdenum	Aids action of some enzymes	None in healthy humans	Unsupplemented total parenteral nutrition support	45 μg	Beans, grains, nuts	Poor growth in laboratory animals; Upper Level is 2 mg/day, based on poor growth in laboratory animals

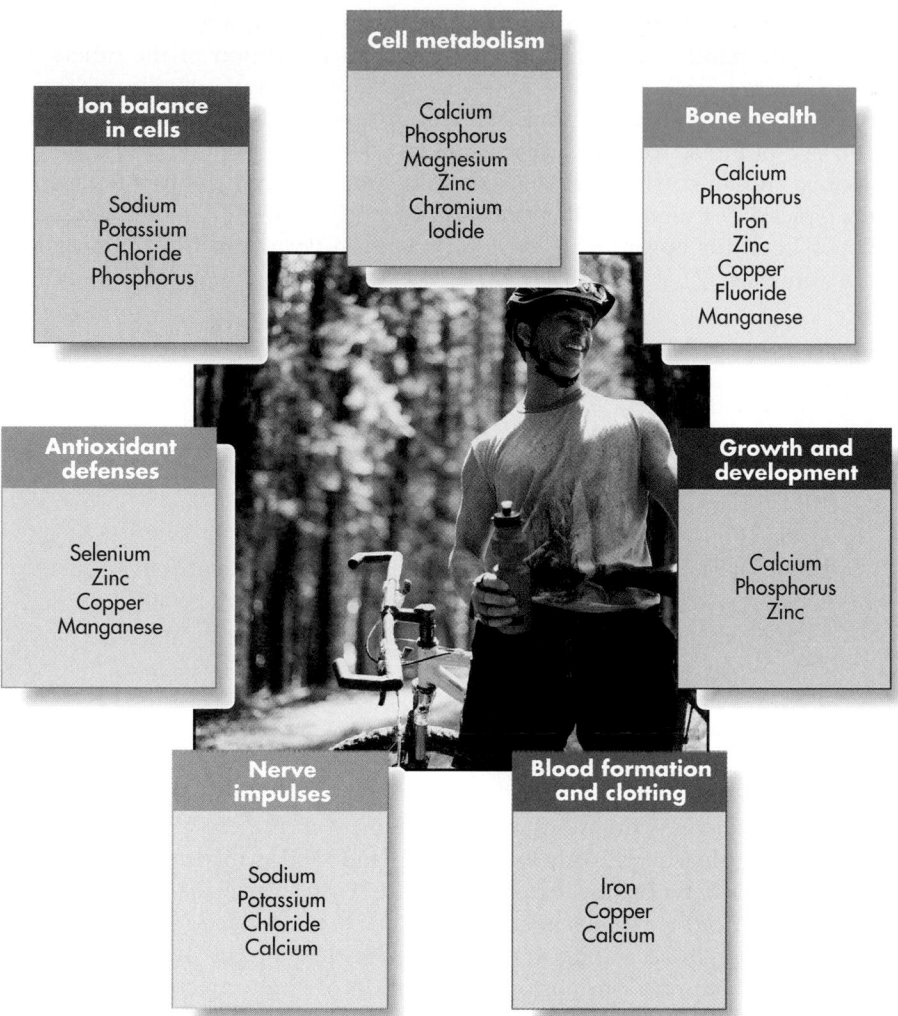

Figure 12-7 | Minerals contribute to many functions in the body. Mineral deficiencies therefore lead to a variety of health problems.

Table 12-4 | A Summary of Ultratrace Minerals for Which Human Needs Have Not Been Definitely Established

Mineral	Proposed Functions	Estimates of Daily Human Needs	Dietary Sources
Boron	Cell membrane function (ion transport), steroid hormone metabolism	1–13 mg	Fruits, leafy vegetables, nuts, beans
Nickel	Amino acid and fatty acid metabolism	25–35 μg	Chocolate, nuts, beans, whole grains
Silicon	Bone formation	25–30 mg	Root vegetables, whole grains
Arsenic	Amino acid metabolism, DNA function	12–25 μg	Fish, grains, cereal products
Vanadium	Mimicry of insulin action	10 μg	Shellfish, mushrooms, black pepper

Deficiency symptoms have been produced mostly in experimental animals. Many trace minerals pose a high risk for toxicity. Any supplement use should not exceed the estimates of human needs listed in this table.

One possibility to consider is that many ultratrace minerals present in tissues are there by accident, and although they don't provide any health benefits, neither do they represent a threat. Most of the current knowledge about the ultratrace elements has come from animal studies, which may suggest possible benefits for humans, but the evidence is tentative at best.

a close interrelation among boron, calcium, and magnesium, but more information is needed to understand how each mineral affects the absorption of the others. Boron acts as a regulator in cell membrane function, such as membrane stability, or acts as the regulator of the movement of cations and anions through the cell membrane. Sources of boron are peanuts, fruits (especially raisins), legumes, potatoes, vegetables, and wine. Coffee and milk, which are low in boron, are other contributors because of the amounts typically consumed. Adults consume about 0.75 to 1.35 mg of boron per day. The Upper Level for boron is 20 mg/day, based on developmental abnormalities in laboratory animals.[10]

Nickel (Ni)

No biochemical function has been clearly defined for nickel for humans, but a variety of deficiency signs have been reported for farm animals and rats. Nickel may function as a cofactor with a variety of enzymes, such as those involved in the breakdown of branched-chain amino acids and odd-chain-length fatty acids.[8] It also may be involved in the metabolism of vitamin B-12 and folic acid during the synthesis of methionine from homocysteine. Nickel is found in chocolate, nuts, legumes, and grains. North Americans have an intake of 69 to 162 μg/day. The Upper Level is 1 mg/day, based on poor weight gain in laboratory animals.[10]

Silicon (Si)

Next to oxygen, silicon is the most abundant element in the earth's crust. If that surprises you, realize that quartz is made of silicon and sand is made of quartz. With all this silicon around, it is obvious that some should find its way into plants, animals, and humans. What is not so obvious is whether people actually need silicon. Studies with laboratory rats and chickens suggest that the answer may be yes. In these animals, silicon has shown some relationship to the formation of connective tissue, especially in the protein portion of bone.[10] There has been some speculative research on silicon and human bone structure, but nothing definitive is known. Silicon can be found in foods such as high-fiber grain products and root vegetables, but knowledge about silicon absorption from foods is limited.

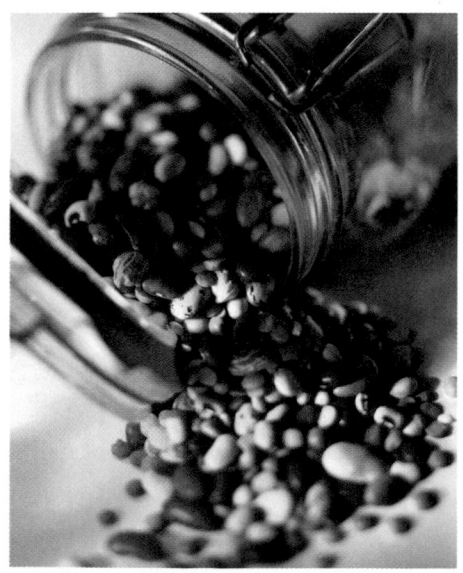

Legumes (beans) are a good source of some ultratrace minerals.

Arsenic (As)

Most people recognize arsenic as a potentially very toxic mineral. Depending on the form of arsenic consumed, absorption varies from 20 to 90%. It is rapidly excreted in the urine and via the bile. Although not clearly established, arsenic is probably biologically active in the metabolism of the amino acid methionine and methyl groups. Another possible role is in the regulation of gene expression to produce certain proteins.[8] Also, arsenic seems to enhance DNA synthesis in white blood cells. For this reason arsenic is being used in some cancer chemotherapy regimens. North Americans consume about 30 μg/day. Fish, grains, and cereal products contribute the most arsenic to the diet.[10]

Vanadium (V)

Vanadium shows pharmacological activity that mimics the actions of insulin, preventing the symptoms of diabetes in diabetic rats; thus, vanadium may have a role in treating human diabetes. Clinical studies with the trace mineral in both type 1 and type 2 diabetes showed some improvement in glucose utilization.[8] Type 2 diabetes patients displayed improved insulin sensitivity. Vanadium is poorly absorbed and is excreted in the urine and bile. Other than vanadium's possible pharmacologic properties in diabetes treatment, a defined biochemical function for humans has not been described. In laboratory animals, it also seems to stimulate the mineralization of bones and teeth and has a variety of other actions. A vanadium deficiency has not been identified in humans. Human diets supply about 6 to 18 μg per day. Vanadium is found in shellfish, mushrooms, parsley, dill, and some prepared foods. The Upper Level is 1.8 mg/day, based on development of kidney damage.[10]

Concept | Check

Chromium may increase the action of the hormone insulin. The amount of chromium found in food depends on soil content. Whole grains, egg yolks, and meat are some of the better sources of chromium. Manganese is a component of bone and many enzymes, including those involved in glucose production. Because our need for it is low, deficiencies are rare. Good food sources of manganese are nuts, oats, tea, and beans. Molybdenum is a component of some enzymes. Deficiencies have appeared only with total parenteral nutrition. Beans, milk and milk products, grains, and nuts are sources of molybdenum. Boron contributes to ion transport across cell membranes, nickel contributes to amino acid metabolism, and silicon contributes to bone metabolism. The roles for some other trace minerals—including arsenic and vanadium—have not been fully established in humans. These minerals are required in such small amounts that diets including a variety of foods and containing some plant protein and whole grains most likely supply adequate amounts.

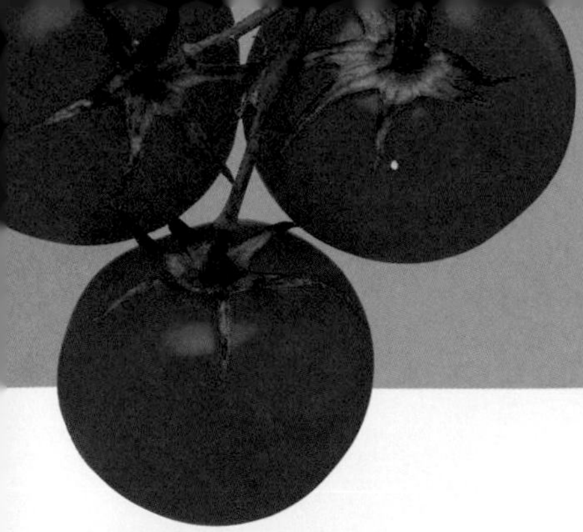

benign Noncancerous; describes tumors that do not spread.

malignant Essentially, malicious; in reference to a tumor, the property of spreading locally and to distant sites.

neoplasm A new and abnormal growth of tissues, which may be benign or cancerous.

carcinoma An invasive malignant tumor derived from the epithelial tissues that cover the body.

sarcoma A malignant tumor arising from connective tissues.

leukemia A malignant neoplasm of blood-forming tissues, the bone marrow.

lymphoma A malignant tumor arising from lymph nodes or other lymph tissues.

Cancer is currently the second leading cause of death for North American adults. Lung, prostate, breast, and colorectal cancers account for slightly over half of all cancers in North America and are the leading cause of cancer death for every racial and ethnic group.[15] The good news is that new cancer cases and cancer deaths for all cancers (except lung cancer in women) have declined in recent years.

What Is Cancer?

Cancer is not a single disease but exists in at least 100 different forms (Figure 12-8). Some of the factors that cause skin cancer may be different from those leading to breast cancer, and treatments for the different varieties of cancer vary with the type of cancer itself. Essentially, cancer is abnormal and uncontrollable cell division. If untreatable or not treated, it leads to death. Most cancers take the form of tumors, although not all tumors are can-

cerous. A tumor is spontaneous new tissue growth that serves no physiological purpose. Tumors can be **benign,** such as a wart that doesn't spread, or **malignant,** such as lung cancer that spreads to surrounding tissues and organs. A malignant **neoplasm** means the same thing as a malignant tumor.

Most cancers fall into one of three groups: carcinomas, sarcomas, and leukemias and lymphomas. **Carcinomas** comprise 80 to 90% of all cancer. They develop from cells that cover the body and affect secretory organs, such as the breast. **Sarcomas** are cancers of connective tissues, such as in bone. **Leukemias** are malignant neoplasms of the blood-forming tissues, the bone marrow. **Lymphomas** are various malignant tumors that are in the lymph nodes or lymphoid tissues.

Benign tumors are enclosed in a membrane that prevents them from spreading. They are dangerous only if they interfere with normal function. For instance, a benign brain tumor can cause illness and death if it blocks blood flow in the brain.

Estimated % of Cancer Deaths for 2004		
Male		**Female**
<1%	Brain	2%
4%	Esophagus and stomach	<1%
32%	Lung	25%
	Breast	15%
3%	Liver	<1%
5%	Pancreas	6%
9%	Leukemia and lymphomas	9%
10%	Colon and rectum	10%
6%	Urinary	
	Ovary	6%
10%	Prostate	
	Uterus and cervix	3%
25%	All others (e.g., oral and skin) (e.g., oral, skin, and bladder)	24%

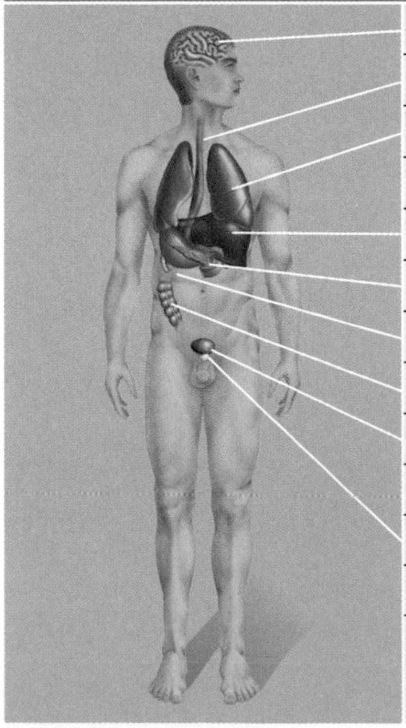

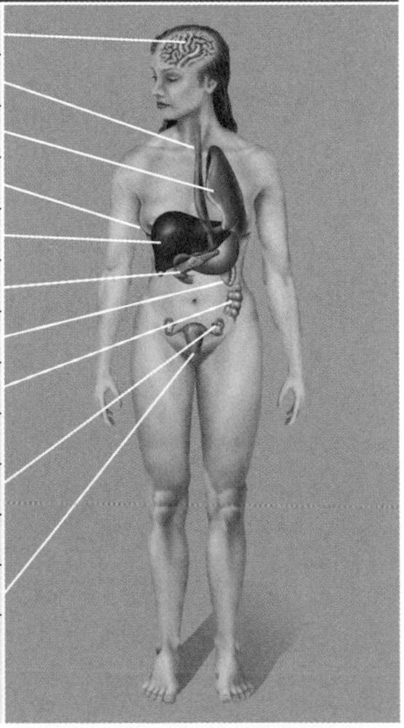

Figure 12-8 | Cancer is actually many diseases. Numerous types of cells and organs are its target. Note that about one-third of all cancers arise from smoking (primarily lung cancer).

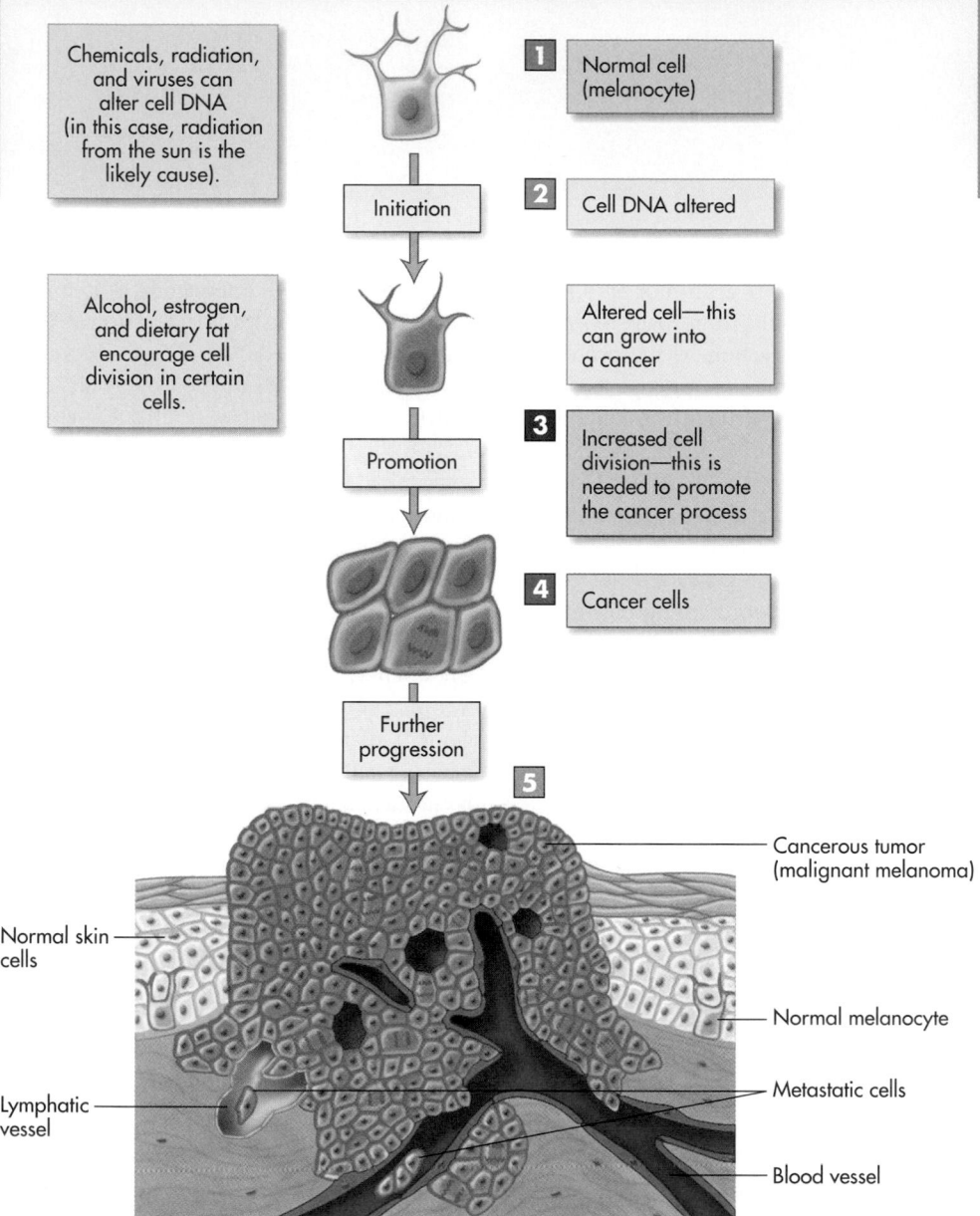

Chemicals, radiation, and viruses can alter cell DNA (in this case, radiation from the sun is the likely cause).

1 Normal cell (melanocyte)

Initiation

2 Cell DNA altered

Alcohol, estrogen, and dietary fat encourage cell division in certain cells.

Altered cell—this can grow into a cancer

Promotion

3 Increased cell division—this is needed to promote the cancer process

4 Cancer cells

Further progression

5

Cancerous tumor (malignant melanoma)

Normal skin cells

Normal melanocyte

Lymphatic vessel

Metastatic cells

Blood vessel

Figure 12-9 | Progression from a normal skin cell (1) to skin cancer through the initiation (2), promotion (3), and progression (4) stages. The ball of cells is a developing tumor. As the mass of cells grows, it can invade surrounding tissues, eventually penetrating into both lymph and blood vessels (5). These vessels carry spreading (metastatic) cancer cells throughout the body, where they can form new cancer sites.

Malignant tumors, on the other hand, are capable of invading surrounding structures, including blood vessels, the lymph system, and nerve tissue. They can **metastasize** to distant sites via the blood or lymph, thereby producing invasive tumors in almost any part of the body (Figure 12-9).

Because leukemia, a cancer found in white blood cells (leukocytes), does not produce a mass, it isn't classified as a tumor; however, it exhibits the fundamental property of rapid and inappropriate growth. Leukemia is still malignant and therefore represents a form of cancer.

Mechanisms of Carcinogenesis

Most cells exist in a homeostatic state; there is a balance between the turning-on and turning-off of cellular replication. Regulation of the cell cycle exists between the gene products that spur replication and gene products that deter replication.

Oncogenes and Other Genes

Genes that produce products that cause a resting cell to divide are referred to as **protooncogenes,** and genes that produce products that prevent cells

metastasize The spreading of disease from one part of the body to another, even to parts of the body that are remote from the site of the original tumor. Cancer cells can spread via blood vessels, the lymphatic system, or direct growth of the tumor.

protooncogenes Genes that cause a resting cell to divide.

455

tumor suppressor genes Genes that prevent cells from dividing.

oncogene A protooncogene out of control.

p53 gene A tumor-suppressor gene that can prevent inappropriate cell division.

telomeres Caps at the end of chromosomes.

telomerase An enzyme that maintains length and completeness of chromosomes.

cancer initiation The stage in the process of cancer development that begins with alterations in DNA, the genetic material in a cell. These alterations may cause the cell to no longer respond to normal physiological controls.

cancer promotion The stage in the cancer process during which cell division increases, in turn decreasing the time available for repair enzymes to act on altered DNA and encouraging cells with altered DNA to develop and grow.

cancer progression The final stage in the cancer process, during which the cancer cells proliferate, forming a mass large enough to significantly affect body functions.

genotoxic carcinogen A compound that directly alters DNA or is converted in cells to metabolites that alter DNA, thereby providing the potential for cancer to develop.

mutation A change in the chemistry of a gene that is perpetuated in subsequent divisions of the cell in which it occurred; a change in the sequence of the DNA base pairs.

from dividing are known as **tumor suppressor genes.** Cancer often results from a lack of suppressor genes or too much action by the protooncogenes. The cancer gene, or **oncogene,** is the protooncogene out of control; it is making dozens or hundreds of copies of itself, and there are no mechanisms to overcome the process. Ultimately, all cancer is genetic, in that defects in specific genes lead to the proliferative growth.

The tumor suppressor genes are the braking mechanisms within a cell, preventing uncontrolled growth. When something goes wrong with these tumor suppressor genes, the oncogenes are free to promote rapid cell growth. One tumor suppressor gene, known as **p53,** can prevent the abnormal growth associated with tumors. Alteration in this gene has been discovered to cause cancers of the ovary, breast, lung, and colon.

There are repair mechanisms within a cell that constantly look for errors in DNA replication and make corrections. Sometimes the repair mechanisms fail, which results in an inherited defect for cancer, such as hereditary colon cancer. Early defects in DNA replication that aren't caught and repaired are likely to predispose the cell to even more errors, thus leading to cancer.

Other agents that play a part in the cell replication process are **telomeres,** caps at the ends of chromosomes. An enzyme called **telomerase** maintains their length and completeness. This enzyme is active when we are young and tapers off as we age. Each time an adult cell divides, the telomeres of the daughter cells are slightly shorter. At some point, telomeres become so short that the genes at the ends of the chromosome can no longer function, and the cell dies. In malignant tumor cells, the telomerase activity increases, and the length of the telomere is maintained, resulting in a cell that can live indefinitely. There seems to be a difference in telomerase activity between normal tissue and cancer tissue. Much more remains to be learned about conditions that promote abnormal telomerase activity and whether this enzyme can become a target in cancer therapy.

Cancer Initiation, Promotion, and Progression

Carcinogenesis, the development of cancer in a body, is a multiple-step event. It starts with the exposure of a cell to a carcinogen, in turn triggering cancer initiation. Subsequently, it is followed by **cancer promotion** and finally **cancer progression** (review Figure 12-9). Initiation can develop spontaneously or can be induced by agents known as **genotoxic carcinogens.** The affected cells can then dictate their own rate of division. Agents that are responsible for carcinogenesis include tobacco, alcohol, radiation, occupational toxins, infections, diet, and drugs (Table 12-5).

A mechanism that can prevent cancer initiation is a family of enzymes in cells that can detoxify and speed up excretion of cancer-producing chemicals. These enzymes are sometimes called phase 2 enzymes. Some dietary phytochemicals increase the amount of these enzymes in the body. The p53 gene, already identified as a tumor suppressor gene, is another way to prevent abnormal growth associated with tumors, because it can postpone cell division, which allows time for damage repair. Enzymes can travel up and down the DNA double helix, repairing broken components and correcting defects. About 99% of the time, the repair enzymes find the damage and correct it before the cell divides again and thus undergoes **mutation.**

The initiation stage of carcinogenesis, during which time DNA is altered, is relatively short, ranging from minutes to days. The promotion state may last for months or years. During this period, the damage is locked into the genetic material in cells. Compounds that increase cell division are called promoters or epigenetic carcinogens. These compounds are thought to promote cancer either by decreasing the time available for repair enzymes to act or by encouraging cells with altered DNA to develop and grow. Some probable promoters are estrogen, alcohol, and possibly a high intake of dietary fat. Bacterial infections in the stomach are also suspected agents. For example, infection with *Helicobacter pylori,* which cause ulcers, may ultimately promote stomach cancer.

The final stage in carcinogenesis, cancer progression, begins with the appearance of cells that grow autonomously (out of control). During the progression phase, these malignant cells proliferate, invade surrounding tissue, and metastasize to other sites. Early in this stage, the immune system may find the altered cells and destroy them. Alternately, the cancer cells may be so defective that their own DNA limits their ability to grow, and they die. If

Table 12-5 | The Cancer Development Process

Cancer Initiation

Process: DNA alteration occurs in this relatively short phase (minutes to days).
Causes:

Radiation: e.g., sun overexposure
    Cross-links double strands of DNA or breaks them into fragments
Chemicals: e.g., aflatoxin (mold from peanuts and cereal grains), benzo(a)pyrene (smoke from charbroiled meat fat). These agents are transformed to highly reactive cancer initiators by **cytochrome P450,** an enzyme system that alters foreign compounds in the body. These metabolites are then able to cause mutations in DNA, RNA, and proteins.
Biological agents: e.g., viruses
    Promote uncontrolled growth of cells by inserting viral DNA or RNA into normal cells, which alters the cell's genes

Cancer Promotion

Process: DNA alterations are "locked" into the genetic material of cells over a period of months to more than 10 years.
Causes:

Long-term excess estrogen exposure
Excess alcohol
Excess dietary fat (controversial)
Bacterial infections: e.g., *Helicobacter pylori*

Cancer Progression

Process: Cells that can grow autonomously appear. These cells spread to surrounding tissue and other sites.
Causes:

Excess energy intake
Lack of early detection
Development of blood supply to the tumor
    The tumor uses newly formed capillaries to grow and spread cancer cells to remote sites in the body.

Anything that increases the rate of cell division decreases the chance that the repair enzymes will find the altered part of the DNA in time to do their work. Once a cell multiplies and incorporates its newly altered DNA into its genetic instructions, the repair enzymes can no longer detect the changes in DNA.

cytochrome P450 A set of enzymes in cells that act on compounds foreign to the body. This action aids in their excretion, but also creates short-lived, highly reactive forms.

nothing impedes cancer cell growth, one or more tumors eventually develop that are large enough to affect body functions, and the signs and symptoms of cancer appear (review Table 12-5).

Is Cancer Environmental or Hereditary?

Inherited mutations cannot account for the dramatic differences in cancer rates around the world. In poorer countries, cancers of the stomach, liver, mouth, esophagus, and uterus are most common, whereas in affluent countries, cancers of the lung, colon-rectum, breast, and prostate gland predominate.

The environmental factors shared by a family can include human papillomavirus infection for cervical cancer, smoking (passive and active) for lung cancer, diet for colon cancer, and *Helicobacter pylori* for stomach cancer. Heritable factors are seen primarily for colorectal, breast, and prostate cancer. Still, the impact of heredity on cancer risk is small; inherited genetic factors account for only 1 to 15% of all the cancers.

Diet and Cancer

Oxidative damage to DNA is likely to cause mutations. This damage can be enhanced by some dietary factors or, in contrast, reduced by enzymes such as those that incorporate the trace mineral selenium. There is evidence that intake of selenium above the RDA has an anticancer effect in humans, but there aren't enough data at this time to make a recommendation as to the extra amount needed.

Excessive energy intakes increase the risk of human cancer. Laboratory animal studies have shown that energy restriction during periods of rapid growth is protective against cancer. No doubt obesity increases the risk of cancers of the uterus, breast, kidney, and possibly the prostate gland, colon, and gallbladder. Excess body fat may affect sex hormone and insulin production, which increases cancer risk, or cancer cells may grow more easily when energy is plentiful.[6]

No link has been found between a low-fat diet and the development of breast cancer, but excess body weight increases the risk. Perhaps certain fatty

People who meet their vitamin C needs may have a lower risk of cancer of the oral cavity, esophagus, stomach, and breast. Whether this benefit is due to vitamin C itself or because these people eat a lot of fruits and vegetables, which provide many other nutrients, is still unknown.

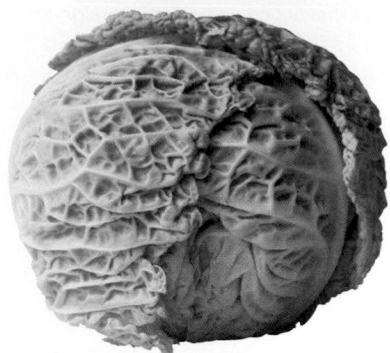

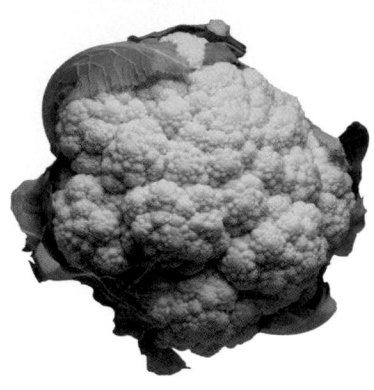

Cruciferous vegetables such as cabbage and cauliflower are rich in cancer-preventing phytochemicals.

acids, such as monounsaturated and polyunsaturated fatty acids in fish and canola oil, are beneficial.

High intakes of vegetables and fruits have been associated with lower risks of many cancers.[4,5,14] The constituents that are protective against cancer have not been identified, but evidence supports the B-vitamin folate as one of the factors. Studies of colorectal cancer show an inverse relationship between folate status and the rate of cancer. An inadequate intake of folate could also influence the risk of mutation.

High intakes of meat and protein products have been associated with an increased risk of prostate cancer. This association might be related to the saturated fat content of the food. In addition, meat cooked at high temperatures over an open flame, such as in charcoal broiling, produces polyaromatic hydrocarbons, one being benzo-[a]pyrene. Benzo-[a]pyrene binds to DNA and produces tumors, such as in the colon.[17]

Excess alcohol consumption increases the risks of upper GI tract cancers. Even moderate alcohol intake seems to increase the risk of cancers of the breast and colon.

Nitrosamines are carcinogenic. Nitrosamines are formed from nitrite, which exists in various foods and is produced endogenously from nitrate in vegetables. Nitrosamine compounds are found in bacon, sausage, hot dogs, beer, cheese, and some nitrite-preserved foods.

Mycotoxins are toxins produced by fungi. Among the many examples is aflatoxin B_1, a component of many moldy foods, such as moldy grain and peanuts. It is classified as a human carcinogen and is thought to cause liver cancer. Drought conditions in Asian and African countries have resulted in the widespread contamination of foods by aflatoxins. Even in the United States, corn has been found with increased carcinogen levels from aflatoxin B_1 because of changing weather conditions, but grain elevator operators and FDA monitor grains for unsafe amounts. Current studies are focusing on various antioxidants that may protect us from environmental carcinogens such as aflatoxins.

Another recent discovery resulting from attempts to find dietary solutions to the prevention of cancer suggests that calcium and vitamin D (or moderate sun exposure) may be part of the answer. Calcium intake is inversely related to cancer, especially colon cancer. It may be that calcium binds free fatty acid and bile acids in the colon so that they are less likely to interact with certain types of intestinal cells, which in turn become cancer.

The hormone form of vitamin D—1,25 $(OH)_2$ vitamin D—has been shown to inhibit the progression of human colorectal cells from cancerous polyps. Vitamin D also has been shown to inhibit rapid colon/rectal cell growth in people with intestinal inflammatory diseases. These combined data suggest a chemopreventive action of vitamin D against colon neoplasms. This action may be the beneficial effect of vitamin D–fortified dairy foods.

Based on our current knowledge of diet and cancer risk, the following guidelines are about all that can be recommended at this time: remain physically active; avoid obesity; engage in regular physical activity that promotes the formation of lean muscle; consume an abundance of fruits, vegetables, and whole grains; consume plenty of low-fat and fat-free dairy products; avoid a high intake of red meat, processed (cured) meats, and animal fat; and avoid excessive use of alcohol (Tables 12-6 and 12-7).[4,5,14,17]

American Institute for Cancer Research Diet and Health Guidelines for Cancer Prevention

1. Choose a diet rich in a variety of plant-based foods.
2. Eat plenty of vegetables and fruits.
3. Maintain a healthy weight and be physically active.
4. Drink alcohol only in moderation, if at all.
5. Select foods low in fat and salt.
6. Prepare and store food safely.
And always remember . . .
Do not use tobacco in any form.

Cancer Warning Signs

Remember also that if a cancer is left untreated, it can spread quickly throughout the body. When this happens, the cancer will much more likely lead to

Table 12-6 | Some Food Constituents Suspected of Having a Role in Cancer

Constituent	Dietary Sources	Action
Possibly Protective*		
Vitamin A	Liver, fortified milk, fruits, vegetables	Encourages normal cell development.
Vitamin D	Fortified milk	Increases production of a protein that suppresses cell growth, such as in the colon.
Vitamin E	Whole grains: vegetable oils: green, leafy vegetables	Prevents formation of nitrosamines and has general antioxidant properties.
Vitamin C	Fruits, vegetables	Can block conversion of nitrites and nitrates to potent carcinogens and likely has general antioxidant properties.
Folate	Fruits, vegetables, whole grains	Encourages normal cell development; especially reduces the risk of colon cancer.
Selenium	Meats, whole grains	Part of antioxidant system that inhibits tumor growth and kills developing cancer cells.
Carotenoids, such as lycopene	Fruits, vegetables	Likely act as antioxidants; some of these possibly influence cell metabolism. Lycopene in particular may reduce the risk of prostate cancer.
Indoles, phenols, and other phytochemical substances	Vegetables, especially cabbage, cauliflower, broccoli, brussels sprouts; garlic; onions; tea	May reduce cancer in the stomach and other organs.
Calcium	Dairy products, green vegetables	Slows cell division in the colon, binds bile acids and free fatty acids, thus reducing colon cancer risk.
Omega-3 fatty acids	Cold-water fish, such as salmon and tuna	May inhibit tumor growth.
Soy products	Tofu, soy milk, tempeh, soy nuts	Phytic acid present possibly binds carcinogens in the intestinal tract; the genistein component possibly reduces growth and metastasis of malignant cells.
Conjugated linoleic acid	Dairy products, meats	May inhibit tumor development and act as an antioxidant.
Fiber-rich foods	Fruits, vegetables, whole-grain breads and cereals, beans, nuts	Colon and rectal cancer risk may be decreased by accelerating intestinal transit and excretion of carcinogens.
Possibly Carcinogenic		
Excessive energy intake	All macronutrients can contribute.	Excess fat mass leading to obesity; linked to increased synthesis of estrogen and other sex hormones; which in excess may themselves increase the risk for cancer. Resulting excess insulin output from creation of an insulin-resistant state is also implicated.
Total fat	Meats, high-fat milk and milk products, animal fats and vegetable oils	The strongest evidence is for excessive saturated and polyunsaturated fat intake. Saturated fat is linked to an increased risk of prostate cancer.
High glycemic load carbohydrates	Cookies, cakes, sugared soft drinks, candy	Insulin surges associated with these foods may increase tumor growth, such as in the colon.
Alcohol	Beer, wine, liquor	Contributes to cancers of the throat, liver, bladder, breast, and colon (especially if the person does not consume enough folate).
Nitrites, nitrates	Cured meats, especially ham, bacon, and sausages	Under very high temperatures will bind to amino acid derivatives to form nitrosamines, which are potent carcinogens.
Aflatoxins	Formed when mold is present on peanuts or grains	May alter DNA structure and inhibit its ability to properly respond to physiologic controls; aflatoxin in particular is linked to liver cancer.
Benzo(a)pyrene and other heterocyclic amines	Charcoal-broiled foods, especially meats	Linked to stomach and colon cancer. To limit this risk, trim fat from meat before cooking, cut barbecuing time by partially cooking meat (such as in a microwave oven), and don't consume blackened parts of meats.

*Many of the actions listed for these possibly protective agents are speculative and have been verified only by experimental animal studies. The best evidence supports obtaining these nutrients and other food constituents from foods. Recently the U.S. Preventive Service Task Force (USPSTF) supported this statement, noting there is no clear evidence that nutrient supplements provide the same benefits.

Table 12-7 | Example of a Diet Intended to Limit the Risk for Cancer—Low in Fat and High in Fruits and Vegetables with Plenty of Calcium

Breakfast
6 oz calcium-fortified orange juice
1 cup ready-to-eat whole-grain breakfast cereal
1 cup 1% milk
1 banana
1 slice whole-wheat toast, jelly, soft margarine
Hot tea

Lunch
Sandwich:
1/2 cup chicken salad served on 1/2 of a bagel or 1 slice of whole-wheat bread
Assorted raw vegetables: carrots, celery, broccoli, chopped lettuce
1 cup 1% milk
Fresh fruit: strawberries, melon, grapes, apple
2 fig cookies

Dinner
3 oz baked fish (e.g., cod, salmon)
Baked potato topped with shredded mozzarella cheese (1/3 cup)
Roasted corn on the cob, soft margarine
Fresh garden salad with low-fat Italian dressing
1 whole-wheat dinner roll
1 scoop lemon ice or orange sherbet
Hot tea

Snack
12-oz can diet cola or apple juice
2 cups popcorn
1/4 cup mixed nuts

Nutrient Breakdown:
2300 kcal
% energy from fat: 25%

death. Thus, early detection is critical. Aids to early detection include the following warning signs (the acronym is CAUTION):

- Change in bowel or bladder habits
- A sore that does not heal
- Unusual bleeding or discharge
- Thickening or lump in the breast or elsewhere
- Indigestion or difficulty in swallowing
- Obvious change in a wart or mole
- Nagging cough or hoarseness

There are still other ways to detect cancer early. Some recommendations are colonoscopy examina-tions for middle-age and older adults, PSA (prostate-specific antigen) tests for men over age 50, Papanicolaou tests (Pap smears) and regular breast examinations (and mammograms starting about age 40 to 50) for women and regular self-examination of testicles for men.[7] Finally, to learn still more about cancer, review these sources of credible cancer information on the Internet:

www.cancer.org American Cancer Society
www.icic.nci.nih.gov CancerNet
www.cancer.med.upenn.edu Oncolink

Summary

1. Six of the trace minerals (iron, zinc, copper, molybdenum, iodide, and selenium) have an RDA. An Adequate Intake has been set for three trace minerals (manganese, chromium, and fluoride).

2. Some trace minerals are difficult to detect in humans, and it is often hard to determine the exact amount of a trace mineral in food. Deficiencies were first observed in small, geographically isolated groups (e.g., selenium deficiency in an area of China) or in people nourished exclusively by total parenteral nutrition that did not contain sufficient trace minerals.

3. Iron is a critical component of hemoglobin, myoglobin, and cytochromes. Iron acts as a cofactor for several enzyme systems. Two-thirds of the body's iron is found in hemoglobin in red blood cells, where its job is to transport oxygen from the lungs to the tissues. A prolonged low intake of iron can lead to decreased production of red blood cells and a lack of oxygen being delivered to the tissues. This condition is called iron deficiency anemia, which results in fatigue upon exertion and apathy as well as decreased learning ability in children.

4. The absorption of iron depends on the body's need for the mineral and on the form of iron in food. The body cannot readily excrete excess iron, but the body has a mucosal block that limits overabsorption. Heme iron from animal foods is better absorbed than nonheme iron obtained from plant sources. The best sources of dietary iron are animal protein, including beef and other dark meats, oysters, and liver.

5. Girls and women have a higher RDA for iron than men because of menstrual blood loss. Even in North America infants and children are often iron deficient.

6. Iron toxicity can occur because of a genetic disorder called hemochromatosis, which causes the overabsorption of iron. Iron poisoning and death can occur when toddlers and young children swallow a large number of iron pills.

7. Zinc functions as a cofactor for many enzyme systems and also stabilizes membranes and other body molecules. Among the processes affected by zinc are growth, antioxidant protection, sexual development, immune function, and taste. A zinc deficiency can result in growth failure, loss of appetite, inadequate mental function, a persistent rash, and decreased immune function.

8. Like iron, the best dietary sources of zinc are found in animal foods. Need drives absorption. And like with iron, a mucosal block in the intestinal cells regulates the amount of zinc that can be absorbed. Calcium and iron in supplement form can interfere with zinc absorption. The richest source of zinc is oysters. Other animal proteins are excellent sources. Plant sources are whole grains, peanuts, and legumes.

9. Copper aids in iron mobilization from body stores. Copper is responsible for the cross-linking in collagen formation and also acts as part of antioxidant enzymes. A copper deficiency can result in a secondary iron deficiency. Copper is found in liver, cocoa, legumes, and whole grains.

10. Selenium acts as a cofactor for the enzyme glutathionine peroxidase, which protects cells against destruction by hydrogen peroxide and free radicals. In some instances, selenium can replace some of the need for vitamin E. Human deficiency is rare in North America. The selenium content of the soil in which a plant is grown greatly affects the selenium content of the plant food. Where the soil is selenium-poor, the inhabitants may experience selenium deficiency. Meat, eggs, fish, and shellfish are sources of selenium. Plant sources include grains and seeds.

11. Iodide forms part of the thyroid hormones, one being thyroxine T_4. A lack of dietary iodide causes an enlarged thyroid gland, known as goiter. The iodide content of the soil in which a plant is grown greatly affects the iodide content of the plant food. Today, iodide deficiency in North America is virtually unknown because of the fortification of table salt with iodide, but deficiency is still a major problem in most parts of the world.

12. Fluoride exposure makes the tooth crystal resistant to dental caries, and fluoride in saliva aids in the remineralization of damaged tooth surfaces. Most North Americans receive fluoride from fluoridated drinking water and toothpaste.

13. Chromium contributes to the action of insulin. Chromium is found in meats and whole grains.

14. Manganese functions in several important enzyme systems, including one that participates in antioxidant protection. Deficiency is rare. Whole grains, legumes, tea, and nuts are food sources.

15. Molybdenum is found in several enzyme systems. Deficiency is rare. Molybdenum is found in plant foods such as legumes and whole grains.

16. Boron contributes to ion transport in cell membranes. Fruits, leafy vegetables, nuts, and beans are sources.

17. Nickel likely participates in amino acid metabolism. Nickel is found in nuts, beans, and whole grains.

18. Silicon is involved in bone formation. Root vegetables and whole grains are sources.

19. Arsenic likely participates in amino acid and DNA metabolism. Fish, grains, and cereal products are sources.

20. Vanadium likely has insulin-like actions in the body. Shellfish and mushrooms are sources.

21. Cancer develops in a multistep fashion in the body. Numerous dietary factors affect the various steps in this process. A diet rich in low-fat and fat-free dairy products, fruits, vegetables, and whole grains likely lessens cancer development in some body tissues. Regular physical activity adds further benefit.

Study Questions

1. What is a balance study, and why is it only a limited tool in evaluating the need for trace minerals?

2. What is anemia? How does a deficiency of vitamins E, K, B-6, folate, and B-12 and the trace minerals iron and copper cause anemia? Describe the specific type of such anemias.

3. Explain three key functions of iron in the human body.

4. What factors increase the absorption of dietary iron?

5. What are some tests used to access iron deficiency anemia? measure iron status? What exactly do these tests measure?

6. Why does zinc affect so many body processes?

7. The fluoridation of drinking water began in the United States in 1945. How else do humans obtain fluoride?

8. Describe the chief function of fluoride, copper, chromium, manganese, boron, nickel, and silicon in the body.

9. Why are animal foods a better source of iron, zinc, and selenium than foods of plant origin?

10. Prior to the 1920s, why was goiter such a health problem for people living in the Great Lakes region of the United States? How was this deficiency disease eventually controlled?

BOOST YOUR STUDY

Check out the *Perspectives in Nutrition: Online Learning Center* www.mhhe.com/wardlawpers7 for quizzes, flash cards, activities, and web links designed to further help you learn about issues surrounding the trace minerals.

Annotated References

1. ADA Reports: Position of the American Dietetic Association: The impact of fluoride on health. *Journal of the American Dietetic Association* 105:1620, 2005.

   The American Dietetic Association reaffirms that fluoride is an important element for all mineralized tissues in the body. Appropriate fluoride intake is beneficial to bone and tooth health.

2. Age-Related Eye Disease Study Research Group: A randomized, placebo-controlled, clinical trial of high-dose supplementation with vitamins C and E and beta-carotene for age-related cataract and vision loss. *Archives of Ophthalmology* 119:1439–1452, 2001.

   Megadose zinc supplements (80 mg/day of zinc oxide) combined with 2 mg/day of copper reduced progression of macular degeneration in people who showed evidence of the disease. The zinc supplements worked even better when provided in combination with 400 IU of vitamin E, 500 mg of vitamin C, and 15 mg of beta-carotene. The authors suggest that adults who have evidence of macular degeneration talk to their physicians about possibly following such a protocol.

3. Burk RF, Leavander OA: Selenium. In Shils ME and others (eds): *Modern nutrition in health and disease.* 10th ed. Philadelphia, PA: Lippincott Williams & Wilkins, 2006.

   Selenium has both known and less well-known functions, such as for thioredoxin, a recently described set of antioxidant enzymes that contain selenium. In some cases, moderately high selenium intakes may help prevent certain diseases, such as cancer.

4. Byers T and others: American Cancer Society guidelines on nutrition and physical activity for cancer prevention: Reducing the risk of cancer with healthy food choices and physical activity. *CA: Cancer Journal for Clinicians* 52:92, 2002.

   A diet low in red and processed meats and rich in fruits, vegetables, and whole grains is advocated as a strategy for reducing cancer risk. Regular physical activity is also important to add.

5. Cancer-fighting foods. *Mayo Clinic Health Letter* 22(12):1, 2004

   Many foods, particularly plant-based foods, might help lower the risk of certain cancers. Unlike individual supplements, foods offer a unique mix of vitamins and minerals, multiple phytochemicals, fiber, and—not least of all—the pleasure of eating.

6. Cotunga N: Obesity, physical activity, and cancer risk. *Today's Dietitian,* p. 14, October 2002.

   Key factors for reducing cancer risk are maintaining a healthy body weight and performing regular physical activity. Avoiding weight gain in adulthood is especially important.

7. Coughlin L: American Cancer Society releases annual guidelines for the early detection of cancer. *American Family Physician* 71(11):2202, 2005.

   The American Cancer Society recommends that breast cancer screening should begin when women are 20 years old, with clinical breast examinations every 3 years until the age of 39. Thereafter, women at average risk should have an annual mammography. Cervical cancer screening should begin 3 years after the onset of vaginal intercourse but no later than 21 years of age. Adults at average risk of developing colorectal cancer should begin screening at 50 years of age. Men at high risk for prostate cancer should begin testing at the age of 45.

8. Eckhert CD: Other trace elements. In Shils ME and others (eds): *Modern nutrition in health and disease.* 10th ed. Philadelphia, PA: Lippincott Williams & Wilkins, 2006.

   At least 18 elements could be considered ultratrace minerals: aluminum, arsenic, boron, bromine, cadmium, chromium, fluoride, germanium, iodine, lead, lithium, molybdenum, nickel, rubidium, selenium, silicon, tin, and vanadium. The role of each in human and laboratory animal physiological systems is reviewed in this chapter.

9. Food and Nutrition Board, Institute of Medicine: *Dietary Reference Intakes for calcium, phosphorus, magnesium, vitamin D, and fluoride.* Washington, DC: National Academy Press, 1997.

   Dietary standards for many major minerals are covered. The rationale used to set RDA or Adequate Intakes and Upper Levels for these nutrients is discussed in detail.

10. Food and Nutrition Board, Institute of Medicine: *Dietary Reference Intakes for vitamin A, vitamin K, arsenic, boron, chromium, copper, iodine, iron, manganese, molybdenum, nickel, silicon, vanadium, and zinc.* Washington, DC: National Academy Press, 2001.

    Dietary standards for many trace minerals are covered. The rationale used to set RDA or Adequate Intakes and Upper Levels for these nutrients is discussed in detail.

11. Food and Nutrition Board, Institute of Medicine: *Dietary Reference Intakes for vitamin C, vitamin E, selenium, and carotenoids.* Washington, DC: National Academy of Sciences, 2000.

    The functions of antioxidant nutrients; how RDA and related standards were determined; and deficiency and toxicity symptoms are explained.

12. Franchini M, Veneri D: Hereditary hemochromatosis. *Hematology* 10(2):145, 2005.

    Hereditary hemochromatosis is a disorder of iron metabolism characterized by progressive tissue iron overload that leads to irreversible organ damage if not treated in time. Transferrin saturation and serum ferritin are still the most reliable tests for the detection of people with hereditary hemochromatosis. Therapeutic phlebotomy is the mainstay of treatment. If phlebotomy is started before the onset of irreversible organ damage, the life expectancy of these patients is similar to that of the normal population.

13. King JC, Cousins, RJ: Zinc. In Shils ME and others (eds): *Modern nutrition in health and disease.* 10th ed. Philadelphia, PA: Lippincott Williams & Wilkins, 2006.

    This chapter presents various subjects relevant to this mineral. Zinc is especially important to cells that have a high turnover, such as immune cells.

14. Liu RH: Potential synergy of phytochemicals in cancer prevention: Mechanism of action. *Journal of Nutrition* 134:347S, 2004.

    No single antioxidant can replace the combination of natural phytochemicals in fruits and vegetables to achieve the health benefits. Antioxidants or bioactive compounds are best acquired through whole-food consumption, not from dietary supplements. Consumption of 5 to 10 servings daily of a wide variety of fruits and vegetables is an appropriate strategy for significantly reducing the risk of chronic diseases such as cancer and to meet nutrient requirements for optimum health.

15. Patel JD and others: Lung cancer in U.S. women. *Journal of the American Medical Association* 291:1763, 2004.

    Lung cancer is the leading cause of cancer death in the United States, including women, and much more so than female breast cancer. It is important that the women who smoke cigarettes (25% of all women) not continue to do so if this health problem is to be conquered.

16. Turnland J: Copper. In Shils ME and others (eds): *Modern nutrition in health and disease.* 10th ed. Philadelphia, PA: Lippincott Williams & Wilkins, 2006.

    Various subjects relevant to this mineral are presented including the diverse roles of copper in the body.

17. Willett WC: Diet and cancer: An evolving picture. *Journal of the American Medical Association* 293(2):233, 2005.

    The relation between red meat consumption and colorectal cancer may not be conclusive, but prudence would suggest that red meat, and processed meats in particular, should be eaten sparingly to minimize risk. When this advice is combined with other healthful diet and lifestyle factors, it appears that approximately 70% of colon cancer can be avoided.

18. Wood RJ, Ronnenberg AG: Iron. In Shils ME and others (eds): *Modern nutrition in health and disease.* 10th ed. Philadelphia, PA: Lippincott Williams & Wilkins, 2006.

    Iron contributes to many functions of body cells, as outlined in this chapter. The need for iron is the driving force behind absorption, especially for nonheme iron.

19. Wright JD and others: Dietary intake of ten key nutrients for public health, United States: 1999–2000. *Advance Data* 334:1, 2003 (April 17).

    Women in general fail to meet iron needs. In contrast, zinc intakes appear adequate across the adult population.

20. Zimmerman MB: Assessing iodine status and monitoring progress of iodized salt programs. *Journal of Nutrition* 134:1673, 2004.

    Despite remarkable progress in the control of iodide deficiency disorders, they remain a significant global health problem. Assessing the severity of the disorders and monitoring the progress of salt iodization programs are cornerstones of a control strategy. Ensuring sustainability of these programs is one of the great remaining challenges in the global fight to eliminate iodide deficiency.

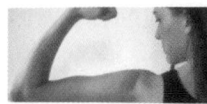

Take | Action

I. Analyze Iron and Zinc Intake in a Sample Vegan Diet

Steve has been a vegan for 2 months. He chose this diet pattern for health reasons, but is his diet really that healthy? His food and beverage intake yesterday was as follows:

Breakfast

Soy milk, 1 cup
Raisin Bran cereal, 1 cup
Banana, 1
Black coffee, 12 oz

Lunch

Sandwich:
    Whole-wheat bread, 2 slices
    Tomato, 1 small
    Bean sprouts, 1/4 cup
    Mayonnaise, 2 tbsp
Granola bar, 1
Orange, 1
Water, 12 oz

Snack

Oatmeal cookies, 3 small
Apple juice, 12 oz

Dinner

Salad:
    Romaine lettuce, 1-1/2 cups
    Carrot, 1 (shredded)
    Cucumber, 1/2 sliced
    Mushrooms, 1/3 cup
    French dressing, 3 tbsp
White bean soup, 2 cups
Whole-wheat crackers, 8
Soy cheese, 1 oz
Hot tea, 12 oz

Snack

Popcorn, 3 cups
Root beer, 12 oz

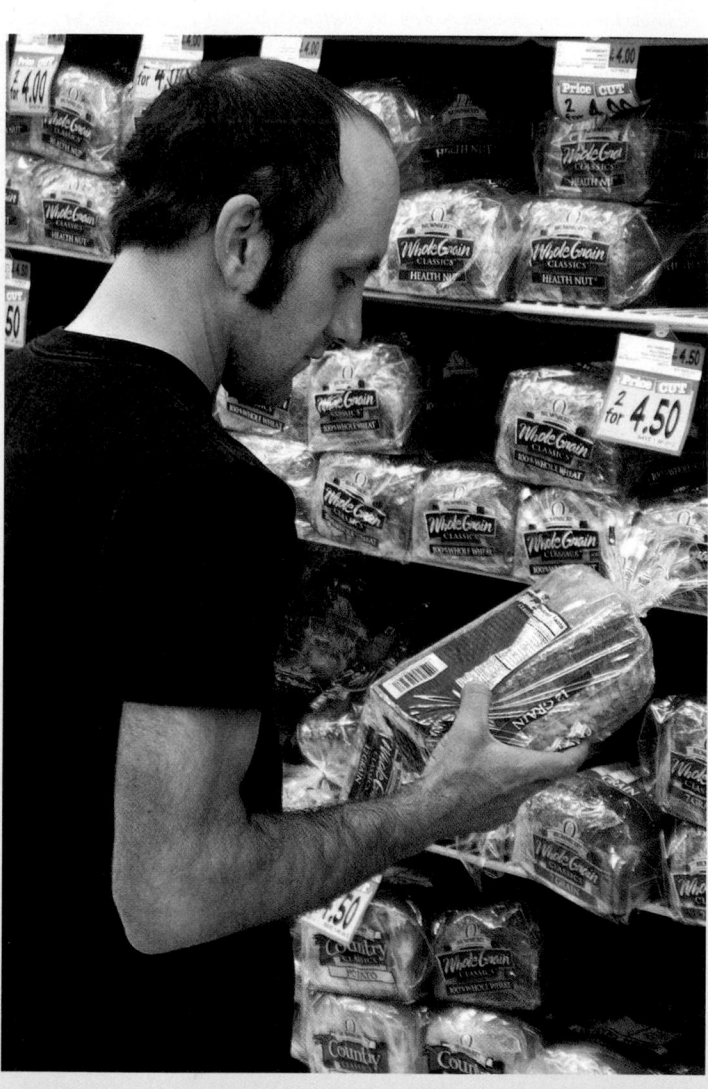

Start by analyzing Steve's iron and zinc intake using Appendix N or the NutritionCalc Plus software. What is your conclusion? Does Steve's diet appear to be a healthy way to eat? What other nutrients may be of concern? Check the analysis for those nutrients also.

II. Check Out Your Municipal Water Supply

Healthy People 2010 set a goal that 75% of people in the United States will be served by community water systems that add sufficient fluoride. Today only about 60% of Americans have access to naturally or artificially fluoridated water. Is your hometown (or college town) water supply fluoridated? To find the answer, check with your local water department. What amount of fluoride is added to drinking water, and how long has this procedure been in operation? You can also check with your family dentist; he or she will know how much fluoride is added to the water in your hometown. If the water supply is not fluoridated, what procedures does your dentist recommend for obtaining sufficient fluoride?

ENERGY BALANCE AND WEIGHT CONTROL

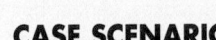

CHAPTER OUTLINE

CASE SCENARIO:

Chris has a hectic schedule. He works full-time at an industrial plant. Three nights a week he attends class at the local community college in pursuit of certification. On weekends he tries to squeeze in studying and time for his family and friends. He has little time to think about what he eats—convenience rules. Unfortunately, over the past few years Chris's weight has been climbing, especially around his waist. Watching television a few nights ago, he saw an infomercial for a product that promises he can eat large portions of tasty foods but not gain weight. Celebrities support the claim that this product allows one to eat at will and not gain weight. This claim—that by taking this product he can eat whatever he wants and never gain weight—is tempting to Chris. What do you think he should do? What advice can you offer Chris for evaluating weight-loss programs?

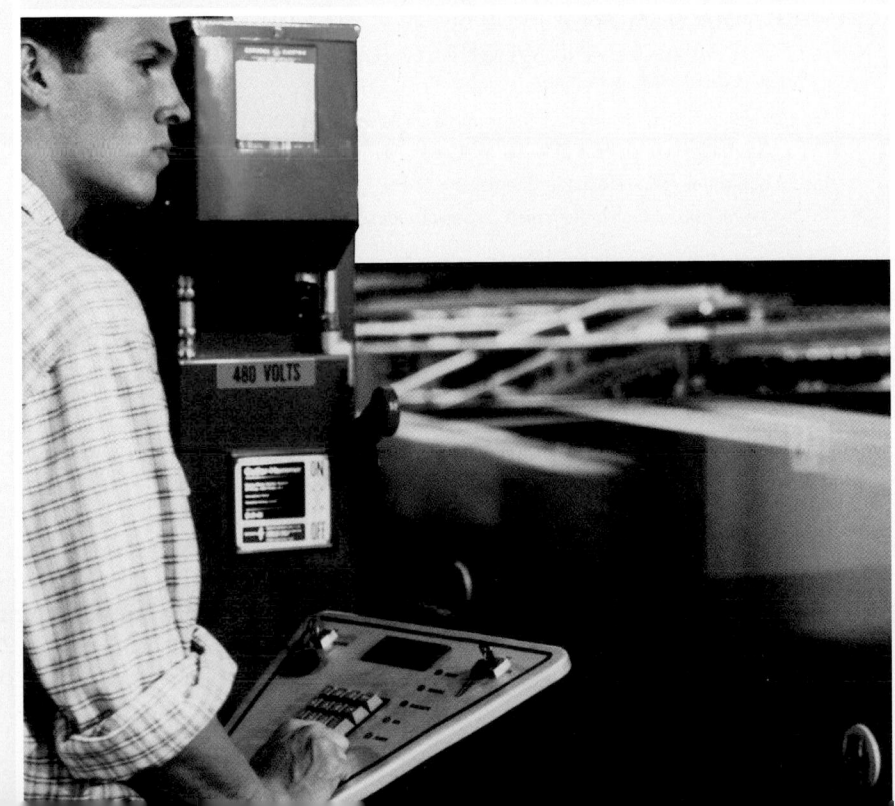

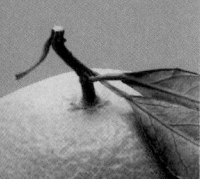

In North America, 29% of men and 44% of women are trying to lose weight. Still, despite all their efforts, the ranks of the obese in North America and worldwide are growing.[9] Recall from Chapter 1 that it is estimated that about 1 billion people in the world are overweight. This problem is increasing not only in the United States but also among affluent people in Brazil, China, India, Russia, the United Kingdom, Germany, and many other countries. Excess weight increases the likelihood of many health problems, such as cardiovascular disease, cancer, hypertension, strokes, certain bone and joint disorders, and type 2 diabetes.[11,19] To some extent regular physical activity can prevent or reduce the risk of these health problems, but lifelong weight control is still an important focus.[10]

For most people, weight-reduction efforts fizzle before people achieve a healthy weight range. Typical popular ("fad") diets are generally monotonous, ineffective, and confusing. They may even endanger some populations, such as children, teenagers, pregnant women, and people with various health disorders. Yet a more logical approach to weight loss is actually very straightforward: (1) Eat less; (2) increase physical activity; and (3) change problematic eating behaviors.[19]

Experts are calling for a national commitment to address the growing weight problem in North America. They suspect that the current trends will not be reversed without a national commitment to weight maintenance and effective new approaches to making our social environment more favorable to maintaining a healthy weight.[2] Chapter 13 discusses these recommendations to help you understand obesity's causes, consequences, and potential treatments. Note that Chapter 17 does the same for child and adolescent obesity.

CHAPTER OBJECTIVES CHAPTER 13 IS DESIGNED TO ALLOW YOU TO:

1. Describe the uses of energy by the body and what constitutes energy balance.
2. Characterize the terms *hunger, appetite,* and *satiety* and outline the internal and external forces involved in satiety regulation.
3. Describe how to establish a healthy weight for a person.
4. Describe various ways to diagnose overweight and obesity.
5. Outline the risks to health posed by overweight and obesity.
6. List and discuss factors affecting energy balance and describe the concept of set point.
7. Describe why and how reduced energy intake, behavior modification, and increased physical activity fit into a weight-loss plan.
8. Evaluate popular weight-reduction diets and determine which are unsafe, doomed to fail, or both.
9. Outline the benefits and hazards of various weight-loss methods for severe obesity.
10. Describe possible reasons and treatments for underweight status.

REFRESH YOUR MEMORY AS YOU BEGIN YOUR STUDY OF ENERGY BALANCE AND WEIGHT CONTROL IN CHAPTER 13, YOU MAY WANT TO REVIEW:
- The concept of energy density and appropriate single serving sizes for foods in Chapter 2
- The causes and consequences of ketosis in Chapter 4
- The fat content of various foods in Chapter 6
- The long-term risks of high-protein diets, especially for some people, in Chapter 7

▌ Energy Balance

This chapter begins with some good news and some bad news. The good news is that if you stay at a healthy body weight, you increase your chances of living a long and healthy life. The bad news is that currently 65% of all North American adults are overweight, significantly more than as recently as the 1980s. Of those, about 45% (30% of the total population) are obese. There is a good chance that any of us could become part of those statistics if we do not pay attention to preventing significant weight gain in adulthood.[4] Gaining more than 10 lb or 2 inches in waist circumference are signals that a reevaluation of diet and lifestyle is in order.

There is no quick cure for overweight, despite what advertisements and infomercials claim. Any success comes from hard work and commitment. Currently, a combination of decrease in energy intake, increase in physical activity, and behavior modification is the most reliable plan for the problem of overweight. And without a doubt, preventing the problem in the first place is the most successful approach of all.[9]

Positive and Negative Energy Balance

Many of us would benefit from paying more attention to the important concept of **energy balance.** Think of energy balance as an equation:

Energy Input = Energy Output
(food intake)　　(metabolism; digestion, absorption, and
　　　　　　　　　transport of nutrients; physical activity)

The relative size (measured in kcals) of the two sides of this equation can influence energy stores, especially the amount of triglyceride stored in adipose tissue (Figure 13-1).[9]

When energy input is greater than energy output, the result is **positive energy balance.** The excess energy consumed is stored, resulting in weight gain. There are some situations in which positive energy balance is necessary. During pregnancy, a surplus of energy is needed to support the developing fetus. Infants and children require a positive energy balance for growth and development. In adults, however, even a small positive energy balance over time can cause body weight to climb.

On the other hand, if energy input is less than energy output, there is an energy deficit, and **negative energy balance** results. Weight loss occurs because the person is in a state of negative energy balance. And even though we think of extra body weight as "fat," this weight loss always involves a reduction in both lean and adipose tissue—just the relative mix differs.

As noted in the introduction, maintaining energy balance—matching energy intake to energy output over the long term—substantially contributes to health and well-being in adults by minimizing the risk of developing many common health problems.[19] Adulthood is often a time of subtle increases in weight gain, which eventually turns into obesity if left unchecked. The process of aging itself does not cause weight gain; rather, weight gain stems from a pattern of excess food intake coupled with limited physical activity and slower metabolism.[9] The following sections look in detail at the factors that affect the energy balance equation.

Energy Intake

Energy needs are met by food intake, represented by the kcals eaten each day. Determining the appropriate amount and type of food to match energy needs over the long run is a challenge for many of us. Our desire to consume food and ability to use it efficiently are evolutionary survival mechanisms. However, because of modern North American food supplies and accessibility, many of us are now too successful in obtaining food energy. The refrigerator has essentially replaced the need to store body fat—food is always at hand.[19] And given the wide availability of food in vending machines, drive-up windows, social gatherings, and fast-food restaurants—combined with larger and larger portions—it is no wonder that the average adult is 8 lb heavier than just 10 years ago. You might say "food hunts man" today. In response to this cultural trend of wide food availability, "defensive eating" (i.e., making careful and conscious food choices, especially in regard to portion size) on a continual basis is important for many of us.[5,15]

How much food energy is contained in a meal? A **bomb calorimeter** can be used to determine the amount of energy in a food. The process is described in Figure 13-2. The bomb calorimeter measures the kcals that can be derived from carbohydrate, fat, protein, and alcohol. Recall that carbohydrates yield about 4 kcal/g, proteins yield about 4 kcal/g, fats yield about 9 kcal/g, and alcohol yields 7 kcal/g. These energy figures

The Growing Overweight/ Obesity Problem

Adults 20 to 74 who are overweight or obese:

1960–1962	**45%**
1971–1974	**47%**
1976–1980	**47%**
1988–1994	**56%**
1999–today	**64.5%**

energy balance The state in which energy intake, in the form of food and beverages, matches energy expended, primarily through basal metabolism and physical activity.

positive energy balance The state in which energy intake is greater than energy expended, generally resulting in weight gain.

negative energy balance The state in which energy intake is less than energy expended, resulting in weight loss.

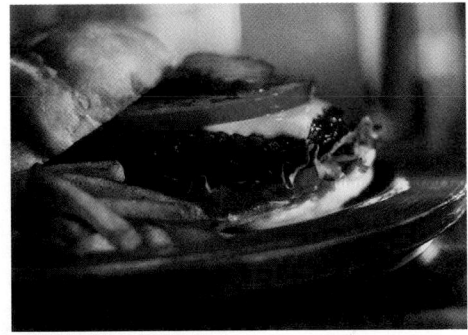

Today we demand food that is immediately available, tastes great, requires little or no preparation, and is served in generous quantities. Of these characteristics, the generous quantities are the most troublesome for many of us. As noted in Chapter 1, a response to serving large quantities might be to share your meal with another person.

bomb calorimeter An instrument used to determine the energy content of a food.

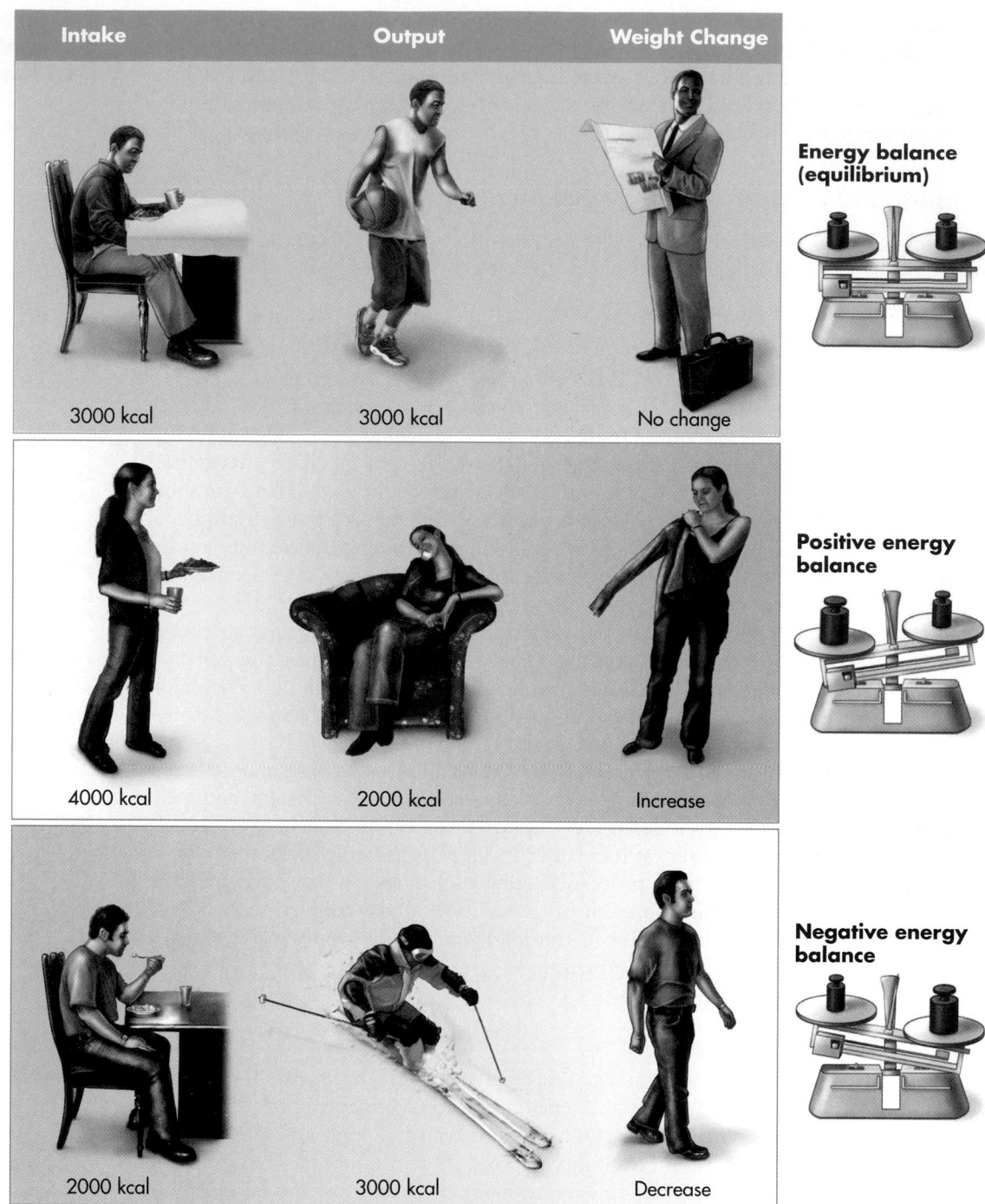

Intake	Output	Weight Change	
3000 kcal	3000 kcal	No change	**Energy balance (equilibrium)**
4000 kcal	2000 kcal	Increase	**Positive energy balance**
2000 kcal	3000 kcal	Decrease	**Negative energy balance**

Figure 13-1 | A model for energy balance—input vs. output. This figure depicts energy balance in practical terms.

have been adjusted for (1) digestibility and (2) substances in food, such as fibrous plant parts that burn in the bomb calorimeter but are unusable by the human body for energy needs. The figures are then rounded to whole numbers. Note, however, that today it is more common to determine the energy content of a food by simply quantifying its carbohydrate, protein, and fat (and possibly alcohol) content. Then the kcal/g factors are used to calculate the total energy content. (Recall that Chapter 1 showed how to do this calculation.)

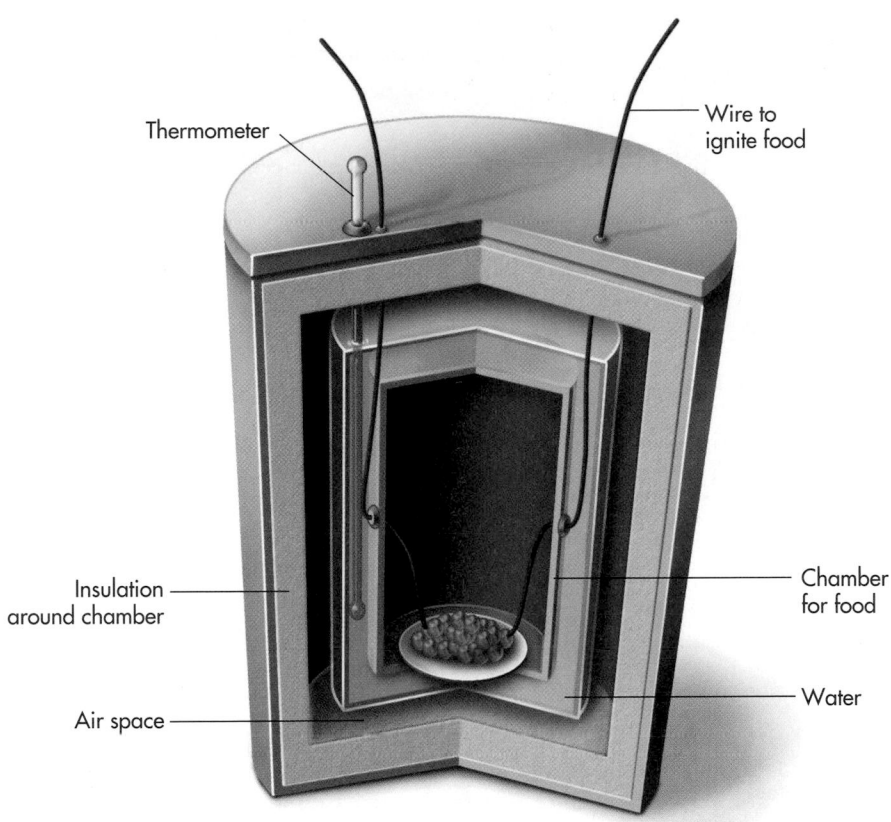

Thermometer

Wire to
ignite food

Insulation
around chamber

Chamber
for food

Air space

Water

Figure 13-2 | Cross-section of a bomb calorimeter. A dried portion of food is burned inside a chamber charged with oxygen and surrounded by water to determine energy content. As the food is burned, it gives off heat, which increases the temperature of the water surrounding the chamber. The increase in water temperature indicates the number of kcal contained in the food, because 1 kcal equals the amount of heat needed to raise the temperature of 1 kg of water by 1°C.

Energy Output

The other side of the energy balance equation is energy output. The body uses energy for three general purposes: basal metabolism; physical activity; and digestion, absorption, and processing of ingested nutrients. A fourth minor form of energy output, known as thermogenesis, refers to energy expended during fidgeting or shivering in response to cold (Figure 13-3).[9]

Basal Metabolism

As covered in Chapter 12, **basal metabolism** (expressed as **basal metabolic rate [BMR]**) represents the minimum amount of energy expended in a fasting state (12 hours or more) to keep a resting, awake body alive in a warm, quiet environment. For a sedentary person, basal metabolism accounts for about 60 to 70% of total energy use by the body. Some of the processes involved include the beating of the heart, respiration by the lungs, and the activity of other organs such as the liver, brain, and kidney.[9] It does not include energy used for physical activity or digestion, absorption, and processing of nutrients recently consumed. If the person is not fasting or completely rested, the term **resting metabolism** is used (expressed as resting metabolic rate [RMR]). An individual's RMR is typically 6% higher than his or her BMR.

To see how basal metabolism contributes to energy needs, consider a 130-lb woman. First, knowing that there are 2.2 lb for every kg, convert her weight into metric units:

$$130 \div 2.2 = 59 \text{ kg}$$

Then, using a rough estimate of basal metabolic rate of 0.9 kcal/kg per hour for an average female (1.0 kcal/kg per hour is used for an average male), calculate her basal metabolic rate:

$$59 \times 0.9 = 53 \text{ kcal/hour}$$

basal metabolism The minimal amount of energy the body uses to support itself in a fasting state when resting and awake in a warm, quiet environment. It amounts to roughly 1 kcal/kg per hour for men and 0.9 kcal/kg per hour for women.

basal metabolic rate (BMR) The rate of energy use (e.g., kcal/min) by the body when at rest and awake in a warm, quiet environment.

resting metabolism The amount of energy the body uses when the person has not eaten in 4 hours and is resting (e.g., 15 to 30 minutes) and awake in a warm, quiet environment. It is roughly 6% higher than basal metabolism due to the less strict criteria for the test; often referred to as *resting metabolic rate (RMR)*.

Figure 13-3 | The components of energy intake and expenditure. This figure incorporates the major variables that influence energy balance. Remember that alcohol is an additional source of energy for some of us (but is not depicted). The size of each component shows the relative contribution of that component to energy balance.

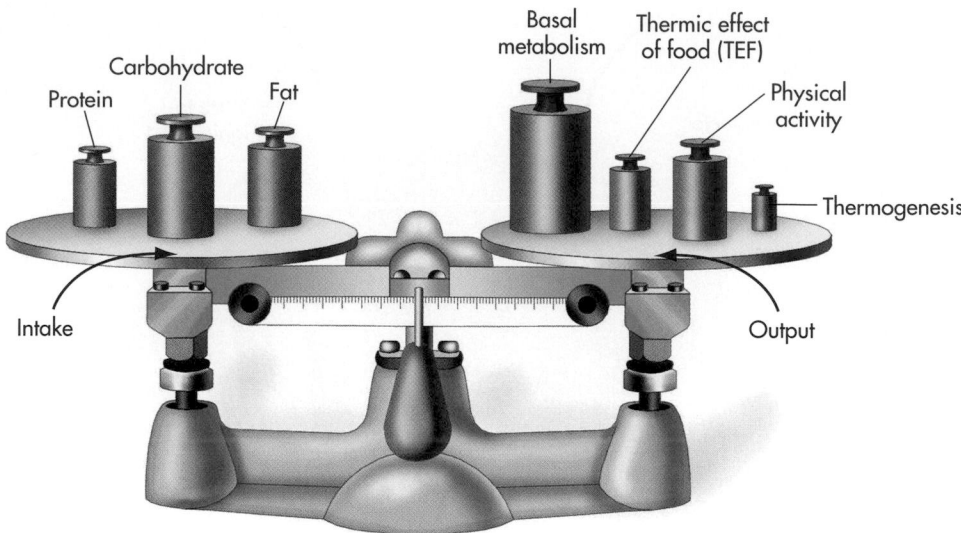

While a person is resting, the percentage of total energy use and corresponding energy use by various organs is approximately as follows:

Brain	19%	265 kcal/day
Skeletal muscle	18%	250 kcal/day
Liver	27%	380 kcal/day
Kidney	10%	140 kcal/day
Heart	7%	100 kcal/day
Other	19%	265 kcal/day

lean body mass Body weight after subtracting fat storage weight. Lean body mass includes organs such as the brain, muscles, and liver as well as blood and other body fluids.

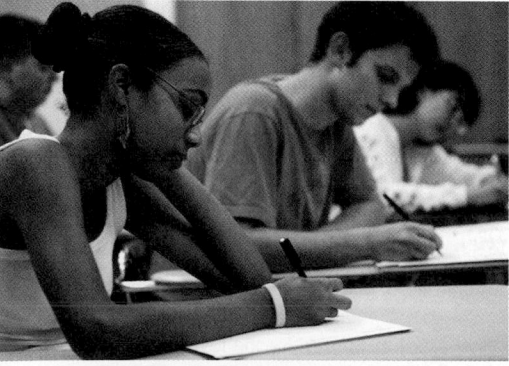

Classwork leads to mental stress but puts little physical stress on the body. Hence, energy needs are only about 1.5 kcal per minute.

Finally, use this hourly basal metabolic rate to find her basal metabolic rate for an entire day:

$$53 \times 24 = 1272 \text{ kcal}$$

These calculations give only an estimate of actual basal metabolism, because it can vary 25 to 30% among individuals. Factors that increase basal metabolism include:

- Greater **lean body mass**
- Larger body surface area
- Male gender (typically more lean body mass compared to females)
- Body temperature (fever or cold environmental conditions)
- Thyroid hormones
- Aspects of nervous system activity (release of norepinephrine)
- Pregnancy
- Caffeine and tobacco use (Still, using smoking to control body weight is not recommended because too many health risks are increased.)

Of those factors, the amount of lean body mass a person has is the most important one.

In contrast to factors that increase basal metabolism, a low-energy intake decreases basal metabolism by about 10 to 20% (about 150 to 300 kcal/day) as the body senses starvation and shifts into a conservation mode. This shift is a barrier to sustained weight loss during dieting that involves an extremely low food intake.[19] In addition, the effects of aging make weight maintenance a challenge. As lean body mass slowly and steadily decreases, basal metabolism declines 1 to 2% for each decade past the age of 30. However, because physical activity aids in maintaining lean body mass, remaining active as we age helps to preserve a high basal metabolism and, in turn, aids in weight control.[10]

Energy for Physical Activity

Physical activity increases energy expenditure above and beyond basal energy needs by as much as 25 to 40%. In choosing to be active or inactive, we determine much of our total energy expenditure for a day. Energy expenditure from physical activity in turn varies widely among people.

Climbing stairs rather than riding the elevator, walking rather than driving to the store, and standing in a bus rather than sitting increase physical activity and, hence, energy use. The alarming rate of and recent increase in obesity in North America are caused in part by our inactivity.[10] Jobs demand less physical activity, and leisure time is often spent slouched before a television or computer.

Thermic Effect of Food (TEF)

In addition to basal metabolism and physical activity, the body uses energy to digest, absorb, and further process the nutrients recently consumed. Energy used for these tasks is referred to as the **thermic effect of food (TEF).** TEF is analogous to a sales tax—it is like being charged about 5 to 10% for the total amount of energy we eat to cover the cost of processing the food eaten. (We may recognize this increase in metabolism as a warming of the body during and right after a meal.) For every 100 kcal needed for basal metabolism and physical activity, we must eat between 105 and 110 kcal. If our daily energy intake was 3000 kcal, TEF would account for 150 to 300 kcal. As with other components of energy output, the total amount can vary somewhat among individuals.[9]

Food composition influences TEF. For example, the TEF value for a protein-rich meal (20 to 30% of the energy consumed) is higher than that of a carbohydrate-rich (5 to 10%) or fat-rich (0 to 3%) meal because it takes more energy to metabolize amino acids into fat than to convert glucose into glycogen or transfer absorbed fat into adipose stores. In addition, large meals result in higher TEF values than the same amount of food eaten over many hours.[9]

Thermogenesis

Thermogenesis represents the increase in nonvoluntary physical activity triggered by cold conditions or overeating. Some examples of nonvoluntary activities include fidgeting, shivering when cold, maintenance of muscle tone, and upholding body posture when not lying down.[9] Studies have shown that some people are able to resist weight gain from overfeeding by inducing thermogenesis, while others are not able to do so to a great extent. Note also that thermogenesis goes by other names: thermoregulation, adaptive thermogenesis, and nonexercise activity thermogenesis (NEAT).

Brown adipose tissue is a specialized form of adipose tissue that participates in thermogenesis. It is found in small amounts in infants. The brown appearance results from its rich blood flow. Brown adipose tissue contributes to thermogenesis by releasing much of the energy from energy-yielding nutrients into the environment as heat. It contains proteins that uncouple energy release with ATP production. Adults have very little brown adipose tissue, and its role in adulthood is unknown. It is thought to mostly be important for thermoregulation in infants, in whom brown adipose tissue contributes as much as 5% of body weight. Hibernating animals also make use of brown adipose tissue so they can generate heat to withstand a long winter.

The contribution of thermogenesis to overall energy expenditure is fairly small. The combination of basal metabolism and TEF accounts for 70 to 80% of energy used by a sedentary person. The remaining 20 to 30% is used mostly for physical activity, with a small amount used for thermogenesis.[9]

thermic effect of food (TEF) The increase in metabolism that occurs during the digestion, absorption, and metabolism of energy-yielding, nutrients. TEF represents 5 to 10% of energy consumed.

The TEF value for alcohol is 20%.

thermogenesis The ability of humans to regulate body temperature within narrow limits (thermoregulation). Two visible examples of thermogenesis are fidgeting and shivering when cold. Other terms used to describe thermogenesis are adaptive thermogenesis and nonexercise activity thermogenesis (NEAT).

brown adipose tissue A specialized form of adipose tissue that produces large amounts of heat by metabolizing energy-yielding nutrients without synthesizing much useful energy for the body. The unused energy is released as heat.

Concept | Check

Energy balance involves matching energy intake with energy output. Energy content of food is expressed in kcals and can be determined using a bomb calorimeter. This analysis yields the 4-9-4-7 estimates for kcals in a gram of carbohydrate, fat, protein, and alcohol.

The body uses energy for four main purposes:

1. Basal metabolism (60 to 70% of total energy output) represents the minimal amount of energy needed to maintain the body at rest. Primary determinants of basal metabolic rate include quantity of lean body mass, amount of body surface, and thyroid hormone concentrations in the bloodstream.
2. Physical activity expenditure (20 to 30% of total energy output) represents energy use for total body cell metabolism above what is needed during rest.

3. Thermic effect of food (5 to 10% of total energy output) represents the energy needed to digest, absorb, and process recently consumed nutrients.
4. Thermogenesis (small, variable percentage of total energy output) includes nonvoluntary, heat-producing activities, such as fidgeting and shivering when cold.

Determination of Energy Use by the Body

The amount of energy a body uses can be measured by both direct and indirect calorimetry or can be estimated based on height, weight, degree of physical activity, and age.

Direct and Indirect Calorimetry

Direct calorimetry measures the amount of body heat released by a person. The subject is put into an insulated chamber, often the size of a small bedroom, and body heat released increases the temperature of a layer of water surrounding the chamber. A kcal, as you recall, is related to the amount of heat required to raise the temperature of water. By measuring the water temperature in the direct calorimeter before and after the body releases heat, scientists can determine the energy expended.

Direct calorimetry works because almost all the energy used by the body eventually leaves as heat. However, few studies use direct calorimetry, mostly because of its expense and complexity.

The most commonly used method of **indirect calorimetry** measures the amount of oxygen a person consumes (Figure 13-4). A predictable relationship exists between the body's use of energy and oxygen. For example, when metabolizing a mixed diet of carbohydrate, fat, and protein—a typical blend of energy-yielding nutrients—the human body needs 1 liter of oxygen to yield about 4.85 kcal of energy.

Instruments to measure oxygen consumption for indirect calorimetry are widely used. They can be mounted on carts and rolled to a hospital bed or carried in backpacks while a person plays tennis or jogs. There are even newly developed handheld instruments (made by Body Gem). Tables showing energy costs of various forms of exercises rely on information gained from indirect calorimetry studies.

Another approach to indirect calorimetry uses **stable isotopes** of oxygen and hydrogen. In this method, a person drinks isotopically labeled water (^2H_2O and $H_2{}^{18}O$). Analysis of urine and blood samples provide data on ^2H and ^{18}O excretion. The labeled oxygen is eliminated from the body as water and carbon dioxide, whereas the hydrogen is eliminated only as water. Subtracting the hydrogen losses from the oxygen losses provides a measure of carbon dioxide output. This ultimate estimate of CO_2 output is then used to calculate energy expenditure, just as is done with oxygen use in indirect calorimetry. ^2H and ^{18}O are stable isotopes of hydrogen and oxygen (therefore, they are nonradioactive); special instruments can measure them in body fluids. This stable isotope method is quite accurate but also very expensive. It is the basis for determining estimated energy requirements for humans (see the next section).

Estimates of Energy Needs

The Food and Nutrition Board has published a number of formulas called Estimated Energy Requirements (EER), to estimate energy needs. Listed here are the formulas for adults (remember to do multiplication and division before addition and subtraction). (Formulas for children, teenagers, pregnant women, and lactating women are listed in Chapters 16 and 17.)

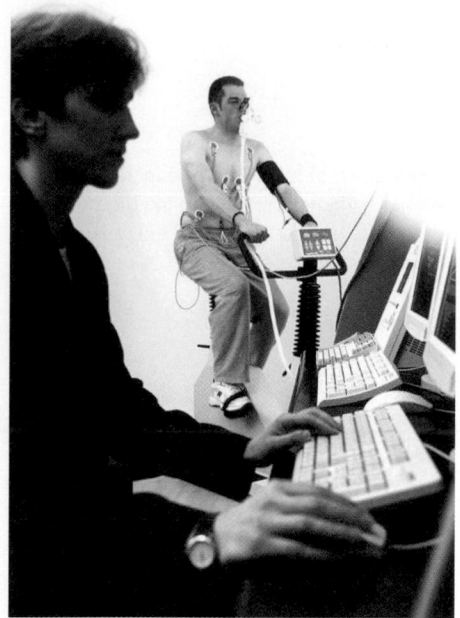

Figure 13-4 | Indirect calorimetry. The method of measuring oxygen use and carbon dioxide output can determine energy use during daily activities.

direct calorimetry A method of determining a body's energy use by measuring heat that is released from the body, usually using an insulated chamber.

indirect calorimetry A method to measure energy use by the body by measuring oxygen uptake. Formulas are then used to convert this gas exchange value into energy use.

stable isotope A specific nonradioactive form of a chemical element. It differs from atoms of other forms (isotopes) of the same element in the number of neutrons in its nucleus. *Stable* means that the isotope is not radioactive, in contrast to some other types of isotopes.

Men 19 years and older

$$EER = 662 - (9.53 \times AGE) + PA \times (15.91 \times WT + 539.6 \times HT)$$

Women 19 years and older

$$EER = 354 - (6.91 \times AGE) + PA \times (9.36 \times WT + 726 \times HT)$$

The variables in the formulas correspond to the following:

EER = Estimated Energy Requirement
AGE = age in years
PA = Physical Activity Estimate (see the accompanying table)
WT = weight in kg (lb ÷ 2.2)
HT = height in meters (inches ÷ 39.4)

Physical Activity (PA) Estimates

Activity Level	PA (Men)	PA (Women)
Sedentary (e.g., no exercise)	1.00	1.00
Low activity (e.g., walks the equivalent of 2 miles per day at 3 to 4 mph)	1.11	1.12
Active (e.g., walks the equivalent of 7 miles per day at 3 to 4 mph)	1.25	1.27
Very active (e.g., walks the equivalent of 17 miles per day at 3 to 4 mph)	1.48	1.45

Practice using the formula for EER. Consider a man who is 25 years old, 5 feet, 9 inches (1.75 meters), 154 lb (70 kg), and has an active lifestyle. His EER is:

$$EER = 662 - (9.53 \times 25) + 1.25 \times (15.91 \times 70 + 539.6 \times 1.75) = 2997$$

You have determined this man's EER to be about 3000 kcal/day. Remember that this is only an estimate; many other factors, such as genetics and hormones, can affect actual energy needs.

A simple method of tracking your energy expenditure, and thus your energy needs, is to use the forms in Appendix G. Begin by taking an entire 24-hour period and listing all activities performed, including sleep. Record the number of minutes spent in each activity; the total should equal 1440 minutes (24 hours). Next, record the energy cost for each activity in kcal per minute following the directions in Appendix G. Multiply the energy cost by the minutes. This figure is the energy expended for each activity. Total all the kcal values. This figure is your estimated energy expenditure for the day.

Concept | Check

Energy use by the body can be measured by direct calorimetry as heat given off and by indirect calorimetry as oxygen used. A person's Estimated Energy Requirement can be estimated based on the following characteristics: gender, height, weight, age, and amount of physical activity.

▌Why Am I Hungry?

Two drives influence our desire to eat and thus take in food energy: **hunger** and **appetite.** These differ dramatically (Figure 13-5). Hunger, our primarily physiological drive to eat, is controlled by internal body mechanisms. Organs such as the liver and brain interact with hormones, hormonelike **(neuroendocrine)** factors, the nervous system, and other aspects of body physiology to influence feeding behavior (Table 13-1).[18] For example, carbohydrate intake induces in the GI tract the release of the hormonelike compound glucagon-like peptide-1 (GLP-1). This release then reduces

---

The Harris-Benedict Equation can be used to determine resting energy expenditure (REE):

Men

REE = 66.5 + (13.8 × WT) + (5 × HT) − (6.8 × AGE)

Women

REE = 655.1 + (9.6 × WT) + (1.9 × HT) − (4.7 × AGE)

The variables in the formulas correspond to the following:

REE = Resting Energy Expenditure
WT = weight in kg (lb ÷ 2.2)
HT = height in cm (inches × 2.54)
AGE = age in years

Rough guidelines for energy needs (in kcals) from MyPyramid are as follows:

Children	Sedentary ⟶	Active
2–3 years	1000 ⟶	1400

Females	Sedentary ⟶	Active
4–8 years	1200 ⟶	1800
9–13	1600 ⟶	2200
14–18	1800 ⟶	2400
19–30	2000 ⟶	2400
31–50	1800 ⟶	2200
51+	1600 ⟶	2200

Males	Sedentary ⟶	Active
4–8 years	1200 ⟶	2000
9–13	1800 ⟶	2600
14–18	2200 ⟶	3200
19–30	2400 ⟶	3000
31–50	2200 ⟶	3000
51+	2000 ⟶	2800

hunger The primarily physiological (internal) drive to find and eat food, mostly regulated by innate cues to eating.

appetite The primarily psychological (external) influences that encourage us to find and eat food, often in the absence of obvious hunger.

neuroendocrine Linked to the combined action of the endocrine glands and the nervous system. Examples include substances released from glands in response to nerve stimulation.

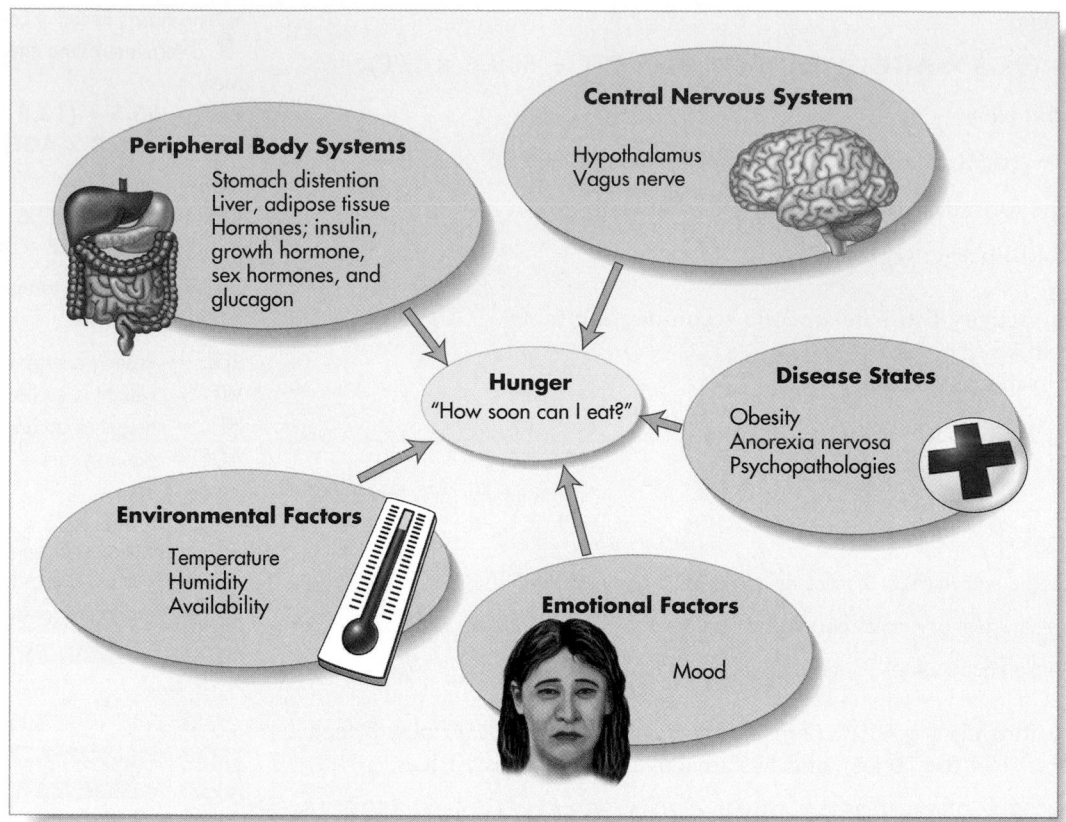

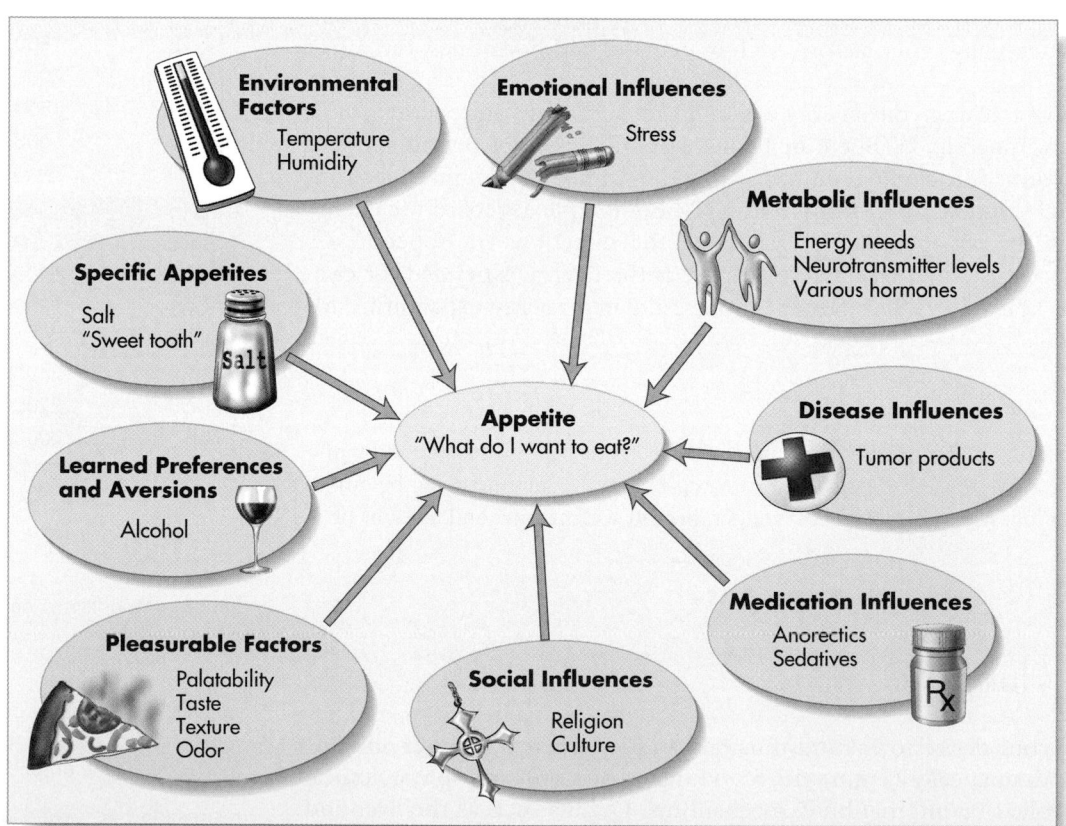

Figure 13-5 | Factors that influence satiety. Although some factors have an impact on both hunger and appetite, internal factors are primarily responsible for hunger, whereas external factors primarily influence appetite. These factors combine to play a role in the complex and interrelated processes that help determine when, what, and how much we eat.

Table 13-1 | Hormones, Neuroendocrine Substances, Medications, and Other Factors That Affect Feeding Behavior†

Increase Food Intake	Decrease Food Intake
Neurotransmitters	
Norepinephrine	Serotonin
Growth hormone releasing hormone	Dopamine
Neuropeptides and Hormones	
Opioids	Cholecystokinin
Galanin	Enterostatin
Neuropeptide Y	Tumor necrosis factor
Agouti-related protein	Glucagon-like peptide-1 (GLP-1)
Orexin-A	Corticotropin releasing hormone
Melanin-concentrating hormone	POMC
Ghrelin	Melanocyte-stimulating hormone
Gastric inhibitory peptide	Melanocortin
	Peptide YY$_{3-36}$
	Amylin
	Adipsin
	Leptin*
Medications	
Corticosteroids	Sibutramine
Some tranquilizers	Amphetamines
Progestins	
Some antidepressants	

†Some of these body hormones may also be used as medications in the future. Many of the neuropeptides are also found in the gastrointestinal tract (see Chapter 3).

*In conjunction with the hormone insulin when both are present in the brain

further food intake. Dr. Peter J. Havel discusses this process in greater detail in the Expert Opinion. Then as macronutrients are absorbed, the liver and surrounding organs communicate with the brain through the two **vagus nerves.** This communication changes subsequent food choices by sending information about the rate of digestion and energy metabolism from the GI tract and the liver to the brain.[18]

Appetite, our primarily psychological drive to eat, is affected by external food choice mechanisms, such as seeing a tempting dessert. Fulfilling either or both drives by eating sufficient food normally brings a state of **satiety,** temporarily halting our desire to continue eating.

Hypothalamus: Key Satiety Regulator

Our bodies have many internal signals to encourage or reduce food intake. The **hypothalamus,** a portion of the brain, is the key integration site for this regulation (Figure 13-6). When stimulated, cells in the feeding centers of the hypothalamus signal us to eat. Then, as we eat, hunger decreases. Eventually, we stop eating as cells in the satiety centers of the hypothalamus are stimulated. Various cues to eat come from other sources, such as groups of cells near the hypothalamus, macronutrients such as glucose in the bloodstream, various hormones and other substances, and **sympathetic nervous system** activity. Overall, as sympathetic nervous system activity decreases, food intake increases. The opposite is also true. Thus, many internal signals both inhibit and encourage food intake.[18]

Chemicals, surgery, and some cancers can destroy the feeding and satiety centers in the hypothalamus. Without satiety-center activity, laboratory animals (and humans) eat their way to obesity. Without feeding-center activity, animals eat little and eventually lose weight.[18]

vagus nerves Nerves arising from the brain that branch off to other organs and are essential for control of speech, swallowing, and gastrointestinal function.

satiety State in which there is no longer a desire to eat; a feeling of satisfaction.

hypothalamus A region at the base of the brain that contains cells that play a role in the regulation of hunger, respiration, body temperature, and other body functions.

sympathetic nervous system Part of the nervous system that regulates involuntary vital functions, including the activity of the heart muscle, smooth muscle, and adrenal glands.

Hypothalamus

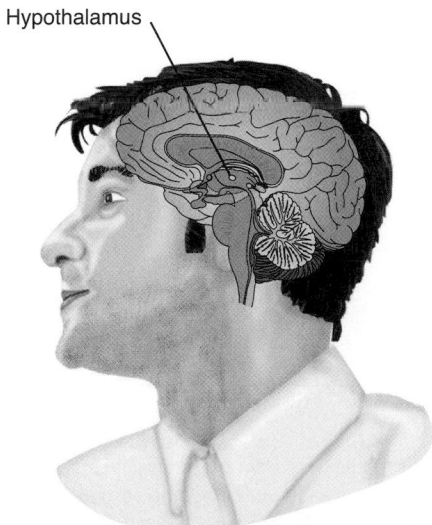

Figure 13-6 | The hypothalamus. This site in the brain does most of the processing of signals regarding food intake.

Satiety Regulation at Other Body Sites

As just mentioned, satiety is controlled by a network of mechanisms spread throughout the body. Satiety is maintained first by the sensory stimulation that food elicits, coupled with the knowledge that a meal was eaten. Second, the effects of nutrient digestion, absorption, and metabolism are felt. The satiety and feeding centers in the hypothalamus communicate and interact with other decision points in the brain, small intestine, and liver. Overall, the process of satiety is very complex.[18]

Dr. Barbara Rolls, an expert in this field, has found that meal-to-meal satiety is influenced by the energy density of foods. Lower-energy-density foods result in the greatest effect. As discussed in Chapter 2, energy density is linked to the total weight of such foods (i.e., water content) and fiber content. Other factors that influence satiety are dietary variety, food particle size, viscosity, glycemic load, palatability, and visual clues such as size and shape. Still, Dr. Rolls suggests that in the long run our eyes might be the most important factor. Thus the practice of recognizing appropriate serving sizes of foods shown in Chapter 2 and training oneself to expect that amount can help control energy intake in the long run.[5] People who have trouble controlling body weight should try to train the eye to expect less food by slowly decreasing serving sizes. Food intake will be reduced as one expects less food but still experiences satiety.[5]

Control of Feeding through Body Composition

Feeding behavior also changes in response to the amount of body fat. When body fat is surgically removed from animals, their food consumption increases. Based on work with genetic forms of obesity in animals, researchers have identified a group of substances that circulate in the blood and communicate the degree of body fatness to the central nervous system. The gene for one such substance in mice and humans has been isolated (called the ob gene). The product produced by the gene has been named **leptin.** Work with one strain of mice suggests that leptin partly decreases the activity of **neuropeptide Y** and other small proteins present in the brain (review Table 13-1).[18] This decrease then reduces food intake. Some people exhibit leptin resistance, in that it doesn't readily bind to its receptors in the brain. This situation then leads to greater hunger than is seen in people who don't have this problem. Only a few people have been found to be truly leptin deficient.

Theoretically, when adipose tissue stores are increasing, leptin (and/or related substances) causes satiety. Conversely, when adipose tissue stores are decreasing, not as much leptin (and/or related substances) is released into the bloodstream, and the desire to eat is enhanced. The main function of leptin is probably energy conservation during periods of inadequate food supply. Low leptin output leads to decreased thyroid gland activity and, thus, a fall in basal metabolism. Leptin-deficient animals also show decreased spontaneous activity, suggesting that they are conserving body energy. Experts suggest that leptin actually may be more important for lessening the effects of starvation than for preventing obesity. Thus, leptin is not there primarily to protect against obesity but, instead, to serve as a signal for low body fat stores.[18]

Because leptin is a protein, it must be injected into the body. Interestingly, not all people treated with leptin have lost significant amounts of weight; some people have even gained weight during the therapy. Currently, the initial excitement over the use of leptin to curb hunger and so contribute to weight loss is waning because clinical trials have not supported its general usefulness. The current hope is that leptin injections will help people limit weight regain after weight loss. There is some evidence that such use of leptin is helpful. (Note that leptin is not available for commercial use at this time.)

Hormones That Affect Satiety

Endorphins, the body's natural opioid painkillers, and hormones, such as high amounts of cortisol, can prod us to eat. The same is true for **ghrelin,** a hormone made by the stomach. On the other hand, other hormones, hormonelike compounds, and

---

leptin A hormone (167 amino acids) made by adipose tissue that influences long-term regulation of fat mass. Leptin also influences reproductive functions as well as other physiological processes such as insulin release.

neuropeptide Y A small protein (36 amino acids) that increases food intake and reduces energy expenditure when injected into the brains of experimental animals.

endorphins Natural body tranquilizers that may be involved in the feeding response and function in pain reduction.

ghrelin A hormone made by the stomach that increases food intake.

still other chemical factors in the body can contribute to the feeling of satiety. With eating, blood concentrations of some digestive hormones, such as cholecystokinin (CCK), increase. This increase, also combined with **gastrointestinal distention,** helps shut off hunger.

Certain parts of the nervous system also contribute to satiety, in part linked to the release of the neurotransmitter histamine. Increased production of **serotonin,** another brain neurotransmitter, has also been linked to intake of various nutrients, especially carbohydrates. High serotonin concentrations in the brain can be calming, induce sleepiness, and reduce food intake.[18] For this reason, medications that prolong serotonin action in the brain are used to treat certain eating disorders (see Chapter 15).

Following the likely influence of gastrointestinal distention, **nutrient receptors** in the small intestine are believed to take over in promoting satiety after a meal. This concept is supported by experiments in which subjects felt satiated when fats or carbohydrates were infused directly into the small intestine. This effect was not reported, however, when the same fats or carbohydrates were infused directly into the bloodstream.

gastrointestinal distention Expansion of the wall of the stomach or intestines due to pressure caused by the presence of gases, food, drink, or other factors. This expansion contributes to a feeling of satiety brought on by food intake.

serotonin A neurotransmitter synthesized from the amino acid tryptophan that affects mood (sense of calmness), behavior, and appetite, and induces sleep.

nutrient receptors Proposed sites in the small intestine that contribute signals to the brain that in turn elicit a feeling of satiety. These receptors are stimulated by nutrient exposure in the lumen of the small intestine.

Nutrients in the Blood That Affect Satiety

Accumulating evidence from both human and animal studies on the regulation of hunger suggests that an underlying hunger for food is never actually absent. After a meal, blood concentrations of macronutrients increase, the brain registers satiety, and hunger is temporarily relieved.[18] Studies suggest that an apolipoprotein on the chylomicrons (apolipoprotein A-IV) also signals satiety to the brain as chylomicrons build up in the blood after a meal.

Several hours after eating, when concentrations of macronutrients in the blood begin to fall, the body must start using energy found in body stores; hunger then returns because satiety is no longer registered by the metabolism of energy-yielding compounds that have been eaten. In other words, feeding signals begin to dominate again.[18]

Does Appetite Regulate What We Eat?

Various feeding and satiety messages from body cells do not single-handedly determine what we eat. Almost everyone has encountered a mouthwatering dessert and devoured it, even on a full stomach. We have an innate taste for sweet and acquire a taste for fat. Appetite can be affected by a variety of external forces, such as environmental and psychological factors as well as social customs (review Figure 13-5).

We often eat because food confronts us. It smells good, tastes good, and looks good. We might eat because it is the right time of day, we are celebrating, or we are trying to overcome the blues. Appetite may not be a biological process, but it does influence food intake. After a meal, memories of pleasant tastes and feelings reinforce appetite. If stress or depression sends you to the refrigerator, you are mostly seeking comfort, not food energy.

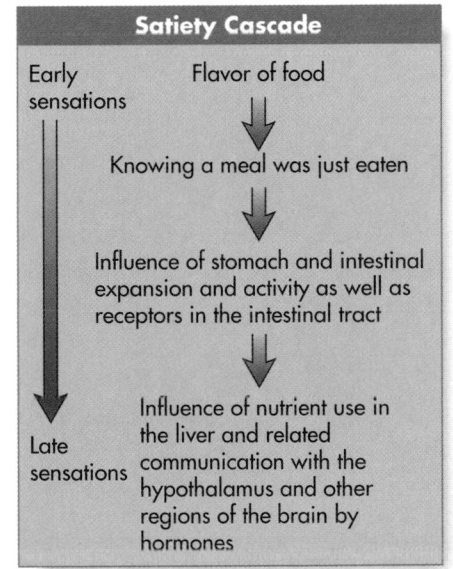

Hunger and Appetite in Perspective

Internal and external signals that drive hunger and appetite generally operate simultaneously and lead us to decide whether to reject or eat a food item. For example, visual and taste stimulation can cause something called *cephalic phase responses* by the body. Saliva flows and digestive hormones and insulin are released in response to seeing, smelling, and initially tasting food, such as a hamburger. The physiological responses prepare the body for the meal. These internal forces are elicited by external cues, again showing the degree to which internal and external forces are intertwined.[18]

The next time you pick up a candy bar or ask for second helpings, remember the physiological influences on eating behavior. Body cells (brain, stomach, intestine, liver,

Social customs, peers, and authority figures can influence the desire to eat. Concern about appearance when on a date can influence the food choices made. A woman concerned about looking "petite" in company may choose a smaller portion of food than when alone. We are also likely to eat more at a meal when with a large group of people than when with a few people or alone, or when someone else is "picking up the check."

and other organs), hormones (such as CCK and ghrelin), neurological components (such as serotonin), and social customs all influence food intake. Where food is ample, appetite—not hunger—mostly triggers eating. Keep track of what triggers your eating for a few days. Is it primarily hunger or appetite? Note as well that this system is not perfect; your body weight can increase (or decrease) over time if you are not careful to balance energy intake with energy output.

Concept | Check

Hunger is the primarily physiological or internal desire to find and eat food. Appeasing it leads to satiety—no further desire to eat exists in that moment. Satiety is influenced by hunger-related (internal) forces in the brain, gastrointestinal tract, adipose tissue, liver, and other organs. Various hormones and neuroendocrine compounds participate. Food intake is also affected by appetite-related (psychological and external) forces such as social custom, time of day, palatability, and presence of others. North Americans probably respond more to external, appetite-related forces than to hunger-related ones in choosing when and what to eat.

Estimation of a Healthy Weight

Numerous methods are used to establish what body weight should be, typically called *healthy weight.* Several tables exist, generally based on weight-for-height. These tables arise from studies of large population groups. When applied to a population, they provide good estimates of weight associated with health and longevity. However, they do not necessarily indicate the healthiest body weight for each individual. Athletes with a large, lean body mass and little body fat are a prime example.

Ideally, family history of weight-related disease and current health conditions, in addition to weight-for-height, should be considered when establishing a healthy weight for an individual. Consideration of the following weight-related conditions is important:[19]

- Hypertension
- Elevated LDL-cholesterol
- Family history of obesity, cardiovascular disease, or certain forms of cancer (e.g., uterus, colon)
- Pattern of fat distribution in the body
- Elevated blood glucose
- Elevated blood triglycerides

On a more practical note, other questions can be pertinent: What is the least one has weighed as an adult for at least a year? What is the largest size clothing one would be happy with? What weight has one been able to maintain during previous diets without feeling constantly hungry? Overall, the individual, under a physician's and/or registered dietitian's guidance, should establish a "personal" healthy weight (or need for weight reduction) based on weight history, fat distribution patterns, family history of weight-related disease, and current health status. This assessment points out how well the person is tolerating any existing excess weight. Thus, current height/weight standards are only a rough guide. Furthermore, a healthy lifestyle may make a more important contribution to a person's health status than the number on the scale. Fit and overweight are not necessarily mutually exclusive (although not often seen together), and nor is thin synonymous with being healthy if the person is not also physically active.

Using Body Mass Index (BMI) to Set Healthy Weight

Over the past 50 years, use of weight-for-height tables issued by the Metropolitan Life Insurance Company have been the typical way healthy weight was established. These tables considered gender and frame size, predicting the weight range at a specific

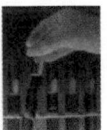

Expert Opinion

Sorting Out Satiety and Weight Regulation: Hormones and Dietary Macronutrients

Peter J. Havel, D.V.M., Ph.D.

Satiety and Short-Term Regulation of Food Intake

Satiety is a condition of satisfaction or gratification with no desire to ingest additional food; it is the state that directly leads to the termination of a meal and determines a meal's size and duration. What triggers the feelings of fullness associated with satiety? First, physical and chemical qualities of the food activate mechano- (stretch) and chemo-receptors in the stomach and upper small intestine. Second, a number of peptide hormones are released in response to the presence of food in the gastrointestinal (GI) tract. Neural signals from stretch receptors, chemo-receptors, and peptide hormone receptors in the liver and GI tract are transmitted to brainstem nuclei via the vagus nerve.

Among many GI tract hormones that are known to decrease hunger and inhibit food intake, cholecystokinin (CCK) and glucagon-like peptide-1 (GLP-1) are the most likely to have a physiological role in satiety. These hormones relay neural signals to the central nervous system. They also can influence satiety indirectly by inhibiting gastric emptying. Together these neural and hormonal signals regulate food intake in the short term, but by themselves they are not sufficient to regulate body weight and body adiposity. For example, in a study in which CCK was repeatedly administered to rats over a period of several weeks, the size of each meal decreased, but meal frequency increased, so overall food intake and body weight were only minimally affected. This finding suggests that the effects of short-term signals, such as GI stretch receptors and CCK, on energy intake are counterbalanced by reduced input from long-term hormonal regulators of energy balance.

Long-Term Regulation of Energy Balance

Long-term energy balance is regulated by several endocrine signals: insulin from the pancreas, leptin produced by adipose cells, and ghrelin (and possibly peptide YY_{3-36}) from the GI tract. These long-term signals act in concert with the short-term signals in the coordinated regulation of energy intake and body adiposity. It has been proposed that the long-term signals determine the sensitivity of the central nervous system to the satiety-inducing effects of the short-term signals. Experimental evidence for this hypothesis indicates that both insulin and leptin increase the sensitivity to CCK, and so its ability to limit meal size in animals. This integration serves to control energy intake to match energy expenditure so that body weight is remarkably stable over time in both humans and other animals. For example, a person who gains 20 lb (~9 kg) of body fat between 20 and 40 years of age is consuming only about 11 kcal/day in excess of energy expenditure (less than a 0.5% mismatch of energy balance). However, larger mismatches of energy intake and expenditure can and do lead to much larger degrees of weight gain and profound obesity.

Insulin

Pancreatic beta cells immediately secrete insulin in response to glucose and amino acids. Insulin concentrations in the bloodstream are inversely related to insulin sensitivity; because increased body fat is a major contributor to insulin resistance, circulating insulin levels are higher in obese people. In addition, insulin levels decrease independently of body weight during fasting. Thus, overall circulating insulin levels and insulin exposure to the brain are proportional to both fat stores and recent energy balance. Insulin is transported to the hypothalamus where it regulates the production of neuropeptides, such as neuropeptide-Y and melanocortins. Insulin also has an important indirect role in long-term energy balance: it regulates leptin production and ghrelin secretion (see the following sections).

Leptin

The hormone leptin, produced by adipose cells, works in the brain to inhibit food intake and increase thermogenesis. It also regulates other endocrine systems (reproductive, thyroid, etc.) involved in adaptation to negative energy balance. Leptin's effects in the central nervous system to inhibit food intake are dependent on a signal pathway that is shared with insulin. Like insulin, leptin production and circulating leptin concentrations are related to both body fat stores and recent energy intake. Leptin levels are proportional to body fat, but leptin levels decrease acutely during fasting or restricted energy intake and increase after refeeding, even if the amount of body fat does not change. These adiposity-independent changes in leptin production primarily relate to changes in insulin-dependent glucose metabolism in adipose cells. The decrease of leptin in times of decreased energy intake helps ensure that when food is scarce, hunger, food-seeking behavior, and an adaptive decrease in energy expenditure are triggered well before body energy

"I can't eat another slice." Have you ever considered the physiological processes involved in feeling full? What role does satiety play in the amount of food you eat, and how does that affect long-term body weight regulation?

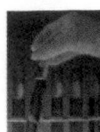

stores become compromised. This appears to be the primary function of leptin in energy balance.

Leptin exists in the body to help manage the threat of starvation, but can it also manage the threat of obesity? Genetic leptin deficiency leads to extreme hunger and massive obesity that are reversed by leptin administration. The leptin deficit induced by dieting suggests that leptin replacement in dieting subjects might help prevent weight regain.

Ghrelin

Endocrine cells in the stomach and upper GI tract produce ghrelin. In contrast to the satiating effects of other GI peptides, ghrelin stimulates food intake. Chronic administration of ghrelin also inhibits fat utilization and induces weight gain in animals, suggesting a role in long-term body weight regulation. Circulating ghrelin levels decrease within 30 minutes after a meal and remain low for up to 3 hours. It is likely that insulin, glucose, and other GI hormones contribute to the inhibition of ghrelin secretion after a meal. Circulating ghrelin levels are lower in obese people compared to people of normal weight, and increase substantially in people who have lost weight through dieting, an effect that predisposes them to future weight regain. Circulating ghrelin levels remain low in patients who have lost weight after Roux-en-Y gastric bypass surgery (discussed later in the chapter), suggesting that lack of an increase in ghrelin levels may contribute to weight loss and weight maintenance after this type of surgery.

Peptide YY$_{3-36}$

Endocrine cells in the colon produce PYY$_{3-36}$ and release it into the bloodstream in response to eating. PYY$_{3-36}$ administration decreases food intake in laboratory animals and humans. Because a relatively short-term (90 minute) infusion of PYY$_{3-36}$ results in a 12-hour reduction of appetite and food intake in humans, it is possible that, unlike most GI peptides that inhibit food intake (e.g., CCK), PYY$_{3-36}$ may function as a medium- to long-term regulator of energy intake. Because PYY$_{3-36}$ levels are reduced in obese individuals and PYY$_{3-36}$ inhibits food intake in both obese and lean subjects, it has been proposed that treatment with PYY$_{3-36}$ may be an effective medical therapy for obesity.

Macronutrients, Satiety, and Energy Balance

There are important differences in the effects of major dietary macronutrients on short-term satiety and long-term energy balance. Dietary fat is energy-dense (9 kcal/g) and so can be overconsumed in the short term. However, fat ingestion also induces greater feelings of fullness due to its effects to delay gastric emptying. Energy consumed in the form of beverages can also be consumed in large quantities, in part because gastric emptying of fluids is rapid. The long-term influence of macronutrients on energy balance and body weight also appears to involve the endocrine signals just discussed. A

number of studies have demonstrated that consumption of low-fat, high-carbohydrate diets results in weight loss in the majority of people, even when portions are not restricted. In contrast, increasing the fat content of the diet almost invariably results in increased energy intake and weight gain in humans and animals.

Circulating leptin concentrations exhibit a nocturnal peak that is largely dependent on insulin responses to meals consumed during the day. High-carbohydrate meals induce larger increases of leptin 4 to 6 hours after the meal than do high-fat meals containing the same amount of energy. The height of the nocturnal leptin peak is reduced when subjects consume high-fat meals. This reduction in leptin output may be an important signal to the CNS in body weight regulation because the amount of leptin released correlates with body weight and body fat loss when a low-fat diet is consumed. However, not all dietary carbohydrates have the same effect. For example, although consuming glucose-sweetened beverages with a meal stimulates insulin and leptin production and induces ghrelin suppression after the meal, these effects are significantly less after consumption of the same meals with fructose-sweetened beverages. The lack of effects of fat and fructose on these endocrine signals of energy balance (insulin, leptin, and ghrelin) suggests an endocrine mechanism by which prolonged consumption of diets high in fat and/or fructose contribute to weight gain and obesity.

Conclusions

Signals from the GI tract, including activation of stretch receptors and the GI hormones CCK and GLP-1, promote sensations of satiety and fullness in order to limit meal size and thereby regulate short-term energy intake. These short-term signals are not sufficient by themselves to regulate energy balance over more prolonged periods of time and therefore are not involved in the long-term control of body weight. The long-term signals—insulin, leptin, ghrelin, and possibly PYY$_{3-36}$—are produced and circulate in proportion to recent energy intake and body adiposity. These long- and short-term signals are integrated such that the long-term signals appear to set the sensitivity of the central nervous system to the satiety-producing effects of the short-term signals. A better understanding of the mechanisms regulating satiety and long-term energy balance will lead to new approaches for managing obesity and its many comorbidities, including diabetes, hypertension, and coronary heart disease.

Dr. Havel is Associate Endocrinologist in the Department of Nutrition at the University of California, Davis. Dr. Havel earned a bachelor of science degree from the University of Washington and doctoral degrees in Veterinary Medicine and Endocrinology, both from University of California, Davis. Dr. Havel's research focuses on the physiology of body weight regulation, carbohydrate and lipid metabolism, and the pathophysiology of obesity and diabetes.

height that was associated with the greatest longevity. The latest table (issued in 1983) and methods for determining frame size can be found in Appendix I.

Currently, **body mass index (BMI)** is the preferred weight-for-height standard (Figure 13-7).[9] Research has shown that body mass index is the weight-for-height standard that is most closely related to body fat content.

Body mass index is calculated as

$$\frac{\text{body weight (in kg)}}{\text{height}^2 \text{ (in meters)}}$$

An alternate method for calculating BMI is

$$\frac{\text{weight (lb)} \times 703}{\text{height}^2 \text{ (inches)}}$$

Table 13-2 lists the BMI for various heights and weights. Health risks from excess weight may begin when the BMI is 25 or more. A healthy weight-for-height is a BMI 18.5 to 24.9. What is your BMI? How much would your weight need to change to yield a BMI of 25? 30? These are general cut-off values for the presence of overweight and obesity, respectively.

The concept of body mass index is convenient to use because the values apply to both men and women. However, any weight-for-height standard is actually a crude measure. Keep in mind, also, that a BMI of 25 to 29.9 is a marker of *overweight* (compared to a standard population) and not necessarily a marker of *overfat*. Many men (especially athletes) have a BMI greater than 25 because of extra muscle tissue. Also, very short adults (under 5 feet tall) may have high BMIs that may not reflect overweight or fatness. For this reason, BMI alone should not be used to diagnose overweight or obesity.

Still, overfat and overweight conditions generally appear together. The focus is on BMI in clinical settings mainly because BMI is easier to measure than total body fat.

A shortcut method for roughly estimating healthy body weight is the pounds per inch of height method. For women, start with 100 lb for the first 5 feet, then add 5 lb for every inch thereafter. To estimate a man's healthy body weight, start with 106 lb for the first 5 feet and then add 6 lb for each inch thereafter. The estimate of weight is then given a ± 10% range. Based on this system, a 6-foot-tall man should weigh about 178 ± 18 lb (106 + [12 × 6 = 178]).

Putting Healthy Weight into Perspective

One current school of thought is to let nature take its course with regard to body weight. According to this proposal, after weight is lost in order to fall within a specific (often unrealistic) height/weight range, people often regain their original weight plus more. In contrast, listening to the body for hunger cues, regularly eating a healthy diet, and remaining physically active (not to be overlooked) eventually helps one maintain an appropriate height/weight value.[19] This concept will be further addressed in the upcoming discussion on treatment for obesity. (It is a cornerstone of the current "size acceptance" movement.) The clearest idea regarding a healthy weight is that it is personal. Weight has to be considered in terms of health, not simply a mathematical calculation.

Concept | Check

Healthy body weight is generally determined in a clinical setting using a body mass index or another weight-for-height standard. Family history and the presence of existing weight-related disease should be considered in determining healthy body weight. Total health and a healthy lifestyle should be the major considerations when determining healthy weight.

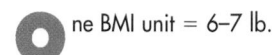

One BMI unit = 6–7 lb.

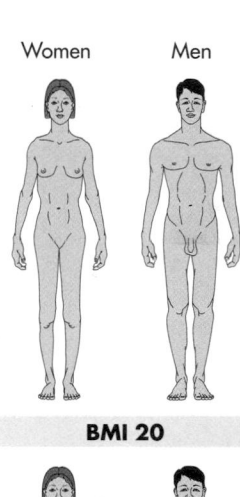

Women   Men

BMI 20

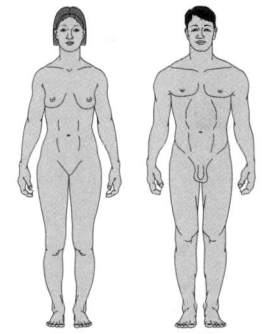

BMI 25

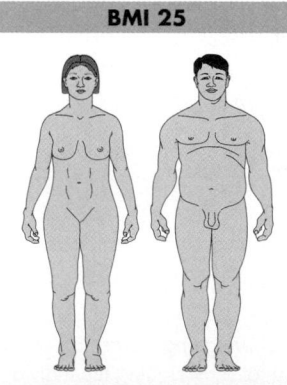

BMI 30

Figure 13-7 | Estimates of body shapes at different BMI values.

Table 13-2 | Body Weight in Pounds According to Height and Body Mass Index (BMI)

Height (Inches)	Healthy BMI						Overweight BMI					Obese BMI		
	19	20	21	22	23	24	25	26	27	28	29	30	35	40
	Body weight (lb)													
58	91	96	100	105	110	115	119	124	129	134	138	143	167	191
59	94	99	104	109	114	119	124	128	133	138	143	148	173	198
60	97	102	107	112	118	123	128	133	138	143	148	153	179	204
61	100	106	111	116	122	127	132	137	143	148	153	158	185	211
62	104	109	115	120	126	131	136	142	147	153	158	164	191	218
63	107	113	118	124	130	135	141	146	152	158	163	169	197	225
64	110	116	122	128	134	140	145	151	157	163	169	174	204	232
65	114	120	126	132	138	144	150	156	162	168	174	180	210	240
66	118	124	130	136	142	148	155	161	167	173	179	186	216	247
67	121	127	134	140	146	153	159	166	172	178	185	191	223	255
68	125	131	138	144	151	158	164	171	177	184	190	197	230	262
69	128	135	142	149	155	162	169	176	182	189	196	203	236	270
70	132	139	146	153	160	167	174	181	188	195	202	207	243	278
71	136	143	150	157	165	172	179	186	193	200	208	215	250	286
72	140	147	154	162	169	177	184	191	199	206	213	221	258	294
73	144	151	159	166	174	182	189	197	204	212	219	227	265	302
74	148	155	163	171	179	186	194	202	210	218	225	233	272	311
75	152	160	168	176	184	192	200	208	216	224	232	240	279	319
76	156	164	172	180	189	197	205	213	221	230	238	246	287	328

Each entry gives the body weight in pounds for a person of a given height and BMI (kg/m²). Pounds have been rounded off. To use the table, find the appropriate height in the far left column. Move across the row to a weight. The number at the top of the column is the BMI for the height and weight.

Healthy weight is currently the preferred term to use for weight recommendations. Older terms, such as *ideal weight* and *desirable weight,* are no longer used in medical literature. However, you still may hear these terms in clinical practice.

Energy Imbalance

If energy intake exceeds output over time, overweight (and often obesity) is a likely result. Often, health problems eventually follow (Table 13-3). In this context, medical and nutrition experts recommend that an individual's cutoff value for obesity should not be based primarily on body weight but, rather, on the total amount of fat in the body, the location of body fat, and the presence or absence of weight-related medical problems.[19]

Estimating Body Fat Content and Diagnosing Obesity

Body fat can range from 2 to 70% of body weight. Desirable amounts of body fat are about 8 to 24% of body weight for men and 21 to 35% for women. In this regard, men with over 24% body fat and women with over about 35% body fat are considered obese. Women need more body fat because some "sex-specific" fat is associated with reproductive functions. This fat is normal and factored into calculations.

To measure body fat content accurately using typical methods, both body weight and body volume of the person must be known. Body weight is easy to measure. Of the typical methods used to estimate body volume, **underwater weighing** is the most accurate. This technique determines body volume using the loss of weight when placed underwater, the relative densities of fat tissue and lean tissue, and a specific mathematical formula. This procedure requires that a subject be totally submerged in a tank

underwater weighing A method of estimating total body fat by weighing the individual on a standard scale and then weighing him or her again submerged in water. The difference between the two weights is used to estimate total body volume.

Table 13-3 | Health Problems Associated with Excess Body Fat

Health Problem	Partially Attributable To
Surgical risk	Increased anesthesia needs as well as greater risk of wound infections (linked to a decrease in immune function)
Pulmonary disease and sleep disorders	Excess weight compresses lungs and pharynx
Type 2 diabetes	Enlarged adipose cells, which poorly bind insulin and poorly respond to the message insulin sends to the cell; increased synthesis of factors (e.g., immune system–related) by enlarged adipose cells that lead to insulin resistance; less synthesis of factors that improve insulin action (e.g., adiponectin) by enlarged adipose cells
Hypertension	Increased miles of blood vessels found in the adipose tissue, increased blood volume, increased sodium retention, and increased resistance to blood flow related to hormones made by adipose cells
Cardiovascular disease (e.g., coronary heart disease and stroke)	Increases in LDL-cholesterol and triglyceride values, low HDL-cholesterol, decreased physical activity, and increased synthesis of blood clotting and inflammatory factors by adipose cells, especially those that are large in size; greater risk for heart failure is also seen, in part due to an altered heart rhythm
Bone and joint disorders (including gout)	Excess pressure put on knee, ankle, and hip joints
Gallstones	Increased cholesterol content of bile
Skin disorders	Trapping of moisture and microorganisms in tissue folds
Various cancers, such as in the kidney, gallbladder, colon and rectum, and uterus (women) and prostate gland (men)	Estrogen production by adipose cells, animal studies suggest excess energy intake encourages tumor development
Shorter stature (in some cases of obesity)	Earlier onset of puberty
Pregnancy risks	More difficult delivery, increased risk of gestational diabetes, and increased needs for anesthesia
Reduced physical agility and increased risk of accidents and falls	Excess weight that impairs movement
Menstrual irregularities and infertility	Hormones produced by adipose cells, such as estrogen
Vision problems	Cataracts and other eye disorders are more often present
Premature death	A variety of risk factors for disease listed in this table
Infections	Reduced immune system activity
Liver damage and eventual failure	Excess fat accumulation in the liver
Erectile dysfunction in men	Low-grade inflammation caused by excess fat mass and reduced function of the cells lining the blood vessels associated with being overweight

The greater the degree of obesity, the more likely and the more serious these health problems generally become. They are much more likely to appear among people who have excess upper-body fat distribution and/or are greater than twice healthy body weight.

of water, and a trained technician needs to direct the procedure (Figure 13-8). **Air displacement** is another method of determining body volume. Body volume is quantified by measuring the space a person takes up inside a measurement chamber, such as the BodPod (Figure 13-9). A further method to measure body volume is to simply submerge a person in a tank and observe the level of the water before and after submersion. The volume of the displaced water is then calculated.

Once body volume is known, it can be used along with body weight to calculate body density. Then, using body density, body fat content finally can be determined. One formula used is:

$$\text{Body density} = \frac{\text{body weight}}{\text{body volume}}$$

$$\% \text{ body fat} = (495 \div \text{body density}) - 450$$

For example, assume that the subject in the underwater weighing tank in Figure 13-8 has a body density of 1.06. The units are g/cm³. The second formula is used to calculate that he has 17% body fat ([495 ÷ 1.06] − 450 = 17).

air displacement A method for estimating body composition that makes use of the volume of space taken up by a body inside a small chamber.

E ven agreed-upon weight standards for BMI are not for everyone. Adult BMIs should not be applied to children and adolescents, frail older people, pregnant and lactating women, and highly muscular individuals. Children and pregnant women have unique BMI standards (see Chapters 16 and 17).

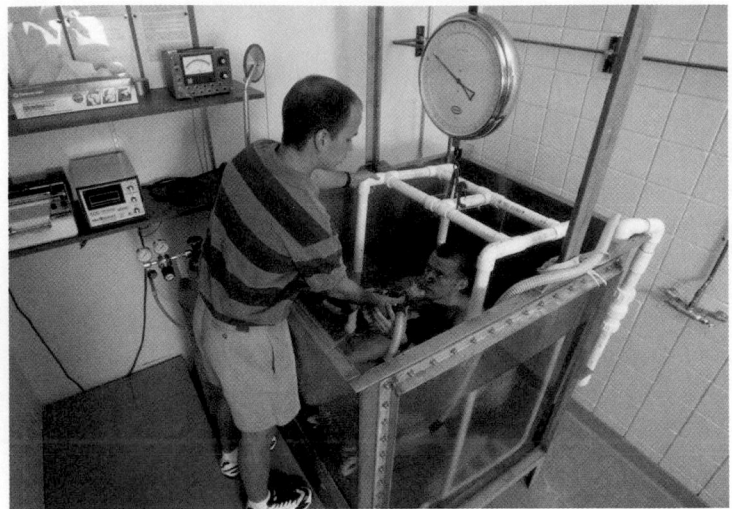

Figure 13-8 | Underwater weighing. In this technique the subject exhales as much air as possible and then holds his or her breath and bends over at the waist. Once the subject is totally submerged, the underwater weight is recorded. Using this value, body volume can be calculated.

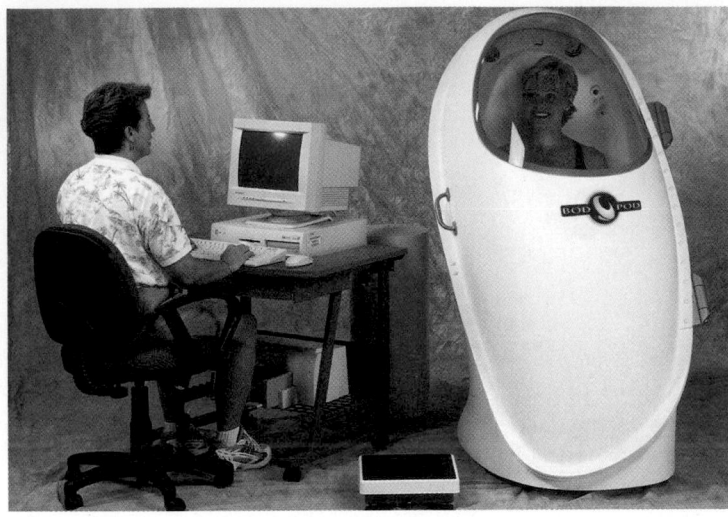

Figure 13-9 | BodPod. This device determines body volume based on the volume of displaced air, measured as a person sits in a sealed chamber for a few minutes.

bioelectrical impedance A method to estimate total body fat that uses a low-energy electrical current. The more fat storage a person has, the more impedance (resistance) to electrical flow will be exhibited.

dual energy X-ray absorptiometry (DEXA) A highly accurate method of measuring body composition and bone mass and density using multiple low-energy X rays.

Another method to assess body fat is to measure total-body electrical conductance when placed in an electromagnetic field (TOBEC). Still another method, near-infrared reactance, exposes the bicep muscle to a beam of near-infrared light. The measuring instrument assesses the interactions of the light beam with fat and lean tissues in the upper arm. After only 2 seconds, this flashlight-size device can give an estimate of body composition. Although convenient and inexpensive, this method is not very accurate.

Skinfold thickness is a common anthropometric method to estimate total body fat content, although there are some limits to its accuracy. Clinicians use calipers to measure the fat layer directly under the skin at multiple sites and then plug these values into a mathematical formula (Figure 13-10).

Bioelectrical impedance also can be used to estimate body fat content. The instrument sends a painless, low-energy electrical current to and from the body via wires and electrode patches to estimate body fat. Researchers surmise that adipose tissue resists electrical flow more than lean tissue does because adipose tissue has a lower electrolyte and water content than lean tissue and so more adipose tissue proportionately means greater electrical resistance. Within a few minutes, bioelectrical impedance analyzers convert body electrical resistance into an approximate estimate of total body fat, as long as body hydration status is normal (Figure 13-11).

Dual energy X-ray absorptiometry (DEXA) is considered the most accurate way to determine body fat, but the equipment is very expensive and not widely available for this use. This X-ray system allows the clinician to divide body weight into three separate components: fat, fat-free soft tissue, and bone mineral. The usual whole-body scan requires about 5 to 20 minutes and the dose of radiation is less than a chest X ray. Obesity, osteoporosis, and other aspects of nutritional health can be investigated using this method (Figure 13-12).

Using Body Mass Index to Define Obesity

BMI offers another way to define obesity (Figure 13-13).[9]

30–39.9	Obese	Increased health risk
40 or greater	Severely obese	Major health risk. Note that the number of North Americans falling into this category is increasing rapidly.

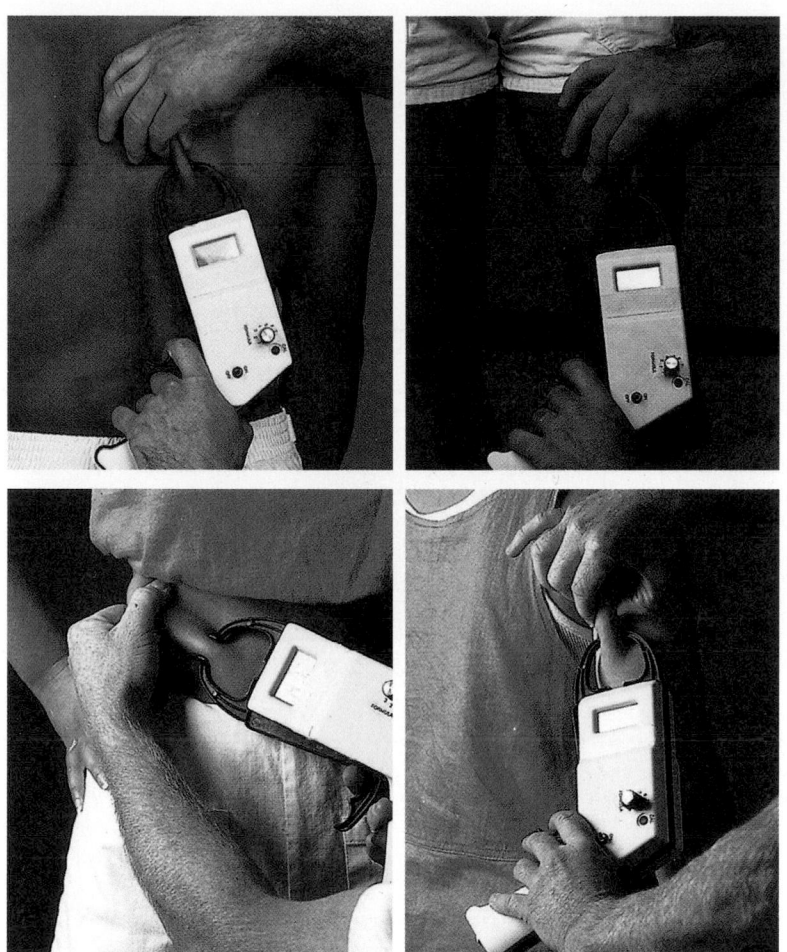

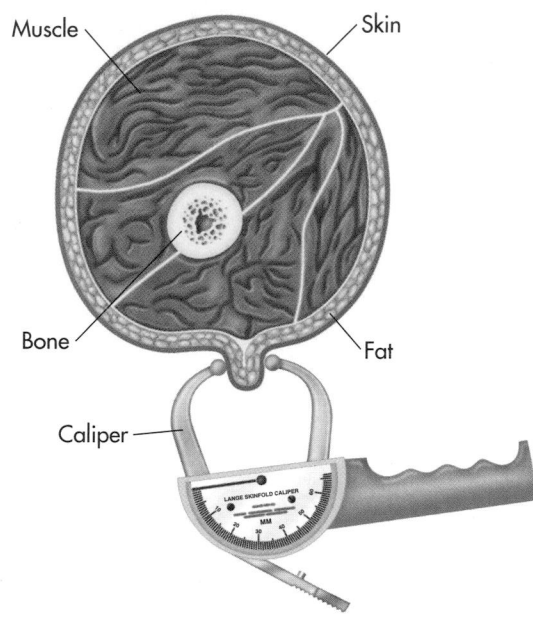

Figure 13-10 | Skinfold measurements. With proper technique and calibrated equipment, skinfold measurements around the body can be used to predict body fat content in about 10 minutes.

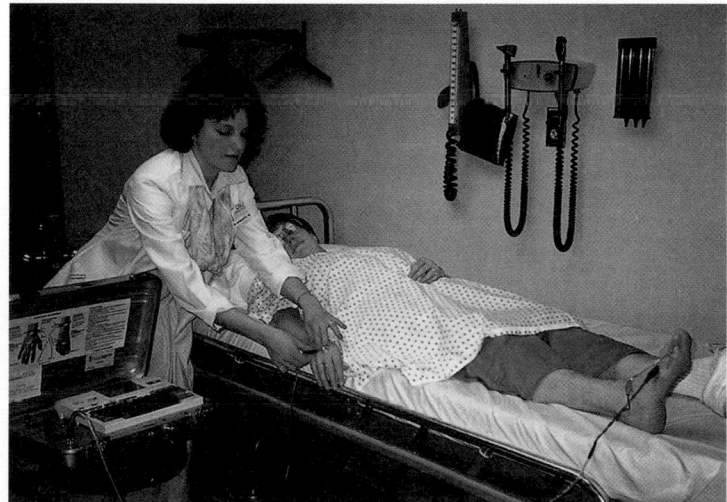

Figure 13-11 | Bioelectrical impedance. This method can estimate total body fat in less than 5 minutes and is based on the principle that fat in the body resists the flow of electricity since it is low in water and electrolytes. The degree of resistance to electrical flow is used to estimate body fatness.

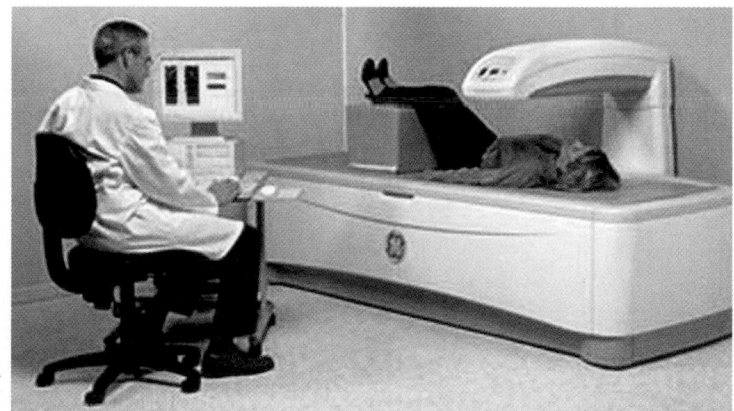

Figure 13-12 | Dual energy X-ray absorptiometry (DEXA). This method measures body fat by releasing small doses of radiation through the body that a detector then quantifies as fat, lean tissue, or bone. The scanner arm moves from head to toe and in doing so can determine body fat as well as bone density. DEXA is currently considered the most accurate method for determining body fat as long as the person is not too obese to fit on the table and/or under the arm of the instrument. The radiation dose is minimal.

Figure 13-13 | Height/weight table based on BMI; the upper ends of the healthy weight ranges correspond to a body mass index of 25.

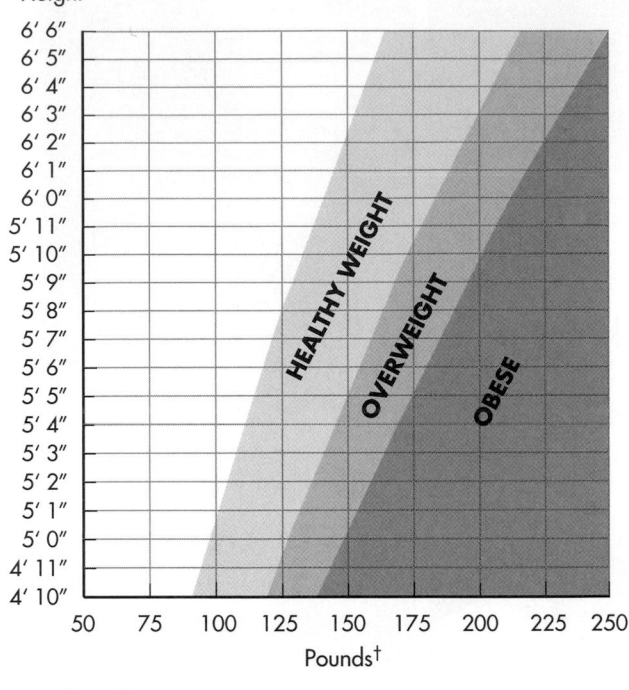

Height*

6′ 6″
6′ 5″
6′ 4″
6′ 3″
6′ 2″
6′ 1″
6′ 0″
5′ 11″
5′ 10″
5′ 9″
5′ 8″
5′ 7″
5′ 6″
5′ 5″
5′ 4″
5′ 3″
5′ 2″
5′ 1″
5′ 0″
4′ 11″
4′ 10″

HEALTHY WEIGHT   OVERWEIGHT   OBESE

50   75   100   125   150   175   200   225   250

Pounds†

* Without shoes.
† Without clothes. The higher weights apply to people with more muscle and bone, such as many men.

Using Body Fat Distribution to Further Evaluate Obesity

Where we store fat, as well as how much, can predict health risks, likely even more than a person's BMI can. Some people store fat in upper-body areas. Others hold fat lower on the body. Excess fat in either place generally spells trouble, but each storage space also has its unique risks. **Upper-body (android) obesity** is more often related to cardiovascular disease, hypertension, and type 2 diabetes.[13] Whereas other adipose cells empty fat directly into general circulation, the fat released from abdominal adipose cells goes straight to the liver by way of the portal vein found there. This process likely interferes with the liver's ability to clear insulin and alters lipoprotein metabolism by the liver. These adipose cells also make substances that increase inflammation in the body as well as increase insulin resistance, blood clotting, and blood vessel constriction. All these changes can lead to long-term health problems.

High blood testosterone (primarily a male hormone) levels apparently encourage upper-body obesity, as does a diet with a high glycemic load, alcohol intake, and smoking. This characteristic male pattern of fat storage appears in an apple shape (large abdomen [pot belly] and thinner buttocks and thighs). Upper body obesity is assessed by simply measuring the waist at the widest point just above the hips when relaxed. A waist circumference more than 40 inches (102 cm) in men and more than 35 inches (88 cm) in women indicates such a shape (Figure 13-14).[9]

Estrogen and progesterone (primarily female hormones) encourage lower-body fat storage and **lower-body (gynecoid or gynoid) obesity.** The small abdomen and much larger buttocks and thighs give a pear-like appearance. After menopause, blood estrogen falls, encouraging upper-body fat distribution in women.

upper-body obesity The type of obesity in which fat is stored primarily in the abdominal area; defined as a waist circumference more than 40 inches (102 centimeters) in men and more than 35 inches (88 centimeters) in women; closely associated with a high risk for cardiovascular disease, hypertension, and type 2 diabetes.

lower-body obesity The type of obesity in which fat storage is primarily located in the buttocks and thigh area.

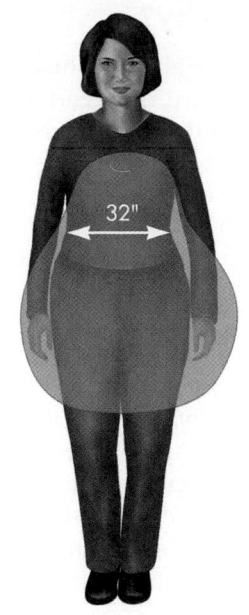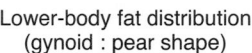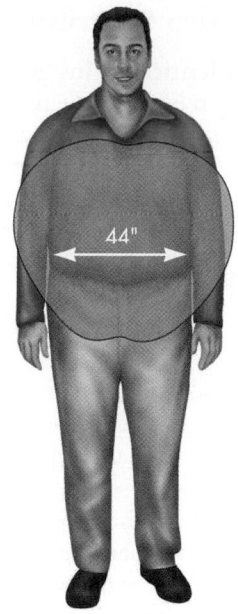

Lower-body fat distribution
(gynoid : pear shape)

Upper-body fat distribution
(android : apple shape)

Figure 13-14 | Body fat distribution, showing upper-body and lower-body locations. The upper-body (android) form brings higher risks for ill health associated with obesity. The woman has a waist circumference of 32 inches. The man has a waist circumference of 44 inches. Thus, the man has upper-body fat distribution but the woman does not, based on a cutoff of 40 inches for men and 35 inches for women.

Concept | Check

Overweight and obesity typically are associated with excessive body fat storage. The risk of health problems related to being overweight especially increases under the following conditions:

- A man's percentage of body fat exceeds 25%; a woman's exceeds about 35%.
- Excess fat is primarily stored in the upper-body region.
- Body mass index (BMI) is 30 or more (calculated as weight in kg divided by height squared in meters).

However, these are merely guidelines. A more individualized approach to assessment is warranted as long as a person is following a healthy lifestyle and has no existing health problems.

Body fat content can be estimated using a variety of methods such as underwater weighing, air displacement, skinfold thickness, bioelectrical impedance, and DEXA. Fat storage distribution further specifies an obese state as either upper body or lower body. Obesity leads to an increased risk for cardiovascular disease, some types of cancer, hypertension, type 2 diabetes, certain bone and joint disorders, and some digestive disorders. The risk for some of these conditions is greater with upper-body fat storage.

Critical | Thinking

Based on what you now know, how would you define the term healthy body weight?

Why Some People Are Obese—Nature Versus Nurture

Both genetic and environmental factors can increase the risk for obesity. Experts in the field are at odds over the relative importance of nature versus nurture.

How Does Nature Contribute to Obesity?

identical twins Two offspring that develop from a single ovum and sperm and, consequently, have the same genetic makeup.

Studies in pairs of **identical twins** give us some insight into the contribution of nature to obesity. Even when identical twins are raised apart, they tend to show similar weight gain patterns, both in overall weight and body fat distribution. Nurture—eating habits and nutrition, which varies between twins who are raised apart—seems to have less to do with obesity than nature does.[9] In fact, research suggests that genes account for up to 40 to 70% of weight differences between people.

We also inherit specific body types. Tall, thin people appear to have an inherently easier time maintaining healthy body weight. Basal metabolism increases as body surface increases, and therefore taller people use more energy than shorter people, even at rest.

Some rats and mice can have a genetic predisposition to obesity if they inherit a "thrifty metabolism"—one that uses energy frugally. This metabolism enables them to store fat more readily than the typical animal. Many of us probably have inherited a thrifty metabolism as well, so that we require less energy metabolism to get through the day. In earlier times, when food supplies were scarce, a thrifty metabolism would have been a built-in safeguard against starvation. Now, with a general abundance of food, people operating in this low gear require much physical activity and wise food choices to prevent obesity. If you think you are prone to weight gain, you likely have inherited a thrifty metabolism.

A child with no obese parent has only a 10% chance of becoming obese. When a child has one obese parent (common in our society), that risk advances up to 40%, and with two obese parents, it soars to 80%. Our genes help determine metabolic rate, fuel use, and differences in brain chemistry—all of which affect body weight.

Does the Body Have a Set Point for Weight?

set point Often refers to the close regulation of body weight. It is not known what cells control this set point or how it actually functions in weight regulation. There is evidence, however, that mechanisms exist that help regulate weight.

The **set-point** theory of weight maintenance proposes that humans have a genetically predetermined body weight or body fat content, which the body closely regulates. Some research suggests that the hypothalamus monitors the amount of body fat in humans and tries to keep that amount constant over time. Recall from earlier in the chapter that the hormone *leptin* forms a communication link between adipose cells and the brain, which allows for some weight regulation.[18]

What evidence supports the set-point theory? In human studies, volunteers who had lost weight through starvation tended to eat in such a way to regain their original weight. In addition, studies in the 1960s using prisoners with no history of obesity

Does the difference in body fat between the grandfathers and the grandsons arise from nature or nurture or both?

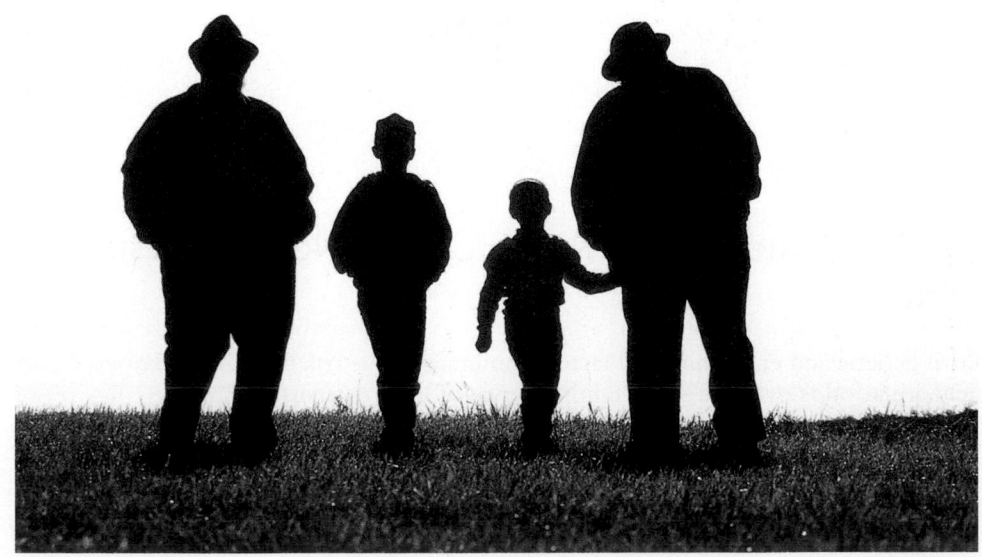

found it was hard for some men to gain weight. Also, after an illness is resolved, a person generally regains lost weight.

Physiological measurements also endorse the set-point theory. For example, when energy intake is reduced, the blood concentration of thyroid hormones falls, which slows basal metabolism. In addition, as weight is lost, the energy cost of weight-bearing activity decreases, so that an activity that burned 100 kcal before weight loss may only burn 80 kcal after weight loss. Furthermore, with weight loss, the body becomes more efficient at storing fat by increasing the activity of the enzyme *lipoprotein lipase*, which takes fat into cells. All these changes protect the body from losing weight.

If a person overeats, basal metabolism tends to increase in the short run, which causes some resistance to weight gain. However, in the long run, resistance to weight gain is much less than resistance to weight loss. When a person gains weight and stays at that weight for a while, the body tends to establish a new set point.

Opponents of the set-point theory argue that weight does not remain constant throughout adulthood—the average person gains weight slowly, at least until old age. Also, if an individual is placed in a different social, emotional, or physical environment, weight can be altered and maintained markedly higher or lower. These arguments suggest that humans, rather than having a set point determined by genetics or the number of adipose cells, actually settle into a particular stable weight based on their circumstances, often referred to as a "settling point."

Overall, the set point is weaker in preventing weight gain than in preventing weight loss.[9] Even with a set point helping us, the odds are in favor of eventual weight gain unless we devote effort to a healthy lifestyle.

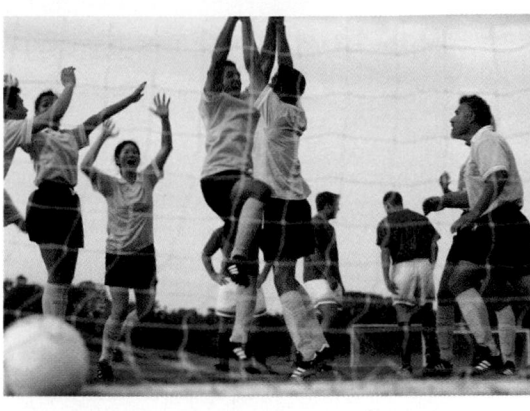

Student life is often full of physical activity. This is not necessarily true for a person's later working life; hence, weight gain is a strong possibility.

Does Nurture Have a Role?

Some researchers would argue that body weight similarities between family members stem more from learned behaviors than from genetic similarities. Even couples (who generally have no genetic link) may behave similarly toward food and eventually assume similar degrees of leanness or fatness. Proponents of nurture pose that environmental factors, such as high-fat diets and inactivity, literally shape us.[9] Consider that our gene pool has not changed much in the past 50 years, but the ranks of obese people have grown in what the U.S. Centers for Disease Control and Prevention describe as epidemic proportions over the last 15 years.

Is poverty associated with obesity? Ironically, the answer is often yes. North Americans of lower socioeconomic status, especially females, are more likely to be obese than those in upper socioeconomic groups. Are cultural expectations or socioeconomic stress (e.g., **food insecurity**) the cause of this increase in obesity in lower socioeconomic classes?

Adult obesity among women is often rooted in childhood obesity. In addition, relative inactivity, periods of stress or boredom, and excess weight gain during pregnancy contribute to female obesity. (Chapter 16 notes that breastfeeding one's infant contributes to loss of some of the excess fat associated with pregnancy.) These patterns suggest both social and genetic links. Male obesity, however, is not strongly linked to childhood obesity and, instead, tends to appear after age 30. This powerful and prevalent pattern suggests a primary role of nurture in obesity, with less genetic influence.

food insecurity A condition of anxiety regarding running out of either food or money to buy more food.

Nature and Nurture Together

Overall, both nature and nurture influence the tendency toward obesity (Table 13-4). The eventual location of fat storage is strongly influenced by genetics. Consider the possibility that obesity is nurture allowing nature to express itself. Some obese people begin life with a slower basal metabolism, maintain an inactive lifestyle, and consume highly refined, energy-dense diets. These people in turn are nurtured into gaining weight, promoting their natural tendency toward obesity.[9]

Table 13-4 | What Encourages Excess Body Fat Stores and Obesity?

Factor	How Fat Storage Is Affected
Age	Excess body fat is more common among adults and middle-aged individuals.
Menopause	Increase in abdominal fat deposition is favored.
Gender	Females generally have more fat.
Positive energy balance	Over a long period, positive energy balance promotes storage of fat.
Composition of diet	Excess energy intake from a high-fat intake, generous alcohol intake, and preference for energy-dense (sugary, fat-rich) foods are likely to contribute to obesity.
Physical activity	Low or decreasing amount of physical activity ("couch potato") affects energy balance and body fat stores.
Basal metabolism	A low value is linked to weight gain.
Thermic effect of food	This is low for some obesity cases.
Increased hunger sensations	Some people especially have trouble resisting the wide food availability typical of modern life, likely linked to the activity of various brain chemicals.
Ratio of fat to lean tissue	A high ratio of fat mass to lean body mass is correlated with weight gain.
Fat uptake by adipose tissue	This is high in some obese individuals and remains high (perhaps even increases) with weight loss.
Variety of social and behavioral factors	Obesity is associated with socioeconomic status; familial conditions; network of friends; busy lifestyles that discourage balanced meals; binge eating; easy availability of inexpensive, "super sized" high-fat fast food; pattern of leisure activities; television time; smoking cessation; excessive alcohol intake; lack of adequate sleep; and number of meals eaten away from home.
Undetermined genetic characteristics	These affect energy balance, particularly via the energy expenditure components, the deposition of the energy surplus as adipose tissue or as lean tissue, and the relative proportion of fat and carbohydrate used by the body.
Race	In some ethnic groups, higher body weight may be more socially acceptable.
Certain medications	Food intake increases.
Childbearing	Women may not lose all weight gained in pregnancy, leading to increased weight gain.
National region	Regional differences, such as high-fat diets and sedentary lifestyles in the Midwest and areas of the South, lead to different rates of obesity in different places.

Still, genes do not fully control destiny. With increased physical activity and decreased food consumption, even those people with a genetic tendency toward obesity can attain a healthier body weight.[20]

The total cost attributable to weight-related disease is about $90 billion annually in the United States. Half of this cost is borne by the taxpayers through Medicare and Medicaid.

Treatment of Overweight and Obesity

Treatment of overweight and obesity should be considered similar to treatment for any chronic disease: it requires long-term lifestyle changes.[19] Too often, however, people view a "diet" as something they go on temporarily, only to resume prior (typically poor) habits once satisfactory results have been achieved. It is mostly for this reason that so many people regain lost weight. Instead, overweight and obese (and as well underweight) people should emphasize healthy, active lifestyles with lifelong dietary modifications (Figure 13-15).[20] The following sections explore why obesity must be regarded as a chronic disease and treated appropriately.

What to Look for in a Sound Weight-Loss Plan

A dieter can try to devise a plan of action by seeking advice from a health professional, such as a registered dietitian, or by consulting current literature. Either way, a sound weight-loss program should especially include these components:[6,8,10]

Rate of Loss

- [ ] Slow and steady weight loss, rather than rapid weight loss, is encouraged.
- [ ] Goal is 1 lb of fat loss per week.
- [ ] A period of weight maintenance for a few months after 10% of body weight is lost.
- [ ] Evaluation of need for further dieting before more weight loss begins.

Flexibility

- [ ] Ability to participate in normal activities (e.g., parties, restaurants).
- [ ] Adaptations to individual habits and tastes.

Intake

- [ ] Nutritional needs are met (except for energy needs).
- [ ] Common foods are included, with no certain foods being promoted as magical.
- [ ] Use of a fortified ready-to-eat breakfast cereal or balanced multivitamin/mineral supplement is recommended, especially when consuming less than 1600 kcal per day.
- [ ] Use MyPyramid as a pattern for food choices.

Behavior Modification

- [ ] Maintenance of healthy lifestyle (and weight) is a key concern; there is a lifetime focus.
- [ ] Changes are reasonable and can be maintained.
- [ ] Social support is encouraged.
- [ ] Plans for relapse so one does not quit after a setback.

Overall Health

- [ ] Screening by a physician is required for people with existing health problems, those over 40 (men) to 50 (women) years of age who plan to substantially increase physical activity, and those who plan to lose weight rapidly.
- [ ] Regular physical activity, proper rest, stress reduction, and other healthy changes in lifestyle are encouraged.
- [ ] Underlying psychological weight issues are addressed, such as depression or marital stress.

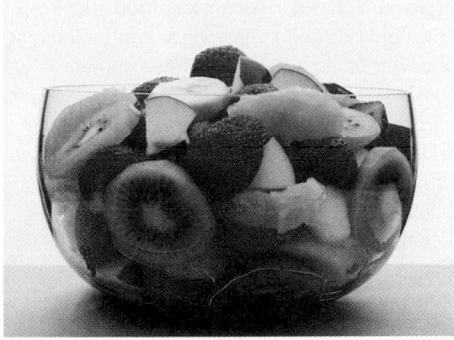

Fruit is a great snack—high nutrient density and low energy density.

Figure 13-15 | Characteristics of a sound weight-loss diet. How many ☑ are part of the diet plan that you may be considering? As noted in the discussion on set point, the body makes numerous physiological adjustments during times of underfeeding or overfeeding that resist weight change. This compensation is most pronounced during times of underfeeding and is why slow, steady weight loss is advocated.[8]

1. Control of energy intake. One recommendation is to decrease energy intake by 100 kcal/day (and increase physical activity by 100 kcal/day). This change should allow for slow and steady weight loss.
2. Increased physical activity.
3. Acknowledgment that maintenance of a healthy weight requires lifelong changes in habits, not simply a short-term weight-loss period.

A one-sided approach that focuses only on restricting energy intake is a difficult plan of action. Instead, adding physical activity and an appropriate psychological component will contribute to success in weight loss and eventual weight maintenance (Figure 13-16).

Weight-Control Objectives from *Healthy People 2010*

- Increase by 40% the proportion of adults who are at a healthy weight (body mass index between 18.5 and 25)
- Reduce by 50% the proportion of adults who are obese (body mass index of 30 or more)
- Reduce by 50% the proportion of children and adolescents who are overweight or obese

Figure 13-16 | Weight-loss triad. The key to weight loss and maintenance can be thought of as a triangle in which the three corners consist of (1) controlling energy intake, (2) performing regular physical activity, and (3) controlling problem behaviors. The three corners of the triangle support each other in that without one corner the triangle becomes incomplete. In the same way, without one of the three keys to weight loss, weight loss and later maintenance become unlikely.

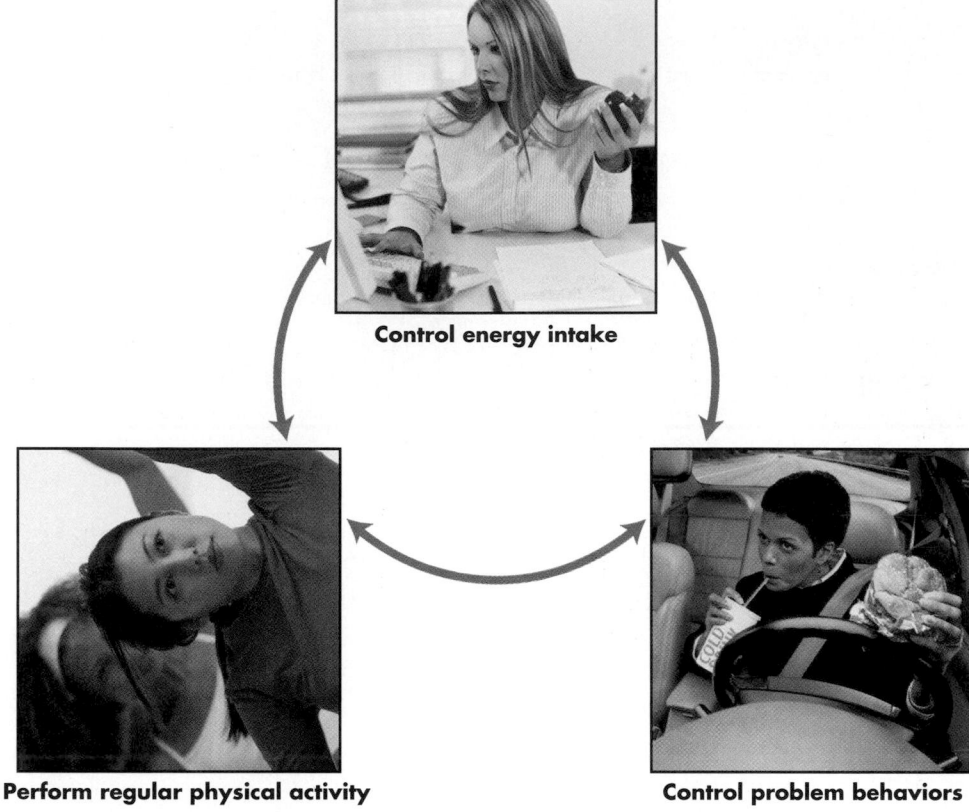

Control energy intake

Perform regular physical activity

Control problem behaviors

As you read brochures, articles, or research reports about specific diet plans, look beyond the weight loss promoted by the diet's advocate to see if the reported weight loss was maintained. If the weight maintenance aspect was missing, then the program was not successful.

Wishful Shrinking—Why Can't Quick Weight Loss Be Mostly Fat?

Rapid weight loss cannot consist primarily of fat loss because a high energy deficit is needed to lose a large amount of adipose tissue. Adipose tissue, which is mostly fat, contains about 3500 kcal/lb. Weight loss as fat includes adipose tissue plus supporting lean tissues and represents approximately 3300 kcal/lb (about 7.2 kcal/g). Therefore, to lose 1 lb of adipose tissue per week, energy intake must be decreased by approximately 500 kcal/day, or physical activity must be increased by 500 kcal/day. Alternately, a combination of both strategies can be used.[9] Diets that promise 10 to 15 lb of weight loss per week cannot ensure that the weight loss is from adipose tissue stores alone. Subtracting enough energy from one's daily intake to lose that amount of adipose tissue simply is not possible. Lean tissue and water, rather than adipose tissue, account for the major part of the weight lost during these dramatic weight-loss programs.

Weight Cycling Is All Too Common

Only about 5% of people who follow commercial diet programs actually lose weight and then remain close to that weight. Typically, one-third of the weight lost during dieting is regained within 1 year of the end of dietary restriction, and almost all weight lost is regained within 3 to 5 years. Some programs have higher success rates than 5%, as do some people who simply lose weight on their own without enrolling in any supervised plan. Overall, however, the statistics are grim. Currently, only the surgical approaches to obesity treatment show routine success in maintaining the weight loss in most people.

Negative health consequences associated with this weight cycling are an increased risk for upper-body fat deposition, profound discouragement and erosion of self-esteem, and possibly a fall in HDL-cholesterol and immune system activity. Nevertheless, experts still encourage obese people to attempt weight loss, with a strong focus on maintaining that lower weight. Still, dieters need to be aware of the trap of today's crash diet, which too often leads to the next month's weight gain. Weight-loss programs that claim you can lose weight and keep it off without changing food intake or increasing physical activity are selling a fantasy. A weight-loss program should be considered successful only when the subjects involved in the process remain at or close to their lower weights.

Weight Loss in Perspective

All these principles point to the importance of preventing obesity. This concept has wide support because conquering the disorder is so difficult.[8] Public health strategies to address the current obesity problem must speak to all age groups. There is a particular need to focus on children and adolescents because patterns of excess weight and sedentary lifestyle developed during youth may form the basis for a lifetime of weight-related illness and increased mortality. In the adult population, attention should be directed toward weight maintenance and increased physical activity.

Concept | Check

Obesity is a chronic disease that necessitates lifelong treatment. Emphasis should be placed especially on preventing obesity, because overcoming this disorder is very difficult. Appropriate weight-loss programs have the following characteristics in common: (1) They meet nutritional needs (except for energy needs); (2) they can adjust to accommodate habits and tastes; (3) they emphasize readily obtainable foods; (4) they promote changing habits that discourage overeating; (5) they encourage regular physical activity; and (6) they help change obesity-promoting beliefs and rally healthy social support.

Control of Energy Intake: The Main Key to Weight Loss and Weight Maintenance

A goal of losing 1 lb or so of stored fat per week may require limiting energy intake to 1200 kcal/day for women and 1500 kcal/day for men. The energy allowance could also be higher for very active people. Keep in mind that in our very sedentary society, decreasing energy intake is vital because it is difficult to burn much energy without ample physical activity. With regard to consuming less energy, some experts suggest consuming less fat (especially saturated fat and *trans* fat), while others suggest consuming less carbohydrate, especially refined (high glycemic load) carbohydrate sources. Protein intakes in excess of what is typically needed by adults are also receiving attention as a weight-loss strategy (especially plant protein sources).[7] Using all these approaches simultaneously is also fine. At this time the low-fat, high-fiber approaches have been the most successful in long-term studies. There is no long-term evidence for the effectiveness of the other approaches.[16] Finding what works for an individual is a process of trial and error. In addition, as shown by Dr. Andrea Buchholz and Dr. Dale Schoeller in their Expert Opinion in Chapter 4, the notion that any type of diet has a "metabolic advantage" (i.e., promotes greater energy use by the body) is nonsense, despite the marketing claims for low-carbohydrate diets.

One way for a dieter to monitor energy intake at the start of a weight-loss program is by reading labels. Label reading is important because many foods are more energy dense than people suppose (Figure 13-17). Another method is to write down food intake for 24 hours and then calculate energy intake from the food table in Appendix N or by using diet analysis software, adjusting future food choices as needed. Because people often underestimate portion size when recording food intake, measuring cups and a food weighing scale can help.

For more information on weight control, obesity, and nutrition, visit the Weight-Control Information Network (WIN) at www.niddk.nih.gov/health/nutrit/win.htm or call 800-WIN-8098. Complete guidelines for weight management are available at www.nhlbi.nih.gov/guidelines/index.htm. Other websites include www.caloriecontrol.org, www.weight.com,www.obesity.org, and www.cyberdiet.com.

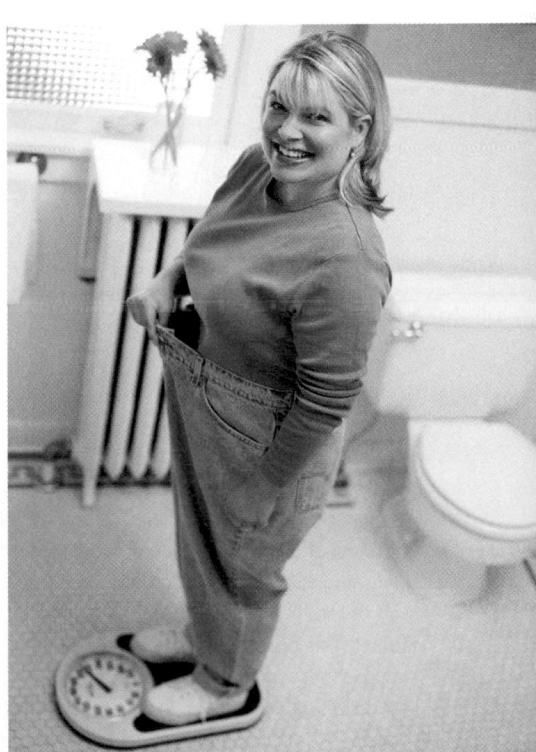

Slow, steady weight loss is one of the characteristics of a sound weight-loss program.

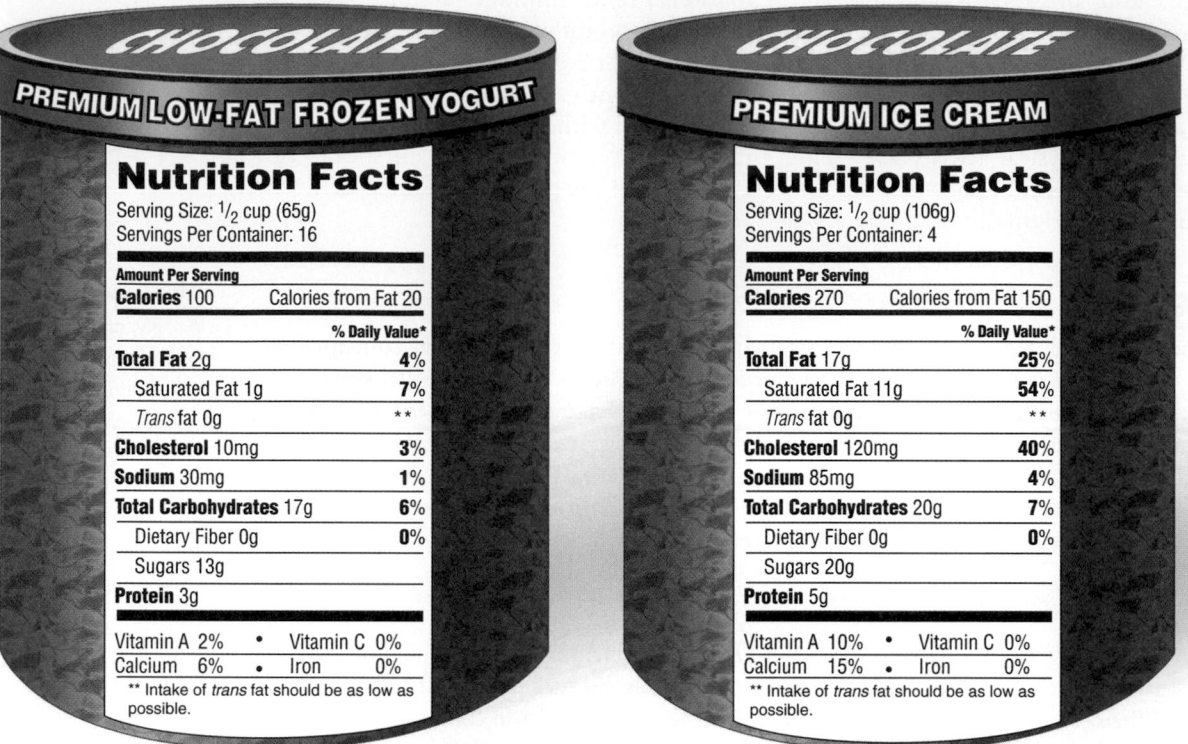

Figure 13-17 | Reading labels helps you choose foods with less energy content. Which of these frozen desserts is the best choice, per 1/2 cup serving, for a person on a weight-loss diet? The % Daily Values are based on a 2000 kcal diet.

Table 13-5 shows how to start reducing energy intake. It is best to consider healthy eating a lifestyle change rather than simply a weight-loss plan. Note also that liquids deserve attention because liquid calories do not stimulate satiety mechanisms to the same extent as solid foods. The corresponding advice from experts is to use beverages that have little or no energy content and limit sugar-sweetened beverages.

Regular Physical Activity: A Second Key to Weight Loss and Especially Important for Later Weight Maintenance

Regular physical activity is very important for everyone, especially people who are trying to lose weight or maintain a lower body weight.[10] Energy use is enhanced. Therefore, it greatly complements a reduction in energy intake for weight loss (but does not substitute for it). Many people rarely do more than sit, stand, and sleep. Obviously, more energy is used during physical activity than at rest. Even expending only 100 to 300 extra kcal/day above and beyond normal daily activity, while controlling energy intake, can lead to a steady weight loss. Furthermore, physical activity has so many other benefits, including a boost for overall self-esteem.

Adding any of the activities in Table 13-6 to one's lifestyle can increase energy output. Duration and regular performance, rather than intensity, are the keys to success with this approach to weight loss. One should search for activities that can be continued over time. In this regard, walking vigorously 3 miles/day can be as helpful as aerobic dancing or jogging, if it is maintained. Moreover, activities of lighter intensity are less likely to lead to injuries. Some resistance exercises such as weight training also

Note that spot-reducing by using diet and physical activity is not possible. "Problem" local fat deposits can be reduced in size, however, using suction lipectomy. Lipectomy means surgical removal of fat. A pencil-thin tube is inserted into an incision in the skin, and the fat tissue, such as that in the buttocks and thigh area, is suctioned. This procedure carries some risks, such as infection; lasting depressions in the skin; and blood clots, which can lead to kidney failure and sometimes death. The procedure is designed to help a person lose about 4 to 8 lb per treatment. Cost is about $1600 per site; total costs range as high as $2600 to $9000.

Table 13-5 | Saving Kcal: Ideas to Help Get Started

Instead of	Try	Number of Kcal Saved
3 oz well-marbled meat (prime rib)	3 oz lean meat (eye of round)	140
1/2 chicken breast, batter-fried	1/2 chicken breast, broiled with lemon	175
1/2 cup beef stroganoff	3 oz lean roast beef (or use a fat-reduced recipe)	210
1/2 cup home-fried potatoes	1 medium baked potato	65
1/2 cup green bean–mushroom casserole	1/2 cup cooked green beans	50
1/2 cup potato salad	1 cup raw vegetable salad	140
1/2 cup pineapple chunks in heavy syrup	1/2 cup pineapple chunks canned in juice	25
2 tbsp bottled French dressing	2 tbsp low-calorie French dressing	150
1/8 9-inch apple pie	1 baked apple, unsweetened	308
1/2 cup ice cream	1/2 cup fat-free ice cream	45
1 danish pastry	1/2 English muffin	150
1 cup sugar-coated corn flakes	1 cup plain corn flakes	60
1 cup whole milk	1 cup 1% low-fat milk	45
7 oz gin and tonic	6 oz wine cooler made with sparkling water	150
1-oz bag potato chips	1 cup plain popcorn	120
1/12 8-inch white layer cake with chocolate frosting	1/12 angel food cake; 10-inch tube	185
12 oz regular beer	12 oz light beer	40

should be added to increase lean body mass and, in turn, fat use (see Chapter 14). And as lean muscle mass increases, so will one's overall metabolic rate. An added benefit of including exercise in a weight-reduction program is maintenance of bone health.

Unfortunately, opportunities to expend energy in our daily lives are diminishing as technology systematically eliminates almost every reason to move our muscles.[2] The easiest way to increase physical activity is to make it an enjoyable part of a daily routine. To start, one might pack a pair of sneakers and walk around the parking lot before coming home after school or work every day. There are also plenty of other simple ways to increase activity of daily living, such as avoiding elevators in favor of stairs, parking the car farther away from the shopping mall, or getting up to change the channels on the television.

A pedometer is a device that monitors activity as steps. Cost is minimal. An often-stated goal for activity is to take at least 10,000 steps/day—typically we take half that many or less. A pedometer tracks this activity.

Behavior Modification: A Third Strategy for Weight Loss

Controlling energy intake, so important to weight loss, also means modifying *problem* behaviors.[6] Only the dieter can decide what behaviors keep him or her from reaching for the wrong foods at the wrong times for the wrong reasons.

What events start (or stop) the action of eating? What factors influence food choices? Psychologists often use terms such as *chain-breaking, stimulus control, cognitive restructuring, contingency management,* and *self-monitoring* when discussing behavior modification (Table 13-7).[19] These factors help place the problem in perspective and organize the intervention strategy into manageable steps.

Chain-breaking separates behaviors that tend to occur together—for example, snacking on chips while watching television. Although these activities do not have to occur together, they often do. Dieters may need to break the chain reaction (see the Take Action at the end of this chapter for more details).

chain-breaking Breaking the link between two or more behaviors that encourage overeating, such as snacking while watching television.

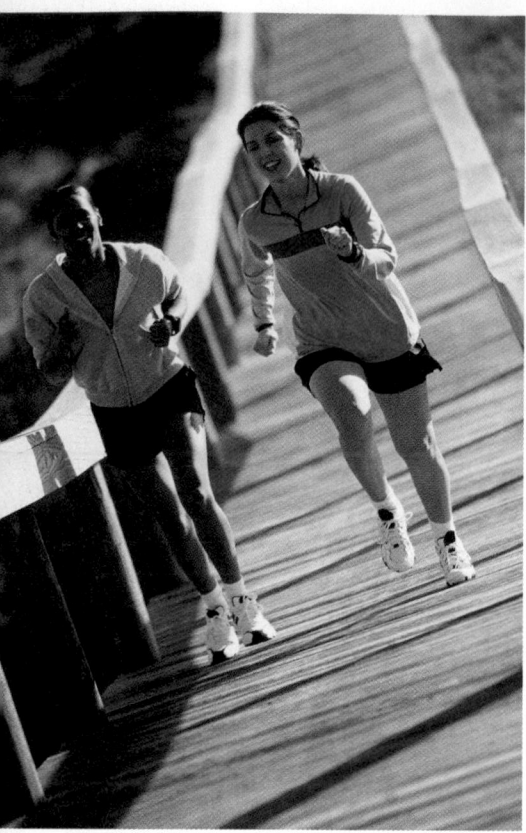

Physical activity complements any diet plan.

Table 13-6 | Approximate Energy Costs of Various Activities, and Specific Energy Costs Projected for a 150-lb (68 kg) Person

Activity	Kcal/kg per Hour	Total kcal/hour	Activity	Kcal/kg per Hour	Total kcal/hour
Aerobics—heavy	8.0	544	Horseback riding	5.1	346
Aerobics—medium	5.0	340	Jogging—medium	9.0	612
Aerobics—light	3.0	204	Ice skating (10 MPH)	5.8	394
Backpacking	9.0	612	Jogging—slow	7.0	476
Basketball—vigorous	10.0	680	Lying—at ease	1.3	89
Cycling (5.5 MPH)	3.0	204	Racquetball—social	8.0	544
Bowling	3.9	265	Roller skating	5.1	346
Calisthenics—heavy	8.0	544	Running or jogging (10 MPH)	13.2	897
Calisthenics—light	4.0	272	Downhill skiing (10 MPH)	8.8	598
Canoeing (2.5 MPH)	3.3	224	Sleeping	1.2	80
Cleaning (female)	3.7	253	Swimming (.25 MPH)	4.4	299
Cleaning (male)	3.5	236	Tennis	6.1	414
Cooking	2.8	190	Volleyball	5.1	346
Cycling (13 MPH)	9.7	659	Walking (2.5 MPH)	3.0	204
Dressing/showering	1.6	106	Walking (3.75 MPH)	4.4	299
Driving	1.7	117	Water skiing	7.0	476
Eating (sitting)	1.4	93	Weight lifting—heavy	9.0	612
Food shopping	3.6	245	Weight lifting—light	4.0	272
Football—touch	7.0	476	Window cleaning	3.5	240
Golf	3.6	244	Writing (sitting)	1.7	118

The values refer to total energy expenditure, including that needed to perform the physical activity plus that needed for basal metabolism, the thermic effect of food, and thermogenesis. Use your diet analysis software for your personal estimate.

stimulus control Altering the environment to minimize the stimuli for eating—for example, removing foods from sight and storing them in kitchen cabinets.

cognitive restructuring Changing one's frame of mind regarding eating—for example, instead of using a difficult day as an excuse to overeat, substituting other pleasures or rewards, such as a relaxing walk with a friend.

contingency management Forming a plan of action to respond to a situation in which overeating is likely, such as when snacks are within arm's reach at a party.

self-monitoring Tracking foods eaten and conditions affecting eating; actions are usually recorded in a diary, along with location, time, and state of mind. This is a tool to help people understand more about their eating habits.

Stimulus control puts one in charge of temptations. Options include pushing tempting food to the back of the refrigerator, removing fat-laden snacks from the kitchen counter, and avoiding the path by the vending machines. Provide a positive stimulus by keeping low-fat snacks available to satisfy hunger/appetite. Note that alcohol and foods offer quick, easy stress relief. Plan healthful alternatives.

Cognitive restructuring changes one's frame of mind. For example, after a hard day, respond with a walk or satisfying talk with a friend instead of a binge. Replace eating reactions to stress with healthful, relaxing alternatives.

Labeling some foods as "off limits" sets up an internal struggle to resist the urge to eat that food. This hopeless battle can keep one feeling deprived and defeated. Managing food choices with the principle of moderation is best. If a favorite food becomes troublesome, place it off limits only temporarily, until it can be enjoyed in moderation.

Contingency management prepares one for potential pitfalls and high-risk situations. Rehearse in advance some appropriate responses to pressures—such as food being passed around at a party.

A **self-monitoring** record can reveal patterns—such as unconscious overeating—that may explain problem eating habits. This record can encourage new habits to counteract unwanted behaviors. Obesity experts note that self-monitoring is the key behavioral tool to use in any weight-loss program.

Overall, it's important to address specific problems, such as snacking, compulsive eating, and mealtime overeating. Behavior modification principles end up as critical

Table 13-7 | Behavior Modification Principles for Weight Loss

Shopping

1. Shop for food after eating—buy nutritious foods.
2. Shop from a list; limit purchases of irresistible "problem" foods. It helps to shop first for fresh foods around the perimeter of the store.
3. Avoid ready-to-eat foods.
4. Put off food shopping until absolutely necessary.

Plans

1. Plan to limit food intake as needed.
2. Substitute periods of physical activity for snacking.
3. Eat meals and snacks at scheduled times; don't skip meals.

Activities

1. Store food out of sight, preferably in the freezer, to discourage impulsive eating.
2. Eat all food in a "dining" area.
3. Keep serving dishes off the table, especially dishes of sauces and gravies.
4. Use smaller dishes and utensils.

Holidays and Parties

1. Drink fewer alcoholic beverages.
2. Plan eating behavior before parties.
3. Eat a low-calorie snack before parties.
4. Practice polite ways to decline food.
5. Don't get discouraged by an occasional setback.

Eating Behavior

1. Put fork down between mouthfuls.
2. Chew thoroughly before taking the next bite.
3. Leave some food on the plate.
4. Pause in the middle of the meal.
5. Do nothing else while eating (for example, reading, watching television).

Reward

1. Plan specific rewards for specific behavior (behavioral contracts).
2. Solicit help from family and friends and suggest how they can help you. Encourage family and friends to provide this help in the form of praise and material rewards.
3. Use self-monitoring records as basis for rewards.

Self-Monitoring

1. Note the time and place of eating.
2. List the type and amount of food eaten.
3. Record who is present and how you feel.
4. Use the diet diary to identify problem areas.

Cognitive Restructuring

1. Avoid setting unreasonable goals.
2. Think about progress, not shortcomings.
3. Avoid imperatives such as *always* and *never*.
4. Counter negative thoughts with positive restatements.

Portion Control

1. Make substitutions, such as a regular hamburger instead of a "quarter pounder" or cucumbers instead of croutons in salads.
2. Think small. Order the entrée and share it with another person. Order a cup of soup instead of a bowl or an appetizer in place of an entrée.
3. Use a to-go container (doggie bag). Ask your server to put half the entrée in a to-go container before bringing it to the table.

Many of us need to become "defensive eaters." Know when to refuse food after satiety registers, and reduce portion sizes.

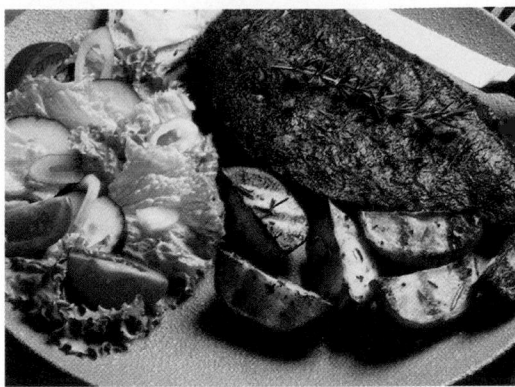

We are faced with many opportunities to overeat. It takes much perseverance to eat sensibly.

Successful weight losers and maintainers from the National Weight Control Registry engage in the following actions:[20]

- Eat a low-fat, high-carbohydrate diet (on average 25% of energy intake as fat).
- Eat breakfast almost every day.
- Self-monitor by regularly weighing themselves and keep a food journal.
- Exercise for a total of about 1 hour/day.
- Eat at restaurants only once or twice per week.

Other recent studies support this approach, especially the last four characteristics.

components of weight reduction and maintenance. Without behavior modification, it is difficult to make the lifelong changes needed to meet weight-control goals.

Relapse Prevention Is Important

A dieter can tolerate an occasional lapse but needs to plan for them.[6] The key is not to overreact, but take charge immediately. Change responses such as "I ate that cookie; I'm a failure" to "I ate that cookie, but I did well to stop after only one!" An occasional cookie is fine; a bag of cookies in one afternoon deserves serious attention. When dieters lapse from their diet plan, newly learned food habits should steer them back toward the plan. Dieters need to learn to avoid the lapse-relapse-collapse trap. Without a strong behavioral program for **relapse prevention** in place, a lapse frequently turns into a relapse. Once a pattern of poor food choices begins, dieters may feel that they have failed and stray further from the plan. As the relapse lengthens, the diet plan collapses, and dieters fall short of their weight-loss goal. Even with a good behavioral plan, a person may fail at a diet. Losing weight is difficult. Overall, maintenance of weight loss is fostered by the "3 *Ms*": motivation, movement, and monitoring.[19]

Social Support Aids Behavioral Change

Healthy social support is helpful in weight control. Helping others understand how they can be supportive can make weight control easier. Family and friends can provide praise and encouragement. A registered dietitian or other weight-control professional can keep dieters accountable and help them learn from difficult situations. Long-term contact with a professional can be quite helpful for later weight maintenance. Groups of individuals attempting to lose weight or maintain losses can provide empathetic support.[19]

relapse prevention A series of strategies used to help prevent and cope with weight-control lapses, such as recognizing high-risk situations and deciding beforehand on appropriate responses.

Critical | Thinking

With regard to readiness to lose weight, what would you say to a young woman who has just had a baby, needs to find a new job, and recently has gone back to school part-time?

Concept | Check

Increasing physical activity in daily life should be part of any weight-loss plan. Daily activity, such as walking and stair climbing, is recommended. Behavior modification can improve conditions for losing weight. One key step is to break behavior chains that encourage overeating, such as snacking while watching television. Another tactic is to modify the environment to reduce temptation; for example, put foods into cupboards to keep them out of sight. In addition, rethinking attitudes about eating—for example, substituting pleasures other than food as a reward for coping with a stressful day—can be important for altering undesirable behavior. Advanced planning to prevent and deal with lapses is vital; as is rallying healthy social support. Finally, careful observation and recording of eating habits can reveal subtle cues that lead to overeating. Overall, weight loss and maintenance are fostered by controlling energy intake, performing regular physical activity, and modifying problem behaviors.

The motivation to lose weight and keep it off generally comes with a proverbial "flip of the switch," in which the desire to lose weight finally becomes more important than the desire to overeat.

Popular Diets—Why All the Commotion?

Many overweight people try to help themselves by using the latest popular (also called fad) diet book. But as you will see, most of these diets do not help, and some can actually harm those who follow them (Table 13-8).

Recently, weight-loss experts came together at the request of USDA to evaluate weight-loss diets. Their conclusion was to forget fads when it comes to dieting. Most of the popular diets are nutritionally inadequate and include certain foods that people would not normally choose to consume in large amounts. The experts stated that eating less of certain foods and becoming more physically active can be much more effective when trying to implement a weight-loss diet. People need a plan that they can live with in the long run because the best predictor of dieting success is long-term adherence to a low-calorie diet.

The goal should be weight control over a lifetime, not immediate weight loss. Every popular diet leads to some immediate weight loss simply because daily energy intake is monitored and monotonous food choices are typically part of the plan. Overall, a traditional moderate diet coupled with regular physical activity is adequate for weight loss.[19]

You may wonder why popular diet books exist at all. Why doesn't the government put a stop to them? Many contain blatant misinformation. However, FDA concerns itself only when products are suspected of doing serious harm, as in the case of earlier forms of liquid protein diets. Classic advice is still valid: "Let the buyer beware." Responsibility rests with the authors and publishers, who want to sell books and earn money. Making outrageous claims sells more books than writing, "Eat less and walk more."

How to Recognize a Dubious Popular Diet

This chapter has already discussed the criteria for evaluating weight-loss programs with regard to their safety and effectiveness. In contrast, dubious popular diets typically share some common characteristics:

1. They promote quick weight loss which is the primary temptation that dieters fall for. This initial weight loss primarily results from water loss and lean muscle mass depletion.
2. They limit food selections and dictate specific rituals, such as eating only fruit for breakfast or cabbage soup every day.
3. They use testimonials from famous people and tie the diet to well-known cities, such as Beverly Hills and New York.
4. They bill themselves as cure-alls. These diets claim to work for everyone, whatever the type of obesity or the person's specific strengths and weaknesses.
5. They often recommend expensive supplements.
6. No attempts are made to change eating habits permanently. Dieters follow the diet until the desired weight is reached and then revert to old eating habits. They are told, for example, to eat rice for a month, lose weight, and then return to old habits.
7. They are generally critical and skeptical of the scientific community. The fact that the medical and dietetics professions cannot provide a quick fix for overweight has led some people to seek advice from those who appear to have the answer.

Probably the cruelest characteristic of these diets is that they essentially guarantee failure for the dieter. The diets are not designed for permanent weight loss. Habits are not changed, and the food selection is so limited that the person cannot follow the diet in the long run. Although dieters assume they have lost fat, they have actually lost mostly muscle and other lean tissue mass. As soon as they begin eating normally again, much of the lost tissue is replaced. In a matter of weeks, most of the lost weight is back. The dieter appears to have failed, when actually the diet has failed. The gain and loss cycle is called weight cycling, or yo-yo dieting. This whole scenario can lead to blame and guilt, challenging the self-worth of the dieter. It can also come with some health costs, such as increased upper-body fat deposition. If someone needs help losing weight, professional help is advised.[19] It is unfortunate that current trends suggest that people are spending more time and money on quick fixes rather than on such professional help.

A well-known example of the effectiveness of monotony contributing to weight loss is the experience of Jared Fogle. He ate primarily Subway sandwiches for 11 months and lost 245 lb. He notes, however, that this is not a miracle diet—it takes a lot of hard work to lead to the success he experienced.

Meal replacement formulas to replace a meal or snack are appropriate to use one to two times per day, if one desires. These are not a magic bullet for weight loss, but have been shown to help some people lose weight.

Table 13-8 | A Summary of Popular Diet Approaches to Weight Control

Approach	Examples	Characteristics	Outcomes
Moderate energy restriction	The Set-Point Diet Slim Chance in a Fat World Weight Watcher's Diet Mary Ellen's Help Yourself Diet Plan The Beyond Diet Staying Thin The Callaway Diet Living without Dieting Volumetrics	Generally 1200 to 1800 kcal/day, with moderate fat intake Reasonable balance of macronutrients Encourage exercise May use behavioral approach	Acceptable if a balanced multi-vitamin and mineral supplement is used and if physician approval is obtained
Restricted carbohydrate	Dr. Atkins New Diet Revolution Calories Don't Count Miracle Diet for Fast Weight Loss Woman Doctor's Diet for Women The Doctor's Quick Weight Loss Diet The Complete Scarsdale Medical Diet	Generally less than 100 g of carbohydrate per day	Ketosis; reduced exercise capacity due to poor glycogen stores in the muscles; excessive animal fat and cholesterol intake; constipation, headaches, halitosis (bad breath), and muscle cramps
Low fat	The Rice Diet Report The Macrobiotic Diet (some versions) The Pritikin Diet Eat More, Weigh Less The 35+ Diet 20/30 Fat and Fiber Fat to Muscle Diet T-Factor Diet Fit or Fat Two-Day Diet The Four Day Wonder Diet Endocrine Control Diet Enter the Zone Protein Power The Five-Day Miracle Diet Healthy for Life Carbohydrate Addicts Diet Sugar Busters South Beach Diet (especially initial phases) The Maximum Metabolism Diet The Pasta Diet The McDougall Plan Ultrafit Diet Stop the Insanity G-Index Diet Outsmarting the Female Fat Cell Foods That Cause You to Lose Weight Lean Bodies Turn Off the Fat Genes	Generally less than 20% of energy intake from fat Limited (or elimination of) animal protein sources; also limited fats, nuts, seeds	Flatulence; possibly poor mineral absorption from excess fiber; limited food choices sometimes leads to deprivation Not necessarily to be avoided, but certain aspects of many of the plans possibly unacceptable
Novelty diets	Dr. Abravenel's Body Type and Lifetime Nutrition Plan (or his other books) Dr. Berger's Immune Power Diet Fit for Life The New Hilton Head Metabolism Diet The Beverly Hills Diet Dr. Debetz Champagne Diet Sun Sign Diet F-Plan Diet Fat Attack Plan Autohypnosis Diet The Princeton Diet The Diet Bible Eat to Succeed The Underburner's Diet Eat to Win Paris Diet Cabbage-Soup Diet Eat Great, Lose Weight Eat Smart Think Smart Scentsational Weight Loss Eat Right 4 Your Type The Greenwich Diet 3 Season Diet Metabolize God's Diet The Weigh Down Diet	Promotes certain nutrients, foods, or combinations of foods as having unique, magical, or previously undiscovered qualities	Malnutrition, no change in habits, which leads to relapse; unrealistic food choices lead to possible bingeing

Types of Popular Diets

Low- or Restricted-Carbohydrate Approaches

The low-carbohydrate diet is currently the most common of the popular diets. Low-carbohydrate intake leads to less glycogen synthesis and therefore less water in the body (about 3 g of water are stored per gram of glycogen). As discussed in Chapter 4, a very-low-carbohydrate intake also forces the liver to produce needed glucose. The source of carbons for this glucose is mostly tissue proteins. (Recall also from Chapter 4 that typical fatty acids can't form glucose.) Thus, a low-carbohydrate diet results in protein tissue loss (which is about 72% water) as well as urinary loss of essential ions such as potassium. Because protein tissue is mostly water, the dieter loses weight very rapidly. When a normal diet is resumed, the protein tissue is rebuilt and the weight is regained.

Low-carbohydrate diets primarily work in the short run because they limit total food intake. And in long-term studies these diets have not shown a distinct advantage compared to diets that simply limit energy intake in general.

Diet plans that use a low-carbohydrate approach are the Dr. Atkins' New Diet Revolution, the Scarsdale Diet, and the Four-Day Wonder Diet. More moderate approaches are found in the various Zone diets (40% of energy intake as carbohydrate), Sugar Busters diet, and the South Beach diet (especially initial phases). When you see a new diet advertisement, look first to see how much carbohydrate it contains. If breads, cereals, fruits, and vegetables are extremely limited, you are probably looking at a low- or restricted-carbohydrate diet.

The popularity of low-carbohydrate diets has already reached its peak. Recent studies show these diets provide no long term advantage over other diet plans.[3] In addition, companies producing foods for these diets have been going bankrupt, as have stores specializing in low-carbohydrate foods.

Low-Fat Approaches

The very-low-fat diet turns out to be a very-high-carbohydrate diet. These diets contain approximately 5 to 10% of energy intake as fat. The most notable are the Pritikin Diet and the Dr. Dean Ornish "Eat More, Weigh Less" diet plans. This approach is not harmful for healthy adults, but it is difficult to follow. People get bored with this type of diet very quickly because they cannot eat many of their favorite foods. These dieters eat primarily grains, fruits, and vegetables, which most people cannot do for very long. Eventually, the person wants some foods higher in fat or protein. These diets are just too different from the typical North American diet for many adults to follow consistently, but may be acceptable for some people.

Novelty Diets

A variety of diets are built on gimmicks. Some novelty diets emphasize one food or food group and exclude almost all others. A rice diet was designed in the 1940s to lower blood pressure; now it has resurfaced as a weight-loss diet. The first phase consists of eating only rice and fruit. Another novelty diet is the egg diet, on which you eat all the eggs you want. On the Beverly Hills Diet, you eat mostly fruit.

The rationale behind these diets is that you can eat only eggs, fruit, or rice for just so long before becoming bored and, in theory, reducing your energy intake. However, chances are that you will abandon the diet entirely before losing much weight.

The most questionable of the novelty diets propose that "food gets stuck in your body." Fit for Life, the Beverly Hills Diet, and Eat Great, Lose Weight are examples. The supposition is that food gets stuck in the intestine, putrefies, and creates toxins that invade the blood and cause disease. In response, recommendations are to not consume meat with potatoes, or consume fruits only after noon. These recommendations make no physiological sense, nor do recommendations for eating according to one's blood type.

Quackery Is Characteristic of Many Popular Diets

Many popular diets fall under the category of quackery—people taking advantage of others. They usually involve a product or service that costs a

People on diets often fall within a non-overweight BMI of 18.5 to 25. Rather than worrying about weight loss, these individuals should be focusing on a healthy lifestyle that allows for weight maintenance. Incorporating necessary lifestyle changes and learning to accept one's particular body characteristics should be the overriding goals. Dieting mania can be viewed as mostly a social problem stemming from unrealistic weight expectations (especially for women) and lack of appreciation for the natural variety in body shape and weight. Not every woman can look like a fashion model, nor can every man look like a Greek god, but all of us can strive for good health and, if physically possible, an active lifestyle.

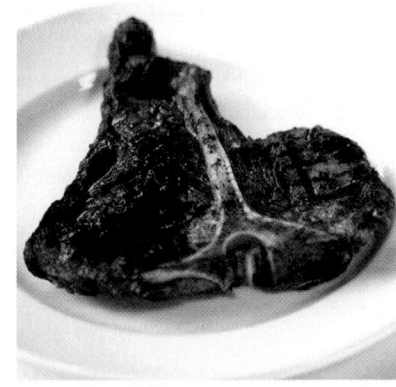

In time, the very-low-carbohydrate, high-protein diets typically leave a person wanting more variety in meals, and so the diets are abandoned. Dropout rates are very high on these diets.

Recently a woman developed liver failure after using a so-called weight-loss aid called usnic acid. Her purchase was via the Internet. Today more than ever, let the buyer beware concerning any purported weight-loss aid not prescribed by a physician.

considerable amount of money. Often, those offering the product or service don't realize that they are promoting quackery because they were victims themselves. For example, they tried the product and by pure coincidence it worked for them, so they wish to sell it to all their friends and relatives.

Numerous other gimmicks for weight loss have come and gone and are likely to resurface.[17] If in the future an important aid for weight loss is discovered, you can feel confident that major journals, such as the *Journal of the American Dietetic Association,* the *Journal of the American Medical Association,* or *The New England Journal of Medicine,* will report it. You don't need to rely on paperback books, infomercials, billboards, or newspaper advertisements for information about weight loss.

Case Scenario| Follow-Up

As you have probably surmised, Chris will just be wasting his money if he buys the product seen in the infomercial. Unfortunately, regulation of the supplement industry currently is woefully lacking. In the future, if there is a meaningful breakthrough in weight loss and weight control, authorities such as the Surgeon General's Office or the National Institutes of Health will make North Americans aware of that fact. At this time, Chris would be better off simply paying more attention to what he is eating and trying to find time for daily physical activity.

Professional Help for Weight Loss

North Americans are willing to try almost anything to shed unwanted pounds. Operation Waistline is a program designed by the U.S. Federal Trade Commission to terminate fraudulent claims being made by weight-loss charlatans with regard to diet products. The program hopes to put an end to the $6 billion spent annually in the United States on counterfeit products. Recently the Enforma Natural Products Corporation had to pay $10 million in response to false claims for its "Fat Trapper" product.

The first professional to see for advice about a weight-loss program is one's family physician. Doctors are best equipped to assess overall health and the appropriateness of weight loss. The physician may then recommend a registered dietitian for a specific weight-loss plan and answers to diet-related questions. Registered dietitians are uniquely qualified to help design a weight-loss plan because they understand both food composition and the psychological importance of food. Exercise physiologists can provide advice about programs to increase physical activity. The expense for such professional interventions is tax deductible in the United States in some cases (see a tax advisor) and often covered by health insurance plans if prescribed by a physician.

Many communities have a variety of weight-loss organizations. These include self-help groups, such as Weight Watchers and Take Off Pounds Sensibly. Other programs, such as Jenny Craig and Medifast, are less desirable for the average dieter. Often, the employees are not registered dietitians or other appropriately trained health professionals. These programs also tend to be expensive because of their requirements for intense counseling or mandatory diet foods and supplements. In addition, the Federal Trade Commission has charged these and other commercial diet-program companies with misleading consumers through unsubstantiated weight-loss claims and deceptive testimonials.

Medications for Weight Loss

People who are candidates for medications for obesity include those with a BMI of 30 or more, or a BMI of 27 to 29.9 with weight-related (i.e., comorbid) conditions, such as type 2 diabetes, cardiovascular disease, hypertension, or excess waist circumference;

those with no contraindications to use of the medication; and those ready to undertake lifestyle change. Success with medications has been shown only in those who also modify their behavior, decrease energy intake, and increase physical activity.[19] Drug therapy alone has not been found to be successful. In addition, if a person has not lost at least 4.4 lb (2 kg) after 4 weeks, it is not likely that the person will benefit from further use of the medication.

Currently three main classes of medications are used.[12] An **amphetamine**-like medication (phenteramine [Fastin or Ionamin]) prolongs the activity of epinephrine and norepinephrine in the brain. This therapy is effective for some people in the short run but has not yet been proven effective in the long run. Most state medical boards currently limit use to 12 weeks unless the person is participating in a medical study using the product. The medication should not be used by pregnant or nursing women or those under 18 years of age.

Sibutramine (Meridia) is a second class of medication that has been approved by FDA for weight loss. It enhances both norepinephrine and serotonin activity in the brain by reducing reuptake of these neurotransmitters by nerve cells. The neurotransmitters then remain active in the brain for a longer period of time and so prolong a sense of reduced hunger. The most common side effects are constipation, dry mouth, insomnia, and a mild increase in blood pressure in some people. Thus, sibutramine should be used with caution in people with a history of hypertension (or cardiovascular disease). Studies have shown that it is effective in helping some people who already eat healthy diets, but just eat too much.[19] The main effect is to moderately reduce appetite so that people eat less. Sibutramine is safe and effective only when combined with a comprehensive weight-control program and when supervised by a physician.

The third class of medication approved by FDA for weight loss is orlistat (Xenical). This medication inhibits lipase enzyme action in the small intestine, reducing fat digestion by about 30%. Orlistat reduces absorption of dietary fat by one-third for about 2 hours when taken along with a meal containing fat. This malabsorbed fat simply is deposited in the feces. *Fat intake has to be controlled,* however, because large amounts of fat in the feces cause numerous side effects, such as gas, bloating, and oily discharge. Interestingly, orlistat use can actually remind the person to follow a fat-controlled diet, because the symptoms resulting from consuming a high-fat meal are unpleasant and quickly develop. Orlistat is taken with each meal containing fat.

Because the malabsorbed fat also carries fat-soluble vitamins into the feces, the person taking orlistat must take a multivitamin and mineral supplement at bedtime. In this way, any micronutrients not absorbed during the day can be replaced; fat malabsorption from the dinner meal will not greatly influence micronutrient absorption in the late evening.

Overall, in skilled hands, prescription medications can aid weight loss in some instances. However, they do not replace the need for reducing energy intake, modifying problem behaviors, and increasing physical activity, both during and after therapy.[14] And more often than not, any weight loss during drug treatment can be attributed mostly to the individual's hard work at balancing energy intake with output.[19]

Treatment of Severe Obesity

Severe (morbid) obesity—weighing at least 100 lb over healthy body weight (or twice one's healthy body weight)—requires professional treatment. Because of the serious health implications of severe obesity, drastic measures may be necessary. Such treatments are recommended only when traditional diets fail. Drastic weight-loss procedures are not without side effects, both physical and psychological, making careful monitoring by a physician necessary.

Very-Low-Calorie Diets

If more traditional diet changes have failed, treating severe obesity with a **very-low-calorie diet (VLCD)** is possible, especially if the person has obesity-related diseases that are not well controlled (e.g., hypertension, type 2 diabetes).[19] Some researchers

amphetamine A group of medications that stimulate the central nervous system and have other effects in the body. Abuse is linked to physical and psychological dependence.

The only two weight-loss medications approved by FDA for long-term use are sibutramine (Meridia) and orlistat (Xenical). Drug companies are working on many other types of medications (e.g., rimonabant) and have high hopes that some of these will prove to be safe and effective for weight loss. In addition, physicians may prescribe medications that are not approved for weight loss per se but can have weight loss as a side effect. Certain antidepressants (e.g., bupropion [Wellbutrin]) are an example.[14] Such an application is termed *off-label,* because the product label does not include weight loss as an FDA-approved use.

very-low-calorie diet (VLCD) Diet that allows a person 400 to 800 kcal per day, often in liquid form. Of this, 120 to 480 kcal is carbohydrate, and the rest is mostly high-quality protein. Also known as *protein-sparing modified fast (PSMF).*

believe that people with body weight greater than 30% above their healthy weight are appropriate candidates. Optifast is one such commercial program. In general, the diet allows a person to consume 400 to 800 kcal/day, often in liquid form. (These diets were previously known as protein-sparing modified fasts.) Of this amount, about 100 to 120 g (400 to 480 kcal) is carbohydrate. The rest is high-quality protein, in the amount of about 70 to 100 g/day (280 to 400 kcal). This low carbohydrate intake often causes ketosis, which may decrease hunger. However, the main reasons for weight loss are the minimal energy consumption and the absence of food choice. About 3 to 4 lb can be lost per week; men tend to lose at a faster rate than women. When physical activity and resistance training augment this diet, a greater loss of adipose tissue occurs. Careful monitoring by a physician is crucial throughout this very restrictive form of weight loss. Major health risks include heart problems and gallstones.

Weight regain remains a nagging problem, especially without a behavioral and physical activity component. If behavioral therapy and physical activity supplement a long-term support program, maintenance of the weight loss is more likely but still difficult. Any program under consideration should include a maintenance plan. Today, antiobesity medications also may be included in this phase of the program.

Gastroplasty

Gastroplasty (gastric bypass surgery, also called stomach stapling) is the primary surgical procedure used today for treating severe obesity.[1] About $1 billion is spent each year for this procedure. The most common and effective surgical approach in the long run is the Roux-en-Y gastric bypass procedure. It works by reducing the stomach capacity to about 30 ml (the volume of one egg or shot glass) and bypassing a short segment of the upper small intestine (Figure 13-18). Weight loss is promoted mainly because overeating of solid foods is now less likely because of reduced ghrelin output and discomfort or vomiting with overeating. It is also necessary to eliminate simple carbohydrates (sugar) from the diet of people who have undergone gastroplasty to avoid *dumping syndrome*. Dumping syndrome is characterized by severe diarrhea, which begins almost immediately following the ingestion of concentrated sugar, such as regular soft drinks, Jell-o, candy, cookies, and other high-sugar foods.

About 75% of people with severe obesity eventually lose 50% or more of excess body weight with this method. In addition, the surgery's success at long-term maintenance often leads to dramatic health improvements, such as reduced blood pressure and elimination of type 2 diabetes. Risk of death from the surgery itself is about 2%, especially if the surgeon has performed less than 20 of the procedures. Risks of this very demanding surgery include bleeding, blood clots, hernias, and severe infections. In the long run, nutrient deficiencies can develop if the person is not adequately treated in the years following the surgery (chewable multivitamin and mineral supplements are often used). Anemia and bone loss might then be the result.

Current patient selection criteria for Roux-en-Y gastroplasty include the following:

- BMI should be greater than 40.
- BMI between 35 and 40 is considered when there are serious obesity-related health concerns.
- Obesity must be present for a minimum of 5 years, with several nonsurgical attempts to lose weight.
- There should be no history of alcoholism or major psychiatric disorders.

The person also must consider that the surgery is costly ($12,000 to $40,000 or more) and may not be covered by medical insurance. In addition, follow-up surgery is often needed after weight loss to correct stretched skin that was previously filled with fat. Furthermore, the surgery necessitates major lifestyle changes, such as the need to plan frequent, small meals. Therefore, the dieter who has chosen this drastic approach to weight loss faces months of difficult adjustments.

Other surgical approaches are vertical-banded gastroplasty, gastric banding procedure, and biliopancreatic diversion. In the vertical-banded gastroplasty, a vertical sta-

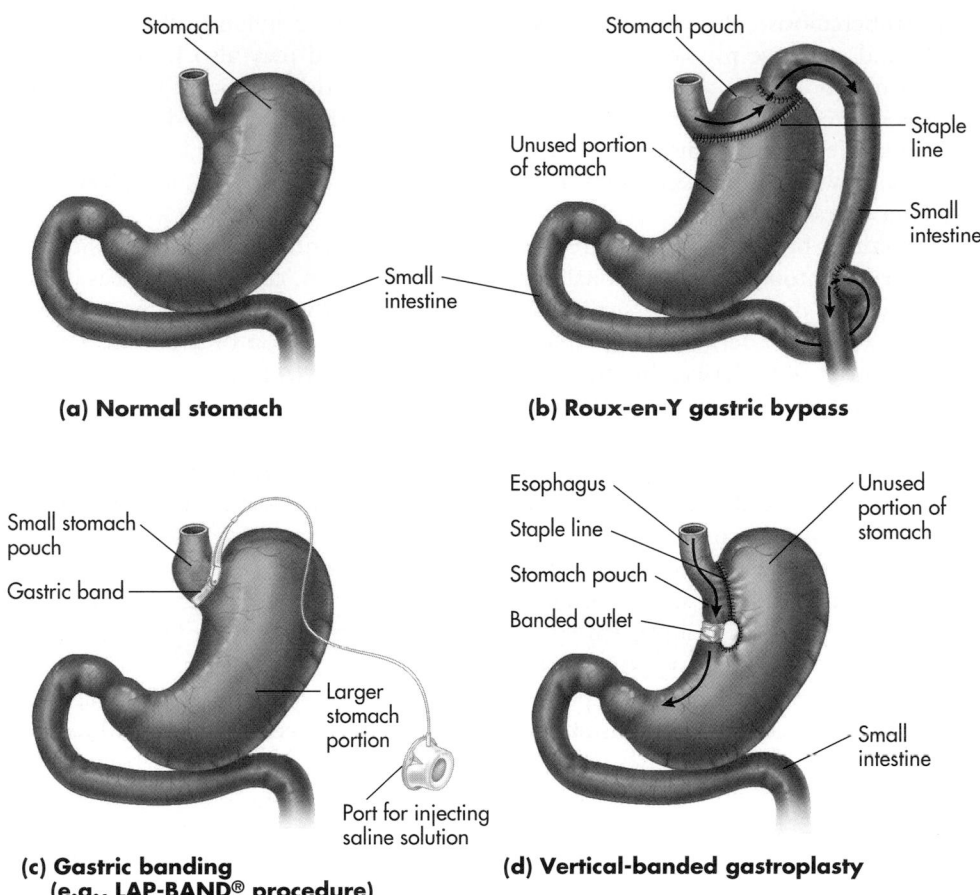

Figure 13-18 | Three of the most common forms of gastroplasty for treatment of severe obesity. The Roux-en-Y procedure *(b)* is the most effective method but is more technically demanding for the surgeon than gastric banding *(c)* or vertical-banded gastroplasty *(d)*. In vertical-banded gastroplasty, the band prevents expansion of the outlet for the stomach pouch.

ple line is made down the length of the stomach to create a small stomach pouch. At the outlet of the pouch, a band is placed to keep the opening from stretching (review Figure 13-18). With gastric banding, a band is placed around the upper portion of the stomach, creating a small stomach pouch (review Figure 13-18). A salt solution can be injected into the band through a port to adjust the size of the pouch over time. In the biliopancreatic diversion (often called duodenal switch), stomach volume is reduced surgically by 75%, and much of the intestinal tract is bypassed. This combination leads to less food consumption and significant nutrient malabsorption. Because of the latter factor, this procedure has yet to gain much acceptance by surgeons for weight loss, whereas the other two procedures are common.

Concept | Check

Severely obese people who have failed to lose weight with conservative weight-loss strategies may consider other options. Their doctors may recommend that they undergo surgery such as reducing the volume of the stomach to approximately 30 ml or following a very-low-calorie diet plan containing 400 to 800 kcal per day. Careful monitoring by a physician is crucial in both cases.

Treatment of Underweight

We frequently hear about the risks of obesity but seldom of **underweight.** In our culture, being underweight is much more socially acceptable than being obese. Underweight can be caused by a variety of factors, such as cancer, infectious disease

underweight A body mass index below 18.5. The cutoff is less precise than for obesity because this condition has been less studied.

(e.g., tuberculosis), digestive tract disorders (e.g., chronic inflammatory bowel disease), and excessive physical activity. Genetic background may also lead to a higher resting metabolic rate, a lean or petite body frame, or both. Significant underweight is also associated with increased death rates, especially when combined with cigarette smoking. Health problems associated with underweight include the loss of menstrual function, low bone mass, complications with pregnancy and surgery, and slow recovery after illness.

Sometimes being underweight requires medical intervention. A physician should be consulted first to rule out hormonal imbalances, depression, cancer, infectious disease, digestive tract disorders, excessive physical activity, and other hidden disease, such as a serious eating disorder (see Chapter 15 for a detailed discussion of eating disorders).

The causes of underweight are not altogether different from the causes of obesity. Internal and external satiety-signal irregularities, the rate of metabolism, hereditary tendencies, and psychological traits can all contribute to underweight.

In growing children, the demand for energy to support physical activity and growth can cause underweight. During growth spurts in adolescence, active children may not take the time to consume enough energy to support their needs. Moreover, gaining weight can be a formidable task for an underweight person. An extra 500 kcal per day may be required to gain weight, even at a slow pace, in part because of the increased expenditure of energy from thermogenesis. In contrast to the weight loser, the weight gainer may need to increase portion sizes.

When underweight requires a specific intervention, one approach for treating adults is to gradually increase their consumption of energy-dense foods, especially those high in vegetable fat. Italian cheeses, nuts, and granola can be good choices because they are low in saturated fat. Dried fruit and bananas are good fruit choices. If eaten at the end of a meal, they don't cause early satiety. The same advice applies to salads and soups. Underweight people should replace such foods as diet soft drinks with healthy energy sources, such as fruit juices and smoothies.

Encouraging a regular meal and snack schedule also aids in weight gain and maintenance. Sometimes people who are underweight have experienced stress at work or have been too busy to eat. Making regular meals a priority may not only help them attain an appropriate weight but also help with digestive disorders, such as constipation, that are sometimes associated with irregular eating times.

Excessively physically active people can reduce activity. If their weight remains low, they can add muscle mass through a resistance training (weight-lifting) program, but they must increase their energy intake to support that physical activity. Otherwise, weight gain will be hindered.

Summary

1. Energy balance considers energy intake and energy output. Negative energy balance occurs when energy output surpasses energy intake, resulting in weight loss. Positive energy balance occurs when energy intake is greater than output, resulting in weight gain.

2. Basal metabolism, the thermic effect of food, physical activity, and thermogenesis account for total energy use by the body. Basal metabolism, which represents the minimum amount of energy used to keep the resting, awake body alive, is primarily affected by lean body mass, surface area, and thyroid hormone concentrations. Physical activity is energy use above that which is expended at rest. The thermic effect of food describes the increase in metabolism that facilitates digestion, absorption, and processing of nutrients recently consumed. Thermogenesis is heat production caused by shivering when cold, fidgeting, and other stimuli. In a sedentary person, about 70 to 80% of energy use is accounted for by basal metabolism and the thermic effect of food.

3. Energy use by the body can be measured directly from heat output or indirectly from oxygen uptake, carbon dioxide output, or both. An Estimated Energy Requirement can be calculated using formulas based on various combinations of body height and weight with degree of physical activity and age.

4. Groups of cells in the hypothalamus and other regions in the brain affect hunger, the primarily internal desire to find and eat food. These cells monitor macronutrients and other substances in the blood and read low amounts as a signal to promote feeding.

5. A variety of external (appetite-related) forces, such as food availability, affect satiety. Hunger cues combine with appetite cues to promote feeding.

6. In North America, the major determinants of food intake are probably appetite-driven forces because food is so readily available. The physiological influences affecting food consumption are often suppressed or ignored.

7. A person of healthy weight generally shows good health and performs daily activities without weight-related problems. A body mass index (weight in kilograms ÷ height^2 in meters) of 18.5 to 25 is one measure of healthy weight, although weight in excess of this value may not lead to ill health. A healthy weight is best determined in conjunction with a thorough health evaluation by a physician.

8. A body mass index of 25 to 29.9 represents overweight. Obesity is defined as a total body fat percentage over 25% (men) or 35% (women), or a body mass index of 30 or more.

9. Fat distribution greatly determines health risks from obesity. Upper-body fat storage, as measured by a waist circumference greater than 40 inches (102 cm) (men) or 35 inches (88 cm) (women), increases the risks of hypertension, cardiovascular disease, and type 2 diabetes more than does lower-body fat storage.

10. A sound weight-loss program emphasizes a wide variety of low-calorie bulky foods; adapts to the dieter's habits; consists of readily obtainable foods; strives to change poor eating habits; stresses regular physical activity; and stipulates the participation of a physician if weight is to be lost rapidly or if the person is over the age of 40 (men) or 50 (women) and plans to perform substantially greater physical activity than usual.

11. A pound of adipose tissue contains about 3500 kcal. Loss or gain of a pound of adipose tissue—the fat itself plus lean support tissue—represents approximately 3300 kcal. Thus, if energy output exceeds intake by about 500 kcal per day, a pound of adipose tissue can be lost per week.

12. Physical activity as part of a weight-loss program should be focused on duration rather than intensity. Ideally, vigorous activity for 60 to 90 minutes should be part of each day.

13. Behavior modification is a vital part of a weight-loss program because the dieter may have many habits that discourage weight maintenance. Specific behavior modification techniques, such as stimulus control and self-monitoring, can be used to help change problem behavior.

14. Medications to blunt appetite, such as phenteramine (Fastin) and sibutramine (Meridia), can aid weight-reduction strategies. Orlistat (Xenical) reduces fat absorption when taken with the meal. Weight-loss drugs are reserved for those who are obese or have weight-related problems, and they must be administered under close physician supervision.

15. The treatment of severe obesity may include surgery to reduce stomach volume to approximately 30 ml (1 oz) or very-low-calorie diets containing 400 to 800 kcal/day. Both of these measures should be reserved for people who have failed at more conservative approaches to weight loss. They also require close medical supervision.

16. Underweight can be caused by a variety of factors, such as excessive physical activity and genetic background. Sometimes being underweight requires medical attention. A physician should be consulted first to rule out underlying disease. The underweight person may need to increase portion sizes and learn to like energy-dense foods. In addition, encouraging a regular meal and snack schedule aids in weight gain as well as weight maintenance.

Study Questions

1. After re-examining the internal and external forces associated with hunger, satiety, and food choices, propose two hypotheses for the development of obesity.

2. Propose two hypotheses for the development of obesity based on the four contributors to energy expenditure.

3. Define a healthy weight in a way that makes the most sense to you.

4. Describe a practical method to define obesity in a clinical setting.

5. What are the two most convincing pieces of evidence that both genetic and environmental factors play significant roles in the development of obesity?

6. List three health problems that obese people typically face. Describe a possible reason why each problem arises.

7. When searching for a sound weight-loss program, what three key characteristics would you look for?

8. Why is the claim for quick, effortless weight loss by any method always misleading?

9. Define the term *behavior modification*. Relate it to the terms *stimulus control*, *self-monitoring*, *chain-breaking*, *relapse prevention*, and *cognitive restructuring*. Give examples of each.

10. Why should the treatment of obesity be viewed as a lifelong commitment rather than just a short episode of weight loss?

BOOST YOUR STUDY

Check out the **Perspectives in Nutrition: Online Learning Center** www.mhhe.com/wardlawpers7 for quizzes, flash cards, activities, and web links designed to further help you learn about energy balance and weight control.

Annotated References

1. Blackburn GL: Solutions in weight control: Lessons from gastric surgery. *American Journal of Clinical Nutrition* 82:248S, 2005.
Surgery is currently the only proven way to achieve significant long-term weight loss, improve obesity-related comorbidities, reduce the risk of premature death, and improve quality of life in a large proportion of obese individuals. Roux-en-Υ gastric bypass, the most widely performed procedure in the United States, achieves significant weight loss in more than 90% of cases of severe obesity.

2. Booth KM and others: Obesity and the built environment. *Journal of the American Dietetic Association* 105:S110, 2005.
Obesity is linked with many features of the "built environment": residence, neighborhood, resources, television, walkability, land use, and

sprawl. Lower socioeconomic status neighbor-hoods are a primary concern, as residents in these areas may have less access to recreational facilities or food stores with healthful, affordable options. In the future, neighborhoods should be designed in ways that promote physical activity.

3. Dansinger ML and others: Comparison of the Atkins, Ornish, Weight Watchers, and Zone diets for weight loss and heart disease risk re-duction: A randomized trial. *Journal of the American Medical Association* 293:43, 2005.

All four popular diets (Atkins, Ornish, Weight Watchers, Zone) are equally effective for helping adults lose weight and reduce cardiac risk fac-tors. Because success in this study directly corre-lated with adherence to the diet, it makes sense to help patients choose the diet that is easiest for them to follow, rather than preferentially en-couraging one diet over any other.

4. Davison KK, Birch LL: Lean and weight stable: Behavioral predictors and psychological corre-lates. *Obesity Research* 12:1085, 2004.

Being at a healthy weight and avoiding large weight fluctuations during adulthood are linked with patterns of healthy eating and regular physi-cal activity, lower dietary restraint, and less re-liance on dieting attempts. These lifestyle be-havioral patterns may emerge during childhood; intervention efforts should focus on this age period.

5. Ello-Martin JA and others: The influence of food portion size and energy density on energy intake: Implications for weight management. *American Journal of Clinical Nutrition* 82:236S, 2005.

Providing older children and adults with larger and larger food portions can lead to significant increases in energy intake. One strategy to ad-dress this effect of portion size is decreasing the energy density of foods. Eating satisfying por-tions of low-energy-dense foods maintains satiety while reducing energy intake.

6. Foster GD and others: Behavioral treatment of obesity. *American Journal of Clinical Nutrition* 82:230S, 2005.

The behavior change process is facilitated through the use of self-monitoring, goal-setting, and prob-lem solving. Behavior therapy can help individuals develop a set of skills (such as eating a low-energy, low-fat diet) to achieve a healthier weight.

7. Hu FB: Protein, body weight, and cardiovascu-lar health. *American Journal of Clinical Nutrition* 82:242S, 2005.

It may be beneficial to partially replace refined carbohydrates with protein sources low in satu-rated fat. Plant sources of protein and fat, such as nuts, legumes, soy, and vegetable oils, may provide even greater health benefits in place of refined carbohydrates and animal products.

8. Hill JO and others: Obesity and the environ-ment: Where do we go from here? *Science* 299: 853, 2003.

A moderate decrease in energy intake (100 kcal) and greater physical activity (100 kcal) are ad-vocated by these authors to achieve the goal of slow weight loss. There is an urgent need to stop the slow weight gain that currently characterizes the fate of most North American adults.

9. Hill JO and others: Obesity: Etiology. In Shils ME and others (eds): *Modern nutrition in health and disease.* 10th ed. Philadelphia, PA: Lippincott Williams & Wilkins, 2006.

Current review of the causes of obesity in our so-ciety. The article points out that obesity is not a simple disease to understand because many fac-tors contribute to its etiology.

10. Jakicic JM and Otto AD: Physical activity con-siderations for the treatment and prevention of obesity. *American Journal of Clinical Nutrition* 82:226S, 2005.

Physical activity is an important component of long-term weight control, and therefore adequate levels of activity should be prescribed to combat the obesity epidemic. Although there is evidence that 30 minutes of moderate-intensity physical activity may improve health outcomes, a growing body of scientific literature suggests that at least 60 minutes of moderate-intensity physical activ-ity may be necessary to maximize weight loss and prevent significant weight regain.

11. Klein S and others: Clinical implications of obe-sity with specific focus on cardiovascular dis-ease. *Circulation* 110:2952, 2004.

Obesity adversely affects cardiac function, in-creases the risk factors for coronary heart disease, and is an independent risk factor for cardiovas-cular disease. The risk of developing coronary heart disease is directly related to obesity related risk factors. In contrast, modest weight loss can affect the entire cluster of cardiovascular disease risk factors simultaneously.

12. Li Z and others: Meta-analysis: Pharmacologic treatment of obesity. *Annals of Internal Medicine* 142(7):532, 2005.

Sibutramine, orlistat, and phentermine, and probably diethylpropion, bupropion, and topi-ramate promote weight loss when given along with recommendations for diet (and other be-havioral and exercise interventions). The amount of extra weight loss attributable to these medications is modest, but still may be clinically significant. Use of each of these medications is reviewed in detail.

13. Lofgren I and others: Waist circumference is a better predictor than body mass index of coro-nary heart disease risk in overweight pre-menopausal women. *Journal of Nutrition* 134:1071, 2004.

Although neither BMI nor waist circumference provides a complete picture of overall risk, the waist circumference classification of the subjects from the present study revealed stronger associa-tions with multiple risk factors for chronic disease. This finding suggests that waist circumference should be used to screen the general population.

14. Moyers SB: Medications as adjunct therapy for weight loss: Approved and off-label agents in use. *Journal of the American Dietetic Association* 105:948, 2005.

Some clinicians prescribe medications not ap-proved for weight loss. These medications are reviewed in the article. Evidence from clinical trials indicates that weight loss resulting from the use of many of these off-label pharmaceutical agents is modest, but still sufficient to diminish cardiovascular risk factors. Medications alone, without behavior modification, are not effective; people who respond to medication typically regain weight when the medication is discontinued.

15. Periera MA and others: The fast-food track to obesity and insulin resistance. *Lancet* 365: 36, 2005.

Participants in this study who reported more than 2 fast-food visits each week gained signifi-cantly more weight and had a twofold increase in insulin resistance, compared with partici-pants who reported fewer than 1 weekly fast-food visit. Thus, the growing use of fast food restau-rants needs to be reexamined by many of us.

16. Ornish D: Was Dr Atkins right? *Journal of the American Dietetic Association* 104: 537, 2004.

The author suggests that the safest way to lose weight in the long run is to focus on reducing fat and refined carbohydrate intake. Whole foods and complex carbohydrates should instead be emphasized.

17. Pittler MH, Ernst E: Dietary supplements for body-weight reduction: A systematic review. *American Journal of Clinical Nutrition* 79:529, 2004.

Evidence for most dietary supplements as aids in reducing body weight is not convincing. None of the reviewed dietary supplements in the article, such as chromium and chitosan, can be recom-mended for over-the-counter use.

18. Smith GP: Control of food intake. In Shils ME and others (eds): *Modern nutrition in health and disease.* 10th ed. Philadelphia, PA: Lippincott Williams & Wilkins, 2006.

The many neurotransmitters and hormones that influence food intake are reviewed by the author. The ways these compounds interact with the brain and GI tract to influence body weight control are highlighted.

19. Wadden TA and others: Obesity: Management. In Shils ME and others (eds): *Modern nutrition in health and disease.* 10th ed. Philadelphia, PA: Lippincott Williams & Wilkins, 2006.

The various tools available to clinicians to help people lose weight are presented by the authors. Concern is also expressed that the effectiveness of these tools, such as recommendations to consume less energy, are being compromised by our cur-rent social environment, and so the latter needs to be addressed as well.

20. Wing RR, Phelan S: Long-term weight loss maintenance. *American Journal of Clinical Nutrition* 82:222S, 2005.

National Weight Control Registry members pro-vide evidence that long-term weight loss mainte-nance is possible and help identify the specific approaches associated with long-term success. The article reviews the habits of these participants, such as regularly eating breakfast, self-monitor-ing weight, and meeting the goal of 60 minutes of physical activity.

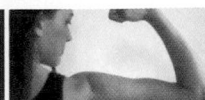

Take | Action

I. A Close Look at Your Weight Status

Determine the following two indices of your body status: body mass index and waist circumference.

Body Mass Index (BMI)

Record your weight in pounds: _____ lb
Divide your weight in pounds by 2.2 to determine your weight in kilograms: _____ kg
Record your height in inches: _____ in
Divide your height in inches by 39.3 to determine your height in meters: _____ m
Calculate your BMI using the following formula:
BMI = _____ kg/ _____ m² = _____

Waist Circumference

Use a tape measure to measure the circumference of your waist (at the navel with stomach muscles relaxed). Circumference of waist = _____ in

Interpretation

1. When BMI is greater than 25, health risks from overweight may begin. It is especially advisable to consider weight loss if your BMI exceeds 30. Does yours exceed 25 (or 30)?
   Yes _____   No _____

2. When a person has a BMI greater than 25 and a waist circumference of more than 40 inches (102 cm) in men or 35 inches (88 cm) in women, there is an increased risk of cardiovascular disease, hypertension, and type 2 diabetes. Does your waist circumference exceed the standard for your gender?
   Yes _____   No _____

3. Do you feel you need to pursue a program of weight loss?
   Yes _____   No _____

Application

From what you've learned in Chapter 13, what habits can you change in patterns of eating and physical activity to lose weight and help ensure maintenance of any loss?

_____

_____

_____

II. An Action Plan to Change or Maintain Weight Status

Now that you have assessed your current weight status, do you feel that you would like to make some changes? Following is a step-by-step guide to behavioral change. This process can be useful even for people who are satisfied with their current weight, because it can be applied to changing exercise habits, self-esteem, and a variety of other behaviors (Figure 13-19).

Becoming Aware of the Problem

By calculating your current weight status, you have already become aware of the problem, if one exists. From here, it is important to find out more information about the cause of the problem and whether it is worth working toward a change.

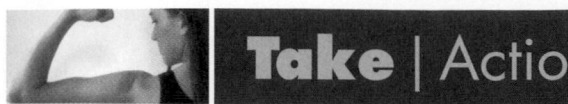

Take | Action

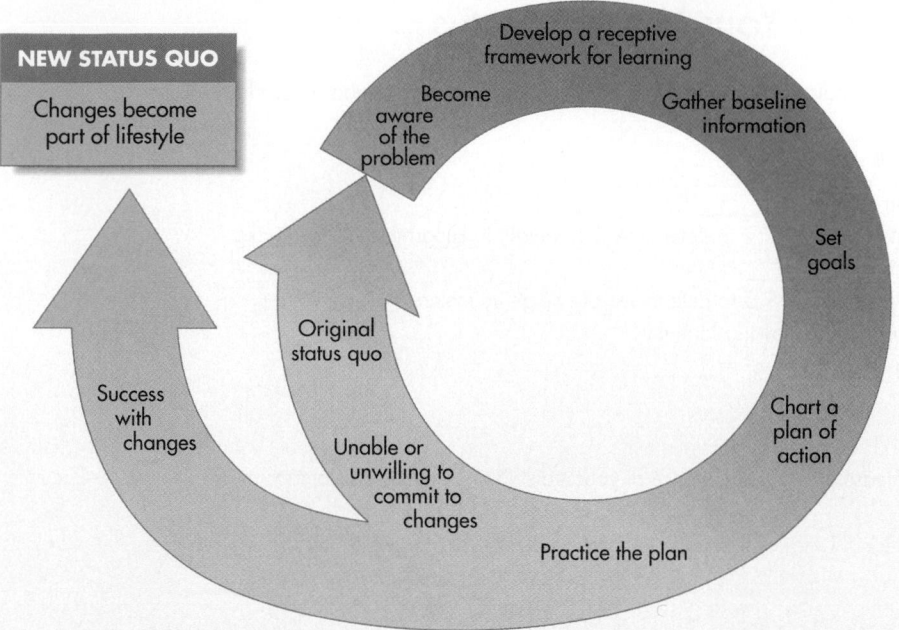

Figure 13-19 A model for behavior change. It starts with awareness of the problem and ends with the incorporation of new behaviors intended to address the problem.

1. Look back at the food diary you completed in Chapter 1. What are the factors that most influence your eating habits? Do you eat out of stress, boredom, or depression? Is volume of food your problem, or do you eat mainly the wrong foods for you? Take some time to assess the root causes of your eating habits.

2. Once you have more information about your specific eating practices, you must decide if it is worth changing these practices. A benefits and costs analysis can be a useful tool in evaluating whether it is worth your effort to make life changes. Use Figure 13-20 as a guide for listing benefits and costs pertinent to your own situation.

Setting Goals

What can you accomplish, and how long will it take? Setting a realistic, achievable goal and allowing a reasonable amount of time to pursue it increase the likelihood of success.

1. Begin by determining the final outcome you would like to achieve. If you are trying to change your eating behaviors to be more healthy, list your reasons for doing so (e.g., overall health, weight loss, self-esteem).

Overall goal:

_____

_____

_____

Reasons to pursue goal:

_____

_____

_____

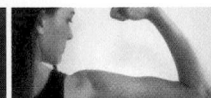

Take | Action

Benefits and Costs Analysis

1 Benefits of changing eating habits?

What do you expect to get, now or later, that you want?
What may you avoid that would be unpleasant?

feel better physically and psychologically
look better

2 Benefits of not changing eating habits?

What do you get to do that you enjoy doing?
What do you avoid having to do?

no need for planning
can eat without feeling guilty

3 Costs involved in changing eating habits?

What do you have to do that you don't want to do?
What do you have to stop doing that you would rather continue doing?

take time to plan meals and shop
must give up some food volume

4 Costs of not changing eating habits?

What unpleasant or undesirable effects are you likely to experience now or in the future?
What are you likely to lose?

creeping weight gain
low self-esteem and poor health

Figure 13-20 | Benefits and costs analysis applied to changing eating habits. This process helps put behavior change into the context of total lifestyle.

---

2. Now list several steps that will be necessary to achieve your goal. Keep in mind, however, that it is generally best to change only a few specific behaviors at first—walking briskly for 60 minutes each day, reducing fat intake, using more whole-grain products, and not eating after 7 P.M. Attempting small and perhaps easier dietary changes first reduces the scope of the problem and increases the likelihood of success.

Steps toward achieving goal:

1. _____

2. _____

3. _____

Note that if you are having trouble deciphering the steps needed to achieve your goal, health professionals are an excellent resource for aid in planning.

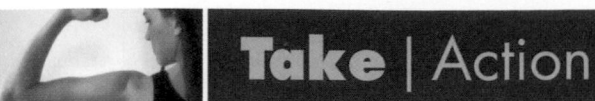

Measuring Commitment

Now that you have collected information and know what is required to reach your goal, you must ask yourself, "Can I do this?" Commitment is an essential component in the success of behavioral change. Be honest with yourself. Permanent change is not quick or easy. Once you have decided that you have the commitment required to see this through, continue on to the following sections.

Making It Official with a Contract

Drawing up a behavioral contract often adds incentive to follow through with a plan. The contract could list goal behaviors and objectives, milestones for measuring progress, and regular rewards for meeting the terms of the contract. After finishing a contract, you should sign it in the presence of some friends. This formality encourages commitment.

Initially, plans should reward positive behaviors, and then they should focus on positive results. Positive behaviors, such as regular physical activity, eventually lead to positive outcomes, such as increased stamina.

Figure 13-21 is a sample contract for increasing physical activity. Keep in mind that this sample contract is only a suggestion; you can add your own ideas as well.

Psyching Yourself Up

Once your contract is in place, you need to psych yourself up. Discouragement from peers and your own temptations to stray from your plan need to be anticipated. Psyching yourself up can enable you to progress toward your goals in spite of others' attitudes and opinions. Everyone benefits from assertiveness when it comes to changing behaviors. The following are a few suggestions. Can you think of any others?

- No one's feelings should be hurt if you say, "No, thank you," firmly and repeatedly when others try to dissuade you from a plan. Tell them you have new diet behavior and your needs are important.
- You don't have to eat a lot to accommodate anyone—your mother, business clients, or the chef. For example, at a party with friends, you may feel you have to eat a lot to participate, but you don't. Another trap is ordering a lot just because someone else is paying for the meal.
- Learn ways to handle put-downs—inadvertent or conscious. An effective response can be to communicate feelings honestly, without hostility. Tell criticizers that they have annoyed or offended you, that you are working to change your habits and would really like understanding and support from them.

Practicing the Plan

Once you've set up a plan, the next step is to implement it. Start with a trial of at least 6 to 8 weeks. Thinking of a lifetime commitment can be overwhelming. Aim for a total duration of 6 months of new activities before giving up. We may have to persuade ourselves more than once of the value of continuing the program. The following are some suggestions to help keep a plan on track:

- *Focus on reducing, but not necessarily extinguishing, undesirable behaviors.* For example, it's usually unrealistic to say, "I'll never eat a certain food again." It's better to say, "I won't eat that *problem* food as often as before."
- *Monitor progress.* Note your progress in a diary and reward yourself according to your contract. While conquering some habits and seeing improvement, you may find yourself quite encouraged, even enthusiastic, about your plan of action. That can give you the impetus to move ahead with the program.
- *Control environments.* In the early phases of behavioral change, try to avoid problem situations, such as parties, coffee breaks, and favorite restaurants. Once new habits are firmly established, you can probably more successfully resist the temptations of these environments.

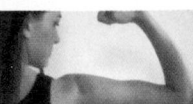

Name *Alan Young*

Goal

I agree to *ride my exercise bike*
                               (specify behavior)

under the following circumstances *for 30 minutes, 4 times per week in the evening*
                               (specify where, when, how much, etc.)

Substitute behavior and/or reinforcement schedule *I will reinforce myself if I've achieved my goal after a month with a weekend off campus with my roommate.*

Environmental planning

In order to help me do this, I am going to (1) arrange my physical and social environment by *buying a new portable CD player*

and (2) control my internal environment (thoughts, images) by *coordinating riding the bike with the first T.V. watching I do in the evening*

Reinforcements

Reinforcements provided by me daily or weekly (if contract is kept):
I will buy myself a new piece of clothing for off campus trip

Reinforcements provided by others daily or weekly (if contract is kept):
at the end of a month if I've completed my goal my parents will buy me a fitness club membership for winter.

Social support

Behavior change is more likely to take place when other people support you. During the quarter/semester please meet with the other person at least three times to discuss your progress.

The name of my "significant helper" is: *Mr. and Mrs. Young*

This contract should include:

1. Baseline data (one week)
2. Well-defined goal
3. Simple method for charting progress (diary, counter, charts, etc.)
4. Reinforcements (immediate and long-term)
5. Evaluation method (summary of experiences, success, and/or new learnings about self).

Figure 13-21 | Alan's behavior contract. Completing such a contract can help generate commitment to behavior change. What would your contract look like?

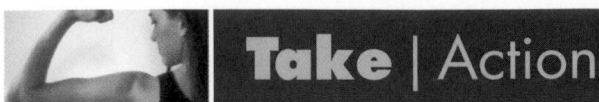

Take | Action

Reevaluating and Preventing Relapse

After practicing a program for several weeks to months, it is important to reassess the original plan. In addition, you may now be able to pinpoint other problem areas for which you need to plan appropriately.

1. Begin by taking a close and critical look at your original plan. Does it actually lead to the goals you set? Are there any new steps toward your goal that you feel capable of adding to your contract? Do you need new reinforcements? It may even be necessary to make a new contract. For permanent change, it is worth this time of reassessment.

2. In practicing your plan over the past weeks or months, you have likely experienced relapses. What triggered these relapses? To prevent a total retreat to your old habits, it is important to set up a plan for such relapses. Do this by identifying high-risk situations, rehearsing a response, and remembering your goals.

You may have noticed a behavior chain in some of your relapses. That is, the relapse may stem from a series of interconnected habitual activities. The way to break the chain is to first identify the activities, pinpoint the weak links, break those links, and substitute other behaviors. Figure 13-22 illustrates a sample behavior chain and a substitute activities list. Consider compiling your own list based on your behavior chains.

Epilogue

If you have used the activities in this section, you are well on your way to permanent behavioral change. Recall that this exercise can be used for a variety of desired changes, including quitting smoking, increasing physical activity, and improving study habits. It is by no means an easy process, but the results can be well worth the effort. Overall, the keys to success are motivation (keeping the problem in the forefront of your mind), having a plan of action, securing the resources and skills needed for success, and looking for help from family, friends, or a group.

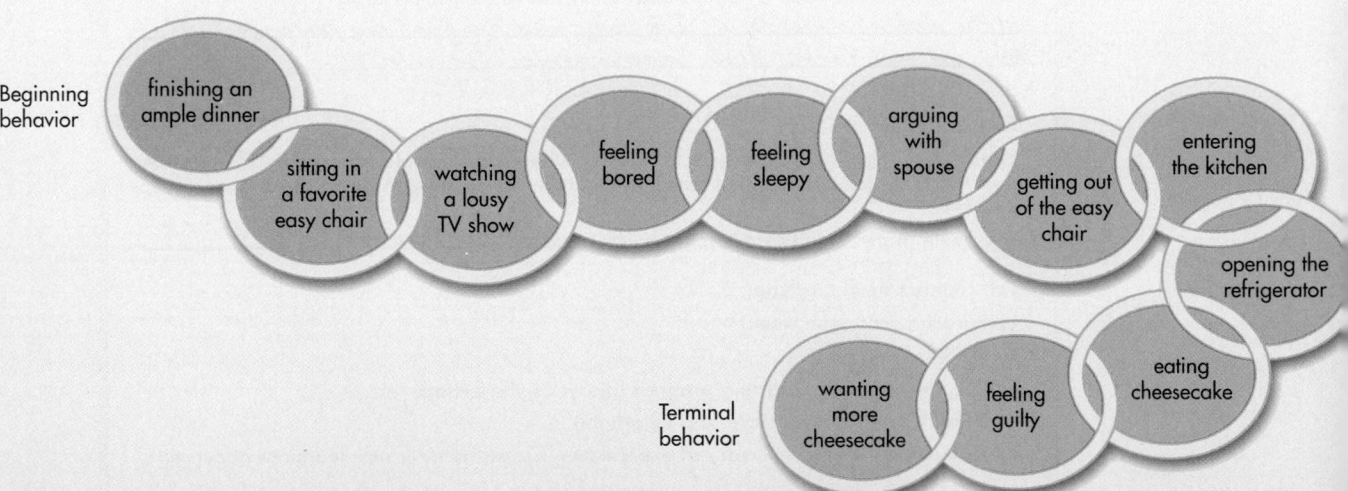

Figure 13-22 | Identifying behavior chains. This is a good tool for understanding more about your habits and pinpointing ways to change wanted habits. The earlier in the chain you substitute a nonfood link, the easier it is to intervene. Four types of behaviors can be substituted in ongoing behavior chain: 1. Fun activities (taking a walk, reading a book); 2. Necessary activities (cleaning a room, balancing your checkbook 3. Incompatible activities (taking a shower); 4. Urge-delaying activities (setting a kitchen timer for 20 minutes before allowing yourself to eat). Overall, using activities to interrupt behavior patterns that lead to inappropriate eating (or inactivity) can be a powerful means of changing ha

NUTRITION: FITNESS AND SPORTS

CHAPTER OUTLINE

CASE SCENARIO:

Marcella is training for a 10K run coming up in 3 weeks. She has read a lot about sports nutrition, especially about the importance of eating a high-carbohydrate diet while in training. She also has been struggling to keep her weight in a range that she feels contributes to better speed and endurance. Consequently, she is trying to eat as little fat as possible. Unfortunately, over the past week her workouts in the afternoon have not met her expectations. Her run times are slower, and she shows signs of fatigue after just 20 minutes into her training program.

Her breakfast yesterday was a large bagel, a small amount of cream cheese, and orange juice. For lunch, she had a small salad with fat-free dressing, a large plate of pasta with tomato marinara sauce and broccoli, and a diet soft drink. For dinner, she had a small broiled chicken breast, a cup of rice, some carrots, and iced tea. Later, she snacked on fat-free pretzels.

What advice would you give Marcella regarding her training diet? Note current strengths and weaknesses. Is her diet likely contributing to her recent fatigue during workouts?

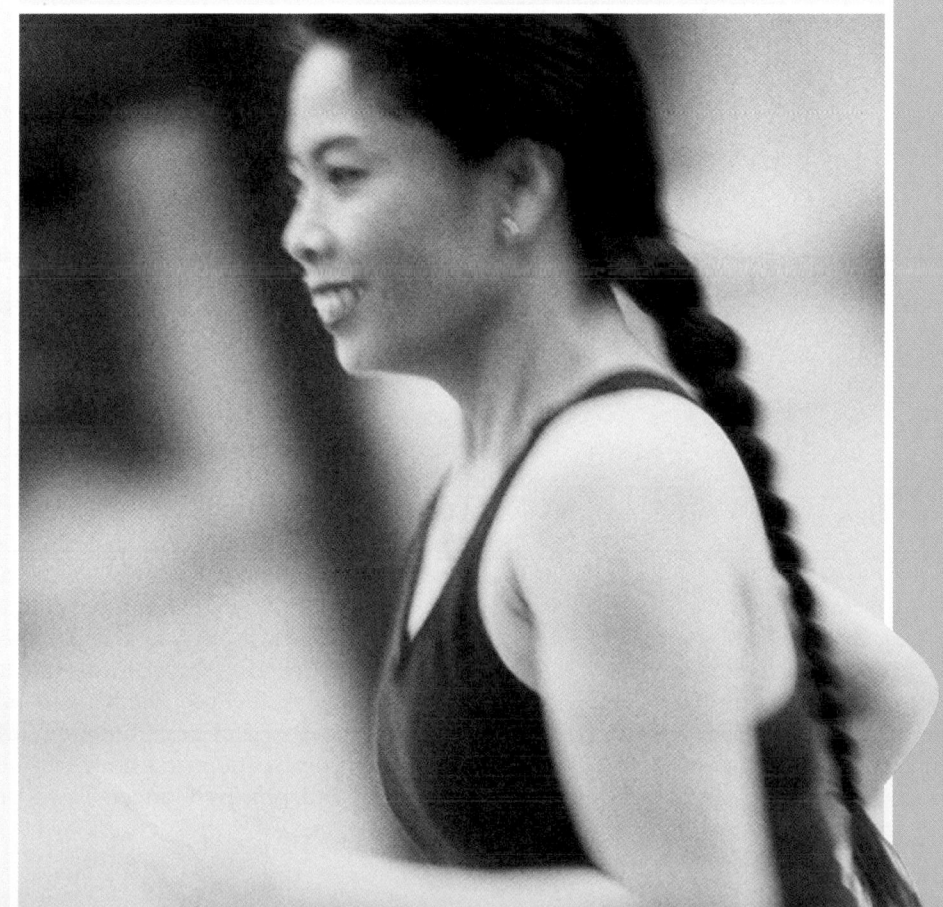

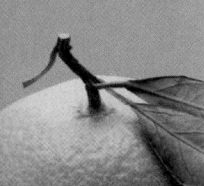

A thletes invest a lot of time and effort in training. Because they often seek ways to enhance their diets to improve performance, athletes make easy targets for purveyors of nutrition misinformation. Most athletes don't want to miss out on any advantage, whether real or perceived, that might give them the winning edge.

Although good eating habits can't substitute for physical training and genetic endowment, proper food and beverage choices are crucial for top-notch performance, contributing to endurance and helping to speed the repair of injured tissues.[19]

Looking at our population in general, experts might disagree on how much carbohydrate, protein, and fat we should consume, but there is no argument over the health benefits of regular physical activity. It is even beneficial for overweight people who remain at that excess weight.[4]

In Chapter 14, you will discover how physical fitness benefits the entire body and how nutrition relates to fitness and sports performance.

The Close Relationship between Nutrition and Fitness

The ability to engage routinely in vigorous physical activity requires good health. Peak performance for physical activity (and exercise) also depends on a diet that supplies all the needed nutrients.[19]

Once muscles have nutrients available to them, what determines the type of fuel they will use? Athletes have a say in that decision, depending on how physically fit they are and how hard they perform. This physical fitness—defined as the ability to perform moderate to vigorous activity without undue fatigue—especially affects fat use by the body. As one's level of physical fitness improves, so does one's ability to mobilize fat stores for energy needs—especially during activities that last for 20 minutes or more.

Beyond affecting fuel use, the benefits of regular physical activity include enhancement of several aspects of heart function, less injury, better sleep habits, and improvement in body composition (less body fat, more muscle mass). Physical activity also can reduce stress and positively affect blood pressure, blood cholesterol, blood glucose

Recall from Chapter 1 how the terms *physical activity* and *exercise* are related. Exercise is physical activity done with the intent to gain health and fitness benefits, whereas physical activity is simply part of day-to-day activities.

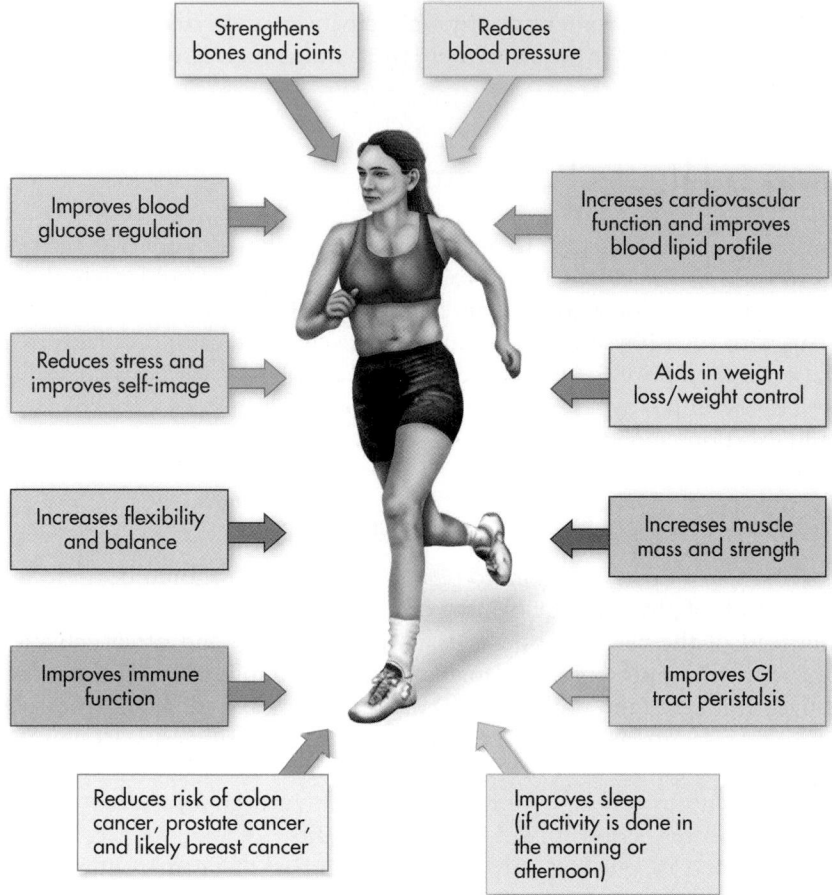

Strengthens bones and joints

Reduces blood pressure

Improves blood glucose regulation

Increases cardiovascular function and improves blood lipid profile

Reduces stress and improves self-image

Aids in weight loss/weight control

Increases flexibility and balance

Increases muscle mass and strength

Improves immune function

Improves GI tract peristalsis

Reduces risk of colon cancer, prostate cancer, and likely breast cancer

Improves sleep (if activity is done in the morning or afternoon)

regulation, and immune function. In addition, physical activity aids in weight control, both by raising resting energy expenditure for a short period of time after exercise and by increasing overall energy expenditure.[3,9,14,16,20] See Figure 14-1 for a further look at these and other benefits of a physically active lifestyle.

Unfortunately, as noted in Chapter 13, many North American adults lead sedentary lives. Most adults do not practice moderate to vigorous physical activity on a regular basis, and about half of all adults quit an exercise program within 3 months. Does this discussion motivate you to assess your activity patterns and improve them as needed?

Healthy People 2010 has set a number of specific objectives for U.S. adults related to physical activity and exercise:

- Reduce by 50% the proportion of adults engaging in no leisure-time physical activity (currently 27% of adults).
- Double the proportion of adults engaging regularly, preferably daily, in moderate exercise for at least 30 minutes per day (currently 45% of adults).
- Increase by 50% the proportion of adults who perform exercises that enhance and maintain muscular strength and endurance (currently 19% of adults).

The *2005 Dietary Guidelines for Americans* recommends three different time goals for physical activity (review Chapter 2).

- 30 minutes/day of moderate-intensity physical activity, in addition to usual activity, for individuals trying to reduce their risk of chronic disease in adulthood. Doing more than 30 minutes or increasing the intensity of the workout could lead to even greater benefits.
- 60 minutes/day of moderate- to vigorous-intensity physical activity to help adults manage body weight and prevent gradual weight gain.

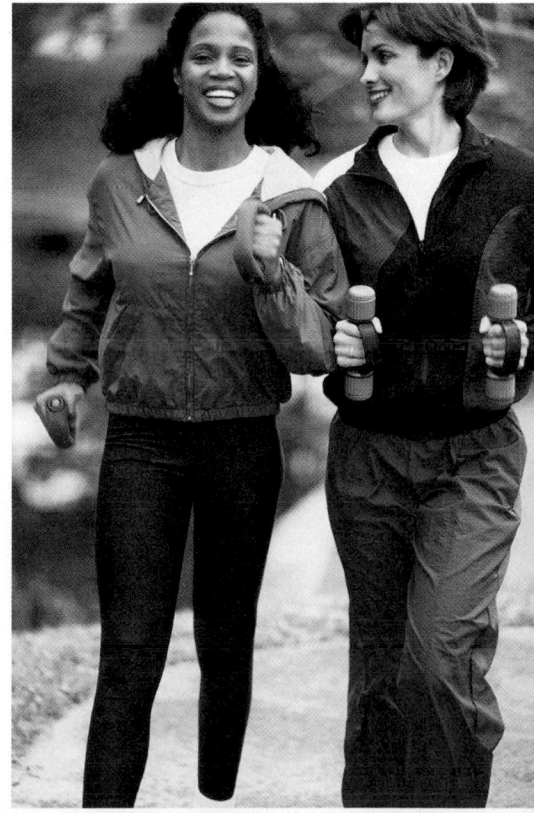

What is the best exercise? One you want to continue to do.

• 90 minutes/day of moderate-intensity physical activity may be needed for some adults to sustain weight loss; at the same time, these individuals also need to monitor their energy intakes.

Designing a Fitness Program

One day in December 2000, Joe Decker:

bicycled 100 miles,
ran 10 miles, hiked 10 miles,
power-walked 5 miles,
kayaked 6 miles,
skied on a NordicTrack 10 miles,
rowed 10 miles, swam 2 miles,
did 3000 abdominal crunches,
did 1100 jumping jacks,
did 1000 leg lifts, did 1100 push-ups.
And he lifted weights for a cumulative total of 278,540 lb.

For his efforts (and pains), he earned a place in the *Guinness Book of World Records* as the fittest man alive.

For healthy people, a gradual increase to a goal of regular physical activity is recommended. Men 40 years of age or older and women 50 years of age or older who have been inactive for many years or who have an existing health problem should discuss their fitness goals with their physician before increasing activity. Health problems that require medical evaluation prior to an exercise program are obesity, cardiovascular disease (or family history of it), hypertension, diabetes (or family history), shortness of breath after mild exertion, and arthritis.

Phase 1: Getting Started Means Getting Going

During the first phase of a fitness program to promote health, you should begin to incorporate short periods of physical activity into your daily routine such as walking, taking the stairs instead of the elevator, house cleaning, gardening, and other activities that cause you to huff and puff a bit. The goal is a total of 30 minutes of this moderate physical activity on most (and preferably all) days. If necessary, these activities can be broken up into increments lasting at least 10 minutes. Experts suggest starting with short intervals and build up to a total of 30 minutes of activity incorporated into each day's tasks.[4] If there is not much time for activity, you can even go for more intensity in the activities over shorter periods to get the same benefits.

The easiest way to increase physical activity is to make it part of a daily routine, similar to other regular activities, such as eating.[11] You do not need to join a gym or attend aerobic classes. Daily activities can meet the Phase 1 goal. Many people find that the best time to exercise is when they need an energy pick-me-up or a break from work. Rather than abandoning an exercise program entirely when obstacles get in the way, strive to use any small periods of available time, such as breaks between classes or coffee breaks at work. Once you reap the benefits of exercise, you will tend to spend more time at it.

Clearly, many activities recommended for Phase 1 are not very vigorous. Although Phase 1 is recommended for people starting an exercise program, fitness experts have not given up on the value of more vigorous physical activity. They're just making concessions to human nature. *Still, most of the possible health benefits from physical activity are seen if this Phase 1 goal is met.*

Phase 2: Achieving and Maintaining Even Greater Physical Fitness

Once you can perform physical activity for 30 minutes per day, turn your attention to more specific exercise activities, such as increasing muscle mass and strength, to reap even more benefits.[18,19]

Warm-up

Begin by doing activities that move the whole torso for 5 to 10 minutes. Start with smaller muscle groups (arms) and work toward larger muscle groups (legs and abdomen).

Do 5 to 10 more minutes of low-intensity exercises, such as walking, slow jogging, or any slow version of anticipated activity. This warms up your muscles so that muscle filaments slide over one another more easily to increase range of motion and decrease the risk of injury.

A term that has been coined recently is *sedentary death syndrome (SeDS)*. The term describes the hazards of being inactive.

Aerobic Workout

Daily aerobic activity is recommended. To start, an aerobic workout prescription considers mode, duration, frequency, intensity, and progression.

Mode: The mode of exercise is the type of exercise prescribed. It must be one that uses large muscle groups in a rhythmic fashion, such as brisk walking, running, lap swimming, or cycling.

Duration: Duration is the amount of time spent in an exercise session. It should generally last at least 20 to 30 minutes, depending on intensity, not counting time for warm-up and cooldown. Ideally, this exercise should be continuous (without stopping), but multiple 10-minute bouts with rest periods in between are also acceptable.

Frequency: The frequency of the exercise describes the number of times that the activity is performed. The frequency of exercise should be at least five times per week. Daily exercising will lead to even further benefits related to physical fitness.

Intensity: Intensity is defined as the level of exertion that indicates the degree of energy expenditure required to sustain the activity. In other words, intensity is used to describe how hard you are working and to what extent you can maintain that intensity over time. Health benefits beyond Phase 1 are especially seen when you can achieve a moderate level of intensity of exercise.

There are a few ways to determine the intensity of exercise. A popular and simple method is to use a percentage of your age-predicted maximum heart rate. To find maximum heart rate, subtract your age from 220. Multiplying maximum heart rate by 0.60 and 0.90 will result in a range of heart rates, sometimes called the *target zone*. For a 20-year-old person beginning an exercise program, maximum heart rate equals 200 beats per minute ($220 - 20 = 200$). Then, (200×0.6) and (200×0.9) yields a target zone of 120 to 180 beats per minute. Measuring heart rate (pulse) is easy: Stop and count your pulse rate for 10 seconds and then multiply that number by 6 to determine your heart rate for one minute. There are also watches available that contain heart rate monitors.

At the initiation of an exercise program, aim for the lower end of the target zone. As you progress and become more physically fit, you can work up to a higher heart rate. As with many of the prediction formulas, calculation of maximum heart rate is just an estimate. Medications, such as those for hypertension and other health conditions, may impact heart rate. If you have health concerns, a physician can help to personalize the target zone.

Another way of determining the intensity of exercise is the Rating of Perceived Exertion scale (RPE). One version includes a range of 1 to 10, with each number corresponding to a subjective feeling of exertion. For example, the number 0 is "nothing at all" (sitting at a table) and the number 10 is considered close to maximal effort or "very, very strong" (all-out sprint) (Figure 14-2).

When using the RPE scale, the goal is to aim for the number 4, which corresponds to the beginning of "somewhat strong." At this point you begin to see significant fitness results. You should be working hard but still be able to talk to an exercise partner (sometimes called the "talk test").

Progression: Progression, the final component, describes how the frequency, intensity, and duration of exercise have increased over a period of time. The first 3 to 6 weeks of your new exercise program are the initiation, or "getting started," phase. This phase corresponds to the time it takes for your body to adapt to the exercise program. The next 5 or 6 months of training are the improvement stage, in which the intensity and duration increase to a point of tapering off. In other words, you notice no further appreciable gains in fitness. This plateau marks the beginning of your maintenance stage.

To help yourself stay with an exercise program, experts recommend the following:

- Start slowly.
- Vary your activities; make it fun.
- Include friends and others.
- Set specific attainable goals and monitor progress.
- Set aside a specific time each day for exercise; build it into your routine, but make it convenient.
- Reward yourself for being successful in keeping up with your goals.
- Don't worry about occasional setbacks; focus on the long-term benefits to your health.

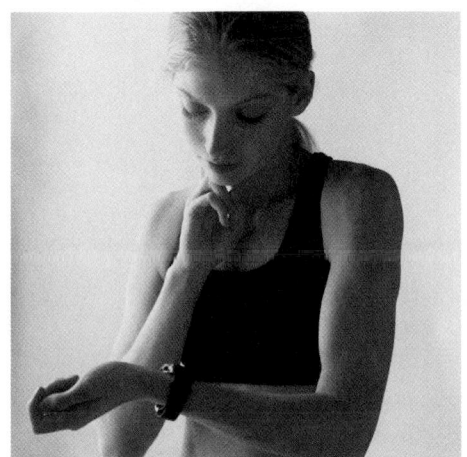

Taking your pulse determines if your exercise output is in the target zone.

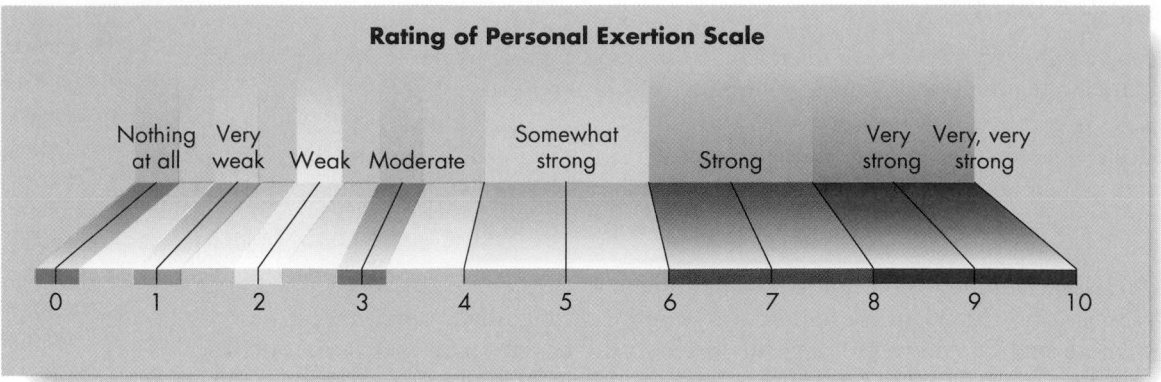

Rating of Personal Exertion Scale

Nothing at all	Very weak	Weak	Moderate		Somewhat strong		Strong		Very strong	Very, very strong	
0	1	2	3	4	5	6	7	8	9		10

Figure 14-2 | A Rating of Perceived Exertion scale (RPE). This version includes a range of 1 to 10, with each number corresponding to a subjective feeling of exertion. An RPE beyond 10 is considered maximal.

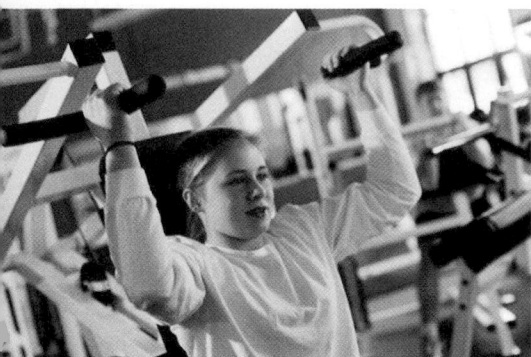

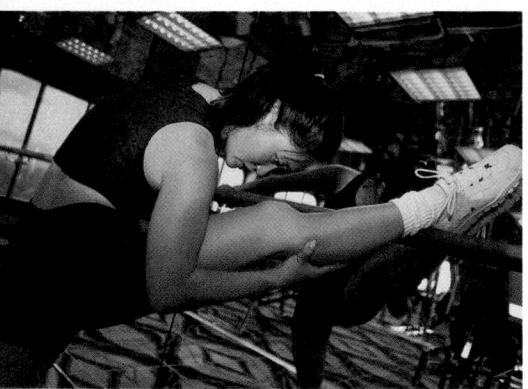

A total fitness plan includes resistance training and stretching after exercise.

At this stage, you evaluate your goals, but need to make no changes to your exercise program in order to maintain the gains already achieved.

Strength-Training Workout

Strength training should be done at least 2, and preferably 3, days per week. To start, a group of 8 to 10 exercises should be performed in a circuit (during the same exercise session) to condition major muscle groups of the upper and lower body. When selecting the proper weight to use, make sure that the weight allows you to perform one or more sets of at least 8 repetitions, but no more than 12. (However, 10 to 15 repetitions is fine for older adults using lighter weights.) Proper form during these exercises is important to avoid injuries. Generally, if more than 12 repetitions can be performed with relative ease, the weight can be increased in moderate increments.

Cooldown

During cooldown, follow a reverse pattern of the warm-up: 5 to 10 minutes of low-intensity activity, and add 5 to 10 minutes of stretching. The same exercises performed during warm-up are appropriate. The cooldown is essential to the prevention of injury and soreness.

Further Considerations

Including several types of enjoyable physical activities in a fitness program may also be helpful. For example, jogging one day might be followed by swimming the next day. Adding variety to a program not only keeps you mentally fresh, but also strengthens different muscle groups and reduces risk of injury. An exercise partner may offer additional motivation.

Vigorous programs for obese people should be non-weight-bearing activities, such as swimming, water aerobics, and bicycling. Note also that even if weight loss does not readily occur, obese people still benefit from regular physical activity.[4]

Whatever activities you choose to include in your fitness program, they should be enjoyable. This way they can become routine. Consider convenience, cost, and options for bad weather so that when motivation wanes, you are not adding further obstacles. Overall, do what you enjoy, but start out small, committing to keeping on track and maintaining reasonable expectations. Positive results may take a month or so to be noticeable.

Energy Sources for Muscle Use

As you learned in Chapter 4, cells can't directly use the energy released from breaking down glucose or triglycerides. Rather, to utilize the chemical energy in foods, body cells must first convert the energy to adenosine triphosphate (ATP).

Adenosine Triphosphate (ATP)—Immediately Usable Energy

The partial breakdown of ATP by cells to yield ADP and P_1 (the abbreviation for inorganic phosphate) releases usable energy for cell functions, including muscle contractions required for locomotion. A resting muscle cell, however, contains just a small amount of ATP, enough to keep the muscle working maximally for about 2 to 4 seconds. To produce more ATP for muscle contraction over extended periods, the body uses **phosphocreatine (PCr),** a high-energy compound that is formed and stored in muscle cells from the amino acid derivative **creatine** (the amino acids glycine, arginine, and methionine participate in its synthesis).[8] Dietary carbohydrates, fats, and proteins are also used as energy sources (Figure 14-3). The breakdown of all these compounds releases enough energy to make more ATP (Table 14-1).

Phosphocreatine: The Initial Resupply of Muscle ATP

During periods of relaxation, muscles synthesize PCr from ATP and creatine and then store this in small amounts. As soon as ADP from the breakdown of ATP begins to accumulate in a contracting muscle, an enzyme is activated that transfers a high-energy P_1 from PCr to ADP, thus reforming ATP (Figure 14-4):

$$PCr + ADP \rightarrow ATP + Cr$$

If no other system for resupplying ATP were available, PCr could probably maintain maximal muscle contractions for about 10 seconds.[19] However, because the energy released from the metabolism of glucose and fatty acids also begins to contribute ATP and thus spares some PCr use, this results in PCr functioning as the major source of energy for all events lasting up to about 1 minute (review Table 14-1).

The main advantage of PCr is that it can be activated instantly and can replenish ATP at rates fast enough to meet the energy demands of the fastest and most powerful sports events, including jumping, lifting, throwing, and sprinting actions. The disadvantage of PCr is that not enough is made and stored in the muscles to sustain a high rate of ATP resupply for more than a few minutes.

Strength-training athletes often use creatine supplements to try to increase muscle mass (see the Nutrition Focus at the end of this chapter for details).

phosphocreatine (PCr) A high-energy compound that can be used to re-form ATP from ADP.

creatine An organic molecule in muscle cells that serves as a part of the high-energy compound creatine phosphate or phosphocreatine.

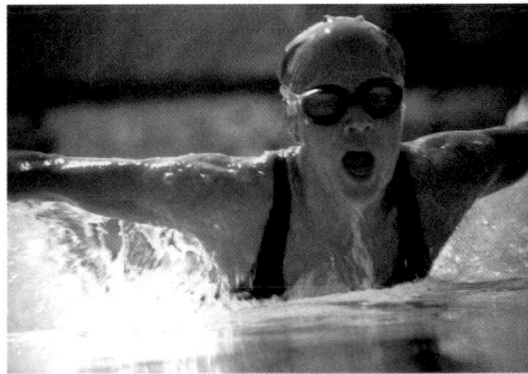

Bursts of muscle activity use a variety of energy sources, including PCr and ATP.

Figure 14-3 | Energy sources for muscular activity. Different fuels are used for ATP synthesis. As shown, ATP can also be synthesized rapidly using phosphocreatine.

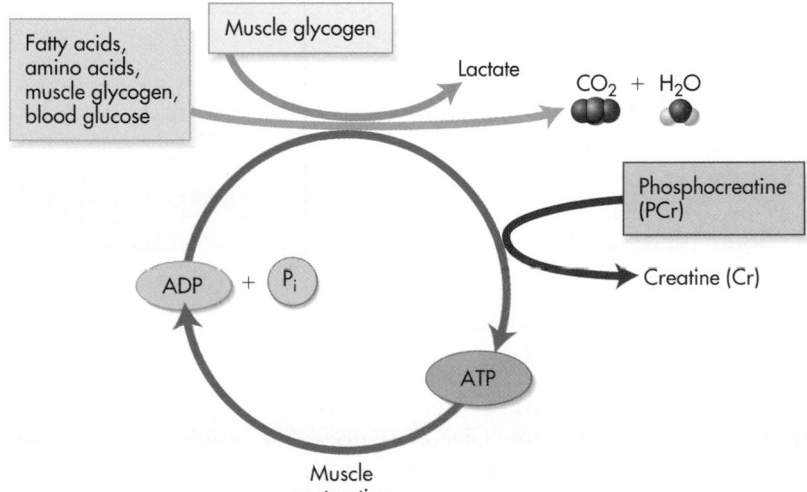

Table 14-1 | Energy Sources Used by Resting and Working Muscle Cells

Source/System*	When in Use	Activity
ATP	At all times	All types
Phosphocreatine (PCr)	All exercise initially; short bursts of exercise thereafter	Shotput, high jump, bench press
Carbohydrate (anaerobic)	High-intensity exercise, especially lasting 30 seconds to 2 minutes	200-yard (about 200-meter) sprint
Carbohydrate (aerobic)	Exercise lasting 2 minutes to 3 hours or more; the higher the intensity (for example, running a 6-minute mile), the greater the use	Basketball, swimming, jogging
Fat (aerobic)	Exercise lasting more than a few minutes; greater amounts are used at lower exercise intensities	Long-distance running, long-distance cycling; much of the fuel used in a brisk 30-minute walk is fat
Protein (aerobic)	Low quantity during all exercise; moderate quantity in endurance exercise, especially when carbohydrate fuel is lacking	Long-distance running

*At any given time, all systems are operating at the same time—just the relative amount of use differs during various activities.

Figure 14-4 | Quick energy for muscle use includes a supply of phosphocreatine (PCr). This can rapidly replenish ATP stores as activity begins. Phosphocreatine can be almost depleted in maximally contracting human forearm muscles in less than 60 seconds. It takes 4 minutes of rest to replenish half the PCr and 7 minutes to replenish 95% of the PCr. Similarly, it takes about 7 minutes of rest to replenish 95% of the PCr depleted with repeated knee extensions against resistance.

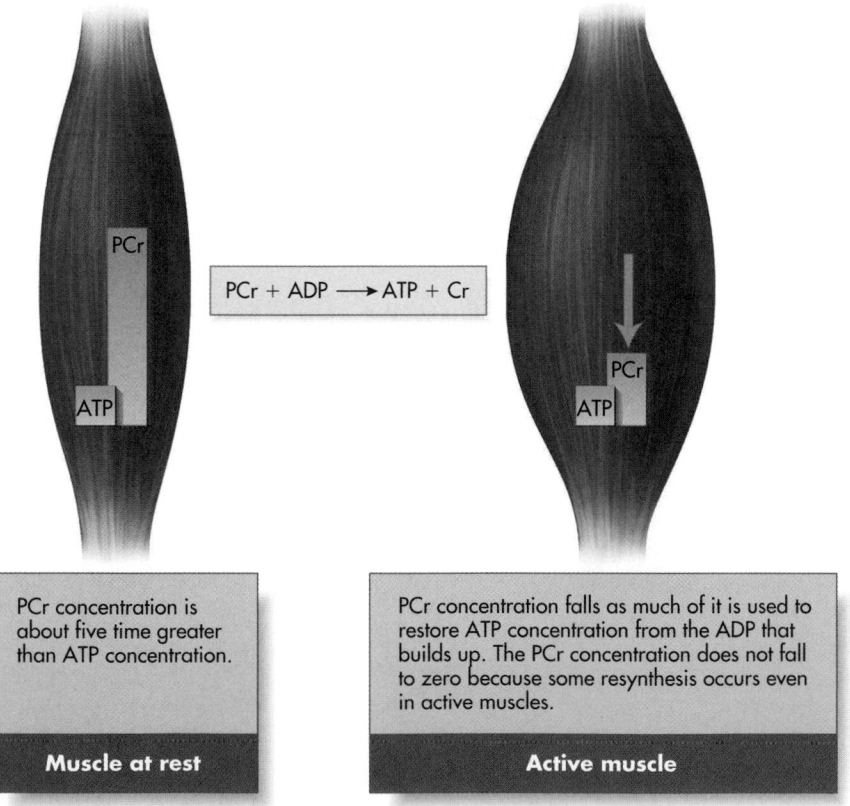

$$PCr + ADP \longrightarrow ATP + Cr$$

PCr concentration is about five time greater than ATP concentration.

Muscle at rest

PCr concentration falls as much of it is used to restore ATP concentration from the ADP that builds up. The PCr concentration does not fall to zero because some resynthesis occurs even in active muscles.

Active muscle

Glucose: Major Fuel for Short-Term, High-Intensity, and Medium-Term Exercise

Recall from Chapter 4 that glucose breaks down during glycolysis, producing the three-carbon compound pyruvate. Glycolysis does not require oxygen, but it only yields a small amount of ATP. If oxygen is present, the pyruvate is metabolized further, yielding much additional ATP.

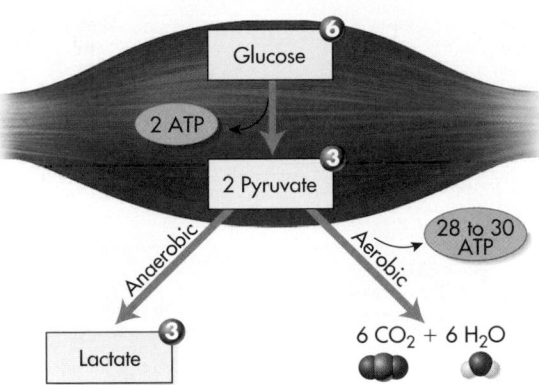

$$ATP \longrightarrow ADP + Pi$$
$$(glucose \longrightarrow glucose\text{-}6\text{-}phosphate)$$

Anaerobic Pathway

When the oxygen supply in muscle is limited (anaerobic state) or when the physical activity is intense (e.g., running 400 meters or swimming 100 meters), pyruvate resulting from glycolysis accumulates in the muscle and is converted to lactate (Figure 14-5). Because the breakdown of 1 glucose to 2 pyruvates yields 2 ATP, glycolysis can resupply some ATP depleted in muscle activity.[8] *Carbohydrate is the only fuel that can be used for this process.* The advantage of the anaerobic pathway is that, other than PCr breakdown, it is the fastest way to resupply ATP in muscle.[19]

Glycolysis provides most of the energy for physical activity from about 30 seconds to 2 minutes after it has started. As you'll see shortly, fat utilization simply can't occur fast enough to meet the ATP demands of short-duration, high-intensity physical activity.[19] If fat were the only available fuel, we would be unable to carry out physical activity more intense than a fast walk or jog.

The anaerobic pathway has three major disadvantages:

- It can't sustain ATP production for long.
- Only about 5% of the energy available from glucose is released during glycolysis.
- The rapid accumulation of lactate from anaerobic glycolysis greatly increases the acidity of muscle cells.

Because high acidity inhibits the activity of key enzymes in glycolysis, anaerobic ATP production soon slows and fatigue sets in. The acidity also leads to a net potassium loss from muscle cells, providing another cause of fatigue.[8] We learn by trial and error an exercise pace that controls muscle lactate concentrations from anaerobic glycolysis.

Most of the lactate that accumulates in active muscle cells is eventually released into the bloodstream. The liver (and to some extent the kidneys) takes up some of the lactate from the blood and resynthesizes it into glucose, an energy-requiring process. This glucose then can reenter the bloodstream, where it is available for cell uptake and breakdown. The heart can also use lactate directly for its energy needs, as can less active muscle cells situated near active ones.

Aerobic Pathway

If there is plenty of oxygen available in muscle (aerobic state) and the physical activity is of moderate to low intensity (e.g., jogging or distance swimming), the bulk of the pyruvate produced by glycolysis in the cytoplasm is shuttled to the mitochondria and further metabolized into carbon dioxide and water in a series of oxygen-requiring reactions. About 95% of the ATP produced from the complete metabolism of glucose is formed aerobically in mitochondria (Figure 14-6).

Although the aerobic pathway supplies ATP more slowly than does the anaerobic pathway, it releases more energy. Furthermore, ATP production via the aerobic pathway can be sustained for hours. Accordingly, this pathway of glucose metabolism

Recall from Chapter 4 that when acids lose a hydrogen ion, as typically happens at the pH of the body, they are given the ending *-ate.* Thus, pyruvic acid is called *pyruvate* and lactic acid is called *lactate* when in the context of body metabolism.

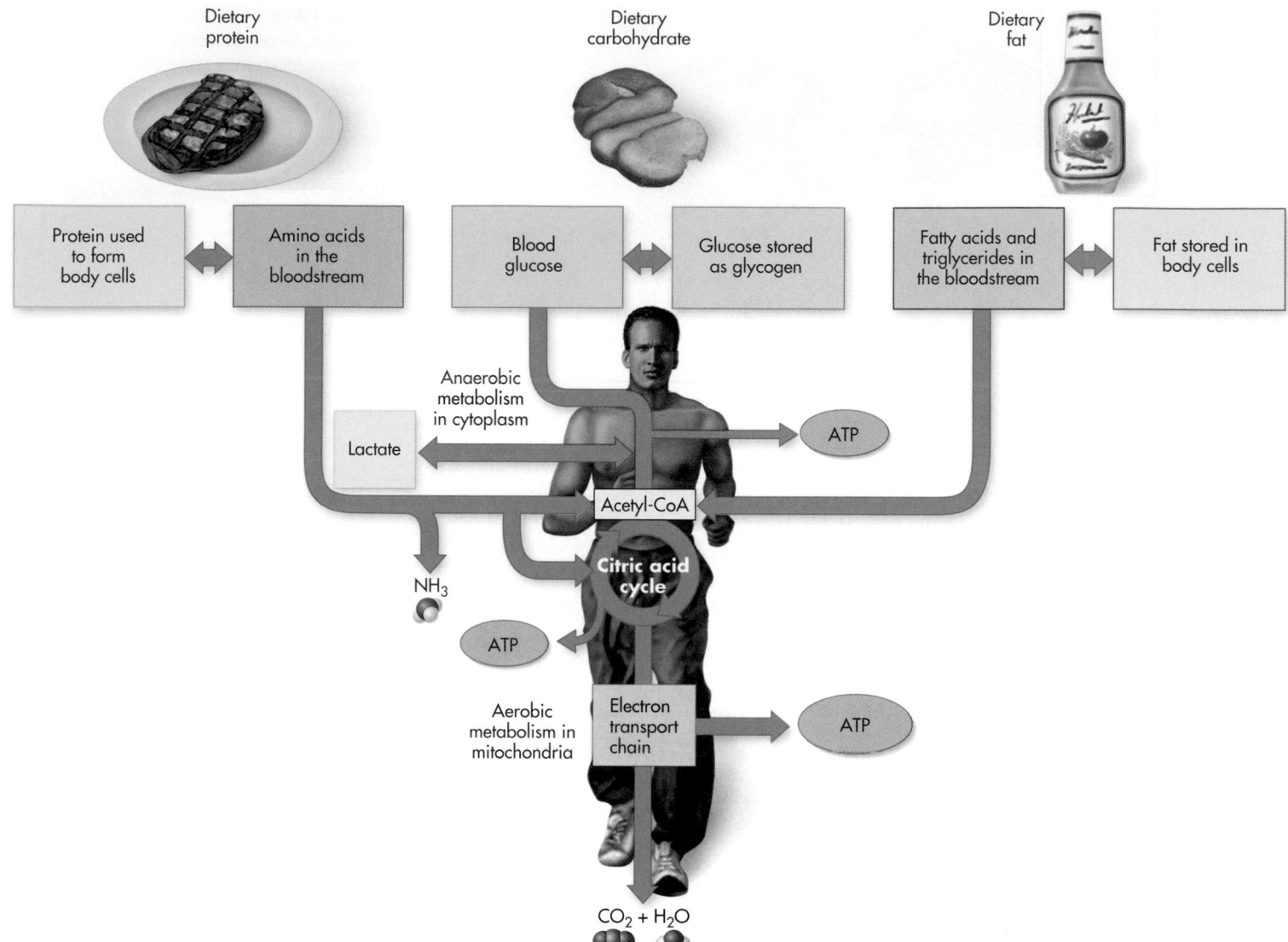

Dietary
protein

Dietary
carbohydrate

Dietary
fat

| Protein used to form body cells | Amino acids in the bloodstream | Blood glucose | Glucose stored as glycogen | Fatty acids and triglycerides in the bloodstream | Fat stored in body cells |

Anaerobic
metabolism
in cytoplasm

Lactate

ATP

Acetyl-CoA

NH_3

Citric acid cycle

ATP

Aerobic
metabolism in
mitochondria

Electron
transport
chain

ATP

$CO_2 + H_2O$

Figure 14-6 | Simplified view of ATP formation from carbohydrate, fat, and protein. Along with phosphocreatine (PCr), all three macronutrients may be used for ATP synthesis, but glucose and fatty acids are primary sources. Glucose may be broken down anaerobically or may undergo complete aerobic metabolism. The products of fatty acid breakdown are channeled into aerobic metabolism (the glycerol that is released as part of the triglyceride is not depicted). Although limited, products of amino acid breakdown also are channeled into the aerobic pathway. Recall from Chapters 10 through 12 that many vitamins and minerals participate in these metabolic pathways.

makes an important energy contribution to sports events lasting from about 2 minutes through 3 or more hours (Figure 14-7).[19]

Glycogen versus Blood Glucose as Muscle Fuel

Glycogen is the temporary storage form of glucose in the liver (about 100 g) and muscles (about 300 g in sedentary people). It is broken down to a form of glucose that in turn can be metabolized by both the anaerobic and aerobic pathways. Glycogen is, in fact, the primary source of glucose for ATP production in muscle cells during fairly intense activities that last for less than about 2 hours. In such activities, the depletion of glycogen in the liver leads to a fall in blood glucose, whereas the depletion of glyco-

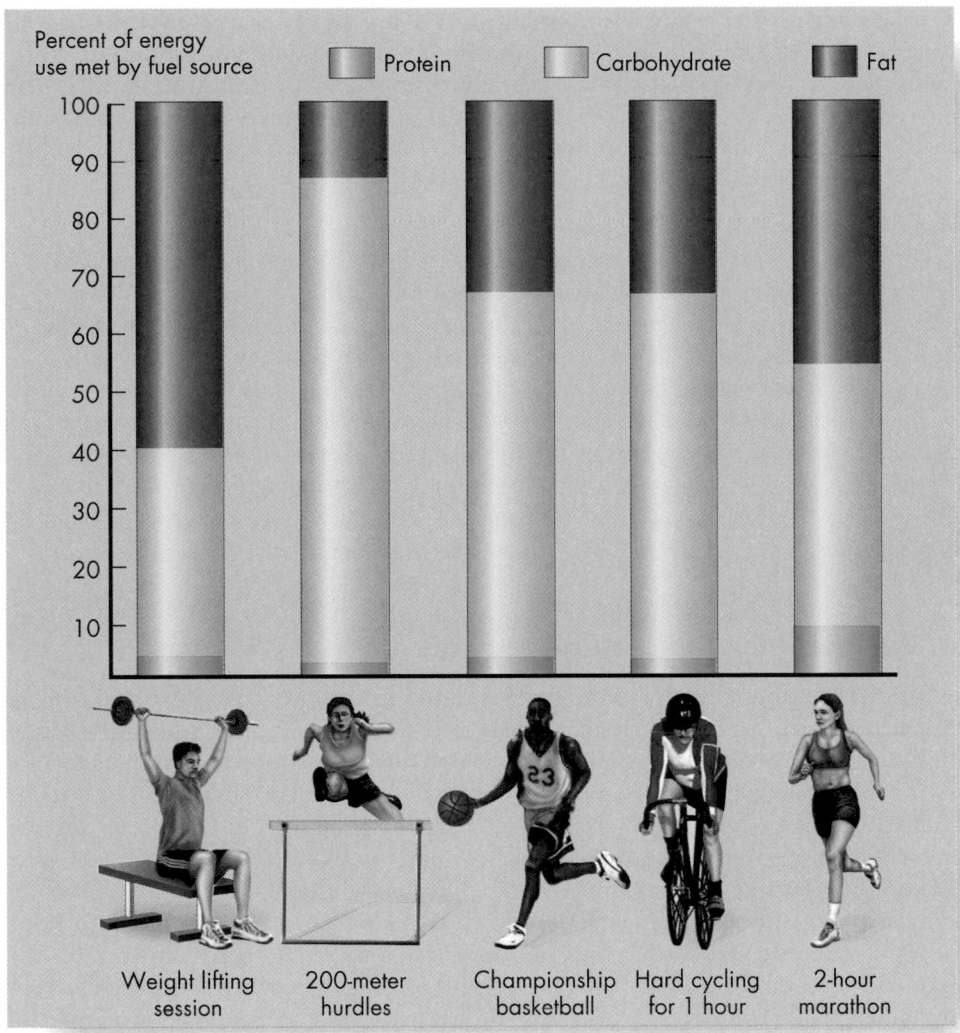

Figure 14-7 | Rough estimates of fuel use during various forms of exercise. With regard to the weight lifting session, carbohydrate use could be somewhat greater and fat use somewhat less if the session is intense and fast-paced (e.g., circuit training). Fat use generally is higher since much of the time spent weight lifting is for rest periods.

gen in the muscles contributes to fatigue.[8] Once these glycogen stores are exhausted, an athlete can continue working at only about 50% of maximal capacity. Athletes call this point of glycogen depletion "hitting the wall," because further exertion is hampered. Thus, when their event will require them to meet or exceed 70% of maximal exertion for more than an hour or so, athletes (e.g., long-distance runners or cyclists) should consider increasing the amount of carbohydrate stored in their muscles. Diets high in carbohydrate can be used to increase muscle glycogen stores—up to double the typical amounts—in advance of competition, thereby forestalling fatigue and improving endurance. A later section in this chapter on carbohydrate needs discusses how to plan such a diet.

As exercise duration increases beyond about 20 to 30 minutes, the maintenance of blood glucose becomes an increasingly important consideration. This can spare the use of muscle glycogen, saving it in the muscle for sudden bursts of effort that may be required, such as a sprint to the finish in a marathon race. A carbohydrate intake of 0.7 g/kg/hour (about 30–60 g/hour) during strenuous endurance exercise, such as cycling that lasts about 1 hour or more, can help maintain adequate blood glucose concentrations, which in turn results in delay of fatigue.[5] A later section on sports drinks discusses this process in more detail.

Without the maintenance of blood glucose during endurance activities, a decline in mental function may also occur (cyclists call this "bonking"). Note however that the fall in blood glucose is related to depletion of liver glycogen, not muscle glycogen, since liver glycogen is used to maintain blood glucose.

Carbohydrate intake is not as important for the muscles in shorter events (e.g., 30 minutes or so) because the muscles do not take up much blood glucose during short-term exercise, relying instead primarily on glycogen stores for carbohydrate fuel. The action of insulin to increase glucose uptake by muscles is blunted by other hormones, such as epinephrine and glucagon, which increase initially during exercise.[19]

Concept | Check

ATP is the main form of energy that cells use. Carbohydrate metabolism to form ATP begins as glucose becomes available from the bloodstream or from glycogen breakdown. Carbohydrate feeding during exercise can also supply glucose. In a muscle cell, each glucose is broken down through a series of steps to yield either lactate or carbon dioxide (CO_2) plus water (H_2O). The breakdown of glucose to carbon dioxide and water is called the aerobic pathway because it requires oxygen. The conversion of glucose to lactate is called the anaerobic pathway because no oxygen is used. This latter process allows the cell to quickly re-form ATP and supports the demand for energy during intense physical activity, as does phosphocreatine (PCr). The aerobic pathway takes longer to supply ATP but provides more energy in the end. This pathway is used more by endurance activities.

Fat: The Main Fuel for Prolonged Low-Intensity Exercise

The majority of stored energy in the body is found in the fatty acids of stored triglycerides. Most of this energy resides in adipose tissue depots, although some is stored in the muscle itself. That stored in muscles is especially used as activity increases from a low to a moderate pace. When fat stores in various adipose tissue depots begin to be broken down for energy, one triglyceride molecule first yields three fatty acids and one glycerol. The free fatty acids are then released into the bloodstream and travel to the muscles. Once fatty acids enter muscle cells, they join with any of those released from intramuscular triglyceride storage.[8] All these fatty acids then move into the mitochondria, using a shuttle system that uses carnitine. Then they are broken down into carbon dioxide and water, using in part the oxygen-requiring electron transport chain that yields much ATP. The rate at which muscles use fatty acids depends on a number of factors:

- *The more trained a muscle, the greater its ability to use fat as a fuel.* After a period of aerobic training, muscle cells contain more and larger mitochondria. These and other changes enable muscle cells to produce more ATP via oxygen-requiring pathways, including the pathway used to burn fat for fuel (Table 14-2).
- *The more fatty acids that are released from adipose tissue stores into the bloodstream, the more fat will be used by the muscles.* Some athletes have attempted to raise their blood concentrations of fatty acids by consuming caffeinated beverages. This practice actually can increase fatty-acid release from adipose tissue and can be helpful to some athletes (see the Nutrition Focus at the end of this chapter).
- *As exercise becomes increasingly prolonged, fat use predominates,* especially when exercise remains at a low or moderate (aerobic) rate. When energy is needed for long-duration exercise or physical labor, there is almost always plenty of fat that can be called on. In comparison, carbohydrate stores are quite limited.

The advantage of fat over other sources of energy is that it provides more "bang for the buck." That is, for a given weight of fuel, fat supplies more than twice as much energy as carbohydrate. The aerobic breakdown of a 6-carbon glucose molecule yields 30 to 32 ATP (ratio of about 5 ATP to 1 carbon), whereas a 16-carbon fatty acid molecule produces 108 ATP (ratio of about 6.8 ATP to 1 carbon).

However, carbohydrate is more efficient than fat in one very important way: the amount of ATP produced per unit of oxygen consumed. It takes 6 O_2 molecules to produce 30 to 32 ATP molecules during the aerobic breakdown of a molecule of glu-

The fatty acids can come from all over the body, not necessarily from depots near the active muscles. *This is why spot reducing does not work.* Exercise can tone the muscles underlying adipose tissue but does not preferentially use those stores. If it did, we would all have lean cheeks and necks, because muscles in that vicinity are regularly used.

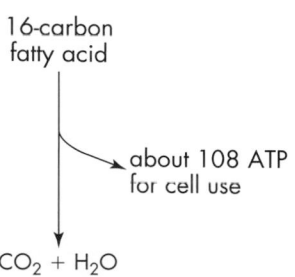

16-carbon
fatty acid

about 108 ATP
for cell use

$CO_2 + H_2O$

ATP yield from aerobic fatty acid utilization.

Table 14-2 | Adaptations to Endurance Exercise in Skeletal Muscle

Changes	Advantage
Increased ability of muscle to store glycogen (high-carbohydrate diet increases this even further)	More glycogen fuel available for the final minutes of an event
Increased triglyceride storage in muscle	Conserves glycogen by allowing for increased fat use
Increased mitochondrial size and number	Conserves glycogen by allowing for increased fat use (even at high exercise outputs)
Increased myoglobin content	Increased oxygen delivery to muscles and increased ability to use fat for fuel

Overall, training allows an athlete to use fat for fuel more readily, which allows the athlete to conserve glycogen for when it is really needed—such as for a burst of speed at the end of a race.

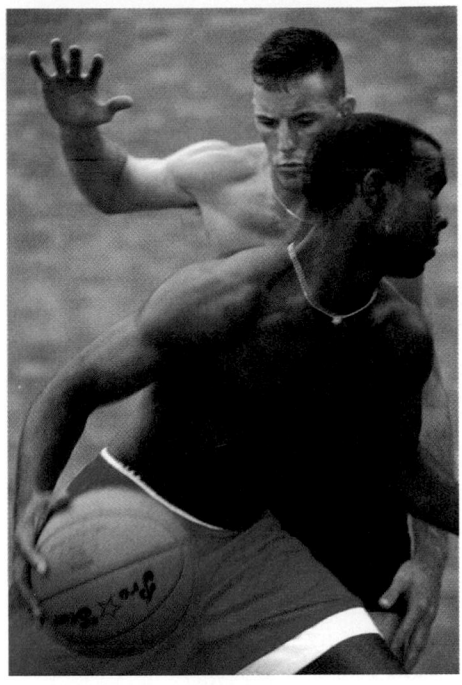

The energy to perform comes from carbohydrate, fat, and protein. The relative mix depends on the pace.

cose (ratio of about 5 ATP to 1 O_2), whereas 23 O_2 molecules are needed to produce 108 ATP molecules from a 16-carbon fatty acid (ratio of about 4.5 ATP to 1 O_2). When an athlete's maximal performance would be limited by the activity of oxygen-requiring pathways (as in competitive endurance exercise), muscle cells also use carbohydrate as an energy source as long as the carbohydrate supply (especially muscle glycogen) lasts.[19]

During very lengthy activities, such as a triathlon, ultramarathon, manual labor in a foundry, or even work at a desk for 8 hours a day, fat supplies about 50 to 90% of the energy required.[19] Overall, keep in mind that the only fuel source we eat that can support intense (anaerobic) activity is carbohydrate. In contrast, slow and steady (aerobic) activity uses primarily fat and carbohydrate.

Protein: A Minor Fuel Source, Primarily for Endurance Exercise

Although amino acids derived from protein can be used to fuel muscles, their contribution is relatively small compared with that of carbohydrate and fat. As a rough guide, only about 5% of the body's general energy needs, as well as the typical energy needs of exercising muscles, is supplied by amino acid metabolism.[8]

However, proteins can contribute significantly to energy needs in endurance exercise, perhaps as much as 15%, especially as glycogen stores in the muscle are exhausted.[8] Most of the energy supplied from protein comes from metabolism of the branched-chain amino acids—leucine, isoleucine, and valine. Because a normal diet provides enough protein to supply ample branched-chain amino acids, protein or amino acid supplements are not needed. In contrast, protein is used for fuel less in resistance exercise (e.g., weight lifting) than for endurance exercise (e.g., running) (review Figure 14-7). The primary muscle fuels for weight lifting are phosphocreatine (PCr) and carbohydrate, with fat providing fuel during the resting stages. Despite this fact, high-protein products such as Pro-Complex, Amino Fuel 2000, High Voltage Protein Drink, and Instant Egg Protein are marketed specifically for weight lifters and bodybuilders and sold in nearly every health-food and fitness store. Instead of consuming supplements like these, consuming high-carbohydrate, moderate-protein foods immediately after a weight-training workout would enhance the anabolic effect of the activity, most likely by increasing the concentrations of insulin and growth hormone in the blood and contributing to protein synthesis.[19] It is impossible to increase muscle mass simply by eating protein, however. Putting physical strain on muscle through strength training or other physical activity is needed.

Concept | Check

Fat is a key aerobic fuel for muscle cells, especially at low to moderate exercise intensities. Training enhances the ability to use fat for fuel, in turn conserving glycogen stores. At rest, muscles burn primarily fat for energy needs. On the other hand, little protein is used to fuel muscles. It supplies roughly 5% of energy needs under most conditions, and perhaps 10 to 15% of energy needs during endurance exercise when glycogen stores have essentially been exhausted.

The Body's Response to Physical Activity

The previous section discussed how muscle cells obtain the ATP energy needed to do work. This section focuses on how muscles and related organs adapt to an increased workload.

Specialized Functions of Skeletal Muscle Fiber Types

The body contains three main types of muscle tissue: skeletal muscle, the type involved in locomotion; smooth muscle, the type found in internal organs except the heart; and cardiac (heart) muscle. Skeletal muscle is composed of three main types of **muscle fibers,** which exhibit distinct functional characteristics:[8]

- Type I (slow twitch—oxidative): Fueled by aerobic metabolism of fat; also called red fibers because of their high myoglobin content.
- Type IIA (fast twitch—oxidative, glycolytic): Fueled by glycolysis using glucose (anaerobic) plus aerobic metabolism of both fat and glucose.
- Type IIX (fast twitch—glycolytic): Fueled by glycolysis using glucose (anaerobic); also called white fibers (in rodents Type IIX fibers are called Type IIB).

Prolonged low-intensity exercise, such as a slow jog, mainly involves use of type I muscle fibers, so the predominant fuel is fat. As exercise intensity increases, type IIA and type IIX fibers are gradually recruited; in turn the contribution of glucose as a fuel increases. Type IIA and type IIX fibers also are important for rapid movements, such as a jump shot in basketball.

The relative proportions of the three fiber types throughout the muscles of the body vary from person to person and are constant throughout each person's life. The individual differences in fiber-type distribution are partially responsible for producing elite marathon runners who could never compete at the same level as sprinters, or elite gymnasts who could never be competitive as long-distance swimmers. Although the proportion of muscle fiber types is largely determined by genetics, appropriate training can develop muscles within limits. For example, aerobic training enhances the capacity of type IIA muscle fibers to produce ATP and may bring about a relative change in size. Overall, great athletes are born, but their genetic potential then must be nurtured by training.[8]

Adaptation of Muscles and Body Physiology to Exercise

With training, muscle strength becomes matched to the muscles' variable work demands. Muscles enlarge after being made to work repeatedly, a response called **hypertrophy.** Certain cells in the muscles gain bulk and improve their ability to work. Conversely, after several days without activity, muscles diminish in size and lose strength, a response called **atrophy.** Both hypertrophy and atrophy are forms of adaptation to the load applied. Thus, many marathon runners have well-developed leg muscles but little arm or chest muscle development.

Repeated aerobic exercise produces beneficial changes in the heart and blood vessels that are responsible for delivering oxygen to the mitochondria of the muscle cells.

The quick, powerful movements of the gymnast rely primarily on type IIA and type IIX muscle fibers. What sort of physiological changes would you expect to occur in a gymnast who has trained diligently for many years?

muscle fiber Essentially a single muscle cell. This is an elongated cell with contractile properties that forms the muscles of the body.

hypertrophy An increase in tissue or organ size.

atrophy A wasting away of tissues or organs.

Because the body needs more oxygen during exercise, it responds to training by producing more red blood cells and expanding total blood volume. Training also leads to an increase in the number of capillaries in muscle tissue; as a result, oxygen can be delivered more easily to muscle cells. Finally, training causes the heart, a muscle itself, to strengthen. Then each contraction empties the heart's chamber more efficiently, so more blood is pumped with each beat. As exercise increases the heart's efficiency, its rate of beating at rest and during submaximal exercise decreases.[19]

Oxygen consumption indicates how hard a person is exercising. The more physically fit a person is, the more work the muscles and body can do and the more oxygen the person can consume. A treadmill test is commonly used to determine a person's $VO_{2\ max}$, which is the maximum amount of oxygen that can be consumed in a unit of time (ml/min). In this test, oxygen consumption is measured as the treadmill speed and/or grade is gradually increased until the subject can no longer increase oxygen use as workload increases. The oxygen consumption measured at this point is $VO_{2\ max}$. Most people can improve their $VO_{2\ max}$ by 15 to 20% or more with training.[8]

Because of individual differences in $VO_{2\ max}$, it is generally best to express exercise intensity as a percentage of $VO_{2\ max}$. The percentage of $VO_{2\ max}$ required for exercise of various intensity is as follows:

- Low intensity (e.g., fast walk)—30 to 50% of $VO_{2\ max}$
- Moderate intensity (e.g., fast jog)—50 to 65% of $VO_{2\ max}$
- High intensity (e.g., 3-hour marathon pace)—70 to 80% of $VO_{2\ max}$
- Very high intensity (e.g., sprints)—85 to 150% of $VO_{2\ max}$

In very-high-intensity activities, the ATP equivalent to the "extra" 50% above 100% of $VO_{2\ max}$ is produced anaerobically from PCr and glycolysis. In terms of fuel sources for muscle cells, fat use peaks as exercise intensity increases (Table 14-3). Carbohydrate use then becomes more important for meeting energy needs.

Exercise output is sometimes expressed in units called metabolic equivalents (METs). One MET is the expenditure of 1 kcal/kg/hr or, on average, 3.5 ml O_2/kg/min. This approximates resting energy expenditure. A brisk walk represents about 4.5 METs of energy expenditure. Exercise prescriptions given to people recovering from a heart attack are often given in MET units.[19]

Power Food: Dietary Advice for Athletes

Athletic training and genetic makeup are two very important determinants of athletic performance. A good diet won't substitute for either factor, but eating well can help enhance and maximize an athlete's potential. On the other hand, poor food choices can seriously reduce performance.

Energy Needs

Athletes need varying amounts of food energy, depending on each athlete's body size, body composition, and the type of training or competition being considered. A small person may need only 1700 kcal/day to sustain normal daily activities without losing

---

ATP (energy) needs dictate the amount of oxygen used by cells: 1.5 or 2.5 ATP molecules are produced from each molecule of oxygen.

VO_{2max} The maximum volume of oxygen that can be consumed per unit of time.

Relative Distribution of Muscle Fiber Types	
	Type 1: Type IIA + Type IIX
Sedentary person	45–50% : 50–55%
Sprinter	20–35% : 65–85%
Marathoner	80% : 20%

Critical | Thinking

Marty started going to the gym about 8 weeks ago. At first, he noticed that he began huffing and puffing about 7 minutes into his aerobic workout. Now, however, he can work out for about 25 minutes without tiring. What is a possible explanation for his ability to work out longer?

Table 14-3 | Fuel Use Estimate Based on Percent of $VO_{2\ max}$

VO_{2max}	Muscle Glycogen	Muscle Triglycerides	Blood Glucose	Free Fatty Acids in the Bloodstream
25%	—	20%	10%	70%
65%	40%	25%	10%	25%
85%	55%	15%	15%	15%

Typical VO_{2max} Values	*ml O_2/kg/min*
Sedentary elderly person	15
Typical middle-aged adult	35–45
Elite athlete	65–75

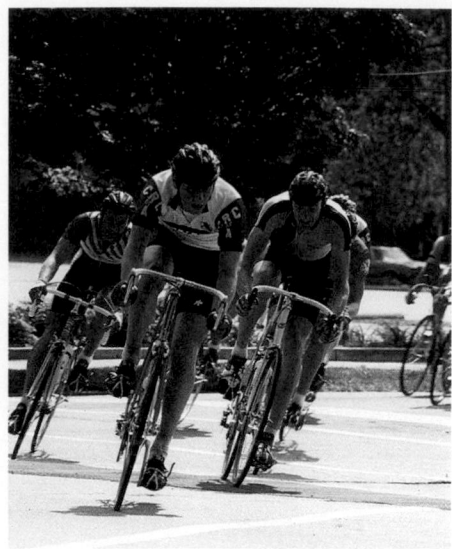

Athletes often expend much energy. In such cases, their resulting increased food and beverage intake should easily provide ample carbohydrate, protein, and other nutrients to support activity.

Review Table 13-6 in Chapter 13, which listed the energy costs of typical forms of physical activity.

body weight; a tall, muscular man may need 4000 kcal/day. These rough estimates can be viewed as starting points that need to be individualized by trial and error for each athlete.

An estimate of the energy required to sustain moderate activity is 5 to 8 kcal/min. The energy required for sports training or competition then has to be added to the energy used just to carry on normal activities. For example, an hour of bowling requires little energy in addition to that required to sustain normal daily living. At the other extreme, a 12-hour endurance bicycle race over mountains can require an additional 4000 kcal/day. Therefore, some athletes may need as much as 7000 kcal/day or more just to maintain body weight while training, whereas others may need 1700 kcal/day or less. If an athlete experiences daily fatigue, the first consideration should be whether that person is consuming enough food. Up to six meals per day may be needed, including one before each workout.

How can we know if an athlete is getting enough energy? Estimating daily intake from a food diary kept by the athlete is one way. Another step is to estimate the athlete's body fat percentage via skinfold measurements, bioelectrical impedance, or underwater weighing (review Chapter 13). Body fat should be the typical amount found for athletes for the specific sport practiced: 5 to 18% for most male athletes and 17 to 28% for most female athletes. The next step is to monitor body weight changes on a daily or weekly basis. If body weight starts to fall, energy intake should be increased; if weight rises because of increases in body fat, the athlete should eat less.[19]

If the body composition test shows that an athlete has too much body fat, the athlete should lower food intake by about 200 to 500 kcal/day while maintaining a regular exercise program until the desirable fat percentage is achieved. Reducing fat intake is the best nutrient-related approach. On the other hand, if an athlete needs to gain weight, increasing food intake by 500 to 700 kcal/day will eventually lead to the needed weight gain. A mix of carbohydrate, fat, and protein is advised, coupled with exercise to make sure this gain is mostly in the form of lean tissue and not fat stores.

Note that wrestlers, boxers, judoists, jockeys, and rowers often try to lose weight before a competition so that they can be certified to compete in a lower weight class. This maneuver helps them gain a mechanical advantage over an opponent of smaller stature. They usually lose this weight before stepping on the scale for weight certification. Athletes can lose up to 22 lb (10 kg) of body weight as water in 1 day by sitting in a sauna, exercising in a plastic sweat suit, or taking diuretic drugs, which speed water loss from the kidneys. Losing as little as 2% of body weight by dehydration, however, can adversely affect endurance performance, especially in hot weather. A pattern of repeated weight loss or gain of more than 5% of body weight by dehydration carries risk of kidney malfunction and heat-related illness. Death is also a possibility.

To prevent future deaths from such weight loss in athletes, the National Collegiate Athletic Association and many states have authorized physicians or athletic trainers to set safe weight and body fat content minimums (e.g., 7% or more of total body weight) for male athletes in weight-class sports (12% or more for females). Under new guidelines, athletes are assigned to weight classes at the beginning of the season and are not allowed to "cut weight" to gain a competitive advantage. (Weight gain in the days after a competition [reflecting regain of body water] can now be no greater than 2 lb.) If athletes, such as wrestlers, wish to compete in a lower weight class and have enough extra fat stores, they should begin a gradual, sustained reduction in energy intake long before the competitive season starts.

Carbohydrate Needs

Anyone who exercises vigorously, especially for more than 1 hour per day on a regular basis, needs to consume a diet that includes moderate to high amounts of carbohydrates. The diet should provide a variety of foods, such as those recommended by MyPyramid. Numerous servings of grains, starchy vegetables, and fruits provide

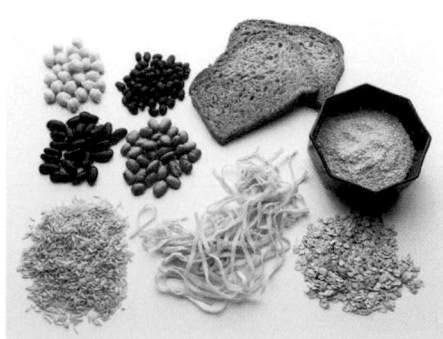

High-carbohydrate foods should form the basis of the athlete's diet.

enough carbohydrate to maintain adequate liver and muscle glycogen stores, especially for replacing glycogen losses from workouts on the previous day. Relatively low-carbohydrate/high-protein diets, such as *The Zone Diet*, are not recommended. Recall that Chapter 13 discussed the Zone Diet. The carbohydrate content of this diet is only 40% of energy intake, rather than the 60% or more that is typically recommended for athletes.[3]

Carbohydrate intake should be at least 5 g/kg of body weight. People engaged in aerobic training and endurance activities (duration 60 minutes or more per day) may need as much as 7 g/kg of body weight. When exercise duration approaches several hours per day, the carbohydrate recommendation increases to up to 10 g/kg of body weight.[2] In other words, triathletes and marathon runners should consider eating close to 500 to 600 g of carbohydrates daily. Even more may be necessary to (1) prevent chronic fatigue and (2) load the muscles and liver with glycogen. Attention to carbohydrate intake is especially important when performing multiple training bouts in a day, such as swim practices, or heavy training on successive days, as in cross-country running. Depletion of carbohydrate ranks just behind depletion of fluid and electrolytes as a major cause of fatigue.

Table 14-4 shows sample menus for diets providing food energy ranging from 1500 to 5000 kcal/day. In addition, the Exchange System described in Appendix E is a very useful tool for planning all types of diets, including high-carbohydrate diets for athletes.

Athletes should obtain at least 60% of total energy needs from carbohydrates (rather than the 50% typical of most North American diets), especially if exercise duration is expected to exceed 2 hours and total energy intake is about 3000 kcal per day or less. Diets providing 4000 to 5000 kcal/day can yield as little as 50% of energy content coming from carbohydrate and still provide sufficient carbohydrate (e.g., 500 to 600 g or so per day).[2]

Note that athletes do not have to give up any specific food when planning a high-carbohydrate diet. The focus is to include more high-carbohydrate foods while moderating concentrated fat sources. Sports nutritionists emphasize the difference between a high-carbohydrate meal and a high-carbohydrate/high-fat meal. Before endurance events such as marathons or triathlons, some athletes seek to increase their carbohydrate reserves by eating foods such as potato chips, french fries, banana cream pie, and pastries. Although such foods provide carbohydrate, they also contain a lot of fat. Better high-carbohydrate food choices include pasta, rice, potatoes, bread, fruit and fruit juices, and many breakfast cereals (check the label for carbohydrate content) (Table 14-5). Sports drinks appropriate for carbohydrate loading, such as GatorLode and UltraFuel, can also help. Consuming a moderate rather than a high amount of fiber during the final day of training is a good precaution to reduce the chances of bloating and intestinal gas during the next day's event.

For athletes who compete in continuous, intense aerobic events lasting more than 60 to 90 minutes (or in shorter events taking place more than once within a 24-hour period), a **carbohydrate-loading** regimen can help maximize the amount of energy stored in the form of muscle glycogen for the event.[19] (Note, however, that this amount of activity applies to few athletes.) In one possible regimen, during the week prior to the event, the athlete gradually reduces the intensity and duration of exercise ("tapering") while simultaneously increasing the percentage of total energy intake supplied by carbohydrate.

For example, consider the carbohydrate-loading schedule of a 25-year-old man preparing for a marathon. His typical energy needs are about 3500 kcal/day. Six days before competition, he completes a final hard workout of 60 minutes. On that day, carbohydrates contribute 45 to 50% of his total energy intake. As he goes through the rest of the week, the duration of his workouts decreases to 40 minutes and then to about 20 minutes by the end of the week. Meanwhile, he increases the amount of carbohydrate in his diet to reach 70 to 80% of total energy intake as the week continues. Total energy intake should decrease as exercise time decreases throughout the week. On the final day before competition, he rests while maintaining the high-carbohydrate intake.

Critical | Thinking

Joe is a wrestler who qualified for the 125-lb weight classification in the annual state high school competition. After a few matches, Joe began to feel dizzy and faint. He was disqualified because he was unable to continue the match. Later, the coach found out that Joe had spent 2 hours in the sauna before weighing in, which had made him dehydrated. What are the consequences of dehydration? What can you suggest as a safer alternative for weight loss?

Appropriate Activities for Carbohydrate Loading

Marathons
Long-distance swimming
Cross-country skiing
30-kilometer runs
Triathlons
Tournament-play basketball
Soccer
Cycling time trials
Long-distance canoe racing

Inappropriate Activities for Carbohydrate Loading

American football games
10-kilometer or shorter runs
Walking and hiking
Most swimming events
Single basketball games
Weight lifting
Most track and field events

carbohydrate loading A process in which a very high carbohydrate intake is consumed for 6 days before an athletic event while tapering exercise duration in an attempt to increase muscle glycogen stores.

Table 14-4 | Sample Daily Menus Based on MyPyramid That Provide Various Total Energy Intakes

1500 kcal Diet	2000 kcal Diet	3000 kcal Diet	4000 kcal Diet	5000 kcal Diet
Breakfast Fat-free milk, 1 cup Cheerios, 1/2 cup Bagel, 1/2 Cherry jam, 2 tsp Margarine, 1 tsp	**Breakfast** Fat-free milk, 1 cup Cheerios, 1 cup Bagel, 1/2 Cherry jam, 1 tbsp Margarine, 1 tsp	**Breakfast** Fat-free milk, 1 cup Cheerios, 2 cups Bagel, 1 Cherry jam, 2 tsp Margarine, 1 tsp Oat bran muffins, 2	**Breakfast** Fat-free milk, 1 cup Cheerios, 2 cups Orange, 1 Bran muffins, 2	**Breakfast** Fat-reduced milk, 1 cup Cheerios, 2 cups Bran muffins, 2 Orange, 1

Lunch
Chicken breast (roasted),
  2 oz
Figs, 1
Fat-free milk, 1/2 cup
Banana, 1
	Lunch
	Chicken breast (roasted),
	  2 oz
	Wheat bread, 2 slices
	Mayonnaise, 1 tsp
	Raisins, 1/4 cup
	Cranberry juice,
	  1 1/2 cups
	Banana, 1
		Lunch
		Chicken breast (roasted),
		  2 oz
		Wheat bread, 2 slices
		Provolone cheese, 1 oz
		Mayonnaise, 1 tsp
		Raisins, 1/3 cup
		Cranberry juice,
		  1 1/2 cups
		Low-fat fruit yogurt, 1 cup
			Snack
			Chopped dates, 3/4 cup
				Snack
				Low-fat yogurt, 1 cup
				Chopped dates, 1 cup

Snack Oatmeal-raisin cookie, 1 Low-fat fruit yogurt, 1 cup	**Snack** Oatmeal-raisin cookies, 3 Low-fat fruit yogurt, 1 cup	**Snack** Banana, 1 Oatmeal-raisin cookies, 3	**Lunch** Romaine lettuce, 1 cup Garbanzo beans, 1 cup Grated carrots, 1/2 cup French dressing, 2 tbsp Macaroni and cheese, 3 cups Apple juice, 1 cup	**Lunch** Apple juice, 1 cup Chicken enchilada, 1 Romaine lettuce, 1 cup Garbanzo beans, 1 cup Shredded carrots, 3/4 cup Chopped celery, 1/2 cup Seasoned croutons, 1 oz French dressing, 2 tbsp Wheat bread, 2 slices Margarine, 1 tbsp

Dinner
Spaghetti w/meatballs,
  1 cup
Romaine lettuce, 1 cup
Italian dressing, 2 tsp
Green beans, 1/2 cup
Cranberry juice, 1 1/2 cups
	Dinner
	Broiled beef sirloin, 3 oz
	Romaine lettuce, 1 cup
	Italian dressing, 2 tsp
	Green beans, 1 cup
	Fat-free milk, 1/2 cup
		Dinner
		Broiled beef sirloin, 3 oz
		Romaine lettuce, 1 cup
		Garbanzo beans, 1 cup
		Italian dressing, 2 tsp
		Spinach pasta noodles,
		  1 1/2 cups
		Margarine, 1 tsp
		Green beans, 1 cup
		Fat-free milk, 1/2 cup
			Snack
			Wheat bread, 2 slices
			Margarine, 1 tsp
			Jam, 2 tbsp
				Snack
				Banana, 1
				Bagel, 1
				Cream cheese, 1 tbsp

18% protein (68 g)
64% carbohydrate (240 g)
19% fat (32 g)
	17% protein (85 g)
	63% carbohydrate (315 g)
	20% fat (44 g)
		17% protein (128 g)
		62% carbohydrate (465 g)
		21% fat (70 g)
			Dinner
			Skinless turkey breast, 2 oz
			Mashed potatoes, 2 cups
			Peas and onions, 1 cup
			Banana, 1
			Fat-free milk, 1 cup
				Dinner
				Fat-reduced milk, 1 cup
				Beef sirloin, 5 oz
				Mashed potatoes, 2 cups
				Spinach pasta noodles,
				  1 1/2 cups
				Grated parmesan cheese,
				  2 tbsp
				Green beans, 1 cup
				Oatmeal-raisin cookies, 3

			Snack Pasta, 1 cup cooked Margarine, 2 tsp Parmesan cheese, 2 tbsp Cranberry juice, 1 cup	**Snack** Cranberry juice, 2 cups Air-popped popcorn, 4 cups Raisins, 1/3 cup
			14% protein (140 g) 61% carbohydrate (610 g) 26% fat (116 g)	14% protein (175 g) 63% carbohydrate (813 g) 24% fat (136 g)

Carbohydrate Loading Regimen

Days before Competition	6	5	4	3	2	1
Exercise time (minutes)	60	40	40	20	20	Rest
Carbohydrate (grams)	450	450	450	600	600	600

This carbohydrate-loading technique usually increases muscle glycogen stores by 50 to 85% over typical conditions (that is, when dietary carbohydrate constitutes only about 50% of total energy intake).

A potential disadvantage of carbohydrate loading is that additional water (about 3 g) is incorporated into the muscles along with each gram of glycogen. Although this water aids in maintaining hydration, for some individuals this additional water weight

Table 14-5 | Grams of Carbohydrate Based on Serving Size of Typical Carbohydrate-Rich Foods

Starches—15 g Carbohydrate per Serving (80 kcal)

One Serving

dry breakfast cereal*, 1/2–3/4 cup	baked potato, 1/4 large
cooked breakfast cereal, 1/2 cup	bagel, 1/4 (4 oz)
cooked grits, 1/2 cup	English muffin, 1/2
cooked rice, 1/3 cup	bread, 1 slice
cooked pasta, 1/3 cup	pretzels, 3/4 oz
baked beans, 1/3 cup	saltine crackers, 6
cooked corn, 1/2 cup	pancake, 4 inches in diameter, 1
cooked/dry beans, 1/2 cup	taco shells, 2 (add 45 kcal)

Vegetables—5 g Carbohydrate per Serving (25 kcal)

One Serving

cooked vegetables, 1/2 cup
raw vegetables, 1 cup
vegetable juice, 1/2 cup
Examples: carrots, green beans, broccoli, cauliflower, onions, spinach, tomatoes, vegetable juice

Fruits—15 g Carbohydrate per Serving (60 kcal)

One Serving

canned fruit or berries, 1/2 cup	grapes (small), 17
fruit juice, 1/2 cup	grapefruit, 1/2
figs (dried), 1 1/2	dates, 3
apple or orange, 1 small	peach, 1
apricots (dried), 8	watermelon cubes, 1 1/4 cups
banana, 1 small	

Milk—12 g Carbohydrate per Serving

One Serving

milk, 1 cup	soymilk, 1 cup
plain low-fat yogurt, 2/3 cup	

Sweets—15 g Carbohydrate per Serving (variable kcal)

One Serving

cake, 2-inch square	ice cream, 1/2 cup
cookies, 2 small	sherbet, 1/2 cup

Modified from *Exchange Lists for Meal Planning* by the American Diabetes Association and American Dietetic Association, 2003, Chicago, American Dietetic Association.

*Note that the carbohydrate content of dry cereal varies widely. Check the labels of the ones you choose and adjust the serving size accordingly.

and related muscle stiffness can detract from their sports performance, making carbohydrate loading inappropriate. Athletes considering a carbohydrate-loading regimen should try it during training (and long before an important competition) to experience its effects on performance. They can then determine whether carbohydrate loading works for them. Note also that consuming carbohydrate during a competition provides about the same advantage as carbohydrate loading prior to the event. In fact, expert advice is currently shifting away from carbohydrate loading and more toward this second method, coupled with a daily diet high in carbohydrate.[19] In addition, remember the importance of the "training effect" discussed on pages 528–529.

Fat Needs

A diet containing up to 35% of energy intake from fat is generally recommended for athletes. Rich sources of monounsaturated fat, such as canola oil, should be emphasized, and saturated fat and *trans* fat intake should be limited.[2]

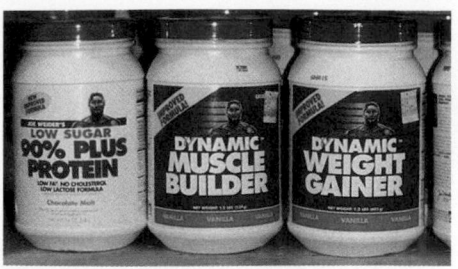

High-protein products, which are often marketed to athletes, are unnecessary in most cases. The same holds true for high-protein bars.

Consuming excessive amounts of protein has drawbacks. As noted in Chapter 7, it increases calcium loss somewhat in the urine. It also leads to increased urine production, possibly compromising body hydration. It also may lead to kidney stones in people with a history of this or other kidney problems. Finally, enough carbohydrate fuel may not be consumed on such a diet, leading to fatigue.

Protein Needs

Typical recommendations for protein intake in the sports nutrition literature for most athletes range from 1.0 to 1.6 g of protein/kg of body weight.[2] This amount is considerably higher than the RDA of 0.8 g/kg of body weight recommended by the Food and Nutrition Board for all adults, including athletes (Table 14-6).

For athletes beginning a strength-training program, some experts recommend up to 1.7 g of protein per kg of body weight.[17] That amount is more than twice the RDA for protein. To date, the value of such an excessive protein intake during the initial phases of strength training has not been supported by sufficient research. In addition, protein intakes above this amount simply result in an increased use of amino acids for energy needs; no further increase in muscle protein synthesis is seen. Note also that energy needs for strength training itself are not the reason for the high protein recommendation, because the fuel used in this activity is primarily phosphocreatine and carbohydrate. The extra protein, theoretically, is required for the synthesis of new muscle tissue brought on by the loading effect of strength training. Once the desired muscle mass is achieved, protein intake need not exceed 1.2 g/kg of body weight.

Table 14-6 summarizes recommended ranges of protein intakes for various types of activity. Any athlete not specifically on a low-calorie regimen can easily meet these protein recommendations simply by eating a variety of foods (review Table 14-4). To illustrate, a 123-lb (53-kg) woman who is performing endurance activity can consume 64 g of protein (53 × 1.2) during a single day by including 3 oz of chicken (one chicken breast), 3 oz of beef (a small, lean hamburger), and two glasses of milk in her diet. Similarly, a 180-lb (77-kg) man who aims to gain muscle mass through strength training needs to consume only 6 oz of chicken (a large chicken breast), 1/2 cup of cooked beans, a 6-oz can of tuna, and three glasses of milk to achieve an intake of 130 g of protein (77 × 1.7) in a day. And for both athletes, these calculations do not even include the protein present in grains or vegetables they will also eat. As you can see, simply by meeting their energy needs, many athletes consume much more protein than is required. Despite marketing claims, protein supplements are an expensive and unnecessary part of a fitness plan.

Athletes who either feel they must significantly limit their energy intake or are vegetarians should specifically determine how much protein they eat. They should make sure to follow a diet that provides at least 1.2 g of protein per kg of body weight per day, the upper recommendation for most athletes.

Vitamin and Mineral Needs

Vitamin and mineral needs are the same or slightly higher for athletes compared with those of sedentary adults. Still, because athletes usually have such high energy intakes, they tend to consume plenty of vitamins and minerals. An exception is athletes con-

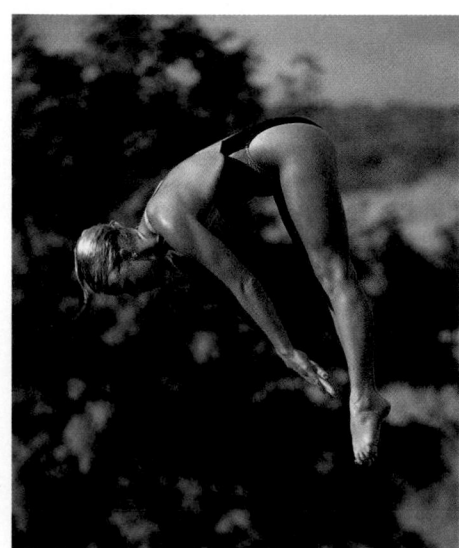

Weight-restricted athletes especially should make sure they are consuming enough protein as well as other essential nutrients.

Table 14-6 | Current Recommendations for Protein Intake Based on kg Body Weight*

Activity Group	g/kg	Amount for a 70-kg Person (g)
Sedentary	0.8	56
Strength trained, maintenance	1.0–1.2	70–84
Strength trained, gain muscle mass	1.5–1.7	105–119
Moderate-intensity endurance activities	1.2	84
High-intensity endurance training	1.6	112

*Calculate kilograms by dividing pounds by 2.2.

Source: Burke L, Deakin V: *Clinical Sports Nutrition*, McGraw-Hill, Roseville NSW2069, Australia, 2000.

suming low-calorie diets (about 1200 kcal or less), such as some female athletes participating in events in which maintaining a low body weight is crucial. These diets may not meet B-vitamin and other micronutrient needs.[10] Vegetarian athletes are also a concern. Such athletes should consume fortified foods such as ready-to-eat breakfast cereals or a balanced multivitamin and mineral supplement.

Athletes' needs for vitamin E and vitamin C may be somewhat greater because of the potential antioxidant protection these nutrients provide; this effect could be especially important in the face of high oxygen use by muscles. Still, as noted by Dr. Priscilla Clarkson in the Expert Opinion, the use of large doses of vitamin E and vitamin C requires more study and is not currently an accepted part of the dietary guidance for athletes. It is more important to follow a diet containing foods rich in antioxidants, such as fruits, vegetables, whole-grain breads and cereals, and vegetable oils. In addition, there is evidence that antioxidant systems in the body increase in activity as exercise training progresses. Oxidative stress produced during exercise might also have benefits, such as for muscle adaptation to exercise, and so trying to block this process may not be advantageous.[12,13]

Iron Deficiency Impairs Performance

Because iron is involved in red blood cell production, oxygen transport, and energy production, a deficiency of this mineral can noticeably detract from optimal athletic performance.[15] The potential causes for iron deficiency in athletes vary. As in the general population, female athletes are most susceptible to low iron status due to monthly menstrual losses. Special diets followed by athletes, such as low-energy and vegetarian (especially vegan) diets, are likely to be low in iron. Distance runners should pay special attention to iron intake, because their intense workouts may lead to gastrointestinal bleeding. Another concern is *sports anemia,* which occurs because exercise causes blood plasma volume to expand, particularly at the start of a training regimen before the synthesis of red blood cells increases. This expansion results in dilution of the blood. In sports anemia, even if iron stores are adequate, blood iron tests may appear low.

Sports anemia is not detrimental to performance, but it is hard to differentiate between sports anemia and true anemia. If iron status is low and not replenished, iron-deficiency anemia and markedly impaired endurance performance can eventually result. True anemia (noted as a reduced blood hemoglobin level) has been found among athletes in some studies (possibly up to about 15% of males and 30% of females), so it is a good idea, especially for adult women athletes, to have their iron status checked at the beginning of a training season and at least once during midseason, and to monitor dietary iron intake.

Any blood test indicating low iron status—sports anemia or not—is cause for follow-up. For some athletes the use of iron supplements may be advisable. However, indiscriminate use of iron supplements is not advised because toxic effects are possible. It is important that physicians investigate the cause of the deficiency because iron deficiency can be caused by blood loss. If caught early, some serious medical conditions can be treated or prevented.

Some studies have suggested that iron deficiency without anemia may also have a negative effect on physical activity and performance.[15] Also, once depleted, iron stores can take months to replenish. For this reason, athletes must be especially careful to meet iron needs.

Calcium Intake Deserves Attention, Especially for Women

Athletes, especially women trying to lose weight by restricting their intake of milk and milk products, can have marginal or low dietary intakes of calcium. This practice compromises optimal bone health. Of still greater concern are women athletes who have stopped menstruating because their arduous exercise training and low body fat content interferes with the normal secretion of reproductive hormones. Disturbing reports

Recall from Chapter 9 that supplement use should not exceed any Upper Levels over the long term. Also, men should be cautious about any use of supplements containing iron.

At one time in his career, long-distance runner Alberto Salazar experienced problems sleeping and performed poorly because of low iron intake and related iron-deficiency anemia.

Expert Opinion

Does Increased Physical Activity Necessitate Antioxidant Supplementation?
Priscilla M. Clarkson, Ph.D.

Adenosine triphosphate (ATP) is the primary fuel that skeletal muscle uses to generate force. A large portion of this ATP is produced in muscle cell mitochondria, specifically the electron transport system. The process of producing ATP in this manner is termed *aerobic metabolism*, where molecular oxygen is reduced (loses two electrons) and combines with hydrogen ions to form metabolic water. About 5% of the oxygen is not fully reduced, resulting in free radicals and reactive oxygen species (ROS), chemicals with unpaired electrons in their outer shell, such as superoxide, hydrogen peroxide, and hydroxyl radicals.

When left unchecked, ROS can wreak havoc by attacking cellular components, especially lipids. The attack on lipids initiates a chain reaction called lipid peroxidation, leading to a generation of more radicals. These processes can result in damage to membranes, proteins, and nucleic acids (e.g., DNA). To neutralize ROS, the body has an elaborate defense system consisting of enzymes such as catalase, superoxide dismutase, and glutathione peroxidase as well as numerous nonenzymatic antioxidants, including beta-carotene, vitamin E, vitamin C, glutathione, ubiquinone (coenzyme Q-10), and flavonoids. All these nonenzymatic antioxidants can be obtained from foods, and some are also synthesized by cells.

Increased physical activity requires muscle to produce more ATP, which in turn requires more oxygen to be used and generates more ROS. Exercise also increases ROS through other means such as increased epinephrine and related compounds as well as production of lactate. In this manner, exercise can produce a temporary imbalance between ROS generation and the ability of antioxidants to counteract them. This imbalance is known as oxidative stress.

Various markers in muscle, blood, and urine have been used to determine oxidative stress in response to exercise. The most common measurements to indicate oxidative stress are by-products of lipid peroxidation that appear in the blood. Changes in status of antioxidant compounds such as glutathione, protein and DNA oxidation products, and antioxidant enzyme activities have also been used. Techniques to directly measure free radicals, used predominantly in in vitro studies, have recently been used with some success to detect free radicals in blood. Of the many studies that used these measures to examine whether exercise increases oxidative stress, most have found increases in oxidative stress in response to intense exercise. However, results from these studies are not consistent in the amount of oxidative stress generated, and some studies found no increase. These equivocal results are likely due to the different levels of training among the subjects, the different exercises and intensities used, and the various measures of oxidative stress employed. The physical outcomes of increased oxidative stress to the person during exercise are unknown, but recent evidence suggests that oxidative stress may contribute to muscle fatigue.

The findings that physical activity increases oxidative stress have led to the concern that regular, strenuous exercise may cause harm to muscles. This idea led to numerous investigations of antioxidant supplementation to reduce oxidative stress in an attempt to determine possible benefits of antioxidant supplements for people who exercise regularly. Early studies that examined whether antioxidant vitamin supplements (mostly vitamins C and/or E) would enhance athletic performance generally concluded that performance was not improved unless there was a preexisting vitamin deficiency. Later research

show that female athletes who do not menstruate regularly have far less dense spinal bones than both nonathletes and female athletes who menstruate regularly. These female athletes are at increased risk for bone fractures during training and competition and for osteoporosis in later life.[7] This combination of risks outweighs the benefits of weight-bearing exercise on bone density. This topic is discussed further in Chapter 15 with respect to the female athlete triad and in Chapter 11, where osteoporosis was reviewed in detail.

Research has clearly documented the importance of regular menstruation to maintain bone mineral density. A woman runner who does not menstruate regularly may also have a higher risk for the development of a **stress fracture.** Thus, female athletes whose menstrual cycles become irregular should consult a physician to determine the cause. Decreasing the amount of training or increasing energy intake and body weight often restores regular menstrual cycles.[20] If irregular menstrual cycles persist, severe bone loss (much of which is not reversible) and osteoporosis can result.[7] Extra calcium in the diet does not necessarily compensate for the effects of menstrual irregularities, but inadequate dietary calcium can make matters worse.

stress fracture A fracture that occurs from repeated jarring of a bone. Common sites include bones of the foot.

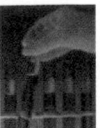

focused on the independent effects of vitamin C or vitamin E supplementation on immune response to exercise or on countering exercise-induced muscle damage. These study results were not consistent in that some studies reported a benefit and other studies reported no effect of antioxidant supplementation. Vitamin C and vitamin E also have been used in combination to determine the effects in reducing muscle damage related to exercise, but here too, the results of studies are equivocal. Supplementation effects of other dietary antioxidants, or combinations of these with vitamin E and vitamin C, have not produced consistent results. It is difficult to make comparisons between the various studies because the type of supplement, dosage, timing of the supplement, intensity of the exercise, and outcome measures differed.

Although exercise can result in oxidative stress, increased oxidative stress is not necessarily harmful. It seems counterintuitive to think that the body's response to exercise, a function essential to life and important for health, would be injurious. In fact, physical training appears to boost the body's natural antioxidant defense system. Several studies have found that training results in increased antioxidant capacity, reduced production of oxidants when at rest, and reduced generation of ROS in the mitochondria, which would increase resistance to subsequent oxidative stress. Moreover, cells have an enhanced repair system related to exercise training. Thus, ROS may serve as signals that stimulate adaptive

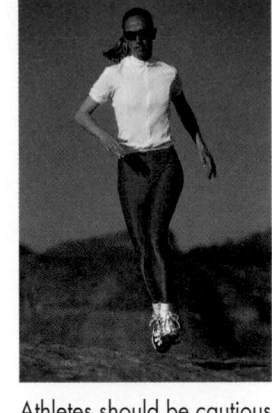

Athletes should be cautious about claims for mega-dose antioxidant supplements. These supplements actually cause more harm than good.

processes. Perhaps the body produces ROS for a reason, that an increase in ROS is not a mistake of metabolism.

The body's natural defense system works to prevent harmful effects of oxidative stress, but some oxidative stress may be necessary to promote training adaptations. It is not known whether strenuous exercise will produce a level of oxidative stress at which the potential risks outweigh the benefits, thus impairing performance and the ability to train effectively. If so, athletes would require antioxidant supplements to restore the balance. Until this information is available, massive interventions with supplements to prevent ROS should be viewed with caution. The antioxidant defense system is a complex interaction and balance of endogenous and exogenous antioxidants. Dramatically increasing selected dietary antioxidants could disrupt this equilibrium and negatively impact the system. A prudent recommendation for athletes in strenuous training is to consume a diet rich in antioxidants and possibly take a balanced multivitamin and mineral supplement (containing no more than the Daily Values listed on the label) to make up for specific diet shortfalls rather than taking supplements that provide high doses of antioxidants.

Dr. Clarkson is Professor of Exercise Science and Associate Dean for Research in the School of Public Health and Health Sciences at the University of Massachusetts–Amherst. She has served as president of the National ACSM and related organizations. She is the 1997 recipient of the National ACSM Citation Award, the 2001 Excellence in Education Award from the Gatorade Sport Science Institute, the National ACSM Honor Award in 2005, and the University of Massachusetts Chancellor's Medal, among other awards. Dr. Clarkson has published over 150 scientific research articles on topics such as how human skeletal muscle responds to environmental challenges.

A Focus on Fluid Needs

Fluid needs for an average adult are about 9 cups per day for women and 13 cups per day for men. Athletes need this amount and generally even more to maintain the body's ability to regulate internal temperature and to keep cool.[5] Most energy released during metabolism appears immediately as heat. Furthermore, heat production in contracting muscles can rise 15 to 20 times above that of resting muscles. Unless this heat is quickly dissipated, **heat exhaustion, heat cramps,** and deadly **heatstroke** may ensue (Figure 14-8).[6] In fact, typically three to five athletes die each year of heatstroke. In 2001, college football players and a professional football player died this way.

Heat exhaustion occurs when heat stress causes loss of body fluid and then depletion of blood volume. Maintaining adequate body fluid is important. As environmental temperature rises above 95°F (35°C), virtually all body heat is lost through the evaporation of sweat from the skin. Sweat rates during prolonged exercise range from 3 to 8 cups (750 to 2000 ml) per hour. However, as the humidity rises, especially

heat exhaustion The first stage of heat-related illness that occurs because of depletion of blood volume from fluid loss by the body. This depletion increases body temperature and can lead to headache, dizziness, muscle weakness, and visual disturbances, among other effects.

heat cramps A frequent complication of heat exhaustion. They usually occur in individuals who have experienced large sweat losses from exercising for several hours in a hot climate and have consumed a large volume of water. The cramps occur in skeletal muscles and consist of contractions for 1 to 3 minutes at a time.

heatstroke A condition in which the internal body temperature reaches 104°F. Sweating generally ceases if left untreated, and blood circulation is greatly reduced. Nervous system damage may ensue, and death is likely. Often the skin of individuals who suffer heatstroke is hot and dry.

Heat Index

Relative Humidity (%)	70°	75°	80°	85°	90°	95°	100°	105°	110°
100	72°	80°	91°	108°					
90	71°	79°	88°	102°	122°				
80	71°	78°	86°	97°	113°	136°			
70	70°	77°	85°	93°	106°	124°	144°		
60	69°	76°	82°	90°	100°	114°	132°	149°	
50	70°	75°	81°	88°	96°	107°	120°	135°	150°
40	68°	74°	79°	86°	93°	101°	110°	123°	137°
30	67°	73°	78°	84°	90°	96°	104°	113°	123°
20	66°	72°	77°	82°	87°	93°	99°	105°	112°
10	65°	70°	75°	80°	85°	90°	95°	100°	105°
0	64°	69°	73°	78°	83°	87°	91°	95°	99°

Air Temperature (°F)

Heat index	Heat disorders possible with prolonged exposure and/or physical activity
80° – 89°	Fatigue
90° – 104°	Sunstroke, heat cramps, and heat exhaustion
105° – 129°	Sunstroke, heat cramps, or heat exhaustion likely and heatstroke possible
130° or higher	Heatstroke/sunstroke highly likely

NOTE: Direct sunshine increases the heat index by up to 15°F

Figure 14-8 | Heat index chart showing associated heat disorders.

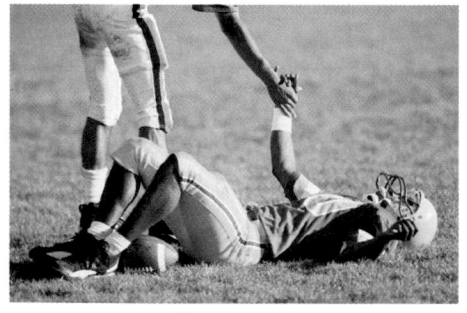

Dehydration, which can lead to illness and death, must be avoided during physical activity.

above 75%, evaporation slows and sweating becomes an inefficient way to cool the body. The result is rapid fatigue, increased work for the heart, and difficulty with prolonged exertion. Clearly, the combination of high heat and humidity (e.g., 95°F and 90% humidity) can be as dangerous as extreme cold.

Increased body temperature associated with dehydration is evident when the amount of water loss only exceeds 2% of body weight, especially in hot weather. This dehydration then leads to a decline in endurance, strength, and overall performance. Wearing football equipment in hot weather can lead to a loss of 2% of body weight in 30 minutes. Marathon runners have been shown to lose 6 to 10% of body weight during a race.

Common symptoms of heat exhaustion include profuse sweating, headache, dizziness, nausea, vomiting, muscle weakness, visual disturbances, and flushing of the skin. A person with heat exhaustion should be taken to a cool environment immediately, and excess clothing should be removed. The body should be sponged with tap water. Fluid replacement, as tolerated, then should suffice to correct the condition.[6]

Heat cramps are a frequent complication of heat exhaustion, but they may appear without other symptoms of dehydration. Cramps usually occur in individuals who have experienced significant sweating from exercising for several hours in a hot climate and who have consumed a large volume of water without replacing sodium losses. It is important not to confuse heat cramps with other forms of muscle cramps, such as those caused by GI tract upset. Heat cramps occur in skeletal muscles, including those of the abdomen and extremities. They consist of a contraction lasting 1 to 3 minutes at a time. The cramp moves down the muscle and is associated with excruciating pain. The best way to prevent heat cramps is to exercise moderately at first and to have adequate salt intake before engaging in long, strenuous activity in the heat, and to not become dehydrated.[6]

Heatstroke can occur when the internal body temperature reaches 104°F or more. Related symptoms include nausea, confusion, irritability, poor coordination, seizures, and coma. Exertional heatstroke results from high blood flow to exercising muscles, which overloads the body's cooling capacity. Sweating generally ceases, and the body temperature may become dangerously high. If left untreated, circulatory collapse, nervous system damage, and death are likely. The death rate from heat stroke is high, approximately 10%.[6]

Many individuals faint during heatstroke, and their skin becomes hot and dry. Cooling the skin with ice packs or cold water is the usual recommended immediate treatment until medical help can be summoned. To decrease the risk of developing heatstroke, athletes should watch for rapid changes in body (2% or more), replace lost fluids, and avoid exercising under extremely hot, humid conditions.

Athletes must avoid becoming dehydrated because dehydration during exercise sets the stage for heat exhaustion, heat cramps, and potentially fatal heatstroke. Fluid intake during exercise, when possible, should be adequate to minimize loss in body weight; following this practice is a good idea even when sweating can go unnoticed, such as when swimming or during the winter.[5]

The recommended fluid status goal is a loss of no more than 2% of body weight during exercise, especially in hot weather. Athletes should first calculate 2% of their body weight and then by trial and error determine how much fluid they must drink to avoid losing more than this amount of weight during exercise. This determination will be most accurate if an athlete is weighed before and after a typical workout. For every 1 lb (1/2 kg) lost, 2 1/2 to 3 cups (about 0.75 liters) of water should be consumed during exercise or immediately afterward. Experts now recommend a total of 2 1/2 to 3 cups (0.75 liters) of water per pound lost, rather than the previous recommendation of 2 cups per pound, because some of the fluid replacement will quickly be lost from increased sweating after exercise and increased urine output. Much of this fluid replacement will have to take place after exercise because it is difficult to consume enough fluid during exercise to prevent weight loss. If weight change can't be monitored, urine color is another measure of hydration status. Urine color should be no more yellow than that of lemonade.[19]

Thirst is a late sign of dehydration and so is not a reliable indicator of an athlete's need to replace fluid during exercise. An athlete who drinks only when thirsty is likely to take 48 hours to replenish fluid loss. After several days of training, an athlete relying on thirst as an indicator can build up a fluid debt that will impair performance.

Fluid Replacement Strategies

The following fluid replacement approach can meet athletes' fluid needs in most cases:[2]

- Freely drink beverages (e.g., water, diluted fruit juice, sports drinks) during the 24-hour period before an event, even if not particularly thirsty.
- Drink 1 1/2 to 2 1/2 cups of fluid (400 to 600 ml) 2 to 3 hours before exercise. This allows time for both adequate hydration and excretion of excess fluid.
- During events lasting more than 30 minutes, consume about 1/2 to 1 1/2 cups (150 to 350 ml) of fluid every 15 to 20 minutes beginning at the start of the exercise. Consuming more than 1 quart (1 liter) per hour can cause discomfort. On hot days, cold drinks are preferable to help cool the body. Again, athletes should not wait until they feel thirsty. In many cases, athletes, especially children and teenagers, need to be reminded to drink.
- Within 4 to 6 hours after exercise, about 2 1/2 to 3 cups of fluid should be consumed for every pound lost. It is also important that weight be restored before the next exercise period. Skipping fluids before or during events will almost certainly impair performance. Note also that because caffeine has a dehydrating effect on the body, fluids containing it should not be part of any hydration plan before, during, or after exercise. Alcoholic beverages also have a diuretic effect.

Use of Sports Drinks

A question that often arises is whether athletes should drink water or a sports-type carbohydrate-electrolyte drink (e.g., All Sport, Exceed Energy Drink, Gatorade, PowerAde, or Amino Force) during competition (Figure 14-9). For sports that require

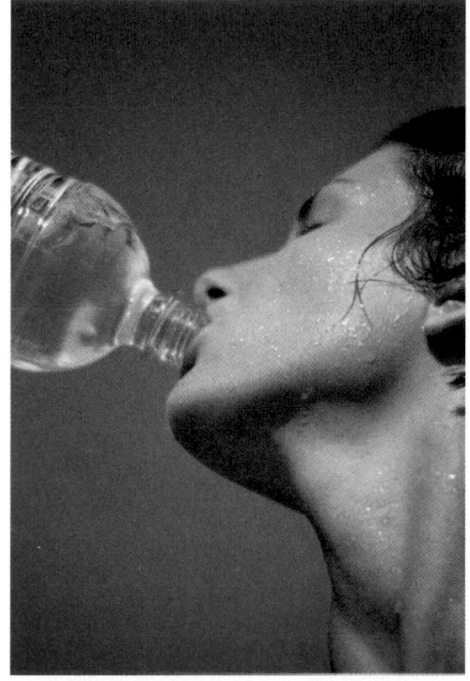

Fluid intake during exercise is important.

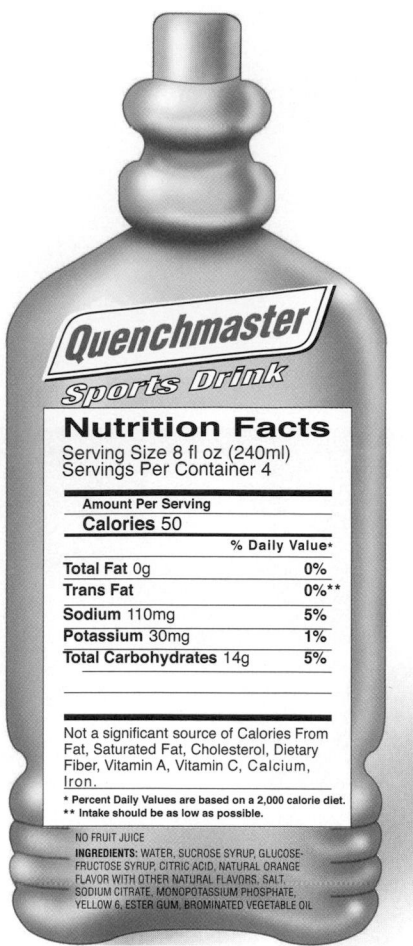

Figure 14-9 | Sports drinks for fluid and electrolyte replacement typically contain simple carbohydrates plus sodium and potassium. The various sugars in this product total 14 g/cup (240 ml) serving. In percentage terms based on weight, the sugar content is about 6% ([14 g sugar per serving ÷ 240 g per serving] × 100 = 5.8%). Sports drinks typically contain about 6 to 8% sugar. This provides ample glucose and other monosaccharides to aid in fueling working muscles, and it is well tolerated. Drinks with a sugar content above 10%, such as soft drinks or fruit juices, may cause stomach distress and so are not recommended.

less than 60 minutes of exertion or when total weight loss is less than 5 to 6 lb, the primary concern is replacing the water lost in sweat because losses of carbohydrate stores and electrolytes (sodium, chloride, potassium, and other minerals) are not usually very great. Although electrolytes are lost in sweat, the quantities lost in brief to moderate duration exercise can be easily replaced later by consuming normal foods such as orange juice, potatoes, and tomato juice. Keep in mind that sweat is about 99% water and only 1% electrolytes and other substances.

When exercise extends beyond 60 minutes, electrolyte (especially sodium) and carbohydrate replacement becomes increasingly important.[5] Use of sports drinks during these longer bouts of exercise—even more so in hot weather—can offer several distinct advantages over water alone.

Water by itself, as you have learned, increases blood volume to allow for efficient cooling and transport of potential cellular fuels and waste products. The addition of carbohydrate to a sports drink supplies glucose to muscles as they become depleted of glycogen and thus can enhance performance when administered during endurance activities (see the later section on carbohydrate replacement). The electrolytes in sports drinks help maintain blood volume, enhance the absorption of water and carbohydrate from the intestine, and stimulate thirst. For these reasons, some experts prefer sports drinks over water for all athletes.

Overall, the decision to use a sports drink hinges primarily on the duration of the activity. As the projected duration of continuous activity approaches 60 minutes or longer, the advantages of a sports drink over plain water clearly emerge. However, athletes should first experiment with sports drinks during practice instead of trying them for the first time during competition.[19]

It is also possible for some athletes to drink too much water. Endurance athletes (especially poorly trained individuals) may compete at relatively low exercise intensities for prolonged periods of time and therefore may not sweat as much as they think they will. Thus, water losses are not very high. In addition, some of these athletes use one-half strength Coca-Cola as their fluid-replacement beverage, which is relatively low in sodium, and they drink this at every rest stop. This combination leads to an eventual fall in blood sodium, which is not desirable (note that a fall in blood sodium can occur in both hot and cold weather). Drinking less fluid, choosing a sports drink containing sodium (usually in the form of sodium chloride), and not gaining weight during the activity can help prevent this problem.[1]

Specialized Dietary Advice for before, during, and after Endurance Exercise

A light meal supplying up to 1000 kcal should be eaten about 2 to 4 hours before an endurance event to top off muscle and liver glycogen stores, prevent hunger during the event, and provide extra fluid. The longer the period before an event, the larger the meal can be, because there will be more time available for digestion. A pre-event meal should consist primarily of carbohydrate (about 200 g), have little fat or fiber, and include a moderate amount of protein (Table 14-7). A meal eaten 1 hour or so before an event should be blended or liquid to promote rapid stomach emptying. Examples are low-fat smoothies, juices, and sports drinks.[19]

Good food choices for a pre-event meal include spaghetti, muffins, bagels, pancakes with fresh fruit topping, oatmeal with fruit, baked potato topped with yogurt or a small amount of sour cream, toasted bread with jam, bananas, apples, oranges, pears, plums, nuts, and low-sugar breakfast cereals with reduced-fat or fat-free milk. Liquid meal-replacement formulas, such as Carnation Instant Breakfast, also can be used. Foods especially rich in fiber should be eaten the previous day to help empty the colon before an event, but they should not be eaten the night before or in the morning before the event. Foods to avoid are those that are fatty or fried, such as sausage, bacon, sauces, and gravies.

Table 14-7 | Convenient Pre-event Meals

Breakfast

Cheerios, 3/4 cup	450 kcal
Reduced-fat milk, 1 cup	82% carbohydrate
Blueberry muffin, 1	(92 g)
Orange juice, 4 oz	
or	
Low-fat fruit yogurt, 1 cup	482 kcal
Plain bagel, 1/2	68% carbohydrate
Apple juice, 4 oz	(84 g)
Peanut butter (for bagel), 1 tbsp	
or	
Whole-wheat toast, 1 slice	507 kcal
Jam, 1 tsp	73% carbohydrate
Apple, 1 large	(98 g)
Reduced-fat milk, 1 cup	
Oatmeal, 1/2 cup (with reduced-fat milk, 1/2 cup)	

Lunch or Dinner

Chili; with beans, 8 oz	900 kcal
Baked potato with sour cream and chives	65% carbohydrate
Chocolate milk shake	(150 g)
or	
Spaghetti noodles, 2 cups	761 kcal
Spaghetti sauce, 1 cup	66% carbohydrate
Reduced-fat milk, 1 1/2 cups	(129 g)
Green beans, 1 cup	
or	
Orange, 1 large	829 kcal
Reduced-fat milk, 1 1/2 cups	70% carbohydrate
Chicken noodle soup, 1 cup	(160 g)
Saltine crackers, 12	
Buttered beans, 1 cup	
Corn, 1 cup	
Angel food cake, 1 slice	

The rule of thumb when timing preactivity meals is to allow 4 hours for a big meal (about 1200 kcal), 3 hours for a moderate meal (about 800 to 900 kcal), 2 hours for a light meal (about 400 to 600 kcal), and an hour or less for a snack (about 300 kcal).

Rule of Thumb for Approximate Pre-event Carbohydrate Intake

Hours Before	Grams per kilogram Body Weight	For a 70-kg Person
1	1	70
2	2	140
3	3	210
4	4	280

Replenishing Fuel during Endurance Exercise

For sporting events that are longer than 60 minutes, consumption of carbohydrate during activity can improve athletic performance because prolonged exercise depletes muscle glycogen stores and low levels of blood glucose lead to fatigue, both physical and mental.[5] Recall that when the supply of energy from carbohydrates runs low, athletes often complain of "hitting the wall," the point at which maintaining a competitive pace seems impossible. One way to overcome this obstacle is to maintain normal blood glucose concentrations by carbohydrate feedings. A general guideline for endurance events is to consume 30 to 60 g of carbohydrate per hour; however, an athlete should experiment during training sessions to establish the level that leads to optimal performance.[5]

In the previous section on fluid needs, you learned that sports drinks are a good source of carbohydrates for endurance events. They supply the necessary fluid, electrolytes, and carbohydrate to keep athletes performing at their best. As an alternative to sports drinks, some athletes have begun to use carbohydrate gels (e.g., PowerGel and Clif Shot) and energy bars (e.g., PowerBar). Check the label on these products to gauge the amount of gel or bar that provides 30 to 60 g of carbohydrate per hour. Gels contain about 25 g of carbohydrate per serving, and depending on the type, popular

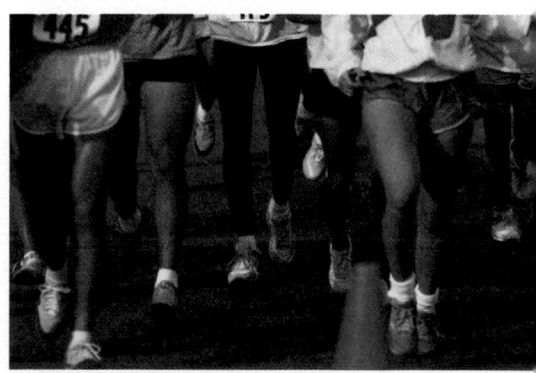

Carbohydrate intake during endurance exercise helps maintain this source of energy for the body.

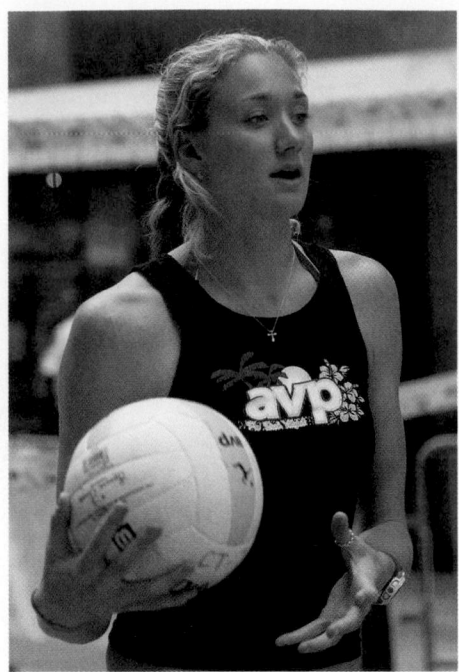

Elite athletes such as Olympic beach volleyball gold medal winner Kerri Walsh are well aware that modifying their diet and training regimen to match up with the specific needs of their sport is key to optimum performance. Replenishing carbohydrate and fluids is especially important when training.

Table 14-8 | Energy and Macronutrient Contents of Popular Energy Bars and Gels

Product	Energy (kcal)	Carbohydrates (g)	Protein (g)	Fat (g)
PowerBar Performance (chocolate)	230	45	10	2
PowerBar ProteinPlus (cookies & cream)	230	38	24	5
PowerBar PowerGel (lemon lime)	110	28	0	0
Luna Bar (cherry-covered chocolate)	180	28	10	4
Clif Bar (chocolate chip)	250	45	10	5
Clif Shot (viva vanilla)	100	24	0	0
Balance Bar (chocolate)	200	22	14	6
Balance Satisfaction (chocolate crisp)	280	47	12	6
Boulder Bar (chocolate)	210	42	10	4

Choosing energy bars is preferable to choosing candy bars and packaged cakes. When used in sports situations, energy bars can be handy. Better yet, however, is to eat a variety of wholesome foods; these offer more health-protective compounds. They are also a less expensive choice, especially for day-to-day snacking.

energy bars range from 2 to 45 g of carbohydrate per serving (Table 14-8). Sports drinks, by comparison, contain about 14 g of carbohydrate per 8-oz serving. The wide range of carbohydrate content in energy bars is due to a variety of marketing trends in the sports supplement industry.

Overall, choosing a bar with about 40 g of carbohydrate and no more than 10 g of protein, 4 g of fat, and 5 g of fiber is recommended. The bars are also typically fortified with vitamins and minerals, often to 100% of the Daily Values. As such, these bars can be seen as a convenient, although somewhat expensive, source of nutrients.

If the athlete prefers solid sources of carbohydrate, fig cookies, Gummy Bears, and jellybeans yield a quick source of glucose with a much lower cost. However, any carbohydrate-containing food, including energy bars and gels, must be accompanied by fluid to ensure adequate hydration.[19]

When regularly consuming energy bars, be aware of your overall micronutrient intake. Many energy bars are fortified with amounts of micronutrients such as vitamin A and iron that could be toxic if several bars are consumed in a day.

Carbohydrate Intake during Recovery from Prolonged Exercise

Carbohydrate-rich foods providing 1 to 2 g of carbohydrate per kg of body weight should be consumed within 2 hours after extended (endurance) exercise, the sooner the better (Table 14-9). Immediately after exercise is when glycogen synthesis is greatest, because the muscles are very insulin-sensitive at this point.[19] This process should then be repeated over the next 2-hour interval. Athletes who are training hard can consume a simple sugar candy, sugared soft drink, fruit or fruit juice, or a sports-type carbohydrate supplement right after training as they attempt to reload their muscles with glycogen. Later, bread, mashed potatoes, and rice can contribute to additional carbohydrate consumption. All these high-glycemic-load carbohydrates especially contribute to glycogen synthesis (recall that Table 5-4 shows the glycemic load of various foods). Adding some rich protein sources may also be considered, with carbohydrate to protein in about a 3:1 ratio. This inclusion is especially useful if the greater food choices allowed help the athlete meet overall energy needs. For a 154-lb (70-kg) athlete, this ratio corresponds to about 70 g of carbohydrate and 25 g of protein in each 2-hour interval. In summary, the following are key factors for achieving the most rapid replenishment of muscle glycogen after exercise: (1) availability of adequate carbohy-

Table 14-9 | Sample Postexercise Meals for Rapid Muscle Glycogen Replacement

Option 1
bagel, 1 regular
peanut butter, smooth, 2 tbsp
fat-free milk, 8 oz
banana, 1 medium
562 kcal, 77 g carbohydrate, 23 g protein, 18 g fat

Option 2
Carnation Instant Breakfast, 1 packet
fat-free milk, 8 oz
banana, 1 medium
peanut butter, 1 tbsp
Blend until smooth
438 kcal, 70 g carbohydrate, 17 g protein, 10 g fat

Option 3
GatorPro, 1.5 cans (11 fl oz per can)
559 kcal, 89 g carbohydrate, 26 g protein, 11 g fat

drate, (2) ingestion of carbohydrate as soon as possible after completion of exercise, and (3) selection of high-glycemic-load carbohydrates.

Fluid and electrolyte intake is also an essential component of an athlete's recovery diet.[2] Replenishing body fluids as quickly as possible is especially important if two workouts a day are performed or if the environment is hot and humid. If food and fluid intake is sufficient to restore weight loss, it generally will also supply enough electrolytes to meet needs during recovery from endurance activities.

Concept | Check

All athletes would do well to follow a well-balanced diet. High-carbohydrate foods should be emphasized and should dominate in pre-event meals. Protein intake above 1.7 g/kg of body weight is not supported by scientific evidence. Most athletes easily consume enough protein from typical food choices. If nutrient supplements are used, dosages generally should not exceed the Upper Level for each nutrient. Fluid should be consumed as liberally as possible before, during, and after an event. Carbohydrate and electrolytes in the fluid help delay fatigue and maintain electrolyte balance when exercise duration exceeds 60 minutes.

Case Scenario| Follow-Up

Marcella is correct in following a high-carbohydrate diet. However, in her effort to minimize her fat intake, she is probably not consuming enough energy, protein, iron, or calcium to support her training routine. She has fallen into the bagel, pasta, and pretzel routine that sports nutritionists warn is not conducive to peak performance. Marcella's performance would improve if she also had a high-protein food at each meal. She could include milk with breakfast and possibly some low-fat yogurt or low-fat cheese at lunch. She should have a carbohydrate/protein snack before her workout, such as half a sandwich with fruit and some water. The sandwich and fruit will help provide her with fuel to support her vigorous training. During her workouts, she could consume a sports drink to meet fluid needs and supply some carbohydrate, or she could consume water along with a few fig cookies or other high-carbohydrate food. In the evenings, she could substitute cheese and crackers for the pretzels to improve protein intake. Overall, it is important for Marcella to fuel her body before, during, and after workouts.

Any nutrition strategies should be tested during practice and trial runs before being used in a meet or key event. An athlete should never try a new food or beverage on the day of competition. Some food items and beverages may not be well tolerated, and the day of competition is not the time to find this out.

Why hasn't fat been mentioned as a way to improve athletic performance during an endurance event? Although it is true that fat is used along with carbohydrate as fuel during prolonged aerobic activity, the processes of digestion, absorption, and metabolism of fat are relatively slow. Therefore, consumption of fat during activity is not likely to translate into better athletic performance.

For more information on sports nutrition, visit the Gatorade Sport Science Institute web page (www.gssiweb.com). For more information on sports medicine, visit www.physsportsmed.com. This home page of *The Physician and Sportsmedicine* journal details current issues in sports medicine, including injury prevention, nutrition, and exercise. Also helpful are the web pages of the American College of Sports Medicine (www.acsm.org), Centers for Disease Control and Prevention (www.cdc.gov/nccdphp/dnpa), and the American Council on Exercise (www.acefitness.org).

NUTRITION FOCUS

Evaluating Ergogenic Aids to Enhance Athletic Performance

ergogenic Work-producing. An ergogenic aid is a mechanical, nutritional, psychological, pharmacological, or physiological substance or treatment that is intended to directly improve exercise performance.

Critical | Thinking

How would you advise someone who was planning to buy a purported "muscle-building" protein supplement? What risks are important to point out?

Extreme diet manipulation to improve athletic performance is not a recent innovation. Thirty years ago, American football players were encouraged on hot practice days to "toughen up" for competition by liberally consuming salt tablets before and during practice and by not drinking water. Now it is widely recognized that this practice can be fatal. Today's athletes are as likely as their predecessors to experiment with artichoke hearts, bee pollen, dried adrenal glands from cattle, seaweed, freeze-dried liver flakes, gelatin, and ginseng. These are just some of the ineffective substances used by athletes in hopes of gaining an **ergogenic** (work-producing) edge.

Today's athletes can benefit from recent scientific evidence documenting the ergogenic properties of a few dietary substances. These ergogenic aids include sufficient water and electrolytes, lots of carbohydrates, and a balanced and varied diet.[19] Protein and amino acid supplements are not among those aids because athletes can easily meet protein needs from foods, as Table 14-4 demonstrated. The use of nutrient supplements should be designed to meet a specific dietary shortcoming, such as an inadequate iron intake. These and other aids, which often have dubious benefits and may pose health risks, must be given close scrutiny before use. The risk-benefit ratio of any ergogenic aid merits careful evaluation.[19]

As summarized in Table 14-10, no scientific evidence supports the effectiveness of many substances touted as performance-enhancing aids. Many are useless; some are dangerous. Athletes should be skeptical of any substance until its ergogenic effect is scientifically verified. FDA has a limited ability to regulate dietary supplements (review Chapter 1), and the manufacturing processes for dietary supplements are not as tightly regulated by FDA as they are for prescription drugs. Some supplements may contain substances that will cause athletes to test positive for various banned substances. This problem was demonstrated in the 2002 Winter Olympics. Recent studies also have called into question the quality control associated with the manufacturing of dietary supplements. Many do not contain the substance and/or the amount listed on the label. These results add yet another worry for the athlete.

The NCAA's Committee on Competitive Safeguards and Medical Aspects of Sports has developed lists of supplements that are permissible and nonpermissible for athletic departments to dispense. Following are key examples:

Permissible	Nonpermissible
Vitamins and minerals	Amino acids
Energy bars (if no more than 30% protein)	Creatine Glycerol
Sports drinks	HMB
Meal replacement drinks such as Ensure Plus or Boost	L-carnitine Protein powders

Even approved substances that have been supported by systematic scientific studies should be used with caution, because the testing conditions may not match those of the intended use. Finally, rather than waiting for a magic bullet to enhance performance, athletes are advised to concentrate their efforts on improving their training routines and sport techniques while consuming well-balanced diets as described throughout this book.

Table 14-10 | An Evaluation of Ergogenic Aids Currently in the Limelight

Substance/Practice	Rationale	Reality
Useful in Some Circumstances		
Creatine	Increase phosphocreatine (PCr) in muscles to keep ATP concentration high	Use of 20 g per day for 5 to 6 days and then a maintenance dose of 2 g per day may improve performance in athletes who undertake repeated bursts of activity, such as in sprinting and weight lifting. Vegetarian athletes may especially show benefits because creatine is low or nonexistent in their diets. Some of the muscle weight gain noted with use results from water contained in muscles. Endurance athletes do not benefit from use. Little is known about the safety of long-term creatine use. Continual use of high doses has led to kidney damage in a few cases (two to date). Cost: $25 to $65 per month.
Sodium Bicarbonate (baking soda)	Counter lactic acid buildup	Partially effective in some circumstances in which lactate is rapidly produced such as wrestling, but induces nausea and diarrhea. The dose used is 300 mgs/kg, given 1 to 3 hours before exercise. Cost: nil.

Table 14-10 | An Evaluation of Ergogenic Aids Currently in the Limelight *(continued)*

Substance/Practice	Rationale	Reality
Useful in Some Circumstances		
Caffeine	Increase use of fatty acids to fuel muscles, promote psychological effects	Drinking two to three 5-ounce cups of coffee (equivalent to 3 to 9 milligrams of caffeine per kilogram of body weight) about 1 hour before events lasting about 5 minutes or longer is useful for some athletes; benefits are less apparent in those who have ample stores of glycogen, are highly trained, or habitually consume caffeine; intake of more than about 600 milligrams (six to eight cups of coffee) elicits a urine concentration illegal under NCAA rules (greater than 15 micrograms per milliliter). A possible side effect is reduced body hydration and shakiness. Cost: $0.08 per 300 mg.
Possibly Useful, Still Under Study		
Beta-hydroxy-beta methylbutyric acid (HMB)	Decrease protein catabolism, causing a net growth-promoting effect	Research in livestock and humans suggests that supplementation with this substance may increase muscle mass. Still, safety and effectiveness of long-term HMB use in humans is unknown. Cost: $100 per month.
Glutamine (an amino acid)	Enhance immune function, preserve lean body mass	Some preliminary studies show decreased occurrence of upper respiratory tract infections in athletes with use. It also may promote muscle growth, but long-term studies are lacking. Protein foods are a rich source of glutamine. Cost: $10 to $20 per month for 1 to 2 g per day.
Branched-chain amino acids (BCAA) (leucine, isoleucine, valine)	Important energy source, especially when carbohydrate stores are depleted	Supplementation of BCAA (10 to 30 g/day) during exercise can increase BCAA in the blood when levels are low due to exercise but there is no consistent evidence of improved performance. Carbohydrate feeding, by delaying use of BCAA as fuel, may negate the need for BCAA supplementation. Preliminary studies show that BCAA use increases muscle mass more than does carbohydrate supplementation alone in swimmers, but there are no studies regarding resistance training. Protein-rich foods (especially dairy proteins) are rich in BCAA. Cost: $20 per month.
Glucosamine	Aid in repair of joint damage	Most of the positive evidence is for repair of knee damage in older people, but a recent large scale trial showed no clear benefit for such use. May be of use to athletes experiencing knee damage, but again reliable evidence is lacking. Cost: $30 per month.
Dangerous or Illegal Substances/Practices		
Anabolic steroids (and related substances, such as androstenedione and tetrahydrogestrinone [THG])	Increase muscle mass and strength	Although effective for increasing protein synthesis, anabolic steroids are illegal in the United States unless prescribed by a physician. They have numerous potential side effects such as premature closure of growth plates in bones (possibly limiting potential height of a teenage athlete), bloody cysts in the liver, increased risk of cardiovascular disease, increased blood pressure, and reproductive dysfunction. Possible psychological consequences include increased aggressiveness, drug dependence (addiction), withdrawal symptoms (such as depression), sleep disturbances, and mood swings (known as "roid rage"). Use of needles for injectable forms adds further health risk. Banned by the International Olympic Committee and many professional sports organizations.
Growth hormone	Increase muscle mass	May increase height; at critical ages may also cause uncontrolled growth of the heart and other internal organs and even death; potentially dangerous; requires careful monitoring by a physician. Use of needles for injections adds further health risk. Banned by the International Olympic Committee.
Blood doping	To enhance aerobic capacity by injecting red blood cells harvested previously from the athlete, or alternately the athlete may use the hormone erythropoietin (Epogen) to increase red blood cell number	May offer aerobic benefit, very serious health consequences are possible, including thickening of the blood, which puts extra strain on the heart, is an illegal practice under Olympic guidelines.
Gamma hydroxybutyric acid (GHB)	Promoted as a steroid alternative for body-building	FDA has never approved it for sale as a medical product; is illegal to produce or sell GHB in the United States. GHB-related symptoms include vomiting, dizziness, tremors, and seizures. Many victims have required hospitalization, and some have died. Clandestine laboratories produced virtually all the chemical accounting for GHB abuse. FDA is working with the U.S. Attorney's office to arrest, indict, and convict individuals responsible for the illegal operations.

Substances that are promoted to athletes but have yet to show any clear ergogenic effects include pyruvic acid (pyruvate), glycerol, ribose, chromium, coenzyme Q-10, medium chain triglycerides, L-carnitine, conjugated linoleic acid (CLA), bovine colostrum, insulin, and amino acids not already mentioned in this section. Any use of these products is not recommended at this time. Note that some of these substances are defined in the glossary.

Summary

1. A gradual increase in regular physical activity is recommended for all healthy persons. A minimum plan includes 30 minutes of physical activity on most (or all) days; 60 to 90 minutes per day provides even more benefit, especially if weight control is an issue. An intense program should begin with warm-up exercises to increase blood flow and warm the muscles and should end with cooldown exercises. Regular resistance activities and stretching add further benefits.

2. Human metabolic pathways extract chemical energy from food and transform it into ATP, the compound that provides energy for body functions.

3. In glycolysis, glucose is broken down into the three-carbon compound pyruvic acid, yielding some ATP. This compound is metabolized further via the aerobic pathway to form carbon dioxide (CO_2) and water (H_2O) or via the anaerobic pathway to form lactic acid.

4. At rest, muscle cells mainly use fat for fuel. For intense exercise of short duration, muscles mostly use phosphocreatine (PCr) for energy. During more sustained intense activity, muscle glycogen breaks down to lactic acid, providing a small amount of ATP. For endurance exercise, both fat and carbohydrate are used as fuels; carbohydrate is used increasingly as activity intensifies. Little protein is used to fuel muscles.

5. $VO_{2\ max}$ is a measure of the maximum volume of oxygen one can consume per unit of time. Oxygen consumption is measured by exercising the subject at an increasing pace and workload until fatigue occurs. The amount of oxygen consumed right before total exhaustion is $VO_{2\ max}$. The value of $VO_{2\ max}$ varies among individuals but usually improves with exercise training.

6. Anyone who exercises regularly should consume a diet that meets energy needs, is moderate to high in carbohydrates and fluid, and is adequate in other nutrients such as iron and calcium.

7. Athletes should consume enough fluid to both minimize loss of body weight and ultimately restore preexercise weight. Sports drinks help replace fluid, electrolyte, and carbohydrate replacement. Their use is especially appropriate when continuous activity lasts beyond 60 minutes.

8. Plenty of carbohydrates should be in the pre-event meal, especially for endurance athletes. High-glycemic-load carbohydrates should be consumed by an athlete within 2 hours after a workout to begin restoration of muscle glycogen stores.

Study Questions

1. How does greater physical fitness contribute to greater overall health? Explain the process.

2. ATP storage in muscle is rapidly depleted once muscle contraction begins. For physical activity to continue, ATP must be resupplied immediately. Describe how resupply occurs after initiation of exercise and at various times thereafter.

3. What is the difference between anaerobic and aerobic exercise? Explain why aerobic metabolism is increased by a regular exercise routine.

4. What is glycogen? How is it used during exercise?

5. Is fat from adipose tissue used as an energy source during exercise? If so, when?

6. What are some typical measures used to assess whether an athlete's energy intake is adequate?

7. List five specific nutrients that athletes need and the appropriate food sources from which these nutrients can be obtained.

8. What conditions might contribute to the inability to get all required nutrients from food, thus requiring use of a multivitamin and mineral supplement?

9. What advice would you give your neighbor, who is planning to run a 5-kilometer (km) race, concerning fluid intake before and during the event?

10. One of your friends, a competitive athlete, asks your opinion about an amino acid supplement sold in a local sporting-goods store. She has read that such supplements can help improve athletic performance. What would you tell her about the general effectiveness of such products?

BOOST YOUR STUDY

Check out the **Perspectives in Nutrition: Online Learning Center** www.mhhe.com/wardlawpers7 for quizzes, flash cards, activities, and web links designed to further help you learn about nutrition as it relates to fitness and sports.

Annotated References

1. Almond CSD and others: Hyponatremia among runners in the Boston Marathon. *The New England Journal of Medicine* 352:1550, 2005.
   Low blood sodium (technically called hyponatremia) is a potential problem if runners drink too much water during a prolonged race. This problem is especially seen in poorly trained runners in comparison to elite athletes. Any fluid replacement needs to be carefully monitored to avoid weight gain during prolonged physical activity.

2. American College of Sports Medicine and others: Nutrition and athletic performance. *Medicine and Science in Sports and Exercise* 32:2130, 2000.
   The athlete who wants to optimize exercise performance needs to follow good nutrition and hydration practices, use supplements and ergogenic aids carefully, minimize severe weight-loss practices, and eat a variety of foods in adequate amounts. The various recommendations for carbohydrate, protein, fat, vitamins, minerals, and fluids in Chapter 14 were taken from this article.

3. Bacon SL and others: Effects of exercise, diet, and weight loss on high blood pressure. *Sports Medicine* 34:307, 2004.

   Even when people with hypertension follow current diet recommendations for that condition, adding physical activity provides a further drop in blood pressure. There is also evidence from this study that numerous other improvements in cardiovascular health result when hypertensive people follow a program of regular physical activity.

4. Blair SN, Church TS: The fitness, obesity, and health equation. *Journal of the American Medical Association* 292:1232, 2004.

   Most of the health benefits from physical activity come with only 30 minutes at a moderate pace performed at least 5 days per week. These results are true for both lean and overweight individuals. Brisk walking, swimming, bicycling, or daily activities such as gardening and house work contribute to meeting this goal.

5. Coyle EF: Fluid and fuel intake during exercise. *Journal of Sports Science* 22:39, 2004.

   Regular fluid and carbohydrate intake are crucial to maintain performance during prolonged physical activity. In the postrecovery period, fluid, carbohydrate, and protein intake deserve the most attention in diet planning. The article provides the scientific support for such advice.

6. Glazer JL: Management of heat stroke and heat exhaustion. *American Family Physician* 71:2133, 2005.

   Heat exhaustion and heatstroke are common and preventable conditions that affect athletes (and other individuals such as older adults). Treatment of heat exhaustion involves putting the person in a cool, shady environment and ensuring adequate hydration. Treating heatstroke is much more complicated, as is outlined in the article.

7. Harber VJ: Energy balance and reproductive function in active women. *Canadian Journal of Applied Physiology* 29:48, 2004.

   It is very important for female athletes engaged in rigorous training programs to meet their energy needs. If not, the resulting negative energy balance will likely lead to a variety of menstrual cycle disturbances that can cause other health problems. The article discusses this issue in detail and provides treatment strategies for problems that may develop.

8. Hunter GR: Physical activity, fitness, and health. In Shils ME and others (eds): *Modern nutrition in health and disease.* 10th ed. Philadelphia, PA: Lippincott Williams & Wilkins, 2006.

   This chapter provides a synthesis of the physiology and related health advantages of regular physical activity.

9. Laaksonen DE and others: Physical activity in the prevention of type 2 diabetes: The Finnish Diabetes Prevention Study. *Diabetes* 54:158, 2005.

   Regular physical activity can substantially reduce the risk of developing type 2 diabetes in high-risk individuals. People who increased their activity from moderate to vigorous amounts reduce their risk of developing type 2 diabetes by 65% compared to people who remained inactive. Even typical low-intensity activities, such as walking, conferred similar benefits in this study.

10. Lukaski HC: Vitamin and mineral status: Effects on physical performance. *Nutrition* 20:632, 2004.

    Physically active people generally consume sufficient vitamins and minerals to support such activity. The clearest indication for use of vitamin and mineral supplements by athletes is to treat existing nutrition deficiencies or to bridge gaps in nutrient intake versus nutrient needs. Use of vitamin and mineral supplements does not improve measures of performance in people consuming adequate diets.

11. Make the most of your exercise minutes. *Consumer Reports on Health,* p. 1, November 2003.

    Key considerations when designing an exercise program are to include alternating bouts of vigorous and easier exercise to give muscles a chance to recover; alternating among exercises to work different muscles; and finding ways to make one's whole day more physically active. The article goes on to provide much guidance surrounding exercise protocols.

12. Nieman DC and others: Vitamin E and immunity after the Kona Triathlon World Championship. *Medicine and Science in Sports and Exercise* 36:1328, 2004.

    Athletes in this study who were provided 800 IU of vitamin E per day for two months before their triathlon event showed a greater degree of whole body oxidant damage compared to athletes who did not consume the supplement. The authors caution that megadose use of vitamin E supplements by athletes promotes lipid oxidation and inflammation during exercise, and so should not be recommended.

13. Powers SK and others: Dietary antioxidants and exercise. *Journal of Sports Sciences* 22:81, 2004.

    After careful review of the scientific literature, the authors could find little evidence for the effectiveness of antioxidant supplements in preventing exercise-related muscle damage. Therefore, they find that antioxidant supplements cannot be recommended at this time for athletes.

14. Ross R and others: Exercise-induced reduction in obesity and insulin resistance in women: A randomized control trial. *Obesity Research* 12:789, 2004.

    Following a regular exercise program for 14 weeks resulted in a reduction in total and abdominal obesity in this study. Adding caloric restriction to the exercise program was associated with even more substantial decrease in those parameters as well as a decrease in insulin resistance.

15. Sinclair LM, Hinton PS: Prevalence of iron deficiency with and without anemia in recreationally active men and women. *Journal of the American Dietetic Association* 105:975, 2005.

    Both male and female athletes are at risk of exhibiting poor iron stores and even iron deficiency anemia, with females being at much higher risk. The authors recommend that athletes be screened for iron deficiency anemia and also have their current state of iron storage tested. Poor iron status can lead to poor work performance and therefore should be avoided.

16. Thompson PD and others: Exercise and physical activity in the prevention and treatment of atherosclerotic cardiovascular disease. *Circulation* 107:3109, 2003.

    The American Heart Association supports the recommendation from the Centers for Disease Control and Prevention (CDC) and the American College of Sports Medicine (ACSM) that individuals should engage in 30 minutes or more of moderate-intensity physical activity (such as brisk walking) on most (preferably all) days of the week. Such activity is beneficial in both the prevention and treatment of cardiovascular disease.

17. Tipton KD, Wolfe RR: Protein and amino acids for athletes. *Journal of Sports Science* 22:65, 2004.

    A well-balanced diet can easily meet the protein needs of athletes. There is no need to consume more than 2 g of protein per kg of body weight, even for strength-training athletes. In fact, an intake of more than 1.7 g of protein per kg of body weight just results in the extra protein being used to meet energy needs.

18. Why everyone needs strength training. *UC Berkeley Wellness Letter,* p. 4, May 2004.

    Strength training is an important part of an overall active lifestyle. One to three sets of 8 to 15 repetitions is sufficient for a specific exercise.

19. Williams MH: *Nutrition for health, fitness, and sport.* 7th ed. Boston: McGraw-Hill, 2005.

    This textbook is excellent for reviewing nutrient needs of athletes as well as learning more about ergogenic aids; it also provides a detailed look at metabolism in exercise.

20. Zanker CL, Cooke CB: Energy balance, bone turnover, and skeletal health in physically active individuals. *Medicine and Science in Sports and Exercise* 36:1372, 2004.

    A physically active lifestyle contributes to maintenance of bone health; however, skeletal problems can result in underweight women who no longer have menstrual periods. The authors stress the importance for women to meet energy needs during exercise in order to avoid this problem. There is even some evidence that the same problem can happen in men who do not meet energy needs, but it is not specifically linked to a sex hormone deficiency, as it is in women. Thus, the key factor in the disturbance of skeletal health is a dietary energy deficit.

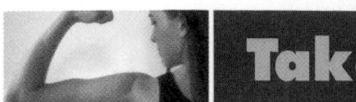

Take | Action

I. Meeting the Protein Needs of an Athlete—A Case Study

Mark is a college student who has been lifting weights at the student recreation center. The trainer at the center recommended a protein drink to help Mark build muscle mass. Answer the questions below about Mark's current food intake and determine whether a protein drink is needed to supplement Mark's diet.

The following is a tally of yesterday's intake. Use Appendix N or NutritionCalc Plus software to calculate Mark's protein intake.

Breakfast	Frosted Mini-Wheats cereal, 2 oz 1% milk, 11/2 cups Orange juice, chilled, 6 oz Glazed yeast doughnut, 1 Brewed coffee, 1 cup
Lunch	Double hamburger with condiments, 1 French fries, 30 Cola, 12 oz Medium apple, 1
Dinner	Frozen lasagna w/meat, 2 pieces 1% milk, 1 cup Looseleaf lettuce, chopped, 1 cup Creamy Italian salad dressing, 2 tsp Medium tomato, 1/2 Whole carrot, raw, 1
Evening snack	Vanilla ice milk, 1 cup Hot fudge chocolate topping, 2 tsp Soft chocolate chip cookies, 2

1. Mark's weight has been stable at 70 kg (154 lb). Determine his protein needs based on the RDA (0.8 g/kg).

    a. Mark's estimated protein RDA: _____

    b. What are the maximum recommendations for protein intake for athletes (see p. 534)? _____

    c. Calculate the maximum protein recommendation for Mark. _____

    _____

2. An analysis of the total energy and protein content of Mark's current diet is 3470 kcal, 125 g of protein (14% of total energy intake supplied by protein). This diet is representative of the food choices and amounts of food that Mark chooses on a regular basis.

    a. What is the difference between Mark's estimated protein needs as an athlete (from question 1) and the amount of protein that his current diet provides? _____

    b. Is his current protein intake inadequate, adequate, or excessive? _____

3. Mark takes his trainer's advice and goes to the supermarket to purchase a protein drink to add to his diet. Four products are available; they contain the following label information.

	Amino Fuel	Joe Weider's Sugar-Free 90% Plus Protein	Joe Weider's Dynamic Muscle Builder	Victory Super Mega Mass 2000
Serving size	3 tbsp	3 tbsp	3 tbsp	1/4 scoop
Kcal	104	110	103	104
Protein (g)	15	24	10	5

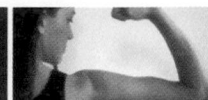

Take | Action

The trainer recommends that Mark add the supplement to his diet two times a day. Mark chooses Joe Weider's Dynamic Muscle Builder.

   a. How much protein would be added to Mark's diet daily from two servings of the supplement alone (prior to mixing it with a beverage)?

   b. Mark mixes the powder with the milk he already consumes at breakfast and dinner. How much protein total would Mark now consume in 1 day? (Add the protein amount from the nutrition analysis to the value from question 3a.)

   c. What is the difference between Mark's estimated protein needs as an athlete and this total value?

4. What is your conclusion—does Mark need the protein supplement?

Answers to Calculations

1a. Mark's estimated protein RDA: 70 kg $\times$ 0.8 g/kg = 56 g.
1b. Maximum recommendation for protein intake for athletes = 1.7 g/kg.
1c. Applied to Mark: 1.7 $\times$ 70 = 119 g.
2a. Difference between Mark's diet and the maximum amount recommended for athletes: 125 − 119 = 6 g.
2b. Mark's current diet is adequate.
3a. Two servings of protein supplement alone = 20 g of protein.
3b. Mark's total protein consumption: 125 g + 20 g = 145 g protein.
3c. Difference between Mark's estimated maximum protein needs as an athlete and total value (from 3b): 145 g − 119 g = 26 g of protein.

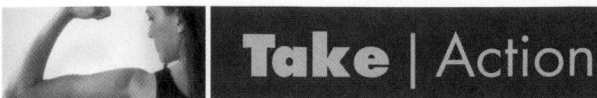

Take | Action

II. How Physically Fit Are You?

The fitness assessments presented here are easy to do and require little equipment. Also included are charts to compare your results to those typical of your peers.

Cardiovascular Fitness: One-Mile Walk

Measure a mile on a running track (usually four laps) or on a little-trafficked neighborhood street (use a car's odometer to get the right distance). With a stopwatch or watch with a second hand, walk the mile as fast as you can. Note the time it took.

Strength: Push-ups

Men: Get up on your toes and hands. Keep your back straight, with hands flat on the floor directly below your shoulders.
 Women: Same position, but you can support your body on your knees if necessary.
 Lower your body, bending your elbows, until your chin grazes the floor. Push back up until your arms are straight. Continue until you can't do any more push-ups (you can rest when in the up position).

Strength: Curl-ups

Lie on the floor on your back with your knees bent, feet flat. Your hands should rest on your thighs. Now squeeze your stomach muscles, push your back flat, and raise your upper body high enough for your hands to touch the tops of your knees. Don't pull with your neck or head, and keep your lower back on the floor. Count how many curl-ups you can do in one minute.

Flexibility: Sit-and-Reach

Place a yardstick on the floor and apply a two-foot piece of tape on the floor perpendicular to the yardstick, crossing at the 15-inch mark. Sit on the floor with your legs extended and the soles of your feet touching the tape at the 15-inch mark, the zero-inch facing you. Your feet should be about 12 inches apart. Put one hand on the other, exhale, and very slowly reach forward as far as you can along the yardstick, lowering your head between your arms. Don't bounce! Note the farthest inch mark you reach. Don't hurt yourself by reaching farther than your body wants to. Relax, and then repeat two more times.
 Now check your results. Want to improve? You know the answer:

- Do aerobic exercise that makes you breathe hard for at least half an hour on almost or all days of the week.
- Lift weights that challenge you two to three times per week.
- Stretch after activity at least a couple of times per week.
- Walk more.

Cardiovascular: One-mile walk (time, in minutes)

	Under 40		Over 40	
	Men	**Women**	**Men**	**Women**
Excellent	13:00 or less	13:30 or less	14:00 or less	14:30 or less
Good	13:01-15:30	13:31–16:00	14:01–16:30	14:31–17:00
Average	15:31-18:00	16:01–18:30	16:31–19:00	17:01–19:30
Below average	18:01-19:30	18:31–20:00	19:01–21:30	19:31–22:00
Poor	19:31 or more	20:01 or more	21:31 or more	22:01 or more

Source: Copper Institute

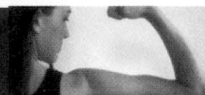

Take | Action

Strength: Push-ups (number completed without rest)

	Men					
Age	**17–19**	**20–29**	**30–39**	**40–49**	**50–59**	**60–65**
Excellent	>56	>47	>41	>34	>31	>30
Good	47–56	39–47	34–41	28–34	25–31	24–30
Above average	35–46	30–39	25–33	21–28	18–24	17–23
Average	19–34	17–29	13–24	11–20	9–17	6–16
Below average	11–18	10–16	8–12	6–10	5–8	3–5
Poor	4–10	4–9	2–7	1–5	1–4	1–2
Very poor	<4	<4	<2	0	0	0
	Women					
Age	**17–19**	**20–29**	**30–39**	**40–49**	**50–59**	**60–65**
Excellent	>35	>36	>37	>31	>25	>23
Good	27–35	30–36	30–37	25–31	21–25	19–23
Above average	21–27	23–29	22–30	18–24	15–20	13–18
Average	11–20	12–22	10–21	8–17	7–14	5–12
Below average	6–10	7–11	5–9	4–7	3–6	2–4
Poor	2–5	2–6	1–4	1–3	1–2	1
Very poor	0–1	0–1	0	0	0	0

Source: topendsports.com

Strength: Curl-ups (number completed in 60 seconds)

	Men					
Age	**18–25**	**26–35**	**36–45**	**46–55**	**56–65**	**65+**
Excellent	>49	>45	>41	>35	>31	>28
Good	44–49	40–45	35–41	29–35	25–31	22–28
Above average	39–43	35–39	30–34	25–28	21–24	19–21
Average	35–38	31–34	27–29	22–24	17–20	15–18
Below average	31–34	29–30	23–26	18–21	13–16	11–14
Poor	25–30	22–28	17–22	13–17	9–12	7–10
Very poor	<25	<22	<17	<9	<9	<7

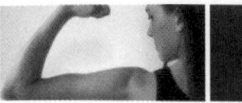

Take | Action

Strength: Curl-ups (number completed in 60 seconds) (con't)

	Women					
Age	**18–25**	**26–35**	**36–45**	**46–55**	**56–65**	**65+**
Excellent	>43	>39	>33	>27	>24	>23
Good	37–43	33–39	27–33	22–27	18–24	17–23
Above average	33–36	29–32	23–26	18–21	13–17	14–16
Average	29–32	25–28	19–22	14–17	10–12	11–13
Below average	25–28	21–24	15–18	10–13	7–9	5–10
Poor	18–24	13–20	7–14	5–9	3–6	2–4
Very poor	<18	<20	<7	<5	<3	<2

Source: topendsports.com

Flexibility: Sit-and-reach (in inches)

	Men	**Women**
Super	> +27	> +30
Excellent	+17–+27	+21–+30
Good	+6–+16	+11–+20
Average	0–+5	+1–+10
Fair	−8––1	−7–0
Poor	−19––9	−14––8
Very poor	< −20	< −15

Source: topendsports.com

These charts are typical charts used by health and fitness experts. For a more thorough assessment of fitness or for development of an exercise plan appropriate for your fitness level, consult a certified personal trainer or other fitness professional.

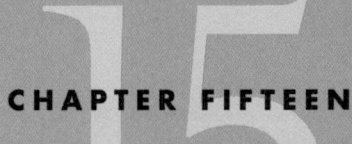

15

EATING DISORDERS: ANOREXIA NERVOSA, BULIMIA NERVOSA, BINGE-EATING DISORDER, AND OTHER CONDITIONS

CHAPTER OUTLINE

CASE SCENARIO:

At age 16, Sarah suddenly became self-conscious about her body when her friends teased her about being overweight. She began exercising to an aerobics video for an hour each day and found that she had success in losing weight; this was just the beginning of her obsession to be thin. Next, Sarah turned to eating less food to lose even more weight and began eliminating certain foods from her diet, such as candy and meat. She increased her water and vegetable intake and chewed sugarless gum to curb her appetite. Once she began dieting, stopping was impossible. She really enjoyed having a high degree of self-control over her body. She was literally obsessed with food and stared at others while they were eating a meal. She occasionally cooked large meals and then refused to eat all but a few bites. By the time Sarah was 19 years old and 5 feet 6 inches tall, her weight had dropped from 150 lb to 85 lb in 20 months. Her family was concerned about her weight status, and demanded that she go to a physician for an evaluation. Sarah was not happy about this idea but believed that her family would stop pestering her if she just went. Sarah did not think she had a problem; she truly thought she was still grotesquely overweight. She did notice, however, that she was intolerant of cold temperatures and was concerned that she had not menstruated in a year.

Does Sarah meet the qualifications to be diagnosed with an eating disorder? What types of therapy do you think the physician will suggest for Sarah? Where could she go for such therapy? What is the likelihood that she will fully recover from her condition?

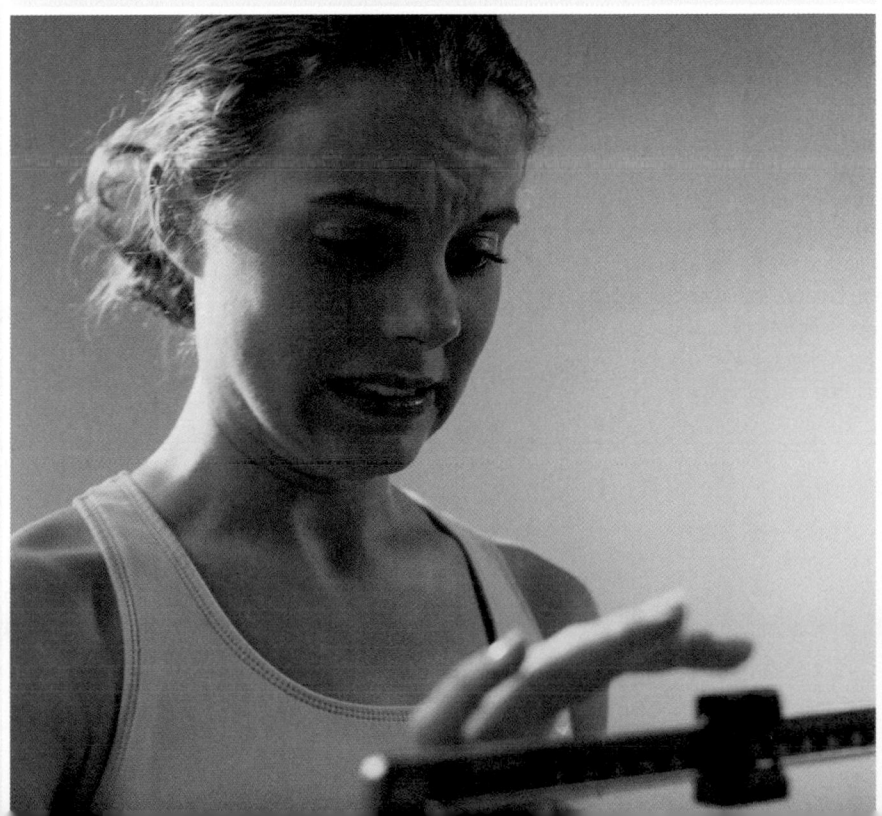

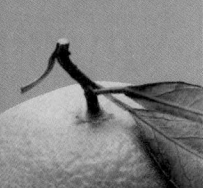

Although obesity is the most common eating disorder in our society, the eating disorders explored in this chapter involve much more severe distortions of the eating process. The eating disorders discussed here are just as serious and can develop into life-threatening conditions if left untreated.[20] What's most alarming about these disorders—such as anorexia nervosa, bulimia nervosa, and binge-eating disorder—is the increasing number of cases reported each year.[2]

Some people are more susceptible to these disorders than others—for genetic, psychological, and physical reasons. Successful treatment of eating disorders, therefore, is complex and must go beyond nutritional therapy.[5] And keep in mind also that eating disorders are not restricted to any socioeconomic class or ethnicity. They can occur at any age in both females and males. This chapter examines the causes and treatments of eating disorders in detail, because they touch many of our lives.

CHAPTER OBJECTIVES CHAPTER 15 IS DESIGNED TO ALLOW YOU TO:

1. Contrast health attitudes toward uses of food with behavior patterns that could lead to unhealthy uses of food.
2. Outline the causes of, effects of, typical persons affected by, and treatment for anorexia nervosa.
3. Outline the causes of, effects of, typical persons affected by, and treatment for bulimia nervosa.
4. Outline the causes of, effects of, typical persons affected by, and treatment for binge-eating disorder.
5. Relate the presence of eating disorders to current social trends.
6. Describe methods to reduce the development of eating disorders, including the use of warning signs to identify early cases.

REFRESH YOUR MEMORY AS YOU BEGIN YOUR STUDY OF EATING DISORDERS, SUCH AS ANOREXIA NERVOSA AND BULIMIA NERVOSA, IN CHAPTER 15, YOU MAY WANT TO REVIEW:

- The role of genetic risk in disease susceptibility in Chapter 1.
- The effects and treatment of osteoporosis in Chapter 11.
- The effects and treatment of iron deficiency anemia in Chapter 12.
- The distinction between hunger and appetite in Chapter 13.
- Calculation of BMI in Chapter 13.
- The effects of neurotransmitters on food intake in Chapter 13.

Early in life, we develop images of "acceptable" and "unacceptable" body types. Of all the attributes that constitute attractiveness, many people view body weight as the most important, partly because we can control our weight somewhat. Fatness is the most dreaded deviation from our cultural ideals of body image, the one most derided and shunned, even among schoolchildren.

From Ordered to Disordered Eating Habits

Eating—a completely instinctive behavior for animals—serves an extraordinary number of psychological, social, and cultural purposes for humans. Eating practices may take on religious meanings; signify bonds within families and ethnic groups; and be a means to express hostility, affection, prestige, or class values. Within the family, providing, preparing, and distributing food may be a means of expressing love, control, or even power.[1]

We are bombarded daily with images of society's "ideal" body. Television programs, billboard advertisements, magazine pictures, movies, and newspapers imply that an ultraslim body will bring happiness, love, and ultimately, success. This fantasy notion is especially ironic given the fact that much of society is becoming fatter. In response, some of us take an extreme approach—the pathological pursuit of weight control or weight loss.

Given the multiple relationships between normal eating and the media's bombardment of the ideal body image, it is not surprising that some people progress from normal eating patterns, to obsessive weight loss behaviors, and then to a full-blown eating disorder.[5]

Food: More Than Just a Source of Nutrients

From birth, we link food with personal and emotional experiences. As infants, we associate milk with security and warmth so the breast or bottle becomes a source of comfort as well as food. As noted in Chapter 1, most people continue to derive comfort and great pleasure from food. This comfort is both a biological and a psychological phenomenon. Food can be a symbol of comfort, but eating can also stimulate the release of certain neurotransmitters (e.g., serotonin) and natural opioids (including endorphins), which produce a sense of calm and euphoria in the human body. Thus, in times of great stress some people turn to food for a druglike, calming effect.

Food is also used as a reward or a bribe. Haven't you heard or spoken something similar to the following comments?

You can have your dessert if you eat five more bites of your vegetables.
You can't play until you clean your plate.
I'll eat the broccoli if you let me watch TV.
If you love me, you'll eat your dinner.

On the surface, using food as a reward or bribe seems harmless enough. Eventually, however, this practice encourages both caregivers and children to use food to achieve goals other than satisfying hunger and nutrient needs. Food may then become much more than a source of nutrients. Regularly using food as a bargaining chip can contribute to abnormal eating patterns. Carried to the extreme, these patterns can lead to **disordered eating.**[2]

Disordered eating can be defined as mild and short-term changes in eating patterns that occur in response to a stressful event, an illness, or a desire to modify the diet for a variety of health and personal appearance reasons. The problem may be no more than a bad habit, a style of eating adapted from friends or family members, or an aspect of preparing for athletic competition. While disordered eating can lead to weight loss or weight gain and to certain nutritional problems, it rarely requires in-depth professional attention. If, however, disordered eating becomes sustained, distressing, or starts to interfere with everyday activities due to physiological changes, professional intervention may be necessary.[1]

Overview of Anorexia Nervosa and Bulimia Nervosa

Given the common practice of dieting in North America, it is not obvious when disordered eating stops and an **eating disorder** begins. Indeed, many eating disorders start with a simple diet. Eating disorders then go on to involve physiological changes associated with food restricting, binge eating, purging, and fluctuations in weight. They also involve a number of emotional and cognitive changes that affect the way a person perceives and experiences his or her body, such as feelings of distress or extreme concern about body shape or weight.[20] Eating disorders are not due to a failure of will or behavior; rather, they are real, treatable medical illnesses in which certain maladaptive patterns of eating take on a life of their own.[18]

The main types of eating disorders are **anorexia nervosa** and **bulimia nervosa.** A third type, **binge-eating disorder,** has been recognized by the psychiatric community since 1994. Currently, scientists are researching whether binge-eating disorder should be included as a diagnosable disease alongside anorexia nervosa and bulimia nervosa.[3] More than 5 million people in North America have one of these disorders; females outnumber males 5 to 1. Eating disorders develop 85% of the time during adolescence or early adulthood, but some reports indicate that their onset can occur during childhood or later in adulthood. Eating disorders frequently co-occur with other psychological disorders such as depression, substance abuse, and anxiety disorders.[20] *People who suffer from eating disorders, especially anorexia nervosa and bulimia nervosa, can experience a wide range of physical health complications, including serious heart conditions and kidney failure, which may even lead to death.* Recognition of eating disorders as important and treatable diseases, therefore, is critical.[5]

Progression from Ordered to Disordered Eating

Attention to hunger and satiety signals; limitation of energy intake to restore weight to a healthful level

↓

Some disordered eating habits begin as weight loss is attempted, such as very restricted eating

↓

Clinically evident eating disorder recognized

disordered eating Mild and short-term changes in eating patterns that occur in relation to a stressful event, an illness, or a desire to modify one's diet for a variety of health and personal appearance reasons.

eating disorder Severe alterations in eating patterns linked to physiological changes. The alterations are associated with food restricting, binge eating, purging, and fluctuations in weight. They also involve a number of emotional and cognitive changes that affect the way a person perceives and experiences his or her body.

anorexia nervosa An eating disorder involving a psychological loss or denial of appetite followed by self-starvation; related in part to a distorted body image and to various social pressures commonly associated with puberty.

bulimia nervosa An eating disorder in which large quantities of food are eaten at one time (binge eating) and then purged from the body by vomiting or by misuse of laxatives, diuretics, or enemas. Alternate means to counteract the excess energy intake are fasting and excessive exercise.

binge-eating disorder An eating disorder characterized by recurrent binge eating and feelings of loss of control over eating that have lasted at least 6 months. Binge episodes can be triggered by frustration, anger, depression, anxiety, permission to eat forbidden foods, and excessive hunger.

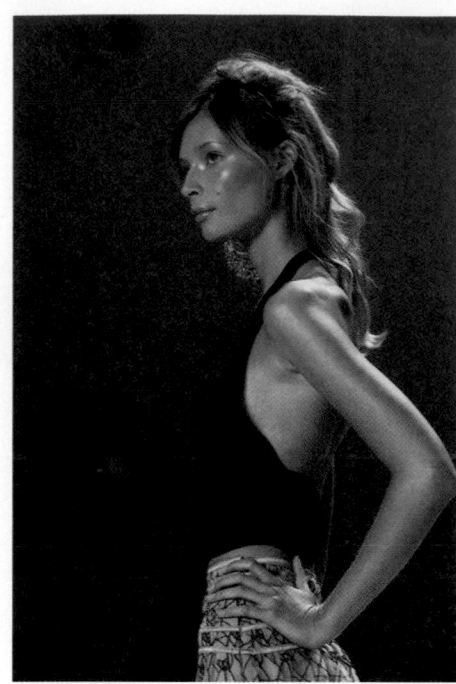

The media and the fashion world bombard us with body images that are unrealistic for most people.

hypergymnasia Exercising more than is required for good physical fitness or maximal performance in a sport; excessive exercise.

ur passion for thinness may have its roots in the Victorian era of the nineteenth century, which specialized in denying "unpleasant" physical realities, such as appetite and sexual desire. Flappers of the 1920s cemented the twentieth century trend for thinness. Since 1922, the BMI values of Miss America winners has steadily decreased; during the last three decades, most winners had a BMI in the underweight range (less than 18.5).

Currently, up to 5% of women in North America develop some form of anorexia nervosa or bulimia nervosa in their lifetimes.[3] This section provides a brief description of the characteristics and diagnoses of these two disorders. Detailed discussion of these and related disorders, including treatment, then follows.

Anorexia nervosa is characterized by extreme weight loss, a distorted body image, and an irrational, almost morbid, fear of obesity and weight gain. Anorexic patients irrationally believe they are fat, even though others constantly comment on their thin physique. Some anorexics realize they are thin but continue to be haunted by certain areas of their bodies that they believe to be fat (such as thighs, buttocks, and stomach). The discrepancy between actual and perceived body shape is an important gauge of the severity of the disease.

Common to both eating disorders, the term *nervosa* refers to disgust with one's body. The term *anorexia* implies a loss of appetite; however, a denial of appetite more accurately describes the behavior of people with anorexia nervosa. Estimating the prevalence of eating disorders is difficult because of underreporting, but approximately 1 in 200 (0.5%)[20] adolescent girls in North America eventually develops anorexia nervosa. This relatively high number may be due to girls' tendency to blame themselves for weight gain associated with puberty. It happens less commonly among adult women and African-American women. Men account for approximately 10% of cases of anorexia nervosa, partly because the ideal image conveyed for men is big and muscular. Among men, athletes are most prone to develop anorexia nervosa, especially those who participate in sports that require weight classes, such as boxers, wrestlers, and jockeys. Other activities that may foster eating disorders in men include swimming, dancing, and modeling.[3]

Bulimia nervosa (*bulimia* means "great [ox] hunger") is characterized by episodes of binge eating followed by attempts to purge the excess energy taken up by the body by vomiting or misuse of laxatives, diuretics, or enemas. Some people use excessive exercise (**hypergymnasia**) to try to burn off a binge's high energy intake. People with bulimia nervosa may be difficult to identify because they keep their binge-purge behaviors secret, and their symptoms are not obvious. Up to 4% of adolescent and college-age women suffer from bulimia nervosa. About 10% of the cases occur in men.[3]

The *Diagnostic and Statistical Manual of Mental Disorders* lists specific criteria for diagnosing eating disorders (Table 15-1). People may exhibit some symptoms of an eating disorder but not enough to enable a medical worker to diagnose the disease. These people may fall under the category Eating Disorders Not Otherwise Specified (EDNOS). One of the categories falling under EDNOS is binge-eating disorder (Table 15-2).[3]

Note that Table 15-1 shows two subcategories for anorexia nervosa: restricting type and binge-eating/purging type. Up to 60% of individuals diagnosed with anorexia nervosa develop a binge and purge pattern. Despite this, their diagnosis is still anorexia nervosa. Bulimia nervosa is a separate condition with distinct criteria.

Over one-third of individuals initially diagnosed with anorexia nervosa may cross over to bulimia nervosa, although the opposite crossover from bulimia nervosa to anorexia nervosa is much less likely. Typically, the crossover between eating disorders occurs within the first five years of the illness. Anorexic persons who perceive their parents as being highly critical are most likely to cross over to bulimia nervosa. In contrast, bulimic individuals who struggle with alcohol abuse are most likely to cross over to anorexia nervosa.

Until recently, most researchers have reported that eating disorders primarily affect middle- and upper-class white women. Now, studies show greater similarities in the rates of body dissatisfaction and disordered eating behaviors across ethnic and cultural groups. Perhaps minorities with eating disorders have been less likely to seek help in the past because of shame, stigma, lack of resources, or language barriers. Also, healthcare workers are less likely to diagnose nonwhites with eating disorders. Although some nonwhite cultures may be more accepting of larger body shapes, mainstream pressures for thinness influence our society as a whole.

Table 15-1 | Diagnostic Criteria for Anorexia Nervosa and Bulimia Nervosa

Anorexia Nervosa

A. Refusal to maintain body weight at or above a minimally normal weight for age and height (e.g., weight loss leading to maintenance of body weight less than 85% of that expected; or failure to make expected weight gain during periods of growth, leading to body weight less than 85% of that expected)

B. Intense fear of gaining weight or becoming fat, even though underweight

C. Disturbance in the way in which one's body weight or shape is experienced, undue influence of body weight or shape on self-evaluation, or denial of the seriousness of the current low body weight

D. In postmenarcheal females, **amenorrhea**—i.e., the absence of at least three consecutive menstrual cycles (A woman is considered to have amenorrhea if her periods occur only following hormone [e.g., estrogen] administration.)

Specify Type

Restricting type: During the current episode of anorexia nervosa, the person has not regularly engaged in binge-eating or purging behavior (such as self-induced vomiting and the misuse of laxatives, diuretics, or enemas).

Binge-eating/purging type: During the current episode of anorexia nervosa, the person has regularly engaged in binge-eating or purging behavior (such as self-induced vomiting and the misuse of laxatives, diuretics, or enemas).

Bulimia Nervosa

A. Recurrent episodes of binge eating. An episode of binge eating is characterized by both of the following:
   1. Eating, in a discrete period of time (e.g., within any 2-hour period), an amount of food that is definitely larger than most people would eat during a similar period of time and under similar circumstances
   2. A sense of lack of control over eating during the episode (e.g., a feeling that one cannot stop eating or control what or how much one is eating)

B. Recurrent inappropriate compensatory behavior to prevent weight gain, such as self-induced vomiting; misuse of laxatives, diuretics, enemas, or other medications; fasting; or excessive exercise

C. The binge eating and inappropriate compensatory behaviors both occur, on average, at least twice a week for 3 months.

D. Self-evaluation is unduly influenced by both body shape and weight.

E. The disturbance does not occur exclusively during episodes of anorexia nervosa.

Specify Type

Purging type: During the current episode of bulimia nervosa, the person has regularly engaged in self-induced vomiting or the misuse of laxatives, diuretics, or enemas.

Nonpurging type: During the current episode of bulimia nervosa, the person has used other inappropriate compensatory behaviors, such as fasting or excessive exercise, but has not regularly engaged in self-induced vomiting or the misuse of laxatives, diuretics, or enemas.

Eating Disorder Not Otherwise Specified (EDNOS)

This category is for disorders of eating that do not meet criteria for any specific eating disorder—for example:

1. For females, all of the criteria for anorexia nervosa are met except that the individual has regular menses.
2. All of the criteria for anorexia nervosa are met except that, despite significant weight loss, the individual's current weight is in the normal range.
3. All of the criteria for bulimia nervosa are met except that the binge eating and inappropriate compensatory mechanisms occur at a frequency of less than twice a week or for a duration of less than 3 months.
4. The regular use of inappropriate compensatory behavior by an individual of normal body weight after eating small amounts of food
5. Repeatedly chewing and spitting out, but not swallowing, large amounts of food
6. Binge-eating disorder (BED): Recurrent episodes of binge eating in the absence of the regular use of inappropriate compensatory behaviors characteristic of bulimia nervosa

Reprinted with permission from the *Diagnostic and Statistical Manual of Mental Disorders*, Fourth Edition (Text Revision) (DSM-IV-TR™). Copyright 2000 American Psychiatric Association.

This table will help you understand the characteristics of anorexia nervosa, bulimia nervosa, and binge-eating disorder. (Table 15-2 on page 558 provides more details on binge-eating disorder.) However, please do not attempt to diagnose these disorders yourself. Instead, use this information to determine whether professional help is needed. Note also that for both anorexia nervosa and bulimia nervosa, all characteristics (A–D or A–E, respectively) must be present to make the diagnosis.

Table 15-3 lists some characteristics of people with anorexia nervosa and bulimia nervosa. Do you know someone who is at risk for these eating disorders? If so, suggest that the person seek a professional evaluation because the sooner treatment begins, the better the chances are for recovery.[19] However, do not try to diagnose eating disorders in your friends or family members. Only a professional can exclude other possible diseases and correctly evaluate the diagnostic criteria required to make a diagnosis of anorexia nervosa or bulimia nervosa. Once an eating disorder is diagnosed, immediate treatment is advisable. As a friend, the best you can do is to encourage an affected

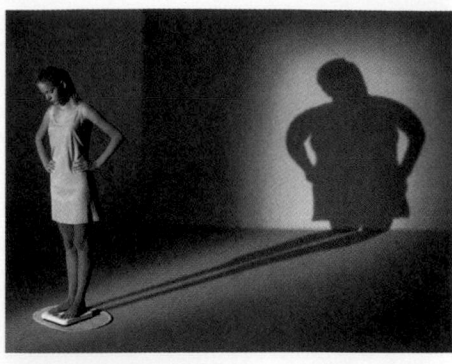

Self-image is an important part of adolescence. For people with eating disorders, the difference between the real and desired body images may be too difficult to accept. See the website www.4women.gov/bodyimage/index.htm.

Table 15-2 | Research Criteria for Binge-Eating Disorder

A. Recurrent episodes of binge eating, an episode being characterized by both of the following:
 1. Eating, in a discrete period of time (e.g., within any 2-hour period), an amount of food that is definitely larger than most people would eat during a similar period of time in similar circumstances
 2. A sense of lack of control during the episodes (e.g., a feeling that one can't stop eating or control what or how much one is eating)
B. During most binge episodes, at least three of the following occur:
 1. Eating much more rapidly than usual
 2. Eating until feeling uncomfortably full
 3. Eating large amounts of food when not feeling physically hungry
 4. Eating alone because of being embarrassed by how much one is eating
 5. Feeling disgusted with oneself, depressed, or very guilty after overeating
C. Marked distress regarding binge eating
D. The binge eating occurs, on average, at least 2 days a week for 6 months.
E. The behavior does not occur only during the course of bulimia nervosa or anorexia nervosa.

Reprinted by permission from the *Diagnostic and Statistical Manual of Mental Disorders,* Fourth Edition (Text Revision) (DSM-IV-TR). American Psychiatric Association, Washington DC, 2000.

Table 15-3 | Typical Characteristics of Anorexic and Bulimic Persons

Anorexia Nervosa	Bulimia Nervosa
• Rigid dieting causing dramatic weight loss, generally to less than 85% of what would be expected for one's age (or BMI of 17.5 or less)	• Secretive binge eating; generally not overeating in front of others
• False body perception—thinking "I'm too fat," even when extremely underweight; relentless pursuit of control	• Eating when depressed or under stress
• Rituals involving food, excessive exercise, and other aspects of life	• Bingeing on a large amount of food, followed by fasting, laxative or diuretic abuse, self-induced vomiting, or excessive exercise (at least twice a week for 3 months)
• Maintenance of rigid control in lifestyle; security found in control and order	• Shame, embarrassment, deceit, and depression; low self-esteem and guilt (especially after a binge)
• Feeling of panic after a small weight gain; intense fear of gaining weight	• Fluctuating weight (±10 lb or 5 kg) resulting from alternate bingeing and fasting
• Feelings of purity, power, and superiority through maintenance of strict discipline and self-denial	• Loss of control; fear of not being able to stop eating
• Preoccupation with food, its preparation, and observing another person eat	• Perfectionism, "people pleaser"; food as the only comfort/escape in an otherwise carefully controlled and regulated life
• Helplessness in the presence of food	• Erosion of teeth, swollen glands
• Lack of menstrual periods after what should be the age of puberty for at least 3 months	• Purchase of syrup of ipecac, a compound sold in pharmacies that induces vomiting
• Possible presence of bingeing and purging practices	

People who exhibit only one or a few of these characteristics may be at risk but probably do not have either disorder. They should, however, reflect on their eating habits and related concerns and take appropriate action such as seeking a careful evaluation by a physician.

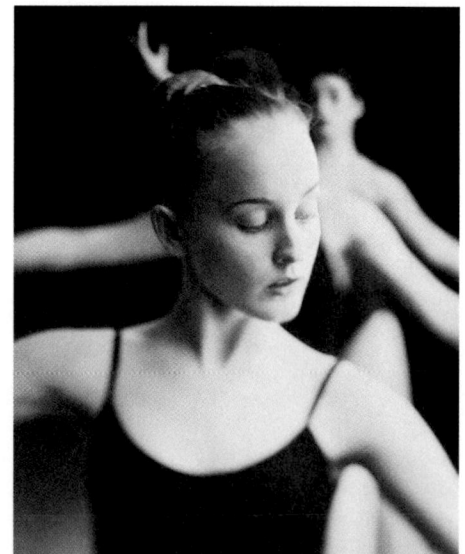

Eating disorders are commonly seen in people who must maintain low body weight, such as ballet dancers.

person to seek professional help. Note that such help is commonly available at student health centers and student guidance/counseling facilities on college campuses.

There are no simple causes of eating disorders, and there are no simple treatments. Stress may have an especially strong role in the development of eating disorders. Drug abuse also is a factor to consider.[6] An underlying commonality seems to be the lack of appropriate coping mechanisms as individuals approach adolescence and young adulthood, coupled with dysfunctional family relationships.

Is There a Genetic Connection to Eating Disorders?

Both anorexia nervosa and bulimia nervosa tend to cluster in families, suggesting that these two eating disorders share common causes. A few research studies have investigated the possible link between genetic factors and the development of eating disorders. These studies have involved a comparison of identical twins with fraternal twins and the incidence of eating disorders. In general, these studies have shown that identical twins have a higher likelihood of developing shared eating disorders than do fraternal twins.[20] This finding indicates that genetics may play a strong role in development of such disorders, because identical twins share the same DNA. However, these studies have not ruled out the impact of the environmental influences in eating disorder development. Identifying genes that cause eating disorders could eventually help in tailoring prevention efforts to those at risk, but affected individuals would still need the same counseling that is part of therapy today.

Anorexia Nervosa

Anorexia nervosa evolves from a dangerous mental state to an often life-threatening physical condition. People suffering from this disorder think they are fat and intensely fear obesity and weight gain. They lose much more weight than is healthful. Although food is entwined in this disease, it stems more from psychological conflict.

Depression is commonly found in conjunction with an eating disorder. In fact, a study done in the 1940s at the University of Minnesota found that depression and obsessional behaviors developed in the subjects during a 6-month period of restricted energy intake. These abnormal behaviors did not reverse immediately after refeeding but, rather, took many weeks to return to normal (see Chapter 20 for details).

About 3 to 10% of people with anorexia eventually die from the disease—from suicide, heart ailments, and infections.[15,20] Anorexia nervosa can worsen the effects of diabetes on the body, especially if too little insulin is injected as a means of increasing glucose excretion in the urine.[18] About one quarter of people with anorexia nervosa recover within 6 years, whereas the rest simply exist with the disease or go on to develop another form of disordered eating or bulimia nervosa. The longer someone suffers from this eating disorder, the poorer the chances are for complete recovery. Prompt and vigorous treatment with close follow-up improves the chances for success.

Anorexia nervosa may begin as a simple attempt to lose weight. A comment from a well-meaning friend, relative, or coach suggesting that the person seems to be gaining weight or is too fat may be all that is needed. The stress of having to maintain a certain weight to look attractive or competent on a job can also lead to disordered eating. Physical changes associated with puberty, the stress of leaving childhood, or the loss of a friend may serve as another trigger. Leaving home for boarding school or college or starting a job can reinforce the desire to appear more "socially acceptable." Still, looking "good" does not necessarily help people deal with anger, depression, low self-esteem, or past experiences with sexual abuse. If these issues are behind the disorder and are not resolved as weight is lost, the individual may intensify efforts to lose weight "to look even better," rather than work through unresolved psychological concerns. The resulting extreme dieting represents a hallmark of anorexia nervosa.[18]

Adolescence is a period of turbulent sexual and social tensions. As teenagers seek to establish separate and independent lives, they often react intensely to how they think others perceive them. At the same time, their bodies are changing, and much of the change is beyond their control. In response to an adolescent's lack of control in life or poor coping mechanisms, dieting may start and then lead to a failure to gain appropriate weight-for-height. This situation may not be readily identified as a problem because the child has not actually lost any weight. Stunting (failure to grow in height) may also occur with a severe decrease in energy intake during a period of growth. If anorexia develops before puberty, sexual maturation and menstruation may be delayed.

A disturbing trend is the attempt to promote eating disorders as a way of life. Some anorexic individuals have personified their illness into a role model named "Ana" who tells them what to eat and mocks them when they don't lose weight. Ana websites reject the serious health risks of anorexic behaviors and instead dispense unsafe "thinspiration" to vulnerable individuals.

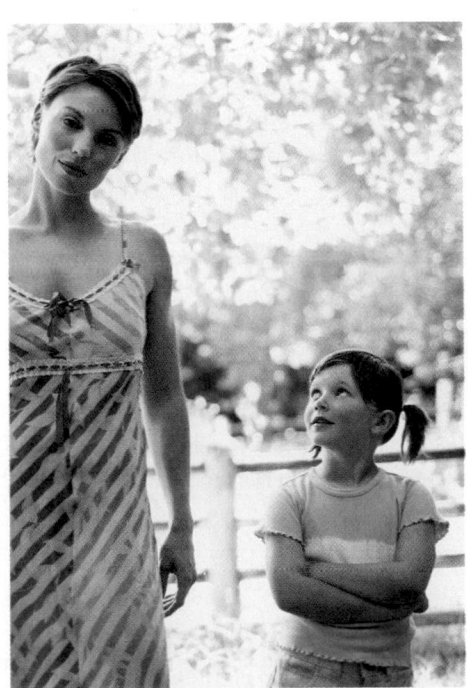

Concern over self-image begins early in life; a focus on good health with regard to body weight should also begin at this time.

Thoughts of an Anorexic Woman

It was the spring of my freshman year of high school, and I had just turned 15. I wanted to get a leading role in the upcoming high school musical, *West Side Story*. I thought I should lose some weight to look more attractive to the student director Shawn, so I decided to give up junk food. The next day my friend Sandra looked at my lunch, spread out neatly on a napkin before me, and squawked, "Dill pickles?! Who brings dill pickles for lunch in a Ziploc plastic bag?" The other girls at the table fell into a fit of hysterics. "Casting for *West Side Story* is coming up," I said, "and I gave up junk food to try to lose a few pounds." One of my friends thought it would be funny to give me an M&M candy—just to smell. Ha, ha. I put it in a little Tupperware container and kept it for days in my backpack as a reminder.

Every once in a while, I did smell it.

For the next few weeks there were times when I would find myself cracking open the refrigerator door and just staring down what I knew to be a deliciously crunchy, crisp, and cold Kit Kat bar in the dairy bin. I didn't eat it though. At the mall with my friends (since at 15, that's about all my parents allowed me to do), Bridgette and Nora wanted to stop and get a Cinnabon. They chided me, but I didn't budge. The Cinnabons smelled so good. But as I sat opposite them in the food court and watched them overdramatize its ooey-gooey goodness, I felt a sense of pride that I could make a decision and stick with it. I could see that they were jealous of my willpower.

When Easter came around, I took a look at the contents of the Easter basket my mom insisted on preparing and turned up my nose at it. I had proven to myself that I could resist temptation . . . why stop now?

I was eventually offered only a minor part in the musical, but I wasn't that disappointed. I was looking so much better as the pounds kept coming off. Every morning, just after going to the bathroom and before getting any breakfast, I would pop onto the scale in my mom's bathroom. One hundred and fifteen pounds and still going. At 5 feet 7 inches, that wasn't too bad.

Also at this time, I started running, and my friend Laura became my running partner. She was getting in shape for the next season of field hockey. After school, we met in the locker room, changed out of our school clothes, and out we went. I had never been much of an athlete—I thought that being part of a team, whether in sports or academics, diluted the excellence I could achieve on my own. Running, however, could just be me and the road—no mediocrity there.

Cheese and butter had made it to the "no" list by the time I was 16 and down to 105 lb. Fat-free was my mantra. In fact, for my 16th birthday, my friends threw a little surprise party for me. Nora, knowing I would put up a fight, made me a cake. "It's your birthday! You can have a piece of cake!" I politely said no, that I would cut it for everyone else, but I really didn't want any. They pestered me and Nora started to feel offended, so finally I took a few bites so she wouldn't burst into tears. It had been so long since I'd had so much sugar. I felt bloated and sick. I ate nothing for the rest of the day, and only 6 saltines, 1 apple, and 2 stalks of celery the next day. Those foods were on the "yes" list. Salads also were okay, but only lettuce with salt and vinegar. I told my parents that the dissections in biology class had given me a distaste for meat, but really, I just didn't want all those calories. For a while, I craved food day and night, but I was getting better and better at holding my ground.

By my senior year, I was skipping lunches altogether, opting instead to hang out in the library and read over my AP Bio text. "Where were you at lunch today?" Bridgette would ask later. "Oh, I had some reading to do. The AP exam is going to be tough." At 100 lb, I was getting closer to finding out what "tough" really meant.

Even though Laura moved out of state, I didn't give up on exercising. Now, the stair stepper in the gym was my favorite. I'd take my microbiology notes, prop them up in front of me, and step-step-step until I had burned 400 kcal. Multitasking felt so efficient. Sometimes I'd go on the stair stepper twice a day. As senior year wore on, though, it got harder and harder to get up in the morning and put on my tennis shoes. And then one morning, in the shower, I just collapsed under the stream of hot water.

I ended up in this hospital bed with an IV tube in my arm. At 92 lb, my body was starving. As it

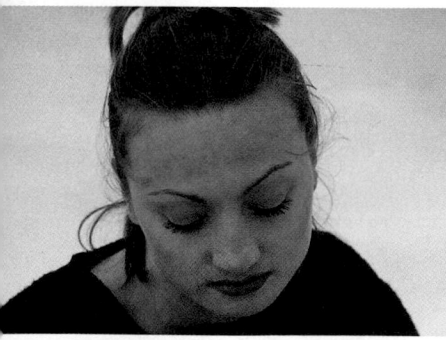

The psychological disease anorexia nervosa can lead to numerous physical problems.

turns out, if you don't give your body any fuel, you start to cannibalize yourself, in a sense. My body had been so hungry, my muscles had been wasting away, and the episode in the shower was due to a problem with my heart. It's a problem I have created . . . not my parents or my distant group of friends . . . just me. My mom was there, next to me, caressing the arm with the IV tube, putting her whole life on hold because of me. Isn't this what I'd wanted—to be in control of my own destiny?

Where do I go from here?

Thoughts of a Bulimic Woman

I am wide awake and immediately out of bed. I think back to the night before, when I made a new list of what I wanted to get done and how I wanted to be. My husband is not far behind me on his way into the bathroom to get ready for work. Maybe I can sneak onto the scale to see what I weigh this morning before he notices me. I am already in my private world. I feel overjoyed when the scale says that I stayed the same weight as I was the night before, and I can feel that slightly hungry feeling. Maybe it will stop today; maybe today everything will change. What were the projects I was going to get done?

We eat the same breakfast, except that I take no butter on my toast, no cream in my coffee, and never take seconds (until Doug gets out the door). Today I am going to be really good, and that means eating certain predetermined portions of food and not taking one more bite than I think I am allowed. I am very careful to see that I don't take more than Doug. I judge myself by his body. I can feel the tension building. I wish Doug would hurry up and leave so I can get going!

As soon as he shuts the door, I try to get involved with one of the myriad responsibilities on my list. I hate them all! I just want to crawl into a hole. I don't want to do anything. I'd rather eat. I am alone; I am nervous; I am no good; I always do everything wrong anyway; I am not in control; I can't make it through the day, I know it. It has been the same for so long. I remember the starchy cereal I ate for breakfast. I am into the bathroom and onto the scale. It measures the same, but I don't want to stay the same! I want to be thinner! I look into the mirror. I think my thighs are ugly and deformed looking. I see a lumpy, clumsy, pear-shaped wimp. There is always something wrong with what I see. I feel frustrated, trapped in this body, and I don't know what to do about it.

I float to the refrigerator knowing exactly what is there. I begin with last night's brownies. I always begin with the sweets. At first I try to make it look like nothing is missing, but my appetite is huge and I resolve to make another batch of brownies. I know there is half of a bag of cookies in the bathroom, thrown out the night before, and I polish them off immediately. I take some milk so my vomiting will be smoother. I like the full feeling I get after downing a big glass. I get out six pieces of bread and toast one side of each in the broiler, turn them over and load them with pats of butter, and put them under the broiler again until they are bubbling. I take all six pieces on a plate to the television and go back for a bowl of cereal and a banana to have along with them. Before the last piece of toast is finished, I am already preparing the next batch of six more pieces. Maybe another brownie or five, and a couple of large bowls full of ice cream, yogurt, or cottage cheese.

My stomach is stretched into a huge ball below my rib cage. I know I'll have to go into the bathroom soon, but I want to postpone it. I am in never-never land. I am waiting, feeling the pressure, pacing the floor in and out of the rooms. Time is passing. Time is passing. It is getting to be time. I wander aimlessly through each of the rooms again, tidying, making the whole house neat and put back together. I finally make the turn into the bathroom. I brace my feet, pull my hair back and stick my finger down my throat, stroking twice, and get up a huge pile of food. Three times, four times, and another pile of food. I can see everything come back. I am so glad to see those brownies because they are so fattening. The rhythm of the emptying is broken and my head is beginning to hurt. I stand up feeling dizzy, empty, and weak. The whole episode has taken about an hour.

From Hall L, Cohn L: *Bulimia—A Guide to Recovery.* Gurze Books: Carlsbad, CA, 1992.

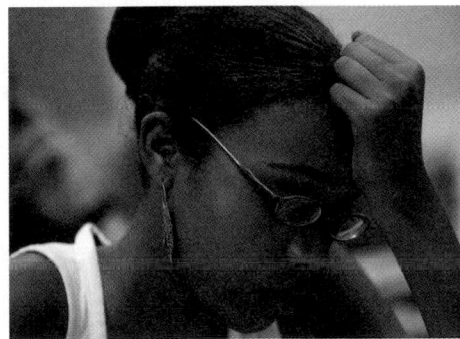

Bulimia nervosa may have an innocent beginning, but can lead to tragic consequences.

By severely limiting energy intake for long periods, adolescent girls and young adult women greatly compromise their nutritional status, impair their reproductive systems, and restrict growth.[10] The harm produced by milder, shorter periods of diet restriction is not clear. Evidence, however, suggests that even moderate diet restriction, if continued, contributes to the risks for various anemias, permanently reduced bone mass, later pregnancy complications, and delivery of a low-birth-weight infant.[12]

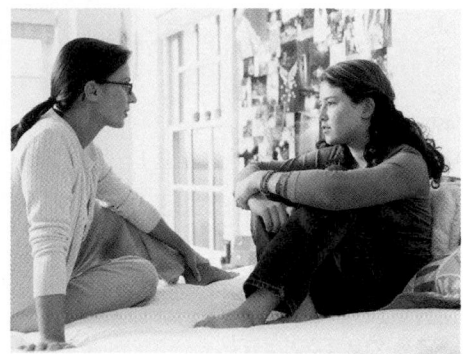

Even well-intentioned parents may place expectations on their children that compound the anxiety often experienced during years of difficult emotional and physiological changes. In response, adolescents and young adults may find comfort in exerting control over their environment through the restrictive behaviors associated with eating disorders.

Parents may not consider a teenager mature enough to make decisions. If the teen disagrees and the situation is very tense, she may turn to purging or starving as a way to show her power: "You may try to control my life, but I can do anything I want with my body."

In the words of one young woman, "I couldn't get angry, because it would be like destroying someone else, like my mother. It felt like she would hate me forever. I got angry through anorexia nervosa. It was my last hope. It's my own body and this was my last-ditch effort."

Teens with chronic illnesses, such as type 1 diabetes or asthma, are at even greater risk for disordered eating.[1] Any evidence of poor weight gain/maintenance or excessive exercise among these individuals is a possible sign of disordered eating.

Extreme dieting is the most important predictor of an eating disorder. (Adolescents expressing concern about their weight should be advised to focus on exercise, which does not appear to impart a risk for subsequent problems.) Once dieting begins, a person developing anorexia nervosa does not stop. The result is a long period of rigidly self-enforced semistarvation, practiced almost with a vengeance, in a relentless pursuit of control. For example, recently, a 19-year-old woman was admitted to the Ohio State University Hospitals with a body weight of 60 lb. She had lost 55 lb in the previous 6 months and was at great risk of impending death. Upon interview, she said she started dieting and could not stop.

Anorexia nervosa may eventually lead to bingeing on large amounts of food in a short time, then purging. Purging occurs primarily through vomiting, but laxatives, diuretics, and enemas are also used. Thus, a person with anorexia nervosa may exist in a state of semistarvation or may alternate periods of starvation with periods of bingeing and purging.[3,16]

Profile of the Typical Person with Anorexia Nervosa

A person with anorexia nervosa refuses to eat enough food to maintain an acceptable weight. This refusal is a common finding of the disease, whether or not other practices, such as binge-purge cycles, appear. The most typical anorexic person is a white female from the middle or upper socioeconomic class. Perhaps her mother also has distorted views of desirable body shape and acceptable food habits. The girl is often described by parents and teachers as responsible, meticulous, and obedient.

The girl is often competitive and often obsessive.[18] At home, she may not allow clutter in her bedroom. Physicians note that after a physical examination, she may fold her examination gown very carefully and clean up the examination room before leaving. Even though such behavior may seem obvious, only a skilled professional can tell the difference between anorexia nervosa and other adolescent complaints, such as delayed puberty, fatigue, and depression.

A common thread underlying many—but not all—cases of anorexia nervosa is conflict within the family structure, typically manifested by an overbearing mother and an emotionally absent father. When family expectations are too high—including those regarding body weight—frustration leads to fighting. Overinvolvement, rigidity, overprotection, and denial are typical daily transactions of such families.

Issues of control are central to the development of anorexia nervosa. The eating disorder can allow an anorexic person to exercise control over an otherwise powerless existence.[5] Losing weight may be the first independent success the person has had. People with anorexia evaluate their self-worth almost entirely in terms of self-control. Some sexually abused children develop anorexia nervosa, believing that if they control their appetite for food, they will feel in control of and can thereby eliminate their shameful feelings. Moreover, food restriction, which arrests development and shuts down sexual impulses, may be a strategy to prevent future victimization and guilt feelings. Often anorexic persons feel hopeless about human relationships and socially isolated because of their dysfunctional families. They focus on food, eating, and weight instead of human relationships.

Early Warning Signs

A person developing anorexia nervosa exhibits important warning signs. At first, dieting becomes the life focus. The person may think, "The only thing I am good at is dieting. I can't do anything else." This innocent beginning often leads to very abnormal self-perceptions and eating habits, such as cutting a pea in half before eating it. Other habits include hiding and storing food and or spreading food around a plate to make it look as if a lot has been eaten. An anorexic person may cook a large meal and watch others eat it while refusing to eat anything. Anorexics may also exercise to the point of obsession, such as doing squats while brushing teeth.

As the disorder progresses, the variety of foods eaten may narrow and be rigidly divided into safe and unsafe ones, with the list of safe foods becoming progressively shorter. For people developing anorexia nervosa, these practices say, "I am in control." These people may be hungry, but they deny it, driven by the belief that good things will happen by just becoming thin enough. For an anorexic person, success is a matter of willpower.

Soon people with anorexia become irritable and hostile and begin to withdraw from family and friends. School performance generally crumbles. They refuse to eat out with family and friends, thinking, "I won't be able to have the foods I want to eat," or "I won't be able to throw up afterward."

Anorexic persons see themselves as rational and others as irrational. They also tend to be excessively critical of themselves and others. Nothing is good enough. Because it cannot be perfect, life appears meaningless and hopeless. A sense of joylessness pervades everything.

As stress increases in the person's life, sleep disturbances and depression are common. Many of the psychological and physical problems associated with anorexia nervosa arise from insufficient energy intake as well as deficiencies of nutrients, such as thiamin and vitamin B-6.[20] For a female, the combination of problems—coupled with lower and lower body weight and fat stores—causes menstrual periods to cease.[13] This sign of the disease may be the first one that a parent notices and represents an additional hallmark of the disease.

Ultimately, an anorexic person eats very little food; 300 to 600 kcal daily is not unusual. In place of food, the person may consume up to 20 cans of diet soft drinks and chew many pieces of sugarless gum each day.

Physical Effects of Anorexia Nervosa

Rooted in the emotional state of the victim, anorexia nervosa produces profound physical effects.[8] The anorexic person often appears to be skin and bones. Body weight less than 85% of that expected is one clinical indicator of anorexia nervosa.[18] This percentage can be calculated using the Metropolitan Life Insurance tables (see Appendix I), but it is important to note that body build and weight history should also be used when estimating an appropriate weight. BMI is a more reliable indicator of the degree of malnourishment; generally, a BMI of 17.5 or less indicates a severe case (review Chapter 13 for more on BMI). For children under age 18, growth charts should be used to assess weight status (see Chapter 17).

This state of semistarvation forces the body to conserve as much energy as possible and results in most of the physical effects of anorexia nervosa (Figure 15-1). Thus, many complications can be ended by returning to a healthy weight, provided the duration of anorexia nervosa has not been too long. Following are predictable effects caused by hormonal responses to and nutrient deficiencies from semistarvation:[3,5,12,20]

Lowered body temperature and cold intolerance caused by loss of insulating fat layer.
Slower metabolic rate caused by decreased synthesis of thyroid hormones.
Decreased heart rate as metabolism slows, leading to easy fatigue, fainting, and an overwhelming need for sleep. Other changes in heart function may also occur, including loss of heart tissue itself and poor heart rhythm.
Iron deficiency anemia, which leads to further weakness.
Rough, dry, scaly, and cold skin from a deficient nutrient intake, which may also show multiple bruises because of the loss of protection from the fat layer normally present under the skin.
Low white blood cell count, which increases the risk of infection and potentially death.

Critical | Thinking

Jennifer is an attractive 13-year-old. However, she's very compulsive. Everything has to be perfect—her hair, her clothes, even her room. Since her body is beginning to mature, she's quite obsessed with having perfect physical features as well. Her parents are worried about her behavior. The school counselor told them to look for certain signs that could indicate an eating disorder. What might those signs be?

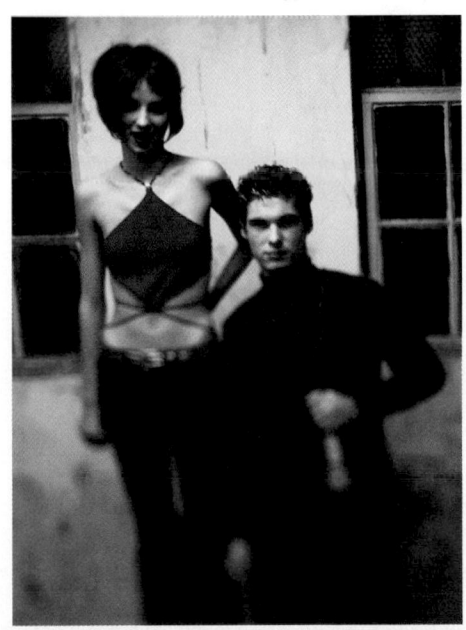

Anorexia nervosa occurs much more frequently in young women than in young men.

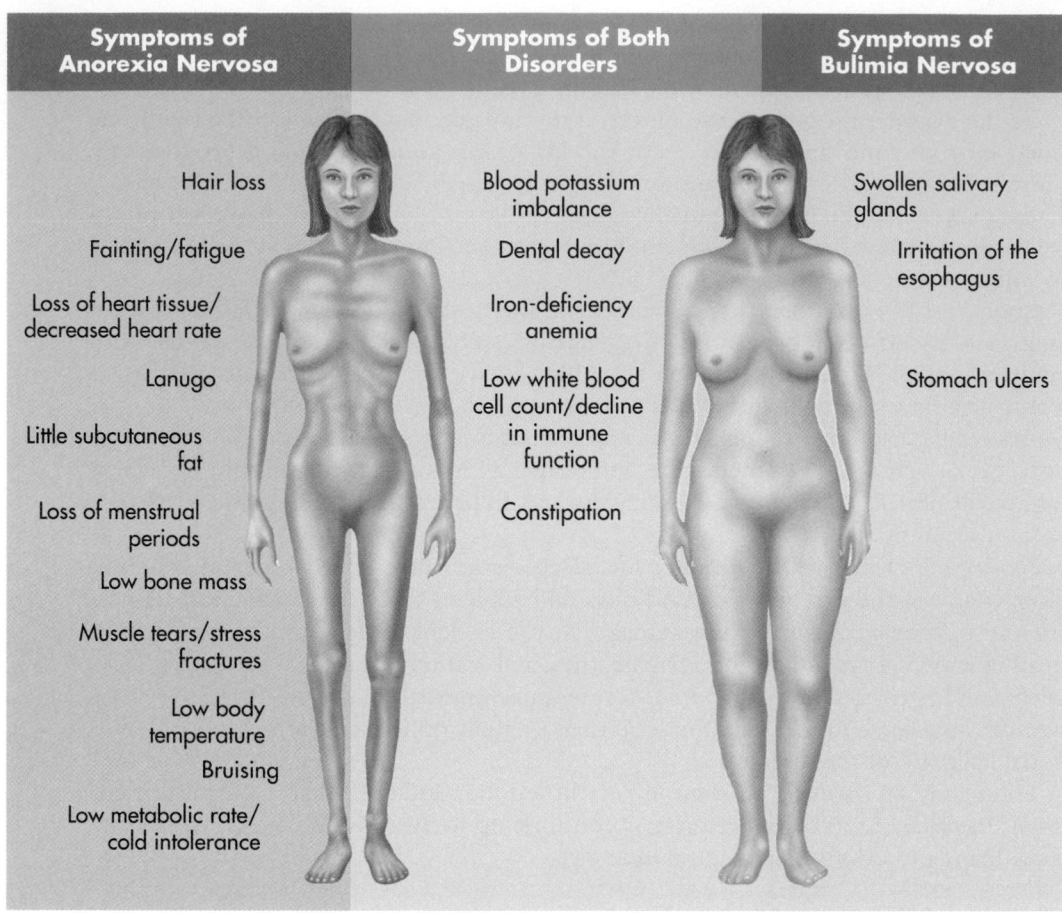

Figure 15-1 | Signs and symptoms of eating disorders. A vast array of physical effects are associated with anorexia nervosa and bulimia nervosa. This figure contains many potential consequences but is not an exhaustive list. These physical effects can also serve as warning signs that a problem exists. Professional evaluation is then indicated.

lanugo Downlike hair that appears after a person has lost much body fat through semistarvation. The hair stands erect and traps air, acting as insulation for the body to compensate for the relative lack of body fat, which usually functions as insulation.

Erika Goodman, a former dancer with the Joffrey Ballet, is now in her fifties and is crippled from osteoporosis resulting from years of restricting food intake to maintain a low body weight. Her food restriction led to irregular or absent menstrual periods for many years.

Abnormal feeling of fullness or bloating, which can last for several hours after eating.

Loss of hair.

Appearance of **lanugo**—downy hairs on the body that trap air, reducing heat loss that occurs with the loss of fat tissue.

Constipation from semistarvation and laxative abuse.

Low blood potassium caused by a deficient nutrient intake, loss of potassium from vomiting, and use of some types of diuretics. Low blood potassium increases the risk of heart rhythm disturbances, another leading cause of death in anorexic people.

Loss of menstrual periods because of low body weight, low body fat content, and the stress of the disease. Accompanying hormonal changes cause a loss of bone mass and increase the risk of osteoporosis later in life.

Changes in neurotransmitter function in the brain, leading to depression.

Eventual loss of teeth caused by acid erosion if frequent vomiting occurs. Until vomiting ceases, one way to reduce this effect on teeth is to rinse the mouth with water right away and brush the teeth as soon as possible. Loss of teeth (along with low bone mass) can be lasting signs of the disease, even if the other physical and mental problems are resolved.

Muscle tears and stress fractures in athletes because of decreased bone and muscle mass.

A person with this disorder is psychologically and physically ill and needs help.[13]

Anorexia nervosa is an eating disorder characterized by semistarvation. It is found primarily—but not exclusively—in adolescent girls, starting at or around puberty. People with anorexia nervosa dwindle essentially to skin and bones but still believe they are fat. Semistarvation produces hormonal changes and nutrient deficiencies that lower body temperature, slow the heart rate, decrease immune response, stop menstrual periods, and contribute to hair, muscle, and bone loss. Anorexia nervosa is a very serious disease that often produces fatal or lifelong consequences.

Treatment of Anorexia Nervosa

People with anorexia often sink into shells of isolation and fear. They deny that a problem exists.[9] Frequently, their friends and family members meet with them to confront the problem in a loving way, called an *intervention*. They present evidence of the problem and encourage immediate treatment. Treatment then requires a multidisciplinary team of experienced physicians, registered dietitians, psychologists, and other health professionals working together.[20] An ideal setting is an eating disorders clinic in a medical center. Outpatient therapy generally begins first and may be extended to 3 to 5 days per week. Day hospitalization (6–12 hours) is another option, as is total hospitalization. Hospitalization is necessary once a person falls below 75% of expected weight, experiences acute medical problems, and/or exhibits severe psychological problems or suicidal risk.[20] Still, even in the most skilled hands at the finest facilities, efforts may fail. The prevention of anorexia nervosa is of utmost importance.

Once a medical team has gained the cooperation and trust of an anorexic patient, the team attempts to work together to restore a sense of balance, purpose, and future possibilities. As previously stated, anorexia nervosa is usually rooted in psychological conflict. However, the anorexic person who has been barely existing in a state of semistarvation cannot focus on much besides food. Dreams and even morbid thoughts about food will interfere with therapy until sufficient weight is regained.

Nutrition Therapy

The first goal of nutrition therapy is to gain the patient's cooperation and trust in order to increase oral food intake. Ideally, weight gain must be enough to raise the metabolic rate to normal and reverse as many physical signs of the disease as possible. Food intake is designed first to minimize or stop any further weight loss. Then the focus shifts to restoring appropriate food habits. After this, the expectation can be switched to slow weight gain. A range of 2 to 3 lb/week is appropriate. Tube feeding and/or total parenteral nutrition support is used only if immediate renourishment is required, because this drastic measure can cause the patient to distrust medical staff.

Energy needs begin at 1000 to 1600 kcal/day in multiple, small meals, and this allocation is increased in 100- to 200-kcal increments every few days as possible until an appropriate rate of weight gain is achieved. This appropriate weight is one in which normal menstruation is restored. An energy distribution of about 50 to 55% carbohydrate, 15 to 20% protein, and 25 to 30% fat is appropriate. This nutrition therapy may ultimately require a daily intake of 3000 to 4000 kcal to attain a goal weight, because the increase in body metabolism and anxiety associated with feeding needs to be accounted for.[17] A multivitamin and mineral supplement will be added, as well as enough calcium to raise intake to about 1500 mg/day. As noted before, nutrient deficiencies are commonly seen in anorexic persons.[20]

Patients need considerable reassurance during the refeeding process because of uncomfortable effects, such as bloating, increase in body heat, and increase in body fat. This process is frightening because these changes can lead to the patient feeling out of

Jennifer continues her pursuit of the perfect thin body into her late teens. She ignores the advice of her parents and the counselor. As a 19-year-old entering college, she is finally beginning to realize that her anorexic behavior might have serious consequences. She has been fluctuating 15 to 20% below her healthy body weight and has been amenorrheic for a few years. She would like to marry someday and have a family. What are some of the health consequences for a person with anorexia nervosa, such as Jennifer?

Some anorexic people use cigarette smoking, which increases metabolic rate, as a way to resist weight gain during nutrition therapy.

A young woman in a self-help group for those with anorexia nervosa explained her feelings to the other group members: "I have lost a specialness that I thought it gave me. I was different from everyone else. Now I know that I'm somebody who's overcome it, which not everybody does."

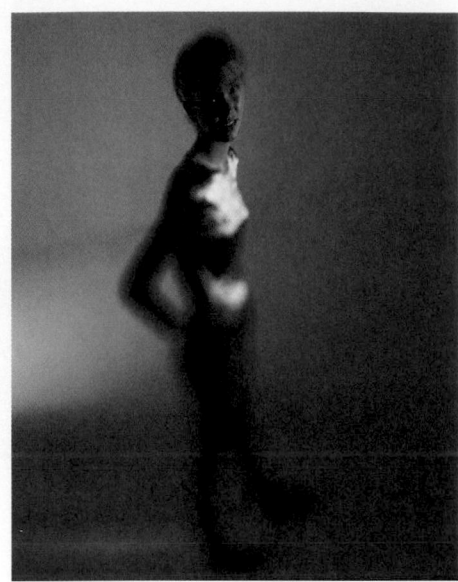

A history of anorexia nervosa can harm physical as well as mental health.

control. Monitoring for rapid changes in electrolytes and minerals in the blood, especially potassium, phosphorus, and magnesium, is critically important as more food is included in the diet.[5]

In addition to helping patients reach and maintain adequate nutritional status, the registered dietitian on the medical team also provides accurate nutrition information throughout treatment, promotes a healthy attitude toward food, and helps the patient learn to eat based on natural hunger and satiety cues. Nutrition therapy with anorexic persons can be frustrating for a dietitian because many anorexic persons are very knowledgeable regarding the energy and fat gram content of most food products. The focus should be on helping these patients identify healthy and adequate food choices that promote weight gain to achieve and maintain a clinically estimated goal weight (e.g., BMI of 20 or more).[1] The medical team also should assure patients that they will not be abandoned after gaining weight.

Because excessive energy expenditure prevents weight gain, professionals must work with anorexic patients to help them moderate their activity. At many treatment centers, patients are placed on moderate bed rest in the early stages of treatment to help promote weight gain.

Experienced professional help is the key. An anorexic patient may be on the verge of suicide and near starvation. In addition, anorexic people are often very clever and resistant. They may try to hide weight loss by wearing many layers of clothes, putting coins in their pockets or underwear, and drinking numerous glasses of water before stepping on a scale.

Psychological and Related Therapy

Once the physical problems of anorexic patients are addressed, the treatment focus shifts to the underlying emotional problems of the disorder. To heal, these patients must reject the sense of accomplishment they associate with an emaciated body and begin to accept themselves at a healthy body weight. If therapists can discover reasons for the disorder, they can develop psychological strategies for restoring normal weight and eating habits. Education about the medical consequences of semistarvation is also helpful. A key aspect of psychological treatment is showing affected individuals how to regain control of other facets of their lives and cope with tough situations. As eating evolves into a normal routine, they can turn to previously neglected activities.

cognitive behavior therapy Psychological therapy in which the person's assumptions about dieting, body weight, and related issues are challenged. New ways of thinking are explored and then practiced by the person. In this way, the person can learn new ways to control disordered eating behaviors and related life stress.

Therapists may use **cognitive behavior therapy,** which involves helping the person confront and change irrational beliefs about body image, eating, relationships, and weight.[5] Underlying issues that may be the cause for the disease, such as sexual abuse, must be identified and addressed by the therapist. Interpersonal therapy is another psychological approach used in anorexia nervosa. Rather than focusing on the patient's eating habits and assumptions about weight and shape, interpersonal therapy formulates the problem in terms of the interpersonal context, usually in one or more of four areas: grief, interpersonal problems (e.g., difficulty forming or maintaining close relationships), interpersonal disputes (e.g., unresolved conflict regarding the expectations of significant others in the person's life), or role transitions (e.g., fear of independence due to lack of self-confidence). Treatment focuses on assisting the patient to change in one or more of these areas.

Family therapy often is important in treating anorexia nervosa, especially for younger patients who still live at home. Family therapy focuses on the role of the illness among family members, the reactions of individual family members, and ways in which their subconscious behavior might contribute to the abnormal eating patterns.[20] Frequently, a therapist finds family struggles at the heart of the problem. As the disorder resolves, patients must relate to family members in new ways to gain the attention that was needed and previously tied to the disease. For example, the family may need to help the young person ease into adulthood and accept its responsibilities as well as its advantages.

Self-help groups for anorexic people, as well as their families and friends, represent nonthreatening first steps into treatment. People can also attend to get a sense of whether they really do have an eating disorder.

Medications are generally not effective in treating the primary symptoms of anorexia nervosa.[20] Fluoxetine (Prozac) and other related antidepressant medications called selective serotonin reuptake inhibitors (SSRIs) may stabilize recovery in patients with anorexia who have attained 85% of their expected body weight. SSRIs work by prolonging serotonin activity in the brain, which in turn regulates mood and feelings of satiety. A variety of other types of pharmacologic agents may have some role in treating mood changes, anxiety, or psychotic symptoms associated with anorexia nervosa (e.g., olanzapine [Zyprexa]) but have limited value in patients unless weight gain is also achieved.[5]

With professional help, many people with anorexia nervosa can lead normal lives. Although they may not be totally cured, they do not have to depend on unusual eating habits to cope with daily problems. They recover a sense of normality in their lives. No universal approach exists because each case is unique. Establishing a strong relationship with either a therapist or another supportive person is an especially important key to recovery. Once anorexic patients feel understood and accepted by another person, they can begin to build a sense of self and exercise some autonomy. As they learn alternative coping mechanisms, recovering patients can leave behind their dysfunctional relationships with food and instead develop healthy personal relationships.[20]

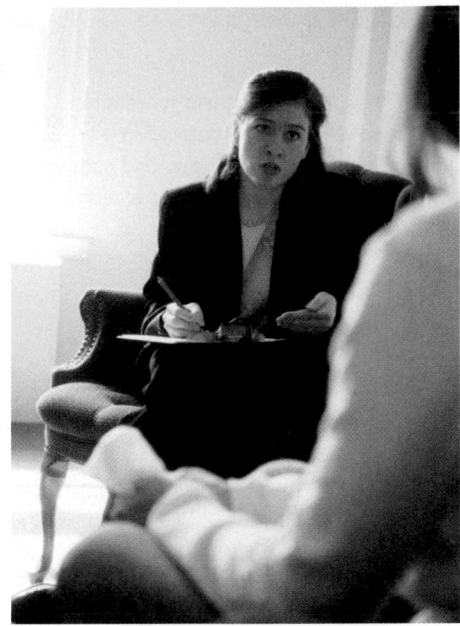

Early treatment for an eating disorder such as anorexia nervosa improves chances of success.

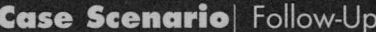

Case Scenario | Follow-Up

Sarah does have the characteristics to be diagnosed with anorexia nervosa because she refuses to maintain a healthy weight-for-height ratio, is at a weight below 85% of that expected, has a distorted view of her appearance, and has had no menstrual periods for over 3 consecutive months.

Sarah would need to be hospitalized initially because of her low BMI of 13.8. While in the hospital, her treatment most likely would consist of moderate bed rest to promote weight gain, and an intake of 1000 to 1600 kcal initially, which is then increased by increments of about 100 to 200 kcal every few days until an acceptable rate of weight gain is achieved.

The goal is for Sarah to achieve a body weight that is at least 90% of an expected weight for her age, such as a BMI of at least 19. This weight goal should also allow for resumption of menstrual periods. The physician would likely prescribe a multivitamin and mineral supplement along with additional supplements of calcium to ensure an intake of about 1500 mg/day. These supplements will correct vitamin and mineral deficiencies that exist, and the calcium will contribute to bone maintenance. A team of health professionals, most likely consisting of a physician, registered dietitian, and psychologist, would provide therapy. Sarah's cooperation would be the most important element for therapy to be successful. She needs to realize she has a problem and that she needs help. The team, especially the psychologist, may use cognitive behavior therapy to help Sarah improve her self-image.

Otherwise, Sarah's outlook for recovery is not good. Even if she is willing to accept the therapy and counseling, relapse is likely to occur. Only about 50% of anorexia nervosa patients have been found to fully recover from the disease. Because Sarah's disordered eating habits have been in place for about 6 years, her problem is deep-rooted. The chances of recovery are greater if a vigorous treatment program is reinforced with close follow-up.

Singer Karen Carpenter's death from complications of anorexia nervosa in 1983 increased awareness of the serious nature of this disease. Currently, the average time for recovery from anorexia nervosa is 7 years; many insurance companies cover only a fraction of the estimated $150,000 cost of treatment.

Concept | Check

To relieve the semistarved condition of most anorexic patients, the initial treatment focuses on moderately increased food intake and slow weight gain. Once these goals are accomplished, psychotherapy can begin to uncover the causes of the disease and help patients develop skills to return to a healthy life. Family therapy can be an important tool in treatment, whereas medications have a limited role.

Bulimia Nervosa

ingeing and purging (via vomiting) in group settings were practiced in pre-Christian Roman times. Bingeing and purging associated with bulimia nervosa are generally practiced in private.

ulimia nervosa is rare in developing countries, which suggests that our culture is an important causal factor.

The binge-purge cycle can lead to a sense of helplessness.

Bulimia nervosa involves episodes of binge eating followed by various means to purge the food. This eating disorder was first described in the medical literature in 1979 and classified as a clinical psychiatric disorder in 1980. It is most common among young adults of college age, although some high school students are also at risk. Susceptible people often have genetic factors and lifestyle patterns that predispose them to becoming overweight, and many try frequent weight-reduction diets as teenagers. Like people with anorexia nervosa, those with bulimia nervosa are usually female and successful. Unlike anorexics, however, they are usually at or slightly above a normal weight.[11] Females with bulimia nervosa are also more likely to be sexually active than those with anorexia nervosa.

The person with bulimia nervosa may think of food constantly. Unlike the anorexic person, who turns away from food when faced with problems, the bulimic person turns toward food in critical situations.[4] Also, unlike those with anorexia nervosa, people with bulimia nervosa recognize their behavior as abnormal.[18] These people often have very low self-esteem and are depressed. Approximately half the people with bulimia nervosa have major depression. Lingering effects of child abuse may be one reason for these feelings. Many bulimic persons report that they have been sexually abused. The world sees their competence, while inside they feel out of control, ashamed, and frustrated.

Bulimic people tend to be impulsive, which may be expressed as thievery, increased sexual activity, drug or alcohol abuse, self-mutilation, or attempted suicide. Some experts have suggested that part of the problem may actually arise from bulimic individuals' inability to control responses to impulse and desire. Some studies have demonstrated that bulimic people tend to come from disengaged families—ones that are loosely organized. In these families, roles for family members are not clearly defined. Rules are very loose and a great deal of conflict exists. In comparison anorexic people tend to have families so actively engaged that roles may be too well defined.[3]

Typical Behavior in Bulimia Nervosa

Many people with bulimic behavior are probably never diagnosed. The strict diagnostic criteria specify that to be classified as having bulimia nervosa, a person must binge and purge at least twice a week for 3 months.[3] People with bulimia nervosa lead secret lives, hiding their abnormal eating habits. Moreover, it is impossible to recognize people with bulimia nervosa simply from their appearance. Because most diagnoses of bulimia nervosa are based on self-reports, current estimates of the number of cases are probably low. The disorder, especially in its milder forms, may be much more widespread than commonly thought.

For intake to qualify as a binge, an atypically large amount of food must be consumed in a short time, and the person must exhibit a lack of control over his or her behavior.[11] Bingeing often alternates with attempts to rigidly restrict food intake. Elaborate food rules are common, such as avoiding all sweets. Thus, eating just one cookie or doughnut may cause bulimic persons to feel they have broken a rule. Feeling like a failure, the bulimic person may then proceed to binge. Usually, this action leads to significant overeating, partly because it is easier to regurgitate a large amount of food than a small amount.

Binge-purge cycles may be practiced daily, weekly, or at longer intervals. A special time is often set aside. Most binge eating occurs at night, when other people are less likely to interrupt, and usually lasts from 1/2 to 2 hours. A binge can be triggered by a combination of hunger from recent dieting, stress, boredom, loneliness, and depression. Bingeing often follows a period of strict dieting and thus can be linked to intense hunger. The binge is not at all like normal eating; once begun, it seems to propel itself. The person not only loses control but generally doesn't even taste or enjoy the food that is eaten during a binge. This separates the practice from simple overeating.

Most commonly, bulimic people consume cakes, cookies, ice cream, and similar high-carbohydrate convenience foods during binges because these foods can be purged relatively easily and comfortably by vomiting. In a single binge, foods supplying up to 3000 kcal or more may be eaten.[5] Purging follows in hopes that no weight will be gained. However, even when vomiting follows the binge, 33 to 75% of the food energy taken in is still absorbed, which causes some weight gain. When laxatives or enemas are used, about 90% of the energy is absorbed, because these products act in the large intestine, beyond the point of most nutrient absorption. Clearly, the belief of bulimic persons that purging soon after bingeing will prevent excessive energy absorption and weight gain is a misconception.

Early in the onset of bulimia nervosa, sufferers often induce vomiting by placing their fingers (or other objects) deep into the throat. In the case of fingers, they may inadvertently bite down on these fingers, such that the resulting bite marks around the knuckles become a characteristic sign of this disorder. Once the disease is established, however, a person can often vomit simply by contracting the abdominal muscles. Vomiting may also occur spontaneously.

Another way bulimic people attempt to compensate for a binge is by engaging in excessive exercise to expend a large amount of energy. Some bulimic people try to estimate the amount of energy eaten in a binge and then exercise to counteract this energy intake. This practice, referred to as "debting," represents an effort to control their weight.[11]

People with bulimia nervosa are not proud of their behavior. After a binge, they usually feel guilty and depressed.[18] Over time, they experience low self-esteem and feel hopeless about their situation (Figure 15-2). Compulsive lying, shoplifting to obtain food, and drug abuse can further intensify these feelings. Bulimic people caught in the act of bingeing by a friend or family member may order the intruder to "get out" and "go away." Sufferers gradually distance themselves from others, spending more and more time preoccupied by and engaging in bingeing and purging.

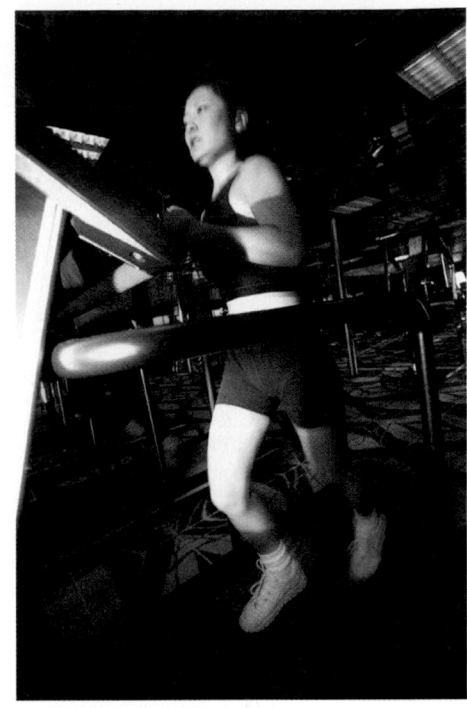

Excessive exercising can be one component of bulimia if it is used as a way to offset the energy intake from a binge. Exercise is considered excessive when it is done at inappropriate times or settings, or when a person does it despite injury or other medical complications.

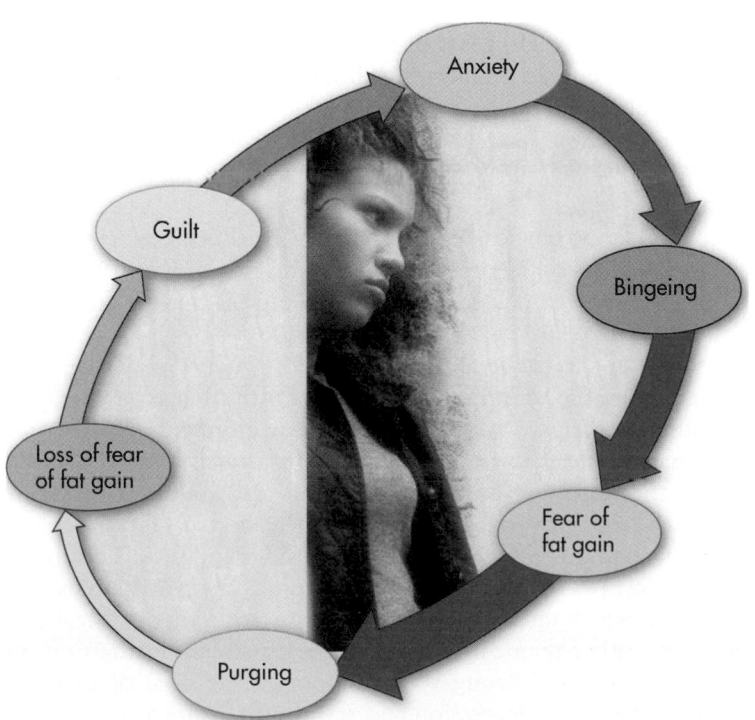

Figure 15-2 | Bulimia nervosa's vicious cycle of obsession.

The November 24, 2005 issue of the *New England Journal of Medicine* (353:2270, 2005) contains an X-ray view of a fork inside a woman's stomach. The woman had an eating disorder and used the fork to induce vomiting.

Health Problems Stemming from Bulimia Nervosa

The vomiting associated with bulimia nervosa is a physically destructive method of purging. Indeed, the majority of health problems associated with bulimia nervosa that are listed here arise from vomiting:[3,7,11]

Repeated exposure of teeth to the acid in vomit causes demineralization, making the teeth painful and sensitive to heat, cold, and acids. Eventually, the teeth may decay severely, erode away from fillings, and finally fall out (Figure 15-3). Dental professionals are sometimes the first health professionals to notice signs of bulimia nervosa. It is important to rinse the mouth with water after any vomiting episode, especially before brushing the teeth.

Blood potassium can drop significantly because of regular vomiting or the use of certain diuretics. This drop can disturb the heart's rhythm and even produce sudden death.

Salivary glands may swell as a result of infection and irritation from persistent vomiting.

Stomach ulcers and tears in the esophagus develop in some cases.

Constipation may result from frequent laxative use.

Ipecac syrup, sometimes used to induce vomiting, is toxic to the heart, liver, and kidneys and can cause accidental poisoning when taken repeatedly.

Overall, bulimia nervosa is a potentially debilitating disorder that can lead to death, usually from suicide, low blood potassium, or overwhelming infections.

Concept | Check

Bulimia nervosa is characterized by episodes of binge eating followed by purging, usually by vomiting. Vomiting is very destructive to the body, often causing severe dental decay, stomach ulcers, irritation of the esophagus, and low blood potassium.

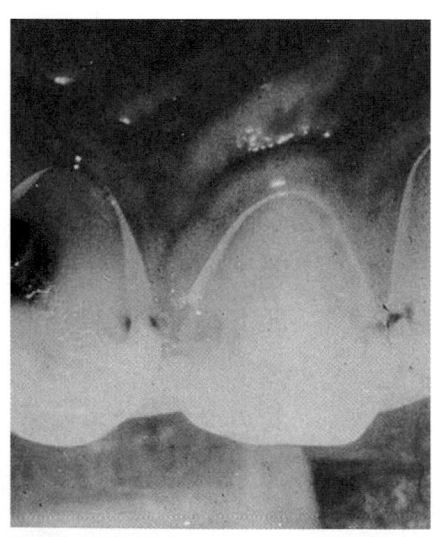

Figure 15-3 | Excessive tooth decay is common in bulimic patients.

Treatment of Bulimia Nervosa

Therapy for bulimia nervosa, as for anorexia nervosa, requires a team of experienced clinicians.[11] Bulimic patients are less likely than those with anorexia to enter treatment in a state of semistarvation. However, if a bulimic patient has lost significant weight, this weight loss must be treated before psychological treatment begins. Although clinicians have yet to agree on the best therapy for bulimia nervosa, they generally agree that treatment should last at least 16 weeks. Hospitalization may be necessary in cases of extreme laxative abuse, regular vomiting, substance abuse, and depression, especially if physical harm is evident.

The first goal of treatment for bulimia nervosa is to decrease the amount of food consumed in a binge session in order to reduce the risk of esophageal tears from related purging by vomiting. A decrease in the frequency of this type of purging will also decrease damage to the teeth.

The primary aim of psychotherapy is to improve patients' self-acceptance and help them to be less concerned about body weight. Cognitive behavior therapy is generally used.[11] Psychotherapy helps correct the all-or-none thinking typical of bulimic persons: "If I eat one cookie, I'm a failure and might as well binge." A patient may be asked to analyze the statement as a scientist would do when testing assumptions. In this way, patient and therapist together examine the validity of food and weight beliefs. The premise of this therapy is that if abnormal attitudes and beliefs can be altered, normal eating will follow. In addition, the therapist guides the person in establishing food habits that will minimize bingeing: avoiding fasting, eating regular meals, and using alternative methods—other than eating—to cope with stressful situations. Group therapy is often useful to foster strong social support. One goal of therapy is to help bulimic persons accept some depression and self-doubt as normal.

Although pharmacological agents should not be used as the sole treatment for bulimia nervosa, studies indicate that some medications may be beneficial in conjunction with other therapies.[11] Fluoxetine (Prozac) is the only antidepressant that has been approved by FDA for use in the treatment of bulimia nervosa, but physicians also may prescribe other forms of SSRI antidepressants, other psychiatric medications, such as imipramine (Tofranil) and lithium carbonate (Lithane), and certain antiseizure medications, such as topiramate (Topamax). This last medication, however, can lead to significant side effects, such as mental confusion.[5]

Nutritional counseling has two main goals: correcting misconceptions about food and reestablishing regular eating habits. Patients are given information about bulimia nervosa and its consequences. Avoiding binge foods and not constantly stepping on a scale may be recommended early in treatment. The primary goal, however, is to develop a normal eating pattern. To achieve this goal, some specialists encourage patients to develop daily meal plans and keep a food diary in which they record food intake, internal sensations of hunger, environmental factors that precipitate binges, and thoughts and feelings that accompany binge-purge cycles. Keeping a food diary not only is an accurate way to monitor food intake but also may help identify situations that seem to trigger binge episodes. With the help of a therapist, patients can develop alternative coping strategies.

In general, the focus is not on stopping bingeing and purging per se but on developing regular eating habits. Once this goal is achieved, the binge-purge cycle should start to break down. Patients are discouraged from following strict rules about healthy food choices because such rules simply mimic the typical obsessive attitudes associated with bulimia nervosa. Rather, encouraging a mature perspective on food intake—that is, regular consumption of moderate amounts of a variety of foods balanced among the food groups—helps patients overcome this disorder.[1]

Setting time limits for finishing meals and snacks is important for people with eating disorders. Many bulimic persons eat very quickly, reflecting their difficulties with satiety. Suggesting that the patient put his or her utensil down after each bite is a behavioral technique that a therapist might try with a recovering bulimic person. (In comparison, many anorexic persons eat in an excessively slow manner—for example, taking 1 hour to eat a muffin cut into tiny, bite-size pieces.)

People with bulimia nervosa must recognize that they are dealing with a serious disorder that can have grave medical complications if not treated. Because relapse is likely, therapy should be long term. People with bulimia nervosa need psychological help because they can be very depressed and are at a high risk for suicide. About 50% of people with bulimia nervosa recover completely from the disorder. Others continue to struggle with it, to varying degrees for the rest of their lives. This fact underscores the need for prevention because treatment is difficult.

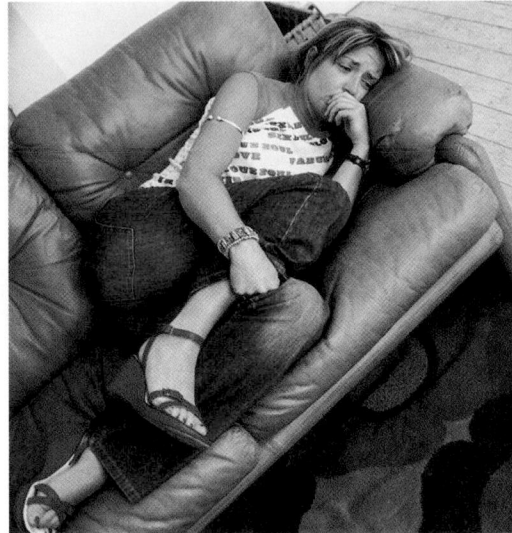

Purging episodes add to the despair felt in people with bulimia nervosa.

The binge-purge cycle can create an initial state of euphoria in the person. Giving up this euphoria has been equated to giving up an addiction. Still, it is important to do so.

Concept | Check

Treatment of bulimia nervosa using nutrition counseling and psychotherapy attempts to restore normal eating habits, to help the person correct distorted beliefs about diet and lifestyle, and to find tools to cope with the stresses of life. Medications such as fluoxetine (Prozac) can aid recovery when added to this regimen.

Eating Disorders Not Otherwise Specified (EDNOS)

EDNOS is a broad category of eating disorders in which individuals have partial syndromes that do not meet the strict criteria for anorexia nervosa or bulimia nervosa.[3] About 50% of people with eating disorders fall into this EDNOS category, especially adolescents. Examples of disordered eating in this category include (1) a woman who meets all the criteria for anorexia nervosa but continues to menstruate; (2) an individual who

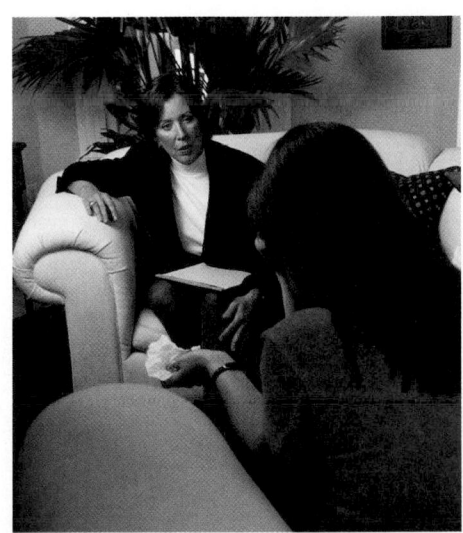

Bulimia nervosa affects many college students. Counselors are aware of this and are available to help.

meets all the criteria for anorexia nervosa but, despite a significant weight loss, has a current weight in the normal range (this could be a person who was once obese); (3) a person who meets all the criteria for bulimia nervosa except that binge eating occurs less than two times a week; (4) a person who meets all the criteria for bulimia nervosa but does not binge (this person might eat normal amounts of food but purges regularly out of fear of weight or fat gain); and (5) a person who repeatedly chews and spits out food but does not swallow it.

Treatment as outlined for anorexia nervosa or bulimia nervosa should be sought in such cases, depending on the specific symptoms exhibited.

Binge-Eating Disorder

EDNOS also includes binge-eating disorder. The typical characteristics for this disorder were listed in Table 15-2. Generally, it can be defined as binge-eating episodes not accompanied by purging (as typifies bulimia nervosa) at least two times per week for at least 6 months. Today health-care professionals recognize binge-eating disorder as a complex and potentially serious problem.[14]

Approximately 30 to 50% of subjects in organized weight-control programs have binge-eating disorder, whereas about 1 to 2% of North Americans in general have this disorder. Many more people in the general population have less severe forms of the disease, but do not meet the formal criteria for diagnosis. The number of cases of binge-eating disorder is far greater than that of either anorexia nervosa or bulimia nervosa. This disorder is also more common among the severely obese and those with a long history of frequent restrictive dieting, although obesity is not a criterion for having binge-eating disorder.

Development and Characteristics of Binge-Eating Disorder

Individuals with binge-eating disorder (about 40% of whom are males) often perceive themselves as hungry more often than normal. They usually started dieting at a young age, began bingeing during adolescence or in their early twenties, and did not succeed in commercial weight-control programs. Almost half of those with severe binge-eating disorder exhibit clinical depression.

Typical binge eaters isolate themselves and eat large quantities of their favorite food or foods readily available. Binge eaters usually consume foods that carry the social stigma of "junk" or "bad" foods—ice cream, cookies, sweets, potato chips, and similar snack foods. Stressful events and feelings of depression or anxiety can trigger this behavior. Giving themselves permission to eat a forbidden food can also precipitate a binge. Other triggers include loneliness, anxiety, self-pity, depression, anger, rage, alienation, and frustration.[14]

In general, people engage in binge eating to induce a sense of well-being and perhaps even numbness, usually in an attempt to avoid feeling and dealing with emotional pain and anxiety. They eat without regard to biological need and often in a recurrent, ritualized fashion. Some people with this disorder eat food continually over an extended period, called *grazing;* others cycle episodes of bingeing with normal eating.[14] For example, someone with a stressful or frustrating job might come home every night and graze until bedtime. Another person might eat normally most of the time but find comfort in consuming large quantities of food when an emotional setback occurs.

Although people with anorexia nervosa and bulimia nervosa exhibit persistent preoccupation with body shape, weight, and thinness, binge eaters do not necessarily share these concerns. Thus, neither purging nor prolonged food restriction is characteristic of binge-eating disorder. Some physicians classify binge-eating disorder as an addiction to food involving psychological dependence. The person becomes attached to the behavior itself and has a drive to continue it, senses only limited control over it, and needs to continue despite negative consequences. Food is used to reduce stress, produce feelings of power and well-being, avoid feelings of intimacy with others, and

Another eating disorder under study is night eating syndrome. In this disorder people eat a lot in the late evening or eat food in order to fall asleep again once awakened in the night. This night eating can contribute to weight gain, so affected persons are urged to seek treatment.

As noted in Chapter 2, spreading one's dietary intake into numerous, small meals over a day does not pose a problem, and even has some health advantages, if overall energy intake remains appropriate.

avoid life problems. Note that obesity and binge eating are not necessarily linked. Not all obese people are binge eaters, and although obesity may result from trying to numb emotional pain with food, it is not necessarily an outcome of binge eating.

Binge-eating disorder is most likely to develop in people who never learned to express and deal appropriately with their feelings. Rather than face their frustration, anger, and pain, they turn to food. The frustration will continue because they never confront the basic problem. Binge eating makes them feel they cannot control the behavior pattern and therefore cannot control their lives. Worse, the binge eating usually increases feelings of guilt, embarrassment, and shame.

Often people who practice binge eating have been shaped by families who do not address and express feelings in healthful ways. The parents nurture and comfort their children with food rather than engage in healthy exchanges of self-disclosure of feelings and potential solutions. Members of such families learn to eat in response to emotional needs and pain instead of hunger. Those who regularly practice binge eating may grow up nurturing others instead of themselves, avoiding their own feelings and taking little time for themselves. Not knowing how to satisfy their personal and emotional needs in more healthful ways, people in these families turn to food.

For some people, frequent dieting beginning in childhood or adolescence is a precursor to binge-eating disorder. During periods when little food is eaten, they get very hungry and obsessive about food. When allowed to eat more food, they feel driven to eat in a compulsive, uncontrolled way. The pattern of strict dieting alternating with binge eating may continue over time.[3]

Help for the Person with Binge-Eating Disorder

People with binge-eating disorder must learn to eat in response to hunger—a biological signal—rather than in response to emotional needs or external factors such as the time of day or the simple presence of food.[14] Counselors often ask binge eaters to record their perceptions of physical hunger throughout the day and at the beginning and end of every meal. These people must learn to respond to a prescribed amount of fullness at each meal. They should initially avoid weight-loss diets because feelings of food deprivation can lead to more disruptive emotions and a greater sense of unmet needs. Diets are likely to encourage more intense problems, such as extreme hunger. Many people with binge-eating disorder may experience difficulty in identifying personal emotional needs and expressing emotions. Because this problem is a common predisposing factor in binge eating, communication issues should be addressed during treatment. Binge eaters often must be helped to recognize their own buried emotions in anxiety-producing situations and then encouraged to share them with their therapist or therapy group. Learning simple but appropriate phrases to say to oneself can help stop bingeing when the desire is strong.

Self-help groups such as Overeaters Anonymous aim to help recovery from binge-eating disorder. The treatment philosophy parallels that of Alcoholics Anonymous and attempts to create an environment of encouragement and accountability to overcome this eating disorder. Dietary advice typically includes avoiding restraint when eating and limiting binge foods. Some experts feel that learning to eat all foods—but in moderation—is an effective goal for binge eaters. This practice can prevent the feelings of desperation and deprivation that come from limiting particular foods. Fluoxetine (Prozac) and related SSRI antidepressants, as well as other psychiatric medications, also have been found to help reduce binge eating in these individuals by decreasing depression. The antiseizure medication topiramate (Topamax) may also be used. Overall, people who have binge-eating disorder are usually unsuccessful in controlling it without professional help.[14]

Other Examples of Disordered Eating

In recent years, another condition—**female athlete triad**—has been recognized as requiring professional treatment. Although this disordered eating pattern shares some characteristics with anorexia nervosa and bulimia nervosa, it has distinctive qualities. Dr. Jackie Berning discusses this condition in detail in the Expert Opinion.

People with binge-eating disorder may come from families with alcoholism or may have suffered sexual abuse. Members of such dysfunctional families often do not know how to deal effectively with emotions. They cope by turning to substances. Family members learn to cover up dysfunctional patterns and learn to nurture the behavior of others at the expense of their own needs.

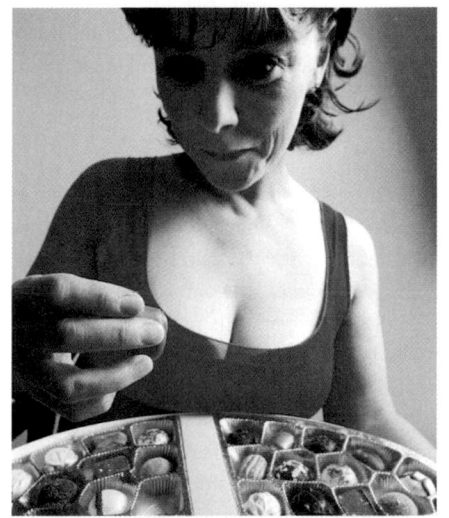

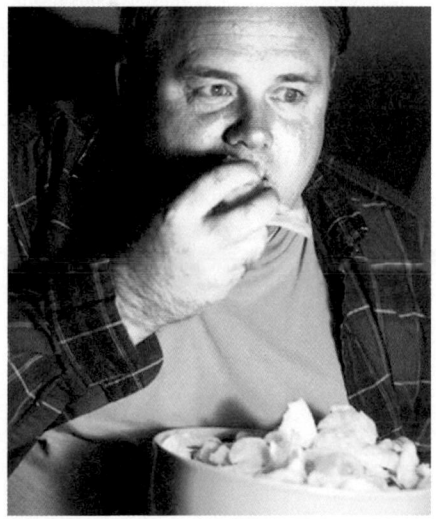

Binge-eating disorder is seen in both men and women. Professional help is advised for people with this disorder.

female athlete triad A condition characterized by disordered eating, lack of menstrual periods, and osteoporosis.

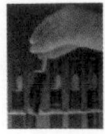

Expert Opinion

The Female Athlete Triad

Jackie Berning, Ph.D., R.D.

For the past 20 years participation in women's sports has surpassed all imagination. Today, women have many more opportunities to participate in high school and collegiate sports as well as the potential to continue their athletic careers in the professional ranks. While these women derive significant health benefits from the physical training associated with sports, they are also at risk for a syndrome of disordered eating, amenorrhea, and bone loss. This triad of disorders is known as the female athlete triad.

Disordered Eating

Disordered eating is a medical term that covers a broad spectrum of eating disorders from poor nutritional habits to the potentially lethal complications of anorexia nervosa and bulimia nervosa. In female athletes, depending on the sport studied, the prevalence of eating disorders ranges from 15 to 62%. Sports that emphasize leanness (such as endurance sports or aesthetic sports) are more likely to have a higher percentage of athletes with eating disorders.

Many female athletes with eating disorders may not meet the strict diagnostic criteria for anorexia nervosa or bulimia nervosa. Instead, they engage in regular energy restriction and fail to meet the energy demands for living and training. The motivation for this energy restriction is multifactorial. The most frequent factor is nutrition misinformation, which is the easiest to address. Dispelling myths and facts about training and diet or offering credible nutrition counseling can place the athlete back on track. Unfortunately, the problem is often more complex. Female athletes in lean profile sports are under intensive pressure from coaches, peers, and judges about body weight and image. This intense pressure and any insensitive comment may play a key role in promoting disordered eating in these young athletes. In other cases, women with established eating disorders might choose to participate in a particular sport to help control her weight.

Amenorrhea

Most amenorrhea seen in female athletes is classified as secondary amenorrhea, because it results from the disease process rather than being a primary cause of the disease itself. Secondary amenorrhea is the loss of menstruation for three or more consecutive cycles in a female who has experienced the onset of menstruation. Between 1 to 44% of female athletes experience amenorrhea. Amenorrhea can be as high as 50% in elite runners and ballet dancers. The cause of the amenorrhea seems to be related to changes in the hypothalamus in the brain, but may be multifactorial. Potential factors include energy restriction, poor eating habits, disordered eating, energy imbalance, rapid weight loss, and increase in training.

Osteoporosis

This risk is related to less estrogen output, and so the athlete loses the protective effect of estrogen on bone. Athletic amenorrhea causes bone loss like that seen in menopause. Numerous studies have shown significant bone loss in amenorrheic athletes. Unfortunately, the bone that is lost is not replaced even if menstrual cycles are resumed. Because many of these young athletes are at a critical age of bone mass, many may never be able to reach their peak bone mass, and because 70% of bone mass is acquired during adolescence and early adulthood, these female athletes are at high risk for hip and spine fractures in later life stages. In addition, amenorrheic athletes are more prone to injury, especially stress fractures.

Prevention of Eating Disorders

A key to developing and maintaining healthful eating behavior is to realize that some concern about diet, health, and weight is normal, as are variations in what we eat, how we feel, and even how much we weigh. For example, most people experience some minimal weight change (up to 2 to 3 lb) throughout the day and even more over the course of a week. A large weight fluctuation or ongoing weight gain or weight loss is more likely to indicate that a problem is present. If you notice a large change in your eating habits, how you feel, or your body weight, it is a good idea to consult your personal physician. Treating physical and emotional problems early helps lead you to peace of mind and good health.

Identifying and Managing the Problem

Members of the sports medicine team, such as registered dietitians, must constantly be aware of the symptoms and signs of female athlete triad. In the athletic culture, episodes of amenorrhea, weight loss, and injuries often may be attributed to some cause other than the female athlete triad. For this reason, it is important for clinicians to obtain and maintain records of amenorrhea among female athletes. Each athlete with amenorrhea should be referred to a physician who can rule out other causes of the amenorrhea, such as pregnancy or thyroid disease. If an athlete appears to be excessively concerned about her weight or dieting or if she presents with marked thinness, obsessive compulsion about training, fine lanugo hair, or erosion of tooth enamel, further investigation or confrontation about the eating disorder is recommended. Finally, a clinician or physician who encounters any athlete with a stress fracture should obtain a menstrual cycle history and baseline nutritional assessment.

Low body weight coupled with excessive exercise can lead to amenorrhea and ultimately female athlete triad.

The management of the athlete presenting with symptoms of the female athlete triad is best accomplished in a multidisciplinary approach including a physician, registered dietitian, psychologist, and athletic trainer. The primary goals of treatment are to control and manage the athlete's eating disorder, to restore normal hormone levels, and to monitor and treat any injuries or other medical complications. Treatment strategies to reach these goals may include a slight reduction (10 to 20%) in the amount of training and a higher energy intake for a 2 to 5% increase in weight. Some amenorrheic athletes who gain weight either by cutting back on training or consuming more energy have a better chance of resuming normal menstrual activity. In addition to weight gain, other factors that need proper attention for normal menstruation are adequate sleep, management of stress, and nutritional intake. Most amenorrheic athletes fear weight gain and must be counseled that an increase in muscle weight could improve their stamina and performance. Calcium supplementation should be implemented in all athletes presenting with amenorrhea. Vegetarianism is another contributing factor to amenorrhea. Vegetarian athletes may be at risk for low energy, protein, and micronutrient intakes because of elimination of food groups such as meat and dairy. Some researchers point out that along with the insufficient energy intake, inadequate amounts of protein may also play a role in the amenorrheic athlete.

Regardless of the cause of the amenorrhea in the female athlete, a qualified nutrition professional can help improve the quality and quantity of the athlete's diet so that normal menstruation has a better chance of resuming. In addition to working individually with the athletes, the registered dietitian should also work with the coach, athletic trainer, physician, and strength and conditioning professional to provide amenorrheic athletes with the best possible environment for maximizing their performance as well as providing a normal, healthy functioning body.

Dr. Berning is a registered dietitian and associate professor at the University of Colorado–Colorado Springs. She specializes in sports nutrition and consults for numerous professional sports teams in the United States. She works extensively with female athletes at the University of Colorado–Boulder and has been involved with counseling amenorrheic athletes for over 15 years. She has coauthored two books and numerous articles and chapters on sports nutrition.

Many people begin to form opinions about food, nutrition, health, weight, and body image prior to or during puberty. Parents, friends, and professionals working with young adults can help form positive habits and appropriate expectations, especially regarding body image.[9] Here is some advice that these people can extend to young adults to help them avoid eating disorders:

- Discourage restrictive dieting, meal skipping, and fasting (except for religious reasons).
- Provide information about normal changes that occur during puberty.
- Correct misconceptions about nutrition, healthy body weight, and approaches to weight loss.
- Carefully phrase any weight-related recommendations and comments.

Not only is treatment of eating disorders far more difficult than prevention, these disorders also have devastating effects on the entire family. For this reason, caregivers and health-care professionals alike must emphasize the importance of an overall healthful diet that focuses on moderation as opposed to restriction and perfection. Restricted diets are especially detrimental to children because they do not supply enough energy to sustain growth. In response, nutritional counseling can assure caregivers that including some sweets and fast food in a child's diet is appropriate (see Chapter 17 for more details).

- Don't overemphasize numbers on a scale. Instead, primarily promote healthful eating irrespective of body weight.
- Encourage normal expression of disruptive emotions.
- Encourage children to eat only when they're hungry.
- Teach the basics of proper nutrition and regular physical activity in school and at home.
- Provide adolescents with an appropriate, but not unlimited, degree of independence, choice, responsibility, and self-accountability for their actions.
- Increase self-acceptance and appreciation of the power and pleasure emerging from one's body.
- Enhance tolerance for diversity in body weight and shape.
- Build respectful environments and supportive relationships.
- Encourage coaches to be sensitive to weight and body-image issues among athletes.
- Emphasize that thinness is not necessarily associated with better athletic performance.

Our society as a whole can benefit from a fresh focus on healthful food practices and a healthful outlook toward food and body weight.

Organizations to Help You Understand More about Eating Disorders

You can gain more insight into eating disorders not only from the technical articles in the references but also from the following resources designed for the lay public:

Academy for Eating Disorders, 6728 McClean Village Dr., McLean, VA 22101; 703-556-9222; www.acadeatdis.org

American Anorexia Bulimia Association, 165 West 46th St., #1108, New York, NY 10036; 212-575-6200; www.aabainc.org/home.html

The National Eating Disorders Organization, 603 Stewart St., Suite 803, Seattle, WA 98101; 206-382-3587 or 800-931-EDAP; www.nationaleatingdisorders.org

Harvard Eating Disorders Centers, 356 Boylston St., Boston, MA 02116; 617-236-7766; www.hedc.org

The National Institute of Mental Health has recently published a concise review of eating disorders (www.nimh.nih.gov/publicat/eatingdisordersmenu.cfm).

Critical | Thinking

Tom, a high school teacher, is concerned about eating disorders. He wants to try to prevent young adults from falling into the discouraging traps of anorexia nervosa and bulimia nervosa. What are some of the topics and issues he should discuss with students in his health classes?

Concept | Check

Food bingeing and grazing without purging are two behaviors characteristic of binge-eating disorder. Emotional disturbances are often at the root of this eating disorder. Treatment addresses deeper emotional issues and endorses avoiding food deprivation and restrictive diets while restoring more normal eating behaviors. The female athlete triad consists of disordered eating, amenorrhea, and osteoporosis, and most commonly affects women in appearance-related and endurance sports. Parents, coaches, teachers, and health professionals need to initiate efforts to prevent and treat this problem.

Summary

1. Anorexia nervosa is most common among high-achieving, perfectionist girls from families marked by conflict, high expectations, rigidity, and denial. The disorder usually starts with dieting in early puberty and proceeds to the near-total refusal to eat. Early warning signs include intense concern about weight gain and dieting as well as abnormal food habits, such as cooking food that they won't allow themselves to eat.

2. Anorexic persons become irritable, hostile, overly critical, and joyless; they tend to withdraw from family and friends. Eventually, anorexia nervosa can lead to numerous physical effects, including a profound decrease in body weight and body fat, a fall in body temperature and heart rate, iron deficiency anemia, a low white blood cell count, hair loss, constipation, low blood potassium, and the loss of menstrual periods. People with anorexia nervosa are in a state of physical illness.

3. Treatment of anorexia nervosa includes increasing food intake to support gradual weight gain. Psychological counseling attempts to help patients establish regular food habits and to find means of coping with the life stresses that led to the disorder. Hospitalization may be necessary as well as use of certain medications.

4. Bulimia nervosa is characterized by secretive bingeing on large amounts of food within a short time span and then purging by vomiting or misuse of laxatives, diuretics, or enemas. Alternately, fasting and excessive exercise may be used. Both men and women are at risk. Vomiting as a means of purging is especially destructive to the body, causing severe tooth decay, stomach ulcers, irritation of the esophagus, low blood potassium, and other problems. Bulimia nervosa poses a serious health problem and is associated with significant risk of suicide.

5. Treatment of bulimia nervosa includes psychological as well as nutritional counseling. During treatment, bulimic persons learn to accept themselves and to cope with problems in ways that do not involve food. Regular eating patterns are developed as these patients begin to plan meals in an informed, healthful manner. Certain medications can be a helpful addition to the regimen.

6. Binge-eating disorder, which is more widespread than either anorexia nervosa or bulimia nervosa, is most common among people with a history of frequent, unsuccessful dieting. Binge eaters typically either binge without purging or graze (i.e., eat continually over extended periods). Thus, this condition falls under the category Eating Disorders Not Otherwise Specified (EDNOS). Emotional disturbances are often at the root of this disordered form of eating. Treatment addresses deeper emotional issues, discourages food deprivation and restrictive diets, and helps restore normal eating behaviors. Certain medications may be a useful addition to this therapy.

Study Questions

1. What are the typical characteristics of a person with anorexia nervosa? What may influence a person to begin rigid, self-imposed dietary patterns?

2. List the detrimental physical and psychological side effects of bulimia nervosa. Describe important goals of the psychological and nutrition therapy used to treat bulimic patients.

3. What is the current thinking concerning medication use for anorexia nervosa and bulimia nervosa?

4. Explain the role of excessive exercise in eating disorders.

5. How might parents significantly contribute to the development of an eating disorder? Suggest an attitude that a parent or an adult friend of yours displayed that may not have been conducive to developing a normal relationship to food.

6. Based on your knowledge of good nutrition and sound dietary habits, answer the following questions:
   a. How can repeated bingeing and purging lead to significant nutrient deficiencies?
   b. How can significant nutrient deficiencies contribute to major health problems in later life?
   c. A friend asks you, the nutrition expert, if it is okay to "cleanse" the body by eating only grapefruit for a week. What is your response?

7. How, in your opinion, has society contributed to the development of various forms of disordered eating? Provide an example.

8. How does binge-eating disorder differ from bulimia nervosa? Describe the factors that contribute to the development and treatment of binge eating disorder.

9. List the three symptoms that constitute the female athlete triad. What is the major health risk associated with loss of menstrual periods in the female athlete?

10. Provide two recommendations to reduce the problem of eating disorders in our society.

> **BOOST YOUR STUDY**
>
> Check out the **Perspectives in Nutrition: Online Learning Center** www.mhhe.com/wardlawpers7 for quizzes, flash cards, activities, and web links designed to further help you learn about eating disorders.

Annotated References

1. ADA Reports: Position of the American Dietetic Association: Nutrition intervention in the treatment of anorexia nervosa, bulimia nervosa, and eating disorders not otherwise specified (EDNOS). *Journal of the American Dietetic Association* 101:810, 2001.

   Eating disorders are complex and serious illnesses, as described in detail in this article. To be effective in treating individuals who suffer from these illnesses, the expert interaction between professionals in many disciplines is required.

2. American Academy of Pediatrics: Identifying and treating eating disorders. *Pediatrics* 111:204, 2003.

   Eating disorders are becoming more common in our society. This article reviews the current diagnostic and treatment options for such disorders.

3. American Psychiatric Association: *Diagnostic and statistical manual of mental disorders.* 4th ed. (text revision) (DSM-IV-TR). Washington, DC: American Psychiatric Association, 2000.

   This manual contains the criteria used in diagnosing an eating disorder. The specific criteria for anorexia nervosa, bulimia nervosa, and binge-eating disorder are provided.

4. Broussard BB: Women's experiences of bulimia nervosa. *Journal of Advanced Nursing* 49:43, 2005.

   Four overall themes characterize living with bulimia nervosa: isolating self, living in fear, being at war with the mind, and pacifying the brain. Bulimic individuals fear being judged by others who might discover their binge-purge cycle, and some fear living without bulimia nervosa because the disease had become such a significant part of their identities.

5. Coughlin JW, Guarda AS: Behavioral disorders affecting food intake: Eating disorders and other psychiatric conditions. In Shils ME and others (eds): *Modern nutrition in health and disease.* 10th ed. Philadelphia, PA: Lippincott Williams & Wilkins, 2006.

   Current review of the causes and treatments of various eating disorders. The specific role of the nutritional professional as part of the treatment team for these disorders is highlighted.

6. Courbasson CM and others: Substance use disorders, anorexia, bulimia, and concurrent disorders. *Canadian Journal of Public Health* 96:102, 2005.

   Individuals, particularly females, who experience substance abuse have a heightened risk for eating disorders; however, treatment facilities typically specialize either in substance abuse or eating disorders and may not be providing appropriate therapy to patients.

7. Frydrych AM and others: Eating disorders and oral health: A review of the literature. *Australian Dental Journal* 50:6, 2005.

   Dentists are sometimes the first health-care professional to recognize an eating disorder in an individual. Repeated vomiting causes tooth destruction and glandular swelling, but there are few protocols in place to assist dentists with referrals for eating disorder therapy.

8. Holtkamp K and others: Depression, anxiety, and obsessionality in long-term recovered patients with adolescent-onset anorexia nervosa. *European Child and Adolescent Psychiatry* 14:106, 2005.

   Anorexia nervosa often is associated with depression, anxiety, and obsessive-compulsive behavior. These traits appear to develop secondary to semistarvation but frequently do not subside even after recovery from anorexia nervosa has occurred.

9. Jackson K: Eating disorders revealed. *Today's Dietitian,* p. 37, March 2004.

   Eating disorders are often hard to recognize because individuals may hide the various practices. This article discusses the many characteristics of eating disorders that can be used in the diagnosis.

10. Kouba S and others: Pregnancy and neonatal outcomes in women with eating disorders. *Obstetrics and Gynecology* 105:255, 2005.

    Pregnant women with past or active anorexia nervosa or bulimia nervosa have a greater risk for delivering infants with low birth weight and small head circumference and who are small for gestational age.

11. Mehler PS: Bulimia nervosa. *The New England Journal of Medicine* 349:875, 2003.

    The combination of cognitive behavior therapy and antidepressant medications provides the best hope for treatment of bulimia nervosa. Nutritional counseling also has a role, such as addressing concerns about specific "forbidden" foods.

12. Miller KK and others: Medical findings in outpatients with anorexia nervosa. *Archives of Internal Medicine* 165:561, 2005.

    Medical problems are typically seen in people with anorexia in our society. Examples are lowered immune system status and bone loss with related history of bone fractures.

13. Pritts SD, Susman J: Diagnosis of eating disorders in primary care. *American Family Physician* 67:297, 2003.

    This article is an excellent review of the diagnosis and stages of treatment of eating disorders. The many physical effects of this disorder also are described.

14. Shanta-Retelny V: Binge eating into obesity. *Today's Dietitian,* p. 34, May 2004.

    Binge-eating disorder is a common problem in people seeking therapy for obesity. The combination of cognitive behavior therapy and certain psychiatric and antiseizure medications cur-
    rently provides the greatest likelihood for successful therapy. Not skipping meals is a key part of the nutrition therapy.

15. Stein D and others: Attempted suicide and self-injury in patients diagnosed with eating disorders. *Comprehensive Psychiatry* 45:447, 2004.

    Individuals with eating disorders have a heightened risk of developing suicidal behavior. Particularly at risk are those who binge and purge; use more than one type of purging method; have a history of drug use, impulse control difficulty, and/or bipolar disorder; and a lengthy history of outpatient and inpatient treatment.

16. Tozzi F and others: Symptom fluctuation in eating disorders: Correlates of diagnostic crossover. *American Journal of Psychiatry* 162:732, 2005.

    Some individuals first diagnosed with anorexia nervosa will experience a crossover to a diagnosis of bulimia nervosa within the first 5 years of their illness. Fewer individuals with bulimia nervosa, however, experience a crossover to anorexia nervosa. Anorexic individuals who perceive high parental criticism and bulimic individuals who struggle with alcohol abuse are most likely to experience a crossover and be diagnosed with a new eating disorder.

17. Van Wymelbeke V and others: Factors associated with the increase in resting energy expenditure during refeeding in malnourished anorexia nervosa patients. *American Journal of Clinical Nutrition* 80:1469, 2004.

    When anorexic patients are fed as part of their treatment, resting energy expenditure increases. Anxiety, physical activity, and cigarette smoking were all linked to resting energy expenditure and contributed to resistance to weight gain.

18. Walsh BT: Eating disorders. In Kasper DL and others (eds.): *Harrison's principles of internal medicine.* New York: McGraw-Hill, 2004.

    This chapter is an excellent review of eating disorders by a noted expert. Both diagnosis and treatment are highlighted.

19. Woods S: Untreated recovery from eating disorders. *Adolescence* 39:361, 2004.

    Some individuals can recover from anorexia nervosa or bulimia nervosa without professional treatment. Among these individuals, those who have the shortest eating disorder duration and most complete recovery have parents who intervened early on in the disorder's progression.

20. Yager J, Andersen AE: Anorexia nervosa. *The New England Journal of Medicine* 353:1441, 2005.

    Detailed depiction of the diagnosis and treatment of anorexia nervosa. Indications for the need for hospitalization are included.

Take | Action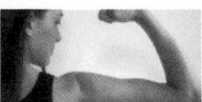

I. Assessing Risk of Developing an Eating Disorder

British investigators have developed a five-question screening tool called the SCOFF Questionnaire for recognizing eating disorders:

1. Do you make yourself <u>S</u>ick because you feel full?

2. Do you lose <u>C</u>ontrol over how much you eat?

3. Have you lost more than <u>O</u>ne stone (about 13 lb) recently?

4. Do you believe yourself to be <u>F</u>at when others say you are thin?

5. Does <u>F</u>ood dominate your life?
   Two or more positive responses suggest an eating disorder.

1. After completing this questionnaire, do you feel that you might have an eating disorder or the potential to develop one?

   _____

   _____

2. Do you think any of your friends might have an eating disorder?

   _____

   _____

3. What counseling and education resources exist in your area or on your campus to help with a potential eating disorder?

   _____

   _____

4. If a friend has an eating disorder, what do you think is the best way to assist him or her in getting help?

   _____

   _____

Source: Morgan JF and others: The SCOFF Questionnaire, *British Medical Journal* 319:1467, 1999.

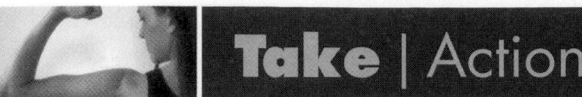 **Take** | Action

II. Helping Prevent Eating Disorders

You have been asked to speak to a junior high school class about eating disorders. What four major points would you make to help prevent disordered eating in this population?

1. _____

2. _____

3. _____

4. _____

Here are points you may consider:

1. Extreme thinness is oversold in the media. Extremely low weight (i.e., BMI of less than 17.5) is generally not healthy.

2. Self-induced vomiting is dangerous. Damage to the teeth, stomach, and esophagus often results.

3. Loss of menstrual periods is a sign of illness. It is important to see a physician about this symptom. Bone deterioration is a common result.

4. Early treatment of eating disorders aids success. These diseases are difficult to treat once firmly established.

16

PREGNANCY AND BREASTFEEDING

CHAPTER OUTLINE

CASE SCENARIO:

Tracey and her husband of 4 years have decided that they are ready to have a child. Tracey has been reading everything she can find on pregnancy because she knows that her prepregnancy health is important to the success of her pregnancy.

She just turned 25 and so is in the recommended childbearing age of 20 to 35 years. She knows she should avoid alcohol: alcohol is particularly toxic to the growing fetus in the first weeks of pregnancy, and she could become pregnant and not know about it right away. Tracey is not a smoker, does not take any medications, and limits her coffee intake to 4 cups a day and soft drink intake to 3 colas per day.

Based on her reading, she has decided to breastfeed her infant and has already inquired about childbirth classes. She has modified her diet to include some extra protein, along with more fruits and vegetables. Recently, she started swimming 5 days a week, and she plans to continue swimming throughout her pregnancy. She has also started taking an over-the-counter vitamin and mineral supplement.

Tracey and her husband think that they have covered all the key areas of prepregnancy care. List a few positive attributes of her current practices. Can you identify some potential problems and what information they may have missed?

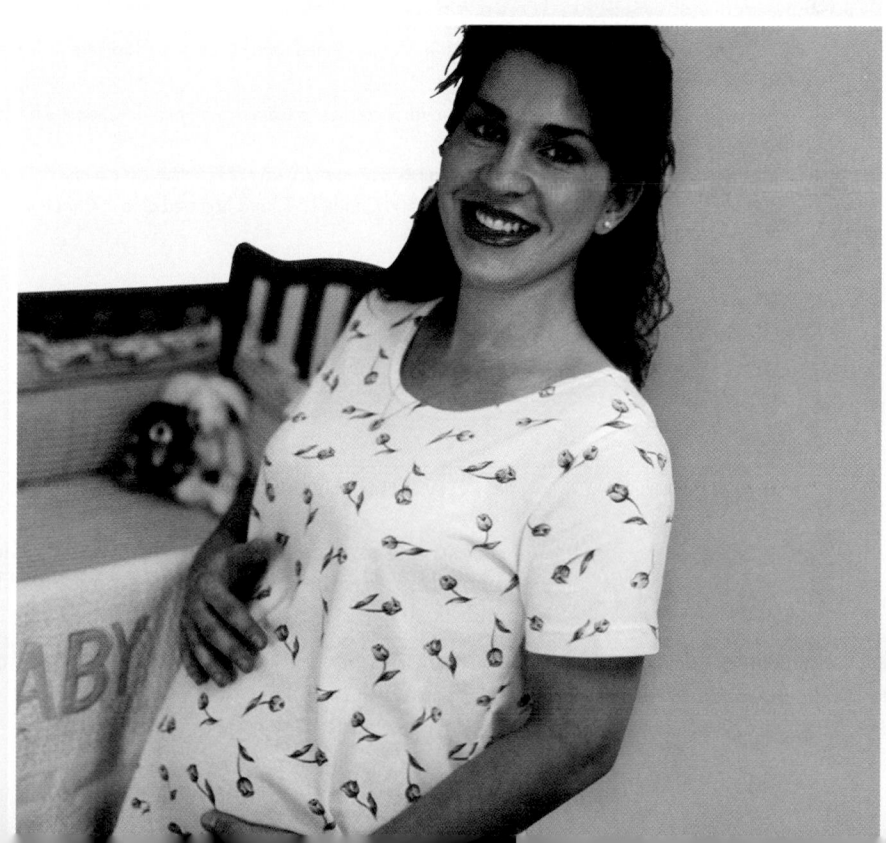

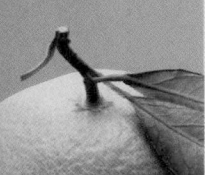

Pregnancy is a very special time. Along with the responsibility of shaping a child's health and personality comes the prospective exhilaration of watching a child develop and grow. Parents-to-be often feel an overriding desire to produce a healthy baby, which can arouse new interest in nutrition and health information. They usually want to do everything possible to maximize their chances of having a robust, lively newborn.

Despite these intentions, the infant mortality rate in North America is higher than that seen in many other industrialized nations. In Canada, about 6.1 of every 1000 infants per year die before their first birthday, whereas in the United States the figure is 6.9. These statistics are alarming for two countries that have such a high per capita expenditure for health care compared to many other countries in the world. And compare these numbers to Sweden, at roughly 3 of every 1000 infants. In addition, in the United States, about 20% of pregnant women receive inadequate prenatal care in the early months of pregnancy. Expectant teenagers are at the highest risk for this problem.

Producing a healthy baby is not just a matter of luck. True, some aspects of fetal and newborn health are beyond our control.[1] Still, conscious decisions about social, health, and nutritional factors during pregnancy significantly affect the baby's future.[5] Choosing to breastfeed the infant adds further benefits.[2] This chapter examines how a woman who eats well during pregnancy and breastfeeding can help her baby to have a healthy start in life.

CHAPTER OBJECTIVES CHAPTER 16 IS DESIGNED TO ALLOW YOU TO:

1. List major physiological changes that occur in the body during pregnancy and how nutrient needs are altered.
2. List factors that predict a successful pregnancy outcome.
3. Specify the optimal weight gain during pregnancy for the normal adult woman.
4. Plan an adequate, balanced meal plan for a pregnant or lactating woman using MyPyramid as a basis.
5. Identify the nutrients that may need to be supplemented during pregnancy and explain the reason for each.
6. Explain the typical discomforts of pregnancy that can be minimized by dietary changes.
7. Describe the physiological processes involved in breastfeeding as well as some advantages of breastfeeding for both the infant and mother.
8. Describe fetal alcohol syndrome and discuss its implications for an infant.

REFRESH YOUR MEMORY AS YOU BEGIN YOUR STUDY OF NUTRITION IN PREGNANCY AND BREASTFEEDING IN CHAPTER 16, YOU MAY WANT TO REVIEW:

- Typical fortification in meal replacement bars in Chapter 1 and ready-to-eat breakfast cereals in Chapter 2.
- Causes and effects of ketosis in Chapter 4.
- The components of the macronutrient classes—carbohydrates, proteins, and lipids—in Chapters 5 to 7, especially omega-3 fatty aids.
- Alcohol content of various beverages in Chapter 8.
- The food sources of folate in Chapter 10, calcium in Chapter 11, and iron and zinc in Chapter 12.
- The calculation of body mass index in Chapter 13.
- Endocrine, reproductive, and immune systems in Appendix C.

▌ Planning for Pregnancy

Because many practices or conditions of the mother can harm the developing fetus, planning for pregnancy is very important. The following are some potentially harmful habits that can be modified when planning to have a baby:[1,3,15,20]

- Lack of enough synthetic folic acid in the diet (at least 3 months before becoming pregnant)
- Any amount of alcohol consumption

Healthy People 2010 includes a goal of increasing to 80% the number of pregnancies that begin with optimal folate status from the current estimate of 21%, in an effort to reduce the occurrence of neural tube defects.

- Use of certain medicines, such as aspirin and related NSAIDs (e.g., ibuprofen [Advil]), as well as typical medicines used to treat the common cold
- Use of illegal drugs, such as marijuana and cocaine
- Any herbal therapies
- Job-related hazards and stresses
- Smoking
- Inadequate intake of other nutrients, such as too little iron, magnesium, and zinc
- Excess vitamin A intake and megadose use of other nutrient supplements
- Heavy caffeine use
- Lack of medical treatment with HIV-positive status or AIDS
- Poor, control of ongoing diabetes or hypertension
- X-ray exposure, including dental X rays

Women need to pay attention to these risks in the months before conception. This precaution is necessary because women often do not suspect they are pregnant during the first few weeks after conception and may not seek medical attention until after the first 2 to 3 months of pregnancy.[3]

Still, even without fanfare, the child-to-be grows and develops daily. For that reason, the health and nutrition habits of a woman who is trying to become pregnant—or has the potential to become pregnant—are particularly important. Although some aspects of fetal and newborn health are beyond control, a woman's conscious decisions about social, health, and nutritional factors affect her infant's health and future. For example, an adequate vitamin and mineral intake at least 8 weeks before conception and then during pregnancy can help prevent birth defects such as neural tube defects (review Figure 10-7 in Chapter 10).[5] Neural tube defects especially have been linked to a folic acid deficiency. Recall from Chapter 10 that neural tube defects develop within 28 days after conception and that adequate folic acid status before and during this part of pregnancy reduces the risk of such defects by about 70%. In addition, because about 50% of pregnancies are unplanned, all women of childbearing age should be aware of the role nutrition plays in the development of a healthy infant, both before and during pregnancy. Following a healthy diet is then very important. The American College of Obstetrics and Gynecology reminds women that it is especially important to meet folic acid needs (400 µg of synthetic folic acid), which is possible if the woman makes careful dietary choices. Alternately, adding a balanced multivitamin and mineral supplement to one's diet is also appropriate for meeting this goal. Dr. Lynn Bailey discusses folic acid and related pregnancy outcomes in greater detail in the Expert Opinion.

Women who have previously given birth to an infant with a neural tube defect such as spina bifida should consult their physician about the need for folic acid supplementation; an intake of 4 mg of synthetic folic acid per day at least one month prior to conception is recommended, but it must be taken under a physician's supervision.

Prenatal Growth and Development

For 8 weeks after conception, a human **embryo** develops from a fertilized **ovum** into a **fetus.** For about another 32 weeks, the fetus continues to develop. When its body finally matures, the infant is born. Until birth, the mother nourishes it via a **placenta,** an organ that forms in her uterus to accommodate the growth and development of the fetus (Figure 16-1).

The specific role of the placenta is to exchange nutrients, oxygen and other gases, and waste products between the mother and the fetus. To accomplish these tasks, the placenta uses all the absorption mechanisms employed by the GI tract (review Chapter 3). Even though the tissues of the placenta and the embryo are "interdigitated," the blood of the fetus and mother never mix. In fact, the fetal blood is separated from the maternal blood by just two layers of cells (5.5 µm). Fetal blood travels from the fetal heart to the placenta by way of two umbilical arteries and returns (nutrient-enriched and waste-free) to the fetus by means of one umbilical vein. In addition, the placenta also is a major site of hormone production during pregnancy. As the pregnancy continues, the placenta enlarges along with the fetus and usually weighs about 1.5 lb (0.7 kg) at delivery.

embryo In humans, the developing in utero offspring from about the beginning of the third week to the end of the eighth week after conception.

ovum The egg cell from which a fetus eventually develops if the egg is fertilized by a sperm cell.

fetus The developing life form from about the beginning of the ninth week after conception until birth.

placenta An organ that forms in the uterus in pregnant women. Through this organ, oxygen and nutrients from the mother's blood are transferred to the fetus and fetal wastes are removed. The placenta also releases hormones that maintain the state of pregnancy.

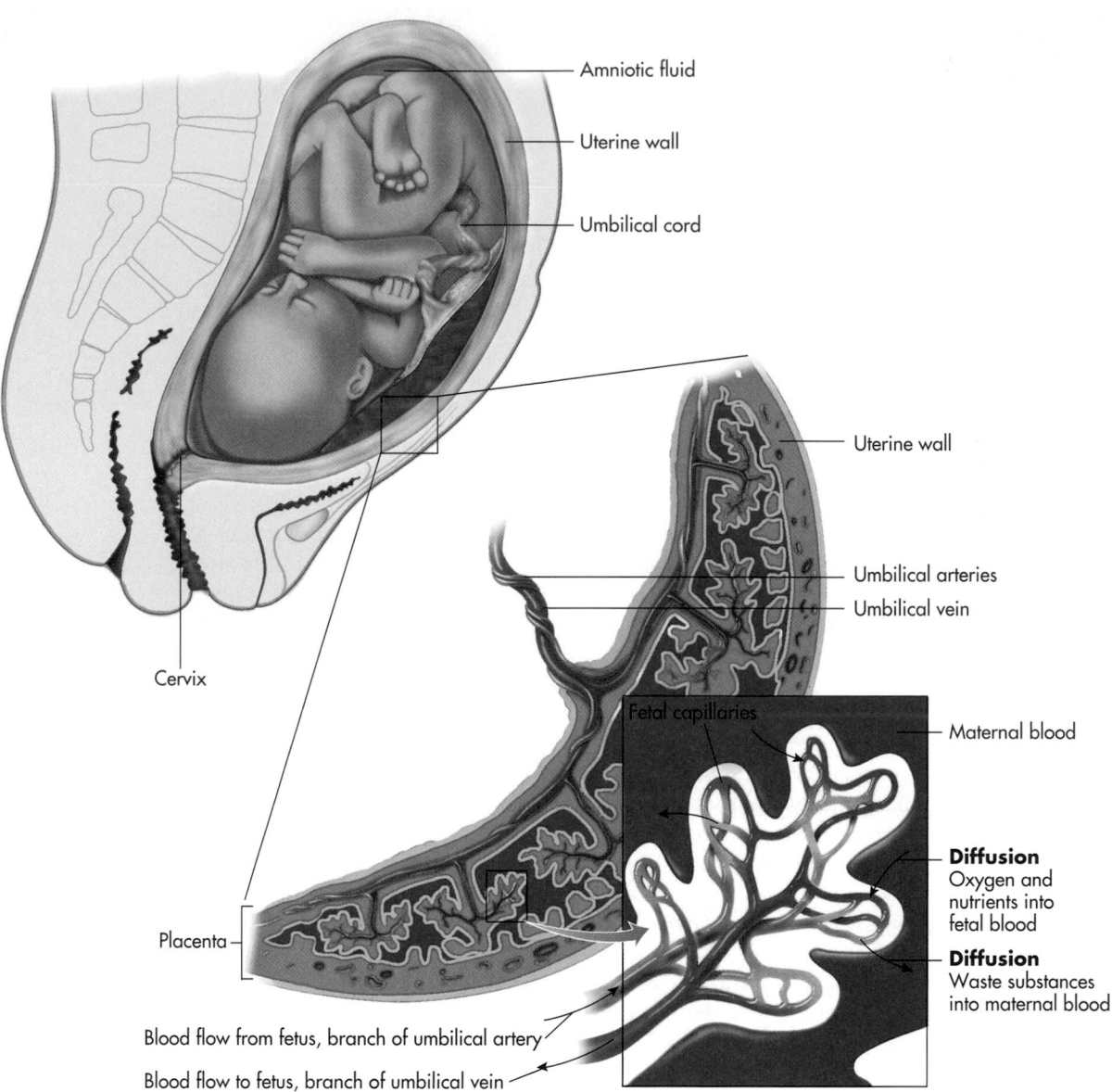

Figure 16-1 | The fetus in relationship to the placenta. The placenta is the organ through which nourishment flows to the fetus. The inset shows how blood circulation of the mother and fetus work together to provide the fetus with oxygen and nutrients while also removing fetal waste products.

Early Growth: The First Trimester Is a Very Critical Time

The formation of the human organism begins when an egg and a sperm unite to form the **zygote** (Figure 16-2). About 30 hours after the egg is fertilized, the zygote reproduces itself by dividing in half. The process of cell division then repeats many times. As the cluster of cells drifts down the fallopian tube to the woman's uterus, several kinds of cells emerge. The entire genetic code is passed to every cell, but each cell uses only a segment of the code to produce proteins. If this partial use did not take place, there would be no different organs or body parts. For example, all cells carry genes that dictate hair color and eye color, but only the cells of the hair follicles and irises respond to that specific information.

On about the fourth day after fertilization, the **conceptus,** now about 128 cells and hollow, arrives in the uterus. By the seventh day, the conceptus implants into the uter-

zygote The fertilized ovum; the cell resulting from the union of an egg cell (ovum) and sperm until it divides.

conceptus A generic term for any developmental stage derived from the fertilized ovum (zygote) until birth. The conceptus includes the extraembryonic membranes as well as the embryo or fetus.

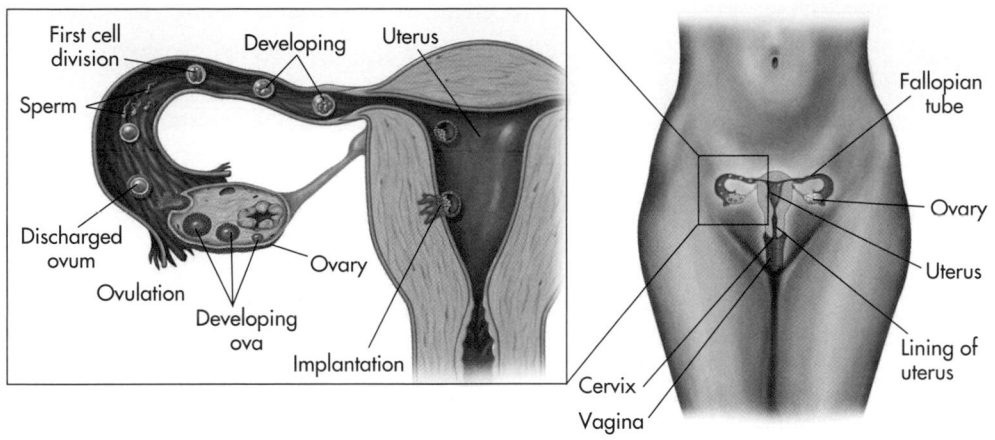

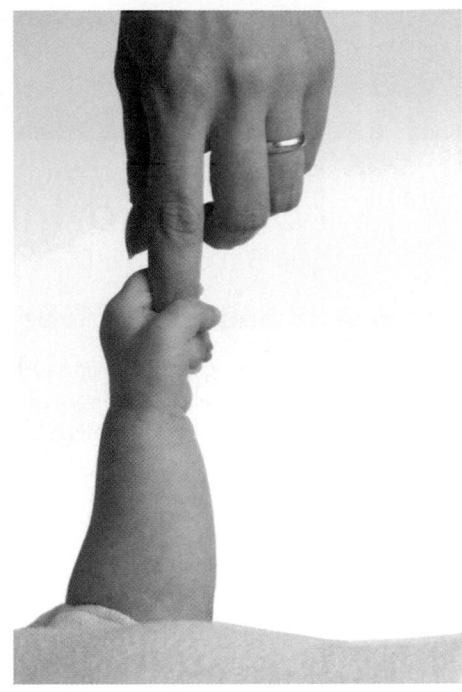

The time to begin thinking about prenatal nutrition is before becoming pregnant. This includes making sure folic acid intake is adequate (400 μg of synthetic folic acid per day) and that any supplemental use of preformed vitamin A does not exceed 100% of the Daily Value (1000 μg RAE or 5000 IU).

Figure 16-2 | After ovulation, the discharged ovum first enters the abdominal cavity and then finds its way into the fallopian tube, where conception, or fertilization, takes place. Sperm cells "swim" up the fallopian tube toward the ovum. Fertilization most often occurs in the outer one-third of the fallopian tube. The ovum also takes an active role in the process of fertilization by attracting and "trapping" sperm with special receptor molecules on its surface. As soon as the head and neck of one spermatozoon enter the ovum (the tail drops off), complex mechanisms in the egg are activated to ensure that no more sperm enter. The 23 chromosomes from the sperm combine with the 23 chromosomes already in the ovum to make up the 46 chromosomes of the conceptus.

ine lining. Two weeks after conception the cell number has increased further, and the conceptus is now termed an embryo. By day 35 of gestation, the heart is beating, and although the embryo is only 8 mm (about 3/8 inch) long, the eyes and so-called limb buds, which ultimately form the arms and legs, are clearly visible. From about the end of the eighth week after conception to its birth about 32 weeks later, the developing offspring is known as a fetus.

For purposes of discussion, the duration of pregnancy—normally, 40 weeks, measured from the first day of the woman's last menstrual period—is commonly divided into three periods, called **trimesters.** Growth begins in the first trimester with a rapid increase in cell number (hyperplasia). This type of growth dominates embryonic and later fetal development. The newly formed cells then begin to grow larger (hypertrophy). Further growth and development then involve mostly hyperplasia with some hypertrophy. By the end of 12 weeks—the first trimester—most organs are formed and the fetus can move (Figure 16-3).

As the embryo or fetus develops, nutritional deficiencies and other insults have the potential to impose damage or risk to organ systems.[11] For example, adverse reactions to medications, high intakes of vitamin A, exposure to radiation, or trauma can alter or arrest the current phase of fetal development, and the effects may last a lifetime (review Figure 16-3). The most critical time for these potential problems is during the first trimester. Most **spontaneous abortions**—premature terminations of pregnancy that occur naturally—happen at this time. Currently, about one-half or more of all pregnancies end in this way, often so early that a woman does not even realize she was pregnant. (An additional 15 to 20% are lost before normal delivery.) Early spontaneous abortions usually result from a genetic defect or fatal error in fetal development. Smoking, alcohol abuse, use of aspirin and NSAIDs, and illicit drug use raise the risk for spontaneous abortion.[5]

A woman should avoid substances that may harm the developing fetus, especially during the first trimester. This caution holds true, as well, for the time when a woman is trying to become pregnant. As previously mentioned, a woman is unlikely to be aware of her pregnancy for at least a few weeks. In addition, the fetus develops so rapidly during the first trimester that if an essential nutrient is not available, the fetus may

trimesters Three 13- to 14-week periods into which the normal pregnancy is somewhat arbitrarily divided for purposes of discussion and analysis (the length of a normal pregnancy is about 40 weeks, measured from the first day of the woman's last menstrual period). Development of the offspring, however, is continuous throughout pregnancy, with no specific physiological characterizations demarcating the transition from one trimester to the next.

spontaneous abortion Cessation of pregnancy and expulsion of the embryo or nonviable fetus prior to 20 weeks gestation. This is the result of natural causes, such as a genetic defect or developmental problem; also called *miscarriage.*

Expert Opinion

Folic Acid Interventions: Public Health Outcomes
Lynn B. Bailey, Ph.D.

Folic Acid and Neural Tube Defects

One of the most exciting recent public health discoveries is that folic acid, a water-soluble vitamin, will significantly reduce the incidence of neural tube defects (NTDs), major birth defects affecting the spinal cord and brain. The key scientific evidence proving that folic acid alone prevents a large percentage of NTDs is evidence from a randomized controlled trial conducted by the Medical Research Council in 1991. This study, confirming numerous observational studies, demonstrated that folic acid supplements taken just prior to conception and during the initial period after conception (periconceptional period) can reduce NTD risk by as much as 70%. The form of the vitamin linked to the reduction in risk for NTDs in the research studies is the monoglutamate form (folic acid), used commercially in supplements and in folic acid–fortified foods.

Metabolically, folate is converted to coenzyme forms required in numerous one-carbon transfer reactions involved in the synthesis of DNA, amino acids, and other essential structural and regulatory compounds required for normal cell division and growth. During the first 28 days of gestation, before most women even know they are pregnant, there is an explosion of new cell division within the embryonic tissue that develops into the spinal cord and brain, a process dependent on an adequate supply of folate.

Folic Acid Fortification

The strong scientific evidence that taking periconceptional folic acid supplements dramatically reduces the risk of NTDs prompted the U.S. Public Health Service in 1992 to recommend that all women of reproductive age consume 400 μg/day of folic acid. Three approaches were recommended: improve dietary habits; fortify foods with folic acid; and take dietary supplements containing folic acid.

Compliance with this 400-μg/day recommendation for folic acid consumption was not good; the majority of women capable of becoming pregnant were not meeting folic acid needs. In response, countries including the United States and Canada now mandate the addition of folic acid to all "enriched" cereal grain products.

In the United States, food fortification was originally proposed by FDA to provide only a portion (100 μg/day) of the recommended dose (400 μg/day) associated with NTD risk reduction and was to be coupled with dietary advice to increase the consumption of folate-rich foods (e.g., orange juice, dark green leafy vegetables). It is now recognized that the estimated daily increase in folic acid consumption due to fortification is approximately twice (~200 μg/day) that originally proposed. This higher-than-expected increase occurred because the food industry added substantially more folic acid to many fortified products than was required by law.

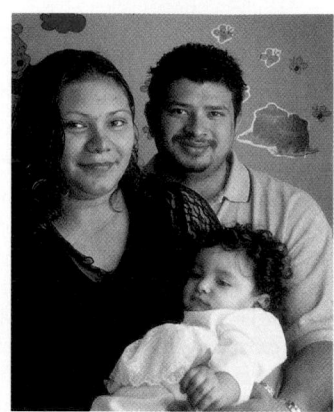

Delivering a healthy baby is more than just luck. Many nutrition- and health-related practices, such as folate intake, need to be considered.

Several thousand food items, including mixed dishes and snack foods, now contain folic acid. The good news is that the widespread consumption of folic acid–fortified foods has resulted in significant increases in blood folate concentrations in all age groups in the United States. It has also been associated with significant reductions in NTDs in both the United States and Canada, demonstrating the successful translation of science into an effective public health policy.

Folic Acid and Heart Defects

This development of widespread folic acid fortification of our food supply now allows researchers to evaluate evidence for an association between

be affected even before evidence of the nutrient deficiency appears in the mother. Still, although a mother's decisions, practices, and precautions during pregnancy contribute to the health of her fetus, she cannot guarantee her fetus good health because some genetic and environmental factors are beyond her control. She and others involved in the pregnancy should not hold an unrealistic illusion of total control.

The quality—rather than the quantity—of nutritional intake is most important during the first trimester. In other words, women should consume the same amount of energy, but the foods chosen should be more nutrient dense.[1] Although some women lose their appetite and feel nauseated during the first trimester, they should be careful to meet nutrient needs as much as possible.

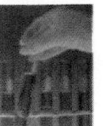

periconceptional folic acid and other common congenital anomalies, including heart defects. Heart defects affect 1 in 110 newborns and account for a third or more of infant deaths due to birth defects, more than for any other congenital anomaly, including NTDs. It is estimated that 6000 deaths attributable to heart defects occur in the United States each year. Research supports the conclusion that taking multivitamins containing folic acid during early pregnancy is associated with a significant risk reduction for heart defects. A randomized controlled trial would allow a comparison between the effect of folic acid alone relative to other vitamins and to a placebo. The resulting data could show a cause-and-effect relationship between folic acid and heart defects. Such a study is required before definitive conclusions and public health recommendations similar to those for NTDs can be made.

Safety Issues Regarding Folic Acid

It is important to address the question of safety of folic acid intake because many of us are consuming more than we have in the past. Based on the Institute of Medicine's thorough consideration of this question, there is no scientific evidence that high intakes of folic acid result in toxic side effects. There is, however, a Tolerable Upper Level for folic acid of 1000 µg/day, based on evidence that high doses of supplemental folic acid in vitamin B-12–deficient individuals (predominantly older adults) may correct the related anemia (often used to diagnose a B-12 deficiency), which may delay diagnosis and treatment and thus allow the progression of the neurological degeneration associated with the B-12 deficiency. This issue is the primary reason that countries outside the United States and Canada have not mandated folic acid fortification.

Some reports suggest that the use of periconceptional folic acid increases the risk of multiple births, a concern because multiple births are associated with more pregnancy complications and are more likely to result in preterm delivery. When the data in these studies were corrected for factors such as the use of reproductive technology and increased maternal age, known to increase the likelihood of multiple births, the association between folic acid

and multiple births was no longer significant. Several recent evaluations of the effect of folic acid fortification on the rate of multiple births in the United States following mandatory folic acid fortification in 1998 led to the conclusion that there was no evidence that multiple births have increased. Women of reproductive age and their health-care providers can support the periconceptional goal of consuming 400 µg/day of folic acid to reduce NTDs without concern that this practice will increase the occurrence of multiple births.

Conclusion

Over the past 20 years, scientific proof of the connection between folic acid and NTDs led to mandatory cereal-product fortification and has ultimately resulted in a significant decline in NTD-affected pregnancies and births in the United States and Canada. Preliminary evidence suggests that folic acid supplementation can also contribute to a reduction in the incidence of *congenital* heart defects. It is no surprise, then, that further programs to educate women and their health-care providers of the benefits of folic acid could result in even fewer NTD-affected births.

Dr. Bailey is Professor in the Food Science and Human Nutrition Department at the University of Florida, Gainesville, Florida. Dr. Bailey received her master of science from Clemson University and her Ph.D. from Purdue University. Dr. Bailey's research area of expertise is folate metabolism, estimation of folate requirements, and factors that influence disease and birth defect risk, including genetic polymorphisms. Dr. Bailey has conducted human metabolic studies over a period of 25 years, generating data that has been instrumental in establishing new dietary intake recommendations for individuals throughout the life cycle, including pregnant women and older adults. Dr. Bailey has received numerous awards for her research, including the 2004 American Society for Nutritional Sciences Centrum Center Award for her accomplishments related to human folate requirements.

Second Trimester

By the beginning of the second trimester, a fetus weighs about 1 oz. Arms, hands, fingers, legs, feet, and toes are fully formed. The fetus has ears and begins to form tooth sockets in its jawbone. Organs continue to grow and mature, and with a stethoscope, physicians can detect the fetus's heartbeat. Most bones are distinctly evident through the body. Eventually, the fetus begins to look more like an infant. It may suck its thumb and kick strongly enough to be felt by the mother. As was shown in Figure 16-3, the fetus can still be affected by exposure to toxins, but not to the degree seen in the first trimester.

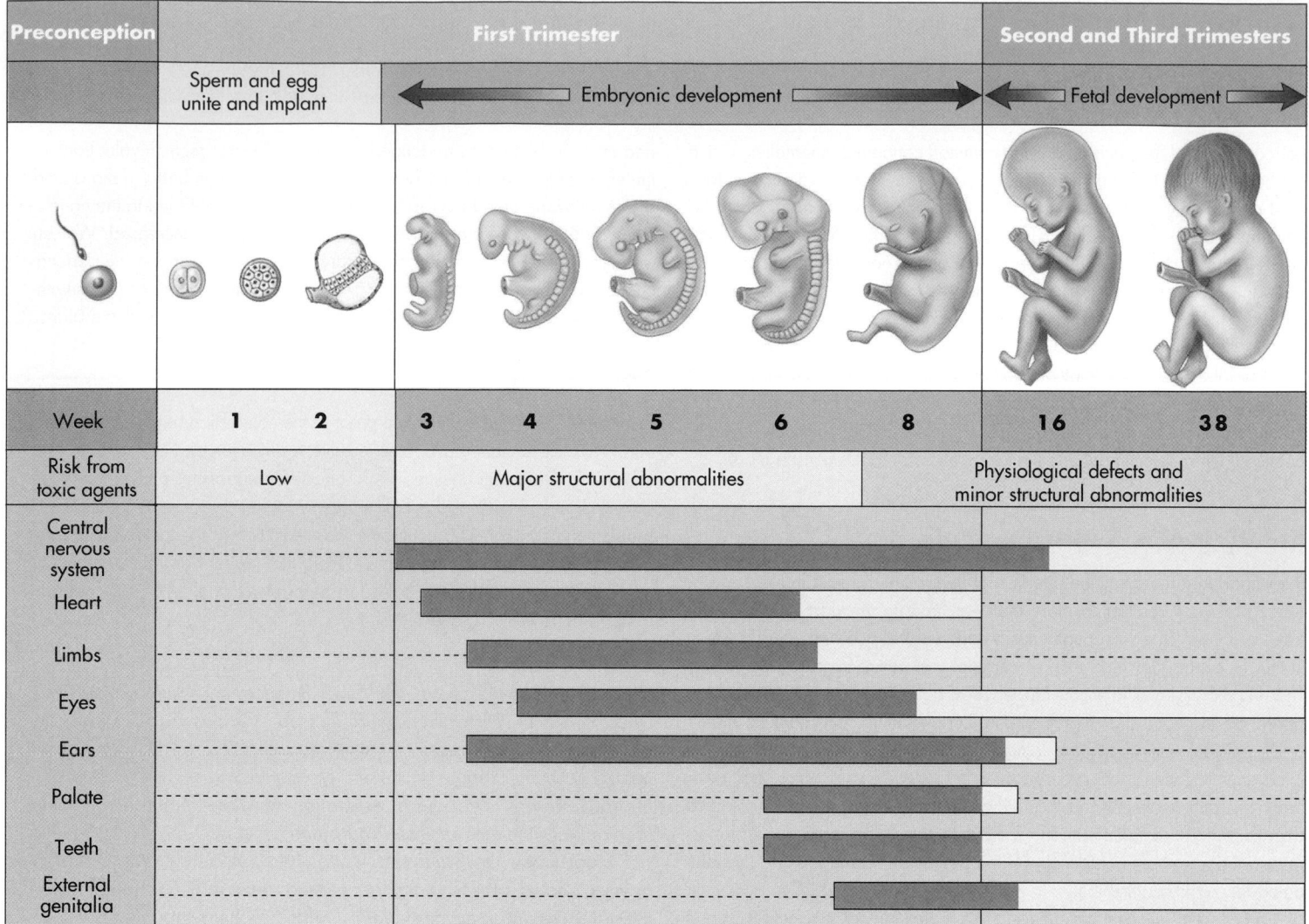

Preconception	First Trimester						Second and Third Trimesters	
	Sperm and egg unite and implant	← Embryonic development →					← Fetal development →	

Week	1	2	3	4	5	6	8	16	38
Risk from toxic agents	Low		Major structural abnormalities					Physiological defects and minor structural abnormalities	
Central nervous system									
Heart									
Limbs									
Eyes									
Ears									
Palate									
Teeth									
External genitalia									

Figure 16-3 | Harmful effects of toxic agents during pregnancy. Vulnerable periods of fetal development are indicated with orange bars. The orange shading indicates the time of greatest risk to the organ. The most serious damage to the fetus from exposure to toxins is likely to occur during the first 8 weeks after conception, two-thirds of the way through the first trimester. As the white bars in the chart show, however, damage to the eyes, brain, and genitals can also occur during the last months of pregnancy.

lactation The period of milk secretion following pregnancy, typically called *breastfeeding*.

During the second trimester, the mother's breast weight increases by approximately 30% because of the development of milk-producing cells and the deposition of 2 to 4 lb of fat for **lactation.** This stored fat serves as a reservoir for the extra energy needed to produce breast milk.[1]

Third Trimester

By the beginning of the third trimester, a fetus weighs about 2 to 3 lb. The third trimester is a crucial time for fetal growth. The fetus will double in length and will multiply its weight by three to four times. An infant who is born after about 26 weeks of

gestation has a good chance of survival if cared for in a nursery for high-risk newborns. However, the infant will not contain the stores of minerals (mainly iron and calcium) and fat that are normally accumulated during the last month of gestation. This and other medical problems, such as a poor ability to suck and swallow, complicate nutritional care for preterm infants. Note also that the fetus takes higher priority than the mother with regard to iron, and will deplete the stores of the mother. If the mother is not meeting her iron needs, she can be severely depleted after delivery.[1]

At 9 months, the fetus usually weighs about 7 to 9 lb (3 to 4 kg) and is about 20 inches (50 cm) long. A soft spot on the top of the head indicates where the skull bones (fontanels) are growing together. The bones finally close by the time the baby is about 12 to 18 months of age.

Definition of a Successful Pregnancy

One common criterion of a successful pregnancy is the protection of the mother's physical and emotional health, so that she can return to her prepregnancy health status. As for the infant, two widely accepted criteria are

- a gestation period longer than 37 weeks
- a birth weight greater than 5.5 lb (2.5 kg)

Sufficient lung development, which is likely to have occurred by 37 weeks' gestation, is critical to the survival of a newborn. The longer the gestation, the greater the ultimate birth weight and maturation state, leading to fewer medical problems.[9]

Low-birth-weight (LBW) infants are those weighing less than 5.5 lb (2.5 kg) at birth. Most commonly, LBW is associated with **preterm** birth. Note that hospital-related costs of caring for low-birth-weight newborns total more than $2 billion per year in the United States, ranging from $20,000 to $200,000 per infant. Compare this amount with an average hospital-related cost of $4300 for a normal delivery and an average of $800 for preventive prenatal care. Full-term and preterm infants who weigh less than the expected weight for their duration of gestation, the result of insufficient growth, are described as **small for gestational age (SGA).** Thus, a full-term infant weighing less than 5.5 lb (2.5 kg) at birth is SGA but not preterm, whereas a preterm infant born at 30 weeks' gestation is probably low birth weight without being SGA. Infants who are SGA are more likely than normal-weight infants to have medical complications, including problems with blood glucose control, temperature regulation, growth, and development in the early weeks after birth.

The newborn's quality of life must also be considered in rating the success of a pregnancy. Overall, the goal of prepregnancy and prenatal care is to ensure that the baby is born healthy, on time, and with the mental, physical, and physiological capabilities to take advantage of whatever life offers, while also protecting the mother's health.[1,3,15]

Concept | Check

To help ensure the optimal health of both the mother and her offspring, adequate nutrition, especially meeting folate needs from a synthetic source starting at least 3 months before pregnancy begins, is vital both before and during pregnancy. Organs and body parts in the offspring begin to develop very soon after conception. The first trimester is a critical period during which inadequate nutrient intake or alcohol and drug use can result in birth defects.

Infants born after 37 weeks of gestation who weigh more than 5.5 lb (2.5 kg) have the fewest medical problems at birth. To reduce infant and maternal medical problems or death, the expectant mother, family, and medical care providers should take the steps necessary to allow the mother to carry the baby in her uterus for the entire 9 months, which in turn contributes to adequate growth. Good nutrition and health practices aid in this goal.

gestation The period of intrauterine development of offspring from conception to birth; in humans, gestation lasts for about 40 weeks after the woman's last menstrual period.

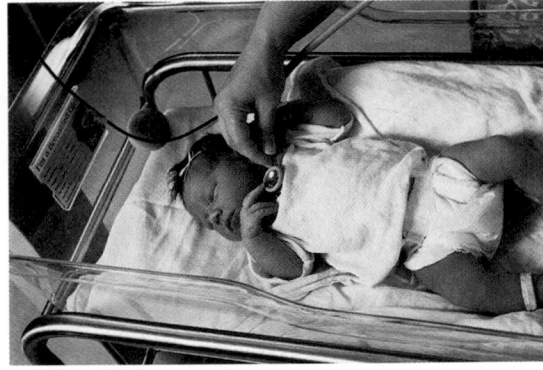

A healthy full-term newborn usually weighs about 7.5 lb and is 20 in. long.

low birth weight (LBW) Referring to any infant weighing less than 2.5 kg (5.5 lb) at birth; most commonly results from preterm birth.

preterm An infant born before 37 weeks of gestation; such an infant is also referred to as *premature.*

small for gestational age (SGA) Referring to infants who weigh less than the expected weight for their length of gestation. This corresponds to less than 2.5 kg (5.5 lb) in a full-term newborn. A preterm infant who is also SGA will most likely develop some medical complications.

A goal of *Healthy People 2010* is to reduce low birth weight and preterm births by one-third.

Studies from Britain suggest that infants who are small for gestational age are likely to develop obesity, diabetes, hypertension, and other health problems during later adult years. Reduced growth of the liver, the pancreas, the kidneys, and other organs during gestation is one possible reason. This increase in health risk is likely to be more pronounced if the infants also fail to gain enough weight in the first year of life.

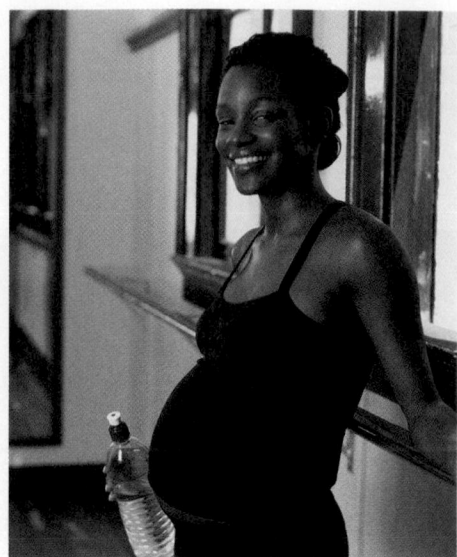

Many women recognize the benefits of remaining active during pregnancy. Health-care providers typically encourage healthy, well-nourished women to engage in moderate exercise as long as increased energy and nutrient needs are met.

The American College of Obstetrics and Gynecology suggests the following guidelines for physical activity during pregnancy:

1. Do not allow heart rate to exceed 140 beats per minute.
2. Avoid exercising in hot, humid weather.
3. Discontinue exercise that causes discomfort or overheating.
4. Drink plenty of liquids to avoid dehydration and overheating.
5. After about the fourth month, don't exercise while lying on your back, because this decreases cardiac output.
6. Avoid an abrupt decrease in exertion. In other words, don't just stop and stand around after a hard workout; rather, continue exercising but at a slow pace, gradually reducing pulse rate.

▌ Increased Nutrient Needs to Support Pregnancy

Pregnancy is a time of increased nutrient needs. Mothers-to-be need individual assessment and counseling, because the nutritional and health status of each woman is different. Still, some general principles are true of most women with regard to increased nutrient needs.[1]

Increased Energy Needs

To support the growth and development of the fetus, pregnant women need to increase their energy intake. Energy needs during the first trimester are essentially the same as for the nonpregnant woman. However, during the second and third trimesters, a pregnant woman must consume approximately 350 to 450 kcal more per day than her prepregnancy needs (the upper end of the range is needed in the third trimester).[1]

This extra energy should be in the form of nutrient-dense foods, not sugary desserts or fat-filled snacks. For example, throughout the day, about six whole-wheat crackers, 1 ounce of cheese, and 1/2 cup of fat-free milk would supply the extra energy (and also some calcium). Although she "eats for two," the pregnant woman must not double her normal energy intake. The eating for two concept refers more appropriately to increased needs for several vitamins and minerals. Micronutrient needs are increased by up to 50% during pregnancy whereas energy needs during the second and third trimesters represent only about a 20% increase.[1]

If a woman is active during her pregnancy, she may need to increase her energy intake by even more than the estimated 350 to 450 kcal per day. Her greater body weight requires more energy for activity. Pregnancy is not the time to begin an intense fitness regimen, but women can generally take part in most low- or moderate-intensity activities during pregnancy. Walking, cycling, swimming, or light aerobics for 30 minutes or more on most days of the week is generally advised and may actually promote an easier delivery.[12] A few types of activities can potentially harm the fetus and should be avoided, especially activities with inherent risk of falls and abdominal trauma. Examples of exercises to avoid, especially during the second and third trimesters, include downhill skiing, weight lifting, soccer, basketball, horseback riding, certain calisthenics (e.g., deep knee bends), any contact sports (e.g., hockey), and scuba diving. Because many women find that they are inactive during the later months, partly because of their increased size, an extra 350 to 450 kcal in their daily diets is usually enough.

Women with high-risk pregnancies, such as those experiencing premature labor contractions, may need to restrict their physical activity. To ensure optimal health for both herself and her infant, a pregnant woman should first consult her physician about physical activity and possible limitations.

Adequate Weight Gain

Adequate weight gain for a mother is one of the best predictors of pregnancy outcome.[9] Her diet should allow for approximately 2 to 4 lb (0.9 to 1.8 kg) of weight gain during the first trimester and then a subsequent weight gain of 0.75 to 1 lb (0.3 to 0.5 kg) weekly during the second and third trimesters. A healthy goal for total weight gain for a woman of normal weight (based on BMI; Table 16-1) averages about 25 to 35 lb (11.5 to 16 kg). Adolescents and African-American women, who often have smaller babies, are strongly advised to aim for the greater amount. Women carrying twins should gain 35 to 45 lb, and those carrying triplets should gain 50 lb (23 kg).[1]

For women with a low BMI (less than 19.8), the goal increases to 28 to 40 lb (12.5 to 18 kg). The goal decreases to 15 to 25 lb (7 to 11.5 kg) for women at a high BMI (26 to 29) and 15 lb (7 kg) (or more) for an obese woman (BMI greater than 29). Figure 16-4 shows why the typical recommendation begins at 25 lb.

Table 16-1 | Recommended Weight Gain in Pregnancy Based on Prepregnancy Body Mass Index (BMI).

Prepregnancy BMI Category	Total Weight Gain*	
	(lb)	(kg)
Low (BMI less than 19.8)	28 to 40	12.5 to 18
Normal (BMI 19.8 to 25.9)	25 to 35	11.5 to 16
High (BMI 26 to 29)	15 to 25	7 to 11.5
Obese (BMI greater than 29)	15 (or more)	7 (or more)

Reprinted with permission from *Nutrition During Pregnancy and Lactation*, Copyright 1992 by the National Academy of Sciences. Courtesy of the National Academy Press, Washington, DC.

*The listed values are for pregnancies with one fetus. Short women (less than 62 in.) should strive for gains at the lower end of the ranges. For women of normal BMI who are carrying twins, the range is 35 to 45 lb (16 to 20 kg). Adolescents within 2 years of beginning menses and African-American women should strive for gains at the upper end of the ranges.

During pregnancy, women in North America are more likely to gain excess weight and make poor food choices than to eat too little.

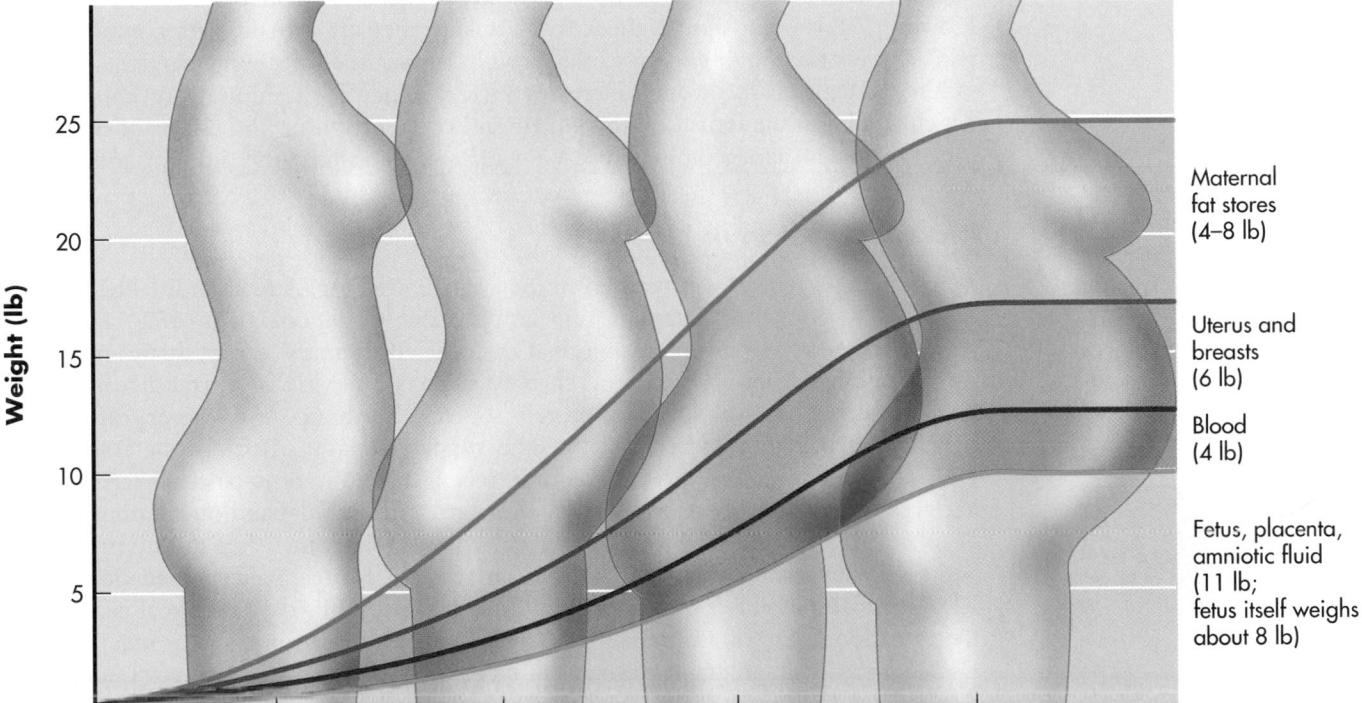

Figure 16-4 | The components of weight gain in pregnancy. A weight gain of 25 to 35 lb is recommended for most women. Note that the various components total about 25 lb.

A weight gain between 25 and 35 lb (11.5 to 16 kg) for a woman starting at normal weight has repeatedly been shown to yield optimal health for both mother and fetus if gestation lasts at least 38 weeks.[1] The weight gain should yield a birth weight of 7.5 lb (3.5 kg). Although some extra weight gain during pregnancy is usually not harmful (about 5 to 10 lb), it can set the stage for a pattern of weight gain during the childbearing years if the mother does not return to her approximate prepregnancy weight.

Weight gain during pregnancy, especially in the teenage years, should generally follow the pattern in Figure 16-4. Weight gain is a key issue in prenatal care and a concern of many mothers-to-be. Remember that inadequate weight gain can cause many

Critical | Thinking

Alexandra wants to have a baby. She has read that it is very important for women to be healthy during pregnancy. However, Jane, her sister, tells her that the time to begin to assess her nutritional and health status is actually before she becomes pregnant. What additional information should Jane give Alexandra?

It is important to note that vitamin A needs increase only by 10%, so a specific focus on this vitamin is not needed. And remember, excess amounts of vitamin A are very harmful to the developing fetus.[5]

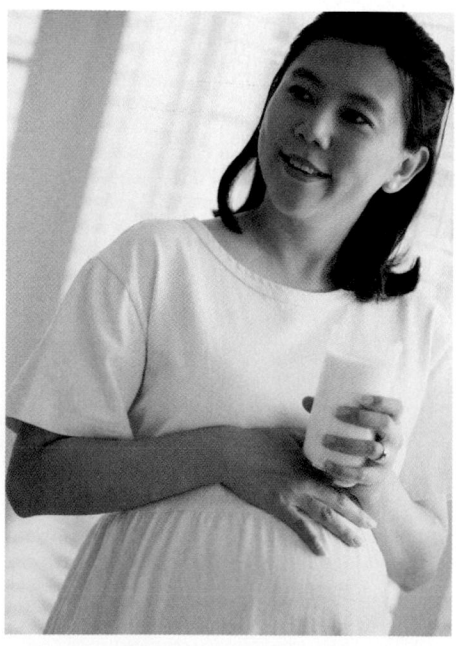

Pregnancy leads to increased nutrient needs for the mother. Meeting these nutrient needs is an important step toward a successful pregnancy.

problems. Many pregnant women keep weekly records of their weight gain to help them adjust their food intake.

If a woman deviates from the desirable pattern, she should make the appropriate adjustment. For example, if a woman begins to gain too much weight during her pregnancy, she should not lose weight to get back on track. Even if a woman gains 35 lb in the first 7 months of pregnancy, she must still gain more during the last 2 months. She should simply slow the increase in weight to parallel the rise on the prenatal weight gain chart. In other words, the sources of the unnecessary calories should be found and minimized. Alternately, if a woman has not gained the desired weight by a given point in pregnancy, she shouldn't gain the needed weight rapidly. Instead, she should slowly gain a little more weight than the typical pattern to meet the goal by the end of the pregnancy. A registered dietitian can help make any needed adjustments.[1]

Increased Protein and Carbohydrate Needs

The RDA for protein increases by an additional 25 g/day during pregnancy. A cup of milk alone contains 8 g. Many nonpregnant women already consume protein in excess of their needs and therefore do not need to increase protein intake any further. However, all women should check to make sure they are actually eating enough protein (as well as enough energy so this protein is not used for energy needs).

The RDA for carbohydrate increases to 175 g/day. This amount prevents ketosis, which can harm the fetus (see the Nutrition Focus section on the effects of many factors on pregnancy outcome). Most women already consume this amount and more.[1]

Increased Vitamin Needs

Vitamin needs generally increase from prepregnancy RDAs/Adequate Intakes by up to 30% for most of the B vitamins, and even greater for vitamin B-6 (45%) and folate (50%). The extra amount of vitamin B-6 and other B vitamins (except folate) needed in the diet is easily met via wise food choices, such as a serving of a typical ready-to-eat breakfast cereal and some animal protein sources. Folate needs, however, often merit specific diet planning and possible vitamin supplementation. Because the synthesis of DNA, and therefore cell division, requires folate, this nutrient is especially crucial during pregnancy. Ultimately, both fetal and maternal growth depend on an ample supply of folate. Red blood cell formation, which requires folate, increases during pregnancy. Serious folate-related anemia therefore can result if folate intake is inadequate. The RDA for folate increases during pregnancy to 600 µg DFE/day. This goal is critical in the nutritional care of a pregnant woman.[3] Increasing folate intakes to meet 600 µg DFE per day for a pregnant woman can be achieved through either dietary sources or a supplemental source of folic acid or a combination of both. Choosing a diet rich in synthetic folic acid, such as from ready-to-eat breakfast cereals or meal replacement bars (look for approximately 50 to 100% of the Daily Value), is especially helpful in meeting folate needs. Recall from Chapter 10 that synthetic folic acid is much more easily absorbed than the various forms of folate found naturally in foods.

Increased Mineral Needs

Mineral needs generally increase during pregnancy, especially the requirements for iodide and iron. Zinc needs also increase. (Calcium needs do not increase but still may deserve special attention because many women have deficient intakes.)[3]

Pregnant women need extra iodide (total of 220 µg/day) for prevention of goiter. Typical iodide intakes are enough if the woman uses iodized salt. Animal proteins or a fortified ready-to-eat breakfast cereal in the diet can easily provide enough extra zinc. Extra iron (total of 27 mg/day) is needed to synthesize the greater amount of hemoglobin needed during pregnancy and to provide iron stores for the fetus. Women often need a supplemental source of iron, especially if they do not consume iron-fortified foods, such as highly fortified breakfast cereals containing close to 100% of the Daily Value for iron (18 mg). Because iron supplements decrease appetite and can cause nausea and constipation, they should be taken between meals or just before going to bed. Milk, coffee, or tea should not be consumed with an iron supplement because these beverages have substances that interfere with iron absorption. Eating foods rich in vitamin C along with nonheme iron-containing foods and iron supplements helps increase iron absorption from those sources.

The consequences of iron-deficiency anemia—especially during the first trimester—can be severe. Negative outcomes include preterm delivery, low-birth-weight infants, and increased risk for fetal death in the first weeks after birth.[1]

Is There an Instinctive Drive during Pregnancy to Consume More Nutrients?

It is a common myth that women instinctively know what to eat during pregnancy. Cravings of the last two trimesters are often related to hormonal changes in the mother or to family traditions. Such "instincts" cannot be trusted, however, based on observations that some women crave nonfood items (called **pica**) such as laundry starch, chalk, cigarette ashes, and soil (clay). This practice can be extremely harmful to the mother and the fetus. Overall, though women may have a natural instinct to consume the right foods in pregnancy, humans are so far removed from living by instinct that relying on our cravings to meet nutrient needs is risky. Nutrition advice by experts is more reliable.[1]

Pregnant women who are not anemic may wait until the second trimester, when pregnancy-related nausea generally lessens, to start iron supplementation if needed.

pica The practice of eating nonfood items, such as dirt, laundry starch, or clay.

Food Plan for Pregnant Women

One approach to a diet that supports successful pregnancy is based on MyPyramid. For an active 24-year-old woman in the first trimester, about 2200 kcal are recommended. The plan should include:

- 3 cups of calcium-rich foods from the milk group, or use of calcium-fortified foods to make up for any gap between calcium intake and need
- 6 ounce-equivalents from the meat & beans group
- 3 cups from the vegetable group
- 2 cups from the fruit group
- 7 ounce-equivalents from the grain group
- 6 teaspoons of vegetable oil

Specifically, choices from the milk group should include low-fat or fat-free versions of milk, yogurt, and cheese. These foods supply extra protein, calcium, and carbohydrate as well as other nutrients. Choices from the meat & beans group should include both animal and vegetable sources. Besides protein, these foods help provide the extra iron and zinc needed. The vegetable and fruit group choices provide a variety of vitamins and minerals. One cup from this combination should be a good vitamin C source, and one cup should be a green vegetable or other rich source of folate. Choices from the grain group should focus on whole-grain and enriched foods. One ounce of a whole-grain ready-to-eat breakfast cereal significantly contributes to meeting many vitamin and mineral needs. Finally, inclusion of plant oils in the diet contributes essential fatty acids. Discretionary calories (up to 300 kcal) can then be added to allow for weight maintenance.

In the second and third trimesters, about 2600 kcal are recommended. The plan should now include:

- 3 cups of calcium-rich foods from the milk group, or use of calcium-fortified foods
- 6 1/2 ounce-equivalents from the meat & beans group
- 3 1/2 cups from the vegetable group

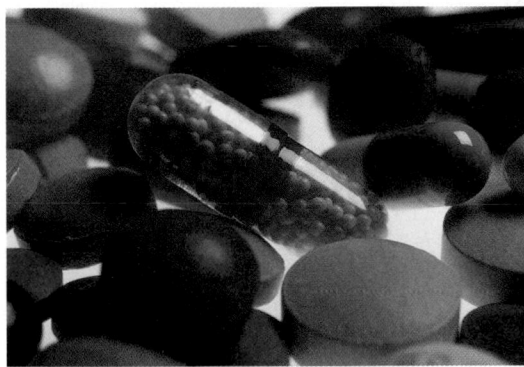

Pregnancy, in particular, is not a time to self-prescribe vitamin and mineral supplements (or medications in general). For example, although vitamin A is a routine component of prenatal vitamins, it is important to note that intakes over three times the RDA for vitamin A have been shown to have toxic effects on the fetus.

- 2 cups from the fruit group
- 8 ounce-equivalents from the grain group
- 7 teaspoons of vegetable oil

Discretionary calories (up to 400 kcal) can then be added. The overall diet should allow for gradual weight gain.

Table 16-2 illustrates one daily menu based on the basic diet plan for women in the second and third trimesters. This menu meets the extra nutrient needs associated with pregnancy. Women who need to consume more than 2600 kcal—and some do for various reasons—should incorporate additional fruits, vegetables, and whole-grain breads and cereals, not poor nutrient sources such as desserts and sugared soft drinks.

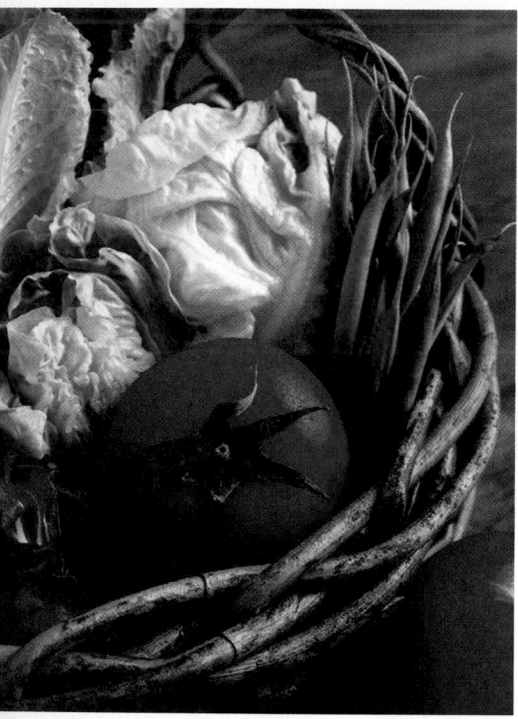

A salad each day provides many nutrients for the prenatal diet.

Table 16-2 | A Sample 2600 kcal Daily Menu That Meets the Nutritional Needs of Most Pregnant and Breastfeeding Women

	Vitamin B-6	Folate	Iron	Zinc	Calcium
Breakfast					
Kellogg's Smart Start cereal, 1 cup	✓	✓	✓	✓	✓
Orange juice, 1 cup		✓			
Fat-free milk, 1 cup	✓				✓
Snack					
Peanut butter, 2 tbsp	✓	✓	✓	✓	
Celery, 2 stalks		✓			
Whole-wheat toast, 1 slice		✓	✓	✓	
Plain low-fat yogurt, 1 cup	✓				✓
Strawberries, 1/2 cup					
Lunch					
Spinach salad, 2 cups with 2 tbsp oil and vinegar dressing		✓			✓
Tomato, 1/2					
Whole-wheat toast, 1 slice		✓	✓	✓	
Provolone cheese, 1 1/2 oz	✓				✓
Snack					
Whole-wheat crackers, 5		✓	✓	✓	
Grape juice, 1 cup					
Dinner					
Lean hamburger, 3 oz, broiled (with condiments)	✓		✓	✓	
Baked beans, 1/2 cup	✓	✓	✓	✓	
Hamburger bun, 1		✓	✓		
Sliced tomato, 1/2					
Cooked broccoli, 1 cup		✓			✓
Soft margarine, 1 tsp					
Iced tea					
Snack					
Granola bar, 2 oz		✓	✓	✓	
Banana, 1/2	✓				
Discretionary calories up to 400 kcal*					

This diet meets nutrient needs for pregnancy and lactation. Lack of a check (✓) indicates a poor source of the nutrient. The vitamin- and mineral-fortified breakfast cereal used in this example makes an important contribution to meeting nutrient needs. Fluids can be added as desired. Total intake of fluids, such as water, should be 10 cups or so per day.

*Amount of discretionary calories will vary based on the actual food choices made within each MyPyramid group.

Use of Prenatal Vitamin and Mineral Supplements

Special supplements formulated for pregnancy are prescribed routinely for pregnant women by most physicians. Some are sold over the counter, whereas others are dispensed by prescription because of their high synthetic folic acid content (1000 μg), which could pose problems for others, such as older people (review Chapter 10). These supplements are very high in iron (27 mg per pill). There is no evidence that use of such supplements causes significant health problems in pregnancy, aside perhaps from the combined amounts of supplementary and dietary vitamin A. During pregnancy, supplemental preformed vitamin A should not exceed 3000 μg RAE/day (15,000 IU per day). Toxicity of vitamin A is linked with **teratogenic** birth defects (review Chapter 9). Toxicity occurs mainly during the first trimester. The primary instances when prenatal supplements especially may contribute to a successful pregnancy are with poor women, teenagers, women with a generally deficient diet, women carrying multiple fetuses, women who smoke or use alcohol or illegal drugs, and vegans. In other cases healthy diets can provide the needed nutrients.[1]

Pregnant Vegetarians

Women who are either lactoovovegetarians or lactovegetarians generally do not face special difficulties in meeting their nutritional needs during pregnancy. Like nonvegetarian women, they should be concerned primarily with meeting vitamin B-6, iron, folate, and zinc needs.

On the other hand, for a vegan, careful diet planning during preconception and pregnancy is crucial to ensure sufficient protein, vitamin D (or sufficient sun exposure), vitamin B-6, iron, calcium, zinc, and especially a supplemental source of vitamin B-12.[1,14,16] The basic vegan diet listed in Chapter 7 should be modified to include more grains, beans, nuts, and seeds to supply the necessary extra amounts of some of these nutrients. And as just mentioned, use of a prenatal multivitamin and mineral supplement also is generally advocated to help fill micronutrient gaps. Note, however, that although these supplements are high in iron, they are not high in calcium (200 mg per pill). If iron and calcium supplements are used, they should not be taken together, to avoid possible competition for absorption.

Concept | Check

Energy needs increase by an average of about 350 to 450 kcal/day during the second and third trimesters of pregnancy. Weight gain should be slow and steady, up to a total of 25 to 35 lb (11.5 to 16 kg) for a woman of normal weight (i.e., prepregnancy BMI of 19.8 to 25.9). Protein and certain vitamin and mineral needs increase during pregnancy. Most important to consider are vitamin B-6, folate, iron, iodide, and zinc. A pregnant woman's diet should be varied and generally follow MyPyramid. A prenatal multivitamin and mineral supplement is commonly prescribed but may not be necessary depending on one's diet and current health status. Taking too many supplements—especially vitamin A—can be hazardous to the fetus.

Effect of Nutritional Status on the Success of Pregnancy

Is this attention to nutrition worth the effort? Yes; evidence shows that the effort is justified. Extra nutrients and energy are used for fetal growth and for changes in the mother's body to accommodate the fetus. Her uterus and breasts grow, the placenta develops, her total blood volume increases, the heart and kidneys work harder, and stores of body fat increase.

Mercury can harm the nervous system of the fetus. FDA warns pregnant women to avoid swordfish, shark, king mackerel, and tile fish because of possible high mercury contamination. Largemouth bass are also implicated. In general, intake of other fish and shellfish should not exceed 12 oz/week. Note also that because canned albacore tuna is a potential mercury source, it should not be consumed in amounts exceeding 6 oz/week.

teratogenic Tending to produce physical defects in a developing fetus.

Because of the nutrient demands of pregnancy coupled with chronic undernutrition, women in many developing countries have a 1 in 20 chance of dying from pregnancy-related causes. In contrast, North American women face a risk of only 1 death from pregnancy-related causes in about every 8000 births. Pregnancy-related death is, in fact, the social indicator with the biggest difference between the developing and industrialized worlds. Smaller differences exist for literacy, life expectancy, and infant mortality. These statistics again show the importance of meeting women's nutrient needs in pregnancy.

Although it is difficult to specify what degree of poor nutrition will affect each pregnancy, a daily diet containing only 1000 kcal has been shown to greatly restrict fetal growth and development.[9] Increased maternal and infant death rates seen in famine-stricken areas of Africa supply further evidence.

Genetic background can explain very little of the observed differences in birth weight in North America. Both environmental factors and nutritional factors are more important. The worse the nutritional condition of the mother at the beginning of pregnancy, the more valuable a good prenatal diet and/or use of prenatal supplements are in improving the course and outcome of her pregnancy.

During World War II, parts of Russia and much of Holland were blockaded. Food supplies were quickly exhausted. The resulting undernutrition greatly affected the birth weights of infants developing in the second or third trimester. Birth defects also occurred more commonly, and the number of new pregnancies fell. As well, the children born in those conditions exhibited a greater risk of mental disorders later in life. After the blockades were lifted, birth weights, subsequent infant health, and the numbers of new pregnancies quickly returned to prewar levels.

At the same time, researchers in Boston noticed that an adequate protein intake was associated with a greater success of pregnancy. It appeared that the mother's diet—not only during pregnancy but also preceding conception—affected the health of both mother and infant. Studies in Toronto then showed that dietary supplements and nutritional counseling improved the health of the pregnant mother and produced a healthier baby. As health improved, complication rates also decreased. Researchers in Great Britain took this one research step further. They showed that height and social class are better predictors of pregnancy outcome than dietary intake during pregnancy. Supporting this finding is a study of middle-class African-American women in Chicago. Even with nutritional supplements, their risk of having LBW infants still exceeded that of middle-class whites, possibly reflecting the effects of poverty on previous generations. This finding suggests that long-term nutritional intake may be critical to pregnancy outcome.

Laboratory animal studies support the importance of diet during pregnancy. Food deprivation in pregnant laboratory animals leads to smaller organ size in the offspring, affecting even the brain, which usually resists nutritional insults. In addition, placentas weigh less, and fewer healthy offspring survive the first weeks of life.

Prenatal Care and Counseling

The chances of producing a healthy baby are maximized with education, an adequate diet, and early and consistent prenatal medical care.[1,5] Also, avoiding the controllable risks discussed in this chapter—especially smoking, over-supplementation with vitamin A, and use of certain medications, illegal drugs, and alcohol—will promote a healthier outcome of pregnancy for both the mother and the baby. If anemia, AIDS, diabetes, or hypertension are present or developing, these conditions must be carefully addressed to minimize complications during pregnancy. Treating ongoing infections is also important, as is avoiding X-ray exposure.

Ideally, women should receive examinations and counseling before becoming pregnant and during pregnancy. Many potential problems that develop during pregnancy can be diagnosed and quickly treated medically.

Food habits cannot be predicted from income, education, or lifestyle. Although some women already have good dietary habits, most can benefit from nutritional advice. All should be reminded of habits that may harm the growing fetus, such as severe dieting or fasting. By focusing on appropriate prenatal care, nutrient intake, and health habits, parents give their fetus—and, later, their infant—the very best chance of thriving.

Several U.S. government programs provide high-quality health care and foods to reduce infant mortality. These programs are designed to alleviate the effects of poverty and insufficient education and nutrient intake. An example of such a program is the

Obesity also increases pregnancy risks, because hypertension and/or diabetes is likely present. These pregnancies require intense monitoring and pose an increased risk of prolonged labor during delivery of the infant as well as a greater risk for birth defects in the infant, primarily because of excess fetal growth.[10]

Women with acquired immune deficiency syndrome (AIDS) may pass the virus that causes this disease to the fetus during pregnancy or the birth process. About one in three infected newborns will develop AIDS symptoms and die within just a few years. Studies show that these odds of mother-infant transmission can be cut significantly if the woman begins taking the drug azidothymidine (AZT) and other related AIDS medications by the fourteenth week of pregnancy. Providing these medications just before birth is helpful as well. Thus, screening pregnant women for AIDS and treating those with AIDS using AZT are currently advocated by some experts.

Special Supplemental Nutrition Program for Women, Infants, and Children (WIC). This program offers health assessments and vouchers for foods that supply high-quality protein, calcium, iron, and vitamins A and C to pregnant women, infants, and children (up to age 5 years) from low-income populations. The WIC program is available in all areas of the United States and has a staff trained to help women have healthy babies.

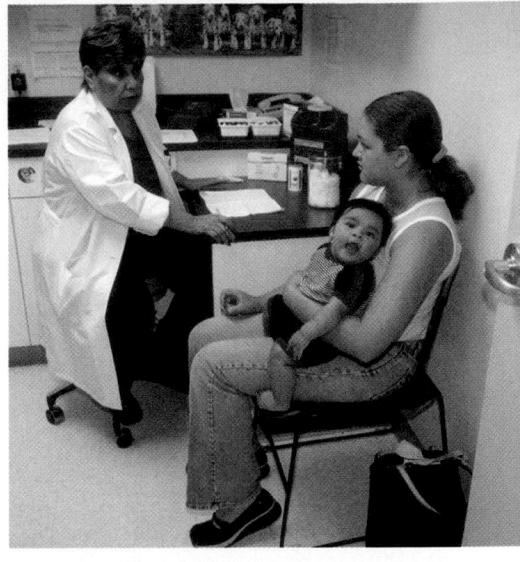

In the United States, low-income pregnant women and their infants (and children) benefit from the nutritional and medical attention provided by the WIC program.

Case Scenario | Follow-Up

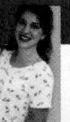

From a dietary standpoint, Tracey is smart to take a close look at her protein intake because needs will increase somewhat during pregnancy. More fruits and vegetables supply extra folate, and her use of an over-the-counter vitamin and mineral supplement ensures that she will have an ample amount. Still, she should discuss this supplement use with her physician. She would probably eventually benefit more from a prenatal supplement, because it will have more iron than over-the-counter multivitamin and mineral supplements. Her diet may not have enough calcium, so she should pay as much attention to consuming extra calcium as she does to consuming protein. Avoiding alcohol is a smart move.

Many experts would say that Tracey is consuming too much caffeine and would be wise to cut back on coffee and caffeine-containing soft drinks to a total of three servings or less per day. Swimming is an excellent choice for exercise, as long as it is not too vigorous. Brisk walking or stationary biking (spinning) are also appropriate.

Concept | Check

Infants born after 37 weeks of gestation and weighing more than 5.5 lb (2.5 kg) have the fewest medical problems at birth. Limiting the factors that increase the risk of having a preterm or small-for-gestational-age infant is a worthwhile goal for individuals and for society as a whole. Such contributing high-risk factors, besides an inadequate diet in general, include low socioeconomic status; closely spaced births; inadequate or absent prenatal care; cigarette smoking; alcohol consumption; aspirin and NSAID use; illegal drug use, such as marijuana and cocaine; teenage pregnancy; obesity; and inadequate prenatal weight gain. Adequate nutrition can reduce the risk of many medical problems in pregnancy.

Physiological Changes of Concern during Pregnancy

During pregnancy, the fetus's needs for oxygen, nutrients, and excretion increase the burden on the mother's lungs, heart, and kidneys. Although a mother's digestive and metabolic systems work very efficiently, some discomfort accompanies the changes her body undergoes to accommodate the fetus.

Heartburn, Constipation, and Hemorrhoids

Hormones (such as progesterone) produced by the placenta relax muscles in both the uterus and the gastrointestinal tract, which often causes heartburn as stomach acid refluxes into the esophagus (review Chapter 3). When reflux occurs, the woman should avoid lying down after eating, eat less fat so that foods pass more quickly from the stomach into the small intestine, and avoid spicy foods she cannot tolerate. She should also consume most liquids between meals to decrease the volume of food in the stomach after meals and thus relieve some of the pressure that encourages reflux. Women with more severe cases may need antacids or related medications.

Critical | Thinking

Hannah, a 16-year-old high school student, has just discovered that she is pregnant. At 5' 3" and 105 lb she is underweight and her typical diet lacks many essential nutrients. For breakfast, she will have coffee and a doughnut, if anything at all. She often skips lunch or eats chips from the vending machine. She then eats a well-rounded dinner with her family. What risks do you see in this situation for Hannah and her baby?

NUTRITION FOCUS

Effects of Other Factors on Pregnancy Outcome

menarche The onset of menstruation. Menarche usually occurs around age 13, 2 or 3 years after the first signs of puberty start to appear.

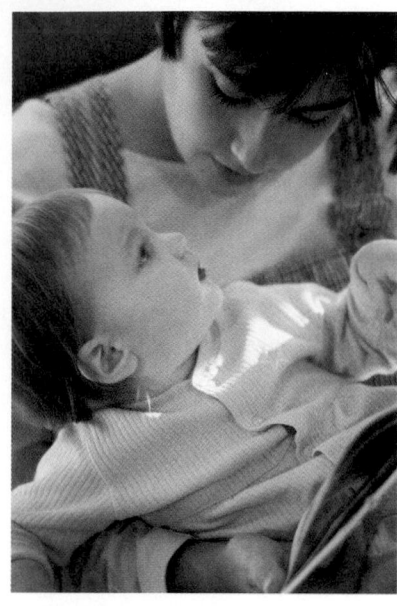

Healthy nutrition, proper prenatal care, and avoiding unsafe behaviors, such as smoking and drugs, are key factors in promoting a successful pregnancy. Too often very young mothers are ill-equipped to cope with the physiological, emotional, and societal pressures of an unplanned pregnancy. These factors contribute to the added risks they face.

Multiple births (i.e., twins) increase the risk for preterm birth.

In North America, maternal death as a result of childbirth is uncommon—only about 11 deaths in every 100,000 live births. The infant mortality rate, however, is much higher: for each 100,000 live births, about 600 to 700 infants die within the first year. The infant death rate among African-Americans is more than double the rates among whites and Hispanics in the United States. Such grim and discomforting statistics can be attributed largely to the current number of teenage pregnancies and to inadequate prenatal care as well as to marginal nutritional health among poor pregnant women. Also, many factors other than nutrition affect the health of mother and fetus.

Low Socioeconomic Status

Several characteristics that are typical of low socioeconomic status, such as poverty, inadequate health care, poor health practices, lack of education, and unmarried status are associated with problems in pregnancy. Currently, in the United States about 31% of all births are to unwed mothers, many of whom are poor.

Closely Spaced and Multiple Births

Siblings born in succession to a mother, with less than a year between birth and subsequent conception, are more likely to be born with low birth weights than are those farther apart in age. The risks of low birth weight, preterm birth, or small size for gestational age are 30 to 40% higher for infants conceived less than 6 months following a birth compared to those conceived 18 to 23 months following a birth. These poor outcomes are probably linked to a lack of enough time for the mother to rebuild nutrient stores that were depleted by the pregnancy.[13]

Teenage Pregnancy

About half a million teenagers give birth in the United States each year, accounting for about 13% of all births. In Canada, the comparable statistics are about half that amount. Teenage pregnancy poses special health problems for both the mother and child. Young women continue maturing into physical adulthood for 5 years after the onset of menstruation (**menarche**). Because the average age for menarche is 13 years in the United States, a woman younger than 18 years is not as physically ready to be pregnant as she will be later. However, by age 16, birth outcomes begin to improve.

Pregnant teens frequently exhibit a variety of other risk factors that can complicate pregnancy and pose a risk to the fetus. For instance, teenagers are more likely than adult women to be underweight at the beginning of pregnancy and to gain too little weight during pregnancy. In addition, their bodies generally lack the maturity needed to carry a fetus safely. Sixteen percent of low-birth-weight infants are born to teenage mothers, even if the mothers receive adequate prenatal care.

Advanced Maternal Age

The risks of low birth weight and preterm delivery increase modestly but progressively with maternal age beyond 35 years (the ideal range is 25 to 35 years). Given close monitoring, however, a woman older than 35 years has an excellent chance of producing a healthy infant. Most women in this age group exhibit typical pregnancy-related problems, which usually are manageable if the woman is under close medical supervision.

Inadequate Prenatal Care

If prenatal care is inadequate, delayed, or absent, untreated maternal nutritional deficiencies can deprive a developing fetus of needed nutrients.[5] In addition, untreated chronic diseases, such as hypertension or diabetes, increase the risk of fetal damage. Without prenatal care, a woman is three times more likely to deliver a low-birth-weight baby—one who will be 40 times more likely to die during the first 4 weeks of life than a normal-birth-weight infant. Although the ideal time to start prenatal care is before conception, about 20% of women in the United States receive no prenatal care throughout the first trimester—a critical time to positively influence the outcome of pregnancy.

Lifestyle Factors

Smoking, use of some medications, alcohol consumption, and illicit drug use during pregnancy all lead to harmful effects. (Use of a sauna or hot tub also can cause problems.) Smoking is linked to preterm birth and low birth weight and appears to increase the risk of birth defects, sudden infant death, and childhood cancer. Problem drugs include aspirin (especially when used heavily), hormone ointments, nose drops and related cold medications, rectal suppositories, weight-control pills, and medications prescribed for previous illnesses.

Marijuana is the most common illegal drug used during the reproductive years. For pregnant women, marijuana use is very risky and potentially can result in reduced blood flow and oxygen to the uterus and placenta and poor fetal growth. Low birth weight and higher risk of premature delivery often are seen in infants whose mothers used marijuana during pregnancy. Cocaine use also has devastating consequences for the developing fetus.

Conclusive evidence shows that repeated consumption of four or more alcoholic drinks at one sitting harms the fetus.[20] Such binge drinking is especially perilous during the first 12 weeks of pregnancy, when critical early developmental events take place in utero. Although scientists don't know whether pregnant women must totally eliminate alcohol use to avoid risk of damage to the fetus, until a safe level can be established women are advised not to drink any alcohol during pregnancy or when there is a chance pregnancy might occur. The embryo (and at later stages, the fetus) has no means of detoxifying alcohol.

Women with chronic alcoholism produce children with a recognizable pattern of malformations called **fetal alcohol syndrome (FAS).**[7] A diagnosis of FAS is based mainly on poor fetal and infant growth, physical deformities (especially of facial features), and mental retardation (Figure 16-5). The infant is frequently irritable and may develop hyperactivity and a short attention span. Limited hand-eye coordination is common. Defects in vision, hearing, and mental processing often develop over time.

Exactly how alcohol causes these defects is not known. One line of research suggests that alcohol, or products produced by the metabolism of alcohol (acetaldehyde), cause faulty movement of cells in the brain during early stages of nerve cell development or block the action of certain brain neurotransmitters. In addition, inadequate nutrient intake, reduced nutrient and oxygen transfer across the placenta, cigarette smoking commonly associated with alcohol intake, drug use, and possibly other factors contribute to the overall result. For more information about fetal alcohol syndrome, visit the website www.cdc.gov/ncbdd/fas/.

Prenatal Ketosis

Ketosis can result from fasting and is not desirable for the growing fetus. Ketone bodies are thought to be poorly used by the fetal brain, implying possible slowing of fetal brain development. Because a pregnant woman can develop significant ketosis after only 20 hours of fasting, experts oppose crash diets or fasting for more than 12 hours during pregnancy. Eating at least 175 g of carbohydrate every day prevents such ketosis. Even nonpregnant women usually eat this amount and more.

Caffeine Consumption

Caffeine decreases the mother's absorption of iron and may reduce blood flow through the placenta. In addition, the fetus is unable to detoxify caffeine. Animal experiments have shown that the risk of spontaneous abortion increases in the first trimester and early in the second trimester with heavy caffeine consumption (greater than 500 mg/day, or the equivalent of about 5 cups of coffee per day). In addition, as caffeine intake increases, so does the risk of delivering a low-birth-weight infant. Heavy caffeine use during pregnancy may also lead to caffeine withdrawal symptoms in the newborn. Researchers advocate that women drink no more than three cups of coffee and no more than four cups of caffeinated soft drinks per day during pregnancy, or when pregnancy is possible. Paying attention to caffeine intake from tea, over-the-counter medicines containing caffeine, and chocolate is also important.

A goal of *Healthy People 2010* is 100% abstinence from alcohol, cigarettes, and illicit drugs by pregnant women.

Pregnant women should recognize that many cough syrups contain alcohol. Cases have been reported of infants with FAS born to mothers who consumed generous amounts of such cough syrups but no other alcoholic beverages.

fetal alcohol syndrome (FAS) A group of irreversible physical and mental abnormalities in the infant that result from the mother's consuming alcohol during pregnancy.

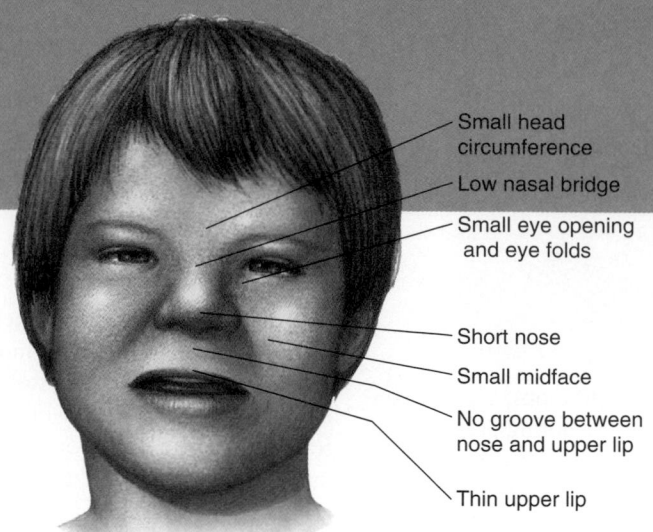

Labels on figure:
- Small head circumference
- Low nasal bridge
- Small eye opening and eye folds
- Short nose
- Small midface
- No groove between nose and upper lip
- Thin upper lip

Figure 16-5 | Fetal alcohol syndrome. The facial features shown are typical of affected children. Additional abnormalities in the brain and other internal organs accompany fetal alcohol syndrome but are not immediately apparent from simply looking at the child. Milder forms of alcohol-induced changes from a lower alcohol exposure to the fetus are known as **fetal alcohol effects.** Affected children exhibit behavior problems without physical effects such as altered facial features.

fetal alcohol effect (FAE) Hyperactivity, attention deficit disorder, poor judgment, sleep disorders, and delayed learning as a result of prenatal exposure to alcohol.

USDA also warns pregnant women (and other people at high risk) to thoroughly cook (e.g., microwave) all ready-to-eat meats, including hot dogs and cold cuts, until they are steaming to reduce risk of listeria infections.

Aspartame Use

Phenylalanine, a component of aspartame (e.g., NutraSweet and Equal), causes concern for some pregnant women. High amounts of phenylalanine in maternal blood disrupt fetal brain development if the mother has a disease known as *phenylketonuria* (review Chapter 4). If the mother does not have this condition, however, it is unlikely that the baby will be affected by moderate aspartame use.

Listeria and Toxoplasmosis Infections

Infection by the bacterium *Listeria monocytogenes* causes mild flulike symptoms, such as fever, headache, and vomiting, about 7 to 30 days after exposure. However, pregnant women, newborn infants, and people with depressed immune function may suffer more severe symptoms, including spontaneous abortion and serious blood infections. In these high-risk people, 25% of infections may be fatal. Because unpasteurized milk, soft cheeses made from raw milk (brie, Camembert, feta, and blue cheeses), and raw cabbage can be sources of *Listeria* organisms, it is especially important that pregnant women (and other people at high risk for infection) avoid these products. Experts advise consuming only pasteurized milk products and cooking meat, poultry, and seafood thoroughly to kill this and other foodborne organisms. It is unsafe in pregnancy to eat any raw meats or other raw animal products, uncooked hot dogs, or any undercooked poultry.

Toxoplasmosis is another infection that causes birth defects, leading to about 3000 such cases per year in the United States. Pregnant women should limit exposure to the organism that causes toxoplasmosis by avoiding contact with cat feces (have someone else clean the cat's litter box or wear gloves), avoiding contact with kittens, bird feces, and garden soil (by wearing garden gloves), and by not eating raw or undercooked meat. Chapter 19 covers foodborne illness, such as *Listeria* and toxoplasmosis infections, in more detail.

Many of the risk factors described in this section are avoidable. The goal of a reduction in maternal and infant deaths requires that more attention be paid to these problems.

Constipation often results as the intestinal muscles relax during pregnancy.[17] It is especially likely to develop late in pregnancy as the fetus competes with the GI tract for space in the abdominal cavity. To offset these discomforts, a woman should perform regular exercise and consume more fluid, fiber, and dried fruits such as prunes (dried plums). The Adequate Intake for fiber in pregnancy is 28 g/day, slightly more than for the nonpregnant woman. Fluid needs are 10 cups/day. These practices can help prevent constipation and a problem that frequently accompanies it, hemorrhoids. Straining during elimination can lead to hemorrhoids, which are already more likely to occur during pregnancy because of other body changes.

A reevaluation of the need and dose of iron supplementation should be considered, because high iron intakes are linked to constipation.

Edema

Placental hormones cause various body tissues to retain fluid during pregnancy. Blood volume also greatly expands during pregnancy. The extra fluid normally causes some swelling (edema). There is no reason to restrict salt severely or use diuretics to limit mild edema. However, the edema may limit physical activity late in pregnancy and occasionally requires a woman to elevate her feet to control the symptoms. Overall, edema generally spells trouble only if it is accompanied by hypertension and the appearance of extra protein in the urine (see the subsequent section titled Pregnancy-Induced Hypertension).

Morning Sickness

About 70 to 85% of pregnant women experience nausea during the early stages of pregnancy. This nausea may be related to the increased sense of smell induced by pregnancy-related hormones circulating in the bloodstream. Although commonly called "morning sickness," pregnancy-related nausea may occur at any time and persist all day. It is often the first signal to a woman that she is pregnant. To help control mild nausea, pregnant women can try the following: avoiding nauseating foods, such as fried or greasy foods; cooking with good ventilation to dissipate nauseating smells; eating saltine crackers or dry cereal before getting out of bed; avoiding large fluid intakes early in the morning; and eating smaller, more frequent meals. Because the iron in prenatal supplements triggers nausea in some women, changing the type of supplement used or postponing use until the second trimester may provide relief in some cases. If a woman thinks her prenatal supplement is related to morning sickness, she should discuss switching to another supplement with her physician.

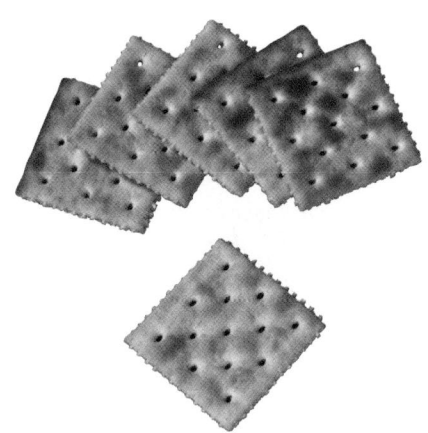

A few saltine crackers upon waking or between meals can help lessen the nausea of morning sickness.

Overall, if a food sounds good to a pregnant woman with morning sickness, whether it is broccoli, soda crackers, or lemonade, she should eat it and eat when she can while also striving to follow her prenatal diet. The American College of Obstetricians and Gynecologists recommends the following for the prevention and treatment of nausea and vomiting of pregnancy:

- History of use of a balanced multivitamin and mineral supplement at the time of conception
- Use of megadoses of vitamin B-6 (10 to 25 mg taken 3 to 4 times a day), especially coupled with the antihistamine doxylamine (10 mg) with each dose. Use of ginger (350 mg taken 3 times per day) may also be helpful in reducing such nausea.

Usually, nausea stops after the first trimester; however, in about 10 to 20% of cases, it can continue throughout the entire pregnancy. In cases of serious nausea, the preceding practices offer little relief. Excessive vomiting can cause dangerous dehydration and must be avoided. When vomiting persists (about 0.5 to 2% of all pregnancies), medical attention is needed.

E xcessive vomiting during pregnancy that leads to dehydration and weight loss is called hyperemesis gravidarum.

Anemia

To supply fetal needs, the mother's blood volume expands to approximately 150% of normal. The number of red blood cells, however, increases by only 20 to 30%, and this increase occurs gradually. As a result, a pregnant woman has a lower ratio of red blood cells to total blood volume in her system. This hemodilution is known as **physiological anemia.** It is a normal response to pregnancy rather than the result of inadequate nutrient intake. If during pregnancy, however, iron stores and/or dietary iron intake are not sufficient to meet needs, any resulting iron-deficiency anemia requires medical attention.

physiological anemia The normal increase in blood volume in pregnancy that dilutes the concentration of red blood cells, resulting in anemia, also called *hemodilution*.

Gestational Diabetes

Hormones synthesized by the placenta decrease the efficiency of insulin and lead to a mild increase in blood glucose, which helps supply energy to the fetus. An excessive rise in blood glucose can lead to **gestational diabetes,** often beginning in weeks 20 to 28, particularly in women who have a family history of diabetes or who are obese. Other risk factors include maternal age over 25 and gestational diabetes in a prior pregnancy. In North America, gestational diabetes develops in about 4% of pregnancies; however, it increases to 7% in the Caucasian population. Today, pregnant women often are screened for diabetes at 24 to 28 weeks by checking for elevated blood glucose concentration 1 to 2 hours after consuming 50 to 100 g of glucose. A woman who develops gestational diabetes needs to implement a special diet that distributes low-glycemic load carbohydrates throughout the day. Sometimes insulin injections are also needed. In addition, regular physical activity helps to control blood glucose.[6]

gestational diabetes A high blood glucose concentration that develops during pregnancy and returns to normal after birth; one cause is the placental production of hormones that antagonize the regulation of blood glucose by insulin.

The primary risk of uncontrolled diabetes during pregnancy is that the fetus can grow quite large.[18] This growth is a result of the oversupply of glucose from maternal circulation coupled with increased production of insulin by the fetus, allowing fetal tissues to take up building materials for growth. The mother may require a cesarean section if the size of the fetus is not compatible with a vaginal delivery. Another threat is that the infant may have low blood glucose at birth because of the tendency to produce extra insulin that began during gestation. Other concerns are the potential for early delivery and increased risk of birth trauma and malformations. Although gestational diabetes often disappears after the infant's birth, it increases the mother's risk of developing diabetes later in life, especially if she fails to maintain a healthy body weight. Recent studies show that infants of mothers with gestational diabetes may also have higher risks of developing obesity and type 2 diabetes as they grow to adulthood. For all these reasons, proper control of gestational diabetes (and any diabetes present in the mother before pregnancy) is extremely important.

Critical | Thinking

Sandy, who is 4 months pregnant, has been having heartburn after meals, constipation, and difficult bowel movements. As a student of nutrition, you understand the digestive system and the role of nutrition in health. What remedies might you suggest to Sandy to relieve her problems?

Pregnancy-Induced Hypertension

Pregnancy-induced hypertension is a high-risk disorder and occurs in about 5 to 7% of pregnancies. In its mild forms, it is also known as *preeclampsia* and, in severe forms, as *eclampsia*. Early symptoms include a rise in blood pressure, excess protein in the urine, edema, changes in blood clotting, and nervous system disorders. Very severe effects, including convulsions, can occur in the second and third trimesters.[19] If not controlled, eclampsia eventually damages the liver and kidneys, and mother and fetus both may die. The populations most at risk for this disorder are women under age 17 or over age 35 and women who have had multiple-birth pregnancies. A family history of pregnancy-induced hypertension in the mother's or father's side of the family, diabetes, African-American race, and a woman's first pregnancy also raise risk. A diet inadequate in vitamin E, vitamin C, calcium, zinc, and other nutrients may also be part of the cause.

pregnancy-induced hypertension A serious disorder that can include high blood pressure, kidney failure, convulsions, and even death of the mother and fetus. Although its exact cause is not known, an adequate diet (especially adequate calcium intake) and prenatal care may prevent this disorder or limit its severity. Mild cases are known as *preeclampsia*; more severe cases are called *eclampsia* (formerly called *toxemia*).

Pregnancy-induced hypertension resolves once the pregnancy ends, making delivery the most reliable treatment for the mother. However, because the problem often begins before the fetus is ready to be born, physicians in many cases must use treatments to prevent the worsening of the disorder. Bed rest and magnesium sulfate are currently the most effective treatment methods, although their effectiveness varies.[19] Magnesium likely acts to relax blood vessels and so leads to a fall in blood pressure. Several other treatments, such as various antiseizure and antihypertensive medications, are under study.

Concept | Check

Heartburn, constipation, hemorrhoids, nausea and vomiting, edema, anemia, and gestational diabetes are possible discomforts and complications of pregnancy. Changes in food habits can often ease these problems. Pregnancy-induced hypertension, with high blood pressure and kidney failure, can lead to severe complications or even death of both the mother and fetus if not treated.

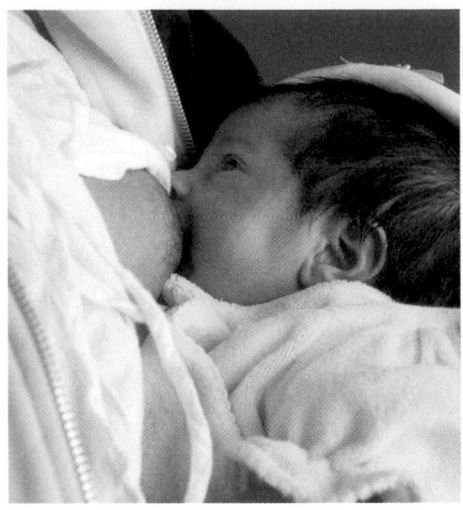

Breastfeeding is the preferred way to feed a young infant.

Breastfeeding

Breastfeeding further fosters the new infant's health and so complements the attention given to diet during pregnancy. The American Dietetic Association and the American Academy of Pediatrics recommend breastfeeding exclusively for the first 6 months, with the continued combination of breastfeeding and infant foods until 1 year.[2] The World Health Organization goes beyond that to recommend breastfeeding (with appropriate solid food introduction; see Chapter 17) for at least 2 years. However, surveys show that only about 70% of North American mothers now begin to breastfeed their infants in the hospital, and at 4 and 6 months only 33% and 20%, respectively, are still breastfeeding their infants. The number falls to 18% at 1 year of age. These statistics refer to Caucasian women; minority women are even less likely to be breastfeeding at these time intervals.

Women who choose to breastfeed usually find it an enjoyable, special time in their lives and in their relationship with their new infant. Although bottle feeding with an infant formula is safe for infants, as discussed in Chapter 17, it does not equal the benefits derived from human milk in all aspects. If a woman doesn't breastfeed her child, breast weight returns to normal very soon after birth.

Many of the benefits of breastfeeding can be found in Table 16-3 and at www.4woman.gov./Breastfeeding/index.htm, sponsored by the U.S. Surgeon General.

Ability to Breastfeed

Almost all women are physically capable of breastfeeding their children (see the later section titled Medical Conditions Precluding Breastfeeding for exceptions). In most cases, problems encountered in breastfeeding are due to a lack of appropriate information. Anatomical problems in breasts, such as inverted nipples, can be corrected during pregnancy. Breast size generally increases during pregnancy and is no indication of success in breastfeeding. Most women notice a dramatic increase in the size and weight of their breasts by the third or fourth day of breastfeeding. If these changes do not occur, a woman needs to speak with her physician or a lactation consultant.

Breastfed infants must be followed closely over the first days of life to ensure that feeding and weight gain are proceeding normally. Monitoring is especially important with a mother's first child, because the mother will be inexperienced with the technique of breastfeeding. Currently, mothers and healthy infants are commonly discharged from the hospital 1 to 2 days after delivery, whereas 20 years ago they stayed in the hospital for 3 or 4 days or longer. One result of such rapid discharge is a decreased period of infant monitoring by health-care professionals. Incidents have been reported of infants developing dehydration and in turn blood clots soon after hospital discharge when breastfeeding did not proceed smoothly. Careful monitoring in this first week by a physician or lactation consultant is advised.

Healthy People 2010 has set a goal of 75% of women breastfeeding their infants at time of hospital discharge, 50% breastfeeding for 6 months, and 25% still breastfeeding at 1 year.

Figure 16-6 | The anatomy of the breast. Many types of cells form a coordinated network to produce and secrete human milk.

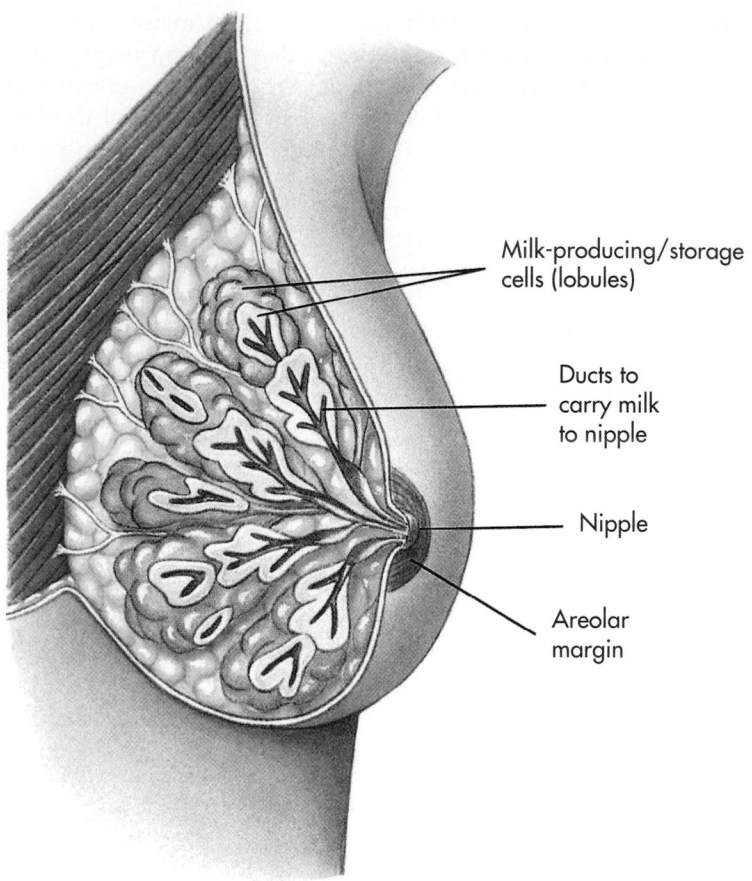

Milk-producing/storage cells (lobules)

Ducts to carry milk to nipple

Nipple

Areolar margin

First-time mothers who plan to breastfeed should learn as much as they can about the process early in their pregnancy.[2] Interested women should learn the proper technique, what problems to expect, and how to respond to them. Overall, breastfeeding is a learned skill, and mothers need knowledge to breastfeed safely, especially with the first child.

Production of Human Milk

lobules Saclike structures in the breast that store milk.

prolactin A hormone secreted by the pituitary gland. It stimulates the synthesis of milk in the breast.

During pregnancy, cells in the breast form milk-producing cells called **lobules** (Figure 16-6). Hormones from the placenta stimulate these changes in the breast. After birth, the mother produces more **prolactin** hormone to maintain the changes in the breast and therefore the ability to produce milk. During pregnancy, breast weight increases by about 1 to 2 lb.

The hormone prolactin also stimulates the synthesis of milk. Infant suckling stimulates prolactin release from the pituitary gland. Milk synthesis then occurs as an infant breastfeeds. The more the infant suckles, the more milk is produced. Because of this, even twins (and triplets) can be breastfed adequately.

Most protein found in human milk is synthesized by breast tissue. Some proteins also enter the milk directly from the mother's bloodstream. These proteins include immune factors (e.g., antibodies) and enzymes. Fats in human milk come from both the mother's diet and those synthesized by breast tissue. The sugar galactose is synthesized in the breast, whereas glucose enters from the mother's bloodstream. Together, these sugars form lactose, the main carbohydrate in human milk.

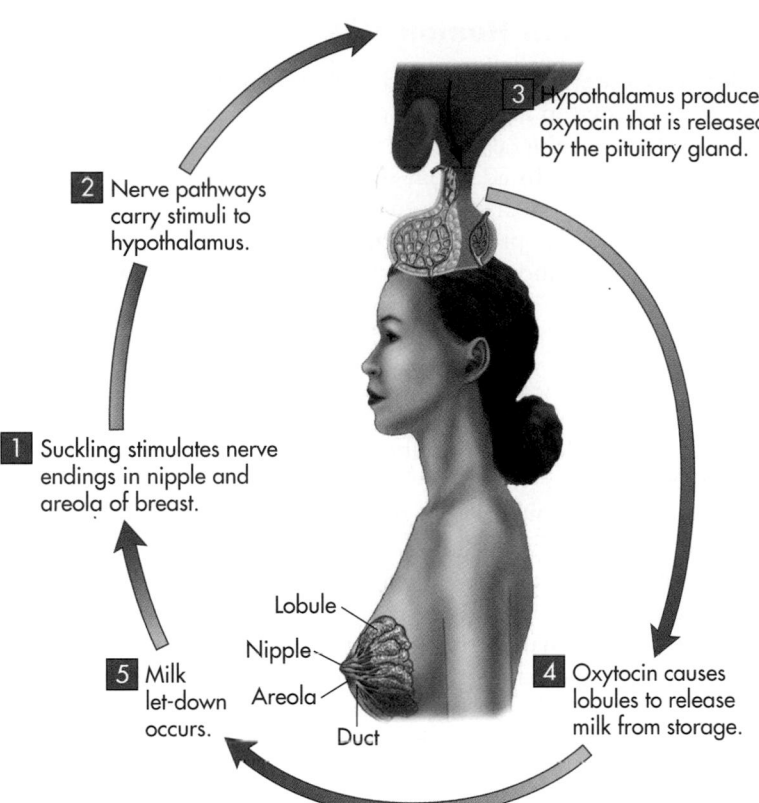

2 Nerve pathways carry stimuli to hypothalamus.

3 Hypothalamus produces oxytocin that is released by the pituitary gland.

1 Suckling stimulates nerve endings in nipple and areola of breast.

Lobule
Nipple
Areola
Duct

5 Milk let-down occurs.

4 Oxytocin causes lobules to release milk from storage.

Figure 16-7 | Let-down reflex. Suckling sets into motion the sequence of events that lead to milk let-down, the flow of milk into ducts of the breast.

Let-Down Reflex

An important brain-breast connection—commonly called the **let-down reflex**—is necessary for breastfeeding. The brain releases the hormone **oxytocin** to allow the breast tissues to let down (release) the milk from storage sites (Figure 16-7). It then travels to the nipple area. A tingling sensation signals the let-down reflex shortly before milk flow begins. If the let-down reflex doesn't operate, little milk is available to the infant. The infant then gets frustrated, which can in turn frustrate the mother.

The let-down reflex is easily inhibited by nervous tension, a lack of confidence, and fatigue. Mothers should be especially aware of the link between tension and a weak let-down reflex. They need to find a relaxed environment in which they can breastfeed.

After a few weeks, the let-down reflex becomes automatic. The mother's response can be triggered just by thinking about her infant or seeing or hearing another infant cry. At first, however, the process can be a bit bewildering. Because she cannot measure the amount of milk the infant takes in, a mother may fear that she is not adequately nourishing the infant.

As a general rule, a well-nourished breastfed infant should (1) have six or more wet diapers per day after the second day of life, (2) show a normal weight gain, and (3) pass at least one or two stools per day that look like lumpy mustard.[2] In addition, softening of the breast during the feeding helps indicate that enough milk is being consumed. Parents who sense that their infant is not consuming enough milk should consult a physician immediately because dehydration can develop rapidly.

It generally takes 2 to 3 weeks to fully establish the feeding routine: infant and mother both feel comfortable, the milk supply meets infant demand, and initial nipple soreness disappears. Establishing the breastfeeding routine requires patience, but the rewards are great. The adjustments are easier if supplemental formula feedings are not introduced until breastfeeding is well established, after at least 3 to 4 weeks. Then it is fine if a supplemental bottle or two of infant formula per day is needed.

let-down reflex A reflex stimulated by infant suckling that causes the release (ejection) of milk from milk ducts in the mother's breasts; also called *milk ejection reflex*.

oxytocin A hormone secreted by the pituitary gland. It causes contraction of the musclelike cells surrounding the ducts of the breasts and the smooth muscle of the uterus.

D isposable diapers can absorb so much urine that it is difficult to judge when they are wet. A strip of paper towel laid inside a disposable diaper makes a good wetness indicator. Alternatively, cloth diapers may be used for a day or two to assess whether nursing is supplying sufficient milk.

Cow's Milk Compared to Human Milk

Energy	Same
Protein	3.2 times higher
Fat	0.2 times lower
Carbohydrate	0.3 times lower
Minerals	3.5 times higher

The fat composition of human milk changes during each feeding. The consistency of milk released initially (fore milk) first resembles that of fat-free milk. It later has a greater fat proportion, similar to whole milk. Finally, the milk released after 10 to 20 minutes (hind milk) is essentially like cream. Infants need to breastfeed long enough (e.g., a total of 20 or more minutes) to get the energy in the rich hind milk to be satisfied between feedings and to grow well.

Nutritional Qualities of Human Milk

Human milk is very different in composition from cow's milk. Unless altered, cow's milk should never be used in infant feeding until the infant is at least 12 months old. Cow's milk is too high in minerals and protein and does not contain enough carbohydrate to meet infant needs. In addition, the major protein in cow's milk (**casein**) is harder for an infant to digest than the major proteins (lactalbumin and other **whey** proteins) in human milk. The proteins in cow's milk also may spur allergies in the infant. Finally, certain compounds in human milk presently under study show other possible benefits for the infant.

Colostrum

At the end of pregnancy the first fluid made by the human breast is **colostrum.** This thick, yellowish fluid may leak from the breast during late pregnancy and is produced in earnest for a few days to a week after birth. Colostrum contains antibodies and immune system cells, some of which pass unaltered through the infant's immature GI tract into the bloodstream.[8] The first few months of life are the only time when we can readily absorb whole proteins across the GI tract. These immune factors and cells protect the infant from some GI tract diseases and other infectious disorders, compensating for the infant's own immature immune system during the first few months of life.

One component of colostrum, the *Lactobacillus bifidus* **factor,** encourages the growth of *Lactobacillus bifidus* bacteria. These bacteria limit the growth of potentially toxic bacteria in the intestine. Overall, breastfeeding promotes the intestinal health of the breastfed infant.

Mature Milk

Human milk composition gradually changes until it achieves the normal composition of mature milk several days after delivery. Human milk looks very different from cow's milk. (Table 17-1 in Chapter 17 provides a direct comparison.) Human milk is thin and almost watery in appearance and often has a slightly bluish tinge. Its nutritional qualities, however, are quite impressive. The overall energy content of human milk is about the same as that of infant formulas (67 kcal/100 ml).

Human milk's whey proteins form a soft, light curd in the infant's stomach and are easy to digest. Some human milk proteins bind iron, reducing the growth of iron-requiring bacteria, some of which can cause diarrhea. Still other proteins offer the important immune protection already noted.

The lipids in human breast milk are high in linoleic acid and cholesterol, which are needed for brain development. Breast milk also contains long-chain omega-3 fatty acids, such as docosahexaenoic acid (DHA). This polyunsaturated fatty acid is used for the synthesis of tissues in the brain and the rest of the central nervous system, and in the retina of the eye.[2]

Human milk composition also allows for adequate fluid status of the infant, provided the baby is exclusively breastfed.[2] A question commonly asked is whether the infant needs additional water, if stressed by hot weather, diarrhea, vomiting, or fever. Providing breastfed infants with up to 4 oz of water a day from a bottle is fine. Note, however, that greater amounts of supplemental water can lead to brain disorders, low blood sodium, and other problems. Thus, extra water should be given only with a physician's guidance.

Food Plan for Women Who Breastfeed

Nutrient needs for a breastfeeding mother change to some extent from those of the pregnant woman in the second and third trimester (see the inside cover of this book). There is a decrease in folate and iron needs and an increase in the need for energy, vitamins A, E, and C, riboflavin, copper, chromium, iodide, manganese, selenium, and zinc. Still, these increased needs of the breastfeeding mother will be met by the general diet plan proposed for pregnant women in the latter stages of pregnancy.[2] Recall that each day this diet plan includes at least:

- 3 cups of calcium-rich foods from the milk group, or use of calcium-fortified foods
- 6 1/2 ounce-equivalents from the meat & beans group
- 3 1/2 cups from the vegetable group
- 2 cups from the fruit group
- 8 ounce-equivalents from the grain group
- 7 teaspoons of vegetable oil

Discretionary calories (up to about 400 kcal) can then be added, depending on the need for slow weight loss or weight maintenance (or even weight gain in some cases).

Table 16-2 provided a menu for such a plan. Substituting a soyburger (veggie burger) for the hamburger in that menu would make this menu plan a practical guide for a lactovegetarian woman as well.

As in pregnancy, a serving of a highly fortified ready-to-eat breakfast cereal (or use of a balanced multivitamin and mineral supplement) is advised to help meet extra nutrient needs. And, as mentioned for pregnant women, breastfeeding mothers should consume fish at least twice a week (or 1 g/day of omega-3 fatty acids from a fish oil supplement) because the omega-3 fatty acids present in fish are secreted into breast milk and are likely to be important for development of the infant's nervous system.

Milk production requires approximately 800 kcal/day. The Estimated Energy Requirement during lactation is an extra 400 to 500 kcal daily above prepregnancy recommendations. The difference between that needed for milk production and the recommended intake—about 300 kcal—may allow a gradual loss of the extra body fat accumulated during pregnancy, especially if breastfeeding is continued for 6 months or more and the woman performs some physical activity.[2]

After giving birth, women are often eager to shed the excess "baby fat." Breastfeeding, however, is no time for crash diets. A gradual weight loss of 1 to 4 lb/ month in the breastfeeding mother is appropriate. At significantly greater rates of weight loss—when energy intake is restricted to less than about 1500 kcal/day— milk output decreases. A reasonable approach for a breastfeeding mother is to eat a balanced diet that supplies at least 1800 kcal/day, has moderate fat content, and includes a variety of dairy products, fruits, vegetables, and whole grains.[2]

To promote the best possible feeding experience for the infant, there are several other dietary factors to consider. Hydration is especially important during breastfeeding; the woman should drink fluids every time her infant breastfeeds. Drinking about 13 cups of fluids per day encourages ample milk production. Poor health habits, such as smoking cigarettes or drinking more than two alcoholic drinks a day, can decrease milk output. (Even less alcohol can have a deleterious effect on milk output in some women.) To avoid exposure to harmful levels of mercury, precautions concerning fish that are likely to contain mercury should extend past pregnancy for the breastfeeding mother. Breastfeeding women also may want to avoid eating peanuts or peanut butter, because several studies have shown that peanut allergens pass into breast milk, potentially increasing the infant's risk for peanut allergy.

Most substances that the mother ingests are secreted into her milk. For this reason, she should limit intake of or avoid all alcohol and caffeine and check all medications with a pediatrician. Some mothers believe that some foods, such as garlic and chocolate, flavor the breast milk and upset the infant. If a woman notices a connection between a food she eats and the infant's later fussiness, she could consider avoiding that food. However, she might experiment again with it later, because infants become fussy for other reasons. Some researchers, on the other hand, feel that the passage of flavors from the mother's diet into her milk affords an opportunity for the infant to learn about the flavor of the foods of its family long before solids are introduced. These researchers suspect that bottle-fed infants are missing significant sensory experiences that, until recent times in human history, were common to all infants.

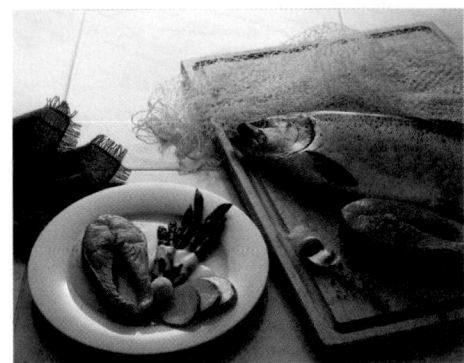

Eating fish at least twice a week will help breastfeeding women ensure that their infants receive important omega-3 fatty acids. It is important, however, to avoid those fish that are likely contaminated with mercury (listed on page 595).

Concept | Check

Recognition of the importance of breastfeeding has contributed to its greater popularity in recent years. Almost all women have the ability to breastfeed. The hormone prolactin stimulates breast tissue to synthesize milk. Some components of human milk come directly from the mother's bloodstream. Infant suckling triggers a let-down reflex, which releases the milk. The more an infant breastfeeds, the more milk is synthesized. The nutrient composition of human milk is very different from that of cow's milk and changes as the infant matures. The first fluid produced, colostrum, is rich in immune factors. The diet for breastfeeding is generally similar to that for pregnancy, except for necessary additional fluids.

reastfeeding provides distinct advantages, but none so great that a woman who decides to bottle-feed should feel she is significantly compromising her infant.

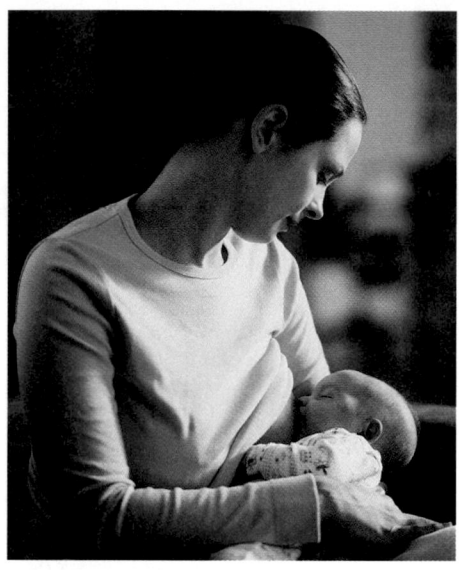

The American Dietetics Association supports breastfeeding as the ideal feeding method for infants. In addition to breastfeeding's nutritional benefits for the infant, ADA also promotes breastfeeding as a public health strategy for improving infant survival rates, decreasing mothers' risks of developing certain diseases, controlling health-care costs, and conserving natural resources.

Breastfeeding Today

As noted already, the vast majority of women are capable of breastfeeding and their infants benefit from it.[2] The many benefits are listed in Table 16-3. Nonetheless, a woman's decision to breastfeed depends on a variety of factors, some of which, you will see, make breastfeeding impractical or undesirable for a woman.

Advantages of Breastfeeding

Just as the milk of all mammals is the perfect nutrition source for the young of that species, human milk is tailored to meet infant nutrient needs for the first 4 to 6 months of life. The possible exceptions are the relative lack of fluoride, iron, and vitamin D. Infant supplements, used under the guidance of a pediatrician, can supply these nutrients and are often recommended, especially vitamin D. The American Academy of Pediatrics recommends that all breastfed infants be given 200 IU of vitamin D/day until they are consuming that much from food, such as at least 2 cups (0.5 liters) of infant formula per day. Some sun exposure also helps in meeting vitamin D needs. Fluoride may be found in the household water supply. If it is not present in adequate amounts or the infant is not receiving tap water, a fluoride supplement should be considered and a dentist consulted. Vitamin B-12 supplements are recommended for the breastfed infant whose mother is a vegan.

Fewer Infections Breastfeeding reduces the infant's overall risk of developing infections, partially because an infant can use the antibodies in human milk.[4,8] Breastfed infants also have fewer ear infections (otitis media) because they do not sleep with a bottle in their mouths. Experts strongly discourage allowing any infants to sleep with a bottle in their mouths, because when that happens, milk can pool in the mouth, back up through the throat, and eventually settle in the ears, creating a growth medium for bacteria. Infant ear infections are a common problem. By avoiding these problems, parents can decrease discomfort for the infant, avoid related trips to the doctor, and

Table 16-3 | Advantages of Breastfeeding

Infant
• Bacteriologically safe
• Always fresh and ready to go
• Provides antibodies while infant's immune system is still immature and provides substances that contribute to maturation of the immune system
• Contributes to maturation of gastrointestinal tract via *Lactobacillus bifidus* factor; decreases incidence of diarrhea and respiratory disease
• Reduces risk of food allergies and intolerances as well as some other allergies
• Establishes habit of eating in moderation, thus decreasing possibility of obesity later in life by about 20%
• Contributes to proper development of jaws and teeth for better speech development
• Decreases ear infections
• May enhance nervous system development (by providing the fatty acid DHA) and eventual learning ability
• May reduce the risk of later developing hypertension and other chronic diseases, such as diabetes

Mother
• Contributes to earlier recovery from pregnancy due to the action of hormones that promote a quicker return of the uterus to its prepregnancy state
• Decreases the risk of ovarian and premenopausal breast cancer
• Potential for quicker return to prepregnancy weight
• Potential for delayed ovulation and therefore reduced chance of pregnancy (short-term benefit, however)

prevent possible hearing loss. Tooth decay from nighttime bottles is another likely consequence of sleeping with a bottle in the mouth (see Chapter 17).

Fewer Allergies and Intolerances Breastfeeding also reduces the chances of some allergies, especially in allergy-prone infants (see Chapter 17). The key time to attain this benefit from breastfeeding is during the first 4 to 6 months of an infant's life. A longer commitment than 4 to 6 months is best, but the first few months are most critical. Breastfeeding for even just the first few weeks is beneficial. Another benefit of breastfeeding is that infants are better able to tolerate human milk than formulas. Formulas sometimes must be switched several times until caregivers find the best one for the infant.

Possible Barriers to Breastfeeding

Widespread misinformation, the mother's need to return to a job, and social reticence all serve as barriers to breastfeeding.

Misinformation Probably the major barriers to breastfeeding are misinformation, such as the idea that one's breasts are too small, and the lack of role models. One positive note has been the widespread increase in the availability of lactation consultants over the past several years. These consultants are a valuable resource for new mothers in the adjustment to breastfeeding. If a woman is interested in breastfeeding, she should find support by talking to women who have experienced it successfully because they can be an invaluable help to the first-time mother. The first-time mother should find a friend she can call on for advice. In almost every community, a group called La Leche League offers classes in breastfeeding and advises women who have problems with it (800-LALECHE or www.lalecheleague.org). Other resources are www.breastfeeding.com, www.breastfeeding.org, and www.nal.usda.gov/wicworks.

Return to an Outside Job Working outside the home can complicate plans to breastfeed. One possibility after a month or two of breastfeeding is for the mother to express and save her own milk. She can use a breast pump or manually express milk into a sterile plastic bottle or nursing bag (used in a disposable bottle system). Saving human milk requires careful sanitation and rapid chilling. It can be stored in the refrigerator for 3 days or be frozen for 3 months. There is a knack to learning how to express milk, but the freedom can be worth it, because it allows others to feed the infant the mother's milk. A schedule of expressing milk and using supplemental formula feedings is most successful if begun after 1 to 2 months of exclusive breastfeeding. After 1 month or so, the baby is well adapted to breastfeeding and probably feels enough emotional security and other benefits from nursing to drink both ways.

Some women can juggle both a job and breastfeeding, but others find it too cumbersome and decide to switch to formula. A compromise—balancing some breastfeedings, perhaps early morning and night, with infant formula feedings during the day—is possible. However, too many supplemental infant formula feedings decrease milk production.

Social Concerns Another barrier for some women is embarrassment about breastfeeding a child in public. Historically our society has stressed modesty and has discouraged public displays of breasts—even for as good a cause as nourishing babies. In the United States, no state or territory has a law prohibiting breastfeeding. However, indecent exposure (including the exposure of women's breasts) has long been a common law or statutory offense. During the 1990s, some individual states, such as Florida and North Carolina, began to clarify the right to breastfeed and to decriminalize public breastfeeding. Since then, several other states have passed similar laws. Women who feel reluctant should be reassured that they do have social support and that breastfeeding can be done very discreetly with little breast exposure.

Although not a nutritional benefit, breastfeeding frees the mother from the time and expense involved in buying and preparing formula and washing bottles. Human milk is ready to go and sterile. This benefit allows the mother to spend more time with her baby.

Frozen human milk should not be thawed in a microwave. The heat can destroy immune factors in the milk and create hot spots that may scald the infant's tongue.

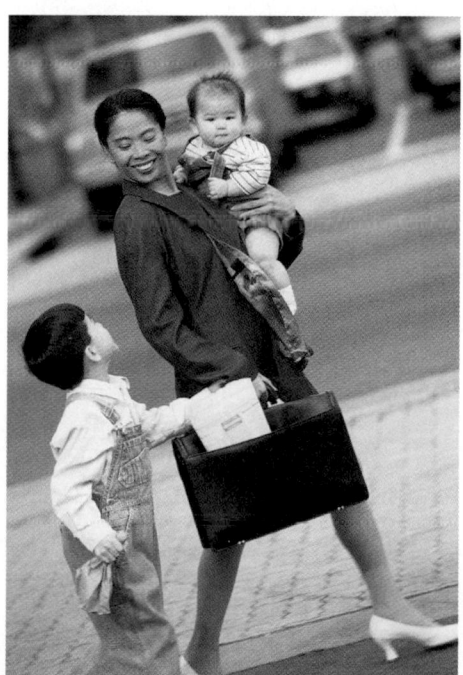

Breastfeeding a baby after returning to work is possible, but requires planning.

reastfeeding mothers should get their physician's permission before embarking on a vigorous exercise program. Breastfeeding women must also take care to drink plenty of fluids before and after workouts and should avoid exercising when fatigued.

Medical Conditions Precluding Breastfeeding Breastfeeding may be ruled out by certain medical conditions in either the infant or mother. For example, breastfeeding may be detrimental to infants with phenylketonuria; the high concentration of phenylalanine in breast milk may overwhelm the impaired ability of these infants to metabolize this amino acid, leading to production of toxic products.

Certain medications, which pass into the milk and adversely affect the nursing infant, are best avoided while breastfeeding. In addition, a woman in North America or other developed regions of the world who has a serious chronic disease (such as tuberculosis, AIDS, or HIV-positive status) or who is being treated with chemotherapy medications should not breastfeed.[2]

Environmental Contaminants in Human Milk

There is some legitimate concern over the levels of various environmental contaminants in human milk. However, the benefits from human milk are very well established and the risks from environmental contaminants are still largely theoretical. Thus, it is probably best to continue with what has been shown to work until sufficiently strong research data contradict it. A few measures a woman could take to counteract some known contaminants are to (1) avoid freshwater fish from polluted waters, (2) carefully wash and peel fruits and vegetables, and (3) remove the fatty edges of meat, because pesticides concentrate in fat. In addition, a woman should not try to lose weight rapidly while nursing (more than 3/4 to 1 lb/week) because contaminants stored in her fat tissue might then enter her bloodstream and affect her milk. If a woman questions whether her milk is safe, especially if she has lived in an area known to have a high concentration of toxic wastes or environmental pollutants, she should consult her local health department.

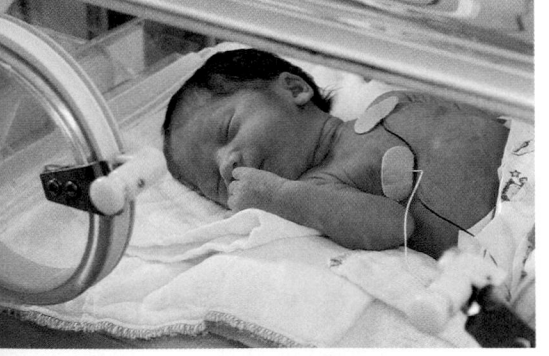

If human milk is used to feed the preterm infant, fortification of the milk with certain nutrients is often needed.

The Breastfeeding of Preterm Infants

There is no universal answer to whether a woman can breastfeed a preterm infant. In some cases, human milk is the most desirable form of nourishment, depending on infant weight and length of gestation. If so, it must usually be expressed from the breast and fed through a tube until the infant's sucking and swallowing reflex develops. This type of feeding demands great maternal dedication. Fortification of the milk with such nutrients as calcium, phosphorus, sodium, and protein is often necessary to match the preterm infant's rapid growth. In other cases, special feeding problems may prevent the use of human milk or necessitate supplementing it with formula. Sometimes total parenteral nutrition (intravenous feeding) is the only option. Working as a team, the pediatrician, neonatal nurses, and registered dietitian must guide the parents in this decision.

Concept | Check

Human milk supplies most of an infant's nutritional needs for the first 6 months, although supplementation with vitamin D, iron, and fluoride may be needed. Breastfeeding is often more convenient than formula feeding. Compared with formula-fed infants, breastfed infants have fewer intestinal, respiratory, and ear infections and are less susceptible to some allergies and food intolerances. Despite the advantages of breastfeeding, a mother may be dissuaded from breastfeeding by misinformation, job responsibilities, and social reticence. A combination of breastfeeding and formula feeding is possible when a mother is regularly away from the infant and is not able to express and store her milk for later use. Breastfeeding is not desirable if a mother has certain diseases or must take medication potentially harmful to the infant. The preterm infant, depending on its condition, may benefit from consuming human milk.

Summary

1. Adequate nutrition is vital during pregnancy to ensure the well-being of both the infant and mother. Poor maternal nutrition and use of some medications, especially during the first trimester, can cause birth defects. Growth restriction and altered development can also occur if these insults happen later in pregnancy.

2. Infants born preterm (before 37 weeks gestation) usually have more medical problems at and following birth than normal infants.

3. A woman typically needs an additional 350 to 450 kcal/day during the second and third trimesters of pregnancy to meet her energy needs. A better measure of meeting energy needs is adequate weight gain. This should occur slowly, reaching a total of 25 to 35 lb (11.5 to 16 kg) in a woman of healthy weight.

4. Protein, carbohydrate, fiber, vitamin, and mineral needs increase during pregnancy. Following MyPyramid is recommended, including whole-grain bread and cereal choices. A supplemental source of iron, in particular, may be needed. Folate nutriture especially should be adequate at the time of conception. Any nutrient supplement use needs to be guided by a physician, because an excess intake of vitamin A and other nutrients during pregnancy can have harmful effects on the fetus.

5. The factors that contribute to poor pregnancy outcome include inadequate health care in general and prenatal care in particular, teenage pregnancy, closely spaced births, smoking, alcohol consumption, illicit drug use (such as cocaine), insufficient carbohydrate intake (less than 175g/day), heavy caffeine use, and various infections, such as *Listeria*.

6. Pregnancy-induced hypertension, gestational diabetes, heartburn, constipation, nausea, vomiting, edema, and anemia are all possible discomforts and complications of pregnancy. Nutrition therapy can help minimize some of these problems.

7. Almost all women are able to breastfeed their infants. The nutrient composition of human milk is very different from that of unaltered cow's milk and is much more desirable. Colostrum, the first fluid produced by the human breast, is very rich in immune factors. Mature milk is rich in protein and in lactose. The diet plan recommended for pregnancy is also appropriate for meeting the nutrient needs of the lactating woman, except that more fluids in general should be consumed.

8. For the infant, the advantages of breastfeeding over formula feeding are numerous, including fewer intestinal, respiratory, and ear infections and fewer allergies and food intolerances. Moreover, breastfeeding is also less expensive and possibly more convenient for the mother than formula feeding. However, an infant can be adequately nourished with formula if the mother chooses not to breastfeed. Breastfeeding is not desirable if the mother has certain diseases or must take medication potentially harmful to the infant. Likewise, breastfeeding is not advised for infants with certain medical conditions, including some preterm infants.

Study Questions

1. Provide three key pieces of advice for parents seeking to maximize their chances of having a healthy infant. Why did you identify those specific factors?

2. Outline current weight-gain recommendations for pregnancy. What is the basis for these recommendations?

3. Identify four key nutrients for which intake should be significantly increased during pregnancy.

4. Why is following MyPyramid advocated to meet the increased nutrient needs of pregnancy?

5. Why does teenage pregnancy receive so much attention these days? At what age do you think pregnancy is ideal? Why?

6. Give three reasons a woman should seriously consider breastfeeding her infant.

7. Describe the physiological mechanisms that stimulate milk production and release. How can knowing about these mechanisms help mothers breastfeed successfully?

8. What guidelines can a woman use to determine whether her breastfed infant is receiving sufficient nourishment?

9. How should the basic food plan suitable for pregnancy be modified during breastfeeding?

10. Where can first-time mothers go for help in establishing successful breastfeeding?

BOOST YOUR STUDY

Check out the **Perspectives in Nutrition: Online Learning Center** www.mhhe.com/wardlawpers7 for quizzes, flash cards, activities, and web links designed to further help you learn about nutrition for pregnant and breastfeeding women.

Annotated References

1. ADA Reports: Position of the American Dietetic Association: Nutrition and lifestyle for a healthy pregnancy outcome. *Journal of the American Dietetic Association* 102:1479, 2002.

    The key components of a healthy lifestyle during pregnancy include appropriate weight gain; consumption of a variety of foods; appropriate and timely vitamin and mineral intake; avoidance of alcohol, tobacco, and other harmful substances; and safe food handling. Vitamin and mineral supplementation is appropriate for some nutrients, particularly in certain situations, such as for vegans.

2. ADA Reports: Position of the American Dietetic Association: Promoting and supporting breastfeeding. *Journal of the American Dietetic Association* 105:810, 2005.

    The American Dietetic Association strongly supports the breastfeeding of infants. This article discusses the benefits from breastfeeding that accrue to the mother and infant as well as dietary considerations that need to be addressed, such as avoiding consumption of species of fish known to contain high amounts of mercury.

3. Allen LH: Multiple micronutrients in pregnancy and lactation: An overview. *American Journal of Clinical Nutrition* 81:1206S, 2005.

    Numerous nutrients contribute to a healthy outcome of pregnancy, including many B vitamins and iron. The author notes that in many cases diet changes allow women to meet these needs, but in some cases supplementation is needed, such as for poor women. Diet changes should begin before pregnancy so a woman has a healthy status in the first weeks when she does not yet know she is pregnant.

4. Bachrach VGR and others: Breastfeeding and the risk of hospitalization for respiratory diseases in infancy: A meta-analysis. *Archives of Pediatrics & Adolescent Medicine* 157:237, 2003.

    Breastfeeding an infant substantially reduces his or her risk of developing respiratory diseases. To achieve this benefit, at least 4 months of exclusive breastfeeding is recommended.

5. Brundage S: Preconception health care. *American Family Physician* 65:2507, 2002.

    Achieving optimal preconception health can help to reduce adverse pregnancy outcomes. It is recommended that women who are planning to become pregnant consume at least 400 μg of synthetic folic acid, get screened and if necessary be treated for any infectious diseases, limit their exposure to environmental toxins, and optimize control of any chronic diseases. In addition, many experts recommend that women planning a pregnancy participate in regular moderate exercise, avoid both obesity and underweight, and steer clear of alcohol, megadoses of vitamin A, and large amounts of caffeine.

6. Crowther CA and others: Effect of treatment of gestational diabetes mellitus on pregnancy outcomes. *The New England Journal of Medicine* 352:2477, 2005.

    This study found that treating gestational diabetes when it develops is important in order to improve the health of the mother, fetus, and ultimately the infant. Diet changes and regular blood glucose monitoring are important parts of the therapy; in some cases insulin injections are also needed to control blood glucose.

7. Eustace LW and others: Fetal alcohol syndrome: A growing concern for health care professionals. *Journal of Obstetrics, Gynecology, and Neonatal Nursing* 32(2):215, 2003.

    The disorders fetal alcohol syndrome and fetal alcohol effect are increasing in the United States. This trend is troubling because consumption of alcohol during pregnancy can harm the fetus irreparably. Currently the amount of alcohol, if any, that can be safely consumed during pregnancy and the exact physiological mechanisms that make alcohol unsafe for the fetus have yet to be identified.

8. Field CJ: The immunological components of human milk and their effect on immune development in infants. *Journal of Nutrition* 135:1, 2005.

    Human milk contains many factors that improve immune function in the infant. This article reviews a number of these quite complex factors.

9. Hulsey TC and others: Maternal prepregnant body mass index and weight gain related to low birth weight in South Carolina. *Southern Medical Journal* 98:411, 2005.

    A healthy weight at conception and adequate weight gain during pregnancy contributed to a substantial reduction in low-birth-weight infants in this study. For example, women with inadequate weight gains had about a 1.5 to 2 times greater risk of delivering a low-birth-weight infant.

10. Kabiru KW, Raynor BD: Obstetric outcomes associated with increase in BMI category during pregnancy. *American Journal of Obstetrics and Gynecology* 191:928, 2004.

    Obesity in pregnant women leads to a high risk for complications in the pregnancy and so requires careful monitoring by the physician. Such complications included gestational diabetes and the need for cesarean deliveries.

11. Keen KL and others: The plausibility of micronutrient deficiencies being a significant contributing factor to the occurrence of pregnancy complications. *Journal of Nutrition* 133:1597S, 2003.

    Numerous studies support the concept that a major cause of pregnancy complications can be suboptimal fetal nutrition. Several observational and intervention studies suggest that diets low in essential vitamins and minerals, such as vitamins A, B-6, and B-12 and the minerals iron, zinc, copper, and magnesium, pose a significant risk for a poor outcome of pregnancy. Improvement in the micronutrient status of the mother when needed may reduce pregnancy complications.

12. Kelly AKW: Practical exercise advice during pregnancy. *The Physician and Sports Medicine* 33(6):24, 2005.

    It is safe for pregnant women to exercise if they are experiencing uncomplicated pregnancies. The author notes that in fact many positive effects of exercise during pregnancy are possible. Most non-weight-bearing exercises (e.g., swimming) and walking are safe for pregnant women. Exercise programs should begin with 15 minutes of exercise three times a week and progress as tolerated. The author discusses how to monitor women as they increase their physical activity.

13. King JC: The risk of maternal nutritional depletion and poor outcomes increases in early or closely spaced pregnancies. *Journal of Nutrition* 133:1732S, 2003.

    An adequate supply of nutrients is probably the single most important environmental factor affecting pregnancy outcome. A short interval between pregnancies or an early pregnancy within 2 years of the onset of menstrual periods increases the risk for preterm birth and growth-retarded infants. Maternal nutrient depletion arising from closely spaced pregnancies is one cause of these poor pregnancy outcomes. Supplementation with food and micronutrients during the interpregnancy period may improve pregnancy outcomes and maternal health among women with early or closely spaced pregnancies.

14. Koebnick C and others: Long-term ovo-lacto vegetarian diet impairs vitamin B-12 status in pregnant women. *Journal of Nutrition* 134:3319, 2004.

    Pregnant women consuming a long-term predominantly vegetarian diet had an increased risk of developing a vitamin B-12 deficiency in this study. Attention to vitamin B-12 intake is thus merited in women who are vegetarians, and this monitoring needs to be done before they become pregnant.

15. Moore VM, Davies MJ: Diet during pregnancy, neonatal outcomes, and later health. *Reproduction, Fertility, and Delivery* 17:341, 2005.

    Animal experiments clearly show that altering the maternal diet before and during pregnancy can induce permanent changes in the offspring birth size, adult health, and life span.

Consequences of inadequate maternal nutrition for the offspring depend on the specific time in gestation that they occur. The authors emphasize the importance of improving diet before a woman becomes pregnant in order to protect her health and the health of her offspring.

16. Pawley N, Bishop NJ: Prenatal and infant predictors of bone health: The influence of vitamin D. *American Journal of Clinical Nutrition* 80:1748S, 2004.

    Women who are vitamin D–deficient during pregnancy deliver infants with disturbed skeletal development and in some cases even with evidence of rickets and fractures. Populations at risk for vitamin D deficiency are those for which, for environmental, cultural, or medical reasons, exposure to sunlight is poor and the dietary intake of vitamin D is low. Especially in these cases, attention to meeting vitamin D needs is very important.

17. Prather CM: Pregnancy-related constipation. *Current Gastroenterology Reports* 6:402, 2004.

Constipation is a common complaint in pregnancy. In most cases, dietary measures such as increased fiber are sufficient to treat the disorder. Any laxative use needs to be reviewed by a physician because some are not appropriate for use during pregnancy.

18. Rosenburg TJ and others: Maternal obesity and diabetes as risk factors for adverse pregnancy outcomes: Differences among four racial/ethnic groups. *American Journal of Public Health* 95:1545, 2005.

    In this large population-based study, obesity and diabetes were clearly associated with adverse pregnancy outcomes: This finding highlights the need for women to control these conditions as best as possible during their childbearing years in order to protect the health of their future infant.

19. Wagner LK: Diagnosis and managements of preeclampsia. *American Family Physician* 70:2317, 2004.

    Preeclampsia is a multisystem disorder of unknown cause. It effects about 5 to 7% of preg-

nancies and is a significant cause of both illness and death in the mother and fetus. Management requires careful monitoring of the mother and fetus once the disorder develops. Currently, magnesium sulfate is the major therapy used, but medications to control related hypertension may also be employed. This article reviews preeclampsia in detail.

20. Welch-Carre E: The neurodevelopmental consequences of prenatal alcohol exposure. *Advances in Neonatal Care* 5:217, 2005.

    Prenatal alcohol exposure and related fetal alcohol syndrome is one of the leading causes of birth defects, developmental disorders, and mental retardation in children. The nervous system of the fetus is particularly vulnerable to alcohol. The author recommends that clinicians provide anticipatory guidance and counseling about alcohol use for women during their childbearing years in order to prevent this disorder.

Take | Action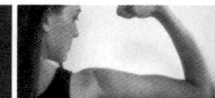

I. Targeting Nutrients Necessary for Pregnant Women

This chapter mentioned that pregnant women may have difficulty meeting their increased needs for folate, vitamin B-6, iron, and zinc. List six foods rich in each of these nutrients next to the appropriate heading below. Refer to Chapters 9 through 12 if necessary.

Nutrient	Foods	Nutrient	Foods
Folate	_____	Iron	_____
	_____		_____
	_____		_____
	_____		_____
	_____		_____
	_____		_____
Vitamin B-6	_____	Zinc	_____
	_____		_____
	_____		_____
	_____		_____
	_____		_____
	_____		_____

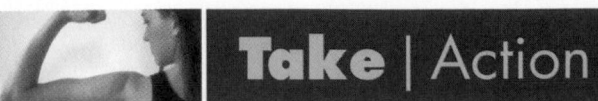

Take | Action

II. Putting Your Knowledge about Nutrition and Pregnancy to Work

A college friend, Angie, tells you that she is newly pregnant. You are aware that she usually likes to eat the following foods for her meals:

Breakfast
Skips this meal, or eats a granola bar
Coffee

Lunch
Sweetened yogurt, 1 cup
Small bagel with cream cheese
Occasional piece of fruit
Regular caffeinated soda, 12 oz

Snack
Chocolate candy bar

Dinner
2 slices of pizza, macaroni and cheese, or 2 eggs with 2 slices of toast
Seldom eats a salad or vegetable
Regular caffeinated soda, 12 oz

Snacks
Pretzels or chips, 1 oz
Regular caffeinated soda, 12 oz

1. Using NutritionCalc Plus software or Appendix N, evaluate Angie's diet for protein, carbohydrate, iron, vitamin B-6, folate, and zinc. How does her intake compare with the recommended amounts for pregnancy?

   _____

   _____

   _____

2. Now redesign Angie's diet and make sure that her intake meets pregnancy needs for carbohydrates, protein, folate, vitamin B-6, and zinc. (Hint: Fortified foods, such as breakfast cereal, are generally nutrient-rich foods, which can more easily help meet her needs.) Increase her iron content as well, but it still may be below the RDA for pregnancy.

   _____

   _____

   _____

17

NUTRITION FROM INFANCY THROUGH ADOLESCENCE

CHAPTER OUTLINE

CASE SCENARIO:

Damon is a 7-month-old boy who has been taken into a clinic for a routine checkup. On examination, he seemed thin, and he plotted on the growth chart at the 25th percentile for weight and the 50th percentile for length. His physician scheduled a follow-up appointment in 3 months. At the 10-month-visit, Damon appeared sluggish. He was again plotted on the growth chart and was now at the 5th percentile for weight but still at the 50th percentile for length.

A registered dietitian interviewed Damon's 16-year-old mother to collect information on his dietary intake. The 24-hour diet recall consisted of two bottles of formula, three bottles of Kool-Aid, and a hot dog. However, the mother was still in school, and at night she often left Damon with the neighbor so that she could go out for a few hours. Thus, she was not aware of all that he ate, because much of her time was spent away from him.

What problems do you think are present in Damon's diet? What potential dangers await Damon if his health status continues along this current growth trend?

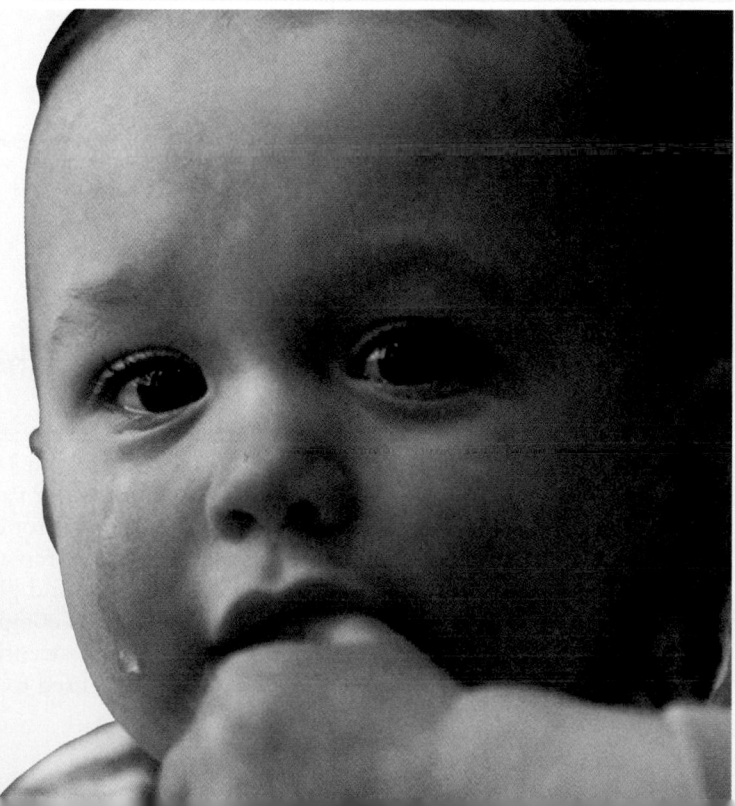

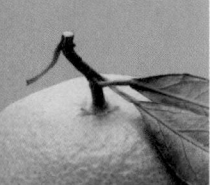

As humans grow through early years into adulthood, our needs for energy and nutrients change. Infants need more energy, protein, vitamins, and minerals per pound of body weight than do adults to support their rapid pace of growth and development.[5] As growth tapers, children need and eat proportionately less. The erratic eating behaviors of young children pose major challenges for parents and other caregivers.[11] In turn, childhood becomes an important time to establish healthful habits, including those related to food choice and physical activity.

Family behaviors wield important influences over the child.[17] Thus, education designed to change children's eating behaviors must be directed simultaneously at the main caregivers. They usually determine what foods are purchased and how those foods are prepared. To help children adopt a lifelong healthy dietary intake, parents and caregivers should provide a variety of foods at home, limit fast food to a few times per week or less, and introduce new foods regularly. Maintaining a pattern of healthful eating (and physical activity) should continue as children grow into teenagers.[4,9,13,20] In exploring all these stages of life, this chapter looks at the key role nutrients play and how food choices should be tailored to meet a child's changing needs.

CHAPTER OBJECTIVES CHAPTER 17 IS DESIGNED TO ALLOW YOU TO:

1. Describe normal growth during infancy and childhood, and state why growth with regard to weight and height is an indicator of the adequacy of an infant's diet.
2. Identify the nutritional needs of infants and children.
3. Explain why infant formula is an acceptable substitute for human milk and why cow's milk is not.
4. Develop an adequate eating plan for an infant or child using food labels and MyPyramid.
5. State why feeding an infant a high-iron food at 6 months is recommended.
6. Explain the rationale—from the standpoint of both nutrition and ongoing physical development—for the delay in feeding an infant solid foods until 4 to 6 months of age.
7. Help parents overcome obstacles associated with children's eating habits.
8. Relate nutrient needs to growth rate in adolescence.
9. Explain some nutrition-related health issues facing children and teenagers today in North America.
10. Distinguish between food allergies and intolerances and provide recommendations for treating both.

REFRESH YOUR MEMORY AS YOU BEGIN YOUR STUDY OF NUTRITION FROM INFANCY THROUGH ADOLESCENCE IN CHAPTER 17, YOU MAY WANT TO REVIEW:

- MyPyramid and the *2005 Dietary Guidelines for Americans* in Chapter 2.
- Diagnosis and treatment of type 2 diabetes in Chapter 5.
- Common sources of saturated fat and *trans* fat in Chapter 6.
- Vegetarianism in the Nutrition Focus in Chapter 7.
- Rich sources of iron and zinc in Chapter 12.
- The concept of body mass index (BMI) and the treatment of obesity in Chapter 13.
- The benefits of regular physical activity in Chapter 14.
- Anorexia nervosa and other eating disorders in Chapter 15.

Nutrition and Child Health: An Introduction

Current trends in nutrition and overall health among children and adolescents in North America have shown both positive and negative results. On a positive note, more children are receiving vaccinations than ever before, fewer teenagers are giving birth, and the poverty rate for children has fallen considerably. In contrast to this good news, the number of children and teenagers with obesity, the metabolic syndrome, and type 2 diabetes is rising, and physical activity in general is on the decline as more time is spent sitting in front of computer screens and television sets.[9,20] Low calcium intakes are also receiving much attention, as soft drinks have replaced much of the milk that children and teenagers used to consume on a daily basis. Whole grains are also in short supply in children's diets.[2,19] This chapter looks at these trends, especially their effects on nutrition and overall health in this age group.

Infant Growth and Physiological Development

During infancy, a child's attitudes toward foods and the whole eating process begin to take shape. If parents and other caregivers practice good nutrition and are flexible, they can lead an infant into lifelong healthful food habits. Such an infant has a good chance both of starting life with the nutrients needed to support brain and body growth spurts and of developing a willingness to try new foods.

These physical and psychological advantages, however, don't guarantee that a child will thrive. Children also need specific attention focused on them; they need to grow in a stimulating environment, and they need a sense of security. For example, children hospitalized for growth failure gain weight more quickly when loving care accompanies needed nutrients.[11]

The Growing Infant

All infants seem to do is eat and sleep. There's a good reason for this. An infant's birth weight doubles in the first 4 to 6 months and triples within the first year. Never again is growth so rapid.[11] Such rapid growth requires a lot of both nourishment and sleep. After the first year, growth is slower; it takes 5 more years to double the weight seen at 1 year. An infant also increases in length in the first year by 50% and then continues to gain height through the teen years. These gains are not necessarily continuous— spurts of growth alternate with plateaus. Height is essentially maximized by age 19, although increases of several inches may occur in the early twenties, especially for boys (Figure 17-1). Head size in proportion to total height shrinks from one-fourth to one-eighth during the climb from infancy to adulthood.

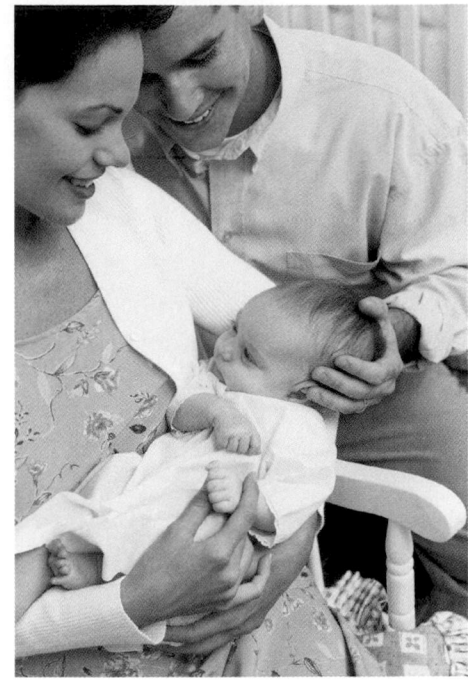

Children benefit from the love and attention of adults.

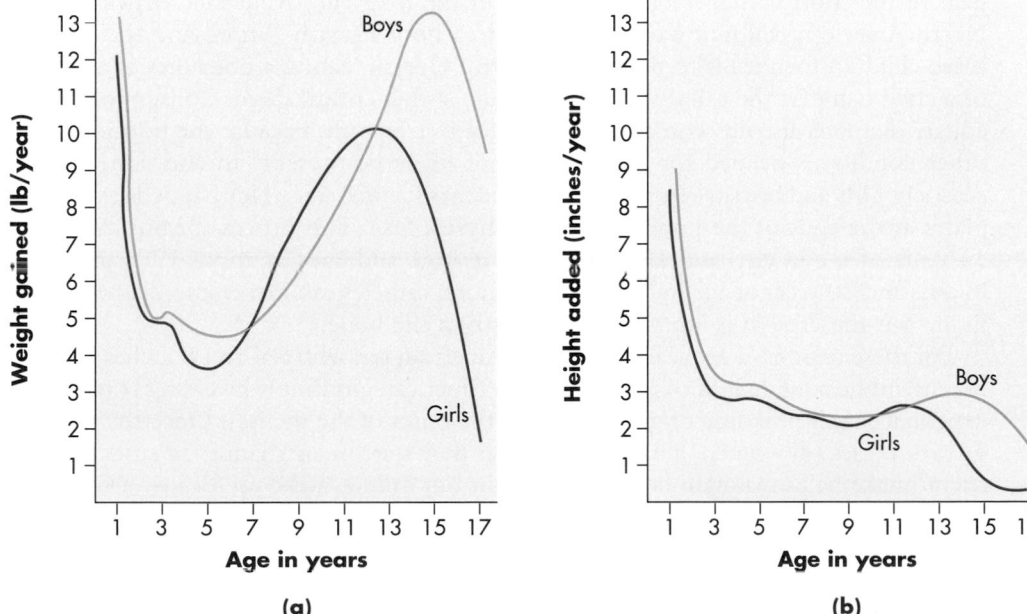

Figure 17-1 | Growth rates. (a) Average gains in weight for girls and boys. (b) Average additions to height for girls and boys. The higher the line in any one year, the greater the amount of annual gain compared with that in other years. Large gains in weight occur in both infancy and puberty, whereas the very high length gain in infancy is never reached again. If graphs such as these were plotted in smaller time segments, they would appear as zigzag lines, rather than smooth lines, reflecting short, periodic spurts in growth in the course of each year.

The human body needs a lot more food to support growth and development than it does to merely maintain its size once growth ceases. When nutrients are missing at critical phases of growth and development, growth slows and may even stop. From observations of Egyptian mummies, we see that infants were about the same size in 300 B.C. as they are today. However, adult mummies are much smaller than adults today. Furthermore, the suits of armor in museum collections of the Middle Ages typically would not fit modern adults. The average height of North American men in 1700 was approximately 5 feet 8 inches, whereas today it is approximately 5 feet 10 inches. These increases suggest that people of earlier times generally ate nutrient-poor diets that did not support the growth we typically experience today.

In countries of the developing world today, about one-third of the children under 5 years of age are short and underweight for their ages. Poor nutrition—called *undernutrition*— is at the heart of the problem. Undernutrition occurs to a lesser extent in North America. The undernourished children are simply smaller versions of nutritionally fit children. In poorer countries, when breastfeeding ceases, children are often fed a high-carbohydrate, low-protein diet. This diet supports some growth but does not allow children to attain their full genetic potential. To grow, children must consume adequate amounts of energy, protein, calcium, iron, zinc, and other nutrients.[1]

Infant development follows a pattern in which body water falls from about 70% at birth to 60% at 1 year. The latter is also the proportion typical in adults. By age 1, a healthy infant's body nitrogen content (and thus protein content) has increased from 2% of body weight at birth to 3%, indicating that the infant has synthesized much new lean tissue.[11]

Effect of Undernutrition on Growth

As with the fetus in utero, the long-term effects of nutritional problems in infancy and childhood depend on the severity, timing, and duration of the nutritional insult to cell processes.

The single best indicator of a child's nutritional status is growth, particularly weight gain in the short run and length (height) in the long run. Mild zinc deficiencies in North American children have been linked to poor growth. Improving the diets of these children then leads to improved growth. Overall, eating a poor diet as an infant or a child hampers the cell division that occurs at that critical stage. Consuming an adequate diet later usually won't compensate for lost growth, because the hormonal and other conditions needed for growth will not likely be present. In addition, growth ceases in girls and boys when the skeleton reaches its final size. This happens as growth plates at the ends of the bones, called **epiphyses,** fuse. This process begins at around 14 years of age in girls and 15 years of age in boys and ends at about 19 years of age in girls and 20 years of age in boys. Furthermore, muscles can increase in diameter later in life but the growth is limited by the length of the bone.[11]

For these reasons, a 15-year-old Central American girl who is 4 feet 8 inches tall cannot attain the adult height of a typical North American girl simply by eating better. Girls experience their peak rate of growth before the onset of the menses. Once the time for growth ceases (in women, about 5 years after they start menstruating), a sufficient nutrient intake helps maintain health and weight but cannot make up for lost growth.

Assessment of Infant Growth and Development

Health professionals assess a child's increases in height and weight by comparing them with typical growth patterns recorded on charts (Figure 17-2). The charts contain 7 to 9 **percentile** divisions, which represent the typical measurements of about 96% of children. A percentile represents the rank of the person among 100 peers matched for age and gender. If a young boy, for example, is at the 90th percentile height for age, he is shorter than 10% (of children) and taller than 89% (of children). A child at the 50th percentile is considered average. Fifty children will be taller than this child; 49 will be shorter.[11]

epiphyses Ends of long bones. The epiphyseal plate—sometimes referred to as the growth plate—is made of cartilage and allows growth of the bone to occur. During childhood, the cartilage cells multiply and absorb calcium to develop into bone.

percentile Classification of a measurement of a unit into divisions of 100 units.

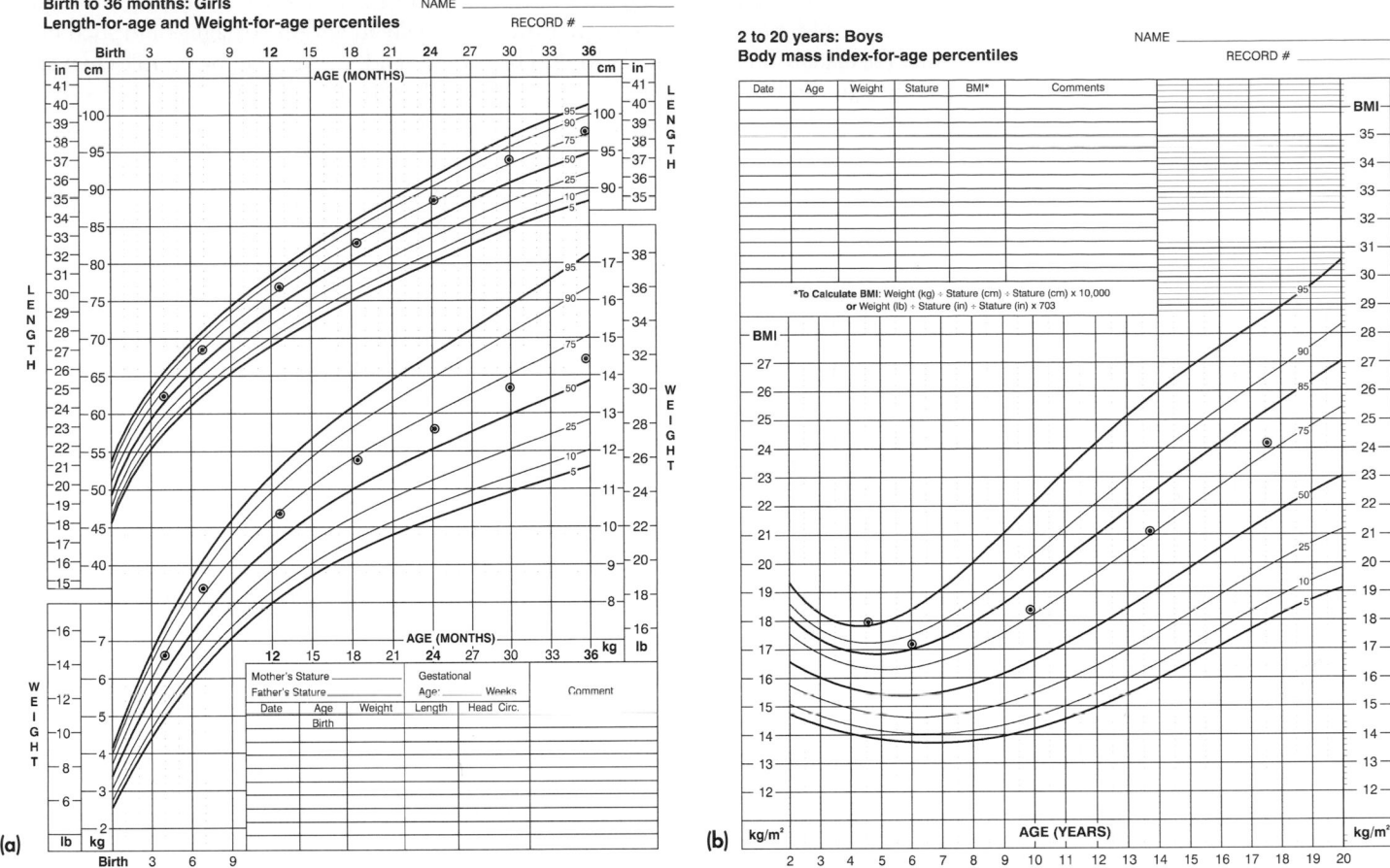

Figure 17-2 | Growth charts for assessment of children in the growing years. The growth of a youngster is plotted to show how the charts are used in health-care settings. (a) Growth charts used to assess length (height) and weight in young girls. A certain weight and length (height) correspond to a percentile value, which is a ranking of the person among 100 peers. This chart shows that at 36 months of age the girl was at the 75th percentile for length and the 62nd percentile for height. (b) Growth charts used to assess weight-for-height relationships in boys ages 2 to 20 years. At 6 years of age the boy was at the 85th percentile for BMI. Today these charts for older children and adolescents typically utilize BMI for the evaluation.

Source: Developed by the National Center for Health Statistics in collaboration with the National Center for Chronic Disease Prevention and Health Promotion (2000). www.cdc.gov/growthcharts. Revised November 21, 2000.

Individual growth charts are available for both males and females. For ages ranging from birth to 36 months, options for growth charts include weight-for-age, length-for-age, weight-for-length, and head circumference-for-age. For males and females who are 2 to 20 years old, growth charts are available to determine weight-for-age and height-for-age; however, the preferred growth chart for children and adolescents is body mass index (BMI)-for-age. For adults, BMI has fixed cutoff points (for example, a BMI of 25 for an adult is considered overweight). As Figure 17-2 shows, this is not true for children, for whom BMI is both gender- and age-specific.

Infants and children should have their growth assessed during regular health checkups. It takes 1 to 3 years for an infant to establish his or her own genetic percentile. Once this figure is established, such as length (height) for age, the child's measurement should then track along that percentile. If the child's growth doesn't keep up with his or her length-for-age percentile, the physician needs to investigate whether a medical or nutritional problem is impeding the predicted growth. Inappropriate weight gain—too little or too much—should also be investigated.[11]

Children under 2 to 3 years of age are measured lying on their backs with knees unflexed so the term *length* is used rather than *height*.

Infants born preterm may catch up in growth in 2 to 3 years. Catching up requires that the child move up in the percentiles—especially in length-for-age—and such movement is usually no cause for alarm. On the other hand, moving up percentiles in weight-for-height can be disturbing if the child approaches the 80th to 90th percentiles. A child at the 85th percentile or above for BMI is considered at risk for overweight. At or above the 95th percentile, the child is considered overweight. At the 95th percentile, the diagnosis of obesity can also be established if the physical exam of the child indicates he or she is truly overfat, which is generally the case at this percentile.

Brain Growth

The brain grows faster in infancy than at any other time of life. To accommodate the growth, an infant's head circumference must be very large in proportion to the rest of the body. The rapid growth stops at about 18 months of age. The rest of the body eventually grows to reach a typical proportion to head size. In early physical checkups, a health professional usually measures the head circumference as another means of assessing growth, especially brain growth. How nutritional status affects brain development and intelligence quotient (IQ) is difficult to measure because scientists haven't figured out how to separate the effects of nature from those of nurture. However, several studies have determined that breastfed infants have higher IQs than do infants who were fed with infant formula.[11] At the same time, studies from Central America suggest that IQ after age 5 years relates more closely to the amount of schooling a child receives than to nutritional intake during childhood.

Adipose Tissue Growth

Since 1970, researchers have speculated that overfeeding during infancy may increase adipose tissue cell numbers. Today, we know that the number of adipose cells can also increase as adulthood obesity develops. Still, if energy intake is limited during infancy to keep down the number of adipose cells, the growth of other organ systems may also be severely restricted. Special concern revolves around body growth and development, especially brain and nervous system development. In addition, most obese infants become normal-weight preschoolers without excessive diet restrictions. For these reasons, it's unwise to greatly restrict diet and especially fat intake in infants. After the first 12 months, fat intake can range from 30 to 40% of energy intake for ages 1 to 3 years and 25 to 35% for older children (and teenagers).[1]

Failure to Thrive

Occasionally, an infant doesn't grow much in the first few months. Physical problems that may contribute to restricted growth range from poor oral cavity development, infections, and heart irregularities to constant diarrhea associated with intestinal problems. However, more than half the infants who fail to thrive have no apparent disease. Sometimes the cause is poor infant-parent interaction that can stem from misinformation, mental depression in the mother, lack of a parent role model, or too little concern about the child's welfare. In general, the problems arise from the parents' inexperience rather than intentional negligence. In addition, many children who fail to thrive have inborn errors of metabolism that are very difficult to diagnose. For example, unusual enzyme deficiencies could lead to poor nutrient absorption and then malnutrition (review the Nutrition Focus in Chapter 4). In all cases a physician should determine the actual cause.[11]

Infants not only need cuddling; they also respond to voices and eye contact, especially at feeding times. New parents need to appreciate the importance of these practices to their infant's well-being. Some parents also may be overcommitted to maintaining a lean child in the hope of preventing future obesity. The result, even though the intention was good, can be failure to thrive.

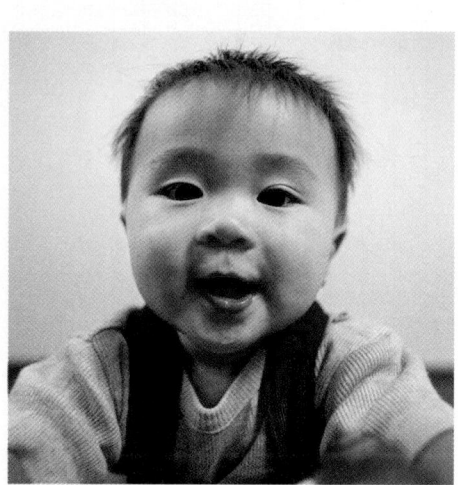

Brain growth is faster in infancy than in any other stage of life. Therefore an infant's head needs to be larger in comparison to the body in order to allow for such growth.

When clinicians encounter an infant who is failing to thrive from a nutritional standpoint, they must first determine whether formula-fed infants are consuming enough energy (see this chapter's section on formula feeding of infants for details). For a breastfed infant, the clinician needs to make sure that sufficient milk intake is taking place. As mentioned in Chapter 16, the child should be breastfeeding about six to eight times a day for about 20 minutes a session and have six to eight wet diapers each day.

C hildren older than 2 years are less likely to experience failure to thrive because they can often get food for themselves. Younger children, for the most part, are limited to what caregivers provide.

Concept | Check

Growth occurs rapidly during infancy: birth weight doubles in about 4 to 6 months and triples within the first year. Lean tissue increases, and the percentage of body water falls during the first year. Undernutrition in childhood can irreversibly inhibit growth and maturation, so that an individual never attains his or her full genetic potential for height. Infant and child growth is assessed by tracking body weight, length (height), and head circumference over time. Body mass index (BMI) is generally used to assess weight for height after 2 years of age. It is not desirable for infants to become obese, although no evidence strongly indicates that obese infants become obese adults. However, severe restriction of energy intake is not recommended for infants because it may slow the growth of organ systems. When infants do not grow properly, their failure to thrive may stem from physical disorders or inadequate care, including inappropriate feeding practices.

Infant Nutritional Needs

Infants' nutritional needs vary as they grow, and these needs differ from adult needs in both amount and proportion (Figure 17-3).[5] Initially, human milk or infant formula (generally using heat-treated cow's milk as a base) supplies needed nutrients. Solid foods are not needed until around 6 months. Even after solid foods are added, the basis of an infant's diet for the first year is still human milk or infant formula. Because of the critical importance of adequate nutrition in infancy and the difficulties encountered in feeding some infants, more time is spent in this chapter on this developmental period than on the later periods of childhood.

Energy

Estimated Energy Requirements (kcals) in infancy are **(89 kcal × weight of infant [kg]) + 75** from 0 to 3 months. From 4 to 6 months, such needs are **(89 kcal × weight of infant [kg]) + 44**; 7 to 12 months **(89 kcal × weight of infant [kg]) − 78**. At 6 months of age, this amount is about 700 kcal daily. Based on body weight comparisons, this amount is two to four times more energy than adults need. Infants need an easy way to get this amount of energy. Either human milk or infant formula is ideal for the first few months. Both are high in fat and supply about 640 kcal per quart of fluid (about 670 kcal per liter; Table 17-1). Later, human milk or infant formula, supplemented by solid foods, can provide even more energy.[5]

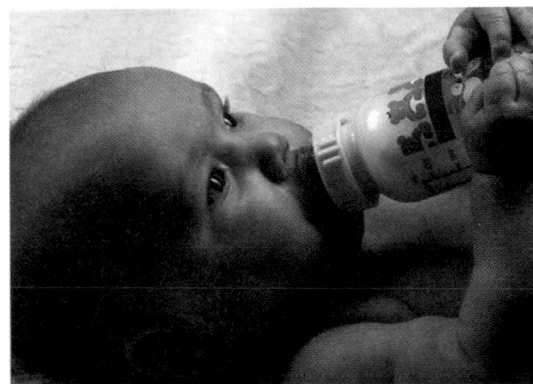

Infants who are formula-fed should remain on formula until 1 year of age.

The infant's high energy needs are primarily driven by its rapid growth and high metabolic rate. The high metabolic rate is caused in part by the ratio of the infant's body surface to its weight. More body surface allows more heat loss from the skin; the body must use extra energy to replace that heat.

Carbohydrate

Carbohydrate needs in infancy are 60 g/day at 0 to 6 months, and 95 g/day at 7 to 12 months. These needs are based on the typical intakes of human milk by breastfed infants and their eventual use of solid foods.

Protein

Daily protein needs in infancy are roughly 1.5 g/kg of body weight/day, or 9.1 g/day for younger infants and 13.5 g/day for older infants. These needs also are based on typical intakes by breastfed infants for 0 to 6 months, and then on the needs for growth

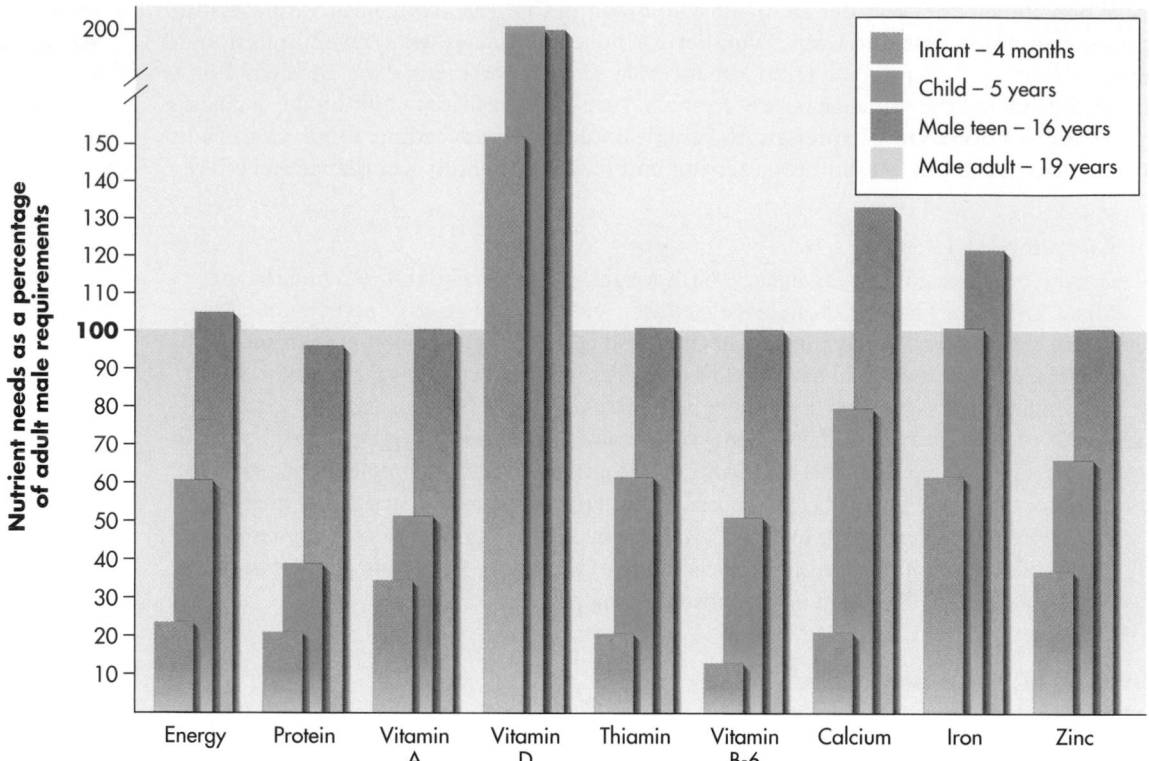

Figure 17-3 | Nutrient needs for infants, children, and teenagers as percentages of those for adult males. Compared with adults, infants' relative energy needs are lower than are their needs for other nutrients, as illustrated by the different heights of the light blue bars. Thus, infants need to obtain relatively larger amounts of nutrients from a smaller intake of food than do adults. This is also true of young children (dark green bars), but to a lesser extent.

of older infants. About half of total protein intake should come from essential amino acids. As with carbohydrate, protein needs are easily satisfied by either human milk or infant formula. Protein intake should not greatly exceed this standard. Excess nitrogen and minerals supplied by high-protein diets would exceed the ability of an infant's kidneys to excrete the resulting metabolic waste products from protein metabolism, thus putting much stress on overall kidney function.[11]

In North America, infant protein deficiency is unlikely except in cases of mistakes in formula preparation, such as when an infant's formula is excessively diluted with water. Protein deficiency may also be induced by elimination diets used to detect food **allergies** (hypersensitivities).[12] As foods are eliminated from the diet, infants may not be offered enough protein to compensate for the high-protein sources no longer present (see the Nutrition Focus in this chapter).

allergy A hypersensitive immune response that occurs when immune bodies produced by us react with a protein we sense as foreign (an antigen).

Fat

Infants need about 30 g of fat per day. The Adequate Intake ranges from 30 to 31 g/day. Essential fatty acids should make up about 15% of total fat intake (about 5 g/day). Both recommendations are again based on the typical intakes of breastfed infants from both human milk and the eventual introduction of solid foods. Fats are an important part of the infant's diet because they are energy-dense and vital to the development of the nervous system. As a concentrated energy source, fat also helps resolve the potential problem of the infant's high energy needs and small stomach capacity. Again, infancy is not an age to greatly restrict fat intake (Figure 17-4).[1]

Table 17-1 | Composition of Human and Cow's Milk and Infant Formulas per Liter (L)

Milk or Formula	Energy (kcal/L)	Protein (g/L)	Fat (g/L)	Carbohydrate (g/L)	Minerals* (g/L)
Milk					
Human milk	750	11	45	70	2
Cow's milk, whole	670	36	36	49	7
Cow's milk, fat-free	360	36	1	51	7
Casein/Whey-Based Formulas					
Similac	680	14	36	71	3
Enfamil	670	15	37	69	3
Carnation	670	16	34	73	3
Soybean Protein-Based Formulas					
ProSobee	670	20	35	67	4
Isomil	680	16	36	68	4
Predigested Protein					
Nutramigen	670	19	26	89	1
Alimentum	680	18	37	68	1
Transition Formulas/Beverages†					
Similac Toddler's Best	670	25	33	75	3
Enfamil Next Step	670	17	33	74	3
Carnation Follow-Up	670	17	27	88	3

At 3 months of age infants typically consume 0.75 to 1 L/day.

*Calcium, phosphorus, and other minerals.

†For use after 6 months of age or later (see label).

Looking at Table 17-1, it is easy to see why fat-free milk products are not recommended for infants—these products do not supply adequate fat and energy to meet needs. Fat-free milk (and reduced fat and whole milk as well) also would provide too much protein and minerals if it were used to meet energy needs.

Two long-chain fatty acids, arachidonic acid (AA) and docosahexaenoic acid (DHA), have very important roles in infant development. The nervous system, especially the brain and eyes, depend on these fatty acids for proper development. During the last trimester, DHA and AA provided by the mother accumulate in the brain and retinas of the eyes in the fetus. Infants who are breastfed are able to continue to acquire these fatty acids from human milk, especially if their mothers are regularly eating fish. Until recently, no infant formulas sold in the United States included AA or DHA, but certain brands with both AA and DHA are now available. These formulas are particulary useful for feeding preterm infants, but they also benefit other infants.[11]

Infants who drink goat's milk need a dietary supplement of folic acid because this milk doesn't supply a sufficient amount of this essential nutrient. Goat's milk is also low in iron, vitamin C, and vitamin D, making it a poor choice for human infants.

Vitamins of Special Interest

As noted in Chapter 9, vitamin K is routinely given by injection to all infants at birth. Formula-fed infants receive the rest of the vitamins they need from the formula. Breastfed infants should be given a vitamin D supplement (200 IU/day) until they are weaned to infant formula and are consuming 500 ml of it.[8] Breastfed infants whose mothers are vegans should receive vitamin B-12 in a supplement form.

Minerals of Special Interest

Infants are born with some internal stores of iron. However, by the time birth weight doubles by 4 to 6 months of age, iron stores are generally depleted. If the mother was iron deficient during the pregnancy, these iron stores will be exhausted even sooner. As you will recall from Chapter 12, iron deficiency anemia can lead to poor mental development in infants. To maintain a desirable iron status in infants, the American

Figure 17-4 | The labels on infant foods, like those on adult foods, contain a Nutrition Facts panel. However, the information provided on infant food labels differs from that on adult food labels, especially with respect to total fat, saturated fat, and cholesterol content (review Figure 2-9 for a comparison). Note also that some cereal brands are fortified with various other micronutrients.

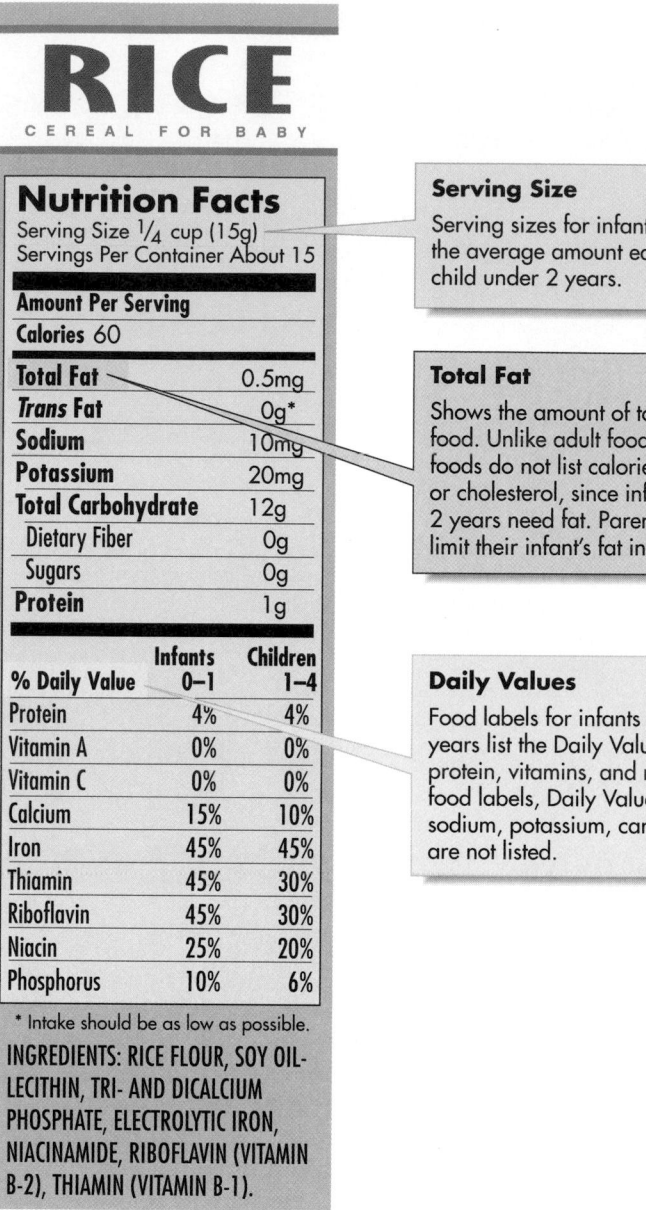

RICE
CEREAL FOR BABY

Nutrition Facts
Serving Size ¼ cup (15g)
Servings Per Container About 15

Amount Per Serving

Calories 60

Total Fat	0.5mg
Trans Fat	0g*
Sodium	10mg
Potassium	20mg
Total Carbohydrate	12g
Dietary Fiber	0g
Sugars	0g
Protein	1g

% Daily Value	Infants 0–1	Children 1–4
Protein	4%	4%
Vitamin A	0%	0%
Vitamin C	0%	0%
Calcium	15%	10%
Iron	45%	45%
Thiamin	45%	30%
Riboflavin	45%	30%
Niacin	25%	20%
Phosphorus	10%	6%

* Intake should be as low as possible.

INGREDIENTS: RICE FLOUR, SOY OIL-LECITHIN, TRI- AND DICALCIUM PHOSPHATE, ELECTROLYTIC IRON, NIACINAMIDE, RIBOFLAVIN (VITAMIN B-2), THIAMIN (VITAMIN B-1).

Serving Size

Serving sizes for infant foods are based on the average amount eaten at one time by a child under 2 years.

Total Fat

Shows the amount of total fat in a serving of the food. Unlike adult food labels, labels on infant foods do not list calories from fat, saturated fat, or cholesterol, since infants and toddlers under 2 years need fat. Parents should not attempt to limit their infant's fat intake.

Daily Values

Food labels for infants and children under 4 years list the Daily Value percentages for protein, vitamins, and minerals. Unlike adult food labels, Daily Values for fat, cholesterol, sodium, potassium, carbohydrate, and fiber are not listed.

Critical | Thinking

Tatiana has been breastfeeding her baby exclusively since he was born 7 months ago. When she and her husband took the baby for his checkup, they were told that he was anemic. They were very surprised, because they thought that human milk contained all the nutrients the baby needed for the first year of life. How might you explain the baby's anemia?

Academy of Pediatrics recommends that formula-fed infants should be given an iron-fortified formula from birth.[11] Low-iron infant formulas are sometimes prescribed to treat infants with various GI tract problems, but their use is discouraged. In contrast, breastfed infants need solid foods to supply extra iron by about 6 months of age. In fact, this need for iron is a major consideration in deciding when to introduce solid foods.[7]

To aid in tooth development, clinicians recommend fluoride supplements for formula-fed infants over 6 months of age if the water supply doesn't contain fluoride.[6] Note that formula manufacturers use fluoride-free water in formula preparation. Parents should consult their dentist for advice on meeting the infant's need for fluoride.

Water

An infant needs about 3 cups (700 to 800 ml) of water per day. Infants typically consume enough human milk or formula to supply this amount. In hot climates, however, supplemental water may be necessary. Furthermore, any conditions that lead to water loss—diarrhea, vomiting, fever, or too much sun—can call for supplemental water.[11]

Infants are easily dehydrated, a condition that has serious effects if not remedied. Dehydration can result in a rapid loss of kidney function, and the infant may then require hospitalization for rehydration. Special fluid-replacement formulas containing electrolytes such as sodium and potassium are available in supermarkets and pharmacies to treat dehydration. A physician should guide any use of these products.

Note that in some stores, bottled water products marketed specifically for infants may be placed alongside infant formulas and electrolyte-replacement solutions. This placement may give parents and caregivers the mistaken impression that bottled water products are appropriate for fluid replacement for infants; they are not and should not be used for such purposes. It is important to remember that excessive fluid can be harmful, especially to the brain.

Overall, it is best to limit supplemental fluids to about 4 oz (120 ml) per day, unless the physician thinks that a greater need exists because of disease or other conditions. In sum, extremes in fluid intake—either too little or too much—can lead to health problems.[11]

Concept | Check

Most nutrient needs in the first 6 months are met by human milk or infant formula. Breastfed infants need a vitamin D supplement; formula-fed infants and breastfed infants may need fluoride supplements after 6 months of age. Infants usually receive enough water from the human milk or formula they drink.

Formula Feeding for Infants

Breastfeeding was covered in detail in Chapter 16. This section focuses on formula feeding. You'll recall that a major advantage of breastfeeding is the provision of immune protection to the infant. Overall, in areas of the world where high standards for water purity and cleanliness are common, formula feeding is a safe alternative for infants (but generally is not as beneficial as breastfeeding).

Formula Composition

Infants cannot tolerate cow's milk as such because of its high protein and mineral content. Cow's milk reflects the growth needs of calves, not of human infants. Thus, cow's milk must be altered by formula manufacturers to be safe for infant feeding. It is important to note that goat's milk, sweetened condensed milk, and evaporated milk also are inappropriate substances for infants. Altered forms of cow's milk, known as infant formulas, are required to conform to strict federal guidelines for nutrient composition and quality. Formulas generally contain lactose and/or sucrose for carbohydrate, heat-treated proteins from cow's milk, and vegetable oils for fat (review Table 17-1).[11] Soy protein–based formulas are available for infants who can't tolerate lactose or the types of proteins found in cow's milk. If the soybean-based formula is not tolerated, the next step is to try a predigested (hydrolyzed) protein formula in which the proteins have been broken down into peptides and amino acids, such as Nutramigen or Alimentum. A variety of other specialized formulas also are available for specific medical conditions. In any case, it is important to use an iron-fortified formula unless a physician recommends otherwise.

Some transition formulas/beverages have been introduced for older infants and toddlers (review Table 17-1). Some of these products are intended for use after 6 months of age if the infant is consuming solid foods, whereas others are intended for use only by toddlers. These transition products are lower in fat than human milk or standard infant formulas; their iron content is higher than that of cow's milk, and their overall mineral content is generally more like that of human milk than cow's milk. According to the manufacturers, the advantages of these transition formulas/beverages over standard formulas for older infants and toddlers include reduced cost and better flavor. Parents should consult their physician with regard to the use of these products.[11]

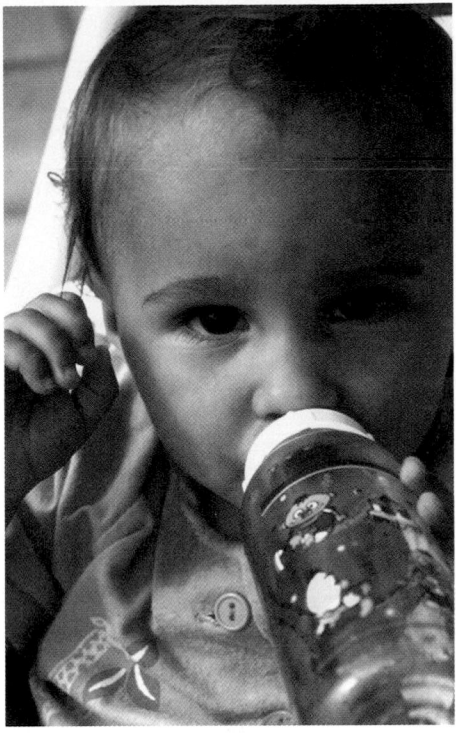

Supplemental fluids should be limited to 4 oz per day unless the infant's physician prescribes a larger amount.

Preterm infants are fed either a specially designed formula or human milk. Total parenteral nutrition may also be required in the initial phase of hospitalization. As noted in Chapter 16, nutrients may be added to human milk to increase its protein, mineral, and energy content. Preterm infants must be fed immediately because their bodies store little fat or carbohydrate. The body composition of a full-term infant includes about 12% fat, whereas the composition of a very preterm infant can include as little as 2% fat.

Parents should consult a physician when choosing an appropriate infant formula. Not all formula-like products are designed for infant use. A 5-month-old girl was admitted to a hospital in Arkansas with symptoms of heart failure, rickets, inflamed blood vessels, and possible nerve damage after being fed Soy Moo (a soy beverage sold in health-food stores) since 3 days of age. The symptoms suggest severe vitamin deficiencies.

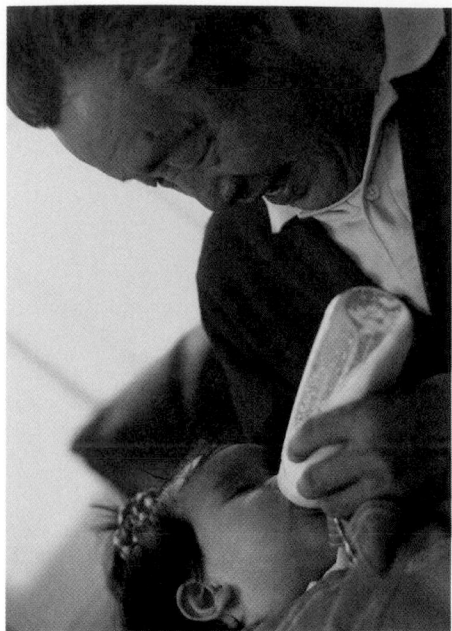

Careful attention during feeding allows the caregiver to notice the infant's signal as to when the feeding should cease.

Formula Preparation

Today, bottles of formula are often prepared one at a time. Some infant formulas come in ready-to-feed form. These are poured into a clean bottle and fed immediately. Room-temperature formula is acceptable for many infants. Otherwise, to warm a bottle of formula, a caregiver can run hot water over it or place it briefly in a pan of simmering water. Note that infant formulas should not be heated in a microwave oven because hot spots may develop, which can burn the infant's mouth and esophagus.

Powdered and concentrated fluid formula preparations are also commonly used. All utensils used in preparing formula from these preparations should be washed and thoroughly rinsed. Powdered or concentrated formulas are poured into a bottle to which clean, cold water is added (following label directions) and then mixed. The formula is then warmed, if desired, and fed immediately to the infant. Hot water from the faucet should not be used to make formula, because it poses a risk for high lead content (see Chapter 19). Cold water poses much less risk.

Refrigerating prepared formula for 1 day is safe. However, formula left over from a feeding should be discarded because it will be contaminated by bacteria and enzymes in the infant's saliva. If well water is used, it should be boiled before making formula for at least the infant's first 3 months of life, and it should be analyzed for excessive concentration of naturally occurring nitrates, which can lead to a severe form of anemia. Note that if nitrates are high in municipal water systems, consumers will be warned (such as in a local newspaper) not to use the water for making infant formula until the concentration falls to a safe amount. Alternately, if water contaminants are a concern, formula can be mixed with bottled nursery water, which is available alongside infant formulas in most supermarkets.

Feeding Technique

Because infants swallow a lot of air as they ingest either formula or human milk, it's important to burp an infant after either 10 minutes of feeding or 1 to 2 oz (30 to 60 ml) from a bottle and again at the end of feeding. Spitting up a bit of milk is normal at this time. Once fed, infants should be placed on their backs, not their stomachs. Infants should not be placed on their stomachs because this sleeping position has been linked to sudden infant death syndrome (SIDS). The Back to Sleep campaign, started in 1994 in the United States, has reduced SIDS by 40%; however, plagiocephaly, otherwise known as flat-head syndrome, has increased as a result. Infant skulls are soft and can take on a different form. Flat-head syndrome can occur if an excessive amount of an infant's life is spent on his or her back, or against a high chair or car seat. In response to this concern, the American Academy of Pediatrics has recommended periodic repositioning of an infant's head while asleep and allowing for time on his or her stomach while awake. In addition, some infants may need to wear specially fitted helmets to correct the shape of their head.[11]

When the infant begins acting full, bottle-feeding should be stopped, even if some milk is left in the bottle. Common cues that signal that an infant has had enough include turning the head away, being inattentive, falling asleep, and becoming playful. Generally, the infant's appetite is a better guide than standardized recommendations concerning feeding amounts. Breastfeeding infants usually have had enough to eat after about 20 minutes. Although it's difficult to tell how much milk breastfed infants are getting, they also give signs when full. By carefully observing bottle-feeding or breastfeeding infants and responding to their cues appropriately, caregivers not only can be assured that the infants' energy needs are being met but also can foster a climate of trust and responsiveness.[5]

Development of Feeding Skills in Older Infants

By 6 to 7 months the infant has learned to grab and transfer objects from one hand to the other (Table 17-2). At about this time, teeth begin to appear, and the infant be-

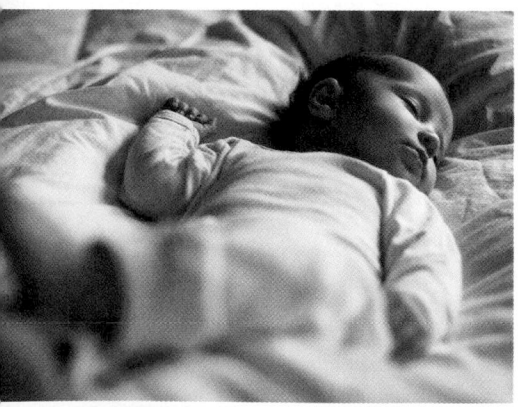

The Back to Sleep campaign advises that infants be placed on their backs for sleeping.

Table 17-2 | Typical Progression of Infant Eating Skills and Solid-Food Introduction*

Age	Feeding Skills	Oral Motor Skills	Types of Food	Suggested Activities
Birth–4 months		Rooting reflex Suckling reflex Swallowing reflex Extrusion reflex	Human milk Infant formula	Breastfeed or bottle-feed
5 months	Is able to grasp objects voluntarily Is learning to reach mouth with hands	Disappearance of extrusion reflex		Possibly introduce thinned cereal if baby not satisfied by breastfeeding or bottle feeding
6 months	Sits with balance while using hands	Transfers food from front of tongue to back	Infant cereal Strained fruit Strained vegetables Egg yolk (if no family history of egg allergy)	Prepare cereal with formula or human milk to a semiliquid texture Use spoon Feed from a dish Advance to 1/3–1/2 cup cereal before adding fruits or vegetables
7 months	Has improved grasp Can transfer objects from hand to hand	Mashes food with lateral movements of jaw Learns side-to-side, or "rotary," chewing Tooth eruption	Infant cereal Strained to junior texture of fruits, vegetables, and meats	Thicken cereal to lumpier texture Sit in high chair with feet supported Introduce cup
8–10 months	Holds bottle without help Drinks from cup Decreases fluid intake and increases solids Coordinates hand-to-mouth movement		Juices (small amounts) Soft, mashed, or minced table foods	Begin finger foods, such as toast or crackers Avoid adding salt, sugar, or fats to food Present soft foods in chunks ready for finger-feeding
10–12 months	Feeds self Holds cup without help	Improved ability to bite and chew	Soft, chopped table foods Whole egg and whole milk (at 1 year of age)	Provide meals in pattern similar to rest of family Use cup at meals

Adapted with permission from *Handbook of Pediatric Nutrition*, 2nd ed., Samour and Athens, p. 87. © 1999, Aspen Publishers, Inc.

*This time line is just an estimate, and individual infants may vary by several months from the ages given. A pediatrician should be consulted if caregivers are concerned about an infant's developmental progress. In general, there is no nutritional reason to begin introducing solid foods before 6 months of age.

gins to handle finger foods with some dexterity. Dry toast, sliced in strips, offers hours of enjoyment.

By age 7 to 8 months infants can push food around on a plate and play with a drinking cup, can hold a bottle, and self-feed a cracker or piece of toast. In mastering these manipulations infants develop self-confidence and self-esteem. It's important that parents be patient and support these early feeding attempts, even though they appear inefficient.

At about 10 months of age, infants practice in earnest self-feeding finger foods and drinking from a cup. Feeding time is often very messy. Food is used as a means to explore the environment. By the first birthday, their bodies have developed sufficiently to accommodate crawling, probably walking, and self-feeding. Although attempts at feeding are still erratic, developing children take great pride in doing more things independently. As children drink from a cup more frequently, fewer bottle feedings and/or breastfeedings are necessary. The added mobility of walking should naturally lead to gradual weaning from the bottle or breast.

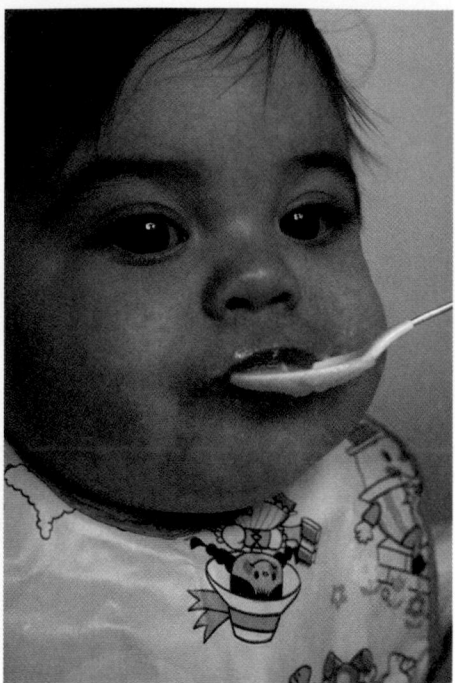

In the early stages of solid food introduction, these foods complement rather than replace human milk or infant formula in the diet.

Parents may believe that the early addition of solid foods will help the infant sleep through the night. Actually, this achievement is a developmental milestone; the amount of food consumed by the infant is irrelevant.

Typical Solid Food Progression, Starting at 6 Months*	
Week 1	Rice cereal
Week 2	Add strained carrots
Week 3	Add applesauce
Week 4	Add oat cereal
Week 5	Add cooked egg yolk
Week 6	Add strained chicken
Week 7	Add strained peas
Week 8	Add plums

*Extending the rice cereal step for a month or so is advised if solid food introduction begins at 4 months of age. Note also that if at any point signs of allergy or intolerance develop, substitute another, similar food item.

Introduction of Solid Foods at about 6 Months of Age

The time to introduce solid foods into an infant's diet hinges on a few important factors:[11]

1. *Nutritional need.* Iron stores are exhausted by about 6 months of age. Either solid foods or iron supplements are then needed to supply iron if the child is breastfed or fed a formula not supplemented with iron. Iron, however, is not the only nutrient low in human milk and unfortified infant formulas. Vitamin D may also deserve attention. Still, before 6 months or so, it's generally unnecessary to add solid foods.
2. *Physiological capabilities.* Infants cannot readily digest starch before 3 months. As they age, their digestive capabilities increase. Kidney function likewise is quite limited until about 4 to 6 weeks of age. Until then, waste products from excessive amounts of dietary protein or minerals are difficult to excrete.
3. *Physical ability.* Three markers indicate that a child is ready for solid foods: (1) the disappearance of the extrusion reflex (thrusting the tongue forward and pushing food out of the mouth), (2) head and neck control, and (3) the ability to sit up with support. These abilities usually occur around 4 to 6 months of age, but they vary with each infant.
4. *Allergy prevention.* An infant's intestinal tract can readily absorb whole proteins from birth until 4 to 5 months of age. Thus, early exposure to many types of proteins—particularly the proteins found in cow's milk and egg whites—may predispose a child to future allergies and other health problems because some types of these proteins may be absorbed intact. For this reason, it's best to minimize the number of different types of proteins in a child's diet, especially during the first 3 months, by focusing exclusively on human milk or infant formula as a nutrient source.[12]

With these considerations in mind—nutritional need, physiological and physical readiness, and allergy prevention—the American Academy of Pediatrics recommends that solid foods not be introduced until about 6 months of age and that infants receive no unaltered cow's milk before 1 year.[5,11]

In general, a child starting solid foods should weigh at least 13 lb (6 kg) and should be drinking more than 32 oz (1 L) of formula daily or breastfeeding more than 8 to 10 times within 24 hours. This description generally applies to 6-month-old infants and to a few 4-month-old infants.

Before 4 to 6 months, infants are not physically mature enough to consume much solid food. Attempts to feed solid foods to infants have sometimes led to forcefeeding with a feeder (a giant syringe) or mixing infant cereal with milk and putting it in a bottle. Even if these are traditional alternatives in your family, there is no reason to carry on these practices. The inconvenience alone should make you consider whether all the effort is worth it. This practice is nutritionally unnecessary, tedious, and possibly dangerous for the infant because it increases the risk of allergies and choking or inhaling food when crying. Only occasionally does a rapidly growing infant—one who consumes more than 32 oz (1 L) of formula daily—really need solid foods at 4 months to meet high energy needs.

Solid Foods That Should Be Fed First

Before 6 months of age, the first solid foods should be iron fortified cereals.[7] A good idea is to offer foods after some breastfeeding or formula feeding, when the edge has been taken off the infant's hunger. This practice aids in early spoon-feeding. Rice cereal is the best cereal to begin with because it's least likely to cause allergies. After the age of 6 months, the first food is not such an important issue. Although yogurt and cottage cheese are well tolerated and their consistencies make them good candidates for early foods, they are not good sources of iron.

Start with teaspoon amounts of a single-ingredient food item, such as rice cereal, and increase the serving size gradually. Once the new food has been fed for about a week without ill effects, another food can be added to the infant's diet. At first, this food can be another type of cereal or perhaps a cooked and strained (or mashed) vegetable, meat, fruit, or egg yolk. It is best to add vegetables before fruits. If fruits are offered first, the infant will prefer the sweet taste and may resist vegetables. Overall, build each feeding step on the previous step, making sure to add only a single ingredient each time.

Waiting about 7 days between new foods is important because it can take that long for evidence of an allergy or intolerance to develop.[11] Symptoms to look for are diarrhea, vomiting, a rash, or wheezing. If one or more of these symptoms appear, the suspected problem food should be avoided for several weeks and then reintroduced in a small quantity. If the problem continues, a physician should be consulted.

It's important not to introduce mixed foods until each component of the mixed food has been given separately. Otherwise, if an allergy or intolerance develops, it will be difficult to identify the offending food. Note that many babies outgrow food sensitivities in childhood. Some foods that commonly cause an allergic response in infants are egg whites, chocolate, nuts, and cow's milk. It's best not to introduce these foods in infancy.[12]

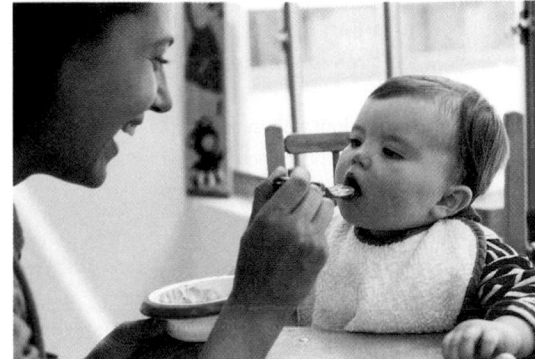

Rice cereal is recommended as the first solid food to be fed to infants.

A variety of strained foods is available for infant feeding at the supermarket. Investigate these and other foods intended for infants the next time you're shopping. Single-food items are more desirable than mixed dinners and desserts, which are less nutrient-dense. Most brands have no added salt, but some fruit desserts contain a lot of added sugar.

As an alternative, plain unseasoned cooked foods—vegetables, fruits, and meats (no seasoning added)—can be ground up in an inexpensive plastic baby food grinder/mill. Another option is to purée a larger amount of food in a blender, freeze it in ice-cube portions, store in plastic bags, and defrost and warm as needed. Careful attention to cleanliness is necessary. Infant foods made at home should be ground before seasonings are added to please the rest of the family. The infant doesn't notice the difference if salt, sugar, or spices are omitted. It's best to introduce infants to a variety of foods, so that by the end of the first year the infant is consuming many foods—milk, meats, fruits, vegetables, and grains.

In the first attempts to introduce solid foods, just getting the food into the infant's mouth proves to be a challenge. The caregiver must proceed slowly. Initially, table foods supplement—rather than replace—formula or human milk. Infants control the situation by signaling when they are hungry and when they have had enough to eat. Self-feeding skills require coordination and can develop only if the infant is allowed to practice and experiment. At 9 to 10 months, the infant's desire to explore, experience, and play with food can also hinder feeding. Presenting new foods for several consecutive days can aid in an infant's acceptance of that food.[5]

Caregivers need to relax and take this phase of infant development in stride. Sloppy, friendly mealtimes actually make for good memories.

To ease efforts in feeding solid foods, consider the following tips:

- Use a baby-sized spoon; a small spoon with a long handle is best.
- Hold the infant comfortably on the lap, as for breastfeeding or bottle feeding, but a little more upright to ease swallowing. When in this position, the infant expects food.
- Put a small dab of food on the spoon tip and gently place it on the infant's tongue.
- Convey a calm and casual approach to the infant, who needs time to get used to food.
- Expect the infant to take only two or three bites of the first meals.

By the end of the first year, finger-feeding becomes more efficient, drinking from a cup improves, and chewing is easier as more teeth erupt. Foods in the diet begin to resemble a balanced diet (Table 17-3).[5] Still, experimentation and unpredictability are to be expected.

A Summary of Infant Feeding Recommendations

Breastfed Infants

- Breastfeed for 6 months or longer, if possible. Then introduce infant formula if and when breastfeeding declines or ceases. Breast milk can also be pumped and placed in a bottle for later use.
- Provide a vitamin D supplement (200 IU/day) (until at least 500 ml of formula is consumed).
- Ask the infant's physician about the need for fluoride, vitamin B-12, and iron supplementation to prevent deficiencies.

Formula-Fed Infants

- Use an iron-fortified infant formula for the first year of life.
- Ask the infant's physician about the need for a fluoride supplement if the water supply is not fluoridated.

All Infants

- Provide a variety of basic, soft foods after 6 months of age, advancing to a varied diet.
- Add iron-fortified cereal at about 6 months of age.

Table 17-3 | A Sample Daily Menu for a 1-Year-Old Child*

Breakfast	Snack
Applesauce, 1–2 tbsp Cheerios, 1/4 cup Whole milk, 1/2 cup	Cheddar cheese, 1/2 oz Wheat crackers, 4 Whole milk, 1/2 cup
Snack	**Dinner**
Hard-cooked egg, 1/2 Wheat toast, 1/2 slice, with 1/2 tsp margarine Orange juice, 1/2 cup	Hamburger (crumbled), 1 oz Mashed potatoes, 1–2 tbsp with 1/2 tsp margarine Cooked carrots (cut in strips, not coins), 1–2 tbsp Whole milk, 1/2 cup
Lunch	**Snack**
Roasted chicken, minced, 1 oz Rice, 1–2 tbsp with 1/2 tsp margarine Cooked peas, 1–2 tbsp Whole milk, 1/2 cup	Banana, 1/2 Oatmeal cookies (no raisins), 2 Whole milk, 1/2 cup

Nutritional Analysis

Total energy (kcal) % energy from	1100
Carbohydrate	40%
Protein	19%
Fat	41%

*This diet is just a start. A 1-year-old may need more or less food. In those cases, serving sizes should be adjusted. The milk can be fed by cup; some can be put into a bottle if the child has not been fully weaned from the bottle. The juice should be fed in a cup.

early childhood caries Tooth decay that results from formula or juice (and even human milk) bathing the teeth as the child sleeps with a bottle in his or her mouth. The upper teeth are mostly affected, because the lower teeth are protected by the tongue; formerly called nursing bottle syndrome and baby bottle tooth decay.

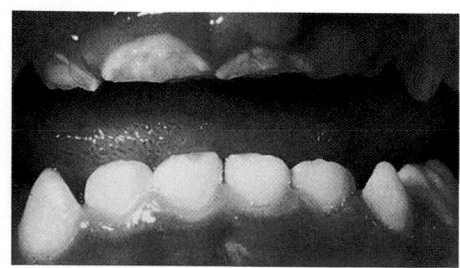

Figure 17-5 | An extreme example of tooth decay caused by early childhood caries. This child was probably put to bed with a bottle. The upper teeth have decayed almost all the way to the gum line.

Weaning from the Breast or Bottle

Around 6 months or so, juices can be offered in a sippy cup with a wide, flat bottom. Drinking from a cup helps prevent **early childhood caries** (Figure 17-5). If an infant drinks continually from a bottle, the carbohydrate-rich fluid bathes the teeth, providing an ideal growth medium for bacteria. Bacteria on the teeth then make acids, which dissolve tooth enamel. Infants should never be put to bed with a bottle or placed in an infant seat with a bottle propped up, because fluid (even milk) pools around the teeth, increasing the likelihood of dental caries. Again, infants need careful attention when being fed, and being propped up with a bottle does not constitute careful attention.[11]

Getting a baby out of the bedtime-bottle habit is difficult. Determined caregivers can either wince through a few nights of their baby's crying or slowly wean the baby away from the bottle with either a pacifier or water (for a week or so).

What Not to Feed an Infant

Following are several foods and practices to avoid when feeding an infant:

- *Honey.* This product may contain spores of *Clostridium botulinum.* The spores can eventually develop into bacteria in the stomach and lead to a foodborne illness known as *botulism.* This illness can be fatal, including in children under 1 year old (see Chapter 19).
- *Very salty and very sweet foods.* Infants don't need a lot of sugar or salt added to their foods. They enjoy bland foods much more than do adults.
- *Excessive infant formula or human milk.* After 6 to 8 months, solid foods should play a greater role in satisfying an infant's increasing appetite. The main reason to switch is that solid foods contain considerably more bioavailable iron than do human milk and low-iron formulas. About 24 to 32 oz (3/4 to 1 L) of human milk or formula daily is ideal after 6 months, with food supplying the rest of the infant's energy needs.

- *Foods that tend to cause choking.* These foods include hot dogs (unless finely cut into sticks, not coin shapes), candy, whole nuts, grapes, coarsely cut meats, raw carrots, popcorn, and peanut butter.
- *Cow's milk, especially low-fat or fat-free cow's milk.* The American Academy of Pediatrics strongly urges parents not to give infants (and children under age 2 as well) fat-reduced, 1%, or fat-free milk.[11] Only after age 2 years can children drink fat-reduced, 1%, or fat-free milk because by then they are consuming enough solid foods to supply energy and fat needs. Before that age, the amount of this milk needed for energy needs would supply too many minerals and in turn could overwhelm the kidneys' ability to excrete the excess. The lower fat intake might also harm nervous system development.
- *Feeding excessive amounts of apple or pear juice.* The fructose and sorbitol contained in these juices can lead to diarrhea because they are slowly absorbed. Also, if fruit juice or related drink products are replacing formula or milk in the diet, the infant may not be receiving adequate amounts of calcium and other minerals that are essential for bone growth. In fact, studies have shown a link between excessive amounts of fruit juice and failure to thrive, GI tract complications, obesity, short stature, and poor dental heath. Thus, these substances should be used sparingly. Infants over the age of 6 months can usually safely consume up to 6 oz of juice in the course of a day, with no more than 2 to 4 oz at a time.[16]

Egg whites should not be fed to children before 1 year of age to prevent the development of allergies.

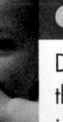

Case Scenario | Follow-Up

Damon's diet is inadequate for a 10-month-old infant because it lacks enough of the nutritious foods his growing body needs to support weight gain. These foods include iron-fortified cereal, puréed infant foods, and appropriate table foods. Damon should stay on the infant formula until 1 year of age and should not be given sugary drinks, nor should these drinks be fed by bottle if used. Damon needs a more energy-dense diet containing a healthful variety of solid foods to provide him with enough energy and essential nutrients to grow and develop.

Concept | Check
Infant formulas generally contain lactose or sucrose, heat-treated proteins from cow's milk, and vegetable oil. Formulas should be fortified with iron. Sanitation is very important in preparing and storing formula. Solid foods should not be added to an infant's diet until the child is both ready for and needs solid food, usually at about 6 months of age. The first solid food can be iron-fortified infant cereals, with very gradual additions of other foods—one at a time each week. Some foods to avoid giving infants in the first year are honey, cow's milk (particularly fat-reduced, 1%, or fat-free milk), very salty or sweet foods, foods that may cause the child to choke, and excessive amounts of fruit juice or related products (e.g., fruit drinks).

Dietary Guidelines for Infant Feeding
In response to various controversies surrounding infant feeding, the American Academy of Pediatrics has issued a number of statements concerning infant diets. The following guidelines are based on these statements:[11]

- *Build to a variety of foods.* For the first months of life, human milk is all an infant needs. When the infant is ready, start adding new foods, one at a time. During the first year, the goal is to teach an infant to enjoy a variety of nutritious foods. A lifetime of healthy eating habits begins with this important first step.

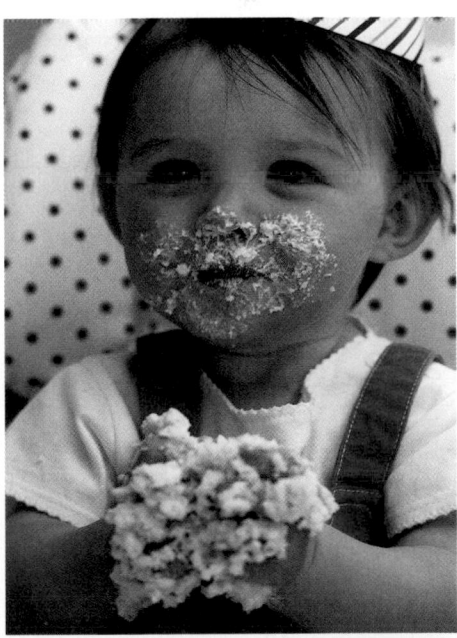

Early feeding attempts should be encouraged, even though they're messy.

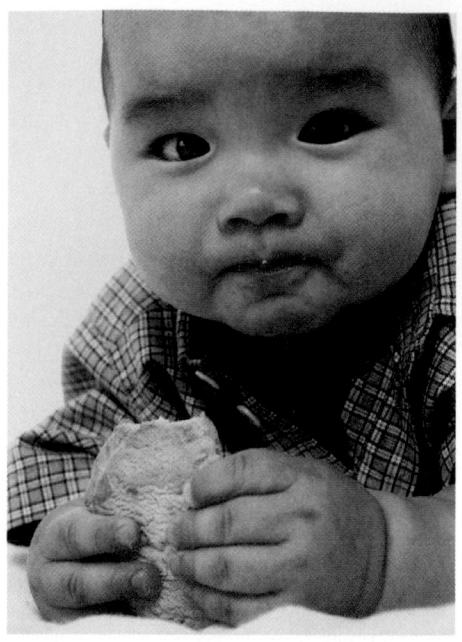

The older infant enjoys finger-feeding.

- *Pay attention to your infant's appetite to avoid overfeeding or underfeeding.* Feed infants when they are hungry. Never force an infant to finish an unwanted serving of food. Watch for signs that indicate hunger or fullness.
- *Infants need fat.* Although fat is the cause of many adult health problems, it's an essential source of energy for growing infants. Fat also helps the nervous system develop.
- *Choose fruits, vegetables, and grains, but don't overdo high-fiber foods.* Although many adults benefit from higher-fiber diets, they are not good for infants. They are bulky, filling, and often low in energy. The natural amounts of fiber and nutrients in fruits, vegetables, and grains are appropriate as part of a healthy infant diet.
- *Infants need sugars in moderation.* Sugars are an additional source of energy for active, rapidly growing infants. Foods such as human milk, fruits, and juices are natural sources of sugars and other nutrients as well. Foods that contain artificial sweeteners should be avoided; they don't provide the energy growing infants need.
- *Infants need sodium in moderation.* Sodium is a necessary mineral found naturally in almost all foods. As part of a healthy diet, infants need sodium for their bodies to work properly.
- *Choose foods containing iron, zinc, and calcium.* Infants need good sources of iron, zinc, and calcium for optimum growth in the first 2 years. These minerals are important for healthy blood, proper growth, and strong bones.

In essence, there is no evidence that very restrictive diets during infancy have positive effects, whereas their hazards are well documented.

Health Problems Related to Infant Nutrition

Parents, other caregivers, and clinicians should be alert for a variety of potential health problems related to infant nutrition, so that corrective action can be taken quickly. In some cases, such problems stem from inappropriate feeding practices and inadequate nutrient intakes, including the following:

- Diet providing insufficient iron
- Absence from the diet of an entire food group from MyPyramid as solid foods are introduced and become the main source of nutrients
- Drinking raw (unpasteurized) milk, which may be contaminated with bacteria or viruses
- Drinking goat's milk, which is low in folate, iron, vitamin C, and vitamin D; if used, it must be pasteurized and given in conjunction with a balanced multivitamin and mineral supplement
- Failure to begin drinking from a cup by 1 year of age
- Continuing to feed from a bottle past 18 months of age
- Intake of supplemental vitamins or minerals above 100% of the appropriate RDA or other nutrient standard
- Drinking large amounts of fruit juice after 6 months of age, especially as a substitute for infant formula or human milk. (Recall that fruit juice is not to be fed at all before 6 months of age.)

The following sections look more closely at five common infant health problems that cause concern for caregivers: colic, diarrhea, milk allergy, iron deficiency anemia, and gastroesophageal reflux. Parents and other caregivers usually need to consult with a physician in dealing with these conditions. The website of the American Academy of Pediatrics (www.aap.org) can also provide useful information.

Colic

The first time an otherwise healthy, well-fed infant has a lengthy, unexplained crying spell, most parents panic. Repeated crying episodes, lasting 3 or more hours that don't respond to typical remedies—such as feeding, holding, or changing diapers—are characteristic of infants who develop **colic.** Colic affects about 10 to 30% of all infants, starting at about 2 to 6 weeks of age and lasting until about 3 months of age, so it is neither uncommon nor abnormal. Colicky infants typically cry during the late afternoon and early evening, and their nighttime sleeping is almost always disturbed by crying spells. In addition, these infants frequently pass gas rectally, clench their fists, draw up their legs, hold the body straight, and want to be held. The only good news is that colic usually goes away after a few months.[11]

Colic generally occurs in the absence of any physical problem in the infant. It tends to be most common in "temperamental" infants—those who are more sensitive, more irritable, more intense, less adaptable, and less consolable than average for their age. In addition, a lack of harmonious interaction between parents and the infant may contribute to the problem. Some researchers have speculated that immature central nervous system mechanisms may cause colic.

Parents can do several things to help reduce excessive crying. For instance, many infants tend to become quiet and alert when held snugly to the shoulder. Parents should also check to see whether the infant is tired or bored or wants to suckle. Some infants can be calmed by rhythmic sounds or movement or with pacifiers.

Breastfeeding of colicky infants should continue. The breastfeeding mother's temporary decrease or cessation in consumption of milk and milk products, caffeine, chocolate, and vegetables such as broccoli and onions may help reduce colic in her infant. Formula-fed infants with severe colic are sometimes helped by changing from a standard formula to a soy-based or predigested protein formula (review Table 17-1) but more often this change provides no relief from the problem. In addition, physicians may prescribe medication to calm colicky infants and reduce gas buildup.[11]

> **colic** Sharp abdominal pain that generally occurs in otherwise healthy infants and is associated with periodic spells of inconsolable crying.

Most parents benefit from the counsel and support of other adults during the anxiety of dealing with a colicky infant, a period of time that may last for several months. Talking with others who have been through similar experiences can help parents improve their tolerance of stress and ability to cope and can increase their confidence in their parenting abilities. Furthermore, to optimize their ability to be sensitive and responsive to their infant, parents need to be well rested and to set aside some time for themselves.

Diarrhea

Diarrhea in infants, characterized by numerous loose stools per day, results from various causes, including bacterial and viral infections. In the United States, about 500 infants die each year of simple dehydration resulting from diarrhea, and about 210,000 are hospitalized for this disorder. Typical symptoms include dry mouth or tongue, few or no tears when crying, no wet diapers for 3 hours or more, irritability and listlessness, and sunken eyes and cheeks. To prevent dehydration, infants with diarrhea should be given plenty of fluids, under the advice of a physician. Specialized electrolyte-replacement fluids, such as Pedialyte, may be recommended for one day or less. These products contain glucose, sodium, potassium, chloride, and water.[11]

Once diarrhea subsides, a bottle-fed infant may be switched to a soy-based, lactose-free formula for a few days, but this change is typically not necessary. The use of a lactose-free formula is intended to allow time for the intestine to produce sufficient lactase enzyme to digest the large amount of lactose typically found in formulas. A breastfed infant should continue at the breast for the duration of the diarrhea.

Milk Allergy

Cow's milk contains more than 40 proteins that can cause allergic reactions in infants. Although some of these proteins are inactivated by heating (scalding) milk, others are very heat stable. A true milk allergy develops in about 1 to 3% of formula-fed infants. Such infants may experience vomiting, diarrhea, blood in the stool, constipation, and other symptoms. If milk allergy is suspected, a formula-fed infant can be switched to a soy-based formula. In 20 to 50% of cases, however, the use of soy formula provides only temporary relief because the soy protein eventually triggers an allergic reaction in some infants. In such cases a predigested-protein formula is necessary (review Table 17-1). If the child is breastfeeding, the mother may experiment with eliminating cow's milk from her diet. Fortunately, milk allergies seldom last beyond 3 years of age.[11]

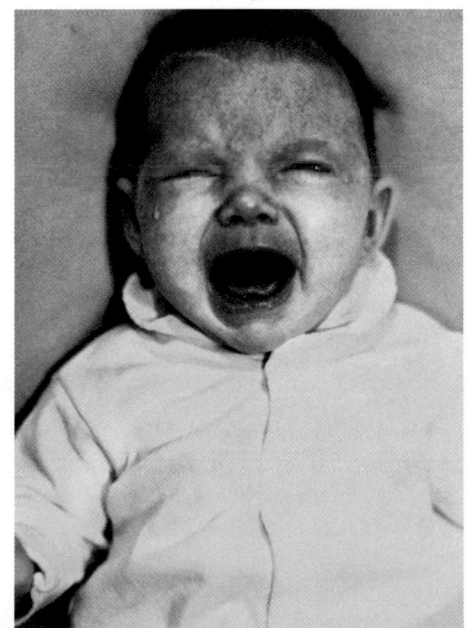

Caring for an inconsolable, colicky infant can cause parents to feel frustrated and helpless.

Iron Deficiency Anemia

Iron deficiency anemia typically occurs in older infants (about 10 to 15% of 1- to 2-year-olds), especially those who consume few solid foods and whose diets are dominated by cow's milk, which both contains little iron and causes intestinal bleeding in young infants. Iron stores are then quickly depleted by the daily need to synthesize new red blood cells. The best way to prevent iron deficiency anemia is to feed the infant an iron-fortified formula beginning at birth, if formula is used. Then start the infant on iron-fortified cereals and meats at about 6 months. Infant formula should also be limited to 16 to 25 oz (500 to 750 ml) daily at this age. If anemia does develop, medicinal iron is used under a physician's guidance.[7]

Gastroesophageal Reflux

Many infants develop gastroesophageal reflux (GER), more commonly known as "spitting up," during their first year of life. In most cases, GER develops before 2 to 3 months of age and usually resolves on its own by the infant's first birthday. The problem arises because the lower esophageal sphincter may not close completely, which allows milk or solid food in the infant's stomach to move back up into the esophagus. The result can be a burning sensation, which causes the infant pain or discomfort. Or the infant might spit up the milk or food. In the majority of cases, GER poses no serious medical concerns. In very rare cases, surgery may be required to remedy the problem.[11]

Concept | Check

Colic is commonly associated with inconsolable crying. It may be helpful for breastfeeding mothers to decrease or avoid intake of milk and milk products, caffeine, chocolate, and certain vegetables, under a physician's guidance. Diarrhea requires additional fluids to prevent dehydration. Infants allergic to proteins in standard cow's milk formula can be switched to an infant formula containing soy protein or predigested protein. Introducing iron-containing solid foods at an appropriate time and avoiding the use of cow's milk during the first year can generally prevent iron deficiency anemia in infants. Any gastroesophageal reflux that develops typically resolves within the first year of life.

Preschool Children: Nutrition Concerns

The rapid growth rate that characterizes infancy tapers off quickly during the subsequent few years. The average annual weight gain is only 4.5 to 6.6 lb (2 to 3 kg), and the average annual height gain is only 3 to 4 in (7.5 to 10 cm) between the ages of 2 and 5 (review Figure 17-1).[11] As a toddler's growth rate tapers off, eating behavior changes. For example, the decreased growth rate leads to a decreased appetite, often called "picky eating," compared with infants. Estimated Energy Requirements (kcals) are now **(89 kcal × weight of child [kg]) − 80** for children 1 to 3 years. Formulas for older preschool children are listed in the section titled School-Age Children: Nutrition Concerns.

Because of the reduced appetite of preschool children, planning a diet that meets their nutrient needs poses a challenge to caregivers.[1] Choosing nutrient-dense foods is particularly important with children who eat relatively little. This is a good time to emphasize some whole grains, fruits, and vegetables without increasing fat and simple sugar intake. A whole-grain ready-to-eat breakfast cereal with limited fat and sugar is an excellent choice.[2] There is no need to decrease fat or simple sugar intake severely, but fatty and sweet food choices should not overwhelm more nutritious ones.[1,16]

The preschool years are the best time for a child to start a healthful pattern of living and eating, focusing on regular physical activity and nutritious food. Parents and other caregivers are role models: if they eat a variety of foods, the children will eat a

Carbohydrate needs in order to supply energy for the central nervous system and to prevent ketosis in childhood are 130 g/day, the same as for adults. The protein needs to allow for growth vary from 1.1 g/kg of body weight/day (13 to 19 g/day) for children 1 to 3 years, to 0.95 g/kg of body weight/day (34 to 52 g/day) for older children. No specific needs for total fat intake have been set, but the diet must contain at least 5 g/day of essential fatty acids (see the inside cover for details). The general recommendation is that total fat intake gradually falls so as to fit into the adult range of 20 to 35% of total energy intake by age 19.

Food Allergies and Intolerances

Adverse reactions to foods—indicated by sneezing, coughing, nausea, vomiting, diarrhea, hives, and other rashes—are broadly classed as food allergies (also called *hypersensitivities*) or **food intolerances.** Allergies involve responses of the immune system designed to eliminate foreign proteins, called **allergens.**[12] The symptoms experienced by susceptible people, such as rapid increase in heart rate and shortness of breath, are the result of this battle. In contrast, the symptoms of food intolerances do not result from a true allergic reaction. Rather, food intolerances are caused by an individual's inability to digest certain food components or by the direct effect of a food component or contaminant on the body. This section examines each process, first allergies and then intolerances, so you can learn how to reduce the risk of suffering from the food you eat.

Food Allergies: Symptoms and Mechanism

Allergic reactions to foods are common and occur more frequently in females than males. Food allergies occur most often during infancy and young adulthood. Experts estimate that up to about 2% of adults and up to about 8% of children are allergic to certain foods. Three types of reactions may occur after the ingestion of problem foods by susceptible people:

- *Classic*—itching, reddening skin, asthma, swelling, choking, and a runny nose
- *GI tract*—nausea, vomiting, diarrhea, intestinal gas, bloating, pain, constipation, and indigestion
- *General*—headache, skin reactions, tension and fatigue, tremors, and psychological problems

Any reaction that is milder than these distinct allergic ones is referred to as a **food sensitivity.**

Allergic reactions vary not only in the body system affected but also in their duration, ranging from seconds to a few days. A generalized, all-systems reaction is called **anaphylactic shock.** This severe allergic response results in low blood pressure and respiratory and GI tract distress. It can be fatal. Overall, allergic reactions result in 30,000 emergency room visits and 150 to 200 deaths per year. A person who is extremely sensitive to a food may not be able to touch the food or even be in the same room where it is being cooked without responding to it. Although any food can trigger anaphylactic shock, the most common culprits are peanuts (actually a legume, not a nut), tree nuts (walnuts, pecans, etc.), shellfish, milk, eggs, soybeans, wheat, and fish. For a small number of people, avoiding foods such as peanuts or shellfish is a matter of life and death.[12]

Almost all food allergies are caused by proteins in milk (also look for casein on the label), eggs (also look for albumin on the label), corn, tree nuts and peanuts, seafood, soy products, and wheat. Other foods frequently identified with adverse reactions include meat and meat products, fruits, and cheese. These foods contain acidlike proteins, usually with a molecular weight between about 10,000 and 70,000, that stimulate the production of antibodies (specifically the **immunoglobulin** (IgE) in susceptible people.

Testing for a Food Allergy

The diagnosis of a food allergy can often be a difficult task (Table 17-4).[12] It requires the participation of a skilled physician. The first step in determining whether a food allergy is present is to record in detail a history of symptoms, time from ingestion to onset of symptoms, duration of symptoms, most recent reaction, quantity and nature of food needed to produce a reaction, and food suspected of causing a reaction. A family history of allergic diseases can also help, because allergic reactions tend to run in families. A physical examination may reveal evidence of an allergy, such as skin diseases and asthma. Various diagnostic tests can rule out other conditions.

The best laboratory test for determining which compounds a person is allergic to is the RAST test. This test estimates the blood concentration of antibodies that bind certain foodborne antigens. (Skin tests can also be used; a drop of antigen is placed under the skin where it has been scratched or punctured. If a person is allergic to the test antigen, a red eruption will develop.)

The next step is to eliminate from the diet for 1 to 2 weeks all tested compounds that appear to cause allergic symptoms, plus all other foods suspected of causing an allergy based on the person's food history. The person generally starts out eating

food intolerance An adverse reaction to food that does not involve an allergic reaction.

allergen A foreign protein, or antigen, that induces excess production of certain immune system antibodies; subsequent exposure to the same protein leads to allergic symptoms. Whereas all allergens are antigens, not all antigens are allergens.

immunoglobulins Proteins found in the blood that are responsible for antibody-mediated immunity and that bind specifically to antigen; also called *antibodies*. Immunoglobulins are produced by certain white blood cells in response to a foreign substance (antigen) in the bloodstream.

People with a history of serious allergic reactions should carry a self-administered form of epinephrine, such as EpiPen, to subside an episode of anaphylactic shock.

food sensitivity A mild reaction to a substance in a food that might be expressed as light itching or redness of the skin.

anaphylactic shock A severe allergic response that results in lowered blood pressure and respiratory and gastrointestinal distress. This reaction can be fatal.

Table 17-4 | Assessment Strategies for Food Allergies

History	Include description of symptoms, time between food ingestion and onset of symptoms, duration of symptoms, most recent allergic episode, quantity of food required to produce reaction, suspected foods, and allergic diseases in other family members.
Physical examination	Look for signs of an allergic reaction (rash, itching, intestinal bloating, etc.).
RAST test	Determine presence of IgE antibodies in blood that bind to antigens tested.
Elimination diet	Establish a diet lacking the suspected offending foods and stay on it for 1 to 2 weeks or until symptoms clear.
Food challenge	Add back small amounts of excluded foods, one at a time, as long as anaphylactic shock is not a possible consequence.
Skin test	Place a sample of the suspected allergen under the skin and watch for an inflammatory reaction.

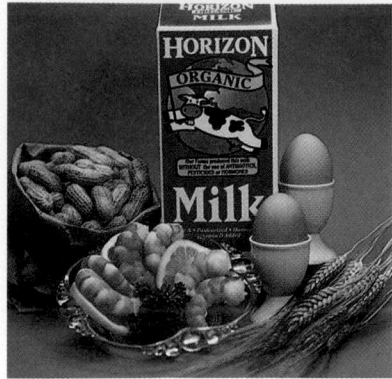

Eggs, wheat, milk, nuts, and seafood pose the greatest risk for food allergies in childhood.

elimination diet A restrictive diet that systematically tests foods that may cause an allergic response by first eliminating them for 1 to 2 weeks and then adding them back one at a time.

prognosis A forecast of the course and end of a disease.

Critical | Thinking

Irene and Chris had a baby 11 months ago. At the last checkup, the doctor told them to start feeding the baby some new solid foods. After 5 days of eating a new food, the baby woke up with a runny nose and vomiting. The doctor told them to stop giving the baby that food. How can the doctor justify his recommendations?

foods to which almost no one reacts, such as rice, vegetables, noncitrus fruits, and fresh meats and poultry. If symptoms are still present, the person can more severely restrict the diet or even use special formula diets that are hypoallergenic.

Once a diet is found that causes no symptoms, called an **elimination diet,** foods that are known not to trigger anaphylactic shock can be added back one at a time.[11] Doses of 1/2 to 1 teaspoon (2.5 to 5 ml) are given at first. The amount is increased until the dose approximates usual intake. Reintroduction should be done using a double-blind approach (review Chapter 1), especially when the reaction has a psychological component or when symptoms are vague or ill defined. Dried foods can be encapsulated and then given to the person. Any reintroduced food that causes significant symptoms to appear is identified as an allergen for the person.

Treating Food Allergies

Once potential allergens are identified, the best treatment is to avoid them, especially for people with zero tolerance. Careful reading of food labels is essential for many allergic people and advisable for all.[12] A major challenge for the clinician treating a person with a food allergy is to make sure that what remains in the diet can still provide essential nutrients. The small food intake of children permits less leeway in removing the offending foods that may contain numerous nutrients. A registered dietitian can help guide the diet-planning process to ensure that the remaining food choices still meet nutrient needs or to guide supplement use, if that is necessary.

If an allergy-prone woman is pregnant or breastfeeding, she should avoid offending foods—such as eggs, shellfish, and peanuts—because allergens can cross the placenta during pregnancy. Allergens are also secreted in her milk. She should work with her

physician and registered dietitian to make sure she still consumes an adequate diet. In addition, when food allergies are common in the family, women are advised to breastfeed their infants exclusively for 6 months. Human milk contains factors that play a role in the maturation of the small intestine. Formula-fed infants, especially those on cow's milk-based formulas, have a greater risk for developing food allergies. Breastfeeding, thus, should continue for as long as possible, preferably to 1 year.[12]

The **prognosis** for food allergies that first appear before 3 years of age is good. About 80% of young children with food allergies outgrow them before 3 years.[11] Parents should be made aware of this prognosis and not assume that the allergy will be long-lived. Food allergies diagnosed after 3 years of age, however, are often more long-lived, but not always. In these cases, about 33% of people outgrow their food allergies within 3 years. For others, the condition may be prolonged; some food allergies can last a lifetime, such as for peanuts, tree nuts, and shellfish. Periodic reintroduction of offending foods can be tried every 6 to 12 months or so to see whether the allergic reaction has decreased. If no symptoms appear, tolerance to the food has developed.

Food Intolerances

Food intolerances are adverse reactions to foods that do not involve allergic mechanisms. Generally, larger amounts of an offending food are required to produce the symptoms of an intolerance than to trigger allergic symptoms. Common causes of food intolerances include

- Constituents of certain foods (e.g., red wine, tomatoes, pineapples) that have a druglike activity, causing physiological effects such as changes in blood pressure

- Certain synthetic compounds added to foods, such as sulfites, food-coloring agents, and monosodium glutamate (MSG)
- Food contaminants, including antibiotics and other chemicals used in the production of livestock and crops as well as insect parts not removed during processing
- Toxic contaminants resulting from the ingestion of improperly handled and prepared foods containing *Clostridium botulinum, Salmonella bacteria,* or other foodborne microorganisms (see Chapter 19)
- Deficiencies in digestive enzymes, such as lactase (see Chapter 5)

Almost everyone is sensitive to one or more of these causes of food intolerance, many of which produce GI tract symptoms.

Sulfites, which are added to foods and beverages as antioxidants, cause flushing, spasms of the airway and a loss of blood pressure in susceptible people. Wine, dehydrated potatoes, dried fruits, gravy, soup mixes, and restaurant salad greens commonly contain sulfites. A reaction to MSG may include an increase in blood pressure, numbness, sweating, vomiting, headache, and facial pressure. MSG is commonly found in restaurant food and many processed foods (e.g., soups). A reaction to tartrazine, a food-coloring additive, includes spasm of the airway, itching, and reddening skin. Tyramine, a derivative of the amino acid tyrosine, is commonly found in "aged" foods, such as cheeses and red wines. This natural food constituent can cause high blood pressure in people taking monoamine-oxidase (MAO) inhibitor medications, which may be prescribed for mental depression.

The basic treatment for food intolerances is to avoid specific offending components. However, total elimination often is not required because people generally are not as sensitive to compounds causing food intolerances as they are to allergens. For instance, a slight amount of sulfites in a glass of wine may be tolerable, whereas a large amount from a chef's salad made with sulfite treated salad greens may cause a reaction.

The American Academy of Allergy and Immunology has a 24-hour toll-free hotline (800-822-2762) to answer questions about food allergies and to help direct people to specialists who treat the problem. Free information on food allergies is available by contacting The Food Allergy & Anaphylaxis Network. The telephone number is (703) 691-3179; the website is www.foodallergy.org.

variety of foods. One possible policy is the one-bite rule: within reason, children should take at least one bite or taste of the foods presented to them. For snacks, parents should select several possibilities of acceptable choices and allow children to choose one; responsibility for food choice ideally should start early.

Helping a Child Choose Nutritious Foods

One way adults can encourage young children to eat nutritious, well-balanced meals is to serve new foods and repeat exposure to them.[11] If a child observes adults and older children eating and enjoying a food, there's a good chance that, most of the time, he or she will eventually accept it. The dinner hour is a good time for children to experience new foods and to develop their own food preferences. Preschool children especially tend to be wary of new foods. One reason is that they have more taste buds, and their taste buds are more sensitive than those of adults. In addition, they have a general distrust of unfamiliar foods. If adults can be patient and persevere, children will build good food habits. Above all, the dinner table should not become a battleground, and using one food as a bribe to eat another—for example, a piece of pie for peas—is strongly discouraged.

Perseverance with children is critical, because it takes effort and commitment to guide them into liking a variety of foods. Be ready for some surprises. Also, if left to

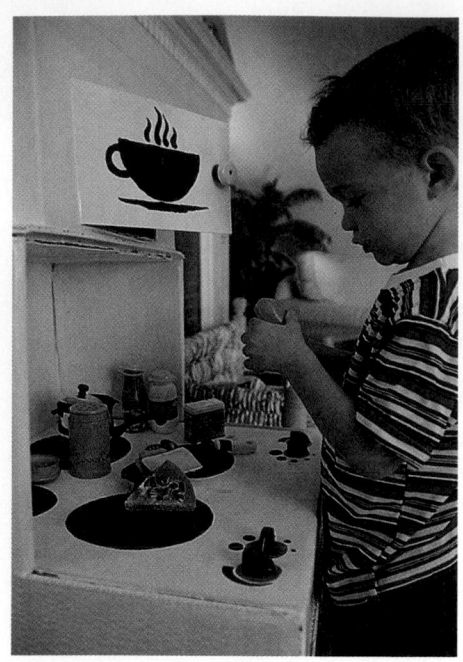

Interest in food starts early in life.

their own devices, preschool children would find a few foods they like and eat them every day. However, by constantly being introduced to new foods, children at this age can expand their nutritional choices, develop an experimental approach, and learn to appreciate a variety of foods. It may take 10 to 15 exposures, but eventually children will accept most foods. A positive outlook by the caregivers helps a lot.[1]

Children generally like certain foods—especially those with crisp textures and mild flavors—and familiar foods. Young children are especially sensitive to hot-temperature foods and tend to reject them.

Parents and other caregivers play a central role in teaching by example.[17] Children more readily learn good table manners alongside others who practice them. The harmony that comes from working at being polite creates a positive environment for learning good nutrition habits. Preschoolers eventually develop skill with spoons and forks and can even use dull knives (Table 17-5). However, it's still a good idea to serve some finger foods. A goal should be to make mealtime a happy, social time, sharing enjoyment of healthful foods. A regular family meal daily—whether breakfast, lunch, or dinner—is an appropriate setting for children to learn about healthful eating and to build good eating habits.

Childhood Feeding Problems

Tensions between parents, or between parents and children, especially during mealtime, often contribute to eating problems. Getting to the root of family problems and creating a more harmonious family atmosphere are important steps toward resolving many

Table 17-5 | Observed Emotional Traits, Eating Behavior, and Food-Related Skills of Preschoolers

Age (years)	Emotional Traits	Eating Behavior	Food-Related Skills
1-2	• Fears new things • Sharing difficult • Requires constant supervision • Enjoys helping but can't be left alone • Curious • Often defiant • Eager for attention	• "Finicky" eater • Holds food in mouth without swallowing • May insist on eating the same food at meal after meal (called a food jag)	• Uses spoon with some skill (especially if hungry) • Can begin to tear, break, snap, and dip foods • Has good control of cup—lifts, drinks, sets it down, holds with one hand • Helps self-feed
3	• The "me too" age—wants to be included in everything • Responds well to options rather than demands • Sharing still difficult • Somewhat rigid about the "right" way to do things	• Eats most foods, except for certain vegetables • Dawdles over food when not hungry • Comments on how foods are served	• Uses spoon in semiadult fashion; may spear with fork • Medium hand muscle development • Feeds self independently, especially if hungry • Can pour milk and juice and serve individual portions from a serving dish if given instructions
4	• Shares well • Needs adult approval and attention—shows off • Understands; needs limits • Follows rules most of the time • Still rigid about the "right" way to do things	• Eating and talking get in the way—prefers to talk • Strong food likes and dislikes • Refuses to eat, to the point of tears	• Uses all eating utensils • Small-finger muscle development • Can wipe, wash, set table, and pour premeasured ingredients • Can peel, spread, cut, roll, and mash foods; cracks eggs
5	• Helpful and cooperative with family chores and routines • Still somewhat rigid about the "right" way to do things • Very attached to parent, home, and family	• Likes familiar foods; prefers most vegetables raw • Latches on to food dislikes of family members and declares these as own	• Fine coordination in fingers and hands • Makes simple breakfast and lunch • Can measure, cut, grind, and grate with some supervision

Modified from M. Sigman-Grant, "Feeding Preschoolers: Balancing Nutritional and Developmental Needs," *Nutrition Today*, July/August 1992, p. 13. Used with permission.

childhood feeding problems. In addition, many parents must be educated as to what to expect of a preschool child and what food-related goals to set (review Table 17-5). Consider some typical complaints and concerns of parents, the causes of the problems, and suggestions for correcting them.

"My Child Won't Eat as Much or as Regularly as He Did as an Infant"

This behavior is typical of preschoolers, because their growth rate slows after infancy; thus, they don't need as much food. Parents often need reminding that a 3-year-old can't be expected to eat as voraciously as an infant or to eat adult-size portions.[1] Table 17-6 shows a general food plan, based on MyPyramid, that is appropriate for preschool and school-age children. Until about 5 years of age, portion sizes in the vegetable group, fruit group, and meat and beans group should be about 1 tablespoon per year of life and can be increased as needed. The same advice does not apply to the grains or milk group, but note that consuming too much milk can leave the diet short on iron. Luckily, normal-weight children have a built-in feeding mechanism, which adjusts hunger to regulate food intake at each stage of growth. If a child is developing and growing normally and the caregiver is providing a variety of healthful foods, all can be confident that the child isn't starving.

A pattern of picky eating is usually just another expression of independence for children, who have a strong desire to establish a self-determined routine. Caregivers should avoid nagging, forcing, and bribing children to encourage eating. Indirectly, these tactics reinforce picky-eating behaviors because of the added attention given to them. Overall, parents should focus on offering a variety of healthy choices and allowing the child to exert some autonomy over the specific type of food and the amount eaten. A child's sudden loss of appetite, however, may be reason for concern because a poor appetite may be a sign of underlying illness.[11]

Parents should also be reminded that food likes and dislikes change rapidly in childhood and are influenced by food temperature, appearance, texture, and taste. Sometimes children object to having foods mixed, as in stews and casseroles, even if they normally like the ingredients separately.

In addition, parents should recognize that this is an important age for children to explore the world around them. Even good eaters are sometimes more interested in exploring than eating. There's room for occasional indulgences, a skipped meal or two, or

Two-year-olds commonly prefer particular foods, but parents needn't worry about this. A child may switch from one specific food focus (often called a jag) to another with equal intensity (older infants may also act this way). If the caregiver continues to offer choices, the child will soon begin to eat a wider variety of foods again, and the specific food focus will disappear as suddenly as it appeared.

Table 17-6 | Food Plan for Preschool and School-Age Children Based on MyPyramid

Food Group	Serving Size	Age 2[2]	Age 5[3]	Age 8[3]	Age 12[3,4]
Grains	ounce	3	5	5	6–7
Vegetables	cup	1	1.5	2	2.5–3
Fruits	cup	1	1.5	1.5	2
Milk	cup	2	2	3	3
Meat & Beans	ounce	2	4	5	5.5–6
Oils	teaspoon	3	4	5	6
Discretionary Calories	kcal	up to 165	up to 170	up to 130	up to 265–290

[1] Log on to www.mypyramid.gov for other ages and other activity levels.
[2] Based on less than 30 minutes of physical activity.
[3] Based on 30–60 minutes of physical activity.
[4] The lower amounts refer to girls.

once in a while "less than ideal" choices. It's eating and lifestyle habits over the course of a month and lifetime that matter. Children master their eating when adults provide opportunities to learn, give support for exploration, and limit inappropriate behavior.

"My Child Is Always Snacking, Yet She Never Finishes Her Meal"

Children have small stomachs. Offering them six or so small meals succeeds better than limiting them to three meals each day. Sticking to three meals a day offers no special nutritional advantages; it's just a social custom. Snacking is fine as long as good dental habits are practiced.[1] When we eat isn't nearly as important as what we eat. If nutritious snacks are readily available, these are good to offer at midmorning or midafternoon when the child becomes hungry (Table 17-7). Fruits and vegetables (fresh, frozen, or juice) and whole-grain breads and crackers are good snack choices. It is important that these snack choices be planned ahead in order to have healthy choices available. Working parents should make sure their children are provided with nutritious snacks to tide them over until dinnertime.

Table 17-7 | Ideas for Nutritious Snacks and Beverages

Snack	Serving Suggestion	Snack	Serving Suggestion	Snack	Serving Suggestion
Fresh raw vegetables	Serve with a dip of cottage cheese or yogurt blended with dried buttermilk dressing.	Ready-to-eat cereals	Use brands low in sugar and containing fiber; serve with raisins.	Parfait	Make with yogurt, fruit, and granola.
Celery	Spread with peanut butter and sprinkle on raisins, shredded carrots, or finely chopped nuts.	Pita bread	Place sliced meat, cheese, lettuce, and tomato in open pocket.	Gelatin	Add fruit or vegetable juice, vegetables, fruits, or cottage cheese.
Bananas	Dip in sweetened yogurt or spread with peanut butter and roll in coconut, chopped nuts, or granola.	English muffins or pita bread	Top with spaghetti sauce, grated cheese, meats; broil or bake and cut in fourths.	Frozen fruit cubes	Freeze puréed applesauce or fruit juice into cubes.
Sliced apples or crackers	Serve with a dip of peanut butter, honey, nuts, raisins, and coconut.	Potato skins	Sprinkle with shredded cheese, broil, and top with yogurt and bacon bits.	Fruit fizz	Add club soda to juice instead of serving soft drinks.
Bagels	Spread with cream cheese or peanut butter and top with chopped bananas, crushed pineapple, or shredded carrots.	Canned chili with beans	Heat and top with onions, lettuce, and tomato; use as dip for Italian or French bread, biscuits, or cornbread.	Fruit shake	Blend milk with fresh fruit (bananas, berries, or a peach) and a dash of cinnamon or nutmeg.
Quick bread or muffins	Make with carrots, zucchini, pumpkin, bananas, nuts, dates, raisins, lemons, squash, or berries.	Kabobs	Make with any combination of fruit, vegetables, and sliced or cubed cooked meat (remove toothpicks before serving).	Yogurt frost	Combine fruit juice and yogurt; add fresh fruit, if desired.
				Hot chocolate	Make hot chocolate or cocoa with milk chocolate and a dash of cinnamon.
Flour tortillas	Spread with refried beans or canned chili with beans, sprinkle with grated cheese and broil; top with chili sauce.	Popcorn	Serve plain or make 3 quarts and sprinkle with 1/4 cup grated cheese and 1/2 tsp garlic or onion salt.	Seeds	Choose shelled sunflower seeds.
				Fish	Put tuna salad on crackers.
				Canned soup	Serve a cup of vegetable or minestrone; nice on a cold winter day.

When a child refuses to eat, it's best not to overreact. Doing so may give the child the idea that eating is a means of getting attention or manipulating a scene. Most children don't starve themselves to any point approaching physical harm. When children refuse to eat, have them sit at the table for a while; if they still aren't interested in eating, remove the food and wait until the next scheduled meal or snack.

"My Child Never Eats Vegetables"

Children generally eat enough fruit but not an adequate amount of vegetables. Everyone dislikes certain foods. Again, the one-bite policy can be used, including for vegetable servings. It takes time for a child to become enthusiastic about a new food; however, with continual exposure and a positive role model, chances are the child may even grow to like it.

Children cannot and should not be forced to eat. They need to develop independence and identities separate from their parents. As already stated, children have to choose for themselves—a practice that should be encouraged. No one food is an essential part of a diet. Hunger is still the best means for getting a child to eat. It may be effective to feed children vegetables at the start of a meal, when they are hungriest. Offer new foods with familiar ones. A platter of raw or lightly cooked carrots, broccoli, green and red peppers, cabbage, and mushrooms eaten as a snack with friends may be accepted. A 4- or 5-year-old child can safely eat raw vegetables without fear of choking. Recall that children often are more sensitive than adults to strong flavors and odors. Nutritious dips, such as small amounts of ranch dressing, "sell" vegetables to many children. Vegetables may acquire more appeal when children help prepare them. And, as with any food, it is important to remember that children are entitled to their own likes and dislikes, too.

Use of Multivitamin and Mineral Supplements

Major scientific groups, such as the American Dietetic Association and the American Society for Clinical Nutrition, believe that multivitamin and mineral supplements are generally unnecessary for healthy children; it's better to emphasize good foods. Fortified ready-to-eat breakfast cereals with milk are especially helpful in closing any gap between current micronutrient intake and needs, such as for vitamin E, folate, and vitamin D. Two micronutrients of particular concern are iron and zinc. These may be lacking in children's diets because children consume such small portions of rich sources, such as animal protein foods. In addition, because the *2005 Dietary Guidelines for Americans* suggests that children over age 2 years follow a diet low in saturated fat and cholesterol, rich sources of iron and zinc may be lacking in their diets. To compensate, parents can search for a whole-grain breakfast cereal that the child likes that also has about 50% of the Daily Value for iron and 25% of the Daily Value for zinc. (These quantities will supply sufficient amounts of both nutrients because the Daily Values are based on the higher needs of adults.) If that's not possible, especially for a child who is ill, who has a very erratic food preference pattern or appetite, or who is on a weight-loss diet, the American Academy of Pediatrics suggests that the child may benefit from a children's multivitamin and mineral supplement not exceeding 100% of Daily Values on the label, especially if these conditions persist.[11] Still, as mentioned many times in this textbook, such a practice does not substitute for an otherwise healthy diet, children included.

If current childhood feeding practices are to become more healthful, the focus should shift to whole-grain breads and cereals, fruits and vegetables, and low-fat milk and milk products.[1,14,20] Caregivers can model this behavior by ordering from the salad bar more often and ordering french fries less often at fast-food restaurants. Children do not need to be severely restricted but, rather, should modify food habits with small changes. Some easy diet changes to begin with are bagels instead of doughnuts, fat-free frozen yogurt instead of ice cream, fat-reduced or 1% milk instead of

Choking is a very preventable hazard for young children. Some suggestions for caregivers include:

- Set a good example at the table by taking small bites and chewing foods thoroughly.
- Insisting that children sit at the table, take their time, and focus on the food during meals and snacks.
- Avoid giving children any foods that are round, firm, sticky, or cut into large chunks. Some examples of foods to avoid are nuts, grapes, raisins, popcorn, peanut butter, and hard pieces of raw fruits or vegetables.

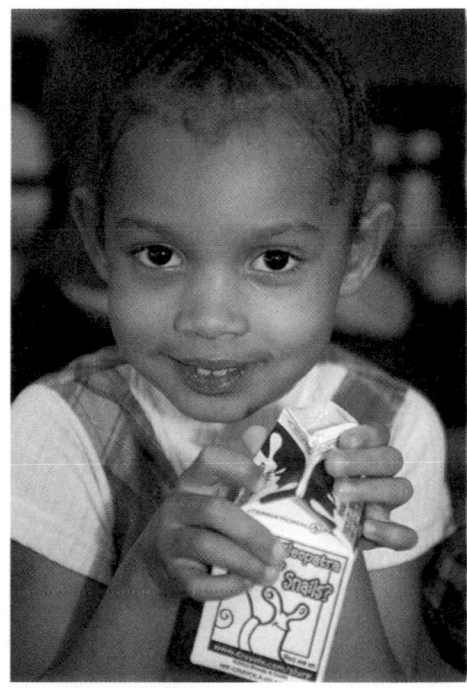

Milk is a nutrient-dense source of protein, calcium, zinc, and other nutrients to support growth. It is especially challenging to meet calcium needs in childhood without regular dairy product consumption (review Chapter 11 for alternative sources of calcium).

Children who follow a totally vegetarian diet should also focus on protein and vitamin B-12 intake.

whole milk, fruit instead of crackers and cheese for snacks, and air-popped popcorn instead of chips.

Other Nutritional Problems in Preschool Children

Three nutrition-related problems found in preschool children are iron deficiency anemia, constipation, and dental caries. Proper diet can help correct or relieve these conditions. Vegetarian diets can also pose problems.

Iron Deficiency Anemia

The best way to prevent iron deficiency anemia in children is to provide foods that are adequate sources of iron. Iron-fortified breakfast cereals and a few ounces of lean meat are convenient means of getting more iron into a child's diet.[1] The high proportion of heme iron in many animal foods allows the iron to be more readily absorbed than is iron from plant foods. Consuming a vitamin C source along with the less readily absorbed iron in plants and supplements aids absorption.

Childhood iron deficiency anemia is most likely to appear in children between the ages of 6 and 24 months.[7] It can lead to decreases in both stamina and learning ability because the oxygen supply to cells decreases. Another effect is lowered resistance to disease. Fortunately, childhood anemia is less common today in North America, probably because of children's use of iron-fortified breakfast cereals. Also deserving of credit in the United States is the Special Supplemental Nutrition Program for Women, Infants, and Children (WIC), sponsored by the U.S. government. This program emphasizes the importance of iron-fortified formulas and cereals and distributes them—along with nutrition education—to low-income parents of infants and preschool children considered to be at nutritional risk.

Constipation

Constipation may be associated with a more serious disease, yet some young children experience constipation that is unrelated to any medical condition. When presented with a constipated child, a physician first has to rule out a medical cause, such as intestinal blockage. And although the most common GI tract symptom that reflects intolerance to cow's milk is diarrhea, chronic constipation may also result. This possibility should be investigated by the physician. Treatment for constipation generally consists of first evacuating the bowels, generally with an enema. The promotion of regular bowel habits then follows, with laxative use as directed by the physician. Several months to years of supportive intervention may be required for effective treatment.

Dietary interventions include eating more fiber and drinking more fluids. Soy milk may also be substituted for cow's milk in the initial stages of treatment. Foods to emphasize for fiber are fruits, vegetables, whole-grain breads and cereals, and beans. The current daily fiber goal for children set by the Food and Nutrition Board varies by age: 1–3 years, 19 g/day; 4–8 years, 25 g/day; 9–13 years, 31 g/day for boys and 25 g/day for girls. After age 13 years, typical adult recommendations are appropriate (see Chapter 5). Currently few children meet this goal.[14] Accompanying fluid recommendations are 4 cups (900 ml) per day for toddlers and about 5 cups (1200 ml) per day for older children.

Dental Caries

A proper diet goes a long way in reducing the risk for dental caries in young children. (Earlier in this chapter it was mentioned that infants are prone to early childhood caries, which can lead to excessive tooth decay.) The following tips can help reduce dental problems in children:

- Begin oral hygiene when teeth start to appear.
- Seek early pediatric dental care.

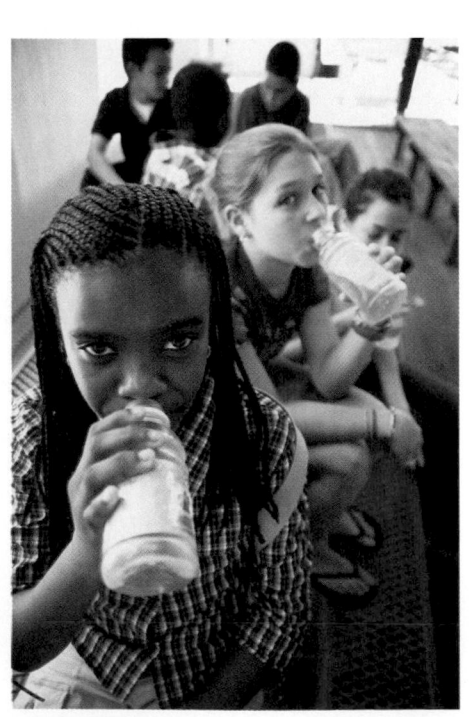

Excessive fruit drink and fruit juice use is another potential problem in preschool (and later adolescent) years. The American Academy of Pediatrics recommends no more than 4 to 6 oz/day for children 1 to 6 years (and 8 to 12 oz/day for ages 7 to 18 years). Sweetened soft drinks should also be limited.

Chapter 5 noted that sugar is not the cause of hyperactivity or antisocial behavior in most children.

- Drink fluoridated water.
- Use small amounts of fluoridated toothpaste twice daily.
- Snack in moderation.
- Have a dentist apply tooth sealants if needed.
- Avoid sticky, high-sugar snacks, especially between meals.
- If toddlers or preschoolers are chewing gum, sugarless gum is the best choice, because it has been shown to reduce the incidence of dental caries.

Chapters 5 and 12 provide a fuller description of diet and dental health. If needed, these discussions will aid in putting this list of recommendations into perspective.

Vegetarianism in Childhood

Vegetarian diets can pose several risks for young children. These risks include the possibility of developing iron deficiency anemia, a deficiency of vitamin B-12, and rickets from a vitamin D deficiency. During the first few years of life, children also may not consume enough energy when following a bulky vegetarian diet. But these known pitfalls are easily avoided by informed diet planning (review the Nutrition Focus in Chapter 7). Diets for children who eat totally vegetarian fare should focus on vitamin B-12, iron, and zinc content, with additional emphasis on vitamin D (or regular sun exposure) and calcium.[1] Some of these dietary inadequacies can be compensated for by increasing oils, nuts, seeds, ready-to-eat breakfast cereals, and fortified soy milk in the diet.

Modifications of Childhood Diets to Reduce Future Disease Risk

Earlier chapters covered the role of diet in development of cardiovascular disease and hypertension and the recommendations concerning diet to reduce the risk for these diseases. Parents sometimes wonder whether similar diet modifications are appropriate and beneficial during childhood.

Diets Designed to Limit Cardiovascular Disease for Children 2 Years of Age and Older

The development of atherosclerosis often begins in childhood. As a result, many experts recommend screening for blood cholesterol in children whose families have histories of early development of cardiovascular disease or high blood cholesterol, and treating children found to have high blood cholesterol with appropriate diet and possibly drug therapy, as discussed in Chapter 6.[3] With regard to diet, children in the United States currently derive about 33% of their energy from fat, with about 13% of energy from saturated fat. The Food and Nutrition Board recommends that fat intake range from 30 to 40% of energy intake for children 1 to 3 years, and 25 to 35% for children 4 to 18 years, so this fat intake is appropriate. However, saturated fat, *trans* fat, and cholesterol intake should be minimized (no set limit). Thus, more work is needed in this regard. These recommendations are consistent with those of the National Cholesterol Education program in the United States and with those from the American Heart Association. An emphasis on plant oils such as canola oil as a major source of fat in the diet helps meet the goals of reduced saturated fat, *trans* fat, and cholesterol intake. In general, it's unnecessary to discourage children from consuming nutrient-dense foods, such as milk and animal proteins, just because they contain some animal fat. The overriding message is moderation in these and other fat sources with a focus on limiting saturated fat, *trans* fat, and cholesterol intake.

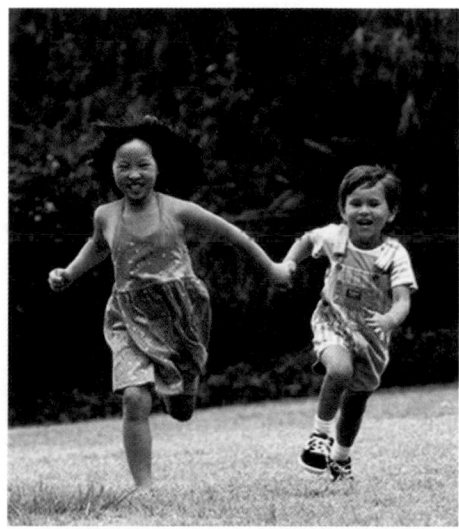

Children benefit from opportunities to be physically active. This contributes to cardiovascular health. The current goal is 60 minutes of such activity each day, the same as for adults. Many children currently are not meeting this goal.

Salt-Restricted Diets

Scientific data neither confirm nor refute the notion that eating less salt (sodium) reduces the risk of future hypertension. Moderation in salt consumption does help build good health habits for the future—especially if the person later develops hypertension

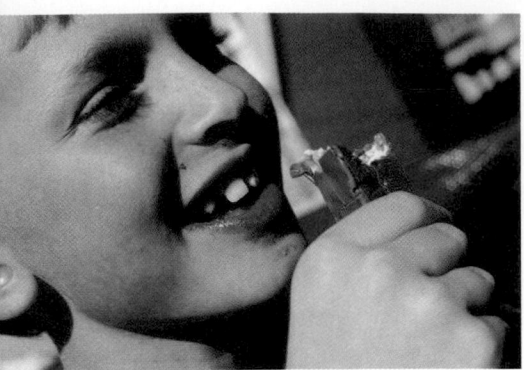

Sweets should be consumed in moderation in childhood but do not have to be avoided altogether.

and needs to eat even less salt. If children become accustomed to less salt, they'll be less inclined to eat very salty foods as adults. This reduction in salt also contributes to better calcium retention in the body, as covered in Chapter 11. If a child with hypertension does not respond to diet and lifestyle therapy, typical antihypertensive medications may be used, but at lower doses than adults require.[9]

Concept | Check

The rapid growth rate of an infant's first year slows during the toddler and preschool years (ages 1 to 5). As a child's appetite decreases, adults need to serve nutrient-dense foods and allow the child to decide how much to eat. Sudden shifts in food preferences are to be expected. Snacking is fine if attention is given to the selection of healthful foods and good dental hygiene. Although children's multivitamin and mineral supplement is usually not needed—a plan following MyPyramid that includes a serving of fortified ready-to-eat breakfast cereal should meet nutrient needs—such use is a reasonable practice. Children need plenty of iron-rich food to prevent iron deficiency anemia and need zinc for growth. Adequate fiber and fluid help prevent constipation. Developing heart-healthy habits after the age of 2 years is advocated, but highly restrictive diets are not appropriate during childhood. Diets for children who eat totally vegetarian fare should focus on meeting needs for protein, vitamin D (or regular sun exposure), vitamin B-12, calcium, iron, and zinc.

▌School-Age Children: Nutrition Concerns

In general, the nutritional concerns and goals applicable to school-age children are the same as those discussed in relation to preschoolers. The MyPyramid for children ages 6–11 years is a good basis for diet planning, with an emphasis on moderating fat and sugar intake and ensuring adequate iron, zinc, and calcium intake (Figure 17-6). Note also that the number of servings increases as age, and so energy needs, increase (review Table 17-6). The Estimated Energy Requirements (kcals) are now **88.5 − (61.9 × Age [y]) + (PA × (26.7 × Weight [kg] + 903 × Height [meters]) + 20** for boys 3 through 8 years. Recall from Chapter 13 that PA stands for physical activity. In this case, PA = 1.00 if the child is sedentary; PA = 1.13 if the child is low active; PA = 1.26 if the child is active; PA = 1.42 if the child is very active. For older boys the formula is the same except that the last value (20) is replaced by the value 25.

For girls ages 3 through 8 years the formula is **135.3 − (30.8 × Age [y]) + (PA × (10.0 × Weight [kg] + 934 × Height [meters]) + 20.** In this case, PA = 1.00 if the child is sedentary; PA = 1.16 if the child is low active; PA = 1.31 if the child is active; PA = 1.56 if the child is very active. For older girls the formula is the same except again the last value (20) is replaced by the value 25. The rest of this major section addresses several nutritional issues of particular concern during the school-age years.

Breakfast, Fat Intake, and Snacks

Once children enter school, their eating patterns become more scheduled and the consumption of regular meals—especially breakfast—becomes an important focus. A fortified ready-to-eat breakfast cereal is typically the greatest source of iron, vitamin A, folic acid, and fiber for children ages 2 to 18.[2] Although there is controversy over the true benefit of breakfast for cognitive ability, children who eat breakfast likely meet their needs for vitamins, minerals, and fiber compared to children not eating breakfast. To influence morning test performance, it currently appears that breakfast must be eaten within a few hours of a test; the rise in blood glucose is thought to enhance performance.

Breakfast menus need not be limited to traditional fare. A little imagination can spark the interest of even the most reluctant child. Instead of conventional breakfast foods, parents can offer leftovers from dinner—pizza, spaghetti, soups, yogurt topped with trail mix, chili with beans, or sandwiches, for starters.

Critical | Thinking

Tim refuses to eat breakfast before school. He doesn't like cereal, toast, or any of the other usual breakfast foods. What can Tim's parents do to ensure that he eats nutritious foods before leaving for school?

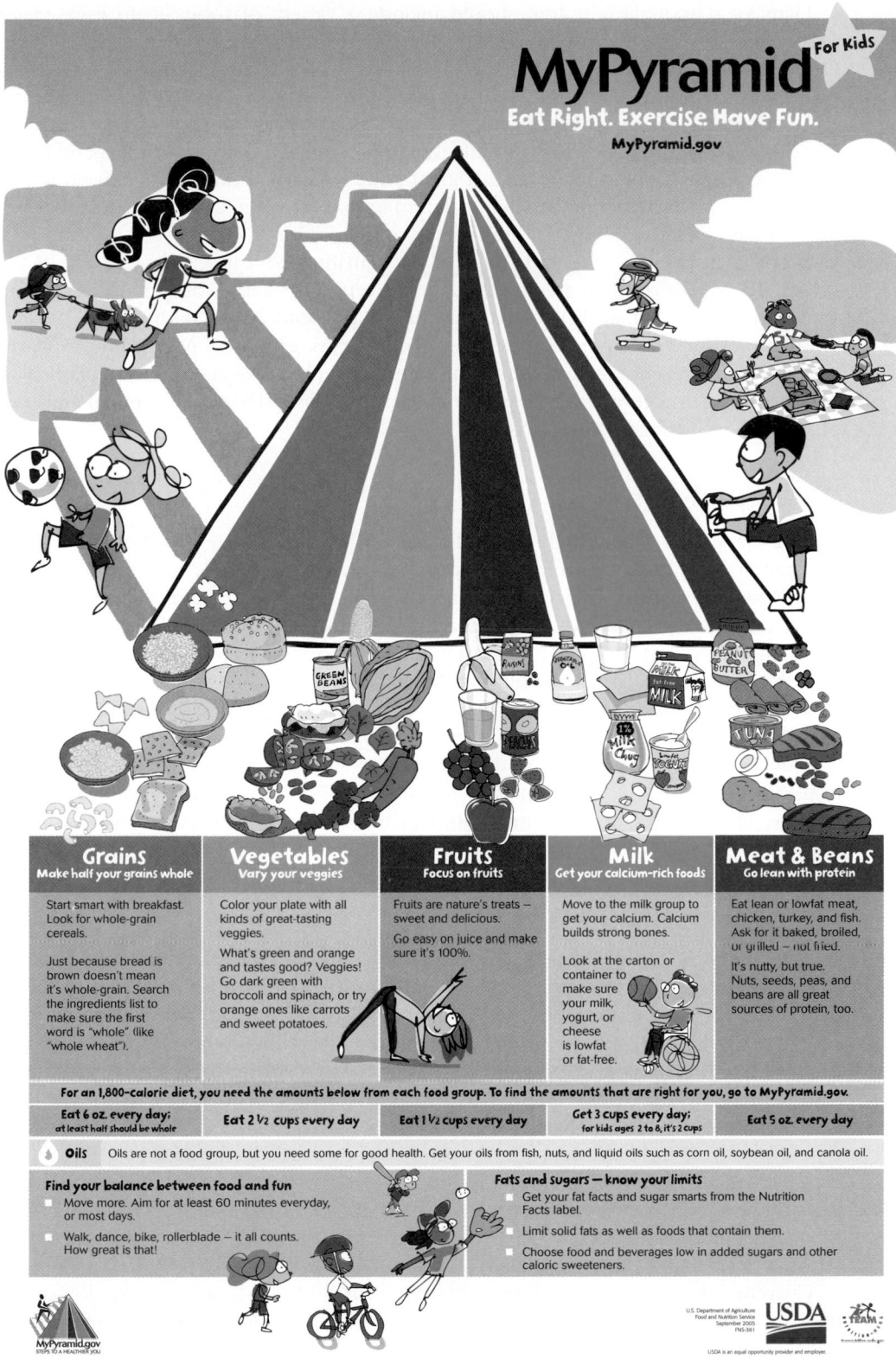

Figure 17-6 | The USDA has created a version of MyPyramid for children ages 6 to 11. The accompanying website (http://mypyramid.gov/kids/index.html) also features kid-friendly resources— such as an interactive MyPyramid Blast Off Game and a meal tracking worksheet—designed to encourage children to make healthier eating and activity choices. This site also contains information and resources that adults can use in educating children about proper nutrition.

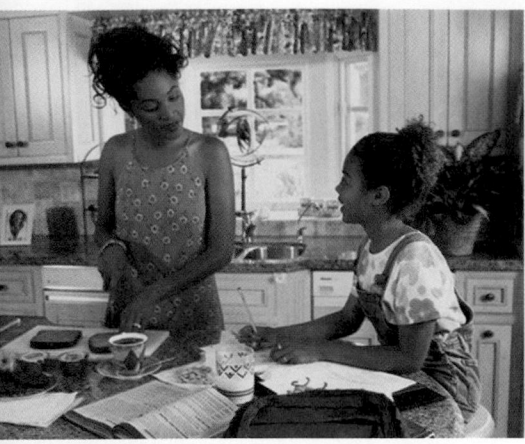

Nutrition education ideally begins in the home as parents and other caregivers provide a healthy, well-balanced diet.

Diets of school-age children should include a variety of foods from each major group, not necessarily excluding any specific food because of its fat content. Overemphasis on fat-reduced diets during childhood has been linked to an increase in eating disorders and encourages an inappropriate "good food, bad food" attitude.

Steering children toward healthful foods, in school and at home, is likely to be more successful if children are exposed to nutrition education. Because children spend much of their younger years in school, it is a great place to learn about positive, healthy eating habits.[17] Such education can help children understand why eating a proper diet will make them feel more energetic, look better, and work more efficiently. One survey of U.S. schoolchildren highlighted the need for nutrition education. On the day of the survey, 40% of the children ate no vegetables, except for potatoes or tomato sauce; 20% ate no fruits. Another study showed that only 2% of about 3300 children 2 to 19 years old had met their recommended servings from the six groups of MyPyramid. Clearly, the diets of many school-age students can stand general improvement, particularly with regard to fruit, vegetable, whole grain, and dairy choices. Drinking minimal amounts of sugared soft drinks is also advised.

Type 2 Diabetes

Type 2 diabetes is generally thought of as an adult condition. As the Nutrition Focus in Chapter 5 explained, it frequently occurs in overweight people who are older than 40. However, recently physicians have noted an alarming increase in the frequency of the disease among children (and teenagers). This increase is primarily due to the rise in obesity in this age group, coupled with minimal physical activity. Up to 85% of children with the disease are overweight at diagnosis. Experts are currently calling for the screening of fasting blood glucose in at-risk children every 2 years, starting at age 10 or at the onset of puberty. Besides obesity and a sedentary lifestyle, other risk factors include having a first- or second-degree relative with the disease, or belonging to a non-White population.[11] Appropriate diet and lifestyle intervention should be implemented, along with the use of medications when necessary. A focus on low glycemic load fruits, vegetables, and whole-grain breads and cereals is especially recommended.

Overweight and Obesity

In the United States, about 15% of school-age children are overweight. The number of cases is currently increasing, especially in minority populations. Obesity is generally diagnosed when a child reaches the 95th percentile for BMI and a physical exam indicates the child is truly overfat, which is usually true for a child who reaches this degree of BMI. In the short run, ridicule, embarrassment, possibly depression, and short stature linked to early puberty are the main consequences of such obesity. In the long run, significant health problems associated with obesity, such as cardiovascular disease, type 2 diabetes, and hypertension, usually will appear in adulthood. However, an increase in these health-related complications has been noted in children. Childhood obesity is a serious health threat, because about 40% of obese children (and about 80% of obese adolescents) become obese adults. Significant weight gain generally begins between ages 5 and 7, during puberty, or during the teenage years.[13]

Current research points to many potential causes of childhood obesity. Recall the nature versus nurture discussion in Chapter 13. Some infants are born with lower metabolic rates; they use energy more efficiently and in turn can more easily save energy intake for fat storage. Studies also suggest, though, that this genetic link accounts for only one-third of individual differences in body weight.

Researchers believe that although diet is still an important factor, inactivity is also a key to the increase in childhood obesity.[19] Today's generation of children now glues itself to the TV for an average of 24 hours a week; many children spend another 10 hours or so playing computer and video games. The American Academy of Pediatrics recommends a limit of 14 hours of TV and video time per week.[11] In addition, exces-

Regular physical activity is an important part of prevention and treatment of weight problems in childhood.

sive snacking, overreliance on fast-food restaurants, parental neglect, the media, lack of safe areas to play, and high-fat/high-energy food choices also contribute to childhood obesity. Sugared soft drinks are especially implicated.[10] Dr. Carol Byrd-Bredbenner discusses these trends in more detail in the Expert Opinion.

The initial approach in treating an obese child is to assess how much physical activity he or she engages in. If a child spends much free time in sedentary activities (such as watching television or playing video games), more physical activities should be encouraged. Both the U.S. government and health professionals recommend 60 minutes or more of moderate to intense physical activity per day for children and adolescents. An overall active lifestyle will help children not only to attain a healthy body weight but also to keep a similar body weight later in life. An increase in physical activity won't just happen; parents and other caregivers need to plan for it. Two good ideas are getting the family together for a brisk walk after dinner and finding an after-school sport the child enjoys.

Moderation in energy intake is important, especially the limitation of high-fat and high-energy foods, such as sugared soft drinks and whole milk. The focus should be more on healthy snacks and foods rich in vitamins and minerals.[1]

Resorting to a weight-loss diet is usually not necessary. As a start, it's best to emphasize changing habits that allow for weight maintenance. Children have an advantage over adults in dealing with obesity; their bodies can use stored energy for growth. Thus, if weight gain can be moderated, increases in height and resulting lean body tissue may reduce the percentage of body weight accounted for as stored fat, yielding a more healthful weight-to-height ratio. Further growth can contribute to success.

If a child is still obese after attaining ultimate adult height, a weight-loss regimen may be necessary, especially after the adolescent growth spurt. Weight loss should be gradual, perhaps 1/2 to 1 lb per week. In addition, the child should be watched closely to ensure that the rate of growth continues to be normal. The child's energy intake shouldn't be so low that gains in height diminish. In addition, medications may be prescribed under a physician's care to reduce food intake (sibutramine [Meridia]) or fat absorption (orlistat [Xenical]). (Older children may even be candidates for obesity-related surgical approaches.)[10]

Obese children often need to find a new way to relate to foods, especially snack foods. An important family rule could be that children are allowed to eat only while sitting at the dining table or in the kitchen. This rule could stop endless hours of snacking in front of the television and make all family members more conscious of when they are eating. It also might be helpful to put portions of snack foods on plates rather than to allow snacking to go on indefinitely, as often happens when children eat directly from a full box of crackers or cookies.

A child's self-esteem is extremely fragile. Obesity itself often affects the child's psyche and mental outlook (e.g., depression). Humiliation doesn't work; it only makes the child feel worse. Support, admiration, and encouragement of the child's efforts at weight control are more effective and should be emphasized.

Finally, it is important to understand that not all children are designed to look like society's ideal. In other words, some children simply weigh more than others. A healthful lifestyle with plenty of physical activity and nutritious foods remains the key concern.

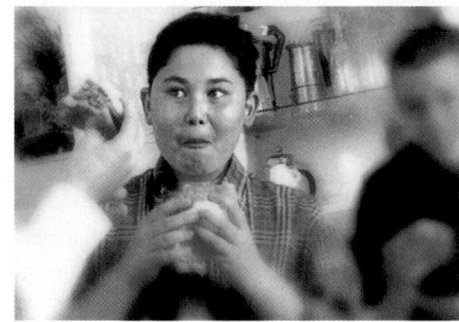

Large portions of foods such as hamburgers and sugared soft drinks served to children are contributing to the obesity and type 2 diabetes epidemics they are experiencing.

To get kids involved in exercise, new physical education classes have been introduced into schools. These classes provide lifelong fitness lessons in such activities as rock climbing, in-line skating, and recreational jogging. These classes help promote activity because they take the focus away from teams and competition, which often discourage and embarrass kids who lack athletic talent.

Concept | Check

The school-age child is advised to follow MyPyramid, moderating choices high in fat and simple sugars. Breakfast is an important meal to refuel the body for a new school day and to help ensure fulfilling nutrient needs for the day. Attention to regular physical activity and healthy diet should help prevent or treat childhood obesity and build a desirable lifestyle pattern for later life.

Are Savvy Marketers Contributing to the Obesity Epidemic in Children?
Carol Byrd-Bredbenner, Ph.D., R.D., F.A.D.A.

In industrialized nations, we have the most nutritious, safe, and abundant food supply of any time in history. So, logically speaking, we should be better nourished and healthier than ever before; but we're not. Diet quality has diminished—soft drink consumption is up, snacking is on the rise, portions are super-sized, the family meal is just about extinct, and children in the United States are getting half their energy intake from added sugar and fat. All these factors and more are playing a role in the escalating obesity epidemic.

Most experts believe that obesigenic or "toxic" environments are at the root of this epidemic because the increase in obesity rates parallels the obesigenic environmental changes seen over the past several decades. Obesigenic environments promote obesity-favoring behaviors by facilitating sedentary behavior with labor-saving devices and sedentary leisure activities; offering easy access to large quantities of affordable, highly palatable, energy-dense foods; and encouraging (advertising) the overconsumption of these foods, which results in the displacement of other, lower-energy but more nutrient-dense foods.

Food advertising messages to eat! eat! eat! have received a great deal of attention lately. Of course marketing affects everyone, but the main concern of policymakers and health professionals is the effect of slick marketing methods targeted to children. This concern is particularly well placed when you consider that children usually cannot tell the difference between advertisements and TV programs until they are age 5 or so. It is only after about age 7 or 8 that children understand that advertisements aim to persuade them to buy a product, and even then, it takes until about age 11 for them to automatically activate thought processes that help them question the validity of an advertisement. Plus, some advertising is so disguised (e.g., advertising games) that it is hard for even some adults to resist.

Why Do Marketers Target Children?

You may wonder why marketers would advertise to children; after all, few of them earn a paycheck. In actuality, children in the United States "control" billions—those under 12 spend $25 billion of their own money annually and influence $200 billion in household spending. Marketers have come to see children as a vast consumer group that can help companies maximize their profits. Marketers reach out to children as soon as they are born! (Some bibs and baby bottles are emblazoned with fast-food or soft-drink logos.)

Where Is Advertising Encountered?

Today, food marketing is similar to surround sound at movie theatres—it is all around us.

Environment: Do a quick Internet image search for a national soft-drink brand or major fast-food chain and see what you discover! You'll find T-shirts, toys (dolls, modeling clay kits), shrink-wrapped cars and buses, hot air balloons, basketball backboards, race cars, umbrellas, children's books that teach math using popular candy brands, and more!

Schools: Visit most schools these days and you'll see food company logos on book covers and educational posters; branded foods sold in the cafeteria and vending machines or as fund-raisers; learning incentives that reward children with a fast-food meal; and promotions for rebate programs sponsored by food companies that provide schools with equipment or cash in return for product labels.

Cross-promotions: A trip down the cereal or cookie aisle at the supermarket is a great place to find examples of cross-promotions—the pairing of a popular spokescharacter like Shrek or a toy with a food. Children's meals at fast-food restaurants often cross-promote menu items and a toy. Cross-promotions help create a positive perception of products and increase brand recognition by young children.

Viral marketing: Tell a friend about a product and you've engaged in viral marketing, which is also called buzz marketing or word of mouth (mouse). Viral marketing is the most basic type of advertising, but in recent years it has become more sophisticated. Marketers now recruit "e-fluentials" (individuals who shape opinions and attitudes of others online) to go to chat rooms and

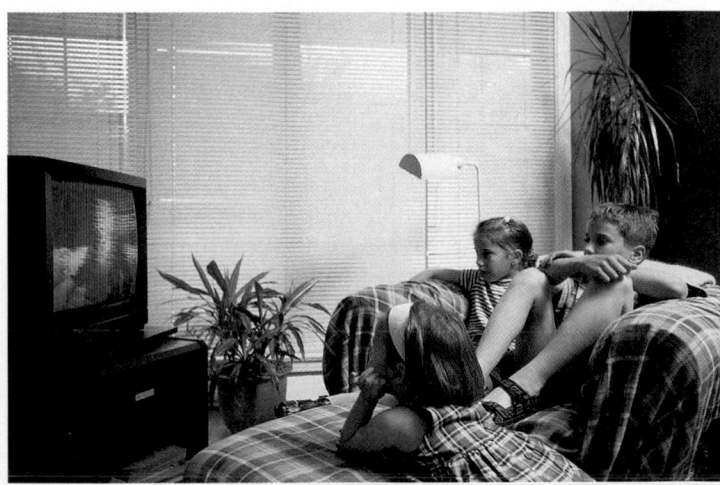

Television has a powerful influence on the eating habits of children.

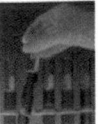

tout a product or post messages on bulletin boards or listservs. Some go to neighborhoods to recruit the kid identified by peers as being the "coolest" (i.e., an influencer) to use their products and give samples to friends.

Websites: Check out the website of a popular candy, soft drink, or snack chip and see how "sticky" they are. These sites use advertainment (a blend of advertising, entertainment, and product branding) to engage visitors and keep them at the website interacting in a positive, fun way with the advertised product. Advertainment might include screen savers, phone ring tones of an advertising jingle, kids' clubs, chat rooms, puzzles, and games. Advertainment is particularly effective because it disguises promotions as games and comics, making it harder for children to be skeptical of advertising messages.

Newspapers, magazines, radio, and television: Open a magazine or channel surf and you will find a wide variety of food advertisements. Despite the rise in all the other types of marketing venues, television remains the favorite of food advertisers. Television advertising is of special concern because children in the United States watch an average of 2 to 3 hours daily and see about 38,000 TV commercials yearly—a quarter of which are for foods or beverages high in sugar or fat. Food marketing on TV is not limited to advertisements; there are product placements, too. Product placement is using a product in the program itself as a prop or part of the storyline. Product placements also can be found in movies (ET's snack of Reese's Pieces boosted product sales 80%) and music (McDonald's is recruiting hip-hop and rap artists to feature the Big Mac in their songs).

Does Food Advertising Affect Food Choices?

It is clear that food advertising is all around us, but does it affect food choices? Most marketing and advertising research is done by food companies and is largely unavailable to outsiders. However, food marketers' spending patterns suggest that advertising works. According to the USDA Economic Research Service's latest estimates, more than $11 billion is spent on food advertising each year—of this, $7 billion is spent on convenience foods, sweets, alcoholic beverages, and restaurants (mostly fast food). A significant amount of this advertising is targeted to children.

Although academic research on the effects of food marketing on children is surprisingly thin and focused mostly on television, we do know this:

Watching TV is associated with increased snacking and poorer quality meals. Families who routinely watch TV during mealtimes eat fewer fruits and vegetables and more pizzas, snack foods, and soft drinks than those families who separate eating and television-watching activities. In addition, foods are requested by children and purchased by parents in the same frequency that they are advertised during children's TV viewing hours.

Advertising increases the number of food purchase requests children make. For many children, their first purchase request occurs in the grocery store around age 2. The most common requests are for breakfast cereals, snacks, beverages, and toys—parents give in to this pester power more than half the time.

Advertising influences food preferences, choices, and intake. Television ads affect kids' breakfast cereal, snack, and beverage preferences and choices and increase their intake of advertised foods. One fast-food chain reported that their toy cross-promotion doubled sales of children's meals.

Advertising affects children's knowledge of nutrition and health. Children who frequently viewed TV believed that to maintain good health they should take advertised medicines, drink soft drinks, and eat fast foods.

So Are Savvy Marketers Contributing to the Obesity Epidemic in Children?

Advertising expenditures and academic research both seem to indicate that advertising does affect food choices. But advertisers argue that their goal is to increase demand for one specific brand—not to increase demand for the food in general. That is, if one fast-food chain steals market share from other brands, its advertisements do not increase intake of competing brands; thus, advertisements do not contribute to obesity. On the other hand, academic research findings indicate that the large expenditures spent on food advertising, which promotes primarily high-calorie foods, does affect food choices, creates desire for advertised foods, and promotes preferences for these foods. At this time, researchers cannot flatly state that food advertising contributes to obesity in children. However, nutrition and health experts from the Food and Agricultural Organization and World Food Organization of the United Nations have concluded that the research evidence is sufficiently strong to state that pervasive marketing of fast foods and other high-calorie foods and beverages are a probable cause of weight gain and obesity in children.

Dr. Byrd-Bredbenner is Professor of Nutrition at Rutgers University. She earned her doctorate at The Pennsylvania State University. Her research focuses on environmental factors that affect dietary choices and health, including advertising, media, nutrition labeling, portion sizes, and food preparation skills. Dr. Byrd-Bredbenner has authored nutrition texts, journal articles, and computer software packages. She has received teaching awards from the American Dietetic Association, Society for Nutrition Education, and U.S. Department of Agriculture.

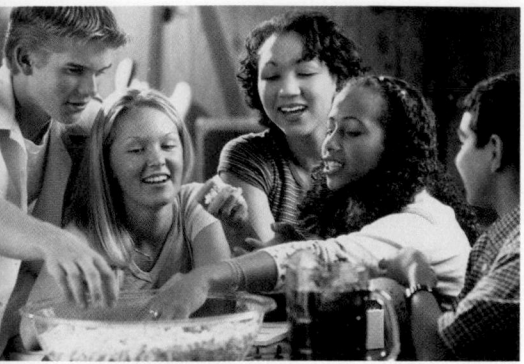

The teenage years are noted for snacking. With reasonable food choices, teenagers can have healthful diets.

The Teenage Years: Nutrition Concerns

Most girls begin a rapid growth spurt between the ages of 10 and 13, and most boys experience rapid growth between the ages of 12 and 15. Nearly every organ in the body grows during these periods. Most noticeable are increases in height and weight and the development of secondary sexual characteristics. Girls usually begin menstruating during this growth spurt, and they grow very little beyond 2 years after menarche. Early-maturing girls may begin their growth spurt as early as age 7 to 8, whereas early-maturing boys may begin growing by age 9 to 10.[11]

During the growth spurt, girls gain about 10 in (25 cm) in height, and boys gain about 12 in (30 cm). Girls also tend to accumulate both lean and fat tissue, whereas boys tend to gain mostly lean tissue. This growth spurt provides about 50% of ultimate adult weight and about 15% of ultimate adult height (review Figure 17-1).

As the growth spurt begins, teenagers begin to eat more. Estimated Energy Requirements are the same as previously listed for older children. If teens choose nutritious food, they can take advantage of their increased hunger and easily satisfy their nutrient needs. As with younger age groups, MyPyramid can provide the basis for meeting these nutrient needs, with the major difference being three servings of milk and milk products (Table 17-8). Following such a plan will meet carbohydrate needs (130 g/day) and protein needs (0.85 g/kg of body weight/day, or 52 g/day for males and 46 g/day for females).

Nutritional Problems and Concerns of Teens

Anorexia nervosa and bulimia nervosa were covered in detail in Chapter 15. Other nutritional problems are more common during the teen years. A survey of high school students showed that only a little over 25% had eaten five servings of fruits and vegetables on the previous day, and they are consuming approximately 25% more sodium than recommended. Another concern is that many teenage girls stop drinking milk, so they may not consume enough calcium to allow for maximal mineralization of bones through their early twenties.[18] Many young women who don't consume enough calcium are likely to develop osteoporosis later, as discussed in Chapter 11.

The Adequate Intake for calcium for both males and females between ages 9 and 18 years is 1300 mg per day, compared with only 800 mg per day for younger children. Three servings per day from the milk group are recommended for all teenagers and

Drinking soft drinks in place of milk causes many teenagers to have inadequate calcium intake. Over the last 20 years soft drinks have been replacing milk as the preferred beverage of adolescents. This trend has been linked to decreased bone mass and increased bone fractures in this age group.

A strictly vegetarian diet must be monitored for adequate energy, protein, iron, vitamin B-12, calcium, and vitamin D (the latter if sun exposure is not sufficient). These nutrients become particularly important in teenagers, because their diets are often already compromised.

Table 17-8 | Food Plan for Teenagers Based on MyPyramid[1,2]

Food Group	Serving Size	Approximate Number of Servings		
		Age 13	Age 16	Age 18
Grains	ounce	6–7	6–10	6–10
Vegetables	cup	2.5–3	2.5–3.5	2.5–3.5
Fruits	cup	2	2–2.5	2–2.5
Milk	cup	3	3	3
Meat & Beans	ounce	5.5–6	5.5–7	5.5–7
Oils	teaspoon	6	6–8	6–8
Discretionary calories	kcal	up to 265–290	up to 265–425	up to 265–425

[1] Assumes 30–60 minutes of physical activity per day. Log on to mypyramid.gov for other ages and levels of physical activity.

[2] Larger amounts refer to boys.

young adults to meet calcium needs. Figure 2-1 in Chapter 2 shows the stark contrast between milk and typical soft drinks with respect to calcium and other nutrients. If milk and milk products are not consumed, alternative calcium sources need to be included. Many teenagers are not meeting their calcium needs.

A further concern is iron deficiency. Iron deficiency anemia sometimes appears in girls after they start menstruating (menarche) and in boys during their growth spurt. About 10% of teenagers have low iron stores or related anemia. Teens who strive to forge an identity by adopting dietary patterns unfamiliar to their families—vegetarianism, for example—may not know enough about the alternate diet pattern to keep from developing health problems, such as iron deficiency anemia. It's important that teenagers choose good food sources of iron, such as lean meats, whole grains, and enriched cereals. Teenage girls, particularly those with heavy menstrual flows, need to eat good sources of iron (or regularly consume an iron supplement). Iron deficiency anemia is a highly undesirable condition for a teen. It can produce increased fatigue and decreased ability to concentrate and learn. School and physical performance may suffer.[11]

Acne is a common teen concern—about 80% of teens experience it. Although it's popularly believed that eating nuts, chocolate, and pizza can make acne worse, scientific studies have failed to show a strong link between any dietary factor and acne. It is important to note that many acne medications contain analogs of vitamin A (e.g., 13-*cis* retinoic acid [Accutane]). Although these treatments can be quite effective, the close supervision by a physician is crucial, because these vitamin A analogs can be toxic. Vitamin A itself is no help in treating acne, and excess amounts of vitamin A or related analogs can cause birth defects. Thus, girls taking these vitamin A medications must not become pregnant.

A Closer Look at the Diets of Teenage Girls

Teenagers in general are apt to adopt fad diets, eat away from home or miss meals completely, and snack a lot. Teenage girls especially are very concerned with weight gain, appearance, and social acceptance. U.S. government statistics reveal that female students are significantly more likely to report current attempts to lose weight (44%) than are male students (15%). Moreover, 27% of female students who considered themselves the right weight report they were currently trying to lose weight. It is important to inform teenage girls that weight gain in the form of increased body fat is to be expected in the adolescent growth spurt.

In an attempt to reach personal goals, teenage girls may eat dangerously little, select just a few items, and frequently skip meals altogether. If their limited food choices then consist of french fries, sugared soft drinks, and pastries, little room is left for foods that are good nutrient sources. Another common practice among teenage girls is having a fat phobia, focusing primarily on foods that are fat-free. However, many teens may not realize that some fat is essential for body functions. This concept is discussed in Chapter 6. The diets of teenage girls often lack adequate sources of folate, calcium, zinc, and vitamins A and C. The common use of diet pills and the increasing number of bulimia nervosa cases further add to these nutritional problems.

Helping Teens Eat More Nutritious Foods

Teenagers face a variety of challenges. They pursue their independence, experience identity crises, seek peer acceptance, and worry about physical appearance. All these factors affect food choice. As noted in the Expert Opinion in this chapter, advertisers take advantage of this situation by pushing a vast array of products—candy, gum, soft drinks, and snacks—at the teenage market. Potato chips and french fries make up more than one-third of the vegetable servings consumed by teens. Additionally, many schools offer french fries on a regular basis, and soft drink machines can be found in school hallways and cafeterias, in turn competing with the school lunch.

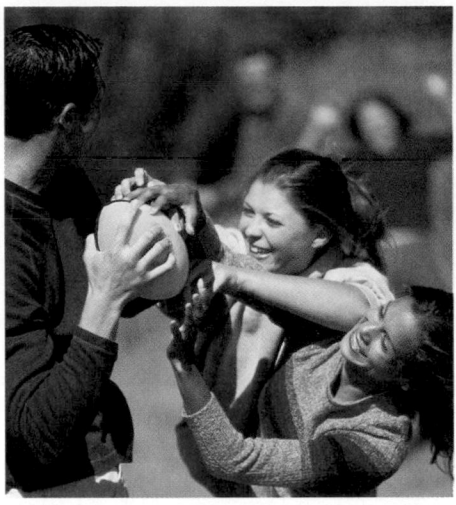

An active lifestyle coupled with a healthy diet should be part of the teen years. Both habits contribute to bone development and bone strength.

Obesity is a growing problem among teenagers, and about 30% of these teenagers have the metabolic syndrome (Syndrome X) discussed in Chapters 5 and 6. If a teen is still obese after attaining ultimate adult height, especially after the adolescent growth spurt, a weight-loss regimen may be necessary. Weight loss should be gradual, perhaps 1 lb/week, and should generally follow the advice in Chapter 13. Weight-loss medications such as sibutramine (Meridia) or orlistat (Xenical) may be prescribed. Obesity-related surgery also may be recommended.[11]

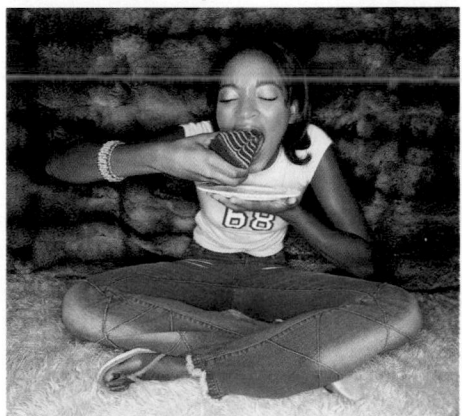

The eating habits of teenage girls can vary widely. Some severely restrict their intake because of the fear of gaining weight, while others use their growing independence to opt almost exclusively for fast-food and fat-laden snacks.

Alcoholism, a significant health problem that may have its roots in the teen years, is covered in detail in Chapter 8. Smoking–another habit that compromises health–also often begins in teen years. Some of this behavior is an attempt to control body weight–not an advisable method.

Clinicians who work with teenagers, including physicians, registered dietitians, and nurses, need to be prepared to discuss and deal with a variety of concerns: sports nutrition, eating disorders, use of steroids, and drug (and alcohol) abuse. Except for substance abuse, these topics usually are not a concern when working with older adult clients.

Teens often don't think about the long-term benefits of good health. They have a hard time relating today's actions to tomorrow's health outcomes. Many teenagers tend to think they can just change habits later; there's no hurry.

Still, healthful teen food habits don't have to include giving up favorite foods. Small portions of fatty foods can complement larger portions of fat-free and reduced-fat dairy products, lean meats, vegetable proteins, fruits, vegetables, and whole-grain products.[2,4,15,20] An example is a plain hamburger with a garden salad (minimize the amount of regular dressing or use a low-fat variety), small order of french fries or chili, and a medium diet soft drink or reduced fat or fat-free milk.

Working with the Teenage Mind-Set

One strategy for working with teenage boys is to stress the importance of nutrition and physical activity for physical development—especially muscular development—and for fitness, vigor, and health. With teenage girls, one approach is to help them understand how to choose nutrient-dense foods and activities that lead to better health while maintaining a healthy weight. For teenagers, it's more effective to focus on the benefits of healthful foods and regular physical activity they can reap right now than to talk about health hazards that may or may not happen later.

Teenage Snacking Practices

Teens often obtain one-fourth to one-third of all their energy and major nutrients from snacks. Unfortunately, studies have found just what you might expect—that teens snack mostly on potato and corn chips, cookies, candies, and ice cream. Key reasons for snacking include an opportunity to get out and socialize with friends, accessibility, hunger, and celebration of a special event. Teenagers can obtain many nutrients from snacking. Even fast-food restaurants offer some good food choices. By choosing wisely and eating in moderation, teens can eat at fast-food restaurants and still consume a healthful diet.[11] Snacks and fast-food restaurants themselves are not the problem; poor food choices are.

Poor dietary habits and exercise formed during teenage years often continue into adulthood, giving rise to an increased risk of chronic diseases, such as cardiovascular disease, osteoporosis, and some types of cancer. Getting this message across to teenagers is an important and challenging task for parents and health professionals.

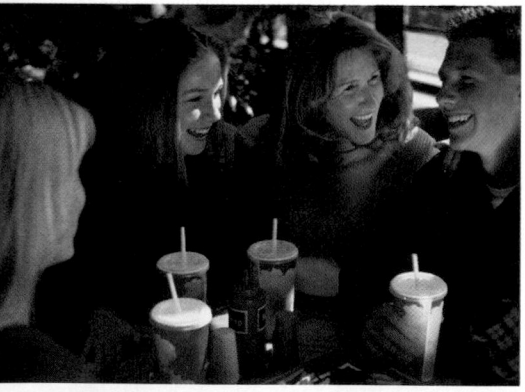

One way to reduce energy intake in a restaurant is to choose water or diet soft drinks in place of regular soft drinks. This will greatly reduce sugar and overall energy intake in the meal or snack, especially considering the large serving sizes typically offered.

Concept | Check

A second period of rapid growth occurs during the teen years. Girls generally start this growth spurt earlier than boys. MyPyramid can direct meal planning. Common nutritional problems in these years arise from poor food choices and include inadequate calcium intake in girls, iron deficiency anemia, and sometimes excessive intake of total fat, saturated fat, and *trans* fat. Because changes occur so rapidly during these years, and in so many areas—psychological, social, and physical—it may be difficult to stress the importance of nutrition to teenagers. Moderation in fat and sugar intake are important goals to consider when choosing snacks.

Summary

1. Growth is very rapid during infancy; birth weight doubles in 4 to 6 months, and length increases by 50% in the first year. An adequate diet, especially in terms of energy as well as the nutrients protein and zinc, is essential to support normal growth. Undernutrition can cause irreversible changes in growth and development. Growth in infants and children can be assessed by measuring body weight, height (or length), and head circumference over time. Growth charts have recently been revised to include a more valid measurement for determining children's growth: body mass index (BMI).

2. Nutrient needs in the first 6 months can be met by human milk or iron-fortified infant formula. Supplementary vitamin D is needed in the first 6 months for breastfed infants, and some infants may need supplemental iron or fluoride after 6 months of age.

3. Infant formulas generally contain lactose or sucrose, heat-treated proteins from cow's milk, and vegetable oil. These formulas may or may not be fortified with iron. Sanitation is very important when preparing and storing formula.

4. Most infants don't need solid foods before 6 months of age. Solid food should not be added to an infant's diet until the nutrients are needed, the GI tract can digest complex foods, the infant has the physical ability to control tongue thrusting, and the risk of developing food allergies has decreased.

5. The first solid food given should be iron-fortified infant cereals or ground meats. Other single foods can be added gradually, at the rate of about one each week. Some foods to avoid giving infants in the first year include honey, cow's milk (especially fat-reduced varieties), very salty or sweet foods, and foods that may cause choking.

6. Introducing iron-containing solid food at the appropriate time and not offering cow's milk until 1 year of age can generally prevent iron deficiency anemia in late infancy.

7. A slower growth rate in preschool years underlies the importance of children's eating nutrient-dense foods and reducing their food serving sizes. Choosing iron-rich foods, such as lean red meats, is important at this age. Portion sizes of 1 tablespoon of each food for each year of life is a good starting point for vegetables, fruits, and meats.

8. Preschoolers should be given some leeway in determining serving size and should be encouraged to try new foods. Highly restrictive diets designed to reduce the risk of cardiovascular disease or hypertension are not recommended for preschoolers or older children unless prescribed by a physician.

9. Obese children and adolescents are more likely to become obese adults and, so, incur greater health risks such as type 2 diabetes. Parents can provide healthful food choices, and children should control portion sizes. When controlled early through diet and exercise interventions, the problem of obesity may correct itself as the child continues to grow in height.

10. During the adolescent growth spurt, both boys and girls have increased needs for iron and calcium. Inadequate calcium intake by teenage girls is a major concern because it can set the stage for the development of osteoporosis later in life. Teenagers generally should moderate their intake of high-fat and sugar-rich foods—especially snacks and fast food, which they often consume in abundance—and should perform regular physical activity.

Study Questions

1. List two factors that limit "catch-up" growth in adulthood when a nutrient-deficient diet has been consumed throughout childhood.

2. Describe how you would assess whether an 8-month-old infant is consuming a healthful diet.

3. Outline three key factors that help determine when to introduce solid foods into an infant's diet.

4. A 3-month-old infant is taken to a clinic with failure to thrive. What are two possible explanations?

5. List three reasons why preschoolers are noted for "picky" eating. For each, describe an appropriate parent response.

6. What three factors are likely to contribute to obesity in a typical 10-year-old child?

7. Compare the guidelines for infant feeding summarized in the chapter with the *2005 Dietary Guidelines for Americans* for children over 2 and adults discussed in Chapter 2. Which guidelines are similar? Do any contradict each other? If so, why?

8. Describe three pros and cons of snacking. What is the basic advice for healthful snacking from childhood through the teenage years?

9. Which two nutrients are of particular concern in planning diets for teenagers? Why does each deserve to be singled out?

10. List three nutrients of concern for a teenage vegetarian.

BOOST YOUR STUDY

Check out the *Perspectives in Nutrition: Online Learning Center* www.mhhe.com/wardlawpers7 for quizzes, flash cards, activities, and web links designed to further help you learn about nutrition for infants and adolescents.

Annotated References

1. ADA Reports: Position of the American Dietetic Association: Dietary guidance for healthy children ages 2 to 11 years. *Journal of the American Dietetic Association* 104:660, 2004.

   MyPyramid combined with the Dietary Guidelines for Americans provide an appropriate blueprint for feeding children. Diets of many children are not following this advice and in turn are contributing to the nutritional problems that are common in childhood and later adulthood.

2. Affenito SG and others: Breakfast consumption by African-American and white adolescent girls correlates positively with calcium and fiber intake and negatively with body mass index. *Journal of the American Dietetic Association* 105:938, 2005.

   Eating breakfast on a regular basis contributes to the overall health of adolescent girls in this study. Breakfast helps girls meet calcium and fiber needs while it also contributes to weight control.

3. AHA Scientific Statement: American Heart Association guidelines for primary prevention of atherosclerotic cardiovascular disease beginning in childhood. *Circulation* 107:1562, 2003.

   It is clear that cardiovascular disease begins in childhood. A healthy diet, regular physical activity, and not smoking are three key ways to forestall the development of cardiovascular disease beginning in childhood. After age 2 it is important to limit saturated fat, trans fat, and cholesterol intake, while especially emphasizing intake of fruits, vegetables, and whole-grain breads and cereals. Rich protein sources such as dairy products, lean meats, fish, and legumes (beans) also deserve attention.

4. Bounds W and others: The relationship of dietary and lifestyle factors to bone mineral indexes in children. *Journal of the American Dietetic Association* 105:735, 2005.

   A primary influence on healthy bone mass parameters in this study was a nutritious diet ample in protein, calcium, phosphorus, vitamin K, magnesium, zinc, energy, and iron. Height and weight were also positively correlated to bone status.

5. Butte N and others: The Start Healthy Feeding Guidelines for Infants and Toddlers. *Journal of the American Dietetic Association* 104:442, 2004.

   Comprehensive guide to the what, when, and how of infant and toddler feeding. A colorful and informative guide to the timing of feeding skills and solid food introduction is included. The general guideline is to introduce solid foods to infants at 6 months of age.

6. Douglas KM and others: A practical guide to infant health. *American Family Physician* 70:2113, 2004.

   If an infant's diet does not provide fluoride (e.g., formula is not mixed with fluoridated water), fluoride should be given after 6 months of age. This article outlines proper and safe instructions. The authors do not recommend fluoride therapy for breastfed infants.

7. Fitch C: Preventing iron deficiency in infants and toddlers. *Today's Dietitian*, p. 32, December 2004.

   The author stresses the need to prevent iron deficiency in infants and toddlers. After 4 to 6 months of age it is important to have a rich source of iron in an infant's diet, such as iron-fortified cereals. Any infant formula used should be iron fortified. Prevention of iron deficiency in toddlers includes limiting cow's milk to 3 cups per day, because it is a poor source of iron.

8. Hatun S and others: Vitamin D deficiency in early infancy. *Journal of Nutrition* 135:279, 2005.

   Prevention of vitamin D deficiencies in infants is essential. The article recommends supplementing the diet of all breastfed infants with vitamin D soon after birth.

9. Hellekson K: Report on the diagnosis, evaluation, and treatment of high blood pressure in children and adolescents. *American Family Physician* 71:1014, 2005.

   Screening for high blood pressure is an important part of regular checkups of children by the child's physician. The latest recommendations for treating high blood pressure if found include a diet rich in vegetables, fruit, and low-fat dairy products; low in salt; and moderate in high-calorie foods and drinks. Regular physical activity is also important, as is weight loss if needed.

10. Kirk S and others: Pediatric obesity epidemic: Treatment options. *Journal of the American Dietetic Association* 105:S44, 2005.

    Reducing energy intake and increasing energy expenditure are important for treating pediatric obesity. Medications and obesity-related surgery may also be employed. The authors stress the importance of involving the family to create a supportive environment as part of the overall therapeutic approach.

11. Kleinmam RE (ed.): *Pediatric nutrition handbook.* Chicago, IL: American Academy of Pediatrics, 2004.

    This book is a comprehensive review of issues surrounding pediatric nutrition. This reference was frequently consulted in the revision of this chapter.

12. Kline DA: Food allergy symptoms and causes. *Today's Dietitian*, p. 10, August 2005.

    This article is an excellent review of the causes and consequences of food allergies. It is often a challenge to help people still follow a balance diet if they have food allergies. Learning how to read labels and substitute foods are two tools that ease such food planning.

13. Koplan JP and others: Preventing childhood obesity: Health in the balance—Executive Summary. *Journal of the American Dietetic Association* 105:131, 2005.

    Preventing childhood obesity involves a healthy eating pattern and regular physical activity. The goal should be achieving and maintaining a healthy body weight. The authors note that many social factors will have to be altered to facilitate this goal, such as providing more outlets for physical activity.

14. Kranz S and others: Dietary fiber intake by American preschoolers is associated with more nutrient-dense diets. *Journal of the American Dietetic Association* 105:221, 2005.

    Children in general would benefit from diets higher in fiber. Improving diet choices in general will allow for this change, including increases in whole grain, fruit, and vegetable content. The healthier the overall diet, the greater number of fiber-rich foods.

15. Lytle L: Nutritional issues for adolescents. *Journal of the American Dietetic Association* 102:S8, 2002.

    Data from large, population-based studies suggest that the typical adolescent's diet places them at increased risk for cardiovascular disease, cancer, osteoporosis, diabetes, and obesity in adulthood. The typical adolescent's diet contains too much total fat, saturated fat, sodium, and soft drinks, and not enough fruits, vegetables, fiber, and calcium.

16. Mrdjenovic G, Levitsky, DA: Nutritional and energetic consequences of sweetened drink consumption in 6- to 13-year-old children. *Journal of Pediatrics* 142:604, 2003.

    Children are not good at regulating overall energy intake in order to compensate for the increased energy coming from sweetened drinks. This lack of regulation results in excess energy intake and overall poor nutrition. Children should have restrictions on sweetened drinks at home and at school, and should be encouraged to drink more water.

17. Patrick H, Nicklas TA: A review of family and social determinants of children's eating patterns and diet quality. *Journal of the American College of Nutrition* 24(2):83, 2005.

    Physical environment has a big influence on the quality of the diets of children as does the influence of the parents. To improve the diets of children, many parameters must be addressed: child, parents, school, and community.

18. Rajeshwari R and others: Longitudinal changes in intake and food sources of calcium from childhood to young adulthood: The Bogalusa Heart Study. *Journal of the American College of Nutrition* 23(4):341, 2005.

Many children are not meeting their calcium needs. Despite a gradual increase in energy intake as children age, calcium intake does not generally increase appreciably. Overall, a greater focus on calcium-rich food choice needs to be made in this age group.

19. Strong WB and others: Evidence-based physical activity for school-age youth. *Journal of Pediatrics* 146:732, 1995.

The authors conclude that school-age children should participate in at least 60 minutes of developmentally appropriate, moderate-to-vigorous physical activity every day. This activity would lead to better weight control, lower blood pressure, and improved muscular health and aerobic fitness.

20. Yoo S and others: Comparison of dietary intakes associated with metabolic syndrome risk factors in young adults: The Bogalusa Heart Study. *American Journal of Clinical Nutrition* 80:841, 2004.

Low fruit and vegetable intake and high sweetened beverage consumption were associated with the metabolic syndrome in this study. Low-fat milk and milk products were found to be protective.

Take | Action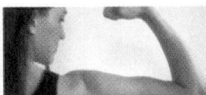

I. Getting Young Bill to Eat

Bill is 3 years old, and his mother is worried about his eating habits. He absolutely refuses to eat vegetables, meat, and dinner in general. Some days he eats very little food. He wants to eat snacks most of the time. His mother wants him to eat a sit down lunch and dinner to make sure he gets all the nutrients he needs. Mealtime is a battle because Bill says he isn't hungry, but his mother wants him to eat everything served on his plate. He drinks five or six glasses of whole milk per day because that is the one food he likes.

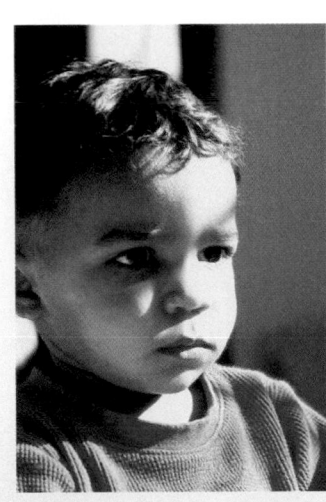

When his mother prepares dinner, she makes plenty of vegetables, boiling them until they are soft, hoping this will appeal to Bill. Bill's dad waits to eat his vegetables last, regularly telling the family that he eats them only because he has to. He also regularly complains about how dinner has been prepared. Bill saves his vegetables until last and usually gags when his mother orders him to eat them. Bill has been known to sit at the dinner table for an hour until the war of wills ends. Bill's mother serves casseroles and stews regularly because they are convenient. Bill likes to eat breakfast cereal, fruit, and cheese and regularly requests these foods for snacks. However, his mother tries to deny his requests so that he will have an appetite for dinner. Bill's mother comes to you and asks you what she should do to get Bill to eat.

Analysis

1   List four mistakes Bill's parents are making that contribute to Bill's poor eating habits.

_____

_____

_____

2. List four strategies they might try to promote good eating habits for Bill.

_____

_____

_____

_____

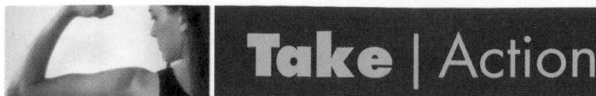

Take | Action

II. Evaluating a Teen Lunch

The following are two typical teen lunches and nutritional information for each:

	Meal 1	Meal 2	
	Cheese pizza, 2 pieces Milk chocolate candy bar, 1 Cola, 20 oz	Large hamburger sandwich with condiments, 1 large French fries, 30 Cola, 20 oz	
	Meal 1	**Meal 2**	**Nutrient Needs for Teens**
Energy (kcal)	990	1000	Males: 3000 Females: 2200
Protein	32	20	Males: 59 Females: 44
Vitamin C (mg)	5	18	Both genders: 45 to 75
Vitamin A (µg RAE)	300	10	Males: 900 Females: 700
Iron (mg)	3	4	Males: 11 Females: 15
Calcium (mg)	545	100	Both genders: 1300

1. Keeping in mind that meals should meet about one-third of nutrient needs, what are the shortcomings and excesses of these meals (i.e., given the nutritional information, compare these meals with one-third the RDA for protein, vitamin C, vitamin A, and iron and the Adequate Intake for calcium)?

   _____

   _____

   _____

2. How would you change these meals to improve balance and to meet the nutrient needs above? (Hint: Use your NutritionCalc Plus software program or Appendix N.)

   _____

   _____

   _____

3. Reflect on your food choices as a teenager. Do you think your meal choices were balanced and varied? Why or why not? What could you have done to improve your nutritional habits at that time?

   _____

   _____

   _____

NUTRITION DURING ADULTHOOD

CHAPTER OUTLINE

CASE SCENARIO:

Frances is a 78-year-old woman who suffers from macular degeneration, osteoporosis, and arthritis. Since her husband died a year ago, she has moved from their family house to a small one-bedroom apartment. Her eyesight is progressively getting worse, making it hard to go to the grocery store or even to cook (for fear of burning herself). She is often lonely; her only son lives 1 hour away and works two jobs, but he visits her as often as he can. Frances has lost her appetite and, as a result, often skips meals during the week. She has resorted to eating mostly cold foods, which are simple to prepare but are seriously limiting variety and palatability in her diet. She is slowly losing weight as a result of her dietary changes and loss of appetite.

Her typical diet usually consists of a breakfast that may include 1 slice of wheat toast with margarine, honey, and cinnamon, and 1 cup of hot tea. If she has lunch, she normally has 1/2 can of peaches, half of a turkey and cheese sandwich, and 1/2 glass of water. For dinner, she might have half of a tuna fish sandwich made with mayonnaise and 1 cup of iced tea. She usually includes one or two cookies at bedtime.

What are the potential consequences of such a poor dietary pattern? What services are available that could help Frances improve her diet and possibly increase her appetite? What other convenience foods could be included in her diet to make it more healthful and more varied?

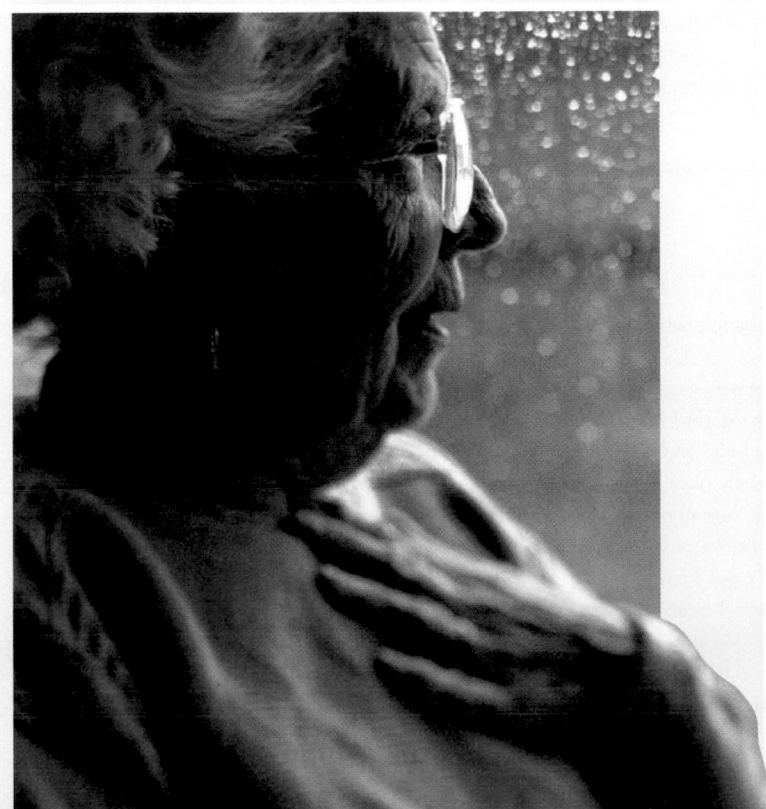

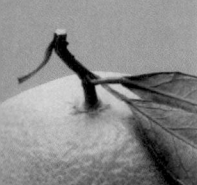

E ating is one of our great pleasures. Guided by common sense and moderation, eating well is also a means to good health. Most of us want a long, productive life, free of illness, yet many people from early middle age onward suffer from obesity, cardiovascular disease, hypertension and strokes, type 2 diabetes, osteoporosis, and other chronic diseases.[1] We can slow the development of, and in some cases even prevent, these diseases by consuming a diet that works against them. The effect of such a diet is most profitable if we begin early and continue throughout adulthood. We serve ourselves best—as individuals and as a nation—by striving to maintain vitality even in the later decades of life. This concept was first explored in Chapter 1 and is discussed again in this chapter, along with the special nutrition needs of older persons.

Keep in mind that present day-to-day health practices can significantly influence health during later life. Although genetics does play a role, as discussed in Chapter 1, many of the health problems that occur with age are not inevitable; they result from diet-related disease processes that influence physical health. Much can be learned from healthy older people whose attention to a healthy diet and physical activity—along with a little luck— keeps them active and vibrant well beyond typical retirement years.[15,18] Successful aging is the goal. Age quickly or slowly— it is partly your choice.

CHAPTER OBJECTIVES CHAPTER 18 IS DESIGNED TO ALLOW YOU TO:

1. Identify how the basic concepts that underlie the *2005 Dietary Guidelines for Americans* relate to adult health.
2. List possible causes of aging.
3. Explain how aging affects nutritional status.
4. List the potential benefits and risks associated with the use of various complementary and alternative medicine practices.
5. Discuss how nutrient needs change as individuals get older.
6. Make recommendations for dietary changes in the prevention and treatment of nutritional problems in older adults.
7. Describe community nutrition services for older persons.

REFRESH YOUR MEMORY AS YOU BEGIN YOUR STUDY OF ADULT NUTRITION ISSUES IN CHAPTER 18, YOU MAY WANT TO REVIEW:

- The effect of genetics on health in Chapter 1.
- Implications of the 1994 Dietary Supplement Health and Education Act in Chapter 1.
- The various body systems in Chapter 3 and Appendix C.
- The sources of fiber in Chapter 5.
- Guidelines for alcohol intake in Chapter 8.
- The dietary sources of vitamin D, the various B-vitamins, and calcium in Chapters 9, 10, and 11, respectively.
- Definition of healthy body weight in Chapter 13.
- The benefits of regular physical activity in Chapter 14.

B esides having other long-lived family members, people who live to 100 years generally:

- Do not smoke or do not drink heavily
- Gain little weight in adulthood
- Eat many fruits and vegetables
- Perform daily physical activity
- Challenge their minds
- Have a positive outlook
- Maintain close friendships
- Are (or were) married (especially true for men)
- Have blood lipoproteins with a large particle size

▌ Nutrition and Adulthood: An Introduction

Health-conscious adults in North America today are typically doing what is within their control to achieve a healthy lifestyle, such as consuming a healthful diet, maintaining a healthy body weight, and following a regimen of regular physical activity. Coupled with avoidance of tobacco products; limitation of or adaptation to stress; adequate sleep; adequate fluid intake; maintaining friendships and optimism; lifelong learning; keeping blood cholesterol, blood glucose, and blood pressure under control; and consultation with health-care professionals on a regular basis, these actions contribute to a healthful, long life.[15] Overall, the key to maximizing health throughout life is for people to establish harmony among their physical, mental, psychological, and social states (see Part 1 in the Take Action section at the end of this chapter).

Based on the needs for various nutrients set by the Food and Nutrition Board, the adult years can be divided into four stages: ages 19 to 30, 31 to 50, 51 to 70, and beyond 70 years of age. The two intervals encompassing ages 19 through 50 are young adulthood; 51 to 70 is middle adulthood; and beyond 70 years of age is older adulthood. Some examples of the dynamic in the nutrition needs of aging are:

- *Calcium*. Needs for this bone-related mineral increase after age 50 for males and females to help counter the harmful effects of accelerated bone loss.
- *Vitamin B-12*. People over the age of 50 should consume foods fortified with vitamin B-12 or take a balanced multivitamin and mineral supplement containing vitamin B-12. Recall from Chapter 10 that about 10 to 30% of older people may have decreased absorption of food-bound vitamin B-12 in part because of reduced acid production by the stomach.
- *Vitamin D*. Compared to the amount of vitamin D needed by individuals of ages 19 to 50, needs increase by 50% for the 51 to 70 age group. Adults over age 70 need *three times more* vitamin D than they did when they were ages 19 to 50. Attention to these differing needs for vitamin D is especially important for people who do not receive regular sun exposure, such as those residing the winter months in the northern United States or Canada. Experts recommend that these older adults be checked yearly for vitamin D status (i.e., be measured for 25-OH vitamin D in the blood).

Overall, attention to healthy nutrition and lifestyle habits is important at all ages.[1] Providing dietary advice for adults ages 19 to 50 years is the focus of the beginning of Chapter 18; the chapter will then look at additional recommendations for adults 51 and older.

As we age, our nutrient needs change. For example, vitamin D needs are higher for persons in older stages of adulthood.

Compression of Morbidity

Although most of us wish for long life, we do not like the thought of failing health in old age. And rightly so! Rather than suffer the ravages of cardiovascular disease, obesity, diabetes, osteoporosis, and other chronic diseases from age 40 to 60 years until death, we should strive to be as free of disease as possible and enjoy vitality throughout even our last decade.[15] **Life expectancy** is at a record high of about 77 years for the general population in North America today, although the span of healthy life is only about 65 years. Thus, an important focus here is not necessarily on living longer but on living healthier.

Striving to have the greatest number of healthy years and the fewest years of illness is often referred to as **compression of morbidity.** In other words, a person tries to compress significant sickness related to aging into the last few years—or months—of life. An example of this concept is illustrated for cardiovascular disease in Figure 18-1. Of the three lines shown, the line on the top depicts rapid deterioration in health; symptoms of cardiovascular disease appear by about age 40, and death occurs at about age 60. In addition, between the ages of 40 and 60 years, symptoms of the disease, and therefore disability, are present.

A healthier lifestyle follows the middle line in Figure 18-1. Here, cardiovascular disease is postponed so that the first symptoms are not apparent until age 60; severe symptoms occur at age 80, with death following a few years later. The line on the bottom is ideal. Disease progresses so slowly that symptoms do not appear during a person's lifetime; therefore, the disease process never hampers activities.

Body cells age no matter what health practices we follow. However, to a considerable extent, you can choose how quickly you age throughout your adult years. In light of the many studies showing the ability even to reverse atherosclerosis, we can say that the rate at which you age is partly your choice.[1]

Although there is little doubt of the benefits of a healthy lifestyle, scientists have also found a strong genetic component to longevity as well as to certain diseases (review Chapter 1). Studies of families, and of twins in particular, provide some support for a genetic contribution to human longevity.

life expectancy The average length of life for a given group of people (usually determined by the year of birth).

compression of morbidity The delay of the onset of disabilities caused by chronic disease.

Keep in mind that extending life without delaying onset of chronic disease prolongs suffering in many cases. In addition, the greater number of disabled years is very costly to all North Americans. For these reasons, prolonging life without compressing the number of disabled years is called the "failure of success."

Figure 18-1 | Compression of morbidity. The goal is to postpone illness until the final days of life. Cardiovascular disease is used as an example. The line on the top shows rapid deterioration in health status, in which symptoms of cardiovascular disease appear by about age 40 and death occurs at about age 60. In addition, between the ages of 40 and 60 years, symptoms of cardiovascular disease—and therefore disability—are present. A healthier lifestyle follows the middle line pattern. Here, cardiovascular disease is postponed, so that the first symptoms are not apparent until age 60; severe symptoms occur at age 80, with death following a few years later. The line on the bottom is the ideal: the disease progresses so slowly that symptoms do not appear during the lifetime; therefore, the disease process never hampers life's activities.

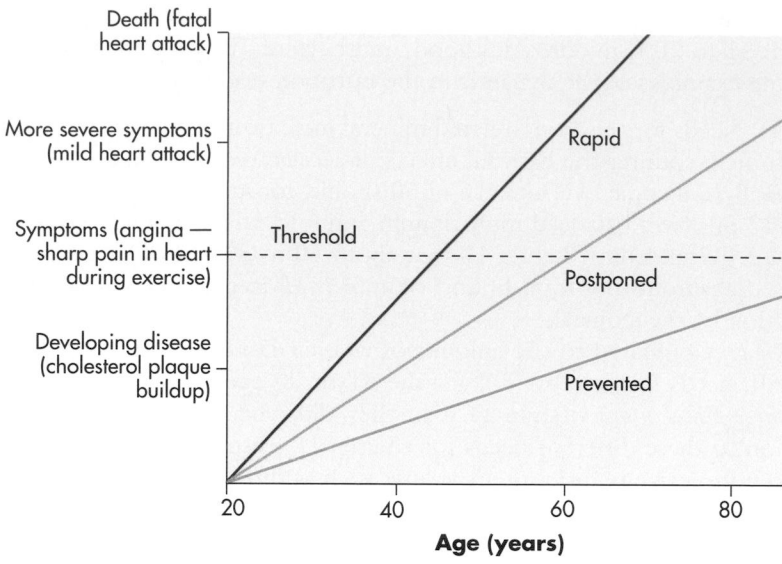

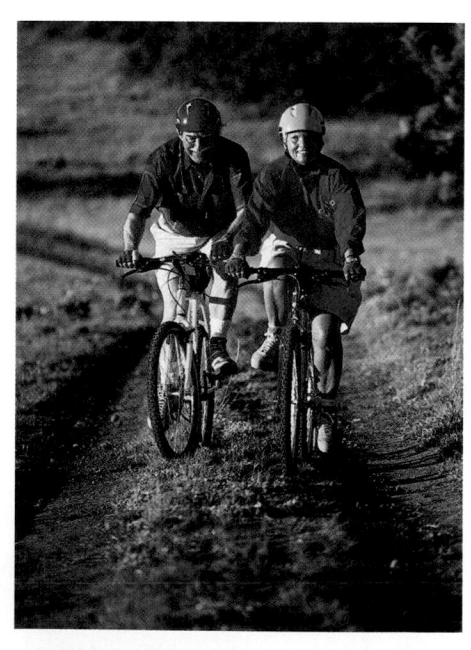

Many adults find that regular physical activity adds an important dimension to their lives. Men over 40 and women over 50 years of age should obtain physician approval before beginning a program of vigorous physical activity. This is especially important for people with evidence of cardiovascular disease, hypertension, or diabetes.

A Diet for the Adult Years

Long-term nutritional health in adulthood is best achieved by following a healthy diet. One blueprint for a healthy diet comes from the *2005 Dietary Guidelines for Americans,* discussed in Chapter 2. Its advice refers to people age 2 years and older and can be summarized into three main points.

1. Consume a variety of nutrient-dense foods and beverages within and among the basic food groups of MyPyramid, while choosing foods that limit the intake of saturated and *trans* fats, cholesterol, added sugars, salt, and alcohol (if used). Foods to emphasize are vegetables, fruits, legumes (beans), whole-grain breads and cereals, and fat-free or low-fat milk or equivalent milk products.
2. Maintain body weight in a healthy range by balancing energy intake from foods and beverages with energy expended. For the latter, engage in at least 30 minutes of moderate-intensity physical activity, above usual activity, at work or home on most days of the week.
3. Practice safe food handling when preparing food. Clean hands, food contact surfaces, and fruits and vegetables before preparation, and cook foods to a safe temperature to kill microorganisms.

You may wonder if, in general, adults in North America are trying to follow many of these recommendations. Since the mid-1950s, they have consumed less saturated fat as more people substitute fat-free and low-fat milk for cream and whole milk. They eat more cheese, however, which is usually a concentrated form of saturated fat. Since 1963, they have eaten less butter, fewer eggs, less animal fat, and more vegetable oils and fish. These changes generally follow the recommendations to reduce the intake of saturated fat and cholesterol in favor of unsaturated fat choices. Today, animal breeders are raising much leaner cattle and hogs than those produced in 1950, which also helps reduce saturated fat intake.

Other aspects of the average adult diet are less promising. The latest nutrition survey of eating habits in the United States shows that the major contributors to energy intake for the average adult diet are sugared soft drinks, white bread, beef, doughnuts, cakes and cookies, whole milk, chicken, cheese, alcoholic beverages, salad dressing, mayonnaise, potatoes, and sugars/syrups/jams. If the trend in diets were truly toward decreasing sugar and saturated fat intake and increasing fiber intake, many of these foods would not appear at the top of the list.

The overriding consideration should be quality and length of life and the impact that dietary changes might have on them. [15,18,20] Adults in general should learn more about risk factors for chronic diseases and do something about each one, when possible.[1]

Concept | Check

A basic plan to promote health and prevent disease includes eating a healthy diet. More specifically, the *2005 Dietary Guidelines for Americans* directs people to eat a variety of foods; maintain healthy weight; choose a diet low in saturated fat and cholesterol and *trans* fat; choose a diet with plenty of vegetables, fruits, legumes (beans), and whole-grain products; use sugars and salt sparingly; and drink little or no alcohol.

Appendix D reviews diet planning guidelines issued by the Canadian government for Canadians. In addition, Chapter 1 discussed *Healthy People 2010*, a U.S. federal agenda aimed at disease prevention and health promotion.

A Closer Look at Middle and Older Adulthood

How long do your family members generally live? Of those who died early in adulthood, can you pinpoint some causes? Do you plan to live longer than your parents did or will? How long will that be? Some basic statistics can help you predict this.

Life Span

Life span refers to the maximum number of years a human can live. As far as we know, life span hasn't changed in recorded time. The longest human life documented to date is 122 years for a woman and 114 years for a man. Genes play a key role in determining longevity, but environment is also important. Note also by comparison that the domestic dog has a life span of 20 years; a rat, 5 years.

life span The potential oldest age a person can reach.

Life Expectancy

Life expectancy is the time an average person born in a specific year, such as 2005, can expect to live. Currently, life expectancy in North America is about 75 years for men and about 80 years for women, with a span of "healthy years" of about 64. Furthermore, if you survive to the age of 80, you can tack on another 7 to 10 years of life expectancy.

Life expectancy hasn't always been this long; for primitive humans, it was about 20 to 35 years. It increased to 40 years in Medieval England and increased to 49 years by the turn of the twentieth century. During the last 80 years, life expectancy for nearly all people has increased, mainly because of changes in the principal causes of death.

In the early 1900s, infectious diseases were the first three causes of death. Vaccines and antibiotics have tremendously lowered the rate of death from these causes. The decline in infant and childhood deaths, coupled with better diets and health care, has allowed more people to age first into maturity and then into older years. Now the principal causes of death in Western societies are related to cardiovascular diseases and cancer diseases that typically surface in middle age (review Table 1-1).

Historically, the trend in the United States, Canada, and other developed nations has been toward an ever older population. For example, during Colonial times, half the U.S. population was over 16 years of age. By 1990, half were over 33. By 2050, half the U.S. population could be over 43, and approximately 20% will be 65 years and older, twice as many as reach 65 today. This age—65 years—is arbitrarily listed as a dividing line for the beginning of later life because at this age a person can currently qualify for full Social Security benefits in the United States. The time at which old age occurs, however, varies for each person according to health and independence.

Among the older population, the group constituting those age 85 years and over is the fastest growing segment. Between 1997 and 2050, the number of people age 85 years and over in the United States is expected to increase from 3.4 million to 19 million. This is

life expectancy The average length of life for a given group of people (usually determined by the year of birth).

Worldwide, the highest average life expectancy is in Japan, 82 years for women and 76 years for men, especially on the island of Okinawa. Researchers suggest that their traditional Okinawan diet based on rice, fish, vegetable protein sources, fruits, vegetables, tea, herbs for seasonings, and small amounts of meat, as well as a generally low energy intake (BMI remains ≈ 21), contributes to this record longevity. Alcohol and salt intake is also minimal.

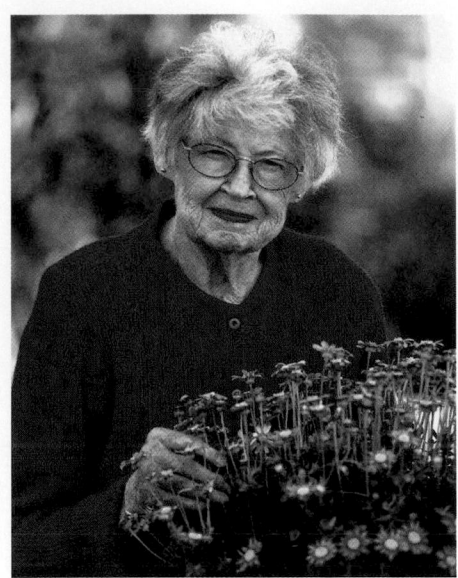

Of all North Americans who have lived to age 65, more than half are now alive.

the first time in history that North America and other Western nations will need to accommodate such a large population of older people. The associated expense will be enormous if a large percentage need special care because of ill health. Even more amazing, 1 million or more people in the United States alone could be over 100 years old in 2050.

The Graying of North America

This "graying" of North America poses some problems. Today, although people older than age 65 account for 13% of the U.S. population, they account for more than 25% of all prescription medications used, 40% of acute care hospital stays, and 50% of the federal health budget. Hip fractures alone cost the nation about $12 billion per year. (Note that regular physical activity reduces such risk.) Of older persons, 65% or more have nutrition-related problems such as cardiovascular disease, type 2 diabetes, hypertension, and osteoporosis.

Postponing these chronic diseases for as long as possible will help people control health-care costs. The more independent, healthy years people live, the better life can be for them and the less they burden the health-care system, which will be increasingly burdened by a growing elderly population. Keep in mind that aging is not a disease. Furthermore, diseases that commonly accompany old age—osteoporosis and atherosclerosis, for example—are not an inevitable part of aging. Many can be prevented or managed. Some people do die of old age, not as a direct result of disease.

The Definition of Aging

One view of aging describes it as processes of slow cell death, beginning soon after fertilization. When we are young, aging is not apparent because the major metabolic activities are geared toward growth and maturation. We produce plenty of active cells to meet physiological needs. During late adolescence and adulthood, the body's major task is to maintain cells. Inevitably, though, cells age and die. Eventually, as more cells die, the body can't adjust to meet all physiological demands, and body functioning begins to decrease (Figure 18-2). Still, organs usually retain enough **reserve capacity** that, for a long time, the body shows no outward disease. Although no symptoms appear, subclinical disease may develop, and if the disease is allowed to progress unchecked, organ function and then body function eventually deteriorate noticeably.

The aging process is clearly illustrated by changes for many people in the function of the enzyme lactase. For some people, lactase activity in the small intestine slows dur-

reserve capacity The extent to which an organ can preserve essentially normal function despite decreasing cell number or cell activity.

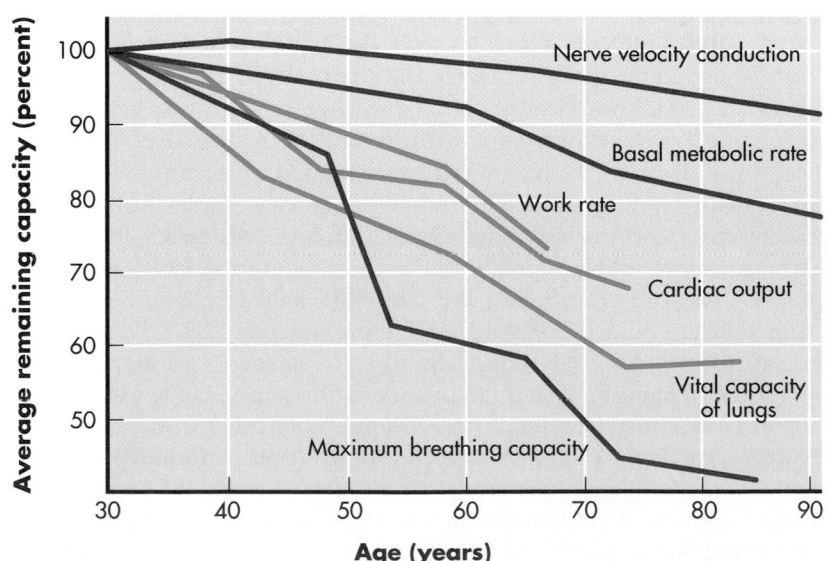

Figure 18-2 | Declines in physiological function seen with aging. The decline in many body functions is especially evident in sedentary people.

ing childhood. Generally, however, clear symptoms of this decline—gas and bloating after milk consumption—do not appear until adulthood. Although lactase output decreases in these cases, perhaps from birth, enough enzyme is present to digest the lactose consumed until adulthood.

Cells age probably because of automatic cellular changes and environmental influences. Even in the most supportive of environments, cell structure and function inevitably change with time. Eventually, cells lose their ability to regenerate the internal parts they need, and they die. This inevitable dying off of deteriorating cells is actually beneficial; researchers have concluded that it likely prevents diseases such as cancer.

Unfortunately, there are negative consequences to this natural cell progression, because as more and more cells in an organ system die, organ function decreases. For example, **kidney nephrons** are continually lost as we age. In some people, this loss leads to eventual kidney failure, but most of us maintain sufficient kidney cells to allow the organ to function throughout life. Again, in aging, there is first a reduction in reserve capacity. Only after the reserve capacity is exhausted does actual organ function noticeably decrease.

The causes of aging are still a mystery. Most likely, the physiological changes of aging are the sum of natural processes, as listed in Table 18-1, and lifestyle practices.[8,10,15,16,18,19,20]

Adopting diet and lifestyle practices that minimize a decline in body function in the adult years is an investment in your future health.[1] You can obtain a free fact sheet from the website for the National Institute on Aging at www.nia.nih.gov or by calling (800) 222-2225. The first Take Action activity in this chapter outlines a comprehensive approach to healthful aging.

Concept | Check

Although life span has not changed, life expectancy has increased dramatically over the past century. An increasing proportion of the North American population is over 65 years of age and will live for decades longer. Avoiding continually rising health-care costs and maximizing satisfaction with life require postponing and minimizing chronic illness. Aging begins early in life and probably results from both automatic cellular changes and environmental influences. A healthy diet can play a role in slowing such processes.

▌Nutritional Implications of Aging

There is more variation in health status among adults over age 50 than in any other age group. This means that chronological age is not useful in predicting physical health status (physiological age). Among people age 70 and over, some are totally independent, healthy people, whereas others are frail and require almost total care. To predict the nutritional problems of an older person, it is necessary to know the extent of physiological change caused by aging and whether the person shows early warning signs for long-term poor nutrition. As you examine how aging affects body systems and how these changes contribute to nutritional health, note the suggested ways to lessen health risks (Table 18-2).

Decreased Appetite and Food Intake

Decreases in body weight are common in adults age 70 and older who may not eat enough to meet energy needs. This phenomenon is a problem for older people in particular because it increases the risk of nutrition-related illness.[9]

Many causes of inadequate food intake in older people are possible. Researchers suggest that biological origins, such as changes in neuroendocrine factors that influence feeding, account for some of this decline (review Chapter 13 for a list of these factors). When older men are underfed in experiments, they do not later increase food

Critical | Thinking

The "fountain of youth" remains a mystery. Many people believe a source exists that can stop the aging process, allowing youth to remain. However, Neil, a history student, asserts that the fountain of youth is not a place or a particular thing but, rather, a combination of diet and lifestyle. How can he justify this claim?

kidney nephrons The units of kidney cells that filter wastes from the bloodstream and deposit them into the urine.

Pharmaceutical companies have begun to market liquid meal-replacement formulas to older adults. Previously, these products were primarily used in hospitals and nursing homes. Many of these products have an unusual taste because of the vitamins and types of proteins that have been added. Older adults can decide if the convenience, cost, and taste make this a wise diet choice.

ven very healthy people have a shortened life expectancy if they are exposed to sufficient environmental stress, such as radiation and certain chemical agents (e.g., industrial solvents). Because cell aging and diseases such as cancer are aggravated by environmental factors, it makes good sense to avoid such risks as excessive sunlight exposure and hazardous chemicals.

Critical | Thinking

Alexis has read several books supporting the idea that reducing one's typical energy intake by 30% can significantly extend one's life. Because she wants to do what is best for her two preschool children, she is thinking about adjusting her family's dietary habits to match this calorie restriction. What should you discuss with Alexis before she proceeds?

glycosylation The process by which glucose attaches to (glycates) other compounds, such as proteins.

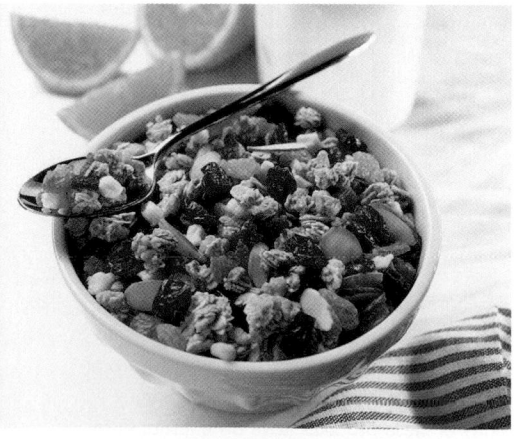

A daily serving of a whole-grain breakfast cereal provides a rich source of vitamins, minerals, and fiber and so contributes to healthy aging.

Table 18-1 | Current Hypotheses about the Causes of Aging

Errors occur in copying the genetic blueprint (DNA).

Once sufficient errors in DNA copying accumulate, a cell can no longer synthesize the major proteins needed to function, and it therefore dies. Damage to DNA in the mitochondria also contributes to the aging process.

Connective tissue stiffens.

Parallel protein strands, found mostly in connective tissue, cross-link to each other. This decreases flexibility in key body components.

Electron-seeking compounds damage cell parts.

Electron-seeking free radicals can break down cell membranes and proteins. The small amount of DNA in mitochondria typically shows this type of damage, and this damage is linked to the aging process. One way to prevent this free radical damage throughout the body is to consume adequate amounts of vitamin E, selenium, and carotenoids.

Hormone function changes.

The blood concentration of many hormones, such as testosterone in men, falls during the aging process. Replacement of this and other hormones is possible, but the resulting risks and benefits are largely unknown.

Glycosylation of proteins.

Blood glucose, when chronically elevated, attaches to (glycates) various blood and body proteins. This action decreases protein function and can encourage immune system attack on such altered proteins.

The immune system loses some efficiency.

The immune system is most efficient during childhood and young adulthood, but with advancing age it is less able to recognize and counteract foreign substances, such as viruses, that enter the body. Nutrient deficiencies, particularly of protein, vitamin E, vitamin B-6, and zinc, also hamper immune function.

Autoimmunity develops.

Autoimmune reactions occur when white blood cells and other immune system components begin to attack body tissues in addition to foreign proteins. Many diseases, including some forms of arthritis, involve this autoimmune response.

Death is programmed into the cell.

Each human cell can divide only about 50 times. Once this total number of divisions occurs, the cell automatically succumbs.

Excess energy intake speeds body breakdown.

Underfed animals, such as spiders, mice, and rats, live longer. Usual energy intake must be reduced by about 30% to see this effect. Currently this approach is the only proven way to substantially slow the aging process.

intake to compensate for reduced food consumption when given the opportunity. Changes in taste and smell may also be important, as are the effects of current medication use. In addition, social aspects play a role in reduced food intake. Many older people live alone, a circumstance that is associated with less food consumption.

To maintain health, older adults need to address the issue of declining weight. Significant weight loss in older people, sometimes termed the "dwindles," increases risk of death. It may also indicate ongoing illness and reduced tolerance to medication or simple withdrawal from life itself.[5,13] Even in apparently healthy older individuals,

Table 18-2 | Typical Physiological Changes of Aging and Recommended Diet and Lifestyle Responses

Physiological Changes	Recommended Responses	Physiological Changes	Recommended Responses
Appetite ⊕	• Monitor weight and strive to eat enough to maintain healthy weight. • Use meal replacement products, such as Boost and Ensure Plus.	Vision ⊕	• Regularly consume sources of carotenoids, vitamin C, vitamin E, and zinc (e.g., fruits, vegetables and whole-grain breads and cereals). • Moderate total fat intake. • Wear sunglasses in sunny conditions. • Avoid tobacco products. • Perform regular physical activity (to lessen insulin resistance). • In the case of diagnosed moderate macular degeneration, talk with a physician about following a protocol of zinc, copper, vitamin E, vitamin C, and beta-carotene supplementation.
Sense of taste and smell ⊕	• Vary the diet. • Experiment with herbs and spices.		
Chewing ability ⊕	• Work with a dentist to maximize chewing ability. • Modify food consistency as necessary. • Eat energy-rich snacks.		
Sense of thirst ⊕	• Consume plenty of fluid each day. • Stay alert for evidence of dehydration (e.g., minimal output or dark-colored urine). Note that dehydration can lead to many problems, especially in older adults.	Lean tissue ⊕	• Meet nutrient needs, especially protein and vitamin D. • Perform regular physical activity, including strength training.
Bowel function ⊕	• Consume enough fiber daily, choosing primarily fruits, vegetables, and whole-grain breads and cereals. • Meet fluid needs.	Cardiovascular function ⊕	• Use diet modifications or physician-prescribed medications to keep blood lipids and blood pressure within desirable ranges. • Stay physically active. • Achieve and maintain a healthy body weight.
Lactase production ⊕	• Limit milk serving size at each use. • Substitute yogurt or cheese for milk. • Use reduced-lactose or lactose-free products. • Seek nondairy calcium sources.	Bone mass ⊕	• Meet nutrient needs, especially calcium and vitamin D (regular sun exposure helps meet needs for vitamin D). • Perform regular physical activity, especially weight-bearing exercise. • Women should consider use of approved osteoporosis medications at menopause. • Remain at a healthy weight (especially avoid unneeded weight loss).
Iron status ⊕	• Include some lean meat and iron-fortified foods in the diet. • Ask physician to monitor blood iron status.		
Liver function ⊕	• Consume alcohol in moderation, if at all. • Avoid consuming excess vitamin A.		
Insulin function ⊕	• Maintain healthy body weight. • Perform regular physical activity. • Limit high glycemic load carbohydrates.	Mental function ⊕	• Meet nutrient needs, especially for vitamin E, vitamin C, vitamin B-6, folate, and vitamin B 12. • Strive for lifelong learning. • Perform regular physical activity. • Obtain adequate sleep.
Kidney function ⊕	• If necessary, work with physician and registered dietitian to modify protein and other nutrients in diet.		
Immune function ⊕	• Meet nutrient needs, especially protein, vitamin E, vitamin B-6, and zinc. • Perform regular physical activity.	Fat stores ⊕	• Avoid overeating. • Perform regular physical activity.
Lung function ⊕	• Avoid tobacco products. • Perform regular physical activity.		

Registered dietitians, physicians, and pharmacists can help with any needed adjustments arising from these problems.

successful weight maintenance may require an increased conscious control over food intake, compared to younger individuals. Adding more spices to food may also stimulate food intake. Consuming energy-dense snacks, such as cheese, nuts, yogurt, oatmeal cookies, and bananas, between meals is also a strategy. When assessing weight in older people, compare present weight with the previous year's weight.

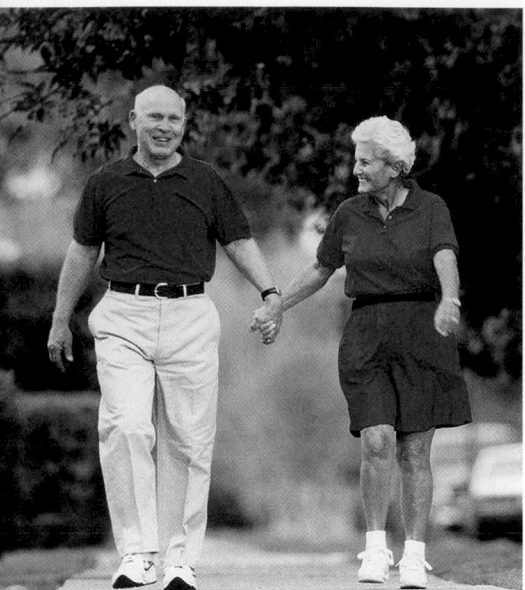

Age is no reason not to continue whatever physical activity is possible. Physical activity contributes to many aspects of good health, including improved functioning of the GI tract.

ostomy A surgically created short circuit in intestinal flow where the end point usually opens from the abdominal cavity rather than the anus, for example, a colostomy.

Incontinence, the inability to control the muscle responsible for retaining urine, affects up to 20% of older adults living at home and about 75% of those in nursing homes. The embarrassment of having to wear adult diapers causes many to avoid fluids (resulting in dehydration and constipation) and to become socially isolated.

Decline in Dental Health

About 30% or more older people in North America have lost all their teeth. Attention to dental hygiene and dental care throughout life greatly lessens this risk. Periodontal (gum) disease commonly causes tooth loss. Replacement dentures enable some people to chew normally, but many older adults—especially men—have denture problems. Solving individual dietary needs requires identifying foods that need to be modified in consistency.[9] When people have problems chewing, nutrient-dense snacks can help. Sometimes just allowing extra time for chewing and swallowing encourages more eating.

Reduced Thirst Sensation

Older adults often partially lose their sense of thirst and in turn don't drink enough fluids. They are then more likely to become dehydrated, a condition that leads to confusion and sometimes hospitalization.[9] In addition, 25% of fluid comes from food. If older adults are not eating enough food, they increase the risk of becoming dehydrated. It is important for older people to consume enough fluids, and if necessary, they should be monitored to ensure they do so.[1] About 9 cups (women) to 13 cups (men) of fluid daily is a good goal. This amount must be adjusted if diuretics are used or in certain other medical conditions, such as the presence of an **ostomy.** Some important signs of dehydration, other than confusion, include dry lips, sunken eyes, increased body temperature, decreased blood pressure, constipation, decreased urine output, and nausea.

Fall in Gastrointestinal Tract Function

The main intestinal problem for older people is constipation (review Chapter 3 for a review of this problem). To keep the intestinal tract performing efficiently, older people should meet fiber needs. The goal for adults over 50 years is 21 g/day for women and 30 g/day for men, unless a physician recommends otherwise. The regular consumption of nuts, fruits, vegetables, beans, and whole-grain breads and cereals provides enough fiber. Fiber medications are generally unnecessary but may be used if overall energy intake does not allow for enough fiber intake. Older persons should also drink more fluid to move along masses that could form from high fiber intake.[1] Physical activity likewise helps promote peristalsis. Because some medications can induce constipation, a physician should be consulted if constipation might be related to a medication. If mineral oil is taken as a laxative, it should always be used with caution—and not at mealtimes—because it binds fat-soluble vitamins and limits their absorption.

Lactase production frequently decreases with age. Chapter 5 listed several options for people with lactose malabsorption and intolerance.

The stomach slows its acid production as people age as well as the synthesis of intrinsic factor. These changes can contribute to poor absorption of vitamin B-12 and eventually to pernicious anemia. Adults age 51 years and older need to meet vitamin B-12 needs with foods or supplements fortified with synthetic vitamin B-12.

Reduced stomach acid production may also hamper iron absorption. Other conditions that affect the body's iron status in particular occur with the regular use of aspirin, which frequently causes blood loss in the stomach, and the use of antacids, which may bind iron. Ulcers and hemorrhoids can also cause blood loss. Careful attention to iron status is necessary in these cases.

Changes in Liver, Gallbladder, and Pancreatic Function

With age, the liver functions less efficiently. When there is a history of significant alcohol consumption, fat buildup in the liver accounts for some decline. Alcohol abuse is a problem among a small but significant group of older individuals who may continue this pattern from earlier in life or develop heavy drinking patterns and alcoholism later. Later development of this problem sometimes arises from the loneliness and social isolation of retirement or loss of a spouse. Alcohol-related sickness is high in older people, so the health consequences of this excess are considerable.[5] Also, older adults are more likely to take medications affected by alcohol intake. If cirrhosis develops, the liver functions even less efficiently, resulting in a reduced ability to detoxify many substances (review Chapter 8). The possibility for vitamin A toxicity in turn increases.

The gallbladder also functions less efficiently as we age. Gallstones may dam up the bile in the gallbladder, causing it to pool and back up into the liver. Gallstones can also interfere with fat digestion by allowing less bile into the small intestine. Obesity is a prime risk factor for gallbladder disease, especially in older women. A low-fat diet or surgery to remove the organ may be necessary for treatment.

Although the digestive function of the pancreas may decline with age, the pancreas has a large reserve capacity. One sign of a failing pancreas is high blood glucose, although this can occur as the result of several conditions. The pancreas may be secreting less insulin or cells may be resisting insulin action—especially muscle cells and, as well, adipose cells in obese people with upper-body fat storage. Another cause can be insufficient chromium intake. Where appropriate, improved nutrient intake, regular physical activity, and weight loss (when needed) can improve insulin action and blood glucose regulation.[1]

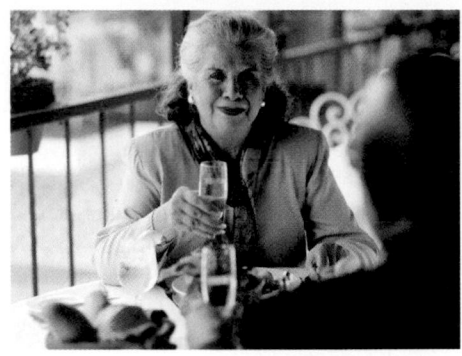

The limit for alcohol intake for older adults is one drink per day.

Decline in Kidney Function

Over time, the kidneys filter wastes more slowly as they lose nephrons (the functional filtration unit). The deterioration significantly decreases the kidneys' ability to excrete the products of protein breakdown, such as urea, and in turn typically requires a reduction in protein intake from habitual amounts to about the RDA or slightly below (0.6 g/kg of body weight).

Reduced Immune Function

With age the immune system often operates less efficiently. Consuming adequate protein, the full gamut of vitamins (especially enough vitamin E and vitamin B-6), and zinc helps maximize the health of the immune system. Recurrent sicknesses and poor wound healing are warning signs of a deficient diet, especially with regard to protein and zinc.[13] Eating too little food in general or too few animal proteins is usually the reason. Older people often eliminate meat from their diet because it's too hard to chew. If necessary, a balanced vitamin and mineral supplement can help bridge gaps in vitamin and mineral intake. On the other hand, overnutrition appears to be equally harmful to the immune system. For example, obesity and excessive fat, iron, and zinc intake can suppress immune function.

Reduced Lung Function

Lung efficiency declines somewhat with age and is especially pronounced in older people who have smoked and continue to smoke tobacco products. Breathing becomes shallower, faster, and more difficult as the amount of active lung tissue decreases. Smoking often leads to emphysema and lung cancer. The decrease in lung efficiency contributes to a general downward spiral in body function; breathing difficulties limit physical activity and endurance and frequently discourage eating.

Besides not smoking, being physically active helps prevent lung problems. People need not lose their capacity to breathe deeply as long as adequate aerobic activity is part of their regular routine.

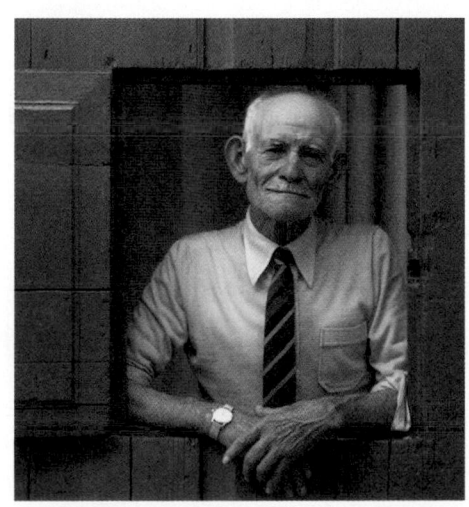

A diet based on vegetables, fruits, pasta, and olive oil as a source of fat—with a small amount of alcohol in the form of red wine—contributes to the many healthy years of life of southern Italians. Their active lifestyle is an additional contributing factor.

Reduced Hearing and Vision

Hearing and vision both decline with age. Hearing impairment occurs mainly in members of industrial societies with urban traffic, aircraft noise, and loud music. Older people may avoid social contacts because they can't hear.

A recent study discussed in Chapter 12 showed that megadose zinc supplements (80 mg/day of zinc oxide with 2 mg of copper oxide) reduced progression of moderate cases of macular degeneration. The zinc supplements worked even better when provided in combination with 400 IU of vitamin E, 500 mg of vitamin C, and 15 mg of beta-carotene. Adults who have evidence of macular degeneration and are considering this protocol should talk to their physician and eyecare specialist first because these supplements can also lead to health problems.

Declining eyesight, frequently caused by retina degeneration, can affect a person's ability to get to a grocery store, locate the foods desired, read labels for nutritional content, and prepare the foods at home. Macular degeneration, one form of failing eyesight in old age, is quite common, affecting about 1.75 million adults in the United States. A major risk factor is cigarette smoking—yet another reason to avoid the habit.

On a positive note, the regular consumption of foods rich in carotenoids—in particular, dark green, leafy vegetables, such as kale, collard greens, spinach, swiss chard, mustard greens, and romaine lettuce—may decrease the risk of developing this form of retina degeneration. These vegetables are rich in lutein and zeaxanthin, two carotenoids found in the portion of the eye subject to damage from age-related changes. Adequate zinc intake is also important. The risk of developing cataracts of the eye is decreased by following a diet rich in fruits and vegetables. Note that eventually such vision losses may make people afraid to socialize, be active, or take care of important routines of daily life, such as shopping.[10]

Decrease in Lean Tissue

Some muscle cells shrink and others are lost as muscles age; some muscles lose their elasticity as they accumulate fat and collagen protein. Lifestyle greatly determines the rate of muscle mass deterioration. As you might predict, an active lifestyle tends to maintain muscle mass, whereas an inactive one encourages its loss.

The loss of muscle mass leads to a decrease in basal metabolism, muscle strength, and energy needs. Furthermore, less muscle mass leads to lower physical activity, which makes the prognosis for maintaining muscle mass even worse. Clearly, it is best to avoid this vicious cycle. Just when all seems lost, though, note that the benefits of exercise are quite striking, especially after the age of 50. Ideally, an active lifestyle should include some resistance activity (weight training) throughout life (Table 18-3).[17]

Physical activity increases muscle strength and mobility, improves balance, eases daily tasks that require some strength, improves sleep, slows bone loss, and increases joint movement, thus reducing injuries. It also has a positive impact on a person's mental outlook.[12,16] However, when older adults stop their strength-training program, gains in muscle strength are quickly lost.

After obtaining a physician's approval to get started, older people can seek out programs to begin strength and aerobic training at community recreation centers or the local YMCA or YWCA. Cardiac rehabilitation centers are another possibility. Most of these organizations have qualified trainers who can help set up a program. Dumbbells are inexpensive and thus ideal for engaging in strength training at home.

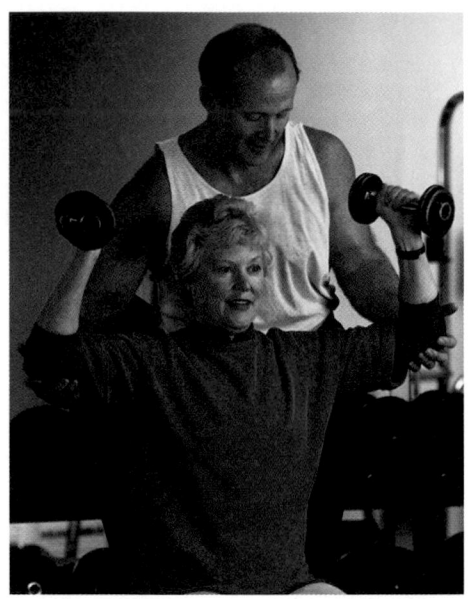

Older people benefit from both aerobic and strength-training exercises. Strength-training (resistance) activity especially helps reverse some of the decline in daily function associated with the muscle loss typically seen in older adulthood. Much of what we associate with old age is due to a lack of a lifetime of such physical activity.

Table 18-3 | Strength Training Recommendations for Older Adults

- Exercises should be performed at least two days per week.
- If weights are used, start with 1 to 2 lb and gradually increase this amount over time.
- Perform exercises that involve the major muscle groups (e.g., arms, shoulders, chest, abdomen, back, hips, and legs) and exercises that enhance grip strength.
- Perform 8 to 15 repetitions of each exercise, then perform a second set.
- Breathe during strength exercises.
- Rest between sets.
- Avoid locking joints in arms and legs.
- Stretch after completing all exercises.
- Stop exercising if pain begins.

Source: National Institute on Aging.

Increases in Fat Stores

As lean tissue decreases with age, the body often takes on more fat. Much of this increase results from overeating and minimal physical activity, although even athletic men and lean women typically gain some degree of midsection fat after the age of 50.

If obesity results, it can raise blood pressure and blood glucose and make walking and performing daily tasks more difficult. Although a small fat gain in adulthood may not compromise health, large gains are problematic.

Reduced Cardiovascular Health

The heart often pumps blood less efficiently in older people, usually because of insufficient physical activity. Poor heart conditioning allows fatty and connective tissues to infiltrate the heart's muscular wall. However, this decline in **cardiac output** is not inevitable with aging and does not occur among older people who remain physically active. In fact, it is thought that the inactive lifestyles of nearly 60% of North American adults may contribute as much to the risk for cardiovascular disease as does smoking a pack of cigarettes per day.[16]

cardiac output The amount of blood pumped by the heart.

Heart attack and stroke, two of the three major causes of death in adults, are caused primarily by atherosclerosis and hypertension. As we age, atherosclerotic plaque accumulates in the arteries, reducing their elasticity, constricting blood flow, and consequently elevating blood pressure.

You already know the main way to limit the buildup of atherosclerotic plaque: keep LDL-cholesterol and the total cholesterol/HDL-cholesterol ratio in the desirable range (review Chapter 6). New evidence shows that a diet very low in fat can cause some plaques to decrease in size. Other studies use diet and medications to lower blood cholesterol, which in turn reduces the amount of plaque in the arteries supplying the heart. These findings suggest that a heart-healthy diet is more important during middle to late adulthood than researchers previously thought. Consuming sufficient vitamin B-6, folate, and vitamin B-12 are also important to avoid elevated blood homocysteine, a likely risk factor for cardiovascular disease.

Much controversy surrounds the treatment for elevated LDL-cholesterol in people over the age of 70. If these people adhere to extremely restrictive diets limited in fat and energy to the point that they can't keep up their weight, or if their diets lack variety, they may become undernourished. Therefore, treating elevated LDL-cholesterol in an older person who has other illnesses, such as chronic lung disease or **dementia,** is probably inappropriate. However, if a healthy 70-year-old who is likely to live another 10 to 15 years has both elevated LDL-cholesterol and evidence of cardiovascular disease, an eating and exercise plan is probably in order to reduce the chance of heart attack.

Hypertension is heavily implicated in both stroke and heart attack in older adults.[4] Blood pressure can be lowered in many people by restricting salt intake. A limit of 1200 mg/day (ages >70) to 1300 mg/day (ages 51 to 70) is recommended, but that diet is difficult to plan and follow for older people who rely on convenience foods. Alternatively, a mild sodium restriction (not to exceed 4000 mg of sodium daily) may be effective for salt-sensitive people but is not so helpful by itself for people whose hypertension is not salt sensitive; it does, however, aid the action of certain diuretics used to treat hypertension. (The Nutrition Focus in Chapter 11 reviews the effects of other nutrients such as calcium and potassium as well as lifestyle interventions on blood pressure.)

We can do much to prevent heart attack and stroke just by eating a balanced diet, walking briskly and otherwise performing regular physical activity, controlling blood pressure, not smoking, and maintaining healthy weight.[18] Regular physical activity and a diet rich in fruits and vegetables are also associated with fewer strokes as adults age, as is a moderate use of alcohol for ischemic strokes.

dementia General persistent loss or decrease in mental function.

Decline in Bone Health

Chapter 11 discussed the decline in bone mass associated with aging. Recall that bone loss in women occurs primarily after menopause. Bone loss in men is slow and steady from middle age throughout later life. Use of bisphosphonate medications is one treatment to lessen bone loss in women, but other medication regimens are also effective (review Chapter 11). For adults in general over age 50, increasing calcium intake to 1200 mg/day (200 mg/day greater than the young adult Adequate Intake) is recommended. Meeting (or slightly exceeding) protein needs is also important, but easy to accomplish.

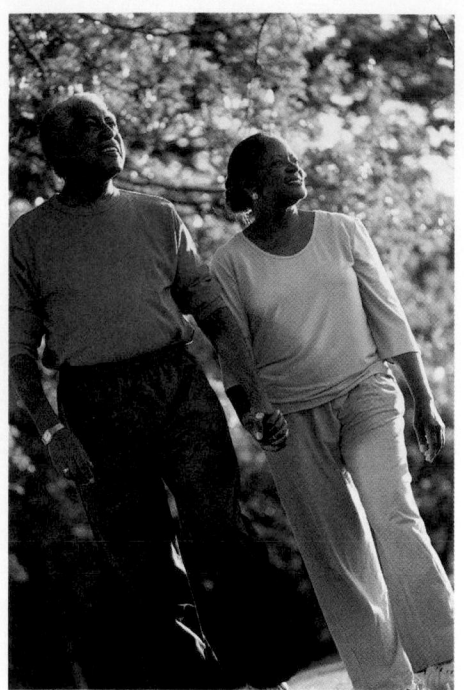

Some sun exposure greatly contributes to vitamin D needs in older people.

G rapefruit juice can increase or decrease the potency of some prescription medications, such as certain blood pressure medications, tranquilizers, antihistamines, blood cholesterol–lowering medications (statins), and others, such as a class of drugs used to treat HIV/AIDS. For this reason, a physician, registered dietitian, or pharmacist should be consulted before grapefruit juice is ingested by people on prescription medications.

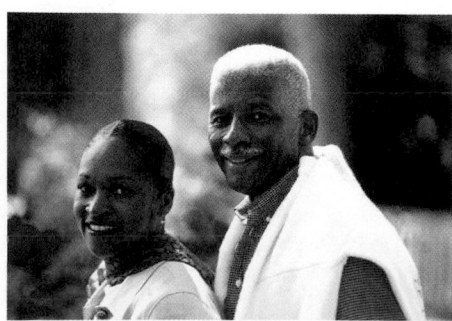

Many older adults are healthy. The goal is to remain that way as long as possible.

Maintaining adequate vitamin D nutriture is also critical, especially if the person experiences little sun exposure (10–15 µg/day [5–10 µg/day greater than the young adult Adequate Intake]). This amount corresponds to 400 to 600 IU/day. Note that the higher recommendation is for adults 70 years and older.

Many older people may suffer from undiagnosed osteomalacia, a condition primarily caused by not enough sun exposure and therefore diminished vitamin D synthesis in the skin. When they can't get regular sun exposure—during the winter or when they are homebound—older people need a dietary (e.g., milk) or supplemental source of vitamin D.

To these two measures, add not smoking and drinking alcohol moderately or not at all. In addition, underweight women are at especially high risk for developing osteoporosis. Performing weight-bearing activity, such as walking, can help preserve bone mass.

Very severe osteoporosis limits the ability of older people to move about, shop, prepare food, and live normally. They eat less and as a result consume fewer nutrients. Older people should also work with their physician to develop a plan for limiting falls. Falls may be caused by the side effects of medication, lack of regular physical activity, gait and balance disorders, impaired vision, and environmental hazards. Protective hip padding can reduce the risk of fracture in individuals who tend to fall.

Other Factors That Influence Nutrient Needs in Aging

Medications and old age often go together. Medications can improve health and quality of life, but some of them also profoundly affect nutrient needs at all ages, including the later years (Table 18-4).[13] Most older adults take prescription drugs; one-quarter of older adults regularly take multiple prescription drugs, called polypharmacy. Many drugs affect appetite or the absorption of nutrients. Often, people must take medications for long periods. These people should work with their physician and pharmacist to coordinate all medications taken. Pharmacists can advise when to take drugs—with or between meals—for maximum effectiveness.

Drug-related nutritional problems include (1) increased need for potassium when certain types of diuretics increase excretion from the body and (2) changes in appetite caused by antidepressant agents or certain antibiotics. Blood loss from the long-term use of aspirin or aspirin-like medications depletes iron reserves and can lead to anemia. People who must take one or more medications for more than just a few weeks should closely watch their diets, eat nutrient-dense foods, and possibly take nutrient supplements to counteract the effects of certain medications. A physician should supervise this last practice, because some supplements can interfere with the function of certain medications. For example, vitamin K can reduce the activity of oral anticoagulants (review Chapter 9).

Depression in Older Adults

Depression occurs in about 12 to 30% of nursing home residents and 17 to 37% of older adults who reside outside of nursing homes. About 15% of persons who are 65 years old or older experience depression. This depression—combined with isolation and loneliness as family and friends die, move away, or become less mobile—frequently contributes to apathetic eating and weight loss.[2] Depression can lead to a continual decline in which poor appetite produces weakness, which leads to even poorer appetite (Figure 18-3). In older adults, the resulting poor nutritional state can produce further mental confusion and increased isolation and loneliness.

If depression is left untreated, it is estimated that 15% of the cases may be fatal (suicide). Depression also may be a sign of an underlying illness, which is another reason

Table 18-4 | Potential Drug-Nutrient Interactions for Some Commonly Used Drugs

Drugs	Uses	Nutrients Affected	Potential Mechanism
Antacids (Maalox)	Reduces stomach acidity	Calcium, vitamin B-12, and iron	Decreased absorption due to altered gastrointestinal pH
Anticoagulants (Coumadin)	Prevents blood clots	Vitamin K	Interference with utilization
Aspirin	Is an anti-inflammatory; reduces pain	Iron	Anemia from blood loss
Cathartics (laxatives)	Induces bowel movement	Calcium and potassium	Poor absorption
Cholestyramine	Reduces blood cholesterol	Vitamins A, D, E, and K	Poor absorption
Cimetidine (Tagamet)	Treats ulcers	Vitamin B-12	Poor absorption
Colchicine	Treats gout	Vitamin B-12, carotenoids, and magnesium	Decreased absorption due to damaged intestinal mucosa
Corticosteroids (prednisone)	Is an anti-inflammatory	Zinc Calcium	Poor absorption Poor utilization
Furosemide (Lasix)	Decreases blood pressure; is a potassium-wasting diuretic	Potassium and sodium	Increased loss
Hydrochlorothiazide	Decreases blood pressure; is a diuretic	Potassium and magnesium	Increased loss; decreased absorption
MAO inhibitors (Parnate)	Is an antidepressant	Tyramine (in aged foods)	High blood pressure caused by limited tyramine metabolism
Tricyclic antidepressants (Elavil)	Is an antidepressant	—	Weight gain from appetite stimulation

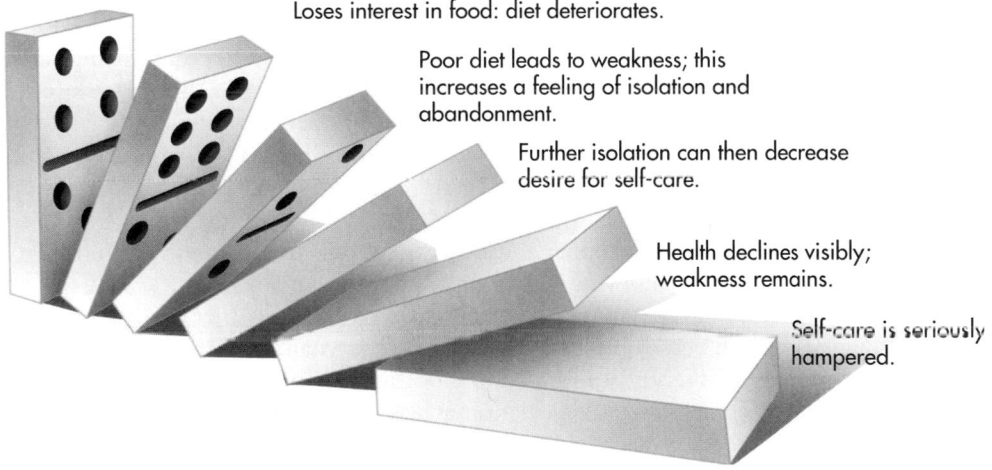

Social isolation; perhaps spouse has died.

Loses interest in food: diet deteriorates.

Poor diet leads to weakness; this increases a feeling of isolation and abandonment.

Further isolation can then decrease desire for self-care.

Health declines visibly; weakness remains.

Self-care is seriously hampered.

Figure 18-3 | The decline of health often seen in older adults. This decline needs to be prevented whenever possible.

that early detection is important in older adults. Depression is often treatable, but medication alone will not help people who are experiencing major life changes such as the death of a spouse. Adequate social support and possibly psychological intervention are also important.[5]

Alcoholism in Older Adults

Alcoholism is a problem in the older population. Approximately two-thirds of these alcohol abusers turn to alcohol much earlier in life and simply continue the habit. About one-third begin later in life because of a variety of factors—more free time, social

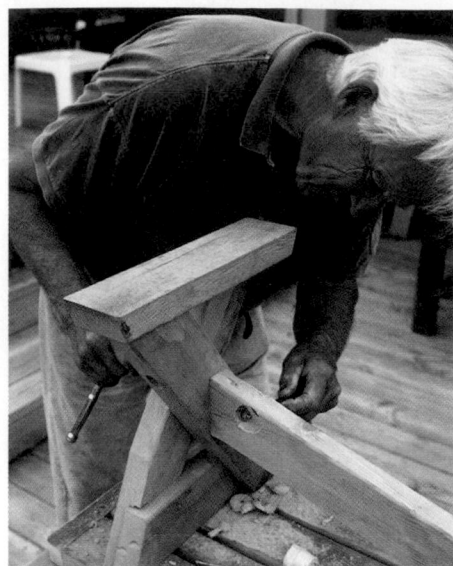

Aging is no reason to withdraw from life. Learning and practicing new skills throughout life is important. Such activities can include perhaps volunteering services to the community or helping one's friends.

Ten Warning Signs of Alzheimer's Disease

1. Recent memory loss that affects job performance
2. Difficulty performing familiar tasks
3. Problems with language
4. Disorientation to time and place
5. Faulty or decreased judgment
6. Problems with abstract thinking
7. Tendency to misplace things
8. Changes in mood or behavior
9. Changes in personality
10. Loss of initiative

events centered around drinking, loneliness, or depression. Some of the symptoms of alcoholism in older persons include trembling hands, sleep problems, memory loss, and unsteady gait; these symptoms can be easily overlooked simply because they are common symptoms of old age in general.

Older adults become intoxicated on a smaller amount of alcohol than when younger because they metabolize alcohol more slowly and have lower amounts of body water in which to dilute the alcohol compared to younger adults. Even small amounts of alcohol can react negatively with various medications that many older persons take. In addition to having adverse effects on the liver, drinking large amounts of alcohol increases the risk of hemorrhagic stroke and may worsen hypertension in older adults. Because drinking large amounts of alcohol produces adverse effects, both men and women over the age of 65 should limit alcohol consumption to no more than one drink per day. Recall from Chapter 8 that one drink per day is defined as 5 oz of wine, 12 oz of beer, or 1.5 oz shot of 80-proof liquor.

Alzheimer's Disease

Alzheimer's disease often takes a terrible toll on the mental and eventual physical health of older people. About 4.5 million adults in the United States have the disease. In general terms, Alzheimer's disease is a type of dementia best described as a progressive brain disorder marked by an inability to remember, reason, or comprehend.[3] The ten warning signs of Alzheimer's disease are listed in the margin. Age is the primary risk factor. Scientists propose various causes, including alterations in cell development or protein production in the brain, strokes, altered composition of lipoproteins in the blood (e.g., apo E4), obesity, poor blood glucose regulation (e.g., diabetes), high blood pressure, and high blood cholesterol. Meeting needs for vitamin E and vitamin C is important. Meeting needs for vitamin B-6, folate, and vitamin B-12 is especially important, because elevated blood homocysteine is also a risk factor. Caregivers should consider several nutrition recommendations in meal preparation. Food intake should be monitored to ensure maintenance of a healthy weight and nutritional state. Other tips are including fish in meals twice per week, minimizing saturated and *trans* fat intake, and making sure meal habits do not pose a health risk (e.g., holding food in one's mouth or forgetting to swallow). Regular physical activity has also been shown to improve mental status in people afflicted by this disease. Four medications have been approved to treat the disease (e.g., donepezil [Aricept]); their effects are modest at best.[11]

Preventive measures for Alzheimer's disease focus on maintaining brain activity through lifelong learning, following a diet rich in fruits and vegetables, and use of ibuprofen.[7] Other earlier "promising" strategies such as estrogen therapy, use of statin medications to lower blood cholesterol, and megadose vitamin E therapy have been shown to be ineffective in recent studies. To find out more about Alzheimer's disease, go to the website for the Alzheimer's Association at www.alz.org or call (800) 272-3900. You can also call the Alzheimer's Disease Education and Referral Center of the National Institute of Aging at (800) 428-4380.

Concept | Check

Nutritional problems common to aging adults relate to both the process of chronic diseases and the normal decrease in organ function that occurs with time. All these organ systems and functions can decrease as we age: appetite; sense of taste, smell, thirst, hearing, and sight; digestion and absorption; liver, gallbladder, pancreatic, kidney, lung, and heart function; and the immune system. In addition, bone mass and muscle mass gradually decrease, the latter largely because of a deficient diet and inactivity. Appropriate dietary changes and regular physical activity can often help reduce the impact of these results of aging.

Complementary and Alternative Medicine Practices

Consumers today may be interested in complementary and alternative medicine (CAM) (also called complementary care and integrative medicine). About 34% of people recently surveyed in the United States used alternative medical practices in the past year, and most of the associated expenses for these often expensive products and services (about $4 billion per year) were paid out-of-pocket. Interest in herbal supplements, however, is currently waning, likely because many people have tried them but have not experienced enough benefit to justify the cost. The majority of the consumers also did not discuss the practice with their primary care physician.

Given the phenomenal advances in medicine over the past decades, what brings people in such numbers to embrace alternative therapies? It may be that many people assume that natural substances are gentler forms of therapy, lacking the harsher side effects of some pharmacological medicines. People may also seek complementary medicine because standard medical treatments didn't work, standard medical treatments had too many adverse effects, they wanted to participate more actively in treatment, or they wanted to combat poor physician communication. The majority of consumers using alternative medicines have illnesses for which conventional medicine cannot offer a cure, such as arthritis, terminal stages of AIDS, and stress-related conditions. These people will almost certainly benefit from the reassurance, hope, and relief that comes with being in a healing situation.

In many instances, self-prescription or healing rituals involve the participants' optimism, commitment, attention, and high expectations for improvement. The mind is a powerful component of treatment, which is proven by the placebo effect. A placebo is a "sugar pill" administered to someone who believes that he or she is being treated with a real medication and subsequently feels better. Many alternative or natural treatments probably have no intrinsic therapeutic value beyond the benefit of the placebo effect. There also are some other ways a traditional remedy may seem to work, such as the natural ups and downs of symptoms, the remission of disease, the possibility that the remedy contains the effective dose of a pharmaceutical medicine or is adulterated with medicines not listed on the label, and the denial of symptoms or mis-representation of effectiveness by people who believe the remedy is effective.

In truth, little scientific evidence is available for physicians and health-care professionals to decipher the positive and negative aspects of natural therapies. Indeed, Western medicine is based on accurate scientific knowledge, which serves as a protective device to prevent harm. On the other hand, alternative therapies often are based on **folk medicine** and have little or no scientific evidence to support them (due to lack of large research trials). Still, health professionals should be aware of the scientific knowledge surrounding some alternative therapies, because clients may express interest in these therapies. Many clients wish physicians would take the time to explain (in simple terms) the nature of the problem; to acknowledge nutritional influences on health, rather than just recommend drugs and surgery as the only approaches for treating illness; to answer questions intelligently about dietary supplements; to be sensitive to mind-body interactions; and to respect questions about alternative practices.

To date, few complementary and alternative therapies have been subjected to scientific scrutiny, and many of the practices are based on presumptions that are unconvincing at best, yet some of the therapies (e.g., acupuncture and chiropractic therapies) show promise in the treatment of certain conditions. The National Institutes of Health in the United States has created the following seven categories of complementary and alternative therapies:

1. *Mind-body interventions:* the use of the mind, such as hypnosis, meditation, biofeedback, and yoga, to enhance health. Integrative medicine teaches health-care providers to focus on the subtle yet complex interactions of mind, body, spirit, community, and environment. *Ayurveda* is a natural healing process from India that includes eating healthful, fresh foods and taking medicinal herbs suited to one's particular mind-body type.
2. *Bioelectrical magnetic therapies:* the use of electrical currents or magnetic fields to promote healing, such as the use of electrical currents to help heal broken bones.
3. *Alternative systems of medical practice:* the use of medicine from another culture, such as

> **folk medicine** A medical treatment based on the beliefs, traditions, or customs of a particular society or ethnic/cultural group.

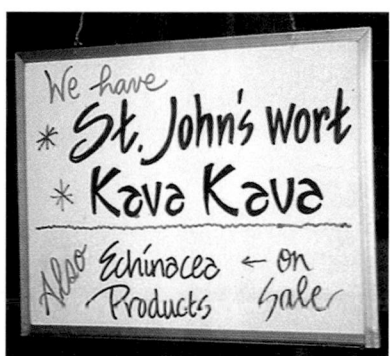

Some herbal products are effective for treating specific medical problems. Follow label instructions carefully. Note potential side effects listed as well as who should not use the product. The best advice is to use these substances only under strict supervision of a physician.

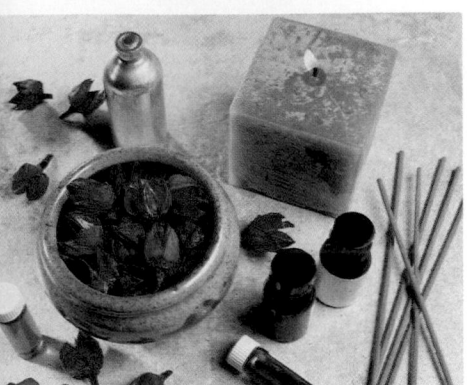

Aromatherapy is typically used to promote relaxation and relieve stress. To date there is little scientific evidence to suggest that aromatherapy can be used to treat or prevent diseases.

chelation The use of medicinal compounds, such as ethylenediaminetetraacetic acid (EDTA), to bind metals and other constituents in the blood.

aromatherapy The use of the vapors of essential oils extracted from flowers, leaves, stalks, fruits, and roots for therapeutic purposes.

Another concern regarding use of herbal and related supplements is the actual content of the active ingredient or ingredients in the product. Recently, many of these products have been tested by independent laboratories and been found to contain either less than or more than the stated label content (see the website www.consumerlabs.com for details).

Native American medicine and Chinese medicine (for example, acupuncture). Acupuncture likely works by stimulating sensory nerves leading to the spinal cord, which leads to a reduction in pain. Acupuncture also may be effective for treating people who experience nausea and vomiting following surgery or chemotherapy, nausea that accompanies pregnancy, pain experienced after certain dental procedures, and recovery from a drug addiction. Typically, a course of treatments should end after 10 sessions if it is not showing benefit. FDA supports the use of acupuncture for such purposes. However, a qualified, certified practitioner must use sterile needles intended for single use and made from nonreactive materials.

4. *Manual healing methods:* the use of the hands to promote healing, such as chiropractic or osteopathic manipulation or massage. FDA recognizes the effectiveness of chiropractic care for the treatment of acute low back pain.

5. *Pharmacologic and biologic treatments:* the use of various substances to treat specific medical problems. This category includes **chelation** therapy.

6. *Herbal medicine:* the use of plants as medicines to treat or prevent disease. By definition, an herb is any plant or part of a plant that is used primarily for medicinal purposes. This category includes **aromatherapy.** Dosage forms include capsules, tablets, extracts or tinctures, powders, dried herbs, teas, creams, and ointments. FDA has established regulations that require the labels of such supplements to include name, quantity, dosage per day, and ingredient amounts.

7. *Diet and nutrition:* the use of foods, vitamins, and minerals to prevent illness and treat disease.

The National Institutes of Health is also sponsoring sites around the United States to study complementary and alternative medicine practices. Thus we may know more about these practices in the future.

The following are a few practical tips on using complementary and alternative medicine practices:

- We often tend to believe what we hear or what close acquaintances tell us. This well-meaning advice does not substitute for scientific verification of safety and effectiveness when it comes to health practices.
- The U.S. federal government provides little regulation regarding nutrient supplements or remedies. "Let the buyer beware" is prudent advice to follow when using these products. Knowledgeable, professional guidance is needed.
- Fraudulent claims for diet- and health-related remedies have always been a part of our culture. It is important to scrutinize carefully the credentials and motives of anyone providing medical or health advice. Phony credentials and bogus practitioners are widespread.
- If it sounds too good to be true, it probably is. The medical community gains nothing by holding back effective cures from the public, despite what the alternative practitioners may say.

Vitamin and Herbal Supplements Are Regulated Loosely by FDA

Unless FDA has evidence that a supplement is inherently dangerous or its label makes illegal claims, FDA will not regulate it closely.[14] FDA is, in fact, prevented from doing so by the Proxmire Amendment to the 1938 Food, Drug, and Cosmetic Act, along with follow-up legislation—the Dietary Supplement Health and Education Act (DSHEA), which was passed in 1994 (and reviewed in Chapter 1). FDA requires a standardized Supplement Facts label on herbs and other related supplements. These labels must list the ingredients, the percent of Daily Value if applicable, common name of the plant, the part of the plant that was used, how much is present in each pill, and a suggested daily dose (Figure 18-4). It is permissible for the labels on such products to claim a benefit related to a classic nutrient-deficiency disease, describe how a nutrient affects human body structure or function (i.e., structure/function claim), and state that general well-being results from consumption of the ingredient or ingredients. On the other hand, a supplement label cannot claim that a product treats, cures, or prevents a disease not completely related to a given nutrient deficiency. For example, an herbal product label can claim that it

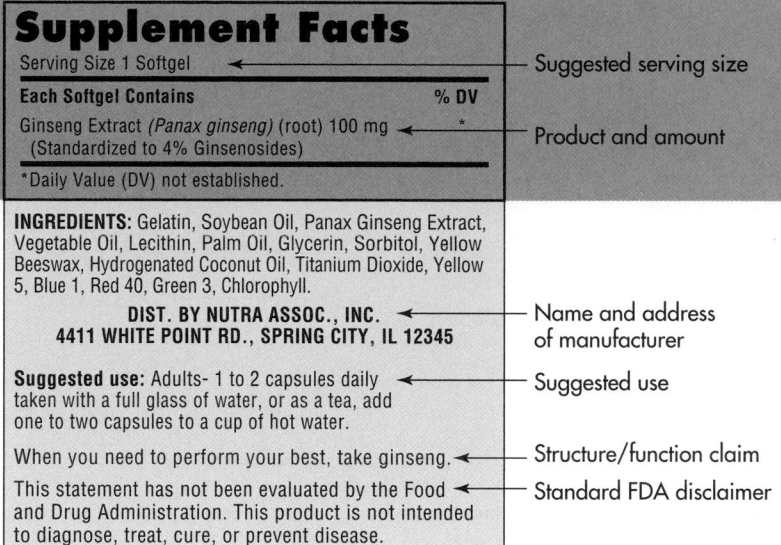

Supplement Facts

Serving Size 1 Softgel ← Suggested serving size

Each Softgel Contains   **% DV**

Ginseng Extract *(Panax ginseng)* (root) 100 mg ← *   ← Product and amount
  (Standardized to 4% Ginsenosides)

*Daily Value (DV) not established.

INGREDIENTS: Gelatin, Soybean Oil, Panax Ginseng Extract, Vegetable Oil, Lecithin, Palm Oil, Glycerin, Sorbitol, Yellow Beeswax, Hydrogenated Coconut Oil, Titanium Dioxide, Yellow 5, Blue 1, Red 40, Green 3, Chlorophyll.

DIST. BY NUTRA ASSOC., INC. ←   ← Name and address
4411 WHITE POINT RD., SPRING CITY, IL 12345   of manufacturer

Suggested use: Adults- 1 to 2 capsules daily ←   ← Suggested use
taken with a full glass of water, or as a tea, add
one to two capsules to a cup of hot water.

When you need to perform your best, take ginseng. ←   ← Structure/function claim

This statement has not been evaluated by the Food ←   ← Standard FDA disclaimer
and Drug Administration. This product is not intended
to diagnose, treat, cure, or prevent disease.

Figure 18-4 | Supplement Facts label on an herbal product. Any nutrients or other food constituents would also be listed if contained in the product.

may help brain function, but not that it cures Alzheimer's disease. The latter would constitute a drug claim. Once in a while, a company will decide to market a supplement as a drug. In that case, the company has to go through the same FDA process mandated for any drug. However, most supplement companies prefer to avoid this whole process and keep their product labels in compliance with DSHEA.

Dietary Supplement Claims

Although structure/function claims do not have to be approved by FDA, manufacturers must have evidence that their marketing statements are truthful and not misleading. In addition, the labels of products bearing such claims must prominently display in boldface type the following disclaimer: **"This statement has not been evaluated by the Food and Drug Administration. This product is not intended to diagnose, treat, cure, or prevent any disease."** Despite this statement, consumers may mistakenly assume FDA has carefully evaluated the products and related claims, as is done for pharmaceuticals and approved health claims.

It is also noteworthy that FDA's requirement for "evidence" for a claim is not a very stringently enforced requirement. In many cases, the evidence used to support a claim is vague or unsubstantiated. However, FDA only ends up challenging a relatively low percentage of these claims. For this reason, some other means are emerging for challenging such claims. Some involve government agencies other than FDA (e.g., the Federal Trade Commission [FTC]). In addition, the supplement industry itself is trying to develop means of self-policing. It will be interesting to see how much impact results from these efforts by government and industry groups. One of the biggest areas of concern is so-called borrowed science. For example, Company A does research on their garlic capsule that shows that this product lowers blood pressure. Company B may also tout this research for their garlic product. However, their product can be prepared quite differently than Company A's product. How do we know that the research on the product of Company A applies to the product of Company B? We don't. This situation discourages many companies from sponsoring research on their products because their competitors might "borrow" their research (many people would call it stealing, not borrowing). Therefore, borrowed science ends up to be a major barrier to much needed research being conducted in the supplement area. How can borrowed science be stopped? FDA can investigate only a limited number of cases, given its budget. Alternatively, lawsuits can be filed by an individual company against the "borrower," but this solution is expensive and time consuming. Another possibility is the emerging government and industry approaches just mentioned, but we'll have to see how effective they will be.

A Closer Look at Herbal Therapy

Throughout history, healers have gone to the garden, forest, and sea to seek herbal remedies. Some natural products may be harmless, others are potentially toxic, and still others may be effective for some problems but dangerous when taken in the wrong dose or by people with certain medical conditions (Table 18-5).[6,14] Herb-drug interactions can be especially severe, such as an increase in the risk of bleeding in a person taking anticoagulant medications. The National Cancer Institute is the world's leader in the search for medicinal compounds in plants. For example, the institute has tested extracts of more than 30,000 plant species for activity against cancer. This work identified some anticancer compounds from flowering plants that have been approved for use in cancer patients.

Critical | Thinking

Jamila went to her local pharmacy yesterday to look for a product to help her stay awake while studying. On the shelves she found a dietary supplement claiming to be a Chinese herbal remedy for sleepiness and fatigue. She thought that because a pharmacy carried the product, it should be safe and should work as indicated on the label.

Is she correct in these assumptions? Are there specific risks associated with taking such herbal remedies?

Table 18-5 | Popular Herbal Remedies, Food Supplements, and Hormones

Herbal and Related Substances	Potential Effects	Side Effects	Who Should Avoid Them
Black cohosh	May reduce postmenopausal symptoms	Nausea, fall in blood pressure	Women taking estrogen, hypertension medications, or aspirin and related drugs
Coenzyme Q-10	Fat-soluble vitamin-like substance with antioxidant properties; some people with chronic conditions, such as heart failure, have low amounts in the body and so may benefit from use	Mild gastrointestinal distress	No specific persons are at risk
Echinacea	May stimulate the immune system and shorten the duration of flulike illnesses; current studies show little or no effect	Nausea, skin irritation, allergic reactions	Anyone with an autoimmune disease or who has allergic reactions to daisies
Feverfew	May reduce the pain and frequency of migraines	Abdominal pain, mouth sores, skin rash	Anyone allergic to ragweed or taking anti-inflammatory drugs, such as aspirin
Garlic	May have antibiotic properties and slightly lower blood cholesterol and blood pressure	In large amounts, burning of the mouth, nausea, sweating, stomach irritation, lightheadedness, reduced blood clotting	Anyone taking anticoagulant medications, such as warfarin, for cardiovascular disease, or AIDS medicines
Ginger	May prevent motion sickness and nausea related to surgery and pregnancy	Gastrointestinal (GI) tract discomfort with high doses on an empty stomach	People with history of gallstones
Ginkgo biloba	May increase the circulation of blood in the body, especially to the brain and lower extremities; evidence is very weak	GI tract upset, headache, irritability, reduced blood clotting	Anyone taking anti-inflammatory or anti-coagulant medications, including vitamin E and aspirin; anyone who has had a stroke or is prone to them
Ginseng	May decrease weakness and fatigue and increase the body's resistance to stress; studies have not confirmed any benefit	Hypertension, asthma attacks, irregular heart beat, insomnia, headache, nervousness, GI tract upset, reduced blood clotting	Anyone taking anti-coagulant medications, such as warfarin; women on hormone replacement therapy; anyone with a chronic GI tract disease; anyone with diabetes
Glucosamine	May decrease joint inflammation and pain associated with osteoarthritis, but a recent, large scale trial showed no such benefit.	GI tract discomfort, which may disappear after 2 weeks	May disrupt blood glucose regulation in people with diabetes
Milk thistle	May have a protective effect on the liver, thought to be due in part to its ability to prevent toxins from contaminating liver cell membranes	Diarrhea	No specific persons are at risk
SAMe	May promote cartilage formation and decreases joint inflammation and pain associated with osteoarthritis; may also act as a mild antidepressant (active ingredient is S-adenosylmethionine)	Mild headaches, which last for short periods of time	Anyone with cardiovascular disease, obsessive compulsive disorder, manic-depression, or addictive tendencies

Other plant-derived compounds are currently being tested for safety and effectiveness in clinical trials but haven't yet been approved.

Traditional knowledge of the healing properties of plants provides leads for such scientists to explore. Any promising compounds they isolate are subjected to rigorous FDA-approved tests to determine safety, effectiveness, and side effects. This controlled testing provides a wealth of information far exceeding that available for most herbal remedies.

The German government publishes a manual that is the most authoritative reference for the use of popular herbal products (*Commission E Monographs*). Unfortunately, little scientific data are available concerning the therapeutic value and safety of the 7000 or so herbs used in traditional medicine, which has been practiced and chronicled primarily by the Chinese. Proponents of Chinese herbal medicine suggest that its safety and efficacy have been well established during its 4000-year his-

Table 18-5 | Popular Herbal Remedies, Food Supplements, and Hormones *(continued)*

Herbal and Related Substances	Potential Effects	Side Effects	Who Should Avoid Them
St. John's wort	Mild antidepressant effect that may work by inhibiting monoamine oxidase (an enzyme in the brain that destroys "feel-good" hormones such as serotonin, epinephrine, and dopamine)	Nausea, fatigue, dry mouth, dizziness, photosensitivity; increases metabolism and removal of many prescription drugs from the body	People taking medications to control depression, HIV, epilepsy, cardiovascular disease, asthma, and to suppress the immune system to keep the body from rejecting a transplanted organ
Saw palmetto	May reduce symptoms of enlarged prostate gland (otherwise known as BPH or benign prostatic hyperplasia) by increasing urinary flow and easing urination; some studies show moderate evidence of effectiveness, while other studies have shown little or no benefit with such use.	Generally uncommon; when taken in large doses: headache, GI tract upset	People taking medication to treat enlarged prostate or BPH; anyone with a chronic GI tract disease
Valerian	May alleviate restlessness and other sleeping disorders that stem from nervous conditions	Headache, morning grogginess, irregular heart beat, GI tract upset (also has a disagreeable odor)	Anyone taking central nervous system depressants, such as sedatives; anyone who drinks alcohol
Hormones			
DHEA	Hormone that when taken orally turns to estrogen and testosterone in the body; few, if any, benefits of supplementation are proven, such as an aid to weight loss or to treat depression; research is ongoing	Masculinization of women, acne, irritability, decreased HDL-cholesterol, possible prostate or breast cancer	Women, due to possible irreversible masculinization qualities
Growth hormone	Hormone that stimulates cell synthesis, such as muscle cells, and overall body growth in children; may be useful in adults who fail to make enough of the hormone	**Carpal tunnel syndrome;** breast development in men; swollen ankles and legs, hypertension, diabetes, cancer	Only available by prescription; requires close physician scrutiny (very expensive)
Melatonin	Hormone that may help people fall asleep faster and reduce jet lag	Reduced ovulation in women, drowsiness, confusion, headache or morning grogginess	Anyone with cardiovascular disease, or anyone of childbearing age
Testosterone	Hormone that affects muscle mass and strength; can reduce menopausal symptoms in women and possibly depression in older men	Masculinization of women, decreased HDL-cholesterol, prostate gland enlargement in men (and possibly increased prostate cancer risk)	Only available by prescription; requires close physician scrutiny; risky in men showing prostate gland enlargement

Note that pregnant or breastfeeding women, children under 2 years old, anyone over the age of 65 years, and anyone with a chronic disease should never take supplements unless under the guidance of a physician.

tory. These individuals also point to the widespread use of herbal therapies in Europe. Still, numerous reports have documented significant health risks associated with the use of some herbal and alternative remedies, sometimes resulting in death. Studies especially implicate germander, pokeroot, sassafras, mandrake, pennyroyal, comfrey, chaparral, yohimbe, lobelia, jin bu huan, kava kava, products containing stephanie and magnolia, senna, hai gen fen, paraguay tea, kombucha tea, tung shueh (Chinese black balls), and willow bark.

There is also a distinct risk that a traditional herbal product may be mislabeled, adulterated with prescription drugs or contaminants (such as lead), or subject to extreme variations in potency. Chinese combination herbs should always be avoided because of the reported cases of adverse health effects and adulteration.

carpal tunnel syndrome A disease in which nerves that travel to the wrist are pinched as they pass through a narrow opening in a bone in the wrist.

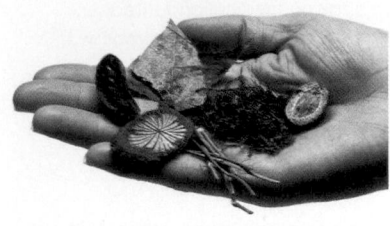

Simply because herbal remedies come from natural sources does not mean they are without health risks. Even those that have been used for centuries may produce harmful effects when combined with standard medications.

A recent concern has been raised with regard to patients who abruptly end alternative medicines at the start of hospital treatments or simply deny that they are involved in alternative therapy. Interactions between alternative therapies and pharmaceutical drugs can be drastic and include complications such as delirium, clotting abnormalities, and rapid heart beat, resulting in the need for intensive care. If these patients had disclosed their treatments, many of the complications could have been prevented. Experts recommend that, if time permits, patients stop taking herbal products for about a week before a scheduled surgery or otherwise take all original supplement containers to the hospital so that the anesthesiologist can evaluate what was taken.

The following are questions that should be asked when evaluating a company's products:

- What forms of production control lab analysis are used to ensure quality, quantity, and reproducibility of the ingredients in individual doses as labeled?
- Is the product labeled with Latin botanical names?
- Does the label have expiration dates and lot numbers, and if so, what is the basis for the labeled expiration dates?
- Does the manufacturer offer a certificate of analysis for each product?
- Has the manufacturer been in business for at least 5 years and have national distribution of the product?

Still, what the label indicates as the active ingredient and the amount of the ingredient that a product claims to contain may or may not be valid, based on the recent analysis of many popular brands of herbal products.

A rational approach to alternative therapy is for people to keep a diary of symptoms, follow only one therapy at a time, check with their physician first before discontinuing a medication, and find out if the alternative practitioner has experience with the medical problem to be treated. Interested consumers might also see if they can enter a study of the substance or procedure in question. In addition, FDA advises anyone who experiences adverse side effects from an herbal remedy to contact a physician. Physicians are encouraged to report such adverse effects to FDA and state and local health departments and consumer protection agencies.

Overall, herbal products should be used with great caution and only in consultation with a person's primary physician. Otherwise, potential side effects may go undiagnosed, or dangerous herb-medicine interactions may develop.[14] Pregnant and nursing women, anyone with a chronic disease, and children under 2 years of age, especially, should not take herbal supplements unless their physicians consent to the practice and monitor them for potential complications.

Some herbalists claim that natural herbs cannot harm people. Scientific evidence strongly contradicts this claim. Indeed, if there's one thing experts agree on, it's this: an herb that has the ability to heal also has the ability, if misused, to harm. In addition, many conditions for which herbs are recommended (such as diabetes and arthritis) are not suitable for self-treatment. For a balanced discussion of herbal remedies, consult the following websites:

Alternative Medicine Foundation
www.amfoundation.org/

The NCCAM Complementary and Alternative Medicine (CAM) Citation Index (CI)
nccam.nih.gov/nccam/resources/cam-ci/

American Botanical Council
www.herbalgram.org/

Complementary and Alternative Medicine Program at Stanford (CAMPS)
scrdp.stanford.edu/camps.html

Center for Complementary and Alternative Medicine Research in Asthma, located at the University of California, Davis
www.camra.ucdovis.edu/

National Institutes of Health Office of Alternative Medicine
altmed.od.nih.gov/

Natural Medicine Comprehensive Database
www.naturaldatabase.com

Nutrient Needs and Dietary Planning in Middle and Older Adulthood

The latest RDAs and related standards for nutrients and energy needs include categories for both men and women who are 51 to 70 years of age and more than 70 years of age. Macronutrient needs do not change from young adults' needs, but needs for some micronutrients do. In addition, because the lifestyle of an active older person can differ considerably from that of a nursing home resident, establishing nutrient needs during these wide age ranges is problematic.

A well-planned diet that follows MyPyramid can meet all nutrient needs for healthy older people within about 1800 kcal, except for probably vitamin D and vitamin B-12. Meeting the vitamin B-12 standard is aided by use of fortified foods, such as ready-to-eat breakfast cereals. The use of a balanced multivitamin and mineral supplement is especially helpful for meeting vitamin D needs if the person does not receive regular sun exposure. Any supplement should be low in or free of iron, because it may have a prooxidant effect. Currently, many nutrition experts recommend a daily balanced multivitamin and mineral supplement for older adults, especially for those 70 years of age and older.

Recommended dietary practices for later years would be to increase the diet's nutrient density and to make sure fiber and fluid intake is adequate.[1] In addition, some protein should come from lean meats to help meet protein, vitamin B-6, vitamin B-12, and zinc needs.

Singles of all ages face logistical problems with food: purchasing, preparing, storing, and using food with minimal waste are challenging. Economy packages of meats and vegetables are normally too large to be useful for a single person. Many singles live in small dwellings, some without kitchens and freezers. Creating a diet to accommodate a limited budget and facilities and a single appetite requires special considerations. Following are some practical suggestions for diet planning for singles:

- If you own a freezer, cook large amounts, divide into portions, and freeze.
- Buy only what you can use; small containers may be expensive, but letting food spoil is also costly.
- Ask the grocer to break open a family-sized package of wrapped meat or fresh vegetables and separate it into smaller units.
- Buy only several pieces of fruit—perhaps a ripe one, a medium-ripe one, and an unripe one—so that the fruit can be eaten over a period of several days.
- Keep a box of dry milk handy to add nutrients to recipes for baked foods and other foods for which this addition is acceptable.

Table 18-6 provides even more ideas.

Nutritional deficiencies and protein-caloric undernutrition have been identified among some aging populations, particularly those in nursing homes or long-term care facilities and those who are hospitalized. These nutritional problems increase the risk for many diseases, including bed sores (pressure ulcers), and compromise recovery from illness and surgery.[13] Friends, relatives, and health-care personnel should look for poor nutrient intake in all older people, including those who live in nursing home settings. Family members have a unique opportunity to make sure nutrient needs are met by looking for weight maintenance based on regular, healthful meal patterns. If problems arise in consuming a healthful diet, registered dietitians can offer professional and personalized advice.

Overall, good nutrition benefits older adults in many ways. Meeting nutrient needs delays the onset of some diseases; improves the management of some existing diseases; hastens recovery from many illnesses; increases mental, physical, and social well-being; and often decreases the need for and length of hospitalization.[1]

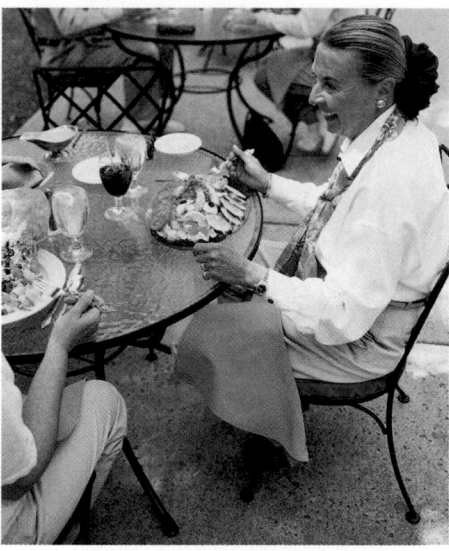

As we age nutrient needs change, but not the need to follow a healthy diet.

If rich calcium sources are not consumed, a person would need a calcium supplement, because typical multivitamin and mineral supplements contain little calcium (about 200 mg). As noted in Chapter 9, providing more calcium than that would greatly increase the pill size.

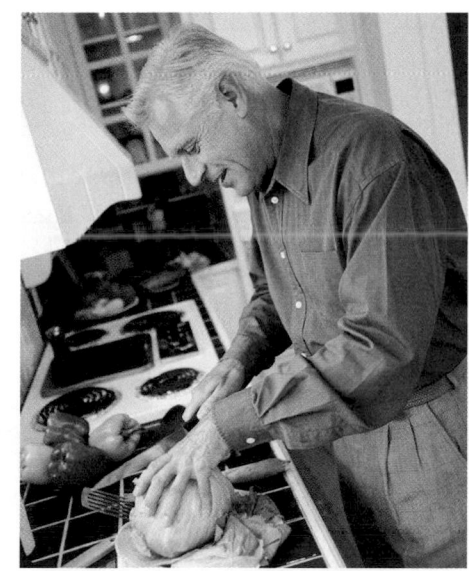

Great attention to food safety is also important for older adults. Chapter 19 provides advice on this topic, such as washing one's hands and work surface before preparing food.

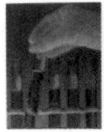

Expert Opinion

Nutrition and Healthy Aging
Katherine Tucker, Ph.D.

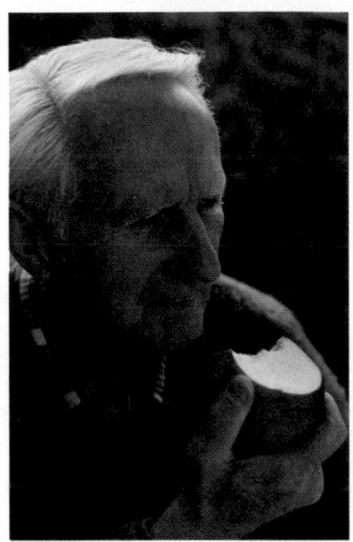

Healthy eating is a key component of healthy aging.

Research continues to confirm the central role of nutrition in maintaining health and independence with age. It is clear that continued physical activity is critical for maintaining weight and lean muscle, and it is generally accepted that a "good" diet is important. What is often less appreciated is that many older adults are at risk of micronutrient inadequacies and that these contribute to a variety of chronic conditions, disability, and loss of independence. Dietary quality is particularly important for older adults. With advancing age, energy requirements and therefore total food intake tend to decrease—but the requirements for most nutrients do not decrease and, in some cases, increase. Surveys show that large segments of the older adult population consume diets with inadequate amounts of protein, vitamins, and minerals and that these deficiencies are associated with risk of chronic disease. Nutrients of particular concern include protein; folate; vitamins B-6, B-12, D, and E; carotenoids; calcium; and magnesium.

Protein

There is a commonly held belief that the U.S. population consumes more than enough protein. Although this statement is certainly true for some segments of the population, it is not always true for older adults. Because of lower efficiency of protein utilization and loss of lean body mass, aging adults have higher protein intake requirements than do younger adults. Until recently, many researchers and physicians recommended that older individuals limit protein intake to protect against bone loss. However, recent studies have demonstrated that both muscle mass and bone mass are better preserved when protein intakes are relatively high. Some scientists currently recommend that individuals over 70 years old consume from 1.0 to 1.25 g/kg/day, which is higher than the current adult RDA of 0.8 g/kg/day.

B vitamins

Several vitamins are inadequately consumed by older adults. Among these, three of the B vitamins have recently received considerable attention due to their importance in prevention of chronic disease. Folate, vitamin B-6, and vi-

tamin B-12 are each involved in methionine metabolism and are required to clear homocysteine, an intermediary amino acid, from the bloodstream and cells in general. Elevated blood concentrations of homocysteine have been associated with risk of cardiovascular disease and stroke and more recently also with bone fracture and cognitive decline. Surveys have regularly shown that large proportions of the older population have both inadequate intake and inadequate blood concentrations of these three vitamins. In the 1990s, the U.S. Food and Drug Administration mandated that all refined grains in the food supply be fortified with folic acid. This change has reduced the prevalence of folate deficiency, but vitamins B-6 and B-12 remain important problems.

Vitamin B-6 is of central importance to protein metabolism and immune function. It is found widely in foods that have not been processed, including whole grains, nuts and seeds, unprocessed meat and fish, legumes, and selected fruits. Although this vitamin has received less attention than folate, it is often inadequately consumed, and some investigators believe the current RDA should be increased for older adults.

With few exceptions, vitamin B-12 is found only in animal-based products. Vitamin B-12 is a particular problem for the older population because for many, a deficiency may exist even when intake appears to be adequate. Up to 40% of the older population may suffer from some degree of stomach inflammation, leading to loss of stomach acid, which is required to separate vitamin B-12 from the protein to which it is bound in food. For this reason, consumption of the RDA for vitamin B-12 does not ensure adequate plasma concentrations. Current recommendations emphasize that older adults obtain vitamin B-12 from fortified breakfast cereals or supplements. Some older individuals will require amounts much higher than the RDA to achieve adequate concentrations.

Vitamin D

Inadequacy of vitamin D is considered by some researchers to be epidemic in the older population. Many older adults do not spend time outside and therefore have limited exposure to sunlight. Further, the abilities of the skin to synthesize vitamin D and of the kidney to convert it to the active form decline with age. Food sources of vitamin D are limited in the U.S. diet, and the major sources—fatty fish and fortified milk—are not widely consumed by older adults. Inadequacy of vitamin D contributes to the high prevalence of low bone mass and osteoporosis and thereby to the incidence of fracture in the older population. This connection is critical because many elders do not recover from the extended bed rest after a hip fracture, which is often the beginning of a downward spiral that leads to loss of muscle mass, loss of mobility, and frequently to death. In addition, vitamin D deficiency has been linked with a variety of other conditions, including immunological and neurological conditions. Just 10 minutes per day of sunlight can make a large difference in vitamin D status. For individuals who cannot get out, supplements are recommended.

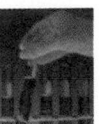

Vitamin E

Current recommendations for vitamin E intake are based on an increasing understanding of the importance of this potent antioxidant in the prevention of age-related declines in a variety of functions. This vitamin is particularly important to immune function and is thereby linked with reductions in infectious disease; there is also evidence of protective effects against cardiovascular disease, cognitive decline, cataract, and cancer. The dietary intake of the majority of the population falls short of recommendations. Vitamin E is another nutrient that is found in large quantities only in selected foods. The major dietary source is vegetable oil. Nuts and seeds have the highest concentrations but are rarely consumed in the U.S. diet. Many older individuals have been persuaded to take vitamin E supplements, but recent studies have identified much stronger protective effects from dietary vitamin E than from supplemental vitamin E, and clinical trials of vitamin E supplements have been disappointing.

Carotenoids

The lack of success of single nutrient supplements has also been seen for other antioxidant nutrients. For example, although beta-carotene from diet has consistently been shown to protect against cardiovascular disease and cancer in dietary studies, randomized trials of beta-carotene supplements failed to show protective effects—and even suggested greater cancer risk in some studies. Dietary intakes of other carotenoids have been shown to have a variety of important antiaging and health protective effects. Specifically, lutein and zeaxanthin (from dark green leafy vegetables, egg yolk, and corn) have been linked with prevention of cataract and age-related macular degeneration, and lycopene (from tomato products) has been linked with prevention of prostate cancer. The evidence suggests that in the case of antioxidants, a variety of nutrients and food chemicals work optimally together and therefore intake should be encouraged from diet rather than from supplements. Diets high in fruit and vegetables, the major sources of carotenoids and other beneficial phytochemicals, are consistently shown to be protective of a wide variety of age-related conditions.

Calcium

Calcium intake is essential to prevent bone loss, particularly among postmenopausal women. Adequate calcium intake is also known to be important for blood pressure regulation and is currently being explored for a possible link with weight maintenance. Few adults meet intake recommendations, particularly older adults, who tend to consume fewer dairy products. Calcium absorption is a complex process, and the capacity for efficient absorption declines with age. Because it is difficult for older adults to meet recommendations from diet, supplements are often recommended. Although there is good evidence that calcium supplements improve bone mineral density and reduce fracture risk, these effects appear to continue only while the supplement is being consumed. Recent studies show that optimal bone health requires many nutrients in addition to calcium and that a good-quality diet may have better long-term protective effects than calcium supplements alone. There are many advantages to consuming calcium-rich foods such as low-fat dairy products, fish (with bones, like sardines or canned salmon), and leafy green vegetables. Improved intakes of such dietary sources should be encouraged because, in addition to calcium, they also tend to include vitamin D, magnesium, potassium, and other important nutrients.

Magnesium

Dietary surveys consistently show that the majority of the adult population falls short of meeting the magnesium intake recommendation. Magnesium is required for numerous metabolic reactions in the body, and although clear deficiency is rarely diagnosed, a constant inadequacy may contribute to a variety of chronic conditions. Sudden death from poor heart rhythm is the best known concern, but general cardiovascular disease, osteoporosis, and diabetes are other conditions that have clearly been linked with low magnesium intake. Like vitamin B-6, magnesium is widespread in an unprocessed food supply, including whole grains, legumes, and fresh vegetables, but is easily lost with processing.

Summary

Much research in the past has focused on the use of single nutrient supplements to prevent specific conditions. The failure of many of those trials with the persistence of evidence of protective effects from diet suggests that we must continue to emphasize good dietary patterns in the population and to work toward improving access to the older population. Current recommendations for the aging population to optimize health and prevent both physical and cognitive decline include a focus on continued physical activity, including resistance training; a nutrient-dense diet that includes plenty of fruit, vegetables, nuts and seeds, whole grains, fish, and low-fat dairy products; and use of fortified breakfast cereals or supplements to ensure adequate vitamin B-12 and D.

Dr. Tucker is Professor of Nutritional Epidemiology at the Friedman School of Nutrition Science and Policy at Tufts University and is Director of the Dietary Assessment and Epidemiology Research Program at the Jean Mayer USDA Human Nutrition Research Center on Aging. Her research focuses on the role of dietary intake and nutritional status in the prevention of chronic diseases in aging populations. She received her Ph.D. in nutritional sciences from Cornell University.

To learn about meal programs for senior citizens in your area, call the *Administration on Aging's Elder Care Locator* (800) 677-1116. For general information on programs for older persons, visit the following websites: *National Institute on Aging,* www.nih.gov/nia/; *American Geriatrics Society,* www.americangeriatrics.org/; and *Administration on Aging,* www.aoa.dhhs.gov/.

Table 18-6 | Guidelines for Healthful Eating in Later Years

- Eat regularly, small frequent meals may be best. Use nutrient-dense foods as a basis for menus.
- Use convenience foods and labor-saving devices.
- Try new foods, new seasonings, and new ways of preparing foods. Don't use just convenience foods and canned goods.
- Keep easy-to-prepare foods on hand for times when you feel tired.
- Have a treat occasionally, perhaps an expensive cut of meat or a favorite fresh fruit.
- Eat in a well-lit or sunny area; serve meals attractively; use foods with different flavors, colors, shapes, textures, and smells.
- Arrange kitchen and eating area so that food preparation and clean-up are easier.
- Eat with friends, relatives, or at a senior center when possible.
- Share cooking responsibilities with a neighbor.
- Use community resources for help in shopping and other daily care needs.
- Stay physically active.
- If possible, take a walk before eating to stimulate appetite.
- When necessary, chop, grind, or blend hard-to-chew foods. Softer protein-rich foods can be substituted for meat when poor dental function limits normal food intake. Prepare soups, stews, cooked whole-grain cereals, and casseroles.
- If your feeding movements are limited, cut the food ahead of time, use utensils with deep sides or handles, and obtain more specialized utensils if needed.

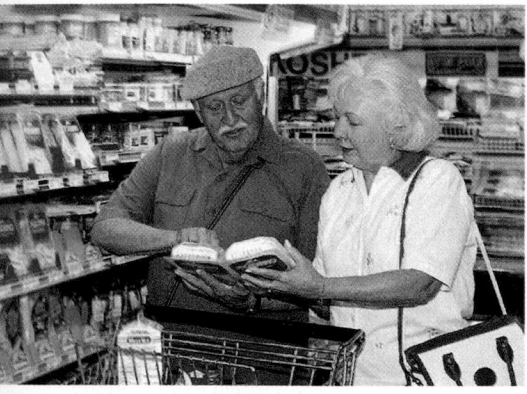

Grocery shopping can become more difficult in one's older years. Assistance from others is often very helpful.

hospice care A facility offering care that emphasizes comfort and dignity in death.

Obtaining enough food may be difficult for some older persons, especially if they are unable to drive and relatives do not live close enough to help with cooking or shopping. For an older person, a request for help may be equated to a loss of independence. Pride, or fear of being victimized by those they hire, may stand in the way of much needed help. In these cases, friends can be a big help. Special transportation arrangements may also be available through a local transit company or taxi service.

Many eligible older people are missing meals and are poorly nourished simply because they don't know of available programs to help them. Irregular meal patterns and weight loss, often caused by difficulties in preparing food, are warning signs that undernutrition may be developing. An effort should be made to identify poorly nourished people and inform them of community services.[5]

Community Nutrition Services for Older Adults

Health-care advice and services for older people can come from clinics, private practitioners, hospitals, and health maintenance organizations. Home health-care agencies, adult day-care programs, adult overnight-care programs, and **hospice care** (for the terminally ill) can provide daily care.

The Nutrition Screening Initiative, a nutrition checklist for health-care workers, family members, and older persons, can be used as a tool to increase health and nutrition awareness and to plan related education of older persons (Figure 18-5). The Nutrition Screening Initiative uses the acronym "DETERMINE" (see page 683) to help identify older people whose health needs require extra attention.

A Nutrition Test for Older Adults

Here's a nutrition check for anyone over age 65. Circle the number of points for each statement that applies. Then compute the total and check it against the nutritional score.

Points	
2	1. The person has a chronic illness or current condition that has changed the kind or amount of food eaten.
3	2. The person eats fewer than two full meals per day.
2	3. The person eats few fruits, vegetables, or milk products.
2	4. The person drinks 3 or more servings of beer, liquor, or wine almost every day.
2	5. The person has tooth or mouth problems that make eating difficult.
4	6. The person does not have enough money for food.
1	7. The person eats alone most of the time.
1	8. The person takes three or more different prescription or over-the-counter drugs each day.
2	9. The person has unintentionally lost or gained 10 pounds within the last 6 months.
2	10. The person cannot always shop, cook, or feed himself or herself.
Total	

Nutritional score:

0–2: Good. Recheck in 6 months.

3–5: Marginal. A local agency on aging has information about nutrition programs for the elderly. The National Association of Area Agencies on Aging can assist in finding help; call (800) 677-1116. Recheck in 6 months.

6 or more: High risk. A doctor should review this test and suggest how to improve nutritional health.

Figure 18-5 | A nutrition checklist for older adults.
Reprinted with permission by the Nutrition Screening Initiative, a project of the American Academy of Family Physicians, the American Dietetic Association, and the National Council on Aging, Inc., and funded in part by a grant from Ross Products Division, Abbott Laboratories.

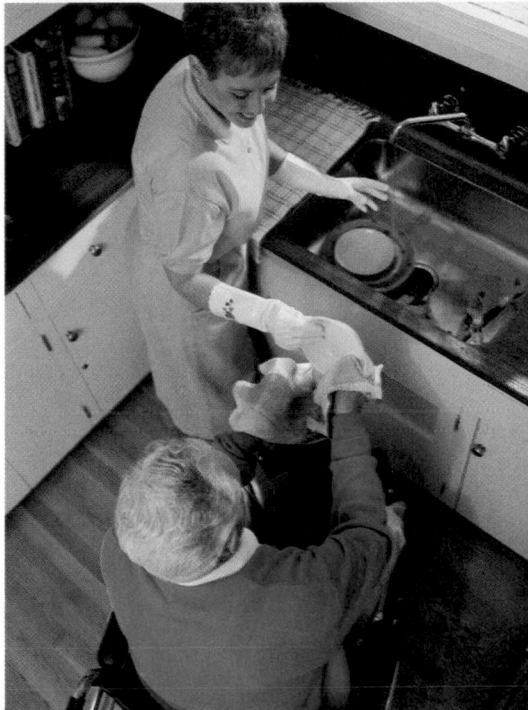

Help is available in most communities to assist older adults in daily tasks. This, in turn, helps older adults meet nutrient needs.

Nutrition programs for people age 60 and over in the United States include congregate meal programs, which provide lunch at a central location, and home-delivered meals (often known as Meals on Wheels if sponsored by the local private or public agencies). About 2.6 million older adults are served each year. Currently about half the people receiving meals use the home-delivered method.

The U.S. government sets specific standards for home-delivered meals and for those served in congregate feeding centers. The meals are designed to provide one-third of RDA/AI. The social aspect often improves appetite and general outlook on life.

Still, congregate meal programs generally provide one meal a day (some provide more) and usually just 5 days per week. Another problem with home-delivered meals is that the one or two meals delivered may never be eaten, and if not eaten on delivery and left at room temperature, they may become unsafe to eat later. Thus, these programs can help older adults but probably don't meet all their nutritional needs.[1]

Determine:

- **D**isease
- **E**ating poorly
- **T**ooth loss or mouth pain
- **E**conomic hardship
- **R**educed social contact and interaction
- **M**ultiple medications
- **I**nvoluntary weight loss or gain
- **N**eed for assistance with self-care
- **E**lder at an advanced age

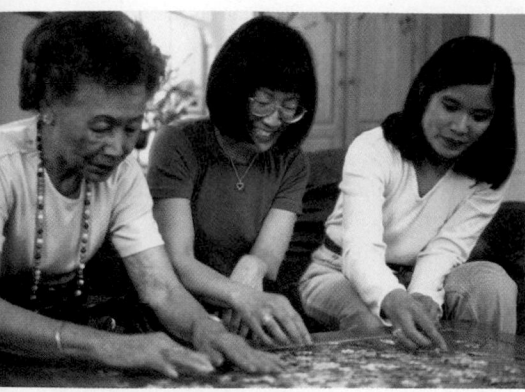

Healthful aging provides many benefits, such as an increased ability to interact with younger family members and friends.

In addition to congregate and home-delivered meals, federal commodity distribution is available in some areas of the United States to low-income older people. Food stamps can benefit older people whose incomes are below the poverty level (see Chapter 20 for details on these programs). Food cooperatives and a variety of clubs, religious, and social organizations provide additional aid.

Concept | Check

Specific nutrient requirements for older adults are only now being extensively studied. Diet plans should be modified for decreased physical abilities, the presence of drug-nutrient interactions, possible depression, and economic constraints. Particular attention should be paid to the opportunity for sun exposure and intake of the vitamins D, B-6, E, folate, and B-12 as well as the minerals calcium and zinc and fiber. A nutrient-dense diet helps meet these needs. Carefully planned multivitamin and mineral supplement use can also help, especially adults 70 years of age and older. In the United States, many nutrition services—such as congregate and home-delivered meals—are available to help the aging population obtain a healthful diet.

Two other websites for organizations that focus on issues surrounding age are:
www.ilcusa.org
www.aging-institute.org

Case Scenario | Follow-Up

Frances could contact a local government office that offers congregate meal programs at a central location. She could inquire about location and available transportation to the site. This meal program would give her social contact with other older persons, which is probably an important element that is missing in her life, and could help alleviate her loneliness. She could also request Meals on Wheels (if available) to provide one hot meal a day, which may be just what she needs to help stimulate her appetite. She could also have groceries delivered to her home if her budget could withstand the extra cost. Other convenience foods that could be included in her diet are milk, assorted nuts, peanut butter, breakfast cereals, canned chicken or deli meats, yogurt, sliced cheese, cottage cheese, calcium-fortified orange juice, canned or frozen fruits and vegetables, and some fresh fruits and vegetables that do not require preparation, such as prewashed lettuce and bananas. A further possibility is a nutrition bar or a liquid nutritional supplement, such as Ensure Plus. The resulting increase in her nutrient intake would help prevent disease in the future and increase her sense of well-being.

Summary

1. Compression of morbidity means delaying symptoms of and disabilities from chronic disease for as many years of life as possible. Most scientists agree upon diet recommendations for the general public, including those provided by the *2005 Dietary Guidelines for Americans*. Such authorities recommend that individuals eat a variety of foods; balance the food eaten with physical activity to maintain or improve weight; choose a diet with plenty of grain products, vegetables, and fruits; choose a diet low in saturated fat and cholesterol; choose a diet moderate in sugars and salt; and limit or avoid alcoholic beverage intake. Regular physical activity is also important, as is safe food preparation.

2. Although maximum life span hasn't changed, life expectancy has increased dramatically over the past century. For many societies, an increasing proportion of the population is over 65 years of age. As health-care costs rise, the goal of delaying disease becomes more important.

3. Aging begins before birth. Cell aging probably results from automatic cellular changes and environmental influences such as DNA damage. Add to this list damage caused by electron-seeking free-radical compounds, high blood glucose, hormonal changes, and alterations in the immune system as possible causes.

4. Nutritional problems of older adults are related to the presence of chronic diseases and to the normal decreases in organ function that occur with time. These include loss of teeth, lessened sensitivity to taste and smell, changes in GI tract function, and deterioration in cardiovascular and bone health. Although disease affects nutritional state, the reverse is also true. Undernutrition adversely affects immune function, allowing for infection.

5. Scientists are only now beginning extensive study of specific nutrient needs for older people. Diet plans should be based on a nutrient-dense approach and individualized for existing health problems, decreased physical abilities, presence of drug-nutrient interactions, possible depression, and economic constraints. Specific nutrients—such as protein, vitamin D, vitamin B-6, folate, vitamin B-12, zinc, and calcium along with fiber and fluid—often deserve special attention in diet planning. A balanced multivitamin and mineral supplement can be used to help meet needs, especially in people age 70 years and older.

6. Health-care workers and family members should use available options for the procurement of food for older adults, especially for those who are nutritionally compromised. Most communities have congregate or home-delivered meal systems, food stamps, and other provisions for those who qualify.

Study Questions

1. List four important points made in the *2005 Dietary Guidelines for Americans* and give an example of why each one may be difficult for older adults to implement. What are some solutions to these barriers?

2. What is the difference between life span and life expectancy?

3. Name two hormones that decline with aging and the functions of each.

4. Describe two hypotheses proposed to explain the causes of aging, and note evidence for each in your daily life experiences.

5. List four organ systems that can decline in function in later years, and list a diet/lifestyle response to help cope with the decline.

6. Defend the recommendation for regular physical activity during older adulthood, including some resistance activity (weight training).

7. How might the nutritional needs of older people differ from those of younger people? How are their needs similar? Be specific.

8. What three resources in a community are widely available to aid older adults in maintaining nutritional health?

9. Describe some warning signs of depression and note a possible nutritional implication as this problem advances.

10. List four warning signs of undernutrition in older people that are part of the acronym DETERMINE. Briefly justify the inclusion of each.

BOOST YOUR STUDY

Check out the *Perspectives in Nutrition: Online Learning Center* www.mhhe.com/wardlawpers7 for quizzes, flash cards, activities, and web links designed to further help you learn about nutrient needs in adulthood.

Annotated References

1. ADA Reports: Position of the American Dietetic Association: Nutrition across the spectrum of aging. *Journal of the American Dietetic Association* 105:616, 2005.

   Behaviors such as a healthful diet, being physically active, and not using tobacco in any form are three keys to healthful aging. The American Dietetic Association supports these practices and encourages older adults to seek medical and nutritional care to treat ongoing health problems such as diabetes and hypertension.

2. Birrer RB and Vermuri SP: Depression in later life: A diagnostic and therapeutic challenge. *American Family Physician* 69.2375, 2004.

   Depression is a common problem in older adulthood. It needs to be addressed because it raises the risk for suicide. Diagnosis and treatment of depression are reviewed in detail in this article.

3. Cummings JL: Alzheimer's disease. *The New England Journal of Medicine* 351:56, 2004.

   This article contains a detailed review of the latest findings on Alzheimer's disease. The au-

   thor notes that delaying the disease should be the main focus, because current medications are not very effective.

4. Dickerson LM, Gibson MV: Management of hypertension in older persons. *American Family Physician* 71:469, 2005.

   Hypertension is a too-common result of the aging process, especially elevated systolic blood pressure. The authors suggest that older people try to combat this trend by following a healthy diet low in sodium and alcohol (if consumed) and as well perform regular physical activity. Typical medications used to treat hypertension in the population are also reviewed.

5. DiMaria-Ghalili RA, Amella E: Nutrition in older adults. *American Journal of Nursing* 105(3):40, 2005.

   Malnutrition in older persons is important to prevent, because it is a bigger risk than over-weight to the health of this population. Risk factors that contribute to malnutrition include a poor diet, limited income, isolation, chronic illness, and various physiological changes that result from aging. These factors in turn can be addressed by appropriate lifestyle interventions reviewed in the article.

6. Fragalis AS: *Popular dietary supplements.* 2nd ed. Chicago, IL: American Dietetic Association, 2003.

   This book provides a comprehensive review of nutrient and herbal supplements. Any use of herbal remedies especially deserves caution; potential benefits and risks in this regard are described.

7. Getting smart about Alzheimer's. *Tufts University Health and Nutrition Letter* 23(3):1, 2005.

   As many as 4.5 million Americans suffer from Alzheimer's disease. Consuming a diet rich in brightly colored fruits and vegetables, which contain many phytochemicals, may prevent the disease. Consuming fish on a regular basis is also important, as is avoiding obesity, exercising regularly, and keeping mentally active. Meeting B vitamin needs is also crucial because many, such as niacin, contribute to brain health.

8. Heilbronn JK, Ravussin E: Calorie restriction and aging: Review of the literature and implications for studies in humans. *American Journal of Clinical Nutrition* 78:361, 2003.

   Calorie restriction has been long known to extend the life span and retard related chronic diseases of rats, mice, fish, flies, and other species. This may be due to a reduction in metabolic rate and oxidative stress, improved insulin sensitivity, and altered nervous system and hormonal activities. Trials are underway to test whether prolonged caloric restriction increases life span or retards the aging process in humans.

9. Litchford MD: Declining nutritional status in older adults. *Today's Dietitian*, p. 12, July 2004.

   The most common causes of declining nutritional status in older adults are poor food choices, failing cognitive status, oral health problems, loss of appetite, and dehydration. Implementing an action plan to treat these problems is important; a registered dietitian can help develop such a plan.

10. Moeller SM and others: Overall adherence to the Dietary Guidelines for Americans is associated with reduced prevalence of early age-related nuclear lens opacities in women. *Journal of Nutrition* 134:1812, 2004.

    A high-quality diet, such as one that follows the Dietary Guidelines for Americans, was shown to prevent or delay the development of lens opacities (i.e., cataracts) in women in this study. Implementing all the recommendations was more helpful than following one or two in isolation, such as just consuming a diet rich in fruits and whole grains.

11. Petersen RC and others: Vitamin E and donepezil for the treatment of mild cognitive impairment. *The New England Journal of Medicine* 352:2379, 2005.

    Megadose vitamin E therapy did not slow development of mild cognitive impairment in this study. This result questions earlier studies that showed a modest but short-lived effect of such therapy. The medication donepezil was somewhat effective, but even this therapy led to only a modest benefit.

12. Rao SS: Prevention of falls in older persons. *American Family Physician* 72:81, 2005.

    Risk factors for falls in older persons—such as muscular weakness, heavy use of medications, old age, impairment of gait and balance, and poor vision—are reviewed in this article. Prevention of falls especially should focus on physical exercise to improve muscular strength and gait as well as a review of all medications used. Having a home inspection by a professional is also helpful to identify physical hazards that can be corrected, such as lack of handrails on stairs.

13. Robertson RG, Montagnini M: Geriatric failure to thrive. *American Family Physician* 70:343, 2004.

    The many factors related to failure to thrive in older adults are reviewed. Use of multiple medications and depression are two common causes that often need to be addressed.

14. Schardt D: Are your supplements safe? *Nutrition Action Healthletter* 30(9):1, 2003.

    This article provides a comprehensive review of popular herbal supplements. It also covers herbs and other substances to avoid because of a high potential for toxicity.

15. Staying well—at your age. *Consumer Reports on Health* 17(9):1, 2005.

    A detailed plan of health promotion and disease prevention as one ages is presented in the article. This plan includes dietary recommendations

(e.g., meeting energy, calcium, iron, and vitamin D needs), aerobic and strength-training physical activities, and appropriate medical screening tests for each decade of adult life.

16. Sisk J: Aging and fit—the shape of things to come. *Today's Dietitian*, p. 34, July 2004.

    Regular physical activity is vital to prevent age-related declines in many aspects of health. A key point is that one is never too old to start an exercise program and achieve health benefits.

17. Szulc P and others: Hormonal and lifestyle determinants of appendicular skeletal muscle mass in men: The MINOS study. *American Journal of Clinical Nutrition* 80:496, 2004.

    In older men, low physical activity, tobacco smoking, thinness, low blood testosterone, and poor vitamin D status were found to be risk factors for reduced muscle mass, termed sarcopenia. Lack of physical activity is especially important to address in order to maintain a healthy amount of muscle mass as one ages.

18. Trichopoulou A and others: Modified Mediterranean diet and survival: EPIC-elderly prospective cohort study. *British Medical Journal* 330:991, 2005.

    A diet characterized by high intakes of vegetables, legumes, fruits, cereals, and unsaturated fats; moderate amounts of fish and alcohol; and low-to-moderate amounts of dairy products and meats lessened the risk of developing cardiovascular disease in people in this study. Total mortality was also reduced, especially so in people who closely adhered to this diet pattern.

19. Trumbo R: Hormone changes in aging adults probed. *Journal of the American Medical Association* 294:663, 2005.

    Hormones that typically decline in aging are testosterone, growth hormone, and thyroid hormone. Replacement of all three is possible, but each carry risks, and so any use needs to be carefully considered by the older person and his or her physician. Growth hormone therapy is very expensive, and so least likely of the three to be administered.

20. Tucker KL and others: The combination of high fruit and vegetables and low saturated fat intakes is more protective against mortality in aging men than is either alone: The Baltimore longitudinal study of aging. *Journal of Nutrition* 135:556, 2005.

    A diet rich in fruits and vegetables and low in saturated fat intakes reduced mortality in aging men in this study. Putting all three recommendations into practice was especially helpful.

I. Am I Aging Healthfully?

Take Control of Your Aging by Dr. William B. Malarkey (Wooster Book Co., Wooster OH, 1999) includes a plan that incorporates various diet and lifestyle factors that are associated with successful aging. Indicate the degree to which you are following such a plan (or alternatively fill this out with a parent or another older relative in mind).

Physical: Do you eat a well-balanced diet, exercise on a regular basis, remain free of illness, abstain from smoking, refrain from drinking alcohol excessively, and experience refreshing sleep?

_____

_____

_____

Intellectual: Are you analytical, do you read regularly, do you learn new things each day, do you engage your mental ability at work (or at school), and do you often reflect on your life?

_____

_____

_____

Emotional: Are you at peace, do you like who you are, are you optimistic, and do you laugh and relax regularly?

_____

_____

_____

Relational: Are you a good listener, do you feel supported by friends, do you attend social functions, do you talk with family members often, and do you feel close to coworkers (or fellow students)?

_____

_____

_____

Spiritual: Do you appreciate nature, give to or serve others, meditate or seek religious worship, and feel life has meaning?

_____

_____

_____

The more of these factors that you include in your life, the more well rounded your plan is for maintaining overall health. Any one of the five areas in which you are not achieving success should show you characteristics to work on in the future.

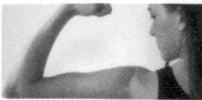

Take | Action

II. Helping Older Adults Eat Better

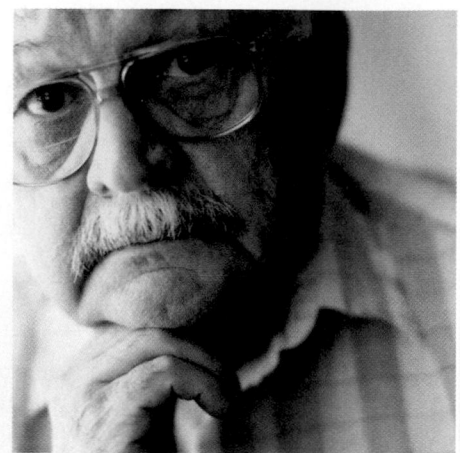

During their lifetimes, most people usually eat meals with families or loved ones. As people reach their older ages, many of them are faced with living and eating alone. In a study of the diets of 4400 older adults in the United States, one man in every five living alone and over age 55 ate poorly. One of four women between the ages of 55 and 64 years followed a low-quality diet. These poor diets can contribute to deteriorating mental and physical health. Consider the following example of the living situation of an older adult.

Neal, a 70-year-old man, lives alone in a home in a local suburban area. His wife died one year ago. He doesn't have many friends; his wife was his primary confidante. His neighbors across the street and next door are friendly, and Neal used to help them with yard projects in his spare time. Neal's health has been good, but he has had trouble with his teeth recently. His diet has been poor, and in the past 3 months his physical and mental vigor have deteriorated. He has been slowly lapsing into a depression and, so, keeps the shades drawn and rarely leaves his house. Neal keeps very little food in the house because his wife did most of the cooking and shopping, and he just isn't that interested in food.

If you were one of Neal's relatives and learned of Neal's situation, what six things could you do or suggest to help improve his nutritional status and mental outlook? Look back through this chapter to get some ideas.

1. _____
2. _____
3. _____
4. _____
5. _____
6. _____

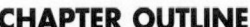

SAFETY OF FOOD AND WATER

CHAPTER OUTLINE

CASE SCENARIO:

Aaron attended a gathering of his officemates on a warm July Saturday. The theme was international dining, and he and his wife were told to bring Argentine beef, a stewlike dish. They followed the recipe and cooking time carefully, removing the dish from the oven at 1 P.M. and keeping it warm by wrapping the pan in a towel. They traveled in their car to the party and set the dish out on the buffet table at 3 P.M. Dinner was to be served at 4 P.M. However, the guests were enjoying themselves so much lounging around the host's pool and drinking ginger beer (also on the menu) that no one began to eat until 6 P.M. Aaron made sure he sampled the Argentine beef that he and his wife made, but his wife did not. He also had some salad, garlic bread, and a sweet dessert made with coconut.

The couple returned home at 11 P.M. and went to bed. About 2 A.M., Aaron knew something was wrong. He had severe abdominal pain and had to make a mad dash to the bathroom. He spent most of the next 3 hours in the bathroom with severe diarrhea. By dawn, the diarrhea had subsided and he had started feeling better. After a few cups of tea and a light breakfast, he was feeling like himself by noon.

What type of foodborne illness did Aaron contract? What precautions for avoiding foodborne illness were ignored by Aaron and the rest of the people at the party? How could this scenario be rewritten to substantially reduce the risk of foodborne illness?

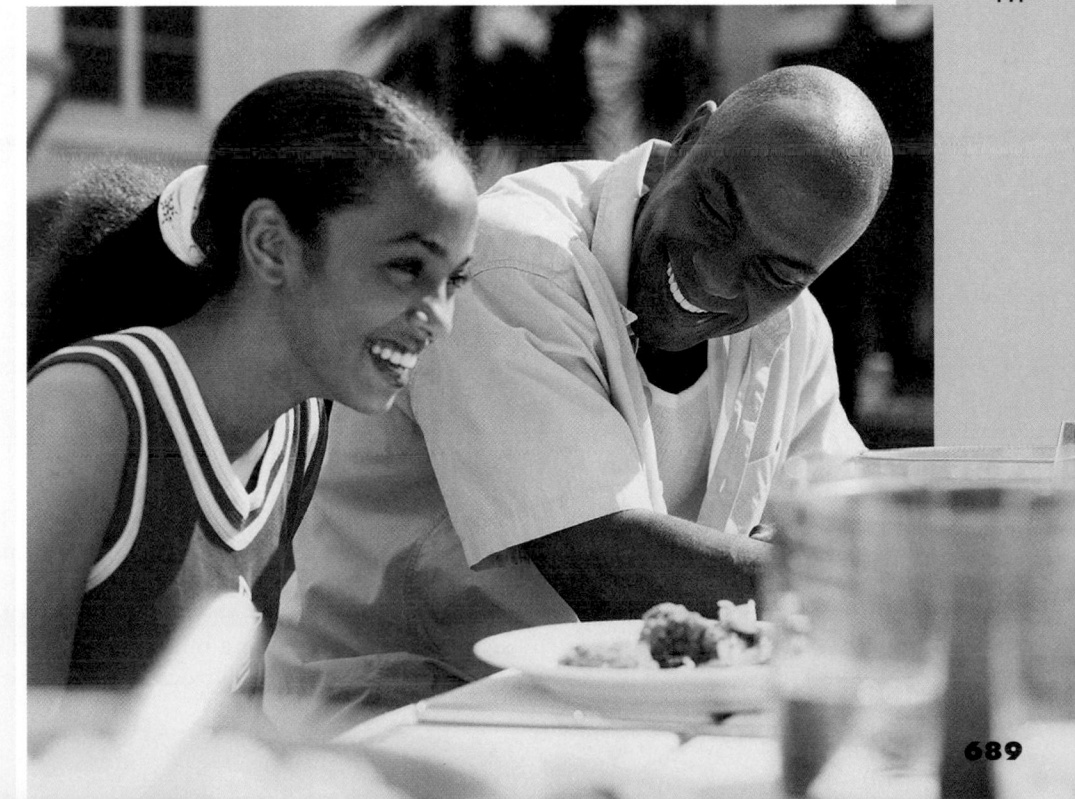

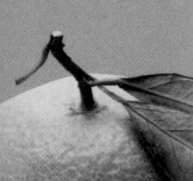

At the turn of the twentieth century, conditions in Chicago's meat-packing industry were sickening. Moldy, spoiled meat was commonly doused with borax to cover up the smell, and glycerine was added to make it look fresh. By 1906, increasing public pressure forced the passage of the first Food and Drug Act in the United States. Federal inspection then safeguarded the public from worm-infested and diseased meat and generally improved food preparation standards.

Today, warnings about the safety of food and water appear everywhere. Attention has turned to more contemporary concerns, such as microbial and chemical contamination. On one hand, we are told to eat more fruits, vegetables, fish, and poultry and to drink more water; on the other hand, we are warned that these may contain dangerous substances, so we still must ask, "How safe is our food and water?"

Scientists and health authorities agree that North Americans enjoy a relatively safe food supply, especially if foods are stored and prepared properly. Our water supply is also generally safe.[2] Over the past 100 or so years, tremendous progress has been made to allow for this. Nonetheless, microorganisms and certain chemicals in foods still can pose a health risk.[1,19] Thus the nutritional and health benefits of food and water must be balanced against any related hazards. Chapter 19 focuses on these food- and water-related hazards—how real they are and how you can minimize their effect on your life. Note that you bear some responsibility for this—government agencies and industry can only do so much.[12] Recall from Chapter 2 that the 2005 Dietary Guidelines for Americans emphasize safe food practices. One goal of *Healthy People 2010* is to reduce by 50% the number of cases of foodborne illness from typical bacterial causes.

CHAPTER OBJECTIVES CHAPTER 19 IS DESIGNED TO ALLOW YOU TO:

1. List some of the types of bacteria, fungi, viruses, and parasites found in food and their common sources.

2. Describe common means by which food and water become contaminated.

3. State conditions that support growth of food microorganisms.

4. Describe the procedures that can be used to limit the risk of foodborne and waterborne illness.

5. Compare and contrast how food-preservation methods, such as pasteurization, canning, irradiation, and aseptic packaging, control the growth of microorganisms in food.

6. Describe the main reasons for using chemical additives in foods, the general classes of additives, and the functions of each class.

7. Identify toxic environmental contaminants in food, related complications of ingestion, and sources.

8. Understand the reasons behind pesticide use, the possible long-term health risks, and the safety limits set for their use.

REFRESH YOUR MEMORY AS YOU BEGIN YOUR STUDY OF FOOD SAFETY IN CHAPTER 19, YOU MAY WANT TO REVIEW:
- The disease phenylketonuria (PKU) in Chapters 4, 5, and 7.
- Alternative sweeteners in Chapter 5.
- Fat substitutes in Chapter 6.
- The causes of cancer in Chapter 12.

Safety of Food and Water: Setting the Stage

During the early stages of urbanization in North America, contaminated water and food—notably, milk—were responsible for many large outbreaks of typhoid fever, septic sore throat, scarlet fever, diphtheria, and other devastating human diseases. These contaminations led to the development of processes for purifying water, treating sewage, and **pasteurizing** milk. Since that time, safe water and milk have become universally available, with only occasional problems from either.[2,3]

pasteurizing The process of heating food products to kill pathogenic microorganisms and reduce the total number of bacteria.

The greatest health risk from food and water today is contamination by **viruses** and **bacteria** and, to a lesser extent, by various forms of **fungi** and **parasites**.[12] These microorganisms can all cause **foodborne illness** and can also cause illness when in the water supply.[3] For example, in one recent case a child died and 50 others became ill from *Escherichia coli (E. coli)* bacteria found in apple juice. In another case, 170 children became ill when their school lunch contained strawberries contaminated by hepatitis A virus. In 1993, 400,000 people in Milwaukee became ill and 100 died from water contaminated with the parasite *Cryptosporidium*.

Even though microbial contamination is the cause of most incidents of food- and water-related illness, North Americans seem more concerned about health risks from chemicals in foods and water. Of U.S. consumers surveyed in a Gallup poll, about 75% said that pesticide contamination was a major concern to them. In the long run, this concern has some merit. On a day-to-day basis, however, it is not very important in North America.[19]

Because microbial contamination of food is by far the more important issue for our day-to-day health, it will be discussed first. Chapter 19 will then cover the use and safety of food additives, concerns over the safety of our water supply, and the risks of pesticides to our health.

What Are the Effects of Foodborne Illness?

According to the U.S. Centers for Disease Control and Prevention, foodborne illness caused 76 million illnesses, 325,000 hospitalizations, and 5000 deaths in the United States in 2002. Hospital costs for foodborne illnesses are estimated at more than $3 billion per year; costs from related lost productivity are estimated at $8 billion per year.[3] Some people are particularly susceptible to foodborne illness, including:[8,9]

- Infants and children
- Older adults
- People with liver disease, diabetes, HIV infection (and AIDS), or cancer
- Pregnant women
- People taking immunosuppressant agents (e.g., transplant patients)

As you can see, foodborne illness has the greatest effect on the most vulnerable people in terms of health status (estimated to be about 30 million people in the United States alone). Some bouts of foodborne illness, especially when coupled with the ongoing health problems, are lengthy and lead to food allergies, seizures, blood poisoning (from **toxins** or microorganisms in the bloodstream), or other illnesses.

Because foodborne illnesses often result from the unsafe handling of food at home, we each bear some responsibility for preventing them.[10,12] Because you can't usually tell by taste, smell, or sight that a particular food contains harmful microorganisms, you might not even be aware that food has caused your distress. In fact, your last case of diarrhea may have been caused by foodborne illness (Table 19-1). Government agencies are also at work on problems regarding food safety, but their work does not substitute for individual safety efforts (Table 19-2).

Why Is Foodborne Illness So Common?

Foodborne illness is carried or transmitted to people by food. Most foodborne illnesses are transmitted through food in which microorganisms are able to grow rapidly. These foods are generally moist, rich in protein, and have a neutral or slightly acidic pH. Unfortunately, this describes many of the foods we eat every day, such as meats, eggs, and dairy products.[2]

Our food industry tries whenever possible to increase the shelf life of food products; however, a longer shelf life allows more time for bacteria in foods to multiply. Some bacteria even grow at refrigeration temperatures. Partially cooked—and some fully cooked—products pose a particular risk because refrigerated storage may only slow, not prevent, bacterial growth.[2]

virus The smallest known type of infectious agent, many of which cause disease in humans. Viruses do not metabolize, grow, or move by themselves. They reproduce only with the aid of a living cellular host. A virus is essentially a piece of genetic material surrounded by a coat of protein.

bacteria Single-cell microorganisms; some produce poisonous substances that cause illness in humans. They contain only one chromosome and lack many organelles found in human cells. Some can live without oxygen and survive by means of **spore** formation.

spores Dormant reproductive cells capable of turning into adult organisms without the help of another cell. Various bacteria and fungi form spores.

fungi Simple parasitic life forms, including molds, mildews, yeasts, and mushrooms. They live on dead or decaying organic matter. Fungi can grow as single cells, like yeast, or as a multicellular colony, as seen with molds.

parasite An organism that lives in or on another organism and derives nourishment from it.

foodborne illness Sickness caused by the ingestion of food containing toxic substances produced by microorganisms.

toxins Poisonous compounds produced by an organism that can cause disease.

Note that some restaurants that will serve requested undercooked food are now warning patrons (on the menu) of the health risks of ordering such foods, particularly with undercooked eggs and meats.

Table 19-1 | Some Examples of Cases of Foodborne Illness

We generally have a safe food supply, but there are occasional instances of foodborne illnesses, such as the incidents listed in this table.

Viruses

• An estimated 6 million oysters from Louisiana were bathed with the Norovirus after ships with ill crew members dumped their sewage overboard. By the time the outbreak was recognized, an estimated 20,000 to 30,000 people had become ill. Another outbreak of the virus was attributed to an infected bakery worker who stirred a vat full of buttercream frosting with his bare hand and arm. In Florida, 83 fraternity members caught the virus from the fraternity house ice machine. During the Gulf War, Norovirus was one of the most common causes of gastroenteritis among U.S. troops. Recently passengers on cruise ships have also contracted Norovirus illness.

• Over 500 adults in the United States contracted hepatitis A after eating raw green onions in a Mexican restaurant. The onions were contaminated during growth in Mexico and were not properly washed by food service workers.

Bacteria

• A previously healthy 5-month-old girl suddenly died at home from contact with a pet iguana infected with *Salmonella*. Unpasteurized juice products were recalled after 57 cases of *Salmonella* illness were reported in California and Colorado. Eight people became ill from *Salmonella* after consuming tiramisu, a dessert that contains raw eggs.

• Six persons were reported ill from a *Shigella* infection after eating chopped, uncooked parsley that was served on chicken sandwiches and in coleslaw. A cruise ship had to return to port when more than 600 people developed shigellosis and one person died.

• The first documented foodborne illness caused by *Listeria* organisms in North America occurred in commercially prepared coleslaw. Later, 48 deaths were associated with soft, Mexican-style cheeses. A listeriosis outbreak associated with undercooked hot dogs and cold cuts resulted in more than 82 illnesses and 17 deaths in 19 states. Another outbreak of *Listeria* sickened at least 120 people and killed 20 in the northeastern United States. Recently 14.5 million pounds of ready-to-eat meat and poultry products were recalled because of possible *Listeria* contamination. A meat-packing firm recalled 27.4 million pounds of turkey and chicken after finding *Listeria* bacteria at the plant.

• The first community outbreak in the United States of *E. coli* O111:H8 sickened 58 teenagers at a cheerleading camp in Texas. The camp salad bar and a communal water barrel were suspected sources of infection. One of the largest *E. coli* O157:H7 outbreaks on record infected more than 1000 people in upstate New York at a county fair. The bacterium was found in infected well water. It killed a 79-year-old man and a 4-year-old girl, and it caused 10 other children to undergo kidney dialysis. Six adults and a 2-year-old child were killed after an *E. coli* outbreak from contaminated drinking water in Canada. The bacteria entered the water supply from animal manure after flooding from a heavy storm. In northeastern Oklahoma, five children were infected with *E. coli* after consuming unpasteurized apple cider. Recently 25 million pounds of hamburger had to be recalled because of potential *E. coli* O157:H7 contamination. A woman died in Columbus, Ohio, after she was infected with *E. coli* O157:H7 bacteria.

• A man in Arkansas developed botulism after eating stew that was cooked and then kept at room temperature for 3 days. He spent 49 days in the hospital—42 of them on mechanical ventilation. Another recent case involved a man who ate hard-boiled eggs that were left in a pickling solution at room temperature for 7 days.

• Since 1992, 17 people in Florida died of *Vibrio vulnificus* infections after eating raw oysters.

• A teenage boy and his father experienced abdominal pain, vomiting, and diarrhea within 30 minutes of eating 4-day-old homemade pesto. The pesto had been reheated and left out a number of times during the 4-day period. It was apparently contaminated with *Bacillus cereus*. As a result, the boy died of liver failure.

Parasites

• A group attending a dinner banquet developed diarrhea 3 to 9 days after eating green onions, which was the likely cause of the outbreak. Eight of 10 stool specimens obtained from the group with foodborne illness were positive for *Cryptosporidium*. Food workers at the restaurant reported they did not consistently wash green onions before using them.

Risks from Seafood

• Four adults became ill with scombroid fish poisoning after eating tuna-spinach salad at a restaurant in Pennsylvania.

• An outbreak of ciguatera fish poisoning involved 17 crew members of a cargo ship that caught, cooked, and ate a barracuda in the Bahamas. All 17 men became ill with nausea, vomiting, abdominal cramps, and diarrhea within hours of eating the fish. Within 2 days, all of the men suffered from muscle pain and weakness, dizziness, and numb or itchy feet, hands, and mouth.

The risk of contracting foodborne illness also is high because of recent consumer trends. First, there is greater consumer interest in eating raw or undercooked animal products. In addition, more people receive medication that suppresses their ability to combat foodborne infectious agents. Another factor is the continuing increase in the number of older adults in the population.

The risk of illness from foodborne microorganisms increases as more of our foods are prepared in kitchens outside the home. Supermarkets have become major food processors over the past decade and now offer a variety of prepared foods from specialty meat shops, salad bars, and bakeries. With the increasing number of two-income

Table 19-2 | U.S. Agencies Responsible for Monitoring the Food Supply

Agency Name	Responsibilities	Methods	How to Contact
United States Department of Agriculture (USDA)	• Enforces wholesomeness and quality standards for grains and produce (while in the field), meat, poultry, milk, eggs, and egg products	• Conducts inspections • Establishes trading • Administers "Safe Handling Label"	www.usda.gov/fsis or www.nal.usda.gov/fnicfoodborne/foodborne.htm or call 1-800-535-4555
Bureau of Alcohol, Tobacco, and Firearms and Explosives (ATF)	• Enforces laws on alcoholic beverages	• Conducts inspections	www.atf.treas.gov
Environmental Protection Agency (EPA)	• Regulates pesticides • Establishes water quality standards	• Approves all U.S. pesticides • Sets pesticide residue limits in food	www.epa.gov
Food and Drug Administration (FDA)	• Ensures safety and wholesomeness of all foods in interstate commerce (except meat, poultry, and processed egg products) • Regulates seafood • Controls product labels	• Conducts inspections • Conducts food sample studies • Sets standards for specific foods	www.fda.gov or call 1-800-FDA-4010
Centers for Disease Control and Prevention (CDC)	• Promotes food safety	• Responds to emergencies concerning foodborne illness • Surveys and studies environmental health problems • Directs/enforces quarantines • Conducts national programs for prevention and control of foodborne and other diseases	www.cdc.gov
National Marine Fisheries Service or NOAA Fisheries	• Monitors domestic and international conservation and management of living marine resources	• Conducts voluntary seafood inspection program • Can use mark to show federal inspection	www.nmfs.noaa.gov
State and local governments	• Promotes milk safety • Monitors food industry within their borders	• Conducts inspections of food-related establishments	Government pages of telephone book

Government agencies responsible for monitoring food safety in Canada and the specific laws followed are listed in Appendix D.

families, more people are looking for convenient, easy-to-prepare, nutritious foods. Supermarkets offer entrées that can be served immediately or reheated. The foods are usually prepared in central kitchens or processing plants and shipped to individual stores.

This centralization of food production by the food-processing and restaurant industry enhances the risk of foodborne illness. If a food product is contaminated in a processing plant, consumers over a wide area can suffer foodborne illness. For example, a malfunction in an ice cream plant in Minnesota resulted in 224,000 suspected cases of *Salmonella* bacterial infections, linked to use of contaminated ice cream mix. At least 4 people died and 700 became ill in Washington and surrounding western states after eating at a chain of fast-food restaurants. The source of the problem was undercooked hamburger contaminated with the bacterium *E. coli* 0157:H7. Note that restaurants generally encounter inspection by local health departments about every 6 months. We must primarily rely on each restaurant to practice good food safety.

Greater consumption of ready-to-eat foods imported from foreign countries is still another cause of increased foodborne illness in North America. In the past, food imports were mostly raw products processed here under strict sanitation standards. Now, however, we import more ready-to-eat processed foods—such as berries from

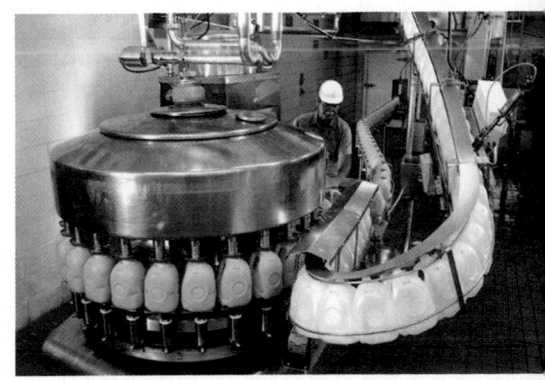

Food contaminated in a central plant can go on to produce illness in people in surrounding states or even across the nation. In the case of juices, shown here, it is only important that they are pasteurized to reduce risk of foodborne illness, especially for the more susceptible of us.

Guatemala and shellfish from Vietnam—some of which are contaminated. U.S. authorities are currently reexamining inspection procedures for these imports.

The use of antibiotics in animal feeds is also increasing the severity of cases of foodborne illness. This antibiotic use encourages bacteria to develop antibiotic-resistant strains, those that can grow even if exposed to typical antibiotic medicines. This issue is currently receiving considerable attention by scientists in the field.

Finally, more cases of foodborne disease are reported now because scientists are more aware of the roles of various players in the process. Every decade the list of microorganisms suspected of causing foodborne illness lengthens.[1] In addition, physicians are more likely to suspect foodborne contaminants as a cause of illness. Furthermore, we now know that food, besides serving as a good growth medium for some microorganisms, simply transmits many others as well. Seafood is receiving greater scrutiny and surveillance by FDA as a cause of foodborne illness. In addition, FDA is conducting a $500,000 campaign to educate U.S. consumers about the risks of eating raw oysters. For more information about these risks, contact FDA's Seafood Hotline at 1-800-FDA-4010 or log on to www.safefood.gov.

▌ Food Preservation: Past, Present, and Future

When traveling to developing countries, it is recommended that you "boil it, peel it, or don't eat it." Ironically, up to 70% of our fruits and vegetables during certain seasons come from these countries. In other words, you do not have to travel to acquire traveler's diarrhea. In response, we should carefully inspect and wash produce, as we would in a foreign country.

irradiation A process in which **radiation** energy is applied to foods, creating compounds (free radicals) within the food that destroy cell membranes, break down DNA, link proteins together, limit enzyme activity, and alter a variety of other proteins and cell functions of microorganisms that can lead to food spoilage. This process does not make the food radioactive.

radiation Literally, energy that is emitted from a center in all directions. Various forms of radiation energy include X-rays and ultraviolet rays from the sun.

aseptic processing A method by which food and container are separately and simultaneously sterilized; it allows manufacturers to produce boxes of milk that can be stored at room temperature.

For centuries, salt, sugar, smoke, fermentation, and drying have been used to preserve food. Ancient Romans used sulfites to disinfect wine containers and preserve wine. For thousands of years, salted fish and meat have fed vast segments of the human population. Most preserving methods work on the principle of decreasing water content. Bacteria need abundant stores of water to grow; yeasts and molds can grow with less water, but some is still necessary. Adding sugar or salt binds water and so decreases the water available to these microbes. The process of drying evaporates off free water.

Decreasing the water content of some high-moisture foods, however, would cause them to lose essential characteristics. To preserve such foods—cucumber pickles, sauerkraut, milk (yogurt), and wine—fermentation has been a traditional alternative. Selected bacteria or yeast are used to ferment or pickle foods. The fermenting bacteria or yeast make acids and alcohol, which minimize the growth of other bacteria and yeast.

Today we can add pasteurization, sterilization, refrigeration, freezing, food **irradiation,** canning, and chemical preservation to the list of food preservation techniques. An additional method of food preservation—**aseptic processing**—simultaneously sterilizes the food and package separately before the food enters the package. Liquid foods, such as fruit juices, are especially easy to process in this manner. With aseptic packaging, boxes of sterile milk and juices can remain on supermarket shelves, free of microbial growth, for many years.

Food irradiation uses minimal doses of radiation in order to control pathogens such as *E. coli* 0157:H7 and *Salmonella*.[14] Even though FDA has permitted irradiation of certain food products for more than a decade, the history of the technology goes back nearly a century, including scientific research, evaluation, and testing. The radiation energy that is used does not make the food radioactive. The energy essentially passes through the food, as in microwave cooking, and no radioactive residues are left behind. However, the energy is strong enough to break chemical bonds, destroy cell walls and cell membranes, break down DNA, and link proteins together. Irradiation thereby controls growth of insects, bacteria, fungi, and parasites in foods.

FDA recently approved the use of irradiation for raw red meat to reduce risk of *E. coli* and other infectious microorganisms. Some food processors are now doing so. Other additions to the approved list are shell eggs and seeds. Prior to this recent approval, the only animal products so treated were pork and chicken. Irradiation also extends the shelf life of spices, dry vegetable seasonings, meats, and fresh fruits and vegetables.

Irradiated food, except for dried seasonings, must be labeled with the international food irradiation symbol, the Radura, and a statement that the product has been treated by irradiation. Foods treated in this way are safe in the opinion of FDA and many other health authorities, including the American Academy of Pediatrics.[14] Although the demand for irradiated foods is still low in the United States, other countries, including Canada, Japan, Italy, and Mexico, all use food irradiation technology widely. Certain consumer groups continually try to block its use in the United States, claiming that irradiation diminishes the nutritional value of food and that it can lead to the formation of harmful compounds, such as carcinogens. Future research should be able to sort out this controversy, but in any case the risk is very low. Keep in mind also that, even when foods, especially meats, have been irradiated, it is still important to follow basic food-safety procedures, because later contamination in food preparation is possible.

This is the Radura, the international label denoting prior irradiation of the food product.

Foodborne Illness: When Undesirable Microorganisms Alter Foods

Most cases of foodborne illness are caused by specific viruses, bacteria, parasites, and fungi. Prions—proteins involved in maintaining nerve cell function—can also turn infectious and lead to diseases such as mad cow disease.[11] Bacteria specifically cause health problems either directly by invading the intestinal wall and producing an *infection* via a toxin contained in the organism, or indirectly by producing a toxin that is secreted into the food, which later harms us (called an *intoxication*). The main way to distinguish an infectious route from an intoxication is time: if symptoms appear in 4 hours or less, it is an intoxication.

Many types of bacteria cause foodborne illness, including *Bacillus, Campylobacter, Clostridium, Escherichia, Listeria, Vibrio, Salmonella,* and *Staphylococcus* (Table 19-3). Bacteria are everywhere: a teaspoon of soil contains about 2 billion bacteria. Luckily, only a small number of bacteria actually pose a threat. In addition, experts speculate that about 70% of cases of foodborne illness go undiagnosed because they result from viral causes, such as Norovirus, and there is no easy way to test for these pathogens.[20] A website coordinating the U.S. efforts on food safety is www.foodsafety.gov. Other useful websites are www.ama-assn.org/foodborne and www.homefoodsafety.org.

A goal of *Healthy People 2010* is to reduce the number of cases of foodborne illness from *Campylobacter, E. coli, Listeria,* and *Salmonella* by 50%.

General Rules for Preventing Foodborne Illness

You can greatly reduce the risk of foodborne illness by following some very important rules. It's a long list, because many risky habits need to be addressed.[3,4,10,12,18]

Purchasing Food

- When shopping, select frozen foods and perishable foods, such as meat, poultry, or fish, last. Always have these products put in separate plastic bags, so that drippings don't contaminate other foods in the shopping cart. Don't let groceries sit in a warm car; this allows bacteria to grow. Take the perishable foods such as meat and egg and dairy products home and promptly refrigerate or freeze them.
- Don't buy or use food from damaged containers that leak, bulge, or are severely dented or from jars that are cracked or have loose or bulging lids. Don't taste or use food that has a foul odor or spurts liquid when the can is opened; the deadly *Clostridium botulinum* toxin may be present.
- Purchase only pasteurized milk and cheese (check the label). This caution is especially important for pregnant women because highly toxic bacteria and viruses that can harm the fetus thrive in unpasteurized milk.
- Purchase only the amount of produce needed for a week's time. The longer you keep fruits and vegetables, the more time is available for bacteria to grow.
- When purchasing precut produce or salads, avoid those that look slimy, brownish, or dry; these are signs of improper holding temperatures.

The World Health Organization's Golden Rules for Safe Food Preparation

1. Choose foods processed for safety.
2. Cook food thoroughly.
3. Eat cooked foods immediately.
4. Store cooked foods carefully.
5. Reheat cooked foods thoroughly.
6. Avoid contact between raw and cooked foods.
7. Wash hands repeatedly.
8. Keep all kitchen surfaces meticulously clean.
9. Protect foods from insects, rodents, and other animals.
10. Use pure water.

The USDA recently simplified these rules into four actions as a part of their Fight BAC! Program (check out www.fightbac.org):

1. Clean. Wash hands and surfaces often.
2. Separate. Don't cross-contaminate.
3. Cook. Cook to proper temperatures.
4. Chill. Refrigerate promptly.

Table 19-3 | Important Microorganisms and Related Factors That Cause Foodborne Illness: Their Sources, Symptoms, and Prevention

Microorganism	Sources	Symptoms	Prevention Methods
Viruses			
Norovirus (Norwalk and Norwalk-like virus), human rotavirus	Found in the human intestinal tract and feces. Contamination occurs: (1) when sewage is used to enrich garden/farm soil (2) by direct hand-to-food contact during the preparation of meals (3) when shellfish are harvested from waters contaminated by sewage.	Onset: 1–2 days. Severe diarrhea, nausea, and vomiting. Respiratory symptoms. Usually lasts 4–5 days but may last for weeks.	• Sanitary handling of foods • Use of pure drinking water • Adequate sewage disposal • Adequate cooking of foods • Good personal hygiene
Hepatitis A virus	Fecal-oral route that contaminates food, beverages, or shellfish.	Onset: 15–50 days. Anorexia, diarrhea, fever, jaundice, and fatigue. May cause liver damage and death.	• Sanitary handling of foods • Use of pure drinking water • Adequate sewage disposal • Thorough cooking of foods
Bacteria			
Campylobacter jejuni	Found on poultry, beef, and lamb and can contaminate meat and milk. Chief food sources are raw poultry and meat and unpasteurized milk.	Onset: 2–5 days after eating, or longer. Diarrhea, abdominal cramping, fever, and sometimes bloody stools. Lasts 2–7 days.	• Thorough cooking of foods • Sanitary food-handling practices • Avoidance of unpasteurized milk
Salmonella species	Found in raw meats, poultry, eggs, fish, sprouts, unpasteurized milk, and products made with these items. Multiplies rapidly at room temperature. The bacteria themselves are toxic.	Onset: 1–3 days after eating. Nausea, fever, headache, abdominal cramps, diarrhea, and vomiting. Can be fatal in infants, the elderly, and the sick.	• Sanitary food-handling practices • Avoidance of any use of unpasteurized raw eggs or undercooked eggs • Thorough cooking of foods • Prompt refrigeration of foods
Shigella species	Transmitted via fecal-oral route and somewhat in food and water.	Onset: 1–3 days. Abdominal cramps, diarrhea, fever, bloody stools.	• Handwashing and sanitary food production
Escherichia coli (0157:H7 and other strains)	Undercooked beef, especially ground beef. Fruits, vegetables, sprouts, and yogurt are also possible sources.	Onset: 1–8 days. Bloody diarrhea, abdominal cramps, kidney failure.	• Thorough cooking, especially of beef • Avoidance of unpasteurized milk, untreated apple cider
Clostridium perfringens	Found throughout the environment. Generally found in meat and poultry dishes. Multiply rapidly in anaerobic conditions when foods are left for extended time at room temperature.	Onset: 8–24 hours after eating (usually 12 hours). Abdominal pain and diarrhea. Symptoms last a day or less, usually mild. Can be more serious in older or ill people.	• Sanitary handling of foods, especially meat and meat dishes, gravies, and leftovers • Thorough cooking and reheating of foods, especially leftovers • Prompt and proper refrigeration
Listeria monocytogenes	Found in soft cheeses made with unpasteurized milk and in unpasteurized milk itself. Resists acid, heat, salt, nitrate, and refrigeration temperatures.	Onset: 9–48 hours for early symptoms; 14–42 days for severe symptoms. Fever, headache, vomiting, and sometimes more severe symptoms. May be fatal.	• Thorough cooking of foods • Sanitary food-handling practices • Avoidance of unpasteurized milk
Staphylococcus aureus	Found in nasal passages and in cuts on skin. Toxin is produced when food contaminated by bacteria is left for extended time at room temperature. Meats, poultry, egg products pose the greatest risk.	Onset: 2–6 hours after eating. Diarrhea, vomiting, nausea, and abdominal cramps. Mimics flu. Lasts 24–36 hours. Rarely fatal.	• Sanitary food-handling practices • Prompt and proper refrigeration of foods • Covering cuts on skin

Table 19-3 | Important Microorganisms and Related Factors That Cause Foodborne Illness: Their Sources, Symptoms, and Prevention *(continued)*

Microorganism	Sources	Symptoms	Prevention Methods
Bacteria *(continued)*			
Clostridium botulinum	Found throughout the environment. However, bacteria produce toxin only in a low-acid, anaerobic environment, such as in canned green beans, mushrooms, spinach, olives, and beef. Honey may carry spores.	Onset: 12–72 hours after eating. Neurotoxic symptoms include double vision, inability to swallow, speech difficulty, and progressive paralysis of the respiratory system. OBTAIN MEDICAL HELP IMMEDIATELY. BOTULISM CAN BE FATAL.	• Use of proper methods for canning low-acid foods • Avoidance of commercial cans of low-acid foods that have leaky seals or are bent, bulging, or broken • Discarding of food if toxin is suspected (off odors are a sign)
Vibrio vulnificus	Raw seafood, especially raw oysters.	Onset: 1–7 days. Diarrhea, fever, weakness, blood infection, death.	• Thorough cooking of seafood
Vibrio cholerae	Human carriers, infected shellfish, contaminated water and food.	Onset: 2–3 days. Vomiting, severe watery diarrhea, which can lead to dehydration and cardiovascular collapse; death.	• Handwashing after using the bathroom
Yersinia enterocolitica	Found throughout the environment; carried in food, water, and feces. Multiply rapidly at both room and refrigerator temperatures. Generally found in raw vegetables, meats, water, and unpasteurized milk.	Onset: 2–3 days. Fever, headache, nausea, diarrhea, and general malaise. Mimics flu and appendicitis. May cause diarrhea in children.	• Thorough cooking • Sanitizing of cutting instruments and cutting boards before preparing foods to be eaten raw • Avoidance of unpasteurized milk and untreated water
Parasites			
Trichinella spiralis	Pork and wild game.	Onset: weeks to months. Muscle weakness, fluid retention in face, fever, flulike symptoms.	• Thorough cooking of pork and wild game
Anisakis	Raw fish.	Onset: 12 hours. Stomach infection, severe stomach pain.	• Thorough cooking of fish
Tapeworms	Raw beef, pork, and fish.	May cause abdominal discomfort, diarrhea.	• Thorough cooking of all animal products • Avoidance of raw fish dishes
Cyclospora cayetanensis	Carried to food via contaminated water; Guatemalan raspberries suspected in recent outbreaks.	Onset: 1–11 days. Prolonged diarrhea, vomiting, muscle aches, fatigue.	• Irradiation (not yet in practice)
Cryptosporidium	Contaminated water (especially fecal material). Large outbreaks have been caused by such contamination of municipal water in Milwaukee, Wisconsin.	Onset: 1–12 days. Diarrhea, vomiting, fever.	• Handwashing • Use of clean or treated water • Use of boiled water if at high risk, such as one who is on immune suppression drugs or has AIDS
Toxoplasma gondii	Raw or undercooked meat, unwashed fruits and vegetables, cat feces.	Onset: 5–20 days. Fever, headache, sore muscles, diarrhea (can be deadly to the fetus of pregnant women).	• Thorough cooking of meats • Adequate washing of raw fruits and vegetables • Handwashing after changing cat litter (avoid cat litter when pregnant)

Table 19-3 | Important Microorganisms and Related Factors That Cause Foodborne Illness: Their Sources, Symptoms, and Prevention *(continued)*

Microorganism	Sources	Symptoms	Prevention Methods
Fungi			
Mycotoxins produced by molds, such as aflatoxin B-1	Found in foods that are relatively high in moisture. Chief food sources are beans and grains.	May cause liver and/or kidney disease.	• Discarding of foods with visible mold • Proper storage of susceptible foods
Ciguatera	Large tropical fish, especially grouper, snapper, and barracuda.	Onset: generally within 6 hours. Diarrhea, abdominal pain, nausea, vomiting, and nerve disorders.	• Avoidance of grouper, amberjack, and barracuda from Caribbean water, especially larger fish
Paralytic shellfish poisoning	Shellfish that have consumed large amounts of dinoflagellate algae (i.e., red tide).	Onset: within 4 hours. Respiratory difficulty.	• Observance of local precautions when harvesting shellfish
Scombroid poisoning	Spoiled fish, especially tuna, mackerel, and mahi-mahi.	Onset: 1–180 minutes. Facial flushing, burning sensation in the mouth, intestinal distress, and headache.	• Avoidance of spoiled fish • Proper refrigeration and prompt use of fresh fish
Prions			
Proteins that help maintain nerve cells. These can turn into infectious prions, leading to diseases such as mad cow disease (bovine spongiform encephalopathy).	Cows, goats, and sheep harboring infectious prions. These are spread from one animal to another if certain by-products of the infected animal (e.g., brains) are used to feed other animals (this process is banned in the United States and Canada). Cooking does not destroy prions.	Onset: 2–30 years. Dementia and psychosis, leading eventually to seizures, blindness, paralysis, and death. Once symptoms begin, death usually occurs within 1 year. At autopsy the person shows numerous holes in the brain.	Three cases of mad cow disease have been confirmed in U.S. cattle, some of which were imported from Canada. (These animals were infected before strict preventive actions were put in place in Canada.) The biggest risk is consumption of meat from cows, goats, and sheep in Europe or Asia. FDA and USDA have banned imports of such animals from Europe.

R egularly cleaning surfaces and equipment with a dilute bleach solution (1:10) is very helpful in reducing the risk of cross-contamination of foods.[13]

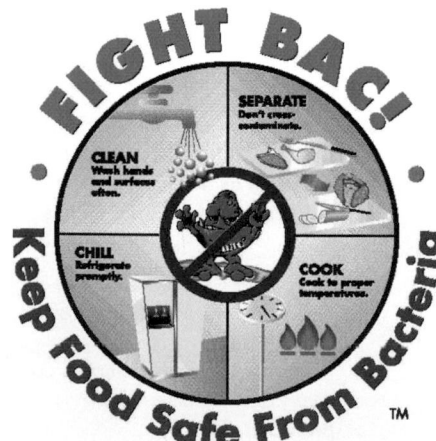

Food safety logo of USDA.

Preparing Food

- Thoroughly wash your hands for 20 seconds with hot, soapy water before and after handling food. This practice is especially important when handling raw meat, fish, poultry, and eggs, after using the bathroom, after playing with pets, or after changing diapers.
- Make sure counters, cutting boards, dishes, and other equipment are thoroughly sanitized and rinsed before use. Be especially careful to use hot, soapy water to wash surfaces and equipment that have come in contact with raw meat, fish, poultry, and eggs as soon as possible to remove *Salmonella* bacteria that may be present. Otherwise, bacteria on the surfaces will infect the next foods that come in contact with the surface, a process called cross-contamination. In addition, replace sponges and wash kitchen towels frequently. (Microwaving sponges for 30 to 60 seconds also helps rid them of live bacteria.)
- If possible, cut foods to be eaten raw on a clean cutting board reserved for that purpose. Then clean this cutting board using hot, soapy water. If the same board must be used for both meat and other foods, cut any potentially contaminated items, such as meat, last. After cutting the meat, wash the cutting board thoroughly.

FDA recommends cutting boards with unmarred surfaces made of easy-to-clean, nonporous materials, such as plastic, marble, or glass. If you prefer a wooden board, make sure it is made of a nonabsorbent hardwood, such as oak or maple, and has no obvious seams or cracks. Then reserve it for a specific purpose; for example, set it aside for cutting raw meat and poultry. Keep a separate wooden cutting board for chopping produce and slicing bread to prevent these products from picking up bacteria from raw meat. Note that many foods are served raw, so any bacteria clinging to them are not destroyed.

Furthermore, FDA recommends that all cutting boards be replaced when they become streaked with hard-to-clean grooves or cuts, which may harbor bacteria. In addition, cutting boards should be sanitized once a week in a dilute bleach solution. Flood the board with the solution, let it sit a few minutes, then rinse thoroughly.

- When thawing foods, do so in the refrigerator, under cold running water, or in a microwave oven. Cook foods immediately after thawing under cold water or in the microwave. Never let frozen foods thaw unrefrigerated all day or night. Also, marinate food in the refrigerator.
- Avoid coughing or sneezing over foods, even when you're healthy. Cover cuts on hands with a sterile bandage. This helps stop *Staphylococcus* from entering food.
- Carefully wash fresh fruit and vegetables under running water to remove dirt and bacteria clinging to the surface, using a vegetable brush if the skin is to be eaten. People have become ill from *Salmonella* that was introduced from melons used in making a fruit salad and from oranges used for fresh-squeezed orange juice. The bacteria were on the outside of the melons and oranges.
- Completely remove moldy portions of food or don't eat the food. *When in doubt, throw the food out.* Mold growth is prevented by properly storing food at cold temperatures and using the food promptly.
- Use refrigerated ground meat and patties in 1 to 2 days and frozen meat and patties within 3 to 4 months.

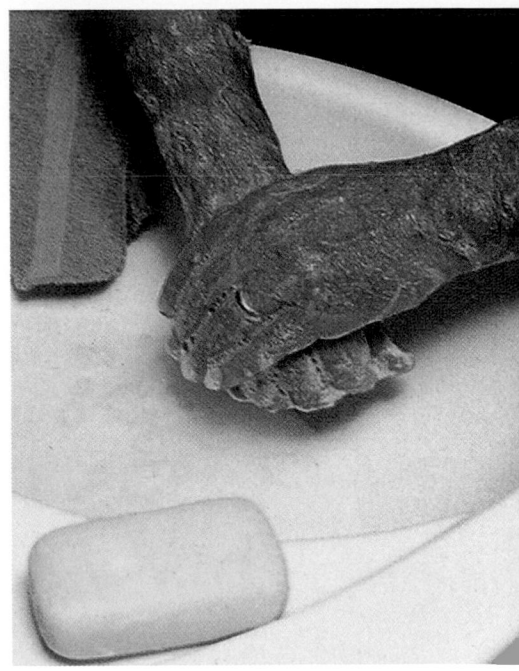

Washing hands thoroughly (for at least 20 to 30 seconds) with hot water and soap should be the first step in food preparation. The four Fs of food contamination are fingers, foods, feces, and flies. Handwashing especially combats the fecal and finger routes.[10]

Cooking Food

- Cook food thoroughly using a bimetallic thermometer to check for doneness, especially for beef and fish (145°F [63°C]), pork (160°F [71°C]), and poultry (165°F [74°C]) (Figure 19-1). Eggs should be cooked until the yolk and white are hard. Alfalfa sprouts and other types of sprouts should be cooked until they are steaming. Cooking is by far the most reliable way to destroy foodborne viruses and bacteria, such as Norovirus and toxic strains of *E. coli*. Freezing only halts viral and bacterial growth. FDA does not recommend that eggs be prepared sunny-side up or over easy.

Many restaurants now include an advisory on menus stating that an increased risk of foodborne illness is associated with eating undercooked eggs. As long as restaurants provide this warning on their menus, however, they are allowed to cook eggs to any temperature requested by the consumer. FDA warns us not to consume homemade ice cream, eggnog, and mayonnaise if made with unpasteurized, raw eggs because of the risk of *Salmonella* foodborne illness. It is safer to use eggs or egg products that have been pasteurized, which kills *Salmonella* bacteria. Overall, a good general precaution is to eat no raw animal products. USDA answers questions about the safe use of animal products (800-535-4555, 10 A.M. to 4 P.M. weekdays, Eastern time).

- Seafood also poses a risk of foodborne illness, especially oysters. Properly cooked seafood should flake easily and/or be opaque or dull and firm. If it's translucent or shiny, it's not done. Raw fish dishes such as sushi, however, can be safe for most people to eat if they are made with very fresh fish that has been commercially frozen and then thawed. The freezing is important to eliminate potential health risks from parasites. FDA recommends that the fish be frozen to an internal temperature of −10° F for 7 days. If you choose to eat uncooked fish, purchase the fish from reputable establishments that have high standards for quality and sanitation. People at high risk for foodborne illness would be wise to avoid raw fish products.

Critical | Thinking

Jon wants to buy a cutting board for his new kitchen. He's been looking at all of the possibilities: plexiglass, plastic, and wood. How would you advise him, so that he can minimize the risk of any foodborne illness from his food preparation?

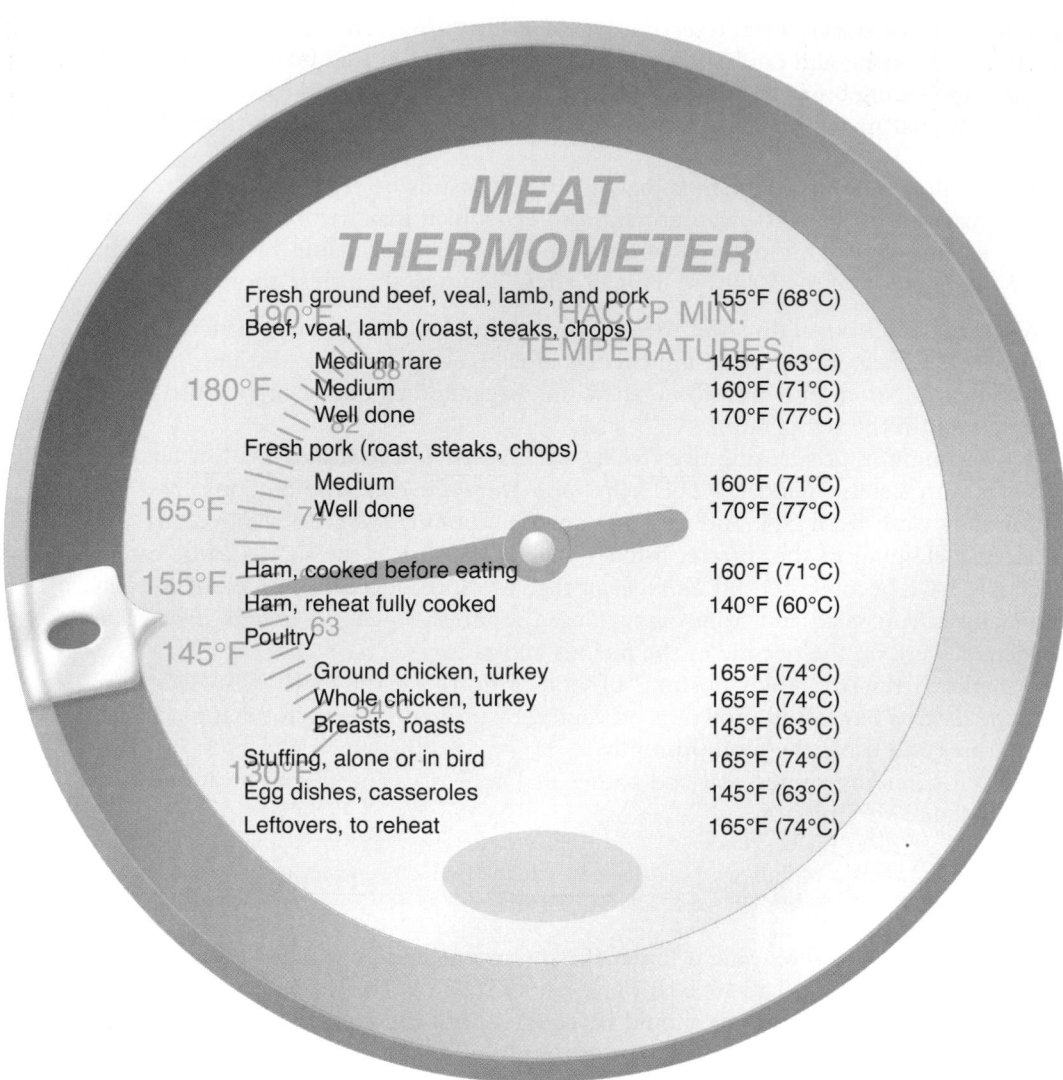

Figure 19-1 | Minimum internal temperatures established by USDA for cooking or reheating foods.

Current Safe Handling Instructions Issued by USDA for Labeling Meat and Poultry Products:

This product was prepared from inspected and passed meat and/or poultry. Some food products may contain bacteria that could cause illness if the product is mishandled or cooked improperly. For your protection, follow these handling instructions.

Keep refrigerated or frozen.
Thaw in refrigerator or microwave.
Keep raw meat and poultry separate from other foods.
Wash working surfaces (including cutting boards), utensils, and hands after touching raw meat or poultry.
Cook thoroughly.
Keep hot foods hot. Refrigerate leftovers immediately or discard.

Safe Handling Instructions for Eggs:

To prevent illness from bacteria: keep eggs refrigerated, cook eggs until yolks are firm, and cook foods containing eggs thoroughly.

- Cook stuffing separately from poultry, or stuff immediately before cooking and then transfer the stuffing to a clean bowl immediately after cooking. Make sure the stuffing reaches 165°F (74°C). *Salmonella* is the major concern with poultry.
- Once a food is cooked, consume it right away, or cool it to 41°F (5°C) within 2 hours. If it is not to be eaten immediately, in hot weather (80°F and above) make sure this cooling is done within 1 hour. Separate the food into as many shallow pans as needed to provide a large surface area for cooling. Be careful not to recontaminate cooked food by contact with raw meat or juices from hands, cutting boards, dirty utensils, or in other ways.
- Serve meat, poultry, and fish on a clean plate—never the same plate that was used to hold the raw product. For example, when grilling hamburgers, don't put cooked burgers on the same plate that was used to carry the raw patties out to the grill.
- For outdoor cooking, cook food completely at the picnic site, with no partial cooking in advance.

Expert Opinion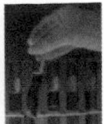

Food Safety—Why Should You Care?

Lydia Medeiros, Ph.D., R.D.

Why does every research journal article on food safety start out quoting statistics about how many illnesses, hospitalizations, and even deaths occur each year because of foodborne illness? It's so common that it's almost becoming a cliché. The reason is that the numbers are shocking. Just think, in a technologically advanced country such as the United States people die from illnesses that could be prevented by simply cooking food adequately or properly washing their hands. But, this information is boring—these are instructions our mothers nagged us about when we were children. And who doesn't wash their hands before handling food? Apparently, plenty of people don't, or if they do they aren't doing it properly. Why else are the statistics on foodborne illness so high?

Could it be that people become confused with too many dos and don'ts—too many rules to follow? As a food safety educator I certainly am asking myself that question. When I began compiling a list of all the behaviors that people should practice to control the most common foodborne illness pathogens, I found almost 60 behaviors scattered among numerous references. After editing the list for vagueness, overlap, and redundancy, our research group asked nationally known experts in food safety to refine the items and associate each behavior to one of 13 pathogens known to cause the majority of foodborne illnesses.

We started to think in the language of the Hazard Analysis Critical Control Point (or HACCP) system, which identifies, first, hazards, and second, control factors that, if practiced, will contain the contamination and growth of foodborne illness pathogens. Of the 29 remaining behaviors on our edited and refined list, we found that each could be organized under just 5 groupings that are control points, like in HACCP. These control factors are: Practice Personal Hygiene, Cook Foods Adequately, Avoid Cross-Contamination, Keep Foods at Safe Temperatures, and Avoid Foods from Unsafe Sources. These control factors can also serve as concise and easy-to-remember educational messages.

As I have applied our research findings to educational programs, I have found that two of the control factors fit well together, as do two others; the last one seems to stand separately. Practice Personal Hygiene and Avoid Cross-Contamination are similar because both involve human behaviors related to cleanliness, whether the hands, the body, or food preparation surfaces are at issue. The differences in the two control factors lie in the microbial pathogens that cause the foodborne illnesses. Practice Personal Hygiene, which focuses on hand cleanliness, is most applicable if the behaviors are practiced before food is touched and when the food is going to be served cold, such as salads. The pathogens controlled best by handwashing are Noroviruses and Norwalk-like viruses, *Shigella* species, and foodborne sources of hepatitis A. Avoiding Cross-Contamination also concerns cleanliness, but the focus is on food preparation utensils, cookware, and food preparation surfaces. The Fight BAC! educational program of the

United States Department of Agriculture is very similar in concept to the research findings of our group with the exception of how cleanliness is taught. Handwashing and food preparation surfaces are combined under the Fight BAC! concept of "CLEAN." We recommend separation of the concept into two control factors because the pathogens best controlled by cleaning and sanitizing food preparation surfaces are *Campylobacter jejuni*, *Salmonella* species, *Toxoplasma gondii*, *Yersinia enterocolitica*, and *Escherichia coli* 0157:H7. This is a very different list from the ones controlled by personal hygiene.

Cook Foods Adequately and Keep Food at Safe Temperatures also have similarities. Both factors focus on controlling temperature of food, except that Cook Foods Adequately is concerned about end-point temperatures of cooking and reheating, whereas Keep Food at Safe Temperatures advocates behaviors associated with holding and storage of cold or hot perishable foods. Foodborne illness pathogens that cause food infections, or illness symptoms due to ingestion of the pathogen itself, are controlled by heat destruction of

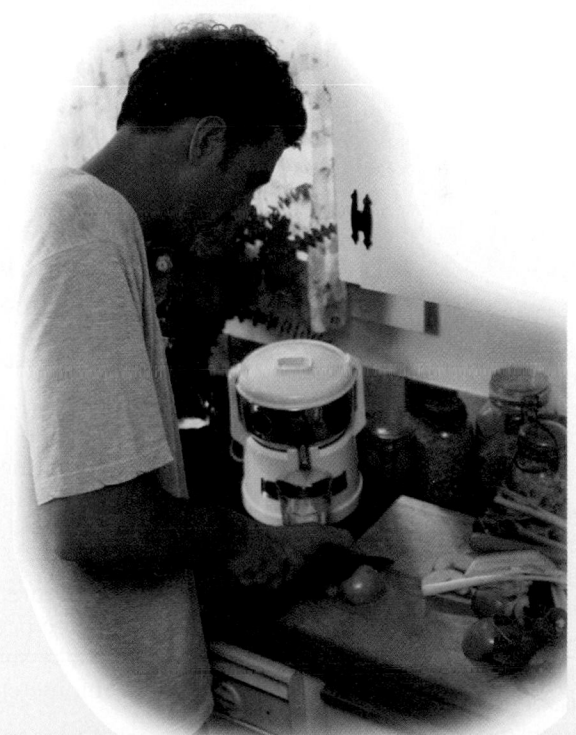

Washing your hands before preparing food is the single best way to limit your risk for foodborne illness.

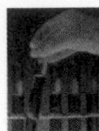

the microorganisms. These are the same pathogens that are also controlled by avoiding cross-contamination. There are, therefore, two ways to control foodborne infections caused by microbial pathogens—by controlling contamination of the food initially or by heating to an adequate temperature, which will result in the destruction of the pathogen. The pathogens best controlled by controlling holding and storage temperatures of foods are somewhat unique among foodborne illness pathogens. These are *Clostridium perfringens, Staphylococcus aureus,* and *Bacillus cereus.* Uniqueness of these pathogens comes from the fact that either they contain spores, which are not destroyed during heating, or they cause illness due to a toxin produced in a temperature-abused food. The toxin causes the illness.

The one remaining control factor is Avoid Foods from Unsafe Sources. These foods include raw eggs, unpasteurized milk or milk products made from raw milk, unpasteurized fruit juices, raw sprouts, and some types of pre-prepared foods served without heating (such as deli salads and hot dogs). For immune-compromised individuals like the elderly, pregnant women, or people with drug- or disease-induced immune suppression, consuming these foods can complicate existing conditions or, in extreme situations, cause death. Certainly, foodborne illness pathogens that are associated with these foods have already been listed for the other control factors, such as *E. coli* 0157:H7 or *Salmonella* species. But for those pathogens, effective consumer behaviors can be used to prevent illnesses in the home. However, for one pathogen—and especially for immune-compromised individuals—avoidance is the most prudent behavior. That pathogen is *Listeria monocytogenes.* (See the *Listeria* section in the chapter for ways to minimize risk.)

With so much to remember about food safety, is there one single message that all people can remember that will control the majority of foodborne illnesses? If there were, that message would be either to practice personal hygiene or wash your hands before you eat or touch foods. For pathogens that cause the most severe illnesses or death, the public health concern clearly remains high; however, the numbers of cases are relatively few and susceptible groups can be targeted for special emphasis in educational programs.

Dr. Medeiros is Associate Professor in the Department of Human Nutrition at The Ohio State University. She is Extension Specialist in Food and Nutrition for The Ohio State University and has an active research program in food safety.

To reduce the risk of bacteria surviving during microwave cooking,

- Cover food with glass or ceramic when possible to decrease evaporation and heat the surface.
- Stir and rotate food at least once or twice for even cooking. Then, allow microwaved food to stand, covered, after heating is completed to help cook the exterior and equalize the temperature throughout.
- Use the oven temperature probe or a meat thermometer to check that food is done. Insert it at several spots.
- If thawing meat in the microwave, use the oven's defrost setting. Ice crystals in frozen foods are not heated well by the microwave oven and can create cold spots, which later cook more slowly.

Storing and Reheating Cooked Food

- Keep foods out of the "danger zone" by keeping hot foods hot and cold foods cold. Hold food below 41°F (5°C) or above 135°F (57°C) (Figure 19-2). Foodborne microorganisms thrive in more moderate temperatures (60°F to 110°F [16°C to 43°C]). Some microorganisms can even grow in the refrigerator. Again, don't leave cooked or refrigerated foods, such as meats and salads, at room temperature for more than 2 hours (or 1 hour in hot weather) because that gives microorganisms an opportunity to grow. Store dry food at 60°F to 70°F (16°C to 21°C).
- Reheat leftovers to 165°F (74°C); reheat gravy to a rolling boil to kill *Clostridium perfringens* bacteria, which may be present. Merely reheating to a good eating temperature isn't sufficient to kill harmful bacteria.
- Store peeled or cut-up produce, such as melon balls, in the refrigerator.
- Make sure the refrigerator stays below 41°F (5°C). Either use a refrigerator thermometer or keep it as cold as possible without freezing milk and lettuce.

Cross-contamination is not only a threat during food preparation, it can also become a problem during food storage. Make sure all foods, including leftovers, are contained and covered in the refrigerator to prevent drippings from uncooked and potentially hazardous foods from tainting other foods. It is a good idea to store foods that are likely to pose risk of foodborne illness on lower shelves of the refrigerator, beneath other foods that are to be eaten raw.

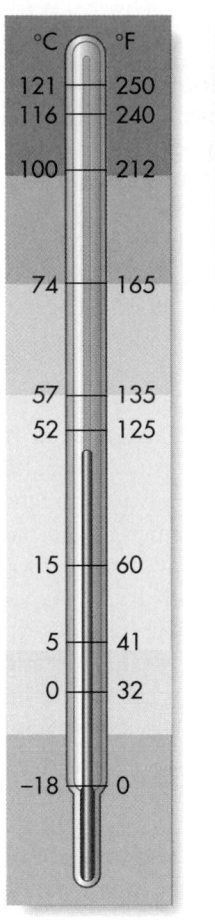
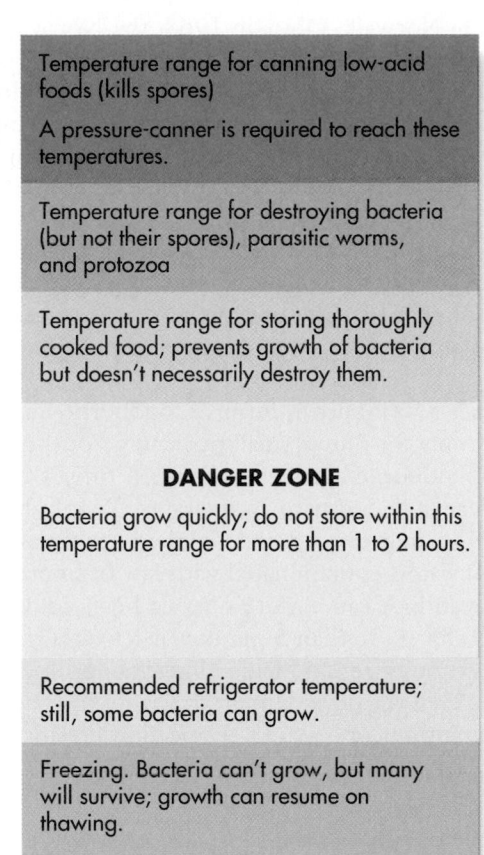

Temperature range for canning low-acid foods (kills spores)

A pressure-canner is required to reach these temperatures.

Temperature range for destroying bacteria (but not their spores), parasitic worms, and protozoa

Temperature range for storing thoroughly cooked food; prevents growth of bacteria but doesn't necessarily destroy them.

DANGER ZONE

Bacteria grow quickly; do not store within this temperature range for more than 1 to 2 hours.

Recommended refrigerator temperature; still, some bacteria can grow.

Freezing. Bacteria can't grow, but many will survive; growth can resume on thawing.

Figure 19-2 | Effects of temperature on microbes that cause foodborne illness. Adapted from *Temperature Guide to Food Safety: Food and Home Notes.* No. 25, Washington DC, June 20, 1977, USDA.

Concept | Check

Viruses and bacteria pose the greatest risk for foodborne illness. In the past, sugar and salt were added to foods, or foods were smoked or dried, to prevent the growth of microorganisms. Today, we know that ensuring cleanliness, keeping hot foods hot and cold foods cold, and cooking foods thoroughly offer additional protection from foodborne illness. Commercial processes, such as pasteurization and irradiation, do the same. Treat all raw animal products, cooked food, and raw fruits and vegetables as potential sources of foodborne illness.

A Closer Look at the Primary Microorganisms That Cause Foodborne Illness

Viruses

Viruses cause more cases of foodborne illness than any other class of microorganisms.[5] Viruses do not metabolize, grow, or move by themselves. Instead, they reproduce within a living host cell and, thus, cannot grow in food once it is harvested or slaughtered. Viruses consist of a protein coat surrounding a nucleic acid core of either DNA or RNA. They have no cell wall. On entering a host cell, a virus takes over the cell's DNA replication processes and causes it to reproduce the virus's genetic material. Generally, the host cell dies in the process and bursts open, releasing new viruses into the surrounding medium. Many viruses cause disease in humans. And, because viruses cannot multiply in foods, they must enter in sufficient amounts through bits of feces that contaminate food.

Rotaviruses are an important cause of diarrhea, mainly in children, leading to about 55,000 hospitalizations per year in the United States. Symptoms appear in 1 to 7 days. Daycare centers are common sites for infections. Thorough, regular handwashing is a necessary practice at these sites, particularly after diaper changing.

First noted in Norwalk, Ohio, in 1968, the Norovirus is a little known but leading cause of stomach and intestinal distress caused by a virus.[20] Norovirus infections usually cause nausea, vomiting, diarrhea, weakness, abdominal pain, loss of appetite, headache, and fever about 24 to 48 hours after exposure. The virus is found in water and foods, and shellfish and salads are most often implicated. Cooking destroys the virus. Noroviruses are probably responsible for about 30 to 40% of all cases of viral intestinal infection in adults and are the leading cause of foodborne illness in general. The infection is typically found in nursing homes and hospitals, restaurants, cruise ships, and events with catered meals. The virus persists because it can survive chlorination and because a low amount of the virus can cause illness. The virus is of most concern for infants, young children, older adults, and people with chronic illnesses. There is no specific treatment.

Hepatitis A is a well-known form of foodborne illness caused by a virus, although this route accounts for only a small percentage of the total number of hepatitis A infections. As a foodborne agent it most often thrives because of unsanitary food handling by carriers of the virus in restaurants. People have also contracted hepatitis A infections from eating raw or undercooked shellfish—clams, oysters, and mussels—harvested from waters contaminated with raw or improperly treated sewage. The virus that causes hepatitis A can endure notable heat, cold, and drying. Cooking foods at 212°F (100°C) for more than 5 minutes inactivates the virus, as does irradiation.

Symptoms of the infection include intestinal problems, weakness, fatigue, jaundice, and sometimes even the development of serious liver disease, requiring hospitalization. Because the symptoms of hepatitis A infection do not usually occur until about 15 to 50 days after eating contaminated food, the source is difficult to identify. It is diagnosed by detection of hepatitis A antibodies. About 30,000 cases are reported annually in the United States.

Raw clams and oysters are particularly risky foods because they are filter feeders, a process that concentrates viruses and toxins present in the water as it is filtered for food. Consumption of these raw shellfish results in the consumption of live viruses and bacteria, too. It is important to buy oysters and clams only from the most reliable sources. By law, shellfish offered for sale must come from licensed beds, but often they do not, so be careful when you either purchase these foods or harvest them yourself. Check with the local health department if you question the safety of waters in an area.

Proper handwashing by food service personnel is especially important in restaurants, day-care centers, hospitals, and other institutions to lessen hepatitis outbreaks. The chlorination of drinking water is a reliable means of destroying the virus.

Recovery from hepatitis A generally occurs of its own accord in 3 to 6 months. This foodborne illness constitutes the only exception to the rule of immunity, because it is the only one in which people infected with the virus are then immune for the rest of their lives.

Bacteria

Bacteria also pose a significant risk for foodborne illness.[1, 2, 9, 13] Bacteria are extremely simple structures. They contain only one chromosome and lack mitochondria, endoplasmic reticulum, golgi body, and lysosomes. Many bacteria are enclosed in a carbohydrate-like capsule, which protects them and aids their adherence to tissues. Some bacteria can survive harsh environmental conditions through spore formation. In the spore state, bacteria can remain stable for months or years.

Certain bacteria can thrive in almost freezing temperatures, whereas others thrive in very high temperatures. The optimum temperature for most disease-causing bacteria is about 98°F (body temperature; 37°C). Bacteria living in the presence of oxygen are called *aerobes*, whereas those living in the absence of oxygen are called *anaerobes*. Those that prefer free oxygen but can live in its absence are called *facultative anaerobes*. Many bacteria produce toxins.

Finding the specific agent that has led to a foodborne illness requires some detective skills. Identifying the agent depends on knowing the food source, the incubation time for and types of symptoms, and the duration of the illness associated with an outbreak. The following sections look at the characteristics of the major contaminants individually.

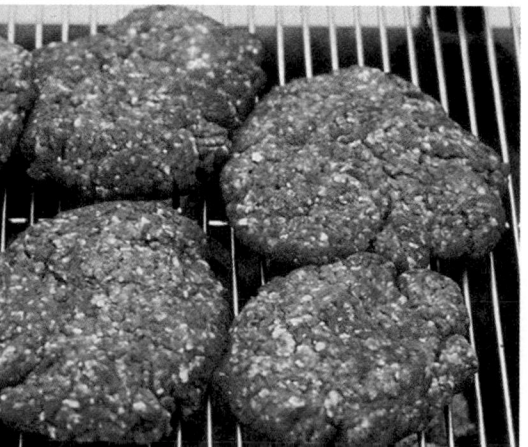

Cook hamburgers to an internal temperature of 160°F (72°C). At this temperature they are brown throughout, the juices run clear, and the inside is hot.

Campylobacter jejuni (C. jejuni)

In recent years, *Campylobacter* has jumped to the top of the list as the number one cause of all domestic bacterial foodborne illnesses, resulting in up to 4 million human infections a year in the United States alone. The bacteria produce a toxin that destroys the mucosal surfaces of the small and large intestines.

Because *C. jejuni* is so difficult to detect in foods, an enormous number of cases of this foodborne illness probably go unreported in this country. Also, most infections are very sporadic and are not associated with a large outbreak, as are other foodborne infections, such as *E. coli* and *Salmonella*. In a study conducted by USDA, more than 90% of the poultry tested was positive for *Campylobacter*.

Symptoms of the illness are acute intestinal inflammation with fever, muscle pain, headache, and diarrhea. During the peak of the disease, 10 or more bowel movements per day are common, and stools are often bloody. Cases are associated with contaminated water, raw or inadequately cooked animal foods, including beef and unpasteurized milk. Poultry, especially chicken, is of most concern. Because this organism grows slowly, the onset of symptoms is delayed, occurring 2 to 5 days after ingesting the contaminated food; it may even take weeks. Older adults, children, and people with weakened immune systems are at particularly high risk.

Treatment uses antibiotic medication, with most people recovering in less than 1 week. Deaths are rare. However, the number of *Campylobacter* infections that are resistant to a class of antibiotics called fluoroquinolones have been on the rise. Antibiotic use in the U.S. poultry industry in fact is the main contributor to this antibiotic resistance. A problem arises when physicians attempt to treat this foodborne illness, because those people infected with the resistant strains are more likely to have severe infections and bloody diarrhea and to be hospitalized. Also, the bacterium is recognized as a major contributing factor to Guillain-Barré syndrome, which is the most common cause of acute paralysis in both children and adults.

Luckily, *Campylobacter* organisms are very sensitive to heat. This trait probably protects most people from infections. Prompt refrigeration, thorough cooking, avoidance of cross-contamination, thorough handwashing, and careful refrigeration of leftovers are important ways to prevent its growth.

Salmonella

There are 2000 strains of *Salmonella* bacteria, many of which cause foodborne illness. *Salmonella* can be killed by normal cooking. Nonetheless, they are responsible for many cases of foodborne illness, up to 23,000 per year in the United States alone, many of which go unreported. Related deaths average 33 per year.

Commonly found in animal and human feces, these bacteria enter food via infected water, contaminated cutting boards, contaminated chicken and other animal products, cracked eggs, and actual bits of feces in food. Ingesting the live bacteria causes the problem. Recent outbreaks of salmonellosis have been traced back to alfalfa sprouts. It is thought that the seeds of these sprouts were contaminated by bird or rodent feces. According to FDA, children, older adults, and persons with weakened immune systems should not eat any raw sprouts, such as alfalfa, mung bean, clover, and radish. Feces from pet reptiles are also sources of *Salmonella* exposure. Infants and young children are at high risk for salmonellosis from indirect or direct contact with reptiles.

Symptoms of *Salmonella* infections include nausea, fever, headache, abdominal cramps, diarrhea, and vomiting, which can develop in 24 to 72 hours. Bed rest and fluids are the only effective treatment, and recovery usually occurs within 2 to 3 days. Deaths are rare. *Salmonella* attacks occur most frequently from consuming eggs, chicken, meat, meat products, custard made with infected eggs, raw milk, and inadequately refrigerated and reheated leftovers. Unpasteurized orange juice and milk may also be contaminated with *Salmonella*. Raw chicken is often contaminated, and undercooked food—including eggs—poses a particular risk. Recently a warning label has been added to egg cartons in an attempt to prevent the up to 66,000 illnesses and

FDA warns us not to consume homemade ice cream, eggnog, and mayonnaise if made with unpasteurized, raw eggs because of the risk of *Salmonella* foodborne illness. Use instead eggs or egg products that have been pasteurized, which kills *Salmonella* bacteria.

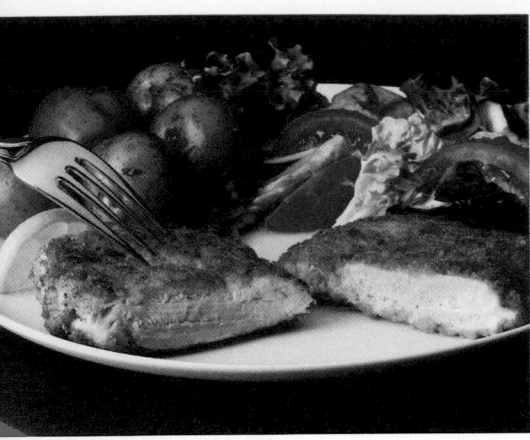

Cook chicken thoroughly to reduce the risk of salmonella infections.

40 deaths per year from eggs contaminated with *Salmonella* inside the shell. The new warning label, shown on page 700, provides instructions for safe handling to help prevent foodborne illness.

Most outbreaks of *Salmonella* infection can be traced to improper food handling. Picnics pose a special challenge, because food is frequently held for hours at a dangerously high temperature (between 41°F and 135°F, or 5°C and 57°C). It takes only about 8 hours for *Salmonella* bacteria to multiply sufficiently to cause illness. Therefore, keep foods above 135°F (57°C) or below 41°F (5°C) to help prevent the growth of *Salmonella* bacteria.

Salmonella also poses a great risk for cross-contamination of foods. To avoid cross-contamination, keep produce, cooked foods, and ready-to-eat foods separate from uncooked meats and raw eggs. Thoroughly clean hands, cutting boards, counters, knives, and other utensils after handling uncooked foods.

Shigella sonnei (S. sonnei)

Foodborne illness caused by the *Shigella* bacterium is a common disease of youngsters in day-care centers, nurseries, and custodial institutions. The infection is transmitted by the fecal-oral route, primarily by way of the hands as well as via food and water. The onset of symptoms usually occurs within 1 to 3 days of being infected. The symptoms include abdominal cramps, diarrhea, fever, and bloody stools. Some carriers of *Shigella* display no symptoms but represent a potential threat to all who come in contact with them. With as little as 10 organisms able to cause an infection, person-to-person transmission is easily accomplished where hygienic conditions are poor.

Although reported infrequently, *Shigella* outbreaks have been associated with raw produce, including green onions, crisp head lettuce, and uncooked, raw parsley. Recent outbreaks have been traced back to raw, chopped parsley that had been cut and stored at room temperature. To avoid contamination from parsley, food handlers should store chopped parsley for short times, keeping it refrigerated, and chop smaller batches. Handwashing and sanitary food production offer the best protection against *Shigella* infections.

Escherichia coli (E. coli)

Escherichia coli (E. coli) is commonly found in the intestinal tract of humans and other animals. Although there are hundreds of benign strains of the bacteria, 0157:H7 and 0111:H8 are especially virulent and cause severe illness. According to the U.S. Centers for Disease Control and Prevention, these *E. coli* bacteria, which are most commonly found in ground beef, kill about 60 people each year and cause illness in an estimated 73,000 more. They are quickly becoming a major threat for foodborne illness, with up to 4% of raw meat products in the United States possibly containing such bacteria.

Children and older adults are most susceptible to the disease. The bacterium is transmitted primarily via contaminated ground beef and roast beef. In response, as previously mentioned, FDA has approved the irradiation of meat to reduce this risk. Although ground beef is the most common source of the *E. coli* bacteria, fruits, vegetables, and drinking water also can harbor the deadly pathogen. Unpasteurized milk, untreated apple cider, salad greens grown in cow manure, cantaloupe, dry-cured salami (because it is not cooked during processing), and many types of sprouts have also been implicated in *E. coli* infections. In one case, fresh apple juice was contaminated with *E. coli* because the apples used to produce the juice had fallen to the ground and had come into contact with animal feces. New methods for apple juice production are being researched; pasteurization is now routine.

After an incubation period of 1 to 8 days, the disease normally lasts 4 to 10 days. The symptoms include severe abdominal cramps, bloody diarrhea, and hemolytic uremic syndrome, a condition that can lead to kidney failure. *E. coli* infection should be investigated as a possible cause in any case of bloody diarrhea.

Recently 19 million pounds of ground beef patties were recalled because of possible *E. coli* 0157:H7 contamination.

Cooking with a meat thermometer and then avoiding recontamination are important ways to prevent this type of foodborne illness. Cider that is not pasteurized or that does not contain preservatives can be heated to a slow simmer until steam rises from the pan before serving or refrigerating to reduce risk.

Clostridium perfringens (C. perfringens)

The bacterium *Clostridium perfringens* lives throughout the environment, especially in soil, the intestines of farm animals and humans, and sewage. It is called the "cafeteria germ," because most foodborne outbreaks caused by this organism are associated with the food service industry or with events where large quantities of food are prepared and served. The symptoms of an infection resemble those of *Salmonella* cases, but the victim usually doesn't vomit. The symptoms occur within 8 to 24 hours of consuming enough live bacteria. Again, bed rest and fluids are the only effective treatment, and recovery usually occurs within a day or so.

C. perfringens thrives in an oxygen-free environment. It forms heat-resistant spores, which become bacteria at temperatures between 70°F and 120°F (21°C and 49°C), and at the same time produces a toxin. The bacteria then can quickly multiply to disease-causing numbers. Foods stored in deep refrigerator pans are especially fertile media for the growth of these bacteria because the centers are isolated from air and they stay warm.

C. perfringens organisms are often found in cooked beef, turkey, gravy, dressing, stews, and casseroles. The best way to prevent their growth is to maintain proper holding temperatures and divide large leftover portions into smaller ones. Be especially careful to cook meats completely and cool them rapidly in small containers. Thoroughly reheat leftover meat to 165°F (74°C) before serving. Always bring leftover gravy to a rolling boil. Refrigerate cold cuts and sliced meats below 41°F or 5°C, and serve them cold.

Listeria monocytogenes (L. monocytogenes)

Listeria monocytogenes is widely distributed in the environment and often enters food from contamination with animal or human feces. It is a very hardy microorganism that resists heat, salt, and acidity much better than many other bacteria. This bacterium survives and even grows at refrigeration temperatures. Because pasteurization destroys *Listeria* organisms, reports of contaminated milk and cheese products suggest that contamination occurred following pasteurization, probably from the addition of unpasteurized milk. Listeriosis in the United States is estimated to kill 500 people a year and causes illness in 2000 more, which means that listeriosis kills 20% of the people it infects.

Listeria infections cause initial symptoms of fever, headache, and vomiting about 9 to 48 hours after exposure. However, newborn infants, pregnant women, and people with depressed immune function may suffer severe symptoms, including meningitis, spontaneous abortion, serious blood infections, and death. It is especially important that pregnant women and other people at high risk avoid products such as unpasteurized or expired milk, uncooked hot dogs, undercooked chicken, fresh paté or meat spreads (canned are fine), Mexican soft cheeses (e.g., queso fresco), and other soft cheeses such as feta, brie, Camembert, and blue-veined cheeses, all of which are suspected of being major sources of *Listeria* infection. USDA also warns pregnant women and other people at high risk to thoroughly cook all ready-to-eat meats, including hot dogs and cold cuts, until they are steaming.

Consuming only pasteurized milk products; cooking meat, poultry, and seafood thoroughly; keeping food refrigerated; and washing fresh produce thoroughly are ways to avoid *Listeria* infection.

Critical | Thinking

Diana had a party at her house for her son's birthday. While cleaning up after the kids had gone home, she realized she had forgotten to put away the potato salad and coleslaw and decided to discard it. However, her husband, Tim, wanted her to just refrigerate it. "After all," he reasoned, "it was only left out for a couple of hours." Why was Diana right in wanting to throw away the leftover unrefrigerated food?

In a recent period of 6 months, more than 45 million pounds of hot dogs, luncheon meats, and other ready-to-eat meat products were recalled because of contamination with potentially deadly *Listeria* bacteria.

A new tool in the battle against foodborne illness is HACCP, or Hazard Analysis and Critical Control Point. This topic was discussed in the Expert Opinion by Dr. Medeiros. As she noted, HACCP is a method of ensuring food safety. Rather than treating the cause after a foodborne illness outbreak has occurred, by applying the principles of HACCP, food handlers critically analyze how they approach food preparation and what conditions may exist that might allow pathogenic microorganisms to enter the food system. Once specific hazards and critical control points (where potential problems can occur) are identified, preventive measures can be used to reduce specific sources of contamination. In this way the food handlers are using HACCP to stop a problem before it starts.

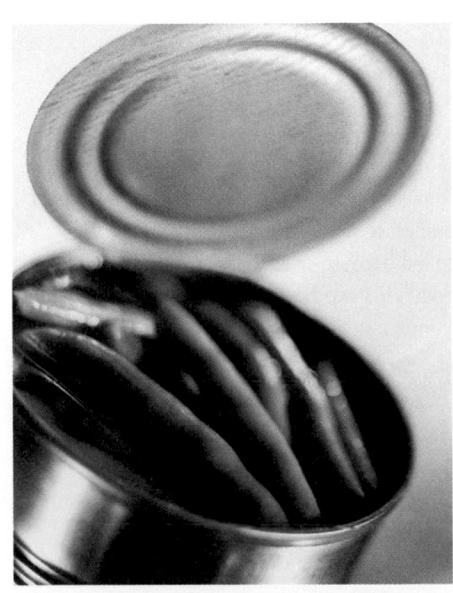

Inspect cans for bulges and foul-smelling liquid as one sign of the presence of the botulism toxin.

Staphylococcus aureus (S. aureus)

The organism *Staphylococcus aureus (S. aureus)* produces toxins as it grows in food. Once ingested, the toxin causes nausea, vomiting, diarrhea, headache, and abdominal cramps. The symptoms usually develop within 2 to 6 hours of eating the contaminated food. People seldom die from the toxin, but they don't develop immunity against future attacks. And, as is true for almost all foodborne illnesses, continued unsafe food handling will result in repeated sickness. Bed rest and fluids are generally the only treatment needed. Recovery usually takes place within 2 to 3 days.

S. aureus bacteria live mainly in the nasal passages and skin sores. These microorganisms enter food when people sneeze and cough over food or handle food while they have open skin sores. Once present in significant numbers in a food, *S. aureus* can make enough toxin to cause human illness in about 4 hours if the food temperature stays near 100°F (38°C). The toxin is undetectable by flavor, odor, and appearance and can even withstand prolonged cooking.

Foods commonly associated with *S. aureus* intoxications are custard, ham, egg salad, cheese, seafood, cream-filled pastries, and milk. A frequent source is whipped cream left standing for hours at room temperature. Keeping these and other foods above 135°F (57°C) or below 41°F (5°C) prevents both the bacteria's growth and further toxin production. To limit the spread of this microorganism, it's important to work with clean hands, working surfaces, and utensils; to direct coughs and sneezes away from food; and to cover skin cuts on hands and arms when handling food.

Clostridium botulinum (C. botulinum)

The *Clostridium botulinum* bacterium can cause botulism, a foodborne illness that can be fatal. This microorganism comes from soil and may exist as a bacterium or spore in any food. As these bacteria multiply in food, they release a deadly toxin. The death rate for botulism receives much public attention; however, only a few cases are reported each year in North America. At one time, botulism was a serious problem in the canning industry, but now adequate heat processing and intact containers have virtually eliminated this danger from North American manufactured canned foods.

The symptoms of botulism appear within 12 to 72 hours of ingesting contaminated food. The toxin blocks acetylcholine release at neuromuscular junctions, causing vomiting, abdominal pain, double vision, dizziness, and acute respiratory failure. The prompt administration of the botulism antitoxin can help prevent the progression of paralysis and reduce the duration of the illness. Sometimes treatment requires intensive care, including mechanical ventilation. The combination of the antitoxin and supportive care has reduced mortality to less than 10%. If the person survives, recovery occurs within 10 days.

C. botulinum grows only in the absence of air, so it thrives primarily in canned food, especially improperly home-canned, low-acid foods, such as string beans, corn, mushrooms, beets, and asparagus. Recently, other foods with oxygen-deprived centers—such as potato salad, sautéed onions, stew, and chopped garlic—have also caused botulism. FDA now requires that chopped garlic in oil be acidified to protect against *C. botulinum*. Consumers should look for a commercially prepared product that contains phosphoric or citric acid. Cured meats also pose a risk for botulism; however, the nitrates and vitamin C used to preserve commercial products inhibit bacterial growth. Botulism has also occurred among Alaskan natives who consume uncooked, fermented fish.

Home-canned foods are the most common sources of botulism. Although the canning process may kill all bacteria and the heat may drive out all oxygen, spores of *C. botulinum* can still survive if the heating is insufficient. When the can or jar cools, the spores germinate into bacteria that produce the toxin. Even foods that were previously thought to be safe due to their acidity, such as tomatoes, require greater care, because new varieties tend to have a higher pH. To ensure the safety of home-canned foods, it is crucial to follow the canning directions exactly. To be safe, always check all cans carefully, even those from commercial facilities. Look for holes, rust on the seams, and swollen sides or tops. Make sure the can sucks in air when opened to indicate that the vacuum was maintained, and make sure the liquid inside is clear, not milky or foul-smelling. If you see any signs of spoilage, return the can to the store or take it to the nearest public health department. Whatever you do, do not taste the food. One green bean can contain enough toxin to kill you. For questions on proper canning techniques, call the Ball Consumer Hotline at 1-800-240-3340.

Botulism also may develop in vivo (inside the living body). Infants between 2 and 9 months of age are at the highest risk because of low stomach acid production. About 250 cases are reported each year. Fortunately, the death rate is low, 1 to 2%. Adults with low stomach acid production are also at risk. Bacteria spores germinate in the stomach and produce the exotoxin. For this reason, honey should not be given to young infants because it can contain the spores of *C. botulinum*.

Parasites

Parasites that enter the body through the intestinal tract include some single-celled protozoans, flukes, nematodes, roundworms, and tapeworms. Although not common in North America, the parasite most apt to be in the food supply is *Trichinella spiralis*.[19] This tiny organism may be present in raw and undercooked pork and pork products, such as sausage. Trichinosis is rare today, probably because people realize that pork must be cooked thoroughly to kill the nematode worm that causes it and because modern sanitary feeding practices have reduced *Trichinella* in hogs. About 20 cases of trichinosis per year are reported in the United States. However, other cases may be unreported. In addition to pork, bear meat and other raw meats are potential sources. It is seldom found in commercial meat.

Trichinosis begins with the consumption of meat containing the **larvae.** The larvae are released during digestion in the small intestine. Within 2 days, the larvae develop into adult nematodes. New larvae are then produced and move into the blood via the intestinal mucosa. The blood carries the larvae to muscle fibers, where they become resident.

In early stages, trichinosis is difficult to diagnose. The symptoms in mild cases develop over weeks to months and are usually thought to be flu. If enough larvae are present, muscle weakness, fever, and fluid retention in the face may eventually result. Thoroughly cooking meat, especially pork, destroys the larvae.

Fungi

Fungi are mostly multicellular organisms. Those of concern in food safety do not infect people, but some mushrooms are intrinsically toxic, and molds growing on foods may produce toxins called **mycotoxins.**[19] Fungi possess cell walls, a nucleus, and a nuclear membrane. They live on dead or decaying organic matter, living together with other organisms either in mutual advantage or as parasites. Fungi can grow as single cells, like yeasts, or as multicellular filamentous colonies, as with molds. They cannot synthesize their own food; rather, they digest their food outside their cell walls and absorb the simpler organic substances for use within the cell.

Most fungi are molds that consist of long, branched threads called *hyphae.* Hyphae form a tangled mass of filaments called *mycelium.* The mold often seen on bread consists of this mycelia.

Fungi require moisture to grow and can obtain water from the medium on which they live or from the atmosphere. When the atmosphere becomes dry, they can go into a resting state or form spores. They can live in a pH range of 2 to 9 and can grow in concentrated salt and sugar solutions. They thrive over a wide temperature range, even in the refrigerator. As spores, fungi can be scattered by the wind or carried by animals. When an airborne spore lands on an appropriate target, such as a ripe peach, the spore germinates and begins to grow, producing the typical mold observed on spoiled fruit.

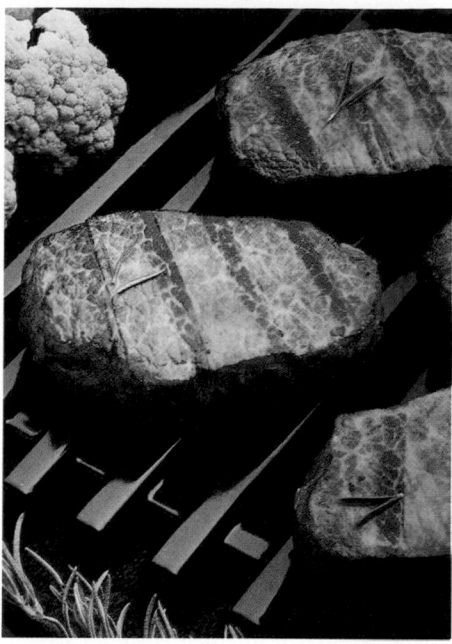

Grill pork to an internal temperature of 160°F (72°C). This eliminates the risk of trichinosis and produces a desirable product.

larva An early developmental stage in the life history of some organisms, such as parasites.

mycotoxins Toxic compounds produced by molds, such as aflatoxin B-1, found on moldy grains.

ad cow disease, or bovine spongiform encephalopathy, is caused by an infectious protein, called a prion, that kills by creating voids in the brain.[11] The human condition, a variant of Creutzfeldt-Jakob disease, causes a form of dementia that has killed about 100 people in Europe who apparently ate contaminated beef. Because of the recent evidence of mad cow disease in Europe, the U.S. government has worked diligently to make sure the cattle here are not exposed. The U.S. government has taken steps to ban beef from Europe since the late 1980s, and has recently banned cattle from Canada. FDA also has implemented a ban on the recycling of animal tissue from ruminant animals (e.g., cows, goats, sheep) for animal feed. These are suspected carriers of the prion. Three cases of mad cow disease have been seen to date in U.S. cattle.

The best-known mycotoxins are the aflatoxins, substances believed to cause liver cancer. Aflatoxin B-1 causes cancer in animals; thus, human exposure is regulated by FDA. The foods most often contaminated with aflatoxins are tree nuts (e.g., walnuts and pecans), peanuts, corn, wheat, and oil seeds, such as cottonseed. FDA considers aflatoxins unavoidable contaminants on foods and therefore has set practical limits for aflatoxins in food and animal feed. Aflatoxins are also present in certain water supply sources, such as pond and ditch water. Some people in China use this type of water for cooking, and they experience a high incidence of liver cancer.

Cooking and freezing halt fungal growth but do not eliminate mycotoxins already produced. Thus, moldy food should not be eaten, or at least not without discarding the moldy portion and much of the surrounding area. Again, when in doubt, throw the food out. Mold growth is prevented by properly storing perishable foods at cold temperatures and using them before evidence of mold growth appears.

Concept | Check

Thoroughly cook all meat, poultry, and fish and other seafood to reduce the risk of foodborne illness from the Norovirus and the bacteria *Campylobacter* and *Salmonella*. In addition, always separate raw meats and poultry products from cooked foods. To prevent foodborne intoxication from *Staphylococcus* organisms, cover cuts on hands and avoid sneezing on foods. To avoid intoxication from *Clostridium perfringens*, rapidly cool leftover foods and thoroughly reheat them. To avoid intoxication from *Clostridium botulinum*, carefully examine canned foods. Overall, don't allow cooked food to stand for more than 1 to 2 hours at room temperature. For other causes of foodborne illness, precautions already mentioned generally apply as well. In addition, consume only pasteurized dairy products and wash all fruits and vegetables; and thoroughly wash your hands with soap and water before and after preparing food and after using the bathroom.

Case Scenario | Follow-Up

Aaron likely contracted *Clostridium perfringens*, based on the fact that he had diarrhea but did not vomit, and the symptoms occurred about 8 hours after consuming the contaminated food. Spores of *Clostridium perfringens* are typically present in meat. Thorough cooking will kill any of the live bacteria present, but the product still may contain spores. These can later germinate if the product is kept in a warm setting for a few hours. The Argentine beef likely contained spores of *Clostridium perfringens*, and these germinated and produced a toxin as the product sat in the car and on the buffet table. Ideally, this product should have remained at room temperature for no longer than 1 hour because the party took place in the summertime. Thus, soon after Aaron and his wife took the Argentine beef out of the oven, it should have been separated into a few smaller pans for speed cooling and then refrigerated. They should have taken these precautions because they knew the food was not going to be served within 1 to 2 hours. Before leaving for the party, they could have recombined the dish into one clean pan. Once they arrived at the party, the food should have been refrigerated again and then thoroughly reheated when it was time to eat. Overall, it is risky to leave perishable items such as meat, fish, poultry, eggs, and dairy products at room temperature for more than 1 to 2 hours.

▌ Food Additives

By the time you see a food on the market shelf, it usually contains substances added to make it more palatable or to increase its nutrient content or shelf life. Manufacturers also add some substances to foods to make them easier to process. Other substances may have accidentally found their way into the foods you buy. All these extraneous substances are known as *additives*, and although some may be beneficial, others, such as sulfites, may be harmful for some people. All purposefully added substances must be evaluated by FDA.[19]

Uses of Food Additives

Most additives are used to limit food spoilage. Food additives such as potassium sorbate are used to maintain the safety and acceptability of foods by retarding the growth of microorganisms implicated in foodborne illness.

Additives are also used to combat some enzymes that lead to undesirable changes in color and flavor in foods but don't cause anything as serious as foodborne illness. This second type of food spoilage occurs when enzymes in a food react to oxygen—for example, when apple and peach slices darken or turn rust color as they are exposed to air. Antioxidants are a type of preservative that slows the action of oxygen-requiring enzymes on food surfaces. These preservatives are not necessarily novel chemicals. They include vitamins E and C and a variety of sulfites.

Without the use of some food additives, it would be impossible to produce massive quantities of foods and safely distribute them nationwide or worldwide, as is now done. Despite consumer concerns about the safety of food additives, many have been extensively studied and prove safe when FDA guidelines for their use are followed.

Intentional versus Incidental Food Additives

Food additives are classified into two types: **intentional food additives** (directly added to foods) and **incidental food additives** (indirectly added as contaminants). Both types of agents are regulated by FDA. Currently, more than 2800 substances are intentionally added to foods. As many as 10,000 other substances enter foods as contaminants. This category includes substances that may reasonably be expected to enter food through surface contact with processing equipment or packaging materials.[19]

The GRAS List

In 1958, all food additives used in the United States and considered safe at that time were put on a **generally recognized as safe (GRAS)** list. Congress established the GRAS list because it believed manufacturers did not need to prove the safety of substances that had been in use for a long time and were already generally regarded as safe. Since that time, FDA has been responsible for proving that a substance does not belong on the GRAS list.[19]

Since 1958, some substances on the list have been reviewed. A few, such as cyclamates, failed the review process and were removed from the list. The additive red dye #3 was banned because it is linked to cancer. Many chemicals on the GRAS list have not yet been rigorously tested, primarily because of expense. These chemicals have received a low priority for testing, mostly because they have long histories of use without evidence of toxicity or because their chemical characteristics do not suggest they are potential health hazards.

When buying food products, especially perishables, check the product date for safety. Four types of dates are commonly used. The *pack date* is the day the product was manufactured. The *pull* or *sell date* indicates the last date the product should be sold. It allows some time for storing food at home before eating. Check the *expiration date* of foods stored at home, because that is the last date the food can safely be consumed. Last, baked goods may have a *freshness date*, indicating that the product may safely be eaten for a short time after the date but may not taste the same.

intentional food additives Additives knowingly (directly) incorporated into food products by manufacturers.

incidental food additives Additives that appear in food products indirectly, from environmental contamination of food ingredients or during the manufacturing process.

generally recognized as safe (GRAS) A list of food additives that in 1958 were considered safe for consumption. Manufacturers were allowed to continue to use these additives, without special clearance, when needed for food products. FDA bears responsibility for proving they are not safe; it can remove unsafe products from the list.

some important definitions:

toxicology	The scientific study of harmful substances
safety	The relative certainty that a substance won't cause injury
hazard	The chance that injury will result from use of a substance
toxicity	The capacity of a substance to produce injury or illness at some dosage

Note that this 100-fold margin of safety is more than 25 times that for vitamin A when you compare the RDA with a potentially toxic dose for pregnant women.

no-observable-effect level (NOEL) The highest dose of an additive that produces no deleterious health effects in animals.

Delaney Clause A clause to the 1958 Food Additives Amendment of the Pure Food and Drug Act in the United States that prevents the intentional (direct) addition to foods of a compound that has been shown to cause cancer in laboratory animals or humans.

Synthetic Compounds

Nothing about a natural product makes it inherently safer than a synthetic product. Consider vitamin E, which is often added to food to prevent rancidity of fats. This chemical is safe when used within certain limits. However, high doses have been associated with health problems, such as interfering with vitamin K activity in the body (review Chapter 9). Thus, even well-known chemicals that we are comfortable using can be toxic in some circumstances and at some concentrations. Many synthetic products also are simply laboratory copies of chemicals that also occur in nature (see the discussion in Chapter 20 on biotechnology for some examples).

Although human endeavors contribute some toxins to foods, such as synthetic pesticides and industrial chemicals, nature's poisons are often even more potent and prevalent. Some cancer researchers suggest that we ingest at least 10,000 times more (by weight) natural toxins produced by plants than we do synthetic pesticide residues. (Plants produce these toxins to protect themselves from predators and disease-causing organisms.) This comparison doesn't make synthetic chemicals any less toxic, but it does put them in a more accurate perspective.

Tests of Food Additives for Safety

Food additives are tested under FDA scrutiny for safety on at least two animal species, usually rats and mice. Scientists determine the highest dose of the additive that produces *no observable effects* in the animals. These doses are proportionately much higher than humans are ever exposed to. The maximum dosage is then divided by at least 100 to establish a margin of safety for human use. The rationale for reducing the **no-observable-effect level (NOEL)** by a 100-fold margin is that we assume humans are at least 10 times more sensitive to food additives than are laboratory animals and that any one person might be 10 times more sensitive than another. This very broad margin ensures that the food additive in question will cause no harmful health effects in humans. In fact, many synthetic chemicals are probably less dangerous at these low doses than are some of the natural compounds in common foods, such as apples or celery.

One important exception applies to the schema for testing intentional food additives: if an additive is shown to cause cancer, even though only in very high doses, no margin of safety is allowed. The food additive cannot be used because it would violate the **Delaney Clause** in the 1958 Food Additive Amendments. This clause prohibits intentionally adding to foods a compound that was introduced after 1958 and causes cancer. Evidence for cancer could come from either laboratory animal or human studies. Very few exceptions to this clause are allowed; the exceptions are discussed in the following section on curing and pickling agents.

Incidental food additives are still another matter altogether. FDA cannot simply ban various industrial chemicals, pesticide residues, and mold toxins from foods, even though some of these contaminants can cause cancer. These products are not purposely added to foods. FDA sets an acceptable level for these substances. Basically, an incidental substance found in a food cannot contribute to more than one cancer case during the lifetimes of 1 million people. If a higher risk exists, the amount of the compound in a food must be reduced until the guideline is met.

Approval for a New Food Additive

Today, before a new food additive can be added to foods, FDA must approve its use. Besides rigorously testing an additive to establish its safety margins, manufacturers must give FDA information that (1) identifies the new additive, (2) gives its chemical composition, (3) states how it is manufactured, and (4) specifies the laboratory methods used to measure its presence in the food supply at the amount of intended use.

Manufacturers must also offer proof that the additive will accomplish its intended purpose in a food, that it is safe, and that it is to be used in no higher amount than

Table 19-4 | Food Additive Categories

Anticaking agents	Flour treating agents	Processing aids: clarifying,
Antimicrobial agents	Formulation aids: carriers,	clouding, catalyst, floccu-
Antioxidants	binders, fillers, plasticizers	lants, filter aids, crystal-
Color and adjuncts	Fumigants	lization inhibitors
Conditioners	Humectants	Propellants
Curing and pickling agents	Leavening	Sequestrants
Dough strengtheners	Lubricants and release	Solvents and vehicles
Drying agents	agents	Stabilizers and thickeners
Emulsifiers	Nonnutritive sweeteners	Surface active agents
Enzymes	Nutritive sweeteners	Surface-finishing agents
Firming agents	Oxidizing and reducing	Synergists
Flavor enhancers	agents	Texturizers
Flavoring agents	pH controllers	

Sugar, salt, corn syrup, and citric acid constitute 98% of all additives (by weight) used in food processing.

needed. Additives cannot be used to hide defective food ingredients, such as rancid oils; to deceive customers; or to replace good manufacturing practices. A manufacturer must establish that the ingredient is necessary for producing a specific food product.

Common Food Additives

A list of food additive categories appears in Table 19-4. Some serve the general function of preservatives: acidic or alkaline agents, antioxidants, antimicrobial agents, curing and pickling agents, and **sequestrants**.[19] The following sections look at some of the specific categories of additives and explain why they are used and what substances are used.

Acidic or Alkaline Agents

Acids, such as calcium lactate, have many uses in foods. As flavor-enhancing agents, they impart a tart taste to soft drinks, sherbets, and cheese spreads. As preservatives, they inhibit microbial growth. As antioxidants, they prevent discoloration and rancidity. They also adjust acid and base balance. Adding acids during food processing reduces the later risk of botulism from eating naturally low-acid vegetables, such as beets.

Alkaline products, such as sodium hydroxide, can alter the texture and flavor of foods, including chocolate. In processing, alkaline products are sometimes used to produce a milder flavor by neutralizing the acids produced during fermentation.

sequestrants Compounds that bind free metal ions. By so doing, they reduce the ability of ions to cause rancidity in foods containing fat.

Alternative Sweeteners

Currently, saccharin (Sweet'n Low), sucralose (Splenda), acesulfame potassium (Sunette), neotame, and tagatose (Naturlose) are the only nonnutritive sweeteners used in foods. (Cyclamate is a nonnutritive sweetener available in Canada.) Because aspartame (NutraSweet) yields some energy, it is considered a nutritive sweetener. Recall from Chapter 5 that the moderate use of these alternative sweeteners is considered safe.

Anticaking Agents

By absorbing moisture, compounds such as calcium silicate, ammonium citrate, magnesium stearate, and silicon dioxide keep table salt, baking powder, powdered sugar, and other powdered food products free flowing. These chemicals prevent the caking and lumping that would make powdered or crystalline products hard to use.

Antimicrobial Agents

Sodium benzoate, sorbic acid, and calcium propionate are common preservatives. Sorbic acid is a potent inhibitor of molds and fungal growth. Calcium propionate, a natural part of some cheeses, inhibits mold growth.

Soft drinks are typical sources of alternative sweeteners for many of us. Moderate use of these products generally poses no health risk for most people.

Antioxidants

Antioxidants as a food preservative help delay food discoloration from oxygen exposure, such as occurs when potatoes are diced. They also help keep fats from turning rancid. Two widely used antioxidants are BHA (butylated hydroxyanisole) and BHT (butylated hydroxytoluene). Alpha-tocopherol (vitamin E), which occurs naturally in nuts, whole grains, and oils, may be added to foods to keep them from becoming rancid. Ascorbic acid (vitamin C), another antioxidant, when added to foods, helps maintain the red color of luncheon meats and other cured foods, and it prevents the formation of cancer-promoting nitrosamines. (Vitamin C is also added to such foods as fruit drinks in order to increase the vitamin content; it is also used as a marketing tool for these products.)

Sulfites, a group of sulfur-based chemicals, are widely used as antioxidants in foods. Some people (1 in 100, according to FDA estimates) are extremely sensitive to sulfites; they may experience shortness of breath, wheezing, and vomiting and may develop hives, diarrhea, abdominal pain, cramps, and dizziness. As a result, FDA now limits the use of sulfites on raw fruits and vegetables—an action directed mainly at salad bars. FDA also requires manufacturers to declare the presence of sulfites on the labels of packaged foods containing at least 10 parts per million (ppm) of sulfites. Labels on wine bottles often contain a sulfite warning.

Colors

Color additives don't improve nutritional qualities, but they can make foods more visually appealing. Food colorings cannot be used to deceive consumers—for example, by covering blemishes, concealing any inferiority, or misleading people in any way. Although colorings are arguably unnecessary additives, manufacturers have satisfied FDA that color is "necessary" for the production of certain foods.

Controversy has surrounded the use of some food colors. Currently, the safety of using tartrazine (FD&C yellow No. 5) is disputed. It has caused allergic symptoms—such as hives, itching, and nasal discharge—in sensitive individuals, especially in people allergic to aspirin. Although few of us are sensitive to tartrazine, FDA requires manufacturers to list FD&C yellow No. 5 on labels of food products containing it. Some red dyes have also raised alarms, and some have been banned. Currently, FDA requires manufacturers to list all forms of synthetic colors on the labels of foods that contain them. Pigments extracted from plant sources are exempted from specific description.

Curing and Pickling Agents

Nitrates and the related chemical group, nitrites, are used as preservatives, especially to prevent the growth of *Clostridium botulinum*. Sodium and potassium nitrates and nitrites are used to preserve meats such as bacon, ham, salami, and hot dogs. Nitrates and nitrites have been used for centuries, in conjunction with salt, to preserve meat. An added effect of nitrates is their reaction with pigments in meat to form a bright pink color. This gives ham, hot dogs, and other cured meats their characteristic appearance.

Nitrate and nitrite consumption from both cured foods and natural vegetables has been associated with the synthesis of nitrosamines in the stomach. Some nitrosamines are cancer-causing agents, particularly for the stomach and esophagus. An increase in colon cancer risk is also under study. The actual risk for stomach or esophageal cancer appears to be low, however, except for people who secrete little stomach acid (some older people, for example).

U.S. government agencies surmise that consumers take for granted a margin of microbial safety gained from nitrate and nitrite use in cured meats. People often serve these meats cold or at least underheated. Consequently, the government agencies have chosen not to ban nitrate or nitrite use in foods but, rather, to change manufacturing practices to lower amounts of preformed nitrosamines and suggest moderation in the use of these food products. Since 1975, there has been an 80% decrease in the amount of nitrites in cured meats.

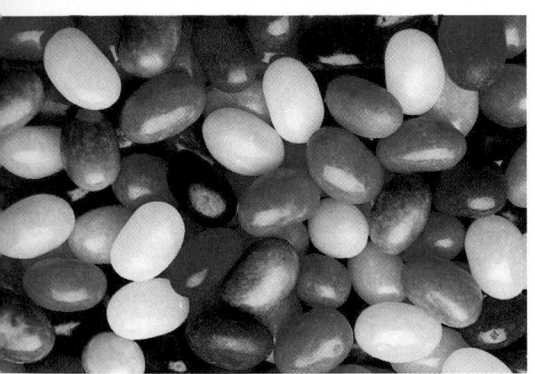

Color additives make some foods more desirable.

You might wonder why, if nitrates and nitrites form chemical substances that can cause cancer, they aren't banned from use in meats by the Delaney Clause. In the United States, USDA regulates the use of chemicals in meats. The laws that govern USDA regulation of foods are different from those that govern FDA regulation. Because of this difference, the Delaney Clause does not apply to USDA actions. Currently, USDA sees no clear threat to public safety from the regulated use of nitrates and nitrites in meats, so no action has been taken. FDA also considers the risk of moderate use to be minimal.

The addition of vitamin C (sodium ascorbate) to cured meats, such as bacon, is one way to reduce the amount of nitrosamines formed in foods. This is a common manufacturing practice. Other antioxidants, such as sodium erythrobate, also inhibit the synthesis of nitrosamines.

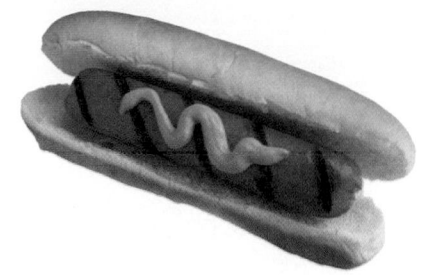

Cured meats derive their pink color from nitrates and nitrites.

Emulsifiers

By distributing and suspending fat in water, emulsifiers improve the uniformity, smoothness, and body of foods such as baked goods, ice cream, and candies. In mayonnaise, for example, egg yolks act as emulsifiers in suspending the acids, such as vinegar or lemon juice, in the oil. Lecithin, derived from soybeans, acts as an emulsifier in chocolate and margarine. Monoglycerides and diglycerides are used as emulsifiers in cake mixes.

Fat Replacements

Fat replacements—such as Paselli SA2, Dur-Low, Oatrim, Sta-Slim 143, Stellar, and Z-trim—are being produced for commercial use. These carbohydrate-based products are an addition to other fat replacement products, such as Olean, discussed in Chapter 6.

Flavors and Flavoring Agents

Both naturally occurring and artificial agents can impart more flavor to foods. These agents include extracts from spices and herbs as well as synthetic agents. You've probably recognized flavors of some spices and of liquid derivatives of onion, garlic, cloves, and peppermint in foods. To meet the demand of industry, manufacturers have developed synthetic flavors that not only taste like natural flavors but also have the advantage of stability. Often artificial flavors, such as butter and banana flavors, have the same chemical composition as the natural flavor.

Flavor Enhancers

Flavor enhancers are substances, such as monosodium glutamate (MSG), that help bring out the natural flavors of foods. Note that the glutamate portion is simply a nonessential amino acid. Glutamate in food provides a substantial, meaty taste known as umami (review Chapter 3). Most people associate MSG with Chinese food, but MSG is widely used in many North American processed foods, such as flavored chips and canned soup. Much of the food prepared for the North American restaurant industry contains MSG. A small percentage of people are sensitive to the glutamate in MSG and, after exposure, experience flushing, chest pain, facial pressure, dizziness, sweating, rapid heart rate, nausea, vomiting, high blood pressure, and headache. The onset of symptoms occurs about 10 to 20 minutes after ingestion and may last from 2 to 3 hours. People who find themselves sensitive to MSG should avoid it. It may be present alone (look for the word *glutamate*) as well as in any isolated protein source (caseinate, texturized vegetable protein, etc.), yeast extract, bouillon, soup stock, and seasonings. Tomatoes, mushrooms, and parmesan cheese are also sources of free glutamate. Fortunately, most of us find that moderate use of MSG or glutamate in foods poses no significant risk to our health.

Infants are more sensitive to MSG than adults, in part because infants have not yet developed a complete blood-brain barrier and so they cannot fully exclude such substances as MSG from the brain.

Humectants

Chemicals such as glycerol, propylene glycol, and sorbitol are added to foods to help retain proper moisture, fresh flavor, and texture. They are often used in candies, shredded coconut, energy (sports) bars, and marshmallows.

Leavening Agents

Air and steam can be used to create a light texture in breads and cakes; however, carbon dioxide bubbles are much more reliable for this purpose. Common leavening agents that produce carbon dioxide gas include yeast, baking powder, and baking soda.

Baking soda must react with acids to generate carbon dioxide. Baking powder can be used in either acid or alkaline conditions.

Maturing and Bleaching Agents

Such compounds as bromates, peroxides, and ammonium chloride hasten the natural aging and whitening processes of milled flour. These compounds shorten the time needed for flour to become usable in baked products. Without these agents, freshly milled flour lacks the qualities necessary to make a stable, elastic dough and requires several months of aging to be useful in baking.

Nutrient Supplements

Vitamin and mineral supplements are added to foods to improve their nutritional quality. Sometimes they replace nutrients lost in processing, as occurs when enriching flour. Vitamin A is added to margarine and some forms of milk and yogurt. Vitamin D is added to some dairy products. Potassium iodide is added to salt, and calcium and folic acid are added to some flours, fruit juices, and other products. Ready-to-eat breakfast cereals often contain a variety of added nutrients.

Stabilizers and Thickeners

Stabilizers and thickeners impart a smooth texture and uniform color and flavor to candies, ice creams and other frozen desserts, chocolate milk, and artificially sweetened beverages. Commonly used substances are pectins, vegetable gums (such as guar gum and carrageenan), gelatins, and agars. They work by absorbing water. Without stabilizers and thickeners, ice crystals form in ice cream and other frozen desserts, and particles of chocolate separate from chocolate milk. Stabilizers are also used to prevent the evaporation and deterioration of flavorings used in cakes, puddings, and gelatin mixes.

Sequestrants

Sequestrants include EDTA and citric acid. They bind many free chemical ions and, by doing so, help preserve food quality by reducing the ability of ions to cause rancidity in products containing fat.

If you are bewildered or concerned about all the additives creeping into your diet, you can easily avoid most of them by emphasizing unprocessed whole foods (Figure 19-3). However, no evidence shows that this practice will necessarily make you healthier. It amounts to a personal decision. Do you have confidence that FDA and food manufacturers are adequately protecting your health and welfare, or do you want to take more personal control by minimizing your intake of compounds not naturally found in foods?

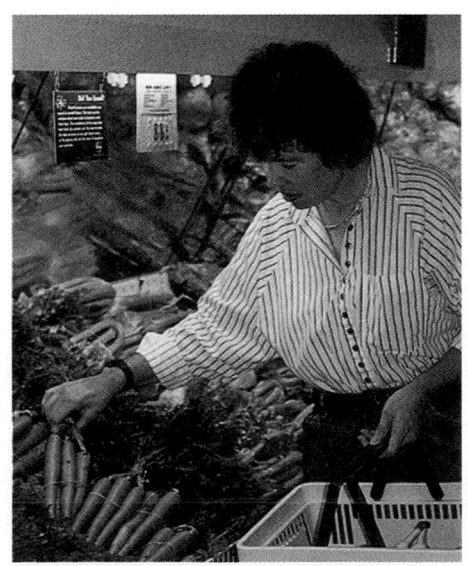
(a)

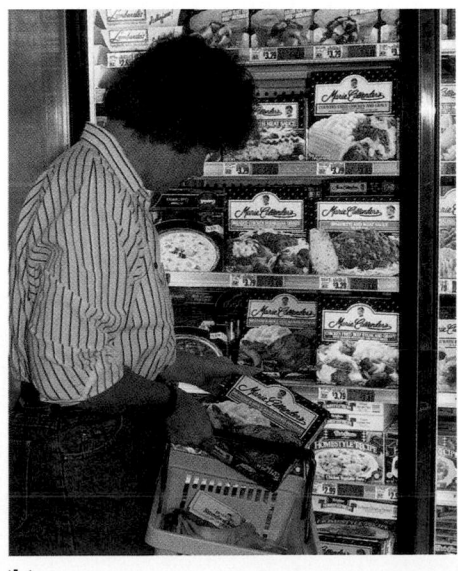
(b)

Figure 19-3 | Depending on food choices, a diet can be either (a) essentially devoid of, or (b) high in food additives.

Risks of Food Additives

If you consume a variety of foods in moderation, the chances of food additives jeopardizing your health are minimal. Pay attention to your body. If you suspect an intolerance or a sensitivity, consult your physician for further evaluation. Remember that in the short run, you are more likely to suffer either from foodborne illness due to poor food-handling practices that allow bacteria to grow in food or from the consumption of raw animal foods containing certain bacteria or viruses than from consuming additives. Excess energy, saturated fat, *trans* fat, cholesterol, salt, and other potential "problem" nutrients in our diets pose the greatest long-term risk.

Critical | Thinking

Recognizing that Joseph is taking a nutrition class, his roommate asks him, "What is more risky: the bacteria that can be present in food or the additives listed on the label of my favorite snack cake?" How should Joseph respond? On what information should he base his conclusions?

Concept | Check

Food additives are used to reduce spoilage from microbial growth, oxygen, metals, and other compounds. Additives are also used to adjust pH, improve flavor and color, leaven, provide nutritional fortification, thicken, and emulsify food components. Additives are classified as intentional (direct), which are purposely added to foods, and incidental (indirect), which turn up in foods from environmental contamination or various manufacturing practices. The amount of an additive allowed in a food is limited to 1/100 of the highest amount that has no observable effect when fed to animals. The Delaney Clause allows FDA to limit intentional addition of cancer-causing compounds to food under its jurisdiction. Also limited by law are the permissible amounts of carcinogens that incidentally enter foods.

Substances That Occur Naturally in Foods and Can Cause Illness

Foods contain a variety of naturally occurring substances that can cause illness. Here are some of the more important examples:[19]

Safrole—found in sassafras, mace, and nutmeg; causes cancer when consumed in high doses.

Solanine—found in potato shoots and green spots on potato skins; inhibits the action of neurotransmitters.

Mushroom toxins—found in some species of mushrooms such as aminita; can cause stomach upset, dizziness, hallucinations, and other neurological symptoms. The more lethal varieties can cause liver and kidney failure, coma, and even death. FDA regulates commercially grown and harvested mushrooms. These are cultivated in concrete buildings or caves. However, there are no systematic controls on individual gatherers harvesting wild species, except in Michigan and Illinois.

Avidin—found in raw egg whites (cooking destroys avidin); binds the vitamin biotin in a way that prevents its absorption, and so a biotin deficiency can develop.

Thiaminase—found in raw fish, clams, and mussels; destroys the vitamin thiamin.

Tetrodotoxin—found in puffer fish (fugu) liver; causes respiratory paralysis.

Oxalic acid—found in spinach, strawberries, sesame seeds, and other foods; binds calcium and iron in the foods, and so limits absorption of these minerals.

Herbal teas—containing senna or comfrey; can cause diarrhea and liver damage.

People have coexisted for centuries with these naturally occurring substances and have learned to avoid some of them and limit intake of others. Today, they pose little health risk. Farmers know potatoes must be stored in the dark so that solanine won't be synthesized. Furthermore, we have developed cooking and food-preparation methods to limit the potency of other substances, such as thiaminase. Spices are used in such small amounts that health risks don't result. Nevertheless, as was noted in the discussion on food additives, it's important to understand that some potentially harmful chemicals in foods occur naturally.

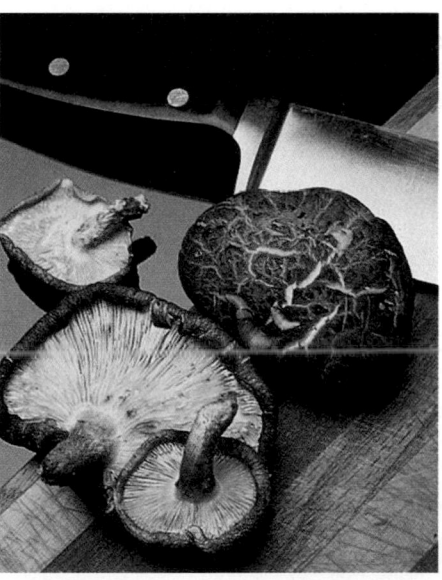

When hunting wild mushrooms, know what you are looking for. Many varieties contain deadly toxins.

Environmental Contaminants in Foods

A variety of environmental contaminants can be found in foods. Table 19-5 in the Nutrition Focus lists ways to limit pesticide residues in the diet. Aside from pesticide residues and products of fungal growth, though, other important contaminants deserve attention.

Lead

Ingesting lead can cause anemia, kidney disease, and damage to the nervous system, which can interfere with nerve impulse conduction. Because lead has a high atomic weight, it is a heavy metal. Many heavy metals are toxic at low doses.

Lead toxicity is a particular problem for children because it is associated with IQ deficits, behavior disorders, slowed growth, impaired hearing, and possibly hypertension and kidney disease later in life.[17] The precise mechanism by which lead affects the brain is not clear; however, because lead is chemically similar to calcium, it can disrupt brain mechanisms that depend on calcium. In addition, lead competes for absorption with iron, which means less oxygen could be carried to the brain. Despite the reduction of lead exposure in children over the past 20 years associated with the decline in leaded gasoline and lead solder used in homes and in the canning industry, approximately 1.7 million children have elevated blood lead. Nearly 900,000 of all children affected are under the age of 6, which is when the brain and central nervous system are most vulnerable. Medical costs for a child with lead intoxication average $2500 per treatment, and most children require two or more treatments.

Exposed children who eat a high-fat diet low in calcium and low in iron absorb more lead than do those who eat a more healthful diet. For children with elevated lead levels, federal experts suggest nutritional and educational intervention, the location of the source of lead (and removal), and medical treatment.

Low-income African-American children who reside disproportionately in inner cities are at an especially increased risk of harmful lead exposure because of the lead-based paint present on the interiors and exteriors of older buildings. As this paint flakes off walls or is abraded from window trim as windows are opened and closed, lead paint chips enter the environment and may be ingested. Regular home cleaning can be a particularly effective way of removing contaminated household dust for those who, unfortunately, are unable to move to lead-free housing.

Approximately 90 to 95% of adult lead exposures occur in the work environment. Occupations that are linked to high blood lead in workers include radiator repair, battery manufacture and recycling, smelting, and construction or remodeling involving lead-based paint.

Other sources of lead include brass fittings on water pumps used in wells, leaded glass or crystal, imported wine from areas where leaded gasoline is still used (especially Eastern Europe), and lead caps on wine bottles in general. Wiping the neck of the bottle with a towel limits this type of exposure. An additional risk is posed by acidic products, such as fruit juice, sauerkraut, and pickled vegetables stored in galvanized, tin, or other metal containers (except stainless steel). Acid can dissolve the metal, and any lead present can then leach into the food product. Foods packaged in ceramic jars from Mexico, some household candlewicks, and certain herbal remedies imported from China and India have also been associated with lead poisoning. Lead is no longer used on commercially produced dishes in the United States. However, many decorative glazes do contain lead—ensure the safety of all containers or dishes used for food storage or serving. Be sure not to use antiques or collectibles, including any made of leaded glass, for food or beverage storage.

Lead can leach from solder joints into copper pipes, so it is important to let tap water run a minute or so before drinking it or cooking with it, especially first thing in the morning or when the water has been off for a few hours. Always start with cold tap

An adequate calcium intake helps reduce risk of lead poisoning. Of course, milk is one rich source of calcium.

Acrylamide is a potential neurotoxin and carcinogen found in deep-fried carbohydrate-rich foods. Acrylamide is a known carcinogen for laboratory animals; however, no studies have been conducted to clearly determine the relationship between acrylamide ingestion and the development of cancer in humans.[6] The average amount of acrylamide consumed by adults is about 70 µg/day. This quantity is above the highest amount recommended in drinking water by the World Health Organization's Guideline Values for Drinking Water Quality, yet significantly below the amount associated with toxicity in laboratory animals. While researchers learn more about the relationship between acrylamide in the food supply and human health, you can act now to lower your intake of acrylamide by consuming fewer carbohydrate-rich fried foods cooked at high temperatures for extended periods of time, such as french fries and potato chips.

water for drinking, cooking, and preparing infant formula, because hot tap water causes greater leaching of lead from solder and pipes than does cold tap water. Lead in drinking water makes up about 20% of the average person's total lead exposure. Laboratories certified by Environmental Protection Agency (EPA) can test drinking water for lead content for about $20 to $50. Softening drinking water is also not advised, because soft water can leach lead from pipes.

Some signs of lead poisoning include tiredness, irritability, muscle and joint pain, headaches, stomach aches and cramps, changes in behavior, and changes in school performance. If you suspect that someone you know has lead poisoning, contact your physician or the local health department. For more information, visit www.epa.gov/lead or call the National Lead Information Center and Clearinghouse at 1-800-424-LEAD.

Dioxin

Dioxin is a chemical that contains chlorine and benzene. It can be created by incinerating chlorine-based material, such as plastics, together with hydrocarbon-based material, such as paper. Dioxins are potent animal toxins with the potential to produce adverse effects on reproduction and development, suppression of the immune system, and cancer. Because dioxin causes cancer and other harmful effects in animals, even in small doses, it probably does so in humans as well. Breast cancer in women is one possibility. EPA characterizes most dioxins as likely human carcinogens. Besides trash-burning incinerators, other sources of dioxin are bottom-feeding fish from the Great Lakes—an area with a great deal of industrial activity and chemical production. Dioxin exposures also include small amounts from breathing air containing trace amounts of particles and in vapor form, from the inadvertent ingestion of soil containing dioxin, and from absorption through the skin contacting air, soil, or water containing small amounts.

For a typical person, dioxin exposure can also occur in the diet through the intake of animal fats. EPA presumes that most dioxin exposure that occurs through the diet is due to dioxin in the environment, which accumulates in the tissues of animals. This dioxin exposure from food is a problem primarily for people who frequently consume fish caught locally. People who eat commercial fish normally eat a variety, and even people who stick to one type of fish don't usually have a problem because fish in interstate commerce generally come from different waters, only a few of which may contain dioxin.

Mercury

FDA first limited another heavy metal, mercury, in foods in 1969 after 120 people in Japan became ill from eating fish contaminated with high amounts. Birth defects in the offspring of some of those people were also blamed on the mercury exposure. The fish most often contaminated is swordfish. Shark may also contain large amounts.[16] Such large predatory fish that live for a long time can accumulate large amounts of mercury. Currently, these species are tested more frequently to ensure that the commercial supply is safe. FDA scientists responsible for seafood agree that these fish are safe for most people, provided they are eaten infrequently (no more than once a week). Because mercury is a neurotoxin, it slows fetal and child development and causes irreversible deficits in brain function. Therefore, pregnant women and women of childbearing age who may become pregnant are advised by FDA not to eat shark, swordfish, king mackerel, and tilefish. Note that other types of fish and seafood, especially smaller, younger varieties, generally contain little mercury. Canned tuna consumption also should be limited to twice a week, though it is much lower in mercury, especially "light" tuna, than the other fish listed.

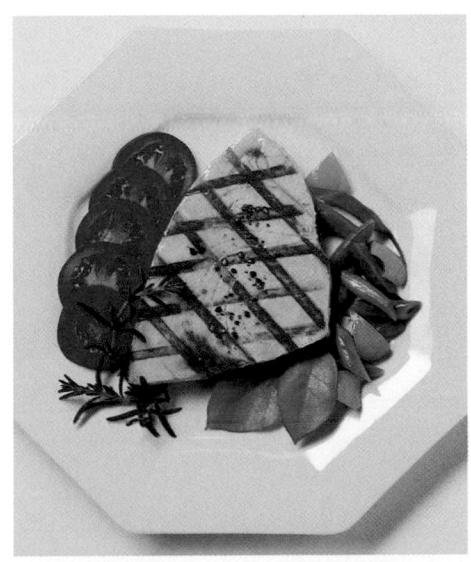

Swordfish is a common source of mercury in our diets. It is best to primarily seek other types of seafoods.

Urethane in Some Alcoholic Beverages

Urethane forms during the fermentation of alcoholic beverages. If the fermented product is heated, as in the production of sherry and bourbon, urethane concentration increases. Although urethane causes cancer in laboratory animals, it's unclear whether it causes cancer in humans. A prudent choice might be to limit the consumption of products such as fruit brandies and sake because these consistently show large amounts of urethane.

Polychlorinated Biphenyls (PCBs)

PCBs were widely used for years in a variety of industrial products; however, because they are linked to liver tumors and reproductive problems in animals, they are no longer produced. FDA has banned their use in machinery associated with food and animal feed since 1977 and has established limits for PCBs in susceptible foods and in paper used for food-packaging material. The most significant food source of PCB residues is fish, primarily freshwater fish, such as coho and chinook salmon from the Great Lakes, and bottom-feeding freshwater species from waters in other industrial areas, such as the Hudson River Valley in New York. Again, a key guideline for fish consumption is variety and moderation when local sources have the potential for contamination.

Cadmium

Cadmium is a natural element in the earth's crust. It is used in the production of batteries, pigments, metal coatings, and plastics. When found in the water or soil it can make its way into our diets, mostly from seafood harvested from water high in cadmium or from plants grown in soil high in cadmium. Still, exposure from the workplace poses the highest risk for cadmium toxicity. Such toxic effects include kidney disease, lung disease (when inhaled), liver disease, and bone deformities. Besides avoiding occupational exposure, the best way to prevent cadmium-related health problems is to consume a wide variety of foods, including seafoods. (Not smoking is also important because tobacco smoke is a common source.)

Protection from Environmental Toxins in Foods

Environmental toxins that cause disease can be present in foods. To reduce exposure, find out which foods pose a risk. In addition, emphasize variety and moderation in food selection. The presence of mercury in swordfish or shark may concern you, but it's normally not a health risk unless your diet is dominated by these fish. The small amount of mercury in most swordfish or shark isn't harmful for most of us if we are exposed to it infrequently. Note also that tips provided in Table 19-5 in the Nutrition Focus for reducing pesticide exposure also apply to reducing exposure to environmental contaminants.

> **Concept** | Check
> A general program to minimize exposure to environmental contaminants includes knowing which foods pose greater risks and consuming a wide variety of foods in moderation.

Our Water Supply: Safety Issues

These days, it is common to see 5-gallon bottles of water being delivered to homes. Grocery store shelves are now stocked with all kinds of bottled waters—more than 700 brands in the United States—ranging from simple plastic jugs containing "pure spring water" to fancier, imported varieties of mineral water in glass bottles. In Europe, bottled water is an institution, as popular as soft drinks are in the United States.

Currently, it is quite fashionable to order a bottle of water at a restaurant or bar. Not only are people looking for alternatives to alcoholic beverages and soft drinks, but they are also attracted to the perceived health value or taste of bottled water. This popular-

*G*enetic alteration of foods such as corn and soybeans has recently created concern, especially in Europe. FDA considers genetically altered products safe if approval for human use has been granted (see Chapter 20 for details).

ity has turned the bottled water industry into a business that rakes in more than $6 billion a year. It is debatable whether spending this much money on bottled water makes any sense.

Bottled Water

Bottled waters vary, depending on the source, use, mineral content, and carbonation. All bottled waters must list the source of the water on the label. This source can include wells, spas, springs, geysers, and quite often, the public water supply. Some bottled water companies add minerals—such as calcium, magnesium, and potassium—to give the water a better taste. FDA sets definitions for terms on the label such as *artesian water, distilled water, purified water, spring water, mineral water,* and others. In essence, the source must be the same one that is listed on the label. Thus, for example, "spring water" must come from an underground spring. The presence of carbon dioxide gas in the water source results in carbonation. Bottled waters from this type of source are said to be naturally sparkling. Other carbonated waters have had carbon dioxide added during bottling. FDA also sets high standards for purity that bottled water producers must meet.

Many people choose bottled water over tap water because they doubt the safety of their public drinking water. Some concern over municipal water supplies is warranted. For example, contamination of the public water supply by the parasite *Cryptosporidium* is possible. This parasite is usually found in lakes and rivers; the typical chlorination procedures used to treat public water supplies do not kill *Cryptosporidium.* This parasite poses little risk to healthy people—other than a case of diarrhea—but it can harm people who have AIDS or other diseases that compromise function of the immune system (such as some forms of cancer therapy or organ transplant therapy).[8] Recently, these high-risk people have, in fact, been advised to boil for at least 1 minute any tap water they use for cooking or drinking to ensure that the parasite is destroyed. Alternatively, individuals can purchase a water filter that screens out *Cryptosporidium* (the National Sanitation Foundation at (800) 673-8010 can provide a list of manufacturers) or use bottled water that is certified to be free of the parasite (contact the supplier if in doubt). Generally, distilled water or that which has undergone reverse osmosis is parasite free.

Monitoring the Safety of Your Water

Under the Safe Water Drinking Act, all public drinking water supplies are monitored for contaminants such as bacteria, various chemicals, and toxic metals (such as lead and mercury). The local municipal water department must mail the results of these tests each year to its consumers. According to the Environmental Protection Agency (EPA), the U.S. water supply ranks among the safest in the world. Nevertheless, this water does sometimes fail to meet the agency's standards for contaminants such as lead and nitrates.[3] Generally, the public will be warned about the latter, because it is dangerous to use nitrate-rich water for mixing infant formulas (review Chapter 17). Some studies indicate that in a year about one in five Americans consumes water that is not up to standards, especially in rural areas. These people could consider using a home water filter or bottled water. The local water department can help a person evaluate whether health risks are worth the cost of home water filters or bottled water.

As a safeguard against contamination, chlorine and ammonia are added to kill bacteria. The addition of such chemicals has raised concern that drinking water may increase rectal and bladder cancer risk, though there is currently no conclusive proof of such risk. If chlorine in tap water does increase cancer risk, the risk is likely extremely small (perhaps two cases of cancer in 1 million people).

If you find the taste of chlorinated tap water unpleasant or are concerned about the possible cancer risk, you can remove the chlorine from tap water by boiling it or by letting a large container filled with water stand uncovered overnight. In both cases, the

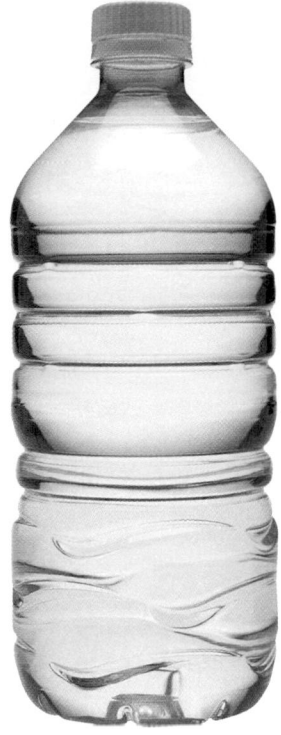

Bottled water is a convenient but relatively expensive source of water. In most cases, tap water is just as healthy a choice to meet our water needs.

chlorine will evaporate, taking its characteristic flavor with it. Alternatively, you can install a filter on the household spigot from which you obtain your water. It should be designed to remove trihalomethanes, common chlorine by-products.

Options Regarding Your Water Source

Keep in mind that by most standards, bottled water ranges from moderately expensive to expensive. In many cases, you are paying for water that is not much different from the water you get from your tap. If you are concerned about the safety of your tap water, you can ask the municipal water department for its most recent test results, or you can have the water tested yourself. A local testing laboratory or state health department can be of service, as can the EPA at (800) 426-4791, if local information is not available (for example, if you have a well). This testing can point out whether there are indeed health risks associated with your water supply. Compared with the cost of bottled water, the testing fee will be insignificant. As noted earlier in the chapter, letting cold water run for a minute or so before taking a drink or before using it in meal preparation is a good way to limit possible lead exposure, especially if the water has been off for more than an hour. In addition, do not use hot tap water for food preparation. For more information, see the website www.epa.gov/safewater.

Concept | Check

Overall, the United States enjoys a very safe water supply. However, people with poor immune status should boil water used for drinking and cooking in order to avoid waterborne illness. Bottled water can also be used if desired.

Pesticides in Food

Pesticides used in food production cause both beneficial and unwanted effects. Most health authorities believe that the benefits outweigh the risks. Pesticides help ensure a safe and adequate food supply and help make foods available at reasonable cost. However, feelings are growing nationwide that pesticides pose avoidable health risks. Consumers have come to assume that synthetic is dangerous and organic is safe. Some researchers believe that this sentiment is grounded in fear and fueled by unbalanced reports. Other researchers say that concern about pesticides is valid and overdue.

Most concern about pesticide residues in food for the average consumer appropriately focuses on chronic rather than acute toxicity because the amounts of residue present, if any, are extremely small. These low concentrations found in foods are not known to produce adverse effects in the short term, although harm has been caused by the high amounts that occasionally result from accidents or misuse.[7] For humans, pesticides pose a danger mainly in their cumulative effects, so their threats to health are difficult to determine. However, growing evidence, including the problems of the contamination of underground water supplies and destruction of wildlife habitats, indicates that North Americans would probably be better off if we reduced our use of pesticides. Both the U.S. government and many farmers are working toward that end (e.g., integrative pest management). Chapter 20 discusses the latest use of biotechnology to reduce pesticide use.

What Is a Pesticide?

Federal law defines a pesticide as any substance or mixture of substances intended to prevent, destroy, repel, or mitigate any pest. The built-in toxic properties of pesticides lead to the possibility that other, nontarget organisms, including humans, might also be harmed. The term *pesticide* tends to be used as a generic reference to many types of products, including insecticides, herbicides, fungicides, and rodenticides. A pesticide product may be chemical or bacterial, natural or synthetic. For agriculture, EPA allows about 10,000 pesticides to be used, containing some 300 active ingredients. About 1.2 billion pounds of pesticides are used each year in the United States, much of which is applied to agricultural crops.

Once a pesticide is applied, it can turn up in a number of unintended and unwanted places. It may be carried in the air and dust by wind currents, remain in soil attached to soil particles, be taken up by organisms in the soil, decompose to other compounds, be taken up by plant roots, enter groundwater, or invade aquatic habitats. Each is a route to the food chain; some are more direct than others.

Why Use Pesticides?

In the United States alone, pests destroy nearly $20 billion of food crops yearly, despite extensive pesticide use. The primary reason for using pesticides is economic—the use of agricultural chemicals increases production and lowers the cost of food, at least in the short run. Many farmers believe that it would be impossible to stay in business without pesticides, which help protect farmers from ruinous losses.

Consumer demands also have changed over the years. At one time, we wouldn't have thought twice about buying an apple with a worm hole; we simply took it home, cut out the wormy part, and ate the apple. Today, consumers find worm holes less acceptable, so farmers rely more and more on pesticides to produce cosmetically attractive fruits and vegetables. On the practical side, pesticides can protect against the rotting and decay of fresh fruits and vegetables. This protection is helpful because our food distribution system doesn't usually permit consumer purchase within hours of harvest. Also, food grown without pesticides can contain naturally occurring organisms that produce carcinogens at concentrations far above current standards for pesticide residues. For example, fungicides help prevent the carcinogen aflatoxin (caused by growth of a fungus) from forming on some crops. Thus, although some pesticides may do little more than improve the appearance of food products, others help keep foods fresher and safer to eat.

How Are Pesticides Regulated?

The responsibility for ensuring that residues of pesticides in foods are below amounts that pose a danger to health is shared by FDA, EPA, and the Food Safety and Inspection Service of USDA in the United States. Table 19-2 listed the roles of various

One of the problems with pesticides is that they create new pests because they destroy the predators (spiders, wasps, and beetles) that naturally keep most plantfeeding insect populations in check. The brown plant hopper, which recently plagued Indonesian rice fields, was not a serious problem before heavy pesticide use began to kill its predators in the early 1970s. In the United States, such major pests as spider mites and the cotton bollworm were merely nuisances until pesticides decimated their predators.

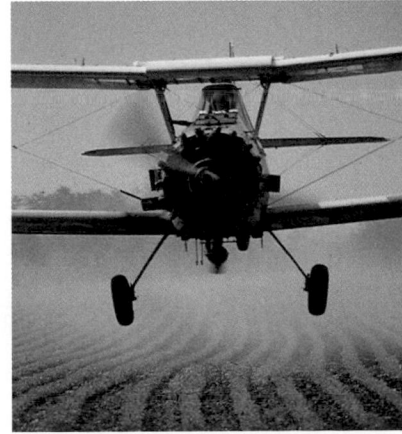

Pesticide use poses a risk-versus-benefit question. Each side has points that deserve to be considered. Rural communities, where exposure is more direct, experience the greatest short-term risk.

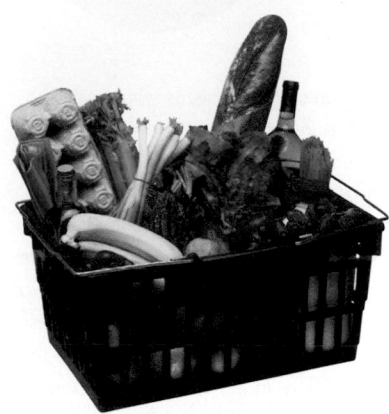

FDA's yearly evaluation of a "market basket" of typical foods (267 food items) shows that pesticide content is minimal in most foods.

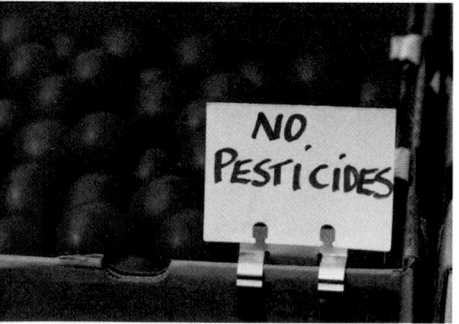

Fruits and vegetables grown without use of pesticides are available and may bear an "organic" label (see Table 2-14 in Chapter 2 for rules regarding the use of the term *organic* on food labels). These products generally are more expensive than those grown using pesticides and typically even contain minor amounts of pesticides. Consumers need to decide if the potential benefits of the products are worth the extra cost.[15]

food protection agencies. FDA is responsible for enforcing pesticide tolerances in all foods except meat, poultry, and certain egg products, which are monitored by USDA. A newly proposed pesticide is exhaustively tested, perhaps over 10 years or more, before it is approved for use. EPA must decide both that the pesticide causes no unreasonable adverse effects on people and the environment and that benefits of use outweigh the risks of using it. However, there is concern about older chemicals registered before 1970, when less stringent testing conditions were permitted. EPA is now asking chemical companies to retest the old compounds using more rigorous tests. Unfortunately, inadequate funding at EPA has hampered the review of older pesticides. The slow pace of this retesting has angered the critics of pesticide use. When weighing whether to approve or cancel a pesticide, EPA considers how much more it would cost the farmer to use an alternative pesticide or process and whether cancellation would decrease productivity. After determining the dollar cost to the farmer, EPA then looks at costs to processors and consumers. Once a pesticide is approved for use, it must follow the margin of safety provisions required of food additives (see the section titled Tests of Food Additives for Safety).

How Safe Are Pesticides?

Dangers from exposure to pesticides through food depend on how potent the chemical toxin is, how concentrated it is in the food, how much and how frequently it's eaten, and the consumer's resistance or susceptibility to the substance. Accumulating information links pesticide use to increased cancer rates in farm communities. For rural counties in the United States, the incidence of lymph, genital, brain, and digestive tract cancers increases with higher-than-average pesticide use. Respiratory cancer cases increase with greater insecticide use. In tests using laboratory animals, scientists have found that some of the chemicals present in pesticide residues cause birth defects, sterility, tumors, organ damage, and injury to the central nervous system. Some pesticides persist in the environment for years.

Still, some researchers argue that the cancer risk from pesticide residues is hundreds of times less than the risk from eating such common foods as peanut butter, brown mustard, and basil. Plants manufacture their own toxic substances to defend themselves against insects, birds, and grazing animals (including humans). When plants are stressed or damaged, they produce even more of these toxins. Because of this plant self-protection, many foods contain naturally occurring chemicals considered toxic, and some are even carcinogenic. Other scientists argue that if natural carcinogens are already in the food supply, then we should reduce the number of added carcinogens whenever possible. In other words, we should do what we can to decrease the problem.

What Testing Is Conducted for Pesticide Residues in Foods?

FDA tests about 20,000 raw products each year for pesticide residues. (A pesticide is considered illegal in this case if it is not approved for use on the crop in question or if the amount used exceeds the allowed tolerance.) The latest FDA studies show no residues in about 60% of samples. Less than 1% of domestic and about 3% of import samples have residues that are continually over tolerance. These findings continue to support previous FDA studies over the past 10 years that pesticide residues in food are generally well below EPA tolerances, and they confirm the safety of the food supply relative to pesticide residues.

What Personal Action Can Be Taken?

We often take risks in our own lives, but we prefer to have a choice in the matter after weighing the pros and cons. With regard to pesticides in food, however, someone else is deciding what is acceptable and what is not. Our only choice is whether to buy or to avoid pesticide-containing foods. In reality it's almost impossible to avoid pesticides entirely, because even organic produce often contains traces of pesticides, probably as the result of cross-contamination from nearby farms.

Short-term studies of the effects of pesticides on laboratory animals cannot precisely pinpoint

Table 19-5 | What You Can Do to Reduce Exposure to Pesticides

FDA's sampling and testing show that pesticide residues in foods do not pose a health hazard. Nevertheless, if you want to reduce dietary exposure to pesticides, follow this advice from the Environmental Protection Agency:

- Consume a wide variety of foods, especially regarding fruits, vegetables, and fish.

- Thoroughly rinse and scrub (with a brush if possible) fruits and vegetables (don't use household soap to clean them because it is not intended for human consumption). Peel them, if appropriate—although some nutrients will be peeled away.

- Remove the outer leaves of leafy vegetables, such as lettuce and cabbage.

- Because residues of some pesticides in animal feed concentrate in the animals' fat, trim fat from meat, poultry, and fish, remove skin (which contains most of the fat) from poultry and fish, and discard fats and oils in broths and pan drippings.

- When fishing, throw back the big fish—the little ones have had less time to take up and concentrate pesticides and other harmful residues. In addition, pay attention to any warnings by local authorities (and on the fishing license) about the high risk for contamination in specific waters or species of fish.

- Avoid lawns, gardens, and flower beds that have recently been treated with pesticides and herbicides. In addition, follow all label directions when using products containing pesticides in or outside the home.

Adapted from Food and Drug Administration: Safety first: Protecting America's food supply, *FDA Consumer*, p. 26, November 1988.

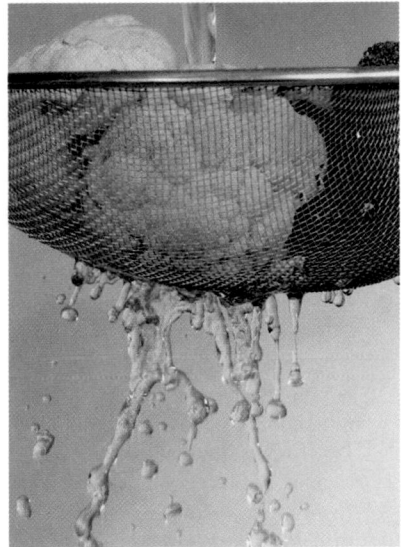

Rinse fruits and vegetables under running water to reduce pesticide exposure.

long-term cancer risks in humans. It should be clearly understood, however, that the presence of minute traces of an environmental chemical in a food does not mean that any adverse effect will result from eating that food.

FDA and other scientific organizations believe that the hazards are comparatively low and in the short run are less dangerous than the hazards of foodborne illness created in our own kitchens. We cannot avoid pesticide risks entirely, but we can limit exposure by following some simple advice (Table 19-5).[7]

We can also encourage farmers to use fewer pesticides to reduce exposure to our foods and water supplies, but we'll have to settle for produce that isn't perfect in appearance or that has been grown with the aid of biotechnology (again, see Chapter 20 for details). Are you concerned enough about pesticides on food to change your shopping habits or take more political action?

Summary

1. Viruses, bacteria, and other microorganisms in food pose the greatest risk for foodborne illness. In the past, salt, sugar, smoke, fermentation, and drying were used to protect against foodborne illness. Today, careful cooking, pasteurization, and keeping hot foods hot and cold foods cold provide additional insurance.

2. Major causes of foodborne illness are the Norovirus and the bacteria *Campylobacter jejuni, Salmonella, Shigella, Staphylococcus aureus,* and *Clostridium perfringens*. In addition, such bacteria as *Clostridium botulinum, Listeria monocytogenes, Yersinia enterocolitica,* and *Escherichia coli* have been found to cause illness.

3. To protect against bacteria, cook susceptible foods thoroughly. In addition, cover cuts on the hands, do not sneeze or cough on foods, avoid contact between raw meat or poultry products and other food products, rapidly cool and thoroughly reheat leftovers, and use only pasteurized dairy products.

4. Cross-contamination commonly causes foodborne illness. It occurs particularly when bacteria on raw animal products contact foods that can support bacterial growth. Because of the risk of cross-contamination, no perishable food should be kept at room temperature for more than 1 to 2 hours (depending on the environmental temperature), especially if it may have come in contact with raw animal products.

5. Treatment for foodborne illness usually includes drinking lots of fluids, avoiding touching food while diarrhea is present, washing hands thoroughly and frequently, and getting bed rest. Botulism, hepatitis A infections, and trichinosis are types of foodborne illness that require prompt medical attention.

6. Food additives are used primarily to extend shelf life by preventing microbial growth and the destruction of food components by oxygen, metals, and other substances. Food additives are classified as those intentionally added to foods and those that incidentally appear in foods. An intentional additive is limited to no more than 1/100 of the greatest amount that causes no observed symptoms in animals. The Delaney Clause allows FDA to ban the use of any intentional food additive under its jurisdiction that causes cancer.
7. Antioxidants, such as BHA, BHT, vitamins E and C, and sulfites, prevent oxygen and enzyme destruction of food products. Emulsifiers suspend fat in water, improving the uniformity, smoothness, and body of foods such as ice cream. Common preservatives include sodium benzoate and sorbic acid, which pre-

vent bacterial growth. Sequestrants bind metals and thus prevent spoilage of food from metal contamination.
8. Toxic substances occur naturally in a variety of foods, such as green potatoes, raw fish, mushrooms, raw soybeans, and raw egg whites. Cooking foods limits their toxic effects in some cases; others are best to avoid altogether, such as toxic mushroom species and the green parts of potatoes.
9. A variety of environmental contaminants can be found in foods. It is helpful to know which foods pose risks and to act accordingly to reduce exposure (e.g., washing fruits and vegetables before use).
10. Overall, the United States enjoys a very safe water supply. However, people with poor immune status should boil water used for drinking and cooking in order to avoid waterborne illness. Bottled water can also be used if desired.

Study Questions

1. Identify three major classes of microorganisms that are responsible for foodborne illness.
2. Which kinds of foods are most likely to be involved in foodborne illness? Why are they targets for contamination?
3. What three trends in food purchasing and production have led to a greater number of cases of foodborne illness in recent years?
4. Why is thoroughly cooking food an important practice for reducing the risk of foodborne illness?
5. List four techniques other than thorough cooking that are important in preventing foodborne illness.
6. Define the term *food additive*, and give examples of four intentional food additives. What are their specific functions in foods? What is their relationship to the GRAS list?
7. Describe the federal process that governs the use of food additives, including the Delaney Clause.
8. Put into perspective the benefits and risks of using additives in food. Point out an easy way to reduce the consumption of food

additives. Do you think use of food additives is worth the effort in terms of maintaining health? Why or why not?
9. Describe four recommendations for reducing the risk of toxicity from environmental contaminants.
10. How do various federal agencies work together to maintain the safety of food?

BOOST YOUR STUDY

Check out the **Perspectives in Nutrition: Online Learning Center** www.mhhe.com/wardlawpers7 for quizzes, flash cards, activities, and web links designed to further help you learn about issues surrounding food and water safety.

Annotated References

1. Acheson DWK: Emerging food pathogens. *Nutrition & the M.D.* 29(3):1, 2003.
   Many diseases known to be transmitted via food have been identified, including illnesses caused by microorganisms, toxins, chemicals, and prions. The actual list of important agents is relatively short. Many of these agents can be considered emerging because they were not recognized until recent times. The article reviews in detail the major agents responsible for foodborne illness.
2. Acheson DWK and Fiore AE: Preventing foodborne illness—what clinicians can do. *The New England Journal of Medicine* 350:437, 2004.
   The food supply in the United States is mostly safe, but more could be done to lessen the risk for developing foodborne illness. This article discusses strategies to do so, as well as summarizes the characteristics of the major organisms that cause foodborne illness.
3. ADA Reports: Position of the American Dietetic Association: Food and water safety. *Journal of the American Dietetic Association* 103:1203, 2003.
   It is the position of the American Dietetic Association that the public has a right to a safe food and water supply. Still, it is estimated that on an annual basis there are 76 million cases of foodborne illness in the United States, with significant economic cost. Thus more work needs to be done with regard to food safety. The safety of drinking water is a lesser concern in general for most consumers, but still deserves consideration as a potential source of illness.
4. Anderson JB and others: A camera's view of consumer food-handling behaviors. *Journal of the American Dietetic Association* 104:186, 2004.
   Improper food handling practices were common in the households studied in this survey.
   Implementing the Fight BAC! Campaign recommendations, such as using a thermometer to test for doneness in meats, would improve food handling practices.
5. Atreya CD: Major foodborne illness causing viruses and current status of vaccines against the disease. *Foodborne Pathogens and Disease* 1(2):89, 2004.
   As many as 67% of cases of foodborne illnesses are caused by viruses. Except for hepatitis A virus, no vaccines are available for the major players, but vaccines may be available in the near future. This article reviews the current progress in this area.
6. Bren L: Turning up the heat on acrylamide. *FDA Consumer*, p. 10, January–February, 2003.
   FDA is currently investigating the risks of acrylamide in our diets, but does not consider the evidence sufficient to warn people about the proposed risk. FDA instead is reemphasizing its

traditional advice to eat a balanced diet, choosing a variety of low-fat and high-fiber grains, fruits, and vegetables.

7. Calvert GM: Health effects of pesticides. *American Family Physician* 69:1613, 2004.

Clear cases of disease from pesticide exposure are seen from acute exposures with high amounts. The true effects of low-dose, chronic exposure has been hard to quantify, but most adults have detectable pesticide levels in their blood. Thus, efforts should be made to reduce pesticide exposure when possible, especially with use in and around the house.

8. Foodborne Illness Primer Work Group: Foodborne illness primer for physicians and other healthcare professionals. *Nutrition in Clinical Care* 7:131, 2004.

Foodborne illness is a serious health problem, primarily for the very young, older adults, and people using immunosuppressive medications. This article provides practical advice on the diagnosis, treatment, and prevention of foodborne illness.

9. Gerner-Smidt P and others: Invasive listeriosis in Denmark 1994–2003: A review of 299 cases with special emphasis on risk factors for mortality. *Clinical Microbiological Infections* 11:618, 2005.

Listeria infections lead to death primarily in older people and people with underlying cases of cancer. It is therefore especially important for these people to be careful of exposure to Listeria.

10. Hillers VN and others: Consumer food-handling behaviors associated with prevention of 13 foodborne illnesses. *Journal of Food Protection* 66:1893, 2003.

Handwashing is highly recommended by experts for the prevention of foodborne illness. The importance of not eating certain foods, such as raw seafood, is another important habit to consider. The use of a thermometer in cooking is also an important practice, as is avoidance of cross-contamination of food products.

11. How now mad cow? *Tufts University Health & Nutrition Letter,* p. 4, May 2004.

After the recent case of mad cow disease in the United States, FDA expanded regulations regarding the feeding and slaughter of cattle. This step goes beyond the already strict regulations put in place in 1997 to limit risk of mad cow disease. Overall, the risk of contracting mad cow disease from meat in the United States remains very low. Still, one could consider avoiding ground meat products, such as hot dogs, and cow brains to further reduce risk because these products are most likely to contain the agent that is linked to the disease.

12. McCabe-Sellers BJ, Beattie SF: Food safety: Emerging trends in foodborne illness surveillance and prevention. *Journal of the American Dietetic Association* 104:1708, 2004.

This article provides a detailed discussion of the prevention of foodborne illness, with suggestions such as paying attention to fresh produce as a source of the primary causative agents—viruses and bacteria. Recommendations for consumers and food handlers are given to reduce risk of foodborne illness, with proper personal hygiene being a major focus.

13. Musher DM, Musher BL: Contagious acute bacterial infections. *The New England Journal of Medicine* 351:2417, 2004.

These authors review the viruses and bacteria associated with foodborne illness. They offer several important recommendations for reducing exposure, including handwashing and use of diluted bleach solutions (1:10) on surfaces when possible.

14. Osterholm MT, Norgan AP: The role of food irradiation in food safety. *The New England Journal of Medicine* 350:1898, 2004.

Irradiation of certain foods such as hamburger greatly reduces the risk for related foodborne illness and so should be employed when useful for a specific food in question. Many government and professional organizations support use of irradiation. Still, proper food handling by manufacturers and consumers remains important, especially because some agents that cause foodborne illness are not susceptible to the radiation doses used.

15. Roche SJ, Keenan MJ: Should we be eating organically grown foods? *Today's Dietitian,* p. 50 September 2003.

Probably the most valid reason for consuming organically grown foods instead of conventionally grown foods is the protection of the environment, farmers, and wildlife from pesticide exposure. Promotion of organic foods, however, must be balanced by the observation that use of pesticides by farmers increases efficiency and is a key reason for the abundance of food available in the United States.

16. Schardt D: Fishing for mercury: Who is at risk? *Nutrition Action Healthletter,* p. 9, March 2003.

People should avoid eating swordfish and shark regularly or at all (because these fish are often high in mercury) and should eat a variety of fish. People who eat locally caught fish should take into account any state and local advisories regarding the fish that are caught in mercury-contaminated lakes, rivers, and streams.

17. Schardt D: Get the lead out—What you don't know can hurt you. *Nutrition Action Healthletter,* p. 1, March 2005.

Reducing lead exposure as much as possible is important to protect your health. There is evidence that hypertension, kidney disease, declines in brain function, and cataracts are linked to lead exposure. Testing your water supply for lead as outlined in the article is one inexpensive way to be alerted to a possible source. Using only cold tap water for cooking is also advised.

18. Sivapalasingam S and others: Fresh produce: A growing cause of outbreaks of foodborne illness in the United States. *Journal of Food Protection* 67:2342, 2004.

Fresh produce such as lettuce, juices, melons, sprouts, and berries have recently been highlighted as sources of agents that lead to foodborne illness. Caution should be used with these items, just as one would with raw meat and dairy products.

19. Taylor SL: Food additives, contaminants, and natural toxicants and their assessment. In Shils ME and others (eds): *Modern nutrition in health and disease.* 10th ed. Philadelphia, PA: Lippincott Williams & Wilkins, 2006.

A variety of naturally occurring toxins are present in our food supply. The mycotoxins from mold are common, as are a variety of toxins present in mushrooms. The author discusses these and other naturally occurring toxins, as well as food additives, and provides advice for minimizing exposure.

20. Widdowson MA and others: Norovirus and foodborne disease, United States, 1991–2000. *Emerging Infectious Diseases* 11:95, 2005.

The Norovirus leads to more causes of foodborne illness than any other agent. What is now needed is better surveillance for this organism so better estimates of actual cases can be made.

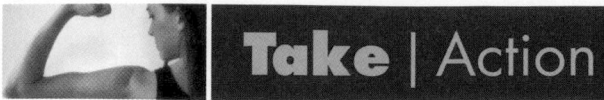

Take | Action

I. Can You Spot the Improper Food Safety Practices?

In this chapter, you learned the following facts: (1) foodborne illness strikes about 76 million of us each year; (2) about 5000 deaths each year are caused by foodborne organisms. Read the following excerpt and find the food safety violations that could lead to illness.

A Local Health Department Inspector Gives the Following Account of His Visit to a Local Diner

As I walked through the kitchen of the Morningside Diner, I noticed that all food handlers washed their hands thoroughly with hot, soapy water before handling the food, especially after handling raw meat, fish, poultry, or eggs. Before preparing raw foods, they also thoroughly washed the cutting boards, dishes, and other equipment. As they used their cutting boards after cutting foods, they wiped them with a damp rag and used them again to cut more food.

When preparing fresh fruits and vegetables, they washed them but were careful to leave a little dirt on for fear of washing important nutrients from the outside. The cooks generally cooked meats to an internal temperature of 180°F (82°C). However, to preserve the flavor, pork was cooked to an internal temperature of 140°F (60°C). Some cooked foods to be served later were cooled to below 41°F (5°C) within 2 hours, and foods such as beef stew were cooled in shallow pans.

The diner served canned foods, even when the cans were dented. When leftovers were reheated, they were raised to an internal temperature of 150°F (66°C) and served immediately. Food handlers took great care to remove moldy portions of food. The cooks prepared stuffing separately from the poultry. The temperature of the refrigerators was approximately 45°F (7°C).

1. List the violations of food safety practices that could contribute to foodborne illness.

   _____
   _____

2. If you were writing a report describing ways to correct these practices, what two key points would you make?

   _____
   _____

II. Take a Closer Look at Food Additives

Evaluate the food label of a convenience food item, either one in the supermarket or one you have available.

1. Write out the list of ingredients.

   _____
   _____

2. Identify the ingredients that you think may be food additives.

   _____
   _____

3. Based on the information available in this chapter, what are the functions and relative safety of these food additives?

   _____
   _____

20

UNDERNUTRITION THROUGHOUT THE WORLD

CHAPTER OUTLINE

CASE SCENARIO:

Jamal traveled to the Philippines with his church group last summer. During their stay, they helped build shelters for people in a village where, a few weeks before, a storm had destroyed several houses. Jamal noticed that many of the children were very short, much shorter than the children in his neighborhood in the United States. His group worked in a remote, low-elevation area where the storm and subsequent flooding had caused the most damage. On several occasions he noticed young mothers crouched on curbs or in doorways, holding their child. These children rarely moved—they appeared pale and listless. In contrast to the children Jamal's group had met at a church in the capital city, most of the children in this village were not active and lively. One evening a nurse from the local clinic came to speak to Jamal's group. She said that many children in this area do not get enough to eat and that health problems were rampant. She considered the recent storm a blessing in disguise, hoping it would spur the Philippine government to send supplies to the village, particularly food and medicines. Jamal is shocked by such a degree of suffering. He wonders why children in the Philippines can be starving to death while many children in his hometown in the United States are overweight.

Should Jamal be surprised by widespread disease and general listlessness of these Philippine children? What nutrients are likely to be deficient in their diets? What other factors contribute to their poor health status?

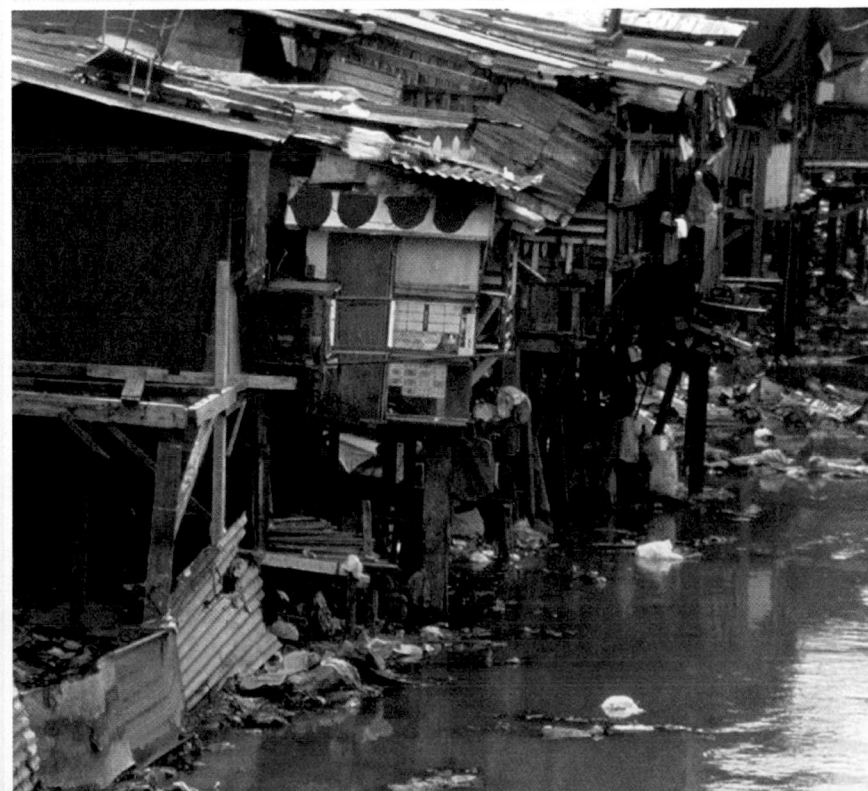

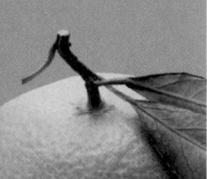

The images are vivid and heartrending. Emaciated children with enormous eyes and stomachs, too weak to cry, stare at us from news photos and television screens. Of the nearly 12 million children under 5 who die each year in developing countries, 55% of the deaths are attributable to undernutrition.[5]

Today, nearly one in six people worldwide is chronically undernourished—too hungry to lead a productive, active life. Over the past 10 years, this problem has become even worse. Throughout the world, the problems of poverty and undernutrition are widespread and growing—despite the fact that there is enough food available to sufficiently feed all of us.[1]

The majority (two-thirds) of undernourished people live in Asia. However, the largest increases in numbers of chronically hungry people currently occur in eastern Africa, particularly in Ethiopia, Sudan, Rwanda, Burundi, Sierra Leone, Kenya, Somalia, Eritrea, and Tanzania. South American countries such as Argentina and Brazil are also experiencing such problems. The eyes of their children haunt us.[20]

Chapter 20 examines the problem of undernutrition and the conditions that create it as well as some possible solutions. If we are to eradicate undernutrition, we all have to understand the problem and assume responsibility for supplying some solutions. Many political leaders and citizens worldwide through their actions contribute directly and indirectly to the economic and social destruction that spawns hunger.[1]

CHAPTER OBJECTIVES CHAPTER 20 IS DESIGNED TO ALLOW YOU TO:

1. Define and characterize the terms *hunger, malnutrition,* and *undernutrition.*

2. Evaluate the consequences of undernutrition during critical periods in a person's life.

3. Examine undernutrition in the United States and highlight several programs established to combat this problem.

4. Examine undernutrition in the developing world and evaluate the major obstacles that hinder a solution.

5. Outline some possible solutions to undernutrition in the developing world.

6. List the worldwide effects of AIDS.

7. Consider how biotechnology may help solve the food shortage and distribution problem in the developing world.

REFRESH YOUR MEMORY AS YOU BEGIN YOUR STUDY OF WORLD HUNGER IN CHAPTER 20, YOU MAY WANT TO REVIEW:

- The health effects of protein-energy malnutrition in Chapter 7.
- The role of vitamin A and rich food sources in Chapter 9.
- The roles of iron, zinc, iodide, and rich food sources in Chapter 12.
- The advantage of breastfeeding to infants in Chapter 16.
- Methods to monitor the adequacy of growth in Chapter 17.

▌ World Hunger: A Continuing Plague

In November 1974, the United Nations World Food Conference proclaimed its bold objective "that within a decade no child will go to bed hungry, that no family will fear for its next day's bread, and that no human being's future and capacities will be stunted by malnutrition." Today, this promise remains unfulfilled: uncertainty regarding the source of one's next meal remains a daily experience for 1 in 6 people in the developing world (800 million to 1.1 billion) and 1 in 10 households in North America.[1]

We must face the reality that the United Nations' members have yet to meet their current pledge to elevate 3 billion people (half of the world's population) out of poverty (living on less than $2 per day). We also have to consider that 45% of the world's income currently goes to the 12% of the world's people who live in rich industrial nations such as the United States and Canada.

▌World Hunger Today

A study of the problem of world hunger and malnutrition today begins with the definition of some key terms.

Hunger is the physiological state that results when not enough food is eaten to meet energy needs. It also describes an uneasiness, a discomfort, a weakness, or a pain caused by lack of food. The medical and social costs of the undernutrition that can result from hunger are high—preterm births, mental disabilities, inadequate growth and development in childhood, poor school performance, decreased work output in adulthood, and chronic disease (Table 20-1). Although malnutrition does occur in North America, it is not due to extreme poverty over a large section of the population. Instead, there are usually specific causes such as an eating disorder, alcoholism, problems in nursing home settings, or homelessness. Also, some degree of moderate malnutrition exists in some of the poorer segments of North American society (i.e., those people earning less than the current poverty level of income).[1] Fortunately, resources such as food banks and food stamps are available to many such people, though sometimes bureaucratic obstacles keep these resources from the people who need them. In addition, a problem known as **food insecurity** categorizes individuals who have anxiety about running out of food or running out of money to buy more food. In 2002,

hunger The primarily physiological (internal) drive to find and eat food, mostly regulated by innate cues to eating.

food insecurity A condition of anxiety regarding running out of either food or money to buy more food.

Table 20-1 | The Realities of Undernutrition Worldwide

- Nearly one in six people worldwide is chronically undernourished—too hungry to lead a productive, active life. This includes one-third of the world's children.

- About 55,000 people die of hunger each day—two-thirds of them are children.

- About 2 billion people in the world suffer from a micronutrient deficiency.

- About 1 billion people in the world have iron deficiency. The same is true for zinc deficiencies.

- Up to 500,000 children are permanently blinded each year simply from lack of vitamin A. About 100 million to 140 million children are deficient in vitamin A.

- About 50 million people worldwide have developed brain damage from maternal iodide deficiency; currently, 2 billion people are at risk for iodide deficiency.

- Residents in developed countries spend more money on pet food, perfumes, and cosmetics than it would take to provide basic education, water, sanitation, health care, and nutrition for all people now deprived of it.

- Every day the world produces enough food to provide about 2400 kcal for each person, generally meeting average calorie needs. A daily intake less than 2100 kcal would not likely sustain an older child or adult, depending on workload.

- Poor women in developing countries face a 50- to 200-fold increased risk of death in pregnancy compared with women in North America.

- In many developing countries, life expectancy of the population is one-half to two-thirds of that of North Americans.

- Almost half of the world's people earn less than $200 a year—many use 80 to 90% of that income to obtain food. About $2000 to $3000 of income each year is needed for a person to reach the life expectancy seen in North America.

- Of the 6.2 billion people in the world, about 1.1 billion drink contaminated water. In India alone, 300,000 children die each year from drinking polluted water.

- About 2 billion people in the world live without proper sanitation, such as reliable toilet facilities.

- Developing countries have 95% of the **AIDS** cases worldwide.

- Developing countries bear 93% of the world's disease burden but use only 11% of the world's health-care resources.

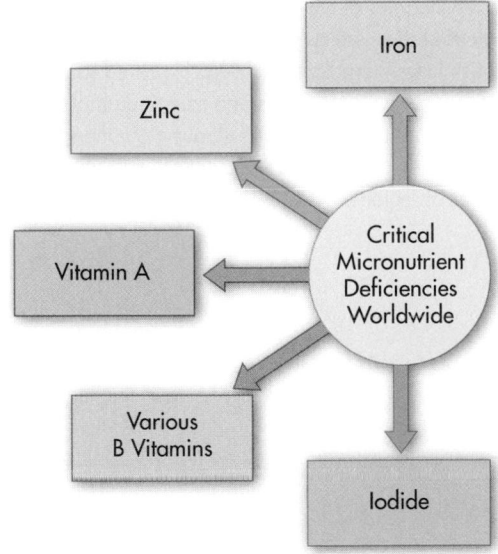

acquired immunodeficiency syndrome (AIDS) A disorder in which a virus (human immunodeficiency virus [HIV]) infects specific types of immune system cells. This leaves the person with reduced immune function and, in turn, defenseless against numerous infectious agents.

over 11% of households in the United States reported that they experienced food insecurity. Of these, 3% reported that they experienced hunger at least one time during that year.[1] Food insecurity is also a problem in Canada.

According to UNICEF (United Nations Children's Fund), the United States ranks 11th out of 16 industrialized countries for child poverty. Fortunately, the United States does have food assistance programs for low-income families, and therefore most children in the United States are shielded from hunger.

Malnutrition is a condition of impaired development or function caused by either a long-term deficiency or excess in energy and/or nutrient intake. When food supplies are low and the population is large, **undernutrition** is common, leading to nutritional deficiency diseases such as goiter (from an iodide deficiency) and xerophthalmia (eye problems caused by poor vitamin A intake). However, when the food supply is ample or overabundant, incorrect food choices coupled with an excessive intake can lead to overnutrition-related chronic diseases; such as type 2 diabetes.

Undernutrition is the most common form of malnutrition among the poor in both developing and developed countries. Currently, about half of the 4 million African children under 5 years of age who die annually are undernourished. Undernutrition is also the primary cause of specific nutrient deficiencies that can result in muscle wasting, blindness, scurvy, pellagra, beriberi, anemia, rickets, goiter, and a host of other problems (Table 20-2).[5]

The most critical micronutrients missing from diets worldwide are iron, vitamin A, iodide, zinc, and various B vitamins (e.g., folate) as well as selenium and vitamin C.[7] About 1 billion people, mostly in the developing world, are affected by iron deficiency. The same is true for zinc deficiencies. With poor iron status, cognitive development will likely be impaired, particularly if prolonged deficiency occurs during early infancy. An estimated 50 million people worldwide also suffer brain damage from preventable maternal iodide deficiency. Although severe vitamin A deficiency, which causes blindness, is on the decline, up to 500,000 preschool-age children are still blinded by it each year. UNICEF reports that the lives of 1 million to 3 million children could be saved annually in the developing world if vitamin A supplements were provided a few times each year. The annual cost per child would be about 6 cents.

Of the 6.2 billion people in the world, about 2 billion may experience episodes of food shortages and be affected by some form of micronutrient malnutrition.[1] Death and disease from infections, particularly those causing acute and prolonged diarrhea or respiratory disease, increase dramatically when the infections occur during a state of chronic undernutrition. Chronic undernutrition leaves many people in the developing world in a continual state of depressed immune function, in turn greatly increasing the risk of death, especially in childhood.[18]

Protein-energy malnutrition (PEM) is a form of undernutrition caused by an extremely deficient intake of energy or protein generally accompanied by an illness. The dramatic results of PEM—kwashiorkor and marasmus—were described in Chapter 7. This chapter focuses on the more subtle effects of a chronic lack of food.

Famine is the extreme form of chronic hunger. Periods of famine are characterized by large-scale loss of life, social disruption, and economic chaos that slows food production. As a result of these extreme events, the affected community experiences a downward spiral characterized by human distress; sales of land, livestock, and other farm assets; migration; division and impoverishment of the poorest families; crime; and the weakening of customary moral codes, as seen in Sudan and Rwanda. In the midst of all this devastation, undernutrition rates soar, infectious diseases such as cholera spread, and many people die.

Special efforts are needed to eradicate the fundamental causes of famine. Causes vary by region and decade, but the most common is crop failure. The most obvious reasons for crop failure are bad weather, war, and civil strife. War deserves a special focus and will be specifically addressed in a separate section on war and political/civil unrest.[11]

---

malnutrition Failing health that results from longstanding dietary practices that do not meet nutritional needs.

undernutrition Failing health that results from a longstanding dietary intake that does not meet nutritional needs.

Blood loss caused by intestinal and blood-borne parasite infections is another common cause of anemia among poor populations, especially when people do not wear shoes. Parasites such as hookworms can easily penetrate the soles of the feet and legs and enter the bloodstream. Although hookworm disease has been largely eradicated through improved sanitation in the United States and other industrialized nations, it continues to plague more than one-eighth of the world's population, mostly in tropical regions.[12]

famine An extreme shortage of food that leads to massive starvation in a population; often associated with crop failures, war, and political unrest.

The Irish potato famine of 1840 to 1850 caused an estimated 2 million deaths and resulted in nearly as many people emigrating to other countries, such as the United States and Canada. More than 3 million people may have perished in the great famine of 1943 in Bengal, India. In 1974, another 1.5 million starved in the country of Bangladesh. China suffered a famine from 1959 to 1961—estimates of mortality range from 16 million to 64 million.

Table 20-2 | Nutrient-Deficiency Diseases That Commonly Accompany Undernutrition

Disease and Key Nutrient Involved	Typical Effects	Foods Rich in Deficient Nutrient	Target Populations for Intervention
Xerophthalmia Vitamin A	Blindness from chronic eye infections, restricted growth, dryness and keratinization of epithelial tissues	Liver, fortified milk, sweet potatoes, spinach, greens, carrots, cantaloupe, apricots	Asia, Africa
Rickets Vitamin D	Poorly calcified bones, bowed legs, other bone deformities	Fortified milk, fish oils, sun exposure	Asia, Africa, and parts of the world where religious dress codes prevent women and children from receiving adequate sun exposure; older adults in developed nations
Beriberi Thiamin	Nerve degeneration, altered muscle coordination, cardiovascular problems	Sunflower seeds, pork, whole and enriched grains, dried beans	Victims of famine in Africa
Ariboflavinosis Riboflavin	Inflammation of tongue, mouth, face and oral cavity, nervous system disorders	Milk, mushrooms, spinach, liver, enriched grains	Victims of famine in Africa
Pellagra Niacin	Diarrhea, dermatitis, dementia	Mushrooms, bran, tuna, chicken, beef, peanuts, whole and enriched grains	Victims of famine in Africa, survivors of war-torn Eastern Europe
Megaloblastic anemia Folate	Enlarged red blood cells, fatigue, weakness	Green leafy vegetables, legumes, oranges, liver	Asia, Africa
Scurvy Vitamin C	Delayed wound healing, internal bleeding, abnormal formation of bones and teeth	Citrus fruits, strawberries, broccoli	Victims of famine in Africa
Iron-deficiency anemia Iron	Reduced work output, retarded growth, increased health risk in pregnancy	Meats, seafood, broccoli, peas, bran, whole-grain and enriched breads	Worldwide
Goiter Iodide	Enlarged thyroid gland in teenagers and adults, possible mental retardation, cretinism	Iodized salt, saltwater fish	South America, Eastern Europe, Africa

Although the nutrients are listed separately to illustrate the important role of each one, often two or more nutrition-deficiency diseases are found in an undernourished person in the developing world.

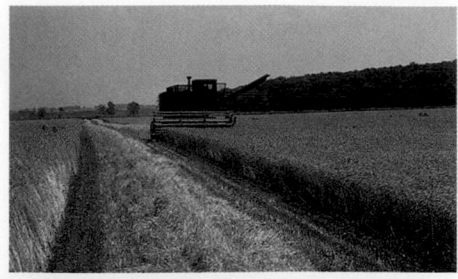

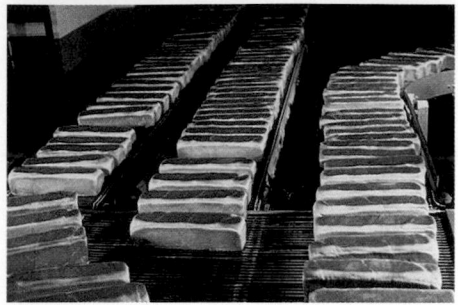

The bounty of food enjoyed in North America relies on rich agricultural resources. Many developing countries do not have such resources to employ.

Critical Life Stages When Undernutrition Is Devastating

Prolonged undernutrition is detrimental to many aspects of human health (Figure 20-1). It is particularly damaging during some periods of growth and old age.

Pregnancy

Undernutrition poses the greatest health risk during pregnancy.[1] Currently about 500,000 women worldwide die each year from complications of pregnancy and childbirth. A pregnant woman needs extra nutrients to meet both her own needs and those of her developing offspring. Nourishing the fetus may deplete maternal stores of nutrients. Maternal iron deficiency anemia is one possible consequence (review Chapter 16).

In Africa, women in their lifetimes give birth, on average, to more than six live babies. Coupled with chronic undernutrition, these high birth rates result in a 1 in 20 chance that a woman will die from pregnancy-related causes. In contrast, North American women face a risk of only 1 death from pregnancy-related causes in about 8000 births. Pregnancy-related death is the social indicator with the biggest difference between the developing and industrialized worlds. Smaller differences exist for literacy, life expectancy, and infant mortality.

Fetal and Infant Stages

The fetus faces major health risks from undernutrition during gestation.[1] To support growth and development of the brain and other body tissues, a growing fetus requires a rich supply of protein, vitamins, and minerals. When these needs are not met, the infant is often born before 37 weeks of gestation, well before the 40 weeks of gestation

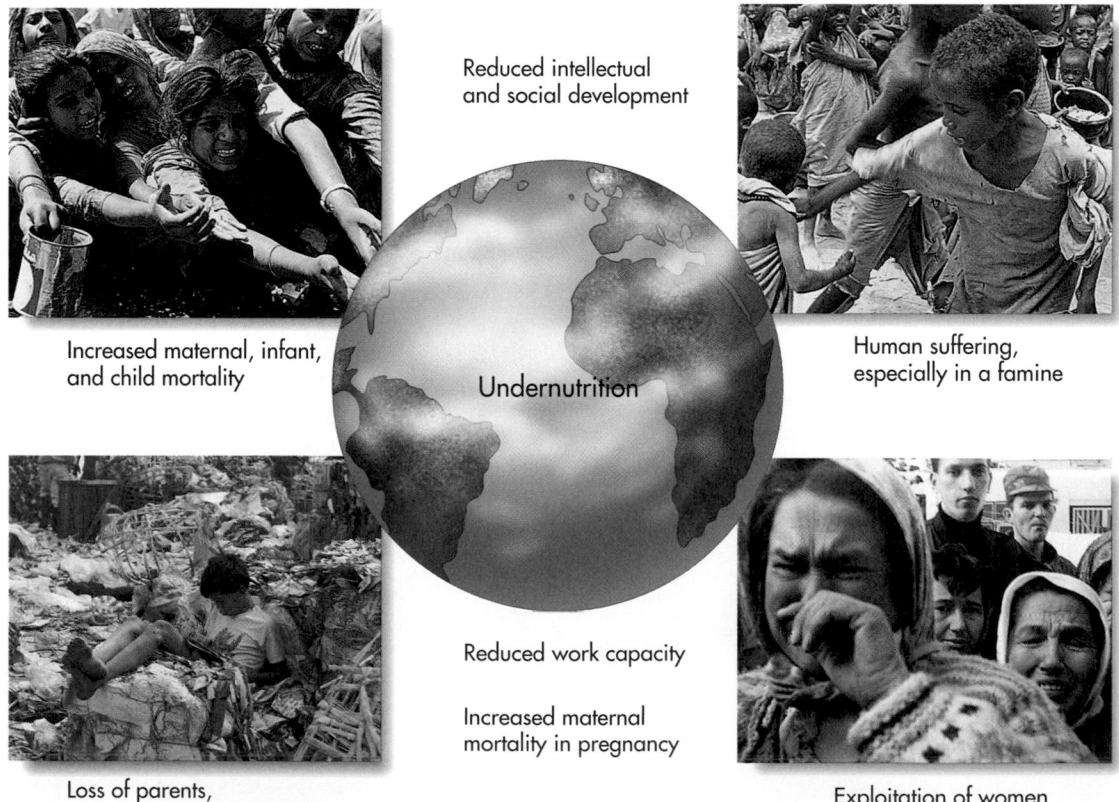

Reduced intellectual and social development

Increased maternal, infant, and child mortality

Human suffering, especially in a famine

Undernutrition

Reduced work capacity

Increased maternal mortality in pregnancy

Loss of parents, especially linked to AIDS

Exploitation of women

Figure 20-1 | Undernutrition affects many aspects of human health and humanity.

that is considered ideal. The consequences of this preterm birth include reduced lung function and a weakened immune system. These conditions not only compromise health but also increase the likelihood of premature death. Long-term problems in growth and development can result if the infant survives. In extreme cases, low-birth-weight infants (about 5.5 lbs [2.5 kg] or less) face 5 to 10 times the normal risk of dying before the age of 1 year, primarily because of reduced lung development. When low birth weight is accompanied by other physical abnormalities, medical intervention can cost $200,000 or more. These costs can be met only in developed countries.

Worldwide, more than 30 million infants are born each year with low birth weight. Currently, about 7% of infants born in the United States and 6% in Canada have low birth weights. In the United States, low birth weight accounts for more than half of all infant deaths and 75% of deaths of infants younger than 1 month old. Whereas undernutrition is a major contributor to low birth weight in developing countries, the primary cause for this problem in industrialized countries is cigarette smoking. Pregnancy during the teenage years, while a girl's body is still growing, contributes to low birth weight in developing and industrialized countries alike.

The percentage of infants born with low birth weight in the United States has been increasing steadily during the past 20 years. One reason is that more twins, triplets, and higher-order multiple births are being born because of improvements in medicine and fertility procedures. Rates of low birth weight also vary by race. About 13% of infants born to African-American women have low birth weights. Among Hispanics in the United States, infants of Mexican origin have the lowest rate of low birth weight (6%), while infants of Puerto Rican heritage have the highest (9%). Among Asian subgroups, low-birth-weight rates range from 5% for infants of Chinese heritage to nearly 9% for Filipino infants.

Childhood

Early childhood, when growth is rapid, is another period when undernutrition is extremely risky. The central nervous system—including the brain—continues to be vulnerable because of rapid growth through early childhood. After the preschool years, brain growth and development slow dramatically until maturity. Nutritional deprivation, especially in early infancy, can lead to permanent brain impairment. Without an effective intervention, it is projected that ongoing undernutrition could leave more than 1 billion children with mental impairment by 2020.

In general, poor children are at the greatest risk for nutritional deprivation and subsequent illness.[16] Stunted growth is an obvious effect, seen in about one-third of children under 5 years of age worldwide. In addition, iron deficiency anemia is much more common among low-income children than children from less deprived families. This deficiency can lead to fatigue upon exertion, reduced stamina, stunted growth, impaired motor development, and learning problems. Undernutrition in childhood can also weaken resistance to infection because immune function decreases when nutrients such as protein, vitamin A, and zinc are very low in a diet. Clearly, undernutrition and illness have a cyclical relationship. Not only does undernutrition lead to illness, but illness, particularly diarrhea and infectious diseases, worsens undernutrition. For this reason, many children in developing countries are dying from the combination of malnutrition and infection. Conversely, when missing nutrients such as vitamin A and zinc are restored to children's diets, improvements in health can be obvious.

Later Years

Older adults, especially older women living alone in poverty, are also at risk for undernutrition. Older adults in general require nutrient-dense foods in amounts dependent on their state of health and degree of physical activity. Because many older adults have

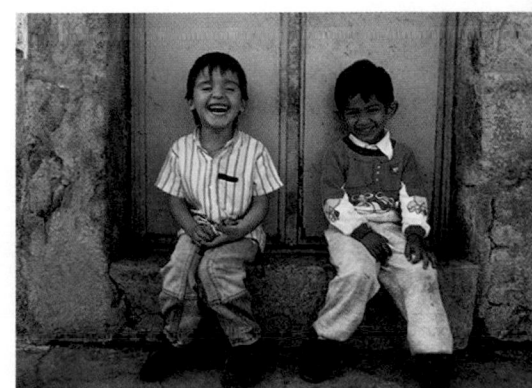

Minimal intakes of protein and zinc limit the growth of children worldwide. About 30% of children in developing countries show evidence of poor growth rates.

fixed incomes and incur significant medical costs, food often becomes a low-priority item. In addition, depression, social isolation, and declining physical and mental health can compound the problem of undernutrition in older adults (review Chapter 18).

General Effects of Semistarvation

In the initial stages, the results of undernutrition from semistarvation are often so mild that physical symptoms are absent and blood tests do not usually detect the slight metabolic changes. Even in the absence of clinical signs and symptoms, however, undernourishment may affect reproductive capacity, resistance to and recovery from disease, and physical activity and work output and may lead to fatigue and behavior problems.[6,16,18] Recall from Chapter 2 that as tissues continue to be depleted of nutrients, blood tests eventually detect biochemical changes, such as a drop in blood hemoglobin concentration. Physical symptoms, such as body weakness, appear with further depletion. Finally, the full-blown symptoms of the predominating deficiency are recognizable, such as when blindness accompanies a vitamin A deficiency.

When a few people in a population develop a severe deficiency, this situation may represent only the "tip of the iceberg." Typically, a much greater number have milder degrees of undernutrition. These deficiencies should not, therefore, be dismissed as trivial, especially in the developing world. It is becoming clear that combined deficiencies of specific vitamins and the minerals iron and zinc can seriously reduce work performance even when they do not cause obvious physical signs and symptoms. This resulting state of ill health, in turn, diminishes the ability of individuals, communities, and even whole countries to perform at peak levels of physical and mental capacity (Figure 20-2).

In addition to their lack of nourishment, the inhabitants of poorer countries must also contend with recurrent infections, poor sanitation, extreme weather conditions, and regular exposure to infectious diseases. They require greater amounts of certain nutrients—especially iron—to combat rampant parasite and other infections. Deficiencies in both iron and zinc can lead to reduced immune function and thereby increase the risk of diseases such as diarrhea and pneumonia.

The effects of hunger are widespread:

- Reduced energy and strength
- Diminished concentration
- Impaired ability to learn
- Lowered productivity
- Worsening of chronic health conditions
- Increased susceptibility to infectious diseases
- Deterioration of mood
- Slowed recovery from illness and injury

Figure 20-2 | The downward spiral of poverty and illness can ultimately end in death (based on World Food Program graphic).

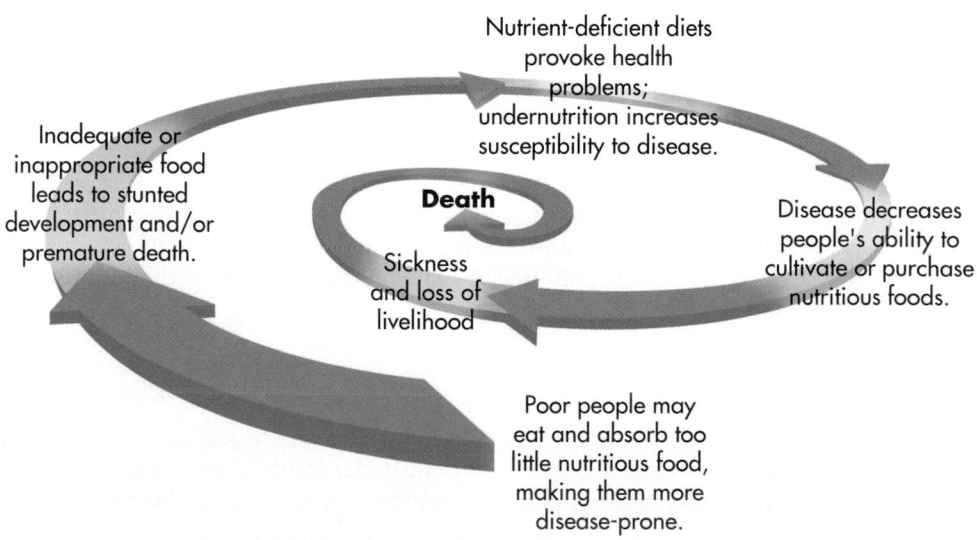

Case Scenario | Follow-Up

Jamal's shock upon encountering the effects of poverty and illness among Philippine children is a natural human response. Sadly, given the conditions in which these children grow up, their listlessness and poor health is hardly surprising. Protein, vitamin A, iron, iodide, and zinc deficiencies contribute to poor growth and depressed immune function. One or more of these deficiencies is likely present in many children in the village. The diets of these children may also be marginal in energy content, further depressing growth and overall health. We know from many nutrition intervention studies that the provision of calories and protein as well as vitamin A, iron, iodide, and zinc—among other micronutrients—can reverse some of this disease pattern and improve health. Still, many children throughout the world exist in a stunted and immune-depressed state associated with their chronically deficient diets.

Concept | Check

Hunger provokes uneasiness and pain when insufficient food is eaten to meet energy needs. Food insecurity is anxiety about running out of food or money to buy more food. Chronic hunger leads to undernutrition, which can cause growth failure in children and physical weakness in adults. Risk of infection increases, and nutrient-deficiency diseases result. The primary cause of undernutrition is poverty. The critical periods for undernutrition occur during pregnancy, infancy, childhood, and old age. Chronic undernutrition decreases work performance, motivation, and immune function. The adverse effects in pregnancy and infancy are quite dramatic, as evidenced by mortality rates much higher than those of healthy populations. Irreversible developmental damage in surviving children is also common.

In the 1940s a group of researchers led by Dr. Ancel Keys examined the general effects of undernutrition on adults. The researchers maintained 32 previously healthy men on a diet that averaged about 1800 kcal daily for 6 months. During this time, the men lost an average of 24% of their body weight. After about 3 months, the participants complained of fatigue, muscle soreness, irritability, intolerance to cold, and hunger pains. They exhibited lack of ambition, self-discipline, and concentration, and they were often moody, apathetic, and depressed. Their heart rate and muscle tone decreased, and they developed edema. When the men were permitted to eat normally again, feelings of recurrent hunger and fatigue persisted even after 12 weeks of rehabilitation. Full recovery required about 8 months. This study tells us much about the general state of undernourished adults worldwide.[13]

Undernutrition in the United States

About 33 million people in the United States (12%) live at or below the poverty level, currently estimated at about $18,400 annually for a family of four (Table 20-3). Of those 33 million, 12 million (37%) are children.

Currently, 8% of Caucasians, 24% of African-Americans, and 23% of Hispanics live in poverty. Many Native Americans are also poor, as are 11% of Asian Americans. (Many Native Americans in Canada also live in poverty.)

The poor often face difficult choices: whether to buy groceries for the family or pay this month's rent; whether to have dental work done or pay the current utility bill; whether to replace clothes the children have outgrown or pay for transportation to apply for a job. Food is one of the few flexible items in a poor person's budget. Whereas housing and utility costs, medical care, and transportation fares are non-negotiable, a person can always eat less. The short-term consequences of eating less may be less dramatic than getting evicted, but the long-term cumulative effects are significant.

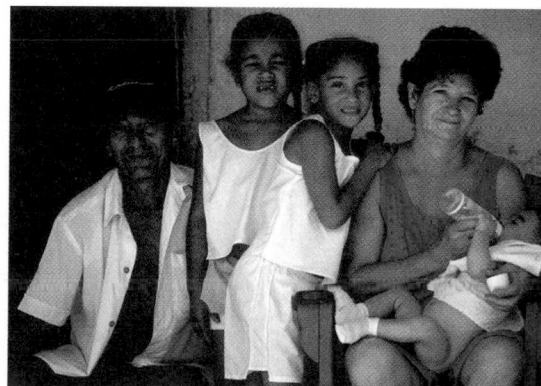

Food insecurity is part of the North American landscape. A safety net of programs exists, but it is porous.

Helping the Hungry in the United States

Until the twentieth century, individuals and a wide variety of charitable, often church-related organizations provided most of the help to poor, undernourished people in the United States. Early programs rarely distributed direct cash payments to poor people because such payments were thought to reduce recipients' motivation to improve their circumstances or change behaviors, such as excessive drinking, that contributed to their poverty. Beginning in the early 1900s, the involvement of local, county, and state governments in providing assistance to the poor has steadily increased.[2]

After observing extensive hunger and poverty during his presidential campaign in the 1960s, John F. Kennedy revitalized the Food Stamp Program, which actually had

Undernutrition in North America is a much more subtle problem than in developing countries. To the untrained eye, undernourished children may just seem skinny when, in fact, their growth is being stunted by insufficient nutrients. More likely, though, today's children from food-insecure households are prone to be overweight. This tendency may be the result of considerable reliance on convenience foods that provide mostly fat and sugar. Also, food-insecure families may buy candies and snack foods as treats when expensive toys and clothing aren't affordable.

Table 20-3 | The Realities of Poverty and Undernutrition in the United States

- About 7% of infants born in the United States are low birth weight. Low birth weight accounts for more than half of all infant deaths and for 75% of deaths of babies under 1 month of age.

- The infant mortality rate in the United States is higher than that of 26 other industrialized countries. Teenage pregnancy contributes to infant mortality in part because young mothers frequently don't meet their nutrient needs.

- Single-parent families constitute about 25% of all families with children. The poverty rate (40%) for the approximately 19 million children in such families is five times higher than that for children in two-parent families.

- About 33 million people in the United States live at or below the poverty level. These poor include about 16% of all children; children, in fact, comprise 37% of the poor. Hunger frequently accompanies poverty.

- A family of four in the United States at the bottom 20% of households has an average income one-fifth of the average income of the top 20% of households.

- In the United States, an estimated 12 million people, or 6.5% of all adults, have experienced homelessness sometime during their lives. An episode of homelessness nearly always lasts for at least 1 week and often for a month or more.

- The Food Stamp Program for low-income people provides each household with $190 per month. About 1 person in 16 currently participates in this program.

- Second Harvest, the largest U.S. food bank, estimates that more than 23 million people, or more than 1 person in 10, rely on food depositories and soup kitchens to feed themselves and their families. Most of these people, the organization reports, are workers who have lost their jobs.

- Food thrown out in U.S. cafeterias, supermarkets, and restaurants could feed 49 million people per year.

begun two decades earlier, and expanded commodity distribution programs. Today the Food Stamp Program for low-income people allows recipients to use an Electronic Benefit Transfer (EBT) card to purchase food and garden seeds—but not tobacco, cleaning items, alcoholic beverages, and nonedible products—at stores authorized to accept them. Each participating household receives about $190 per month, on average. Currently about 21 million people in the United States participate in this program (Table 20-4).

The U.S. Congress established the School Breakfast Program in 1965 as politicians became aware of the number of hungry children coming to school. School breakfast and lunch programs still enable low-income students—8.4 million for breakfast and 27 million for lunch—to receive meals free or at reduced cost if certain income guidelines are met (under $23,920 to $34,040, respectively, for annual income of a family of four). In the same year, the U.S. Congress funded group noontime (called *congregate*) meals and home-delivered meals for all citizens over 60 years of age, regardless of income (donations are requested, however). Both remain active programs, serving about 1 million meals each day, but they still do not reach all who need help. In addition, in 1972 the Special Supplemental Nutrition Program for Women, Infants, and Children (WIC) was authorized. This program provides food vouchers and nutrition education to low-income pregnant and lactating women and their young children. Today, it serves about 7.6 million people.

Between 1969 and 1971, some already large federal food programs were expanded and others were created. For example, the Food Stamp Program served only 2 million people in 1968, but by 1971 it was serving 11 million. The National School Lunch Program, which served only 2 million poor children before 1970, was serving 8 million children by 1971. Soon after, the School Breakfast Program, a pilot program for children living in impoverished areas, became available nationally. And, as just mentioned, in 1972 the Special Supplemental Nutrition Program for Women, Infants, and Children (WIC) began.

Table 20-4 | Some Current Federally Subsidized Programs That Supply Food for People in the United States

Program	Eligibility	Description
Food Stamp Program	Low-income families	Electronic Benefit Transfer (debit) cards are given to purchase food at grocery stores; the amount is based on size of household and income.
The Emergency Food Assistance Program (TEFAP)	Low-income families	Nutrition assistance is provided to needy Americans through distribution of USDA food commodities.
Commodity Supplemental Food Program	Certain low-income populations, such as pregnant women, children until the age of 6 years, and seniors	USDA surplus foods are distributed by county agencies; not found in all states; may be based on nutritional risk.
Special Supplemental Nutrition Program for Women, Infants, and Children (WIC)	Low-income pregnant/lactating women, infants, and children less than 5 years old at nutritional risk	Coupons are given to purchase milk, cheese, fruit juice, cereal, infant formula, and other specific food items at grocery stores; includes nutrition education component.
National School Lunch Program	Low-income children of school age	Free or reduced-price lunch is distributed by the school; meal follows USDA pattern based on MyPyramid; cost for the child depends on family income. For students who do not participate in the lunch program, special milk program may be available.
School Breakfast Program	Low-income children of school age	Free or reduced-price breakfast is distributed by the school; meal follows USDA pattern; cost for the child depends on family income.
Child and Adult Care Food Program	Children enrolled in organized child-care programs and seniors in adult-care programs; income guidelines are the same as those for the School Lunch Program	Reimbursement is given for meals supplied to children at the site; meals must follow USDA guidelines based on MyPyramid.
Congregate Meals for the Elderly	Age 60 or over (no income guidelines)	Free noon meal is furnished at a site; meal follows specific pattern based on one-third of nutrient needs.
Home-Delivered Meals	Age 60 or over, homebound	Noon meal is delivered at no cost or for a donation at least 5 days a week. Sometimes additional meals for later consumption are delivered at the same time; often referred to as "Meals on Wheels."
Summer Food Service Program	Residence in a low-income neighborhood or participation in a program	Free, nutritious meals and snacks are given to children in a low-income area at a central site, such as a school or a community center during long school vacations.
Food Distribution Program on Indian Reservations	Low-income American Indian and non-Indian households on reservations; members of federally recognized tribes	Distribution of monthly food packages; includes nutrition education component; alternative to Food Stamp Program.

Sometimes, severe undernutrition due to involuntary hunger does occur in the United States. More often, though, Americans experience periodic episodes of hunger and food insecurity. Unemployment, medical and housing expenses, and even occasional holiday shopping can cause a household to be hungry or food insecure.[1]

Government food assistance programs are like a safety net—they are strong, yet porous. Privately funded programs have stepped in to take an important role in state and federal efforts to combat hunger and related food insecurity in the United States. There are currently more than 150,000 charitable food providers (such as food banks

The availability of cooking facilities affects nutrient intake among the poor. Without cooking facilities, people may buy expensive convenience foods that require no preparation. These typically highly processed snack foods provide energy but are often lacking in nutrients.

and food pantries) helping to cope with this problem. They serve about 23 million Americans. Many low-income U.S. households rely on food pantries, and a recent survey found that slightly more than two of every three people requesting such emergency food assistance were members of families—children and their parents.

Socioeconomic Factors Related to Undernutrition

In the United States, persistent hunger and food insecurity are largely associated with two interrelated conditions: poverty and homelessness. Thus, the economic, social, and political changes that lead to an increase in the number of poor or homeless people also tend to intensify the problem of undernutrition.

Poverty

Underemployment leads to poverty. An overabundance of unskilled manual laborers exists throughout North America. Many such people (and families) suffer hardships when layoffs occur seasonally or because of changes in the economy. Contrary to common perceptions, the parents in most poor families are working—nearly two in three families contain at least one worker. Often, however, the jobs available to untrained adults are in the service sectors, such as the food service and retail industries, which pay minimum wage and may not offer health and other benefits to employees. Even when one or both parents work at these low-paying jobs, their families may still be left with the choice of either paying rent or buying groceries.

Another primary factor contributing to poverty has been the dramatic increase in the number of single-parent families in the United States, the result of high rates of divorce and out-of-wedlock births. Currently, there are about 4 million single-parent families. The poverty rate (40%) for the approximately 19 million children in single-parent families is five times higher than the rate for children in two-parent families.

Homelessness

Homelessness is much more evident now than in 1980 because the economics of poverty and undernutrition has changed in an important way. The economic status of the working poor has declined because affordable housing is harder for them to find. Due to the nation's rising affluence, higher-income tenants have bid up the prices of the apartments in some cities beyond the financial resources of poorer tenants. The U.S. government considers housing costs, which include rent and utilities, to be affordable if they make up no more than 30% of a family's income. A recent U.S. government report stated that 1 in 8 low-income families pay more than half their incomes for housing or live in dilapidated units. These families, although not homeless, are likely to experience undernutrition without direct food assistance. Families with children currently account for about 43% of the homeless. An estimated 12 million people in the United States, or 1 in 15 of all adults, have experienced homelessness sometime during their lives. This statistic rises to about 1 in 7 when it includes people who have moved into someone else's residence during periods when they had nowhere else to live. Moreover, the continuing changes in the economic circumstances they face could force such low-income families into homelessness, at least temporarily.

Other important causes of homelessness include unemployment, personal crises, and widespread release of mentally ill patients from mental institutions in the 1980s. The abuse of alcohol and crack cocaine is another notable cause. Up to 85% of all homeless people in large cities in the United States abuse alcohol or drugs or have a mental illness. Most people with such problems are unable to find and hold employment; without support from family or friends, they and their dependents will probably become homeless.

Homeless children suffer higher rates of many medical problems than do other children, some of which include:

Upper respiratory tract infections
Scabies and lice
Tooth decay
Ear and skin infections
Diaper rash
Eye infections
Developmental delays
Trauma-related injuries

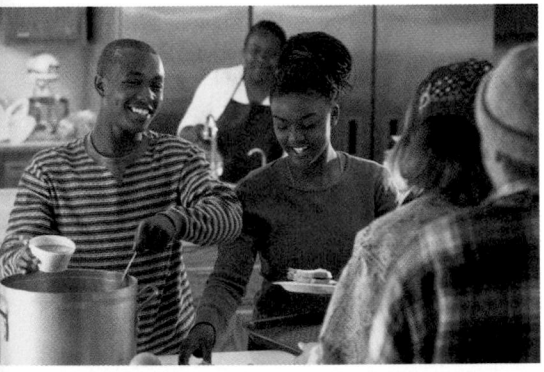

Food pantries and soup kitchens are important sources of nutrients for a growing number of people in the United States. Consider volunteering some of your time to a local program.

Possible Solutions to Poverty and Hunger in the United States

Few people would dispute the importance of supporting physically and mentally challenged adults and the multitude of poor children in the United States. The debate begins when able-bodied adults are receiving public aid. Many of these people have extenuating circumstances or have dug such a deep financial hole for themselves that it is difficult to get out. The United States has enough resources to feed every citizen; government-funded food assistance programs have helped to alleviate some problems of undernutrition in the United States. The question is, *Can government programs provide a permanent solution to poverty and undernutrition . . . and should they?*

Private emergency food network systems are also important to consider, but are not sufficient to meet all food needs in the United States. Furthermore, most of the donated items are limited in nutritional value. By necessity, processed and canned grocery items predominate, rather than fresh or frozen fruits and vegetables or protein-rich foods such as milk.

Some observers believe that publicly funded assistance programs have self-propagated—that they provide an incentive for poor, single women to have more children, because more children entitle a family to more benefits. New welfare reform laws have addressed this issue by requiring able-bodied adults to get jobs and by limiting future direct support to 5 years in a lifetime. It is up to each state to determine how to implement this work requirement and establish exceptions for certain situations, as in the case of disability, short-term downturns in the economy, or other overwhelming hardships.

Many states are improving child care, teaching parenting skills, and expanding job opportunities as they help people end their dependence on welfare payments. Nationwide, the number of people on welfare has fallen 60% since 1992, but recently the number has stabilized and in some states has increased slightly.

Despite even the highest motivation, the outlook is bleak for many people who attempt to gain independence from assistance programs. Teen pregnancy may have cut short the education or vocational training of one or both parents, thwarting efforts to earn adequate income. Often, the expense of reliable and safe child care far exceeds the meager income from a minimum-wage job. Illness of either the parents or children may prevent the adults from holding steady employment. Poor communication skills, inability to relocate, and a lack of economic reserves also complicate financial independence. Regardless of how wasteful government assistance appears to some people, it will probably always be necessary to some extent.

Many people in the United States consider an increase in individual responsibility to be a critical goal. Government programs cannot easily fix poverty and the resulting hunger that stem from irresponsible individual behavior. Government programs can, however, help reduce or prevent the poverty that results largely from lack of education or opportunity.

Because long-term undernutrition—especially among children—has both individual and societal consequences, everyone in the United States is affected by this problem, either directly or indirectly.[1] The next few years are likely to bring further changes in both government and private assistance programs, demanding new initiatives. As the welfare system is further reformed and government programs are redesigned, it is likely that some individuals will suffer. The hope is that these new approaches will lead to long-term progress and the eventual relief of poverty and hunger.

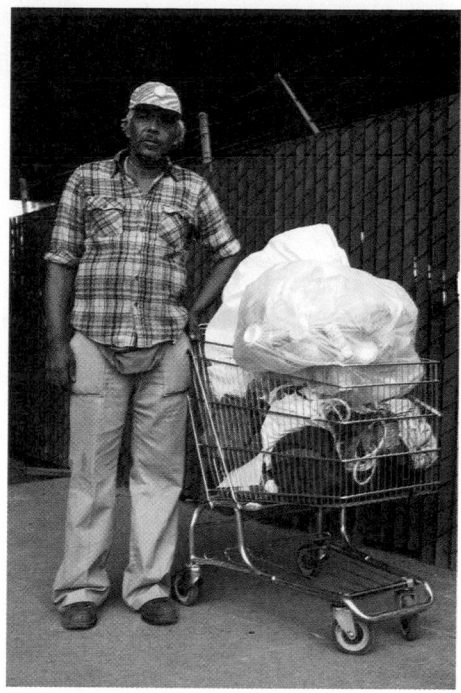

Homelessness can be the result of many problems, including poverty.

One goal of *Healthy People 2010* is to increase food security among U.S. households from the current 88% to 94%. Another is to reduce growth retardation to 5% among low-income children under age 5. For the latest thinking on food insecurity in the United States see the March 2006 issue of the Journal of the American Dietetic Association (106: 446, 2006).

Concept | Check

In response to reports of widespread poverty and hunger during the 1960s, the U.S. Congress established several food assistance programs and substantially increased funding for already existing programs. Largely as a result of these federal programs, undernutrition had decreased substantially by the mid-1970s. The presence of poverty, homelessness, and undernutrition is influenced by economic, cultural, and individual factors as well as government policies. The serious questions about the long-term effectiveness of many government assistance programs are causing major changes in their program design. All citizens can help reduce the problem of undernutrition.

Undernutrition in the Developing World

Undernutrition in the developing world is also tied to poverty, and any true solution must address this issue. However, these countries have a multitude of problems so complex and interrelated that they cannot be treated separately. Programs that have proved immensely helpful in the United States (and throughout the rest of North America) are only a starting point in this context. The following major obstacles stand in the way of easy solutions:[5, 11, 15, 17, 20]

- Extreme imbalances in the food/population ratio in different regions of a country
- War and political/civil unrest, especially in Africa
- The rapid depletion of natural resources, such as farmland, fish, and water
- The disease AIDS, especially in sub-Saharan Africa and Asia
- High external (foreign) debt, much of which is owed to developed nations
- Poor **infrastructure,** especially poor housing, sanitation and storage facilities, education, communications, and transportation systems

Each problem deserves individual consideration (Figure 20-3).

infrastructure The basic framework of a system or organization. For a society, this includes roads, bridges, telephones, and other basic technologies.

Food/Population Ratio

The world has 6.2 billion inhabitants. Currently, population growth exceeds economic growth in much of the developing world, and as a result, poverty is increasing. This disrupts the balance in the food/population ratio, tipping it toward food shortages. If we want to ensure a decent life for a widening segment of humanity, many experts suggest that the growth in the earth's most vulnerable populations should slow. If not, by 2050 the world may have 1 to 3 billion more people than it does today—most of them in countries where the average person earns less than $2 per day. Currently in Africa's poorest countries, nearly 65% of people live on less than $1 per day. Unless a catastrophe occurs, more than 9 of 10 infants in the next generation will be born in the poorest parts of the world.

More than three-quarters of people in the world live in developing countries, and more than half live in Asia. A recent United Nations report on worldwide hunger revealed that almost two-thirds of the world's undernourished live in Asia and the Pacific Rim. The world's food supplies also are not distributed equally among consumers. Gross disparities exist between developed and developing countries, among the rich and the poor within countries, and even within families (males may be fed before females).

Figure 20-3 | Many factors contribute to undernutrition in the developing world. Any solutions to the problem must take these factors into consideration.

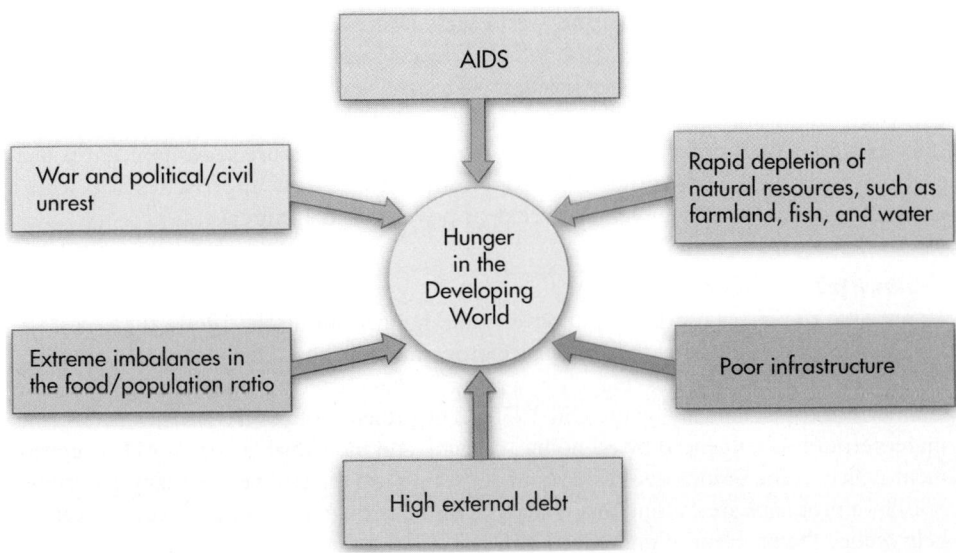

Still, economists estimate that world food production will, in fact, continue to increase more rapidly than world population in the near future, allowing the food/population ratio to increase through the year 2020. This increase will come at a high cost, however, in terms of the water, fertilizer, and pesticides needed to allow for this production. Overall, in the short run, the primary problem appears not to be food production but distribution and use, especially in poverty-stricken areas of developing nations.

Eventually, though, food production will begin to lag behind population growth. Most good farmland in the world is already in use, and because of poor farming practices or competing land-use demands, the number of farmable acres worldwide decreases annually. For many reasons, sustainable world food output—an amount that doesn't deplete the earth's resources—is now running well behind food consumption. This discrepancy suggests that food production in less-developed countries will barely keep up with population growth and will soon lag behind.

Birth control programs, an obvious brake on population expansion, have been effective in developed countries but relatively ineffective in many developing countries that could really benefit from them. Among women, family planning and contraceptive use worldwide has increased to 60% today, up from 10% in 1969. If the United Nations, voluntary organizations, and governments had not started promoting family planning and contraceptive use, the population today might be as high as 7 or 8 billion. However, women (and men) in many developing countries are still lacking adequate access to contraceptives. Organizations such as Population Services International are trying to keep distribution costs low and make the products available to as many people as possible by subsidizing condoms and oral contraceptives to areas such as Bangladesh.

Promoting breastfeeding also contributes to the goal of birth control. Although it is not a completely reliable method of contraception, exclusively breastfeeding an infant lessens ovulation, thereby lowering the likelihood of fertilization, for an average of six months. (Women who do not breastfeed generally begin to ovulate within a month or so after giving birth.) When childbirths are more widely spaced, not only do fewer total births occur, but the mother has a longer chance to recover from pregnancy, and the infant receives feeding priority for a longer time. One possible exception to the healthful nature of breastfeeding occurs, however, when mothers are infected with the **human immunodeficiency virus (HIV).** The risk of transferring the virus through human milk is about 10%. Depending on the circumstances, this risk may outweigh the benefits of breastfeeding.

Experience with family planning programs in developing countries and historical changes in birth rates in many developed countries suggest an important conclusion: generally, only when people have enough to eat and are financially secure do they feel confident that having fewer children will still result in enough surviving sons and/or daughters to provide for their care in later years. Increasing per capita income and improving education, especially for women in developing nations, are currently considered to be the most likely long-term solutions to excessive population growth. In the last few years this effort has led to a decline in family size in Brazil, Egypt, India, and Mexico. A major concern is whether there are enough resources worldwide to raise per capita income and provide enough education to slow population growth.

Concept | Check

Currently, world food production is sufficient to meet the energy needs of the world's population. Despite these adequate food resources, undernutrition continues to exist because of poverty, politics, and unequal food distribution. In addition, projected population growth may soon overwhelm food production. Most scientists and world leaders recommend limiting population growth, especially in developing countries where birth rates are high.

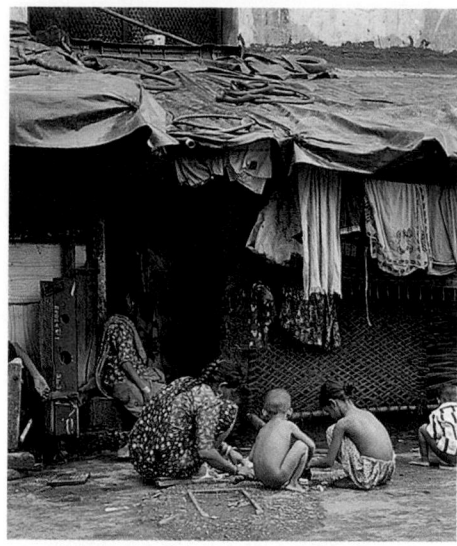

Poverty aggravates the problem of hunger in the developing world.

Whether the earth can yield enough food for all people has been a long-standing question. As early as 1798, English clergyman and political economist Thomas Malthus proposed a rather pessimistic view of our prospects. He said the population would increase in a **geometric ratio**—2, 4, 8, 16, 32, and so on. Meanwhile, at best, the food supply would increase only in an **arithmetic ratio**—2, 4, 6, 8, 10, and so on. This prediction means that while the food/population ratio might begin at 2/2, eventually the population will grow to 32 while food supplies will only increase to feed 10. However, eminent British scientists at the time pointed out that scientific advances in agriculture would greatly increase food production. In fact, their predictions have proved true, to an extent. The aptly named "population explosion" is currently undermining this progress in the developing world.

geometric ratio A series of numbers wherein the division of each number by the one to the left of it yields the same answer.

arithmetic ratio A series of numbers wherein the difference between each number is the same.

human immunodeficiency virus (HIV) The virus that leads to acquired immunodeficiency syndrome (AIDS).

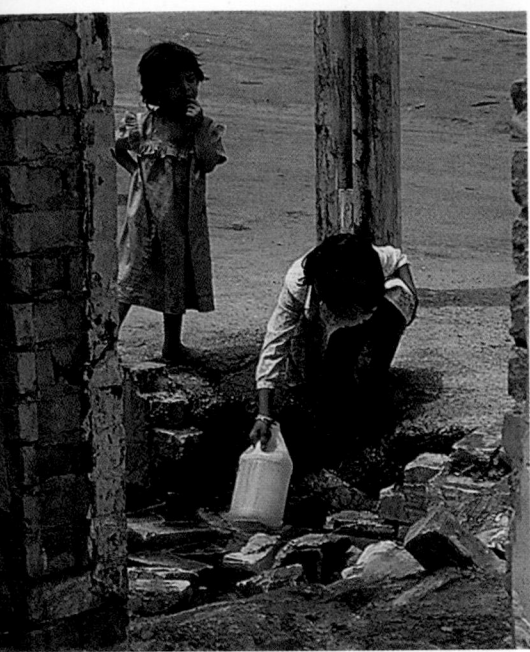

Homes and infrastructure are often damaged during times of war and political unrest.

The recent conflicts in the Darfur region of Sudan have led to high rates of death and undernutrition among people displaced by war.[11]

green revolution Increases in crop yields accompanying the introduction of new agricultural technologies in less-developed countries, beginning in the 1960s. The key technologies were high-yielding, disease-resistant strains of rice, wheat, and corn; greater use of fertilizer and water; and improved cultivation practices.

War and Political/Civil Unrest

The Millennium Summit of the United Nations pledged to "spare no effort to free our peoples from the scourge of war." Against that background stands the reality that worldwide military spending has doubled over the past 20 years. In the twentieth century, deadly weapons of war took an enormous toll on civilians living in poor, politically vulnerable, war-torn nations. Although Africa has been ravaged by economic decay and famine for years, military spending in Africa more than doubled in the 1970s and held firm through the 1990s. Currently, less than one-half of 1% of the world's yearly production of goods and services is devoted to economic development assistance, whereas approximately 6% goes to military expenditures.

Aside from the economic impact of military spending, civil disruptions and wars are setting back the progress of the poor and contributing to massive undernutrition. All but two of the major conflicts in 2000 took place in the developing world. War-related famine affects at least 20 million people in southern and northeastern Africa. The border war between Ethiopia and neighboring Eritrea has had a tremendous negative impact on food resources. A World Bank official stated that the food shortage in Ethiopia is a problem that will persist until political changes are made. Currently, 12.4 million people in Ethiopia, Eritrea, Djibouti, Kenya, Somalia, and Zimbabwe are at risk for food shortages. Other conflicts continue between Congo (formerly Zaire) and the Republic of Congo as well as in Angola and Sudan, where millions have been put at risk of starvation. In the capital of war-torn Iraq, Baghdad, child malnutrition nearly doubled between 2002 and 2003. Disruptions in infrastructure from bombing and looting limit the safety of water, and as a result, health officials have observed a 250% increase in cases of diarrhea. Furthermore, health facilities needed to cope with undernutrition and dehydration have been damaged and looted throughout Baghdad and the surrounding area. Overall, most people in war-torn areas are without sufficient shelter, clothing, food, or means of obtaining them. Worldwide, this entire problem is projected to worsen over the next 15 years.

Even when food is available, political divisions may impede its distribution to the point that undernutrition will plague many people for years to come. Especially during emergencies, programs designed to help the poor have been undermined by unstable administration, corruption, and political influence. During such political chaos, relief agencies are often caught between warring factions and the people they are trying to help. This dilemma occurred in the mid-1990s in Zaire, where Rwandan refugee camps fell under the control of a militant group. The rebels controlled the food coming into the camps and would not allow relief agencies to do their work.

During the 1960s and 1970s, the problem of undernutrition in developing countries was perceived as a technical one: how to produce enough food for the growing world population. The problem is now seen as largely political: how to achieve cooperation among and within nations so that gains in food production and infrastructure are not wiped out by war. The best answer lies in a combination of approaches—finding technical solutions to help with the problems of chronic hunger and poverty and resolving political crises that have pushed developing nations into a state of acute hunger and chaos.

Rapid Depletion of Natural Resources

As we quickly deplete the earth's resources, population control grows increasingly critical. Agriculture production is approaching its limits in many areas worldwide. Environmentally unsustainable farming methods are undermining food production, especially in developing countries.

The **green revolution** was a phenomenon that began in the 1960s when crop yields rose dramatically in some countries, such as the Philippines, India, and Mexico (countries in Africa did not benefit because climates were not compatible with the crops used). The increased use of fertilizers and irrigation and the development of superior crops through careful plant breeding made this boost in agricultural production possible.[8] Many of the technologies associated with the green revolution have now achieved their potential. Rice yields, for example, have not increased significantly since the release of superior varieties in 1966. (Actually, the green revolution was intended as a stopgap measure until world leaders could control population growth.)

Future gains in productivity may be much harder to accomplish because of the existence of less productive farmland. Until the introduction of another superior strain of rice or other grain, developing countries will not benefit greatly from recent, more modest breakthroughs in biotechnology (see the Nutrition Focus section on use of biotechnology).

Areas of the world that remain uncultivated or ungrazed are mostly too rocky, steep, infertile, dry, wet, or inaccessible to sustain farming. Nearly all irrigation water available worldwide is currently being used, and groundwater supplies are becoming depleted at rapid rates in many regions. An eventual water shortage is projected to increase war and civil unrest in arid areas of the world, such as Northern Africa and the Middle East. China, which has more than 20% of the world's irrigated land, is also plagued with a growing scarcity of fresh water. In the future, billions of people will face ongoing water shortages.

The prospects of obtaining substantially more food from the oceans are also poor. In recent years, the amount of fish caught worldwide has leveled off. Fish was once considered the poor person's protein, but this option is no longer available because farming of fish currently does not come close to compensating for the degree of reduction in wild fish populations.[15]

Clearly, we can exploit the earth's resources only so far—the world population probably cannot continue to expand as it does today without the potential for serious famine and death. The Food and Agriculture Organization (FAO) of the United Nations works on this principle: "The fight to ensure that all people have enough nutritious food to eat is worthy of our greatest efforts, but it must be fought with the full recognition that it cannot be won unless agricultural, fishery, and forestry production returns to the earth as much as—or more than—it takes." Thus, if food production is to keep up with the expanding population, immediate action is needed to protect the earth's already deteriorated environment from further destruction.

Inadequate Shelter and Sanitation

When people die from undernutrition in developing countries, other factors, such as inadequate shelter and sanitation, almost always contribute. Poor sanitation along with undernutrition particularly raises the risk of infection (Figure 20-4). For example, the 1994 plague in Surat (northwest India), linked mainly to unsanitary housing conditions, killed almost 5000 people and sparked the panicked exodus of another half a million.

Inadequate and deteriorating shelters threaten the lives of more than 500 million people today. Many of the 15 million annual deaths of children—half of them under 5 years old—in developing countries could be prevented by improving the standards of environmental hygiene. Urban populations of some developing countries are currently growing at an annual rate of 5 to 7%. Such a skewed population distribution will result in more poverty. The current urban explosion is the result of both high birth rates and continuing migration of people to the cities from rural areas. People go to the cities to find employment and resources that the countryside can no longer provide. Worldwide, 38% of people lived in urban areas in 1975. The figure is now about 50% and is expected to reach 70% by 2050. Nine of the world's 10 largest cities will be in poor countries 20 years from now. Currently 12 of the world's 15 most polluted cities are in Asia alone.

In developing countries, the poor make up most of the urban population, and their needs for housing and community services often go beyond available governmental resources. Most of these urban poor live in overcrowded, self-made shelters that lack a safe and adequate water supply and are only partially served by public utilities. The

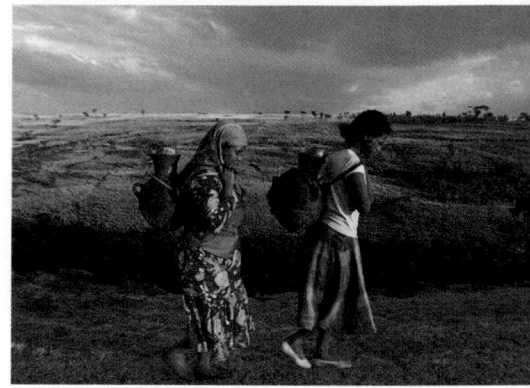

Lasting gains have come slowly in the world's battle against undernutrition.

In Brazil, migrants displaced by multinational land developers have flooded from the north and northeast into Rio de Janeiro and São Paulo, attracted by the prospect of jobs. There they have built shantytowns next to apartment towers and affluent suburbs, but the jobs do not materialize, and urban poverty simply replaces rural impoverishment.

Figure 20-4 | Nutritional status and overall food supply combine with a variety of environmental factors to influence the risk of infection and the ultimate outcome.

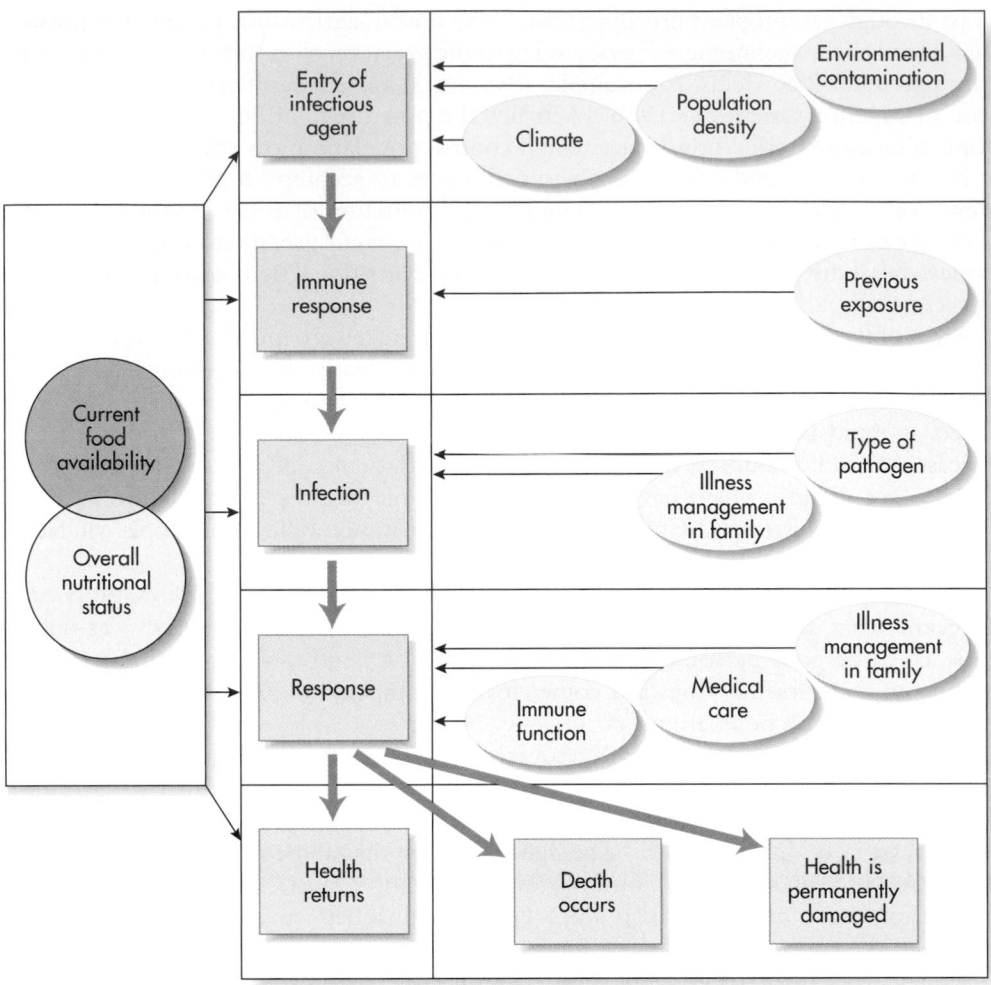

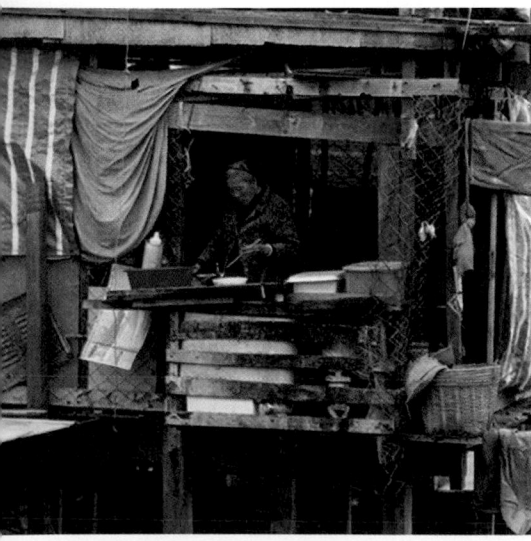

Inadequate sanitation facilities and the consumption of contaminated water cause the majority of all diseases. About 1 billion people in developing countries lack access to a safe water supply.

shantytowns and ghettos of the developing world are often worse than the rural areas the people left behind. Because the urban poor need cash to purchase food, they often subsist on diets that are even more meager than the homegrown rural fare. Making matters worse, haphazard shelters often lack facilities to protect food from spoilage or damage by insects and rodents. This inability to protect food supplies in some developing countries leads to the loss of as much as 40% of all perishable foods.

The shift from rural to urban life takes its greatest toll on infants and children. Infants are often weaned early from the breast to infant formula, partly because the mother must find employment and partly because she may be influenced by advertisements depicting images of sophisticated, formula-feeding women. Unfortunately, because infant formulas are relatively expensive, poor parents may try to conserve the formula by either overdiluting the mixture or using too little to meet the infant's needs. Because the water supply may not be safe, the prepared formula is also likely to be contaminated with bacteria. Human milk, in contrast, is much more hygienic, readily available, and nutritious. It also provides infants with immunity to some ailments. Promoting breastfeeding is important when it is safe for the infant (review the earlier discussion of AIDS, HIV, and breastfeeding).

Overall, the single most effective health advantage for people, wherever they live, is a safe and convenient water supply.[17] Inadequate sanitation and the consumption of contaminated water cause 75% of all diseases and more than one-third of all deaths in developing countries. The World Health Organization (WHO) estimates that 1.1 billion people, about one-sixth of all people, have an unsafe and inadequate water supply. In addition, up to 90% of the diseases seen in developing countries may be attributed to contaminated water.

Poor sanitation, another example of inadequate infrastructure in the developing world, creates a critical public health problem. Human feces, rotting garbage, and associated insect and rodent infestations are potent sources of disease organisms commonly seen in urban areas of the developing world. Two of the most dangerous substances encountered in routine daily living are human urine and feces. The inability to dispose of the massive numbers of dead people (and dead animals) resulting from civil wars causes additional sanitation problems. In some developing countries, diarrheal diseases account for as many as one-third of all deaths in children under 5 years of age. WHO estimates that even with improvements in housing, 2 billion people in the world still lack proper sanitation facilities.

High External Debt

Since the 1970s many developing countries have become trapped in a cycle of borrowing repeatedly from foreign countries and international banks. Servicing these external debts, which now total about $2.5 trillion, has brought several countries to the verge of economic collapse. About $6 billion is owed to the United States. The external debt of Latin America represents 45% of the area's gross regional output of goods and services.

Many African nations also carry large debt burdens—currently, $350 billion. This problem is made worse by recent drops in prices for the raw commodities they export, higher prices for imported oil, and embezzlement of funds by high-ranking officials. To make up the difference between export income and import expenses, countries have been forced to borrow millions of dollars from international banks. Although the African debts are much smaller in absolute terms than those of Brazil, Argentina, and Mexico, for example, the actual burden is greater when national incomes and export earnings are considered. Nearly half the money African nations earn from exports goes to paying off the continent's multibillion-dollar debt. Much of the rest goes to fund imports of machinery, concrete, trucks, and consumer goods from developed countries. Little is left for domestic programs, necessitating cutbacks that translate into fewer resources to counter already widespread undernutrition.

The Group of Eight—consisting of the world's most industrialized nations—is planning to forgive some external debt owed by developing countries. The $40 billion that has been promised should end the external debt of 18 countries, including some in Africa and South America. The debt repayment depends on the developing country's agreement to practice good governance and to use the money saved to support health care, education, and infrastructure improvements.

Concept | Check

War and civil strife, along with a decline in the world's natural resources, contribute to the difficulty of ending undernutrition in many developing countries. In addition, substandard housing conditions, impure water, and inadequate sanitation worldwide increase the risk for infection and disease. Infection then combines with undernutrition to compromise further the health of impoverished people. Finally, many developing countries are burdened by extremely high external debts, which severely limit their ability to implement programs to reduce undernutrition.

The Impact of AIDS Worldwide

Currently, about 40 million people around the world are infected with the human immunodeficiency virus (HIV) or have gone on to develop AIDS from the infection. The male to female ratio is about 1:1, but the disease is now increasing faster in women than men.[20] About 20 million people worldwide have died from AIDS.

An individual can be infected with HIV through contact with bodily fluids including blood, semen, vaginal secretions, and human milk. Thus the virus can be transmitted through sexual contact, through blood-to-blood contact, and from a mother to an infant during pregnancy, delivery, or breastfeeding. The virus has a very limited ability to exist outside the body.

Once infected with HIV, the individual is said to be HIV-positive. If untreated, the viral disease progresses over the next few years, and the individual develops symptoms of opportunistic infections such as diarrhea, lung disease, weight loss, and a form of

The face of AIDS is quickly becoming the face of a child. About 500,000 deaths of children in subsharan Africa in 2004 were linked to AIDS. (Compare that to about 300 deaths of children linked to AIDS in developed countries during the same year.)

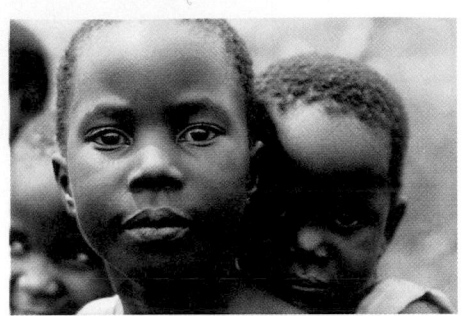

A particularly sad consequence of AIDS in Africa is the number of AIDS orphans, children whose parents have both died of AIDS. The United Nations has estimated that there will be 20 million AIDS orphans in Africa by the year 2010.

Can eating a balanced diet prevent AIDS? The answer, unfortunately, is no. Healthy eating does not cure the disease, but it can help to lessen the impact of infections associated with AIDS. Poor nutritional status, such as for vitamin A and vitamin E, contributes to a quicker onset of symptoms such as body wasting and fever and to a more rapid demise. In fact, daily use of a multivitamin and mineral supplement has been shown in some studies to reduce disease progression in people with HIV infections and AIDS.[10] Overall maintenance of nutritional status should be an integral part of the treatment for AIDS.[3]

cancer. Once individuals have developed these symptoms, they are said to have AIDS. Without treatment, an individual will likely die from AIDS within 4 to 5 years.

In Africa, particularly sub-Saharan countries, HIV is rampant throughout the entire population, both men and women. This region contains nearly 70% of the world's HIV-positive people. In most areas of sub-Saharan Africa, AIDS is reducing life expectancy by one-half, especially if the person also has tuberculosis. Note also that in 2004 about 500,000 deaths of children in sub-Saharan Africa were linked to AIDS. (Compare that to about 300 deaths of children linked to AIDS in developed countries in the same year.) In many countries, AIDS is also creating orphans, an estimated 3.7 million worldwide (660,000 in South Africa alone).

North America also has an AIDS problem. In the United States alone, it is estimated that about 1 million people (1 in every 280 persons) are infected with HIV, many of whom are unaware of their infections. (Recent reports show 1 in every 100 persons in New York City is infected with HIV.) About 450,000 people in the United States have died from the disease since it surfaced in the early 1980s, and each year about 50,000 new cases are reported. HIV affects a greater percentage of minority populations in the United States.

Although no vaccine is available to prevent AIDS, the latest antiviral drugs can significantly slow the progression of the disease. However, there are many barriers to the use of these drugs in the developing world. For example, the newest therapies require a person to take at least three different drugs in the form of about 14 pills each day. Just a few missed doses can significantly reduce the effectiveness of the drugs and result in faster disease progression. Another barrier is economic: a typical drug regimen can cost approximately $14,000 per year, not including unforeseen hospital stays. Certain drug companies and governments are working to lower the cost of AIDS drugs for developing nations, or even provide them at no cost. Still, in many cases, the drugs remain out of reach to the people who need them. It has been suggested that developed nations should step in and cover most or all of the costs. The United Nations is spearheading an effort to raise the $8 to $10 billion needed to fight the disease.

The main goal for addressing the problem of AIDS in the developing world is prevention of new cases through education regarding safer sex and the importance of clean needles, and through other behavior-linked approaches. Providing AIDS drugs to pregnant women is also important. If a woman begins taking AIDS drugs such as zidovudine (AZT) by the fourteenth week of pregnancy, the risk of transferring the virus to her offspring is greatly reduced. Providing the drug immediately before birth also helps.

The devastating effects of AIDS on our civilization have been very rapid when measured by earth's scale of time. And the true costs to society—other than the cost of human lives—have yet to emerge.[19] The very nature of the disease is likely to inflict significant human devastation worldwide, partly because its primary route of transmission—sexual activity—is basic human behavior. A recent study warns us that 57 countries risk major HIV outbreaks. Reported HIV cases are increasing rapidly in Africa, the Indian subcontinent, Southeast Asia, China, the Caribbean, Russia, and much of Eastern Europe.

Behind the mind-boggling statistics on AIDS are less obvious costs to businesses, families, schools and universities, and society in general. For example, worker productivity will plummet because AIDS victims produce less and demand more, especially in the latter stages of the disease. Business productivity drops even further when relatives take time away from work and school to care for family members afflicted with AIDS. Furthermore, AIDS demands a considerable amount of family income. Hard-pressed families, who have to devote much of their income to doctors and medicines, have little left for living expenses. Other family members must struggle to keep up with daily duties because they must care for orphans left behind in the disease's wake. To learn more about AIDS, check out the website www.unaids.org.

Concept | Check

Currently, about 40 million people around the world are infected with the human immunodeficiency virus (HIV) or have gone on to develop acquired immunodeficiency syndrome (AIDS) from the infection. The virus can be transmitted through sexual contact, through blood-to-blood contact, or from a mother to a baby during pregnancy, delivery, and breastfeeding. Without treatment, an individual once infected will likely die from AIDS within 4 to 5 years. The main hope for currently addressing the problem of AIDS in the developing world is prevention of new cases.

Reducing Undernutrition in the Developing World

As you have probably guessed, greatly reducing undernutrition in the developing world will be complicated and will take considerable time to accomplish (Figure 20-5). Today, it is a common practice for the more affluent nations to supply famine areas

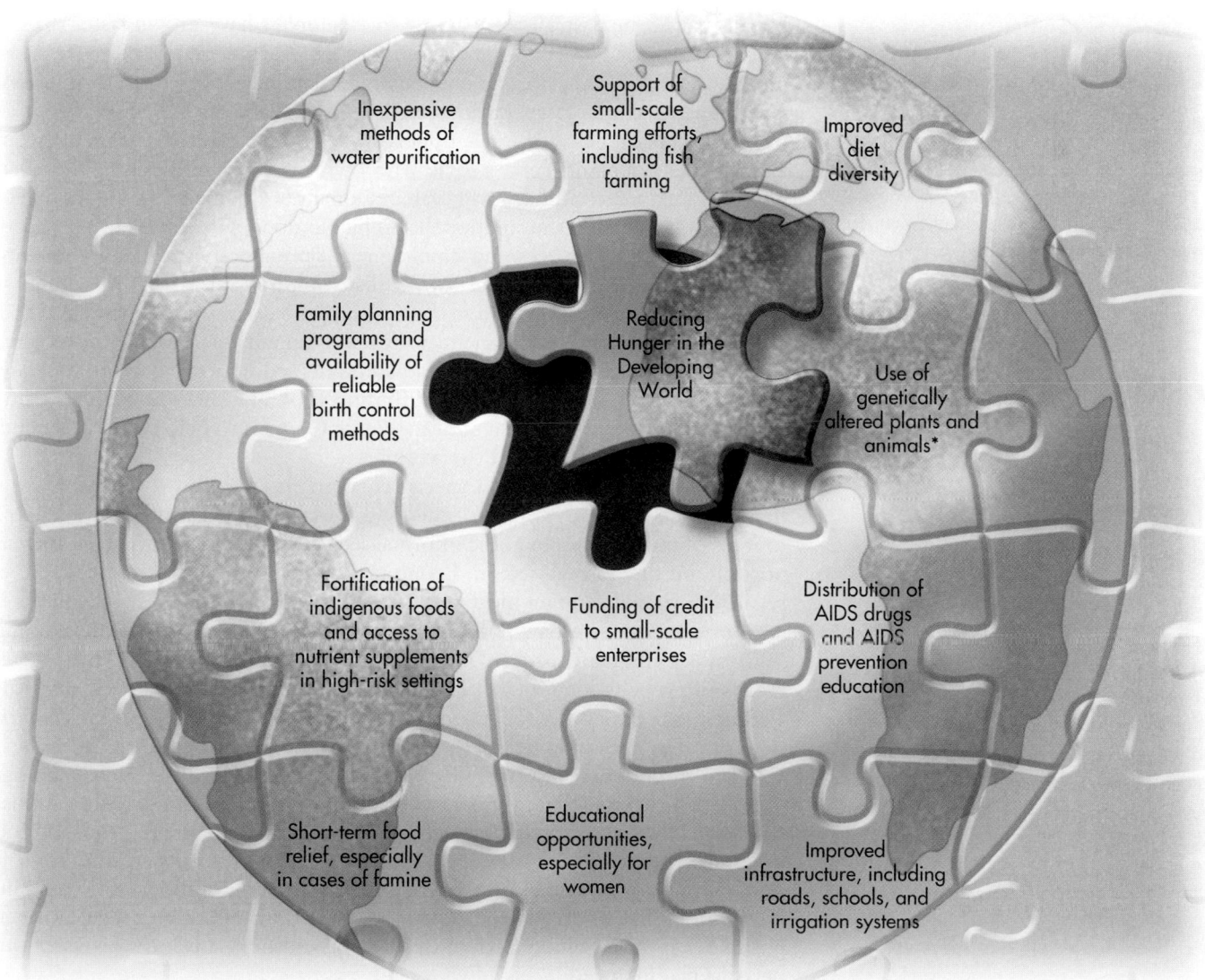

Figure 20-5 | Possible solutions to the puzzle of hunger in the developing world. Putting all the pieces together employs the action steps that contribute to meeting the overall goal. *The Nutrition Focus section in this chapter discusses the genetic alteration of plants and animals in detail.

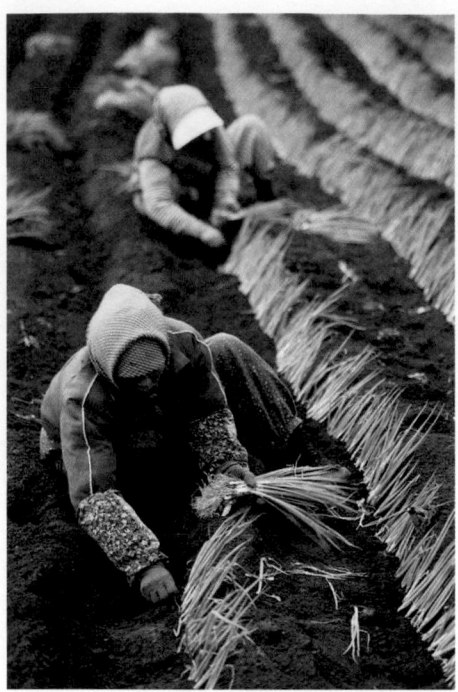

Food security is fostered by communities raising and distributing locally grown food. Dr. Hugo Melgar-Quiñonez and Dr. Ana Claudia Zubieta discuss this further in their Expert Opinion.

Critical | Thinking

Stan has read about various relief efforts to help undernourished people in developing countries, especially the emergency food aid programs for famine-ravaged areas. Many of these efforts appear to be only temporary, and he wonders what long-range approaches might help alleviate the problem of undernutrition. What suggestions would you give Stan about possible long-term solutions for undernutrition in developing countries?

with direct food aid. However, direct food aid is not a long-term solution. Although it reduces the number of deaths from famine, it can also reduce incentives for local production by driving down prices. In addition, the affected countries may have little or no means of transporting the food to the people who need it most, and the donated foods may not be culturally acceptable.

In the short run, there is no choice—aid must be given because people are starving. Still, improving the infrastructure for poor people, especially rural people, needs to be the long-term focus. This future-minded approach is necessary because the most significant factor affecting the undernutrition of people in impoverished areas of the world is their reliance on outside sources for basic needs. Their dependence makes them constantly vulnerable.

Three basic approaches to counteract micronutrient deficiencies are suggested: increase diversity of the food supply; fortify specific foods with nutrients; and provide nutrient supplementation for individuals when necessary.[1,4,10]

Development Tailored to Local Conditions Is Important

Recall that in the past 40 years, world food supplies have grown faster than the population. Thus, the increase in undernutrition during this period has been caused by an increase in the number of people cut off from their share of this supply. Millions of farmers are losing access to resources they need to be self-reliant. There is a growing realization that unless economic opportunities can be created as part of a plan for sustainable development, rural people who own no land will flock to the overcrowded cities. In response, careful, small-scale regional development is one option.

For the most part, the solution lies in helping people meet their own needs and directing them to resources and employment opportunities rather than simply giving them resources. Experience has shown that the provision of credit—along with training, food storage facilities, and marketing support—allows rural people to actively participate in their own development, which will benefit their families and communities.

One U.S. program, the Peace Corps, has helped improve conditions in developing nations by providing education, distributing food and medical supplies, and building structures for local use. The aim of the Peace Corps is to help create independent, self-sustaining economies around the world.

Impoverished women are a special concern. In addition to working longer hours than men do, they grow most of the food for family consumption and make up three-fourths of the labor force in the informal sector of the economy and an increasing proportion in the formal sector. Economic opportunities for women and education regarding family planning must be augmented. Of the 3 billion people in the world living on less than $2 a day, 70% are women. Moreover, among the developing world's 900 million illiterate people, women outnumber men 2 to 1. Thus, an important means of propelling nations out of poverty is to end the cycle of female neglect.

Suitable technologies for processing, preserving, marketing, and distributing nutritious local staples also need to be encouraged, so that small farmers can flourish. Education on how to use these foods to create healthful diets, such as preparing vitamin A–rich vegetables, adds further benefit. Supplementing indigenous foods with nutrients that are in short supply, such as iron, various B vitamins, zinc, and iodide, also deserves consideration. One current program involves adding iron to sugar in various parts of the world. The Nutrition Focus section examines the role of biotechnology in improving nutrient quality and other plant and animal characteristics, another possible positive step in lessening undernutrition. In addition, advances in water purification need to be employed.

Promoting extensive land ownership may also be one part of the solution. Increasing the availability of food is one of its many advantages. If food resources are concentrated among a minority of people, as often happens with unequal land ownership, food is not likely to be equally distributed unless efficient transportation systems are in place. Inequitable distribution then proves to be a very difficult problem to resolve.

Raising the economic status of impoverished people by employing them is as important as expanding the food supply. If an increase in food supply is achieved without an accompanying rise in employment, there may be no long-term change in the number of undernourished people. Although food prices may fall with increased mechanization, use of fertilizers, and other modern technologies, it needs to be realized that these advances can also displace people from jobs, a result that worsens rather than helps the population.

Some Concluding Thoughts

Today, the economic loss from undernutrition is staggering, and the amount of human pain and suffering is incalculable. With all the international relief efforts and assistance from governments and private organizations combined, we are still failing in our battle against undernutrition.[20]

Life is not necessarily fair, but the aim of civilization should be to make it more so. The world has both enough food and the technical expertise to end hunger. What is lacking is the concerted political will to do so.

Ultimately, the depletion of world resources, the massive debt incurred by poorer countries, and the toll taken in human lives affect the world economy and well-being. The resulting instability can go on to affect the developing world, as has been apparent in recent years.

Concept | Check

Overall, one important solution to undernutrition in the developing world lies in providing sufficient employment so that people can purchase the food their families need. Providing access to land and other food production resources will also counteract undernutrition. Development programs must be sensitive to regional conditions to ensure that the new technologies introduced do not intensify existing problems for the poorest people.

Alleviating Food Insecurity and Hunger

Hugo Melgar-Quiñonez, M.D., Ph.D., and Ana Claudia Zubieta, Ph.D.

Food *security* is defined as access by all people at all times to enough food for an active and healthy life, including the ready availability of nutritionally adequate and safe foods and the ensured ability to acquire acceptable foods in socially acceptable ways. On the other hand, food *insecurity* is defined as the limited or uncertain availability of nutritionally adequate and safe foods and the limited or uncertain ability to acquire acceptable foods in socially acceptable ways. The degree of food insecurity of a given population is associated with

- factors related to "having sufficient food"
- factors that influence the types and diversity of the food supply
- psychological issues, such as anxiety, stress, and conflicts, caused by deprivation and restricted choice of foods
- social and cultural influences concerning the means used for the acquisition of foods
- periodic climatic changes, which can vary in duration
- environmental disasters, such as drought or floods
- political and social instability

Also important are available assets and resources, market dynamics, resource allocation within households, and nutritional and health-care practices that affect the way families and communities guarantee stable access to food. Finally, limited diversity of foods produced, poor postharvest practices, soil infertility, land tenure conflicts, and lack of agricultural knowledge deserve consideration.

Why This Attention to Food Insecurity?

Food insecurity has long been a concern of world leaders, as evidenced by the Universal Declaration of Human Rights: "Everyone has the right to a standard of living adequate for the health and well-being of himself and of his family, including food." At the 1996 World Food Summit, representatives from many different countries reaffirmed "the right of everyone to have access to safe and nutritious food, consistent with the right to adequate food and the fundamental right of everyone to be free from hunger." Nevertheless, the most recent figures on food insecurity and hunger by the United Nations' Food and Agriculture Organization (FAO) estimate that worldwide, more than 850 million people do not have enough to eat. Moreover, in "The State of Food Insecurity in the World," the FAO reports that despite a decrease in the number of hungry people in developing countries during the first half of the 1990s, there was a substantial increase of almost 4 million hungry people per year during the second half of that decade.

Food insecurity is associated with major health problems because of its direct impact on the nutritional status of individuals. Even though food-insecure families may have access to enough food to meet energy requirements, they typically struggle with severe micronutrient deficiencies. This paradox demonstrates the challenge these families face in not only obtaining adequate quantities of food but also foods of high nutritional quality. With iron, for example, which is present in a variety of plant and animal foods, some forms are better absorbed than others (heme versus nonheme iron, respectively) and certain dietary factors can enhance or decrease iron's absorption (ascorbic acid versus phytate, respectively). Zinc is another important micronutrient contained in protein-rich foods such as meat, fish and shellfish, and whole grains. It is possible for zinc deficiency to occur in the absence of overt malnutrition. This deficiency can be observed in populations who have poor quality diets (limited animal protein) or who eat traditional foods that impair zinc bioavailability because of high phytate content (e.g., maize, beans, and rice). Iron and zinc deficiencies are usually associated with depletion of other micronutrients and can lead to multiple severe health problems, such as anemia, growth and cognitive retardation, and impaired immune function. Moreover, micronutrient deficiencies can affect the scholastic performance and productivity of individuals and communities.

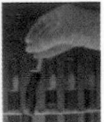

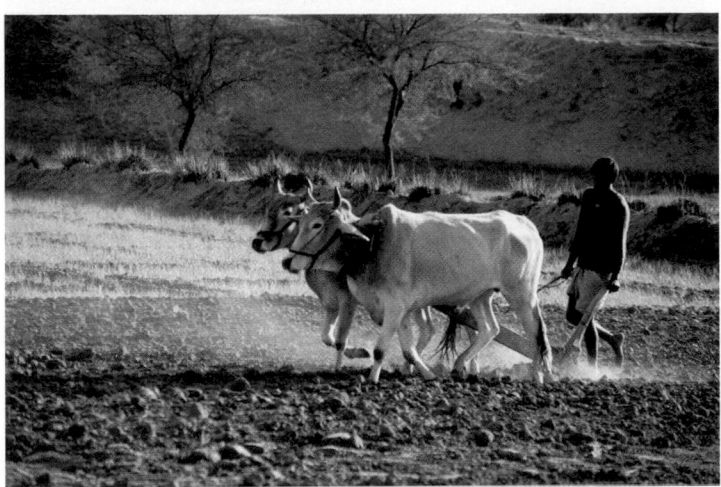

Local production of food is one step in conquering global food insecurity.

Conquering Food Insecurity—What Works?

It is well recognized that the only sustainable approach to decreasing such micronutrient deficiencies are food-based strategies that include the diversification of food production at the household level, promotion of a micronutrient-rich food intake, and development of local techniques for food fortification with one or more nutrients. Community-implemented food-based strategies are also seen as a sustainable approach to decreasing food insecurity. In contrast, attempts to improve nutrition status based on supplementation and fortification have been shown to have serious limitations as long-term solutions.

Although it is often stated that food-based interventions must replace supplements in the long run, remarkably little attention has been paid to the development of appropriate, sustainable, and effective programs. However, there are some examples of success in this area, shown in studies conducted in developing countries and indigenous populations in Canada. For example, in rural Kenya, small increases in the availability of animal source foods have shown to enhance the intake of essential micronutrients, with a related improvement in nutritional status and cognitive development of schoolchildren. In addition, sound policies and higher investments targeting key areas such as access to markets, agricultural productivity, water management, infrastructure, and communication can strengthen food security and reduce malnutrition across the developing world.

Given the complex causes of food insecurity, it is essential that researchers and policymakers incorporate local perceptions, attitudes, and expertise in their research and program design. This practice will positively affect the accuracy of the data gathered as well as the outcome of interventions. Community participation is now considered to be the key to successful community development programs. Consequently, in recent years many international development projects have begun to include more active community involvement in problem identification and project planning. Participatory approaches emphasize the need to modify the practices and attitudes of outside experts and extension workers toward the communities they serve so that better dialogue is established between external agencies and the local people. This approach would also provide a strong foundation for empowering communities to assume greater roles in developing and implementing future interventions.

Dr. Melgar-Quiñonez is Assistant Professor in the Department of Human Nutrition at The Ohio State University. He received his medical and doctoral degrees from the Friedrich Schiller University, Jena, Germany. He and his research group have conducted research in food security with Latino immigrant families in the United States as well as in rural and urban areas in several Latin American countries (Bolivia, Brazil, Colombia, Ecuador, Guatemala, and Mexico), Africa (Burkina Faso and Ghana), and Asia (Philippines). Dr. Zubieta is a postdoctoral research associate in the Department of Human Nutrition at The Ohio State University. She received her Ph.D. degree in nutrition from the University of California, Davis. She has participated in several community nutrition studies in Latin America and in other developing countries (Bolivia, Botswana, Ecuador, Guatemala, Kenya, and Mexico).

NUTRITION FOCUS

The Role of Biotechnology in Expanding Worldwide Food Availability

biotechnology A collection of processes that involve the use of biological systems for altering and, ideally, improving the characteristics of plants, animals, and other forms of life.

The American Dietetic Association recently supported the use of biotechnology for combating undernutrition worldwide (*Journal of the American Dietetic Association* 106: 285, 2006).

genetic engineering Manipulation of the genetic makeup of any organism with recombinant DNA technology.

recombinant DNA technology A test tube technology that rearranges DNA sequences in an organism by cutting the DNA, adding or deleting a DNA sequence, and rejoining DNA molecules with a series of enzymes.

genetically modified organism (GMO) Any organism created by genetic engineering.

transgenic Organism that contains genes originally present in another organism.

The ability of humans to manipulate nature has enabled us to improve the production and yield of many important foods. Traditional **biotechnology** is almost as old as agriculture. The first farmer to improve his stock by selectively breeding the best bull with the best cows was implementing biotechnology in a simple sense. The first baker to use yeast to make bread rise took advantage of biotechnology.

By the 1930s, biotechnology made possible the selective breeding of better plant hybrids. As a result, corn production in the United States quickly doubled. Through similar methods, agricultural wheat was crossed with wild grasses to confer more desirable properties, such as greater yield, increased resistance to mildew and bacterial diseases, and tolerance to salt or adverse climatic conditions.

Another type of biotechnology uses hormones rather than breeding. In the last decade, Canadian salmon have been treated with a hormone that allows them to mature three times faster than normal—without changing the fish in any other way. In general terms, biotechnology can be understood as the use of living things—plants, animals, bacteria—to manufacture products.

The New Biotechnology

The new biotechnology used in agriculture includes several methods that directly modify products. It differs from traditional methods because it more directly changes some of the genetic material (DNA) of organisms to improve characteristics.[9] Crossbreeding plants or animals is no longer the only tool. Development of the new process, called **genetic engineering,** began in the 1970s. The field now features a wide range of cell and subcell techniques for the synthesis and placement of genetic material in organisms (Figure 20-6). This process of **recombinant DNA technology** allows access to a wider gene pool, and it permits faster and more accurate production of new and more useful microbial, plant, and animal species. Conventional breeding is inefficient and has inconsistent results; biotechnology utilizes genetic material more precisely. Scientists select the traits they want and genetically engineer or introduce the gene that produces the desired trait into plants or animals

(now called a **genetically modified organism [GMO]** or **transgenic**). It is important to note, however, that the genetic engineering does not replace conventional breeding practices; both work together.

Already, genetic engineering of agricultural products has allowed us to make use of new types of seeds, growth hormones, and microbial inoculants to stop pests and frost damage. Biotechnology is also used to develop drought-tolerant crops as well as to detect *Listeria* and other microorganisms that cause foodborne illness. Scientists are engineering plants that grow with the use of fewer pesticides, and new forms of potatoes that can be stored longer without preservatives. In addition, biotechnology can allow scientists to create fruits and grains with greater amounts of nutrients such as beta-carotene (e.g., "golden rice") and vitamins E and C. Researchers are also examining ways to modify the fatty-acid makeup of vegetable oils. Because biotechnology is being used cautiously and conservatively, these early benefits of the new biotechnology will strike us as only subtly different. The ultimate benefits, however, could be important if foods eaten by people in the developing world can be so enhanced.

Few consumers in the United States realize that currently about 40% of all corn and 90% of all soybeans produced in the United States have been genetically engineered to resist certain insects, thereby reducing pesticide use, and/or survive when sprayed with herbicides that kill surrounding weeds. Some papaya plants have been genetically engineered for viral resistance.

Genetic modification of corn has received a lot of media attention. Corn can be genetically altered by inserting a gene from the bacterium *Bacillus thuringiensis,* usually referred to as the Bt gene, into the corn DNA. The gene allows the corn plant to make a protein that is lethal to certain caterpillars that destroy the plant. The Bt protein in the corn, however, is present in the plant in very low concentrations and has no effect on humans—it is digested along with the other proteins in corn. For many years organic farmers have used the Bt bacteria as a dust on plants in order to destroy pests. (Dusting crops, however, does not change the DNA of the plant.)

FDA is confident that currently approved varieties of genetically engineered foods are safe to

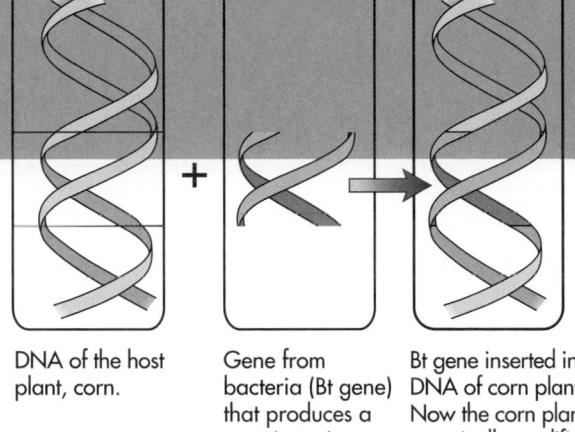

DNA of the host plant, corn.

Gene from bacteria (Bt gene) that produces a protein toxic to the European corn borer.

Bt gene inserted into DNA of corn plant. Now the corn plant is genetically modified. It makes the Bt toxin and, so, is resistant to the European corn borer.

Figure 20-6 | Biotechnology involves various techniques for transferring foreign DNA into an organism. In this diagram, a sample of DNA is cleaved out of a larger DNA fragment and inserted into the DNA of a host cell. Thus, the host cell contains new genetic information, with the potential of providing the cell with new capabilities. For corn, this could mean resistance to the European corn borer. The corn plant is now referred to as a genetically modified organism (GMO). In another application, bacteria can be engineered to produce the human form of the hormone insulin.

consume. A controversy arose over use of StarLink corn in 2000. In this case, the GMO corn variety was approved for animal feed but not human consumption, yet it found its way into some corn products, such as taco shells. Food manufacturers are not currently required to disclose the GMO content on food labels. Some manufacturers, however, have promoted their products as being "GMO-free" on labels. A recent study showed that even these foods typically have GMO content. In fact, 70% of processed foods contain at least one GMO ingredient.[14] So it is not surprising that when Gerber Products Co. tried to introduce a line of GMO-free baby foods, they found that they could not produce products from raw materials currently available.

FDA does not believe that labeling of GMO products is needed because the products pose no health risk. Public response to use of GMO biotechnology, nevertheless, has been mixed. Even the scientific community has conflicting opinions about this technology, with supporters as convinced about the benefits as opponents are of the risks. The biggest debate in the United States surrounds the potential environmental hazards of introducing genes from one species to another. Some challengers even question the actual reduction in pesticide use that accompanies the cultivation of GMO crops. Although the use of GMOs may reduce the need for environmentally harmful activities, such as spraying crops with pesticides, critics point out that seeds produced with additional insecticide potential will lead to rapid insect resistance because the insecticides are continuously emitted. Use of traditional pesticides involves prudent application, in part to avoid insect resistance. In addition, accidental release of genetically modified animals, such as fish, may go on to harm wild varieties.

Although the risks of biotechnology may appear to be momentarily negligible, they may be cumulative and therefore of concern in the long run. In addition, will allergens, such as those found in peanuts, eggs, milk, wheat, and shellfish, be added to genetically engineered foods that previously did not contain them? Evidence of this contamination has been seen in soybeans. Note, however, that FDA carefully examines all products developed with this technology and will enforce labeling of potential allergens that may be newly present in food altered by biotechnology.

The public has long been opposed to processes perceived as harmful to the environment, such as producing unnatural products. Because food reserves are high in the United States, Canada, and Europe, some people question the need to increase food production. Skepticism surrounds unnatural products, as exemplified by Western Europe's ban of hormones used in beef and milk production and of nearly all GMO foods. Some North Americans support this stance. Citizens believe the increase in the food supply is not worth the risks.

Role of the New Biotechnology in the Developing World

Whether applications of genetic engineering will help to significantly reduce undernutrition in the developing world remains to be seen. Unless price cuts accompany the increased production, only landowners and suppliers of biotechnology will enjoy the benefits. Small farmers may benefit if they can afford to purchase the GMO seeds. This point deserves emphasis: the person who cannot afford to buy enough food today will still face that same predicament in the future.

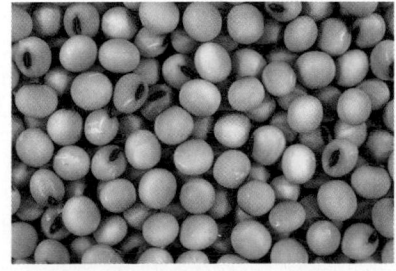

Both traditional plant breeding and biotechnology have produced high-yielding and disease-resistant plant varieties, such as with corn.

Soybeans are a common GMO food in the marketplace (80% of the total).

As with most innovations, the more successful farmers—often those with large farms—will adopt the new biotechnology first. Therefore, the present trend toward fewer and larger farms will continue in the developing world, a movement that undermines the solution to one of the most pressing undernutrition issues there. Furthermore, biotechnology does not promise dramatic increases in the production of most grains and cassava, the primary food resources in developing parts of the world.

With the introduction of drought- and pest-resistant as well as self-fertilizing crops, agricultural biotechnology may help to lessen world hunger. Perhaps the most promising potential of genetically modified foods today lies within the realm of plant breeding for micronutrients. Developing countries will then have a tool to treat and prevent selected nutrient deficiencies among their populations if they have access to farming resources to augment the micronutrient composition of crops.[9] In addition, greater yields for indigenous plants, such as tomatoes that tolerate high soil salinity, are another hopeful outcome. Biotechnology will likely be a useful tool against the complex scourge of world undernutrition. Improved crops produced by this technology, together with political and other efforts, can contribute to the battle of worldwide undernutrition.

Critical | Thinking

Bobbie is in a debate class and has been assigned to argue the biotechnologist's side of genetic engineering. Help her come up with a list of arguments in favor of biotechnology. What would the list look like if Bobbie were on the opposing side?

Summary

1. Poverty is commonly linked to chronic or periodic undernutrition. Malnutrition can occur when the food supply is either scarce or abundant. The resulting deficiency conditions and degenerative diseases contribute to poor health.

2. Undernutrition is the most common form of malnutrition in developing countries. It results from inadequate intake, absorption, or use of nutrients or food energy. Many deficiency conditions consequently appear, and infectious diseases thrive because the immune system cannot function properly.

3. The greatest risk of undernutrition occurs during critical periods of growth and development: gestation, infancy, and childhood. Low birth weight is a leading cause of infant deaths worldwide. Many developmental problems are caused by nutritional deprivation during critical periods of brain growth. People in their later years are also at great risk.

4. Undernutrition diminishes both physical and mental capabilities. In poor countries, this situation is worsened by recurrent infections, unsanitary conditions, extreme weather, inadequate shelter, and exposure to diseases.

5. In North America, famine is not seen but food insecurity and undernutrition remain problems. Soup kitchens, food stamps, the school lunch and breakfast programs, and the Special Supplemental Nutrition Program for Women, Infants, and Children (WIC) have focused on improving the nutritional health of poor and at-risk people. When adequately funded, these programs have proved effective in reducing undernutrition. The need to reduce out-of-wedlock pregnancies remains a national priority because single parents and their children are much more likely to live in poverty.

6. Multiple factors contribute to the problem of undernutrition in the developing world. In densely populated countries, food resources, as well as the means for distributing food, may be inadequate. Farming methods often encourage erosion, which deprives the soil of valuable nutrients and thereby hampers future efforts to grow food. Limited water availability hinders food production. Naturally occurring devastation from droughts, excessive rainfall, fire, crop infestation, and human causes—such as urbanization, war and civil unrest, debt, poor sanitation, and AIDS—all contribute to the major problem of undernutrition.

7. Proposed solutions to world undernutrition must consider multiple interacting factors, many of which are thoroughly embedded in cultural traditions. Family planning efforts, for example, may not succeed until life expectancy increases. Through education, efforts should be made to upgrade farming methods, improve crops, limit pregnancies, encourage breastfeeding when it is safe to do so, and improve sanitation and hygiene.

8. Direct food aid is only a short-term solution. In what may appear to be a step backward, many experts recommend more sustainable subsistence-level farming. Small-scale industrial development is another way to create meaningful employment and purchasing power for vast numbers of the rural poor. Various biotechnology applications may also prove beneficial.

Study Questions

1. Describe the difference between malnutrition and undernutrition.
2. Describe in a short paragraph any evidence of undernutrition that you saw while you were growing up, such as on television. What are/were the likely roots of these problems?
3. What do you believe are the major factors contributing to undernutrition in wealthy nations such as the United States? What are some solutions to this problem?
4. What three points would you make to a group of seventh-grade girls concerning the economic perils of teen pregnancy and parenting?
5. Personal responsibility is a common theme in political circles. How does it relate to the problem of undernutrition in the United States? Does it apply to all causes of the problem?
6. Outline how war and civil unrest in developing countries have worsened problems of chronic hunger over the past few years.
7. How important is population control in addressing the problem of world hunger now and in the future? Support your answer with three main points.
8. Why is solving the problem of undernutrition a key factor in the development of the full potential of developing countries?
9. Discuss how infrastructure could influence the causes and solutions of chronic hunger in a developing nation.
10. Name three nutrients that are often lacking in the diets of undernourished people. What effects can be expected with each deficiency?

BOOST YOUR STUDY

Check out the **Perspectives in Nutrition: Online Learning Center** www.mhhe.com/wardlawpers7 for quizzes, flash cards, activities, and web links designed to further help you learn about issues surrounding world hunger.

Annotated References

1. ADA Reports: Position of the American Dietetic Association: Assessing world hunger, malnutrition, and food security. *Journal of the American Dietetic Association* 103:1046, 2003.

   It is the position of the American Dietetic Association that access to adequate amounts of safe, nutritious, and culturally appropriate foods is a fundamental human right. It is important to encourage programs and practices that combat hunger and malnutrition, increase food security, promote self-sufficiency, and are environmentally and economically sustainable.

2. ADA Reports: Position of the American Dietetic Association: Child and adolescent food and nutrition programs. *Journal of the American Dietetic Association* 103:887, 2003.

   The current food programs targeted at low-income households, such as the Food Stamp Program, have gone a long way to increasing the nutrient intake of children and adolescents. It is important that these food programs are supported by adequate funding.

3. ADA Reports: Position of the American Dietetic Association and Dietitians of Canada: Nutrition intervention in the care of persons with human immunodeficiency virus infection. *Journal of the American Dietetic Association* 104:1425, 2004.

   Meeting nutrient needs is very important to maintain the best health possible in people with HIV infections and AIDS.

4. Ash DM and others: Randomized efficacy trial of a micronutrient-fortified beverage in primary school children in Tanzania. *American Journal of Clinical Nutrition* 77:891, 2003.

   Fortifying beverages with micronutrients is one strategy to help reduce micronutrient deficien-
cies in developing countries. Such practices have been shown to reduce the risk of nutrient deficiencies. (Other recent studies also support the efficacy of this practice: Journal of Nutrition 133:1834, 2003, and Journal of Nutrition 133:1339, 2003.)

5. Black RE and others: Why are 10 million children dying each year? *The Lancet* 361:2226, 2003.

   More than 10 million children die each year, mostly from preventable causes. Undernutrition is the underlying cause of a substantial portion of these childhood deaths.

6. Brown KH: Diarrhea and malnutrition. *Journal of Nutrition* 133:328S, 2003.

   Undernutrition increases the risk of severe diarrheal disease. Prevention strategies include promotion of breastfeeding to prevent diarrheal disease, continued feeding during illness, and supplementation with selected micronutrients to prevent infections and reduce their severity.

7. Darton-Hill I and others: Micronutrient deficiencies and gender: Social and economic costs. *American Journal of Clinical Nutrition* 81:1198S, 2005.

   Micronutrient deficiencies in developing countries, such as for vitamin A, iodide, iron, and zinc, lead to health problems, especially in females. Addressing these micronutrient deficiencies is important in order to improve economic status at the personal, community, and national level in developing countries.

8. Davies PW: Historical perspective from the green revolution to the gene revolution. *Nutrition Reviews* 61(6):S124, 2003.

   Improved strains of plants can be achieved through traditional plant breeding and direct
genetic manipulation. Greater application of both technologies is needed to attain the full benefits with regard to an increase in food production.

9. Dunford M: The GM food debate. *Today's Dietitian*, p. 12, June 2004.

   The genetic engineering of foods has both risks and benefits, and both are described in this article.

10. Fawzi W and others: Studies of vitamins and minerals and HIV transmission and disease progression. *Journal of Nutrition* 135:938, 2005.

    Daily use of a multivitamin and mineral supplement has been shown to be helpful in a few studies and may be especially helpful to reduce disease progression, because nutrient deficiencies are common in people with HIV infections and AIDS.

11. Grandesso F and others: Mortality and malnutrition among populations living in South Darfur, Sudan. *Journal of the American Medical Association* 293:1490, 2005.

    The recent conflicts in the Darfur region of Sudan have led to high rates of death and undernutrition among people displaced by war. This article describes what has been seen numerous times in the last 50 years—undernutrition and related death is a typical casualty of war.

12. Hoetz, PJ and others: Hookworm infection. *The New England Journal of Medicine* 351:799, 2004.

    An estimated 740 million cases of hookworm infections exist in the world, primarily in the tropics and subtropics. Excellent medications are available to treat the disease and should be made widely available.

13. Kalm LM, Semba RD: They starved so that others be better fed: Remembering Ancel Keys

and the Minnesota experiment. *Journal of Nutrition* 135:1347, 2005.

Detailed and interesting account of the semi-starvation studies conducted in the 1940s by Ancel Keys and colleagues. These experiments were conducted to better understand the effects of semistarvation that many peoples in World War II were experiencing and to determine how best to safely refeed semistarved individuals.

14. Palmer S: GE foods under the microscope. *Today's Dietitian*, p. 34, May 2005.

About 70% of all processed foods sold in the United States contain substances that have undergone some genetic alteration. This article explores some of the benefits and concerns regarding the use of this fairly recent technology in our food supply.

15. Pauly D, Watson R: Counting the last fish. *Scientific American*, p. 43, July 2003.

Overfishing has led to declines in certain fish populations worldwide. Better management of fish harvest is needed to prevent further aggravations.

16. Pelletier DL, Frongillo EA: Changes in child survival are strongly associated with changes in malnutrition in developing countries. *Journal of Nutrition* 133:107, 2003.

Considerable evidence suggests that undernutrition affects human performance, overall health and survival, physical growth, cognitive development, reproduction, physical work capacity, and risks for many chronic diseases. Efforts to reduce undernutrition worldwide are important if we are to reduce overall mortality.

17. Perkins S: Crisis on tap? Pollution and burgeoning populations stress Earth's water resources. *Science News* 162:42, 2002 (July).

Approximately one-third of the world's population lives in areas of water scarcity. Included in this estimate are 450 million people who live in areas of severe water stress.

18. Scrimshaw NS: Historical concepts of interactions, synergism, and antagonism between nutrition and infection. *Journal of Nutrition* 133:316S, 2003.

Maintaining nutritional health is important for proper functioning of the immune system, thereby reducing the risk of infectious diseases.

19. Steinbrook R: After Bangkok—Expanding the global response to AIDS. *The New England Journal of Medicine* 351:738, 2004.

The advances in treatment of AIDS have largely benefited developed countries. There is an urgent need to provide the benefits to people infected with AIDS in the developing world.

20. Yach D and others: The global burden of chronic diseases: Overcoming impediments to prevention and control. *Journal of the American Medical Association* 291:2616, 2004.

Nutrient deficiencies are common in the developing world. Such areas also experience the greatest burden of deaths from diarrhea, HIV and AIDS, and various childhood diseases. There needs be more attention to this enormous problem in the developing world.

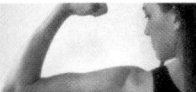 **Take** | Action

I. Fighting World Undernutrition on a Personal Level

If you want to do something about world and domestic undernutrition, consider the following activities. It is a noble act to try to make a difference, even if you make just one small step. As with any change in behavior, do not try to do too many things at once. Try one or two activities that represent your commitment to solving this problem.

1. Volunteer at a local soup kitchen or homeless shelter for a period of time (1 month, for example). What insights could you gain?

2. Coordinate the efforts of a campus organization to donate some money to a voluntary agency that does antihunger work, such as the following:

Bread for the World
50 F Street, NW, Suite 500
Washington, DC 20001

Oxfam America
PO Box 1211
Albert Lea, MN 56007-1211

Save the Children Foundation
54 Wilton Rd
Westport, CT 06880

CARE
650 First Ave.
New York, NY 10016

Second Harvest
35 E Wacker Dr. #2000
Chicago, IL 60601

3. Make a contribution of nonperishable foods to the ongoing offering at a place of worship near you. If such an offering does not exist, start one.

4. Get on a food recovery program's mailing list, and read its newsletters for information on upcoming fund-raisers and other activities; become involved.

5. Participate in food drives organized by local grocery stores by contributing food or services. Food-drive organizers may need volunteers to transport the donations from the store to a food pantry. Pay special attention to events around World Food Day, October 16.

II. Joining the Battle against Undernutrition

Imagine that you recently spent your summer vacation in a developing country and saw evidence of undernutrition and hunger. Then imagine that you are now asking a large corporation to support your efforts to ease hunger and suffering in this area. Develop a two-paragraph statement outlining why it is important to address hunger issues in this area. Include how you think a large corporation could assist you in your efforts.

appendix A

CHEMISTRY: A TOOL FOR UNDERSTANDING NUTRITION

You have already completed at least one basic high school and/or college course in chemistry; consequently, this appendix serves only to review key chemistry principles that arise in the study of nutrition. The study of human nutrition requires a basic awareness of and familiarity with general chemistry, organic chemistry, and biochemistry. This appendix provides fundamental concepts regarding atoms, molecules, chemical bonds, pH, organic compounds, and biochemical structures. An understanding of basic chemistry may make the study of nutrition easier and more interesting. It helps connect nutrient characteristics with the structural and chemical attributes of the individual components of food (Table A-1).

One concept to keep in mind is that the physical and chemical properties of almost anything—whether atoms, molecules, or organisms—are intimately related to its structure. A basic knowledge of chemical structures can help you visualize important fundamental concepts in nutrition.

Properties of Matter and Mass

All living and nonliving things are composed of matter. Matter exists in three states: solid, liquid, or gas. An example of a solid is ice, a liquid is water, and a gas is steam. Two characteristics of matter are (1) it has mass and (2) it occupies space (volume). Mass is related to the amount of force it takes to move an object—it takes less force to move a paper clip than a pencil; therefore, the clip has less mass. Volume is related to the amount of space an object occupies—a pint of water occupies less space than a gallon; therefore, a pint has a smaller volume. Both these properties depend on how much of the substance there is.

Another property of matter is density. Density is defined as the mass of an object divided by its volume:

$$\text{Density} = \frac{\text{Mass}}{\text{Volume}}$$

Density is independent of how much matter is available. The density of water in a lake is the same as in a cup. Density is commonly expressed in units of grams per cubic centimeter (g/cm^3). Table A-2 lists the densities of several common substances.

You can use density to compare objects. Using the density of pure water as a comparison ($1.0\ g/cm^3$), lean body tissue has a density of about $1.1\ g/cm^3$. The density of body fat in comparison is about $0.9\ g/cm^3$. Substances that are less dense than water are buoyant (they tend to float), whereas substances that are more dense than water sink. The next time you are at the swimming pool, note the density of men and women. Women tend to have more body fat, so they float; men are generally more muscular (have more lean tissue), so they tend to sink deeper in the water. This physical property is used to determine the amount of body fat stored in a person (see Chapter 13).

Table A-1 | Periodic Table of the Elements

Key:
- Atomic Number
- Symbol
- Atomic Mass (Atomic Weight)

Example: 1 / H / 1.00794

Main-Group Elements · Transitional Metals · Inner-transitional Metals

Period	1 IA	2 IIA	3 IIIB	4 IVB	5 VB	6 VIB	7 VIIB	8 VIIIB	9 VIIIB	10 VIIIB	11 IB	12 IIB	13 IIIA	14 IVA	15 VA	16 VIA	17 VIIA	18 VIIIA
1	1 H 1.00794																	2 He 4.002602
2	3 Li 6.941	4 Be 9.012182											5 B 10.811	6 C 12.011	7 N 14.00674	8 O 15.9994	9 F 18.998403	10 Ne 20.1797
3	11 Na 22.989768	12 Mg 24.3050											13 Al 26.981539	14 Si 28.0855	15 P 30.973762	16 S 32.066	17 Cl 35.4527	18 Ar 39.948
4	19 K 39.0983	20 Ca 40.078	21 Sc 44.955910	22 Ti 47.88	23 V 50.9415	24 Cr 51.9961	25 Mn 54.93805	26 Fe 55.847	27 Co 58.93320	28 Ni 58.69	29 Cu 63.546	30 Zn 65.39	31 Ga 69.723	32 Ge 72.61	33 As 74.92159	34 Se 78.96	35 Br 79.904	36 Kr 83.80
5	37 Rb 85.4678	38 Sr 87.62	39 Y 88.90585	40 Zr 91.224	41 Nb 92.90638	42 Mo 95.94	43 Tc (98)	44 Ru 101.07	45 Rh 102.90550	46 Pd 106.42	47 Ag 107.8682	48 Cd 112.411	49 In 114.82	50 Sn 118.710	51 Sb 121.75	52 Te 127.60	53 I 126.90447	54 Xe 131.29
6	55 Cs 132.90543	56 Ba 137.327	57 La* 138.9055	72 Hf 178.49	73 Ta 180.9479	74 W 183.85	75 Re 186.207	76 Os 190.2	77 Ir 192.22	78 Pt 195.08	79 Au 196.96654	80 Hg 200.59	81 Tl 204.3833	82 Pb 207.2	83 Bi 208.98037	84 Po (209)	85 At (210)	86 Rn (222)
7	87 Fr (223)	88 Ra (226)	89 Ac** (227)	104 Rf (261)	105 Db (262)	106 Sg (263)	107 Bh (262)	108 Hs (265)	109 Mt (267)	110 xxx (269)	111 xxx (272)	112 xxx (277)						

*Lanthanides

58 Ce 140.115	59 Pr 140.90765	60 Nd 144.24	61 Pm (145)	62 Sm 150.36	63 Eu 151.965	64 Gd 157.25	65 Tb 158.92534	66 Dy 162.50	67 Ho 164.93032	68 Er 167.266	69 Tm 168.93421	70 Yb 173.04	71 Lu 174.967

**Actinides

90 Th 232.0381	91 Pa (231)	92 U 238.0289	93 Np (237)	94 Pu (244)	95 Am (243)	96 Cm (247)	97 Bk (247)	98 Cf (251)	99 Es (252)	100 Fm (257)	101 Md (258)	102 No (259)	103 Lr (262)

Elements 110, 111, 112 have yet to be named.

A-2

Table A-1 concluded

Key to Abbreviations

Name	Symbol	Name	Symbol	Name	Symbol	Name	Symbol
Actinium	Ac	Europium	Eu	Mercury	Hg	Scandium	Sc
Aluminum	Al	Fermium	Fm	Molybdenum	Mo	Seaborgium	Sg
Americium	Am	Fluorine	F	Neodymium	Nd	Selenium	Se
Antimony	Sb	Francium	Fr	Neon	Ne	Silicon	Si
Argon	Ar	Gadolinium	Gd	Neptunium	Np	Silver	Ag
Arsenic	As	Gallium	Ga	Nickel	Ni	Sodium	Na
Astatine	At	Germanium	Ge	Niobium	Nb	Strontium	Sr
Barium	Ba	Gold	Au	Nitrogen	N	Sulfur	S
Berkelium	Bk	Hafnium	Hf	Nobelium	No	Tantalum	Ta
Beryllium	Be	Hahnium	Ha	Osmium	Os	Technetium	Tc
Bismuth	Bi	Hassium	Hs	Oxygen	O	Tellurium	Te
Bohrium	Bh	Helium	He	Palladium	Pd	Terbium	Tb
Boron	B	Holmium	Ho	Phosphorus	P	Thallium	Tl
Bromine	Br	Hydrogen	H	Platinum	Pt	Thorium	Th
Cadmium	Cd	Indium	In	Plutonium	Pu	Thulium	Tm
Calcium	Ca	Iodine	I	Polonium	Po	Tin	Sn
Californium	Cf	Iridium	Ir	Potassium	K	Titanium	Ti
Carbon	C	Iron	Fe	Praseodymium	Pr	Tungsten	W
Cerium	Ce	Krypton	Kr	Promethium	Pm	Uranium	U
Cesium	Cs	Lanthanum	La	Protactinium	Pa	Vanadium	V
Chlorine	Cl	Lawrencium	Lw	Radium	Ra	Xenon	Xe
Chromium	Cr	Lead	Pb	Radon	Rn	Ytterbium	Yb
Cobalt	Co	Lithium	Li	Rhenium	Re	Yttrium	Y
Copper	Cu	Lutetium	Lu	Rhodium	Rh	Zinc	Zn
Curium	Cm	Magnesium	Mg	Rubidium	Rb	Zirconium	Zr
Dubnium	Db	Manganese	Mn	Ruthenium	Ru		
Dysprosium	Dy	Meitnerium	Mt	Rutherfordium	Rf		
Einsteinium	Es	Mendelevium	Md	Samarium	Sm		
Erbium	Er						

Table A-2 | Densities of Some Selected Substances

Example	Density	State
Oxygen	1.31	Gas g/l
Olive oil	0.92	Liquids g/ml (g/cm³)
Water	1.00	
Sucrose	1.59	Solids g/cm³
Salt	2.16	

Physical and Chemical Properties of Substances

Every substance has a characteristic set of physical and chemical properties. Physical properties can be determined without altering the chemical composition of the substance. Ice melts at 1°C. Sugar melts at 186°C. Melting and boiling points are common examples of physical properties.

chemical reaction An interaction between two chemicals that changes both participants.

Chemical properties, such as whether the compound is an acid or a base, determine the changes that a substance undergoes in **chemical reactions.** Other substances affect the chemical properties of a substance. A chemical change or reaction is a process whereby the composition of one or more substances is changed. What actually takes place is affected by the chemical properties of the participants. For example, given the right conditions, exposing glucose to oxygen causes it to break down to carbon dioxide and water.

$$C_6H_{12}O_6 \quad + \quad 6O_2 \quad \rightarrow \quad 6CO_2 \quad + \quad 6H_2O$$

Glucose $\qquad$ Oxygen $\qquad$ Carbon dioxide $\qquad$ Water

Units

The SI units (*Systeme International d'Unités*) used for scientific measurements designate a specific metric unit. The units used most frequently in nutrition are mass (kilogram), length (meter), temperature, and amount of substance. Prefixes indicate decimal fractions or multiples of the various units. For example, *kilo* means 1×10^3 and 1 *milli* is 1×10^{-3}.

Celsius A centigrade measure of temperature. For conversion: (degrees in Fahrenheit − 32) × 5/9 = °C (degrees in Celsius × 9/5) + 32 = °F.

The temperature scale commonly used in scientific studies is the **Celsius** scale. On this scale, water freezes at 0°Celsius (32°Fahrenheit). Water boils at 100°C (212°F). Normal body temperature is 37.0°C (98.6°F). For English-metric conversions for length, weight, temperature, and volume (amount) see Appendix L.

Calories and Joules

Energy is measured in calories or joules. A calorie is the amount of energy required to raise the temperature of 1 gram of water 1 degree C. The SI unit of energy is the joule (J). A mass of 1 g moving at a velocity of 1 m/s possesses the energy equivalent of 1 J. A calorie or joule is not a large amount of energy, so kilocalories (kcal) and kilojoules (kJ) are widely used in nutrition chemistry, biology, and biochemistry. In terms of the joule, 1 kcal = 4.184 kJ.

Scientific Notation

In science, very large and very small numbers frequently must be used, but they are awkward because large numbers have a long string of trailing zeros and small numbers have a long string of leading zeros. A more convenient way to express these numbers is to use the power of 10, or scientific notation.

In scientific notation, a number is expressed as a product of a coefficient multiplied by a power of 10. The coefficient is a number equal to or greater than 1 but less than 10. The power of 10 is the exponent. In other words:

$$a \times 10^b$$

where a is the coefficient and b is the exponent.

$$6.02217 \times 10^{23} = 602,217,000,000,000,000,000,000$$

$$2.99161 \times 10^{-23} = 0.0000000000000000000000299161$$

In the previous examples, the positive exponent for the number indicates that the number is very large, while the negative exponent indicates a very small number.

Atoms

The smallest unit of matter that can undergo a chemical change is called an **atom.** An element is composed of atoms of only one kind. For example, the element carbon is composed of just carbon atoms. There are more than 100 different elements.

Atomic Structure

The center of the atom is for the most part a nucleus containing two (subatomic) particles: **protons,** which carry a positive charge, and **neutrons,** with no charge. Usually the mass of the proton equals the mass of the neutron. Adding the number of protons and neutrons together equals the atomic mass of the atom. An atom of carbon containing 6 protons and 6 neutrons has an atomic mass of 12. The atomic mass of nitrogen is 14 and the atomic mass of oxygen is 16.

The atomic number is equal to the number of protons in the nucleus. What are the atomic numbers of hydrogen, carbon, nitrogen, and oxygen?

Surrounding the nucleus of the atom are negatively charged subatomic particles called **electrons.** The nucleus is actually surrounded by an electron cloud. Electrons have about 2000 times less mass than the mass of protons or neutrons. Thus, all the mass of an atom essentially is located within the nucleus. The structure of an atom can therefore be pictured as a very tiny, highly dense nuclear core surrounded by a cloud of electrons. The number of electrons in an atom equals the number of protons, so the net charge is zero.

Electrons surrounding the nucleus have a somewhat peculiar, nonintuitive (contrary to what would be expected) behavior. For instance, it's impossible to know precisely where any given electron is located at any given moment. It is only possible to define a volume of space where the electron is most likely to be found. This volume has a specific distribution of electron density in space and is called an orbital. An orbital is a volume of space. Each orbital has its own characteristic energy and shape. Different orbitals have different energies.

Orbitals of similar energy are grouped together into energy levels. The energy levels are assigned coordinate numbers—1, 2, 3, etc.—that increase as one moves away from the nucleus. Energy level 1 contains only one orbital, an s orbital. This orbital can hold a maximum of two electrons. Energy level 2 contains an s orbital and a p orbital; the s orbital can contain up to 2 electrons, and the p orbital up to 6. Energy level 3 contains an s orbital, a p orbital and a d orbital. As before, the s orbital and p orbital can hold up to 2 and 6 electrons respectively, while the d orbital can contain as many as 10. Thus each energy level can hold a maximum of 2, 8, 18, or 32 electrons, depending on the number of orbitals, and any energy level can hold less than the maximum number of electrons.

Atoms tend to exist in the lowest possible energy state. Thus electrons tend to occupy orbitals at low energy levels before filling orbitals at higher energy levels. The first

---

To change a number greater than 1 into scientific notation, move the decimal point to the left until the number is greater than 1 but less than 10. This number is the coefficient. The number of places that the decimal is moved becomes the exponent of 10. To change a number less than 1 into scientific notation, move the decimal point to the right until the number is greater than 1 but less than 10. This number is the coefficient. The number of places that the decimal is moved is again the exponent of 10, but this time a negative sign is placed in front of it.

atom Smallest combining unit of an element. An atom contains protons, neutrons, and electrons.

proton The part of an atom that is positively charged.

neutron The part of an atom that has no charge.

electron A part of an atom that is negatively charged. Electrons orbit the nucleus.

Hydrogen has an atomic mass of 1 because it has 1 proton and no neutrons.

Table A-3 | Atoms Commonly Present in Organic Molecules

Atom	Symbol	Atomic Number	Atomic Mass	Energy Level 1	Energy Level 2	Energy Level 3	Number of Chemical Bonds to Attain Electron Stability
Hydrogen	H	1	1	1	0	0	1
Carbon	C	6	12	2	4	0	4
Nitrogen	N	7	14	2	5	0	3
Oxygen	O	8	16	2	6	0	2
Sulfur	S	16	32	2	8	6	2

Only the electrons in the outermost energy level (if it is incomplete) can participate in chemical reactions to form chemical bonds. The outermost electrons of an atom are known as its valence electrons.

isotope An alternate form of a chemical element. It differs from other atoms of the same element in the number of neutrons in its nucleus.

energy level outside the nucleus has room for just two electrons. When that is full, the next energy level away from the nucleus is available for electrons, and there is room for 8 electrons. For example, hydrogen has one electron in energy level 1. Carbon has 2 electrons in energy level 1 and 4 in energy level 2. In energy level 3, there is room for 8 electrons. Sulfur, with an atomic number of 16, has 2 electrons in the first energy level, 8 in the second, and 6 in the third (Table A-3).

An atom tends to bond with other atoms that will fill its outermost energy level and produce a number of valence electrons equal to the noble gas that is the farthest to the right in its row in the periodic table (e.g., helium and argon). For instance, a hydrogen atom, with only a single electron, will react with other atoms that provide another electron and fill the energy level with two electrons, the same number of electrons as in the noble gas helium.

Isotopes and Atomic Weight

All the atoms of an element have the same number of protons in the nucleus, but the number of neutrons in the nuclei of elements such as carbon, nitrogen, and oxygen may vary. All elements have such varieties, called **isotopes,** that differ from each other only in the number of neutrons and, consequently, atomic mass. Most hydrogen atoms have only one proton, but isotopic forms can have one or two neutrons. Some isotopes are radioactive, but most are not. Tritium, a radioactive isotope of hydrogen, has one proton and two neutrons. Carbon nuclei can contain five, six, seven, or eight neutrons.

Isotopes are distinguished by adding the number of protons and neutrons together and writing the resultant sum as a superscript to the left of the symbol for the element. For example, a carbon nuclei with six protons and six neutrons is written as ^{12}C. The isotope containing seven neutrons is labeled ^{13}C, and the isotope containing eight neutrons is labeled ^{14}C. Note that because all these atoms have six protons, they are all carbon atoms. However, because they possess different numbers of neutrons, they represent isotopes of carbon. All isotopes of an element behave the same way chemically.

Atomic weight actually takes into account that an element is a mixture of isotopes. If all carbon were ^{12}C, the atomic weight would be the same as its atomic mass, 12. But because some carbon exists as ^{13}C and ^{14}C, the atomic weight is slightly higher, 12.011. The atomic weight is based on the relative abundance of the various isotopes.

Although the ordinary chemical behavior of different isotopes of the same element is virtually identical, the radiochemical behavior is sometimes different. Isotopes exhibit such differences in physical behavior because they decay (break down) to more stable isotopes by giving off nuclear particles of ionizing radiation. Certain unstable isotopes (radioisotopes) are in an obvious process of decay. Every element has at least one such radioisotope. These radioisotopes have a physical half-life, which is the time required for 50% of its atoms to decay to a more stable state. Isotopes such as ^{32}P (Phosphorus) emit radiation that can be measured by instruments such as Geiger counters and scintillation counters. The isotope ^{14}C decays more rapidly than other isotopes of carbon.

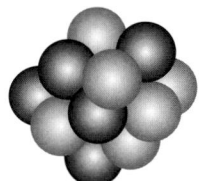

^{12}Carbon
6 Protons
6 Neutrons
6 Electrons

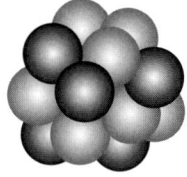

^{13}Carbon
6 Protons
7 Neutrons
6 Electrons

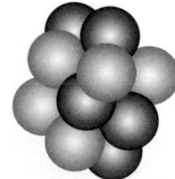

^{14}Carbon
6 Protons
8 Neutrons
6 Electrons

Other isotopes are not radioactive but can still be traced in bodily fluids or tissues using other types of instruments. Examples include ^{13}C and ^{15}N; these are called stable isotopes because they decay very slowly and do not emit radiation.

Isotope "markers," such as ^{32}P and ^{13}C, have a practical use, because they can be used to trace nutrients as they follow various chemical pathways in the body. For example, researchers can "mark" a glucose molecule with a radioactive carbon atom (^{14}C). This marking allows the researchers to see where the carbons of glucose are distributed in the body, and it helps indicate what chemical transformations glucose undergoes when metabolized. Such studies have demonstrated that glucose can become part of the lipid stored in adipose cells, or form CO_2 (detected as $^{14}CO_2$) that is exhaled. Isotope techniques are widely used in nutrition research.

Atomic and Molar Mass

Atoms are very small. One ^{12}C atom has a mass of 1.993×10^{-23}g. The units used to quantify atomic mass are called atomic mass units (amu). The carbon amu is calculated by dividing the mass of a carbon atom by 1.6605×10^{-24}, which is essentially the mass of one proton or neutron. By performing this calculation on ^{12}C, you will find that the mass of a carbon atom is 12 amu. The amu for each element is listed in the bottom portion of each entry in the periodic table. Each amu is based on comparing the element's mass to that of ^{12}C.

You are familiar with counting units, such as the number of sticks in a package of chewing gum. In chemistry, the unit for counting atoms, ions (an electrically charged atom), and molecules (a combination of atoms) is the mole. A mole is defined as the amount of matter that contains as many objects (things) as the number of atoms in 12 g of ^{12}C. The number of atoms in 12 g of ^{12}C is

$$12 \text{ g } ^{12}C \times \frac{1 \text{ atom}}{1.993 \times 10^{-23}\text{g } ^{12}C} = 6.023 \times 10^{23} \text{ atoms}$$

It is not their weight but the *number* of molecules that determines the physiological effect of a substance. Therefore, the number of "objects" in a mole of carbon (or any other substance) is 6.02×10^{23}, which is called Avogadro's number. For example:

$$1 \text{ mol } ^{12}C \text{ atoms} = 6.02 \times 10^{23} \text{ } ^{12}C \text{ atoms}$$

$$1 \text{ mol of water molecules} = 6.02 \times 10^{23} \text{ } H_2O \text{ molecules}$$

$$1 \text{ mol } NO_3^- \text{ ions} = 6.02 \times 10^{23} \text{ } NO_3^- \text{ ions}$$

A single ^{12}C atom has a mass of 12 amu, but a single ^{24}Mg is twice as massive, 24 amu. Because a mole always has the same number of particles, a mole of Mg is twice as massive as a mole of ^{12}C atoms. A mole of carbon weighs 12 g; a mole of Mg weighs 24 g. The same number that refers to the mass of a single atom of an element (in amu) also represents the mass (in g) of 1 mol of atoms of that element. For example, one ^{12}C atom weighs 12 amu. One mol ^{12}C weighs 12 g. One ^{24}Mg atom weighs 24 amu, and 1 mol ^{24}Mg weighs 24 g.

The mass in g of 1 mole of a substance is called its molar mass. The molar mass (in g) of any substance is always numerically equal to its formula weight (in amu). For example, one H_2O molecule weighs 18.0 amu, and 1 mol of H_2O weighs 18.0 g. One NaCl molecule weighs 58.5 amu, and 1 mol of NaCl weighs 58.5 g.

Molecules, Covalent Bonds, Hydrogen Bonds, and Ions and Ionic Compounds

Molecules

Molecules are formed through the interaction of the electrons in the outermost orbitals (valence electrons) of two or more electrons. When electrons are shared, chemical **bonds** are formed. The term **compound** refers to molecules composed of more

Dalton is another term used to indicate atomic mass, such as for proteins, DNA, and RNA. One Dalton is equivalent to one amu.

molecule A group of atoms chemically linked together—that is, tightly connected by attractive forces (see also *compound*).

bond A sharing of electrons, charges, or attractions linking two atoms.

compound A group of different types of atoms bonded together in definite proportion (see also *molecule*). Not all chemical compounds exist as molecules. Some compounds are made up of ions attracted to each other, such as Na^+Cl^- (table salt).

Ethanol

Molecular
formula

C_2H_6O

Structural
formula

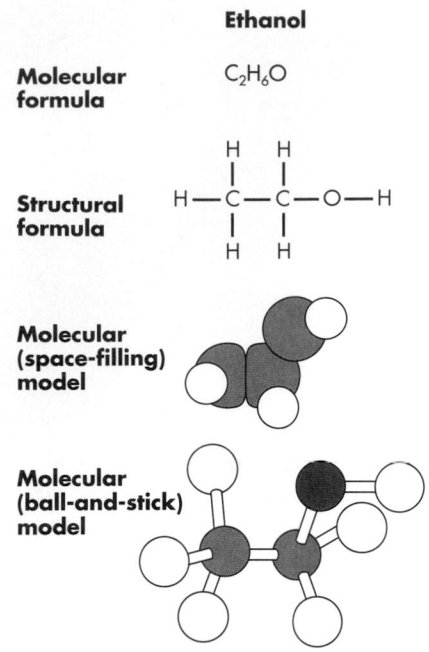

Molecular
(space-filling)
model

Molecular
(ball-and-stick)
model

Figure A-1 | Examples of the molecular and structural formulas and the molecular models of ethanol. The space-filling model gives a more realistic feeling of the space occupied by the atoms. On the other hand, the ball-and-stick type shows the bonds and bond angles more clearly.

---

covalent bond A union of two atoms formed by the sharing of electrons.

---

than one element. Water is a compound. Each molecule (or compound) possesses its own properties, such as color, taste, and density.

Hydrogen can form just one chemical bond because it has room for just one electron in its orbital of two electrons, in turn yielding a noble gas electron configuration. Carbon can form four chemical bonds, nitrogen three, and oxygen two (review Table A-3).

A molecular formula gives the elemental composition of a molecule or compound. This formula consists of the symbols of the atoms in the molecule plus a subscript denoting the number of each type of atom.

A structural formula shows how the atoms are arranged with respect to each other. As an extension, molecular and ball-and-stick models approximate the shape of the molecule (Figure A-1).

When molecules combine with each other, atoms do not increase or decrease in number. Atoms present in starting materials must be present in the products. For example, compare the number of oxygen atoms in glucose and the oxygen itself to the number in the products of the reaction (18 vs. 18). This example also illustrates the process of conservation of mass.

$$C_6H_{12}O_6 + 6\ O_2 \rightarrow 6\ CO_2 + 6\ H_2O$$

Covalent Bonds

When atoms share their valence electrons, a **covalent bond** is formed (Figure A-2). The electrons shared between atoms are bonding electrons; these represent the adhesive that holds the atoms together in molecular form.

When two identical atoms share electrons, such as in the formation of hydrogen gas (H_2) or oxygen gas (O_2), the covalent bond is very strong because the electrons are shared equally. This equal distribution between the atoms makes the molecule nonpolar. Consider the simple compound methane (CH_4). Hydrogen has one valence electron and its outermost (only) orbital can hold a maximum of two electrons. Carbon has four electrons in its outermost energy level or valence shell, and that shell can hold a maximum of eight electrons. Both carbon and hydrogen fill their valence shells to the maximum by sharing electrons with each other. Notice that each hydrogen in methane contains two electrons and that the carbon atom ends up with eight electrons. A good way to look at this is that the hydrogen atoms share one pair of electrons, whereas the carbon atoms share four pairs of electrons (review Figure A-2).

Guidelines that govern the formation of covalent bonds are as follows:

1. The valence shell of each element must have room to accommodate additional electrons.

Figure A-2 Covalent bonds. | In each of the four bonds, one electron of the carbon is shared with the electron of a hydrogen atom in a single, sausage-shaped molecular orbital encompassing the two nuclei. Methane is the simplest organic molecule. Even the largest organic molecules are held together by strong covalent bonds like these.

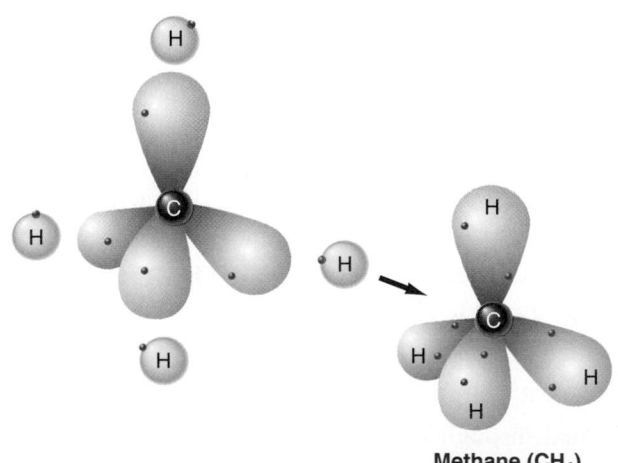

Methane (CH_4)

2. Second-row nonmetallic elements of the periodic table (e.g., carbon, nitrogen, and oxygen) and hydrogen typically fill their outermost energy levels by sharing the necessary number of electrons with another element.

3. Third-row nonmetals and those beyond this point in the periodic table (e.g., phosphorus and sulfur) frequently attain stability by giving up electrons in the outermost energy level rather than adding them. Phosphorus, for example, typically makes five bonds to attain stability instead of the three that are needed to have the electron configuration of the noble gas argon (18 electrons).

A single covalent bond forms when two atoms share one electron pair. A double covalent bond forms when two atoms share two electron pairs.

When electrons spend approximately equal time around each atom nucleus, the bond is called a nonpolar covalent bond. These are the strongest covalent bonds. If the two nuclei are not equally attractive to electrons, their atoms can form a polar covalent bond in which the electrons spend more time orbiting the more attractive nucleus. For example, when hydrogen bonds with oxygen, the electrons are more attracted to the oxygen nucleus and orbit that nucleus more than they do the hydrogen nucleus. Electrons carry a negative charge, which makes the oxygen region of the molecule slightly negative and the hydrogen region slightly positive. The Greek letter delta (δ) is used to symbolize a charge less than that of one electron or proton. A slightly negative region of a molecule is shown as δ⁻ and a slightly positive region is shown as δ⁺. A molecule such as this is called a dipole because it has two charged ends.

When two different atoms form a covalent bond, the bonding electrons are never shared equally. Consider again the H–O bond in water. It is unreasonable to expect that the hydrogen nucleus (containing one proton) and the oxygen nucleus (containing eight protons) have identical forces of attraction for the shared electron pair. In addition, other factors come into play, such as how many energy levels each atom has, how many electrons are in each, and the distance the shared electrons are from each nucleus. All these factors lead to an unequal sharing of electrons in a covalent bond between different atoms.

The ability of an atom in a molecule to attract electrons is called electronegativity. Elements toward the top right corner of the periodic table have the highest electronegativity, and those toward the bottom left have the lowest (electronegativity generally increases from left to right in a row of the periodic table, and decreases going down a column; the difference in the electronegativities of bonded atoms can be used to determine the polarity of a bond). Metals have low electronegativity, whereas nonmetals have relatively high electronegativity. Oxygen and nitrogen have the highest electronegativities of the elements typically found in compounds important to nutrition. The electronegativity values of atoms determine the type of chemical bond formed. If the electronegativity values are not very different, a covalent bond is formed. If the electronegativity of two bonding atoms differs greatly, electron transfer occurs to yield an ionic bond, as in Na^+Cl^- (see the subsequent section on ions and ionic compounds).

Hydrogen Bonds

Water, and most other molecules containing an O—H or N—H bond, exhibit a particularly strong interaction called hydrogen bonding (Figure A-3). In this case, the hydrogen atom of one molecule is attracted to a nonbonded electron pair (called a lone pair) of a highly electronegative atom on a neighboring molecule, such as oxygen. Water molecules are attracted to each other by hydrogen bonds. This attraction is responsible for many of the biologically important properties of water. Hydrogen bonds, such as those found in large proteins and DNA, help to hold the molecule together. These molecules fold or twist into three-dimensional shapes due in part to the action of hydrogen bonds. Hydrogen bonds are usually symbolized by a dotted line between the atoms: —C—O · · · H—N—. Hydrogen bonds are the weakest of all chemical bonds.

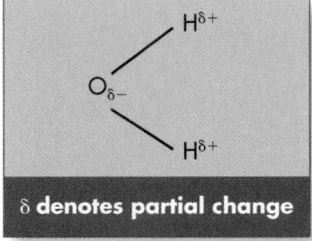

δ denotes partial change

Water is a good example of a dipole compound. The oxygen atom pulls electrons from the two hydrogen atoms toward its side of the water molecule, so that the oxygen side is more negatively charged than the hydrogen side of the molecule. Water, the most abundant molecule in the body, serves as a good solvent because of the nature of its basic structure.

Polar molecules are weakly attracted both to ions and to other polar molecules. The positive end of the molecule can align itself with an anion or with the negative end of another molecule. These attractive forces, called, respectively, ion-dipole and dipole-dipole forces, are much weaker than covalent bonds individually, but when there are many of them, they make a significant contribution to the total energy of a collection of molecules. Water, for instance, has a much higher boiling point than expected because the molecules are held together by such forces.

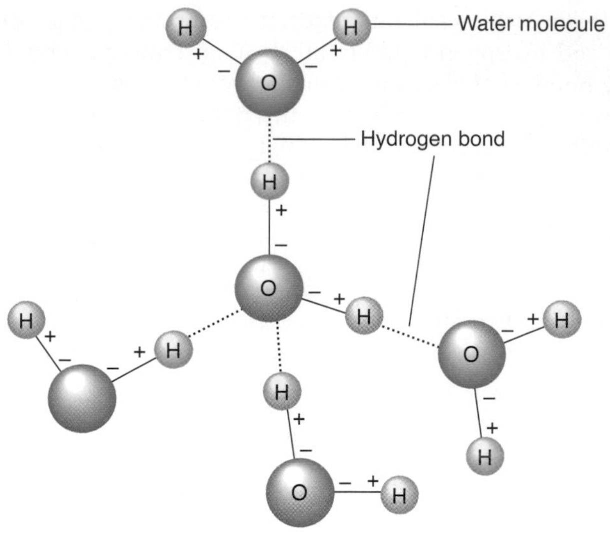

Figure A-3 | Hydrogen bonds between water molecules. The oxygen atoms of water molecules are weakly joined together by the attraction of the electronegative oxygen for the positively charged hydrogen. These weak bonds are called hydrogen bonds.

ionic bond A union between two atoms formed by an attraction of a positive ion to a negative ion, as seen in table salt (NA^+Cl^-).

Water molecules that surround ions attract other water molecules to form hydration spheres around each ion. This mechanism makes ions and numerous molecules soluble in water.

Ions and Ionic Compounds

Atoms that have an equal number of positively charged protons and negatively charged electrons are electrically neutral. Atoms or molecules that have positive or negative charges are called ions. **Ionic bonds** result when one or more valence electrons from one atom are completely transferred to another atom or molecule. Elements that have one to three valence electrons have a tendency to give up electrons, and those with four to seven valence electrons have a tendency to accept electrons. The electrons are not shared. In both cases the elements are giving up or taking on electrons to achieve the electron configuration of the closest noble gas. Take the case of sodium chloride. One atom loses electrons, so that its number of electrons becomes smaller than its number of protons; thus, it becomes positively charged as Na^+ in sodium chloride. Now, sodium has the same number of electrons as neon. The other atom gains electrons, so its number of electrons is greater than its number of protons; it becomes negatively charged as Cl^- in sodium chloride. Now, chloride has the same number of electrons as argon.

Positively charged ions are called cations; they move toward the negative pole in an electric field. An atom with more electrons than protons is negatively charged and is known as an anion; it moves to the positive pole. NaCl is an example of an ionic compound. Note the name change that occurs when an element gains an electron to become a negative ion; the suffix becomes –*ide*.

These charged atoms, where electron(s) have been added or removed, are collectively known as ions. Sodium (Na^+), potassium (K^+), and calcium (Ca^{2+}) are found in the body as cations. Chloride (Cl^-) is a common anion in the body. See Table A-4 for a more complete list of common ions found in the body.

Ionic bonds are weaker than polar covalent bonds. Ionic compounds easily separate when dissolved in water. Table salt (NaCl) is obvious when poured out of the salt shaker, but when the salt is stirred into a cup of water it disappears. It *dissociates*. The polar water's negative side (oxygen) is attracted to the Na^+, and the positive side (hydrogen) is attracted to Cl^-.

Salts

Salts are substances composed of cations and anions. Table salt is NaCl. The Na^+ and Cl^- are attracted to each other by electrostatic force, and the resulting ionic compound is known chemically as sodium chloride. Salts are formed by the interaction of acids and bases in a neutralization reaction. Water is also formed in such a reaction. In

Table A-4 | Important Ions in the Human Body

Common Ion	Symbol	Some Functions
Calcium	Ca^{2+}	Component of bones and teeth; necessary for blood clotting, muscle contraction, and nerve transmission
Sodium	Na^+	Helps maintain membrane potentials (electrical charge differences across a membrane) and water balance
Potassium	K^+	Helps maintain membrane potentials
Hydrogen	H^+	Helps maintain acid-base balance
Hydroxide	OH^-	Helps maintain acid-base balance
Chloride	Cl^-	Helps maintain acid-base balance
Bicarbonate	HCO_3^-	Helps maintain acid-base balance
Ammonium	NH_4^+	Helps maintain acid-base balance
Phosphate	PO_4^{3-}	Component of bones and teeth; involved in energy exchange and acid-base balance
Iron	Fe^{2+}	Necessary for red blood cell formation and function
Magnesium	Mg^{2+}	Necessary for enzyme function
Iodide	I^-	Part of the thyroid hormones
Fluoride	F^-	Strengthens bones and teeth

this type of reaction, hydrogen ions of an acid are replaced by the positive ions of a base, and a salt forms. For example, when hydrochloric acid reacts with sodium hydroxide, table salt is produced:

$$HCl \quad + \quad NaOH \quad \rightarrow \quad NaCl \quad + \quad H_2O$$

Hydrochloric acid	Sodium hydroxide	Salt	Water
	(Neutralization reaction)		

The formula for salts can be misleading. For example, NaCl suggests that table salt exists as a discrete entity containing one sodium ion and one chloride ion. An inspection of the chemical structure of table salt shows that it is actually a three-dimensional stack of layers—much like having a ream of paper with all the pages glued together (Figure A-4).

Salts separate to form positively and negatively charged ions when dissolved in water. Substances that dissolve in water and conduct electricity are called electrolytes. (A solute that produces ions in solution forms an electrolytic solution that conducts an electrical current.) Sodium (Na^+), potassium (K^+), calcium (Ca^{2+}), chloride (Cl^-), magnesium (Mg^{2+}), phosphate (PO_4^{3-}), and bicarbonate (HCO_3^-) are various electrolytes commonly found in the body.

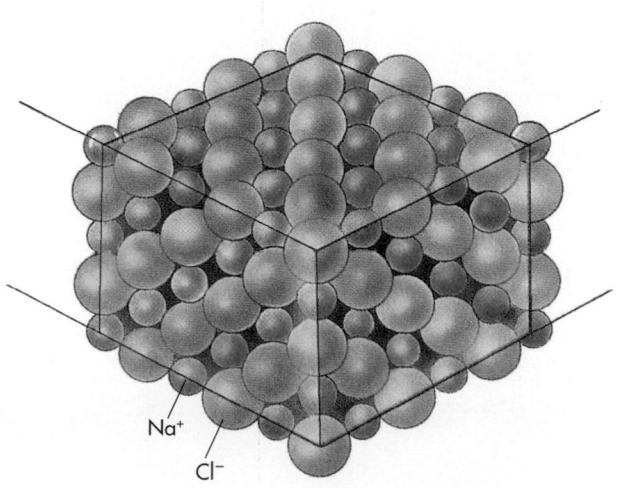

Figure A-4 | Molecules of sodium chloride (table salt) in typical cube-shape formation.

Water molecules of two hydrogens and one oxygen are held together by polar covalent bonds. Although these are strong bonds, a *small* proportion of them break, releasing a hydrogen ion and a hydroxide ion. The hydrogen ion (a proton) is transferred to another oxygen in a water molecule, forming a *hydronium ion*. This means that a pair of water molecules can act as an acid and a base, because water self-ionizes, forming hydronium ions and hydroxide ions:

$$2H_2O \longleftrightarrow H_3O^+ + OH^-$$
Water   Hydronium ion   Hydroxide ion

For simplicity, ionized water will be represented by H^+ and OH^-:

Acids, Bases, and the pH Scales

You have a pretty good idea of what acids and bases are. You know that lemon juice is an acid and drain cleaners are strong bases.

A solution that has a higher concentration of protons (H^+) is said to be acidic, and one that is lower is basic, or alkaline. An acid is defined as a substance that can ionize and release protons (H^+) into solution. It is a proton donor.

Any substance that releases protons (hydrogen ions) when in water is an acid. For example, hydrogen chloride (HCl) forms hydrogen and chloride ions (H^+ and Cl^-) in solution and therefore is an acid.

$$HCl \rightarrow H^+ + Cl^-$$

Figure A-5 lists several common acids and bases. A base is a negatively charged ion or a molecule that ionizes to produce an anion. This then can combine with a proton (H^+), removing it from solution. This base is a proton acceptor. Any substance that can accept hydrogen ions while in water is a base.

Many bases can function as proton acceptors by releasing hydroxide ions (OH^-) when dissolved in water. Most strong bases release OH^- into solution. The OH^- combines with H^+ to form water.

$$NaOH \rightarrow Na^+ + OH^-$$
Sodium hydroxide   Sodium ion   Hydroxide ion

$$OH^- + H^+ \rightarrow H_2O$$
Hydroxide ion   Hydrogen ion   Water

Figure A-5 | pH scale. The diagonal line indicates the proportionate number of hydrogen ions to hydroxide ions. Any pH value above 7 is basic, and any pH value below 7 is acidic.

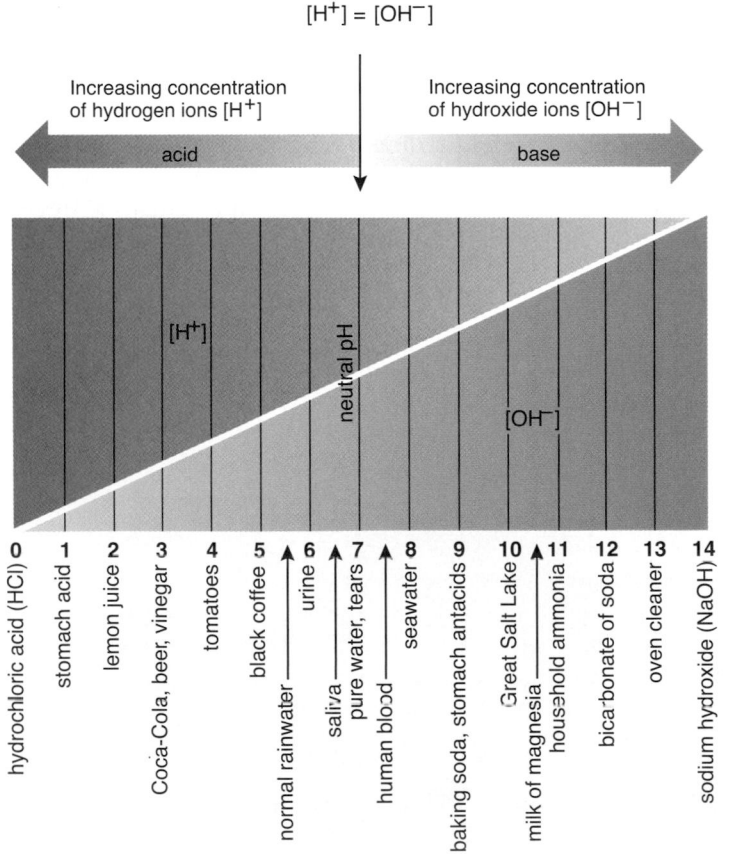

pH

Acidity is expressed in terms of pH, a measure of the molarity (the ratio of solute per liter of solution) of H^+. Molarity is expressed by square brackets, so the molarity of H^+ is symbolized as $[H^+]$. pH is defined as the negative logarithm of the hydrogen ion molarity (concentration), or $pH = -\log [H^+]$. The pH unit is the H^+ concentration of a solution. Pure water has a neutral pH because it contains equal amounts of hydrogen (hydronium) and hydroxyl ions. The pH scale runs from 0 to 14 (review Figure A-5).

Because pH is a negative logarithmic scale, a solution with a pH of 4 has an **acidic pH** that is 10 times greater than that of a solution with a pH of 5, and is 100 times more acidic than a solution with a pH of 6. These numbers may be confusing because they are inversely related to the hydrogen ion concentration: A solution with a high hydrogen ion concentration has a low pH number. A solution with a low hydrogen concentration has a high pH number. Acid solutions have a pH of less than 7. Basic, or **alkaline pH,** solutions have a pH greater than 7.

A slight disruption of pH can seriously disturb normal physiological functions, so it is important the body be able to control pH. Blood normally has a pH range from 7.35 to 7.45. Any deviations from this range can cause dizziness, fainting, coma, paralysis, or death.

Acids and bases are classified as strong or weak. Strong acids and strong bases dissociate completely when dissolved in water. Consequently, they release all their hydrogen ions or hydroxide ions when dissolved. In general, the more completely an acid or a base dissociates, the stronger it is. Hydrochloric acid, for example, is a strong acid because it completely dissociates in water.

Weak acids only partially dissociate in water. Consequently, they release only some of their acidic hydrogens. For example, when acetic acid ($CH_3C\overset{\overset{O}{\|}}{}\!\!-OH$, the principal component of vinegar) dissolves in water, it dissociates only partially.

$$CH_3\overset{\overset{O}{\|}}{C}-OH \longleftrightarrow CH_3\overset{\overset{O}{\|}}{C}-O^- + H^+$$

| Acetic acid | Acetate ion | Proton |

The equilibrium lies far to the left, so that only a small fraction of the acetic acid in the vinegar is dissociated into acetate ions and protons.

Most weak bases release hydroxide into solution by reacting with the water itself. For example, ammonia (NH_3) reacts with water to form NH_4^+ and OH^-.

$$NH_3 + H_2O \longleftrightarrow NH_4^+ + OH^-$$

| Ammonia | Water | Ammonium ion | Hydroxide ion |

Buffers

Many of the biochemical reactions that occur in living tissues require tight control of pH. To prevent changes in the H^+ concentration in the body and to control the pH, a system of buffers is maintained. These buffers are ions and molecules that stabilize the pH of a solution. In the blood (plasma), the pH is maintained by the carbonic acid–bicarbonate buffer system. The acid is formed by the combination of water and carbon dioxide. Carbonic acid separates into bicarbonate ion (HCO_3^-) and the hydrogen ion (H^+).

$$HCO_3^- + H^+ \longleftrightarrow H_2CO_3 \longleftrightarrow H_2O + CO_2$$

| Bicarbonate | Hydrogen ion | Carbonic acid | Water | Carbon dioxide |

acidic pH A pH less than 7. Lemon juice has an acidic pH.

alkaline pH A pH greater than 7. Baking soda in water yields an alkaline pH.

The kidneys also play a buffering role in the body by absorbing or releasing H^+ or HCO_3^-, depending on the acid-base balance in the person. In fact, much of the excess acid leaves the body via the urine (urine has an acid pH). Thus, the kidneys and lungs keep this buffering system functioning and, in turn, are key to acid-base balance in the body.

The reaction can go either way. The direction depends on the concentration of ions on either side of the arrows. For example, if an acid were released into the blood plasma (more H^+ in solution), the reaction would be driven to the right. The carbon dioxide produced could then be exhaled via the lungs. Acids that are present in the plasma come from cellular activities, but despite the increase in H^+ ions by these activities, the blood plasma pH hardly changes; it is essentially constant. The buffer, bicarbonate, accomplishes this. It is constantly formed to maintain normal pH.

Free Radicals

You are aware that atoms tend to share electron pairs when forming chemical bonds, and there is a tendency to share enough electrons to completely fill the valence shell so as to form a noble gas configuration. A consequence is that atoms or elements are rarely found with unpaired electrons. But when a molecule with an extra electron does arise, it is called a free radical. An example is the superoxide anion. Oxygen is composed of two oxygen atoms (O_2); if an electron is added, it becomes superoxide, or $O_2^{\bullet-}$. The dot signifies an unpaired electron.

Superoxide and other free radicals are reactive, primarily because they contain an unpaired electron. Free radicals seek an electron by attacking and removing electrons from other compounds, such as at the location where hydrogens are attached to carbon. This not only damages the other molecule but transforms it into a free radical.

$$R^\bullet + -CH_2 \rightarrow RH^+ - CH^{-\bullet}$$

Free radicals are also formed when a covalent bond breaks and each atom or molecule fragment recovers the electron originally used to make the bond. In this case, energy—usually in the form of sunlight, ultraviolet radiation, or heat—is used to break the bond.

$$A - B + \text{energy} \rightarrow A^\bullet + B^\bullet$$

Because free radicals are reactive, they can generate thousands of other free radicals within minutes in a chain-reaction process. The reactivity of free radicals sometimes produces detrimental effects in living systems. For instance, the development of cardiovascular disease and some types of cancer, such as skin and lung cancer, is probably promoted by free radicals. However, some normal physiological functions in the body involve free radical formation; for example, free radicals are used by various white blood cells to kill invading bacteria.

The body has a number of mechanisms, such as antioxidants, for neutralizing free radicals. Antioxidants are substances that react with and neutralize free radical forms of oxygen and nitrogen. The enzyme superoxide dismutase (SOD) converts superoxide into oxygen and hydrogen peroxide. One form of SOD contains the minerals copper and zinc, whereas another form contains manganese. Other antioxidants obtained from the diet are vitamin E and various phytochemicals.

Some substances are used extensively in the food industry to trap free radicals or prevent their formation. This use allows for increased storage time of food by decreasing chemical breakdown. These substances are part of a class of food additives called preservatives (see Chapter 19). Vitamin E added to cooking oils protects $C=C$ bonds by trapping free radicals.

Organic Chemistry

Organic compounds contain carbon in combination with other elements, such as hydrogen, oxygen, and nitrogen. Carbon compounds are associated with living things, but why carbon? It is because carbon forms very stable covalent bonds, such as single, double, and even triple bonds. Carbon also forms these bonds with many other atoms.

Carbon atoms can even form rings and chains by bonding to other carbons. Variation in the length of the chains, and their atomic configurations, allows the formation of a wide variety of molecules. Organic molecules generally also contain hydrogen.

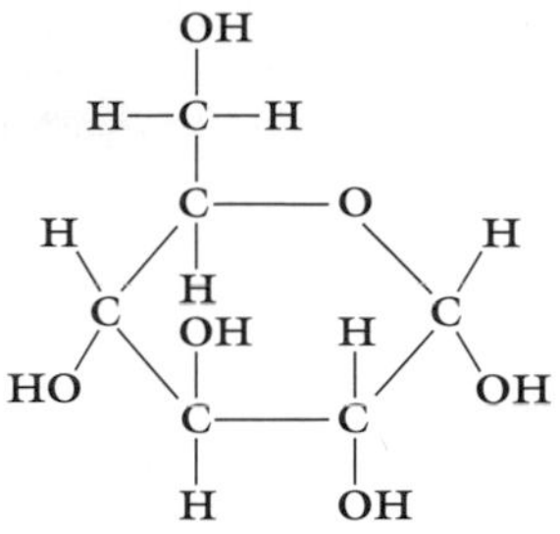

Cyclic and Chain Compounds

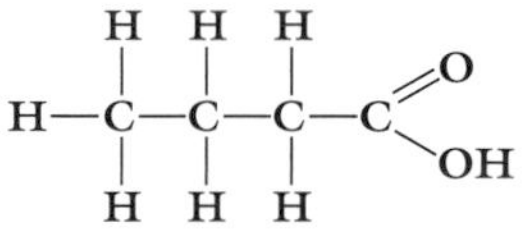

Cyclic organic compounds are common forms of hydrocarbons. Note the diagram of butyric acid (a chain) in the margin and compare that to the structure of glucose, which is a ring. Even though the two compounds are only carbon, oxygen, and hydrogen, each conveys a very different property. Some ring structures are referred to as aromatic compounds.

Hydrocarbons as chains or rings provide the backbone of many groups of compounds that make up important organic nutrients. Other groups are attached to these backbones. They usually contain atoms of oxygen, nitrogen, phosphorus, and sulfur. The functional or reactive groups provide the unique chemical properties of organic molecules. Classes of organic molecules are known by their functional groups.

Glucose

Butyric acid

A Closer Look at Functional Groups

Several important organic compounds contain a functional group called a carbonyl group (C=O). The carbonyl group is the parent compound for ketones, aldehydes, and many related groups. Table A-5 has a list of all these compounds that are important to nutrition.

Ketones are organic compounds in which the carbonyl group occurs in the interior of a carbon chain and is therefore flanked by carbon atoms. Body fat that is breaking down at a rapid rate produces ketones (C—C̈—C), some of which are removed from the body by way of the urine (review Chapter 4).

Aldehydes (—C̈—H) are organic compounds that contain a carbonyl group to which at least one hydrogen atom is attached. This active group is found in one important form of vitamin A. As an aldehyde, it plays a central role in vision.

Many of the most common substances in both foods and the body contain carboxylic acids. A carboxylic acid (—C̈—OH) contains the carbonyl group with an OH group attached. These acids are widely distributed in tissues and natural products. Vinegar contains acetic acid. Citrus fruits contain citric acid, and vitamin C is ascorbic acid.

The carboxyl group is an acid because it can donate a H^+ (proton) to a solution. A very common acid formed in muscle cells is lactic acid. When lactic acid ionizes, it releases the H^+ and becomes lactate. Because both forms of the acid (ionized and non-ionized) are in solution, the proportion depends on the pH of the solution.

An alcohol has the carbon-oxygen bond, but the O is also bonded to a single hydrogen. This leaves only a single bond between the carbon and oxygen, forming an —OH or hydroxide group (ROH).

An ester (R—C̈—O—C) is an organic compound that has an O—C group attached to a carbonyl group. An ester is the product of a reaction between a carboxylic acid and an alcohol. The formation of lipids called triglycerides involves the formation of ester bonds.

The carbonyl portion of a compound such as an ester is called an acyl group. Thus, removal of the hydroxyl group (OH) from an organic acid forms an acyl group.

Two sulfur atoms (S—S), each attached to a carbon, produce a disulfide group. This group is important to the structural characteristics of certain proteins.

Table A-5 | Typical Chemical Groups Found in Nutrients

Functional Group	Name	Typically Found In	Example
—OH	Hydroxide	Alcohols	CH_2—OH
—C=O | H	Aldehyde	Sugars	CH_3C=O | H
C—C=O | C	Ketone	Ketones	CH_3C=O | CH_3
—C=O | OH	Carboxyl	Acids	CH_3C=O | OH
—S—S—	Disulfide	Proteins	—CH_2—S—S—CH_2—
—C=O |	Carbonyl	Aldehydes, ketones, carboxylic acids, amides	$(CH_3)_2C$=O
| —C—NH_2 |	Amine	Proteins	CH_3—NH_2
—C=O | NH_2	Amide	Vitamins	—CH_2C=O | NH_2
O— | –O—P=O | O—	Phosphate	High-energy compounds	O— | —CH_2—O—P=O | O—CH_2-
—C=O | O—C	Ester	Triglycerides	(structure)
O ‖ —O—C—CH_2-	Acyl	Triglycerides	(structure)

A single carbon with an amine (also called amino) group attached (—NH_2) is a component of all amino acids.

Isomerism

Molecules that have identical chemical formulas but different structures are called **isomers.** A simple example is two compounds with the formula C_2H_6O.

$$CH_3CH_2OH \qquad CH_3OCH_3$$

Ethanol   Methyl ether

isomers Different chemical structures for compounds that share the same chemical formula.

Both these compounds can be harmful. However, there are intake levels at which ethanol produces no toxic symptoms (i.e., the amount in a small glass of wine), but at which methyl ether would cause very toxic effects. This fact illustrates an important point about isomers: because they have different structures, they can have different *chemical* properties.

The difference in properties between two isomers can be great (as in the preceding example) or very subtle, but the differences are there and are detectable. There are different types of isomerism, but only two of the common types will be briefly reviewed in this section: structural isomers and stereoisomers.

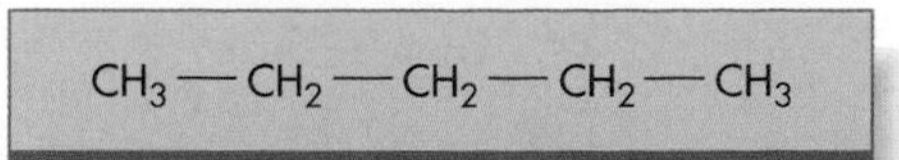

Structural Isomers

Isomers in which the number and kinds of bonds differ are called structural isomers. Molecules containing chains of carbon atoms typically have many structural isomers. Any variation in the way the chain is branched gives rise to a new isomer. For example, pentane (C_5H_{12}) has three isomers, as shown in the margin.

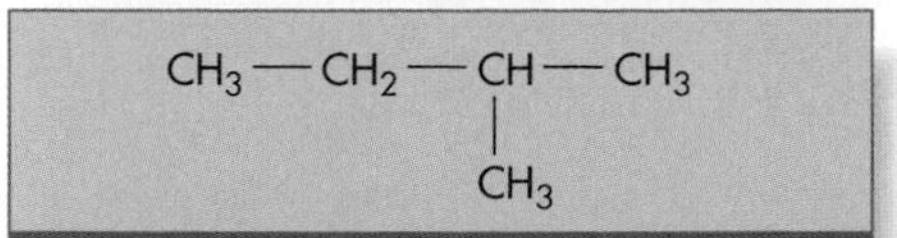

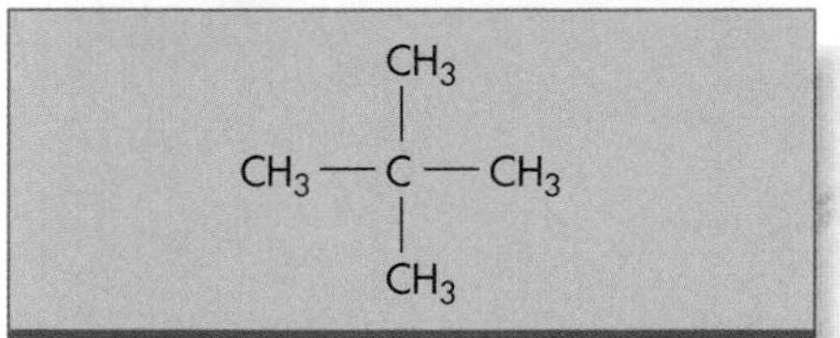

Stereoisomers

Stereoisomers have the same number and types of chemical bonds but with different spatial arrangements (different configurations in space). Molecules containing double bonds illustrate stereoisomers. Because there is no freedom to rotate around a C=C bond, molecules containing such bonds frequently exhibit stereoisomerism. For example, hydrogens or various chemical compounds can be located on the same side of the bond (*cis* configuration) or on opposite sides of the double bond (*trans* configuration).

Consider oleic acid and its isomer elaidic acid (Figure A-6a). Oleic acid is a *cis* isomer, or the form found naturally in food. With food-processing technology, such as hydrogenation, some *cis* bonds of fatty acids are converted to *trans* bonds. When vegetable oils are converted to vegetable fats, such as in margarine or shortening, some of the *trans* isomers are formed. The *trans* isomer elaidic acid is not the natural form. Isomers of these types (i.e., *cis* and *trans*) are called geometric isomers.

Describing each stereoisomerism depends on which way the functional groups are arranged with respect to each other. If there are two isomers, D stands for dextro or right-handed, and L stands for levo or left-handed, such as alanine in D-alanine and L-alanine (Figure A-6b). Stereoisomers that can't be superimposed on their mirror images are called optical isomers. Optical isomers can be identified from each other by their reaction to polarized light. One solution of an isomer that rotates the plane of polarized light to the right is dextrorotary. And the solution of its optical isomer rotates the plane of light to the left and, so, is levorotary.

The difference between two stereoisomers is "fit." This difference is important because the molecule has to fit an enzyme in order to make the chemical reaction proceed. For example, human enzymes use only L-amino acids (building blocks of protein) and D-sugars to build compounds. D-amino acids and L-sugars just won't function as such in the body. It is rather like trying to wear the left-hand glove on the right hand and do anything that requires manual skill.

A carbon atom with four different atoms or groups of atoms attached is described as being chiral (also called asymmetric). A molecule with one chiral carbon can have two stereoisomers, such as alanine (see Figure A-6b). When two or more (n) chiral carbons are present, there can be 2^n stereoisomers. Some stereoisomers are mirror images of each other, while others are not.

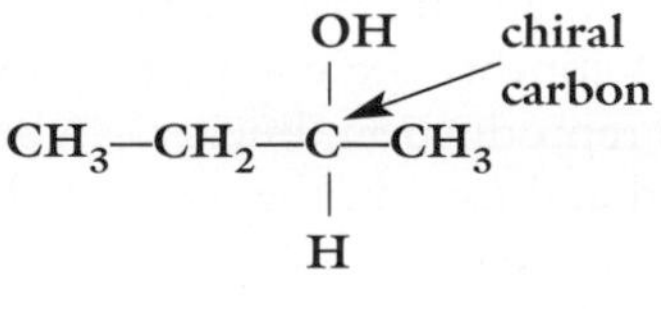

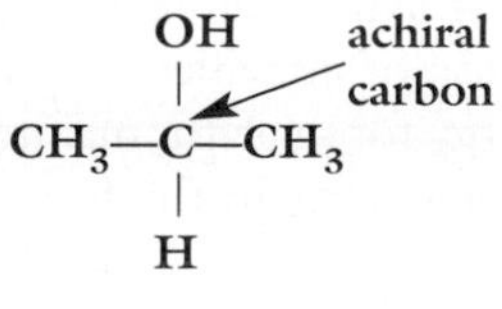

CH₃—CH₂—C—CH₃ — OH (chiral carbon) / H

CH₃—C—CH₃ — OH (achiral carbon) / H

Pentane

$CH_3 - CH_2 - CH_2 - CH_2 - CH_3$

Neopentane

$CH_3 - CH_2 - CH - CH_3$ with CH_3 below

Isopentane

$CH_3 - C - CH_3$ with CH_3 above and CH_3 below

cis configuration A form seen in compounds with double bonds, such as fatty acids, in which the hydrogens on both ends of the double bond lie on the same side of the plane of that bond.

trans configuration Compound in which the hydrogens lie opposite each other across a carbon-carbon double bond.

Generous intakes of *trans* isomers of fatty acids are associated with an increased risk of cardiovascular disease (see Chapter 6).

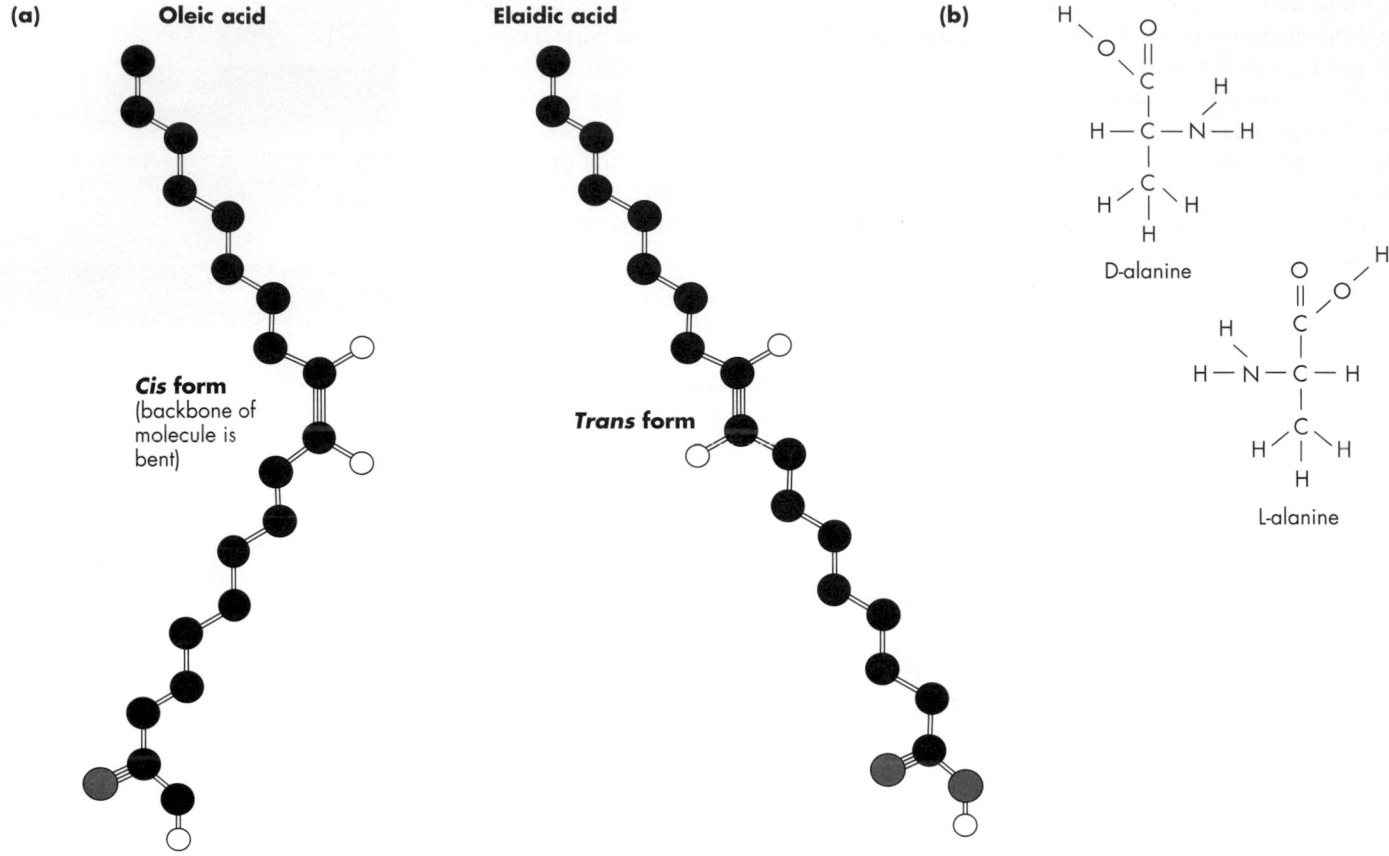

Figure A-6 | (a) *Cis* and *trans* isomers of fatty acids. *Cis* forms are the most common forms in unprocessed foods. (b) Optical isomers of alanine—an amino acid. The L isomer is the most commonly found amino acid in nature.

In living organisms, many molecules are chiral.

When compounds have more than one chiral center, the "RS" system of naming is used, rather than the D and L system. Every chiral carbon is designated either *R* or *S,* based on specific rules.

This RS terminology is important to understanding vitamin E chemistry. It is now known that vitamin E as alpha-tocopherol has three chiral centers, and so has eight different stereoisomers ($2^3 = 8$). All three are found in synthetic preparations. The three chiral centers are identified as 2, 4, and 8 as related to the position on the tail of the molecule (see Chapter 9). The RRR isomer (i.e., R form at all of the 3 chiral centers on the phytal tail) is the natural form. A transfer protein in the liver only recognizes the R form of the chiral center at the 2 position. Of all the eight combinations of R and S in the phytal tail of synthetic vitamin E, the only biologically active ones are RRR, RSR, RSS, RRS, because they all have the R form in the 2 position.

Biochemistry

The study of the chemistry or molecular basis of life and the reactions, structures, and composition of living materials is known as biochemistry. Biochemical reactions are possible because of enzymes. Living organisms convert the energy they extract from food into energy for growth, maintenance, and reproduction. Energy can be stored for future use. The energy in the food is converted and used in the form of chemical en-

Isomers of Vitamin E

RRR and SRR isomers of vitamin E. Of the two, only the RRR isomer contributes to vitamin E needs.

ergy contained in adenosine triphosphate (ATP). The fact that living organisms can self-replicate depends on deoxyribonucleic acid (DNA) and the genetic code. All forms of life store and transmit genetic information in the form of DNA.

Approximately 98.5% of the body's weight is composed of the elements oxygen, carbon, hydrogen, nitrogen, calcium, and phosphorus. Elements such as iron, zinc, and copper are present in trace amounts in the body, but that doesn't mean they are unimportant. For instance, iron combines with a blood protein to form hemoglobin, an oxygen carrier. Hemoglobin transports oxygen from the lungs to the tissues and assists in returning carbon dioxide from the tissues to the lungs for removal.

Water is the most abundant chemical in the body, making up to about 70% of human tissue. Other important classes of compounds in the body are the proteins, carbohydrates, lipids, and nucleic acids.

Biochemical Reactions

All the biochemical reactions that occur in the body are described as metabolism. The intermediate compounds in metabolism are termed *metabolites*. Metabolic reactions that build (synthesize) complex molecules are described as anabolic. An example is the synthesis of protein from amino acids. The reactions that break down (degrade) larger molecules into smaller ones are described as catabolic. An example is starch breaking down to glucose molecules.

Carbohydrates

Carbohydrates are aldehydes with hydroxyl groups and ketones, containing carbon, hydrogen, and oxygen with the general formula CH_2O. (There are twice as many hydrogen atoms as carbon and oxygen atoms.) The suffix *-ose* indicates a sugar. *Hexose* refers to a 6-carbon monosaccharide. There are three structural isomers of hexose: galactose, glucose, and fructose. All have the same formula, $C_6H_{12}O_6$, but the arrangement of their individual atoms differs slightly.

Di- and *polysaccharides* are assembled by a condensation reaction. Water is a byproduct of the reaction. In contrast, hydrolysis, or the splitting by the addition of water, digests di- and polysaccharides to smaller sugar units (for details, see the later section entitled Important Chemical Reactions Related to the Study of Nutrition).

The simplest carbohydrates are monosaccharides. When two monosaccharides are chemically bonded, they form a disaccharide, or double sugar. The table sugar sucrose is an example of a disaccharide, formed from glucose and fructose.

Polysaccharides are many monosaccharides joined by covalent bonds. Plant starch and cellulose are examples of polysaccharides. Some starches have thousands of glucose subunits. In animals, carbohydrate is stored as an animal starch called glycogen, found in liver and muscle tissue.

Lipids

Lipids are a class of nonpolar compounds that are grouped according to solubility in organic solvents. They don't readily dissolve in water because most are nonpolar or hydrophobic.

Simple lipids include fatty acids and steroids. The lipid cholesterol serves as the precursor (parent) for the steroid hormones, such as testosterone, estrogen, and progesterone. Complex lipids include triglycerides (often referred to as *triacylglycerols*), which are esters of glycerol and fatty acids. Phospholipids are composed of glycerol, phosphoric acid, and long-chain fatty acids; sphingolipids are composed of sphingosine, phosphoric acid, long-chain fatty acids, and choline; and glycosphingolipids are composed of sphingosine, fatty acids, and carbohydrates.

Triglycerides represent fuel found in food and stored in adipose tissues. Phospholipids are part polar and part nonpolar, which allows them to interact with water and function as emulsifiers. Sphingophospholipids make up the material surrounding nerves. Glycosphingolipids are structural material for brain and nerve tissue. These complex lipids can be hydrolyzed to yield fatty acids.

Prostaglandins are a special type of fatty acid produced by almost all organs in the body and have specific regulatory functions. They are all derived from certain dietary (essential) fatty acids (see Chapter 6 and Appendix B).

Proteins

Proteins are polymers of amino acids. Twenty common amino acids are incorporated into the great variety of body proteins. Although the amino acids contain an amine (amino)

$$\begin{array}{c} \text{O} \\ \parallel \end{array}$$

group (NH_2) and a carboxylic acid group ($-C-OH$), each has a distinctive structure (Figure A-7). Proteins typically contain many atoms, such as carbon, nitrogen, sulfur, hydrogen, and oxygen.

The genetic information found in DNA in the nucleus of the cell is the code book for constructing a protein. The sequence of amino acids in a protein follows the DNA code for synthesizing the protein. This protein can be made over and over again because of the code carried in the person's genes.

Nucleic Acids (DNA and RNA)

Nucleic acids include DNA (deoxyribonucleic acid), RNA (ribonucleic acid), and the subunits from which they are formed, called nucleotides. The nucleotide is made of three components: a 5-carbon pentose sugar, a phosphate group, and a nitrogenous base (Figure A-8). There are two kinds of nitrogenous base: purines (double ring) and pyrimidines (single ring).

The sugar contained in RNA is ribose. The pyrimidine bases in ribonucleic acids are uracil and cytosine, and the purine bases are guanine and adenine. RNA is a single polynucleotide strand, not a double strand like DNA.

DNA found in the nucleus of the cell is the basis of the genetic code. The sugar in DNA deoxyribose can be covalently bonded to the purine bases adenine and guanine and to the pyrimidine bases cytosine and thymine (Figure A-9). These four types of nucleotides can produce the long chain that makes up a single strand of DNA. The DNA is a two-stranded sugar phosphate chain that twists around in such a way to form a helix. The bases project into the center of the helix, forming a staircase structure. The two strands are held together by hydrogen bonds (Figure A-10).

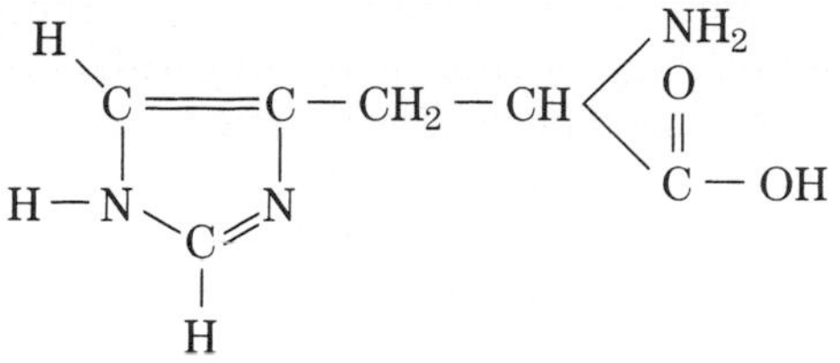

Histidine (His)
(essential)

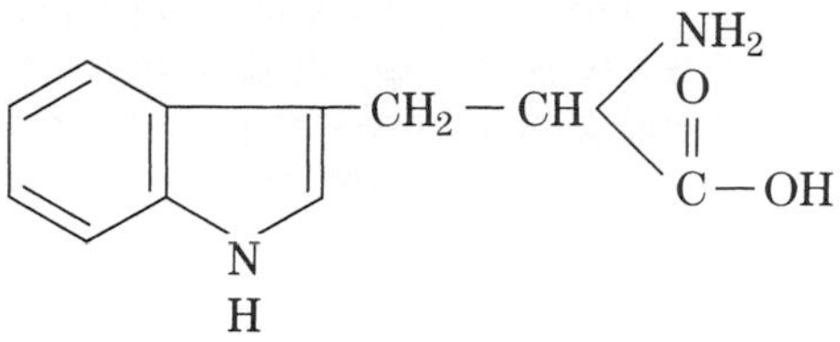

Tryptophan (Trp)
(essential)

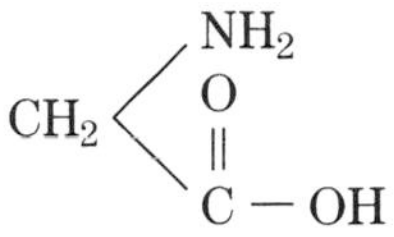

Glycine (Gly)

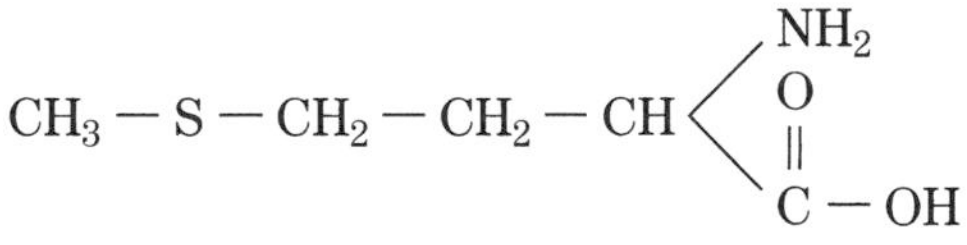

Methionine (Met)
(essential)

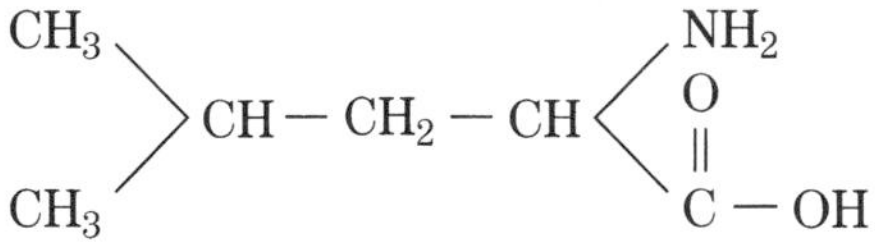

Leucine (Leu)
(essential)

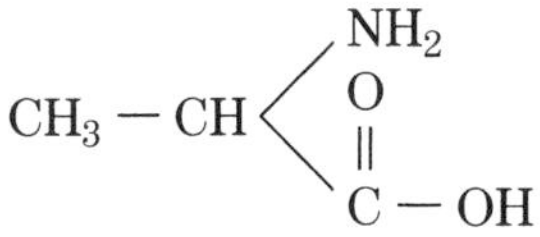

Alanine (Ala)

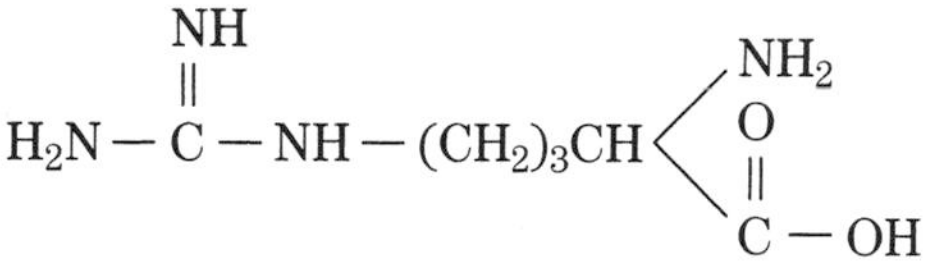

Arginine (Arg)
(essential)

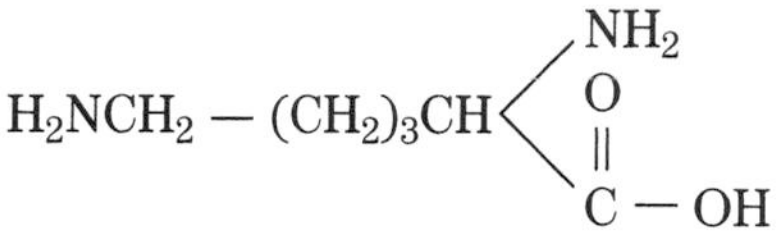

Lysine (Lys)
(essential)

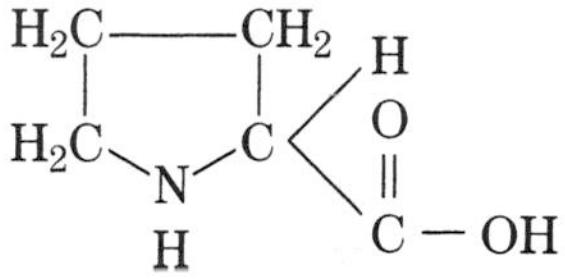

Proline (Pro)

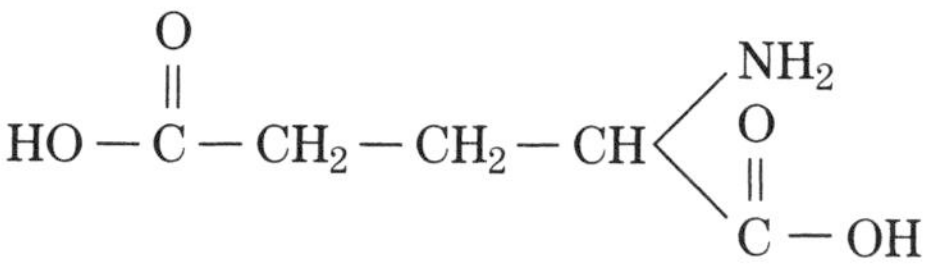

Glutamic Acid (Glu)

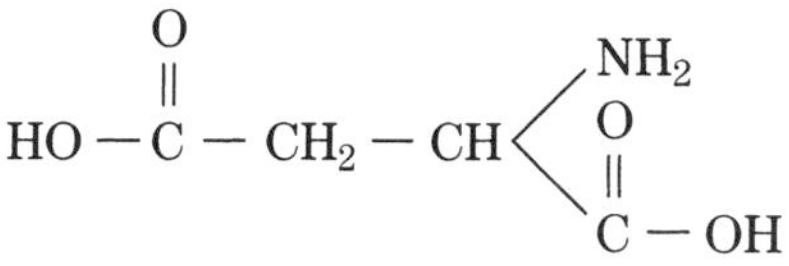

Aspartic Acid (Asp)

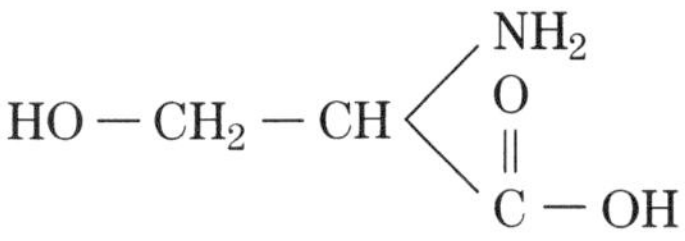

Serine (Ser)

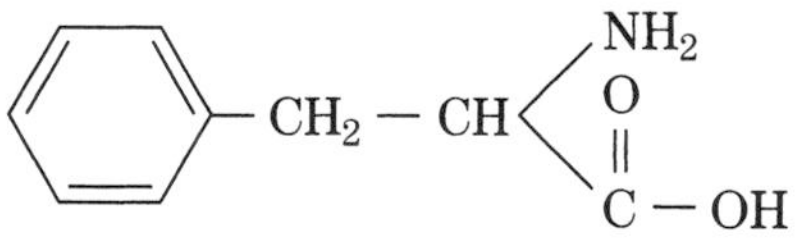

Phenylalanine (Phe)
(essential)

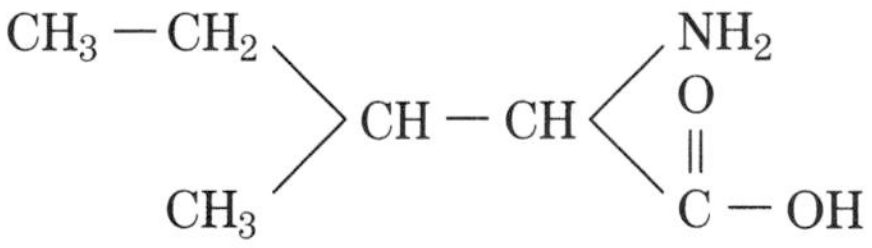

Isoleucine (Ile)
(essential)

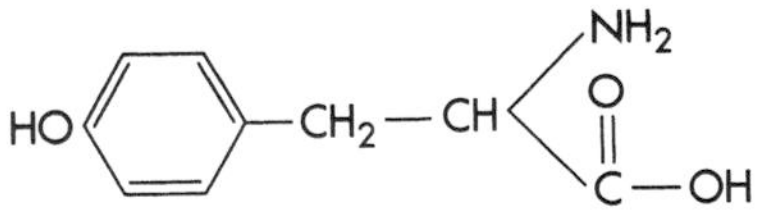

Tyrosine (Tyr)

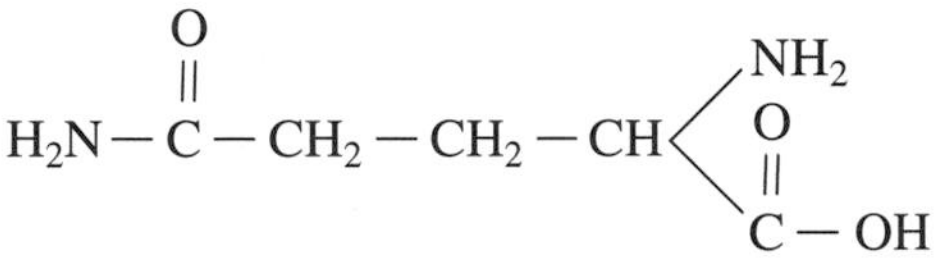

Glutamine (Gln)

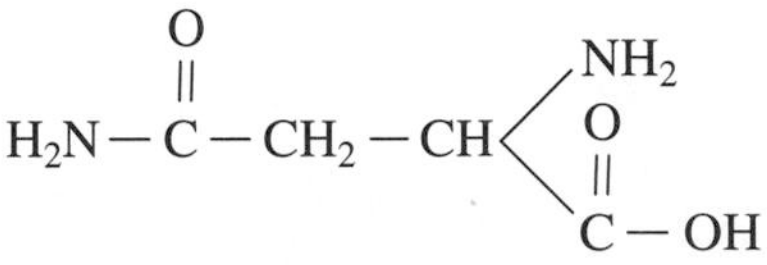

Asparagine (Asn)

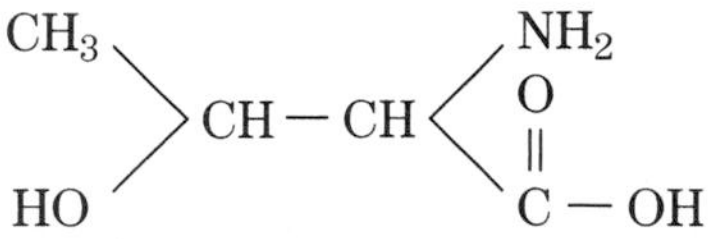

Threonine (Thr)
(essential)

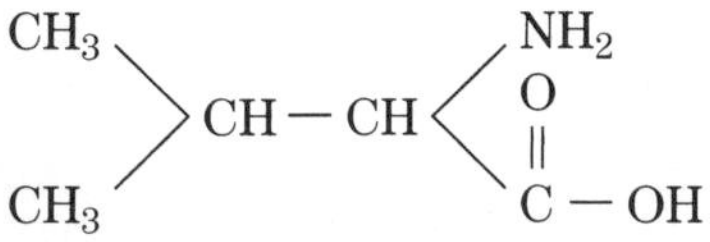

Valine (Val)
(essential)

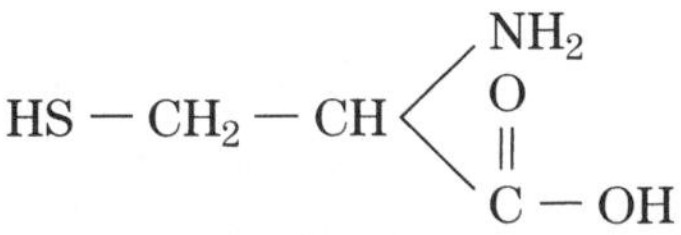

Cysteine (Cys)

Figure A-7 | The 20 common amino acids in foods.

(a)

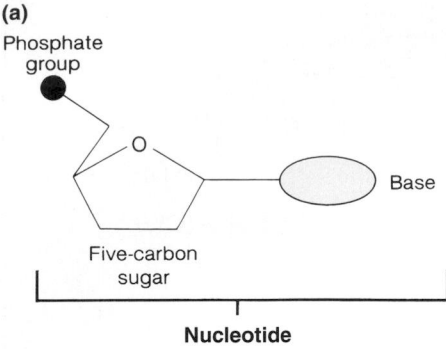

Nucleotide

(b)

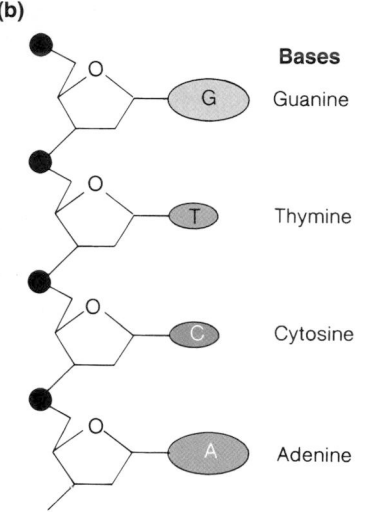

Bases

G Guanine

T Thymine

C Cytosine

A Adenine

Figure A-8 | (a) The general structure of a nucleotide. (b) A polymer of nucleotides, or polynucleotide, is formed by sugar-phosphate bonds between nucleotides.

DNA always contains an equal number of purine and pyrimidine bases. And there is a relationship called complementary base pairing—adenine pairs only with thymine, and guanine pairs only with cytosine. (In RNA adenine pairs with uracil.)

Although there are only four bases, the number of sequences of bases is endless. The total human genome consists of billions of base pairs making up about 35,000 genes. The applications of this knowledge can lead to genetic screening for breast cancer and, in the future, are likely to help produce drugs to treat obesity and inborn errors of metabolism.

During replication, the helix uncoils and separates, so that each chain or strand serves as a template for the synthesis of its complementary chain. This step is important for cell division. Each daughter cell receives DNA containing one strand of the original molecule and one new strand.

RNA, another nucleic acid, takes its instructions from DNA. There are three types of RNA: ribosomal RNA, transfer RNA, and messenger RNA. Ribosomal RNA forms part of the structure of ribosomes in the cell; this is where proteins are synthesized. Messenger RNA contains the code for the synthesis of a specific protein transcribed from DNA. Transfer RNA decodes the genetic message in RNA and assembles the amino acids for the protein assembly line (see Chapter 7 for details). The process is called translation.

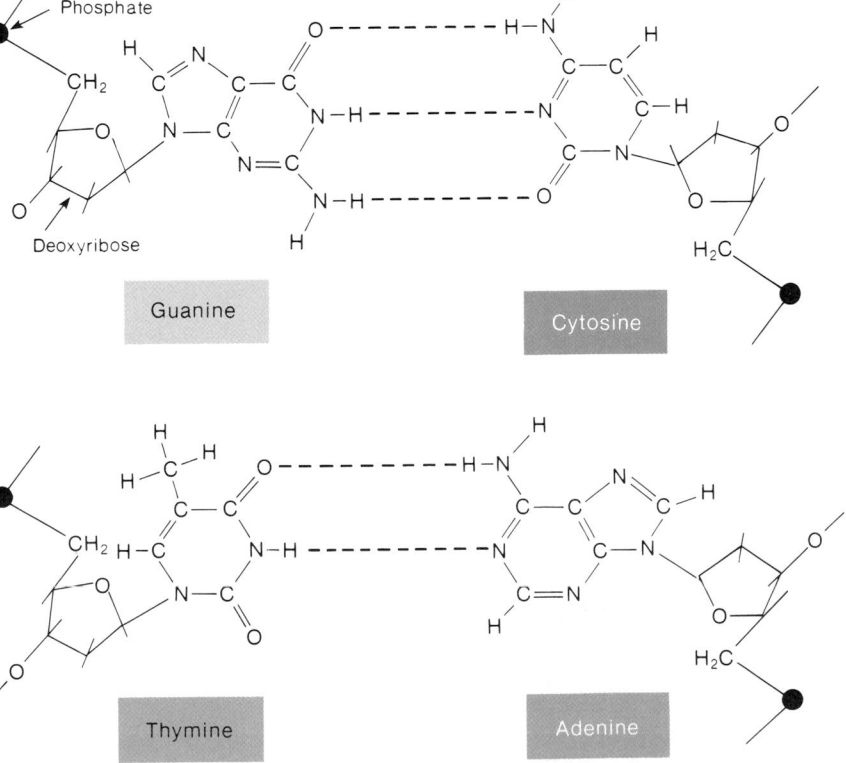

Figure A-9 | The four nitrogenous bases in deoxyribonucleic acid (DNA). Notice that hydrogen bonds can form between guanine and cytosine and between thymine and adenine.

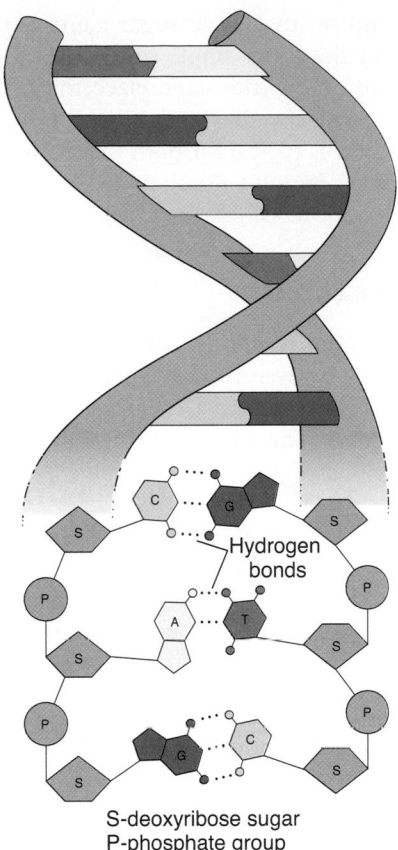

Figure A-10 | The double-helix structure of DNA. The two strands are held together by hydrogen bonds between complementary bases in each strand.

Important Chemical Reactions Related to the Study of Nutrition

One of the most important properties of chemical compounds is the type of reactions they undergo. Chemical reactions are responsible for vision, thinking, movement, and everything else that occurs in the human body.

In a chemical reaction, a compound or set of compounds (the reactants) is converted into another compound or set of compounds (the products), accompanied by the absorption or release of energy, which is typically heat in biological processes. In effect, the reactants reshuffle their atoms to form products. Clearly, then, no atoms lose their identity during a chemical reaction, and no atoms are gained, lost, or converted to another kind of atom during the course of chemical activity.

Chemists have grouped reactions according to their similarities in chemical behavior. Some of these reactions are performed over and over within each cell. Following is a brief overview of some important reaction types.

Condensation Reactions

A condensation reaction occurs when two molecules join together to form a larger molecule and water is released. The two-reactant molecules typically contain hydroxyl groups, meaning that there are two OH groups. A simple example is the condensation of glucose and galactose to make lactose and water.

$$C_6H_{12}O_6 \quad + \quad C_6H_{12}O_6 \quad \rightarrow \quad C_{12}H_{22}O_{11} \quad + \quad H_2O$$

Glucose   Galactose   Lactose   Water

One –OH group on the single sugar gains a proton and forms a water molecule. The OH group on the other single sugar loses a proton and forms a bond with the other molecule—in exactly the same place that the water molecule leaves. Note that this is an overall description of what happens, not how it happens. In addition, keep in mind that although it is typical for both molecules to contain an –OH group in a condensation reaction, it is not a requirement for the reaction. A condensation reaction can occur where only one of the reactants contains an –OH group.

Hydrolysis Reactions

Hydrolysis reactions are reactions that occur when water is added to a compound. In biological systems, hydrolysis reactions are very frequently the reverse of condensation reactions. That is, water is added to a large molecule, which results in the formation of two smaller molecules. This can be illustrated by the hydrolysis of lactose.

$$C_{12}H_{22}O_{11} + H_2O \rightarrow C_6H_{12}O_6 + C_6H_{12}O_6$$

Lactose   Water   Glucose   Galactose

Oxidation and Reduction Reactions

Oxidation-reduction (redox) reactions are important in nutrition science because they release energy from food during oxidation and synthesize carbohydrates, fatty acids, and other organic compounds during reduction. Redox reactions follow three rules:

1. No oxidation reaction takes place without something being reduced at the same time, and no reduction takes place without something being oxidized.
2. Oxidation is the loss of electrons.
3. Reduction is the gain in electrons.

A simple redox reaction involving iron is as follows:

$$Fe^{3+} + e^- \longleftrightarrow Fe^{2+}$$

A biochemical redox reaction involving the coenzyme form of riboflavin occurs as follows:

$$FAD \longleftrightarrow FADH_2$$
+2H / −2H

Chapters 4, 10, and 12 provide more information about coenzymes, cofactors, and oxidation-reduction reactions.

Energy and Enzymatic Reactions

Enzymes are large proteins with varying amino acid composition that behave as organic **catalysts.** They are highly specific. Enzymes help a reaction to proceed by lowering the "energy of activation" so that the reaction can go faster (Figure A-11). Enzymes lower this energy barrier between the reactants and the products. Some of the enzyme reactions that occur in the cell require coenzymes (vitamins) at the active site to make the reaction go, whereas many others don't. Fortunately, an enzyme isn't consumed by the reaction, so it can be used over and over.

Common Chemical Structures

Most compounds in the body are composed of carbon, hydrogen, and oxygen, with carbon often being the predominant atom. Some commonly encountered combinations of atoms, called functional groups, have been given specific names because they appear in

---

Many important compounds in cells are formed through condensation reactions, and the breakdown of many compounds into smaller fragments occurs via hydrolysis reactions.

In organic chemistry oxidation is the loss of hydrogen (or gain of oxygen).

In organic chemistry reduction is the gain of hydrogen (or loss of oxygen).

catalyst A compound that speeds reaction rates but is not altered by the reaction.

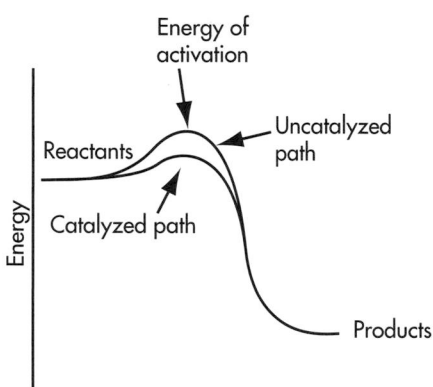

Figure A-11 | Enzymes and other catalysts accelerate chemical reactions by reducing the energy barrier to the reactions. Reactant molecules free in solution can react only if they meet in just the right orientation and with enough energy. An enzyme holds its substrate molecules in the right orientation to react and exerts forces on them that cause chemical bonds to break and form. In this way, an enzyme lowers the energy barrier that substrates must pass and, so, increases their reaction rates.

many molecules. You need to be familiar with them, for they are the most important features in many of our nutrients. The important ones were listed in Table A-5. You will be using these names and studying these structures throughout this course.

The Drawing of Chemical Structures

Chemists have developed a shorthand notation for writing chemical formulas, called skeletal structures. In skeletal structures, neither carbon atoms nor the hydrogens bonded to the carbon atoms are expressly shown. What are shown are the bonds between the carbon atoms and the position of all atoms other than carbon and hydrogen. Keep in mind that there are carbon atoms at the apices of every angle in the structure (with the appropriate number of hydrogens attached to the carbon) and at the terminal end of the sticks. By way of illustration, look at a skeletal structure of propane ($CH_3CH_2CH_3$).

The advantage of using skeletal structures is that it allows for a clear representation of complex molecules without cluttering up the picture. This notation will be used throughout the text. It is handy when large structures, such as fatty acids, have to be represented.

$$CH_2$$
$$CH_3 \quad CH_3$$
Propane   Skeletal structure
of propane

appendix B

DETAILED DEPICTIONS OF GLYCOLYSIS, CITRIC ACID CYCLE, ELECTRON TRANSPORT CHAIN, CLASSES OF EICOSANOIDS, AND HOMOCYSTEINE METABOLISM

The following illustrations are provided to help you better visualize the changes in chemical structures throughout the metabolic processes described. These figures reflect greater scientific detail than the more simplified versions in Chapter 4, Chapter 6, and Chapter 10.

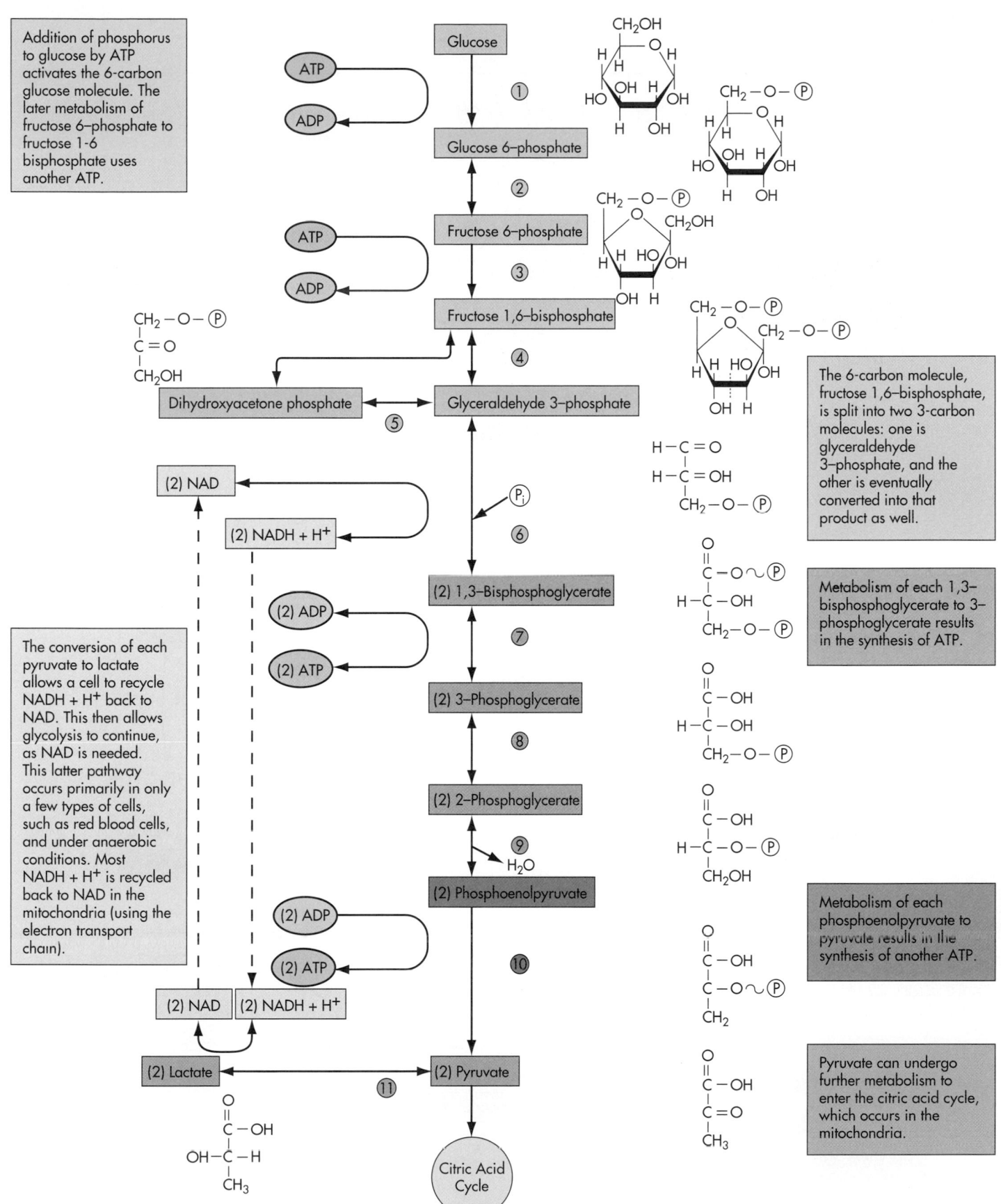

Figure B-1 | Detailed depiction of the individual chemical reactions that comprise glycolysis—glucose to pyruvate. Glycolysis takes place in the cytosol of the cell. The enzymes in the cytosol that participate at the following steps are (1) hexokinase, (2) phosphohexose isomerase, (3) phosphofructokinase, (4) aldolase, (5) phosphotriose isomerase, (6) glyceraldehyde-3-phosphate dehydrogenase, (7) phosphoglycerate kinase, (8) phosphoglycerate mutase, (9) enolase, and (10) pyruvate kinase. Sometimes (11) lactate dehydrogenase is used to recycle NADH + H$^+$ back to NAD (anaerobic glycolysis). P$_i$ represents a phosphate group.

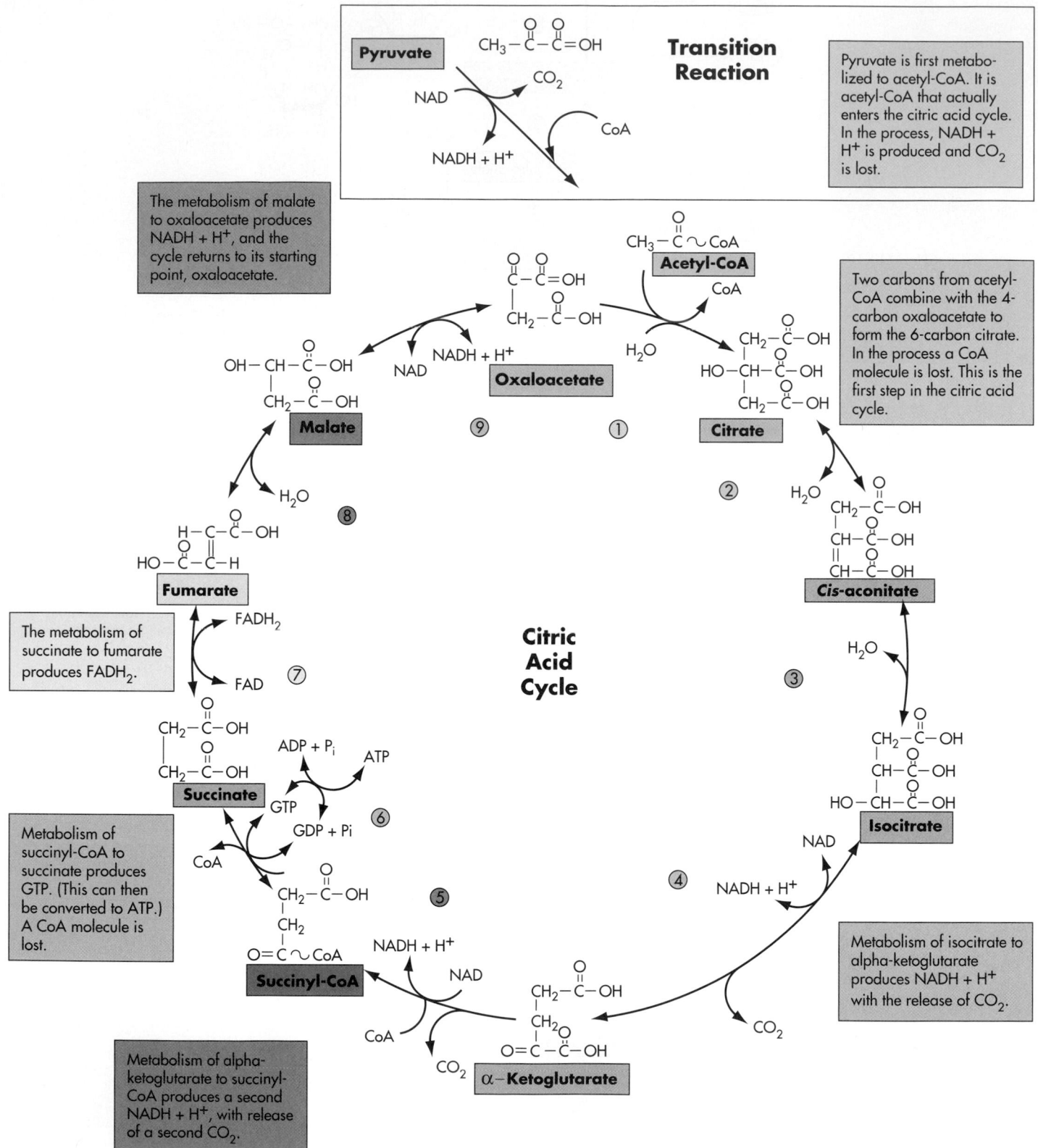

Figure B-2 | Detailed depiction of conversion of pyruvate to acetyl-CoA in the transition reaction and the individual chemical reactions of the citric acid cycle. Conversion of pyruvate to acetyl-CoA uses an enzyme complex that includes pyruvate dehydrogenase. The enzymes used in the citric acid cycle at the following steps are (1) citrate synthase, (2) aconitase, (3) aconitase, (4) isocitrate dehydrogenase, (5) alpha-ketoglutarate dehydrogenase, (6) succinate thiokinase, (7) succinate dehydrogenase, (8) fumarase, and (9) malate dehydrogenase. CoA stands for coenzyme A, which is made from the vitamin pantothenic acid (see Chapter 10 for the chemical structure). Note that the CO_2 molecules lost during one turn of the citric acid cycle are not those from the carbons donated by acetyl-CoA. Instead, the carbons are broken off the portion of the citrate molecule derived from oxaloacetate.

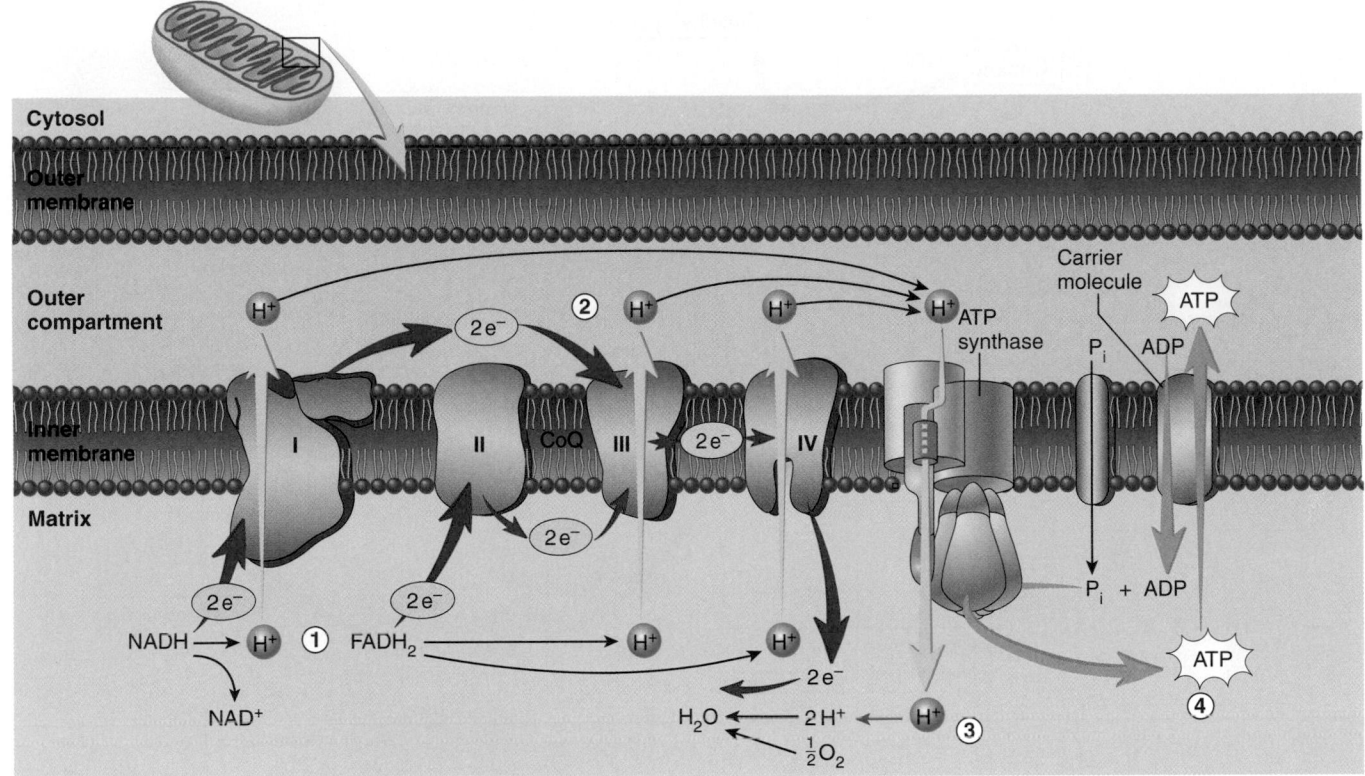

1. NADH or FADH$_2$ transfer their electrons to the electron transport chain.

2. As the electrons are separated by coenzyme Q (CoQ) and move through the electron transport chain, some of their energy is used to pump hydrogen ions into the outer compartment.

3. The hydrogen ions diffuse back into the inner compartment through special channels (ATP synthase) that couple the hydrogen ion movement with the production of ATP. The electrons, hydrogen ions, and oxygen combine to form water.

4. ATP is transported out of the inner compartment by a carrier molecule that exchanges ATP for ADP. A different carrier molecule moves phosphate into the inner compartment.

Figure B-3 | Detailed depiction of the electron-transport chain. NADH + H$^+$ and FADH$_2$ transfer their hydrogen ions and electrons to electron carriers located on the inner mitochondrial membrane. The electrons and hydrogen ions combine with oxygen to form water (H$_2$O). The energy yielded by the entire process is used to generate ATP. Each NADH+H$^+$ in the mitochondria releases enough energy to form the equivalent of 2.5 ATP, while each FADH$_2$ releases enough energy to form the equivalent of 1.5 ATP.

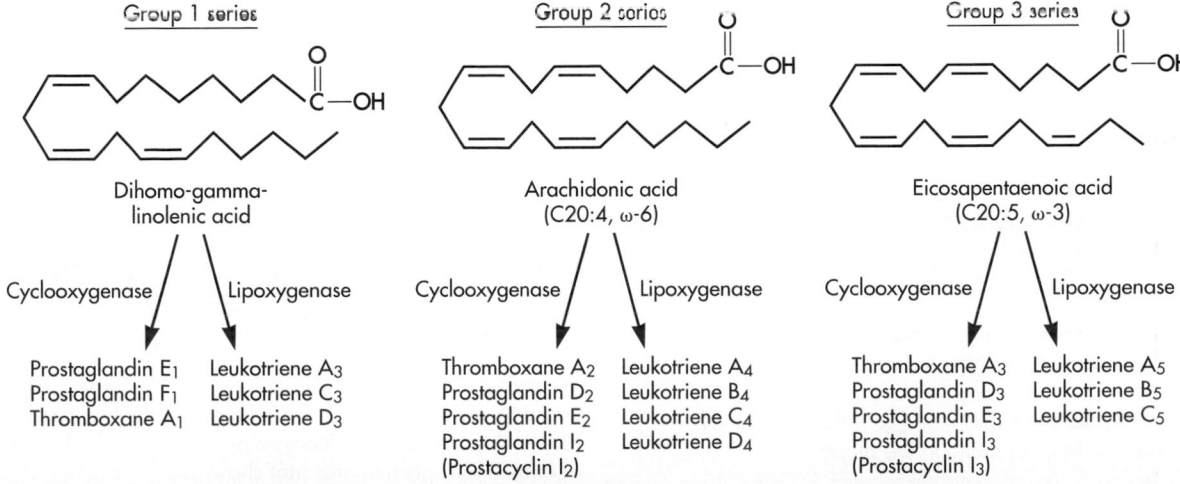

Figure B-4 | Examples of eicosanoids from the three major groups. The parent fatty acid produces profound difference in how eicosanoids across the three groups act in the body (e.g., thromboxane A$_1$ vs. A$_2$ vs. A$_3$).

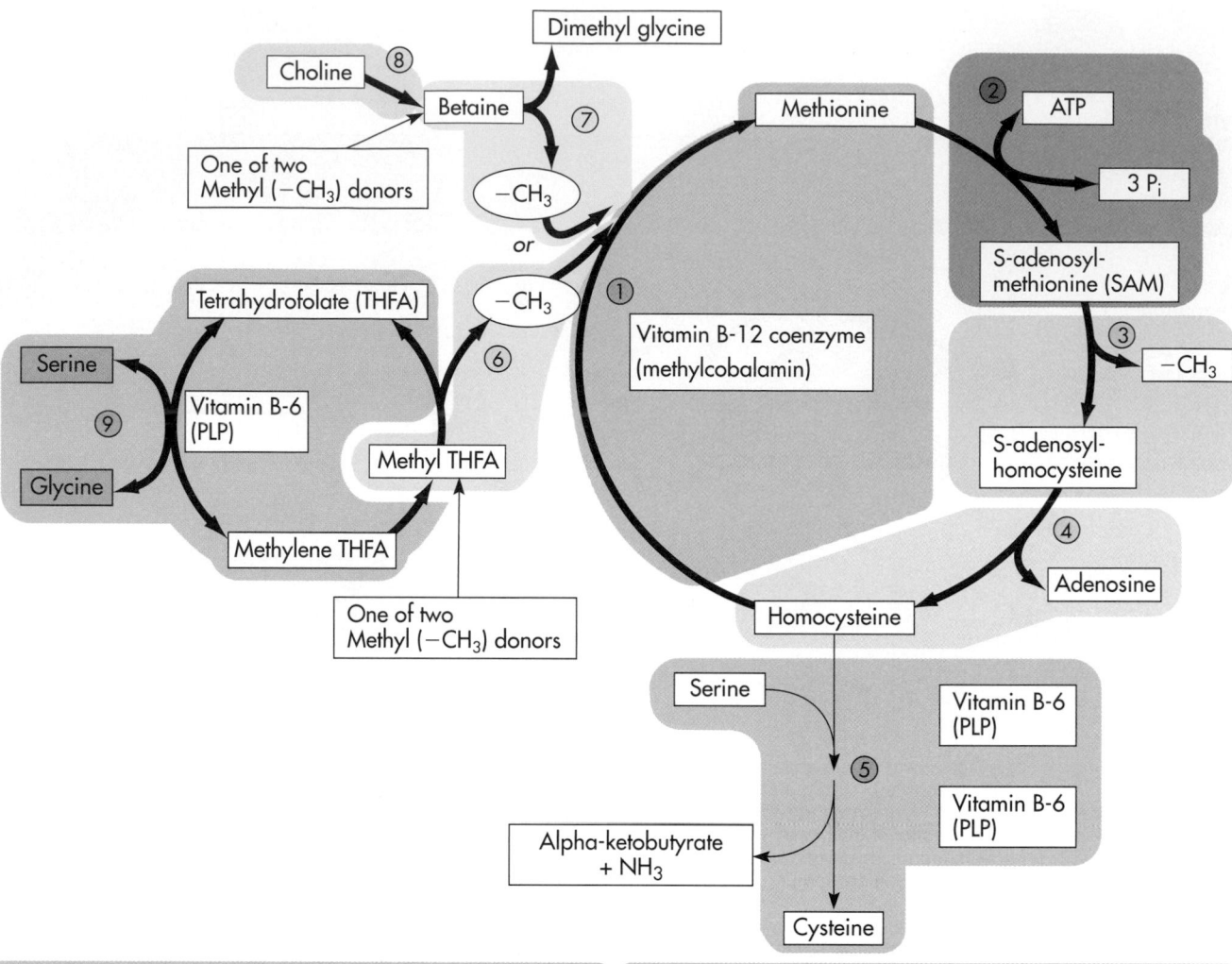

① With the aid of the vitamin B-12 coenzyme (methylcobalamin), the methyl group (−CH₃) is transferred from the folate coenzyme, methyl THFA, to homocysteine to form methionine. Another important function of this reaction is to make the resulting tetrahydrafolate coenzyme available to participate in DNA synthesis.

② Methionine can be converted to S-adenosyl-methionine (SAM) with the addition of adenosine from ATP. The three phosphate groups are removed.

③ S-adenosyl-methionine is converted to S-adenosyl homocysteine by removal of the −CH₃, which is donated to a variety of methyl group acceptors.

④ S-adenosyl homocysteine is converted back to homocysteine with the removal of adenosine.

Overall, this cycle, especially step ①, helps control the concentration of homocysteine in the blood.

⑤ With the aid of vitamin B-6 coenzyme PLP, homocysteine is used to make the nonessential amino acid cysteine. The nonessential amino acid serine contributes part of its carbon skeleton to homocysteine. This is another pathway that helps control blood homocysteine concentration.

⑥ Either methyl tetrahydrofolate or

⑦ Betaine is a donor of a methyl group to form methionine.

⑧ The betaine is derived from choline.

⑨ Note that the serine-glycine reaction is reversible in conjunction with THFA and methylene THFA. Here is another example of vitamin B-6 in action as PLP.

In summary, the coenzymes of vitamin B-12, folate, and vitamin B-6, along with choline, work together as a team to control the amount of homocysteine in the blood. The vitamin riboflavin also participates (not shown).

Figure B-5 | Detailed diagram of folate, vitamin B-12, vitamin B-6, and choline metabolism in relation to homocysteine metabolism. Note that step 9 (serine → glycine) is the major source of methyl groups for this overall pathway.

appendix C

HUMAN PHYSIOLOGY: A TOOL FOR UNDERSTANDING NUTRITION

This appendix explores the various systems in the body beyond the digestive system, focusing specifically on how these systems relate to the study of human nutrition. This focus will set the stage for investigating the various nutrients associated with human nutrition. Before that process can begin, however, it is important to review the processes taking place in a human cell.

The Cell: Structure and Function

The cell is the basic structural and functional unit of life. Living organisms are made of many different kinds of cells specialized to perform particular functions, and all cells are derived from preexisting cells. In the human body, the trillions of cells all have certain basic characteristics that are alike. All cells have compartments, particles, or filaments that perform specialized functions; these structures are called organelles. There are at least 15 different organelles, but this section discusses only eight. The numbers preceding the names of the cell structures correspond to the structures illustrated in Figure C-1.

1. Cell (Plasma) Membrane

There is an outside and inside to every cell, as defined by the cell (plasma) membrane. This membrane holds in the cellular contents and regulates the direction and flow of substances into and out of the cell. Cell-to-cell communication also occurs by way of this membrane. Some cells can even penetrate another cell membrane and so invade that cell.

The cell membrane is a lipid bilayer (or double membrane) of **phospholipids** with their water-soluble (polar) heads facing into the interior of the cell and out to the exterior of the cell. The water-insoluble (nonpolar) tails are tucked into the interior of the cell membrane (Chapter 6 reviews phospholipids in detail and Appendix A reviews the concept of polar and nonpolar compounds).

Cholesterol is a fat-soluble component of the membrane, so it is embedded within the bilayer. This cholesterol provides rigidity and thus stability to the membrane.

There are also various proteins embedded in the membrane. Proteins provide structural support, act as transport vehicles, and function as enzymes that affect chemical processes within the membrane. Some proteins are open channels that allow water-soluble substances to pass into and out of the cell. Proteins on the outside surface of the membrane act as receptors, snagging essential substances the cell needs and drawing them into the cell. Other proteins act as gates, opening and closing to control the flow of various particles into and out of the cell.

> **phospholipid** Any of a class of fat-related substances that contain phosphorus, fatty acids, and a nitrogen-containing base. The phospholipids are an essential part of every cell.

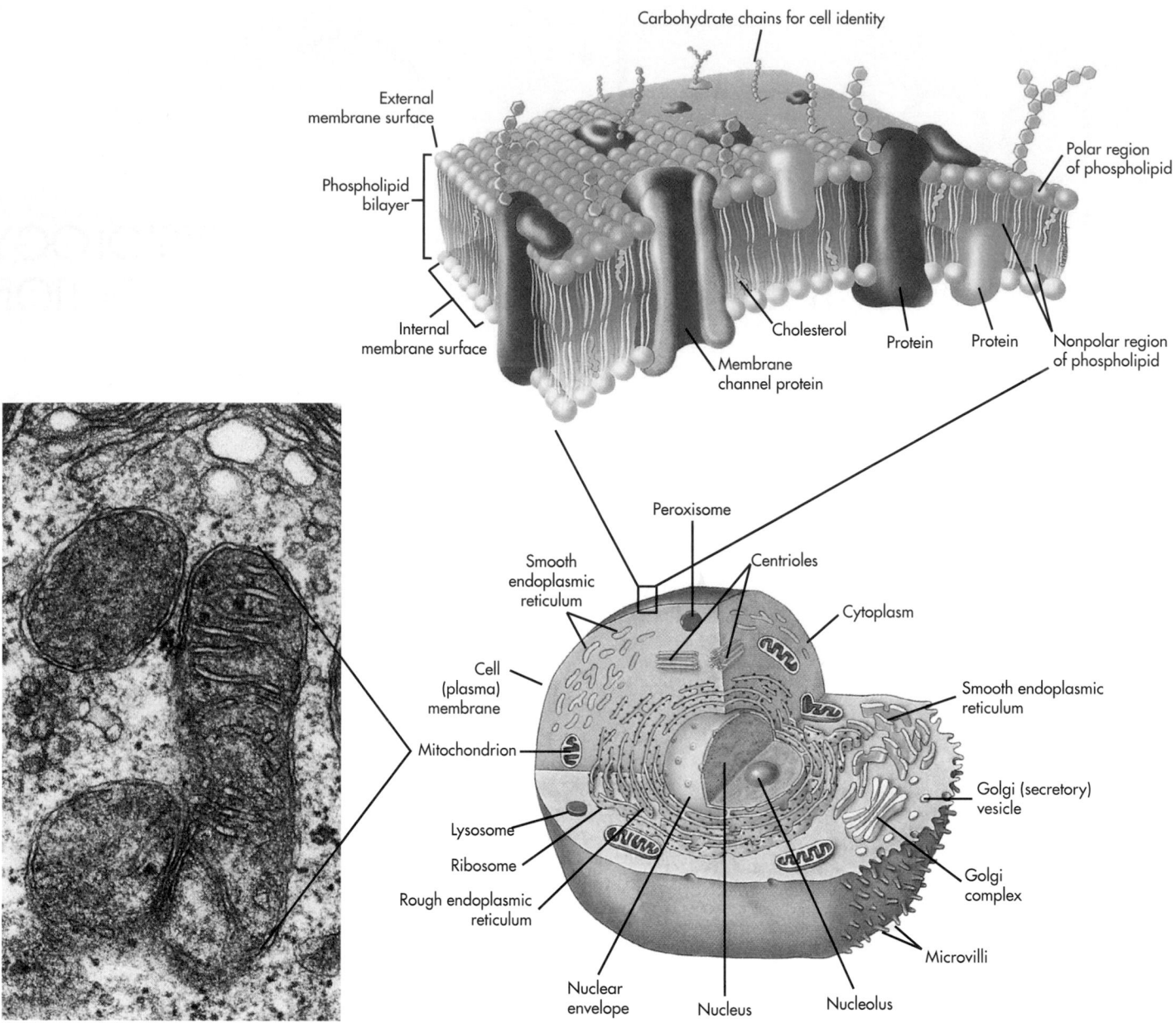

Figure C-1 | An animal cell. Almost all human cells contain these various organelles. Shown in greater detail are mitochondria and the cell membrane. Note: Not all cells have microvilli. The nuclear envelope encloses the nucleus. The centrioles participate in cell division.

glycocalyx Projections of proteins on the microvilli; they contain enzymes to digest protein and carbohydrate.

organelles Compartments, particles, or filaments that perform specialized functions within a cell.

In addition to the lipid and protein, the membrane also contains carbohydrates that mark the exterior of the cell, called the **glycocalyx.** These carbohydrates are combined either with proteins or fats and provide a delivery service for sending messages to the cell's organelles. The structures also provide distinct identification for a cell. In addition, they detect invaders and initiate defensive actions. In sum, these carbohydrates provide tags that are important to cellular identity and interaction.

Included within the cell membrane are **organelles.** They carry out vital roles in cell functions. Some structures allow the cell to replicate itself, others provide energy, and others destroy the cell when it is worn out. Still other organelles produce and secrete products destined for other cells.

2. Cytoplasm

The **cytoplasm** is the fluid material and organelles within the cell, not including the nucleus. (The **cytosol** is the fluid surrounding the organelles.) A small amount of ATP energy for use by the cell can be produced by glycolysis reactions that occur in the cytoplasm. This contributes to our survival, because it is the key process in red blood cell energy metabolism; it is called anaerobic metabolism because it doesn't require oxygen.

3. Mitochondria

Mitochondria are sometimes called "power plants," or the powerhouse of the cell. These organelles are capable of converting the energy in our energy-yielding nutrients (carbohydrate, protein, and fat) to a form that cells can use, again ATP. This is an aerobic process that uses the oxygen we inhale, and water, enzymes, and other compounds (see Chapter 4 for details). With the exception of red blood cells, all cells contain mitochondria; only the size, shape, and numbers vary.

Mitochondria have a double membrane and this characteristic is key to overall mitochondrial function. Within the inner membrane, the electron transport chain and ATP synthesis take place. In the inner matrix of the mitochondria, the citric acid cycle, B-oxidation of fatty acids, and the transition reaction involving pyruvate take place.

The biochemical pathways that operate in the mitochondrial matrix are also capable of synthesizing cell components, such as the **carbon skeletons** needed to produce amino acids. These will eventually become cellular protein.

4. Cell Nucleus

The **cell nucleus** is surrounded by its own double membrane. The nucleus controls actions that occur in the cell, using the hereditary material known as deoxyribonucleic acid (DNA). DNA is the "code book" that contains directions for making substances the cell needs. It consists of genes on **chromosomes.** This code book remains in the nucleus of the cell, but conveys its information to other cell organelles by way of a similar molecule called **ribonucleic acid (RNA).** The RNA has the responsibility of *transcribing* the information of the DNA and moving out through pores in the nuclear membrane to the cytoplasm. The RNA then carries the code to protein-synthesizing sites called **ribosomes.** There, the RNA code is *translated* into a specific protein (see Chapter 7 for details on protein synthesis). With the exception of the red blood cell, all cells have one or more nuclei.

The **nucleoli** are areas within the nucleus of the cell containing a combination of protein and RNA. This is where RNA is produced for export to the cytoplasm.

DNA has the secondary task of cell replication. DNA is a double-stranded molecule, and when the cell begins to divide, each strand is separated and an identical copy of each is made. Thus, each new DNA molecule contains one new strand of DNA and one strand from the original DNA. In this way, the genetic code is preserved from one cell generation to the next. The mitochondria contain their own DNA, so they reproduce themselves independently of the nucleus.

The transport of proteins, vitamins, and other material from the cytoplasm to the nucleus also occurs through pores in the nuclear membrane, as just mentioned. These small molecules serve a variety of functions, including the activation (or inactivation) of certain parts of the DNA.

5. Endoplasmic Reticulum (ER)

The outer membrane of the cell nucleus is continuous with a network of tubes called the **endoplasmic reticulum (ER).** The ER is found in two types: rough and smooth. The rough endoplasmic reticulum has ribosomes bound to it, whereas the smooth does not. As noted earlier, ribosomes are the sites where proteins are synthesized.

---

cytoplasm The fluid and organelles (except the nucleus) in a cell.

cytosol The water-based phase of the cytoplasm; excludes organelles such as mitochondria.

mitochondria The main sites of energy production in a cell. They also contain the pathway for oxidizing fat for fuel, among other metabolic pathways.

carbon skeleton What remains of an amino acid after the amino group has been removed.

cell nucleus An organelle bound by its own double membrane and containing chromosomes, the genetic information for cell protein synthesis.

chromosome A single, large DNA molecule and its associated proteins containing many genes; stores and transmits genetic information.

ribonucleic acid (RNA) The single-stranded nucleic acid involved in the transcription of genetic information and translation of that information into protein structure.

ribosomes Cytoplasmic particles that mediate the linking together of amino acids to form proteins; attached to endoplasmic reticulum as bound ribosomes, or suspended in cytoplasm as free ribosomes.

nucleolus Center for production of ribosomes within the cell nucleus.

endoplasmic reticulum (ER) An organelle in the cytoplasm composed of a network of canals running through the cytoplasm. Rough ER contains ribosomes. Smooth ER contains no ribosomes.

Many of these proteins play a central role in human nutrition. The smooth ER is involved in lipid synthesis, detoxification of toxic substances, and calcium storage and release in the cell.

6. Golgi Complex

Golgi complex The cell organelle near the nucleus that processes newly synthesized protein for secretion or distribution to other organelles.

secretory vesicles Membrane-bound vesicles produced by the Golgi apparatus; contain proteins and other compounds to be secreted by the cell.

lysosome A cell organelle that contains digestive enzymes for use inside the cell for turnover of cell parts.

apoptosis A process that occurs over time in which enzymes in a cell set off a series of events that disable numerous cell functions, eventually leading to cell death.

peroxisome Cell organelle that uses oxygen to remove hydrogens from compounds. This produces hydrogen peroxide (H_2O_2), which breaks down into O_2 and H_2O.

hydrogen peroxide Chemically, H_2O_2.

The **Golgi complex** is a packaging site for proteins and lipids that are used in the cytoplasm or exported from the cell. The Golgi complex consists of sacs within the cytoplasm in which products of the rough endoplasmic reticulum are received, processed, separated according to function and destination, and "packaged" in **secretory vesicles** for secretion by the cell.

7. Lysosomes

Lysosomes are the cell's digestive system. They are sacs that contain enzymes for the digestion of foreign material. Sometimes known as "suicide bags," they are responsible for digesting worn-out or damaged cells. They carry out **apoptosis,** or programmed cell death, which occurs naturally or is associated with illness or infections. Certain cells that are associated with immunity contain many lysosomes.

8. Peroxisomes

Peroxisomes contain enzymes that detoxify harmful chemicals. **Hydrogen peroxide** (H_2O_2) is formed as a result of such enzyme action. Peroxisomes contain a protective enzyme called *catalase,* which prevents excessive accumulation of hydrogen peroxide in the cell, which would be very damaging. Peroxisomes also play a minor role in metabolizing one possible source of energy for cells—alcohol.

The remainder of this appendix looks at the body systems. Keep in mind that these systems depend on the cell functions just discussed.

Integumentary System

integumentary Having to do with the skin, hair, glands, and nails; the largest organ in the body.

epidermis The outermost layer of the skin, composed of epithelial layers.

dermis The second, or deep, layer of the skin, under the epidermis.

decubitus ulcers Chronic ulcers (also called bedsores) that appear in pressure areas of the skin over a body prominence. These sores develop when people are confined to bed or immobilized.

The first system to examine is the one you are most familiar with, the **integumentary** system, which is made up of dissimilar elements, such as the skin, hair, various glands, and nails. The largest organ in the body, the skin, consists of two principal layers, the **epidermis** and the **dermis** (Figure C-2). The epidermis is the layer of skin composed largely of dead cells, which are used for protection from environmental pathogens, toxins, injury, and water. We don't want to absorb water through the skin, nor do we want water to readily escape the body.

The dermis is a deeper and thicker layer of skin, with an extensive network of blood vessels, sweat glands, oil-secreting glands, nerve endings, and hair follicles. When people are confined to bed for long periods of time, **decubitus ulcers,** also called bedsores, may develop because of restricted blood flow to the dermis. This lack of blood causes cells to die and open wounds to develop—a potentially life-threatening situation. Adequate intakes of protein, vitamin A, vitamin C, and zinc intake may help prevent this problem.

The appearance of the skin, hair, and nails is clinically important because it can indicate nutritional deficiencies. For instance, hot, dry skin is an obvious sign of dehydration due to inadequate water intake. (Other signs and symptoms of nutrient deficiencies, as manifested by the skin, are described in Chapters 5, 6, 7, 9, 10, 11, and 12 as the functions of individual nutrients are explained.)

The skin plays a vital role in temperature regulation. Heat produced by the body's metabolic processes, especially the processes that occur in muscle, must be removed before cells are damaged. Heat is removed from the body through the skin. And when we are cold, we warm ourselves by shivering, because muscle contractions generate heat.

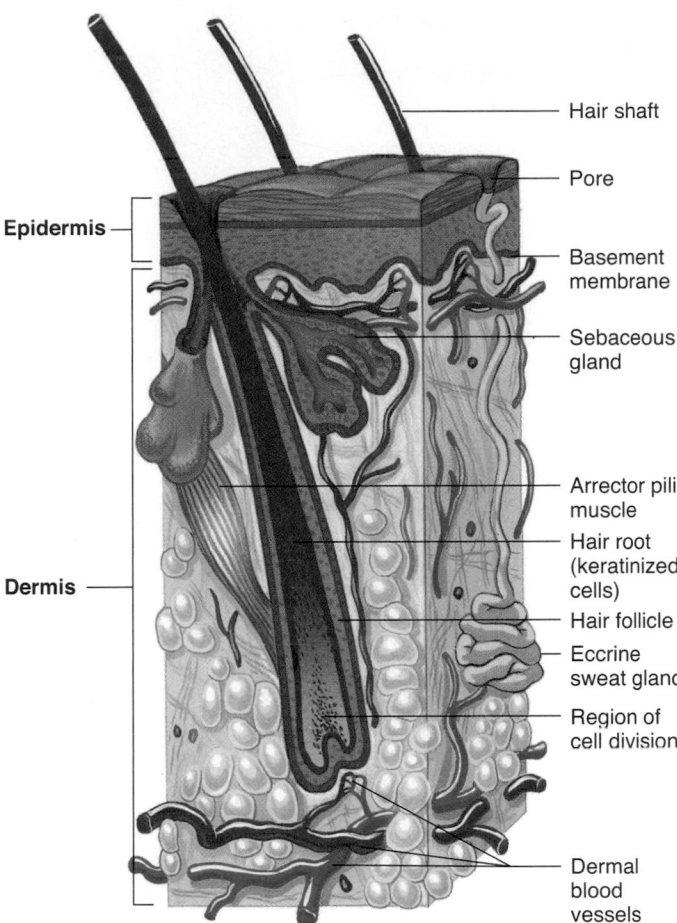

Figure C-2 | Cross-section of the skin. This is the major organ of the integumentary system.

Hair shaft

Pore

Epidermis

Basement membrane

Sebaceous gland

Arrector pili muscle

Dermis

Hair root (keratinized cells)

Hair follicle

Eccrine sweat gland

Region of cell division

Dermal blood vessels

An important nutrient, vitamin D, can be obtained from our diet, but the skin can also make it from a cholesterol derivative located in the skin. There is more detail about this process in Chapter 9.

The sweat glands produce perspiration, or sweat, which helps evaporate fluids to cool the body and excrete certain wastes. Mammary glands within the breasts are modified sweat glands designed to secrete milk to feed a newborn.

Skeletal System

Approximately 206 bones make up the skeletal system; this is the rigid framework to which the soft tissues and organs of the body are attached. Each bone is an organ that participates in the overall functioning of the skeleton. Bones that make up the skull and vertebral column protect the brain and spinal cord from injury. Likewise, the rib cage protects the heart, lungs, liver, and spleen from external damage. Bones have attachment sites for skeletal muscles, ligaments, and tendons. (Bones attached to muscles allow body movement when muscles contract.) Blood cell formation, known as **hematopoiesis,** takes place within the marrow of some bones. Bones also are a storehouse for minerals such as calcium, phosphorus, magnesium, sodium, and fluoride. Rather than being considered dried, dead tissues, bones are metabolically active and constantly adapting to a changing environment.

Long bones, such as those found in the arms and legs, consist of two types of body tissue: cortical and trabecular (Figure C-3). **Cortical bone** is hard and dense. It forms a protective shell on the exterior of the bone. **Trabecular bone** is found within the

hematopoiesis The production of blood cells.

cortical bone Dense, compact bone that constitutes the outer surface and shafts of bone; also called compact bone. Cortical bone makes up 75 to 80% of total bone mass.

trabecular bone The spongy, inner matrix of bone found primarily in the spine, pelvis, and ends of bones; also called cancellous bone. Trabecular bone makes up 20 to 25% of total bone mass.

Figure C-3 | Diagram of a long bone. The epiphysis, consisting of trabecular bone, is surrounded by a layer of cortical bone. The epiphyseal line indicates that the bone has completed growth. The production of blood cells occurs in the porous chambers of trabecular bone. The collagen material, the structural material of bone, is observed by the open flap. The skeletal system provides a reserve of calcium and phosphorus for day-to-day needs when dietary intake is inadequate.

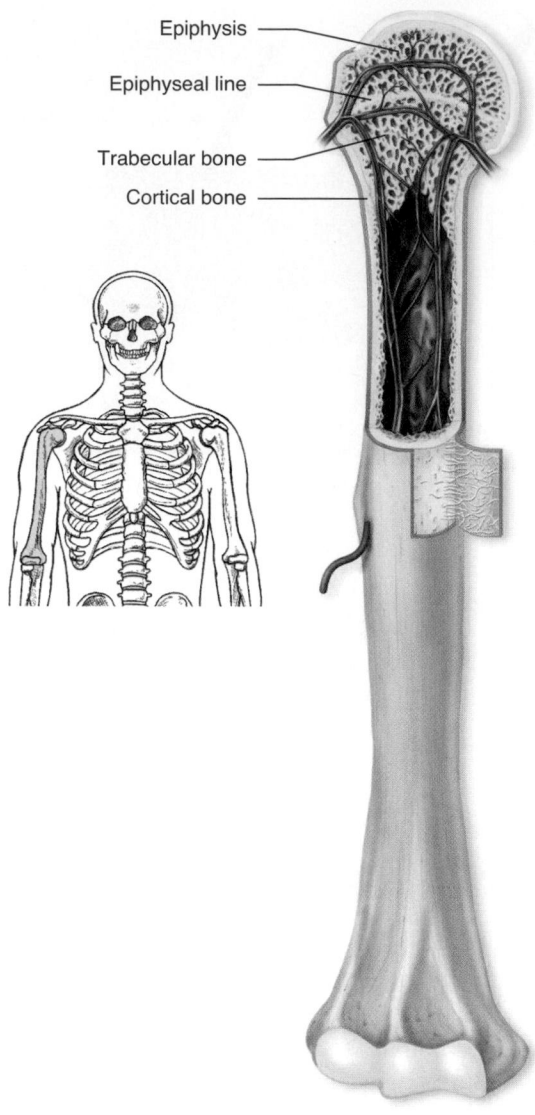

Epiphysis

Epiphyseal line

Trabecular bone

Cortical bone

epiphysis The end of a long bone. The epiphyseal plate—sometimes referred to as the growth plate—is made of cartilage and allows growth of the bone to occur. During childhood, the cartilage cells multiply and absorb calcium to develop into bone.

epiphyseal plate A cartilage-like layer in the long bone. It functions in linear growth.

epiphyseal line A line that replaces the epiphyseal plate when bone growth is complete.

collagen The major protein of the material that holds together the various structures of the body.

hydroxyapatite A compound, composed primarily of calcium and phosphate, that is deposited into the bone protein matrix to give bone strength and rigidity $(Ca_{10}[PO_4]_6OH_2)$.

cortical bone at the ends of long bones and in the vertebrae. The shaft of the long bones is a cylinder of cortical bone surrounding a central cavity containing the marrow (review Chapter 11).

At the end of the long bone is the **epiphysis,** consisting of trabecular bone covered by cortical bone. The epiphysis is strong and allows for the attachment of tendons and ligaments. Red bone marrow is made of trabecular bone and is the source of red blood cells as well as white blood cells and platelets. In children, just behind the epiphysis is the **epiphyseal plate.** This area of bone is responsible for linear growth. When linear growth is complete, an **epiphyseal line** replaces the plate.

Bones are constructed from several types of cells under the influence of a variety of growth factors. These factors stimulate the formation of **collagen,** a type of flexible protein matrix, which forms the basic shape of bone. Minerals—principally, calcium and phosphorus—are embedded in the matrix, which give the bone strength. **Hydroxyapatite,** the name of the calcium phosphorus salt deposited in the protein matrix, constitutes about 85% of minerals in bone and makes it possible for the bone to resist compression and bending.

Calcification (also called ossification) of bone varies from bone to bone, but most bones mature (are ossified) by ages 17 to 25. However, some bones, such as the sternum (breast bone), may not complete growth until age 30-plus years.

Bone is constantly **remodeled** throughout life. Formation and **resorption** of bone occur because of the continual activity of **osteoblasts** and **osteoclasts.** Osteoblasts are bone-building cells and osteoclasts are bone resorbing cells. In the first 20 or so years of life, bone formation is greater than resorption. By age 50 or 60, resorption is greater than deposition and bone diseases are likely to occur. Exercise promotes bone deposition, whereas a lack of exercise results in bone loss.

Bone deposition (ossification) and bone resorption (dissolution) also maintain homeostasis of calcium and phosphorus in the blood. Three hormones control the process: the vitamin D hormone ($1,25(OH)_2$ vitamin D or calcitriol), calcitonin, and parathyroid hormone (PTH).

Other hormones are involved in bone maintenance, such as growth hormone; thyroid hormones; sex hormones, especially estrogen; and adrenocorticoid hormones. In addition, vitamins A, K, and C perform important jobs in bone metabolism. More information about bones can be found in Chapters 9, 10, 11, and 14, which cover vitamins, minerals, and exercise.

Muscular System

The functions of the muscular system are to provide movement and to generate body heat. Most of the energy released by a muscle cell during physical exercise is in the form of heat. **Muscle fibers** respond when stimulated by motor **neurons** (nerve cells). A muscle cell converts the chemical energy in ATP into the mechanical energy of muscle contraction.

There are three types of muscle tissue: **smooth, cardiac,** and **skeletal.** Smooth muscle fibers have a single nucleus and function in involuntary movements within internal organs. Cardiac muscle fiber is **striated** (striped) with a single nucleus. The stripes in muscle fibers are caused by the arrangement of alternating dark and light contractile proteins (**myosin** and **actin**). This type of muscle performs the involuntary rhythmic contractions of the heart. Skeletal muscle, also containing striated muscle fibers, has several nuclei and is involved in voluntary movements. Skeletal muscle is attached to bone by **tendons.** (Note that Chapter 14 also discusses some specific muscle fiber types.)

Skeletal Muscle

Skeletal muscle fibers are actually long cells with the same organelles that are found in other cells. However, unlike most other cells, skeletal muscle cells possess an excellent supply of fuel in the form of glycogen, the body's storage form of the sugar glucose.

Skeletal muscles contract when stimulated by motor neurons. Motor neurons can stimulate several muscle fibers simultaneously. A single muscle fiber is not a very efficient machine. The activation of numerous muscle fibers by multiple motor neurons results in increased muscle strength as the number of fibers stimulated by neurons increases.

Muscle Contraction

As previously mentioned, within muscle fibers are the dark and light stripes called striations. Each muscle cell, when viewed in the electron microscope, contains subunits called **myofibrils.** The myofibrils are the source of the light and dark bands or stripes. The importance of these structures is the presence of unique proteins, actin and myosin. The functioning structure of the myofibril is the **sarcomere,** the contracting unit.

When a muscle fiber is stimulated by a neuron to contract, one of the first events to occur is the release of large amounts of calcium from storage in the smooth endoplasmic reticulum (also called sarcoplasmic reticulum). This is the "on" switch. The presence of calcium allows the two main proteins, myosin and actin, to get ready to slide into each other and set the **power stroke** in motion. Of course, energy is required to carry out the muscle contraction. Here is where ATP plays the key role (Figure C-4).

remodeling The constant building and breakdown of bone throughout life.

resorption The loss of a substance by physiologic or pathologic means.

osteoblasts Cells in bone that secrete mineral and bone matrix.

osteoclasts Bone cells that arise originally from a type of white blood cell. Osteoclasts secrete substances that lead to bone erosion. This erosion can set the stage for subsequent bone mineralization.

muscle fiber Component of a muscle cell.

neuron The structural and functional unit of the nervous system, consisting of cell body, dendrites, and axon.

smooth muscle Muscle tissue under involuntary control; found in the GI tract, artery walls, respiratory passages, the urinary tract, and the reproductive tract.

cardiac muscle Muscle tissue that makes up the walls of the heart; produces rhythmical involuntary contractions.

skeletal muscle Muscle tissue responsible for voluntary body movements.

myosin A thick filament protein that connects with actin to cause a muscle contraction.

actin A protein in muscle fiber that, together with myosin, is responsible for contraction.

tendon Dense connective tissue that attaches a muscle to a bone.

myofibrils A bundle of contractile fibers within a muscle cell.

sarcomere A portion of a muscle fiber that is considered the functional unit of a myofibril.

power stroke Movement of the thick filament alongside the thin filament in a muscle cell, causing muscle contraction.

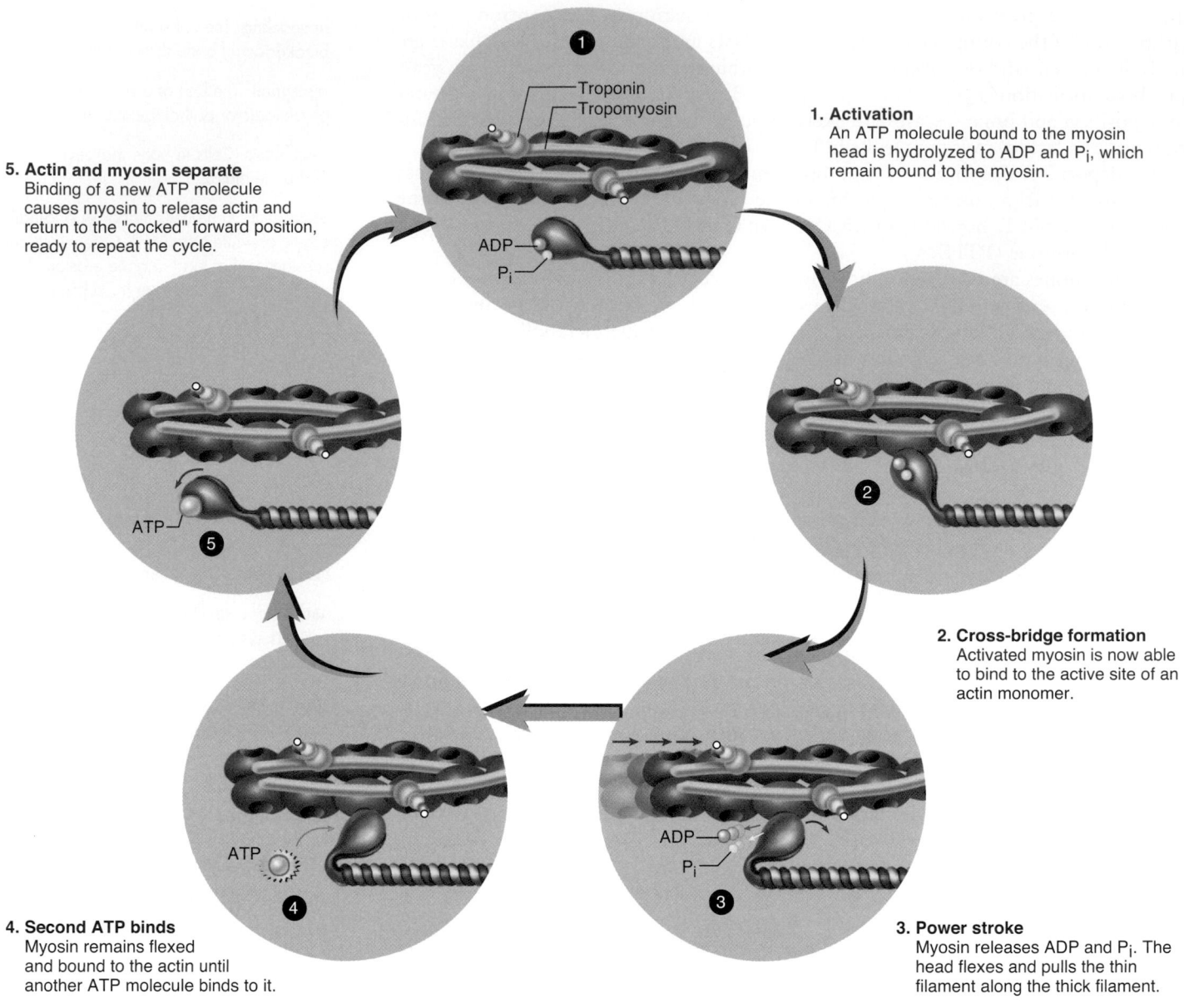

1. Activation
An ATP molecule bound to the myosin head is hydrolyzed to ADP and P_i, which remain bound to the myosin.

5. Actin and myosin separate
Binding of a new ATP molecule causes myosin to release actin and return to the "cocked" forward position, ready to repeat the cycle.

2. Cross-bridge formation
Activated myosin is now able to bind to the active site of an actin monomer.

4. Second ATP binds
Myosin remains flexed and bound to the actin until another ATP molecule binds to it.

3. Power stroke
Myosin releases ADP and P_i. The head flexes and pulls the thin filament along the thick filament.

Figure C-4 | Muscle contraction. In Step 1, or activation, an ATP is bound to the myosin head (purple) and is split into ADP and P_i. Troponin and tropomyosin are proteins that participate in this process. During Step 2, the activated myosin can now bind to the actin (the red beads). In Step 3, the myosin head releases the ADP and P_i. The head flexes and pulls the thin filament along the thick filament. This is the *power stroke*. In Step 4, the myosin remains bound to the actin until another ATP binds to the myosin. The new ATP causes the myosin to release the actin, so that it can get ready for another cycle, Step 5. Actin and myosin separate, which leads to muscle relaxation. The white dot in this figure is calcium, a nutrient required for muscle action.

Another ATP is needed to release the actin from the myosin. This is the end of the contraction. As the muscle moves to the "off" position the calcium is transported back to storage, the muscle fiber relaxes, and it gets ready for another contraction.

The reason that muscle action occurs at all is due to the essential nutrient calcium. When the muscle is relaxed, there is very little calcium in the cytoplasm of the muscle cell because calcium is in storage. However, when the muscle is ready to go to work, as directed by the motor neuron, calcium is moved out of storage, which sets the stage for the power stroke. And, when the contraction ends, the calcium is released from the muscle fibers and goes back into storage.

Cardiac and Smooth Muscle

Cardiac muscle and smooth muscle, although similar in many ways to skeletal muscle in their use of calcium as an off/on switch, operate under involuntary control.

In cardiac muscle, the stimulation occurs automatically by a group of muscle cells. These cells initiate the heartbeat and set the heart rate under control of the brain and the influence of certain hormones.

Smooth muscles are found in the lungs, blood vessels, GI tract, and other internal organs. In the GI tract, they produce important contractions in peristalsis (see Chapter 3 for details).

Circulatory System

The circulatory system is made up of two separate systems: the cardiovascular system and the lymphatic system. The cardiovascular system consists of the heart and blood vessels. The lymphatic system consists of lymphatic vessels, lymph, and a number of lymph tissues.

One organ vital to our existence is the heart, a four-chambered pump that keeps blood continuously circulating around the body. It takes about 1 minute for blood to leave the heart, circulate to all tissues in the body, and return to the heart. When we are exercising strenuously, the blood can circulate at a rate of six times per minute.

The cells that make up the tissues of the body need a constant supply of water, oxygen, and nutrients. In addition, the body needs ATP energy, which in turn comes from the breakdown of energy nutrients within the cells. The blood carries oxygen from the lungs to all organs in the body. The blood also carries nutrients from the digestive tract to all tissues and to storage sites when nutrients are not needed immediately for energy, growth, or repair. Waste materials produced by cells must be removed by way of the skin, lungs, kidneys, and digestive tract. This, too, is a function of the cardiovascular system. The delivery of hormones to their target cells, the maintenance of a constant body temperature, and the distribution of white blood cells to protect against invading pathogens are all performed by the blood and circulatory systems without our ever being aware of any specific action. The circulatory system has chemical means to prevent excessive loss of blood from damaged vessels. It uses the clotting process (see Chapter 9).

Blood Constituents

Red blood cells, known as **erythrocytes,** are carriers of oxygen to all tissues and play a role in the return of carbon dioxide to the lungs. The white blood cells, known as **leukocytes,** function as part of the immune system. They protect the body from invading pathogens. The blood is able to clot because of platelets and other clotting factors. The liquid part of blood is known as **plasma.** In contrast, **serum** is the fluid that results after the blood is first allowed to clot before being centrifuged; this will not contain the blood-clotting factors.

Heart Structure

The heart has two sides, left and right. The right side is closest to your right arm; likewise, the left side is closest to your left arm. The upper part of the heart has left and right **atria,** which empty simultaneously into the lower part of the heart, the left and right **ventricles.**

Blood travels in blood vessels from the left side of the heart, through the **aorta** to major **arteries.** Arteries become smaller and smaller until they are so tiny they are classified as **arterioles.** The blood flows from the arterioles into microscopic, weblike structures called **capillaries.** Capillaries are just one cell layer thick and have pores that

A unique feature of smooth muscle is its ability to stretch. By the end of pregnancy, the smooth muscle in the uterus can be stretched up to eight times its prepregnant length.

erythrocyte A mature red blood cell. It has no nucleus and a life span of about 120 days; contains hemoglobin, which transports oxygen and carbon dioxide.

leukocyte A white blood cell.

plasma The fluid, noncellular portion of the circulating blood. This includes the blood serum plus all blood-clotting factors. In contrast, serum is the fluid that results after the blood is first allowed to clot before being centrifuged; this does not contain the blood-clotting factors.

serum The portion of the blood fluid remaining after (1) the blood is allowed to clot and (2) the red and white blood cells and other solid matter are removed by centrifugation.

atria The two upper chambers of the heart, which receive venous blood.

ventricles The two lower chambers of the heart, which contain blood to be pumped from the heart.

aorta The major blood vessel of the body leaving from the left ventricle.

artery A blood vessel that carries blood away from the heart.

capillary A microscopic blood vessel that connects an arteriole and a venule; the functional unit of the circulatory system.

vein A blood vessel that conveys blood to the heart.

systemic circuit The part of the circulatory system concerned with the flow of blood from the left ventricle to the body and back to the right atrium.

venule A tiny vessel that carries blood from the capillary to a vein.

allow oxygen, water, and other nutrients to leave the blood for surrounding cells and that allow waste and other products of cellular metabolism to enter the blood. There are few cells in the body that aren't close to a capillary. Larger blood vessels are not porous, so blood cannot escape these vessels. Only in the capillaries can the blood discharge and recover substances associated with nearby cells.

As the blood exits the capillaries, it flows into tiny **venules,** which enlarge and become **veins,** returning the blood to the right side of the heart. The route from the left side of the heart to the capillaries and then back to the right side of the heart is called the **systemic circuit** of blood (Figures C-5, C-6 and C-7).

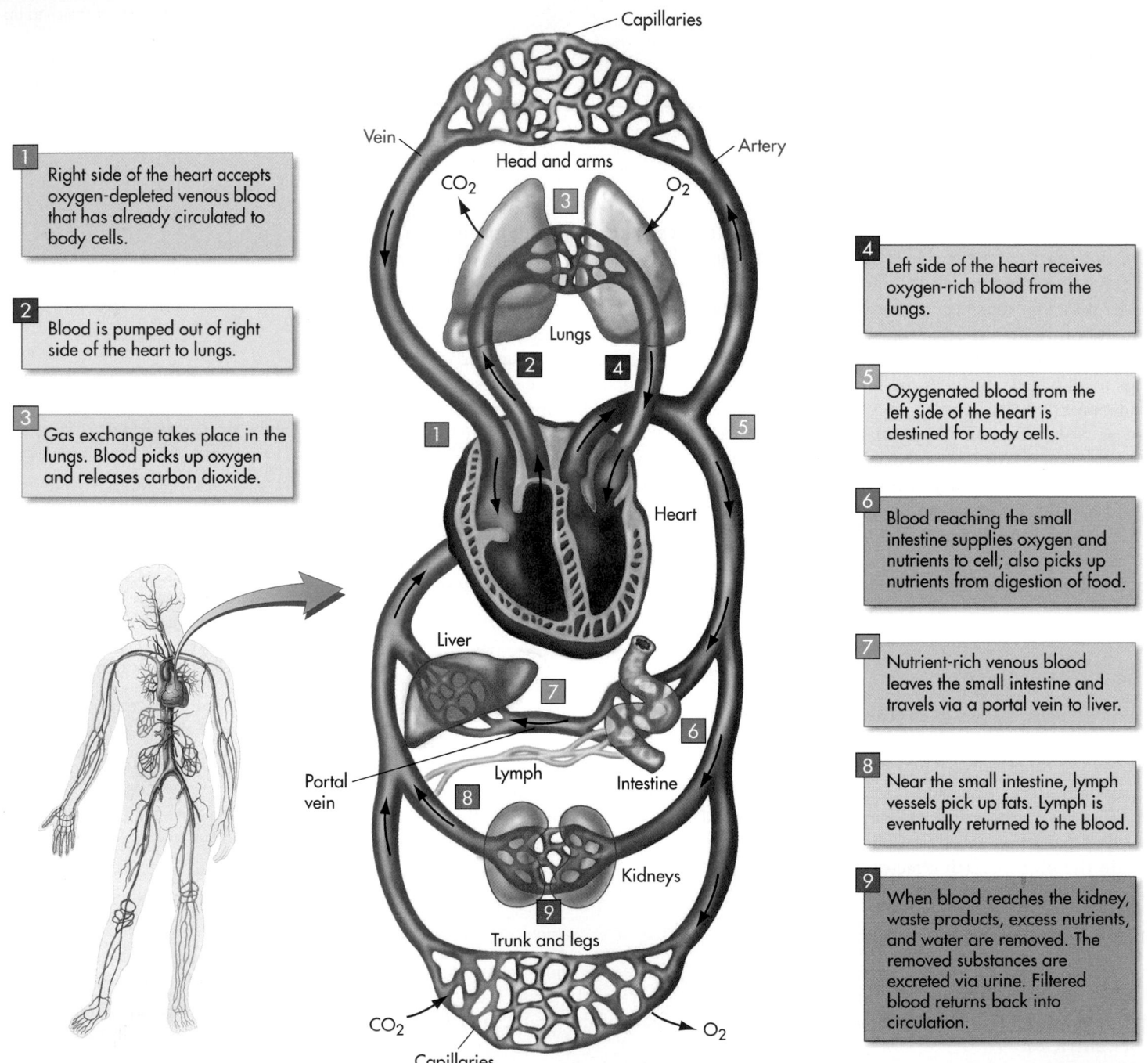

1. Right side of the heart accepts oxygen-depleted venous blood that has already circulated to body cells.

2. Blood is pumped out of right side of the heart to lungs.

3. Gas exchange takes place in the lungs. Blood picks up oxygen and releases carbon dioxide.

4. Left side of the heart receives oxygen-rich blood from the lungs.

5. Oxygenated blood from the left side of the heart is destined for body cells.

6. Blood reaching the small intestine supplies oxygen and nutrients to cell; also picks up nutrients from digestion of food.

7. Nutrient-rich venous blood leaves the small intestine and travels via a portal vein to liver.

8. Near the small intestine, lymph vessels pick up fats. Lymph is eventually returned to the blood.

9. When blood reaches the kidney, waste products, excess nutrients, and water are removed. The removed substances are excreted via urine. Filtered blood returns back into circulation.

Figure C-5 | Blood circulation through the body. This figure shows the paths that blood takes from the heart to the lungs (Steps 1–3), back to the heart (Step 4), and through the rest of the body (Steps 5–9). The red color indicates blood that is richer in oxygen; blue is for blood carrying more carbon dioxide. Keep in mind that arteries and veins go to all parts of the body.

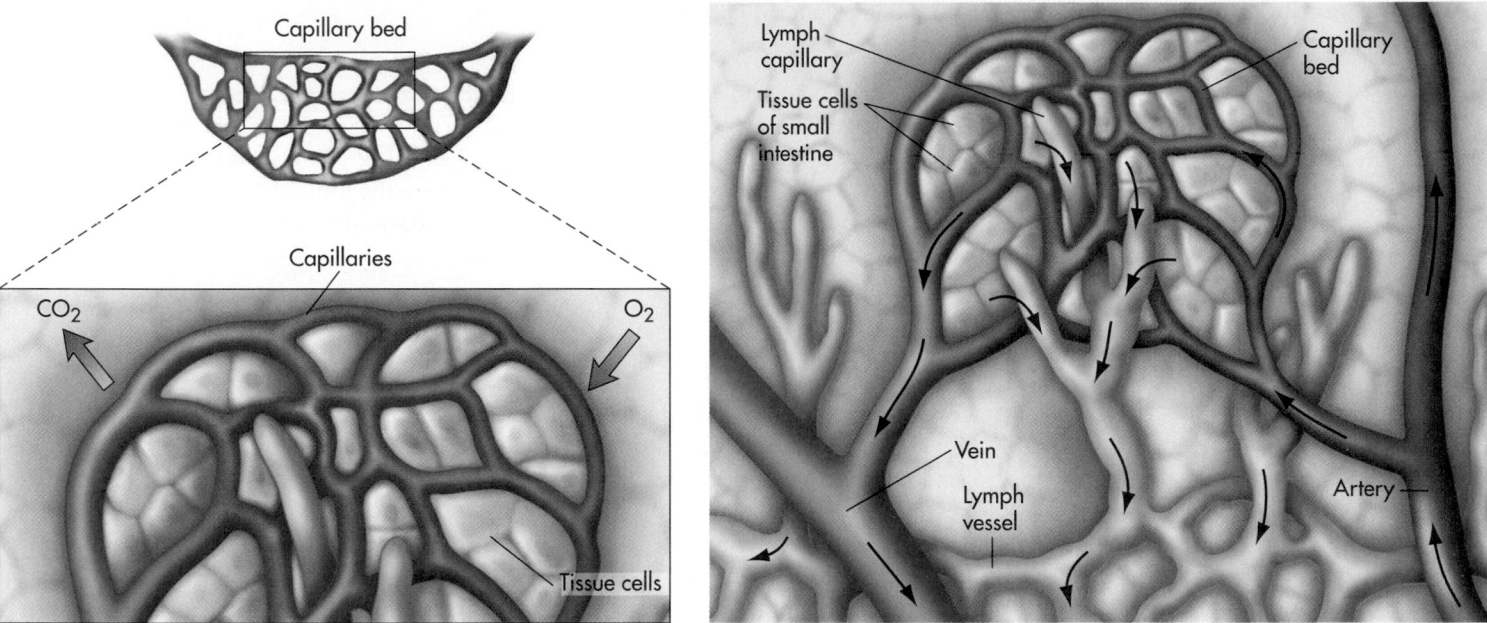

Figure C-6 | Capillary and lymph vessels. (*a*) Exchange of oxygen and nutrients for carbon dioxide and waste products occurs between the capillaries and the surrounding tissue cells. (*b*) Lymph vessels are also present in capillary beds, such as in the small intestine. Lymph vessels in the small intestine are also called **lacteals.** Note that the lymph vessels are blind-ended.

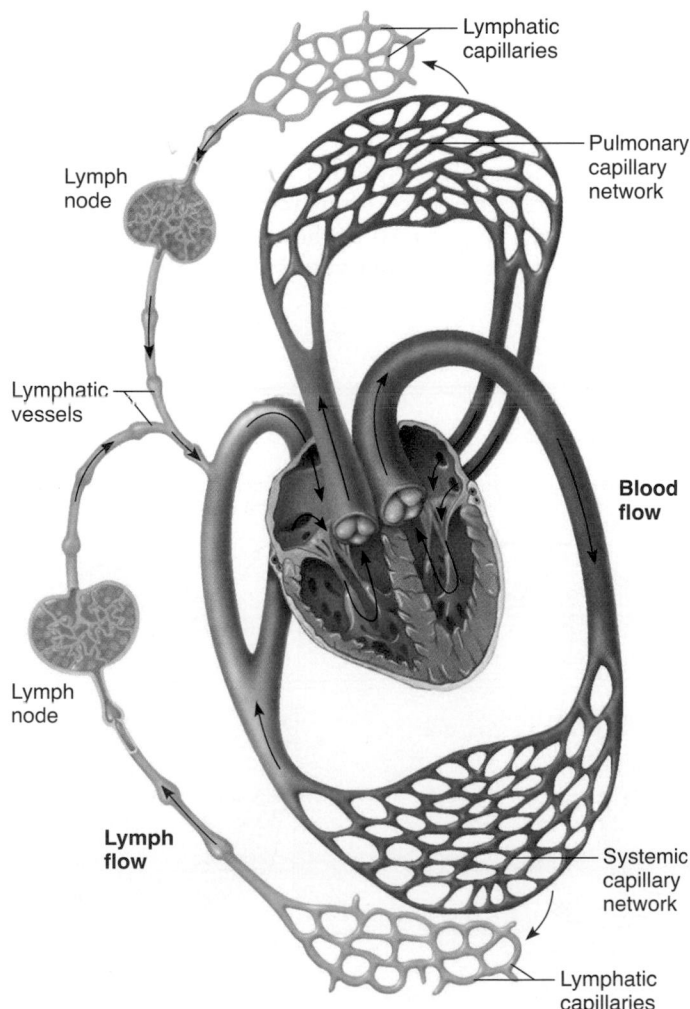

Figure C-7 | Lymph. As lymph moves through the lymphatic system, it encounters lymph nodes, containing immune cells that destroy invading pathogens. Lymph also carries dietary fat and fat-soluble nutrients from the digestive tract to the blood, utilizing the thoracic duct.

The flow of blood through the circulatory system is measured by pressure in millimeters of mercury. The average arterial (artery) pressure is about 100 mm Hg, whereas the average venous pressure is only 2 mm Hg. To guarantee return flow back to the heart, blood is moved through the veins by the contraction of skeletal muscles. There are also valves in the veins that prevent a backflow of blood.

Flow of Materials between Capillaries and Cells

As the blood flows from the arterioles into the capillaries, the hydrostatic pressure generated by the force of the heart's contraction causes fluid to flow into spaces around the surrounding cells, called the **extracellular fluid (ECF)** (Figure C-8). Some of this fluid returns to the capillaries and some enters another nearby vessel called a **lymphatic vessel.**

Oxygen and nutrients leave the capillaries and enter the ECF and are then delivered to cells by one of the mechanisms mentioned in Chapter 3: passive and facilitated diffusion, active transport, and pinocytosis. Cellular products plus waste substances are collected in the ECF and are either released to the capillaries that connect to the venules or channeled into the lymph vessels. Oxygen travels to the cell by diffusing from the blood into the extracellular fluid and then in through the cell membrane. Carbon dioxide exits the cell and goes to the blood in the same way. This is one of two important gas exchange activities in the body and is often referred to as internal respiration.

The right atrium of the heart receives dark red venous blood from the body, which is then pumped into the right ventricle. The right ventricle pumps blood through the pulmonary arteries to the capillaries in the lungs. The lungs then return the freshly oxygenated blood to the left atrium of the heart via the pulmonary veins. This route is known as **pulmonary circulation.**

As the blood moves through the pulmonary capillaries, carbon dioxide is released for expiration, and the inhaled oxygen is taken up by the blood. This is the other site for gas exchange in the body, often referred to as external respiration. The oxygenated blood (now a bright red) in the atrium is pumped to the left ventricle. The blood is pumped out of the left ventricle and through the aorta to the systemic circuit.

extracellular fluid (ECF) Fluid present outside the cells; it includes intravascular and interstitial fluids; represents about one-third of all body fluid.

lymphatic vessel A vessel that carries lymph.

pulmonary circulation The system of blood vessels from the right ventricle of the heart to the lungs and back to the left atrium of the heart.

Figure C-8 | Distribution of body fluids. The intracellular compartment contains fluid in the cell, which is free to move into the extracellular compartment. The extracellular compartment contains the fluid between the cell and the capillary, called the interstitial fluid. The extracellular fluid also includes the fluid within blood and lymph vessels. This figure shows the fluid (plasma) from the blood moving freely between cells and capillaries through the interstitial fluid.

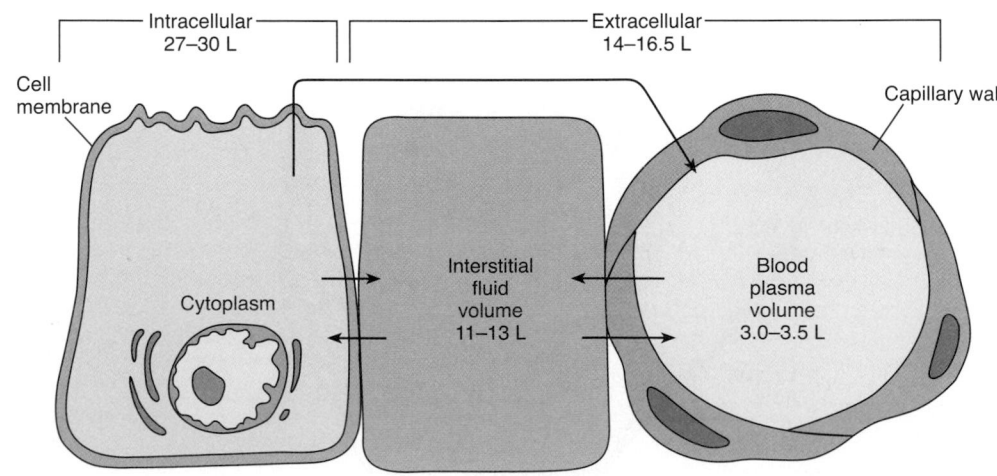

Other Circulatory Systems

One specific capillary bed does not send blood back to the heart but, rather, directs it toward the liver. This is the **portal system** of the GI tract, composed of veins draining blood from the capillaries of the intestine and stomach. These veins empty into a large **portal vein,** which acts as a direct pipeline to the liver. (The brain also has a portal system.)

The heart also has its own circulatory system. Coronary vessels supply blood to meet cardiac needs. These arteries are particularly susceptible to damage by deposits of cholesterol and other lipids in the artery wall. This accumulation of cholesterol can lead to coronary heart disease. There is more about this disease in Chapter 6.

Lymphatic System

The lymphatic system is closely related to the immune system in that both provide us with defense against pathogenic invaders. As the lymphatic system collects fluid from tissues, it picks up microorganisms as well. The fluid passes through many **lymph nodes** as it makes its way back to the bloodstream. In the nodes is an abundant collection of white blood cells ready to detect pathogens in the lymph fluid and quickly destroy them. The lymphatic system consists of lymph vessels, lymph fluid, lymph nodes, and lymphatic tissue, with its population of immune cells.

The interstitial or extracellular fluid (fluid surrounding the cell) contains many components that are too large to pass through holes in the capillaries, so they are blocked from returning directly to the bloodstream. Therefore, they take an indirect route via the lymphatic system back to general circulation (review Figure C-7).

Lymph also serves as the passageway by which fat-soluble nutrients are absorbed from the GI tract and carried into the bloodstream. Lymph also contains bacteria, viruses, cellular trash, and cancer cells on their way to invade some distant site. Lymph generates immune cells, called **lymphocytes,** that combat these invaders (see the next section on the immune system).

At the terminal end of the capillaries, the fluid released from the capillaries into the venules is less than the amount of fluid entering the capillaries from the arterioles. The missing 15% of fluid represents the extracellular fluid that is returned to the vascular system via the lymphatic system. This fluid is subsequently delivered to the lymphatic system by way of specialized capillaries called lymph capillaries. Blood plasma and fluid in the tissues are constantly being interchanged. The fluid, which is now called **lymph,** enters these porous vessels and consists of extracellular fluid and proteins too large to squeeze back into the capillaries.

In addition to microorganisms, the lymph contains absorbed dietary fat. The absorption of fats occurs only in the **lacteals,** which are lymphatic capillaries of the small intestine, not the portal vein. From the lacteals, lymph is directed into larger vessels, called **lymph ducts,** and is moved toward the heart by the action of skeletal muscle contractions and other body movements.

As the lymph makes its way back to the heart, it encounters clusters of lymph nodes containing phagocytic cells, lymphocytes, and mobile **macrophages,** which help destroy invading pathogens and filter the lymph. **T lymphocytes** and **B lymphocytes** are found in these nodes and are major players in immunity (see the section titled Immune System). When you are ill and seek medical attention, do you ever wonder why your physician checks the lymph glands in your neck for swelling? Swelling means the lymph nodes are in combat against an invading pathogen.

The spleen, thymus gland, and tonsils are considered lymphoid organs. The spleen contains phagocytes, which filter out foreign substances and destroy worn-out red blood cells. The thymus gland is important in immunity during childhood. Tonsils protect against invaders that are inhaled or eaten.

portal system A general term that describes veins in the GI tract that convey blood from capillaries in the intestines and portions of the stomach to the liver.

portal vein A large vein that leaves from the intestine and stomach and connects to the liver.

lymph node A small structure located along the course of the lymph vessels.

lymphocyte A class of white blood cells involved in the immune system, generally comprising about 25% of all white blood cells. There are several types of lymphocytes with diverse functions, including antibody production, allergic reactions, graft rejections, tumor control, and regulation of the immune system.

lymph The clear, plasmalike fluid that flows through lymph vessels.

lacteal A small lymphatic duct within a villus of the small intestine.

lymph duct A large lymphatic vessel that empties lymph into the circulatory system.

macrophage Any large mononuclear phagocytic cell that is found in the tissues and is derived from a monocyte in the blood. Besides functioning as important phagocytes, macrophages secrete numerous cytokines and act as antigen-presenting cells.

T lymphocyte A type of white blood cell that recognizes intracellular antigens (e.g., viral antigens in infected cells), fragments of which move to the cell surface. T lymphocytes originate in the bone marrow but must mature in the thymus gland.

B lymphocyte A type of white blood cell that recognizes antigens (e.g., bacteria) present in extracellular sites in the body and is responsible for antibody-mediated immunity. B lymphocytes originate and mature in the bone marrow and are released into the blood and lymph.

Eventually, the lymph empties into the thoracic duct and the right lymphatic duct, then into veins that enter the right atrium of the heart, and finally into general circulation (review Figure C-7). There is further discussion of transport of lipid substances in the lymph system in Chapter 6.

Immune System

The cells that carry out immune functions are known collectively as the immune system. Unlike other systems in the body, they do not exist as anatomically connected organs, but rather as separate collections of cells throughout the body. They provide defense against invading pathogens—microorganisms, or substances capable of producing disease. They discriminate between "self" and "nonself." They are very sensitive indicators of the body's nutritional status. The most numerous of the immune system cells are the leukocytes.

Our body constantly wages war against disease-producing microorganisms such as bacteria, viruses, fungi, and parasites; or substances capable of producing disease such as toxins from snake venom; or allergens, which trigger allergic reactions via **antigen** release; or cancer cells (Figure C-9). The most common invaders are bacteria, which are one-cell organisms with a cell wall in addition to a plasma membrane, and viruses, which are nucleic acids surrounded by a protein coat. Viruses can't multiply by themselves because they lack ribosomes for protein synthesis, so they survive by taking over a cell and instructing the host to produce the proteins and energy they need for survival.

antigen Any foreign substance, generally large in size, that induces a state of sensitivity and/or resistance to microbes or toxic substances after a lag period; substance that stimulates a specific aspect of the immune system.

Leukocytes and Macrophages

Leukocytes, also known as white blood cells, are produced in the bone marrow and may undergo further development in tissues outside the marrow. They travel via the blood and enter into tissues where they function. They are classified by their structure and the affinity for certain types of dye. For example, the monocyte has a single, prominent nucleus. Another type of immune cell takes up the red dye eosin and so is called an eosinophil. There are five general types of leukocytes, which are listed in Table C-1 along with a brief description of their functions.

Macrophages are found in almost all tissues of the body. They are derived from one kind of leukocyte, the monocyte. When a monocyte leaves the blood and enters into a

Table C-1 | Types and Functions of Leukocytes

Leukocyte	Function
Neutrophil	Phagocytizes bacteria. Forms highly toxic compounds that destroy bacteria.
Eosinophil	Phagocytizes antigen-antibody complex, allergy-causing antigens, inflammatory chemicals. Attacks parasites, such as worms.
Basophil	Secretes histamine, a vasodilator, thus increasing blood flow to tissues. Secretes heparin, which prevents blood clotting.
Lymphocytes	Natural killer cells attack cells infected with viruses or that have turned cancerous. B lymphocytes present antigens and activate other cells of the immune system. Can become plasma cells that secrete antibodies. Serve as memory cells in humoral immunity. T lymphocytes destroy foreign cells, regulate the immune response, and serve as memory cells in cellular immunity.
Monocytes	Differentiate into numerous types of macrophages. Macrophages phagocytize pathogens, dead neutrophils, and cellular debris. They present antigens and activate other cells of the immune system.

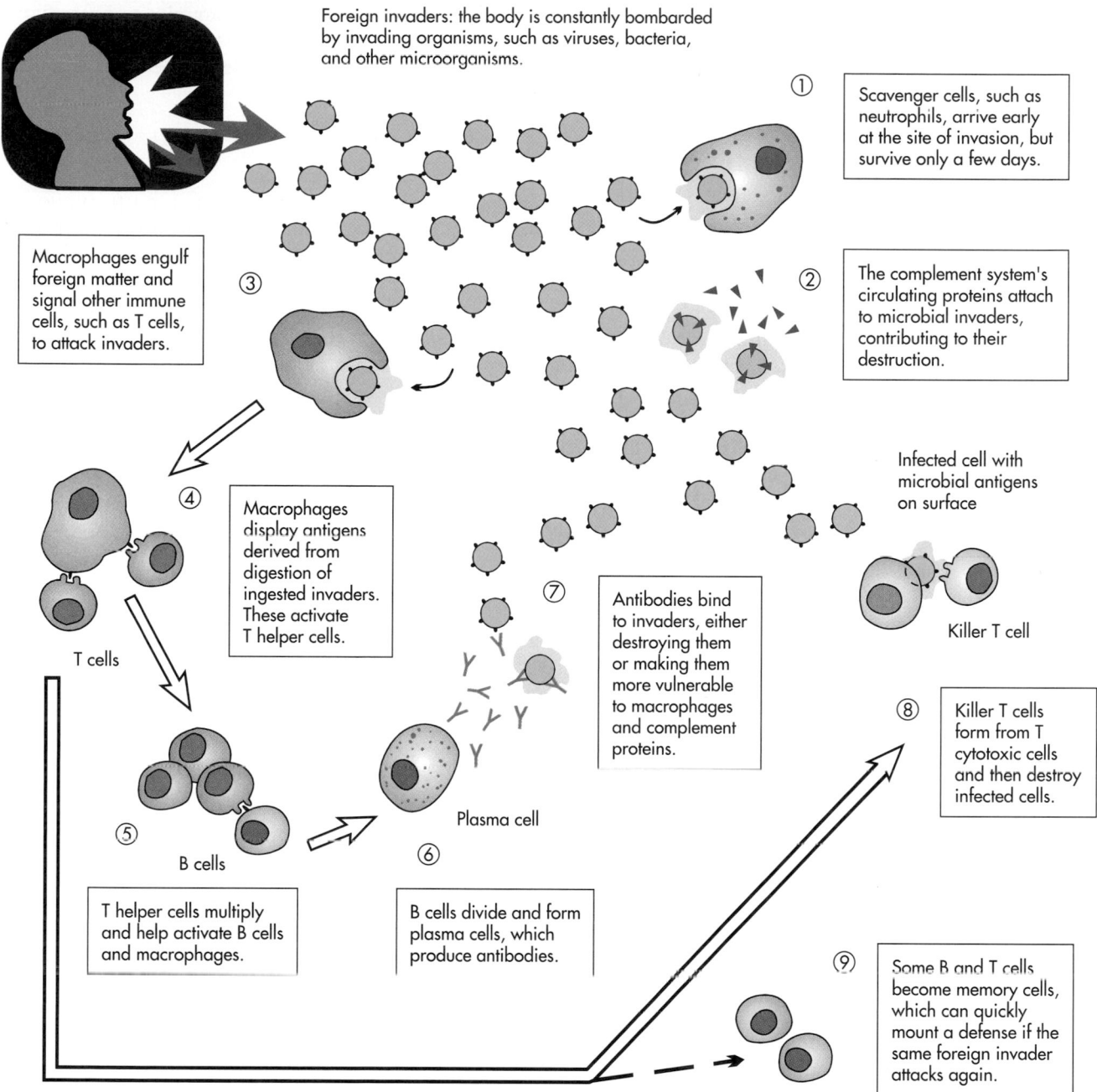

Foreign invaders: the body is constantly bombarded by invading organisms, such as viruses, bacteria, and other microorganisms.

① Scavenger cells, such as neutrophils, arrive early at the site of invasion, but survive only a few days.

Macrophages engulf foreign matter and signal other immune cells, such as T cells, to attack invaders.

③

② The complement system's circulating proteins attach to microbial invaders, contributing to their destruction.

Infected cell with microbial antigens on surface

④ Macrophages display antigens derived from digestion of ingested invaders. These activate T helper cells.

T cells

⑦ Antibodies bind to invaders, either destroying them or making them more vulnerable to macrophages and complement proteins.

Killer T cell

⑧ Killer T cells form from T cytotoxic cells and then destroy infected cells.

Plasma cell

⑤ B cells

T helper cells multiply and help activate B cells and macrophages.

⑥ B cells divide and form plasma cells, which produce antibodies.

⑨ Some B and T cells become memory cells, which can quickly mount a defense if the same foreign invader attacks again.

Figure C-9 | Biological warfare. The body commands a wide assortment of defenders to reduce the danger of infection and help guard against repeat microbial infections. The ultimate target of all immune response is an antigen, commonly a foreign protein from a bacterium or other microbe.

tissue, it is transformed into a macrophage. At birth, the baby is already supplied with macrophages, which continue to develop throughout life. They are strategically located throughout the body to phagocytize foreign material.

Mast cells are produced in the bone marrow and found in almost all tissues and organs. They release histamine and the other chemicals that are involved in inflammation.

Other participants in the immune system are **cytokines,** a complicated group of protein messengers that are produced by various cells throughout the body. They regulate the host cells' function and growth.

mast cell Tissue cell that releases histamine and other chemicals involved in inflammation.

cytokine A protein secreled by a cell that regulates the activity of neighboring cells.

There are two types of immunity: nonspecific, or natural, immunity and specific, or acquired, immunity. The nonspecific immunity protects against foreign invaders without having to recognize the specific appearance of the invaders, whereas specific immunity is acquired.

Nonspecific Immunity

Nonspecific immunity is an array of mechanisms that are present at birth and do not require any activation. They are barriers such as the skin and the **mucous membranes** of the GI tract, reproductive system, urinary tract, and respiratory tract. The **mucus** produced by these tissues traps invaders. Internally, other forms of nonspecific immunity include phagocytic cells, which can swallow bacteria and other harmful substances and ultimately destroy them. Acid produced by the stomach (HCl) can destroy ingested pathogens. Inflammation is a local response to infection or injury. The purpose is to destroy or inactivate foreign invaders and begin the process of repair. Fever is also an internal defense mechanism. It seems to aid in the recovery process by reducing the amount of iron in the blood, which in turn reduces bacterial activity. Fever also seems to be associated with an increase in **interferons.** Viral infections are subject to short-term control by this group of proteins released by infected cells. Interferons are receiving a lot of attention today as potent weapons against cancers, hepatitis C, and other diseases.

Specific Immunity

Specific immunity involving the lymphocytes is directed at specific molecules. When nonspecific immunological defenses fail to halt an invasion by pathogens or by toxins produced by pathogens, another mechanism comes into action. This mechanism is based on the action of antibodies, lymphocytes, and other cells of the immune system and is known as **antibody-mediated immunity,** or humoral immunity.

Recall that antigens are molecules that are generally large in size and foreign to the body. A given molecule can have a number of antigenic determinant sites that stimulate the production of various antibodies. When we successfully fight off an invader, chemicals called **antibodies** have been in action. Antibodies are highly specific proteins produced by B lymphocytes in response to antigens. Antigens are detected as dangerous intruders. They are detected because the immune system can identify molecules that are "self"—they belong to *me* personally—from "nonself" molecules. (Recall that one role of the carbohydrates found on the cell membrane is to identify "self.")

The lymphocytes that produce antibodies, designated B lymphocytes, are produced in the bone marrow. These B lymphocytes wage war against bacterial infections as well as some viral infections and even a few parasites. B lymphocytes (or B cells) and antibodies, also known as **immunoglobulins,** come in five major classifications. These bind to the antigen on the invader and begin a process of attack. This antibody-antigen interaction soon produces **plasma cells,** which results in the production of more antibody proteins to continue the attack. A person can produce as many different antibodies as there are exposures to specific antigens. It is estimated that there are 100 million trillion antibody molecules per person, representing a few million species of antigens.

Memory cells are then produced by B cells and provide active immunity. Once you have been exposed to an antigen, you develop active immunity. Obviously, this is the basis of vaccinations; an inactivated pathogen is injected and the body develops immunity to that pathogen.

The blood also contains a group of proteins called **complement** proteins. Complement proteins are released into the area of infection and attach to the target pathogen to be destroyed. The antibody-antigen combination does not cause the destruction of the pathogenic invaders, but it does identify them so that they can be attacked by nonspecific immune processes such as the complement proteins.

---

nonspecific immunity Defenses that stop the invasion of pathogens; requires no previous encounter with a pathogen.

mucous membranes Membranes that line passageways open to the exterior environment; also called mucosae.

mucus A thick fluid secreted by glands throughout the body. It contains a compound that has both a carbohydrate and a protein nature. It acts as both a lubricant and a means of protection for cells.

interferons A group of proteins released by virus-infected cells that bind to other cells, stimulating synthesis of antiviral proteins that in turn inhibit viral multiplication.

specific immunity The function of lymphocytes directed at specific antigens.

antibody-mediated immunity Specific immunity provided by B lymphocytes; also known as humoral immunity.

antibodies Blood proteins that inactivate foreign proteins found in the body. This helps prevent and control infections.

immunoglobulins Proteins found in the blood that are responsible for antibody-mediated immunity and that bind specifically to antigen; also called *antibodies*. Immunoglobulins are produced by certain white blood cells in response to a foreign substance (antigen) in the bloodstream.

plasma cells A form of B lymphocytes that produce about 2000 antibodies per second.

memory cells B lymphocytes that remain after an infection to convey long-lasting or permanent immunity.

complement A series of blood proteins that participate in a complex reaction cascade following stimulation by an antigen-antibody complex on the surface of a bacterial cell. Various activated complement proteins can enhance phagocytosis, contribute to inflammation, and destroy bacteria.

Complement proteins attach to the pathogenic invader and drill holes in its membrane, thus leading to its destruction. (The hole in the wall allows water to flow into the cell, causing the cell to burst.)

T lymphocytes (T cells) directly attack and destroy specific cells, which are identified by specific antigens on the cell surface. T lymphocytes produce **cell-mediated immunity** because they actually are in contact with the enemy cell. T cells must be first activated in the thymus gland.

The actual T lymphocytes that are killers are known as **cytotoxic T cells.** They recognize the infected cell and attach themselves through a CD8 receptor. There are also **helper T cells.** They attach to an infected cell through the CD4 receptor. They promote phagocytic activity. Together the cytotoxic and helper T cells bind to the infected cell and lead to the cell's destruction. You may have heard of CD4 cells because they are markers for AIDS. When the disease progresses, the CD4 count decreases as the virus attacks helper T cells (and macrophages).

Most of the information concerning the relationship of nutrition to immunity comes from studies in poor countries of the developing world, where children die of infectious diseases secondary to malnutrition. Protein-energy malnutrition deficiencies of vitamins and minerals and an inadequate intake of certain fatty acids seriously alter immune function. There is more information about how individual nutrients make it possible to support an immune response in Chapters 9 through 12.

Allergies are types of immune responses. One type of allergic response is almost immediate. The symptoms are produced by B lymphocytes exposed to an allergen, as demonstrated by a runny nose, red eyes, and itchy skin (dermatitis). The culprit is **histamine,** an altered form of the common amino acid histidine. This type of immune response can be treated by antihistamine drugs. Allergies are further discussed with eicosanoids in Chapter 6 and adolescent nutrition in Chapter 17.

Delayed hypersensitivity, an abnormal T cell response, can occur as late as 72 hours after exposure. The best known example of this type of immune response is contact dermatitis caused by coming in contact with poison ivy, poison oak, or poison sumac.

A final type of immunity is known as autoimmunity. Here the immune system fails to recognize "self," thinking a normal cell is an antigen. The immune system then goes on the attack by activating T lymphocytes and the production of antibodies by B lymphocytes, which kills the cell. In other words, the defense mechanisms are confused and attack the body rather than invaders. There are at least 40 autoimmune diseases. Some well-known examples include rheumatoid arthritis, type 1 diabetes, and multiple sclerosis.

Respiratory System

In order to produce sufficient energy to meet body needs, there must be oxygen present to help convert food energy into ATP. When oxygen is supplied to the tissues, carbon dioxide is produced and removed from the body by the combined actions of the cardiovascular and respiratory systems.

The organs of the respiratory system are the nose, pharynx, larynx, trachea, bronchi, and lungs. *Respiration* refers to breathing and to the exchange of gases between the blood and other tissues. The respiratory tract features the **alveoli** (plural) in the lungs. These are tiny structures where one form of gas exchange takes place, described previously as external respiration (Figure C-10). The **alveolus** (singular), the basic functional unit of respiration, allows oxygen to be recovered from inhaled air and loads it onto red blood cells for transport to target tissues throughout the body. Simultaneously, carbon dioxide in the blood is released into the lungs and ultimately exhaled into the air.

Air reaches the lungs from the nasal cavity and the mouth by first passing through the **pharynx** to the **larynx.** The larynx is open to the trachea during breathing but closes during swallowing. The **trachea** is a tube that connects the larynx to the **bronchial tree.** The bronchial tree is located in the lungs and looks like a tree with

cell-mediated immunity A process in which T lymphocytes come in actual contact with the invading cells in order to destroy them.

cytotoxic T cells Type of T cells that interact with the infected host cell through special receptor sites on the T cell surface.

helper T cells Type of T cells that interact with macrophages and secrete substances to signal an invading pathogen; stimulates B lymphocytes to proliferate.

histamine A breakdown product of the amino acid histidine that stimulates acid secretion by the stomach and has other effects on the body, such as contraction of smooth muscles, increased nasal secretions, relaxation of blood vessels, and changes in constriction of airways.

alveoli, alveolus The basic functional units of the lungs.

pharynx The organ of the digestive tract and respiratory tract located at the back of the oral and nasal cavities.

larynx The structure located between the pharynx and trachea that contains the vocal cords.

trachea The airway leading from the larynx to the bronchi.

bronchial tree The bronchi and the branches that stem out to bronchioles.

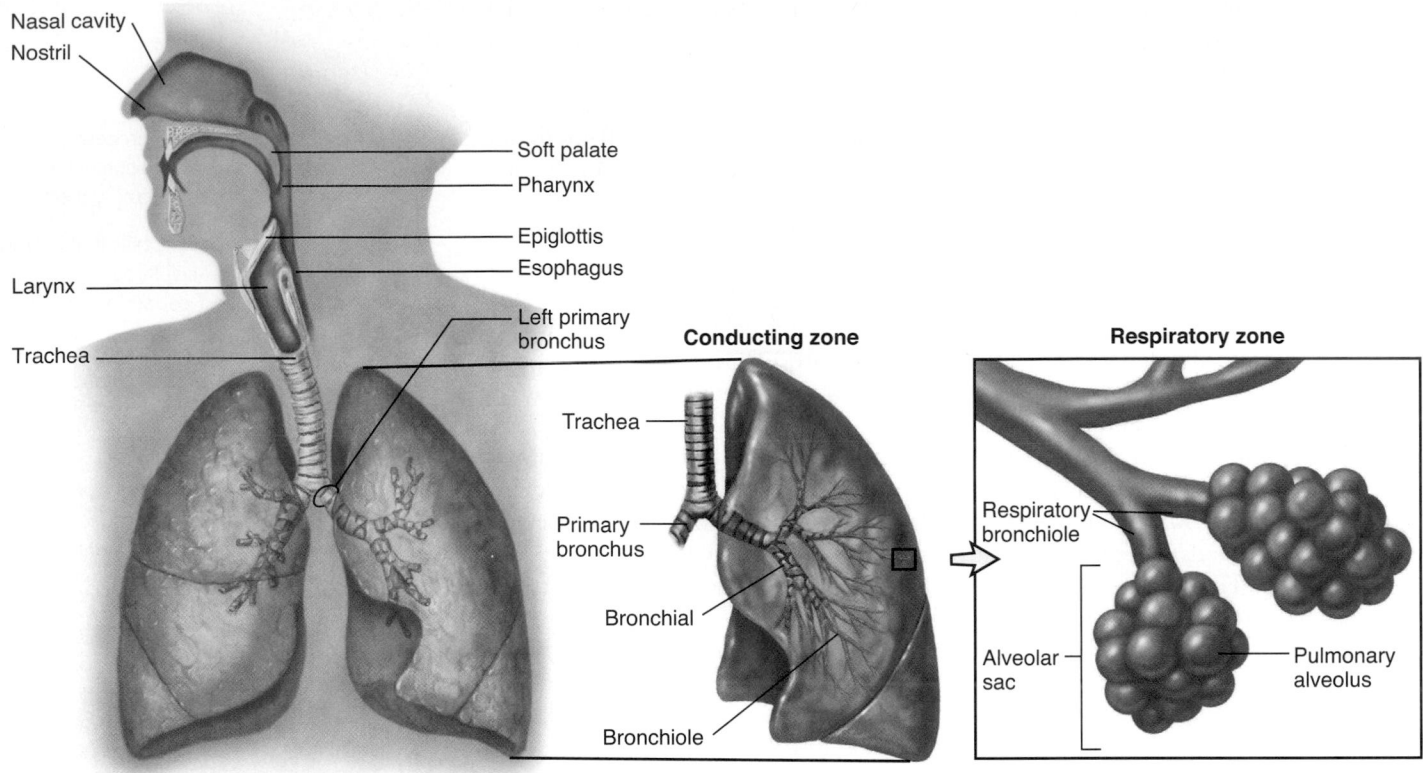

Figure C-10 | Anatomy of the respiratory system. Air enters through the nose and mouth and is conducted into bronchioles of the lungs. Gas exchange occurs in the alveoli.

bronchioles The smallest division of the bronchi.

branches. The branches on this tree get smaller and smaller the farther out they go from the tree trunk (the trachea) into lung tissue until finally they turn into **bronchioles,** the location of the pulmonary alveoli.

The distance across the alveoli is two cells thick; one cell for the alveoli plus one cell for the pulmonary capillaries. Gas exchange allows CO_2 and O_2 to diffuse easily between the blood and lungs. There is an estimated 300 million alveoli in the lungs, providing a tremendous surface area for the diffusion of gases.

Another aspect of respiration is the discharge of water through the lungs. This process is obvious on a cold day when the breath we exhale turns to ice crystals, and we can see vapor forming around the mouth and nose. Of course, such water loss is much more extensive during hot, humid weather when the body loses heat via the lungs.

Nervous System

homeostasis A series of adjustments that prevent change in the internal environment in the body.

central nervous system (CNS) The brain and spinal cord portions of the nervous system.

peripheral nervous system (PNS) The nerves of the central nervous system that lie outside the brain and spinal cord.

The nervous system is a regulatory system controlling a variety of body functions. It can detect changes occurring in various organs and take corrective action when needed to maintain the constancy of the internal environment, **homeostasis.** The nervous system regulates activities that occur almost instantaneously, such as muscle contractions and perception of danger.

The nervous system consists of the **central nervous system (CNS)** and the **peripheral nervous system (PNS).** The central nervous system contains the brain and spinal cord. The peripheral nervous system, with its nerves coming from the central nervous system, branch out to all organs of the body.

The basic structural and functional unit of the nervous system is the neuron—a cell that responds to electrical and chemical signals, conducts electrical impulses, and

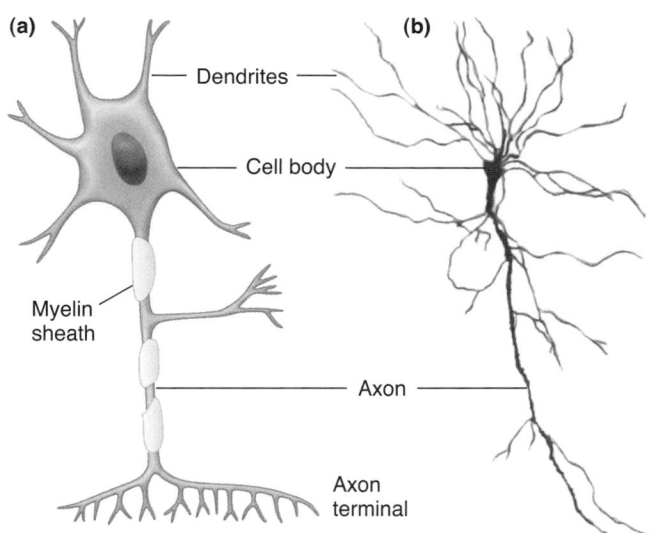

(a)
- Dendrites
- Cell body
- Myelin sheath
- Axon
- Axon terminal

(b)

Figure C-11 | (*a*) An illustration of a neuron or nerve cell, showing the cell body with dendrites and the axon. The axon releases the neurotransmitters. (*b*) How a neuron looks under a light microscope.

releases chemical regulators (Figure C-11). Neurons allow us to perceive what is occurring in our environment, engage in learning, store vital information in memory, and control the body's voluntary actions. Incoming information to the body depends on sensory receptors, such as visual, auditory, smell, and tactile receptors.

Neurons can't produce new cells, although some can regenerate parts of their structures. Loss of nerve tissue causes loss of important functions. A spinal cord injury is likely to cause permanent paralysis.

Neuroglia (glial cells) protect neurons and aid in their function. They are far more abundant than neurons. For example, one group of neuroglia wraps nerves in a protective myelin sheath, a job associated with vitamin B-12 (review Figure C-11). This sheath acts like an insulating material, isolating one nerve conduction pathway from the others. Another group of neuroglia phagocytizes pathogens and disposes of cellular debris in the CNS.

Each neuron contains a cell body with a nucleus and rough endoplasmic reticulum, **dendrites,** and an **axon.** Information (electrical or chemical stimuli) enters the cell through the dendrites and/or the cell body, and the output of electrical impulses leaves by way of the axon.

By now, you may be wondering about the term *nerve*. A **nerve** is a bundle of axons located outside the CNS. Nerves contain axons of both sensory and motor neurons.

Axons end close to, or may be in physical contact with, the next neuron. In most cases, however, the electrical signal at the end of the axon is converted to a chemical signal called a **neurotransmitter** that is released into the gap (Figure C-12). The transmission from neuron to neuron or from neuron to muscle cell is by way of these neurotransmitters. The space between one neuron and the next is known as a **synapse.** Neurotransmitters that bridge the gap are derived from common nutrients found in foods (review Chapter 11 for more details). There are a variety of neurotransmitters—**dopamine, norepinephrine, acetylcholine,** and **serotonin** are just a few.

The body's fight or flight mechanism—the ability to survive a threat—depends on the **adrenergic** effect provided by adrenergic neurons secreting **epinephrine** and norepinephrine. The adrenergic effect stimulates the heart to beat faster, constricts blood vessels to raise blood pressure, increases breathing, and promotes the breakdown of glycogen in the liver. These changes are essential to survival, because they make it possible to provide plenty of glucose, our basic muscle fuel, instantly when there is an emergency and muscles need to respond quickly. **Cholinergic** effects usually produce the opposite response of adrenergic effects.

The brain has a tremendous metabolic rate; the blood that it requires accounts for 20% of the total cardiac output. This translates into 750 ml of blood per minute being pumped through the brain, yielding a steady supply of oxygen and glucose. Any

dendrite A relatively short, highly branched nerve cell process that carries electrical activity to the main body of the nerve cell.

axon The part of a nerve cell that conducts impulses away from the main body of the cell.

nerve A bundle of nerve cells outside the central nervous system.

neuroglia (glial cells) Specialized support cells of the central nervous system.

neurotransmitter A compound made by a nerve cell that allows for communication between it and other cells.

synapse The space between the end of one nerve cell and the beginning of another nerve cell.

dopamine A type of neurotransmitter in the central nervous system that leads to feelings of euphoria, among other functions; it is also used to form norepinephrine, another neurotransmitter molecule.

norepinephrine A neurotransmitter released from nerve endings, and a hormone produced by the adrenal gland in times of stress.

acetylcholine A neurotransmitter released from nerve endings.

serotonin A neurotransmitter synthesized from the amino acid tryptophan that affects mood (sense of calmness), behavior, and appetite and induces sleep.

epinephrine A hormone produced by the adrenal gland in times of stress. It may also have neurotransmitter functions, such as in the brain.

adrenergic Relating to the actions of epinephrine and norepinephrine.

cholinergic Relating to the actions of acetylcholine.

Figure C-12 | Transmission of the message from one neuron to another neuron or other cell relies on neurotransmitters. Vesicles containing neurotransmitters fuse with the membrane of the neuron, and the neurotransmitter is released into the synapse. The neurotransmitter then binds to the receptors on the nearby neuron (or cell). In this way, the message is sent from one neuron to another, or to the cell that ultimately performs the action directed by the message.

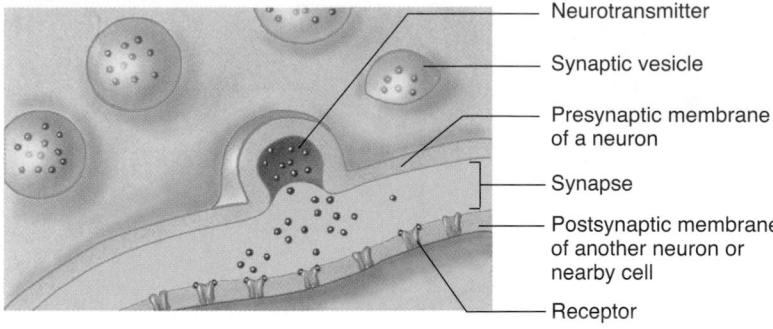

- Neurotransmitter
- Synaptic vesicle
- Presynaptic membrane of a neuron
- Synapse
- Postsynaptic membrane of another neuron or nearby cell
- Receptor

The most important nutrient for continued efficient brain function is carbohydrate in the form of glucose. Should the diet fail to deliver enough carbohydrate that can form glucose, the body will synthesize it in sufficient amounts to provide for the needs of the brain. Alternately, the brain will use an alternative fuel called ketone bodies, but this is not healthy for the body over the long term (review Chapter 4).

interruption in the supply of these two substances is life-threatening. The brain also generates waste materials that are promptly removed by this high blood flow rate.

All the various structures that make up the nervous system are related to a person's nutritional status. For example, most of the axons of the CNS and PNS are covered by myelin. Vitamin B-12 plays a key role in the formation of myelin.

The transmission of information through the nervous system depends on nutrients obtained from the diet: calcium, sodium, and potassium. The sodium ion (Na^+) (mostly extracellular) and the potassium ion (K^+) (mostly intracellular) located on either side of the axon membrane exchange places as they flow through ion channels in response to electrical stimulation. This is how an electrical signal is transmitted. They are later pumped back to their previous location.

Calcium allows the release of neurotransmitters from the axon of a neuron. As we have seen, the neurotransmitter carries the signal to the next neuron as it jumps the synapse. Fortunately, a calcium-deficient diet will never have a major effect on nerve transmission; the body can always find enough calcium to keep the nervous system functioning. There are, however, rare instances when a deficiency of calcium causes tetany. (More about tetany appears in Chapter 11.)

Other nutrients required for the nervous system are various amino acids. One amino acid we obtain from dietary protein, tryptophan, is converted to serotonin by neurons. This neurotransmitter has a variety of behavioral effects. Varying the amount of dietary tryptophan controls the amount of serotonin produced by neurons. The amino acid tyrosine can be converted to dopamine and norepinephrine.

The GI tract has its own separate nervous system. The sight or smell of food, or one's emotions, can signal muscle cells and glands to prepare the way for food and turn on digestive processes (Chapter 3 has more details).

Endocrine System and Hormones

Endocrine glands secrete regulatory substances, hormones, into the blood for distribution to target tissues or organs. The endocrine gland that secretes a hormone is responding to the need to restore homeostasis. This section is by no means a complete exploration of all the body's hormones but concentrates on those that affect nutrition (Figure C-13).

Some hormones control metabolic functions, such as appetite, and the transport of substances through cell membranes. Others control growth, and still others are responsible for sex and reproduction. Of all these hormones, some are described as "local," in that they function in the immediate vicinity of their production. There are also many interrelationships between hormones and the nervous system. For example, the adrenal gland and the pituitary gland respond to neural stimuli.

Some hormones from the pituitary gland control the secretion of other endocrine glands. And, as mentioned in the previous section, a substance such as norepinephrine secreted as a neurotransmitter can act as a hormone.

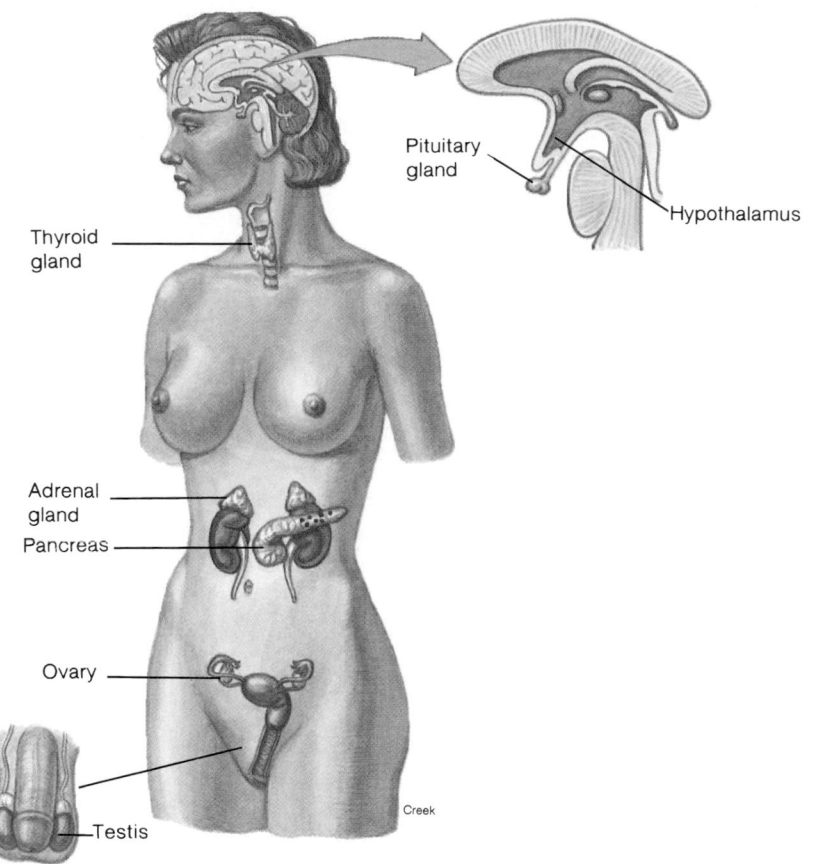

Figure C-13 | The major endocrine glands. Note the location of some of the endocrine glands. These glands secrete a variety of hormones.

Chemical Classification of Hormones

General hormones are classified according to chemical categories: **steroids, glycoproteins, polypeptides,** and **amines.**

Steroid hormones are lipid substances synthesized from cholesterol (Table C-2). The glycoproteins are long chains of amino acids (100 or more) bound to carbohydrate (Table C-3). Follicle-stimulating hormone (FSH), luteinizing hormone (LH), thyroid-stimulating hormone (TSH), and several other pituitary hormones are such hormones and are referred to as **tropic hormones** because they stimulate the secretion of another hormone and usually stimulate the growth of the associated gland. For example, TSH stimulates the production of the thyroid hormone. Another group of hormones are polypeptide chains made of fewer than 100 amino acids per chain (Table C-4). Amines are hormones synthesized from the amino acids tyrosine and tryptophan (Table C-5).

steroids A group of hormones and related compounds that are derivatives of cholesterol.

glycoprotein A protein containing a carbohydrate group.

polypeptide Fifty to 2000 or more amino acids bonded together.

amines Can refer to hormones made of one or a few amino acids.

tropic hormone A hormone that stimulates the secretion of another secreting gland.

Table C-2 | Steroid Hormones

Hormone	Gland	Target	Effect	Role in Nutrition
Testosterone	Testes, adrenal glands	Reproductive organs	Reproduction, secondary sexual development	Muscle growth
Estrogens, progesterone	Ovaries, adrenal glands	Reproductive organs	Reproduction, secondary sexual characteristics	Maintenance of bone
Cortisol	Adrenal glands	Liver	Glucocorticoid activity	Metabolism of protein, carbohydrate, fat
Aldosterone	Adrenal glands	Kidney	Mineral-corticoid activity	Electrolyte balance

Table C-3 | Glycoprotein Hormones

Hormone	Gland	Target	Effect	Role in Nutrition
FSH, LH, TSH	Pituitary gland	Variety of organs	Stimulation of target organ to produce its own hormone	None directly

Table C-4 | Polypeptide Hormones

Hormone	Gland	Target	Effect	Role in Nutrition
Antidiuretic hormone	Pituitary gland	Kidney	Water retention, vasoconstriction	Maintenance of proper blood volume
Prolactin (tropic hormone)	Pituitary gland	Mammary gland	Milk production; in males, indirect enhancement of testosterone secretions	Nourishment of newborn
Oxytocin	Pituitary gland	Uterus and mammary glands	Contraction of uterus, mammary secretions	Milk production
Insulin	Pancreas	Fat and muscle cells	Decreased blood glucose concentration	Storage of glucose as glycogen, increased fat storage, increased amino acid uptake by cells
Glucagon	Pancreas	Liver	Increased blood glucose concentration	Release of glucose from liver stores, increased fat mobilization
ACTH (adrenocorticotropic hormone)	Pituitary gland	Adrenal glands	Secretion of glucocorticoids	Secretion of adrenal cortical hormones
Growth hormone (tropic hormone)	Pituitary gland	Most cells	Promotion of amino acid uptake by cells	Promotion of protein synthesis and growth, increased fat utilization for energy
Parathyroid hormone	Parathyroid glands	Intestinal tract, kidneys	Increased blood calcium	Release of calcium from bone into blood
Calcitonin	Thyroid gland	Bone	Inhibition of breakdown of bone, stimulation of calcium excretion by kidneys	Reduced blood calcium concentration
Leptin	No gland, just adipose tissue	Hypothalamus	Targeting of satiety center	Decreased appetite

Table C-5 | Amine Hormones

Hormone	Gland	Target	Effect	Role in Nutrition
Epinephrine, norepinephrine*	Adrenal glands	Heart, blood vessels, brain, lungs	Increased metabolic rate	Release of glucose into the blood, fat mobilization
Thyroid hormones	Thyroid gland	Most organs	Increased oxygen consumption, growth, brain development, development of CNS in fetus	Protein synthesis, increased metabolic rate
Melatonin	Pineal gland	Specific neurons	Maintenance of body (circadian) rhythms, sleep	Scavenging of atoms and molecules that are highly reactive and dangerous

*Norepinephrine also functions as a neurotransmitter, depending on location in the body. Epinephrine is suspected of doing the some, such as in the brain.

There are also special hormones that regulate the digestive tract. These are discussed in Chapter 3.

Interesting Features of Hormones

The steroid and thyroid hormones can be taken in pill form because they are not digested in the GI tract; thus, they can be absorbed into the body in their active state. All the other hormones are deactivated when taken by mouth because their biological activity is destroyed by digestive enzymes. That is why the hormone insulin must be taken by injection to bypass the digestive tract.

Some hormones must undergo chemical changes before they can function. For example, vitamin D synthesized in the skin and/or obtained from food is converted to an active hormone by the kidneys and liver.

Neural and Endocrine Regulation

Whether a chemical is acting as a hormone or a neurotransmitter, the target cell must have a receptor protein to combine with it. This causes a change in the target cell (Chapter 3 provides a fuller discussion of this concept). This also means that there must be a mechanism to turn off the action. Hormones are subject to control by an off switch. For example, when the blood glucose concentration has been returned to normal by the action of the hormone insulin, insulin production is turned off. If it were not, the person would experience decreasing glucose concentrations until the concentration dropped so low that the person would go into shock and die.

Urinary System

The urinary system is composed of two kidneys located on the back of the abdominal wall, one on each side of the vertebral column (Figure C-14). Each is connected to the urinary bladder by a **ureter.** The bladder is emptied by way of the **urethra.**

Each bean-shaped kidney has an outer section called the cortex and an inner section called the medulla. The medulla is composed of cone-shaped pyramid structures, which empty waste materials into a funnel-shaped tube ending in the ureter. Ureters carry urine from the kidneys to the bladder for temporary storage. Blood flows through the kidneys at a rate of about 120 ml/minute.

Kidney Functions

The kidneys regulate the composition of the blood (plasma) and the interstitial fluid, known together as the extracellular fluid. This regulation is accomplished by filtering the blood and forming urine, which is basically the filtrate. As a result of kidney action and the formation of urine, the volume of blood plasma is controlled, and blood pressure is maintained. The kidneys remove metabolic waste and foreign chemicals from the blood, and they maintain a certain concentration of electrolytes such as Na^+, K^+, and HCO_3^- (bicarbonate) in the plasma. The kidneys constantly monitor the composition of the blood and produce hormones to maintain homeostasis. For example, the kidneys produce the hormone **erythropoietin,** which is responsible for the synthesis of red blood cells. The kidneys convert a form of vitamin D into its active hormone form. During times of fasting, the kidneys can produce glucose from amino acids.

Kidney Structure

Each kidney is enclosed in a fatty, fibrous sack that protects it from external physical damage. Examined microscopically, the functional unit of the kidney, the **nephron,** is disclosed. Nephrons extend through the renal cortex and the renal medulla. There are

In most cases, a single gland secretes a single hormone, but in a few cases, a gland secretes more than one hormone. In addition, sometimes a hormone is produced by more than one gland.

ureter A tube that transports urine from the kidney to the urinary bladder.

urethra The tube that transports urine from the urinary bladder to the outside of the body.

Together with the lungs, the kidneys maintain the pH of the blood.

erythropoietin A hormone secreted mostly by the kidneys that enhances red blood cell synthesis and stimulates red blood cell release from bone marrow.

nephron The functional unit of the kidney.

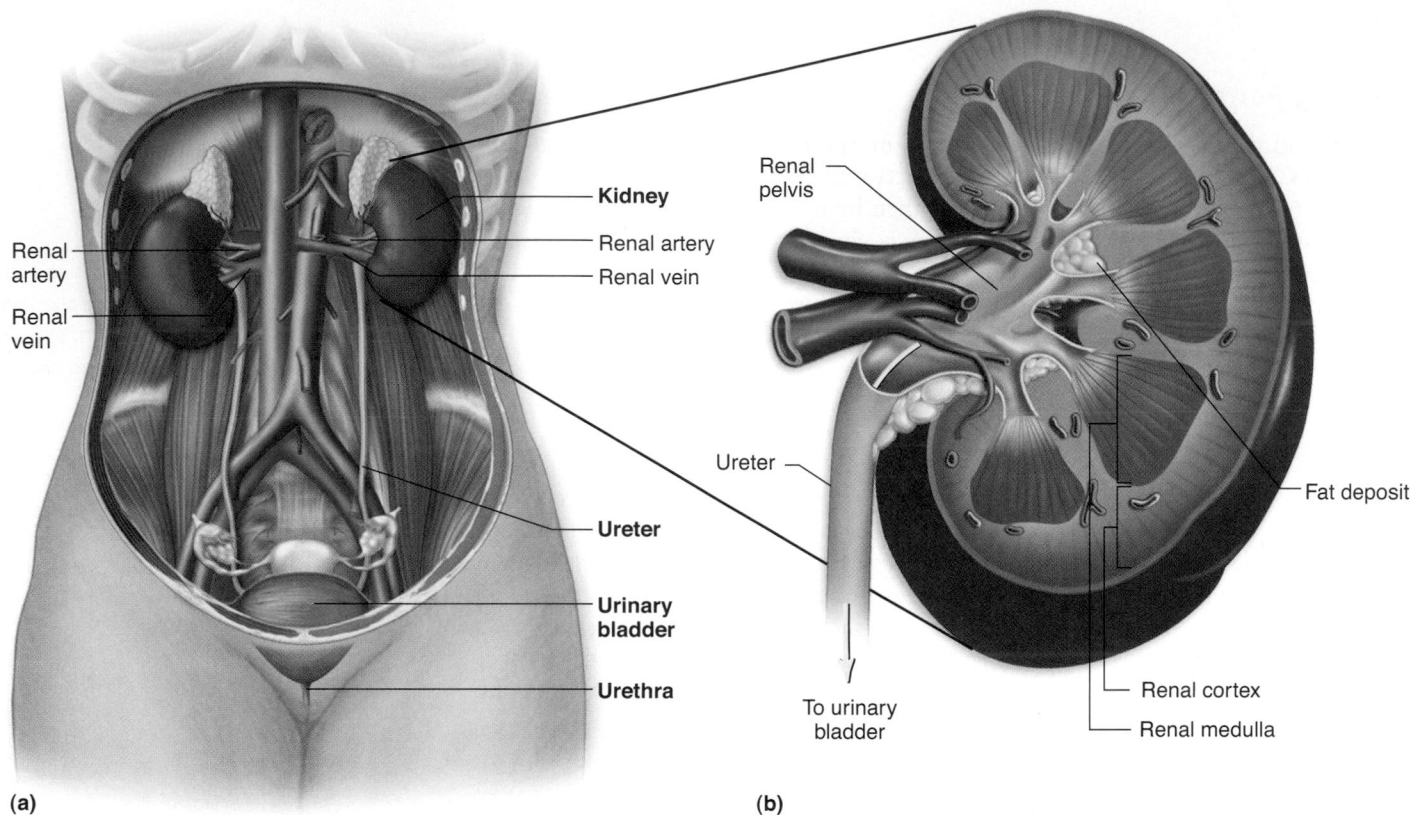

(a)

(b)

Figure C-14 | Organs of the urinary system. (*a*) The urinary system of the female. The male's urinary system is the same, except that the urethra extends through the penis. (*b*) A cross section of the kidney. The kidneys are bean-shaped organs located on either side of the spinal column and filter waste from the blood, which is then stored in the bladder as urine. The kidneys are connected to the urinary bladder by ureters. The outer section of the kidney is the cortex, the inner section is the medulla. The functional unit of the kidney, the nephron, loops through the cortex and medulla, and the fluid that flows through these tiny structures is separated so that the waste is removed from the blood into collecting ducts and drains into the renal pelvis. Thus the urine exits by way of the ureter to the bladder. The remaining fluid is returned to the circulatory system to maintain the normal composition of the blood.

glomerulus The capillaries in the kidney that filter waste products from the blood.

more than 1 million nephrons per kidney. The nephron consists of small tubules allied with small blood vessels. The tiny capillary filtration unit, the **glomerulus,** is held in a small capsule (Bowman's capsule). The glomerulus filters large amounts of fluid from the blood, removing the dissolved waste and excess fluid to form urine, which leaves by way of the tubules. The remaining fluid is returned to the blood.

This ingenious mechanism constantly adjusts the composition of the blood. In doing so the essential components are recovered and returned to general circulation, waste products and excess water are removed, and unneeded nutrients (ones in which storage compartments are full or there are no storage facilities) are flushed away by the urine.

Reproductive System

Reproduction is a fundamental property of all living things. We die, but our genes live on in our progeny. In humans, both ova and sperm, called gametes (sex cells), contain 23 chromosomes. The fertilized egg contains 46 chromosomes (23 from each parent) and is programmed to produce a new human. At conception, the instructions for the developing embryo are all present. Through the actions of the female reproductive organs, supported by hormonal secretions, a human is produced about 40 weeks after conception, providing that essential nutrients are present and no genetic defects are encountered. The most precarious time during pregnancy is during the development of the embryo (the first 13 weeks), when a woman is least likely to know she is pregnant.

The male reproductive organs consist of the scrotum (containing the testes), the penis, the urethra, the seminal vesicles, and the prostate. The female reproductive organs consist of the ovaries, uterus, and vagina (review Figure C-14).

In addition to reproduction, the sex hormones stimulate bone growth and the closure of the epiphyseal plate, thus causing the cessation of bone growth. Estrogens protect against bone loss. The sex hormone testosterone stimulates protein synthesis, such as muscle growth and bone growth.

Puberty, or the onset of adult sex life, takes place during early adolescence. **Menarche,** the term used to describe the onset of menstruation, occurs usually between the ages of 11 and 16 in females. In the male, sexual maturation occurs somewhat later and is initiated by hormonal secretions from the brain.

The female reproductive system is discussed in Chapter 16 in more detail.

menarche The onset of menstruation. Menarche usually occurs around age 13, 2 or 3 years after the first signs of puberty start to appear.

appendix D
DIETARY ADVICE FOR CANADIANS

Recommended Nutrient Intake (RNI) The Canadian version of RDA published in 1990.

Excellent World Wide Web resources for Canadians are Health Canada (**www. hc-sc.gc.ca**), Dietitians of Canada (**www. dietitians.ca**), and the National Institute of Nutrition (**www.nin.ca**).

The information in this appendix includes advice on dietary patterns as well as regulations that apply to food labeling. Previous **RNIs** for nutrients have been replaced by the Dietary Reference Intakes (DRIs) that apply to Canadian and U.S. citizens. These are listed on the inside cover. Both Canadian and American scientists worked on the various DRI committees, coming up with a set of harmonized Dietary Reference Intakes for both countries.

Summary of the Nutrition Recommendations for Canadians

The latest Nutrition Recommendations of the Scientific Review Committee of the Office of Nutrition Policy and Promotion suggest that the Canadian diet should supply:

- essential nutrients in the amounts specified in the updated Recommended Nutrient Intakes (RNIs);
- sufficient energy to maintain a healthy weight when balanced with physical activity (energy intakes for adults should not be lower than 1800 kilocalories in order to meet RNIs);
- no more than 30% of energy as fat and no more than 10% of energy as saturated fat;
- at least 55% energy as carbohydrates;
- less sodium than is now used;
- no more than 5% of energy as alcohol, or 2 drinks per day (whichever is less), with no alcohol during pregnancy;
- no more caffeine than the equivalent of four regular cups of coffee per day; and
- water containing no less than 1 mg/litre of fluoride.

In essence, suggested actions toward healthful eating as listed in Canada's Guidelines for Healthy Eating include the following:

- Enjoy a VARIETY of foods.
- Emphasize cereals, breads, other grain products, vegetables, and fruit.
- Choose lower-fat dairy products, leaner meats, and foods prepared with little or no fat.
- Achieve and maintain a healthful body weight by enjoying regular physical activity and healthy eating.
- Limit salt, alcohol, and caffeine.

The *Canadian Food Guide* is a guide to help Canadians make wise food choices (Figure D-1). The rainbow side of the Food Guide places foods into four groups: grain products; vegetables and fruit; milk products; and meat and meat alternatives. The rainbow includes information about the types of foods to choose from each food group for healthy eating.

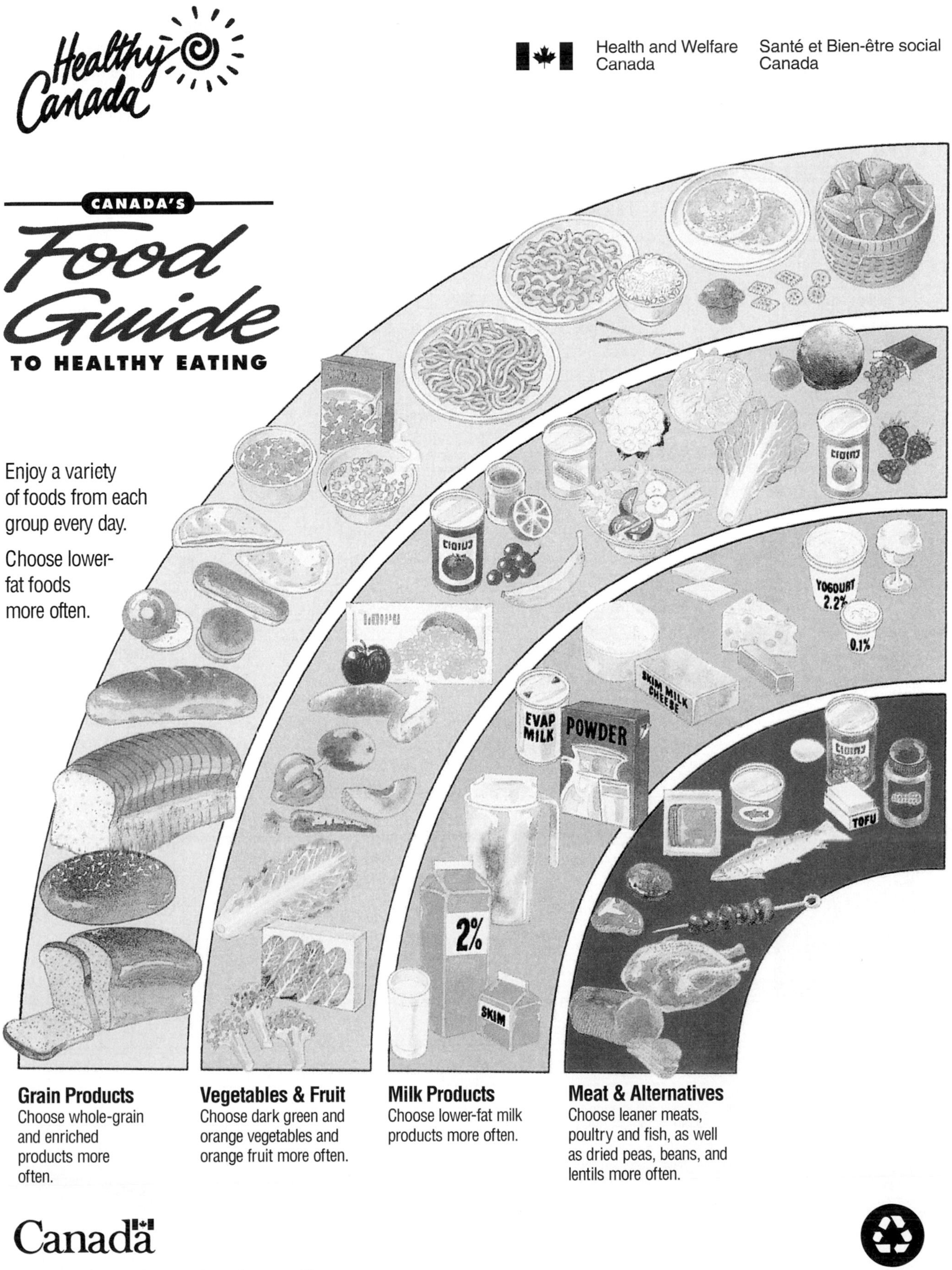

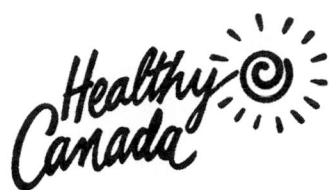

Healthy Canada
Health and Welfare Canada
Santé et Bien-être social Canada
CANADA'S
Food Guide
TO HEALTHY EATING
Enjoy a variety of foods from each group every day.
Choose lower-fat foods more often.
EVAP MILK
POWDER
SKIM MILK CHEESE
YOGOURT 2.2%
0.1%
2%
SKIM
TOFU
Grain Products
Choose whole-grain and enriched products more often.
Vegetables & Fruit
Choose dark green and orange vegetables and orange fruit more often.
Milk Products
Choose lower-fat milk products more often.
Meat & Alternatives
Choose leaner meats, poultry and fish, as well as dried peas, beans, and lentils more often.
Canada

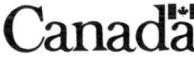

Figure D-1 | Canadian Food Guide to Healthy Eating.

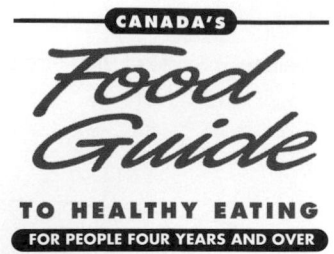

CANADA'S
Food Guide
TO HEALTHY EATING
FOR PEOPLE FOUR YEARS AND OVER

Different People Need Different Amounts of Food

The amount of food you need every day from the four food groups and other foods depends on your age, body size, activity level, whether you are male or female and if you are pregnant or breastfeeding. That's why the Food Guide gives a lower and higher number of servings for each food group. For example, young children can choose the lower number of servings, while male teenagers can go to the higher number. Most other people can choose servings somewhere in between.

Grain Products
5–12
SERVINGS PER DAY

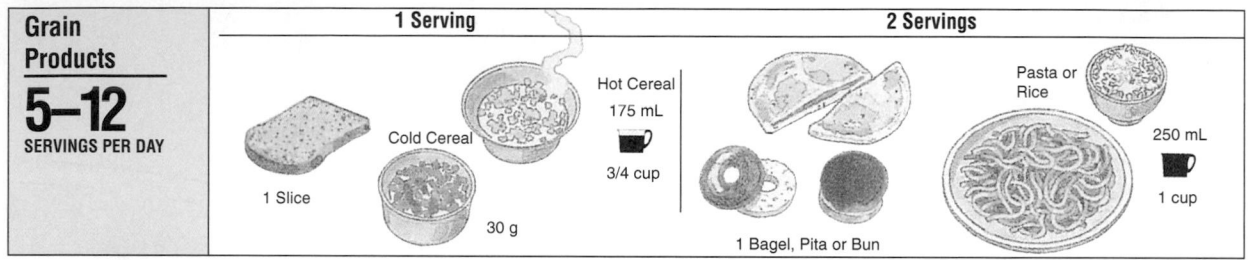

Vegetables & Fruit
5–10
SERVINGS PER DAY

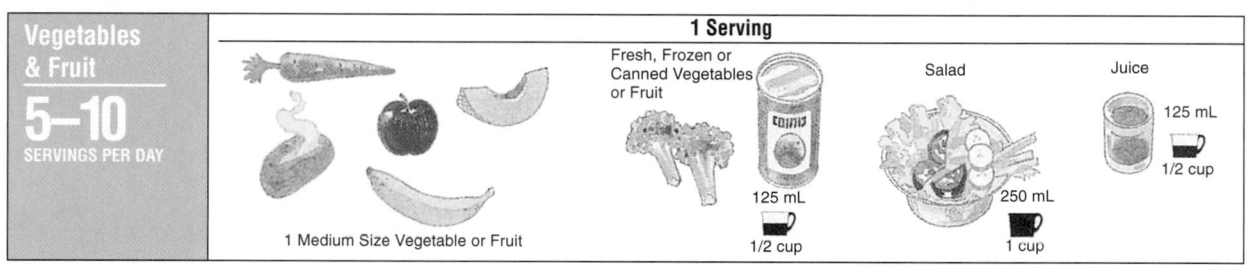

Milk Products
SERVINGS PER DAY
Children 4–9 years: 2–3
Youth 10–16 years: 3–4
Adults: 2–4
Pregnant & Breast-feeding Women: 3–4

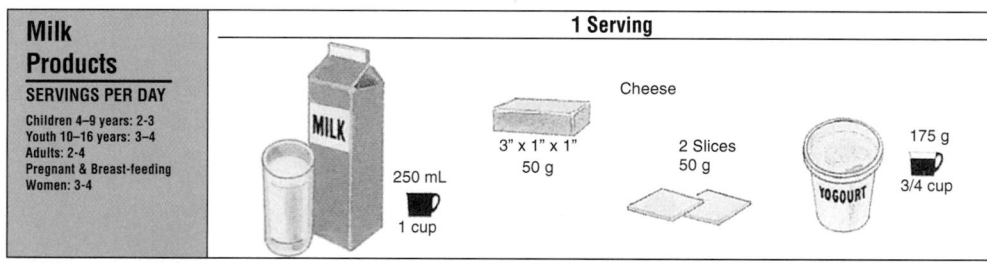

Other Foods

Taste and enjoyment can also come from other foods and beverages that are not part of the four food groups. Some of these foods are higher in fat or Calories, so use these foods in moderation.

Meat & Alternatives
2–3
SERVINGS PER DAY

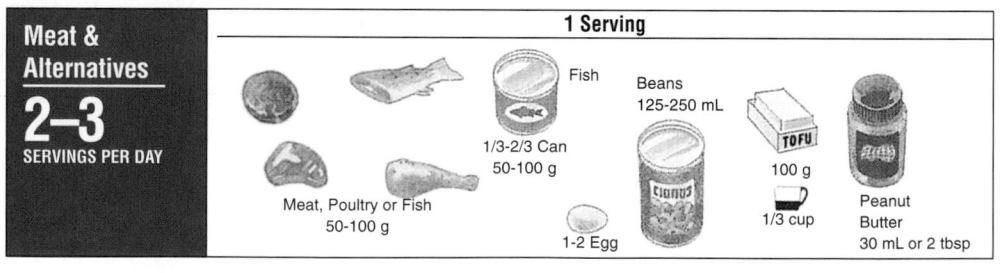

Enjoy eating well, being active, and feeling good about yourself. That's   VITALITE 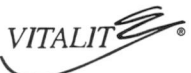 ®

© Minister of Supply and Services Canada 1992   Cat. No. H39-252 / 1992E   No changes permitted. Reprint permission not required.
ISBN 0-662-19648-1

Figure D-1 | Canadian Food Guide to Healthy Eating.

The bar side of the Food Guide helps Canadians decide how much they need from each group every day. The guide gives a range for the number of servings for each food group, since different people need different amounts of food. The Food Guide also shows serving sizes for different foods.

The bar side of the Food Guide also tells how other foods that are not part of the four food groups can have a role in healthy eating. Because some of these "other foods" are higher in fat or calories, the Food Guide recommends using these foods in moderation.

Nutrition Labels

The former Canadian Nutrition Label is shown here. Consumers have now started to see more information about the nutritional value of most prepackaged food under new labeling requirements that were published on January 1, 2003. The new regulations require most food labels to carry a mandatory *Nutrition Facts* table listing Calories and 13 key nutrients.

HOW TO READ THE FORMER CANADIAN NUTRITION LABEL

Nutrition information is expressed per **suggested serving**. The serving size will vary according to food type and brand. Consider this fact when comparing foods.

Gives the calorie content (Cal)

Indicates the quantity of naturally occurring and added sugars as well as dietary fibre

Indicates the level of sodium from salt and all other sources

Vitamins and minerals are expressed as a percentage of the highest recommended amount

millilitres: 5 mL = 1 teaspoon

kilojoules: metric unit of energy 1 Cal = 4.18kJ

grams: 28 g = 1 ounce

LASAGNA
Nutrition Information
per 275 g serving
(1 cup/250 mL)

Energy	275	Cal
	1140	kJ
Protein	19	g
Fat	7	g
Polyunsaturates	0.8	g
Monounsaturates	1.9	g
Saturates	2.5	g
Cholesterol	46	mg
Carbohydrate	34	g
Starch	29	g
Sugars	5	g
Dietary Fibre	0.2	g
Sodium	850	mg
Potassium	675	mg

Percentage of Recommended Daily Intake

Thiamine	20%
Riboflavin	19%
Niacin	18%
Calcium	12%
Iron	28%

The New Canadian Nutrition Label

As noted on page A-59, new regulations published on January 1, 2003, make nutrition labeling mandatory on most food labels using a new format. The regulations also update requirements for nutrient content claims and permit, for the first time in Canada, diet-related health claims for foods.

How to Read the Latest Canadian Nutrition Label

The Regulations provide for the optional declaration of the number of Calories both from fat and from saturates plus *trans*. Recommendations on the % of Calories from fat apply to the total diet rather than to an individual food. Therefore, inclusion of the % of Calories from fat in the Nutrition Facts table may be confusing and is not permitted.

The Nutrition Facts table provides information on saturated and *trans* fatty acids which have been shown to raise serum cholesterol levels. The declaration of the other groups of fatty acids, mono-unsaturates, omega-3 and omega-6 polyunsaturates, is optional unless claims are made, in which case all three must be declared.

Potassium is not included as a mandatory nutrient of the Nutrition Facts table because it is not considered to be a nutrient of general public health importance. The declaration of potassium, however, is mandatory when a claim is made for the sodium or salt content of a food which contains an added potassium salt.

Daily Value is a comparison standard comprised of
(a) vitamin or mineral amounts referred to in the definition of a recommended daily intake for that vitamin or mineral
(b) nutrient amounts referred to in the definition of reference standard for that nutrient

Serving size is stipulated for various foods.

The amount of vitamins and minerals is expressed as a percentage of the Daily Value per serving of stated size.

Nutrition Facts
Per 1 cup (264g)

Amount	% Daily Value
Calories 260	
Fat 13g	**20%**
Saturated Fat 3g + Trans Fat 2g	**25%**
Cholesterol 30mg	
Sodium 660mg	**28%**
Carbohydrate 31g	**10%**
Fibre 0g	**0%**
Sugars 5g	
Protein 5g	
Vitamin A 4%	Vitamin C 2%
Calcium 15%	Iron 4%

There is also a Canadian Nutrition Label for children under two years of age.

Nutrition Facts
Per 1 jar (126 mL)

	Amount
Calories	110
Fat	0g
Sodium	10 mg
Carbohydrate	27g
Fibre	4g
Sugars	18g
Protein	0g
% Daily Value	
Vitamin A 6%	Vitamin C 45%
Calcium 2%	Iron 2%

Recommended Daily Intakes and Reference Standards

Below are the **Recommended Daily Intakes** and **Reference Standards** used on Nutrition Labels for persons 2 years of age and older.*†‡

Dietary Constituent	Amount	Dietary Constituent	Amount
Fat	**65 g**	Folacin	220 µg
The sum of saturated fatty		Vitamin B$_{12}$	2 µg
acids and *trans* fatty acids	**20 g**	Pantothenic acid or	
Cholesterol	**300 mg**	pantothenate	7 mg
Carbohydrate	**300 g**	Vitamin K	**80 mg**
Fibre	**25 g**	Biotin	**30 µg**
Sodium	**2400 mg**	Calcium	1100 mg
Chloride	**3400 µg**	Phosphorus	1100 mg
Potassium	**3500 mg**	Magnesium	250 mg
Vitamin A	1000 RE	Iron	14 mg
Vitamin D	5 µg	Zinc	9 mg
Vitamin E	10 mg	Iodide	160 µg
Vitamin C	60 mg	Selenium	**50 µg**
Thiamin, thiamine or vitamin B$_1$	1.3 mg	Copper	**2 mg**
Riboflavin or vitamin B$_2$	1.6 mg	Manganese	**2 mg**
Niacin	23 NE	Chromium	**120 µg**
Vitamin B$_6$	1.8 mg	Molybdenum	**75 µg**

*RE = retinol equivalents

†NE = niacin equivalents

‡Together these constitute the Daily Values used on the new Canadian Nutrition Label. Note that Reference Standards are bolded.

Approved Nutrient Content Claims

Below is a sample of approved nutrient content claims for food labels.

Energy

- *Free of energy:* The food provides less than 5 Calories or 21 kilojoules per reference amount and serving of stated size.
- *Low in energy:* The food provides 40 Calories or 167 kilojoules or less per reference amount and serving of stated size.
- *Reduced in energy:* The food is processed, formulated, reformulated or otherwise modified so that it provides at least 25% less energy per reference amount of a similar food.
- *Lower in energy:* The food provides at least 25% less energy per reference amount of a similar food.
- *Source of energy:* The food provides at least 100 Calories or 420 kilojoules per reference amount and serving of stated size.
- *More energy:* The food provides at least 25% more energy, totalling at least 100 more Calories or 420 more kilojoules per reference amount of a similar food.

Protein

- *Low in protein:* The food contains no more than 1 g of protein per 100 g of the food.
- *Source of protein:* The food has a protein rating of 20 or more, as determined by official method FO-1, *Determination of Protein Rating,* October 15, 1981, (*a*) per reasonable daily intake; or (*b*) per 30 g combined with 125 mL of milk, if the food is a breakfast cereal.

- *Excellent source of protein:* The food has a protein rating of 40 or more, as determined by official method FO-1, *Determination of Protein Rating,* October 15, 1981, (*a*) per reasonable daily intake; or (*b*) per 30 g combined with 125 mL of milk, if the food is a breakfast cereal.
- *More protein:* The food (*a*) has a protein rating of 20 or more, as determined by official method FO-1, *Determination of Protein Rating,* October 15, 1981, (i) per reasonable daily intake, or (ii) per 30 g combined with 125 mL of milk, if the food is a breakfast cereal; and (*b*) contains at least 25% more protein, totalling at least 7 g more, per reasonable daily intake compared to the reference food of the same food group or the similar reference food.

Fat

- *Free of fat:* The food contains less than 0.5 g of fat per reference amount and serving of stated size.
- *Low in fat:* The food contains 3 g or less of fat per reference amount and serving of stated size and, if the reference amount is 30 g or 30 mL or less, per 50 g.
- *Reduced in fat:* The food is processed, formulated, reformulated or otherwise modified so that it contains at least 25% less fat than the reference amount of a similar food.
- *Lower in fat:* The food contains at least 25% less fat per reference amount of the food, than the reference amount of the reference food of the same food group.
- *100% fat-free:* The food (*a*) contains less than 0.5 g of fat per 100 g; (*b*) contains no added fat.
- *No added fat:* (1) The food contains no added fats or oils set out in Division 9, or added butter or ghee, or ingredients that contain added fats or oils, or butter or ghee.
- *Free of saturated fatty acids:* The food contains less than 0.2 g saturated fatty acids and less than 0.2 g *trans* fatty acids per reference amount and serving of stated size.
- *Low in saturated fatty acids:* (1) The food contains 2 g or less of saturated fatty acids and *trans* fatty acids combined per reference amount and serving of stated size. (2) The food provides 15% or less energy from the sum of saturated fatty acids and *trans* fatty acids.
- *Reduced in saturated fatty acids:* The food is processed, formulated, reformulated or otherwise modified, without increasing the content of *trans* fatty acids, so that it contains at least 25% less saturated fatty acids per reference amount of the food than the reference amount of the similar reference food.
- *Lower in saturated fatty acids:* The food contains at least 25% less saturated fatty acids and the content of *trans* fatty acids is not higher per reference amount of the food, than the reference amount of the reference food of the same food group.
- *Free of* trans *fatty acids:* The food contains less than 0.2 g of *trans* fatty acids per reference amount and serving of stated size.
- *Reduced in* trans *fatty acids:* The food is processed, formulated, reformulated or otherwise modified, without increasing the content of saturated fatty acids, so that it contains at least 25% less *trans* fatty acids per reference amount of the food than the reference amount of the similar reference food.
- *Lower in* trans *fatty acids:* The food contains at least 25% less *trans* fatty acids and the content of saturated fatty acids is not higher per reference amount of the food compared to the reference amount of a similar food.
- *Source of omega-3 polyunsaturated fatty acids:* The food contains 0.3 g or more of omega-3 polyunsaturated fatty acids per reference amount and serving of stated size.
- *Source of omega-6 polyunsaturated fatty acids:* The food contains 2 g or more of omega-6 polyunsaturated fatty acids per reference amount and serving of stated size.

Cholesterol

- *Free of cholesterol:* The food contains less than 2 mg of cholesterol per reference amount and serving of stated size.
- *Low in cholesterol:* The food contains 20 mg or less of cholesterol per reference amount and serving of stated size (if the reference amount is 30 g or 30 mL or less, per 50 g.)
- *Reduced in cholesterol:* The food is processed, formulated, reformulated or otherwise modified so that it contains at least 25% less cholesterol per reference amount of a similar food.
- *Lower in cholesterol:* The food contains at least 25% less cholesterol per reference amount of a similar food.

Sodium or Salt

- *Free of sodium or salt:* The food contains less than 5 mg of sodium per reference amount and serving of stated size.
- *Low in sodium or salt:* The food contains 140 mg or less of sodium per reference amount and serving of stated size.
- *Reduced in sodium or salt:* (1) The food is processed, formulated, reformulated or otherwise modified so that it contains at least 25% less sodium per reference amount of a similar food.
- *Lower in sodium or salt:* The food contains at least 25% less sodium per reference amount of the food.
- *No added sodium or salt:* The food contains no added salt, other sodium salts, or ingredients that contain sodium that functionally substitute for added salt.
- *Lightly salted:* The food contains at least 50% less added sodium than the sodium added to a similar reference food.

Sugars

- *Free of sugars:* The food contains less than 0.5 mg of sugars per reference amount and serving of stated size.
- *Reduced in sugars:* The food is processed, formulated, reformulated or otherwise modified so that it contains at least 25% less sugars, totalling at least 5 g less per reference amount of the food.
- *Lower in sugars:* The food contains at least 25% less sugars, totalling at least 5 g less per reference amount of the food.
- *No added sugars:* (1) The food contains no added sugars, no ingredients containing added sugars or ingredients that contain sugars that functionally substitute for added sugars.

Fibre

- *Source of fibre:* (1) The food contains 2 g or more (*a*) of fibre per reference amount and serving of stated size, if no fibre or fibre source is identified in the statement or claim; or (*b*) of each identified fibre or fibre from an identified fibre source per reference amount and serving of stated size, if a fibre or fibre source is identified in the statement or claim.
- *High source of fibre:* The food contains 4 g or more (*a*) of fibre per reference amount and serving of stated size, if no fibre or fibre source is identified in the statement or claim; or (*b*) of each identified fibre or fibre from an identified fibre source per reference amount and serving of stated size, if a fibre or fibre source is identified in the statement or claim.
- *Very high source of fibre:* The food contains 6 g or more (*a*) of fibre per reference amount and serving of stated size, if no fibre or fibre source is identified in the statement or claim; or (*b*) of each identified fibre or fibre from an identified fibre source

per reference amount and serving of stated size, if a fibre or fibre source is identified in the statement or claim.

- *More fibre:* The food contains at least 25% more fibre, totalling at least 1 g more, if no fibre or fibre source is identified in the statement or claim, or at least 25% more of an identified fibre or fibre from an identified fibre source, totalling at least 1 g more, if a fibre or fibre source is identified in the statement or claim compared to reference amount of a similar food.

Light and Lean

- *Light in energy or fat:* The food meets the conditions set out for the subject "reduced in energy" or "reduced in fat."
- *Lean:* The food (*a*) is meat or poultry that has not been ground, a marine or fresh water animal or a product of any of these; and (*b*) contains 10% or less fat.
- *Extra lean:* The food (*a*) is meat or poultry that has not been ground, a marine or fresh water animal or a product of any of these; and (*b*) contains 7.5% or less fat.

Approved Health Claims for Nutrition Labels

If a manufacturer follows specific guidelines addressing both the nutrients noted in the claim as well as guidelines pertaining to other nutrients in a food, the following health claims can be made.

- A healthy diet containing foods high in potassium and low in sodium may reduce the risk of high blood pressure, a risk factor for stroke and heart disease.
- A healthy diet with adequate calcium and vitamin D, and regular physical activity, help to achieve strong bones and may reduce the risk of osteoporosis.
- A healthy diet low in saturated and trans fats may reduce the risk of heart disease.
- A healthy diet rich in a variety of vegetables and fruit may help reduce the risk of some types of cancer.
- Foods very low in starch and fermentable sugars can make the following health claims:
  - Won't cause cavities;
  - does not promote tooth decay;
  - does not promote dental caries; or
  - is non-cariogenic.

appendix E

THE EXCHANGE SYSTEM: A HELPFUL MENU-PLANNING TOOL

The **Exchange System** is a valuable tool for roughly estimating the energy, protein, carbohydrate, and fat content of a food or meal. This tool organizes many details of the nutrient composition of foods into a manageable framework. By using the Exchange System, you can plan daily menus to fall roughly within specific percentages of macronutrients without having to look up or memorize the nutrient values of numerous foods, so the time you spend now becoming familiar with the Exchange System will pay dividends in the future.

In the Exchange System, individual foods are placed into three broad groups: carbohydrate, meat and meat substitutes, and fat. Within these groups are lists that contain foods of similar macronutrient composition: various types of milk, fruits, vegetables, starch, other carbohydrates, meat and meat substitutes, and fat. These lists are designed so that when the proper serving size is observed, each food on a list provides about the same amount of carbohydrate, protein, fat, and energy. This equality allows the exchange of foods on each list, hence the term *Exchange System*.

The Exchange System was originally developed for planning diabetic diets. Diabetes is easier to control if the person's diet has about the same composition day after day. If a certain number of **exchanges** from each of the various lists is eaten each day, that regularity is easier to achieve. However, because the Exchange System provides a quick way to estimate the energy, carbohydrate, protein, and fat content in any food or meal, it is a valuable menu-planning tool.

Becoming Familiar with the Exchange System

To use the Exchange System, you must know which foods are on each list and the serving sizes for each food.

Table E-1 gives the serving sizes for foods on each exchange list as well as the carbohydrate, protein, fat, and energy content per exchange. Note that the meat and milk lists are divided into subclasses, which vary in fat content and, hence, in the amount of energy they provide. Foods on the meat and fat lists contain essentially no carbohydrate; those on the fruit and fat lists lack appreciable amounts of protein; and those on the vegetable, fruit, and other carbohydrates lists contain essentially no fat. You need to study Table E-1 and Figure E-1 to become familiar with the exchange lists, the sizes of the exchanges (that is, serving sizes) on each list, and the amounts of carbohydrate, protein, fat, and energy per exchange.

Before you can turn a group of exchanges into a daily meal plan, you must be aware of which foods are on each exchange list (Figure E-1). The entire U.S. Exchange System is presented in Appendix F, which you should consult frequently while exploring the system to discover its various peculiarities. For example, the starch list includes

Exchange System A system for classifying foods into numerous lists based on the foods' macronutrient composition and establishing serving sizes, so that one serving of each food on a list contains the same amount of carbohydrate, protein, fat, and energy content.

exchange The serving size of a food on a specific exchange list.

Table E-1 | Nutrient Composition of Exchange System Lists (2003 Edition)

Groups/Lists	Household Measures*	Carbohydrate (g)	Protein (g)	Fat (g)	Energy (kcal)
Carbohydrate Group					
Starch	1 slice, 3/4 cup raw, or 1/2 cup cooked	15	3	1 or less†	80
Fruit	1 small/medium piece	15	—	—	60
Milk	1 cup				
Fat-free/very low-fat		12	8	0–3†	90
Reduced-fat		12	8	5	120
Whole		12	8	8	150
Other carbohydrates	Varies	15	Varies	Varies	Varies
Nonstarchy vegetables	1 cup raw or 1/2 cup cooked	5	2	—	25
Meat and Meat Substitutes Group	**1 oz**				
Very lean		—	7	0–1	35
Lean		—	7	3	55
Medium-fat		—	7	5	75
High-fat		—	7	8	100
Fat Group	**1 tsp**	**—**	**—**	**5**	**45**

*Just an estimate; see exchange lists for actual amounts.

†Calculated as 1 g for purposes of energy contribution.

Reproduction of the exchange lists in whole or in part, without permission of The American Dietetic Association or the American Diabetes Association, Inc. is a violation of federal law. This material has been modified from *Exchange Lists for Meal Planning*, which is the basis of a meal planning system designed by a committee of the American Diabetes Association and The American Dietetic Association. While designed primarily for people with diabetes and others who must follow special diets, the exchange lists are based on principles of good nutrition that apply to everyone. Copyright © 2003 by the American Diabetes Association and the American Dietetic Association.

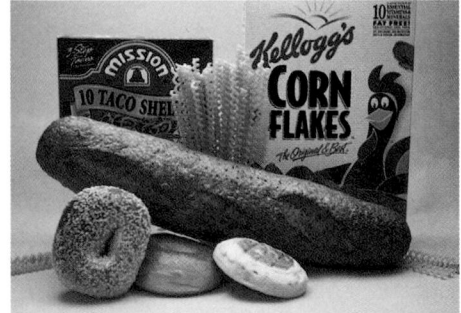
Starch exchange choices

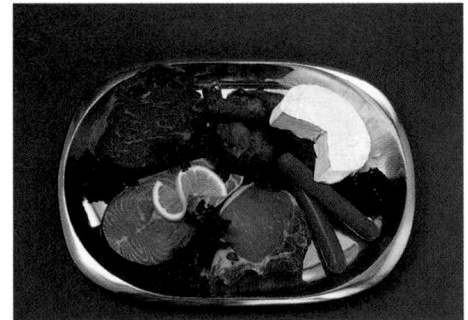
Meat and meat substitutes exchange choices

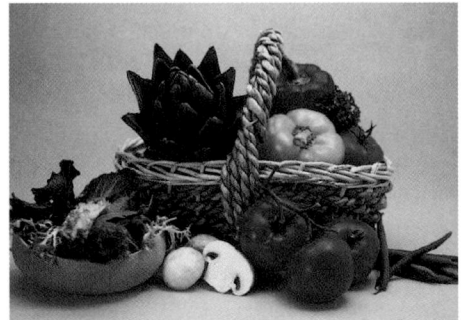
Vegetable exchange choices

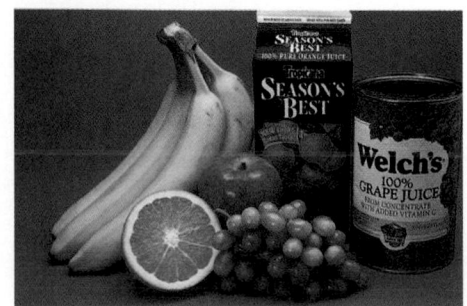
Fruit exchange choices

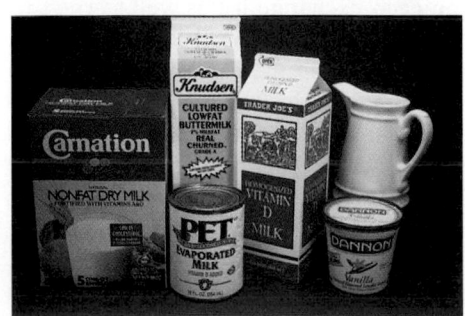
Milk exchange choices

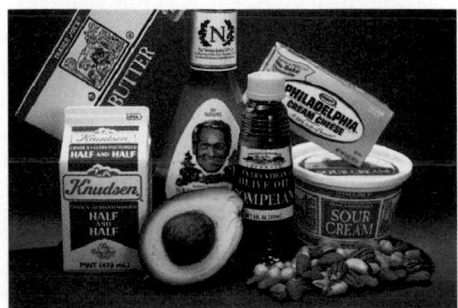
Fat exchange choices

Figure E-1 | Foods arranged according to the Exchange System lists.

not only bread, dry cereal, cooked cereal, rice, and pasta, but also baked beans, corn on the cob, and potatoes. These foods are not identical to those composing the grain group in MyPyramid. The Exchange System is not concerned with the origin of a food, whether animal or vegetable. It is primarily concerned with the macronutrients carbohydrate, protein, and fat in each food on a specific list. For example, the carbohydrate composition of potatoes resembles that of bread more than that of broccoli, although potatoes are vegetables. In addition, several foods on the meat and meat substitutes list are not meats. The list of other carbohydrates includes jam, angel food cake, fat-free frozen yogurt, and foods such as frosted cake that count as both other carbohydrate exchanges and fat exchanges. Bacon appears in the fat list rather than the high-fat meat category.

Free foods (essentially calorie-free) include bouillon, diet soda, coffee, tea, dill pickles, and vinegar as well as herbs and spices. Most vegetables, such as cabbage, celery, mushrooms, lettuce, and zucchini, also can be considered free foods; their minimal energy contribution need not count in the calculations when they are eaten in moderation (1 to 2 servings per meal or snack).

Using the Exchange System to Develop Daily Menus

Use the Exchange System to plan a 1-day menu. Target an energy content of 2000 kcal, with 55% derived from carbohydrates (1100 kcal), 15% from protein (300 kcal), and 30% from fat (600 kcal). These specifications can be translated into 2 low-fat milk exchanges, 3 vegetable exchanges, 5 fruit exchanges, 11 starch exchanges, 4 lean meat exchanges, and 6 fat exchanges (Table E-2). Note that this example is only one of many possible combinations; the Exchange System offers great flexibility.

Table E-3 arbitrarily separates these exchanges into breakfast, lunch, dinner, and a snack. Breakfast includes 1 reduced-fat milk exchange, 2 fruit exchanges, 2 starch exchanges, and 1 fat exchange. This total corresponds to 3/4 cup of a ready-to-eat breakfast cereal, 1 cup of reduced-fat milk, 1 slice of bread with 1 tsp margarine, and 1 cup of orange juice.

Lunch consists of 2 fat exchanges, 4 starch exchanges, 1 vegetable exchange, 1 reduced-fat milk exchange, and 2 fruit exchanges. This total translates into one slice of bacon with 1 teaspoon mayonnaise on two slices of bread, with tomato—in other words, a bacon and tomato sandwich. You can also add lettuce to the sandwich. Lettuce can be considered a free vegetable choice. Add to this meal a 9-inch banana (1 exchange = 1 small banana), 1 cup of reduced-fat milk, and 6 graham crackers (2 1/2 inches by 2 1/2 inches). Later, add a snack of 3/4 oz of pretzels for another starch exchange.

Table E-2 | Possible Exchange Patterns That Yield 55% of Energy as Carbohydrate, 30% as Fat, and 15% as Protein for Energy Intakes Greater Than 2000 kcal

kcal/Day Exchange List	1200*	1600*	2000	2400	2800	3200	3600
Milk (reduced-fat)	2	2	2	2	2	2	2
Vegetable	3	3	3	4	4	4	4
Fruit	3	4	5	6	8	9	9
Starch	5	8	11	13	15	18	21
Meat (lean)	4	4	4	5	6	7	8
Fat	2	4	6	8	10	11	13

This is just one set of options. More meat could be included if less milk were used, for example.

*Energy intakes of 1200 and 1600 kcal contain 20% of energy as protein and 50% energy as carbohydrate to allow for greater flexibility in diet planning.

Table E-3 | Sample 1-Day 2000 kcal Menu Based on the Exchange System Plan*

Breakfast	
1 reduced-fat milk exchange	1 cup reduced-fat milk (some on cereal)
2 fruit exchanges	1 cup orange juice
2 starch exchanges	3/4 cup ready-to-eat breakfast cereal, 1 piece whole-wheat toast
1 fat exchange	1 tsp soft margarine on toast

Lunch	
4 starch exchanges	2 slices whole-wheat bread, 6 graham crackers (2 1/2 inches by 2 1/2 inches)
2 fat exchanges	1 slice bacon, 1 tsp mayonnaise
1 vegetable exchange	1 sliced tomato
2 fruit exchanges	1 banana (9 inches)
1 reduced-fat milk exchange	1 cup reduced-fat milk

Snack	
1 starch exchange	3/4 oz pretzels

Dinner	
4 lean meat exchanges	4 oz lean steak (well trimmed)
2 starch exchanges	1 medium baked potato
1 fat exchange	1 tsp soft margarine
2 vegetable exchanges	1 cup cooked broccoli
1 fruit exchange	1 kiwi fruit
	Coffee (if desired)

Snack	
2 starch exchanges	1 bagel
2 fat exchanges	2 tbsp regular cream cheese

*The target plan was a 2000 kcal energy intake, with 55% from carbohydrate, 15% from protein, and 30% from fat. Computer analysis indicates that this menu yielded 2040 kcal, with 53% from carbohydrate, 16% from protein, and 31% from fat—in close agreement with the targeted goals.

Dinner consists of 4 lean meat exchanges, 1 fruit exchange, 2 vegetable exchanges, 1 fat exchange, and 2 starch exchanges. This total corresponds to a 4-oz broiled steak (meat only, no bone), 1 medium baked potato (1 exchange = 1 small baked potato) with 1 tsp of margarine, 1 cup of broccoli, and 1 kiwi fruit. Coffee (if desired) is not counted, because it contains no appreciable energy.

Finally, you can have a snack containing 2 starch exchanges and 2 fat exchanges. This total translates into 1 bagel with 2 tbsp of regular cream cheese.

This 1-day menu is only one of many that are possible with the exchange lists. Apple juice could replace the orange juice; two apples could be exchanged for the banana. The choices are endless. Notice that an exchange diet is much easier to plan if you use individual foods, as was done here; however, the Exchange System tables list some combination foods to help you (see Appendix F). Using combination foods, such as pizza or lasagna, however, makes it more difficult to calculate the number of exchanges in a serving. For instance, lasagna typically has meat exchanges, vegetable exchanges, and starch exchanges. With practice, you will be able to tackle such complex foods (Figure E-2). For now, using individual foods makes learning the Exchange System much easier. Finally, you might want to prove to yourself that the food choices listed in Table E-3 really meet the exchange plan. This demonstration will give you practice turning exchanges into actual food servings.

Exchange List	Total Exchanges to Be Consumed Daily	Exchanges Consumed at Each Meal		
		Breakfast	Lunch	Dinner
MILK				
VEGETABLE				
FRUIT				
STARCH				
MEAT AND SUBSTITUTES				
FAT				

Figure E-2 | Record the Exchange System pattern you have chosen in the left column. Then distribute the exchanges throughout the day, noting the food to be used and the serving size.

appendix F

Milk Exchange List

Fat-Free and Low-Fat Milk

(12 g carbohydrate, 8 g protein, 0–3 g fat, 90 kcal)

1 cup	fat-free, ½%, and 1% milk and buttermilk
⅓ cup	powdered (fat-free dry, before adding liquid)
½ cup	canned, evaporated fat-free milk
1 cup	buttermilk made from fat-free or low-fat milk
1 cup	soy milk (low-fat or fat-free)
⅔ cup (6 oz)	yogurt made from fat-free milk (plain, unflavored)
⅔ cup (6 oz)	yogurt, fat-free, flavored, sweetened with nonnutritive sweetener and fructose

Reduced-Fat Milk

(12 g carbohydrate, 8 g protein, 5 g fat, 120 kcal)

1 cup	2% milk
1 cup	soy milk
¾ cup	yogurt plain, low-fat (added milk solids)
1 cup	sweet acidophilus milk

Whole Milk

(12 g carbohydrate, 8 g protein, 8 g fat, 150 kcal)

1 cup	whole milk
½ cup	evaporated whole milk
1 cup	goat's milk
1 cup	kefir
1 cup	yogurt, plain (made from whole milk)

*The exchange lists are the basis of a meal planning system designed by a committee of the American Diabetes Association and the American Dietetic Association. While designed primarily for people with diabetes and others who must follow special diets, the exchange lists are based on principles of good nutrition that apply to everyone. Copyright © 2003 by the American Diabetes Association and the American Dietetic Association.

Vegetable Exchange List

(5 g carbohydrate, 2 g protein, 0 g fat, 25 kcal)
1 vegetable exchange equals:

½ cup cooked vegetables or vegetable juice
1 cup raw vegetables

artichoke
artichoke hearts
asparagus
beans (green, wax, Italian)
bean sprouts
beets
broccoli
brussels sprouts
cabbage
carrots
cauliflower
celery

cucumber
eggplant
green onions or scallions
greens (e.g., collard)
kohlrabi
leeks
mixed vegetables (without corn,
    peas, or pasta)
mushrooms
okra
onions
pea pods

peppers (all varieties)
radishes
salad greens (all varieties)
sauerkraut
spinach
squash (summer)
tomato (fresh, canned, sauce)
tomato/vegetable juice
turnips
water chestnuts
watercress
zucchini

Fruit Exchange List

Fruit

(15 g carbohydrate, 0 g protein, 0 g fat, 60 kcal)
1 fruit exchange equals:

1 (4 oz)	apple, unpeeled (small)
4 rings	apple, dried
½ cup	applesauce (unsweetened)
4 (5½ oz)	apricots, fresh
8 halves	apricots, dried
½ cup	apricots, canned
1 (4 oz)	banana (small)
¾ cup	blackberries
¾ cup	blueberries
⅓ melon (11 oz)	cantaloupe (small)
1 cup cubes	cantaloupe
12 (3 oz)	cherries
½ cup	cherries, canned
3	dates
2 (3½ oz)	figs, fresh (large)
1½	figs, dried
½ cup	fruit cocktail
½ (11 oz)	grapefruit (large)
¾ cup	grapefruit sections, canned
17 (3 oz)	grapes (small)
1 slice (10 oz)	honeydew melon (or 1 cup cubes)
1 (3½ oz)	kiwi
¾ cup	mandarin orange sections
½ (5½ oz)	mango (or ½ cup)
1 (5 oz)	nectarine (small)
1 (6½ oz)	orange (small)
½ (8 oz)	papaya (or 1 cup cubes)

1 (4 oz)	peach, fresh (medium)
½ cup	peaches, canned
½ (4 oz)	pear, fresh
½ cup	pear, canned
¾ cup	pineapple, fresh
½ cup	pineapple, canned
2 (5 oz)	plums (small)
½ cup	plums, canned
3	plums, dried (prunes)
2 tbsp	raisins
1 cup	raspberries
1¼ cups	strawberries (raw, whole)
2 (8 oz)	tangerines (small)
1 slice (13½ oz)	watermelon (or 1¼ cups cubes)

Fruit Juice

½ cup	apple juice/cider
⅓ cup	cranberry juice cocktail
1 cup	cranberry juice cocktail, reduced-calorie
⅓ cup	fruit juice blends, 100% juice
⅓ cup	grape juice
½ cup	grapefruit juice
½ cup	orange juice
½ cup	pineapple juice
⅓ cup	prune juice

Starch Exchange List

(15 g carbohydrate, 3 g protein, 0–1 g fat, 80 kcal)
1 starch exchange equals:

Bread

¼ (1 oz)	bagel
2 slices (1½ oz)	bread, reduced-calorie
1 slice (1 oz)	bread, white, whole-wheat, pumpernickel, or rye
4 (⅔ oz)	bread sticks, crisp, 4 inch × ½ inch
½	English muffin
½ (1 oz)	hot dog or hamburger bun
¼	naan, 8 inch × 2 inch
1	pancake, 4 inch across × ¼ inch thick
½	pita, 6 inches across
1 slice (1 oz)	raisin bread, unfrosted
1 (1 oz)	roll, plain (small)
1	tortilla, corn, 6 inches across
1	tortilla, flour, 6 inches across
⅓	tortilla, flour, 10 inches across
1	waffle, 4 inches square or across, reduced-fat

Cereals and Grains

½ cup	bran cereal
½ cup	bulgur
½ cup	cereal, cooked
¾ cup	cereal, unsweetened, ready-to-eat
3 tbsp	cornmeal (dry)
⅓ cup	couscous
3 tbsp	flour (dry)
¼ cup	granola, low-fat
¼ cup	Grape-Nuts
½ cup	grits
½ cup	kasha
⅓ cup	millet
¼ cup	muesli
½ cup	oats
⅓ cup	pasta
1½ cups	puffed cereal
⅓ cup	rice, white or brown
½ cup	Shredded Wheat
½ cup	sugar-frosted cereal
3 tbsp	wheat germ

Starchy Vegetables

⅓ cup	baked beans
½ cup	corn
½ (5 oz)	corn on the cob (large)
1 cup	mixed vegetables with corn, peas, or pasta
½ cup	peas, green
½ cup	plantain
½ cup or	
½ medium (3 oz)	potato, boiled
¼ large (3 oz)	potato, baked with skin
½ cup	potato, mashed
1 cup	squash, winter (acorn, butternut, pumpkin)
½ cup	yam, sweet potato, plain

Crackers and Snacks

8	animal crackers
3	graham crackers, 2½-inch square
¾ oz	matzoh
4 slices	melba toast
24	oyster crackers
3 cups	popcorn (popped, no fat added or low-fat microwave)
¾ oz	pretzels
2	rice cakes, 4 inches across
6	saltine-type crackers
15–20 (¾ oz)	snack chips, fat-free (tortilla, potato)
2–5 (¾ oz)	whole-wheat crackers, no fat added

Dried Beans, Peas, and Lentils

(Counts as 1 starch exchange plus 1 very lean meat exchange)

½ cup	beans and peas (garbanzo, pinto, kidney, white, split, black-eyed)
⅔ cup	lima beans
½ cup	lentils
3 tbsp	miso

Starchy Foods Prepared with Fat

(Counts as 1 starch exchange plus 1 fat exchange)

1	biscuit, 2½ inches across
½ cup	chow mein noodles
1 (2 oz)	corn bread, 2-inch cube
6	crackers, round butter type
1 cup	croutons
1 cup (2 oz)	French-fried potatoes (oven-baked) (see also the fast-foods list)
¼ cup	granola
⅓ cup	hummus

Starchy Foods Prepared with Fat (continued)

⅕ (1 oz)	muffin, 5 oz
3 cups	popcorn, microwaved
3	sandwich crackers, cheese or peanut butter filling
9–13 (¾ oz)	snack chips (potato, tortilla)
⅓ cup	stuffing, bread (prepared)
2	taco shell, 6 inches across
1	waffle, 4-inch square or across
4–6 (1 oz)	whole-wheat crackers, fat added

Other Carbohydrates Exchange List

One exchange equals 15 g carbohydrate, or 1 starch, or 1 fruit, or 1 milk.

Exchanges per Serving

1/12th cake (about 2 oz)	angel food cake, unfrosted	2 carbohydrates
2-inch square (about 1 oz)	brownie, unfrosted (small)	1 carbohydrate, 1 fat
2-inch square (about 1 oz)	cake, unfrosted	1 carbohydrate, 1 fat
2-inch square (about 2 oz)	cake, frosted	2 carbohydrates, 1 fat
2	cookies, fat-free (small)	1 carbohydrate
2 (about ⅔ oz)	cookies or sandwich cookies with creme filling (small)	1 carbohydrate, 1 fat
¼ cup	cranberry sauce, jellied	1½ carbohydrates
1 (about 2 oz)	cupcake, frosted (small)	2 carbohydrates, 1 fat
1 (1½ oz)	doughnut, plain cake (medium)	1½ carbohydrates, 2 fats
3¾ inches across (2 oz)	doughnuts, glazed	2 carbohydrates, 2 fats
1 bar (1⅓ oz)	Energy, sport or breakfast bar	2 carbohydrates, 1 fat
1 bar (2 oz)	Energy, sport or breakfast bar	3 carbohydrates, 1 fat
½ cup (3½ oz)	fruit cobbler	3 carbohydrates, 1 fat
1 bar (3 oz)	fruit juice bars, frozen, 100% juice	1 carbohydrate
1 roll (¾ oz)	fruit snacks, chewy (puréed fruit concentrate)	1 carbohydrate
1 tbsp	honey	1 carbohydrate
1 tbsp	sugar	1 carbohydrate
1½ tbsp	fruit spread, 100% fruit	1 carbohydrate
½ cup	gelatin, regular	1 carbohydrate
3	gingersnaps	1 carbohydrate
1 bar (1 oz)	granola or snack bar (regular and low-fat)	1½ carbohydrates
½ cup	ice cream, low-fat	1½ carbohydrates
½ cup	ice cream	1 carbohydrate, 2 fats
½ cup	ice cream, light	1 carbohydrate, 1 fat
½ cup	ice cream, fat-free, no sugar added	1 carbohydrate
1 tbsp	jam or jelly, regular	1 carbohydrate
1 cup	milk, chocolate, whole	2 carbohydrates, 1 fat
⅙ pie	pie, fruit, 2 crusts (8 inches across)	3 carbohydrates, 2 fats
⅛ pie	pie, pumpkin or custard (8 inches across)	2 carbohydrates, 2 fats
½ cup	pudding, regular (made with reduced-fat milk)	2 carbohydrates
½ cup	pudding, sugar-free (made with fat-free milk)	1 carbohydrate
1 can (10–11 oz)	reduced-calorie meal replacement (shake)	1½ carbohydrates, 0–1 fat
1 cup	rice milk, low-fat or fat-free, plain	1 carbohydrate
1 cup	rice milk, low-fat, flavored	1½ carbohydrates
¼ cup	salad dressing, fat-free	1 carbohydrate
½ cup	sherbet, sorbet	2 carbohydrates
½ cup	spaghetti or pasta sauce, canned	1 carbohydrate, 1 fat
1 cup (8 oz)	sports drinks	1 carbohydrate
1 tbsp	sugar	1 carbohydrate
1 (2½ oz)	sweet roll or Danish	2½ carbohydrates, 2 fats
2 tbsp	syrup, light	1 carbohydrate
1 tbsp	syrup, regular	1 carbohydrate
5	vanilla wafers	1 carbohydrate, 1 fat
⅓ cup	yogurt, frozen, fat-free	1 carbohydrate
1 cup	yogurt, low-fat with fruit	3 carbohydrates, 0–1 fat

Meat and Meat Substitutes Exchange List

Very Lean Meat and Substitutes List

(0 g carbohydrate, 7 g protein, 0–1 g fat, and 35 kcal)
One very lean meat exchange equals:

Poultry
1 oz   chicken or turkey (white meat, no skin), Cornish hen (no skin)

Fish
1 oz   fresh or frozen cod, flounder, haddock, halibut, trout; tuna, fresh or canned in water

Shellfish
1 oz   clams, crab, lobster, scallops, shrimp, imitation shellfish

Game
1 oz   duck or pheasant (no skin), venison, buffalo, ostrich

Cheese with 1 g or less fat per oz
¼ cup   fat-free or low-fat cottage cheese
1 oz   fat-free cheese

Other
1 oz   processed sandwich meats with 1 g or less fat per oz, such as deli thin, shaved meats, chipped beef, turkey, ham
2   egg whites
¼ cup   egg substitute, plain
1 oz   hot dogs with 1 g or less fat per oz
1 oz   kidney (high in cholesterol)
1 oz   sausage with 1 g or less fat per oz

Counts as one very lean meat and one starch exchange:

½ cup   dried beans, peas, lentils (cooked)

Lean Meat and Substitutes List

(0 g carbohydrate, 7 g protein, 3 g fat, and 55 kcal)
One lean meat exchange equals:

Beef
1 oz   USDA Select or Choice grades of lean beef trimmed of fat, such as round, sirloin, and flank steak; tenderloin; roast (rib, chuck, rump); steak (T-bone, porterhouse, cubed), ground round

Pork
1 oz   lean pork, such as fresh ham; canned, cured, or boiled ham; Canadian bacon; tenderloin, center loin chop

Lamb
1 oz   roast, chop, leg

Veal
1 oz   lean chop, roast

Poultry
1 oz   chicken, turkey (dark meat, no skin), chicken white meat (with skin), domestic duck or goose (well drained of fat, no skin)

Fish
1 oz   herring (uncreamed or smoked)
6   oysters (medium)
1 oz   salmon (fresh or canned), catfish
2   sardines (canned, medium)
1 oz   tuna (canned in oil, drained)

Game
1 oz   goose (no skin), rabbit

Cheese
¼ cup   4.5%–fat cottage cheese
2 tbsp   grated Parmesan
1 oz   cheeses with 3 g or less fat per oz

Other
1½ oz   hot dogs with 3 g or less fat per oz
1 oz   processed sandwich meat with 3 g or less fat per oz, such as turkey pastrami or kielbasa
1 oz   liver, heart (high in cholesterol)

Medium-Fat Meat and Substitutes List

(0 g carbohydrate, 7 g protein, 5 g fat, and 75 kcal)
One medium-fat meat exchange equals:

Beef
1 oz   most beef products (ground beef, meatloaf, corned beef, short ribs, prime grades of meat trimmed of fat, such as prime rib)

Pork
1 oz   top loin, chop, Boston butt, cutlet

Lamb
1 oz   rib roast, ground

Veal
1 oz   cutlet (ground or cubed, unbreaded)

Poultry
1 oz   chicken dark meat (with skin), ground turkey or ground chicken, fried chicken (with skin)

Fish

1 oz	any fried fish product

Cheese (with 5 g or less fat per oz)

1 oz	feta
1 oz	mozzarella
¼ cup (2 oz)	ricotta

Other

1	egg (high in cholesterol, limit to 3 per week)
1 oz	sausage with 5 g or less fat per oz
¼ cup	tempeh
4 oz (½ cup)	tofu

High-Fat Meat and Substitutes List

(0 g carbohydrate, 7 g protein, 8 g fat, and 100 kcal)
One high-fat meat exchange equals:

Pork

1 oz	spareribs, ground pork, pork sausage

Cheese

1 oz	all regular cheeses, such as American, cheddar, Monterey Jack, Swiss

Other

1 oz	processed sandwich meats with 8 g or less fat per oz, such as bologna, pimento loaf, salami
1 oz	sausage, such as bratwurst, Italian, knockwurst, Polish, smoked
1	hot dog (turkey or chicken) (10 per pound)
3 slices	bacon (20 slices per pound)

Counts as one high-fat meat plus one fat exchange:

1	hot dog (beef, pork, or combination) (10 per pound)

Fat Exchange List

Monounsaturated Fats List

(5 g fat and 45 kcal)
One exchange equals:

2 tbsp (1 oz)	avocado (medium)
1 tsp	oil (canola, olive, peanut)
	olives:
8	ripe, black (large)
10	green, stuffed (large)
6 nuts	almonds, cashews

6 nuts	mixed (50% peanuts)
10 nuts	peanuts
4 halves	pecans
½ tbsp	peanut butter, smooth or crunchy
1 tbsp	sesame seeds
2 tsp	tahini or sesame paste

Polyunsaturated Fats List

(5 g fat and 45 kcal)
One exchange equals:

	margarine:
1 tsp	stick, tub, or squeeze
1 tbsp	lower-fat (30 to 50% vegetable oil)
	mayonnaise:
1 tsp	regular
1 tbsp	reduced-fat
4 halves	nuts, walnuts, English
1 tsp	oil (corn, safflower, soybean)

	salad dressing:
1 tbsp	regular
2 tbsp	reduced-fat
	Miracle Whip Salad Dressing:
2 tsp	regular
1 tbsp	reduced-fat
1 tbsp	seeds: pumpkin, sunflower

Saturated Fats List

(5 g fat and 45 kcal)
One exchange equals:

1 slice	bacon, cooked (20 slices per pound)
1 tsp	bacon, grease

	butter:
1 tsp	stick
2 tsp	whipped
1 tbsp	reduced-fat

2 tbsp (½ oz)	chitterlings, boiled		sour cream:
	cream cheese:	2 tbsp	regular
1 tbsp (½ oz)	regular	3 tbsp	reduced-fat
2 tbsp (1 oz)	reduced-fat		
1 tsp	shortening or lard		

Free Foods List

A *free food* is any food or drink that contains less than 20 kcal or less than 5 g of carbohydrate per serving. Foods with a serving size listed should be limited to three servings per day. Foods listed without a serving size can be eaten as often as you like.

Fat-Free or Reduced-Fat Foods

1 tbsp (½ oz)	cream cheese, fat-free	1 tbsp	salad dressing, fat-free
1 tbsp	creamers, nondairy, liquid		nonstick cooking spray
2 tsp	creamers, nondairy, powdered	1 tbsp	salad dressing, fat-free or low-fat, Italian
1 tbsp	mayonnaise, fat-free	2 tbsp	salad dressing, fat-free, Italian
1 tsp	mayonnaise, reduced-fat	1 tbsp	sour cream, fat-free, reduced-fat
4 tbsp	margarine, fat-free	1 tbsp	whipped topping, regular
1 tsp	margarine, reduced-fat	2 tbsp	whipped topping, light or fat-free
1 tbsp	Miracle Whip, fat-free		
1 tsp	Miracle Whip, reduced-fat nonstick cooking spray		

Sugar-Free Foods

1 candy	candy, hard, sugar-free	2 tsp	jam or jelly, light
	gelatin dessert, sugar-free		sugar substitutes*
	gelatin, unflavored	2 tbsp	syrup, sugar-free
	gum, sugar-free		

Drinks

	bouillon, broth, consommé		coffee
	bouillon or broth, low-sodium		diet soft drinks, sugar-free
	carbonated or mineral water		drink mixes, sugar-free
	club soda		tea
1 tbsp	cocoa powder, unsweetened		tonic water, sugar-free

Condiments

1 tbsp	catsup	2 slices	pickles, sweet (bread and butter)
	horseradish	¾ oz	pickles, sweet (gherkin)
	lemon juice	¼ cup	salsa
	lime juice	1 tbsp	soy sauce, regular or light
	mustard	1 tbsp	taco sauce
1 tbsp	pickle relish		vinegar
1½	pickles, dill (medium)	2 tbsp	yogurt

*Sugar substitutes, alternatives, or replacements that are approved by the Food and Drug Administration (FDA) are safe to use. Common brand names include:
Equal (aspartame)
Splenda (sucralose)
Sprinkle Sweet (saccharin)
Sweet One (acesulfame K)
Sweet-10 (saccharin)
Sugar Twin (saccharin)
Sweet 'N Low (saccharin)

Seasonings

flavoring extracts
garlic
herbs, fresh or dried
pimento

spices
Tabasco or hot pepper sauce
wine, used in cooking
Worcestershire sauce

Combination Foods List

	Entrées	Exchanges per Serving
1 cup (8 oz)	tuna noodle casserole, lasagna, spaghetti with meatballs, chili with beans, macaroni and cheese	2 carbohydrates, 2 medium-fat meats
2 cups (16 oz)	chow mein (without noodles or rice)	1 carbohydrate, 2 lean meats
½ cup (3½ oz)	tuna or chicken salad	½ carbohydrate, 2 lean meats, 1 fat
	Frozen Entrées and Meals	
generally 14–17 oz	dinner-type meal	3 carbohydrates, 3 medium-fat meats, 3 fats
3 oz	meatless burger, soy-based	½ carbohydrate, 2 lean meats
3 oz	meatless burger, vegetable and starch-based	1 carbohydrate, 1 lean meat
¼ of 12-inch (6 oz)	pizza, cheese, thin crust	2 carbohydrates, 2 medium-fat meats, 1 fat
¼ of 12-inch (6 oz)	pizza, meat topping, thin crust	2 carbohydrates, 2 medium-fat meats, 2 fats
1 (7 oz)	pot pie	2½ carbohydrates, 1 medium-fat meat, 3 fats
8–11 oz	entrée or meal with less than 340 kcal	2–3 carbohydrates, 1–2 lean meats
	Soups	
1 cup	bean	1 carbohydrate, 1 very lean meat
1 cup (8 oz)	cream (made with water)	1 carbohydrate, 1 fat
6 oz prepared	instant	1 carbohydrate
8 oz prepared	instant with beans/lentils	2½ carbohydrates, 1 very lean meat
½ cup (4 oz)	split pea (made with water)	1 carbohydrate
1 cup (8 oz)	tomato (made with water)	1 carbohydrate
1 cup (8 oz)	vegetable beef, chicken noodle, or other broth-type	1 carbohydrate

Fast-Foods

		Exchanges per Serving
1 (5–7 oz)	burritos with beef	3 carbohydrates, 1 medium-fat meat, 1 fat
6	chicken nuggets	1 carbohydrate, 2 medium-fat meats, 1 fat
1 each	chicken breast and wing, breaded and fried	1 carbohydrate, 4 medium-fat meats, 2 fats
1	chicken sandwich, grilled	2 carbohydrates, 3 very lean meats
6 (5 oz)	chicken wings, hot	1 carbohydrate, 3 medium-fat meats, 4 fats
1	fish sandwich/tartar sauce	3 carbohydrates, 1 medium-fat meat, 3 fats
1 medium serving (5 oz)	French fries	4 carbohydrates, 4 fats
1	hamburger (regular)	2 carbohydrates, 2 medium-fat meats
1	hamburger (large)	2 carbohydrates, 3 medium-fat meats, 1 fat
1	hot dog with bun	1 carbohydrate, 1 high-fat meat, 1 fat
1	individual pan pizza	5 carbohydrates, 3 medium-fat meats, 3 fats
¼ 12-inch (about 6 oz)	pizza, cheese, thin crust	2½ carbohydrates, 2 medium-fat meats
¼ 12-inch (about 6 oz)	pizza, meat, thin crust	2½ carbohydrates, 2 medium-fat meats, 1 fat
1 (5 oz)	soft-serve cone (small)	2½ carbohydrates, 1 fat
1 sub (6 inches)	submarine sandwich	3 carbohydrates, 1 vegetable, 2 medium-fat meats, 1 fat
1 (3–3½ oz)	taco, hard or soft shell	1 carbohydrate, 1 medium-fat meat, 1 fat

appendix G

DIETARY INTAKE AND ENERGY EXPENDITURE ASSESSMENT

Although it may seem overwhelming at first, it is actually very easy to track the foods you eat. One tip is to record foods and beverages consumed as soon as possible after the actual time of consumption.

I. Fill in the food record form that follows. This appendix contains a blank copy (see the completed example in Table G-1). Then, to estimate the nutrient values of the foods you are eating, consult food labels and the food composition table in this book (Appendix N), or use the nutrition software package available with this book. If these resources do not have the serving size you need, adjust the value. If you drink ½ cup of orange juice, for example, but a table has values only for 1 cup, halve all values before you record them. Then, consider pooling all the same food to save time; if you drink a cup of 1% milk three times throughout the day, enter your milk consumption only once as 3 cups. As you record your intake for use on the nutrient analysis form that follows, consider the following tips:

- Measure and record the amounts of foods eaten in portion sizes of cups, teaspoons, tablespoons, ounces, slices, or inches (or convert metric units to these units).
- Record brand names of all food products, such as "Quick Quaker Oats."
- Measure and record all those little extras, such as gravies, salad dressings, taco sauces, pickles, jelly, sugar, catsup, and margarine.
- For beverages
  —List the type of milk, such as whole, skim, 1%, evaporated, chocolate, or reconstituted dry.
  —Indicate whether fruit juice is fresh, frozen, or canned.
  —Indicate type for other beverages, such as fruit drink, fruit-flavored drink, Kool-Aid, and hot chocolate made with water or milk.
- For fruits
  —Indicate whether fresh, frozen, dried, or canned.
  —If whole, record number eaten and size with approximate measurements (such as 1 apple—3 in. in diameter).
  —Indicate whether processed in water, light syrup, or heavy syrup.
- For vegetables
  —Indicate whether fresh, frozen, dried, or canned.
  —Record as portion of cup, teaspoon, or tablespoon, or as pieces (such as carrot sticks—4 in. long, ½ in. thick).
  —Record preparation method.
- For cereals
  —Record cooked cereals in portions of tablespoon or cup (a level measurement after cooking).
  —Record dry cereal in level portions of tablespoon or cup.

—If margarine, milk, sugar, fruit, or something else is added, measure and record amount and type.

- For breads
  —Indicate whether whole wheat, rye, white, and so on.
  —Measure and record number and size of portion (biscuit—2 in. across, 1 in. thick; slice of homemade rye bread—3 in. by 4 in., ¼ in. thick).
  —Sandwiches: list *all* ingredients (lettuce, mayonnaise, tomato, and so on).
- For meat, fish, poultry, and cheese
  —Give size (length, width, thickness) in inches or weight in ounces after cooking for meat, fish, and poultry (such as cooked hamburger patty—3 in. across, ½ in. thick).
  —Give size (length, width, thickness) in inches or weight in ounces for cheese.
  —Record measurements only for the cooked, edible part—without bone or fat that is left on the plate.
  —Describe how meat, poultry, or fish was prepared.
- For eggs
  —Record as soft or hard cooked, fried, scrambled, poached, or omelet.
  —If milk, butter, or drippings are used, specify kinds and amount.
- For desserts
  —List commercial brand or "homemade" or "bakery" under brand.
  —Purchased candies, cookies, and cakes: specify kind and size.
  —Measure and record portion size of cakes, pies, and cookies by specifying thickness, diameter, and width or length, depending on the item.

Time	Minutes Spent Eating	M or S*	H† (0–3)	Activity While Eating	Place of Eating	Food and Quantity	Others Present	Reason for Choice

*M or S: Meal or snack

†H: Degree of hunger (0 = none; 3 = maximum)

Table G-1 One Day's Food Record—This Activity Can Help You Understand More about Your Food Habits

Time	Minutes Spent Eating	M or S*	H† (0–3)	Activity While Eating	Place of Eating	Food and Quantity	Others Present	Reason for Choice
7:10 A.M.	15	M	2	Standing, fixing lunch	Kitchen	orange juice, 1 cup Crispix, 1 cup Reduced-fat milk, ½ cup Sugar, 2 tsp Black coffee	—	Health Habit Health Taste Habit
10:00 A.M.	4	S	1	Sitting, taking notes	Classroom	Diet cola, 12 oz	Class	Weight control
12:15 P.M.	40	M	2	Sitting, talking	Student union	Chicken sandwich with lettuce and mayonnaise (3 oz chicken, 2 slices of bread, 2 tsp mayonnaise) Pear, 1 medium Reduced-fat milk, 1 cup	Friends	Taste Health Health
2:30 P.M.	10	S	1	Sitting, studying	Library	Regular cola, 12 oz	Friend	Hunger
6:30 P.M.	35	M	3	Sitting, talking	Kitchen	Pork chop, 1 Baked potato, 1 Margarine, 2 tbsp Lettuce and tomato salad, 1½ cups Ranch dressing, 2 tbsp Peas, ½ cup Whole milk, 1 cup Cherry pie, 1 small piece Ice tea, 12 oz	Boyfriend	Convenience Health Taste Health Taste Health Habit Taste Health
9:10 P.M.	10	S	2	Sitting, studying	Living room	Apple, 1 Glass mineral water, 1	—	Weight control Weight control

*M or S: Meal or snack

†H: Degree of hunger (0 = none; 3 = maximum)

II. Now complete the nutrient analysis form as shown, using your food record. A blank copy of this form is printed in this appendix for your use. Note that the diet analysis software available with this book will create such a table for you if you simply enter all food eaten.

Nutrient Analysis Form (Sample)

Name	Quantity	kcal	Protein (g)	Carbohydrates (g)	Fiber (g)	Total fat (g)	Monounsaturated fat (g)	Polyunsaturated fat (g)	Saturated fat (g)	Cholesterol (g)	Calcium (mg)	Iron (mg)
Egg bagel, 3 5 in. diameter	1	180	7.45	34.7	0.748	1.00	0.286	0.400	0.171	44.0	20.0	2.10
Jelly	1 tbsp	49.0	0.018	12.7	—	0.018	0.005	0.005	0.005	—	2.00	0.120
Orange juice, prepared fresh or frozen	1½ cups	165	2.52	40.2	1.49	0.210	0.037	0.045	0.025	—	33.0	0.411
Cheeseburger, McDonald's	2	636	30.2	57.0	0.460	32.0	12.2	2.18	13.3	80.0	338	5.68
French fries, McDonald's	1 order	220	3.00	26.1	4.19	11.5	4.37	0.570	4.61	8.57	9.10	0.605
Cola beverage, regular	1½ cups	151	—	38.5	—	—	—	—	—	—	9.00	0.120
Pork loin chop, broiled, lean	4 oz	261	36.2	—	—	11.9	5.35	1.43	4.09	112	5.67	1.04
Baked potato with skin	1	220	4.65	51.0	3.90	0.200	0.004	0.087	0.052	—	20.0	2.75
Peas, frozen, cooked	½ cup	63.0	4.12	11.4	3.61	0.220	0.019	0.103	0.039	—	19.0	1.25
Margarine, regular or soft, 80% fat	20 g	143	0.160	0.100	—	16.1	5.70	6.92	2.76	—	5.29	—
Iceberg lettuce, chopped	2 cups	14.6	1.13	2.34	1.68	0.212	0.008	0.112	0.028	—	21.2	0.560
French dressing	2 oz	300	0.318	3.63	0.431	32.0	14.2	12.4	4.94	—	7.10	0.227
Reduced fat milk	1 cup	121	8.12	11.7	—	4.78	1.35	0.170	2.92	22.0	297	0.120
Graham crackers	2	60.0	1.04	10.8	1.40	1.46	0.600	0.400	0.400	—	6.00	0.367
Totals		2584	99.0	300	17.9	112	44.1	24.8	33.4	266	792	15.4
RDA or related nutrient standard*		2900	58	130	38						1000	8
% of nutrient needs			89	170	230	47						79	193

Abbreviations: g = grams, mg = milligrams, μg = micrograms

*Values from inside cover. The values listed are for a male age 19 years. Note that number of kcal is just a rough estimate. It is better to base energy needs on actual energy output.

†In RAE units. Table values generally are in RE units today because the food values have not been updated to reflect the latest vitamin A standards. RAE equal RE for foods with preformed vitamin A, such as for the pork chop, but RAE are only about half the RE listed for foods with provitamin A carotenoids, such as for the peas (see Chapter 9 for details).

‡Amounts refer to actual folate content rather than dietary folate equivalents (DFE). This difference is important to consider if the food contains added synthetic folic acid as part of enrichment or fortification. Any such folic acid is absorbed about twice as much as the folate present naturally in foods. So the total contribution of folate in the food in comparison to human needs will be greater than if all the folate was naturally in the food product. Nutrient analysis tables have yet to be updated to reflect the dietary folate equivalents of products (see Chapter 10 for more details).

Nutrient Analysis Form (Sample) cont'd

Magnesium (mg)	Phosphorus (mg)	Potassium (mg)	Sodium (mg)	Zinc (mg)	Vitamin A (RE)	Vitamin C (mg)	Vitamin E (mg)	Thiamin (mg)	Riboflavin (mg)	Niacin (mg)	Vitamin B-6 (mg)	Folate (µg)	Vitamin B-12 (µg)
18.0	61.0	65.0	300	0.612	7.00	—	1.80	2.58	0.197	2.40	0.030	16.3	0.065
0.720	1.00	16.0	4.00	—	0.200	0.710	0.016	0.002	0.005	0.036	0.005	2.00	—
36.0	60.0	711	3.00	0.192	28.5	145	0.714	0.300	0.060	0.750	0.165	163	
45.8	410	314	1460	5.20	134	4.10	0.560	0.600	0.480	8.66	0.230	42.0	1.82
26.7	101	564	109	0.320	5.00	12.5	0.203	0.122	0.020	2.26	0.218	19.0	0.027
3.00	46.0	4.00	15.0	0.049	—	—	—	—	—	—	—	—	—
34.0	277	476	88.2	2.54	3.15	0.454	0.405	1.30	0.350	6.28	0.535	6.77	0.839
55.0	115	844	16.0	0.650	—	26.1	0.100	0.216	0.067	3.32	0.701	22.2	—
23.0	72.0	134	70.0	0.750	53.4	7.90	0.400	0.226	0.140	1.18	0.090	46.9	—
0.467	4.06	7.54	216	0.041	199	0.028	2.19	0.002	0.006	0.004	0.002	0.211	0.017
10.1	22.4	177	10.1	0.246	37.0	4.36	0.120	0.052	0 034	0.210	0.044	62.8	—
5.81	3.63	7.03	666	0.045	0.023	—	15.9	—	—	—	0.006	—	—
33.0	232	377	122	0.963	140	2.32	0.080	0.095	0.403	0.210	0.105	12.0	0.888
6.00	20.0	36.0	86.0	0.113	—	—	—	0.020	0.030	0.600	0.011	1.80	—
298	1425	3732	3165	11.7	607	204	22.5	5.52	1.79	25.9	2.14	395	3.65
400	700	4700	1500	11	900†	90	15	1.2	1.3	16	1.3	400‡	2.4
75	204	80	210	106	67	226	150	450	138	162	160	99	152

Nutrient Analysis Form

Name	Quantity	kcal	Protein (g)	Carbohydrates (g)	Fiber (g)	Total fat (g)	Monounsaturated fat (g)	Polyunsaturated fat (g)	Saturated fat (g)	Cholesterol (g)	Calcium (mg)	Iron (mg)
Totals												
RDA or related nutrient standard*												
% of nutrient needs												

*Values from inside cover. Note that number of kcals is just a rough estimate. It is better to base energy needs on actual energy output.

†Use RAE values, even though food table is based on RE units.

‡Use DFE values, even though the food is based on total folate content, irrespective of natural or synthetic source.

Nutrient Analysis Form cont'd

Magnesium (mg)	Phosphorus (mg)	Potassium (mg)	Sodium (mg)	Zinc (mg)	Vitamin A (RE)	Vitamin C (mg)	Vitamin E (mg)	Thiamin (mg)	Riboflavin (mg)	Niacin (mg)	Vitamin B-6 (mg)	Folate (µg)	Vitamin B-12 (µg)
						†							‡	

III. Complete the following table as you summarize your dietary intake.

Percentage of kcal from Protein, Fat, Carbohydrate, and Alcohol

Intake

Protein (P): _____ g/day × 4 kcal/g = (P) _____ kcal/day
Fat (F): _____ g/day × 9 kcal/g = (F) _____ kcal/day
Carbohydrate (C): _____ g/day × 4 kcal/g = (C) _____ kcal/day
Alcohol (A): = (A) _____ kcal/day*
Total kcal (T)/day = (T) _____ kcal/day

Percentage of kcal from protein:

$\frac{(P)}{(T)} \times 100 = $ _____ %

Percentage of kcal from fat:

$\frac{(F)}{(T)} \times 100 = $ _____ %

Percentage of kcal from carbohydrate:

$\frac{(C)}{(T)} \times 100 = $ _____ %

Percentage of kcal from alcohol:

$\frac{(A)}{(T)} \times 100 = $ _____ %

NOTE: The four percentages can total 99, 100, or 101, depending on the way in which figures were rounded off earlier.

*To calculate how many kcal in a beverage are from alcohol, look up the beverage in Appendix N. Determine how many kcal are from carbohydrate (multiply carbohydrate grams times 4), fat (fat grams times 9), and protein (protein grams times 4). The remaining kcal are from alcohol.

IV. Use the table on the following page to again record your food intake for one day, placing each food item in the correct category of MyPyramid, with the correct number of servings (see pages 58–59 in Chapter 2). Note that a food such as toast with soft margarine contributes to two categories—namely, to the grain group and to the oils group. You can expect that many food choices will contribute to more than one group. Indicate the number of servings from the MyPyramid that each food yields.

Indicate the Number of Servings from MyPyramid That Each Food Yields

Food or Beverage	Amount Eaten	Milk	Meat & Beans	Fruits	Vegetables	Grains	Oils
Group totals							
Recommended servings							
Shortages in numbers of servings							

V. Evaluation. Are there weaknesses suggested in your nutrient intake that correspond to missing servings in MyPyramid? Consider replacing the missing servings to improve your nutrient intake.

VI. For the same day you keep your food record also keep a 24-hour record of your activities. Include sleeping, sitting, and walking as well as the obvious forms of exercise. Calculate your energy expenditure for these activities using Table 13-6 in Chapter 13 or the software available with this book. Try to substitute a similar activity if your particular activity is not listed. Calculate the total kcal you used for the day. Following is an example of an activity record and a blank form for your use. Ask your professor whether you are to turn in the form or the activity printout from the software.

Weight (kg)*: 70 kg

Activity	Time (Minutes): Convert to Hours	Column 1 kcal/kg/hr (from Table 13-6)	Energy Cost Column 2 (Column 1 × Time)	Column 3 (Column 2 × Weight in kg)
Brisk walking	(60 min) 1 hr	4.4	(× 1) = 4.4	(× 70) = 308

*lb/2.2

Weight (kg)*:

Activity	Time (Minutes): Convert to Hours	Column 1 kcal/kg/hr (from Table 13-6)	Energy Cost Column 2 (Column 1 × Time)	Column 3 (Column 2 × Weight in kg)

Total kcal used (add all items listed in column 3)

*lb/2.2

appendix H

FATTY ACIDS, INCLUDING OMEGA-3 FATTY ACIDS, IN FOODS

Chain Length, Number, and Site of Double Bonds for Common Fatty Acids

Common Name of Fatty Acid	Number of Carbon Atoms and Number and Site of Double Bond(s), Counting from Methyl End ($-CH_3$) if Appropriate
Saturated Fatty Acids (No Double Bonds)	
Formic	1
Acetic	2
Propionic	3
Butyric	4
Valeric	5
Caproic	6
Caprylic	8
Capric	10
Lauric	12
Myristic	14
Palmitic	16
Stearic	18
Unsaturated Fatty Acids	
Oleic	18:1 (9-10) ω-9
Linoleic	18:2 (6-7, 9-10) ω-6
Alpha-linolenic	18:3 (3-4, 6-7, 9-10) ω-3
Arachidonic	20:4 (6-7, 9-10, 12-13, 15-16) ω-6
Eicosapentaenoic	20:5 (3-4, 6-7, 9-10, 12-13, 15-16) ω-3
Docosahexaenoic	22:6 (3-4, 6-7, 9-10, 12-13, 15-16, 18-19) ω-3

Fatty Acid Composition of Selected Foods*

						Fatty Acid[†]				
	Saturated					Unsaturated				
Food Item	<C12:0	C12:0	14:0	C16:0	C18:0	C18:1 ω-9	C18:2 ω-6	C18:3 ω-3	C20:5 ω-3	C22:6 ω-3
Fats and Oils		Lauric Acid	Myristic Acid	Palmitic Acid	Stearic Acid	Oleic Acid	Linoleic Acid	Alpha-Linolenic Acid	EPA[‡]	DHA[‡]
Beef tallow	—	0.90	3.70	24.9	18.9	36.0	3.1	0.60	—	—
Butter	7.0	2.20	8.10	21.3	9.8	20.4	1.8	1.20	—	—
Cocoa butter	—	—	0.10	25.4	33.2	32.6	2.8	0.10	—	—
Corn oil	—	—	—	11.0	2.0	25.0	58.0	0.70	—	—
Cottonseed oil	—	—	0.80	22.7	2.3	17.0	51.5	0.20	—	—
Lard	0.1	0.20	1.30	23	15.2	40.9	9.7	1.10	—	—
Olive oil	—	—	—	11.0	2.5	72.5	7.5	0.60	—	—
Palm kernel oil	7	47.00	16.40	8.1	2.8	11.4	1.6	—	—	—
Palm oil	—	0.10	1.00	43.5	4.3	36.6	9.1	0.20	—	—
Safflower oil	—	—	—	4.2	1.9	14.4	74.6	—	—	—
Shortenings	0.2	0.10	1.60	23.0	15.2	41.0	9.7	1.10	—	—
Margarine, stick	—	—	0.20	9.7	6.0	36.0	24.3	1.10	—	—
Margarine, tub	—	—	0.100	8.7	5.0	37.3	24.6	1.10	—	—
Canola oil	—	—	—	4.0	1.8	56.0	20.3	9.30	—	—
Soybean oil	—	—	—	14.0	4.0	29.0	45.0	3.00	—	—
Coconut oil	14.0	45.00	17.00	8.2	3.0	6.0	1.8	—	—	—
Peanut oil	—	—	0.100	9.5	2.2	44.8	32.0	—	—	—
Cod liver oil	—	—	3.6	10.6	2.8	20.6	0.9	0.9	6.9	11.0
Menhaden oil	—	—	8.0	15.1	3.8	14.6	2.2	1.5	13.2	4.9
Meat, Fish, and Poultry										
Beef, lean only, uncooked	—	0.04	0.50	4.0	2.1	6.5	0.4	0.16	—	—
Chicken, white meat, cooked	—	0.03	0.01	2.1	0.7	3.5	2.1	0.10	0.01	0.05
Salmon, coho, cooked	—	—	0.18	0.8	0.3	1.7	0.2	0.40	0.40	1.40
Tuna, light, canned in water	—	—	0.02	0.2	0.1	0.1	—	0.02	0.05	0.20
Nuts and Seeds										
Walnuts	—	—	—	4.4	1.6	8.8	38	9	—	—
Flaxseeds	—	—	—	1.8	1.4	6.9	4.3	18.1	—	—

From USDA Nutrient Database for Standard Reference, Release 13.

*Only major fatty acids are presented.

[†]All values represent grams per 100 g edible portion.

[‡]EPA eicosapentaenoic acid
DHA docosahexaenoic acid } fish oil fatty acids

appendix I

THE 1983 METROPOLITAN LIFE INSURANCE COMPANY HEIGHT-WEIGHT TABLE AND DETERMINATION OF FRAME SIZE

1983 Metropolitan Life Insurance Company Height-Weight Table*†

Women					Men				
Height		Frame			Height		Frame		
Ft.	In.	Small	Medium	Large	Ft.	In.	Small	Medium	Large
4	10	102–111	109–121	118–131	5	2	128–134	131–141	138–150
4	11	103–113	111–123	120–134	5	3	130–136	133–143	140–153
5	0	104–115	113–126	122–137	5	4	132–138	135–145	142–156
5	1	106–118	115–129	125–140	5	5	134–140	137–148	144–160
5	2	108–121	118–132	128–143	5	6	136–142	139–151	146–164
5	3	111–124	121–135	131–147	5	7	138–145	142–154	149–168
5	4	114–127	124–138	134–151	5	8	140–148	145–157	152–172
5	5	117–130	127–141	137–155	5	9	142–151	148–160	155–176
5	6	120–133	130–144	140–159	5	10	144–154	151–163	158–180
5	7	123–136	133–147	143–163	5	11	146–157	154–166	161–184
5	8	126–139	136–150	146–167	6	0	149–160	157–170	164–188
5	9	129–142	139–153	149–170	6	1	152–164	160–174	168–192
5	10	132–145	142–156	152–173	6	2	155–168	164–178	172–197
5	11	135–148	145–159	155–176	6	3	158–172	167–182	176–202
6	0	138–151	148–162	158–179	6	4	162–176	171–187	181–207

Reprinted courtesy of Metropolitan Life Insurance Company, *Statistical Bulletin.*

Permission granted courtesy of Metropolitan Life Insurance Company, *Statistical Bulletin.*

*Based on a weight-height mortality study conducted by the Society of Actuaries and the Association of Life Insurance Medical Directors of America, Metropolitan Life Insurance Medical Directors of America, Metropolitan Life Insurance Company, revised 1983.

†Weights at ages 25 to 59 based on lowest mortality. Height includes 1-in. heel. Weight for women includes 3 lb for indoor clothing. Weight for men includes 5 lb for indoor clothing.

Using the Metropolitan Life Insurance Table to Estimate Healthy Weight

The Metropolitan Life Insurance table is a common method for estimating healthy weight. The table lists for any height the weight that is associated with a maximum life span. The table does not tell the healthiest weight for a living person; it simply lists the weight associated with longevity.

Criticisms of this table stem from the inclusion of some people and the exclusion of others. For example, only policyholders of life insurance are included. In addition, smokers are included, but anyone over the age of 60 is excluded. Weight is measured only at the time of purchase of insurance, and there is no follow-up. All these factors contribute to the fact that this table is to be used only as a rough screening tool; not meeting the exact recommendations should not be cause for alarm.

To diagnose overweight or obesity using the table, calculate the percentage of the Metropolitan Life Insurance table weight. Use the midpoint of a weight range for a specific height.

$$\frac{(\text{Current wt.} - \text{wt. from table})}{\text{Weight from table}} \times 100$$

Example:

$$\frac{140 - 120}{120} \times 100 = 17\% \text{ over standard}$$

Overweight can be defined as weighing at least 10% more than the weight listed on the table. Obesity weighs in at 20% more than that listed on the table. Moreover, this measure of obesity comes in degrees. Whereas mild obesity carries little health risk, severe obesity raises overall health risk twelvefold.

Degrees of Obesity

% over Healthy Body Weight	Form of Obesity
20–40%	Mild
41–99%	Moderate
100%+	Severe

Determining Frame Size

Method 1

Height is recorded without shoes.

Wrist circumference is measured just beyond the bony (styloid) process at the wrist joint on the right arm, using a tape measure.

The following formula is used:

$$r = \frac{\text{Height (cm)}}{\text{Wrist circumference (cm)}}$$

Frame size can be determined as follows:[†]

Males	Females
$r > 10.4$ small	$r > 11$ small
$r = 9.6$–10.4 medium	$r = 10.1$–11 medium
$r < 9.6$ large	$r < 10.1$ large

[†]From Grant JP: *Handbook of total parenteral nutrition.* Philadelphia: WB Saunders, 1980.

Method 2

The patient's right arm is extended forward, perpendicular to the body, with the arm bent so the angle at the elbow forms 90 degrees, with the fingers pointing up and the palm turned away from the body. The greatest breadth across the elbow joint is measured with a sliding caliper along the axis of the upper arm, on the two prominent bones on either side of the elbow. This measurement is recorded as the elbow breadth. The following tables give elbow breadth measurements for medium-framed men and women of various heights. Measurements lower than those listed indicate a small frame size; higher measurements indicate a large frame size.

Men[‡]		Women	
Height in 1″ Heels	Elbow Breadth	Height in 1″ Heels	Elbow Breadth
5′2″–5′3″	2½–2⅞″	4′10″–4′11″	2¼–2½″
5′4″–5′7″	2⅝–2⅞″	5′0″–5′3″	2¼–2½″
5′8″–5′11″	2¾–3″	5′4″–5′7″	2⅜–2⅝″
6′0″–6′3″	2¾–3¼″	5′8″–5′11″	2⅜–2⅝″
6′4″ and over	2⅞–3¾″	6′0″ and over	2½–2¾″

appendix J
NUTRITION CALCULATIONS

Conversions are mathematical techniques that are useful to express the same quantity in different measurements. This section will walk you step by step through a few basic conversions that are important to understand when studying human nutrition.

Begin with 2.2 pounds and 1 kilogram; they are equivalent. Each represents the same weight but is expressed in different units. Below is the conversion factor to change pounds to kilograms and kilograms to pounds.

$$\frac{2.2\ \text{lb}}{1\ \text{kg}} \quad \text{or} \quad \frac{1\ \text{kg}}{2.2\ \text{lb}}$$

Because these factors equal 1, they can be multiplied by a number without changing the measurement value. This allows the units to be changed.

Here are some examples of problems that are commonly seen when studying nutrition.

Example 1: Convert the weight of 150 lb to kg.

Step 1: Choose the conversion factor in which the unit you are seeking is on top.

$$\frac{1\ \text{kg}}{2.2\ \text{lb}}$$

Step 2: Multiply 150 pounds by the factor

$$150\ \cancel{\text{lb}} \times \frac{1\ \text{kg}}{2.2\ \cancel{\text{lb}}} = \frac{150\ \text{kg}}{2.2} = 59\ \text{kg}$$

Example 2: Convert 1/2 cup to an approximate number of milliliters for use in a recipe.

Step 1: The conversion factor is

$$\frac{1\ \text{cup}}{240\ \text{ml}} \quad \text{or} \quad \frac{240\ \text{ml}}{1\ \text{cup}}$$

Step 2: Multiply 1/2 cup by the conversion factor.

$$^{1}/_{2}\ \cancel{\text{cup}} \times \frac{240\ \text{ml}}{1\ \cancel{\text{cup}}} = 120\ \text{ml}$$

Example 3: Suppose that for one day in your diet you consumed 290 g of carbohydrate, 60 g of fat, 70 g of protein, and 15 g of alcohol. Calculate the energy intake for the day as well as the percentage of carbohydrate, fat, protein, and alcohol in the day's diet.

Step 1: Calculate the total energy intake. Begin by multiplying the grams of car-bohydrate, fat, protein, and alcohol by the number of kcal that each gram yields.

$$\text{Carbohydrate: } 290 \text{ g} \times \frac{4 \text{ kcal}}{g} = 1160 \text{ kcal}$$

$$\text{Fat: } 60 \text{ g} \times \frac{9 \text{ kcal}}{g} = 540 \text{ kcal}$$

$$\text{Protein: } 70 \text{ g} \times \frac{4 \text{ kcal}}{g} = 280 \text{ kcal}$$

$$\text{Alcohol: } 15 \text{ g} \times \frac{7 \text{ kcal}}{g} = 105 \text{ kcal}$$

Step 2: Add all the values together for total energy intake.

$$1160 + 540 + 280 + 105 = 2085 \text{ total kcal}$$

Step 3: Calculate the percentage of total carbohydrate by multiplying the grams of carbohydrate by the energy yield and total energy factor.

$$290 \text{ g} \times \frac{4 \text{ kcal}}{g} \times \frac{100\%}{2085 \text{ kcal}} = 56\% \text{ carbohydrate}$$

Step 4: Calculate the percentage of total fat by multiplying the grams of fat by the energy yield and total energy factor.

$$60 \text{ g} \times \frac{9 \text{ kcal}}{g} \times \frac{100\%}{2085 \text{ kcal}} = 26\% \text{ fat}$$

Step 5: Calculate the percentage of total protein by multiplying the grams of protein by the energy yield and total energy factor.

$$70 \text{ g} \times \frac{4 \text{ kcal}}{g} \times \frac{100\%}{2085 \text{ kcal}} = 13\% \text{ protein}$$

Step 6: Calculate the percentage of total alcohol by multiplying the grams of alcohol by the energy yield and total energy factor.

$$15 \text{ g} \times \frac{7 \text{ kcal}}{g} \times \frac{100\%}{2085 \text{ kcal}} = 5\% \text{ alcohol}$$

Example 4: How many grams of saturated fat are contained in a 3-oz hamburger? A 5-oz hamburger contains 8.5 g of saturated fat.

Step 1: The conversion factor for grams of saturated fat is

$$\frac{8.5 \text{ g saturated fat}}{5\text{-oz hamburger}}$$

Step 2: Multiply 3-oz hamburger by the conversion factor.

$$3 = \text{oz hamburger} \times \frac{8.5 \text{ g saturated fat}}{5\text{-oz hamburger}} = \frac{3 \times 8.5 \text{ g}}{5} = \frac{25.5}{5}$$

$$= 5 \text{ g of saturated fat}$$

Conversions are also useful when you are working with nutrient units. Two common units you will encounter are sodium and folate. The conversion factor to change milligrams of sodium to milligrams of salt, and milligrams of salt to milligrams of sodium is

$$\frac{1000 \text{ mg sodium}}{2500 \text{ mg salt}} \quad \text{or} \quad \frac{2500 \text{ mg salt}}{1000 \text{ mg sodium}}$$

To convert micrograms of synthetic folate in supplements and enriched foods to Dietary Folate Equivalents (micrograms DFE), use this conversion factor:

$$\frac{1 \text{ μg synthetic folic acid}}{1.7 \text{ μg DFE}} \quad \text{or} \quad \frac{1.7 \text{ μg DFE}}{1 \text{ μg synthetic folic acid}}$$

For naturally occurring folate, assign each microgram of food folate a value of 1 microgram DFE:

$$\frac{1 \text{ μg food folate}}{1 \text{ μg DFE}} \quad \text{or} \quad \frac{1 \text{ μg DFE}}{1 \text{ μg food folate}}$$

Example 5: A frozen pepperoni pizza contains 2200 mg of salt. How much sodium is in the pizza?

Step 1: Choose the conversion factor with the unit you are seeking on top.

$$\frac{1000 \text{ mg sodium}}{2500 \text{ mg salt}}$$

Step 2: Multiply 2200 mg of salt by the conversion factor.

$$2200 \text{ mg salt} \times \frac{1000 \text{ mg sodium}}{2500 \text{ mg salt}} = 880 \text{ mg of sodium}$$

Example 6: If a ready-to-eat breakfast cereal contains 200 μg of synthetic folic acid, how many μg of folate in the product are in DFE units?

Step 1: Choose the conversion factor with the unit you are seeking on top.

$$\frac{1.7 \text{ μg DFE}}{1 \text{ μg synthetic folic acid}}$$

Step 2: Multiply 200 μg of synthetic folic acid by the conversion factor.

$$200 \text{ μg synthetic folic acid} \times \frac{1.7 \text{ μg DFE}}{1 \text{ μg synthetic folic acid}}$$

$$= 340 \text{ μg DFE}$$

Example 7: An orange has 50 μg of food folate. How many μg of folate in DFE does the orange contain?

Step 1: Choose the conversion factor with the unit you are seeking on top.

$$\frac{1 \text{ μg DFE}}{1 \text{ μg food folate}}$$

Step 2: Multiply 50 μg of food folate by the conversion factor.

$$50 \text{ μg food folate} \times \frac{1 \text{ μg DFE}}{1 \text{ μg food folate}} = 50 \text{ μg DFE}$$

appendix K

Consider the following reliable sources of food and nutrition information:

Journals That Regularly Cover Nutrition Topics

American Family Physician*
American Journal of Clinical Nutrition
American Journal of Epidemiology
American Journal of Medicine
American Journal of Nursing
*American Journal of Obstetrics
 and Gynecology*
American Journal of Physiology
American Journal of Public Health
American Scientist
Annals of Internal Medicine
Annual Reviews of Medicine
Annual Reviews of Nutrition
Archives of Disease in Childhood
Archives of Internal Medicine
British Journal of Nutrition
BMJ (British Medical Journal)
Cancer
Cancer Research
Circulation
Diabetes

Diabetes Care
Disease-a-Month
FASEB Journal
FDA Consumer*
Food Chemical Toxicology
Food Engineering
Gastroenterology
Geriatrics
Gut
Human Nutrition: Applied Nutrition
Human Nutrition: Clinical Nutrition
*Journal of the American College of
 Nutrition**
*Journal of the American Dietetic
 Association**
Journal of the American Geriatric Society
*JAMA (Journal of the American Medical
 Association)*
Journal of Applied Physiology
*Journal of the Canadian Dietetic
 Association**
Journal of Clinical Investigation
Journal of Food Service

Journal of Food Technology
*JNCI (Journal of the National Cancer
 Institute)*
Journal of Nutrition
Journal of Nutritional Education*
Journal of Nutrition for the Elderly
Journal of Pediatrics
Lancet
Mayo Clinic Proceedings
Medicine & Science in Sports and Exercise
Nature
The New England Journal of Medicine
Nutrition
Nutrition Reviews
Nutrition Today*
Pediatrics
The Physician and Sports Medicine
Postgraduate Medicine*
Proceedings of the Nutrition Society
Science
Science News*
Scientific American*

The majority of these journals are available in college and university libraries or in a specialty library on campus, such as one designated for health services or home economics. As indicated, a few journals will be filed under their abbreviations rather than the first word in their full name. A reference librarian can help you locate any of these sources. The journals with an asterisk (*) are ones you may find especially interesting and useful because of the number of nutrition articles presented each month or the less technical nature of the presentation.

Magazines for the Consumer That Cover Nutrition Topics

Men's Health
Better Homes and Gardens

Good Housekeeping
Health

Parents
Self

Textbooks and Other Sources for Advanced Study of Nutrition Topics

Groff JL, Gropper SS: *Advanced human nutrition and metabolism*. Belmont, CA: Wadsworth, 2005.

International Life Sciences Institute: *Present knowledge in nutrition*. 8th ed. Washington DC: The Nutrition Foundation, 2001.

Mahan LK, Escott-Stump S: *Krause's food, nutrition, and diet therapy*. 11th ed. Philadelphia: W.B. Saunders, 2004.

Murray RK and others: *Harper's biochemistry*. 26th ed. New York: McGraw-Hill, 2003.

Schils ME, and others: *Modern nutrition in health and disease*. 10th ed. Philadelphia: Lippincott, 2006.

Stipanuk MH: *Biochemical and physiological aspects of human nutrition*. Philadelphia: W.B. Saunders, 2000.

Newsletters That Cover Nutrition Issues on a Regular Basis

American Institute for Cancer Research Newsletter
American Institute for Cancer Research (AICR) 1759 R St. N.W. Washington, DC 20009
www.aicr.org

Dairy Council Digest
National Dairy Council
10255 West Higgins Road, Suite 900
Rosemont, IL 60018
www.nationaldairycouncil.org

Nutrition Close-Up
Egg Nutrition Center
1819 H St. N.W., No. 510
Washington, DC 20009
(free)
www.enc-online.org

Environmental Nutrition
52 Riverside Dr.
New York, NY 10024
www.environmentalnutrition.com

Food and Nutrition News
National Cattlemen's Beef Association
444 Michigan Ave.
Chicago, IL 60611
(free)
www.beef.org

Harvard Medical School Health Letter
Department of Continuing Education
25 Shattuck St.
Boston, MA 02115
www.hms.harvard.edu/news/index.html

Mayo Clinic Health Letter
P.O. Box 53889
Boulder, CO 80322-3889
www.mayohealth.org

National Council Against Health Fraud Newsletter (NCAHF)
P.O. Box 1276
Loma Linda, CA 92354
www.ncahf.org

Nutrition Action Healthletter
1875 Connecticut Ave.
Washington, DC 20009-5728
www.cspinet.org

Nutrition Forum
George Stickley Co.
210 Washington Square
Philadelphia, PA 19106
www.quackwatch.com

Tufts University Diet & Nutrition Letter
P.O. Box 420235
Palm Coast, FL 32142
www.healthletter.tufts.edu

University of California at Berkeley Wellness Letter
P.O. Box 420148
Palm Coast, FL 32142
magazines.enews.com/magazines/vcbw

Professional Organizations with a Commitment to Nutrition Issues

American Academy of Pediatrics
P.O. Box 1034
Evanston, IL 60204
www.aap.org

American Cancer Society
90 Park Ave.
New York, NY 10016
www.cancer.org

American College of Sports Medicine
P.O. Box 1440
Indianapolis, IN 46204
www.acsm.org

American Dental Association
211 E. Chicago Ave.
Chicago, IL 60611
www.ada.org

American Diabetes Association
2 Park Ave.
New York, NY 10016
www.diabetes.org

American Dietetic Association
120 S. Riverside Plaza
Suite 2000
Chicago, IL 60606
www.eatright.org

American Geriatrics Society
770 Lexington Ave.
Suite 400
New York, NY 10021
www.americangeriatrics.org

American Heart Association
7272 Greenville Ave.
Dallas, TX 75231
www.americanheart.org

American Medical Association
Nutrition Information Section
535 N. Dearborn St.
Chicago, IL 60610
www.ama-assn.org

American Public Health Association
1015 Fifteenth St. N.W.
Washington, DC 20005
www.apha.org

American Society for Clinical Nutrition
9650 Rockville Pike
Bethesda, MD 20014
www.faseb.org/ajcn

American Society for Nutritional Sciences
9650 Rockville Pike
Bethesda, MD 20014
www.asns.org

The Canadian Diabetes Association
15 Toronto St.
Suite 1001
Toronto, Ontario M5C 2E3 Canada
www.diabetes.ca

The Canadian Dietetic Association
480 University Ave.
Suite 601
Toronto, Ontario M5G 1V2 Canada
www.dietitians.ca

The Canadian Society for Nutritional
  Sciences
Department of Foods and Nutrition
University of Manitoba
Winnipeg, Manitoba, R3T 2N2 Canada
www.hc-sc.gc.ca

Environmental Working Group (EWG)
1718 Connecticut Ave., N.W. Suite 600
Washington, DC 20009
www.ewg.org

Food and Nutrition Board
National Research Council
National Academy of Sciences
2101 Constitution Ave. N.W.
Washington, DC 20418
www.nas.edu

Institute of Food Technologies
221 N. LaSalle St.
Chicago, IL 60601
www.ift.org

National Council on the Aging
1828 L St. N.W.
Washington, DC 20036
www.ncoa.org

National Institute of Nutrition
1335 Carling Ave.
Suite 210
Ottawa, Ontario K1Z OL2 Canada
www.nin.ca/En/home.html

National Osteoporosis Foundation
1150 Seventeenth St. N.W., Suite 500
Washington, DC 20036
www.nof.org

Society for Nutrition Education
7150 Winton Drive Suite 300
Indianapolis, IN 46268
www.sne.org

Professional or Lay Organizations Concerned with Nutrition Issues

Bread for the World Institute
50 F Street, N.W., Suite 500
Washington, DC 20001
www.bread.org

California Council Against Health Fraud,
  Inc.
P.O. Box 1276
Loma Linda, CA 92354
www.ncahf.org

Children's Foundation
1420 New York Ave. N.W.
Suite 800
Washington, DC 20005
www.childrenfoundation.com

Food Research and Action Center
  (FRAC)
1875 Connecticut Ave. N.W. #540
Washington, DC 20009
www.frac.org

Institute for Food and Development
  Policy
1885 Mission St.
San Francisco, CA 94103
www.foodfirst.org

La Leche League International, Inc.
9616 Minneapolis Ave.
Franklin Park, IL 60131
www.lalecheleague.org

March of Dimes Birth Defects
  Foundation
(National Headquarters)
1275 Mamaroneck Ave.
White Plains, NY 10605
www.modimes.org

National WIC Association (NWA)
2001 S Street, N.W., Suite 580
Washington, DC 20009
www.nwica.org

Overeaters Anonymous (OA)
2190 190th St.
Torrance, CA 90504
www.overeatersanonymous.org

Oxfam America
26 West St.
Boston, MA 02111
www.oxfamamerica.org

Local Resources for Advice on Nutrition Issues

Registered dietitians (R.D.s or in Canada
also RDNs) in health care, city,
county, or state agencies as well as in
private practice
Cooperative extension agents in county
extension offices
Nutrition faculty affiliated with
departments of food and
nutrition, home economics, and
dietetics

Government Agencies Concerned with Nutrition Issues or That Distribute Nutrition Information

United States
The Consumer Information
  Center
Department 609K
Pueblo, CO 81009
www.pueblo.gsa.gov

Food and Drug Administration (FDA)
5600 Fishers Lane
Rockville, MD 20852
www.fda.gov

Food and Nutrition Information and
  Education Resources Center
National Library of Congress
Beltsville, MD 20705
www.nal.usda.gov

Human Nutrition Research Division
Agricultural Research Center
Beltsville, MD 20705
www.usda.gov

National Center for Health Statistics
3700 East-West
Hyattsville, MD 20782
www.cdc.gov/nchs

National Heart, Lung, and Blood
  Institute
9000 Rockville Pike, Building 31,
  Room 4A21
Bethesda, MD 20892
www.nhlbi.nih.gov

National Institute on Aging
Information Office
Building 31, Room 5C35
Bethesda, MD 20205
www.nih.gov/nia

Office of Cancer Communications
National Cancer Institute
Building 31, Room 10A18
90 Rockville Pike
Bethesda, MD 20205
www.nci.nih.gov

MyPyramid
USDA, Center for Nutrition Policy
and Promotion
www.mypyramid.gov

USDA, Agricultural Research Service
6505 Belcrest Rd., Room 344
Hyattsville, MD 20782
www.usda.gov

USDA, Food Safety & Inspection
Service
Room 1180 South, 14th and
Independence Ave. S.W.
Washington, DC 20250
www.usda.gov

U.S. Government Printing Office
The Superintendent of Documents
Washington, DC 20402
www.gpo.gov

Canada
Canadian Food Inspection Agency
59 Camelot Dr.
Nepean, Ontario K1A OY9
www.inspection.gc.ca

Health and Welfare Canada
Canadian Government Publishing Center
Minister of Supply and Services
Ottawa, Ontario K1A 0S9
www.hc-sc.gc.ca

Nutrition Programs
446 Jeanne Mance Building
Tunney's Pasture
Ottawa, Ontario K1A 1B4
www.hc-sc.gc.ca

Nutrition Services
P.O. Box 488
Halifax, Nova Scotia B3J 3R8
www.fns.usda.gov

United Nations
Food and Agriculture Organization (FOA)
North American Regional Office
1001 22nd St. N.W.
Washington, DC 20437

or

Via della Terma di Caracella
0100 Rome, Italy
www.fao.org

World Health Organization (WHO)
1211 Geneva 27
Switzerland
www.who.org

Trade Organizations and Companies That Distribute Nutrition Information

American Institute of Baking
P.O. Box 1148
Manhattan, KS 66502
www.aibonline.org

American Meat Institute
P.O. Box 3556
Washington, DC 20007
www.meatami.com

Beech-Nut Nutrition Corporation
Booth 1414
Checkerboard Square
St. Louis, MO 63164
www.beech-nut.com/index.htm

Best Foods
Consumer Service Department
Division of CPC International
International Plaza
Englewood Cliffs, NJ 07632
www.bestfoods.com

Campbell Soup Co.
Food Service Products Division
Campbell Plaza
Camden, NJ 08103
www.campbellsoups.com

The Dannon Company, Inc.
120 White Plains Rd.
Tarrytown, NY 10591-5536
www.dannon.com

Del Monte Foods
One Market Plaza
San Francisco, CA 94105
www.delmonte-international.com

General Mills
P.O. Box 1113
Minneapolis, MN 55440
www.generalmills.com

Gerber Products Co.
445 State St.
Fremont, MI 49413
www.gerber.com

H.J. Heinz
Consumer Relations
P.O. Box 57
Pittsburgh, PA 15230
www.heinzbaby.com

Idaho Potato Commission
P.O. Box 1968
Boise, ID 83701
www.idahopotatoes.com

Kellogg Company
Department of Home Economics
Services
Battle Creek, MI 49016
www.kellog.com

Kraft General Foods
Three Lakes Dr.
Northfield, IL 60093
www.kraftfoods.com

Mead Johnson Nutritionals
2404 Pennsylvania Ave.
Evansville, IN 47721
www.meadjohnson.com

National Dairy Council
10255 W. Higgins Rd.
Rosemont, IL 60018-4233
www.nationaldairycoun.org

The NutraSweet Kelco
Company
1751 Lake Cook Rd.
Deerfield, IL 60015
**www.nutrasweetkelco.com/
default.htm**

Pillsbury Company
1177 Pillsbury Building
608 Second Ave. S.
Minneapolis, MN 55402
www.pillsbury.com

Ross Laboratories
Director of Professional
Services
625 Cleveland Ave.
Columbus, OH 43216
www.ross.com

Sunkist Growers, Inc.
14130 Riverside Dr.
Sherman Oaks, CA 91423
www.sunkist.com/index.html

Vitamin Nutrition Information Service
(VNIS)
Hoffmann-LaRoche
340 Kingsland Ave.
Nutley, NJ 07110
www.rocheusa.com

appendix L

ENGLISH-METRIC CONVERSIONS AND METRIC AND HOUSEHOLD UNITS

Metric-English Conversions

Length

English (USA)	Metric
inch (in.)	= 2.54 cm, 25.4 mm
foot (ft)	= 0.30 m, 30.48 cm
yard (yd)	= 0.91 m, 91.4 cm
mile (statute) (5280 ft)	= 1.61 km, 1609 m
mile (nautical) (6077 ft, 1.15 statute mi)	= 1.85 km, 1850 m

Metric	English (USA)
millimeter (mm)	= 0.039 in (thickness of a dime)
centimeter (cm)	= 0.39 in
meter (m)	= 3.28 ft, 39.37 in
kilometer (km)	= 0.62 mi, 1091 yd, 3273 ft

Weight

English (USA)	Metric
grain	= 64.80 mg
ounce (oz)	= 28.35 g
pound (lb)	= 453.60 g, 0.45 kg
ton (short—2000 lb)	= 0.91 metric ton (907 kg)

Metric	English (USA)
milligram (mg)	= 0.002 grain (0.000035 oz)
gram (g)	= 0.04 oz (1/28 of an oz)
kilogram (kg)	= 35.27 oz, 2.20 lb
metric ton (1000 kg)	= 1.10 tons

Volume

English (USA)	Metric
cubic inch	= 16.39 cc
cubic foot	= 0.03 m^3
cubic yard	= 0.765 m^3
teaspoon (tsp)	= 5 ml
tablespoon (tbsp)	= 15 ml
fluid ounce	= 0.03 liter (30 ml)*
cup (c)	= 237 ml
pint (pt)	= 0.47 liter
quart (qt)	= 0.95 liter
gallon (gal)	= 3.79 liters

Metric	English (USA)
milliliter (ml)	= 0.03 oz
liter (L)	= 2.12 pt
liter	= 1.06 qt
liter	= 0.27 gal

Metric and Other Common Units

Unit/Abbreviation	Other Equivalent Measure
milligram/mg	1/1000 of a gram
microgram/µg	1/1,000,000 of a gram
deciliter/dl	1/10 of a liter (about 1/2 cup)
milliliter/ml	1/1000 of a liter (5 ml is about 1 tsp)
International Unit/IU	Crude measure of vitamin activity generally based on growth rate seen in animals

1 liter ÷ 1000 = 1 milliliter or 1 cubic centimeter (10^{-3} liter)

1 liter ÷ 1,000,000 = 1 microliter (10^{-6} liter)

*Note: 1 ml = 1 cc

Fahrenheit-Celsius Conversion Scale

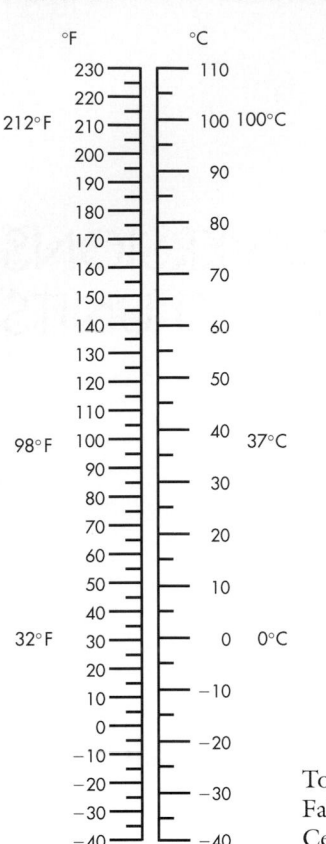

Household Units

3 teaspoons	= 1 tablespoon
4 tablespoons	= ¼ cup
5⅓ tablespoons	= ⅓ cup
8 tablespoons	= ½ cup
10⅔ tablespoons	= ⅔ cup
16 tablespoons	= 1 cup
1 tablespoon	= ½ fluid ounce
1 cup	= 8 fluid ounces
1 cup	= ½ pint
2 cups	= 1 pint
4 cups	= 1 quart
2 pints	= 1 quart
4 quarts	= 1 gallon

To convert temperature scales:
Fahrenheit to Celsius °C = (°F − 32) × 5/9
Celsius to Fahrenheit °F = 9/5 (°C) + 32

appendix M

ESTIMATED AVERAGE REQUIREMENTS
FOR NUTRIENTS

Estimated Average Energy Requirements Set by the Food and Nutrition Board, Institute of Medicine, National Academies

Life Stage Group	CHO (g/d)	PROT (g/kg/d)	Vitamin A (μg/d)	Vitamin C (mg/d)	Vitamin E (mg/d)	Thiamin (mg/d)	Riboflavin (mg/d)	Niacin (mg/d)	Vitamin B-6 (mg/d)
Children									
1–3 y	100	0.88	210	13	5	.4	.4	5	.4
4–8 y	100	0.76	275	22	6	.5	.5	6	.5
Males									
9–13 y	100	0.76	445	39	9	.7	.8	9	.8
14–18 y	100	0.73	630	63	12	1.0	1.1	12	1.1
19–30 y	100	0.66	625	75	12	1.0	1.1	12	1.1
31–50 y	100	0.66	625	75	12	1.0	1.1	12	1.1
51–70 y	100	0.66	625	75	12	1.0	1.1	12	1.4
> 70 y	100	0.66	625	75	12	1.0	1.1	12	1.4
Females									
9–13 y	100	0.76	420	39	9	.7	.8	9	.8
14–18 y	100	0.71	485	56	12	.9	.9	11	1.0
19–30 y	100	0.66	500	60	12	.9	.9	11	1.1
31–50 y	100	0.66	500	60	12	.9	.9	11	1.1
51–70 y	100	0.66	500	60	12	.9	.9	11	1.3
> 70 y	100	0.66	500	60	12	.9	.9	11	1.3
Pregnancy									
≤ 18 y	135	0.88	530	66	12	1.2	1.2	14	1.6
19–30 y	135	0.88	550	70	12	1.2	1.2	14	1.6
31–50 y	135	0.88	550	70	12	1.2	1.2	14	1.6
Lactation									
≤ 18 y	160	1.05	880	96	16	1.2	1.3	13	1.7
19–30 y	160	1.05	900	100	16	1.2	1.3	13	1.7
31–50 y	160	1.05	900	100	16	1.2	1.3	13	1.7

NOTE: This information taken from the various DRI reports (see www.nap.edu).

Folate (μg/d)	Vitamin B-12 (μg/d)	Copper (μg/d)	Iodine (μg/d)	Iron (mg/d)	Magnesium (mg/d)	Molybdenum (μg/d)	Phosphorus (mg/d)	Selenium (μg/d)	Zinc (mg/d)
120	.7	260	65	3.0	65	13	380	17	2.2
160	1.0	340	65	4.1	110	17	405	23	4
250	1.5	540	73	5.9	200	26	1055	35	7
330	2.0	685	95	7.7	340	33	1055	45	8.5
320	2.0	700	95	6	330	34	580	45	9.4
320	2.0	700	95	6	350	34	580	45	9.4
320	2.0	700	95	6	350	34	580	45	9.4
320	2.0	700	95	6	350	34	580	45	9.4
250	1.5	540	73	5.7	200	26	1055	35	7
330	2.0	685	95	7.9	300	33	1055	45	7.5
320	2.0	700	95	8.1	255	34	580	45	6.8
320	2.0	700	95	8.1	265	34	580	45	6.8
320	2.0	700	95	5	265	34	580	45	6.8
320	2.0	700	95	5	265	34	580	45	6.8
520	2.2	785	160	23	355	40	1055	49	10.5
520	2.2	800	160	22	290	40	580	49	9.5
520	2.2	800	160	22	300	40	580	49	9.5
450	2.4	985	209	7	300	50	1055	59	11.6
450	2.4	1000	209	6.5	255	50	580	59	10.4
450	2.4	1000	209	6.5	265	50	580	59	10.4

appendix N

FOOD COMPOSITION TABLE

The following table of nutrient values of foods represents a small portion of the database found in the NutritionCalc Plus 2.0 diet analysis program available from McGraw-Hill. The nutrient data in the software and in this appendix comes from the ESHA Research database. Some nutrient or food component values for some foods are not included in the database because no *accurate* data values exist. The nutrient or component may in fact be present in the food, but insufficient laboratory analyses have been performed to establish an accurate value. These missing values are indicated by a – (dash) in the appropriate nutrient columns.

Name-brand foods often have missing values because manufacturers are only required to analyze for nutrients that must appear on Nutrition Facts labels and only to the level of accuracy required by the nutrition labeling regulations. All missing nutrient or food component values are clearly marked in the table. You are encouraged to refer to the NutritionCalc Plus 2.0 technical support website (mhhe.com/support) for links to nutrient data sites provided by food manufacturers and restaurants not found in this appendix.

The following is a list of abbreviations used in the Food Composition Table:

Abbreviation Key

Unit/Amt = Unit Amount
Wt (g) = Weight in grams
Energy (kcal) = kilocalories
Prot (g) = Protein
Carb (g) = Carbohydrate
Fiber (g) = Dietary fiber
Fat (g) = Total fat
Sat (g) = Saturated fat
Mono (g) = Monounsaturated fat
Poly (g) = Polyunsaturated fat
Chol (mg) = Cholesterol
Vit A (RE) = Vitamin A
Thia (mg) = Thiamin
Ribo (mg) = Riboflavin
Niac (mg NE) = Niacin
Vit B-6 (mg) = Vitamin B-6
Vit B-12 (µg) = Vitamin B-12
Fol (µg) = Folate
Vit C (mg) = Vitamin C
Vit D (IU) = Vitamin D
Vit E (mg AT) = Vitamin E
Cal (mg) = Calcium

Iron (mg) = Iron
Magn (mg) = Magnesium
Phos (mg) = Phosphorus
Pota (mg) = Potassium
Sodi (mg) = Sodium
Zinc (mg) = Zinc
Wat (%) = Water
Alco (g) = Alcohol
Caff (g) = Caffeine

g = gram
mg = milligram
µg = microgram
mg AT = milligrams of alpha
   tocopheral
mg NE = milligrams of Niacin
   Equivalents
oz = ounce
lb = pound
Tbs = tablespoon
tsp = teaspoon

PAGE KEY: A-108 Beverage and Beverage Mixes A-110 Other Beverages A-110 Beverages, Alcoholic A-112 Candies and Confections, Gum A-116 Cereals, Breakfast Type A-120 Cheese and Cheese Substitutes A-122 Dairy Products and Substitutes A-124 Desserts A-130 Dessert Toppings A-130 Eggs, Substitutes, and Egg Dishes A-132 Ethnic Foods A-136 Fast Foods/Restaurants A-150 Fats, Oils, Margarines, Shortenings, and Substitutes A-150 Fish, Seafood, and Shellfish A-152 Food Additives A-152 Fruit, Vegetable, or Blended Juices A-154 Grains, Flours, and Fractions A-154 Grain Products, Prepared and Baked Goods

Code	Food Name	Unit/ Amt	Wt (g)	Energy (kcal)	Prot (g)	Carb (g)	Fiber (g)	Fat (g)	Sat (g)	Mono (g)	Poly (g)	Chol (mg)	Vit A (RE)
BEVERAGE AND BEVERAGE MIXES													
Carbonated Drinks													
4794	Lemonade, cnd, Country Time	1 cup	247	90	0	23	0	0	0.0	0.0	0.0	—	0
20055	Soda, 7 Up	1 cup	240	100	0	26	0	0	0.0	0.0	0.0	0	0
20207	Soda, 7 Up, diet	1 cup	240	0	0	0	0	0	0.0	0.0	0.0	0	0
20006	Soda, club	1 cup	237	0	0	0	0	0	0.0	0.0	0.0	0	0
20147	Soda, Coca Cola/Coke	1 cup	246	103	0	27	0	0	0.0	0.0	0.0	0	0
443	Soda, cola, caff free	12 fl-oz	372	156	0	40	0	0	0.0	0.0	0.0	0	0
4796	Soda, Dr Pepper	1 cup	246	100	0	27	0	0	0.0	0.0	0.0	—	0
4797	Soda, Dr Pepper, diet	1 cup	246	0	0	0	0	0	0.0	0.0	0.0	—	0
20530	Soda, fruit punch	1 cup	251	117	0	32	0	0	0.0	0.0	0.0	—	0
20031	Soda, grape	1 cup	248	107	0	28	0	0	0.0	0.0	0.0	0	0
20032	Soda, lemon lime	1 cup	246	98	0	26	0	0	0.0	0.0	0.0	0	0
20271	Soda, Mountain Dew	1 cup	240	113	0	31	0	0	0.0	0.0	0.0	0	0
20272	Soda, Mountain Dew, diet	1 cup	240	0	0	0	0	0	0.0	0.0	0.0	0	0
20161	Soda, Mr Pibb	1 cup	249	97	0	26	0	0	0.0	0.0	0.0	0	0
20029	Soda, orange	1 cup	248	119	0	31	0	0	0.0	0.0	0.0	0	0
20166	Soda, Pepsi	1 cup	240	100	0	27	0	0	0.0	0.0	0.0	0	0
20167	Soda, Pepsi, diet	1 cup	240	0	0	0	0	0	0.0	0.0	0.0	0	0
20009	Soda, root beer	1 cup	246	101	0	26	0	0	0.0	0.0	0.0	0	0
20454	Soda, root beer, diet, w/nutrasweet	1 cup	240	0	0	0	0	0	0.0	0.0	0.0	0	—
20163	Soda, Sprite	1 cup	249	96	0	26	0	0	0.0	0.0	0.0	0	0
4815	Soda, Squirt	1 cup	246	100	0	27	0	0	0.0	0.0	0.0	—	0
Coffee and Substitutes													
20312	Coffee Substitute, inst, dry	1 tsp	3	10	0	3	—	0	0.0	0.0	0.0	0	0
20592	Coffee, cappuccino, w/lowfat milk, tall	1.5 cup	244	110	8	11	0	4	2.5	—	—	15	80
20639	Coffee, cappuccino, w/whole milk, tall	1.5 cup	244	140	7	11	0	7	4.5	—	—	30	60
20439	Coffee, espresso, prep at restaurant	1 cup	237	5	0	0	0	0	0.2	0.0	0.2	0	0
20659	Coffee, latte, iced, w/lowfat milk, tall	1.5 cup	392	90	7	10	0	3	2.0	—	—	15	60
20023	Coffee, reg, inst, prep w/water	1 cup	238	5	0	1	0	0	0.0	0.0	0.0	0	0
Dairy Mixed Drinks and Mixes													
44	Drink, carob, prep f/dry mix w/milk	1 cup	256	192	8	22	1	8	4.6	2.0	0.5	26	69
14	Drink, chocolate, dry mix	2.5 tsp	22	75	1	20	1	1	0.4	0.2	0.0	0	0
40	Drink, strawberry, dry mix	2.5 tsp	22	85	0	22	0	0	0.0	0.0	0.0	0	0
12	Hot Cocoa, dry mix	3 tsp	28	113	2	24	1	1	0.7	0.4	0.0	2	0
48	Hot Cocoa, prep f/dry mix w/water	1 cup	275	151	2	32	1	2	0.9	0.5	0.0	3	1
62057	Instant Breakfast, French vanilla, dry mix, pkt	1 ea	36	130	4	27	0	0	0.0	0.0	0.0	3	350
101	Instant Breakfast, prep w/1% milk	1 cup	281	233	15	36	0	3	1.8	—	—	14	469
25	Instant Breakfast, prep w/2% milk, pwd	1 cup	281	253	15	36	0	5	3.1	—	—	24	469
26	Instant Breakfast, prep w/whole milk	1 cup	281	280	15	36	0	9	5.3	—	—	38	630
30	Malted Milk, chocolate, dry mix	3 tsp	21	79	1	18	1	1	0.5	0.2	0.1	0	1

Thia (mg)	Ribo (mg)	Niac (mg NE)	Vit B6 (mg)	Vit B12 (µg)	Fol (µg)	Vit C (mg)	Vit D (IU)	Vit E (mg AT)	Cal (mg)	Iron (mg)	Magn (mg)	Phos (mg)	Pota (mg)	Sodi (mg)	Zinc (mg)	Wat (%)	Alco (g)	Caff (g)
—	—	—	—	—	—	0.0	—	—	—	—	—	—	—	90	—	91	0.00	0.00
—	—	—	—	0.00	—	0.0	—	—	—	—	—	45	—	50	—	89	0.00	0.00
0.00	0.00	—	0.00	0.00	—	0.0	—	—	—	—	—	—	—	35	—	100	0.00	0.00
0.00	0.00	0.00	0.00	0.00	0.0	0.0	—	0.0	12	0.01	2.4	0	5	50	0.2	100	0.00	0.00
0.00	0.00	0.00	0.00	0.00	0.0	0.0	0.0	0.0	7	0.07	2.5	36	2	5	0.0	89	0.00	30.67
0.00	0.00	0.00	0.00	0.00	0.0	0.0	—	0.0	11	0.07	3.7	48	4	15	0.0	89	0.00	0.00
—	—	—	—	—	—	0.0	—	—	—	—	—	—	—	35	—	89	0.00	27.20
—	—	—	—	—	—	0.0	—	—	—	—	—	—	—	35	—	—	0.00	27.20
—	—	—	—	—	—	0.0	—	—	0	0.00	—	0	13	10	—	—	0.00	0.00
0.00	0.00	0.00	0.00	0.00	0.0	0.0	—	0.0	7	0.20	2.5	0	2	37	0.2	89	0.00	0.00
0.00	0.00	0.03	0.00	0.00	0.0	0.0	—	0.0	5	0.17	2.5	0	2	27	0.1	90	0.00	0.00
—	—	—	—	0.00	—	0.0	—	—	0	0.00	—	0	—	47	—	87	0.00	36.66
—	—	—	—	0.00	—	0.0	—	—	0	0.00	—	0	—	23	—	100	0.00	36.66
0.00	0.00	0.00	0.00	0.00	0.0	0.0	0.0	0.0	—	—	—	29	14	7	—	90	0.00	27.00
0.00	0.00	0.00	0.00	0.00	0.0	0.0	—	0.0	12	0.15	2.5	2	5	30	0.2	88	0.00	0.00
—	—	—	—	0.00	—	0.0	—	—	0	0.00	—	35	—	23	—	88	0.00	24.67
—	—	—	—	0.00	—	0.0	—	—	0	0.00	—	27	5	23	—	—	0.00	24.00
0.00	0.00	0.00	0.00	0.00	0.0	0.0	—	0.0	12	0.11	2.5	0	2	32	0.2	89	0.00	0.00
—	—	—	—	0.00	—	—	—	—	—	—	—	—	—	30	—	100	0.00	0.00
—	—	—	—	—	—	0.0	—	—	—	—	—	0	0	23	—	89	0.00	0.00
—	—	—	—	—	—	0.0	—	—	—	—	—	—	—	15	—	89	0.00	0.00
—	—	—	—	—	—	0.0	—	—	0	0.00	—	—	—	0	—	0	0.00	0.00
—	—	—	—	—	—	2.4	—	—	250	0.00	—	—	—	110	—	—	0.00	90.00
—	—	—	—	—	—	2.4	—	—	250	0.00	—	—	—	105	—	—	0.00	90.00
0.00	0.41	12.34	0.00	0.00	2.4	0.5	—	0.0	5	0.31	189.6	17	273	33	0.1	98	0.00	502.44
—	—	—	—	—	1.2	—	—	—	250	0.00	—	—	—	100	—	—	0.00	90.00
0.00	0.00	0.56	0.00	0.00	0.0	0.0	—	0.0	10	0.10	7.2	7	72	5	0.0	99	0.00	61.97
0.10	0.44	0.34	0.10	1.08	12.8	0.0	—	0.1	251	0.63	25.6	205	335	118	0.9	84	0.00	0.00
0.00	0.02	0.10	0.00	0.00	1.5	0.2	—	0.0	8	0.68	21.2	28	128	45	0.3	1	0.00	7.78
0.00	0.01	0.01	0.00	0.00	0.0	0.1	0.0	0.0	1	0.10	0.2	1	1	8	0.0	0	0.00	0.00
0.02	0.15	0.17	0.02	0.37	0.0	0.5	—	0.2	40	0.34	23.5	89	202	143	0.4	2	0.00	5.09
0.03	0.20	0.21	0.03	0.49	0.0	0.5	—	0.2	60	0.46	33.0	118	269	195	0.6	86	0.00	5.48
0.30	0.14	5.00	0.40	0.60	99.7	27.0	0.0	6.8	250	4.50	79.7	100	249	95	3.0	—	0.00	0.00
0.40	0.47	5.48	0.52	1.53	117.7	30.9	100.0	5.4	406	4.86	118.5	392	731	267	4.1	79	0.00	0.00
0.40	0.47	5.48	0.52	1.50	117.7	30.9	100.0	5.5	403	4.86	118.5	390	726	264	4.1	78	0.00	0.00
0.40	0.46	5.46	0.51	1.50	117.7	30.7	100.0	5.5	396	4.86	117.1	386	721	262	4.1	77	0.00	0.00
0.03	0.03	0.41	0.02	0.03	10.7	0.3	1.0	0.0	13	0.47	14.7	37	130	53	0.2	1	0.00	7.76

PAGE KEY: A-108 Beverage and Beverage Mixes | A-110 Other Beverages | A-110 Beverages, Alcoholic A-112 Candies and Confections, Gum A-116 Cereals, Breakfast Type
A-120 Cheese and Cheese Substitutes A-122 Dairy Products and Substitutes A-124 Desserts A-130 Dessert Toppings A-130 Eggs, Substitutes, and Egg Dishes A-132 Ethnic Foods
A-136 Fast Foods/Restaurants A-150 Fats, Oils, Margarines, Shortenings, and Substitutes A-150 Fish, Seafood, and Shellfish A-152 Food Additives
A-152 Fruit, Vegetable, or Blended Juices A-154 Grains, Flours, and Fractions A-154 Grain Products, Prepared and Baked Goods

Code	Food Name	Unit/ Amt	Wt (g)	Energy (kcal)	Prot (g)	Carb (g)	Fiber (g)	Fat (g)	Sat (g)	Mono (g)	Poly (g)	Chol (mg)	Vit A (RE)
Fruit Flavored Drinks													
20004	Drink, breakfast, orange, prep f/pwd	1 cup	248	122	0	31	0	0	0.0	0.0	0.0	0	191
20385	Drink, cherry, swtnd, prep	8 fl-oz	254	60	0	16	0	0	0.0	0.0	0.0	0	0
20737	Drink, fruit punch	8 fl-oz	252	110	0	29	—	0	0.0	0.0	0.0	0	—
20176	Drink, fruit punch, non carbonated	12 fl-oz	360	200	0	50	0	0	0.0	0.0	0.0	0	—
20761	Drink, Island Punch	1 cup	252	110	0	27	—	0	0.0	0.0	0.0	0	—
20045	Drink, lemonade, prep f/pwd	1 cup	266	112	0	29	0	0	0.0	0.0	0.0	0	0
20746	Drink, pink lemonade	8 fl-oz	252	110	0	26	—	0	0.0	0.0	0.0	0	—
20123	Juice Drink, citrus fruit, calc fort	1 cup	240	112	1	28	0	0	0.0	0.0	0.0	0	1
20744	Juice Drink, raspberry peach	1 cup	252	120	0	29	—	0	0.0	0.0	0.0	0	—
793	Juice, apple	8 fl-oz	236	110	0	29	0	0	0.0	0.0	0.0	0	—
1853	Juice, grape	8 fl-oz	236	150	0	38	0	0	0.0	0.0	0.0	0	—
794	Juice, grapefruit	8 fl-oz	236	120	0	29	0	0	0.0	0.0	0.0	0	—
1854	Juice, orange	8 fl-oz	236	120	0	29	0	0	0.0	0.0	0.0	0	—
3128	Juice, prune, cnd	1 cup	256	182	2	45	3	0	0.0	0.1	0.0	0	1
6504	Juice, tomato, cnd	1 cup	243	50	2	10	2	0	0.0	0.0	0.0	0	100
6507	Juice, vegetable, cnd	1 cup	243	50	2	10	2	0	0.0	0.0	0.0	0	400
OTHER BEVERAGES													
38405	Drink, atole, cornmeal	1 cup	245	206	4	40	1	4	2.2	1.1	0.3	14	33
38362	Drink, horchata de arroz, rice beverage, Mexican	1 cup	245	100	0	25	0	0	0.0	0.0	0.0	0	0
20589	Drink, sugar cane, Puerto Rico	1 cup	240	164	0	42	0	0	0.0	0.0	0.0	0	0
Teas													
20495	Tea, bag	1 ea	2	0	0	0	0	0	0.0	0.0	0.0	0	0
20014	Tea, brewed w/tap water	1 cup	237	2	0	1	0	0	0.0	0.0	0.0	0	0
20538	Tea, Cool Drink, can/btl	1 cup	248	82	0	22	0	0	0.0	0.0	0.0	0	0
20681	Tea, green, sweetened, btl	1 cup	252	100	0	25	—	0	0.0	0.0	0.0	0	—
20894	Tea, herbal, Cranberry Cove, brewed	1 cup	237	0	0	0	0	0	0.0	0.0	0.0	0	0
20853	Tea, herbal, Echinacea Complete Care, brewed	1 cup	237	0	0	0	0	0	0.0	0.0	0.0	0	0
20899	Tea, herbal, Sleepytime, brewed	1 cup	237	0	0	0	0	0	0.0	0.0	0.0	0	0
30451	Tea, iced, 100%, inst, pwd	2 tsp	1	0	0	0	0	0	0.0	0.0	0.0	0	0
20724	Tea, iced, w/lemonade	8 fl-oz	252	110	0	28	0	0	0.0	0.0	0.0	0	—
Water													
20051	Water, btld	1 cup	237	0	0	0	0	0	0.0	0.0	0.0	0	0
20041	Water, municipal	1 cup	237	0	0	0	0	0	0.0	0.0	0.0	0	0
BEVERAGES, ALCOHOLIC													
34066	Beer, amber ale	12 fl-oz	356	169	2	14	—	0	0.0	0.0	0.0	0	—
22500	Beer, can/btl, 12 fl oz	12 fl-oz	356	139	1	11	0	0	0.0	0.0	0.0	0	0
34053	Beer, Light	12 fl-oz	353	105	1	5	0	0	0.0	0.0	0.0	0	—
22685	Beer, non alcoholic, Near	12 fl-oz	356	32	1	5	0	0	0.0	0.0	0.0	0	0
22671	Bourbon, 80 proof	1 fl-oz	28	64	0	0	0	0	0.0	0.0	0.0	0	0
22513	Brandy, 80 proof	1 fl-oz	28	64	0	0	0	0	0.0	0.0	0.0	0	0
22514	Gin, 80 proof	1 fl-oz	28	64	0	0	0	0	0.0	0.0	0.0	0	0
22547	Liqueur, Amaretto, 1 shot	1 ea	30	106	0	13	0	0	0.0	0.0	0.0	0	0
34052	Malt Beverage, Zima	12 fl-oz	353	185	0	21	0	0	0.0	0.0	0.0	0	—
22555	Mixed Drink, Bacardi cocktail	1 ea	63	117	0	6	0	0	0.0	0.0	0.0	0	0

PAGE KEY: A-158 Granola Bars, Cereal Bars, Diet Bars, Scones, and Tarts   A-158 Meals and Dishes   A-162 Meats   A-168 Nuts, Seeds, and Products   A-170 Poultry   A-172 Salad Dressings, Dips, and Mayonnaise   A-172 Salads   A-174 Sandwiches   A-176 Sauces and Gravies   A-176 Snack Foods—Chips, Pretzels, Popcorn   A-178 Soups, Stews, and Chilis   A-180 Spices, Flavors, and Seasonings   A-182 Sports Bars and Drinks   A-182 Supplemental Foods and Formulas   A-184 Sweeteners and Sweet Substitutes   A-184 Vegetables and Legumes   A-198 Weight Loss Bars and Drinks   A-200 Miscellaneous

Thia (mg)	Ribo (mg)	Niac (mg NE)	Vit B6 (mg)	Vit B12 (µg)	Fol (µg)	Vit C (mg)	Vit D (IU)	Vit E (mg AT)	Cal (mg)	Iron (mg)	Magn (mg)	Phos (mg)	Pota (mg)	Sodi (mg)	Zinc (mg)	Wat (%)	Alco (g)	Caff (g)
0.00	0.21	2.53	0.25	0.00	0.0	73.2	—	0.0	126	0.01	2.5	47	60	10	0.0	87	0.00	0.00
—	—	—	—	0.00	—	6.0	—	—	0	0.00	—	0	0	0	—	94	0.00	0.00
—	—	—	—			0.0	—	—	—	—	—	—	—	10	—	88	0.00	0.00
—	—	—	—	0.00		65.0	—	—	—	—	—	0	0	45	—		0.00	0.00
—	—	—	—			—	—	—	—	—	—	—	—	10	—	89	0.00	0.00
0.00	0.00	0.00	0.00	0.00	0.0	34.0	—	0.0	29	0.05	2.7	3	3	19	0.1	89	0.00	0.00
—	—	—	—			0.0								10		90	0.00	0.00
0.05	0.02	0.31	0.05		5.2	79.8	0.0	0.1	316	0.21	16.7	20	196	4	0.1	88	0.00	0.00
—	—	—	—			0.0	—	—	—	—	—	—	—	10	—	88	0.00	0.00
—	—	—	—			—	—	—	—	—	—	—	—	10	—	88	0.00	0.00
—	—	—	—				—	—	—	—	—	—	—	10	—	84	0.00	0.00
—	—	—	—				—	—	—	—	—	—	—	0	—	87	0.00	0.00
—	—	—	—				—	—	—	—	—	—	—	0	—	—	0.00	0.00
0.03	0.18	2.00	0.56	0.00	0.0	10.5	—	0.3	31	3.01	35.8	64	707	10	0.5	81	0.00	0.00
—	—	—	—			72.0	—	—	20	0.72	—	—	430	750	—	94	0.00	0.00
—	—	—	—			60.0	—	—	40	0.72	—	—	520	620	—	94	0.00	0.00
0.12	0.23	0.81	0.07	0.36	6.4	0.9	—	0.1	140	0.67	24.2	117	185	55	0.6	80	0.00	0.00
0.00	0.00	0.14	0.00	0.00	0.4	0.1	—	0.0	12	0.34	3.5	5	6	7	0.1	89	0.00	0.00
0.07	0.03	0.05	0.00	0.00	0.0	0.0	—	0.0	12	2.25	8.0	5	39	42	0.2	81	0.00	0.00
—	—	—	—	—	—	0.0	—	—	0	0.00	—	—	25	0	—	—	0.00	55.00
0.00	0.02	0.00	0.00	0.00	11.8	0.0	—	0.0	0	0.05	7.1	2	88	7	0.0	100	0.00	47.36
—	—	—	—	—	—	0.0	—	—	0	0.00	—	73	38	33	—	—	0.00	11.00
—	—	—	—			0.0	—	—	—	—	—	—	—	10	—	90	0.00	18.00
—	—	—	—			0.0	—	—	0	0.00	—	—	30	0	—	100	0.00	0.00
—	—	—	—	—	—	35.0	—	—	0	0.00	—	—	—	0	7.5	100	0.00	0.00
—	—	—	—			0.0	—	—	0	0.00	—	—	30	0	—	100	0.00	0.00
—	—	—	—			0.0	—	—	0	0.00	—	—	45	0	—	—	0.00	40.00
—	—	—	—			0.0	—	—	—	—	—	—	—	10	—	89	0.00	18.00
0.00	0.00	0.00	0.00	0.00	0.0	0.0	—	0.0	2	0.01	2.4	0	0	2	0.0	100	0.00	0.00
0.00	0.00	0.00	0.00	0.00	0.0	0.0	—	0.0	5	0.00	2.4	0	0	5	0.0	100	0.00	0.00
—	—	—	—	—	—	—	—	—	—	—	—	—	—	44	—	—	18.65	0.00
0.01	0.09	1.83	0.15	0.07	21.4	0.0	—	0.0	14	0.07	21.4	50	96	14	0.0	93	12.82	0.00
0.03	0.03	1.40	—	—	—	—	—	—	11	—	—	—	59	11	—	98	14.11	0.00
0.01	0.09	1.61	0.18	0.07	21.4	0.0	—	0.0	25	0.03	32.1	110	89	18	0.0	98	1.07	0.00
0.00	0.00	0.00	0.00	0.00	0.0	0.0	—	0.0	0	0.00	0.0	1	1	0	0.0	67	9.28	0.00
0.00	0.00	0.00	0.00	0.00	0.0	0.0	—	0.0	0	0.00	0.0	1	1	0	0.0	67	9.28	0.00
0.00	0.00	0.00	0.00	0.00	0.0	0.0	—	0.0	0	0.00	0.0	1	1	0	0.0	67	9.28	0.00
0.00	0.00	0.01	0.00	0.00	0.0	0.0	0.0	0.0	0	0.01	0.5	1	4	2	0.0	30	7.73	0.00
0.03	0.03	0.87	—	—	—	—	—	—	38	—	—	—	51	20	—	—	16.94	0.00
0.00	0.00	0.02	0.00	0.00	1.2	1.0	0.0	0.0	2	0.05	1.2	3	12	11	0.0	68	13.72	0.00

PAGE KEY: A-108 Beverage and Beverage Mixes   A-110 Other Beverages   A-110 Beverages, Alcoholic   A-112 Candies and Confections, Gum   A-116 Cereals, Breakfast Type   A-120 Cheese and Cheese Substitutes   A-122 Dairy Products and Substitutes   A-124 Desserts   A-130 Dessert Toppings   A-130 Eggs, Substitutes, and Egg Dishes   A-132 Ethnic Foods   A-136 Fast Foods/Restaurants   A-150 Fats, Oils, Margarines, Shortenings, and Substitutes   A-150 Fish, Seafood, and Shellfish   A-152 Food Additives   A-152 Fruit, Vegetable, or Blended Juices   A-154 Grains, Flours, and Fractions   A-154 Grain Products, Prepared and Baked Goods

Code	Food Name	Unit/ Amt	Wt (g)	Energy (kcal)	Prot (g)	Carb (g)	Fiber (g)	Fat (g)	Sat (g)	Mono (g)	Poly (g)	Chol (mg)	Vit A (RE)
34057	Mixed Drink, bloody mary, prep f/recipe	1 ea	209	46	1	7	1	0	0.0	—	—	0	117
22538	Mixed Drink, daiquiri, 6.8 fl oz can	1 ea	207	259	0	33	0	0	0.0	0.0	0.0	0	0
34058	Mixed Drink, gin & tonic, prep f/recipe	1 ea	232	160	0	8	0	0	0.0	0.0	0.0	0	0
22556	Mixed Drink, high ball	1 ea	160	105	0	0	0	0	0.0	0.0	0.0	0	0
22569	Mixed Drink, Irish coffee, 1 fl oz	1 ea	26	26	0	1	0	1	0.8	0.4	0.0	5	15
22568	Mixed Drink, Long Island iced tea	1 ea	125	119	0	9	0	0	0.0	0.0	0.0	0	0
22566	Mixed Drink, Mai Tai	1 ea	126	305	0	29	0	0	0.0	0.0	0.1	0	0
22557	Mixed Drink, margarita	1 ea	77	170	0	11	0	0	0.0	0.0	0.0	0	0
22571	Mixed Drink, Mexican eggnog/rompope	4 fl-oz	122	203	5	19	0	7	2.8	2.3	0.7	184	102
22561	Mixed Drink, pina colada	1 ea	141	245	1	32	0	3	2.3	0.1	0.0	0	0
22683	Mixed Drink, screwdriver cocktail	1 ea	213	182	1	18	0	0	0.0	0.0	0.0	0	14
22567	Mixed Drink, tequila sunrise	1 ea	172	189	1	15	0	0	0.0	0.0	0.0	0	17
22534	Mixed Drink, whiskey sour mix, btld	4 fl-oz	124	108	0	26	0	0	0.0	0.0	0.0	0	0
22593	Rum, 80 proof	1 fl-oz	28	64	0	0	0	0	0.0	0.0	0.0	0	0
22515	Tequila, 80 proof	1 fl-oz	28	64	0	0	0	0	0.0	0.0	0.0	0	0
22594	Vodka, 80 proof	1 fl-oz	28	64	0	0	0	0	0.0	0.0	0.0	0	0
22670	Whiskey, 80 proof	1 fl-oz	28	64	0	0	0	0	0.0	0.0	0.0	0	0
22577	Wine, all table types	6 fl-oz	177	136	0	6	0	0	0.0	0.0	0.0	0	0
22608	Wine, cooking, red	1 fl-oz	30	20	0	3	0	0	0.0	0.0	0.0	0	0
22609	Wine, cooking, white	1 fl-oz	30	20	0	3	0	0	0.0	0.0	0.0	0	0
22681	Wine, cooler	1 cup	227	113	0	13	0	0	0.0	0.0	0.0	0	0
22509	Wine, dry, sherry	1 fl-oz	29	20	0	0	—	0	0.0	0.0	0.0	0	0
20076	Wine, non alcoholic	4 fl-oz	116	7	1	1	0	0	0.0	0.0	0.0	0	0
22501	Wine, red	6 fl-oz	177	127	0	3	0	0	0.0	0.0	0.0	0	0
22600	Wine, rice, Japanese	1 fl-oz	29	39	0	1	0	0	0.0	0.0	0.0	0	0
22511	Wine, Sweet Vermouth	1 fl-oz	30	46	0	4	—	0	0.0	0.0	0.0	0	0
CANDIES AND CONFECTIONS, GUM													
23017	Baking Chips, milk chocolate	1.5 oz	43	228	3	25	1	13	6.1	5.6	0.3	10	21
90704	Candy Bar, 3 Musketeers, 0.8 oz bar	1 ea	23	94	1	17	0	3	1.5	1.0	0.1	2	3
23125	Candy Bar, 5th Avenue, 2 oz bar	1 ea	57	273	5	36	2	14	3.8	6.0	1.9	3	8
23049	Candy Bar, Almond Joy, 1.7 oz	1 ea	48	231	2	29	2	13	8.5	2.5	0.6	2	4
90678	Candy Bar, Baby Ruth, 1.2 oz bar	1 ea	34	158	2	21	1	9	4.2	2.2	1.1	1	1
90653	Candy Bar, Butterfinger, 1.6 oz bar	1 ea	45	216	3	33	1	9	4.6	2.2	1.1	0	0
23116	Candy Bar, Caramello, 1.6 oz bar	1 ea	45	210	3	29	1	10	5.8	2.4	0.3	12	28
23118	Candy Bar, carob, 3 oz bar	1 ea	85	459	7	48	3	27	24.7	0.4	0.3	3	0
23099	Candy Bar, crisped rice, chocolate chip, 1 oz bar	1 ea	28	115	1	21	1	4	1.5	1.1	1.0	0	100
4196	Candy Bar, dark chocolate, 1.5 oz bar	0.5 ea	42	230	2	25	4	14	9.0	—	—	3	0
4198	Candy Bar, dark chocolate, w/almonds, 1.5 oz bar	0.5 ea	42	230	3	23	4	15	8.0	—	—	3	0
91519	Candy Bar, Heath, bites	15 pce	39	207	2	25	1	12	6.1	3.4	1.0	7	18
23060	Candy Bar, Kit Kat, 1.5 oz bar	1 ea	43	220	3	27	0	11	7.6	2.5	0.4	5	10
23061	Candy Bar, Krackel, 1.5 oz bar	1 ea	43	218	3	27	1	11	6.8	2.7	0.2	5	9
23037	Candy Bar, Mars almond, 1.76 oz bar	1 ea	50	234	4	31	1	12	3.6	5.3	2.0	8	8
92633	Candy Bar, milk chocolate, 0.6 oz bar	1 ea	17	90	1	10	0	5	3.5	—	—	5	0
90687	Candy Bar, Milky Way, 1.9 oz bar	1 ea	54	228	2	39	1	9	4.2	3.2	0.3	8	10
23035	Candy Bar, Mounds, 1.9 oz bar	1 ea	54	262	2	32	2	14	11.1	0.2	0.1	1	0
23062	Candy Bar, Mr. Goodbar, 1.75 oz bar	1 ea	50	267	5	27	2	16	7.0	4.1	2.2	5	17
23133	Candy Bar, Nestle Crunch, 1.4 oz bar	1 ea	40	207	2	26	1	10	6.0	3.4	0.3	5	6

Thia (mg)	Ribo (mg)	Niac (mg NE)	Vit B6 (mg)	Vit B12 (µg)	Fol (µg)	Vit C (mg)	Vit D (IU)	Vit E (mg AT)	Cal (mg)	Iron (mg)	Magn (mg)	Phos (mg)	Pota (mg)	Sodi (mg)	Zinc (mg)	Wat (%)	Alco (g)	Caff (g)
0.00	0.00	0.03	0.00	0.00	2.4	23.6	0.0	0.0	19	1.07	2.2	4	52	558	0.0	94	1.38	0.00
0.00	0.00	0.02	0.00	0.00	2.1	2.7	0.0	0.0	0	0.01	2.1	4	23	83	0.1	75	19.90	0.00
0.00	0.00	0.00	0.00	0.00	0.0	0.0	0.0	0.0	3	0.03	0.9	2	1	7	0.1	88	18.56	0.00
0.00	0.00	0.00	0.00	0.00	0.0	0.0	0.0	0.0	6	0.02	1.2	2	3	25	0.1	90	15.09	0.00
0.00	0.00	0.03	0.00	0.00	0.1	0.0	1.8	0.0	3	0.00	1.1	3	12	2	0.0	86	1.63	—
0.00	0.00	0.02	0.00	0.00	1.3	3.2	0.0	0.0	4	0.05	1.8	12	14	6	0.0	83	12.14	0.00
0.00	0.00	0.05	0.00	0.00	1.2	1.0	0.0	0.0	3	0.09	2.4	6	24	11	0.1	54	27.56	0.00
0.00	0.00	0.03	0.00	0.00	1.2	1.0	0.0	0.0	2	0.05	1.4	4	15	4	0.0	62	18.50	0.00
0.03	0.20	0.07	0.07	0.55	18.0	0.6	43.7	0.5	106	0.54	11.1	136	125	42	0.7	69	7.48	0.00
0.03	0.02	0.17	0.05	0.00	16.5	6.9	0.0	0.1	11	0.27	10.6	10	100	9	0.2	65	13.89	0.00
0.14	0.02	0.34	0.07	0.00	74.9	66.5	0.0	0.3	15	0.18	17.1	29	326	2	0.1	83	15.10	0.00
0.07	0.02	0.33	0.09	0.00	18.2	33.3	0.0	0.1	10	0.46	11.7	17	179	7	0.1	80	18.68	0.00
0.01	0.00	0.00	0.00	0.00	0.0	3.3	—	0.0	2	0.14	1.2	7	35	126	0.1	78	0.00	0.00
0.00	0.00	0.00	0.00	0.00	0.0	0.0	—	0.0	0	0.02	0.0	1	1	0	0.0	67	9.28	0.00
0.00	0.00	0.00	0.00	0.00	0.0	0.0	—	0.0	0	0.00	0.0	1	1	0	0.0	67	9.28	0.00
0.00	0.00	0.00	0.00	0.00	0.0	0.0	—	0.0	0	0.00	0.0	1	0	0	0.0	67	9.28	0.00
0.00	0.00	0.00	0.00	0.00	0.0	0.0	—	0.0	0	0.00	0.0	1	1	0	0.0	67	9.28	0.00
0.00	0.02	0.12	0.03	0.01	1.8	0.0	—	0.0	14	0.62	15.9	23	149	11	0.1	87	16.45	0.00
0.30	0.30	0.30	—	0.00	—	0.3	—	—	2	0.30	—	4	24	180	—	88	3.59	0.00
0.30	0.30	0.30	—	0.00	—	0.3	—	—	2	0.30	—	4	26	180	—	88	3.59	0.00
0.00	0.01	0.10	0.02	0.00	2.7	4.1	0.0	0.0	13	0.62	11.9	15	102	19	0.1	90	8.81	0.00
0.00	0.00	0.01	0.00	0.00	0.3	0.0	—	0.0	2	0.11	2.9	4	26	2	0.0	89	2.72	0.00
0.00	0.00	0.11	0.01	0.00	1.2	0.0	—	0.0	10	0.46	11.6	17	102	8	0.1	98	0.00	0.00
0.00	0.05	0.14	0.05	0.01	3.5	0.0	—	0.0	14	0.75	23.0	25	198	9	0.2	88	16.45	0.00
0.00	0.00	0.00	0.00	0.00	0.0	0.0	—	0.0	1	0.02	1.7	2	7	1	0.0	78	4.69	0.00
0.00	0.00	0.05	0.00	0.00	0.1	0.0	—	0.0	2	0.07	2.7	3	28	3	0.0	72	4.59	0.00
0.05	0.12	0.15	0.01	0.25	5.1	0.0	—	0.9	80	1.00	26.8	88	158	34	0.9	2	0.00	8.51
0.00	0.02	0.05	0.00	0.03	0.0	0.1	—	0.2	19	0.17	6.6	21	30	44	0.1	6	0.00	1.80
0.07	0.05	2.21	0.05	0.10	20.4	0.2	—	1.5	41	0.68	35.2	80	197	128	0.6	2	0.00	2.83
0.00	0.07	0.23	0.02	0.05	—	0.3	—	0.0	31	0.61	31.8	54	122	68	0.4	8	0.00	—
0.02	0.02	0.94	0.01	0.00	10.5	0.0	—	0.6	15	0.23	24.8	47	121	73	0.4	5	0.00	1.36
0.05	0.02	1.39	0.05	0.00	15.0	0.0	—	0.8	16	0.34	37.6	61	179	97	0.5	1	0.00	2.26
0.01	0.18	0.51	0.01	0.28	—	0.8	0.0	0.1	97	0.49	19.1	68	155	55	0.4	7	0.00	1.80
0.09	0.15	0.87	0.10	0.85	17.9	0.4	—	1.0	258	1.10	30.6	107	538	91	3.0	2	0.00	0.00
0.15	0.17	2.00	0.20	0.00	39.7	0.0	—	0.0	6	1.78	13.6	38	48	79	0.2	7	0.00	—
—	—	—	—	—	—	0.0	—	—	0	1.08	—	—	—	0	—	—	0.00	—
—	—	—	—	—	—	0.0	—	—	20	1.08	—	—	—	0	—	—	0.00	—
0.00	0.03	0.03	0.00	—	0.4	0.3	—	0.0	34	0.30	2.3	28	82	96	0.0	1	0.00	0.00
0.05	0.09	0.20	0.00	0.23	6.0	0.0	—	0.1	53	0.43	15.7	57	98	23	0.0	2	0.00	5.94
0.01	0.07	0.10	0.01	0.25	2.6	0.3	—	0.0	67	0.44	5.5	52	138	83	0.2	1	0.00	—
0.01	0.15	0.46	0.02	0.18	4.5	0.3	—	3.9	84	0.55	36.0	117	162	85	0.6	4	0.00	2.00
—	—	—	—	—	—	0.0	—	—	32	0.14	—	—	—	15	—	5	0.00	3.96
0.01	0.11	0.18	0.02	0.17	3.2	0.5	—	0.7	70	0.40	18.3	78	130	129	0.4	6	0.00	4.30
0.00	0.00	0.00	0.00	0.00	0.0	0.4	—	0.1	11	1.12	0.0	0	173	78	0.0	9	0.00	9.15
0.07	0.07	1.71	0.02	0.15	18.9	0.4	—	1.6	55	0.68	23.3	81	195	20	0.5	0	0.00	8.93
0.12	0.21	1.57	0.15	0.15	31.4	0.1	—	0.4	67	0.20	23.0	80	137	53	0.6	1	0.00	9.52

PAGE KEY: A-108 Beverage and Beverage Mixes   A-110 Other Beverages   A-110 Beverages, Alcoholic   A-112 Candies and Confections, Gum   A-116 Cereals, Breakfast Type   A-120 Cheese and Cheese Substitutes   A-122 Dairy Products and Substitutes   A-124 Desserts   A-130 Dessert Toppings   A-130 Eggs, Substitutes, and Egg Dishes   A-132 Ethnic Foods   A-136 Fast Foods/Restaurants   A-150 Fats, Oils, Margarines, Shortenings, and Substitutes   A-150 Fish, Seafood, and Shellfish   A-152 Food Additives   A-152 Fruit, Vegetable, or Blended Juices   A-154 Grains, Flours, and Fractions   A-154 Grain Products, Prepared and Baked Goods

Code	Food Name	Unit/ Amt	Wt (g)	Energy (kcal)	Prot (g)	Carb (g)	Fiber (g)	Fat (g)	Sat (g)	Mono (g)	Poly (g)	Chol (mg)	Vit A (RE)
92654	Candy Bar, Payday, snack size, 0.7 oz bar	1 ea	20	90	2	10	—	5	0.5	—	—	0	—
23137	Candy Bar, peanut, 1.4 oz bar	1 ea	40	207	6	19	2	13	1.9	6.6	4.2	0	0
91513	Candy Bar, Reese's Nutrageous, 0.6 oz bar	2 ea	34	176	4	18	1	11	3.0	4.3	2.8	1	2
23036	Candy Bar, Skor, toffee bar, 1.4 oz bar	1 ea	40	212	1	24	1	13	7.5	3.7	0.5	21	57
23040	Candy Bar, Snickers, 2 oz bar	1 ea	57	265	5	37	1	11	4.2	4.7	1.5	8	22
23146	Candy Bar, Symphony, milk chocolate, 1.5 oz bar	1 ea	43	226	4	25	1	13	7.8	3.4	0.3	10	20
90705	Candy Bar, Twix, caramel, 2.06 oz two bar pkg	1 ea	58	291	3	38	1	14	5.2	7.8	0.5	3	15
92221	Candy Bar, Twix, chocolate fudge cookie bar, 3.6 oz bar	1 ea	100	550	7	56	3	33	5.0	14.3	12.5	6	11
23151	Candy Bar, Whatchamacallit, 1.7 oz bar	1 ea	48	238	4	30	1	11	8.2	1.8	0.4	6	19
92658	Candy Bar, Zero, 0.6 oz bar	1 ea	17	70	1	12	—	2	1.5	—	—	0	—
23085	Candy, Almond Roca	1 pce	11	48	1	7	0	2	1.1	0.6	0.2	1	2
4148	Candy, Bit O Honey, Nestle	6 pce	40	160	1	32	0	3	2.0	0.8	0.2	0	0
92707	Candy, caramel, Sugar Daddy, lrg	1 ea	48	200	1	43	0	2	1.0	—	—	0	0
23015	Candy, caramels	1 pce	10	39	0	8	0	1	0.7	0.1	0.0	1	0
92374	Candy, cotton	2.1 oz	60	220	3	56	—	0	0.0	0.0	0.0	0	—
23078	Candy, fondant, chocolate cvrd	2 pce	28	102	1	22	0	3	1.5	0.9	0.1	0	1
92647	Candy, Good N Plenty, snack size box	1 ea	17	60	0	14	0	0	0.0	0.0	0.0	0	0
23409	Candy, gumdrops	1.5 oz	43	168	0	42	0	0	0.0	0.0	0.0	0	0
23412	Candy, gummy worms, pces	10 pce	74	293	0	73	0	0	0.0	0.0	0.0	0	0
23031	Candy, hard, all flvrs	1 pce	6	24	0	6	0	0	0.0	0.0	0.0	0	0
92653	Candy, hard, lollipop	1 ea	17	60	0	16	0	0	0.0	0.0	0.0	0	0
23472	Candy, jawbreakers, Everlasting Gobstoppers, Willy Wonka	6 pce	16	59	0	15	—	0	0.0	0.0	0.0	—	—
23033	Candy, jellybeans, sml	10 pce	11	41	0	10	0	0	0.0	0.0	0.0	0	0
23063	Candy, Kisses, milk chocolate	6 pce	28	145	2	17	1	9	5.2	2.8	0.3	6	16
52154	Candy, licorice, black, vines/ropes	4 pce	40	140	1	33	0	0	0.0	0.0	0.0	0	0
52155	Candy, licorice, red, vines/ropes	4 pce	40	140	1	34	0	0	0.0	0.0	0.0	0	0
92644	Candy, malt choc, Whoppers	9 ea	20	90	1	15	0	4	3.0	—	—	0	0
23047	Candy, milk chocolate peanut	1.5 oz	43	219	4	26	1	11	4.4	4.7	1.8	4	11
92642	Candy, Milk Duds	7 ea	21	90	1	15	0	4	1.0	—	—	0	—
23193	Candy, mints, After Eight	5 pce	41	147	1	31	1	6	3.4	1.8	0.2	0	1
23225	Candy, mints, peppermint, Breath Saver	1 pce	2	10	0	2	0	0	0.0	0.0	0.0	—	—
92657	Candy, Nibs, licorice	9 ea	12	35	0	9	—	0	0.0	0.0	0.0	0	0
92201	Candy, nougat, 0.5 oz pce	1 ea	14	56	0	13	0	0	0.2	0.0	0.0	0	0
23021	Candy, peanuts, milk chocolate cvrd	1.5 oz	43	221	6	21	2	14	6.2	5.5	1.8	4	14
23088	Candy, peanuts, yogurt cvrd	1.5 oz	43	230	6	18	2	16	6.9	4.8	3.1	0	0
90803	Candy, pralines, prep f/recipe	1 pce	40	174	1	22	1	10	2.7	—	—	10	30
23517	Candy, raisins, chocolate cvrd	35 pce	40	160	1	27	2	7	4.0	—	—	0	2
23089	Candy, raisins, yogurt cvrd	1.5 oz	43	167	2	31	1	5	4.3	0.1	0.1	0	0
92643	Candy, Sixlets	6 ea	38	170	1	29	0	7	5.0	—	—	0	0
23485	Candy, Skittles, original bite size candies, 2.17 oz pkg	1 ea	62	249	0	56	0	3	0.5	1.8	0.1	0	0
23144	Candy, Starburst, fruit chews	1 pce	5	20	0	4	0	0	0.1	0.2	0.2	0	0
92705	Candy, Sugar Babies	30 ea	44	180	0	41	0	2	0.0	—	—	0	0
4149	Candy, SweeTarts, reg	8 pce	15	60	0	14	0	0	0.0	0.0	0.0	0	0
90806	Candy, taffy, prep f/recipe	1 pce	34	99	1	17	0	3	1.0	—	—	4	—
92769	Candy, Tootsie Roll	6 pce	40	155	1	35	0	1	0.4	0.8	0.1	1	0

PAGE KEY: A-158 Granola Bars, Cereal Bars, Diet Bars, Scones, and Tarts   A-158 Meals and Dishes   A-162 Meats   A-168 Nuts, Seeds, and Products   A-170 Poultry   A-172 Salad Dressings, Dips, and Mayonnaise   A-172 Salads   A-174 Sandwiches   A-176 Sauces and Gravies   A-176 Snack Foods—Chips, Pretzels, Popcorn   A-178 Soups, Stews, and Chilis   A-180 Spices, Flavors, and Seasonings   A-182 Sports Bars and Drinks   A-182 Supplemental Foods and Formulas   A-184 Sweeteners and Sweet Substitutes   A-184 Vegetables and Legumes   A-198 Weight Loss Bars and Drinks   A-200 Miscellaneous

Thia (mg)	Ribo (mg)	Niac (mg NE)	Vit B6 (mg)	Vit B12 (µg)	Fol (µg)	Vit C (mg)	Vit D (IU)	Vit E (mg AT)	Cal (mg)	Iron (mg)	Magn (mg)	Phos (mg)	Pota (mg)	Sodi (mg)	Zinc (mg)	Wat (%)	Alco (g)	Caff (g)
—	—	—	—	—	—	—	—	—	—	—	—	—	—	65	—	13	0.00	0.00
0.03	0.05	3.14	0.05	0.00	29.8	0.0	—	1.6	31	0.37	43.7	122	162	62	1.6	2	0.00	0.00
0.05	0.02	1.77	0.02	—	19.0	0.2	—	0.4	23	0.41	23.1	60	124	48	0.4	2	0.00	—
0.00	0.03	0.05	0.00	0.10	1.2	0.2	—	0.0	52	0.23	4.0	24	61	126	0.1	2	0.00	—
0.02	0.07	2.03	0.05	0.09	15.3	0.0	—	0.9	60	0.68	40.8	108	183	129	1.4	6	0.00	4.53
0.03	0.15	0.14	0.01	0.17	—	0.9	0.0	0.1	107	0.38	23.4	88	186	43	0.5	1	0.00	28.06
0.07	0.10	0.43	0.00	0.17	11.1	0.2	—	1.1	53	0.46	18.7	64	110	113	0.6	4	0.00	1.75
0.14	0.20	1.11	0.03	0.33	9.0	1.0	—	2.7	130	1.30	46.0	147	309	266	0.9	2	0.00	10.00
0.05	0.10	1.19	0.01	0.18	8.7	0.4	—	0.6	57	0.54	13.5	67	146	144	0.2	3	0.00	4.82
—	—	—	—	—	—	—	—	—	—	—	—	—	—	35	—	—	0.00	—
0.00	0.01	0.15	0.00	0.00	3.3	0.0	—	0.2	16	0.10	4.9	19	34	20	0.1	5	0.00	—
0.00	0.10	0.01	0.00	0.07	1.6	0.0	—	0.4	20	0.11	2.8	18	50	120	0.1	8	0.00	0.00
—	—	—	—	—	—	0.0	—	—	20	0.00	—	—	—	65	—	—	0.00	0.00
0.00	0.02	0.02	0.00	0.00	0.5	0.1	—	0.3	14	0.00	1.7	12	22	25	0.0	8	0.00	0.00
—	—	—	—	—	—	—	—	—	—	—	—	—	—	0	—	—	0.00	0.00
0.00	0.01	0.15	0.00	0.00	0.3	0.0	—	0.1	5	0.43	17.6	27	47	7	0.1	8	0.00	1.12
—	—	—	—	—	—	0.0	—	—	0	0.11	—	—	—	40	—	—	0.00	0.00
0.00	0.00	0.00	0.00	0.00	0.0	0.0	—	0.0	1	0.17	0.4	0	2	19	0.0	1	0.00	0.00
0.00	0.00	0.00	0.00	0.00	0.0	0.0	—	0.0	2	0.30	0.7	1	4	33	0.0	1	0.00	0.00
0.00	0.00	0.00	0.00	0.00	0.0	0.0	—	0.0	0	0.01	0.2	0	0	2	0.0	1	0.00	0.00
—	—	—	—	—	—	0.0	—	—	0	0.00	—	—	—	10	—	5	0.00	0.00
—	—	—	—	—	—	—	—	—	—	—	—	—	—	1	—	8	0.00	0.00
0.00	0.00	0.00	0.00	0.00	0.0	0.0	—	0.0	0	0.00	0.2	0	4	6	0.0	6	0.00	0.00
0.01	0.09	0.09	0.00	0.10	2.3	0.1	—	0.4	54	0.38	17.0	61	109	23	0.4	1	0.00	6.96
—	—	—	—	—	—	0.0	—	—	0	0.00	—	—	—	60	—	15	0.00	—
—	—	—	—	—	—	0.0	—	—	0	0.00	—	—	—	20	—	12	0.00	0.00
—	—	—	—	—	—	0.0	—	—	40	0.18	—	—	—	65	—	—	0.00	—
0.03	0.07	1.74	0.03	0.07	16.2	0.2	—	1.1	43	0.49	32.3	99	148	20	1.0	2	0.00	4.67
—	—	—	—	—	—	—	—	—	—	—	—	—	—	40	—	6	0.00	—
0.01	0.01	0.11	0.00	0.00	0.4	0.0	—	0.2	9	0.62	18.5	23	69	5	0.2	6	0.00	8.19
—	—	—	—	—	—	—	—	—	—	—	—	—	0	0	—	0	0.00	0.00
—	—	—	—	—	—	0.0	—	—	0	0.00	—	—	—	60	—	25	0.00	0.00
0.00	0.01	0.07	0.00	0.00	0.7	0.0	—	0.4	4	0.07	4.5	8	15	5	0.1	2	0.00	0.00
0.05	0.07	1.80	0.09	0.18	3.4	0.0	—	1.5	44	0.56	40.8	90	213	17	1.0	2	0.00	9.35
0.14	0.09	2.48	0.07	0.18	49.9	0.1	—	2.3	64	0.93	35.0	113	202	24	0.8	4	0.00	0.00
0.05	0.02	0.11	0.01	0.02	2.5	0.2	4.8	0.4	20	0.34	13.4	33	67	40	0.4	17	0.00	0.00
—	—	—	—	—	—	1.0	—	—	16	3.00	—	—	—	40	—	10	0.00	—
0.05	0.07	0.33	0.07	0.12	3.9	0.9	—	0.6	48	0.56	10.3	55	236	19	0.2	10	0.00	0.00
—	—	—	—	—	—	0.0	—	—	40	0.00	—	—	—	55	—	1	0.00	—
0.00	0.00	0.00	0.00	0.00	0.0	41.2	—	0.3	0	0.00	0.6	1	6	10	0.0	4	0.00	0.00
0.00	0.00	0.00	0.00	0.00	0.0	2.6	—	0.0	0	0.00	0.1	0	0	3	0.0	7	0.00	0.00
—	—	—	—	—	—	0.0	—	—	20	0.00	—	—	—	40	—	—	0.00	—
—	—	—	—	—	—	0.0	—	—	0	0.00	—	—	—	0	—	—	0.00	—
0.00	0.01	0.10	0.00	0.00	1.3	0.0	1.0	0.6	9	0.01	9.1	16	19	152	0.1	34	0.00	0.00
0.01	0.02	0.07	0.00	0.00	3.6	0.0	—	0.3	14	0.31	8.8	23	46	18	0.2	7	0.00	2.79

PAGE KEY: A-108 Beverage and Beverage Mixes   A-110 Other Beverages   A-110 Beverages, Alcoholic   A-112 Candies and Confections, Gum   A-116 Cereals, Breakfast Type
A-120 Cheese and Cheese Substitutes   A-122 Dairy Products and Substitutes   A-124 Desserts   A-130 Dessert Toppings   A-130 Eggs, Substitutes, and Egg Dishes   A-132 Ethnic Foods
A-136 Fast Foods/Restaurants   A-150 Fats, Oils, Margarines, Shortenings, and Substitutes   A-150 Fish, Seafood, and Shellfish   A-152 Food Additives
A-152 Fruit, Vegetable, or Blended Juices   A-154 Grains, Flours, and Fractions   A-154 Grain Products, Prepared and Baked Goods

Code	Food Name	Unit/ Amt	Wt (g)	Energy (kcal)	Prot (g)	Carb (g)	Fiber (g)	Fat (g)	Sat (g)	Mono (g)	Poly (g)	Chol (mg)	Vit A (RE)
4144	Candy, Treasures, peanut butter	4 pce	43	240	3	22	1	16	7.0	—	—	5	0
4143	Candy, Treasures, w/caramel	3 pce	35	170	1	22	0	9	5.0	—	—	5	0
23082	Chewing Gum, stick	1 pce	3	7	0	2	0	0	0.0	0.0	0.0	0	0
23369	Fruit Leather, cherry	1 oz	28	105	0	23	0	2	0.7	0.9	0.0	0	—
91256	Fudge, plain	1.5 oz	43	188	0	27	0	9	6.0	—	—	11	10
23007	Marshmallows	4 ea	29	92	1	23	0	0	0.0	0.0	0.0	0	0
92226	Snack, crisped rice, peanut butter, 3.6 oz bar	1 ea	100	443	6	71	2	16	5.3	6.0	3.0	3	250

CEREALS, BREAKFAST TYPE

Cereals, Cooked and Dry

Code	Food Name	Unit/ Amt	Wt (g)	Energy (kcal)	Prot (g)	Carb (g)	Fiber (g)	Fat (g)	Sat (g)	Mono (g)	Poly (g)	Chol (mg)	Vit A (RE)
40055	Cereal, hot, breakfast pilaf, ckd	0.5 cup	140	170	6	30	6	3	—	—	—	0	0
40179	Cereal, hot, Cream Of Rice, ckd w/water & salt	1 cup	244	127	2	28	0	0	0.0	0.1	0.1	0	0
38497	Cereal, hot, Farina, enrich, prep w/water & salt	1 cup	233	119	4	26	1	0	0.0	0.1	0.0	0	0
40186	Cereal, hot, Maltex, ckd w/water & salt	1 cup	249	189	6	39	2	1	0.2	0.1	0.4	0	0
40239	Cereal, hot, Maypo, ckd w/water & salt	1 cup	240	170	6	32	5	2	0.4	0.6	0.5	0	701
40138	Cereal, hot, multigrain, ckd	1 cup	246	202	7	40	4	2	0.3	0.5	1.1	0	116
38500	Cereal, hot, oat bran, prep w/water & salt	1 cup	219	94	4	16	4	2	0.4	0.7	0.8	0	4
40072	Cereal, hot, oatmeal, plain, inst, fort, prep w/water	0.75 cup	177	97	4	17	3	2	0.3	0.5	0.6	0	285
40190	Cereal, hot, Roman Meal, plain, ckd w/water & salt	1 cup	241	147	7	33	8	1	0.1	0.1	0.4	0	0
40188	Cereal, hot, wheat, plain, ckd w/water & salt	1 cup	240	122	4	26	1	0	0.0	0.1	0.0	0	0
40191	Cereal, hot, Wheatena, ckd w/water & salt	1 cup	243	143	5	29	5	1	0.2	0.2	0.6	0	1
40089	Grits, corn, inst, plain, prep w/water f/pkt	1 ea	137	93	2	21	1	0	0.0	0.0	0.1	0	0
38455	Grits, corn, white, dry	0.25 cup	42	150	3	33	1	0	0.0	0.0	0.0	0	20
38571	Grits, hominy, yellow, quick, dry	0.25 cup	37	125	3	29	2	1	0.2	0.2	0.3	0	21

Cereals, Ready To Eat

Code	Food Name	Unit/ Amt	Wt (g)	Energy (kcal)	Prot (g)	Carb (g)	Fiber (g)	Fat (g)	Sat (g)	Mono (g)	Poly (g)	Chol (mg)	Vit A (RE)
54234	Cereal, 100% Bran	0.33 cup	29	83	4	23	8	1	0.1	—	—	0	150
40095	Cereal, All-Bran	0.5 cup	30	78	4	22	9	1	0.2	0.2	0.6	0	158
40258	Cereal, Alpha-Bits, 1.1 oz svg	1 ea	32	130	3	27	1	2	0.0	—	—	0	150
40098	Cereal, Apple Jacks	1 cup	30	117	1	27	1	1	0.1	0.2	0.3	0	42
40278	Cereal, Banana Nut Crunch	1 cup	59	249	5	44	4	6	0.8	—	—	0	150
40394	Cereal, Basic 4	1 cup	55	202	4	42	3	3	0.4	1.0	1.1	0	118
61203	Cereal, bran flakes	0.75 cup	30	96	3	24	5	1	0.1	0.1	0.3	0	225
40032	Cereal, Cap'N Crunch	0.75 cup	27	108	1	23	1	2	0.4	0.3	0.2	0	4
40297	Cereal, Cheerios	1 cup	30	111	4	22	4	2	0.4	0.6	0.2	0	150
40325	Cereal, Chex, corn	1 cup	30	112	2	26	0	0	0.1	0.1	0.1	0	140
40333	Cereal, Chex, rice	1.25 cup	31	117	2	27	0	0	0.1	0.1	0.1	0	155
40335	Cereal, Chex, wheat	1 cup	30	104	3	24	3	1	0.1	0.1	0.2	0	90
40414	Cereal, Cinnamon Grahams	0.75 cup	30	113	2	26	1	1	0.2	0.3	0.3	0	150
40126	Cereal, Cinnamon Toast Crunch	0.75 cup	30	127	2	24	1	3	0.5	1.5	1.0	0	150
61272	Cereal, Coco Roos, chocolate	0.75 cup	30	122	1	26	1	1	0.3	0.6	0.1	0	397
40102	Cereal, Cocoa Krispies	0.75 cup	31	118	2	27	1	1	0.6	0.1	0.1	0	153
40257	Cereal, Cocoa Pebbles	0.75 cup	29	115	1	25	0	1	1.1	—	—	0	150
40425	Cereal, Cocoa Puffs	1 cup	30	117	1	26	1	1	0.2	0.5	0.2	0	0
40103	Cereal, Complete Oat Bran Flakes	0.75 cup	30	105	3	23	4	1	0.2	0.5	0.3	0	235
40324	Cereal, Cookie Crisp	1 cup	30	117	1	26	0	1	0.2	0.4	0.2	0	145
61214	Cereal, corn flakes, plain	1 cup	28	101	2	24	1	0	0.0	0.0	0.0	0	216
40206	Cereal, Corn Pops	1 cup	31	118	1	28	0	0	0.1	0.1	0.1	0	144

PAGE KEY: A-158 Granola Bars, Cereal Bars, Diet Bars, Scones, and Tarts   A-158 Meals and Dishes   A-162 Meats   A-168 Nuts, Seeds, and Products   A-170 Poultry
A-172 Salad Dressings, Dips, and Mayonnaise   A-172 Salads   A-174 Sandwiches   A-176 Sauces and Gravies   A-176 Snack Foods—Chips, Pretzels, Popcorn
A-178 Soups, Stews, and Chilis   A-180 Spices, Flavors, and Seasonings   A-182 Sports Bars and Drinks   A-182 Supplemental Foods and Formulas
A-184 Sweeteners and Sweet Substitutes   A-184 Vegetables and Legumes   A-198 Weight Loss Bars and Drinks   A-200 Miscellaneous

Thia (mg)	Ribo (mg)	Niac (mg NE)	Vit B6 (mg)	Vit B12 (µg)	Fol (µg)	Vit C (mg)	Vit D (IU)	Vit E (mg AT)	Cal (mg)	Iron (mg)	Magn (mg)	Phos (mg)	Pota (mg)	Sodi (mg)	Zinc (mg)	Wat (%)	Alco (g)	Caff (g)
—	—	—	—	—	—	0.0	—	—	40	0.36	—	—	—	80	—	—	0.00	—
—	—	—	—	—	—	0.0	—	—	40	0.00	—	—	—	60	—	—	0.00	—
0.00	0.00	0.00	0.00	0.00	0.0	0.0	0.0	0.0	0	0.00	0.0	0	0	0	0.0	3	0.00	0.00
0.00	0.00	0.00	—	—	—	—	—	—	7	0.07	—	—	46	56	—	—	0.00	0.00
—	—	—	—	—	—	0.0	—	—	0	0.18	—	—	—	42	—	—	0.00	0.00
0.00	0.00	0.01	0.00	0.00	0.3	0.0	—	0.0	1	0.07	0.6	2	1	23	0.0	16	0.00	0.00
0.43	0.44	6.90	0.52	—	119.0	14.9	—	—	344	5.17	28.0	102	185	406	0.5	4	0.00	0.00
—	—	—	—	—	—	0.0	—	—	20	1.44	—	—	—	15	—	—	0.00	0.00
0.00	0.00	0.98	0.07	0.00	7.3	0.0	0.0	0.0	7	0.49	7.3	41	49	422	0.4	88	0.00	0.00
0.15	0.10	1.80	0.01	0.00	53.6	0.0	0.0	0.0	9	11.00	7.0	30	33	128	0.2	87	0.00	0.00
0.25	0.10	2.36	0.07	0.00	29.9	0.0	0.0	1.1	22	1.78	57.3	177	266	189	1.9	81	0.00	0.00
0.70	0.79	9.35	0.93	2.77	12.0	28.3	0.0	0.2	130	8.38	52.8	247	211	259	1.5	83	0.00	0.00
0.38	0.46	4.42	0.46	0.00	17.2	0.0	0.0	3.4	69	5.40	66.4	184	138	2	0.9	79	0.00	0.00
0.25	0.07	0.20	0.02	0.00	11.0	0.0	0.0	0.1	24	2.11	65.7	180	151	101	1.2	89	0.00	0.00
0.25	0.31	3.59	0.37	0.00	76.1	0.0	0.0	0.2	99	7.67	40.7	96	94	80	0.8	86	0.00	0.00
0.23	0.11	3.07	0.10	0.00	24.1	0.0	0.0	0.4	29	2.11	108.5	214	301	198	1.8	83	0.00	0.00
0.47	0.23	5.76	0.01	0.00	4.8	0.0	0.0	0.0	5	9.60	4.8	24	31	324	0.2	88	0.00	2.40
0.02	0.05	1.33	0.05	0.00	21.9	0.0	0.0	1.3	15	1.36	51.0	146	187	578	1.7	85	0.00	0.00
0.15	0.18	2.21	0.05	0.00	46.6	0.0	0.0	0.0	8	7.96	9.6	29	38	288	0.2	82	0.00	0.00
—	—	—	—	—	—	0.0	—	—	0	0.36	—	—	35	0	—	14	0.00	0.00
0.18	0.14	1.59	0.09	0.00	57.0	0.0	—	0.1	1	1.51	14.8	46	62	1	0.3	12	0.00	0.00
0.37	0.43	5.00	0.50	0.00	100.0	0.0	0.0	—	22	8.10	80.6	236	275	121	3.7	3	0.00	0.00
0.68	0.81	4.44	3.59	5.63	393.0	6.0	51.0	0.4	117	5.28	108.6	345	306	73	3.7	2	0.00	0.00
—	—	—	—	—	—	0.0	—	—	100	2.70	—	—	—	210	—	—	0.00	0.00
0.50	0.38	4.61	0.44	1.37	93.0	13.8	38.1	0.0	8	4.17	16.5	38	36	142	1.5	3	0.00	0.00
0.37	0.41	5.00	0.50	1.50	99.7	0.1	40.1		21	16.20	48.4	183	171	253	1.5	4	0.00	0.00
0.30	0.34	3.90	0.38	1.14	78.7	0.0	31.4	0.6	196	3.51	40.2	232	155	316	3.0	7	0.00	0.00
0.37	0.43	5.00	0.50	1.50	99.9	0.0	39.9	0.3	17	8.10	64.2	152	185	220	1.5	4	0.00	0.00
0.43	0.47	5.71	0.56	0.00	420.1	0.0	0.0	0.2	4	5.15	15.1	45	54	202	4.3	2	0.00	0.00
0.54	0.50	5.76	0.66	1.42	200.1	6.0	39.9	0.1	122	10.31	39.3	132	209	213	4.6	4	0.00	0.00
0.37	0.43	5.01	0.50	1.50	200.1	6.0	0.0	0.1	100	9.00	8.4	22	25	288	3.8	2	0.00	0.00
0.38	0.43	5.17	0.51	1.54	206.8	6.2	41.2	0.0	103	9.30	9.3	35	30	292	3.9	3	0.00	0.00
0.23	0.25	3.00	0.30	0.89	240.0	3.6	24.0	0.2	60	8.69	24.0	90	113	267	2.4	2	0.00	0.00
0.37	0.43	5.01	0.50	1.50	99.9	6.0	39.9	0.1	100	4.50	8.1	20	44	237	3.8	3	0.00	0.00
0.37	0.43	5.01	0.50	1.50	99.9	6.0	39.9	0.3	100	4.50	8.1	80	43	206	3.8	3	0.00	0.00
0.40	0.44	5.28	0.52	1.59	105.9	15.9	—	0.1	21	4.76	10.8	42	53	201	0.2	3	0.00	1.20
0.46	0.69	4.96	1.01	2.15	197.5	15.0	40.3	0.1	40	6.88	11.8	32	61	197	1.5	3	0.00	1.54
0.37	0.43	5.00	0.50	1.50	100.0	0.0	40.0	—	3	1.79	10.7	23	42	157	1.5	3	0.00	—
0.37	0.43	5.01	0.50	1.50	99.9	6.0	0.0	0.1	100	4.50	8.1	20	50	171	3.8	3	0.00	0.60
1.64	1.79	21.00	2.09	6.03	403.5	63.0	42.0	12.7	16	18.89	45.0	105	120	210	15.6	3	0.00	0.00
0.37	0.43	5.01	0.50	1.50	99.9	6.0	39.9	0.1	100	4.50	8.4	40	27	178	3.8	2	0.00	0.60
0.37	0.43	5.00	0.50	1.50	100.0	0.0	40.0	0.1	1	5.40	4.5	15	33	266	0.1	4	0.00	0.00
0.37	0.43	4.98	0.50	1.51	102.0	6.0	50.2	0.0	5	1.91	2.2	10	26	120	1.5	3	0.00	0.00

PAGE KEY: A-108 Beverage and Beverage Mixes   A-110 Other Beverages   A-110 Beverages, Alcoholic   A-112 Candies and Confections, Gum   A-116 Cereals, Breakfast Type   A-120 Cheese and Cheese Substitutes   A-122 Dairy Products and Substitutes   A-124 Desserts   A-130 Dessert Toppings   A-130 Eggs, Substitutes, and Egg Dishes   A-132 Ethnic Foods   A-136 Fast Foods/Restaurants   A-150 Fats, Oils, Margarines, Shortenings, and Substitutes   A-150 Fish, Seafood, and Shellfish   A-152 Food Additives   A-152 Fruit, Vegetable, or Blended Juices   A-154 Grains, Flours, and Fractions   A-154 Grain Products, Prepared and Baked Goods

Code	Food Name	Unit/ Amt	Wt (g)	Energy (kcal)	Prot (g)	Carb (g)	Fiber (g)	Fat (g)	Sat (g)	Mono (g)	Poly (g)	Chol (mg)	Vit A (RE)
40205	Cereal, Cracklin' Oat Bran	0.75 cup	55	225	5	39	6	8	2.3	4.6	1.2	0	252
4354	Cereal, Cranberry Almond Crunch	1 cup	55	210	4	43	3	3	0.0	—	—	0	150
40017	Cereal, crispy rice	1 cup	28	111	2	25	0	0	0.0	0.0	0.0	0	372
40040	Cereal, Crispy Wheaties 'N Raisins	1 cup	55	183	4	45	5	1	0.2	0.1	0.4	0	150
61179	Cereal, Familia	1 cup	122	473	12	90	10	8	0.9	3.9	2.0	0	2
61303	Cereal, Fiber 7	3.6 oz	100	353	14	78	14	1	0.3	0.2	0.6	0	106
40130	Cereal, Fiber One	0.5 cup	30	59	2	24	14	1	0.1	0.1	0.4	0	0
40218	Cereal, Froot Loops	1 cup	30	118	2	26	1	1	0.5	0.1	0.2	0	142
61306	Cereal, frosted flakes	0.75 cup	30	116	1	27	1	0	0.1	0.0	0.1	0	218
40043	Cereal, Frosted Mini Wheats	1 cup	51	173	5	41	5	1	0.2	0.1	0.5	0	0
60932	Cereal, Frosted Oats	0.75 cup	28	111	2	23	1	2	0.4	0.5	0.3	0	178
40256	Cereal, Fruit & Bran, peaches raisins & almonds, svg	1 cup	55	190	4	42	6	3	0.0	—	—	0	150
40266	Cereal, Fruity Pebbles	0.75 cup	27	108	1	24	0	1	0.2	—	—	0	150
60964	Cereal, Go Lean	0.75 cup	40	114	10	23	8	1	0.2	0.2	0.4	0	1
40245	Cereal, Golden Crisp	0.75 cup	27	107	1	25	0	0	0.1	—	—	0	150
40299	Cereal, Golden Grahams	0.75 cup	30	112	2	25	1	1	0.2	0.4	0.4	0	150
40009	Cereal, granola, 100% Natural, honey raisin oats	0.5 cup	51	225	5	34	3	9	3.6	3.8	1.1	1	1
40048	Cereal, granola, homemade, w/oats & wheat germ	0.5 cup	61	299	9	32	5	15	2.8	4.7	6.5	0	1
40277	Cereal, Grape Nuts	0.5 cup	58	208	6	47	5	1	0.2	0.2	0.7	0	150
40265	Cereal, Grape Nuts Flakes	0.75 cup	29	106	3	24	3	1	0.2	0.2	0.5	0	150
60969	Cereal, Harmony	3.6 oz	100	365	11	79	4	2	0.5	0.8	0.6	0	273
40004	Cereal, Harvest Oat Flakes	0.75 cup	29	109	3	23	2	1	0.2	0.4	0.4	0	2
61344	Cereal, Healthy Fiber, multigrain flakes	0.75 cup	28	100	3	23	4	0	0.0	0.0	0.0	0	20
60958	Cereal, Heart to Heart	1 oz	28	99	4	22	4	1	0.3	0.3	0.3	0	323
40293	Cereal, Honey Bunches Of Oats, almond	0.75 cup	31	126	2	24	1	3	0.3	—	—	0	150
40427	Cereal, Honey Graham Oh!s	0.75 cup	27	111	1	23	1	2	0.5	0.4	0.2	0	177
40264	Cereal, Honeycomb	1.33 cup	29	115	2	26	1	1	0.2	—	—	0	150
40134	Cereal, Just Right	1 cup	43	160	3	36	2	1	0.1	0.2	0.8	0	294
40410	Cereal, Kaboom	1.25 cup	30	115	3	24	2	1	0.3	0.3	0.4	0	150
40010	Cereal, Kix	1.33 cup	30	113	2	26	1	1	0.2	0.2	0.2	0	154
40011	Cereal, Life, plain	0.75 cup	32	120	3	25	2	1	0.3	0.5	0.5	0	1
40300	Cereal, Lucky Charms	1 cup	30	114	2	25	2	1	0.2	0.3	0.3	0	150
40124	Cereal, Mueslix, five grain muesli	1 cup	82	289	6	63	6	5	0.7	2.0	1.8	0	747
40449	Cereal, Oat Bran O's	0.75 cup	28	100	3	23	3	0	0.0	0.0	0.0	0	20
40302	Cereal, Oatmeal Raisin Crisp	1 cup	55	204	5	45	4	2	0.4	0.7	0.6	0	0
54233	Cereal, Oreo O's	0.75 cup	27	112	1	22	1	2	0.4	—	—	0	150
40216	Cereal, Product 19	1 cup	30	100	2	25	1	0	0.1	0.1	0.2	0	216
40018	Cereal, puffed rice	1 cup	14	54	1	12	0	0	0.0	0.0	0.0	0	0
40209	Cereal, raisin bran	1 cup	61	195	5	47	7	2	0.3	0.3	0.9	0	155
40210	Cereal, Rice Krispies	1.25 cup	33	119	2	28	0	0	0.1	0.1	0.1	0	153
40420	Cereal, Rice Krispies Treats	0.75 cup	30	122	1	26	0	2	0.4	0.9	0.2	0	152
40020	Cereal, Shredded Wheat, biscuits	1 ea	21	72	2	17	2	0	0.1	0.1	0.2	0	0
40068	Cereal, Smacks	0.75 cup	27	104	2	24	1	0	0.1	0.2	0.2	0	153
40211	Cereal, Special K	1 cup	31	117	7	22	1	0	0.1	0.1	0.2	0	230
40413	Cereal, Toasty O's	1 cup	30	112	3	22	3	2	0.4	0.7	0.6	0	375
40412	Cereal, Tootie Fruities	1 cup	32	125	2	28	1	1	0.3	0.3	0.2	0	218

PAGE KEY: A-158 Granola Bars, Cereal Bars, Diet Bars, Scones, and Tarts   A-158 Meals and Dishes   A-162 Meats   A-168 Nuts, Seeds, and Products   A-170 Poultry   A-172 Salad Dressings, Dips, and Mayonnaise   A-172 Salads   A-174 Sandwiches   A-176 Sauces and Gravies   A-176 Snack Foods—Chips, Pretzels, Popcorn   A-178 Soups, Stews, and Chilis   A-180 Spices, Flavors, and Seasonings   A-182 Sports Bars and Drinks   A-182 Supplemental Foods and Formulas   A-184 Sweeteners and Sweet Substitutes   A-184 Vegetables and Legumes   A-198 Weight Loss Bars and Drinks   A-200 Miscellaneous

Thia (mg)	Ribo (mg)	Niac (mg NE)	Vit B6 (mg)	Vit B12 (μg)	Fol (μg)	Vit C (mg)	Vit D (IU)	Vit E (mg AT)	Cal (mg)	Iron (mg)	Magn (mg)	Phos (mg)	Pota (mg)	Sodi (mg)	Zinc (mg)	Wat (%)	Alco (g)	Caff (g)
0.41	0.47	5.67	0.56	1.71	112.8	17.6	45.0	0.8	23	2.03	67.7	179	248	157	1.7	3	0.00	0.00
—	—	—	—	—	—	0.0	—	—	0	1.79	—	—	—	190	—	—	0.00	0.00
0.51	0.58	6.92	0.68	0.07	88.2	14.8	—	0.0	5	0.69	11.8	31	27	206	0.5	2	0.00	0.00
0.75	0.85	10.01	1.00	3.02	200.2	0.0	40.2	0.3	0	7.48	42.4	140	227	251	7.5	7	0.00	0.00
0.38	0.67	2.20	0.11	0.34	19.5	0.7	—	1.4	211	3.39	386.7	411	603	61	2.3	2	0.00	0.00
0.52	0.60	7.05	0.69	2.11	141.0	4.2	—	1.0	71	2.53	144.0	327	460	53	2.9	3	0.00	0.00
0.37	0.43	5.01	0.50	1.50	99.9	6.0	0.0	0.2	100	4.50	60.0	150	232	129	3.8	4	0.00	0.00
0.68	0.57	7.26	1.10	2.11	105.6	14.1	37.5	0.1	4	6.11	9.9	34	36	150	5.7	3	0.00	0.00
0.73	0.81	9.68	0.97	1.45	96.9	14.5	38.7	0.0	0	4.36	2.4	10	20	194	0.1	3	0.00	0.00
0.37	0.41	5.00	0.50	1.50	100.0	0.0	0.0	0.3	16	14.78	60.2	150	173	5	1.6	6	0.00	0.00
0.28	0.50	5.90	0.58	0.00	448.0	7.1	0.0	0.1	7	5.32	17.4	68	52	242	4.4	2	0.00	0.00
—	—	—	—	—	—	0.0	—	—	20	5.40	—	—	—	260	—	—	0.00	0.00
0.37	0.41	5.00	0.50	1.50	99.9	0.0	40.0	—	1	1.79	5.1	16	30	158	1.5	3	0.00	0.00
0.14	0.05	1.29	0.12	0.00	25.6	0.0	—	0.2	56	2.00	66.0	190	370	66	0.3	2	0.00	0.00
0.37	0.41	5.00	0.50	1.50	99.9	0.0	40.0	—	4	1.79	16.5	37	34	40	1.5	3	0.00	0.00
0.37	0.43	5.01	0.50	1.50	99.9	6.0	39.9	0.1	350	4.50	8.1	200	50	268	3.8	3	0.00	0.00
0.12	0.11	0.80	0.07	0.10	14.1	0.4	0.0	0.5	59	1.24	48.9	152	250	19	1.0	4	0.00	0.00
0.44	0.18	1.28	0.18	0.00	50.6	0.7	0.0	3.6	48	2.58	106.8	279	328	13	2.5	5	0.00	0.00
0.37	0.41	5.00	0.50	1.50	99.8	0.0	40.0	—	20	16.20	58.0	139	178	354	1.2	4	0.00	0.00
0.37	0.43	5.00	0.50	1.50	100.0	0.0	40.0	0.1	11	8.10	29.9	88	99	140	1.2	3	0.00	0.00
2.73	1.54	18.20	1.82	7.59	727.0	55.0	73.0	24.5	1091	16.39	44.0	182	166	645	13.6	3	0.00	0.00
0.07	0.10	0.69	0.05	0.00	11.1	0.0	0.0	0.5	16	0.87	32.4	102	99	204	0.8	2	0.00	0.00
0.15	0.17	2.00	0.20	0.60	40.0	0.0	—	—	0	0.72	—	—	100	15	—	5	0.00	0.00
0.15	0.05	0.51	1.73	5.15	343.6	25.8	—	11.6	15	1.84	85.1	25	85	1	1.3	3	0.00	0.00
0.37	0.41	5.00	0.50	1.50	100.1	0.0	40.0	—	11	8.10	21.4	60	70	187	0.3	3	0.00	0.00
0.43	0.50	5.90	0.58	0.00	420.1	7.1	0.0	0.2	3	5.30	0.0	38	42	162	4.4	3	0.00	0.00
0.37	0.43	5.00	0.50	1.50	100.0	0.0	40.0	—	5	2.70	10.7	27	35	215	1.5	2	0.00	0.00
0.30	0.34	3.91	0.38	1.15	80.0	0.0	—	1.8	11	12.68	26.7	83	95	264	0.7	3	0.00	0.00
0.37	0.43	5.01	0.50	1.50	200.1	6.0	39.9	0.1	100	8.10	15.9	80	63	285	3.8	2	0.00	0.00
0.37	0.43	5.01	0.50	1.50	200.1	6.3	42.3	0.1	150	8.10	8.1	40	35	267	3.8	2	0.00	0.00
0.40	0.46	5.50	0.55	0.00	416.0	0.0	0.0	0.2	112	8.94	30.7	133	91	164	4.1	4	0.00	0.00
0.37	0.43	5.01	0.50	1.50	200.1	6.0	39.9	0.1	100	4.50	15.9	60	57	203	3.8	2	0.00	0.00
0.75	0.83	9.84	0.99	3.27	196.8	0.8	0.0	8.9	67	8.93	82.0	215	369	107	7.5	8	0.00	0.00
0.15	0.17	2.00	0.20	0.60	40.0	0.0	—	—	0	0.72	—	—	90	90	—	3	0.00	0.00
0.37	0.41	5.01	0.50	1.49	100.1	6.1	0.0	1.4	20	4.51	40.2	100	200	216	3.8	6	0.00	0.00
0.37	0.41	5.00	0.50	1.50	99.9	0.0	40.0	—	5	1.79	14.9	32	49	128	1.5	2	0.00	
1.50	1.71	20.01	2.06	6.00	399.9	61.2	39.3	13.5	5	18.09	15.9	40	50	207	15.3	3	0.00	
0.05	0.03	0.49	0.00	0.00	21.6	0.0	0.0	0.0	1	0.40	4.2	17	16	1	0.2	4	0.00	0.00
0.38	0.43	5.17	0.51	1.54	103.7	0.4	41.5	0.4	29	4.63	83.0	259	372	362	1.5	8	0.00	0.00
0.87	0.79	7.09	0.92	2.00	151.1	6.4	40.9	0.0	5	2.65	9.6	39	39	319	0.5	4	0.00	0.00
0.38	0.41	5.09	0.50	1.50	204.0	6.0	40.5	0.1	3	1.86	6.9	24	24	189	0.2	3	0.00	0.00
0.05	0.01	1.09	0.05	—	10.5	0.0	0.0	—	9	0.68	35.7	75	74	1	0.5	5	0.00	0.00
0.37	0.43	5.00	0.50	1.50	101.3	6.1	40.0	0.1	6	0.34	15.9	46	41	50	0.4	2	0.00	0.00
0.52	0.58	7.13	1.98	6.05	399.9	21.0	50.0	4.7	9	8.36	19.2	68	61	224	0.9	3	0.00	0.00
0.37	0.43	5.00	0.50	0.00	99.9	15.0	40.0	0.2	40	8.10	32.1	100	94	284	3.8	4	0.00	0.00
0.37	0.43	5.00	0.50	1.50	99.8	15.0	40.0	0.3	100	4.50	8.0	20	39	149	3.8	3	0.00	0.00

PAGE KEY: A-108 Beverage and Beverage Mixes   A-110 Other Beverages   A-110 Beverages, Alcoholic   A-112 Candies and Confections, Gum   A-116 Cereals, Breakfast Type   A-120 Cheese and Cheese Substitutes   A-122 Dairy Products and Substitutes   A-124 Desserts   A-130 Dessert Toppings   A-130 Eggs, Substitutes, and Egg Dishes   A-132 Ethnic Foods   A-136 Fast Foods/Restaurants   A-150 Fats, Oils, Margarines, Shortenings, and Substitutes   A-150 Fish, Seafood, and Shellfish   A-152 Food Additives   A-152 Fruit, Vegetable, or Blended Juices   A-154 Grains, Flours, and Fractions   A-154 Grain Products, Prepared and Baked Goods

Code	Food Name	Unit/ Amt	Wt (g)	Energy (kcal)	Prot (g)	Carb (g)	Fiber (g)	Fat (g)	Sat (g)	Mono (g)	Poly (g)	Chol (mg)	Vit A (RE)
40021	Cereal, Total, wheat	0.75 cup	30	97	3	22	3	1	0.2	0.1	0.3	0	150
40128	Cereal, Uncle Sam	1 cup	55	237	9	36	11	6	0.7	1.1	4.6	0	0
40307	Cereal, Wheaties	1 cup	30	107	3	24	3	1	0.2	0.3	0.3	0	150
40362	Cereal, whole grain, w/raisins, all nat	0.5 cup	50	195	4	41	3	3	0.7	0.8	0.5	0	1
CHEESE AND CHEESE SUBSTITUTES													
Natural Cheeses													
47855	Cheese, blue, 1" cube	1 ea	17	61	4	0	0	5	3.2	1.3	0.1	13	35
47859	Cheese, brie, 1" cube	1 ea	17	57	4	0	0	5	3.0	1.4	0.1	17	30
47861	Cheese, camembert, 1" cube	1 ea	17	51	3	0	0	4	2.6	1.2	0.1	12	41
47863	Cheese, cheddar, 1" cube	1 ea	17	69	4	0	0	6	3.6	1.6	0.2	18	46
1551	Cheese, cheddar, fat free, 1" cube	1 ea	28	40	8	1	0	0	0.0	0.0	0.0	3	60
1525	Cheese, cheddar, five peppercorn, 1" cube	1 ea	28	110	7	1	0	9	5.0	—	—	30	60
1008	Cheese, cheddar, shredded	0.25 cup	28	114	7	0	0	9	6.0	2.7	0.3	30	77
47864	Cheese, cheddar, slice, 1 oz	1 ea	28	114	7	0	0	9	6.0	2.7	0.3	30	77
47865	Cheese, colby, 1" cube	1 ea	17	68	4	0	0	6	3.5	1.6	0.2	16	47
1010	Cheese, colby, shredded	0.25 cup	28	111	7	1	0	9	5.7	2.6	0.3	27	77
47866	Cheese, colby, slice, 1 oz	1 ea	28	112	7	1	0	9	5.7	2.6	0.3	27	77
47871	Cheese, feta, 1" cube	1 ea	17	45	2	1	0	4	2.5	0.8	0.1	15	21
47873	Cheese, fontina, 1" cube	1 ea	15	58	4	0	0	5	2.9	1.3	0.2	17	40
1078	Cheese, goat, hard	3.6 oz	100	452	31	2	0	36	24.6	8.1	0.8	105	494
1080	Cheese, goat, soft	3.6 oz	100	268	19	1	0	21	14.6	4.8	0.5	46	293
1054	Cheese, gouda	1 oz	28	101	7	1	0	8	5.0	2.2	0.2	32	47
47881	Cheese, limburger, 1" cube	1 ea	18	59	4	0	0	5	3.0	1.5	0.1	16	61
47884	Cheese, monterey jack, 1" cube	1 ea	17	64	4	0	0	5	3.3	1.5	0.2	15	35
1017	Cheese, monterey jack, shredded	0.25 cup	28	105	7	0	0	9	5.4	2.5	0.3	25	58
47885	Cheese, monterey jack, slice, 1 oz	1 ea	28	106	7	0	0	9	5.4	2.5	0.3	25	58
1553	Cheese, mozzarella, fat free, 1" cube	1 ea	28	40	8	1	0	0	0.0	0.0	0.0	3	60
47891	Cheese, muenster, 1" cube	1 ea	18	64	4	0	0	5	3.3	1.5	0.1	17	52
1021	Cheese, muenster, shredded	0.25 cup	28	104	7	0	0	8	5.4	2.5	0.2	27	84
1075	Cheese, parmesan, grated	1 Tbs	5	22	2	0	0	1	0.9	0.4	0.1	4	6
1061	Cheese, parmesan, hard, 1" cube	1 ea	10	40	4	0	0	3	1.7	0.8	0.1	7	11
1510	Cheese, pepper jack, 1" cube	1 ea	28	110	7	1	0	9	5.0	—	—	30	60
47899	Cheese, provolone, 1" cube	1 ea	17	60	4	0	0	5	2.9	1.3	0.1	12	41
47900	Cheese, provolone, slice, 1 oz	1 ea	28	100	7	1	0	8	4.8	2.1	0.2	20	69
1064	Cheese, ricotta, whole milk	0.25 cup	62	108	7	2	0	8	5.1	2.2	0.2	32	76
13348	Cheese, string, mozzarella, sticks, 1 oz	1 ea	28	50	8	1	0	2	1.0	—	—	5	40
47911	Cheese, sweitzer, 1" cube	1 ea	15	57	4	1	0	4	2.7	1.1	0.1	14	34
47908	Cheese, Swiss, 1" cube	1 ea	15	57	4	1	0	4	2.7	1.1	0.1	14	34
1027	Cheese, Swiss, shredded	0.25 cup	27	103	7	1	0	8	4.8	2.0	0.3	25	61
47912	Cheese, Swiss, slice, 1 oz	1 ea	28	108	8	2	0	8	5.0	2.1	0.3	26	64
1508	Cottage Cheese	0.5 cup	114	100	13	4	0	4	3.0	—	—	15	60
1047	Cottage Cheese, 1% fat	0.5 cup	113	81	14	3	0	1	0.7	0.3	0.0	5	12
1014	Cottage Cheese, 2% fat	0.5 cup	113	102	16	4	0	2	1.4	0.6	0.1	9	25
47848	Cottage Cheese, fat free, small curd	0.5 cup	126	90	12	8	0	0	0.0	0.0	0.0	10	40
1015	Cream Cheese	2 Tbs	29	101	2	1	0	10	6.4	2.9	0.4	32	108
1452	Cream Cheese, fat free	2 Tbs	29	28	4	2	0	0	0.3	0.1	0.0	2	81
1083	Cream Cheese, soft	2 Tbs	30	100	2	1	0	10	7.0	—	—	30	60

PAGE KEY: A-158 Granola Bars, Cereal Bars, Diet Bars, Scones, and Tarts   A-158 Meals and Dishes   A-162 Meats   A-168 Nuts, Seeds, and Products   A-170 Poultry   A-172 Salad Dressings, Dips, and Mayonnaise   A-172 Salads   A-174 Sandwiches   A-176 Sauces and Gravies   A-176 Snack Foods—Chips, Pretzels, Popcorn   A-178 Soups, Stews, and Chilis   A-180 Spices, Flavors, and Seasonings   A-182 Sports Bars and Drinks   A-182 Supplemental Foods and Formulas   A-184 Sweeteners and Sweet Substitutes   A-184 Vegetables and Legumes   A-198 Weight Loss Bars and Drinks   A-200 Miscellaneous

Thia (mg)	Ribo (mg)	Niac (mg NE)	Vit B6 (mg)	Vit B12 (µg)	Fol (µg)	Vit C (mg)	Vit D (IU)	Vit E (mg AT)	Cal (mg)	Iron (mg)	Magn (mg)	Phos (mg)	Pota (mg)	Sodi (mg)	Zinc (mg)	Wat (%)	Alco (g)	Caff (g)
2.10	2.42	26.43	2.81	6.42	477.0	60.0	39.9	13.5	1104	22.35	39.3	89	103	192	17.5	3	0.00	0.00
1.25	1.45	8.97	0.52	0.00	29.2	33.8	—	0.4	52	2.22	113.3	206	245	113	2.1	4	0.00	0.00
0.75	0.85	9.98	1.00	3.00	200.1	6.0	39.9	0.2	0	8.10	32.1	100	111	218	7.5	3	0.00	0.00
0.15	0.09	0.93	0.07	0.05	12.0	0.3	0.0	0.9	30	1.32	42.5	134	204	118	1.0	4	0.00	0.00
0.00	0.07	0.18	0.02	0.20	6.2	0.0	—	0.0	91	0.05	4.0	67	44	241	0.5	42	0.00	0.00
0.00	0.09	0.05	0.03	0.28	11.1	0.0	—	0.0	31	0.09	3.4	32	26	107	0.4	48	0.00	0.00
0.00	0.07	0.10	0.03	0.21	10.5	0.0	2.0	0.0	66	0.05	3.4	59	32	143	0.4	52	0.00	0.00
0.00	0.05	0.00	0.00	0.14	3.1	0.0	2.0	0.0	123	0.11	4.8	87	17	106	0.5	37	0.00	0.00
—	—	—	—	—	—	—	—	—	400	—	—	—	—	220	—	63	0.00	0.00
—	—	—	—	—	—	0.0	—	—	200	0.00	—	—	—	180	—	36	0.00	0.00
0.00	0.10	0.01	0.01	0.23	5.1	0.0	3.4	0.1	204	0.18	7.9	145	28	175	0.9	37	0.00	0.00
0.00	0.10	0.01	0.01	0.23	5.1	0.0	3.4	0.1	204	0.18	7.9	145	28	176	0.9	37	0.00	0.00
0.00	0.05	0.01	0.00	0.14	3.1	0.0	—	0.0	118	0.12	4.5	79	22	104	0.5	38	0.00	0.00
0.00	0.10	0.02	0.01	0.23	5.1	0.0	—	0.1	194	0.20	7.3	129	36	171	0.9	38	0.00	0.00
0.00	0.10	0.02	0.01	0.23	5.1	0.0	—	0.1	194	0.21	7.4	130	36	171	0.9	38	0.00	0.00
0.02	0.14	0.17	0.07	0.28	5.4	0.0	—	0.0	84	0.10	3.2	57	11	190	0.5	55	0.00	0.00
0.00	0.02	0.01	0.00	0.25	0.9	0.0	—	0.0	82	0.02	2.1	52	10	120	0.5	38	0.00	0.00
0.14	1.19	2.40	0.07	0.11	4.0	0.0	—	0.3	895	1.87	54.0	729	48	346	1.6	29	0.00	0.00
0.07	0.37	0.43	0.25	0.18	12.0	0.0	—	0.2	140	1.89	16.0	256	26	368	0.9	61	0.00	0.00
0.00	0.09	0.01	0.01	0.43	6.0	0.0	2.7	0.1	198	0.07	8.2	155	34	232	1.1	41	0.00	0.00
0.00	0.09	0.02	0.01	0.18	10.4	0.0	—	0.0	89	0.01	3.8	71	23	144	0.4	48	0.00	0.00
0.00	0.07	0.01	0.00	0.14	3.1	0.0	—	0.0	128	0.11	4.6	76	14	92	0.5	41	0.00	0.00
0.00	0.10	0.02	0.01	0.23	5.1	0.0	—	0.1	211	0.20	7.6	125	23	151	0.8	41	0.00	0.00
0.00	0.10	0.02	0.01	0.23	5.1	0.0	—	0.1	211	0.20	7.7	126	23	152	0.9	41	0.00	0.00
—	—	—	—	—	—	—	—	—	400	—	—	—	—	220	—	63	0.00	0.00
0.00	0.05	0.01	0.00	0.25	2.1	0.0	—	0.0	125	0.07	4.7	82	23	110	0.5	42	0.00	0.00
0.00	0.09	0.02	0.01	0.41	3.4	0.0	—	0.1	203	0.11	7.6	132	38	177	0.8	42	0.00	0.00
0.00	0.01	0.00	0.00	0.10	0.5	0.0	—	0.0	55	0.03	1.9	36	6	76	0.2	21	0.00	0.00
0.00	0.02	0.02	0.00	0.11	0.7	0.0	2.9	0.0	122	0.07	4.5	71	9	165	0.3	29	0.00	0.00
—	—	—	—	—	—	0.0	—	—	200	0.00	—	—	—	170	—	36	0.00	0.00
0.00	0.05	0.02	0.00	0.25	1.7	60.0	—	0.0	129	0.09	4.8	84	23	149	0.5	41	0.00	0.00
0.00	0.09	0.03	0.01	0.40	2.8	0.0	—	0.1	214	0.15	7.9	141	39	248	0.9	41	0.00	0.00
0.00	0.11	0.05	0.02	0.20	7.4	0.0	—	0.1	128	0.23	6.8	98	65	52	0.7	72	0.00	0.00
—	—	—	—	—	—	0.0	—	—	200	0.00	—	—	—	220	—	58	0.00	0.00
0.00	0.03	0.00	0.00	0.50	0.9	0.0	6.6	0.1	119	0.02	5.7	85	12	29	0.7	37	0.00	0.00
0.00	0.03	0.00	0.00	0.50	0.9	0.0	6.6	0.1	119	0.02	5.7	85	12	29	0.7	37	0.00	0.00
0.01	0.07	0.01	0.01	0.89	1.6	0.0	11.9	0.1	214	0.05	10.3	153	21	52	1.2	37	0.00	0.00
0.01	0.07	0.02	0.01	0.94	1.7	0.0	12.5	0.1	224	0.05	10.8	161	22	54	1.2	37	0.00	0.00
—	—	—	—	—	—	0.0	—	—	100	0.00	—	—	—	400	—	80	0.00	0.00
0.01	0.18	0.14	0.07	0.70	13.6	0.0	—	0.0	69	0.15	5.7	151	97	459	0.4	82	0.00	0.00
0.02	0.20	0.15	0.09	0.80	14.7	0.0	—	0.0	78	0.18	6.8	171	108	459	0.5	79	0.00	0.00
—	—	—	—	—	—	0.0	—	—	80	0.00	—	—	—	450	—	—	0.00	0.00
0.00	0.05	0.02	0.00	0.11	3.8	0.0	—	0.1	23	0.34	1.7	30	35	86	0.2	54	0.00	0.00
0.00	0.05	0.05	0.00	0.15	10.7	0.0	—	0.0	54	0.05	4.1	126	47	158	0.3	76	0.00	0.00
—	0.02	—	—	0.00	—	0.0	—	—	20	0.00	0.0	40	40	100	0.0	56	0.00	0.00

PAGE KEY: A-108 Beverage and Beverage Mixes   A-110 Other Beverages   A-110 Beverages, Alcoholic   A-112 Candies and Confections, Gum   A-116 Cereals, Breakfast Type
A-120 Cheese and Cheese Substitutes   A-122 Dairy Products and Substitutes   A-124 Desserts   A-130 Dessert Toppings   A-130 Eggs, Substitutes, and Egg Dishes   A-132 Ethnic Foods
A-136 Fast Foods/Restaurants   A-150 Fats, Oils, Margarines, Shortenings, and Substitutes   A-150 Fish, Seafood, and Shellfish   A-152 Food Additives
A-152 Fruit, Vegetable, or Blended Juices   A-154 Grains, Flours, and Fractions   A-154 Grain Products, Prepared and Baked Goods

Code	Food Name	Unit/ Amt	Wt (g)	Energy (kcal)	Prot (g)	Carb (g)	Fiber (g)	Fat (g)	Sat (g)	Mono (g)	Poly (g)	Chol (mg)	Vit A (RE)
Process Cheese and Cheese Substitutes													
1001	Cheese Product, American, cold pack	1 oz	28	94	6	2	0	7	4.4	2.0	0.2	18	48
1376	Cheese Product, monterey, past, proc, slice	1 pce	21	70	4	1	0	5	3.0	—	—	20	20
48288	Cheese Substitute	3.6 oz	100	141	22	9	0	1	0.8	0.4	0.0	6	10
48332	Cheese, American, past, proc, fat free, 1" cube	1 ea	16	24	4	2	0	0	0.1	0.0	0.0	2	70
48314	Cheese, American, past, proc, low fat, 1" cube	1 ea	18	32	4	1	0	1	0.8	0.4	0.0	6	11
1096	Cheese, American, past, proc, low fat, shredded	1 cup	113	203	28	4	0	8	5.0	2.3	0.3	40	67
1092	Cheese, mozzarella, imit	0.25 cup	28	70	3	7	0	3	1.0	1.8	0.5	0	123
47918	Cheese, pimento, past, proc, 1" cube	1 ea	18	66	4	0	0	5	3.4	1.6	0.2	16	46
48311	Cottage Cheese Substitute, soy	1 cup	225	340	28	16	0	18	2.6	4.0	10.3	0	9
DAIRY PRODUCTS AND SUBSTITUTES													
Creams and Substitutes													
54390	Cream Substitute, light	1 cup	242	167	2	22	0	8	2.2	4.9	1.0	0	1
506	Cream Substitute, pwd	1 tsp	2	11	0	1	0	1	0.6	0.0	0.0	0	0
500	Cream, half & half	2 Tbs	30	39	1	1	0	3	2.1	1.0	0.1	11	30
54384	Cream, half & half, fat free	1 Tbs	15	9	0	1	0	0	0.1	0.1	0.0	1	2
501	Cream, light	1 Tbs	15	29	0	1	0	3	1.8	0.8	0.1	10	28
502	Cream, whipping, heavy	2 Tbs	30	103	1	1	0	11	6.9	3.2	0.4	41	124
503	Cream, whipping, heavy, whipped	2 Tbs	15	52	0	0	0	6	3.4	1.6	0.2	20	62
54262	Creamer, non-dairy	1 Tbs	17	20	0	2	0	1	0.0	0.5	0.0	0	0
54315	Creamer, soy milk, plain	1 Tbs	15	15	0	1	0	1	0.0	—	—	0	0
504	Sour Cream, cultured	2 Tbs	29	62	1	1	0	6	3.8	1.7	0.2	13	52
54383	Sour Cream, fat free	3.6 oz	100	74	3	16	0	0	0.0	0.0	0.0	9	74
505	Sour Cream, imitation, cultured	2 Tbs	29	60	1	2	0	6	5.1	0.2	0.0	0	0
Milks and Non-Dairy Milks													
7	Buttermilk, low fat, cultured	1 cup	245	98	8	12	0	2	1.3	0.6	0.1	10	17
17	Eggnog	1 cup	254	343	10	34	0	19	11.3	5.7	0.9	150	117
81	Milk Substitute, fluid, w/hydrog veg oil	1 cup	244	149	4	15	0	8	1.9	4.9	1.2	0	0
4	Milk, 1%, w/add vit A & D	1 cup	244	102	8	12	0	2	1.5	0.7	0.1	12	142
2	Milk, 2%, w/add vit A & D	1 cup	244	122	8	11	0	5	3.1	1.4	0.2	20	134
18	Milk, chocolate, 2%, cmrcl	1 cup	250	180	8	26	1	5	3.1	1.5	0.2	18	138
59	Milk, chocolate, nonfat/skim	1 cup	250	144	9	27	1	1	0.7	0.3	0.0	4	142
173	Milk, evaporated	2 Tbs	32	40	2	3	0	2	1.5	0.4	0.1	10	0
23	Milk, goat	1 cup	244	168	9	11	0	10	6.5	2.7	0.4	27	142
1	Milk, whole, 3.25%	1 cup	244	146	8	11	0	8	4.6	2.0	0.5	24	70
66	Milk, whole, dry pwd	1 Tbs	8	40	2	3	0	2	1.3	0.6	0.1	8	21
20584	Rice Milk	1 cup	245	144	3	28	2	2	0.3	0.5	1.1	0	0
20033	Soy Milk	1 cup	245	127	11	12	3	5	0.6	0.9	1.9	0	152
20920	Soy Milk, chocolate	1 cup	250	140	5	23	0	4	0.0	—	—	0	100
20493	Tea, rice	1 cup	245	144	3	28	2	2	0.3	0.5	1.1	0	0
Yogurt													
2425	Yogurt, banana creme, lowfat, 6 oz ctn	1 ea	170	170	5	33	0	2	1.0	—	—	10	150
2836	Yogurt, cherry, fruit on the bottom, 8 oz ctn	1 ea	227	220	9	42	1	2	1.0	—	—	10	0
2574	Yogurt, coffee, nonfat, 8 oz ctn	1 ea	227	207	12	40	0	0	0.2	0.1	0.0	4	4
72088	Yogurt, fruit, nonfat	1 cup	245	230	11	47	0	0	0.3	0.1	0.0	5	7
2426	Yogurt, plain custard	1 cup	227	130	15	19	0	0	0.0	0.0	0.0	5	0

Thia (mg)	Ribo (mg)	Niac (mg NE)	Vit B6 (mg)	Vit B12 (µg)	Fol (µg)	Vit C (mg)	Vit D (IU)	Vit E (mg AT)	Cal (mg)	Iron (mg)	Magn (mg)	Phos (mg)	Pota (mg)	Sodi (mg)	Zinc (mg)	Wat (%)	Alco (g)	Caff (g)
0.00	0.12	0.01	0.03	0.36	1.4	0.0	—	0.2	141	0.23	8.5	113	103	274	0.9	43	0.00	0.00
—	—	—	—	—	—	0.0	—	—	100	0.00	—	—	—	280	—	—	0.00	0.00
0.02	0.47	0.15	0.12	1.23	8.0	0.0	—	0.0	552	0.91	35.0	499	336	1239	3.3	64	0.00	0.00
0.00	0.07	0.02	0.00	0.18	4.3	0.0	—	0.0	110	0.03	5.8	150	46	244	0.5	57	0.00	0.00
0.00	0.07	0.00	0.00	0.14	1.6	0.0	—	0.0	123	0.07	4.3	149	32	257	0.6	59	0.00	0.00
0.02	0.43	0.09	0.09	0.87	10.2	0.0	—	0.3	773	0.49	27.1	935	203	1616	3.8	59	0.00	0.00
0.00	0.12	0.09	0.00	0.23	3.1	0.0	0.6	0.6	172	0.10	11.6	165	129	194	0.5	47	0.00	0.00
0.00	0.05	0.00	0.00	0.11	1.4	0.4	—	0.1	107	0.07	3.8	130	28	250	0.5	39	0.00	0.00
0.00	0.31	1.12	0.15	0.00	49.5	0.0	—	1.4	423	12.60	513.0	500	448	45	3.9	71	0.00	0.00
0.00	0.00	0.00	0.00	0.00	0.0	0.0	—	0.7	2	1.36	0.0	182	428	145	0.1	86	0.00	0.00
0.00	0.00	0.00	0.00	0.00	0.0	0.0	—	0.0	0	0.01	0.1	8	16	4	0.0	2	0.00	0.00
0.00	0.03	0.01	0.00	0.10	0.9	0.3	—	0.1	32	0.01	3.0	29	39	12	0.2	81	0.00	0.00
0.00	0.03	0.01	0.00	0.07	0.6	0.1	—	0.0	14	0.00	2.4	23	31	22	0.1	86	0.00	0.00
0.00	0.01	0.00	0.00	0.02	0.3	0.1	—	0.1	14	0.00	1.4	12	18	6	0.0	74	0.00	0.00
0.00	0.02	0.00	0.00	0.05	1.2	0.2	15.5	0.3	19	0.00	2.1	18	22	11	0.1	58	0.00	0.00
0.00	0.01	0.00	0.00	0.02	0.6	0.1	7.8	0.2	10	0.00	1.0	9	11	6	0.0	58	0.00	0.00
—	—	—	—	—	—	0.0	—	—	0	0.00	—	—	25	0	—	82	0.00	0.00
—	—	—	—	—	—	0.0	—	—	0	0.00	—	—	—	5	—	—	0.00	0.00
0.00	0.03	0.01	0.00	0.09	3.2	0.3	—	0.2	33	0.01	3.2	24	41	15	0.1	71	0.00	0.00
0.03	0.15	0.07	0.01	0.30	11.0	0.0	—	0.0	125	0.00	10.0	95	129	141	0.5	81	0.00	0.00
0.00	0.00	0.00	0.00	0.00	0.0	0.0	—	0.2	1	0.10	1.7	13	46	29	0.3	71	0.00	0.00
0.07	0.37	0.14	0.07	0.54	12.2	2.5	—	0.1	284	0.11	27.0	218	370	257	1.0	90	0.00	0.00
0.09	0.47	0.27	0.12	1.13	2.5	3.8	—	0.5	330	0.50	48.3	277	419	137	1.2	74	0.00	0.00
0.02	0.20	0.00	0.00	0.00	0.0	0.0	—	0.7	81	0.94	14.6	181	278	190	2.9	88	0.00	0.00
0.05	0.44	0.23	0.09	1.07	12.2	0.0	126.8	0.0	290	0.07	26.8	232	366	107	1.0	90	0.00	0.00
0.10	0.44	0.21	0.09	1.12	12.2	0.5	104.8	0.1	285	0.07	26.8	229	366	100	1.0	89	0.00	0.00
0.09	0.40	0.31	0.10	0.85	12.5	2.2	100.0	0.1	285	0.60	32.5	255	422	150	1.0	84	0.00	5.00
0.09	0.34	0.28	0.10	0.87	13.6	2.3	100.0	0.1	292	0.68	45.5	265	486	121	1.2	85	0.00	7.50
0.00	0.10	0.05	0.01	0.05	2.5	0.0	25.0	0.0	80	0.00	7.6	60	95	30	0.2	76	0.00	0.00
0.11	0.34	0.68	0.10	0.17	2.4	3.2	29.3	0.2	327	0.11	34.2	271	498	122	0.7	87	0.00	0.00
0.10	0.44	0.25	0.09	1.07	12.2	0.0	98.7	0.1	276	0.07	24.4	222	349	98	1.0	88	0.00	0.00
0.01	0.10	0.05	0.01	0.25	3.0	0.7	25.0	0.0	73	0.03	6.8	62	106	30	0.3	2	0.00	0.00
0.09	0.02	1.86	0.17	0.00	3.4	0.0	—	1.3	15	0.50	53.6	96	50	86	0.8	86	0.00	—
0.15	0.11	0.70	0.23	2.99	39.2	0.0	39.2	(3.3)	93	2.70	61.2	135	304	135	1.1	88	0.00	0.00
—	0.50	—	—	3.00	24.0	0.0	120.0	—	300	1.44	—	—	350	75	0.6	—	0.00	—
0.09	0.02	1.86	0.17	0.00	3.4	0.0	—	1.3	15	0.50	53.6	96	50	86	0.8	86	0.00	—
—	—	—	—	—	—	0.0	80.0	—	200	0.00	—	150	260	80	—	76	0.00	0.00
—	—	—	—	—	—	0.0	—	—	300	0.00	—	—	480	150	—	77	0.00	0.00
0.10	0.47	0.25	0.10	1.24	24.7	1.8	2.3	0.0	404	0.20	38.7	318	518	155	2.0	76	0.00	0.00
0.10	0.43	0.25	0.10	1.14	22.1	1.7	—	0.1	372	0.17	36.8	292	475	142	1.8	75	0.00	0.00
0.15	0.50	—	—	—	—	0.0	—	—	400	0.00	32.0	300	550	220	—	84	0.00	0.00

PAGE KEY: A-108 Beverage and Beverage Mixes   A-110 Other Beverages   A-110 Beverages, Alcoholic   A-112 Candies and Confections, Gum   A-116 Cereals, Breakfast Type
A-120 Cheese and Cheese Substitutes   A-122 Dairy Products and Substitutes   A-124 Desserts   A-130 Dessert Toppings   A-130 Eggs, Substitutes, and Egg Dishes   A-132 Ethnic Foods
A-136 Fast Foods/Restaurants   A-150 Fats, Oils, Margarines, Shortenings, and Substitutes   A-150 Fish, Seafood, and Shellfish   A-152 Food Additives
A-152 Fruit, Vegetable, or Blended Juices   A-154 Grains, Flours, and Fractions   A-154 Grain Products, Prepared and Baked Goods

Code	Food Name	Unit/ Amt	Wt (g)	Energy (kcal)	Prot (g)	Carb (g)	Fiber (g)	Fat (g)	Sat (g)	Mono (g)	Poly (g)	Chol (mg)	Vit A (RE)
2000	Yogurt, plain, low fat, 12g prot/8 oz	1 cup	245	154	13	17	0	4	2.5	1.0	0.1	15	34
71587	Yogurt, soy, vanilla, 6 oz ctn	1 ea	170	120	4	23	1	2	0.0	—	—	0	10
7546	Yogurt, tofu	1 cup	262	246	9	42	1	5	0.7	1.0	2.7	0	10
2015	Yogurt, vanilla, low fat	1 cup	245	208	12	34	0	3	2.0	0.8	0.1	12	29

DESSERTS

Brownies and Bars

Code	Food Name	Unit/ Amt	Wt (g)	Energy (kcal)	Prot (g)	Carb (g)	Fiber (g)	Fat (g)	Sat (g)	Mono (g)	Poly (g)	Chol (mg)	Vit A (RE)
47100	Bar, apple cinnamon, fruit & oatmeal, 1.3 oz pce	1 ea	37	136	2	26	1	3	0.4	1.0	0.2	0	261
23171	Bar, Rice Krispie, 1 oz pce	1 ea	28	107	1	20	0	3	0.6	1.3	0.8	0	85
62904	Brownie, cmrcl prep, square, lrg, 2 3/4" x 7/8"	1 ea	56	227	3	36	1	9	2.4	5.0	1.3	10	11
47019	Brownie, prep f/recipe, 2" square	1 ea	24	112	1	12	1	7	1.8	2.6	2.3	18	46

Cakes & Cheesecakes

Code	Food Name	Unit/ Amt	Wt (g)	Energy (kcal)	Prot (g)	Carb (g)	Fiber (g)	Fat (g)	Sat (g)	Mono (g)	Poly (g)	Chol (mg)	Vit A (RE)
46004	Cake, angel food, cmrcl prep, 1/12 pce	1 pce	28	73	2	16	0	0	0.0	0.0	0.1	0	0
46102	Cake, applesauce, w/icing	1 pce	108	399	3	69	1	13	2.7	5.9	4.0	20	39
46103	Cake, banana, w/o icing	1 pce	87	262	3	46	1	8	1.6	3.6	2.1	32	83
46262	Cake, carrot, buttercream frosted	1 pce	71	280	2	36	1	15	3.5	—	—	35	100
46062	Cake, chocolate, prep f/rec, w/o frosting 9" whl or 1/12 pce	1 pce	95	340	5	51	2	14	5.2	5.7	2.6	55	39
46120	Cake, chocolate, w/fluffy white icing, prep f/recipe, slice	1 pce	91	280	3	43	1	11	2.7	—	—	23	50
46118	Cake, chocolate, w/vanilla icing, 1/12 piece	1 pce	103	367	3	53	1	17	4.3	—	—	23	52
46005	Cake, coffee, cinnamon, w/crumb topping prep f/mix, 1/8 pce	1 pce	56	178	3	30	1	5	1.0	2.2	1.8	27	20
42721	Cake, Ding Dongs, w/cream filling, Hostess	1 ea	80	368	3	45	2	19	11.0	4.0	1.2	14	—
46205	Cake, fruit, cmrcl prep	1 pce	43	139	1	26	2	4	0.5	1.8	1.4	2	3
45562	Cake, funnel	1 pce	90	278	7	29	1	14	2.7	4.4	6.3	63	58
46000	Cake, gingerbread, prep f/rec, 1/9 of 8" square	1 pce	74	263	3	36	1	12	3.1	5.3	3.1	24	10
46108	Cake, graham cracker	1 pce	45	159	3	22	0	7	1.6	3.2	1.6	33	66
46111	Cake, lemon, w/icing	1 pce	109	385	3	71	1	11	1.9	4.8	3.4	34	62
46070	Cake, pineapple upside down, prep f/rec, 1/9th of 8" square	1 pce	115	367	4	58	1	14	3.4	6.0	3.8	25	75
71261	Cake, pound, w/butter, cmrcl prep, 1/10 pce	1 pce	30	116	2	15	0	6	3.5	1.8	0.3	66	47
46077	Cake, shortcake, biscuit type, prep f/recipe	3.6 oz	100	346	6	48	1	14	3.8	6.0	3.6	3	19
46116	Cake, spice, w/icing	1 pce	109	368	5	62	1	12	3.2	5.9	1.9	50	39
46115	Cake, sponge, chocolate, w/o icing	1 pce	66	197	5	36	1	4	1.4	1.5	0.5	139	62
46455	Cake, yellow, prep f/dry mix, 2" x 3" pce	1 pce	55	150	2	27	0	4	1.0	2.5	0.0	0	0
46012	Cake, yellow, w/chocolate icing, cmrcl prep, 1/8 of 18 oz	1 pce	64	243	2	35	1	11	3.0	6.1	1.4	35	21
62352	Cheesecake, cherry	1 ea	113	330	6	27	1	22	13.0	—	—	100	300
49001	Cheesecake, no bake, prep f/dry mix, 1/12 of 9"	1 pce	99	271	5	35	2	13	6.6	4.5	0.8	29	99
46426	Cupcake, chocolate, w/frosting, low fat	1 ea	43	131	2	29	2	2	0.5	0.8	0.2	0	0

Cookies

Code	Food Name	Unit/ Amt	Wt (g)	Energy (kcal)	Prot (g)	Carb (g)	Fiber (g)	Fat (g)	Sat (g)	Mono (g)	Poly (g)	Chol (mg)	Vit A (RE)
90634	Cookie Crumbs, chocolate wafer	1 cup	112	485	7	81	4	16	4.7	5.4	4.7	2	3
62910	Cookie Crumbs, vanilla wafer, lower fat	1 cup	80	353	4	59	2	12	3.1	5.2	3.1	41	6
47073	Cookie, almond	2 ea	20	103	2	10	1	6	1.0	3.4	1.6	9	41
47074	Cookie, applesauce	2 ea	36	132	2	23	1	4	0.9	2.0	1.2	9	42
47746	Cookie, biscotti, chocolate	1 ea	30	120	1	15	2	6	3.0	—	—	20	0
90163	Cookie, biscuit, arrowroot	1 ea	5	22	0	4	0	1	0.2	0.4	0.1	0	0
90164	Cookie, biscuit, tea	1 ea	5	22	0	4	0	1	0.2	0.4	0.1	0	0
90637	Cookie, chocolate chip bar, prep w/marg f/recipe, 2" square	1 ea	32	156	2	19	1	9	2.6	3.3	2.7	10	50
47031	Cookie, chocolate chip, enrich, higher fat, cmrcl, med 2.25"	1 ea	10	49	1	6	0	2	0.8	1.3	0.1	0	0
42726	Cookie, chocolate chip, refrig dough	1 ea	28	127	1	18	1	6	1.8	2.5	0.5	—	—

PAGE KEY: A-158 Granola Bars, Cereal Bars, Diet Bars, Scones, and Tarts A-158 Meals and Dishes A-162 Meats A-168 Nuts, Seeds, and Products A-170 Poultry A-172 Salad Dressings, Dips, and Mayonnaise A-172 Salads A-174 Sandwiches A-176 Sauces and Gravies A-176 Snack Foods—Chips, Pretzels, Popcorn A-178 Soups, Stews, and Chilis A-180 Spices, Flavors, and Seasonings A-182 Sports Bars and Drinks A-182 Supplemental Foods and Formulas A-184 Sweeteners and Sweet Substitutes A-184 Vegetables and Legumes A-198 Weight Loss Bars and Drinks A-200 Miscellaneous

Thia (mg)	Ribo (mg)	Niac (mg NE)	Vit B6 (mg)	Vit B12 (μg)	Fol (μg)	Vit C (mg)	Vit D (IU)	Vit E (mg AT)	Cal (mg)	Iron (mg)	Magn (mg)	Phos (mg)	Pota (mg)	Sodi (mg)	Zinc (mg)	Wat (%)	Alco (g)	Caff (g)
0.10	0.51	0.28	0.11	1.37	27.0	2.0	—	0.1	448	0.20	41.7	353	573	172	2.2	85	0.00	0.00
—	—	—	—	—	—	0.0	—	—	500	0.72	—	—	—	20	—	—	0.00	0.00
0.15	0.05	0.62	0.05	0.00	15.7	6.5	—	0.8	309	2.77	104.8	100	123	92	0.8	78	0.00	0.00
0.10	0.49	0.25	0.10	1.29	27.0	2.0	—	0.0	419	0.17	39.2	331	537	162	2.0	79	0.00	0.00
0.23	0.49	5.80	0.57	0.00	116.1	0.2	0.0	0.0	10	0.46	8.2	34	49	85	0.2	15	0.00	0.00
0.10	0.10	1.30	0.12	0.00	27.5	3.9	0.0	0.4	2	0.50	4.2	12	12	123	0.1	13	0.00	0.00
0.14	0.11	0.95	0.01	0.03	26.3	0.0	—	0.1	16	1.25	17.4	57	83	175	0.4	14	0.00	1.12
0.02	0.05	0.23	0.01	0.03	7.0	0.1	—	0.7	14	0.43	12.7	32	42	82		13	0.00	—
0.02	0.14	0.25	0.00	0.01	9.9	0.0	—	0.0	40	0.15	3.4	9	26	212	0.0	33	0.00	0.00
0.11	0.11	0.99	0.05	0.05	5.2	0.9	3.5	1.8	20	1.28	10.1	45	137	163	0.2	20	0.07	0.00
0.14	0.17	1.16	0.20	0.07	11.5	2.9	3.1	1.2	26	1.11	15.5	50	168	181	0.3	33	0.10	0.00
0.05	0.07	0.40	—	—	8.0	0.0	—	—	20	0.72	—	—	—	230	—	—	0.00	0.00
0.12	0.20	1.08	0.03	0.15	25.6	0.2	—	1.5	57	1.52	30.4	101	133	299	0.7	24	0.00	—
0.10	0.12	0.82	0.01	0.07	29.3	0.1	2.9	0.9	18	0.93	10.8	41	64	207	0.3	36	0.00	—
0.12	0.12	0.94	0.01	0.09	33.4	0.2	4.6	0.9	23	1.02	11.3	47	61	232	0.3	28	0.00	—
0.09	0.10	0.85	0.02	0.07	26.9	0.1	—	0.1	76	0.80	10.1	120	63	236	0.3	30	0.00	0.00
—	—	—	—	—	—	—	—	—	3	1.84	—	—	—	241	—	12	0.00	0.00
0.01	0.03	0.34	0.01	0.00	8.6	0.2	—	0.4	14	0.88	6.9	22	66	116	0.1	25	0.00	0.00
0.23	0.31	1.86	0.05	0.23	13.6	0.4	—	2.4	128	1.86	17.7	137	155	117	0.6	42	0.00	0.00
0.14	0.11	1.28	0.14	0.03	24.4	0.1	—	1.8	53	2.13	51.8	40	325	242	0.3	28	0.00	0.00
0.05	0.10	0.61	0.01	0.09	5.2	0.1	7.2	1.0	51	0.75	6.9	52	50	189	0.3	28	0.07	0.00
0.07	0.11	0.73	0.03	0.11	6.0	1.5	4.4	1.6	67	0.81	5.9	154	53	359	0.2	22	0.00	0.00
0.18	0.18	1.37	0.03	0.09	29.9	1.4	—	1.5	138	1.70	14.9	94	129	367	0.4	32	0.00	0.00
0.03	0.07	0.38	0.00	0.07	12.3	0.0	—	0.2	10	0.40	3.3	41	36	119	0.1	25	0.00	0.00
0.31	0.27	2.56	0.02	0.07	53.0	0.2	—	2.0	205	2.53	16.0	143	106	506	0.5	28	0.00	0.00
0.12	0.18	1.12	0.03	0.11	9.1	0.1	8.7	2.2	76	1.50	13.4	209	136	281	0.4	27	0.17	0.00
0.10	0.20	0.73	0.05	0.25	14.2	0.9	15.8	0.4	21	1.66	19.7	89	98	42	0.6	30	0.00	4.59
—	—	—	—	—	—	0.0	—	—	12	0.54	—	90	45	240	—	—	0.00	0.00
0.07	0.10	0.80	0.01	0.10	14.1	0.0	—	1.5	24	1.33	19.2	103	114	216	0.4	22	0.00	—
—	—	—	—	—	—	1.2	—	—	60	1.08	—	—	—	250	—	—	0.00	0.00
0.11	0.25	0.49	0.05	0.31	29.7	0.5	—	1.1	170	0.46	18.8	232	209	376	0.5	44	0.00	0.00
0.01	0.05	0.31	0.00	0.00	6.5	0.0	—	0.8	15	0.66	10.8	79	96	178	0.2	23	0.00	0.86
0.23	0.30	3.20	0.05	0.10	68.3	0.0	—	0.8	35	4.48	59.4	148	235	650	1.2	4	0.00	7.84
0.21	0.25	2.48	0.05	0.10	48.0	0.0	—	0.2	38	1.89	11.2	83	78	250	0.3	5	0.00	0.00
0.05	0.07	0.50	0.00	0.01	4.1	0.0	0.8	1.6	15	0.51	14.9	35	44	47	0.2	6	0.00	0.00
0.07	0.05	0.37	0.02	0.01	3.1	0.4	1.0	0.7	27	0.72	11.4	47	74	78	0.2	19	0.00	0.00
—	—	—	—	—	—	0.0	—	—	0	0.72	—	—	—	30	—	—	0.00	—
0.01	0.01	0.17	0.00	0.00	5.0	0.0	—	0.0	2	0.12	0.9	6	5	19	0.0	4	0.00	0.00
0.01	0.01	0.17	0.00	0.00	5.0	0.0	—	0.0	2	0.12	0.9	6	5	19	0.0	4	0.00	0.00
0.05	0.05	0.43	0.02	0.02	10.6	0.1	—	0.9	12	0.79	17.6	32	72	116	0.3	6	0.00	5.11
0.01	0.01	0.23	0.00	0.00	6.3	0.0	—	0.2	4	0.36	4.8	12	15	30	0.1	4	0.00	1.10
—	—	—	—	—	—	—	—	—	—	—	—	—	—	88	—	10	0.00	—

PAGE KEY: A-108 Beverage and Beverage Mixes   A-110 Other Beverages   A-110 Beverages, Alcoholic   A-112 Candies and Confections, Gum   A-116 Cereals, Breakfast Type   A-120 Cheese and Cheese Substitutes   A-122 Dairy Products and Substitutes   A-124 Desserts   A-130 Dessert Toppings   A-130 Eggs, Substitutes, and Egg Dishes   A-132 Ethnic Foods   A-136 Fast Foods/Restaurants   A-150 Fats, Oils, Margarines, Shortenings, and Substitutes   A-150 Fish, Seafood, and Shellfish   A-152 Food Additives   A-152 Fruit, Vegetable, or Blended Juices   A-154 Grains, Flours, and Fractions   A-154 Grain Products, Prepared and Baked Goods

Code	Food Name	Unit/ Amt	Wt (g)	Energy (kcal)	Prot (g)	Carb (g)	Fiber (g)	Fat (g)	Sat (g)	Mono (g)	Poly (g)	Chol (mg)	Vit A (RE)
43660	Cookie, chocolate sandwich	3 ea	33	150	2	23	2	6	0.5	3.5	2.0	0	0
47041	Cookie, chocolate wafer	2 ea	12	52	1	9	0	2	0.5	0.6	0.5	0	0
50962	Cookie, chocolate, fudge stripes	3 ea	32	159	2	21	1	8	5.1	—	—	2	5
47183	Cookie, cinnamon, Teddy Grahams	22 ea	28	120	2	22	—	4	1.0	—	—	—	—
50971	Cookie, creme sandwich, sug free	3 ea	28	120	1	21	2	6	1.3	—	—	1	0
47733	Cookie, Do-Si-Dos	3 ea	36	170	3	22	1	8	1.0	—	—	0	0
47012	Cookie, fig bar	2 ea	32	111	1	23	1	2	0.4	1.0	0.9	0	3
47043	Cookie, fortune	3 ea	24	91	1	20	0	1	0.2	0.3	0.1	0	0
47324	Cookie, fudge brownie, sugar free	1 ea	24	79	1	18	0	0	0.1	0.1	0.0	0	0
47044	Cookie, fudge, cake type	1 ea	21	73	1	16	1	1	0.2	0.4	0.1	0	0
47045	Cookie, gingersnap	4 ea	28	116	2	22	1	3	0.7	1.5	0.4	0	0
47077	Cookie, granola	1 ea	13	60	1	9	1	2	1.6	0.2	0.2	0	0
47737	Cookie, lemon drop	3 ea	33	160	2	20	0	8	2.0	—	—	0	0
43676	Cookie, lemon sandwich	3 ea	33	469	2	23	2	6	0.5	3.5	2.0	0	0
47109	Cookie, molasses, med	1 ea	15	64	1	11	0	2	0.5	1.1	0.3	0	0
47161	Cookie, newton, fig	2 ea	31	116	2	19	2	3	1.0	1.0	0.0	0	—
47252	Cookie, Nutter Butter sandwich	2 ea	28	130	3	19	1	6	1.0	2.5	1.0	5	—
47496	Cookie, oatmeal raisin, home style	1 ea	26	107	1	17	1	4	0.8	1.3	0.3	3	1
47052	Cookie, oatmeal, refrig dough	2 ea	32	136	2	19	1	6	1.5	3.4	0.8	8	3
50948	Cookie, peanut butter	2 ea	28	134	2	16	1	7	1.5	—	—	0	0
47079	Cookie, pecan sandies	1 ea	15	75	1	10	0	4	0.9	2.0	0.5	3	2
47061	Cookie, raisin, soft type	2 ea	30	120	1	20	0	4	1.0	2.3	0.5	1	2
47734	Cookie, Samoas	2 ea	28	160	2	17	2	9	6.0	—	—	0	0
47665	Cookie, shortbread	1 ea	15	75	1	10	0	4	0.9	2.0	0.5	3	2
47011	Cookie, snickerdoodle, prep f/recipe	1 ea	20	80	1	12	0	3	2.1	—	—	9	25
50941	Cookie, sugar	2 ea	28	127	1	18	0	6	1.2	—	—	0	0
47738	Cookie, Tagalongs	2 ea	28	150	3	13	2	10	4.0	—	—	0	0
47739	Cookie, Thin Mints	4 ea	28	140	1	18	1	8	2.0	—	—	0	0
47740	Cookie, Trefoils	5 ea	32	160	2	20	0	8	1.0	—	—	0	0
47715	Cookie, vanilla sandwich	5 ea	43	210	2	30	1	10	2.5	—	—	5	0
47513	Cookie, wedding cake	1 ea	10	53	0	7	0	3	0.5	—	—	0	0
47026	Crackers, animal	10 ea	12	56	1	9	0	2	0.4	1.0	0.2	0	0
50966	Crackers, animal, frosted	1 ea	56	282	2	38	1	14	8.3	—	—	0	0
Doughnuts													
45630	Doughnut, buttermilk, glazed	1 ea	64	270	3	35	0	13	3.0	—	—	15	0
71335	Doughnut, cake, holes	1 ea	14	59	1	7	0	3	0.5	1.3	1.1	5	5
62914	Doughnut, cream puff, choc, custard filled, prep f/rec 3.5 x 2	1 ea	112	293	7	27	1	18	4.6	7.3	4.4	142	234
45508	Doughnut, eclair, chocolate, custard filled, prep f/rec, 5 x 2	1 ea	100	262	6	24	1	16	4.1	6.5	3.9	127	209
71343	Doughnut, glazed, enrich, lrg, 4 1/4"	1 ea	75	302	5	33	1	17	4.4	9.6	2.2	4	3
45507	Doughnut, jelly filled, 3 1/2" oval	1 ea	85	289	5	33	1	16	4.1	8.7	2.0	22	15
71856	Doughnut, plain, wheat free	1 ea	54	154	8	19	0	5	1.5	—	—	33	4
Frozen Desserts													
46110	Cake, ice cream, chocolate roll, 12 oz whl or 1/10 pce	1 pce	34	101	1	14	0	5	2.1	1.8	0.8	15	22
90721	Frozen Dessert Pop, 1.75 fl oz bar	1 ea	52	37	0	10	0	0	0.0	0.0	0.0	0	0
23050	Frozen Dessert Pop, double stick	1 ea	128	92	0	24	0	0	0.0	0.0	0.0	0	0
23051	Frozen Dessert, slushy	1 cup	193	247	1	63	0	0	0.0	0.0	0.0	0	0
23114	Frozen Dessert, snow cone	1 ea	190	243	1	62	0	0	0.0	0.0	0.0	0	0

PAGE KEY: A-158 Granola Bars, Cereal Bars, Diet Bars, Scones, and Tarts A-158 Meals and Dishes A-162 Meats A-168 Nuts, Seeds, and Products A-170 Poultry A-172 Salad Dressings, Dips, and Mayonnaise A-172 Salads A-174 Sandwiches A-176 Sauces and Gravies A-176 Snack Foods—Chips, Pretzels, Popcorn A-178 Soups, Stews, and Chilis A-180 Spices, Flavors, and Seasonings A-182 Sports Bars and Drinks A-182 Supplemental Foods and Formulas A-184 Sweeteners and Sweet Substitutes A-184 Vegetables and Legumes A-198 Weight Loss Bars and Drinks A-200 Miscellaneous

Thia (mg)	Ribo (mg)	Niac (mg NE)	Vit B6 (mg)	Vit B12 (μg)	Fol (μg)	Vit C (mg)	Vit D (IU)	Vit E (mg AT)	Cal (mg)	Iron (mg)	Magn (mg)	Phos (mg)	Pota (mg)	Sodi (mg)	Zinc (mg)	Wat (%)	Alco (g)	Caff (g)
—	—	—	—	—	—	0.0	—	—	40	1.08	—	—	—	105	—	—	0.00	—
0.01	0.02	0.34	0.00	0.00	7.3	0.0	—	0.1	4	0.47	6.4	16	25	70	0.1	4	0.00	0.83
—	—	—	—	—	—	0.0	—	—	14	0.61	—	—	—	128	—	—	0.00	—
—	—	—	—	—	—	—	—	—	—	—	—	—	—	170	—	—	0.00	—
0.07	0.07	0.75	—	—	16.5	0.0	—	—	4	0.38	—	—	—	67	—	1	0.00	0.00
—	—	—	—	—	—	0.0	—	—	0	0.36	—	—	—	105	—	—	0.00	0.00
0.05	0.07	0.60	0.01	0.02	11.2	0.1	—	0.2	20	0.93	8.6	20	66	112	0.1	16	0.00	0.00
0.03	0.02	0.43	0.00	0.00	15.8	0.0	—	0.0	3	0.34	1.7	8	10	66	0.0	8	0.00	0.00
0.01	0.02	0.38	0.00	0.00	—	0.0	—	0.0	4	0.43	7.3	17	40	106	0.1	14	0.00	—
0.05	0.03	0.25	0.00	0.01	9.0	0.0	—	0.1	7	0.51	6.7	17	29	40	0.1	12	0.00	0.00
0.05	0.07	0.91	0.02	0.00	24.4	0.0	—	0.3	22	1.78	13.7	23	97	183	0.2	5	0.00	0.00
0.07	0.02	0.23	0.05	0.00	10.5	0.1	—	0.0	9	0.37	13.1	46	47	43	0.2	3	0.00	0.00
—	—	—	—	—	—	0.0	—	—	0	0.72	—	—	—	150	—	8	0.00	0.00
—	—	—	—	—	—	0.0	—	—	40	1.08	—	—	—	80	—	5	0.00	0.00
0.05	0.03	0.44	0.01	0.00	13.4	0.0	—	0.0	11	0.95	7.8	14	52	69	0.1	6	0.00	0.00
—	—	—	—	—	—	—	—	—	—	0.69	—	—	78	116	—	—	0.00	0.00
—	—	—	—	—	—	—	—	—	—	0.72	—	—	55	110	—	0	0.00	0.00
0.07	0.03	0.44	—	—	—	0.0	—	—	8	0.58	—	—	60	98	—	11	0.00	0.00
0.07	0.05	0.60	0.00	0.00	11.2	0.0	—	0.8	10	0.68	9.0	33	47	94	0.2	15	0.00	0.00
0.05	0.05	1.20	—	—	17.4	0.0	—	—	10	0.62	—	—	—	114	—	8	0.00	0.00
0.05	0.05	0.50	0.00	0.00	1.4	0.0	0.9	0.5	5	0.40	2.6	16	15	68	0.1	4	0.00	0.00
0.05	0.05	0.58	0.01	0.00	9.6	0.1	—	0.7	14	0.68	6.3	25	42	101	0.1	13	0.00	0.00
—	—	—	—	—	—	2.4	—	—	0	0.72	—	—	—	45	—	—	0.00	0.00
0.05	0.05	0.50	0.00	0.00	1.4	0.0	0.9	0.5	5	0.40	2.6	16	15	68	0.1	4	0.00	0.00
0.05	0.03	0.40	0.00	0.00	13.6	0.1	2.7	0.1	8	0.46	2.1	10	23	75	0.1	18	0.00	0.00
0.05	0.02	0.67	—	—	14.8	0.0	—	—	12	0.63	—	—	—	86	—	9	0.00	0.00
—	—	—	—	—	—	0.0	—	—	0	0.72	—	—	—	85	—	—	0.00	0.00
—	—	—	—	—	—	0.0	—	—	200	—	—	—	—	80	—	—	0.00	0.00
—	—	—	—	—	—	0.0	—	—	0	0.36	—	—	—	90	—	—	0.00	0.00
—	—	—	—	—	—	0.0	—	—	20	1.08	—	—	—	125	—	1	0.00	0.00
—	—	—	—	—	—	0.0	—	—	0	0.23	—	—	—	15	—	—	0.00	0.00
0.03	0.03	0.43	0.00	0.00	12.9	0.0	—	0.0	5	0.34	2.2	14	12	49	0.1	4	0.00	0.00
—	—	—	—	—	—	0.0	—	—	5	0.62	—	—	—	141	—	—	0.00	0.00
—	—	—	—	—	—	0.0	—	—	60	1.08	—	—	—	290	—	19	0.00	0.00
0.02	0.02	0.25	0.00	0.03	7.3	0.0	—	0.3	6	0.27	2.8	38	18	76	0.1	21	0.00	0.00
0.12	0.30	0.88	0.07	0.37	48.2	0.3	—	2.3	71	1.32	16.8	120	131	377	0.7	52	0.00	2.24
0.11	0.27	0.80	0.05	0.34	43.0	0.3	—	2.0	63	1.17	15.0	107	117	337	0.6	52	0.00	2.00
0.27	0.15	2.14	0.03	0.07	36.8	0.1	—	0.3	32	1.52	16.5	70	81	256	0.6	25	0.00	0.00
0.27	0.11	1.82	0.09	0.18	57.8	0.0	—	0.4	21	1.50	17.0	72	67	249	0.6	36	0.00	0.00
0.02	133.86	0.10	0.02	0.00	19.9	9.6	0.0	0.0	57	0.40	8.2	84	132	—	—	—	0.00	0.00
0.03	0.07	0.30	0.00	0.07	2.3	0.1	3.5	0.3	42	0.50	9.1	40	57	45	0.2	39	0.02	—
0.00	0.00	0.00	0.00	0.00	0.0	0.0	—	0.0	0	0.00	0.5	0	2	6	0.0	80	0.00	0.00
0.00	0.00	0.00	0.00	0.00	0.0	0.0	—	0.0	0	0.00	1.3	0	5	15	0.0	80	0.00	0.00
0.00	0.00	0.00	0.00	0.00	0.0	1.9	—	0.0	4	0.31	1.9	2	6	42	0.0	67	0.00	0.00
0.00	0.00	0.00	0.00	0.00	0.0	1.9	—	0.0	4	0.30	1.9	2	6	42	0.0	67	0.00	0.00

PAGE KEY: A-108 Beverage and Beverage Mixes   A-110 Other Beverages   A-110 Beverages, Alcoholic   A-112 Candies and Confections, Gum   A-116 Cereals, Breakfast Type   A-120 Cheese and Cheese Substitutes   A-122 Dairy Products and Substitutes   A-124 Desserts   A-130 Dessert Toppings   A-130 Eggs, Substitutes, and Egg Dishes   A-132 Ethnic Foods   A-136 Fast Foods/Restaurants   A-150 Fats, Oils, Margarines, Shortenings, and Substitutes   A-150 Fish, Seafood, and Shellfish   A-152 Food Additives   A-152 Fruit, Vegetable, or Blended Juices   A-154 Grains, Flours, and Fractions   A-154 Grain Products, Prepared and Baked Goods

Code	Food Name	Unit/ Amt	Wt (g)	Energy (kcal)	Prot (g)	Carb (g)	Fiber (g)	Fat (g)	Sat (g)	Mono (g)	Poly (g)	Chol (mg)	Vit A (RE)
2032	Frozen Dessert, sundae, hot fudge	1 ea	158	284	6	48	0	9	5.0	2.3	0.8	21	62
2045	Frozen Yogurt Cone, chocolate, sml	1 ea	78	168	4	24	1	7	4.2	2.3	0.4	1	37
2044	Frozen Yogurt Sandwich	1 ea	85	181	4	32	0	4	2.3	1.3	0.4	1	37
72125	Frozen Yogurt, chocolate	1 cup	174	221	5	38	4	6	4.0	1.7	0.2	23	70
625	Frozen Yogurt, vanilla, lowfat	0.5 cup	106	200	9	31	0	4	2.5	—	—	65	40
72188	Ice Cream Bar, Fudgsicle	1 ea	61	90	3	16	1	2	1.0	—	—	5	0
72187	Ice Cream Bar, Fudgsicle, fat free	1 ea	51	65	3	14	1	0	0.2	—	—	2	0
2113	Ice Cream Cone, chocolate, small	1 ea	78	173	3	25	1	7	4.4	2.2	0.4	18	62
2092	Ice Cream Cone, chocolate dipped	1 ea	78	187	3	24	1	10	5.7	2.9	0.5	29	77
2093	Ice Cream Cone, vanilla, small	1 ea	78	166	3	21	0	8	5.0	2.4	0.4	32	86
2087	Ice Cream Sandwich	1 ea	59	144	3	22	1	6	3.2	1.7	0.4	20	53
2051	Ice Cream, chocolate, soft serve	1 cup	173	355	6	48	1	17	10.3	4.8	0.6	43	147
71814	Ice Cream, neapolitan	0.5 cup	65	130	2	16	0	7	4.0	—	—	25	40
71810	Ice Cream, rocky road	0.5 cup	65	160	3	19	1	8	4.5	—	—	25	40
2053	Ice Cream, strawberry, imit	0.5 cup	66	132	2	16	0	7	5.9	0.4	0.1	0	0
2004	Ice Cream, vanilla	0.5 cup	66	133	2	16	0	7	4.5	2.0	0.3	29	79
72119	Ice Cream, vanilla, fat free	3.6 oz	100	138	4	30	1	0	0.0	0.0	0.0	0	202
2052	Ice Cream, vanilla, imit	0.5 cup	66	132	2	16	0	7	5.9	0.4	0.1	0	0
2020	Milk Shake, chocolate, fast food	1 cup	166	211	6	34	3	6	3.8	1.8	0.2	22	45
2482	Milk Shake, vanilla, fountain type	1 cup	166	224	5	35	0	8	4.9	2.3	0.3	32	80
2011	Sherbet, orange	0.5 cup	74	107	1	22	2	1	0.9	0.4	0.1	0	8
Fruit Desserts													
49005	Apple Brown Betty	0.75 cup	155	268	4	47	3	8	4.2	—	—	16	53
49019	Cobbler, berry	1 cup	217	507	6	94	4	13	2.9	5.6	4.1	2	23
49023	Crisp, cherry	1 cup	246	704	6	113	3	27	4.7	12.3	8.6	2	250
49015	Strudel, apple	1 pce	71	195	2	29	2	8	1.5	2.3	3.8	4	5
Gelatin Desserts													
23052	Gelatin, prep f/dry mix w/water	0.5 cup	135	84	2	19	0	0	0.0	0.0	0.0	0	0
Pastries and Sweet Rolls													
42363	Buns, honey	1 ea	65	270	3	35	1	13	3.0	—	—	0	0
45523	Croissant, cheese, med	1 ea	57	236	5	27	1	12	6.1	3.7	1.4	32	120
71042	Danish, cinnamon nut, 4 1/4"	1 ea	65	280	5	30	1	16	3.8	8.9	2.8	30	6
71041	Danish, raisin nut, 4 1/4"	1 ea	65	280	5	30	1	16	3.8	8.9	2.8	30	6
42746	Danish, strawberry swirl	1 ea	62	254	3	37	1	11	3.0	3.6	4.4	0	0
45549	Dumpling, apple	1 ea	190	672	7	85	3	35	6.9	15.2	10.7	0	8
45515	Fritter, apple	1 ea	24	87	1	8	0	6	1.2	2.4	1.6	20	13
45593	Pastry, apple cinnamon	1 ea	52	205	2	37	1	5	0.9	3.1	1.4	0	100
45594	Pastry, brown sugar cinnamon	1 ea	50	219	3	32	1	9	1.0	3.6	4.6	0	100
45572	Pastry, cheese danish	1 ea	71	266	6	26	1	16	4.8	8.0	1.8	11	26
45595	Pastry, cherry	1 ea	52	204	2	37	1	5	0.9	3.0	1.6	0	100
45601	Pastry, chocolate fudge, frosted	1 ea	52	201	3	37	1	5	1.0	2.7	1.1	0	100
45782	Pastry, s'mores	1 ea	52	204	3	36	1	5	1.5	3.1	0.9	0	100
Pastry, Pie, Dessert Crusts, and Cones													
45500	Crust, pie, graham cracker, prep f/rec, bkd, 9" or 1/8 pce	1 pce	30	148	1	19	0	7	1.6	3.4	2.1	0	61
45535	Crust, pie, rtb, enrich, fzn, 9" whl or 1/8 pce	1 pce	18	82	1	8	0	5	0.8	2.2	2.0	0	0

PAGE KEY: A-158 Granola Bars, Cereal Bars, Diet Bars, Scones, and Tarts A-158 Meals and Dishes A-162 Meats A-168 Nuts, Seeds, and Products A-170 Poultry
A-172 Salad Dressings, Dips, and Mayonnaise A-172 Salads A-174 Sandwiches A-176 Sauces and Gravies A-176 Snack Foods—Chips, Pretzels, Popcorn
A-178 Soups, Stews, and Chilis A-180 Spices, Flavors, and Seasonings A-182 Sports Bars and Drinks A-182 Supplemental Foods and Formulas
A-184 Sweeteners and Sweet Substitutes A-184 Vegetables and Legumes A-198 Weight Loss Bars and Drinks A-200 Miscellaneous

Thia (mg)	Ribo (mg)	Niac (mg NE)	Vit B6 (mg)	Vit B12 (µg)	Fol (µg)	Vit C (mg)	Vit D (IU)	Vit E (mg AT)	Cal (mg)	Iron (mg)	Magn (mg)	Phos (mg)	Pota (mg)	Sodi (mg)	Zinc (mg)	Wat (%)	Alco (g)	Caff (g)
0.05	0.30	1.07	0.12	0.64	9.5	2.4	19.0	0.7	207	0.57	33.2	228	395	182	0.9	60	0.00	1.58
0.07	0.18	0.68	0.05	0.18	4.7	0.5	—	0.2	99	0.97	30.8	116	197	84	0.6	53	0.00	—
0.03	0.15	0.34	0.05	0.18	7.3	0.5	—	0.1	95	0.34	12.0	98	151	57	0.4	52	0.00	0.00
0.07	0.31	0.23	0.07	0.11	20.9	11.7	—	0.2	174	0.80	43.5	155	407	110	0.5	71	0.00	5.21
—	—	—	—	—	—	0.0	—	—	250	0.00	—	—	—	55	—	—	0.00	0.00
—	—	—	—	—	—	0.0	—	—	80	0.36	—	—	—	65	—	65	0.00	—
—	—	—	—	—	—	0.5	—	—	81	0.46	—	—	—	48	—	66	0.00	—
0.03	0.12	0.36	0.02	0.27	4.3	0.4	6.2	0.3	88	0.49	17.3	83	168	46	0.4	54	0.00	2.33
0.03	0.18	0.34	0.03	0.25	3.8	0.4	3.7	0.2	88	0.46	18.2	83	161	61	0.6	52	0.00	2.33
0.03	0.18	0.28	0.03	0.28	3.9	0.4	3.7	0.1	95	0.23	11.5	82	151	65	0.5	58	0.00	0.00
0.02	0.11	0.18	0.02	0.18	4.8	0.3	2.4	0.1	60	0.28	12.7	64	122	36	0.4	48	0.00	—
0.07	0.27	0.21	0.05	0.63	9.4	1.1	6.9	0.5	206	0.66	37.3	184	384	89	1.0	58	0.00	5.19
—	—	—	—	—	—	2.0	0.0	—	60	0.00	—	—	—	55	—	61	0.00	—
—	—	—	—	—	—	0.0	0.0	—	60	0.36	—	—	—	65	—	—	0.00	—
0.02	0.15	0.07	0.03	0.38	1.3	0.3	0.0	0.1	90	0.07	10.0	71	144	49	0.7	61	0.00	0.00
0.02	0.15	0.07	0.02	0.25	3.3	0.4	22.9	0.2	84	0.05	9.2	69	131	53	0.5	61	0.00	0.00
0.05	0.25	0.14	0.05	0.44	7.0	0.0	—	0.0	149	0.00	21.0	150	302	97	1.1	64	0.00	0.00
0.02	0.15	0.07	0.03	0.38	1.3	0.3	0.0	0.1	90	0.07	10.0	71	144	49	0.7	61	0.00	0.00
0.10	0.40	0.27	0.07	0.56	8.3	0.7	57.7	0.2	188	0.51	28.3	170	333	161	0.7	72	0.00	1.65
0.05	0.25	0.20	0.05	0.49	7.4	9.0	—	0.1	172	0.38	19.6	135	247	86	0.8	70	0.00	0.00
0.01	0.07	0.05	0.01	0.09	5.2	4.3	—	0.0	40	0.10	5.9	30	71	34	0.4	66	0.00	0.00
0.23	0.14	2.01	0.07	0.01	32.4	0.3	8.2	0.3	74	1.98	16.4	51	150	309	0.4	61	0.00	0.00
0.31	0.28	2.55	0.07	0.05	12.8	12.4	—	2.8	181	2.39	19.7	134	189	260	0.5	47	0.00	0.00
0.20	0.25	1.98	0.14	0.14	16.1	2.7	—	4.3	153	3.50	19.7	323	219	836	0.4	40	0.00	0.00
0.02	0.01	0.23	0.02	0.15	19.9	1.2	—	1.0	11	0.30	6.4	23	106	191	0.1	44	0.00	0.00
0.00	0.00	0.00	0.00	0.00	1.4	0.0	—	0.0	4	0.02	1.4	30	1	101	0.0	84	0.00	0.00
—	—	—	—	—	—	0.0	—	—	0	0.36	—	—	—	160	—	—	0.00	0.00
0.30	0.18	1.23	0.03	0.18	42.2	0.1	—	0.8	30	1.23	13.7	74	75	316	0.5	21	0.00	0.00
0.14	0.15	1.49	0.07	0.14	53.9	1.1	—	0.5	61	1.16	20.8	72	62	236	0.6	20	0.00	0.00
0.14	0.15	1.49	0.07	0.14	53.9	1.1	—	0.5	61	1.16	20.8	72	62	236	0.6	20	0.00	0.00
—	—	—	—	—	—	0.0	—	—	20	1.08	—	—	—	170	—	16	0.00	0.00
0.40	0.30	3.53	0.05	0.00	11.2	1.6	—	4.5	13	3.11	16.6	76	130	10	0.5	33	0.00	0.00
0.03	0.05	0.31	0.01	0.05	2.9	0.3	—	0.7	13	0.34	3.0	22	34	10	0.1	37	0.00	0.00
0.15	0.17	1.98	0.20	0.00	41.6	0.0	—	0.0	12	1.82	5.7	28	47	174	0.3	12	0.00	0.00
0.15	0.17	2.00	0.20	0.00	40.0	0.0	—	0.0	16	1.79	8.0	32	68	214	0.6	10	0.00	0.00
0.12	0.18	1.41	0.02	0.11	42.6	0.1	—	0.2	25	1.13	10.6	77	70	320	0.5	31	0.00	0.00
0.15	0.17	1.98	0.20	0.00	41.6	0.0	—	0.0	15	1.82	8.3	44	59	220	0.6	12	0.00	0.00
0.15	0.15	1.98	0.20	0.00	52.0	0.0	—	0.0	20	1.82	15.1	44	82	203	0.3	12	0.00	—
0.15	0.15	1.98	0.20	0.00	52.0	0.0	—	0.0	15	1.82	10.9	39	65	199	0.2	12	0.00	—
0.02	0.05	0.63	0.00	0.00	7.2	0.0	—	0.7	6	0.64	5.4	19	26	171	0.1	4	0.00	0.00
0.05	0.07	0.43	0.00	0.00	12.6	0.0	—	0.4	3	0.36	2.9	10	18	104	0.1	21	0.00	0.00

PAGE KEY: A-108 Beverage and Beverage Mixes   A-110 Other Beverages   A-110 Beverages, Alcoholic   A-112 Candies and Confections, Gum   A-116 Cereals, Breakfast Type   A-120 Cheese and Cheese Substitutes   A-122 Dairy Products and Substitutes   A-124 Desserts   A-130 Dessert Toppings   A-130 Eggs, Substitutes, and Egg Dishes   A-132 Ethnic Foods   A-136 Fast Foods/Restaurants   A-150 Fats, Oils, Margarines, Shortenings, and Substitutes   A-150 Fish, Seafood, and Shellfish   A-152 Food Additives   A-152 Fruit, Vegetable, or Blended Juices   A-154 Grains, Flours, and Fractions   A-154 Grain Products, Prepared and Baked Goods

Code	Food Name	Unit/ Amt	Wt (g)	Energy (kcal)	Prot (g)	Carb (g)	Fiber (g)	Fat (g)	Sat (g)	Mono (g)	Poly (g)	Chol (mg)	Vit A (RE)
Pies													
48004	Pie, apple, cmrcl prep, w/enrich flour, 8" whl or 1/6 pce	1 pce	117	277	2	40	2	13	4.4	5.1	2.6	0	39
48023	Pie, banana cream, no bake, prep f/mix, 9" whl or 1/8 pce	1 pce	92	231	3	29	1	12	6.4	4.2	0.7	27	92
48025	Pie, blueberry, cmrcl prep, 8" whl or 1/6 pce	1 pce	117	271	2	41	1	12	2.0	5.0	4.1	0	55
48005	Pie, cherry, cmrcl prep, 8" whl or 1/6 pce	1 pce	117	304	2	47	1	13	3.0	6.8	2.4	0	68
48031	Pie, chocolate cream, cmrcl prep, 8" whl or 1/6 pce	1 pce	113	344	3	38	2	22	5.6	12.6	2.7	6	0
71646	Pie, key lime, w/o topping, 10" whl or 1/8 pce	1 pce	113	420	6	55		20	12.0	—	—	20	40
48177	Pie, lemon, 4 oz svg	1 ea	113	320	3	50	2	12	3.0	—	—	40	0
48040	Pie, peach, 8" whl or 1/6 pce	1 pce	117	261	2	38	1	12	1.8	5.0	4.4	0	19
48012	Pie, pecan, cmrcl prep, 8" whl or 1/6 pce	1 pce	113	452	5	65	4	21	4.0	12.1	3.6	36	59
48000	Pie, pumpkin, cmrcl prep, 8" whl or 1/6 pce	1 pce	109	229	4	30	3	10	1.9	4.4	3.4	22	613
48130	Pie, rhubarb, 9" or 1/8 pce	1 pce	118	316	3	48	2	13	3.6	—	—	3	18
48185	Pie, strawberry, 3.7 oz svg	1 ea	106	310	2	50	1	12	3.0	—	—	0	0
Puddings, Custards, and Pie Fillings													
2659	Custard, chocolate, prep f/dry mix w/2% milk	0.5 cup	136	116	4	18	1	3	1.7	0.8	0.1	10	68
48001	Pie Filling, apple, cnd	0.5 cup	128	129	0	33	1	0	0.0	0.0	0.0	0	0
48015	Pie Filling, cherry, cnd	0.5 cup	132	152	0	37	1	0	0.0	0.0	0.0	0	26
48017	Pie Filling, lemon	0.5 cup	133	463	6	93	1	9	2.2	3.8	1.9	175	125
48044	Pie Filling, pumpkin, cnd	0.5 cup	135	140	1	36	11	0	0.1	0.0	0.0	0	1120
58203	Pudding, all flvrs, not choc, inst, low cal, dry mix	3.6 oz	100	342	1	82	1	1	0.2	0.2	0.3	0	0
2649	Pudding, rice, prep f/dry mix w/2% milk	0.5 cup	144	160	5	30	0	2	1.4	0.6	0.1	9	68
2653	Pudding, tapioca, prep f/dry mix w/2% milk	0.5 cup	141	148	4	28	0	2	1.4	0.6	0.1	8	68
2764	Pudding, vanilla, fat free, 4 oz snack cup	1 ea	113	104	2	23	0	0	0.2	0.0	0.0	2	35
56331	Roll, yorkshire pudding, prep f/recipe, 1.5 oz svg	1 pce	42	87	3	10	0	4	1.8	1.7	0.3	32	27
DESSERT TOPPINGS													
46037	Frosting, chocolate, creamy, 16 oz can	1.328 oz	38	149	0	24	0	7	2.1	3.4	0.8	0	0
46038	Frosting, coconut nut, rte, 16 oz can	1.328 oz	38	155	1	20	1	9	2.6	4.6	1.3	0	0
46323	Frosting, cream cheese, rte	2 Tbs	35	150	0	24	0	6	1.5	—	—	0	0
46330	Frosting, lemon creme, rte	2 Tbs	35	150	0	24	0	6	1.5	—	—	0	0
46336	Frosting, strawberry creme, rte	2 Tbs	35	150	0	24	0	6	1.5	—	—	0	0
54308	Syrup, caramel	2 Tbs	39	100	1	25	0	0	0.0	0.0	0.0	0	0
23437	Syrup, chocolate	2 Tbs	39	100	1	24	—	0	0.0	0.0	0.0	0	0
54312	Syrup, raspberry	2 Tbs	38	100	0	25	0	0	0.0	0.0	0.0	0	0
23069	Topping, butterscotch	2 Tbs	41	103	1	27	0	0	0.0	0.0	0.0	0	11
23070	Topping, caramel	2 Tbs	41	103	1	27	0	0	0.0	0.0	0.0	0	11
23014	Topping, chocolate fudge	2 Tbs	38	133	2	24	1	3	1.5	1.5	0.1	1	2
92528	Topping, hot fudge	1 Tbs	19	70	1	10	—	2	1.0	—	—	5	—
23071	Topping, marshmallow cream, 7 oz jar	1 ea	198	639	2	157	0	1	0.1	0.2	0.1	0	0
23163	Topping, pineapple	2 Tbs	42	108	0	28	0	0	0.0	0.0	0.0	0	1
23164	Topping, strawberry	2 Tbs	42	108	0	28	0	0	0.0	0.0	0.0	0	1
510	Topping, whipped cream, pressurized	2 Tbs	8	19	0	1	0	2	1.0	0.5	0.1	6	14
565	Topping, whipped, lite, Cool Whip	2 Tbs	9	20	0	2	0	1	1.0	0.0	0.0	0	0
EGGS, SUBSTITUTES, AND EGG DISHES													
19525	Egg Substitute, liquid	0.25 cup	63	53	8	0	0	2	0.4	0.6	1.0	1	23
7736	Egg Substitute, Scramblers, fzn	0.25 cup	57	39	7	2	0	0	—	—	—	2	62
19507	Egg Whites, raw	0.625 cup	152	79	17	1	0	0	0.0	0.0	0.0	0	0

PAGE KEY: A-158 Granola Bars, Cereal Bars, Diet Bars, Scones, and Tarts   A-158 Meals and Dishes   A-162 Meats   A-168 Nuts, Seeds, and Products   A-170 Poultry   A-172 Salad Dressings, Dips, and Mayonnaise   A-172 Salads   A-174 Sandwiches   A-176 Sauces and Gravies   A-176 Snack Foods—Chips, Pretzels, Popcorn   A-178 Soups, Stews, and Chilis   A-180 Spices, Flavors, and Seasonings   A-182 Sports Bars and Drinks   A-182 Supplemental Foods and Formulas   A-184 Sweeteners and Sweet Substitutes   A-184 Vegetables and Legumes   A-198 Weight Loss Bars and Drinks   A-200 Miscellaneous

Thia (mg)	Ribo (mg)	Niac (mg NE)	Vit B6 (mg)	Vit B12 (µg)	Fol (µg)	Vit C (mg)	Vit D (IU)	Vit E (mg AT)	Cal (mg)	Iron (mg)	Magn (mg)	Phos (mg)	Pota (mg)	Sodi (mg)	Zinc (mg)	Wat (%)	Alco (g)	Caff (g)
0.02	0.02	0.31	0.03	0.00	31.6	3.7	—	1.8	13	0.52	8.2	28	76	311	0.2	52	0.00	0.00
0.09	0.12	0.64	0.02	0.18	19.3	0.5	—	1.5	67	0.41	11.0	154	104	267	0.3	51	0.00	0.00
0.00	0.03	0.34	0.03	0.00	31.6	3.2	—	1.2	9	0.34	5.8	27	58	380	0.2	52	0.00	0.00
0.02	0.02	0.23	0.05	0.00	31.6	1.1	—	0.9	14	0.56	9.4	34	95	288	0.2	46	0.00	0.00
0.03	0.11	0.76	0.01	0.00	14.7	0.0	—	3.1	41	1.21	23.7	77	144	154	0.3	44	0.00	0.00
—	—	—	—	—	—	0.0	—	—	150	0.72	—	—	—	200	—	—	0.00	0.00
—	—	—	—	—	—	0.0	—	—	20	0.72	—	—	—	330	—	—	0.00	0.00
0.07	0.03	0.23	0.02	0.00	33.9	1.1	—	1.1	9	0.57	7.0	26	146	316	0.1	54	0.00	0.00
0.10	0.14	0.28	0.01	0.10	38.4	1.2	—	0.4	19	1.17	20.3	87	84	479	0.6	19	0.00	0.00
0.05	0.17	0.20	0.05	0.28	26.2	1.1	—	1.1	65	0.86	16.4	77	168	307	0.5	58	0.00	0.00
0.18	0.14	1.53	0.01	0.00	36.3	3.8	0.8	1.1	46	1.30	11.4	35	166	197	0.2	45	0.00	0.00
—	—	—	—	—	—	9.0	—	—	20	1.08	—	—	—	300	—	—	0.00	0.00
0.05	0.20	0.15	0.05	0.44	6.8	1.2	49.0	0.1	171	0.40	27.2	133	248	71	0.7	80	0.00	1.36
0.01	0.00	0.03	0.01	0.00	0.0	0.1	—	0.0	5	0.37	2.5	9	57	56	0.1	73	0.00	0.00
0.02	0.01	0.18	0.05	0.00	5.3	4.8	—	0.3	15	0.31	9.2	20	139	24	0.1	71	0.00	0.00
0.09	0.25	0.56	0.07	0.34	18.9	14.1	—	1.2	29	1.12	8.3	88	99	108	0.6	18	0.00	0.00
0.01	0.15	0.50	0.20	0.00	47.2	4.7	—	1.1	50	1.42	21.6	61	186	281	0.4	71	0.00	0.00
0.00	0.00	0.00	0.00	0.00	0.0	0.0	—	0.1	19	0.23	7.0	2179	47	4232	0.0	4	0.00	0.00
0.10	0.20	0.63	0.05	0.34	5.8	1.0	48.3	0.1	151	0.52	18.7	125	187	157	0.5	73	0.00	0.00
0.03	0.20	0.10	0.05	0.34	5.6	1.0	48.5	0.1	148	0.07	16.9	116	188	171	0.5	75	0.00	0.00
—	—	—	—	—	—	0.3	—	—	86	0.05	—	115	123	241	—	76	0.00	0.00
0.03	0.07	—	0.02	0.41	3.8	0.4	—	—	55	0.37	—	—	67	248	0.3	57	0.00	0.00
0.00	0.00	0.03	0.00	0.00	0.4	0.0	—	0.6	3	0.52	7.9	30	74	69	0.1	17	0.00	0.75
0.00	0.00	0.07	0.01	0.00	0.8	0.1	—	0.6	5	0.20	7.2	24	70	73	0.2	21	0.00	0.00
—	—	—	—	—	—	0.0	—	—	0	0.00	—	—	—	70	—	14	0.00	0.00
—	—	—	—	—	—	0.0	—	—	0	0.00	—	—	—	70	—	14	0.00	0.00
—	—	—	—	—	—	0.0	—	—	0	0.00	—	—	—	70	—	14	0.00	0.00
—	—	—	—	—	—	0.0	—	—	20	0.00	—	—	—	105	—	33	0.00	0.00
—	—	—	—	—	—	0.0	—	—	0	0.36	—	—	—	25	—	35	0.00	7.00
—	—	—	—	—	—	0.0	—	—	0	0.00	—	—	—	5	—	31	0.00	0.00
0.00	0.03	0.01	0.00	0.03	0.8	0.1	—	0.0	22	0.07	2.9	19	34	143	0.1	32	0.00	0.00
0.00	0.03	0.01	0.00	0.03	0.8	0.1	—	0.0	22	0.07	2.9	19	34	143	0.1	32	0.00	0.00
0.02	0.10	0.14	0.02	0.10	1.9	0.0	—	0.9	38	0.60	24.3	64	171	131	0.3	22	0.00	2.66
—	—	—	—	—	—	—	—	—	—	—	—	—	—	80	—	25	0.00	—
0.00	0.00	0.15	0.00	0.00	2.0	0.0	—	0.0	6	0.43	4.0	16	10	159	0.1	20	0.00	0.00
0.01	0.00	0.03	0.00	0.00	0.9	1.3	—	0.0	3	0.05	2.6	1	18	18	0.0	33	0.00	0.00
0.00	0.00	0.07	0.00	0.00	2.6	5.8	—	0.0	3	0.11	1.7	2	22	9	0.0	33	0.00	0.00
0.00	0.00	0.00	0.00	0.01	0.2	0.0	—	0.0	8	0.00	0.8	7	11	10	0.0	61	0.00	0.00
—	—	—	—	—	—	0.0	—	—	0	0.00	—	0	0	0	—	66	0.00	0.00
0.07	0.18	0.07	0.00	0.18	9.4	0.0	—	0.2	33	1.32	5.6	76	207	111	0.8	83	0.00	0.00
0.17	0.40	0.00	0.12	1.76	—	0.0	—	—	19	0.62	—	59	95	122	0.7	83	0.00	0.00
0.00	0.67	0.15	0.00	0.14	6.1	0.0	0.0	0.0	11	0.11	16.7	23	248	252	0.0	88	0.00	0.00

PAGE KEY: A-108 Beverage and Beverage Mixes   A-110 Other Beverages   A-110 Beverages, Alcoholic   A-112 Candies and Confections, Gum   A-116 Cereals, Breakfast Type
A-120 Cheese and Cheese Substitutes   A-122 Dairy Products and Substitutes   A-124 Desserts   A-130 Dessert Toppings   A-130 Eggs, Substitutes, and Egg Dishes   A-132 Ethnic Foods
A-136 Fast Foods/Restaurants   A-150 Fats, Oils, Margarines, Shortenings, and Substitutes   A-150 Fish, Seafood, and Shellfish   A-152 Food Additives
A-152 Fruit, Vegetable, or Blended Juices   A-154 Grains, Flours, and Fractions   A-154 Grain Products, Prepared and Baked Goods

Code	Food Name	Unit/ Amt	Wt (g)	Energy (kcal)	Prot (g)	Carb (g)	Fiber (g)	Fat (g)	Sat (g)	Mono (g)	Poly (g)	Chol (mg)	Vit A (RE)
19600	Egg Yolks, raw	0.25 cup	61	196	10	2	0	16	5.8	7.1	2.6	750	238
19539	Eggs, deviled	1 ea	31	63	4	0	0	5	1.2	1.7	1.5	122	50
19510	Eggs, hard bld, lrg	1 ea	50	78	6	1	0	5	1.6	2.0	0.7	212	85
19516	Eggs, scrambled, prep f/one lrg egg butter & milk	1 ea	61	101	7	1	0	7	2.2	2.9	1.3	215	89
19509	Eggs, whole, lrg, fried	1 ea	46	92	6	0	0	7	2.0	2.9	1.2	210	93
19501	Eggs, whole, raw, lrg	1 ea	50	74	6	0	0	5	1.5	1.9	0.7	212	70
19535	Omelette, one egg w/cheese & ham	1 ea	78	156	11	2	0	11	4.5	4.4	1.4	198	133
19536	Omelette, Spanish	1 ea	145	178	8	6	1	14	3.4	5.9	3.0	220	211
19544	Omelette, w/sausage, one egg	1 ea	95	167	11	2	0	13	3.9	5.2	1.9	267	149

ETHNIC FOODS

Italian Foods

Code	Food Name	Unit/ Amt	Wt (g)	Energy (kcal)	Prot (g)	Carb (g)	Fiber (g)	Fat (g)	Sat (g)	Mono (g)	Poly (g)	Chol (mg)	Vit A (RE)
16260	Dinner, chicken, alfredo, w/broccoli, fzn, Healthy Choice	1 ea	326	300	25	34	2	7	3.0	—	—	50	20
56128	Dish, ravioli, cheese, w/tomato sauce, svg	1 ea	250	341	15	38	2	15	6.4	5.0	1.9	162	236
53432	Sauce, marinara	0.5 cup	127	120	2	20	2	4	1.0	—	—	0	50

Mexican Foods

Code	Food Name	Unit/ Amt	Wt (g)	Energy (kcal)	Prot (g)	Carb (g)	Fiber (g)	Fat (g)	Sat (g)	Mono (g)	Poly (g)	Chol (mg)	Vit A (RE)
90856	Beans, refried, fat free, cnd	0.5 cup	130	110	7	21	6	0	0.0	0.0	0.0	0	0
9096	Beans, refried, original, cnd	0.5 cup	128	100	6	18	5	2	1.0	—	—	0	0
9095	Beans, refried, spicy, cnd	0.5 cup	128	100	6	18	6	2	1.0	—	—	0	0
82019	Burrito, bean & cheese, ckd	1 ea	142	300	9	46	4	9	4 5	—	—	15	40
3770	Chicle, fresh, pulp	1 cup	241	200	1	48	13	3	0.5	1.3	0.0	0	14
7931	Chili Peppers, jalapeno, fresh	1 ea	14	4	0	1	0	0	0.0	0.0	0.0	0	11
45777	Dessert, Churro	1 ea	26	116	1	12	0	7	2.0	4.1	0.9	2	6
70150	Dinner, burrito, beef & bean, w/salsa, fzn	1 ea	305	540	24	62	8	22	9.2	8.8	1.8	49	81
1753	Dinner, enchilada & tamale, beef, combination ckd f/fzn	1 ea	312	450	10	56	9	20	8.0	—	—	30	150
56124	Dish, fajitas, beef	1 ea	223	399	23	36	3	18	5.5	7.6	3.5	45	43
56123	Dish, fajitas, chicken	1 ea	223	363	20	44	5	12	2.3	5.5	3.1	39	65
3634	Guava, fresh	0.5 cup	82	56	2	12	4	1	0.2	0.1	0.3	0	51
5224	Jicama, fresh	1 cup	120	46	1	11	—	0	0.0	0.0	0.1	0	2
20122	Mixed Drink, pina colada, non alcoholic, mix	1 ea	30	32	0	7	0	1	0.5	0.0	0.0	0	0
3199	Passion Fruit, purple, fresh	1 ea	18	17	0	4	2	0	0.0	0.0	0.1	0	23
3745	Plantain, fresh, med	1 ea	179	218	2	57	4	1	0.3	0.1	0.1	0	200
56122	Quesadilla	1 ea	54	183	6	18	1	10	3.5	3.4	2.2	13	41
42185	Rolls, Mexican, bolillo	1 ea	117	307	10	61	2	2	0.5	0.2	0.6	1	4
53676	Salsa	2 Tbs	30	10	0	2	0	0	0.0	0.0	0.0	0	0
53207	Salsa, chunky, restaurant style	2 Tbs	30	10	0	1	0	0	0.0	0.0	0.0	0	0
27127	Salsa, garden pepper, med	2 Tbs	31	10	0	2	0	0	0.0	0.0	0.0	0	10
53642	Salsa, green chili, mild	2 Tbs	30	8	0	1	0	0	—	—	—	0	14
53584	Salsa, hot, cnd	2 Tbs	32	5	0	2	0	0	0.0	0.0	0.0	0	20
53645	Salsa, picante, med	2 Tbs	30	8	0	1	0	0	—	—	—	0	14
53647	Salsa, ranchera, hot	2 Tbs	30	9	0	2	0	0	—	—	—	0	36
53686	Salsa, restaurant style	62 g	62	30	2	6	2	0	0.0	0.0	0.0	0	20
4017	Salsa, rstd garlic	68 g	68	30	2	6	2	0	0.0	0.0	0.0	0	20
53643	Salsa, suprema, med	2 Tbs	30	8	0	1	0	0	—	—	—	0	10
27123	Salsa, thick 'n chunky, med	2 Tbs	30	10	0	3	0	0	0.0	0.0	0.0	0	20
53640	Salsa, thick 'n chunky, med	2 Tbs	30	8	0	1	0	0	—	—	—	0	18
53245	Salsa, verde, med	2 Tbs	29	10	0	2	—	0	0.0	0.0	0.0	0	0
53103	Sauce, enchilada, green	1 cup	250	187	4	13	4	14	8.1	3.9	1.2	43	156

PAGE KEY: A-158 Granola Bars, Cereal Bars, Diet Bars, Scones, and Tarts A-158 Meals and Dishes A-162 Meats A-168 Nuts, Seeds, and Products A-170 Poultry A-172 Salad Dressings, Dips, and Mayonnaise A-172 Salads A-174 Sandwiches A-176 Sauces and Gravies A-176 Snack Foods—Chips, Pretzels, Popcorn A-178 Soups, Stews, and Chilis A-180 Spices, Flavors, and Seasonings A-182 Sports Bars and Drinks A-182 Supplemental Foods and Formulas A-184 Sweeteners and Sweet Substitutes A-184 Vegetables and Legumes A-198 Weight Loss Bars and Drinks A-200 Miscellaneous

Thia (mg)	Ribo (mg)	Niac (mg NE)	Vit B6 (mg)	Vit B12 (μg)	Fol (μg)	Vit C (mg)	Vit D (IU)	Vit E (mg AT)	Cal (mg)	Iron (mg)	Magn (mg)	Phos (mg)	Pota (mg)	Sodi (mg)	Zinc (mg)	Wat (%)	Alco (g)	Caff (g)
0.10	0.31	0.00	0.20	1.17	88.7	0.0	65.3	1.6	78	1.65	3.0	237	66	29	1.4	52	0.00	0.00
0.01	0.15	0.01	0.05	0.31	12.7	0.0	15.0	0.6	15	0.34	2.9	50	37	50	0.3	70	0.00	0.00
0.02	0.25	0.02	0.05	0.56	22.0	0.0	—	0.5	25	0.60	5.0	86	63	62	0.5	75	0.00	0.00
0.02	0.27	0.05	0.07	0.46	18.3	0.1	21.0	0.5	43	0.73	7.3	104	84	171	0.6	73	0.00	0.00
0.02	0.23	0.03	0.07	0.63	23.5	0.0	17.2	0.6	27	0.91	6.0	96	68	94	0.6	69	0.00	0.00
0.02	0.23	0.03	0.07	0.63	23.5	0.0	17.3	0.5	26	0.92	6.0	96	67	70	0.6	76	0.00	0.00
0.10	0.31	0.60	0.11	0.61	17.0	0.1	—	0.8	113	0.81	12.4	179	145	372	1.2	67	0.00	0.00
0.07	0.36	0.81	0.17	0.50	29.7	19.0	—	2.0	60	1.15	16.2	142	269	170	0.8	80	0.00	0.00
0.12	0.36	0.69	0.12	0.79	23.1	0.4	52.4	1.0	64	1.07	12.1	156	162	294	1.1	72	0.00	0.00
—	—	—	—	—	—	12.0	—	—	100	1.79	—	—	—	530	—	—	0.00	0.00
0.31	0.43	2.95	0.18	0.38	30.3	9.4	—	2.1	172	3.09	32.9	220	405	574	1.5	72	0.00	0.00
—	—	—	—	0.00	—	1.2	—	—	0	0.72	—	—	—	480	—	—	0.00	0.00
—	—	—	—	—	—	0.0	—	—	40	2.70	—	—	—	460	—	77	0.00	0.00
—	—	—	—	—	—	0.0	—	—	40	1.98	—	—	—	510	—	78	0.00	0.00
—	—	—	—	—	—	0.0	—	—	40	1.98	—	—	—	630	—	78	0.00	0.00
—	—	—	—	—	—	0.0	—	—	40	0.72	—	—	—	690	—	—	0.00	0.00
0.00	0.05	0.47	0.09	0.00	33.7	35.4	—	0.6	51	1.92	28.9	29	465	29	0.2	78	0.00	0.00
0.01	0.00	0.15	0.07	0.00	6.6	6.2	—	0.1	1	0.10	2.7	4	30	0	0.0	92	0.00	0.00
0.03	0.02	0.37	0.00	0.00	1.2	0.0	—	1.0	2	0.33	1.7	8	8	7	0.1	23	0.00	0.00
0.49	0.44	5.69	0.31	1.08	134.4	20.1	—	1.6	144	5.53	70.7	350	685	881	3.6	63	0.00	0.00
—	—	—	—	—	—	0.0	—	—	150	1.79	—	—	—	1530	—	—	0.00	0.00
0.38	0.30	5.40	0.37	2.05	23.0	26.8	—	1.7	84	3.75	37.6	238	479	316	3.5	65	0.00	0.00
0.43	0.33	6.11	0.37	0.10	41.8	36.8	—	1.7	101	3.31	48.2	188	534	343	1.6	65	0.00	0.00
0.05	0.02	0.88	0.09	0.00	40.4	188.3	—	0.6	15	0.20	18.1	33	344	2	0.2	81	0.00	0.00
0.01	0.02	0.23	0.05	0.00	14.4	24.2	—	0.5	14	0.72	14.4	22	180	5	0.2	90	0.00	0.00
0.00	0.00	0.03	0.00	0.00	3.5	1.5	0.0	0.0	3	0.05	2.3	7	21	2	0.0	75	0.00	0.00
0.00	0.01	0.27	0.01	0.00	2.5	5.4	—	0.0	2	0.28	5.2	12	63	5	0.0	73	0.00	0.00
0.09	0.10	1.23	0.54	0.00	39.4	32.9	—	0.3	5	1.07	66.2	61	893	7	0.3	65	0.00	0.00
0.12	0.14	1.09	0.03	0.05	5.8	14.7	—	1.0	132	1.21	13.4	107	77	230	0.6	35	0.00	0.00
0.69	0.46	6.59	0.03	0.00	41.1	0.0	0.3	0.1	14	3.80	22.1	90	98	7	0.8	37	0.00	0.00
—	—	—	—	—	—	2.4	—	—	0	0.00	—	—	55	115	—	92	0.00	0.00
—	—	—	—	—	—	0.0	—	—	0	0.00	—	—	—	140	—	95	0.00	0.00
—	—	—	—	—	—	0.0	—	—	0	0.00	—	—	—	240	—	91	0.00	0.00
—	—	—	—	—	—	4.1	—	—	5	0.28	—	—	—	175	—	92	0.00	0.00
—	—	—	—	—	—	2.4	—	—	0	0.00	—	—	95	170	—	92	0.00	0.00
—	—	—	—	—	—	2.5	—	—	4	0.01	—	—	—	150	—	92	0.00	0.00
—	—	—	—	—	—	1.3	—	—	5	0.03	—	—	—	171	—	91	0.00	0.00
—	—	—	—	—	—	1.2	—	—	0	0.36	—	—	—	420	—	85	0.00	0.00
—	—	—	—	—	—	1.2	—	—	20	0.00	—	—	—	460	—	—	0.00	0.00
—	—	—	—	—	—	1.5	—	—	3	0.01	—	—	—	166	—	92	0.00	0.00
—	—	—	—	—	—	0.0	—	—	0	0.00	—	—	—	230	—	88	0.00	0.00
—	—	—	—	—	—	4.4	—	—	6	0.05	—	—	—	160	—	92	0.00	0.00
—	—	—	—	—	—	0.0	—	—	0	0.00	—	—	—	95	—	91	0.00	0.00
0.09	0.15	2.92	0.18	0.14	13.3	23.1	0.0	0.9	77	1.17	41.4	118	540	30	0.6	87	0.00	0.00

PAGE KEY: A-108 Beverage and Beverage Mixes   A-110 Other Beverages   A-110 Beverages, Alcoholic   A-112 Candies and Confections, Gum   A-116 Cereals, Breakfast Type   A-120 Cheese and Cheese Substitutes   A-122 Dairy Products and Substitutes   A-124 Desserts   A-130 Dessert Toppings   A-130 Eggs, Substitutes, and Egg Dishes   A-132 Ethnic Foods   A-136 Fast Foods/Restaurants   A-150 Fats, Oils, Margarines, Shortenings, and Substitutes   A-150 Fish, Seafood, and Shellfish   A-152 Food Additives   A-152 Fruit, Vegetable, or Blended Juices   A-154 Grains, Flours, and Fractions   A-154 Grain Products, Prepared and Baked Goods

Code	Food Name	Unit/ Amt	Wt (g)	Energy (kcal)	Prot (g)	Carb (g)	Fiber (g)	Fat (g)	Sat (g)	Mono (g)	Poly (g)	Chol (mg)	Vit A (RE)
53102	Sauce, enchilada, red	1 cup	250	321	3	10	2	31	16.7	10.1	2.8	91	349
53224	Sauce, taco, thick & smooth, med	1 Tbs	16	10	0	2	0	0	0.0	0.0	0.0	0	0
91932	Seasoning, fajita	0.25 tsp	1	0	0	0	0	0	0.0	0.0	0.0	0	—
57531	Taco, sml	1 ea	171	369	21	27	—	21	11.4	6.6	1.0	56	139
56113	Tamale, w/meat	1 ea	70	134	6	11	1	7	2.6	3.1	1.0	19	14
5445	Tomatillo, fresh, med	1 ea	34	11	0	2	1	0	0.0	0.1	0.1	0	4
42023	Tortilla, corn, med, 6"	1 ea	26	57	1	12	2	1	0.1	0.2	0.4	0	0
90646	Tortilla, flour, 6"	1 ea	32	100	3	16	1	2	0.6	1.2	0.5	0	0
66017	Tostada, bean & cheese	1 ea	144	223	10	27	—	10	5.4	3.1	0.7	30	73
56645	Tostada, beef & cheese	1 ea	163	315	19	23	—	16	10.4	3.3	1.0	41	83
Asian Foods													
7084	Bean Cakes, Japanese style	1 ea	32	130	2	16	1	7	1.0	2.9	2.6	0	0
6459	Bean Sprouts, cnd, svg	1 ea	83	12	1	2	1	0	0.0	—	—	0	0
5654	Broccoli, stir fried	1 cup	156	44	5	8	5	1	0.1	0.0	0.3	0	216
1717	Dinner, stir fry, chicken & veg, oriental, fzn, Healthy Choice	1 ea	337	360	19	57	5	6	2.0	—	—	25	350
70455	Dish, beef, oriental style	1 ea	227	300	10	45	2	7	3.0	—	—	51	100
56094	Dish, chop suey, beef, w/noodles	1 cup	220	421	22	31	—	24	4.7	8.3	9.2	43	103
56234	Dish, chop suey, pork, w/noodles	1 cup	220	448	22	31	4	27	4.8	7.7	12.8	48	19
57618	Dish, chow mein, pork, w/noodles	1 cup	220	448	22	31	4	27	4.8	7.7	12.8	48	19
56238	Dish, chow mein, shrimp, w/noodles	1 cup	220	272	17	24	3	13	1.9	3.1	6.9	82	15
2999	Dish, duck curry, Thai, prep f/recipe, svg	1 ea	277	316	17	5	1	25	8.3	—	—	72	77
56288	Dish, egg foo yung, pork	1 ea	86	124	8	4	1	8	2.1	3.0	2.3	167	86
1991	Dish, green curry chicken, Thai, prep f/recipe, svg	1 ea	386	614	23	18	5	54	42.6	—	—	53	846
1998	Dish, peanut chicken w/rice, Thai, prep f/recipe, svg	1 ea	309	272	19	26	3	11	2.3	—	—	36	351
2998	Dish, potstickers, veal, Thai, prep f/recipe, svg	1 ea	244	647	27	99	4	14	5.0	—	—	58	26
2995	Dish, spring roll, vegetable, Thai, prep f/recipe	1 pce	63	158	4	20	1	7	0.9	—	—	3	140
2996	Dish, sweet noodles, Thai, prep f/recipe, svg	1 ea	142	339	14	37	2	15	2.4	—	—	121	66
3249	Java Plum, fresh	3 ea	9	5	0	1	—	0	—	—	—	0	0
7503	Miso	1 cup	275	547	32	73	15	17	3.1	3.4	8.8	0	22
7508	Natto	1 cup	175	371	31	25	9	19	2.8	4.3	10.9	0	0
38048	Pasta, chow mein noodles, dry	1 cup	45	237	4	26	2	14	2.0	3.5	7.8	0	0
5121	Peas, edible pod, fresh	10 ea	34	14	1	3	1	0	0.0	0.0	0.0	0	37
5666	Peas, snow, pods, stir fried	1 cup	165	69	5	12	4	0	0.1	0.0	0.1	0	21
5665	Peas, snow, pods, stmd	1 cup	165	69	5	12	4	0	0.1	0.0	0.1	0	23
38082	Rice, brown, med grain, ckd	0.5 cup	98	109	2	23	2	1	0.2	0.3	0.3	0	0
38021	Rice, wild, ckd	1 cup	164	166	7	35	3	1	0.1	0.1	0.3	0	0
38289	Rice, wild, dry	1 cup	160	571	24	120	10	2	0.2	0.3	1.1	0	3
1985	Salad, chicken, broiled, Thai, prep f/recipe, svg	1 ea	403	257	24	25	2	7	1.9	—	—	60	139
1987	Sauce, coconut, Thai, prep f/recipe, svg	1 ea	126	65	2	13	2	1	0.1	—	—	0	207
1999	Sauce, peanut, Thai, prep f/recipe, svg	0.75 cup	199	412	18	19	4	33	6.6	—	—	0	37
53461	Sauce, plum, rts	2 Tbs	38	70	0	16	0	0	0.1	0.1	0.2	0	2
53357	Sauce, sweet & sour, rts	2 Tbs	33	40	0	8	0	1	0.1	0.2	0.4	0	5
53004	Sauce, teriyaki, rts	1 Tbs	18	15	1	3	0	0	0.0	0.0	0.0	0	0
5253	Seaweed, agar, fresh	0.5 cup	40	10	0	3	0	0	0.0	0.0	0.0	0	0
50181	Soup, won ton	1 cup	241	182	14	14	1	7	2.3	3.0	1.0	53	99
91818	Sushi, California roll	1 ea	198	292	8	49	3	3	1.0	—	—	3	90

PAGE KEY: A-158 Granola Bars, Cereal Bars, Diet Bars, Scones, and Tarts   A-158 Meals and Dishes   A-162 Meats   A-168 Nuts, Seeds, and Products   A-170 Poultry   A-172 Salad Dressings, Dips, and Mayonnaise   A-172 Salads   A-174 Sandwiches   A-176 Sauces and Gravies   A-176 Snack Foods—Chips, Pretzels, Popcorn   A-178 Soups, Stews, and Chilis   A-180 Spices, Flavors, and Seasonings   A-182 Sports Bars and Drinks   A-182 Supplemental Foods and Formulas   A-184 Sweeteners and Sweet Substitutes   A-184 Vegetables and Legumes   A-198 Weight Loss Bars and Drinks   A-200 Miscellaneous

Thia (mg)	Ribo (mg)	Niac (mg NE)	Vit B6 (mg)	Vit B12 (µg)	Fol (µg)	Vit C (mg)	Vit D (IU)	Vit E (mg AT)	Cal (mg)	Iron (mg)	Magn (mg)	Phos (mg)	Pota (mg)	Sodi (mg)	Zinc (mg)	Wat (%)	Alco (g)	Caff (g)
0.07	0.12	0.74	0.14	0.10	17.0	20.3	0.0	1.6	55	0.62	20.0	76	336	36	0.3	82	0.00	0.00
—	—	—	—	—	—	0.0	—	—	0	0.36	—	—	40	125	—	85	0.00	0.00
—	—	—	—	—	—	—	—	—	—	—	—	—	—	130	—	—	0.00	0.00
0.15	0.43	3.21	0.23	1.03	68.4	2.2	—	1.9	221	2.41	70.1	203	474	802	3.9	58	0.00	0.00
0.17	0.14	2.49	0.09	0.17	4.5	1.0	—	0.3	24	1.41	20.7	67	140	84	0.9	64	0.00	0.00
0.00	0.00	0.62	0.01	0.00	2.4	4.0	—	0.1	2	0.20	6.8	13	91	0	0.1	92	0.00	0.00
0.01	0.01	0.38	0.05	0.00	1.3	0.0	—	0.1	21	0.31	18.7	82	48	12	0.3	46	0.00	0.00
0.17	0.09	1.13	0.01	0.00	33.3	0.0	—	0.1	41	1.07	7.0	40	50	204	0.2	30	0.00	0.00
0.10	0.33	1.32	0.15	0.68	43.2	1.3	—	1.2	210	1.88	59.0	117	403	543	1.9	66	0.00	0.00
0.10	0.55	3.15	0.23	1.16	75.0	2.6	—	—	217	2.86	63.6	179	572	896	3.7	62	0.00	0.00
0.07	0.05	0.55	0.01	0.00	9.1	0.0	0.0	1.2	3	0.67	6.1	21	58	1	0.2	23	0.00	0.00
—	—	—	—	0.00	—	14.2	—	—	10	0.25	—	—	—	20	—	96	0.00	0.00
0.09	0.18	0.93	0.23	0.00	88.5	123.4	0.0	0.7	75	1.37	39.0	103	505	42	0.6	91	0.00	0.00
—	—	—	—	—	—	4.8	—	—	40	2.70	—	—	—	600	—	—	0.00	0.00
—	—	—	—	—	—	18.0	—	—	60	2.70	—	—	—	1220	—	—	0.00	0.00
0.36	0.37	5.73	0.38	1.67	43.8	20.1	—	1.8	39	4.19	54.2	262	519	950	3.5	63	0.00	0.00
0.77	0.43	6.23	0.41	0.41	41.8	20.2	—	2.7	45	3.29	52.8	249	489	848	2.6	62	0.00	0.00
0.77	0.43	6.23	0.41	0.41	41.8	20.2	—	2.7	45	3.29	52.8	249	489	848	2.6	62	0.00	0.00
0.23	0.23	4.46	0.18	0.58	45.1	9.4	—	1.3	58	3.42	51.2	220	391	710	1.3	74	0.00	0.00
0.15	0.25	4.46	0.23	0.28	8.9	5.0	10.2	0.6	72	2.94	77.8	204	742	602	1.7	80	0.00	0.00
0.12	0.25	0.79	0.14	0.40	22.3	3.2	—	1.1	27	0.81	11.9	105	157	131	0.9	75	0.00	0.00
0.15	0.17	7.65	0.49	0.23	57.0	91.5	7.1	2.0	65	7.82	140.7	331	866	889	2.6	74	0.00	0.00
0.21	0.11	8.25	0.47	0.14	66.1	67.3	5.1	1.7	42	2.66	48.0	191	344	901	1.2	81	0.00	0.00
0.87	0.72	12.23	0.21	0.57	145.1	1.8	5.1	1.4	106	6.73	50.2	238	329	1020	2.9	41	0.00	0.00
0.18	0.14	1.87	0.02	0.00	31.7	0.9	8.2	1.3	58	1.77	11.9	42	75	263	0.4	49	0.00	0.00
0.07	0.09	1.01	0.14	0.56	15.2	4.6	50.8	1.6	277	2.92	40.1	170	176	377	1.3	50	0.00	0.00
0.00	0.00	0.01	0.00	0.00	—	1.3	—	—	2	0.01	1.4	2	7	1	0.0	83	0.00	0.00
0.27	0.63	2.49	0.55	0.21	52.2	0.0	—	0.0	157	6.84	112.0	437	578	10252	7.0	43	0.00	0.00
0.28	0.33	0.00	0.23	0.00	14.0	22.8	—	0.0	380	15.05	201.2	304	1276	12	5.3	55	0.00	0.00
0.25	0.18	2.68	0.05	0.00	40.5	0.0	—	1.6	9	2.13	23.4	72	54	198	0.6	1	0.00	0.00
0.05	0.02	0.20	0.05	0.00	14.3	20.4	—	0.1	15	0.70	8.2	18	68	1	0.1	89	0.00	0.00
0.21	0.12	0.93	0.25	0.00	55.1	84.2	0.0	0.6	71	3.43	39.6	87	330	7	0.4	89	0.00	0.00
0.21	0.12	0.93	0.23	0.00	58.4	84.2	0.0	0.6	71	3.43	39.6	87	330	7	0.4	89	0.00	0.00
0.10	0.00	1.29	0.15	0.00	3.9	0.0	—	0.2	10	0.51	42.9	75	77	1	0.6	73	0.00	0.00
0.09	0.14	2.10	0.21	0.00	42.6	0.0	—	0.4	5	0.98	52.5	134	166	5	2.2	74	0.00	0.00
0.18	0.41	10.77	0.62	0.00	152.0	0.0	—	1.3	34	3.14	283.2	693	683	11	9.5	8	0.00	0.00
0.15	0.15	10.36	0.56	0.25	29.1	27.3	8.6	0.7	38	2.00	48.7	208	511	1637	1.1	85	0.00	0.00
0.05	0.05	0.85	0.02	0.00	6.9	5.0	0.0	0.1	33	0.74	17.2	27	319	82	0.2	85	0.00	0.00
0.09	0.14	10.18	0.44	0.00	55.1	2.2	0.0	6.4	40	2.13	107.8	297	544	3376	2.1	60	0.00	0.00
0.00	0.02	0.38	0.02	0.00	2.3	0.2	—	0.1	5	0.55	4.6	8	99	205	0.1	54	0.00	0.00
0.00	0.00	0.07	0.00	0.00	0.7	0.0	—	0.1	6	0.28	2.3	3	22	116	0.0	71	0.00	0.00
0.00	0.00	0.23	0.01	0.00	3.6	0.0	—	0.0	4	0.31	11.0	28	40	690	0.0	68	0.00	0.00
0.00	0.00	0.01	0.00	0.00	34.0	0.0	—	0.3	22	0.74	26.8	2	90	4	0.2	91	0.00	0.00
0.40	0.25	4.59	0.20	0.40	18.8	3.4	—	0.4	31	1.75	20.6	153	316	543	1.1	84	0.00	0.00
—	—	—	—	—	—	4.8	—	—	20	1.08	—	—	—	952	—	—	0.00	0.00

PAGE KEY: A-108 Beverage and Beverage Mixes   A-110 Other Beverages   A-110 Beverages, Alcoholic   A-112 Candies and Confections, Gum   A-116 Cereals, Breakfast Type   A-120 Cheese and Cheese Substitutes   A-122 Dairy Products and Substitutes   A-124 Desserts   A-130 Dessert Toppings   A-130 Eggs, Substitutes, and Egg Dishes   A-132 Ethnic Foods   A-136 Fast Foods/Restaurants   A-150 Fats, Oils, Margarines, Shortenings, and Substitutes   A-150 Fish, Seafood, and Shellfish   A-152 Food Additives   A-152 Fruit, Vegetable, or Blended Juices   A-154 Grains, Flours, and Fractions   A-154 Grain Products, Prepared and Baked Goods

Code	Food Name	Unit/ Amt	Wt (g)	Energy (kcal)	Prot (g)	Carb (g)	Fiber (g)	Fat (g)	Sat (g)	Mono (g)	Poly (g)	Chol (mg)	Vit A (RE)
91814	Sushi, cucumber roll	6 pce	85	120	3	25	2	1	0.0	—	—	0	50
92378	Sushi, krab roll	6 pce	112	150	7	30	2	1	0.0	—	—	3	60
56313	Sushi, w/veg & fish	3 oz	85	119	5	24	1	0	0.1	0.1	0.1	6	70
6880	Sweetpotatoes, fresh, cubes	1 cup	133	114	2	27	4	0	0.0	0.0	0.0	0	1886
6206	Vegetables, Japanese style, fzn	0.5 cup	127	78	2	8	2	5	2.3	—	—	12	96
6208	Vegetables, Japanese style, stir fry, fzn	0.5 cup	116	35	2	7	2	0	0.0	—	—	0	74
57294	Vegetables, oriental style, stir fry, fzn	0.5 cup	54	41	2	7	0	1	0.1	—	—	0	38
6646	Vegetables, pepper style, stir fry, fzn	0.5 cup	54	15	0	3	0	0	0.0	—	—	0	23
6592	Vegetables, teriyaki, marinated/seasoned, fzn	1.25 cup	110	100	2	7	2	7	1.0	—	—	0	500
6460	Waterchestnuts, slices, cnd	100 g	100	50	1	12	5	0	0.0	—	—	0	0
5222	Watercress, fresh, chpd	1 cup	34	4	1	0	0	0	0.0	0.0	0.0	0	160
49116	Wrappers, egg roll, 7" square	1 ea	32	93	3	19	1	0	0.1	0.1	0.2	3	1

FAST FOODS/RESTAURANTS

Generic Fast Food

Code	Food Name	Unit/ Amt	Wt (g)	Energy (kcal)	Prot (g)	Carb (g)	Fiber (g)	Fat (g)	Sat (g)	Mono (g)	Poly (g)	Chol (mg)	Vit A (RE)
56654	Cheeseburger, double, double bun, reg, w/condiments & veg	1 ea	228	650	30	53	—	35	12.8	12.6	6.4	93	84
56648	Cheeseburger, lrg, plain	1 ea	185	609	30	47	—	33	14.8	12.7	2.4	96	185
66015	Cheeseburger, reg, w/condiments & veg	1 ea	154	359	18	28	—	20	9.2	7.2	1.5	52	91
6175	Dish, corn, cob, w/butter	1 ea	146	155	4	32	—	3	1.6	1.0	0.6	6	51
6185	Dish, mashed potatoes	0.5 cup	121	100	3	20	—	1	0.6	0.4	0.4	2	15
17187	Fish, fillet, brd/batter fried	3 oz	85	197	12	14	0	10	2.4	2.2	5.3	29	9
42353	French Toast, w/butter	2 pce	135	356	10	36	0	19	7.7	7.1	2.4	116	138
66007	Hamburger, reg, plain	1 ea	90	274	12	31	—	12	4.1	5.5	0.9	35	0
2022	Milk Shake, strawberry, fast food	1 cup	283	320	10	53	1	8	4.9	2.2	0.3	31	74
2024	Milk Shake, vanilla, fast food	1 cup	166	185	6	30	0	5	3.1	1.4	0.2	18	63
56639	Nachos, w/cheese	7 pce	113	346	9	36	—	19	7.8	8.0	2.2	18	154
6176	Onion Rings, breaded, fried, svg	8 pce	78	259	3	29	—	15	6.5	6.3	0.6	13	2
45122	Pancakes, w/butter & syrup	1 ea	116	260	4	45	1	7	2.9	2.6	1.0	29	41
5463	Potatoes, hash browns	0.5 cup	72	151	2	16	—	9	4.3	3.9	0.5	9	3
6173	Salad, potato	0.333 cup	95	108	1	13	—	6	1.0	1.6	2.9	57	28
56623	Salad, tossed, veg, w/o dressing	1.5 cup	207	33	3	7	—	0	0.0	0.0	0.1	0	236
56601	Sandwich, breakfast, egg bacon, w/biscuit	1 ea	150	458	17	29	1	31	8.0	13.4	7.5	352	108
56602	Sandwich, breakfast, egg ham, w/biscuit	1 ea	192	442	20	30	1	27	5.9	11.0	7.7	300	240
56600	Sandwich, breakfast, egg, w/biscuit	1 ea	136	373	12	32	1	22	4.7	9.1	6.4	245	181
56606	Sandwich, croissant, w/egg & cheese	1 ea	127	368	13	24	—	25	14.1	7.5	1.4	216	282
56607	Sandwich, croissant, w/egg, cheese & bacon	1 ea	129	413	16	24	—	28	15.4	9.2	1.8	215	142
66031	Sandwich, english muffin, w/cheese & sausage	1 ea	115	393	15	29	1	24	9.9	10.1	2.7	59	104
56604	Sandwich, ham, w/biscuit	1 ea	113	386	13	44	1	18	11.4	4.8	1.0	25	33

A&W Restaurants

Code	Food Name	Unit/ Amt	Wt (g)	Energy (kcal)	Prot (g)	Carb (g)	Fiber (g)	Fat (g)	Sat (g)	Mono (g)	Poly (g)	Chol (mg)	Vit A (RE)
81303	Cheeseburger	1 ea	191	500	28	43	3	24	9.0	—	—	90	200
81305	Cheeseburger, deluxe, w/bacon	1 ea	278	600	32	44	4	33	12.0	—	—	110	250
81319	Dish, french fries, cheese, svg	1 ea	170	390	4	50	4	19	5.0	—	—	5	0
81352	Frozen Dessert, Oreo, med, A&W Polar Swirl	1 ea	397	833	16	125	2	30	11.7	—	—	54	350
81330	Frozen Dessert, sundae, hot fudge, A&W	1 ea	189	350	8	54	1	11	6.0	—	—	30	150
81311	Hamburger	1 ea	177	460	26	39	3	22	8.0	—	—	75	40
81314	Hot Dog, cheese, w/bun	1 ea	126	320	11	25	1	20	7.0	—	—	40	20
81315	Hot Dog, chili & cheese, w/bun	1 ea	154	350	13	27	2	21	8.0	—	—	45	40

PAGE KEY: A-158 Granola Bars, Cereal Bars, Diet Bars, Scones, and Tarts   A-158 Meals and Dishes   A-162 Meats   A-168 Nuts, Seeds, and Products   A-170 Poultry   A-172 Salad Dressings, Dips, and Mayonnaise   A-172 Salads   A-174 Sandwiches   A-176 Sauces and Gravies   A-176 Snack Foods—Chips, Pretzels, Popcorn   A-178 Soups, Stews, and Chilis   A-180 Spices, Flavors, and Seasonings   A-182 Sports Bars and Drinks   A-182 Supplemental Foods and Formulas   A-184 Sweeteners and Sweet Substitutes   A-184 Vegetables and Legumes   A-198 Weight Loss Bars and Drinks   A-200 Miscellaneous

Thia (mg)	Ribo (mg)	Niac (mg NE)	Vit B6 (mg)	Vit B12 (µg)	Fol (µg)	Vit C (mg)	Vit D (IU)	Vit E (mg AT)	Cal (mg)	Iron (mg)	Magn (mg)	Phos (mg)	Pota (mg)	Sodi (mg)	Zinc (mg)	Wat (%)	Alco (g)	Caff (g)
—	—	—	—	—	—	0.0	—	—	0	0.36	—	—	—	90	—	65	0.00	0.00
—	—	—	—	—	—	0.0	—	—	0	0.36	—	—	—	240	—	—	0.00	0.00
0.14	0.03	1.51	0.07	0.17	7.9	2.0	—	0.3	13	1.19	13.7	56	112	48	0.4	65	0.03	0.00
0.10	0.07	0.74	0.28	0.00	14.6	3.2	—	0.3	40	0.81	33.2	63	448	73	0.4	77	0.00	0.00
0.05	0.09	0.37	0.10	0.00	35.4	44.4	—	—	40	0.69	21.6	50	179	320	—	—	0.00	0.00
—	—	—	—	—	—	32.4	—	—	31	0.70	15.1	42	191	439	—	—	0.00	0.00
—	—	—	—	0.00	—	5.6	—	—	33	0.27	—	—	—	281	—	—	0.00	0.00
—	—	—	—	0.00	—	9.1	—	—	3	0.10	—	—	—	9	—	—	0.00	0.00
—	—	—	—	0.00	—	21.0	—	—	20	0.00	—	—	—	510	—	—	0.00	0.00
—	—	—	—	0.00	—	0.0	—	—	3	0.27	—	—	—	12	—	86	0.00	0.00
0.02	0.03	0.07	0.03	0.00	3.1	14.6	—	0.3	41	0.07	7.1	20	112	14	0.0	95	0.00	0.00
0.17	0.11	1.74	0.00	0.00	27.5	0.0	—	0.0	15	1.08	6.4	26	26	183	0.2	29	0.00	0.00
0.56	0.43	8.34	0.27	2.06	91.2	2.7	—	2.0	169	4.71	36.5	349	390	921	4.1	47	0.00	0.00
0.47	0.56	11.17	0.28	2.52	74.0	0.0	22.2	—	91	5.46	38.9	422	644	1589	5.6	39	0.00	0.00
0.31	0.23	6.38	0.15	1.23	64.7	2.3	—	1.3	182	2.65	26.2	216	229	976	2.6	55	0.00	0.00
0.25	0.10	2.18	0.31	0.00	43.8	6.9	—	—	4	0.87	40.9	108	359	29	0.9	72	0.00	0.00
0.10	0.05	1.45	0.28	0.05	9.7	0.5	—	—	25	0.56	21.8	67	356	275	0.4	79	0.00	0.00
0.09	0.09	1.78	0.09	0.93	14.5	0.0	—	—	15	1.78	20.4	145	272	452	0.4	54	0.00	0.00
0.57	0.50	3.92	0.05	0.36	72.9	0.1	—	—	73	1.88	16.2	146	177	513	0.6	51	0.00	0.00
0.33	0.27	3.72	0.05	0.88	53.1	0.0	10.8	0.5	63	2.40	18.9	103	145	387	2.0	38	0.00	0.00
0.12	0.55	0.50	0.11	0.87	8.5	2.3	22.6	0.4	320	0.31	36.8	283	515	235	1.0	74	0.00	0.00
0.07	0.30	0.31	0.09	0.60	8.3	1.3	60.6	0.1	203	0.15	20.0	170	290	136	0.6	75	0.00	0.00
0.18	0.37	1.53	0.20	0.81	10.2	1.2	—	—	272	1.27	55.4	276	172	816	1.8	40	0.00	0.00
0.07	0.09	0.87	0.05	0.11	51.6	0.5	—	0.3	69	0.80	14.8	81	122	405	0.3	37	0.00	0.00
0.20	0.28	1.69	0.05	0.11	25.5	1.7	—	0.7	64	1.30	24.4	238	125	552	0.5	50	0.00	0.00
0.07	0.00	1.07	0.17	0.00	7.9	5.5	—	0.1	7	0.47	15.8	69	267	290	0.2	60	0.00	0.00
0.07	0.10	0.25	0.14	0.10	23.8	1.0	—	—	13	0.68	7.6	53	256	312	0.2	79	0.00	0.00
0.05	0.10	1.13	0.17	0.00	76.6	48.0	—	—	27	1.29	22.8	81	356	54	0.4	96	0.00	0.00
0.14	0.23	2.40	0.14	1.02	60.0	2.7	—	2.0	189	3.74	24.0	238	250	999	1.6	47	0.00	0.00
0.67	0.60	2.00	0.27	1.19	65.3	0.0	—	2.3	221	4.55	30.7	317	319	1382	2.2	55	0.00	0.00
0.30	0.49	2.15	0.10	0.62	57.1	0.1	—	3.3	82	2.90	19.0	388	238	891	1.0	50	0.00	0.00
0.18	0.37	1.50	0.10	0.76	47.0	0.1	—	—	244	2.20	21.6	348	174	551	1.8	45	0.00	0.00
0.34	0.34	2.19	0.11	0.86	45.1	2.2	—	—	151	2.19	23.2	276	201	889	1.9	44	0.00	0.00
0.69	0.25	4.13	0.15	0.68	66.7	1.3	—	1.3	168	2.25	24.1	186	215	1036	1.7	38	0.00	0.00
0.50	0.31	3.48	0.14	0.02	38.4	0.1	—	1.7	160	2.72	22.6	554	197	1433	1.6	28	0.00	0.00
—	—	—	—	—	—	2.4	—	—	150	4.50	—	—	—	870	—	—	0.00	0.00
—	—	—	—	—	—	6.0	—	—	200	5.40	—	—	—	1390	—	—	0.00	0.00
—	—	—	—	—	—	18.0	—	—	40	0.00	—	—	—	880	—	—	0.00	0.00
—	—	—	—	—	—	0.0	—	—	467	4.19	—	—	—	646	—	—	0.00	—
—	—	—	—	—	—	0.0	—	—	200	0.36	—	—	—	140	—	60	0.00	—
—	—	—	—	—	—	2.4	—	—	100	4.50	—	—	—	690	—	—	0.00	0.00
—	—	—	—	—	—	1.2	—	—	60	1.44	—	—	—	920	—	—	0.00	0.00
—	—	—	—	—	—	1.2	—	—	80	1.79	—	—	—	1080	—	—	0.00	0.00

PAGE KEY: A-108 Beverage and Beverage Mixes A-110 Other Beverages A-110 Beverages, Alcoholic A-112 Candies and Confections, Gum A-116 Cereals, Breakfast Type A-120 Cheese and Cheese Substitutes A-122 Dairy Products and Substitutes A-124 Desserts A-130 Dessert Toppings A-130 Eggs, Substitutes, and Egg Dishes A-132 Ethnic Foods A-136 Fast Foods/Restaurants A-150 Fats, Oils, Margarines, Shortenings, and Substitutes A-150 Fish, Seafood, and Shellfish A-152 Food Additives A-152 Fruit, Vegetable, or Blended Juices A-154 Grains, Flours, and Fractions A-154 Grain Products, Prepared and Baked Goods

Code	Food Name	Unit/ Amt	Wt (g)	Energy (kcal)	Prot (g)	Carb (g)	Fiber (g)	Fat (g)	Sat (g)	Mono (g)	Poly (g)	Chol (mg)	Vit A (RE)
81317	Hot Dog, w/bun	1 ea	90	280	11	22	1	17	6.0	—	—	35	20
81341	Ice Cream Float, root beer, med	1 ea	467	330	4	70	0	4	2.5	—	—	15	100
81348	Milk Shake, chocolate, med, A&W	1 ea	475	700	11	100	2	29	18.1	—	—	125	312
81358	Milk Shake, vanilla, med, A&W	1 ea	475	719	12	97	0	31	18.8	—	—	134	250
81343	Potatoes, french fries, sml svg	1 ea	113	313	4	45	4	13	3.3	—	—	0	0
81310	Sandwich, chicken, grilled	1 ea	262	430	37	37	4	15	3.5	—	—	90	40
Arby's													
42433	Biscuit, w/butter	1 ea	82	280	5	27	0	17	4.0	—	—	0	—
9008	Cheese, mozzarella sticks, 4.8 oz svg	1 ea	137	470	18	34	2	29	14.0	—	—	60	—
9011	Chicken, finger, 4 pack	1 ea	192	640	31	42	0	38	8.0	—	—	70	—
9009	Onion, petals	4 oz	113	410	4	43	2	24	3.5	—	—	0	—
8986	Potatoes, french fries, curly, med svg	1 ea	128	400	5	50	4	19	4.5	—	—	0	0
8997	Salad, caesar	1 ea	223	90	7	8	3	4	2.5	—	—	10	—
52074	Salad, garden	1 ea	349	70	4	14	6	1	0.0	—	—	0	518
8988	Sandwich, beef melt, w/cheddar	1 ea	150	320	16	36	2	14	6.0	—	—	45	—
69045	Sandwich, beef, Arby Q	1 ea	186	360	16	40	2	14	4.0	—	—	70	—
69055	Sandwich, beef, philly & swiss cheese, submarine	1 ea	311	670	36	46	4	40	16.0	—	—	75	—
56341	Sandwich, chicken, breast fillet	1 ea	208	550	24	47	2	30	5.0	—	—	90	—
69095	Sandwich, chicken, cordon bleu	1 ea	242	630	34	47	2	35	8.0	14.4	12.6	120	—
69046	Sandwich, chicken, grilled, deluxe	1 ea	252	450	29	37	2	22	4.0	—	—	110	88
69043	Sandwich, French dip, submarine	1 ea	285	410	28	43	2	16	9.0	—	—	45	—
56342	Sandwich, ham swiss, hot	1 ea	170	340	23	35	1	13	4.5	—	—	90	40
8992	Sandwich, roast beef swiss	1 ea	360	780	37	74	6	40	14.0	—	—	80	—
56336	Sandwich, roast beef, regular	1 ea	157	330	21	35	2	14	7.0	—	—	45	0
53256	Sauce, Arbys, pkt	1 ea	14	15	0	4	0	0	0.0	0.0	0.0	0	—
9025	Sauce, honey mustard, dipping	1 oz	28	130	0	5	0	12	1.5	—	—	10	—
Boston Market													
52109	Cole Slaw, svg	1 ea	430	310	7	29	10	22	3.0	—	—	20	—
57529	Dish, macaroni & cheese, svg	1 ea	192	280	13	33	1	11	6.0	—	—	30	—
7390	Dish, mashed potatoes, homestyle, svg	1 ea	173	210	4	30	2	9	5.0	—	—	25	—
57528	Dish, mashed potatoes, w/gravy, homestyle, svg	1 ea	201	230	4	32	3	9	5.0	—	—	25	—
57530	Dish, pot pie, chicken, original, svg	1 ea	425	750	26	57	2	46	14.0	—	—	110	—
53541	Gravy, chicken, 1 oz svg	1 ea	28	15	0	2	0	0	0.0	—	—	0	—
52104	Salad, caesar, svg	1 ea	269	470	14	17	3	40	9.0	—	—	35	—
1143	Sandwich, marinated grilled chicken	1 ea	284	670	42	45	2	36	6.0	—	—	105	—
50299	Soup, chicken noodle, hearty, svg	1 cup	190	100	6	8	0	4	1.5	—	—	30	—
7391	Spinach, creamed, svg	1 ea	181	260	9	11	2	20	13.0	—	—	55	—
Burger King													
56352	Cheeseburger	1 ea	136	370	20	31	2	18	9.0	—	—	55	60
57001	Cheeseburger, double	1 ea	197	570	35	32	2	34	17.0	—	—	110	100
56355	Cheeseburger, Whopper	1 ea	303	780	34	55	4	47	17.0	—	—	105	150
57000	Cheeseburger, Whopper Jr	1 ea	180	460	21	33	2	27	10.0	—	—	60	80
9087	Chicken, Tenders, 4 pce svg	1 ea	62	170	11	10	0	9	3.0	—	—	25	0
42429	French Toast, sticks, svg	1 ea	112	390	6	46	2	20	4.5	—	—	0	0
56351	Hamburger	1 ea	123	320	18	30	2	14	6.0	—	—	45	20
56354	Hamburger, Whopper	1 ea	278	680	29	53	4	39	12.0	—	—	80	100

PAGE KEY: A-158 Granola Bars, Cereal Bars, Diet Bars, Scones, and Tarts   A-158 Meals and Dishes   A-162 Meats   A-168 Nuts, Seeds, and Products   A-170 Poultry   A-172 Salad Dressings, Dips, and Mayonnaise   A-172 Salads   A-174 Sandwiches   A-176 Sauces and Gravies   A-176 Snack Foods—Chips, Pretzels, Popcorn   A-178 Soups, Stews, and Chilis   A-180 Spices, Flavors, and Seasonings   A-182 Sports Bars and Drinks   A-182 Supplemental Foods and Formulas   A-184 Sweeteners and Sweet Substitutes   A-184 Vegetables and Legumes   A-198 Weight Loss Bars and Drinks   A-200 Miscellaneous

Thia (mg)	Ribo (mg)	Niac (mg NE)	Vit B6 (mg)	Vit B12 (µg)	Fol (µg)	Vit C (mg)	Vit D (IU)	Vit E (mg AT)	Cal (mg)	Iron (mg)	Magn (mg)	Phos (mg)	Pota (mg)	Sodi (mg)	Zinc (mg)	Wat (%)	Alco (g)	Caff (g)
—	—	—	—	—	—	0.0	—	—	40	1.44	—	—	—	710	—	—	0.00	0.00
—	—	—	—	—	—	0.0	—	—	150	0.36	—	—	—	120	—	—	0.00	0.00
—	—	—	—	—	—	0.0	—	—	281	1.69	—	—	—	200	—	—	0.00	—
—	—	—	—	—	—	0.0	—	—	438	1.69	—	—	—	212	—	—	0.00	0.00
—	—	—	—	—	—	19.6	—	—	0	0.00	—	—	—	465	—	—	0.00	0.00
—	—	—	—	—	—	6.0	—	—	100	3.59	—	—	—	1080	—	—	0.00	0.00
0.23	0.14	3.00	—	—	—	0.0	—	—	40	0.00	—	—	130	780	—	—	0.00	0.00
—	—	—	—	—	—	1.2	—	—	400	0.72	—	—	—	1330	—	—	0.00	0.00
—	—	—	—	—	—	0.0	—	—	20	2.70	—	—	—	1590	—	—	0.00	0.00
—	—	—	—	—	—	0.0	—	—	40	0.72	—	—	—	300	—	—	0.00	0.00
0.07	0.09	2.57	—	0.00	—	15.5	—	—	0	1.86	—	—	934	993	0.8	41	0.00	0.00
—	—	—	—	—	—	42.0	—	—	200	1.79	—	—	—	170	—	—	0.00	0.00
0.17	0.20	1.26	—	—	—	42.0	—	—	80	1.44	—	—	635	45	0.9	—	0.00	0.00
—	—	—	—	—	—	0.0	—	—	80	2.70	—	—	—	850	—	—	0.00	0.00
0.25	0.37	9.00	—	—	—	4.8	—	—	80	3.59	—	—	456	1530	—	—	0.00	0.00
0.44	0.72	13.89	—	—	—	9.0	—	—	300	2.70	—	—	646	1850	5.9	—	0.00	0.00
0.23	0.56	9.17	0.38	—	18.4	3.6	—	—	80	1.79	30.6	184	336	1160	0.2	—	0.00	0.00
0.44	0.68	10.97	—	—	—	1.2	—	—	200	0.89	—	—	499	1820	2.4	—	0.00	0.00
0.34	0.31	14.89	—	—	—	1.2	—	—	60	2.70	—	—	722	1050	—	—	0.00	0.00
0.36	0.87	15.55	—	—	—	1.2	—	—	80	4.50	—	—	679	1200	—	—	0.00	0.00
0.81	0.37	7.80	0.31	—	26.0	1.2	—	—	150	2.70	31.0	405	382	1450	0.9	—	0.00	0.00
—	—	—	—	—	—	2.4	—	—	200	2.70	—	—	—	1690	—	—	0.00	0.00
—	—	—	—	—	—	0.0	—	—	60	3.59	16.2	122	427	890	3.8	—	0.00	0.00
—	—	—	—	—	—	1.2	—	—	0	0.00	—	—	28	180	—	—	0.00	0.00
—	—	—	—	—	—	0.0	—	—	0	0.00	—	—	—	160	—	—	0.00	0.00
—	—	—	—	—	—	—	—	—	—	—	—	—	—	230	—	—	0.00	0.00
—	—	—	—	—	—	—	—	—	—	—	—	—	—	890	—	—	0.00	0.00
—	—	—	—	—	—	—	—	—	—	—	—	—	—	590	—	74	0.00	0.00
—	—	—	—	—	—	—	—	—	—	—	—	—	—	780	—	—	0.00	0.00
—	—	—	—	—	—	—	—	—	—	—	—	—	—	1530	—	—	0.00	0.00
—	—	—	—	—	—	—	—	—	—	—	—	—	—	180	—	89	0.00	0.00
—	—	—	—	—	—	—	—	—	—	—	—	—	—	1070	—	—	0.00	0.00
—	—	—	—	—	—	—	—	—	—	—	—	—	—	810	—	—	0.00	0.00
—	—	—	—	—	—	—	—	—	—	—	—	—	—	500	—	89	0.00	0.00
—	—	—	—	—	—	—	—	—	—	—	—	—	—	740	—	—	0.00	0.00
—	—	—	—	—	—	0.0	—	—	150	2.70	—	—	—	750	—	—	0.00	0.00
—	—	—	—	—	—	0.0	—	—	250	4.50	—	—	—	1020	—	—	0.00	0.00
—	—	—	—	—	—	9.0	—	—	250	5.40	—	—	—	1390	—	—	0.00	0.00
—	—	—	—	—	—	4.8	—	—	150	3.59	—	—	—	740	—	—	0.00	0.00
—	—	—	—	—	—	0.0	—	—	0	0.36	—	—	—	420	—	—	0.00	0.00
—	—	—	—	—	—	0.0	—	—	60	1.79	—	—	—	440	—	—	0.00	0.00
—	—	—	—	—	—	0.0	—	—	80	2.70	—	—	—	530	—	—	0.00	0.00
—	—	—	—	—	—	9.0	—	—	100	5.40	—	—	—	940	—	—	0.00	0.00

PAGE KEY: A-108 Beverage and Beverage Mixes   A-110 Other Beverages   A-110 Beverages, Alcoholic   A-112 Candies and Confections, Gum   A-116 Cereals, Breakfast Type   A-120 Cheese and Cheese Substitutes   A-122 Dairy Products and Substitutes   A-124 Desserts   A-130 Dessert Toppings   A-130 Eggs, Substitutes, and Egg Dishes   A-132 Ethnic Foods   A-136 Fast Foods/Restaurants   A-150 Fats, Oils, Margarines, Shortenings, and Substitutes   A-150 Fish, Seafood, and Shellfish   A-152 Food Additives   A-152 Fruit, Vegetable, or Blended Juices   A-154 Grains, Flours, and Fractions   A-154 Grain Products, Prepared and Baked Goods

Code	Food Name	Unit/ Amt	Wt (g)	Energy (kcal)	Prot (g)	Carb (g)	Fiber (g)	Fat (g)	Sat (g)	Mono (g)	Poly (g)	Chol (mg)	Vit A (RE)
56999	Hamburger, Whopper Jr	1 ea	167	410	18	32	2	23	7.0	—	—	50	40
9041	Onion Rings, lrg	1 ea	137	480	7	60	5	23	6.0	—	—	0	0
56362	Sandwich, Big Fish	1 ea	263	710	24	67	4	38	14.0	—	—	50	20
56360	Sandwich, chicken	1 ea	224	660	25	53	3	39	8.0	—	—	70	20
9057	Sandwich, chicken tenders	1 ea	148	450	14	37	2	27	5.0	—	—	30	40
Carl's Junior													
91433	Burrito, breakfast	1 ea	185	480	27	26	2	30	13.0	—	—	465	150
91404	Cheeseburger, Western Bacon	1 ea	225	650	32	63	2	30	12.0	—	—	80	40
91419	Chicken, nuggets, Chicken Stars, svg	1 ea	90	280	12	15	0	19	4.5	—	—	40	0
91421	Dish, baked potato bacon cheese, Great Stuff	1 ea	411	630	20	76	6	29	7.0	—	—	35	150
91406	Hamburger, Jr	1 ea	134	330	18	34	1	13	5.0	—	—	45	0
91403	Hamburger, Super Star	1 ea	345	790	42	49	2	46	14.0	—	—	130	100
91414	Potatoes, french fries, svg	1 ea	92	290	5	37	3	14	3.0	—	—	0	0
91425	Salad, garden, Salad To Go	1 ea	137	50	3	4	2	2	1.5	—	—	10	600
91407	Sandwich, chicken, bbq, charbroiled	1 ea	199	280	25	37	2	3	1.0	—	—	60	60
91411	Sandwich, chicken, crispy, bacon swiss	1 ea	291	720	32	66	3	36	10.0	—	—	75	80
91413	Sandwich, fish, Carl's Catch	1 ea	201	510	18	50	1	27	7.0	—	—	80	60
Chick-Fil-A													
69188	Chicken, breast, fillet, brd	1 ea	105	230	23	10	0	11	2.5	—	—	60	40
52139	Salad, carrot raisin, sml	1 ea	91	130	1	22	2	5	1.0	—	—	0	1700
52135	Salad, Chick-N-Strips	1 ea	315	340	30	19	3	16	5.0	—	—	85	600
69152	Sandwich, chicken	1 ea	170	410	28	38	1	16	3.5	—	—	60	40
69183	Wrap, chicken caesar, Cool Wrap	1 ea	227	460	38	51	3	11	6.0	—	—	85	150
69182	Wrap, chicken, spicy	1 ea	225	390	31	51	3	7	3.5	—	—	70	40
Chili's Grill&Bar													
4822	Dinner, chicken, platter, Guiltless Grill	0.5 ea	326	282	19	42	2	4	1.5	—	—	29	368
4826	Salad, chicken, w/dressing	1 ea	445	272	29	27	6	5	1.0	—	—	47	416
4825	Sandwich, chicken, Guiltless Grill	1 ea	553	527	44	70	11	8	2.0	—	—	43	620
Dairy Queen													
56372	Cheeseburger, double, homestyle	1 ea	219	540	35	30	2	31	16.0	—	—	115	150
16287	Dinner, chicken, strip, basket, w/gravy	1 ea	415	1000	35	102	5	50	13.0	—	—	55	40
2131	Frozen Dessert, banana split, Royal Treats	1 ea	369	510	8	96	3	12	8.0	—	—	30	200
2352	Frozen Dessert, Misty Slush, med	1 ea	595	290	0	74	0	0	0.0	0.0	0.0	0	0
2368	Frozen Dessert, oreo, med, Dairy Queen Blizzard	1 ea	326	640	12	97	1	23	11.0	—	—	45	250
56368	Hamburger, homestyle	1 ea	138	290	17	29	2	12	5.0	—	—	45	40
56374	Hot Dog	1 ea	99	240	9	19	1	14	5.0	—	—	25	20
2222	Ice Cream Cone, chocolate, med	1 ea	198	340	8	53	0	11	7.0	—	—	30	150
2143	Ice Cream Cone, vanilla, med	1 ea	213	355	9	57	0	10	6.5	—	—	32	161
2134	Ice Cream Sandwich, Dairy Queen	1 ea	85	200	4	31	1	6	3.0	—	—	10	40
2348	Ice Cream, chocolate, soft serve, Dairy Queen	0.5 cup	94	150	4	22	0	5	3.5	—	—	15	100
2224	Milk Shake, chocolate, med, Dairy Queen	1 ea	539	770	17	130	0	20	13.0	—	—	70	400
56383	Onion Rings, svg	1 ea	113	320	5	39	3	16	4.0	—	—	0	0
71690	Sandwich, bbq beef	1 ea	142	300	16	37	2	9	3.5	—	—	35	40
Dennys													
1125	Biscuit, w/sausage gravy, svg	1 ea	198	398	8	45	0	21	6.0	—	—	12	0
25238	Breakfast, Country Slam	1 ea	510	1000	41	61	1	66	21.0	—	—	467	300
1077	Breakfast, sausage supreme skillet	1 ea	425	857	27	29	8	62	19.0	—	—	466	490

PAGE KEY: A-158 Granola Bars, Cereal Bars, Diet Bars, Scones, and Tarts   A-158 Meals and Dishes   A-162 Meats   A-168 Nuts, Seeds, and Products   A-170 Poultry   A-172 Salad Dressings, Dips, and Mayonnaise   A-172 Salads   A-174 Sandwiches   A-176 Sauces and Gravies   A-176 Snack Foods—Chips, Pretzels, Popcorn   A-178 Soups, Stews, and Chilis   A-180 Spices, Flavors, and Seasonings   A-182 Sports Bars and Drinks   A-182 Supplemental Foods and Formulas   A-184 Sweeteners and Sweet Substitutes   A-184 Vegetables and Legumes   A-198 Weight Loss Bars and Drinks   A-200 Miscellaneous

Thia (mg)	Ribo (mg)	Niac (mg NE)	Vit B6 (mg)	Vit B12 (μg)	Fol (μg)	Vit C (mg)	Vit D (IU)	Vit E (mg AT)	Cal (mg)	Iron (mg)	Magn (mg)	Phos (mg)	Pota (mg)	Sodi (mg)	Zinc (mg)	Wat (%)	Alco (g)	Caff (g)
—	—	—	—	—	—	4.8	—	—	80	3.59	—	—	—	520	—	55	0.00	0.00
—	—	—	—	—	—	0.0	—	—	150	0.00	—	—	—	690	—	—	0.00	0.00
—	—	—	—	—	—	0.0	—	—	80	3.59	—	—	—	1200	—	—	0.00	0.00
—	—	—	—	—	—	0.0	—	—	80	2.70	—	—	—	1330	—	—	0.00	0.00
—	—	—	—	—	—	3.6	—	—	60	1.79	—	—	—	680	—	—	0.00	0.00
—	—	—	—	—	—	0.0	—	—	350	2.70	—	—	—	750	—	—	0.00	0.00
—	—	—	—	—	—	1.2	—	—	200	4.50	—	—	—	1430	—	—	0.00	0.00
—	—	—	—	—	—	0.0	—	—	20	1.08	—	—	—	330	—	47	0.00	0.00
—	—	—	—	—	—	36.0	—	—	150	4.50	—	—	—	1700	—	—	0.00	0.00
—	—	—	—	—	—	2.4	—	—	60	3.59	—	—	—	480	—	—	0.00	0.00
—	—	—	—	—	—	9.0	—	—	100	5.40	—	—	—	910	—	—	0.00	0.00
—	—	—	—	—	—	21.0	—	—	0	1.08	—	—	—	170	—	36	0.00	0.00
—	—	—	—	—	—	15.0	—	—	80	0.72	—	—	—	60	—	93	0.00	0.00
—	—	—	—	—	—	4.8	—	—	80	2.70	—	—	—	830	—	—	0.00	0.00
—	—	—	—	—	—	6.0	—	—	250	3.59	—	—	—	1610	—	—	0.00	0.00
—	—	—	—	—	—	2.4	—	—	150	1.79	—	—	—	1030	—	51	0.00	0.00
—	—	—	—	—	—	0.0	—	—	40	1.08	—	—	—	990	—	—	0.00	0.00
—	—	—	—	—	—	3.6	—	—	20	0.36	—	—	—	90	—	—	0.00	0.00
—	—	—	—	—	—	6.0	—	—	150	1.08	—	—	—	680	—	—	0.00	0.00
—	—	—	—	—	—	0.0	—	—	100	2.70	—	—	—	1300	—	—	0.00	0.00
—	—	—	—	—	—	0.0	—	—	400	3.59	—	—	—	1540	—	—	0.00	0.00
—	—	—	—	—	—	4.8	—	—	200	3.59	—	—	—	1150	—	—	0.00	0.00
—	—	—	—	—	—	16.5	—	—	86	4.00	—	—	—	1642	—	—	0.00	0.00
—	—	—	—	—	—	16.0	—	—	36	4.00	—	—	—	1475	—	—	0.00	0.00
—	—	—	—	—	—	26.0	—	—	306	9.00	—	—	—	2923	—	—	0.00	0.00
—	—	—	—	—	—	3.6	—	—	250	4.50	—	—	—	1130	—	—	0.00	0.00
—	—	—	—	—	—	9.0	—	—	60	4.50	—	—	—	2510	—	—	0.00	0.00
—	—	—	—	—	—	15.0	—	—	250	1.79	—	—	—	180	—	—	0.00	—
—	—	—	—	—	—	0.0	—	—	0	0.00	—	—	—	30	—	—	0.00	0.00
—	—	—	—	—	—	1.2	—	—	400	2.70	—	—	—	500	—	—	0.00	—
—	—	—	—	—	—	3.6	—	—	60	2.70	—	—	—	630	—	56	0.00	0.00
—	—	—	—	—	—	3.6	—	—	60	1.79	—	—	—	730	—	55	0.00	0.00
—	—	—	—	—	—	1.2	—	—	250	1.79	—	—	—	160	—	—	0.00	—
—	—	—	—	—	—	2.6	—	—	269	1.94	—	—	—	172	—	—	0.00	0.00
—	—	—	—	—	—	0.0	—	—	80	1.08	—	—	—	140	—	51	0.00	—
—	—	—	—	—	—	0.0	—	—	100	0.72	—	—	—	75	—	—	0.00	—
—	—	—	—	—	—	2.4	—	—	600	2.70	—	—	—	420	—	—	0.00	—
—	—	—	—	—	—	0.0	—	—	20	1.44	—	—	—	180	—	—	0.00	0.00
—	—	—	—	—	—	0.0	—	—	60	2.70	—	—	—	610	—	—	0.00	0.00
—	—	—	—	—	—	0.0	—	—	10	0.18	—	—	—	1267	—	—	0.00	0.00
—	—	—	—	—	—	0.0	—	—	70	4.13	—	—	—	2727	—	—	0.00	0.00
—	—	—	—	—	—	22.8	—	—	180	2.88	—	—	—	1700	—	—	0.00	0.00

PAGE KEY: A-108 Beverage and Beverage Mixes   A-110 Other Beverages   A-110 Beverages, Alcoholic   A-112 Candies and Confections, Gum   A-116 Cereals, Breakfast Type   A-120 Cheese and Cheese Substitutes   A-122 Dairy Products and Substitutes   A-124 Desserts   A-130 Dessert Toppings   A-130 Eggs, Substitutes, and Egg Dishes   A-132 Ethnic Foods   A-136 Fast Foods/Restaurants   A-150 Fats, Oils, Margarines, Shortenings, and Substitutes   A-150 Fish, Seafood, and Shellfish   A-152 Food Additives   A-152 Fruit, Vegetable, or Blended Juices   A-154 Grains, Flours, and Fractions   A-154 Grain Products, Prepared and Baked Goods

Code	Food Name	Unit/ Amt	Wt (g)	Energy (kcal)	Prot (g)	Carb (g)	Fiber (g)	Fat (g)	Sat (g)	Mono (g)	Poly (g)	Chol (mg)	Vit A (RE)
17277	Chicken, breast, grilled, svg	1 ea	170	219	26	16	0	6	1.0	—	—	67	60
25249	Chicken, buffalo wings	1 ea	35	71	8	0	0	4	1.4	—	—	42	15
25248	Dish, appetizer sampler, w/chicken mozzarella onion & sauce	1 ea	482	1405	47	124	4	80	24.0	—	—	75	30
10432	Dish, fish & chips, w/tartar sauce, svg	1 ea	255	732	30	48	3	47	7.0	—	—	105	0
38655	French Toast, cinnamon swirl, w/o topping & margarine, svg	1 ea	341	1030	23	124	4	49	21.0	—	—	280	370
52144	Hamburger, classic	1 ea	312	673	37	42	3	40	15.0	—	—	106	200
12199	Hamburger, w/cheese, classic	1 ea	369	836	47	43	3	53	19.0	—	—	137	210
19548	Omelette, ham 'n cheddar, Dennys	1 ea	397	743	36	24	2	55	10.0	—	—	657	580
19547	Omelette, ultimate, Dennys	1 ea	482	780	31	29	4	62	14.0	—	—	639	540
38657	Onion Rings, basket	1 ea	255	824	11	83	1	50	12.0	—	—	14	30
25250	Quesadilla, chicken	1 ea	454	827	50	43	2	55	23.0	—	—	181	630
12195	Sandwich, club	1 ea	312	718	32	62	3	38	7.0	—	—	75	60
Dominos Pizza													
91365	Breadsticks	1 ea	37	116	3	18	1	4	0.8	—	—	0	4
91369	Chicken, buffalo wings	1 ea	25	50	6	2	0	2	0.6	—	—	26	8
56386	Pizza, cheese, hand tossed, 12"	2 pce	159	375	15	55	3	11	4.8	—	—	23	131
91360	Pizza, Hawaiian feast, hand tossed, 12"	2 pce	204	450	21	58	3	16	7.2	—	—	41	173
91361	Pizza, pepperoni feast, hand tossed, 12"	2 pce	196	534	24	56	3	25	10.9	—	—	57	175
91357	Pizza, veggie feast, hand tossed, 12"	2 pce	203	439	19	57	4	16	7.1	—	—	34	181
Dunkin' Donuts													
50720	Chowder, clam, New England, svg	1 ea	227	200	10	16	0	10	3.0	—	—	30	100
45742	Doughnut, Bismark	1 ea	80	310	4	42	1	14	4.0	—	—	0	0
45700	Doughnut, cake, chocolate	1 ea	59	210	3	19	1	14	3.0	—	—	0	0
45695	Doughnut, cake, old fash	1 ea	60	280	3	24	1	19	4.0	—	—	0	0
45708	Doughnut, raised, glazed	1 ea	46	160	3	23	1	7	2.0	—	—	0	0
42636	Fritter, apple	1 ea	95	300	5	41	2	13	3.0	—	—	0	0
69090	Sandwich, ham cheese, croissant	1 ea	192	710	33	29	0	32	13.0	—	—	85	100
50722	Soup, cream of broccoli, svg	1 ea	227	200	8	17	0	11	6.0	—	—	25	200
45749	Turnover, apple	1 ea	109	350	5	49	2	15	4.0	—	—	0	0
El Pollo Loco													
28110	Chicken, strips, svg	1 ea	213	558	41	48	0	25	5.0	—	—	76	0
49103	Frozen Dessert, banana split	1 ea	425	717	12	107	3	28	11.0	—	—	56	80
4012	Guacamole, 1.8 oz svg	1 ea	50	52	0	5	0	3	0.0	—	—	0	30
1655	Salad, garden, reg	1 ea	113	105	5	7	1	7	3.0	—	—	15	60
1656	Salad, tostada	1 ea	397	304	29	28	4	11	3.0	—	—	57	190
28104	Salsa, avocado	28.35 g	28	12	0	1	0	1	0.0	—	—	0	5
7204	Taco, chicken, soft	1 ea	128	238	17	15	0	12	4.0	—	—	74	120
49112	Tortilla, corn, 6"	1 ea	28	70	1	14	1	1	0.0	—	—	0	30
Hardees													
9280	Cheeseburger	1 ea	124	313	16	26	1	14	7.0	—	—	40	—
56412	Hamburger	1 ea	110	265	14	26	1	10	4.0	—	—	35	—
9286	Potatoes, french fries, Crispy Curls, reg svg	1 ea	96	340	5	41	0	18	4.0	—	—	0	—
6146	Potatoes, french fries, reg svg	1 ea	113	340	4	45	0	16	2.0	—	—	0	—
56418	Sandwich, roast beef, regular	1 ea	123	310	17	26	2	16	6.0	—	—	43	—

PAGE KEY: A-158 Granola Bars, Cereal Bars, Diet Bars, Scones, and Tarts   A-158 Meals and Dishes   A-162 Meats   A-168 Nuts, Seeds, and Products   A-170 Poultry   A-172 Salad Dressings, Dips, and Mayonnaise   A-172 Salads   A-174 Sandwiches   A-176 Sauces and Gravies   A-176 Snack Foods—Chips, Pretzels, Popcorn   A-178 Soups, Stews, and Chilis   A-180 Spices, Flavors, and Seasonings   A-182 Sports Bars and Drinks   A-182 Supplemental Foods and Formulas   A-184 Sweeteners and Sweet Substitutes   A-184 Vegetables and Legumes   A-198 Weight Loss Bars and Drinks   A-200 Miscellaneous

Thia (mg)	Ribo (mg)	Niac (mg NE)	Vit B6 (mg)	Vit B12 (µg)	Fol (µg)	Vit C (mg)	Vit D (IU)	Vit E (mg AT)	Cal (mg)	Iron (mg)	Magn (mg)	Phos (mg)	Pota (mg)	Sodi (mg)	Zinc (mg)	Wat (%)	Alco (g)	Caff (g)
—	—	—	—	—	—	1.2	—	—	10	1.08	—	—	—	880	—	—	0.00	0.00
—	—	—	—	—	—	2.4	—	—	16	1.29	—	—	—	462	—	—	0.00	0.00
—	—	—	—	—	—	6.6	—	—	440	2.88	—	—	—	5305	—	—	0.00	0.00
—	—	—	—	—	—	0.0	—	—	0	1.44	—	—	—	1335	—	—	0.00	0.00
—	—	—	—	—	—	0.0	—	—	180	6.48	—	—	—	675	—	—	0.00	0.00
—	—	—	—	—	—	10.8	—	—	130	4.50	—	—	—	1142	—	—	0.00	0.00
—	—	—	—	—	—	10.8	—	—	340	4.50	—	—	—	1595	—	—	0.00	0.00
—	—	—	—	—	—	6.6	—	—	290	3.05	—	—	—	1518	—	—	0.00	0.00
—	—	—	—	—	—	37.8	—	—	90	3.59	—	—	—	1360	—	—	0.00	0.00
—	—	—	—	—	—	4.8	—	—	40	1.25	—	—	—	2173	—	—	0.00	0.00
—	—	—	—	—	—	54.0	—	—	640	1.79	—	—	—	1982	—	—	0.00	0.00
—	—	—	—	—	—	13.2	—	—	120	4.32	—	—	—	1666	—	—	0.00	0.00
—	—	—	—	—	—	0.1	—	—	6	0.87	—	—	—	152	—	—	0.00	0.00
—	—	—	—	—	—	0.1	—	—	6	0.31	—	—	—	175	—	—	0.00	0.00
—	—	—	—	—	—	0.0	—	—	187	2.99	—	—	—	776	—	—	0.00	0.00
—	—	—	—	—	—	1.9	—	—	274	3.29	—	—	—	1102	—	51	0.00	0.00
—	—	—	—	—	—	0.1	—	—	279	3.40	—	—	—	1349	—	44	0.00	0.00
—	—	—	—	—	—	1.3	—	—	279	3.44	—	—	—	987	—	53	0.00	0.00
—	—	—	—	—	—	3.6	—	—	150	2.70	—	—	—	1050	—	—	0.00	0.00
—	—	—	—	—	—	2.4	—	—	0	0.72	—	—	—	260	—	—	0.00	0.00
—	—	—	—	—	—	3.6	—	—	0	1.44	—	—	—	270	—	—	0.00	—
—	—	—	—	—	—	1.2	—	—	0	1.08	—	—	—	350	—	—	0.00	0.00
—	—	—	—	—	—	1.2	—	—	0	0.36	—	—	—	200	—	—	0.00	0.00
—	—	—	—	—	—	0.0	—	—	0	1.44	—	—	—	320	—	—	0.00	0.00
—	—	—	—	—	—	24.0	—	—	250	2.70	—	—	—	1840	—	—	0.00	0.00
—	—	—	—	—	—	18.0	—	—	250	0.36	—	—	—	1050	—	83	0.00	0.00
—	—	—	—	—	—	2.4	—	—	0	0.72	—	—	—	340	—	—	0.00	0.00
—	—	—	—	—	—	0.0	—	—	100	2.70	—	—	—	1876	—	—	0.00	0.00
—	—	—	—	—	—	22.2	—	—	270	1.98	—	—	—	310	—	—	0.00	0.00
—	—	—	—	—	—	4.2	—	—	40	0.73	—	—	—	282	—	—	0.00	0.00
—	—	—	—	—	—	6.6	—	—	110	0.36	—	—	—	99	—	—	0.00	0.00
—	—	—	—	—	—	22.8	—	—	180	3.24	—	—	—	1175	—	—	0.00	0.00
—	—	—	—	—	—	7.2	—	—	0	0.18	—	—	—	204	—	92	0.00	0.00
—	—	—	—	—	—	10.2	—	—	181	1.62	—	—	—	631	—	—	0.00	0.00
—	—	—	—	—	—	0.0	—	—	10	0.36	—	—	—	35	—	42	0.00	0.00
—	—	—	—	—	—	—	—	—	—	—	—	—	—	895	—	—	0.00	0.00
—	—	—	—	—	—	—	—	—	—	—	—	—	—	663	—	—	0.00	0.00
—	—	—	—	—	—	—	—	—	—	—	—	—	—	950	—	—	0.00	0.00
—	—	—	—	—	—	—	—	—	—	—	—	—	—	390	—	41	0.00	0.00
—	—	—	—	—	—	—	—	—	—	—	—	—	—	804	—	—	0.00	0.00

PAGE KEY: A-108 Beverage and Beverage Mixes   A-110 Other Beverages   A-110 Beverages, Alcoholic   A-112 Candies and Confections, Gum   A-116 Cereals, Breakfast Type   A-120 Cheese and Cheese Substitutes   A-122 Dairy Products and Substitutes   A-124 Desserts   A-130 Dessert Toppings   A-130 Eggs, Substitutes, and Egg Dishes   A-132 Ethnic Foods   A-136 Fast Foods/Restaurants   A-150 Fats, Oils, Margarines, Shortenings, and Substitutes   A-150 Fish, Seafood, and Shellfish   A-152 Food Additives   A-152 Fruit, Vegetable, or Blended Juices   A-154 Grains, Flours, and Fractions   A-154 Grain Products, Prepared and Baked Goods

Code	Food Name	Unit/ Amt	Wt (g)	Energy (kcal)	Prot (g)	Carb (g)	Fiber (g)	Fat (g)	Sat (g)	Mono (g)	Poly (g)	Chol (mg)	Vit A (RE)
56404	Sandwich, sausage egg, w/biscuit	1 ea	156	617	19	44	—	41	12.9	—	—	224	—
56403	Sandwich, sausage, w/biscuit	1 ea	114	553	13	44	—	36	11.0	—	—	30	—
In-N-Out Burgers													
81119	Potatoes, french fries	1 ea	125	400	7	54	2	18	5.0	—	—	0	0
Jack in the Box													
56434	Cheeseburger	1 ea	116	300	14	31	2	13	6.0	—	—	40	40
15162	Chicken, strips, 5 pce svg	1 ea	150	360	27	24	1	17	3.0	—	—	80	40
62548	Dish, fish & chips	1 ea	281	780	19	86	6	39	9.0	—	—	45	20
56433	Hamburger	1 ea	104	250	12	30	2	9	3.5	—	—	30	0
2163	Milk Shake, chocolate, med, Jack in the Box	1 ea	332	630	11	85	1	27	16.0	—	—	85	150
2165	Milk Shake, vanilla, med, Jack in the Box	1 ea	332	610	12	73	0	31	18.0	—	—	95	150
56446	Onion Rings, svg	1 ea	120	450	7	50	3	25	5.0	—	—	0	40
56448	Salad, side	1 ea	86	50	2	3	1	3	1.5	—	—	10	75
69035	Sandwich, chicken	1 ea	164	400	15	38	3	21	3.0	—	—	40	40
56377	Taco	1 ea	90	170	7	12	2	10	3.5	—	—	15	60
Jamba Juice													
81280	Breadsticks, pizza, w/add prot, svg	1 ea	76	230	9	33	2	6	1.5	—	—	5	60
81227	Smoothie, Banana Berry, Jamba Juice	16 fl-oz	475	270	2	66	3	2	0.0	—	—	0	20
81245	Smoothie, Coldbuster, Jamba Juice	16 fl-oz	476	280	3	65	3	2	0.0	—	—	5	700
81266	Smoothie, Orange Dream Machine, Jamba Juice	16 fl-oz	504	410	15	84	1	2	1.0	—	—	5	80
81253	Smoothie, PowerBoost	16 fl-oz	519	280	4	67	6	1	0.0	—	—	0	600
81283	Smoothie, Razzmatazz, Jamba Juice	16 fl-oz	490	300	2	72	3	1	0.0	—	—	0	20
81362	Smoothie, strawberry banana	8 fl-oz	240	124	1	29	1	0	0.0	0.0	0.0	0	0
Kentucky Fried Chicken													
42331	Biscuit, buttermilk	1 ea	57	190	2	23	0	10	2.0	—	—	0	0
15163	Chicken, breast, original rec	1 ea	161	380	40	11	0	19	6.0	—	—	145	0
56451	Cole Slaw, svg	1 ea	130	190	1	22	3	11	2.0	—	—	5	250
6152	Corn, cob, large	1 ea	162	150	5	26	7	3	1.0	—	—	0	0
56453	Potatoes, mashed, w/gravy, svg	1 ea	136	130	2	18	1	4	1.0	—	—	0	20
6188	Potatoes, wedges, svg	1 ea	102	240	5	30	3	12	3.0	—	—	0	0
Long John Silvers													
91388	Cheese, cheesesticks, brd, fried, 0.5 oz ea	3 ea	45	140	4	12	1	8	2.0	—	—	10	40
56477	Cornbread, hush puppies, svg	1 ea	23	60	1	9	1	2	0.5	—	—	0	0
56461	Fish, batter dipped, reg, 3.3 oz	1 pce	92	230	11	16	0	13	4.0	—	—	30	0
69030	Sandwich, fish, batter dipped	1 ea	177	440	17	47	3	21	5.0	—	—	40	60
19108	Shrimp, battered	1 ea	14	45	2	3	0	3	1.0	—	—	15	0
McDonalds													
69009	Cheeseburger	1 ea	119	326	15	33	2	15	6.2	5.2	1.5	42	—
69010	Cheeseburger, Big Mac	1 ea	219	572	26	47	3	31	10.9	11.3	8.5	79	—
69012	Cheeseburger, Quarter Pounder	1 ea	199	535	30	39	2	29	13.8	12.1	2.6	96	—
15174	Chicken, nuggets, McNuggets, 4 pce svg	4 pce	72	190	10	13	1	11	2.5	—	—	35	0
47147	Cookie, McDonaldland, pkg	1 ea	57	230	3	38	1	8	2.0	—	—	0	0
19579	Eggs, scrambled, svg	1 ea	102	160	13	1	0	11	3.5	—	—	425	150
2171	Frozen Dessert, sundae, hot fudge, low fat	1 ea	179	340	8	52	1	12	9.0	—	—	30	100
69008	Hamburger	1 ea	105	270	13	32	2	10	3.6	4.1	1.3	27	—
69011	Hamburger, Quarter Pounder	1 ea	171	438	27	38	2	20	8.3	9.4	2.1	68	—
2169	Milk Shake, vanilla, sml, McDonalds	1 ea	293	360	11	59	0	9	6.0	—	—	40	60

Thia (mg)	Ribo (mg)	Niac (mg NE)	Vit B6 (mg)	Vit B12 (µg)	Fol (µg)	Vit C (mg)	Vit D (IU)	Vit E (mg AT)	Cal (mg)	Iron (mg)	Magn (mg)	Phos (mg)	Pota (mg)	Sodi (mg)	Zinc (mg)	Wat (%)	Alco (g)	Caff (g)
—	—	—	—	—	—	—	—	—	—	—	—	—	—	1359	—	—	0.00	0.00
—	—	—	—	—	—	—	—	—	—	—	—	—	—	1305	—	—	0.00	0.00
—	—	—	—	—	—	0.0	—	—	20	1.79	—	—	—	245	—	—	0.00	0.00
—	—	—	—	—	—	0.0	—	—	150	3.59	—	—	180	840	—	—	0.00	0.00
—	—	—	—	—	—	1.2	—	—	0	1.79	—	—	430	970	—	—	0.00	0.00
—	—	—	—	—	—	15.0	—	—	20	2.70	—	—	1060	1740	—	—	0.00	0.00
—	—	—	—	—	—	0.0	—	—	100	3.59	—	—	155	610	—	—	0.00	0.00
—	—	—	—	—	—	0.0	—	—	350	0.36	—	—	720	330	—	—	0.00	—
—	—	—	—	—	—	0.0	—	—	400	0.00	—	—	730	320	—	64	0.00	0.00
—	—	—	—	—	—	18.0	—	—	40	2.70	—	—	150	780	—	30	0.00	0.00
—	—	—	—	—	—	0.0	—	—	80	0.72	—	—	160	75	—	—	0.00	0.00
—	—	—	—	—	—	4.8	—	—	100	2.70	—	—	200	770	—	—	0.00	0.00
—	—	—	—	—	—	0.2	—	—	100	1.08	40.4	168	235	390	1.4	66	0.00	0.00
0.37	0.25	3.00	0.03	0.00	80.0	4.8	0.0	0.8	80	2.70	8.0	20	130	450	0.3	—	0.00	0.00
0.05	0.10	0.80	0.60	0.11	16.0	9.0	0.0	0.4	80	0.72	24.0	40	540	35	0.3	—	0.00	0.00
0.23	0.14	2.00	0.30	0.00	100.0	684.0	0.0	10.1	60	0.72	40.0	60	800	15	7.5	—	0.00	0.00
0.23	0.25	0.80	0.11	0.47	60.0	78.0	100.0	0.0	400	0.72	32.0	300	540	230	0.6	—	0.00	0.00
2.70	2.89	34.00	3.59	4.80	360.0	198.0	240.0	12.1	600	1.44	240.0	80	810	30	7.5	—	0.00	0.00
0.05	0.17	4.00	0.69	0.11	100.0	36.0	0.0	0.0	80	1.08	24.0	60	570	45	0.3	—	0.00	0.00
—	—	—	—	—	—	60.0	—	—	0	0.89	—	—	475	10	—	—	0.00	0.00
—	—	—	—	—	—	0.0	—	—	0	0.72	—	—	—	580	—	36	0.00	0.00
—	—	—	—	—	—	0.0	—	—	0	1.79	—	—	—	1150	—	55	0.00	0.00
—	—	—	—	—	—	24.0	—	—	40	0.00	—	—	—	300	—	—	0.00	0.00
—	—	—	—	—	—	6.0	—	—	60	1.08	—	—	—	10	—	—	0.00	0.00
—	—	—	—	—	—	2.4	—	—	0	0.36	—	—	—	380	—	—	0.00	0.00
—	—	—	—	—	—	3.6	—	—	20	1.79	—	—	—	830	—	—	0.00	0.00
—	—	—	—	—	—	0.0	—	—	100	0.72	—	—	—	320	—	—	0.00	0.00
—	—	—	—	—	—	0.0	—	—	20	0.36	—	—	—	200	—	43	0.00	0.00
—	—	—	—	—	—	4.8	—	—	20	1.79	—	—	—	700	—	54	0.00	0.00
—	—	—	—	—	—	9.0	—	—	60	3.59	—	—	—	1120	—	—	0.00	0.00
—	—	—	—	—	—	1.2	—	—	0	0.00	—	—	—	125	—	43	0.00	0.00
0.34	0.18	4.82	0.09	1.57	30.9	0.4	—	0.1	219	1.75	29.8	179	234	739	2.4	45	0.00	0.00
0.40	0.43	7.94	0.37	2.77	59.1	0.7	—	0.1	278	3.06	54.8	298	399	1062	4.7	51	0.00	0.00
0.23	0.51	8.06	0.18	3.48	31.8	0.6	—	0.4	356	2.02	51.7	364	444	1176	5.6	48	0.00	0.00
—	—	4.92	—	0.20	—	0.0	—	0.9	9	0.70	16.4	191	202	360	0.7	51	0.00	0.00
—	—	2.03	—	—	—	0.0	—	1.0	20	1.79	11.3	71	63	250	0.4	13	0.00	0.00
0.07	0.50	0.05	0.11	1.11	44.0	0.0	—	0.9	40	1.08	10.0	172	126	170	1.1	—	0.00	0.00
—	—	—	—	—	—	1.2	—	—	250	0.72	—	—	—	170	—	59	0.00	—
0.31	0.07	4.55	0.10	1.17	29.4	0.3	—	0.1	130	1.77	25.2	112	204	502	2.0	45	0.00	0.00
0.27	0.34	7.94	0.25	2.83	37.6	0.5	—	0.1	149	2.96	41.0	207	385	640	5.2	49	0.00	0.00
—	—	—	—	—	—	1.2	—	—	350	0.36	—	327	534	250	—	—	0.00	0.00

PAGE KEY: A-108 Beverage and Beverage Mixes   A-110 Other Beverages   A-110 Beverages, Alcoholic   A-112 Candies and Confections, Gum   A-116 Cereals, Breakfast Type
A-120 Cheese and Cheese Substitutes   A-122 Dairy Products and Substitutes   A-124 Desserts   A-130 Dessert Toppings   A-130 Eggs, Substitutes, and Egg Dishes   A-132 Ethnic Foods
A-136 Fast Foods/Restaurants   A-150 Fats, Oils, Margarines, Shortenings, and Substitutes   A-150 Fish, Seafood, and Shellfish   A-152 Food Additives
A-152 Fruit, Vegetable, or Blended Juices   A-154 Grains, Flours, and Fractions   A-154 Grain Products, Prepared and Baked Goods

Code	Food Name	Unit/ Amt	Wt (g)	Energy (kcal)	Prot (g)	Carb (g)	Fiber (g)	Fat (g)	Sat (g)	Mono (g)	Poly (g)	Chol (mg)	Vit A (RE)
48136	Pie, apple	1 ea	77	260	3	34	1	13	3.5	—	—	0	—
6156	Potatoes, french fries, sml svg	1 ea	68	210	3	26	2	10	1.5	—	—	0	0
57764	Salad, chef, shaker	1 ea	206	150	17	5	2	8	3.5	—	—	95	300
56479	Salad, garden, shaker	1 ea	149	100	7	4	2	6	3.0	—	—	75	150
81097	Sandwich, chicken, crisp deluxe	1 ea	219	537	27	49	3	26	4.6	8.2	12.0	64	—
81098	Sandwich, chicken, grilled, McGrill	1 ea	213	422	31	39	3	16	3.1	4.5	8.2	70	—
69013	Sandwich, Filet O Fish	1 ea	141	415	16	40	2	21	4.7	6.4	10.1	45	—
49141	Sandwich, ham egg cheese, w/bagel	1 ea	218	550	26	58	2	23	8.0	—	—	255	150
69006	Sandwich, sausage cheese, w/muffin	1 ea	112	360	13	26	1	23	8.0	—	—	45	40
69007	Sandwich, sausage egg cheese, w/muffin	1 ea	162	440	19	27	1	28	10.0	—	—	255	100
69004	Sandwich, sausage egg, w/biscuit	1 ea	162	490	16	31	1	33	10.0	—	—	245	60
42747	Sweet Roll, cinnamon	1 ea	95	390	6	50	2	18	5.0	—	—	65	80
Olive Garden													
4836	Breadsticks	1 ea	50	140	5	26	—	2	0.0	—	—	0	—
4832	Dinner, chicken giardino	1 ea	611	460	36	59	—	8	3.0	—	—	60	—
4834	Dinner, shrimp primavera	1 ea	535	603	44	84	—	13	2.0	—	—	275	—
Pizza Hut													
92495	Chicken, wings, mild, 2 pce svg	2 pce	53	110	11	1	0	7	2.0	—	—	70	60
57787	Pizza, cheese, 6"	1 pce	63	160	7	18	1	7	3.0	—	—	15	40
56489	Pizza, cheese, med, 12"	1 pce	99	240	12	30	2	8	4.5	—	—	25	60
57372	Pizza, ham, med, 12"	1 pce	98	220	12	29	2	6	3.0	—	—	20	60
57383	Pizza, Meat Lover's, pan, med, 12"	1 pce	123	340	15	29	2	19	7.0	—	—	35	60
56482	Pizza, pepperoni, pan, med, 12"	1 pce	102	290	11	29	2	15	5.0	—	—	25	60
57376	Pizza, pork, med, 12"	1 pce	111	270	13	30	3	11	5.0	—	—	25	60
57377	Pizza, sausage, Italian, med, 12"	1 pce	111	290	13	30	2	12	6.0	—	—	30	60
57382	Pizza, Veggie Lovers, pan, med, 12"	1 pce	119	260	10	30	2	12	4.0	—	—	15	80
Subway													
91790	Chili, con carne	1 cup	240	310	17	28	9	14	5.0	—	—	35	150
91784	Chowder, clam, New England	1 cup	240	140	5	19	7	4	1.0	—	—	15	150
91786	Chowder, potato cheese	1 cup	240	210	7	22	2	10	7.0	—	—	25	300
52119	Salad, chicken, breast, rstd	1 ea	303	140	16	12	3	3	1.0	—	—	45	150
52115	Salad, club	1 ea	322	150	17	12	3	4	1.5	—	—	35	150
69119	Sandwich, beef steak cheese, w/white, 6"	1 ea	256	390	24	48	5	14	5.0	—	—	35	100
69125	Sandwich, chicken breast, rstd, w/white, 6"	1 ea	236	320	23	47	5	5	2.0	—	—	45	60
69115	Sandwich, ham, w/white, 6"	1 ea	232	290	18	46	4	5	1.5	—	—	25	60
69129	Sandwich, meatball, w/white, 6"	1 ea	287	530	24	53	6	26	10.0	—	—	55	150
69121	Sandwich, roast beef, w/white, 6"	1 ea	222	290	19	45	4	5	2.0	—	—	20	60
69137	Sandwich, turkey breast, w/ ham, w/white, 6"	1 ea	232	290	20	46	4	5	1.5	—	—	25	60
69111	Sandwich, turkey, w/white, 6"	1 ea	222	280	18	46	4	4	1.5	—	—	20	60
69109	Sandwich, veggie delite, w/white, 6"	1 ea	166	230	9	44	4	3	1.0	—	—	0	60
Taco Bell													
56519	Burrito, bean	1 ea	198	370	14	55	8	10	3.5	—	—	10	100
57678	Burrito, chicken, grilled, Stuft	1 ea	325	680	35	76	7	26	7.0	—	—	70	100
57677	Burrito, chili cheese	1 ea	156	390	16	40	3	18	9.0	—	—	40	150
45585	Dessert, cinnamon twists, svg	1 ea	35	160	1	28	0	5	1.0	—	—	0	0
57665	Gordita, beef, supreme	1 ea	153	310	14	30	3	16	7.0	—	—	35	100
56533	Nachos, svg	1 ea	99	320	5	33	2	19	4.5	—	—	5	0

PAGE KEY: A-158 Granola Bars, Cereal Bars, Diet Bars, Scones, and Tarts   A-158 Meals and Dishes   A-162 Meats   A-168 Nuts, Seeds, and Products   A-170 Poultry
A-172 Salad Dressings, Dips, and Mayonnaise   A-172 Salads   A-174 Sandwiches   A-176 Sauces and Gravies   A-176 Snack Foods—Chips, Pretzels, Popcorn
A-178 Soups, Stews, and Chilis   A-180 Spices, Flavors, and Seasonings   A-182 Sports Bars and Drinks   A-182 Supplemental Foods and Formulas
A-184 Sweeteners and Sweet Substitutes   A-184 Vegetables and Legumes   A-198 Weight Loss Bars and Drinks   A-200 Miscellaneous

Thia (mg)	Ribo (mg)	Niac (mg NE)	Vit B6 (mg)	Vit B12 (µg)	Fol (µg)	Vit C (mg)	Vit D (IU)	Vit E (mg AT)	Cal (mg)	Iron (mg)	Magn (mg)	Phos (mg)	Pota (mg)	Sodi (mg)	Zinc (mg)	Wat (%)	Alco (g)	Caff (g)
0.18	0.10	1.41	0.02	0.00	8.3	24.0	—	1.4	20	1.08	6.5	35	63	200	0.2	—	0.00	0.00
—	—	—	—	—	—	9.0	—	0.8	9	0.36	26.5	88	468	135	0.3	41	0.00	0.00
—	—	—	—	—	—	15.0	—	—	150	1.44	—	—	—	740	—	—	0.00	0.00
—	—	—	—	—	—	15.0	—	—	150	1.08	—	—	—	120	—	—	0.00	0.00
0.34	0.40	11.18	0.28	0.72	63.5	0.7	—	1.5	171	2.69	61.3	353	449	1424	2.2	51	0.00	0.00
0.37	0.36	11.31	0.28	0.69	57.5	0.6	—	0.9	175	2.39	59.6	343	505	1240	1.2	58	0.00	0.00
0.30	0.18	3.13	0.05	1.51	29.6	0.4	—	1.6	154	0.92	38.1	185	276	663	0.8	43	0.00	0.00
—	—	—	—	—	—	0.0	—	—	200	4.50	—	—	—	1490	—	—	0.00	0.00
—	—	—	—	—	15.7	0.0	—	0.7	200	1.79	21.7	156	191	740	1.5	—	0.00	0.00
—	—	—	—	—	30.0	0.0	—	1.1	250	2.70	26.0	273	250	890	2.1	52	0.00	0.00
—	—	3.76	—	—	25.7	0.0	—	1.5	80	2.70	19.4	475	258	1010	1.5	49	0.00	0.00
—	—	—	—	—	—	—	—	—	60	1.44	—	—	—	310	—	20	0.00	0.00
—	—	—	—	—	—	—	—	—	—	—	—	—	—	270	—	—	0.00	0.00
—	—	—	—	—	—	—	—	—	—	—	—	—	—	1180	—	—	0.00	0.00
—	—	—	—	—	—	—	—	—	—	—	—	—	—	1220	—	—	0.00	0.00
—	—	—	—	—	—	0.0	—	—	0	0.72	—	—	—	320	—	—	0.00	0.00
—	—	—	—	—	—	0.0	—	—	100	1.44	—	—	—	310	—	—	0.00	0.00
—	—	—	—	—	—	1.2	—	—	200	1.44	—	—	—	520	—	47	0.00	0.00
—	—	—	—	—	—	6.0	—	—	150	1.79	—	—	—	550	—	—	0.00	0.00
—	—	—	—	—	—	6.0	—	—	150	2.70	—	—	—	750	—	—	0.00	0.00
—	—	—	—	—	—	2.4	—	—	150	2.70	—	—	—	560	—	—	0.00	0.00
—	—	—	—	—	—	3.6	—	—	150	1.79	—	—	—	640	—	—	0.00	0.00
—	—	—	—	—	—	3.6	—	—	150	1.79	—	—	—	660	—	—	0.00	0.00
—	—	—	—	—	—	9.0	—	—	150	2.70	—	—	—	470	—	—	0.00	0.00
—	—	—	—	—	—	12.0	—	—	60	—	—	—	—	900	—	—	0.00	0.00
—	—	—	—	—	—	0.0	—	—	60	1.79	—	—	—	900	—	86	0.00	0.00
—	—	—	—	—	—	0.0	—	—	200	0.00	—	—	—	1010	—	—	0.00	0.00
—	—	—	—	—	—	30.0	—	—	40	1.08	—	—	—	800	—	—	0.00	0.00
—	—	—	—	—	—	30.0	—	—	40	18.00	—	—	—	1110	—	—	0.00	0.00
—	—	—	—	—	—	24.0	—	—	150	8.10	—	—	—	1210	—	—	0.00	0.00
—	—	—	—	—	—	21.0	—	—	60	5.40	—	—	—	1000	—	—	0.00	0.00
—	—	—	—	—	—	21.0	—	—	60	3.59	—	—	—	1270	—	—	0.00	0.00
—	—	—	—	—	—	27.0	—	—	150	5.40	—	—	—	1360	—	—	0.00	0.00
—	—	—	—	—	—	21.0	—	—	60	6.30	—	—	—	910	—	—	0.00	0.00
—	—	—	—	—	—	21.0	—	—	60	3.59	—	—	—	1220	—	—	0.00	0.00
—	—	—	—	—	—	21.0	—	—	60	3.59	—	—	—	1010	—	—	0.00	0.00
—	—	—	—	—	—	21.0	—	—	60	3.59	—	—	—	510	—	—	0.00	0.00
—	—	—	—	—	—	4.8	—	—	200	2.70	—	—	—	1200	—	—	0.00	0.00
—	—	—	—	—	—	6.0	—	—	300	3.59	—	273	—	1950	—	—	0.00	0.00
—	—	—	—	—	—	0.0	—	—	300	1.79	—	—	—	1080	—	—	0.00	0.00
—	—	—	—	—	—	0.0	—	—	0	0.36	—	—	—	150	—	—	0.00	0.00
—	—	—	—	—	—	4.8	—	—	150	2.70	—	—	—	590	—	—	0.00	0.00
—	—	—	—	—	—	0.0	—	—	80	0.72	—	—	—	530	—	40	0.00	0.00

PAGE KEY: A-108 Beverage and Beverage Mixes A-110 Other Beverages A-110 Beverages, Alcoholic A-112 Candies and Confections, Gum A-116 Cereals, Breakfast Type A-120 Cheese and Cheese Substitutes A-122 Dairy Products and Substitutes A-124 Desserts A-130 Dessert Toppings A-130 Eggs, Substitutes, and Egg Dishes A-132 Ethnic Foods A-136 Fast Foods/Restaurants A-150 Fats, Oils, Margarines, Shortenings, and Substitutes A-150 Fish, Seafood, and Shellfish A-152 Food Additives A-152 Fruit, Vegetable, or Blended Juices A-154 Grains, Flours, and Fractions A-154 Grain Products, Prepared and Baked Goods

Code	Food Name	Unit/ Amt	Wt (g)	Energy (kcal)	Prot (g)	Carb (g)	Fiber (g)	Fat (g)	Sat (g)	Mono (g)	Poly (g)	Chol (mg)	Vit A (RE)
56531	Pizza, Mexican	1 ea	216	550	21	46	7	31	11.0	—	—	45	150
57685	Quesadilla, cheese	1 ea	142	490	19	39	3	28	13.0	—	—	55	100
57689	Quesadilla, chicken	1 ea	184	540	28	40	3	30	13.0	—	—	80	150
56537	Salad, taco, w/salsa & shell	1 ea	533	790	31	73	13	42	15.0	—	—	65	300
53604	Sauce, border, mild, 1 oz svg	1 ea	28	5	0	1	0	0	0.0	0.0	0.0	0	60
56524	Taco	1 ea	78	170	8	13	3	10	4.0	—	—	25	60
56525	Taco, soft, beef	1 ea	90	191	9	19	2	9	4.1	—	—	23	55
56689	Taco, soft, chicken	1 ea	99	190	14	19	1	6	2.5	—	—	30	20
56528	Tostada	1 ea	170	250	11	29	7	10	4.0	—	—	15	100
Taco Johns													
57576	Burrito, bean, w/cheese	1 ea	187	380	15	53	10	12	5.0	—	—	15	—
57577	Burrito, beefy	1 ea	187	430	22	41	8	20	9.0	—	—	55	—
49127	Dessert, churros	1 ea	55	230	2	31	1	11	2.0	—	—	10	—
57585	Dish, chimi platter, beef & bean	1 ea	422	760	27	88	9	34	11.0	—	—	50	—
57586	Enchilada, double	1 ea	422	720	37	54	11	40	18.0	—	—	105	—
57589	Mexi Rolls	1 ea	213	480	20	33	3	30	10.0	—	—	50	—
57593	Nachos, svg	1 ea	142	380	6	38	1	23	6.0	—	—	10	—
57596	Taco Burger, w/cheese	1 ea	142	280	14	28	3	12	5.0	—	—	35	—
57600	Taco, crispy	1 ea	94	180	9	13	3	10	4.0	—	—	25	—
57601	Taco, soft shell	1 ea	113	220	11	21	4	10	5.0	—	—	25	—
Taco Time													
7141	Beans, refritos, svg	1 ea	201	326	18	44	13	10	5.0	—	—	22	44
56542	Burrito, bean, soft	1 ea	193	380	16	58	13	10	4.0	—	—	15	—
56621	Burrito, chicken, crisp	1 ea	150	422	17	32	2	25	8.0	—	—	54	—
56541	Burrito, meat, crispy	1 ea	163	552	34	39	7	30	10.0	—	—	58	—
56543	Burrito, meat, soft	1 ea	193	491	31	48	12	21	8.0	—	—	56	—
56620	Burrito, veggie	1 ea	321	491	21	70	10	16	6.0	—	—	24	—
56550	Cheeseburger, taco	1 ea	215	633	31	48	7	36	10.0	—	—	66	—
56551	Chimichanga, meat	1 ea	349	768	37	62	12	43	18.0	—	—	89	—
45586	Empanada, berry	1 ea	113	387	5	66	3	12	1.0	5.0	6.0	2	16
2488	Frozen Dessert, Choco Taco	1 ea	113	310	3	37	1	17	10.0	—	—	20	40
1696	Gordita, taco meat	1 ea	227	470	18	44	4	24	7.0	—	—	35	150
56554	Nachos, svg	1 ea	301	680	26	61	11	38	19.0	—	—	78	—
50979	Quesadilla, cheese	1 ea	93	205	11	17	1	11	6.0	—	—	30	—
56556	Salad, taco, w/o dressing, reg	1 ea	215	479	30	30	7	28	11.0	—	—	63	—
56545	Taco, crisp	1 ea	115	295	22	16	5	17	7.0	—	—	48	—
56674	Taco, fish	1 ea	231	470	19	32	2	29	8.0	—	—	60	—
56655	Taco, soft, value	1 ea	150	316	24	23	5	15	7.0	—	—	48	—
56856	Tostada, w/bean	1 ea	138	211	10	26	7	8	4.0	—	—	15	—
56548	Tostada, w/meat	1 ea	219	447	35	33	12	21	9.0	—	—	61	—
1705	Wrap, chicken, classic	1 ea	494	813	29	101	6	33	11.0	—	—	67	—
Wendy's													
56570	Cheeseburger, jr	1 ea	129	310	17	34	2	12	6.0	—	—	45	60
56571	Cheeseburger, w/bacon, jr	1 ea	165	380	20	34	2	19	7.0	—	—	55	80
15176	Chicken, nuggets, 5 pce svg	1 ea	75	220	11	13	0	14	3.0	—	—	35	0
50311	Chili, sml svg	1 ea	227	200	17	21	5	6	2.5	—	—	35	150
56579	Dish, baked potato bacon cheese	1 ea	380	580	18	79	7	22	6.0	—	—	40	100

PAGE KEY: A-158 Granola Bars, Cereal Bars, Diet Bars, Scones, and Tarts   A-158 Meals and Dishes   A-162 Meats   A-168 Nuts, Seeds, and Products   A-170 Poultry   A-172 Salad Dressings, Dips, and Mayonnaise   A-172 Salads   A-174 Sandwiches   A-176 Sauces and Gravies   A-176 Snack Foods—Chips, Pretzels, Popcorn   A-178 Soups, Stews, and Chilis   A-180 Spices, Flavors, and Seasonings   A-182 Sports Bars and Drinks   A-182 Supplemental Foods and Formulas   A-184 Sweeteners and Sweet Substitutes   A-184 Vegetables and Legumes   A-198 Weight Loss Bars and Drinks   A-200 Miscellaneous

Thia (mg)	Ribo (mg)	Niac (mg NE)	Vit B6 (mg)	Vit B12 (μg)	Fol (μg)	Vit C (mg)	Vit D (IU)	Vit E (mg AT)	Cal (mg)	Iron (mg)	Magn (mg)	Phos (mg)	Pota (mg)	Sodi (mg)	Zinc (mg)	Wat (%)	Alco (g)	Caff (g)
—	—	—	—	—	—	6.0	—	—	350	3.59	—	—	—	1030	—	—	0.00	0.00
—	—	—	—	—	—	0.0	—	—	500	1.44	—	—	—	1150	—	—	0.00	0.00
—	—	—	—	—	—	2.4	—	—	500	1.79	—	—	—	1380	—	—	0.00	0.00
—	—	—	—	—	—	21.0	—	—	400	6.30	—	—	—	1670	—	—	0.00	0.00
—	—	—	—	—	—	0.0	—	—	0	0.00	—	—	—	210	—	—	0.00	0.00
—	—	—	—	—	—	2.4	—	—	60	1.08	—	—	—	350	—	—	0.00	0.00
—	—	—	—	—	—	2.2	—	—	91	1.63	—	—	—	564	—	—	0.00	0.00
—	—	—	—	—	—	1.2	—	—	100	1.08	—	—	—	550	—	—	0.00	0.00
—	—	—	—	—	—	4.8	—	—	150	1.44	—	—	—	710	—	—	0.00	0.00
—	—	—	—	—	—	—	—	—	—	—	—	—	—	830	—	—	0.00	0.00
—	—	—	—	—	—	—	—	—	—	—	—	—	—	870	—	—	0.00	0.00
—	—	—	—	—	—	—	—	—	—	—	—	—	—	120	—	—	0.00	0.00
—	—	—	—	—	—	—	—	—	—	—	—	—	—	1930	—	—	0.00	0.00
—	—	—	—	—	—	—	—	—	—	—	—	—	—	2090	—	—	0.00	0.00
—	—	—	—	—	—	—	—	—	—	—	—	—	—	1270	—	—	0.00	0.00
—	—	—	—	—	—	—	—	—	—	—	—	—	—	970	—	—	0.00	0.00
—	—	—	—	—	—	—	—	—	—	—	—	—	—	600	—	—	0.00	0.00
—	—	—	—	—	—	—	—	—	—	—	—	—	—	270	—	—	0.00	0.00
—	—	—	—	—	—	—	—	—	—	—	—	—	—	470	—	—	0.00	0.00
0.23	0.15	1.00	0.37	0.00	13.2	3.0	—	—	218	3.03	—	256	340	525	2.0	—	0.00	0.00
—	—	—	—	—	—	—	—	—	—	—	—	—	—	—	—	—	0.00	0.00
—	—	—	—	—	—	—	—	—	—	—	—	—	—	795	—	—	0.00	0.00
—	—	—	—	—	—	—	—	—	—	—	—	—	—	—	—	—	0.00	0.00
—	—	—	—	—	—	—	—	—	—	—	—	—	—	—	—	—	0.00	0.00
—	—	—	—	—	—	—	—	—	—	—	—	—	—	643	—	—	0.00	0.00
—	—	—	—	—	—	—	—	—	—	—	—	—	—	—	—	—	0.00	0.00
—	—	—	—	—	—	—	—	—	—	—	—	—	—	—	—	—	0.00	0.00
0.15	0.20	2.00	0.05	—	20.0	10.0	—	—	84	3.00	—	56	170	1	0.0	—	0.00	0.00
—	—	—	—	—	—	0.0	—	—	60	0.72	—	—	—	100	—	—	0.00	—
—	—	—	—	—	—	12.0	—	—	150	3.59	—	—	—	940	—	—	0.00	0.00
—	—	—	—	—	—	—	—	—	—	—	—	—	—	—	—	—	0.00	0.00
—	—	—	—	—	—	—	—	—	—	—	—	—	—	255	—	—	0.00	0.00
—	—	—	—	—	—	—	—	—	—	—	—	—	—	—	—	—	0.00	0.00
—	—	—	—	—	—	—	—	—	—	—	—	—	—	—	—	—	0.00	0.00
—	—	—	—	—	—	—	—	—	—	—	—	—	—	660	—	—	0.00	0.00
—	—	—	—	—	—	—	—	—	—	—	—	—	—	599	—	—	0.00	0.00
—	—	—	—	—	—	—	—	—	—	—	—	—	—	215	—	—	0.00	0.00
—	—	—	—	—	—	—	—	—	—	—	—	—	—	—	—	—	0.00	0.00
—	—	—	—	—	—	—	—	—	—	—	—	—	—	1688	—	—	0.00	0.00
—	—	—	—	—	—	3.6	—	—	150	3.59	—	—	230	820	—	49	0.00	0.00
—	—	—	—	—	—	9.0	—	—	150	3.59	—	—	320	890	—	—	0.00	0.00
—	—	—	—	—	—	1.2	—	—	20	0.72	—	—	190	480	—	48	0.00	0.00
—	—	—	—	—	—	2.4	—	—	80	1.79	—	—	470	870	—	—	0.00	0.00
—	—	—	—	—	—	42.0	—	—	200	3.59	—	—	1410	950	—	—	0.00	0.00

PAGE KEY: A-108 Beverage and Beverage Mixes A-110 Other Beverages A-110 Beverages, Alcoholic A-112 Candies and Confections, Gum A-116 Cereals, Breakfast Type A-120 Cheese and Cheese Substitutes A-122 Dairy Products and Substitutes A-124 Desserts A-130 Dessert Toppings A-130 Eggs, Substitutes, and Egg Dishes A-132 Ethnic Foods A-136 Fast Foods/Restaurants A-150 Fats, Oils, Margarines, Shortenings, and Substitutes A-150 Fish, Seafood, and Shellfish A-152 Food Additives A-152 Fruit, Vegetable, or Blended Juices A-154 Grains, Flours, and Fractions A-154 Grain Products, Prepared and Baked Goods

Code	Food Name	Unit/ Amt	Wt (g)	Energy (kcal)	Prot (g)	Carb (g)	Fiber (g)	Fat (g)	Sat (g)	Mono (g)	Poly (g)	Chol (mg)	Vit A (RE)
56580	Dish, baked potato broccoli cheese	1 ea	411	480	9	81	9	14	3.0	—	—	5	350
71834	Frozen Dessert, Frosty, dairy, jr	1 ea	113	170	4	28	0	4	2.5	—	—	20	80
2177	Frozen Dessert, Frosty, dairy, med	1 ea	298	440	11	73	0	11	7.0	—	—	50	200
56574	Hamburger, Big Bacon Classic	1 ea	282	570	34	46	3	29	12.0	—	—	100	150
71831	Potatoes, french fries, med, svg	1 ea	142	390	4	56	6	17	3.0	—	—	0	0
52080	Salad, caesar, w/o dressing, side	1 ea	99	70	7	2	1	4	2.0	—	—	15	450
56588	Salad, taco, supremo, w/o chips	1 ea	495	360	27	29	8	17	9.0	—	—	65	500
69059	Sandwich, chicken, grilled	1 ea	188	300	24	36	2	7	1.5	—	—	55	40

FATS, OILS, MARGARINES, SHORTENINGS, AND SUBSTITUTES

Fat Substitutes

Fats and Oils, Animal

Code	Food Name	Unit/ Amt	Wt (g)	Energy (kcal)	Prot (g)	Carb (g)	Fiber (g)	Fat (g)	Sat (g)	Mono (g)	Poly (g)	Chol (mg)	Vit A (RE)
8000	Butter, salted	1 Tbs	14	100	0	0	0	11	7.2	2.9	0.4	30	98
8003	Fat, bacon grease	1 tsp	4	39	0	0	0	4	1.7	1.9	0.5	4	0
8107	Fat, lard	1 Tbs	13	115	0	0	0	13	5.0	5.8	1.4	12	0

Fats and Oils, Vegetable

Code	Food Name	Unit/ Amt	Wt (g)	Energy (kcal)	Prot (g)	Carb (g)	Fiber (g)	Fat (g)	Sat (g)	Mono (g)	Poly (g)	Chol (mg)	Vit A (RE)
8084	Oil, canola	1 Tbs	14	124	0	0	0	14	1.0	8.2	4.1	0	0
8009	Oil, corn, salad or cooking	1 Tbs	14	120	0	0	0	14	1.8	3.8	7.4	0	0
8008	Oil, olive, salad or cooking	1 Tbs	14	119	0	0	0	14	1.8	10.0	1.4	0	0
90965	Oil, veg, pure	1 Tbs	14	120	0	0	0	14	1.5	6.0	6.0	0	0

Margarines and Spreads

Code	Food Name	Unit/ Amt	Wt (g)	Energy (kcal)	Prot (g)	Carb (g)	Fiber (g)	Fat (g)	Sat (g)	Mono (g)	Poly (g)	Chol (mg)	Vit A (RE)
8490	Margarine, soft, safflower oil	1 Tbs	14	100	0	0	0	11	1.0	8.0	2.0	0	100

Shortenings

Code	Food Name	Unit/ Amt	Wt (g)	Energy (kcal)	Prot (g)	Carb (g)	Fiber (g)	Fat (g)	Sat (g)	Mono (g)	Poly (g)	Chol (mg)	Vit A (RE)
8007	Shortening, household, hydrog soybean & cttnsd oil	1 Tbs	13	113	0	0	0	13	3.2	5.7	3.3	0	0

FISH, SEAFOOD, AND SHELLFISH

Code	Food Name	Unit/ Amt	Wt (g)	Energy (kcal)	Prot (g)	Carb (g)	Fiber (g)	Fat (g)	Sat (g)	Mono (g)	Poly (g)	Chol (mg)	Vit A (RE)
19049	Clams, bkd/brld, sml	15 ea	150	210	23	5	0	11	1.9	4.4	2.9	60	223
19151	Crab, imit	3 oz	85	99	11	11	0	1	0.1	0.1	0.3	42	6
17002	Fish Sticks, heated f/fzn, 4" x 1" x 1/2"	1 ea	28	76	4	7	0	3	0.9	1.4	0.9	31	9
17179	Fish, catfish, channel, fillet, bkd/brld, farmed	3 oz	85	129	16	0	0	7	1.5	3.5	1.2	54	13
17090	Fish, haddock, fillet, bkd/brld	3 oz	85	95	21	0	0	1	0.1	0.1	0.3	63	16
70260	Fish, halibut, battered, fzn	3 ea	113	330	13	22	0	21	3.0	8.0	1.5	20	—
17049	Fish, mackerel, Atlantic, fillet, bkd/brld	3 oz	85	223	20	0	0	15	3.6	6.0	3.7	64	46
17121	Fish, orange roughy, fillet, bkd/brld	3 oz	85	76	16	0	0	1	0.0	0.5	0.0	22	20
17093	Fish, perch, ocean, Atlantic, fillet, bkd/brld	3 oz	85	103	20	0	0	2	0.3	0.7	0.5	46	12
17171	Fish, salmon, pink, fillet, bkd/brld	3 oz	85	127	22	0	0	4	0.6	1.0	1.5	57	35
17068	Fish, sole, fillet, bkd/brld	3 oz	85	100	21	0	0	1	0.3	0.2	0.5	58	11
71139	Fish, sturgeon, filled, bkd/brld mixed species 4.5" x 2" 1/8" x 7/8"	3 oz	85	115	18	0	0	4	1.0	2.1	0.8	65	224
17101	Fish, tuna, bluefin, fillet, bkd/brld	3 oz	85	156	25	0	0	5	1.4	1.7	1.6	42	644
19056	Lobster, bkd/brld	1 ea	125	146	25	2	0	4	2.0	1.1	0.2	96	60
19061	Scallops, bkd/brld	4 ea	100	134	20	3	0	4	0.7	1.5	1.2	40	46
19065	Shrimp, bkd/brld, w/margarine & salt, med	2 ea	10	16	2	0	0	1	0.1	0.2	0.2	18	9
19401	Shrimp, cocktail	1 cup	230	218	28	21	5	3	0.5	0.4	1.0	196	72
70702	Shrimp, popcorn, breaded, fzn	20 ea	112	270	11	28	1	13	2.0	5.0	2.0	35	0

PAGE KEY: A-158 Granola Bars, Cereal Bars, Diet Bars, Scones, and Tarts   A-158 Meals and Dishes   A-162 Meats   A-168 Nuts, Seeds, and Products   A-170 Poultry   A-172 Salad Dressings, Dips, and Mayonnaise   A-172 Salads   A-174 Sandwiches   A-176 Sauces and Gravies   A-176 Snack Foods—Chips, Pretzels, Popcorn   A-178 Soups, Stews, and Chilis   A-180 Spices, Flavors, and Seasonings   A-182 Sports Bars and Drinks   A-182 Supplemental Foods and Formulas   A-184 Sweeteners and Sweet Substitutes   A-184 Vegetables and Legumes   A-198 Weight Loss Bars and Drinks   A-200 Miscellaneous

Thia (mg)	Ribo (mg)	Niac (mg NE)	Vit B6 (mg)	Vit B12 (µg)	Fol (µg)	Vit C (mg)	Vit D (IU)	Vit E (mg AT)	Cal (mg)	Iron (mg)	Magn (mg)	Phos (mg)	Pota (mg)	Sodi (mg)	Zinc (mg)	Wat (%)	Alco (g)	Caff (g)
—	—	—	—	—	—	72.0	—	—	200	4.50	—	—	1400	510	—	—	0.00	0.00
—	—	—	—	—	—	0.0	—	—	150	0.72	—	—	290	100	—	—	0.00	—
—	—	—	—	—	—	0.0	—	—	400	1.44	—	—	770	260	—	—	0.00	—
—	—	—	—	—	—	15.0	—	—	200	5.40	—	—	580	1460	—	—	0.00	0.00
—	—	—	—	—	—	3.6	—	—	20	1.44	—	—	770	340	—	—	0.00	0.00
—	—	—	—	—	—	21.0	—	—	150	1.08	—	—	280	250	—	—	0.00	0.00
—	—	—	—	—	—	27.0	—	—	350	3.59	—	—	950	1090	—	—	0.00	0.00
—	—	—	—	—	—	9.0	—	—	80	2.70	—	—	430	740	—	—	0.00	0.00
0.00	0.00	0.00	0.00	0.01	0.4	0.0	7.8	0.3	3	0.00	0.3	3	3	81	0.0	16	0.00	0.00
0.00	0.00	0.00	0.00	0.00	0.0	0.0	—	0.0	0	0.00	0.0	0	0	6	0.0	0	0.00	0.00
0.00	0.00	0.00	0.00	0.00	0.0	0.0	—	0.1	0	0.00	0.0	0	0	0	0.0	0	0.00	0.00
0.00	0.00	0.00	0.00	0.00	0.0	0.0	—	2.4	0	0.00	0.0	0	0	0	0.0	0	0.00	0.00
0.00	0.00	0.00	0.00	0.00	0.0	0.0	—	1.9	0	0.00	0.0	0	0	0	0.0	0	0.00	0.00
0.00	0.00	0.00	0.00	0.00	0.0	0.0	—	1.9	0	0.09	0.0	0	0	0	0.0	0	0.00	0.00
—	—	—	—	—	—	0.0	—	3.0	0	0.00	—	—	—	0	—	0	0.00	0.00
—	—	—	—	—	—	0.0	—	—	0	0.00	—	—	—	90	—	19	0.00	0.00
0.00	0.00	0.00	0.00	0.00	0.0	0.0	—	0.1	0	0.00	0.0	0	0	0	0.0	0	0.00	0.00
0.12	0.30	2.96	0.10	82.93	26.9	21.8	6.0	3.1	84	24.69	16.2	301	559	202	2.4	72	0.00	0.00
0.02	0.10	1.91	0.15	1.77	1.7	0.0	—	0.1	36	0.33	39.8	131	209	52	0.3	72	0.00	0.00
0.03	0.05	0.60	0.01	0.50	12.0	0.0	1.9	0.1	6	0.20	7.0	51	73	163	0.2	46	0.00	0.00
0.36	0.05	2.14	0.14	2.38	6.0	0.7	—	1.1	8	0.69	22.1	208	273	68	0.9	72	0.00	0.00
0.02	0.03	3.94	0.28	1.17	11.1	0.0	—	0.4	36	1.14	42.5	205	339	74	0.4	74	0.00	0.00
																48	0.00	0.00
0.14	0.34	5.82	0.38	16.15	1.7	0.3	—	1.6	13	1.34	82.5	236	341	71	0.8	53	0.00	0.00
0.10	0.15	3.10	0.28	1.96	6.8	0.0	—	0.5	32	0.20	32.3	218	327	69	0.8	69	0.00	0.00
0.10	0.10	2.06	0.23	0.98	8.5	0.7	—	1.4	117	1.00	33.2	236	298	82	0.5	73	0.00	0.00
0.17	0.05	7.25	0.20	2.94	4.3	0.0	—	1.1	14	0.83	28.1	251	352	73	0.6	70	0.00	0.00
0.07	0.10	1.85	0.20	2.13	7.7	0.0	—	0.6	15	0.28	49.3	246	293	89	0.5	73	0.00	0.00
0.07	0.07	8.59	0.20	2.13	14.5	0.0	—	0.5	14	0.76	38.3	230	310	59	0.5	70	0.00	0.00
0.23	0.25	8.96	0.44	9.25	1.7	0.0	—	1.1	9	1.11	54.4	277	275	43	0.7	59	0.00	0.00
0.00	0.07	1.29	0.09	3.77	13.6	0.0	7.0	1.3	75	0.47	42.5	225	428	492	3.5	74	0.00	0.00
0.00	0.05	1.33	0.17	1.75	18.5	3.5	4.0	1.7	30	0.34	68.0	266	392	231	1.2	71	0.00	0.00
0.00	0.00	0.28	0.00	0.12	0.3	0.2	14.0	0.1	6	0.28	4.5	25	23	21	0.1	68	0.00	0.00
0.10	0.10	4.30	0.25	1.26	47.7	25.7	147.2	3.5	91	3.76	59.4	307	576	1129	1.6	75	0.00	0.00
—	—	—	—	—	—	0.0	—	—	40	1.44	—	—	—	610	—	—	0.00	0.00

PAGE KEY: A-108 Beverage and Beverage Mixes   A-110 Other Beverages   A-110 Beverages, Alcoholic   A-112 Candies and Confections, Gum   A-116 Cereals, Breakfast Type
A-120 Cheese and Cheese Substitutes   A-122 Dairy Products and Substitutes   A-124 Desserts   A-130 Dessert Toppings   A-130 Eggs, Substitutes, and Egg Dishes   A-132 Ethnic Foods
A-136 Fast Foods/Restaurants   A-150 Fats, Oils, Margarines, Shortenings, and Substitutes   A-150 Fish, Seafood, and Shellfish   A-152 Food Additives
A-152 Fruit, Vegetable, or Blended Juices   A-154 Grains, Flours, and Fractions   A-154 Grain Products, Prepared and Baked Goods

Code	Food Name	Unit/ Amt	Wt (g)	Energy (kcal)	Prot (g)	Carb (g)	Fiber (g)	Fat (g)	Sat (g)	Mono (g)	Poly (g)	Chol (mg)	Vit A (RE)
FOOD ADDITIVES													
ALGINATES													
Bases and Preps													
54032	Prep, consomme, chicken style, w/o msg, vgtrn, dry mix	1 cup	246	522	21	76	—	15	2.0	—	—	1	—
Chemicals													
Colors, Flavors, and Aromas													
26624	Flavor, vanilla extract	1 tsp	4	12	0	1	0	0	0.0	0.0	0.0	0	0
Gums, Fibers, Starches, Pectins, Emulsifiers													
30000	Cornstarch	1 Tbs	8	30	0	7	0	0	0.0	0.0	0.0	0	0
Ingredient Sweeteners													
Nutraceuticals													
Nutritional Additives													
JUICE—100% FRUIT, VEGETABLE, OR BLENDED													
3008	Juice, apple, unswtnd, cnd/btld	1 cup	248	117	0	29	0	0	0.0	0.0	0.1	0	0
3455	Juice, grapefruit, pink, fresh	1 cup	247	96	1	23	0	0	0.0	0.0	0.1	0	109
3090	Juice, orange, fresh	1 cup	248	112	2	26	0	0	0.1	0.1	0.1	0	50
3561	Juice, orange, fzn, conc	2.2 oz	63	110	1	27	0	0	0.0	0.0	0.0	0	0
Fruits													
3001	Apples, fresh, lrg, 3 1/4"	1 ea	212	110	1	29	5	0	0.1	0.0	0.1	0	13
3147	Applesauce, swtnd, unsalted, cnd	1 cup	255	194	0	51	3	0	0.1	0.0	0.1	0	5
3157	Apricots, fresh, whole	1 ea	35	17	0	4	1	0	0.0	0.1	0.0	0	67
3016	Avocado, avg, fresh	1 ea	201	322	4	17	13	29	4.3	19.7	3.7	0	28
3020	Banana, fresh, med, 7" to 7 7/8" long	1 ea	118	105	1	27	3	0	0.1	0.0	0.1	0	7
3029	Blueberries, fresh	0.5 cup	68	39	1	10	2	0	0.0	0.0	0.1	0	4
3026	Boysenberries, fresh	0.5 cup	72	31	1	7	4	0	0.0	0.0	0.2	0	16
3036	Cherries, sweet, fresh	1 ea	7	4	0	1	0	0	0.0	0.0	0.0	0	0
3191	Currants, red, fresh	1 cup	112	63	2	15	5	0	0.0	0.0	0.1	0	4
3676	Figs, fresh, lrg, 2 1/2"	1 ea	64	47	0	12	2	0	0.0	0.0	0.1	0	9
3203	Gooseberries, fresh	0.5 cup	75	33	1	8	3	0	0.0	0.0	0.2	0	22
3818	Grapefruit, pink, fresh, 3 3/4"	0.5 ea	123	52	1	13	2	0	0.0	0.0	0.0	0	143
3820	Grapefruit, red, fresh, 3 3/4"	0.5 ea	123	52	1	13	2	0	0.0	0.0	0.0	0	143
3638	Kiwi, fresh	1 cup	177	108	2	26	5	1	0.1	0.1	0.5	0	14
3067	Lemon Peel, fresh	1 Tbs	6	3	0	1	1	0	0.0	0.0	0.0	0	0
3071	Limes, peeled, fresh, 2"	1 ea	67	20	0	7	2	0	0.0	0.0	0.0	0	3
71769	Mandarin Oranges, fresh, med, 2 3/8"	1 ea	84	45	1	11	2	0	0.0	0.1	0.1	0	57
71774	Mandarin Oranges, w/light syrup, cnd	1 cup	252	154	1	41	2	0	0.0	0.0	0.1	0	212
3221	Mango, fresh, whole	0.5 ea	104	67	1	18	2	0	0.1	0.1	0.1	0	79
3076	Melon, cantaloupe, fresh, med, 5"	1 ea	552	188	5	45	5	1	0.3	0.0	0.4	0	1866
71102	Melon, honeydew, fresh, 5 1/4"	1 ea	1000	360	5	91	8	1	0.4	0.0	0.6	0	60
3309	Mulberries, fresh	10 ea	15	6	0	1	0	0	0.0	0.0	0.0	0	0
3215	Nectarines, fresh, 2 1/2"	1 ea	136	60	1	14	2	0	0.0	0.1	0.2	0	46
3082	Oranges, fresh, med, 2 5/8"	1 ea	131	62	1	15	3	0	0.0	0.0	0.0	0	29
3720	Papaya, fresh, lrg, 5 3/4" x 3 1/"4	1 ea	380	148	2	37	7	1	0.2	0.1	0.1	0	418
3096	Peaches, fresh, med, w/o skin, 2 1/2"	1 ea	98	38	1	9	1	0	0.0	0.1	0.1	0	31
3103	Pears, fresh, bartlett, med	1 ea	166	96	1	26	5	0	0.0	0.0	0.0	0	3
71114	Pineapple, chunks, w/juice, cnd, not drained	0.5 cup	124	75	1	20	1	0	0.0	0.0	0.0	0	5

PAGE KEY: A-158 Granola Bars, Cereal Bars, Diet Bars, Scones, and Tarts   A-158 Meals and Dishes   A-162 Meats   A-168 Nuts, Seeds, and Products   A-170 Poultry   A-172 Salad Dressings, Dips, and Mayonnaise   A-172 Salads   A-174 Sandwiches   A-176 Sauces and Gravies   A-176 Snack Foods—Chips, Pretzels, Popcorn   A-178 Soups, Stews, and Chilis   A-180 Spices, Flavors, and Seasonings   A-182 Sports Bars and Drinks   A-182 Supplemental Foods and Formulas   A-184 Sweeteners and Sweet Substitutes   A-184 Vegetables and Legumes   A-198 Weight Loss Bars and Drinks   A-200 Miscellaneous

Thia (mg)	Ribo (mg)	Niac (mg NE)	Vit B6 (mg)	Vit B12 (µg)	Fol (µg)	Vit C (mg)	Vit D (IU)	Vit E (mg AT)	Cal (mg)	Iron (mg)	Magn (mg)	Phos (mg)	Pota (mg)	Sodi (mg)	Zinc (mg)	Wat (%)	Alco (g)	Caff (g)
—	—	—	—	—	—	—	—	—	—	—	—	—	492	46494	—	—	0.00	0.00
0.00	0.00	0.01	0.00	0.00	0.0	0.0	—	0.0	0	0.00	0.5	0	6	0	0.0	53	1.49	0.00
0.00	0.00	0.00	0.00	0.00	0.0	0.0	—	0.0	0	0.03	0.2	1	0	1	0.0	8	0.00	0.00
0.05	0.03	0.25	0.07	0.00	0.0	2.2	—	0.0	17	0.92	7.4	17	295	7	0.1	88	0.00	0.00
0.10	0.05	0.49	0.10	0.00	24.7	93.9	0.0	0.1	22	0.49	29.6	37	400	2	0.1	90	0.00	0.00
0.21	0.07	0.99	0.10	0.00	74.4	124.0	—	0.1	27	0.50	27.3	42	496	2	0.1	88	0.00	0.00
0.00	—	0.00	0.00	—	10.0	78.0	—	0.0	20	0.00	—		430	5	—	53	0.00	0.00
0.03	0.05	0.18	0.09	0.00	6.4	9.8	—	0.4	13	0.25	10.6	23	227	2	0.1	86	0.00	0.00
0.02	0.07	0.47	0.07	0.00	2.5	4.3	—	0.5	10	0.88	7.6	18	156	8	0.1	80	0.00	0.00
0.00	0.00	0.20	0.01	0.00	3.1	3.5	—	0.3	5	0.14	3.5	8	91	0	0.1	86	0.00	0.00
0.12	0.25	3.49	0.51	0.00	162.8	20.1	—	4.2	24	1.11	58.3	105	975	14	1.3	73	0.00	0.00
0.03	0.09	0.77	0.43	0.00	23.6	10.3	—	0.1	6	0.31	31.9	26	422	1	0.2	75	0.00	0.00
0.02	0.02	0.28	0.03	0.00	4.1	6.6	—	0.4	4	0.18	4.1	8	52	1	0.1	84	0.00	0.00
0.00	0.01	0.46	0.01	0.00	18.0	15.1	—	0.8	21	0.44	14.4	16	117	1	0.4	88	0.00	0.00
0.00	0.00	0.00	0.00	0.00	0.3	0.5	—	0.0	1	0.01	0.7	1	15	0	0.0	82	0.00	0.00
0.03	0.05	0.10	0.07	0.00	9.0	45.9	—	0.1	37	1.12	14.6	49	308	1	0.3	84	0.00	0.00
0.03	0.02	0.25	0.07	0.00	3.8	1.3	—	0.1	22	0.23	10.9	9	148	1	0.1	79	0.00	0.00
0.02	0.01	0.23	0.05	0.00	4.5	20.8	—	0.3	19	0.23	7.5	20	148	1	0.1	88	0.00	0.00
0.05	0.03	0.25	0.07	0.00	16.0	38.4	—	0.2	27	0.10	11.1	22	166	0	0.1	88	0.00	0.00
0.05	0.03	0.25	0.07	0.00	16.0	38.4	—	0.2	27	0.10	11.1	22	166	0	0.1	88	0.00	0.00
0.05	0.03	0.60	0.10	0.00	44.2	164.1	—	2.6	60	0.55	30.1	60	552	5	0.2	83	0.00	0.00
0.00	0.00	0.01	0.00	0.00	0.8	7.7	—	0.0	8	0.05	0.9	1	10	0	0.0	82	0.00	0.00
0.01	0.00	0.12	0.02	0.00	5.4	19.5	—	0.1	22	0.40	4.0	12	68	1	0.1	88	0.00	0.00
0.05	0.02	0.31	0.07	0.00	13.4	22.4	—	0.2	31	0.12	10.1	17	139	2	0.1	85	0.00	0.00
0.12	0.10	1.12	0.10	0.00	12.6	49.9	—	0.3	18	0.93	20.2	25	197	15	0.6	83	0.00	0.00
0.05	0.05	0.60	0.14	0.00	14.5	28.7	—	1.2	10	0.12	9.3	11	161	2	0.0	82	0.00	0.00
0.23	0.10	4.05	0.40	0.00	115.9	202.6	—	0.3	50	1.15	66.2	83	1474	88	1.0	90	0.00	0.00
0.37	0.11	4.17	0.87	0.00	190.0	180.0	—	0.2	60	1.70	100.0	110	2280	180	0.9	90	0.00	0.00
0.00	0.01	0.09	0.00	0.00	0.9	5.5	0.0	0.1	6	0.28	2.7	6	29	2	0.0	88	0.00	0.00
0.05	0.03	1.52	0.02	0.00	6.8	7.3	—	1.0	8	0.37	12.2	35	273	0	0.2	88	0.00	0.00
0.10	0.05	0.37	0.07	0.00	39.3	69.7	—	0.2	52	0.12	13.1	18	237	0	0.1	87	0.00	0.00
0.10	0.11	1.27	0.07	0.00	144.4	234.8	—	2.8	91	0.37	38.0	19	977	11	0.3	89	0.00	0.00
0.01	0.02	0.79	0.01	0.00	3.9	6.5	—	0.7	6	0.25	8.8	20	186	0	0.2	89	0.00	0.00
0.01	0.03	0.25	0.05	0.00	11.6	7.0	—	0.2	15	0.28	11.6	18	198	2	0.2	84	0.00	0.00
0.11	0.01	0.34	0.09	0.00	6.2	11.8	—	0.0	17	0.34	17.4	7	152	1	0.1	84	0.00	0.00

PAGE KEY: A-108 Beverage and Beverage Mixes   A-110 Other Beverages   A-110 Beverages, Alcoholic   A-112 Candies and Confections, Gum   A-116 Cereals, Breakfast Type   A-120 Cheese and Cheese Substitutes   A-122 Dairy Products and Substitutes   A-124 Desserts   A-130 Dessert Toppings   A-130 Eggs, Substitutes, and Egg Dishes   A-132 Ethnic Foods   A-136 Fast Foods/Restaurants   A-150 Fats, Oils, Margarines, Shortenings, and Substitutes   A-150 Fish, Seafood, and Shellfish   A-152 Food Additives   A-152 Fruit, Vegetable, or Blended Juices   A-154 Grains, Flours, and Fractions   A-154 Grain Products, Prepared and Baked Goods

Code	Food Name	Unit/ Amt	Wt (g)	Energy (kcal)	Prot (g)	Carb (g)	Fiber (g)	Fat (g)	Sat (g)	Mono (g)	Poly (g)	Chol (mg)	Vit A (RE)
3112	Pineapple, fresh	1 ea	472	227	3	60	7	1	0.0	0.1	0.2	0	28
3121	Plums, fresh, 2 1/8"	1 ea	66	30	0	8	1	0	0.0	0.1	0.0	0	22
3197	Pomegranate, fresh, 3 3/8"	1 ea	154	105	1	26	1	0	0.1	0.1	0.1	0	15
3202	Raisins, golden, seedless, packed cup	0.25 cup	41	125	1	33	2	0	0.1	0.0	0.1	0	0
3209	Rhubarb, fresh, diced	0.5 cup	61	13	1	3	1	0	0.0	0.0	0.1	0	6
3134	Strawberries, fresh, whole	1 cup	144	46	1	11	3	0	0.0	0.1	0.2	0	3
3087	Tangelo, fresh, 2 3/8"	1 ea	96	45	1	11	2	0	0.0	0.0	0.0	0	21
3717	Tangerines, fresh, lrg, 2 1/2"	1 ea	98	52	1	13	2	0	0.0	0.1	0.1	0	67
3143	Watermelon, fresh, slice, 1/16 melon	1 pce	286	86	2	22	1	0	0.0	0.1	0.1	0	160
GRAINS, FLOURS, AND FRACTIONS													
38650	Dish, wheat pilaf, dry mix	2 oz	57	184	6	42	5	1	0.2	0.1	0.4	0	7
28018	Flour, all purpose, self-rising, bleached, enrich	0.25 cup	30	100	3	22	0	0	0.0	0.0	0.0	0	0
38030	Flour, all purpose, white, bleached, enrich	0.25 cup	31	114	3	24	1	0	0.0	0.0	0.1	0	0
46086	Flour, cake, white, enrich, unsifted	0.25 cup	34	124	3	27	1	0	0.0	0.0	0.1	0	0
38032	Flour, whole wheat	0.25 cup	30	102	4	22	4	1	0.1	0.1	0.2	0	0
38017	Oats, old fash, dry	0.5 cup	40	148	5	27	4	3	0.4	0.8	0.9	0	0
38575	Oats, steel cut, Irish style, dry	0.25 cup	40	148	5	27	4	3	0.4	0.8	0.9	0	0
2730	Tapioca, dry	1.5 tsp	6	20	0	5	0	0	0.0	0.0	0.0	0	0
38027	Wheat, bulgur, dry	0.25 cup	35	120	4	27	6	0	0.1	0.1	0.2	0	0
38026	Wheat, germ, tstd	1 cup	113	432	33	56	17	12	2.1	1.7	7.5	0	11
38068	Wheat, sprouted	1 cup	108	214	8	46	1	1	0.2	0.2	0.6	0	0
GRAIN PRODUCTS, PREPARED AND BAKED GOODS													
Bagels													
71165	Bagel, egg, 3"	1 ea	57	158	6	30	1	1	0.2	0.2	0.4	14	19
8846	Bagel, plain, classic, 4 oz svg	1 ea	112	296	11	60	3	2	—	—	—	0	0
Biscuits													
42001	Biscuit, buttermilk, prep f/recipe, 2 1/2"	1 ea	60	212	4	27	1	10	2.6	4.2	2.5	2	14
71195	Biscuit, plain, prep f/recipe, 2 1/2"	1 ea	60	212	4	27	1	10	2.6	4.2	2.5	2	14
42205	Biscuit, whole wheat	1 ea	63	199	6	30	5	7	1.7	3.0	2.2	2	14
Breads and Rolls													
71024	Bread Crumbs, white, soft, enrich	1 cup	45	120	3	23	1	1	0.3	0.3	0.6	0	0
71021	Bread, 7 grain, slice	1 pce	26	65	3	12	2	1	0.2	0.4	0.2	0	0
42052	Bread, Boston brown, cnd, slice	1 pce	45	88	2	19	2	1	0.1	0.1	0.3	0	11
42042	Bread, cracked wheat, slice, reg	1 pce	25	65	2	12	1	1	0.2	0.5	0.2	0	0
71207	Bread, French, slice, lrg	1 pce	96	263	8	50	3	3	0.6	1.2	0.7	0	0
42049	Bread, oatmeal, slice	1 pce	27	73	2	13	1	1	0.2	0.4	0.5	0	1
42007	Bread, pita, white, enrich, lrg, 6 1/2"	1 ea	60	165	5	33	1	1	0.1	0.1	0.3	0	0
42051	Bread, raisin, enrich, slice	1 pce	26	71	2	14	1	1	0.3	0.6	0.2	0	0
57235	Bread, rye, mild	1 pce	32	70	3	13	4	0	0.0	—	—	0	0
42003	Bread, sourdough starter	1 cup	250	359	17	70	5	2	0.2	—	—	1	38
42012	Bread, wheat, slice	1 pce	25	65	2	12	1	1	0.2	0.4	0.2	0	0
42138	Bread, white, prep w/2% milk f/recipe, slice	1 pce	42	120	3	21	1	2	0.5	0.5	1.2	1	10
71020	Bread, whole grain, slice	1 pce	26	65	3	12	2	1	0.2	0.4	0.2	0	0
71939	Bread, wraps, thin thin	1 ea	35	110	4	21	0	1	0.0	—	—	0	0
42036	Breadsticks, plain, 7 5/8" x 5/8"	1 ea	10	41	1	7	0	1	0.1	0.4	0.4	0	0

PAGE KEY: A-158 Granola Bars, Cereal Bars, Diet Bars, Scones, and Tarts   A-158 Meals and Dishes   A-162 Meats   A-168 Nuts, Seeds, and Products   A-170 Poultry   A-172 Salad Dressings, Dips, and Mayonnaise   A-172 Salads   A-174 Sandwiches   A-176 Sauces and Gravies   A-176 Snack Foods—Chips, Pretzels, Popcorn   A-178 Soups, Stews, and Chilis   A-180 Spices, Flavors, and Seasonings   A-182 Sports Bars and Drinks   A-182 Supplemental Foods and Formulas   A-184 Sweeteners and Sweet Substitutes   A-184 Vegetables and Legumes   A-198 Weight Loss Bars and Drinks   A-200 Miscellaneous

Thia (mg)	Ribo (mg)	Niac (mg NE)	Vit B6 (mg)	Vit B12 (µg)	Fol (µg)	Vit C (mg)	Vit D (IU)	Vit E (mg AT)	Cal (mg)	Iron (mg)	Magn (mg)	Phos (mg)	Pota (mg)	Sodi (mg)	Zinc (mg)	Wat (%)	Alco (g)	Caff (g)
0.37	0.15	2.30	0.51	0.00	70.8	170.9	—	0.1	61	1.32	56.6	38	543	5	0.5	86	0.00	0.00
0.01	0.01	0.28	0.01	0.00	3.3	6.3	—	0.2	4	0.10	4.6	11	104	0	0.1	87	0.00	0.00
0.05	0.05	0.46	0.15	0.00	9.2	9.4	—	0.9	5	0.46	4.6	12	399	5	0.2	81	0.00	0.00
0.00	0.07	0.46	0.12	0.00	1.2	1.3	—	0.0	22	0.74	14.4	47	308	5	0.1	15	0.00	0.00
0.00	0.01	0.18	0.00	0.00	4.3	4.9	—	0.2	52	0.12	7.3	9	176	2	0.1	94	0.00	0.00
0.02	0.02	0.56	0.07	0.00	34.6	84.7	—	0.4	23	0.60	18.7	35	220	1	0.2	91	0.00	0.00
0.07	0.03	0.27	0.05	0.00	28.8	51.1	—	0.2	38	0.10	9.6	13	174	0	0.1	87	0.00	0.00
0.05	0.03	0.37	0.07	0.00	15.7	26.2	—	0.2	36	0.15	11.8	20	163	2	0.1	85	0.00	0.00
0.09	0.05	0.50	0.12	0.00	8.6	23.2	—	0.1	20	0.68	28.6	31	320	3	0.3	91	0.00	0.00
0.17	0.10	2.47	0.11	0.00	12.1	1.2	0.0	0.3	23	1.10	10.8	49	213	645	0.6	9	0.00	0.00
0.15	0.10	1.60	—	—	40.0	0.0	—	—	60	1.44	—	—	35	400	—	16	0.00	0.00
0.25	0.15	1.84	0.00	0.00	57.2	0.0	—	0.0	5	1.45	6.9	34	33	1	0.2	12	0.00	0.00
0.31	0.15	2.32	0.00	0.00	63.7	0.0	—	0.0	5	2.50	5.5	29	36	1	0.2	13	0.00	0.00
0.12	0.05	1.90	0.10	0.00	13.2	0.0	—	0.2	10	1.15	41.4	104	122	2	0.9	10	0.00	0.00
0.21	0.05	0.33	0.03	0.00	19.5	0.0	0.0	0.3	19	1.86	107.9	183	143	1	1.3	9	0.00	0.00
0.21	0.05	0.33	0.03	0.00	19.5	0.0	0.0	0.3	19	1.86	107.9	183	143	1	1.3	9	0.00	0.00
—	—	—	—	—	—	0.0	—	—	0	0.00	—	0	0	0	—	—	0.00	0.00
0.07	0.03	1.78	0.11	0.00	9.4	0.0	—	0.0	12	0.86	57.4	105	144	6	0.7	9	0.00	0.00
1.88	0.93	6.32	1.11	0.00	397.8	6.8	0.0	18.1	51	10.27	361.6	1295	1070	5	18.8	6	0.00	0.00
0.23	0.17	3.32	0.28	0.00	41.0	2.8	—	0.1	30	2.30	88.6	216	183	17	1.8	48	0.00	0.00
0.31	0.12	1.96	0.05	0.09	50.2	0.3	—	0.1	7	2.26	14.2	48	39	288	0.4	33	0.00	0.00
0.47	0.31	3.96	0.00	0.00	0.1	0.1	0.0	0.0	14	3.32	0.4	71	80	510	0.0	34	0.00	0.00
0.20	0.18	1.76	0.01	0.05	36.6	0.1	—	0.8	141	1.74	10.8	98	73	348	0.3	29	0.00	0.00
0.20	0.18	1.76	0.01	0.05	36.6	0.1	—	0.8	141	1.74	10.8	98	73	348	0.3	29	0.00	0.00
0.15	0.11	2.20	0.12	0.07	13.0	0.2	10.1	1.3	155	1.69	56.9	199	200	210	1.2	28	0.00	0.00
0.20	0.15	1.97	0.03	0.00	49.9	0.0	—	0.1	68	1.67	10.3	45	45	306	0.3	36	0.00	0.00
0.10	0.09	1.12	0.09	0.01	30.7	0.1	—	0.1	24	0.89	13.8	46	53	127	0.3	38	0.00	0.00
0.00	0.05	0.50	0.03	0.00	4.9	0.0	—	0.1	32	0.93	28.3	50	143	284	0.2	47	0.00	0.00
0.09	0.05	0.92	0.07	0.00	15.2	0.0	—	0.1	11	0.69	13.0	38	44	134	0.3	36	0.00	0.00
0.50	0.31	4.55	0.03	0.00	142.1	0.0	—	0.3	72	2.43	25.9	101	108	585	0.8	34	0.00	0.00
0.10	0.05	0.85	0.01	0.00	16.7	0.0	—	0.1	18	0.73	10.0	34	38	162	0.3	37	0.00	0.00
0.36	0.20	2.77	0.01	0.00	64.2	0.0	—	0.2	52	1.57	15.6	58	72	322	0.5	32	0.00	0.00
0.09	0.10	0.89	0.01	0.00	27.6	0.0	—	0.1	17	0.75	6.8	28	59	101	0.2	34	0.00	0.00
0.15	0.14	3.00	0.30	0.89	80.0	0.0	—	—	100	1.79	60.0	—	—	70	2.2	47	0.00	0.00
1.00	1.35	10.68	0.30	0.31	508.7	0.5	35.2	0.1	123	6.17	42.9	358	522	57	1.9	64	0.00	0.00
0.10	0.07	1.02	0.01	0.00	22.8	0.0	—	0.1	26	0.82	11.5	38	50	132	0.3	37	0.00	0.00
0.17	0.15	1.50	0.01	0.02	38.2	0.1	—	0.4	24	1.25	8.0	48	61	151	0.3	35	0.00	0.00
0.10	0.09	1.12	0.09	0.01	30.7	0.1	—	0.1	24	0.89	13.8	46	53	127	0.3	38	0.00	0.00
—	—	—	—	—	—	0.0	—	—	40	1.44	—	—	—	190	—	—	0.00	0.00
0.05	0.05	0.52	0.00	0.00	16.2	0.0	—	0.1	2	0.43	3.2	12	12	66	0.1	6	0.00	0.00

PAGE KEY: A-108 Beverage and Beverage Mixes   A-110 Other Beverages   A-110 Beverages, Alcoholic   A-112 Candies and Confections, Gum   A-116 Cereals, Breakfast Type   A-120 Cheese and Cheese Substitutes   A-122 Dairy Products and Substitutes   A-124 Desserts   A-130 Dessert Toppings   A-130 Eggs, Substitutes, and Egg Dishes   A-132 Ethnic Foods   A-136 Fast Foods/Restaurants   A-150 Fats, Oils, Margarines, Shortenings, and Substitutes   A-150 Fish, Seafood, and Shellfish   A-152 Food Additives   A-152 Fruit, Vegetable, or Blended Juices   A-154 Grains, Flours, and Fractions   A-154 Grain Products, Prepared and Baked Goods

Code	Food Name	Unit/ Amt	Wt (g)	Energy (kcal)	Prot (g)	Carb (g)	Fiber (g)	Fat (g)	Sat (g)	Mono (g)	Poly (g)	Chol (mg)	Vit A (RE)
42020	Buns, hamburger	1 ea	43	120	4	21	1	2	0.5	0.5	0.8	0	0
42021	Buns, hot dog/frankfurter	1 ea	43	120	4	21	1	2	0.5	0.5	0.8	0	0
42649	Cornbread, homestyle, prep f/dry mix, 2" x 3" pce	1 pce	52	150	3	26	1	4	1.0	1.5	1.0	5	0
42015	Croissant, butter, med	1 ea	57	231	5	26	1	12	6.6	3.1	0.6	38	120
45520	Dumpling, plain	1 ea	32	40	1	7	0	1	0.3	0.4	0.3	1	4
43512	Matzoh Balls	3 ea	42	58	2	7	0	2	0.5	0.8	0.5	44	20
71886	Pretzels, soft, garlic	1 ea	120	320	9	66	2	1	0.0	—	—	0	0
42018	Rolls, dinner, brown & serve, browned	1 ea	28	84	2	14	1	2	0.5	1.0	0.3	0	0
42158	Rolls, dinner, prep f/recipe w/2% milk, 2 1/2"	1 ea	35	111	3	19	1	3	0.6	1.0	0.7	12	32
42022	Rolls, hard, 3 1/2"	1 ea	57	167	6	30	1	2	0.3	0.6	1.0	0	0
71358	Rolls, hoagie, whole wheat, med	1 ea	94	250	8	48	7	4	0.8	1.1	2.0	0	0
71359	Rolls, submarine, whole wheat, med	1 ea	94	250	8	48	7	4	0.8	1.1	2.0	0	0
Bread Crumbs, Croutons, Breading Mixes & Batters													
42004	Bread Crumbs, plain, grated, dry	1 Tbs	7	27	1	5	0	0	0.1	0.1	0.1	0	0
42016	Croutons, plain, dry	0.25 cup	8	31	1	6	0	0	0.1	0.2	0.1	0	0
Crackers													
43503	Cracker Crumbs, graham, plain	1 cup	84	355	6	65	2	8	1.3	3.4	3.2	0	0
71273	Crackers, cheese, 1" square	30 ea	30	151	3	17	1	8	2.8	3.6	0.7	4	9
11712	Crackers, club style	1 ea	7	32	1	5	0	1	0.3	—	—	0	0
11745	Crackers, ea, Town House	5 ea	16	83	1	9	0	5	0.9	—	—	0	1
47253	Crackers, graham, honey	3 ea	21	92	2	16	1	3	0.7	—	—	0	0
43535	Crackers, matzoh, egg, svg	1 oz	28	111	3	22	1	1	0.2	0.2	0.1	24	4
43509	Crackers, melba toast, plain, pce, 3 3/4" x 1 3/4" x 1/8"	1 pce	5	20	1	4	0	0	0.0	0.0	0.1	0	0
70963	Crackers, original, svg	5 ea	16	79	1	10	0	4	0.6	2.8	0.3	0	0
43506	Crackers, saltines	4 ea	12	51	1	9	0	1	0.2	0.8	0.1	0	0
43581	Crackers, wheat, original	16 ea	29	136	2	20	1	6	0.9	2.0	0.4	0	0
Muffins													
44585	English Muffin, traditional	1 ea	57	130	5	26	2	0	0.0	—	—	0	0
44515	Muffin, plain, prep f/recipe w/2% milk	1 ea	57	169	4	24	2	6	1.2	1.6	3.3	22	23
42295	Popover, unenrich, dry mix, 6 oz pkg	1 ea	170	631	18	121	—	7	1.7	3.4	1.4	0	0
Pancakes, French Toast, and Waffles													
45033	Crepe, suzette	1 ea	66	159	4	16	0	9	3.8	3.2	1.3	83	81
42156	French Toast, prep f/recipe w/2% milk	1 pce	65	149	5	16	1	7	1.8	2.9	1.7	75	84
45192	Pancakes, buttermilk	1 ea	43	99	3	16	0	3	0.6	1.3	0.9	5	73
45152	Waffles, buttermilk egg, 7" prep f/dry mix	1 ea	81	230	6	37	2	7	1.0	3.5	2.5	10	0
Pasta													
57411	Dish, ravioli, beef, square, preckd	9 pce	146	300	14	40	1	8	3.8	—	—	77	—
92216	Dish, tortellini, cheese filled	1 cup	108	332	15	51	2	8	3.9	2.2	0.5	45	42
91205	Pasta, acini di pepe, enrich, dry, all brands	3.6 oz	100	364	14	74	3	1	0.4	—	—	0	0
38365	Pasta, egg noodles	0.75 cup	68	200	8	33	1	4	1.0	—	—	40	0
38580	Pasta, elbow twist, semolina, dry	0.75 cup	56	201	7	41	2	1	0.3	0.2	0.8	0	0
91211	Pasta, lasagna noodles, enrich, dry, all brands	3.6 oz	100	364	14	74	3	1	0.4	—	—	0	0
38102	Pasta, macaroni noodles, enrich, ckd	1 cup	140	197	7	40	2	1	0.1	0.1	0.4	0	0
38551	Pasta, rice noodle, ckd	0.5 cup	88	96	1	22	1	0	0.0	0.0	0.0	0	0
38105	Pasta, shells, sml, enrich, ckd	0.5 cup	58	81	3	16	1	0	0.1	0.0	0.2	0	0
38118	Pasta, spaghetti noodles, enrich, ckd	0.5 cup	70	99	3	20	1	0	0.1	0.1	0.2	0	0

PAGE KEY: A-158 Granola Bars, Cereal Bars, Diet Bars, Scones, and Tarts   A-158 Meals and Dishes   A-162 Meats   A-168 Nuts, Seeds, and Products   A-170 Poultry   A-172 Salad Dressings, Dips, and Mayonnaise   A-172 Salads   A-174 Sandwiches   A-176 Sauces and Gravies   A-176 Snack Foods—Chips, Pretzels, Popcorn   A-178 Soups, Stews, and Chilis   A-180 Spices, Flavors, and Seasonings   A-182 Sports Bars and Drinks   A-182 Supplemental Foods and Formulas   A-184 Sweeteners and Sweet Substitutes   A-184 Vegetables and Legumes   A-198 Weight Loss Bars and Drinks   A-200 Miscellaneous

Thia (mg)	Ribo (mg)	Niac (mg NE)	Vit B6 (mg)	Vit B12 (µg)	Fol (µg)	Vit C (mg)	Vit D (IU)	Vit E (mg AT)	Cal (mg)	Iron (mg)	Magn (mg)	Phos (mg)	Pota (mg)	Sodi (mg)	Zinc (mg)	Wat (%)	Alco (g)	Caff (g)
0.17	0.14	1.78	0.02	0.09	47.7	0.0	—	0.0	59	1.42	9.0	27	40	206	0.3	35	0.00	0.00
0.17	0.14	1.78	0.02	0.09	47.7	0.0	—	0.0	59	1.42	9.0	27	40	206	0.3	35	0.00	0.00
—	—	—	—	—	—	0.0	—		9	0.49	—	90	40	280	—	35	0.00	0.00
0.21	0.14	1.25	0.02	0.09	50.2	0.1	—	0.5	21	1.15	9.1	60	67	424	0.4	23	0.00	0.00
0.05	0.05	0.41	0.00	0.01	1.8	0.1	—	0.1	45	0.43	3.0	28	20	66	0.1	72	0.00	0.00
0.02	0.07	0.31	0.01	0.09	4.5	0.0	—	0.3	6	0.43	3.3	26	22	13	0.2	72	0.00	0.00
—	—	—	—	—	—	0.0	—	—	20	2.16	—	—	—	830	—	—	0.00	0.00
0.14	0.09	1.12	0.01	0.01	27.4	0.0	—	0.1	33	0.87	6.4	32	37	146	0.2	32	0.00	0.00
0.14	0.14	1.21	0.01	0.05	31.5	0.1	—	0.3	21	1.03	6.7	44	53	145	0.2	29	0.00	0.00
0.27	0.18	2.42	0.01	0.00	54.1	0.0	—	0.2	54	1.87	15.4	57	62	310	0.5	31	0.00	0.00
0.23	0.14	3.46	0.18	0.00	28.2	0.0	—	0.8	100	2.26	79.9	211	256	449	1.9	33	0.00	0.00
0.23	0.14	3.46	0.18	0.00	28.2	0.0	—	0.8	100	2.26	79.9	211	256	449	1.9	33	0.00	0.00
0.07	0.02	0.44	0.00	0.01	7.2	0.0	—	0.0	12	0.33	2.9	11	13	49	0.1	7	0.00	0.00
0.05	0.01	0.40	0.00	0.00	9.9	0.0	—	0.0	6	0.31	2.3	9	9	52	0.1	6	0.00	0.00
0.18	0.25	3.46	0.05	0.00	38.6	0.0	—	0.3	20	3.13	25.2	87	113	508	0.7	4	0.00	0.00
0.17	0.12	1.39	0.17	0.14	45.6	0.0	—	0.0	45	1.42	10.8	65	44	298	0.3	3	0.00	0.00
—	—	—	—	—	—	0.0	—	—	2	0.15	—	—	—	70	—	7	0.00	0.00
—	—	—	—	—	—	0.2	—	—	4	0.47	—	—	—	155	—	—	0.00	0.00
—	—	—	—	—	—	0.0	—	—	17	0.73	—	—	—	114	—	3	0.00	0.00
0.21	0.18	1.44	0.01	0.05	6.8	0.0	—	0.3	11	0.76	6.8	42	43	6	0.2	6	0.00	0.00
0.01	0.00	0.20	0.00	0.00	6.2	0.0	—	0.0	5	0.18	3.0	10	10	41	0.1	5	0.00	0.00
0.03	0.05	0.61	0.00	0.00	9.6	0.0	—	—	24	0.64	3.2	48	15	124	0.2	3	0.00	0.00
0.00	0.05	0.62	0.00	0.00	16.7	0.0	—	0.1	8	0.68	2.6	12	18	129	0.1	5	0.00	0.00
0.09	0.09	1.15	0.02	—	12.2	0.0	—	—	23	1.07	15.1	60	56	168	—	2	0.00	0.00
—	—	—	—	—	—	0.0	—	—	80	1.08	—	—	—	250	—	43	0.00	0.00
0.15	0.17	1.32	0.01	0.09	29.1	0.2	—	1.0	114	1.36	9.7	87	69	266	0.3	38	0.00	0.00
0.17	0.03	1.76	0.07	0.14	42.5	0.2	—	1.8	54	1.38	42.5	170	170	1541	1.5	12	0.00	0.00
0.07	0.17	0.60	0.03	0.23	10.7	3.0	21.1	0.6	45	0.75	8.3	69	86	74	0.4	56	0.00	0.00
0.12	0.20	1.05	0.05	0.20	27.9	0.2	—	0.7	65	1.09	11.0	76	87	311	0.4	55	0.00	0.00
0.10	0.11	1.47	0.15	0.43	22.1	0.6	—	0.0	15	1.32	7.7	145	44	225	0.3	47	0.00	0.00
—	—	—	—	—	—	0.0	—	—	43	1.50	—	450	130	900	—	—	0.00	0.00
—	—	—	—	—	—	—	—	—	119	2.10	—	—	—	400	—	—	0.00	0.00
0.34	0.33	2.91	0.05	0.17	79.9	0.0	—	0.2	164	1.62	22.7	229	96	372	1.1	30	0.00	0.00
0.80	0.44	5.36	—	—	214.0	0.0	—	—	18	3.21	53.7	141	144	5	1.2	10	0.00	0.00
—	—	—	—	—	—	0.0	—	—	0	1.79	—	—	—	140	—	—	0.00	0.00
0.49	0.20	3.33	0.07	0.00	10.3	0.0	—	0.1	12	1.61	—	105	—	3	0.7	11	0.00	0.00
0.80	0.44	5.36	—	—	214.0	0.0	—	—	18	3.21	53.7	141	144	5	1.2	10	0.00	0.00
0.28	0.14	2.33	0.05	0.00	107.8	0.0	—	0.1	10	1.96	25.2	76	43	1	0.7	66	0.00	0.00
0.01	0.00	0.05	0.00	0.00	2.6	0.0	—	—	4	0.11	2.6	18	4	17	0.2	74	0.00	0.00
0.11	0.05	0.95	0.01	0.00	44.3	0.0	—	0.0	4	0.80	10.3	31	18	1	0.3	66	0.00	0.00
0.14	0.07	1.16	0.01	0.00	53.9	0.0	—	0.0	5	0.98	12.6	38	22	1	0.4	66	0.00	0.00

PAGE KEY: A-108 Beverage and Beverage Mixes   A-110 Other Beverages   A-110 Beverages, Alcoholic   A-112 Candies and Confections, Gum   A-116 Cereals, Breakfast Type   A-120 Cheese and Cheese Substitutes   A-122 Dairy Products and Substitutes   A-124 Desserts   A-130 Dessert Toppings   A-130 Eggs, Substitutes, and Egg Dishes   A-132 Ethnic Foods   A-136 Fast Foods/Restaurants   A-150 Fats, Oils, Margarines, Shortenings, and Substitutes   A-150 Fish, Seafood, and Shellfish   A-152 Food Additives   A-152 Fruit, Vegetable, or Blended Juices   A-154 Grains, Flours, and Fractions   A-154 Grain Products, Prepared and Baked Goods

Code	Food Name	Unit/ Amt	Wt (g)	Energy (kcal)	Prot (g)	Carb (g)	Fiber (g)	Fat (g)	Sat (g)	Mono (g)	Poly (g)	Chol (mg)	Vit A (RE)
Rice													
38013	Rice, white, long grain, ckd	1 cup	158	205	4	45	1	0	0.1	0.1	0.1	0	0
Stuffing and Mixes													
38491	Baking Mix, dry, Bisquick	0.33 cup	40	162	3	24	1	6	1.6	2.5	0.5	0	0
42037	Stuffing, bread, prep f/dry mix	0.5 cup	100	178	3	22	3	9	1.7	3.8	2.6	0	125
Tortillas and Taco/Tostada Shells													
42359	Taco Shells	2 ea	27	130	2	18	2	6	1.0	3.8	1.2	0	0
Granola Bars, Cereal Bars, Diet Bars, Scones, and Tarts													
53227	Bar, cereal, mixed berry	1 ea	37	137	2	27	1	3	0.6	1.9	0.4	0	150
23100	Bar, granola, almond, hard	1 ea	24	117	2	15	1	6	3.0	1.8	0.9	0	1
47591	Bar, granola, cinnamon	2 ea	42	180	4	29	2	6	0.5	—	—	0	0
63342	Bar, granola, fruit & nut	3.6 oz	100	397	8	77	5	6	0.7	0.2	4.8	0	28
47592	Bar, granola, oats 'n honey	2 ea	42	180	4	29	2	6	0.5	—	—	0	0
23059	Bar, granola, plain, hard	1 ea	24	115	2	16	1	5	0.6	1.1	3.0	0	4
42071	Scones	1 ea	42	150	4	19	1	6	2.0	2.6	1.3	49	69
MEALS AND DISHES													
Canned Meals and Dishes													
92620	Dish, ravioli, beef, w/meat sauce, cnd	1 cup	212	260	11	39	5	7	3.0	—	—	10	100
FROZEN OR REFRIGERATED MEALS AND DISHES													
Frozen/Refrigerated Breakfasts													
70830	Eggs, scrambled, low fat	1 ea	170	240	12	18	2	13	3.0	—	—	40	225
70826	Sandwich, breakfast, sausage egg cheese, w/biscuit	1 ea	156	460	16	37	3	28	11.0	—	—	115	0
Frozen/Refrigerated Children's Meals													
Frozen/Refrigerated Dinners													
70023	Dinner, beef noodles, w/veg, fzn	1 ea	298	407	14	59	3	14	4.8	5.6	2.4	31	312
11118	Dinner, beef, pot roast, fzn, Healthy Choice	1 ea	312	300	20	41	8	6	2.0	—	—	40	250
15957	Dinner, chicken & noodles, homestyle, ckd f/fzn	1 cup	340	390	12	44	7	19	7.0	—	—	50	700

Thia (mg)	Ribo (mg)	Niac (mg NE)	Vit B6 (mg)	Vit B12 (µg)	Fol (µg)	Vit C (mg)	Vit D (IU)	Vit E (mg AT)	Cal (mg)	Iron (mg)	Magn (mg)	Phos (mg)	Pota (mg)	Sodi (mg)	Zinc (mg)	Wat (%)	Alco (g)	Caff (g)
0.25	0.01	2.32	0.15	0.00	91.6	0.0	—	0.1	16	1.89	19.0	68	55	2	0.8	68	0.00	0.00
0.20	0.15	1.67	—	—	—	0.0	—	—	60	1.39	—	—	50	499	—	—	0.00	0.00
0.14	0.10	1.48	0.03	0.00	39.0	0.0	—	1.4	32	1.09	12.0	42	74	543	0.3	65	0.00	0.00
—	—	—	—	—	—	0.0	—	—	40	0.72	—	—	63	190	—	2	0.00	0.00
0.37	0.40	4.98	0.51	0.00	40.0	0.0	—	0.0	14	1.80	9.6	36	70	110	1.5	14	0.00	0.00
0.07	0.01	0.14	0.00	0.00	2.8	0.0	—	0.4	8	0.58	19.1	54	64	60	0.4	3	0.00	0.00
—	—	—	—	—	—	0.0	—	—	0	1.08	—	—	—	160	—	—	0.00	0.00
0.49	0.43	5.11	0.80	0.00	160.0	0.0	—	1.1	36	5.30	85.0	243	238	251	1.9	7	0.00	0.00
—	—	—	—	—	—	0.0	—	—	0	1.08	—	—	—	160	—	—	0.00	0.00
0.05	0.02	0.38	0.01	0.00	5.6	0.2	—	0.3	15	0.72	23.8	68	82	72	0.5	4	0.00	0.00
0.15	0.15	1.21	0.02	0.10	7.9	0.1	6.7	0.7	80	1.32	7.1	74	49	171	0.3	27	0.00	0.00
0.15	0.17	4.00	—	—	60.0	0.0	—	—	40	1.79	—	—	—	1070	—	—	0.00	0.00
—	—	—	—	—	—	4.8	—	—	40	0.72	—	—	—	620	—	73	0.00	0.00
—	—	—	—	—	—	0.0	—	—	150	1.79	—	—	—	1060	—	46	0.00	0.00
0.25	0.25	3.44	0.20	0.87	38.0	16.5	—	1.3	116	2.02	43.5	210	466	2756	2.3	68	0.00	0.00
—	—	—	—	—	—	18.0	—	—	20	1.79	—	—	—	600	—	—	0.00	0.00
0.27	0.28	5.69	—	—	—	0.0	—	—	60	1.79	—	—	374	1080	—	—	0.00	0.00

PAGE KEY: A-108 Beverage and Beverage Mixes   A-110 Other Beverages   A-110 Beverages, Alcoholic   A-112 Candies and Confections, Gum   A-116 Cereals, Breakfast Type   A-120 Cheese and Cheese Substitutes   A-122 Dairy Products and Substitutes   A-124 Desserts   A-130 Dessert Toppings   A-130 Eggs, Substitutes, and Egg Dishes   A-132 Ethnic Foods   A-136 Fast Foods/Restaurants   A-150 Fats, Oils, Margarines, Shortenings, and Substitutes   A-150 Fish, Seafood, and Shellfish   A-152 Food Additives   A-152 Fruit, Vegetable, or Blended Juices   A-154 Grains, Flours, and Fractions   A-154 Grain Products, Prepared and Baked Goods

Code	Food Name	Unit/ Amt	Wt (g)	Energy (kcal)	Prot (g)	Carb (g)	Fiber (g)	Fat (g)	Sat (g)	Mono (g)	Poly (g)	Chol (mg)	Vit A (RE)
446	Dinner, egg roll, w/fried rice & chicken, ckd f/fzn	1 ea	241	330	12	51	5	9	3.0	—	—	60	200
70151	Dinner, enchilada, cheese, w/beans & rice, fzn	1 ea	340	515	19	71	14	18	7.8	6.7	2.3	32	121
1756	Dinner, fish, sticks, ckd f/fzn	1 ea	187	290	11	33	4	13	4.5	—	—	30	100
70766	Dinner, meatloaf, Swanson	1 ea	468	640	24	65	6	31	14.0	—	—	45	60
11071	Dinner, steak, salisbury, Swanson	1 ea	461	610	34	46	10	33	17.0	—	—	80	150
57293	Dinner, stir fry, teriyaki veg, fzn	1 cup	108	92	4	17	1	1	0.3	—	—	1	175
16912	Dinner, turkey, breast, traditional, fzn, Healthy Choice	1 ea	298	290	22	40	5	4	2.0	—	—	45	80

Frozen/Refrigerated Dishes

Code	Food Name	Unit/ Amt	Wt (g)	Energy (kcal)	Prot (g)	Carb (g)	Fiber (g)	Fat (g)	Sat (g)	Mono (g)	Poly (g)	Chol (mg)	Vit A (RE)
56668	Corn Dog	1 ea	175	460	17	56	—	19	5.2	9.1	3.5	79	61
16167	Dish, chicken & noodles, casserole, Swanson	1 ea	284	300	18	36	2	9	3.0	—	—	50	20
70749	Dish, fish & chips, Swanson	1 ea	156	350	16	38	4	15	4.5	—	—	30	40
16163	Dish, pot pie, chicken, Swanson	1 ea	198	410	10	43	2	22	9.0	—	—	25	200
16915	Dish, pot pie, turkey, Swanson	1 ea	198	400	10	42	3	21	8.0	—	—	25	100
57845	Dish, rice bowl, chicken & veg	1 ea	340	360	21	56	3	5	1.5	—	—	25	—
52165	Dish, rice bowl, chicken, sweet & sour	1 ea	340	360	17	65	2	3	0.5	—	—	30	—
83063	Dish, rice bowl, fried	1 ea	340	450	18	77	6	8	0.5	—	—	0	700
57140	Dish, tortellini, three cheese, fzn	2.9 oz	81	250	11	37	2	7	3.5	—	—	35	0

Frozen/Refrigerated Dinners/Dishes—Vegetarian

Code	Food Name	Unit/ Amt	Wt (g)	Energy (kcal)	Prot (g)	Carb (g)	Fiber (g)	Fat (g)	Sat (g)	Mono (g)	Poly (g)	Chol (mg)	Vit A (RE)
8869	Corn Dog, vegetarian	1 ea	71	159	8	22	1	4	0.5	1.2	2.5	0	0

Prepared Generic or Homemade Meals and Dishes

Code	Food Name	Unit/ Amt	Wt (g)	Energy (kcal)	Prot (g)	Carb (g)	Fiber (g)	Fat (g)	Sat (g)	Mono (g)	Poly (g)	Chol (mg)	Vit A (RE)
7037	Beans, baked, prep f/recipe	1 cup	253	382	14	54	14	13	4.9	5.4	1.9	13	0
56258	Chicken, liver, chopped, w/egg & onion	1 cup	208	472	27	6	1	37	11.2	15.2	7.2	753	4581
11013	Dish, beef curry	1 cup	236	436	27	13	3	31	7.0	14.5	7.4	69	367
56195	Dish, chicken & noodles, w/cream sauce	1 cup	224	320	22	32	1	11	3.2	4.3	2.5	81	100
56200	Dish, chicken & noodles, w/tomato sauce	1 cup	224	291	20	31	2	9	2.1	3.8	2.5	74	143
15904	Dish, chicken cacciatore	1 cup	244	459	42	13	2	26	6.3	9.7	7.2	128	132
56213	Dish, chicken dumplings	1 cup	244	372	26	22	1	19	5.1	7.8	4.6	89	52
56287	Dish, egg foo young, chicken	1 ea	86	121	8	4	1	8	1.9	2.8	2.3	167	87
56110	Dish, egg roll, w/o meat	1 ea	64	101	3	10	1	6	1.2	2.9	1.3	30	16
11000	Dish, goulash, beef	1 cup	249	270	33	7	1	12	3.2	4.3	2.5	84	31
56239	Dish, jambalaya, shrimp	1 cup	243	310	27	28	1	9	1.8	3.8	2.8	181	133
56140	Dish, meatballs, Swedish, w/cream sauce	1 cup	246	406	31	17	1	23	9.5	9.0	1.3	163	94
56180	Dish, pork & potatoes, w/gravy	1 cup	252	255	21	21	2	10	3.2	4.3	1.1	57	1
56100	Dish, spaghetti w/meatballs, prep f/recipe	1 cup	248	362	18	28	3	18	4.8	—	—	65	164
57523	Dish, spring roll, fresh	1 ea	64	113	5	9	1	6	1.4	3.0	1.3	37	16
11008	Dish, stroganoff, beef	1 cup	256	408	26	16	1	27	10.6	7.9	6.3	85	99
56130	Dish, tortellini, meat	1 cup	190	373	25	33	1	15	5.4	5.7	2.1	240	134
56215	Dish, turkey & stuffing	1 cup	200	273	35	19	1	5	1.4	1.7	1.3	105	19
56242	Gumbo, w/rice, New Orleans style	1 cup	244	193	14	17	2	8	1.6	2.6	2.7	40	63
56150	Hash, beef	1 cup	190	312	21	21	2	16	4.9	5.7	3.3	57	0
56231	Pie, shepherds, w/beef	1 cup	243	278	17	32	3	9	2.6	4.0	1.7	37	78

Pizza

Code	Food Name	Unit/ Amt	Wt (g)	Energy (kcal)	Prot (g)	Carb (g)	Fiber (g)	Fat (g)	Sat (g)	Mono (g)	Poly (g)	Chol (mg)	Vit A (RE)
56995	Pizza, bagel, cheese & pepperoni, fzn	2 pce	22	52	3	6	1	2	0.8	—	—	4	20
56993	Pizza, bagel, cheese, extra, fzn	4 pce	88	190	11	24	3	6	2.0	—	—	10	80
81030	Pizza, Canadian bacon, fzn	1 ea	195	440	17	50	2	19	3.5	—	—	15	0

Thia (mg)	Ribo (mg)	Niac (mg NE)	Vit B6 (mg)	Vit B12 (µg)	Fol (µg)	Vit C (mg)	Vit D (IU)	Vit E (mg AT)	Cal (mg)	Iron (mg)	Magn (mg)	Phos (mg)	Pota (mg)	Sodi (mg)	Zinc (mg)	Wat (%)	Alco (g)	Caff (g)
—	—	—	—	—	—	0.0	—	—	40	1.08	—	—	—	1270	—	—	0.00	0.00
0.31	0.27	2.21	0.33	0.18	112.4	6.0	—	1.8	289	4.36	99.1	414	645	1967	2.7	66	0.00	0.00
—	—	—	—	—	—	3.6	—	—	60	1.79	—	—	—	820	—	—	0.00	0.00
—	—	—	—	—	—	18.0	—	—	150	5.40	—	—	—	1870	—	73	0.00	0.00
—	—	—	—	—	—	4.8	—	—	200	5.40	—	—	—	1620	—	74	0.00	0.00
—	—	—	—	—	—	10.2	—	—	73	0.58	—	—	—	717	—	—	0.00	0.00
0.44	0.25	6.00	—	—	—	36.0	—	—	20	1.44	—	270	540	460	—	—	0.00	0.00
0.28	0.69	4.15	0.09	0.43	103.2	0.0	—	0.7	102	6.17	17.5	166	262	973	1.3	47	0.00	0.00
—	—	—	—	—	—	0.0	—	—	200	3.59	—	—	—	940	—	76	0.00	0.00
—	—	—	—	—	—	1.2	—	—	150	1.44	—	—	—	930	—	54	0.00	0.00
—	—	—	—	—	—	1.2	—	—	20	1.79	—	—	—	780	—	—	0.00	0.00
—	—	—	—	—	—	2.4	—	—	20	1.79	—	—	—	700	—	62	0.00	0.00
—	—	—	—	—	—	—	—	—	—	—	—	—	—	1020	—	—	0.00	0.00
—	—	—	—	—	—	—	—	—	—	—	—	—	—	620	—	—	0.00	0.00
—	—	—	—	—	—	3.6	—	—	150	6.30	—	—	—	1090	—	—	0.00	0.00
—	—	—	—	—	—	0.0	—	—	0	0.00	—	—	—	300	—	30	0.00	0.00
0.10	0.05	0.00	—	—	—	0.0	—	—	12	0.64	—	113	66	527	0.2	49	0.00	0.00
0.34	0.11	1.02	0.23	0.00	121.4	2.8	—	1.3	154	5.03	108.8	276	906	1068	1.8	65	0.00	0.00
0.18	1.79	4.19	0.63	18.23	734.3	17.9	—	2.5	41	8.32	28.1	365	256	92	4.5	66	0.00	0.00
0.18	0.34	5.42	0.47	3.04	20.3	24.6	—	5.9	44	4.23	59.0	292	978	802	6.1	68	0.00	0.00
0.25	0.34	4.94	0.20	0.37	14.6	0.8	—	0.9	132	2.36	42.0	237	276	139	2.0	71	0.00	0.00
0.27	0.23	5.73	0.31	0.20	16.5	11.8	—	2.1	34	2.90	47.2	177	478	658	1.9	72	0.00	0.00
0.18	0.31	13.98	0.72	0.43	16.5	14.8	29.3	3.0	61	3.02	56.1	305	690	247	3.1	66	0.44	0.00
0.23	0.31	9.32	0.30	0.31	11.0	1.9	—	0.9	128	2.50	34.5	261	297	244	1.9	72	0.00	0.00
0.05	0.23	0.88	0.11	0.34	22.3	3.1	—	1.1	27	0.81	11.4	96	136	132	0.8	76	0.00	0.00
0.07	0.10	0.80	0.05	0.05	13.4	2.9	—	0.9	14	0.81	9.1	38	97	274	0.3	70	0.00	0.00
0.15	0.31	5.73	0.46	3.25	21.3	8.7	14.9	1.8	18	3.57	45.6	336	698	225	5.3	78	0.00	0.00
0.28	0.10	4.76	0.21	1.17	12.2	16.9	—	2.3	104	4.38	63.6	300	439	370	1.7	72	0.00	0.00
0.30	0.52	6.57	0.31	2.41	20.2	2.7	—	0.3	124	3.19	43.4	326	573	407	5.5	70	0.00	0.00
0.56	0.25	5.90	0.50	0.52	16.4	14.9	—	0.3	22	1.73	40.6	262	821	651	2.4	78	0.00	0.00
0.25	0.30	4.38	0.28	0.94	67.7	16.3	16.9	2.5	92	3.32	43.7	173	479	1133	3.4	71	0.00	0.00
0.15	0.12	1.27	0.09	0.11	9.9	2.1	—	0.8	15	0.82	10.0	57	124	274	0.5	66	0.00	0.00
0.18	0.38	4.51	0.28	2.60	20.2	1.8	—	2.4	92	3.64	40.4	308	556	677	4.9	72	0.00	0.00
0.46	0.56	4.48	0.21	0.89	29.1	0.0	—	1.1	178	3.11	28.1	290	231	437	2.2	61	0.00	0.00
0.23	0.31	13.10	0.44	0.36	28.7	2.9	—	0.6	43	2.27	47.5	293	403	511	2.5	70	0.00	0.00
0.20	0.15	4.51	0.20	2.41	45.6	13.5	—	1.4	71	2.60	40.1	152	446	542	15.2	83	0.00	0.00
0.15	0.20	3.74	0.49	1.79	16.5	7.1	—	1.2	19	2.46	36.4	204	587	470	5.0	69	0.00	0.00
0.20	0.18	3.90	0.58	1.25	21.1	16.4	—	1.3	40	2.18	46.9	193	764	312	3.9	75	0.00	0.00
—	—	—	—	—	—	2.2	—	—	25	0.36	—	—	38	162	—	—	0.00	0.00
—	—	—	—	—	—	9.0	—	—	150	0.72	—	—	150	490	—	—	0.00	0.00
—	—	—	—	—	—	0.0	—	—	150	3.59	—	—	—	1160	—	—	0.00	0.00

PAGE KEY: A-108 Beverage and Beverage Mixes A-110 Other Beverages A-110 Beverages, Alcoholic A-112 Candies and Confections, Gum A-116 Cereals, Breakfast Type A-120 Cheese and Cheese Substitutes A-122 Dairy Products and Substitutes A-124 Desserts A-130 Dessert Toppings A-130 Eggs, Substitutes, and Egg Dishes A-132 Ethnic Foods A-136 Fast Foods/Restaurants A-150 Fats, Oils, Margarines, Shortenings, and Substitutes A-150 Fish, Seafood, and Shellfish A-152 Food Additives A-152 Fruit, Vegetable, or Blended Juices A-154 Grains, Flours, and Fractions A-154 Grain Products, Prepared and Baked Goods

Code	Food Name	Unit/ Amt	Wt (g)	Energy (kcal)	Prot (g)	Carb (g)	Fiber (g)	Fat (g)	Sat (g)	Mono (g)	Poly (g)	Chol (mg)	Vit A (RE)
56782	Pizza, cheese, for one, fzn	1 ea	184	497	21	48	4	24	—	—	—	40	—
56781	Pizza, deluxe, for one, fzn	1 ea	234	582	23	51	4	32	10.0	9.0	3.0	20	245
56779	Pizza, pepperoni, for one, fzn	1 ea	191	546	20	50	4	30	9.0	7.0	2.0	20	263
70898	Pizza, pepperoni, fzn, svg	1 ea	146	432	16	42	3	22	7.0	10.0	3.4	22	61
56778	Pizza, sausage, for one, fzn	1 ea	213	571	23	49	4	32	10.0	7.0	3.0	20	272
57178	Pizza, supreme, fzn, 1/5 of 12"	1 pce	130	300	14	30	3	14	6.0	—	—	30	60
MEATS													
Beef													
10820	Beef, average of all cuts, ckd, 1/8" trim	3 oz	85	247	22	0	0	17	6.6	7.2	0.6	74	0
10095	Beef, average of all cuts, ckd, choice, 1/4" trim	3 oz	85	274	22	0	0	20	8.0	8.6	0.7	75	0
10099	Beef, average of all cuts, ckd, prime, 1/4" trim	3 oz	85	274	22	0	0	20	8.1	8.6	0.7	71	0
10097	Beef, average of all cuts, ckd, select, 1/4" trim	3 oz	85	247	22	0	0	17	6.7	7.2	0.6	73	0
10705	Beef, average of all cuts, lean, ckd, 1/4" trim	3 oz	85	184	25	0	0	8	3.2	3.5	0.3	73	0
47441	Beef, chuck, ground, extra lean, raw	4 oz	113	130	22	0	0	5	2.0	2.0	0.5	60	0
10740	Beef, cubed patty	1 ea	91	251	15	2	0	20	8.1	—	—	64	11
58115	Beef, ground, hamburger, bkd, 10% fat	3 oz	85	182	23	0	0	9	3.7	4.0	0.3	73	0
58120	Beef, ground, hamburger, bkd, 15% fat	3 oz	85	204	22	0	0	12	4.6	5.3	0.4	77	0
58125	Beef, ground, hamburger, bkd, 20% fat	3 oz	85	216	21	0	0	14	5.9	6.1	0.4	77	0
58110	Beef, ground, hamburger, bkd, 5% fat	3 oz	85	148	23	0	0	5	2.5	2.4	0.3	62	0
10051	Beef, jerky, lrg pce	1 ea	20	81	7	2	0	5	2.1	2.2	0.2	10	0
53688	Beef, meat stick, spicy	0.63 oz	18	100	4	1	1	8	3.0	—	—	25	0
11019	Beef, meatballs	4 ea	112	240	19	7	0	14	5.1	6.3	0.7	93	21
11020	Beef, patty, brd, 3.6 oz	1 ea	101	216	17	6	0	13	4.6	5.7	0.7	84	19
11487	Beef, porterhouse steak, brld, 1/8" trim	3 oz	85	253	20	0	0	19	7.2	8.2	0.7	60	0
11407	Beef, prime rib, brld, 1/8" trim	3 oz	85	301	21	0	0	24	9.8	10.3	0.8	71	0
11386	Beef, rib pot roast, brld, 1/8" trim	3 oz	85	287	18	0	0	23	9.4	9.8	0.9	68	0
11015	Beef, ribs, w/bbq sauce	3 oz	85	148	18	2	0	7	2.6	2.9	0.3	52	16
11815	Beef, roast, Italian style, deli meat	2 oz	57	60	11	1	0	1	0.5	—	—	20	0
11681	Beef, roast, lean, rstd	3 oz	85	169	24	0	0	7	2.8	3.0	0.2	66	0
11680	Beef, roast, rstd	3 oz	85	227	22	0	0	15	5.8	6.3	0.5	68	0
10737	Beef, salisbury steak, patty, ckd, 3 oz	1 ea	85	280	12	5	0	23	10.7	—	—	59	7
11678	Beef, steak, brld/bkd	3.6 oz	100	255	28	0	0	15	5.9	6.3	0.5	83	0
11679	Beef, steak, lean, brld/bkd	3.6 oz	100	199	30	0	0	8	3.1	3.3	0.3	81	0
10049	Beef, stew meat, ckd	0.75 cup	105	322	29	0	0	22	8.5	9.4	0.8	106	0
10050	Beef, stew meat, lean, ckd	0.75 cup	105	248	33	0	0	12	4.5	5.2	0.4	107	0
10806	Beef, T-bone steak, brld, 0" trim	3 oz	85	210	21	0	0	14	5.2	6.1	0.5	51	0
10805	Beef, T-bone steak, brld, 1/4" trim	3 oz	85	260	20	0	0	19	7.6	8.6	0.7	55	0
11491	Beef, T-bone steak, brld, 1/8" trim	3 oz	85	238	21	0	0	17	6.4	7.3	0.6	53	0
10933	Beef, tenderloin, filet mignon, rstd, 1/8" trim	3 oz	85	276	20	0	0	21	8.3	8.7	0.9	72	0
10908	Beef, top round steak, brsd, 1/8" trim	3 oz	85	202	29	0	0	9	3.2	3.5	0.4	77	0
10943	Beef, top sirloin steak, raw, 1/8" trim	4 oz	113	228	23	0	0	14	5.8	6.2	0.5	53	0
11014	Beef, w/bbq sauce	1 cup	263	457	56	8	1	21	7.9	9.0	1.1	160	49
11016	Beef, w/sweet & sour	1 cup	252	336	16	28	2	18	6.1	7.2	2.6	54	33
10846	Beef, whole rib, brld, 1/8" trim	3 oz	85	287	19	0	0	23	9.2	9.7	0.8	70	0

PAGE KEY: A-158 Granola Bars, Cereal Bars, Diet Bars, Scones, and Tarts | A-158 Meals and Dishes | A-162 Meats | A-168 Nuts, Seeds, and Products A-170 Poultry
A-172 Salad Dressings, Dips, and Mayonnaise A-172 Salads A-174 Sandwiches A-176 Sauces and Gravies A-176 Snack Foods—Chips, Pretzels, Popcorn
A-178 Soups, Stews, and Chilis A-180 Spices, Flavors, and Seasonings A-182 Sports Bars and Drinks A-182 Supplemental Foods and Formulas
A-184 Sweeteners and Sweet Substitutes A-184 Vegetables and Legumes A-198 Weight Loss Bars and Drinks A-200 Miscellaneous

Thia (mg)	Ribo (mg)	Niac (mg NE)	Vit B6 (mg)	Vit B12 (µg)	Fol (µg)	Vit C (mg)	Vit D (IU)	Vit E (mg AT)	Cal (mg)	Iron (mg)	Magn (mg)	Phos (mg)	Pota (mg)	Sodi (mg)	Zinc (mg)	Wat (%)	Alco (g)	Caff (g)
—	—	—	—	—	—	—	—	2.0	—	—	48.0	386	342	—	4.0	46	0.00	0.00
0.30	0.81	3.52	0.25	2.00	80.0	0.0	—	2.0	332	2.56	61.0	480	498	1367	5.0	53	0.00	0.00
0.25	0.70	2.57	0.20	2.00	97.0	0.0	—	4.0	336	2.03	53.0	443	416	1353	4.0	45	0.00	0.00
0.33	0.34	3.60	0.14	0.82	68.6	2.8	—	1.6	220	3.51	35.0	302	289	902	2.2	42	0.00	0.00
0.30	0.76	2.84	0.23	2.00	109.0	0.0	—	4.0	371	2.27	60.0	505	456	1363	0.0	48	0.00	0.00
—	—	—	—	—	—	0.0	—	—	150	1.44	—	—	—	690	—	—	0.00	0.00
0.07	0.18	3.16	0.28	2.09	6.0	0.0	—	0.2	8	2.27	19.6	177	271	54	5.1	53	0.00	0.00
0.07	0.18	3.03	0.27	2.04	6.0	0.0	10.2	0.1	9	2.19	18.7	169	260	52	4.9	50	0.00	0.00
0.07	0.18	3.64	0.31	2.07	6.8	0.0	—	0.2	8	2.07	20.4	168	295	53	4.6	51	0.00	0.00
0.07	0.18	3.11	0.28	2.07	6.0	0.0	—	0.1	9	2.25	19.6	174	269	53	5.1	52	0.00	0.00
0.09	0.20	3.50	0.31	2.25	6.8	0.0	—	0.1	8	2.53	22.1	198	306	57	5.9	59	0.00	0.00
—	—	5.00	—	2.40	—	0.0	—	—	0	1.79	—	—	—	65	4.5	—	0.00	0.00
0.10	—	—	—	—	—	8.0	—	—	17	1.89	—	—	—	53	—	58	0.00	0.00
0.02	0.15	4.44	0.30	2.13	5.1	0.0	—	0.3	11	2.46	17.9	164	255	52	5.7	61	0.00	0.00
0.02	0.15	4.19	0.28	2.11	5.1	0.0	—	0.4	15	2.32	17.0	158	243	54	5.5	59	0.00	0.00
0.03	0.14	3.94	0.28	2.10	6.0	0.0	—	0.4	20	2.19	16.2	152	230	57	5.3	58	0.00	0.00
0.02	0.15	4.69	0.30	2.13	5.1	0.0	—	0.3	7	2.58	18.7	169	268	49	5.8	65	0.00	0.00
0.02	0.02	0.34	0.03	0.20	26.5	0.0	—	0.1	4	1.07	10.1	81	118	438	1.6	23	0.00	0.00
—	—	—	—	—	—	0.0	—	—	0	0.72	—	—	—	350	—	23	0.00	0.00
0.07	0.28	4.17	0.15	1.72	12.4	0.6	—	0.1	45	2.10	23.3	167	306	138	3.8	62	0.00	0.00
0.07	0.25	3.75	0.12	1.54	11.2	0.6	—	0.1	40	1.89	21.0	151	276	124	3.4	62	0.00	0.00
0.09	0.18	3.46	0.30	1.83	6.0	0.0	—	0.2	7	2.32	19.6	159	273	54	3.9	53	0.00	0.00
0.07	0.15	3.46	0.28	2.50	6.0	0.0	—	0.2	11	1.89	18.7	151	282	54	4.9	47	0.00	0.00
0.05	0.14	2.35	0.20	2.46	5.1	0.0	—	0.2	9	1.86	16.2	155	263	54	4.3	49	0.00	0.00
0.05	0.12	2.61	0.20	2.19	5.8	1.3	—	0.3	12	2.08	19.9	150	295	204	4.1	66	0.00	0.00
—	—	—	—	—	—	0.0	—	—	0	1.08	—	—	—	360	—	73	0.00	0.00
0.07	0.18	3.42	0.28	2.17	6.9	0.0	10.2	0.1	5	2.19	22.3	191	321	57	5.5	62	0.00	0.00
0.07	0.17	3.06	0.27	2.03	6.1	0.0	10.2	0.2	6	1.98	19.6	173	290	53	4.8	56	0.00	0.00
0.07	—	—	—	—	—	4.0	—	—	51	1.20	—	—	—	621	—	—	0.00	0.00
0.09	0.21	4.57	0.38	2.45	8.3	0.0	12.0	0.1	9	2.61	25.4	209	365	61	5.2	55	0.00	0.00
0.10	0.23	5.26	0.46	2.53	9.3	0.0	12.0	0.1	9	2.75	28.8	228	411	66	5.9	60	0.00	0.00
0.07	0.25	3.10	0.30	2.58	7.3	0.0	12.6	0.2	11	3.27	21.6	231	265	66	7.9	50	0.00	0.00
0.07	0.28	3.35	0.31	2.76	8.2	0.0	12.6	0.1	11	3.73	24.6	259	291	70	9.3	56	0.00	0.00
0.09	0.20	3.63	0.31	1.86	6.0	0.0	—	0.2	4	2.84	20.4	169	257	57	4.0	58	0.00	0.00
0.07	0.18	3.36	0.28	1.80	6.0	0.0	—	0.2	6	2.63	18.7	157	240	57	3.7	52	0.00	0.00
0.09	0.18	3.51	0.30	1.85	6.0	0.0	—	0.2	7	2.41	20.4	164	286	56	4.0	55	0.00	0.00
0.07	0.21	2.54	0.20	2.08	6.8	0.0	—	0.2	8	2.65	18.7	173	282	48	3.4	48	0.00	0.00
0.05	0.20	3.09	0.23	2.23	7.7	0.0	—	0.1	4	2.69	20.4	183	271	38	3.7	55	0.00	0.00
0.07	0.10	6.78	0.62	1.19	12.5	0.0	—	0.4	27	1.67	23.8	212	357	59	4.0	66	0.00	0.00
0.15	0.40	8.10	0.61	6.76	17.9	4.0	—	0.9	36	6.44	61.6	463	913	632	12.7	66	0.00	0.00
0.11	0.18	2.61	0.31	1.59	12.7	21.6	—	1.2	27	2.69	33.7	151	336	930	3.9	74	0.00	0.00
0.07	0.14	2.77	0.23	2.46	5.1	0.0	—	0.2	9	1.86	17.0	152	268	54	4.5	48	0.00	0.00

Code	Food Name	Unit/ Amt	Wt (g)	Energy (kcal)	Prot (g)	Carb (g)	Fiber (g)	Fat (g)	Sat (g)	Mono (g)	Poly (g)	Chol (mg)	Vit A (RE)
Game Meats													
40559	Bison, ground, raw	4 oz	113	253	21	0	0	18	7.7	7.1	0.8	79	0
14009	Bison, rstd	3 oz	85	122	24	0	0	2	0.8	0.8	0.2	70	0
40565	Deer, ground, raw	4 oz	113	178	25	0	0	8	3.8	1.5	0.4	91	0
40551	Deer, rstd	3 oz	85	134	26	0	0	3	1.1	0.7	0.5	95	0
40560	Elk, ground, raw	4 oz	113	195	25	0	0	10	3.9	2.8	0.5	75	0
14014	Elk, rstd	3 oz	85	124	26	0	0	2	0.6	0.4	0.3	62	0
14068	Rabbit, brd, ckd	3.6 oz	100	245	28	6	0	11	2.9	4.0	2.8	86	0
14013	Venison, rstd	3 oz	85	134	26	0	0	3	1.1	0.7	0.5	95	0
Goat													
Lamb													
40354	Lamb, Austl, average of all cuts, ckd, 1/8" trim	3 oz	85	218	21	0	0	14	6.8	5.7	0.6	74	—
13628	Lamb, average of all cuts, ckd, choice, 1/8" trim	3 oz	85	230	22	0	0	15	6.3	6.5	1.1	82	0
13669	Lamb, ground, ckd	3.6 oz	100	283	25	0	0	20	8.1	8.3	1.4	97	0
Lunchmeats and Sausages													
13250	Frank, beef, fat free	1 ea	50	39	7	3	0	0	0.1	0.1	0.0	15	0
57967	Frank, beef, rducd fat	1 ea	49	120	6	0	0	10	4.5	—	—	25	0
13283	Frankfurter, beef	3.6 oz	100	326	13	2	0	29	12.3	14.0	1.4	64	0
13284	Frankfurter, beef & pork	3.6 oz	100	331	12	3	0	30	10.9	14.1	2.9	52	0
58290	Frankfurter, beef, low fat	1 cup	151	352	18	2	0	29	12.2	14.8	0.9	60	0
13318	Frankfurter, beef, low fat	1 ea	50	80	6	7	0	2	1.0	—	—	15	0
13260	Frankfurter, chicken	1 ea	45	116	6	3	0	9	2.5	3.8	1.8	45	18
13274	Frankfurter, low sod	1 ea	57	180	7	1	0	16	6.9	7.8	0.8	35	0
13012	Frankfurter, turkey	1 ea	45	102	6	1	0	8	2.7	2.5	2.2	48	0
13325	Hot Dog, fat free	1 ea	50	36	6	2	0	0	0.1	0.1	0.1	14	0
13000	Lunchmeat, beef, thin slice	1 oz	28	42	5	0	0	2	0.8	0.9	0.1	20	0
13177	Lunchmeat, bologna, beef	1 oz	28	90	3	1	0	8	3.6	4.3	0.3	18	0
58284	Lunchmeat, bologna, beef, low fat	1 cup	138	282	16	7	0	20	7.5	8.9	0.7	61	0
10439	Lunchmeat, bologna, beef, slice	1 pce	38	100	5	1	0	8	3.5	—	—	20	0
11829	Lunchmeat, bologna, chicken, slice	1 pce	38	100	4	1	0	9	2.5	—	—	45	20
13251	Lunchmeat, bologna, fat free, 1 oz svg	1 pce	28	22	4	2	0	0	0.1	0.1	0.0	7	0
13245	Lunchmeat, chicken breast, honey glazed, slice	1 oz	28	31	6	1	0	0	0.1	0.2	0.1	15	0
13257	Lunchmeat, chicken breast, oven rstd, fat free, slice	1 oz	28	24	5	0	0	0	0.0	0.0	0.0	12	0
58149	Lunchmeat, chicken breast, oven rstd, 1 oz slice	1 pce	28	20	5	0	0	0	0.0	0.0	0.0	10	—
58167	Lunchmeat, ham, brown sugar, deli, 0.8 oz slice	2 pce	45	60	8	4	0	1	0.0	—	—	10	0
13262	Lunchmeat, ham, extra lean, 5% fat, sliced	1 cup	135	148	23	4	0	4	1.2	1.7	0.5	65	0
11819	Lunchmeat, ham, smkd, deli meat	2 oz	57	60	9	2	0	2	0.5	—	—	30	0
58199	Lunchmeat, roast beef, choice, deli, 0.8 oz slice	2 pce	45	50	9	0	0	2	0.5	—	—	25	0
13114	Lunchmeat, turkey breast, oven rstd, fat free, slice	1 oz	28	24	4	1	0	0	0.1	0.1	0.0	9	0
13255	Lunchmeat, turkey breast, smkd, fat free, slice	1 oz	28	23	4	1	0	0	0.1	0.0	0.0	9	0
13020	Pastrami, turkey, slices	1 oz	28	35	5	1	0	1	0.3	0.4	0.3	19	1
13201	Salami, hard, slice	1 oz	28	104	7	0	0	8	3.1	4.2	0.8	27	2
58014	Salami, Italian, pork	3 oz	85	361	18	1	0	31	11.1	15.5	3.1	68	0
13025	Salami, turkey, ckd, 1 oz slice	2 pce	57	86	9	0	0	5	1.6	1.8	1.4	43	1
13182	Sausage, beef, smokies	1 ea	43	127	5	1	0	11	4.8	5.5	0.4	27	0

PAGE KEY: A-158 Granola Bars, Cereal Bars, Diet Bars, Scones, and Tarts   A-158 Meals and Dishes   A-162 Meats   A-168 Nuts, Seeds, and Products   A-170 Poultry   A-172 Salad Dressings, Dips, and Mayonnaise   A-172 Salads   A-174 Sandwiches   A-176 Sauces and Gravies   A-176 Snack Foods—Chips, Pretzels, Popcorn   A-178 Soups, Stews, and Chilis   A-180 Spices, Flavors, and Seasonings   A-182 Sports Bars and Drinks   A-182 Supplemental Foods and Formulas   A-184 Sweeteners and Sweet Substitutes   A-184 Vegetables and Legumes   A-198 Weight Loss Bars and Drinks   A-200 Miscellaneous

Thia (mg)	Ribo (mg)	Niac (mg NE)	Vit B6 (mg)	Vit B12 (μg)	Fol (μg)	Vit C (mg)	Vit D (IU)	Vit E (mg AT)	Cal (mg)	Iron (mg)	Magn (mg)	Phos (mg)	Pota (mg)	Sodi (mg)	Zinc (mg)	Wat (%)	Alco (g)	Caff (g)
0.15	0.25	5.57	0.40	2.02	12.5	0.0	—	0.3	12	2.95	21.5	205	348	75	4.9	64	0.00	0.00
0.09	0.23	3.16	0.34	2.43	6.8	0.0	—	0.3	7	2.91	22.1	178	307	48	3.1	67	0.00	0.00
0.62	0.33	6.46	0.52	2.11	4.5	0.0	—	0.5	12	3.30	23.8	228	374	85	4.8	71	0.00	0.00
0.15	0.50	5.71	0.31	2.70	4.0	0.0	—	0.2	6	3.79	20.4	192	285	46	2.3	65	0.00	0.00
0.14	0.28	5.55	0.37	2.42	7.9	0.0	—	0.3	14	3.11	24.9	221	365	90	6.1	69	0.00	0.00
—	—	—	—	5.53	7.7	0.0	—	0.0	4	3.08	20.4	153	279	52	2.7	66	0.00	0.00
0.10	0.15	6.55	0.30	5.65	9.5	0.0	12.0	1.4	35	3.26	24.3	212	291	103	2.2	52	0.00	0.00
0.15	0.50	5.71	0.31	2.70	4.0	0.0	—	0.2	6	3.79	20.4	192	285	46	2.3	65	0.00	0.00
0.10	0.28	4.63	0.31	2.44	—	—	—	—	14	1.63	18.7	166	256	65	4.0	59	0.00	0.00
0.09	0.21	5.57	0.11	2.19	16.2	0.0	—	0.1	14	1.63	20.4	164	270	61	4.0	56	0.00	0.00
0.10	0.25	6.69	0.14	2.60	19.0	0.0	—	0.2	22	1.78	24.0	201	339	81	4.7	55	0.00	0.00
—	—	—	—	—	—	0.0	—	—	10	0.98	9.5	64	234	464	1.2	78	0.00	0.00
—	—	—	—	—	—	0.0	—	—	0	0.72	—	—	—	360	—	64	0.00	0.00
0.05	0.10	2.30	0.10	1.38	3.6	0.0	—	0.2	21	1.51	3.0	88	168	1037	2.3	53	0.00	0.00
0.18	0.11	2.51	0.10	1.17	3.6	0.0	—	0.2	12	1.22	10.1	87	169	1132	2.0	52	0.00	0.00
0.07	0.15	3.47	0.15	2.10	6.0	1.5	—	0.3	12	1.74	16.6	288	195	1572	3.0	64	0.00	0.00
—	—	—	—	—	—	2.4	—	—	0	0.36	—	—	—	400	—	66	0.00	0.00
0.02	0.05	1.38	0.14	0.10	1.8	0.0	0.0	0.1	43	0.89	4.5	48	38	616	0.5	58	0.00	0.00
0.02	0.05	1.37	0.07	0.87	2.3	0.0	—	0.1	11	0.81	1.7	50	95	177	1.2	57	0.00	0.00
0.01	0.07	1.86	0.10	0.12	3.6	0.0	—	0.3	48	0.82	6.3	60	81	642	1.4	63	0.00	0.00
—	—	—	—	—	—	0.0	—	—	8	0.46	10.5	81	236	487	0.6	79	0.00	0.00
0.01	0.05	1.21	0.10	0.73	3.1	0.0	—	0.1	3	0.58	5.4	48	122	401	1.1	69	0.00	0.00
0.00	0.02	0.68	0.05	0.40	3.7	0.0	9.1	—	3	0.38	4.0	31	48	334	0.6	54	0.00	0.00
0.07	0.14	3.45	0.20	1.92	6.9	1.4	—	0.3	12	1.37	16.6	246	203	1628	2.5	65	0.00	0.00
—	—	—	—	—	—	0.0	—	—	0	0.36	—	—	—	340	—	60	0.00	0.00
—	—	—	—	—	—	1.2	—	—	40	0.72	—	—	—	350	—	60	0.00	0.00
—	—	—	—	—	—	0.0	—	—	4	0.25	6.2	43	44	274	0.3	78	0.00	0.00
—	—	—	—	—	1.1	0.0	—	—	3	0.31	10.2	82	93	408	0.2	70	0.00	0.00
—	—	—	—	—	—	0.0	—	—	3	0.37	10.2	73	90	352	0.2	76	0.00	0.00
—	—	—	—	—	—	—	—	—	—	—	—	—	—	240	—	77	0.00	0.00
—	—	—	—	—	—	0.0	—	—	0	0.36	—	—	—	490	—	—	0.00	0.00
1.25	0.30	6.75	0.62	1.00	5.4	0.0	—	0.4	12	1.08	23.0	294	472	1493	2.6	74	0.00	0.00
—	—	—	—	—	—	0.0	—	—	0	0.36	—	—	—	430	—	74	0.00	0.00
—	—	—	—	—	—	0.0	—	—	0	1.08	—	—	—	250	—	—	0.00	0.00
—	—	—	—	—	—	0.0	—	—	3	0.31	7.7	66	58	338	0.2	76	0.00	0.00
—	—	—	—	—	—	0.0	—	—	3	0.21	8.5	69	62	310	0.2	78	0.00	0.00
0.01	0.07	1.00	0.07	0.07	1.4	4.6	—	0.1	3	1.19	4.0	57	98	278	0.6	72	0.00	0.00
0.15	0.07	1.42	0.11	0.52	0.9	0.0	17.6	—	3	0.51	6.0	51	101	560	0.9	38	0.00	0.00
0.79	0.28	4.76	0.46	2.38	1.7	0.0	—	0.2	9	1.28	18.7	195	289	1607	3.6	35	0.00	0.00
0.23	0.17	2.25	0.23	0.56	5.7	0.0	13.3	0.1	23	0.70	12.5	151	122	569	1.3	72	0.00	0.00
—	—	—	—	—	4.7	0.0	—	—	5	0.75	6.5	99	74	416	1.3	56	0.00	0.00

PAGE KEY: A-108 Beverage and Beverage Mixes   A-110 Other Beverages   A-110 Beverages, Alcoholic   A-112 Candies and Confections, Gum   A-116 Cereals, Breakfast Type
A-120 Cheese and Cheese Substitutes   A-122 Dairy Products and Substitutes   A-124 Desserts   A-130 Dessert Toppings   A-130 Eggs, Substitutes, and Egg Dishes   A-132 Ethnic Foods
A-136 Fast Foods/Restaurants   A-150 Fats, Oils, Margarines, Shortenings, and Substitutes   A-150 Fish, Seafood, and Shellfish   A-152 Food Additives
A-152 Fruit, Vegetable, or Blended Juices   A-154 Grains, Flours, and Fractions   A-154 Grain Products, Prepared and Baked Goods

Code	Food Name	Unit/ Amt	Wt (g)	Energy (kcal)	Prot (g)	Carb (g)	Fiber (g)	Fat (g)	Sat (g)	Mono (g)	Poly (g)	Chol (mg)	Vit A (RE)
58242	Sausage, chicken & beef, smkd, pieces	1 cup	138	408	26	0	0	33	9.9	14.1	6.5	97	43
13021	Sausage, pepperoni, beef & pork, slice, 1 3/8" x 1/8"	1 pce	6	26	1	0	0	2	0.9	1.0	0.1	6	0
58353	Sausage, pork, link, USDA, ckd f/fzn	3.6 oz	100	267	20	0	0	20	5.5	8.7	2.3	98	15
13184	Sausage, smokies, links	1 ea	43	130	5	1	0	12	4.0	5.7	1.2	27	0
58232	Sausage, turkey, ckd	3.6 oz	100	196	24	0	0	10	2.3	3.0	2.7	92	15
Pork and Ham													
27096	Bacon Bits	1 Tbs	7	24	3	0	0	1	0.5	0.7	0.2	5	0
92207	Bacon, cured, microwv	1 pce	8	38	3	0	0	3	0.9	1.2	0.3	9	1
92208	Bacon, cured, pan fried	1 pce	8	42	3	0	0	3	1.0	1.4	0.4	9	1
28143	Canadian Bacon, 2 oz svg	1 ea	56	68	9	1	—	3	1.0	1.4	0.3	27	0
12118	Pork, avg of retail cuts, leg shoulder & loin, lean, ckd	3 oz	85	180	25	0	0	8	2.9	3.7	0.6	73	2
12309	Pork, avg of retail cuts, leg shoulder loin & sparerib, ckd	3 oz	85	232	23	0	0	15	5.3	6.5	1.2	77	2
12240	Pork, avg of retail cuts, loin & shoulder blade, ckd	3 oz	85	214	24	0	0	13	4.5	5.6	1.0	73	2
12311	Pork, avg of retail cuts, loin & shoulder blade, lean, ckd	3 oz	85	179	25	0	0	8	2.8	3.6	0.6	72	2
12184	Pork, chop, blade loin, brld	3 oz	85	272	19	0	0	21	7.9	9.1	1.9	73	2
12081	Pork, chop, breaded, brld/bkd, 3.6 oz svg	1 ea	100	259	25	6	0	14	5.1	6.2	1.5	72	2
12192	Pork, chop, center loin, brld	3 oz	85	204	24	0	0	11	4.1	5.0	0.8	70	3
12126	Pork, chop, w/bbq sauce	1 ea	116	209	23	3	0	11	3.7	4.9	1.2	65	23
12243	Pork, cured ham, dinner 3 oz slice, add wtr	1 ea	84	83	14	0	0	3	1.0	1.5	0.3	41	0
12307	Pork, cured ham, lean, 8% fat, rstd	1 cup	140	231	31	1	0	11	3.7	5.2	1.5	80	0
12099	Pork, ground, ckd	3 oz	85	253	22	0	0	18	6.6	7.9	1.6	80	2
12010	Pork, ribs, spareribs, brsd	3 oz	85	338	25	0	0	26	9.5	11.5	2.3	103	3
12060	Pork, roast, top loin, rstd	3 oz	85	192	25	0	0	10	3.5	4.5	0.7	66	2
92798	Pork, shred, w/original bbq sauce, ckd	0.25 cup	56	90	6	11	0	2	0.5	—	—	15	40
12900	Pork, sweet & sour	3 oz	85	87	6	9	1	3	0.8	1.2	0.9	14	12
12237	Pork, tenderloin, chop, brld	3 oz	85	171	25	0	0	7	2.5	2.8	0.6	80	2
Veal													
11531	Veal, avg of all cuts, ckd	3 oz	85	196	26	0	0	10	3.6	3.7	0.7	97	0
Variety Meats and By-Products													
10472	Beef, liver, brsd	3 oz	85	162	25	4	0	4	1.4	0.6	0.5	337	8042
Meat Substitutes, Soy Tofu and Vegetable													
27044	Bacon Bits, meatless	1 Tbs	7	33	2	2	1	2	0.3	0.4	0.9	0	0
7509	Bacon Substitute, vegetarian, strips	3 ea	15	46	2	1	0	4	0.7	1.1	2.3	0	1
7732	Beef Substitute, vegetarian, burger	0.25 cup	55	60	9	2	1	2	0.3	0.5	1.1	0	0
7558	Beef Substitute, vegetarian, fillet	1 ea	85	246	20	8	5	15	2.4	3.7	7.9	0	0
7561	Beef Substitute, vegetarian, patty	1 ea	56	110	12	4	3	5	0.8	1.2	2.6	0	0
7547	Chicken Substitute, vegetarian	1 cup	168	376	40	6	6	21	3.1	4.6	12.2	0	0
7549	Fish Sticks Substitute, vegetarian	1 ea	28	81	6	3	2	5	0.8	1.2	2.6	0	0
92148	Hot Dog Substitute	1 ea	70	163	14	5	3	10	1.4	2.7	5.5	0	0
7550	Hot Dog Substitute, vegetarian	1 ea	51	102	10	4	2	5	0.8	1.2	2.6	0	0
7551	Lunchmeat Substitute, vegetarian, 0.5 oz slice	1 pce	14	26	2	1	0	2	0.2	0.3	0.6	0	0
90626	Sausage Substitute, vegetarian, breakfast slices, 1 oz	1 ea	28	72	5	3	1	5	0.8	1.3	2.6	0	0
7564	Tempeh	0.5 cup	83	160	15	8	—	9	1.8	2.5	3.2	0	0
7519	Tofu, dried, fzn, 0.6 oz svg	1 pce	17	82	8	2	1	5	0.7	1.1	2.9	0	9
7522	Tofu, fermented & salted, block	3 oz	85	99	7	4	0	7	1.0	1.5	3.8	0	14
90040	Tofu, fermented & salted, w/calc sulfate, block, 0.4 oz	1 ea	11	13	1	1	0	1	0.1	0.2	0.5	0	2

PAGE KEY: A-158 Granola Bars, Cereal Bars, Diet Bars, Scones, and Tarts   A-158 Meals and Dishes   A-162 Meats   A-168 Nuts, Seeds, and Products   A-170 Poultry
A-172 Salad Dressings, Dips, and Mayonnaise   A-172 Salads   A-174 Sandwiches   A-176 Sauces and Gravies   A-176 Snack Foods—Chips, Pretzels, Popcorn
A-178 Soups, Stews, and Chilis   A-180 Spices, Flavors, and Seasonings   A-182 Sports Bars and Drinks   A-182 Supplemental Foods and Formulas
A-184 Sweeteners and Sweet Substitutes   A-184 Vegetables and Legumes   A-198 Weight Loss Bars and Drinks   A-200 Miscellaneous

Thia (mg)	Ribo (mg)	Niac (mg NE)	Vit B6 (mg)	Vit B12 (µg)	Fol (µg)	Vit C (mg)	Vit D (IU)	Vit E (mg AT)	Cal (mg)	Iron (mg)	Magn (mg)	Phos (mg)	Pota (mg)	Sodi (mg)	Zinc (mg)	Wat (%)	Alco (g)	Caff (g)
0.05	0.17	5.59	0.23	0.51	5.5	0.0	—	0.7	15	1.49	19.3	153	192	1408	2.4	56	0.00	0.00
0.02	0.00	0.30	0.01	0.09	0.3	0.0	0.5	0.0	1	0.07	1.0	10	17	98	0.2	31	0.00	0.00
0.73	0.23	2.79	0.28	0.88	1.0	0.0	—	0.7	9	1.14	19.0	190	239	540	2.8	59	0.00	0.00
—	—	—	—	—	—	0.0	—	—	4	0.50	7.3	103	77	433	0.9	56	0.00	0.00
0.07	0.25	5.71	0.31	1.23	6.0	0.7	—	0.2	22	1.49	21.0	202	298	665	3.9	65	0.00	0.00
—	—	—	—	—	—	0.0	—	—	2	0.20	4.6	43	39	224	0.3	35	0.00	0.00
0.03	0.01	0.75	0.02	0.11	0.2	0.0	—	0.0	1	0.10	2.3	36	37	155	0.3	16	0.00	0.00
0.03	0.01	0.91	0.02	0.10	0.2	0.0	—	0.0	1	0.10	2.8	44	47	192	0.3	12	0.00	0.00
—	—	—	—	—	—	0.8	—	—	3	0.50	10.6	—	156	569	1.0	73	0.00	0.00
0.72	0.28	4.40	0.37	0.63	0.9	0.3	—	0.2	18	0.93	22.1	202	319	50	2.5	60	0.00	0.00
0.64	0.28	4.19	0.34	0.64	5.1	0.3	—	0.2	21	0.93	20.4	197	301	53	2.5	55	0.00	0.00
0.72	0.28	4.21	0.34	0.62	5.1	0.3	10.2	0.2	20	0.83	20.4	193	308	48	2.2	57	0.00	0.00
0.74	0.28	4.46	0.37	0.63	5.1	0.3	—	0.4	19	0.91	22.1	199	321	48	2.4	60	0.00	0.00
0.55	0.25	3.49	0.31	0.70	3.4	0.6	—	0.3	25	0.79	18.7	180	293	60	2.9	52	0.00	0.00
0.81	0.30	4.75	0.41	0.62	5.8	0.5	12.0	0.4	24	1.00	26.8	240	400	415	2.2	52	0.00	0.00
0.91	0.23	4.46	0.36	0.62	5.1	0.3	—	0.3	28	0.68	21.3	197	304	49	1.9	58	0.00	0.00
0.73	0.28	4.90	0.36	0.64	5.0	1.9	—	0.5	19	1.30	24.1	221	373	860	2.4	65	0.00	0.00
0.60	0.18	3.93	0.31	0.40	—	0.0	—	—	4	1.01	16.9	203	221	1018	1.7	75	0.00	0.00
1.02	0.38	7.44	0.49	0.94	4.2	0.0	—	0.4	11	1.96	26.6	347	507	1939	3.7	66	0.00	0.00
0.60	0.18	3.57	0.33	0.46	5.1	0.6	10.2	0.2	19	1.10	20.4	192	308	62	2.7	53	0.00	0.00
0.34	0.31	4.65	0.30	0.92	3.4	0.0	—	0.3	40	1.57	20.4	222	272	79	3.9	40	0.00	0.00
0.51	0.25	4.36	0.31	0.46	6.8	0.3	—	0.3	4	0.68	19.6	183	291	37	1.9	59	0.00	0.00
—	—	—	—	—	—	0.0	—	—	0	0.72	—	—	—	380	—	—	0.00	0.00
0.20	0.07	1.37	0.15	0.12	3.9	7.4	10.2	0.4	11	0.54	12.9	56	145	316	0.6	77	0.00	0.00
0.81	0.31	4.30	0.43	0.82	5.1	0.9	—	0.3	4	1.17	29.8	247	378	54	2.5	61	0.00	0.00
0.05	0.27	6.78	0.25	1.34	12.8	0.0	—	0.3	19	0.98	22.1	203	276	74	4.0	57	0.00	0.00
0.15	2.91	14.90	0.86	60.02	215.2	1.6	—	0.4	5	5.55	17.9	423	299	67	4.5	59	0.00	0.00
0.03	0.00	0.10	0.00	0.07	8.9	0.1	—	0.5	7	0.05	6.7	15	10	124	0.1	8	0.00	0.00
0.66	0.07	1.12	0.07	0.00	6.3	0.0	—	1.0	3	0.36	2.9	10	26	220	0.1	49	0.00	0.00
0.12	0.10	1.96	0.23	1.13	—	0.0	—	—	4	1.73	—	56	25	269	0.4	71	0.00	0.00
0.93	0.75	10.19	1.27	3.56	86.7	0.0	—	2.9	81	1.70	19.6	382	510	416	1.2	45	0.00	0.00
0.50	0.34	5.59	0.67	1.34	43.7	0.0	—	1.0	16	1.17	10.1	193	101	308	1.0	58	0.00	0.00
1.14	0.40	2.44	1.17	3.66	127.7	0.0	—	4.5	59	5.48	28.6	563	91	1191	1.2	59	0.00	0.00
0.31	0.25	3.35	0.41	1.17	28.6	0.0	—	1.1	27	0.56	6.4	126	168	137	0.4	45	0.00	0.00
0.31	0.57	2.20	0.05	1.63	54.6	0.0	—	1.3	23	0.99	12.6	241	69	330	0.8	58	0.00	0.00
0.56	0.61	8.15	0.50	1.22	39.8	0.0	—	1.0	17	0.92	9.2	175	76	219	0.6	58	0.00	0.00
0.56	0.03	1.55	0.11	0.56	14.0	0.0	—	0.4	6	0.25	3.2	62	28	100	0.2	65	0.00	0.00
0.66	0.10	3.13	0.23	0.00	7.3	0.0	—	0.6	18	1.03	10.1	63	65	249	0.4	50	0.00	0.00
0.05	0.30	2.19	0.18	0.07	19.9	0.0	—	0.0	92	2.24	67.2	221	342	7	0.9	60	0.00	0.00
0.07	0.05	0.20	0.05	0.00	15.6	0.1	—	0.0	62	1.64	10.0	82	3	1	0.8	6	0.00	0.00
0.12	0.09	0.31	0.07	0.00	24.7	0.2	—	0.0	39	1.67	44.2	62	64	2443	1.3	70	0.00	0.00
0.01	0.00	0.03	0.00	0.00	3.2	0.0	—	0.0	135	0.21	6.4	8	8	316	0.2	70	0.00	0.00

PAGE KEY: A-108 Beverage and Beverage Mixes A-110 Other Beverages A-110 Beverages, Alcoholic A-112 Candies and Confections, Gum A-116 Cereals, Breakfast Type A-120 Cheese and Cheese Substitutes A-122 Dairy Products and Substitutes A-124 Desserts A-130 Dessert Toppings A-130 Eggs, Substitutes, and Egg Dishes A-132 Ethnic Foods A-136 Fast Foods/Restaurants A-150 Fats, Oils, Margarines, Shortenings, and Substitutes A-150 Fish, Seafood, and Shellfish A-152 Food Additives A-152 Fruit, Vegetable, or Blended Juices A-154 Grains, Flours, and Fractions A-154 Grain Products, Prepared and Baked Goods

Code	Food Name	Unit/ Amt	Wt (g)	Energy (kcal)	Prot (g)	Carb (g)	Fiber (g)	Fat (g)	Sat (g)	Mono (g)	Poly (g)	Chol (mg)	Vit A (RE)
NUTS, SEEDS, AND PRODUCTS													
4572	Almond Butter	1 cup	250	1582	38	53	9	148	14.0	95.9	31.0	0	0
4507	Coconut, fresh, shredded	1 cup	80	283	3	12	7	27	23.8	1.1	0.3	0	0
4559	Coconut, milk, cnd	2 Tbs	28	56	1	1	0	6	5.3	0.3	0.1	0	0
4575	Coconut, tstd f/dried	2 Tbs	9	55	0	4	1	4	3.9	0.2	0.0	0	0
4571	Nuts, almonds, dry rstd, salted, whole	22 ea	28	169	6	5	3	15	1.1	9.5	3.6	0	0
4549	Nuts, almonds, dry rstd, unsalted, whole	1 cup	138	824	30	27	16	73	5.6	46.4	17.5	0	0
4620	Nuts, almonds, oil rstd, salted	22 ea	28	172	6	5	3	16	1.2	9.9	3.8	0	0
4505	Nuts, almonds, oil rstd, unsalted	22 ea	28	172	6	5	3	16	1.2	9.9	3.8	0	0
4642	Nuts, beechnuts, dried	2 oz	57	327	4	19	2	28	3.2	12.4	11.4	0	0
4536	Nuts, Brazil, dried, lrg	6 ea	28	186	4	3	2	19	4.3	7.0	5.8	0	0
4750	Nuts, Brazil, dried, unblanched, shelled	1 cup	140	918	20	17	10	93	21.2	34.4	28.8	0	0
4519	Nuts, cashews, dry rstd, salted	0.25 cup	34	197	5	11	1	16	3.1	9.4	2.7	0	0
4621	Nuts, cashews, dry rstd, unsalted	0.25 cup	34	197	5	11	1	16	3.1	9.4	2.7	0	0
4596	Nuts, cashews, oil rstd, salted	0.25 cup	32	189	5	10	1	16	2.8	8.4	2.8	0	0
4622	Nuts, cashews, oil rstd, unsalted	0.25 cup	32	188	5	10	1	16	2.8	8.4	2.8	0	0
63431	Nuts, filberts, whole	1 cup	135	848	20	23	13	82	6.0	61.6	10.7	0	3
4513	Nuts, hazelnuts, whole	1 cup	135	848	20	23	13	82	6.0	61.6	10.7	0	3
4516	Nuts, macadamia, dried	11 ea	28	204	2	4	2	21	3.4	16.7	0.4	0	0
4595	Nuts, mixed, w/o peanuts, oil rstd, salted	0.25 cup	36	221	6	8	2	20	3.3	11.9	4.1	0	0
4594	Nuts, mixed, w/o peanuts, oil rstd, unsalted	0.25 cup	36	221	6	8	2	20	3.3	11.9	4.1	0	1
4592	Nuts, mixed, w/peanuts, dry rstd, salted	0.25 cup	34	203	6	9	3	18	2.4	10.8	3.7	0	0
4591	Nuts, mixed, w/peanuts, dry rstd, unsalted	0.25 cup	34	203	6	9	3	18	2.4	10.8	3.7	0	1
4593	Nuts, mixed, w/peanuts, oil rstd, salted	0.25 cup	36	219	6	8	3	20	3.1	11.3	4.7	0	0
4533	Nuts, mixed, w/peanuts, oil rstd, unsalted	0.25 cup	36	219	6	8	4	20	3.1	11.3	4.7	0	1
4541	Nuts, peanuts, dry rstd, salted	30 ea	30	176	7	6	2	15	2.1	7.4	4.7	0	0
4756	Nuts, peanuts, dry rstd, unsalted	30 ea	30	176	7	6	2	15	2.1	7.4	4.7	0	0
4763	Nuts, peanuts, oil rstd, salted	30 ea	27	162	8	4	3	14	2.3	7.0	4.1	0	0
4755	Nuts, peanuts, oil rstd, unsalted	32 ea	28	163	7	5	2	14	1.9	6.8	4.4	0	0
4542	Nuts, peanuts, oil rstd, unsalted, chpd	1 cup	133	773	35	25	9	66	9.1	32.5	20.7	0	0
4699	Nuts, peanuts, Spanish, oil rstd, salted	0.5 cup	74	426	21	13	7	36	5.6	16.2	12.5	0	0
4665	Nuts, peanuts, Spanish, oil rstd, unsalted	1 cup	147	851	41	26	13	72	11.1	32.4	25.0	0	0
4517	Nuts, peanuts, Spanish, raw	0.25 cup	36	208	10	6	3	18	2.8	8.1	6.3	0	0
4578	Nuts, pecans, halves	1 cup	108	746	10	15	10	78	6.7	44.1	23.3	0	6
4624	Nuts, pine	10 ea	1	7	0	0	0	1	0.1	0.2	0.3	0	0
4525	Nuts, walnuts, black, dried, chpd	1 cup	125	772	30	12	8	74	4.2	18.8	43.8	0	5
4626	Peanut Butter, chunky	2 Tbs	32	188	8	7	3	16	2.6	7.9	4.7	0	0
4576	Peanut Butter, chunky, unsalted	2 Tbs	32	188	8	7	3	16	2.6	7.9	4.7	0	0
4627	Peanut Butter, creamy	2 Tbs	32	188	8	6	2	16	3.3	7.6	4.4	0	0
63338	Peanut Butter, creamy, rducd fat	3.6 oz	100	520	26	36	5	34	7.4	16.2	10.3	0	0
4636	Peanut Butter, creamy, unsalted	2 Tbs	32	188	8	6	2	16	3.3	7.6	4.4	0	0
62939	Peanut Butter, crunchy, rducd fat	2 Tbs	36	190	8	15	2	12	2.5	—	—	0	0
4747	Peanut Butter, rducd fat	1 Tbs	16	81	4	5	1	5	1.0	2.8	1.6	0	—
62949	Peanut Butter, w/grape jelly, Goober	3 Tbs	53	230	7	24	2	13	2.0	—	—	0	0
4777	Seeds, flax/linseed	1 cup	155	763	30	53	43	53	5.0	10.6	34.8	0	0
4545	Seeds, sunflower, kernels, dried	1 cup	144	821	33	27	15	71	7.5	13.6	47.1	0	9

Thia (mg)	Ribo (mg)	Niac (mg NE)	Vit B6 (mg)	Vit B12 (µg)	Fol (µg)	Vit C (mg)	Vit D (IU)	Vit E (mg AT)	Cal (mg)	Iron (mg)	Magn (mg)	Phos (mg)	Pota (mg)	Sodi (mg)	Zinc (mg)	Wat (%)	Alco (g)	Caff (g)
0.33	1.52	7.19	0.18	0.00	162.5	1.8	—	65.0	675	9.25	757.5	1308	1895	1125	7.6	1	0.00	0.00
0.05	0.01	0.43	0.03	0.00	20.8	2.6	—	0.2	11	1.94	25.6	90	285	16	0.9	47	0.00	0.00
0.00	0.00	0.18	0.00	0.00	4.0	0.3	—	0.2	5	0.93	13.0	27	62	4	0.2	73	0.00	0.00
0.00	0.00	0.05	0.02	0.00	0.8	0.1	—	0.1	2	0.31	8.5	20	51	3	0.2	1	0.00	0.00
0.01	0.23	1.09	0.03	0.00	9.4	0.0	—	7.4	75	1.27	81.1	139	211	96	1.0	3	0.00	0.00
0.10	1.19	5.30	0.17	0.00	45.5	0.0	—	35.9	367	6.21	394.7	675	1029	1	4.9	3	0.00	0.00
0.02	0.21	1.03	0.02	0.00	7.7	0.0	—	7.4	82	1.03	77.7	132	198	96	0.9	3	0.00	0.00
0.02	0.21	1.03	0.02	0.00	7.7	0.0	—	7.4	82	1.03	77.7	132	198	0	0.9	3	0.00	0.00
0.17	0.20	0.50	0.38	0.00	64.1	8.8	—	—	1	1.38	0.0	0	577	22	0.2	7	0.00	0.00
0.17	0.00	0.07	0.02	0.00	6.2	0.2	—	1.6	45	0.68	106.6	206	187	1	1.2	3	0.00	0.00
0.86	0.05	0.40	0.14	0.00	30.8	1.0	—	8.0	224	3.40	526.4	1015	923	4	5.7	3	0.00	0.00
0.07	0.07	0.47	0.09	0.00	23.6	0.0	—	0.3	15	2.05	89.1	168	194	219	1.9	2	0.00	0.00
0.07	0.07	0.47	0.09	0.00	23.6	0.0	—	0.3	15	2.05	89.1	168	194	5	1.9	2	0.00	0.00
0.11	0.07	0.56	0.10	0.00	8.1	0.1	—	0.3	14	1.97	88.7	173	205	100	1.7	2	0.00	0.00
0.11	0.07	0.56	0.10	0.00	8.1	0.1	—	0.3	14	1.97	88.7	173	205	4	1.7	3	0.00	0.00
0.87	0.15	2.43	0.75	0.00	152.6	8.5	—	20.3	154	6.34	220.1	392	918	0	3.3	5	0.00	0.00
0.87	0.15	2.43	0.75	0.00	152.6	8.5	—	20.3	154	6.34	220.1	392	918	0	3.3	5	0.00	0.00
0.34	0.05	0.69	0.07	0.00	3.1	0.3	—	0.2	24	1.04	36.9	53	104	1	0.4	1	0.00	0.00
0.18	0.17	0.70	0.05	0.00	20.2	0.2	—	3.0	38	0.93	90.4	162	196	110	1.7	3	0.00	0.00
0.18	0.17	0.70	0.05	0.00	20.2	0.2	—	2.2	38	0.93	90.4	162	196	4	1.7	3	0.00	0.00
0.07	0.07	1.61	0.10	0.00	17.1	0.1	—	3.7	24	1.26	77.1	149	204	229	1.3	2	0.00	0.00
0.07	0.07	1.61	0.10	0.00	17.1	0.1	—	2.1	24	1.26	77.1	149	204	4	1.3	2	0.00	0.00
0.18	0.07	1.79	0.09	0.00	29.5	0.2	—	2.6	38	1.13	83.4	165	206	149	1.8	2	0.00	0.00
0.18	0.07	1.79	0.09	0.00	29.5	0.2	—	2.1	38	1.13	83.4	165	206	4	1.8	2	0.00	0.00
0.12	0.02	4.05	0.07	0.00	43.5	0.0	—	2.3	16	0.68	52.8	107	197	244	1.0	2	0.00	0.00
0.12	0.02	4.05	0.07	0.00	43.5	0.0	—	2.1	16	0.68	52.8	107	197	2	1.0	2	0.00	0.00
0.01	0.01	3.73	0.11	0.00	32.4	0.2	—	1.9	16	0.40	47.5	107	196	86	0.9	1	0.00	0.00
0.07	0.02	4.00	0.07	0.00	35.3	0.0	—	1.9	25	0.50	51.8	145	191	2	1.9	2	0.00	0.00
0.34	0.14	18.98	0.34	0.00	167.6	0.0	—	9.2	117	2.43	246.1	688	907	8	8.8	2	0.00	0.00
0.23	0.05	10.97	0.18	0.00	92.6	0.0	0.0	5.4	74	1.67	123.5	284	570	318	1.5	2	0.00	0.00
0.46	0.11	21.95	0.37	0.00	185.2	0.0	—	10.9	147	3.34	247.0	569	1141	9	2.9	2	0.00	0.00
0.25	0.05	5.80	0.12	0.00	87.6	0.0	—	2.7	39	1.42	68.6	142	272	8	0.8	6	0.00	0.00
0.70	0.14	1.25	0.23	0.00	23.8	1.2	—	1.5	76	2.73	130.7	299	443	0	4.9	4	0.00	0.00
—	—	—	—	0.00	—	0.0	—	—	0	0.05	—	—	—	0	—	2	0.00	0.00
0.07	0.15	0.58	0.73	0.00	38.8	2.1	—	2.2	76	3.90	251.2	641	654	2	4.2	5	0.00	0.00
0.02	0.03	4.38	0.12	0.00	29.4	0.0	0.0	2.0	14	0.61	51.2	102	238	156	0.9	1	0.00	0.00
0.02	0.03	4.38	0.12	0.00	29.4	0.0	—	2.0	14	0.61	51.2	102	238	5	0.9	1	0.00	0.00
0.01	0.02	4.28	0.17	0.00	23.7	0.0	—	2.9	14	0.60	49.3	115	208	147	0.9	2	0.00	0.00
0.27	0.05	14.60	0.31	0.00	60.0	0.0	—	6.7	35	1.89	170.0	369	669	540	2.8	1	0.00	0.00
0.01	0.02	4.28	0.17	0.00	23.7	0.0	—	2.9	14	0.60	49.3	115	208	5	0.9	2	0.00	0.00
—	—	5.00	0.11	0.00	24.0	0.0	—	—	0	0.72	60.0	—	—	220	0.9	—	0.00	0.00
—	—	2.07	—	0.00	—	—	—	—	6	0.31	—	59	115	89	—	3	0.00	0.00
—	—	—	—	0.00	—	0.0	—	—	0	0.36	—	—	—	160	—	—	0.00	0.00
0.25	0.25	2.17	1.44	0.00	430.9	2.0	—	0.5	308	9.64	561.1	772	1056	53	6.5	9	0.00	0.00
3.29	0.36	6.48	1.11	0.00	326.9	2.0	—	49.7	167	9.75	509.8	1015	992	4	7.3	5	0.00	0.00

PAGE KEY: A-108 Beverage and Beverage Mixes   A-110 Other Beverages   A-110 Beverages, Alcoholic   A-112 Candies and Confections, Gum   A-116 Cereals, Breakfast Type
A-120 Cheese and Cheese Substitutes   A-122 Dairy Products and Substitutes   A-124 Desserts   A-130 Dessert Toppings   A-130 Eggs, Substitutes, and Egg Dishes   A-132 Ethnic Foods
A-136 Fast Foods/Restaurants   A-150 Fats, Oils, Margarines, Shortenings, and Substitutes   A-150 Fish, Seafood, and Shellfish   A-152 Food Additives
A-152 Fruit, Vegetable, or Blended Juices   A-154 Grains, Flours, and Fractions   A-154 Grain Products, Prepared and Baked Goods

Code	Food Name	Unit/ Amt	Wt (g)	Energy (kcal)	Prot (g)	Carb (g)	Fiber (g)	Fat (g)	Sat (g)	Mono (g)	Poly (g)	Chol (mg)	Vit A (RE)
4597	Seeds, sunflower, kernels, dry rstd, salted	0.25 cup	32	186	6	8	3	16	1.7	3.0	10.5	0	0
4551	Seeds, sunflower, kernels, dry rstd, unsalted	0.25 cup	32	186	6	8	4	16	1.7	3.0	10.5	0	0
4546	Seeds, sunflower, kernels, oil rstd, unsalted	1 cup	135	799	27	31	14	69	9.5	10.9	46.3	0	1
4552	Seeds, sunflower, oil rstd, salted	0.25 cup	34	200	7	8	4	17	2.4	2.7	11.6	0	0
63261	Soy Nuts, wheat free	1.8 oz	50	241	20	14	6	11	1.7	—	—	1	4
POULTRY													
Chicken—BBQ, Breaded, Fried, Glazed, Grilled, Raw													
15064	Chicken, breast & wing, white meat, brd, fried	3 oz	85	258	19	10	1	15	4.1	6.4	3.5	77	30
81202	Chicken, breast, fillet, grilled	1 ea	85	100	20	1	0	2	—	—	—	45	0
81186	Chicken, breast, oven rstd, fat free, 0.75 oz slice	2 pce	42	33	7	1	0	0	0.1	0.1	0.0	15	0
15921	Chicken, breast, sweet & sour	1 ea	131	118	8	15	1	3	0.5	0.9	1.4	23	22
15915	Chicken, breast, teriyaki	3 oz	85	118	18	4	0	2	0.6	0.7	0.6	55	11
15057	Chicken, broiler/fryer, breast, w/o skin, fried	3 oz	85	159	28	0	0	4	1.1	1.5	0.9	77	6
15004	Chicken, broiler/fryer, breast, w/o skin, rstd	3 oz	85	140	26	0	0	3	0.9	1.1	0.7	72	5
15039	Chicken, broiler/fryer, breast, w/o skin, stwd	3 oz	85	128	25	0	0	3	0.7	0.9	0.6	65	5
15013	Chicken, broiler/fryer, breast, w/skin, batter fried	3 oz	85	221	21	8	0	11	3.0	4.6	2.6	72	17
15003	Chicken, broiler/fryer, breast, w/skin, flour fried	3 oz	85	189	27	1	0	8	2.1	3.0	1.7	76	13
15001	Chicken, broiler/fryer, breast, w/skin, rstd	3 oz	85	168	25	0	0	7	1.9	2.6	1.4	71	23
15113	Chicken, broiler/fryer, dark meat, w/skin, batter fried	3 oz	85	253	19	8	0	16	4.2	6.4	3.8	76	26
15079	Chicken, broiler/fryer, dark meat, w/skin, flour fried	3 oz	85	242	23	3	0	14	3.9	5.7	3.3	78	26
15080	Chicken, broiler/fryer, dark meat, w/skin, rstd	3 oz	85	215	22	0	0	13	3.7	5.3	3.0	77	51
15903	Chicken, buffalo wings, w/bone, spicy	1 pce	16	49	4	0	0	3	0.9	1.3	0.9	13	9
15063	Chicken, drumstick & thigh, dark meat, brd, fried	3 oz	85	247	17	9	1	15	4.1	6.3	3.6	95	38
81198	Chicken, ground, raw	4 oz	113	150	18	0	0	9	2.5	—	—	75	0
15243	Chicken, nuggets	4 pce	73	207	12	11	0	13	4.0	6.2	1.6	44	22
15902	Chicken, patty, brd, ckd	1 ea	75	213	12	11	0	13	4.1	6.4	1.7	45	22
15136	Chicken, roasting, dark meat, w/o skin, raw	4 oz	113	128	21	0	0	4	1.1	1.3	1.0	82	20
15134	Chicken, roasting, light meat, w/o skin, raw	4 oz	113	124	25	0	0	2	0.4	0.5	0.5	65	9
49158	Chicken, tenders, breast meat, fat free, bkd	3 ea	85	120	13	16	2	0	0.0	0.0	0.0	30	0
49171	Chicken, tenders, breast, ckd f/fzn	3 ea	85	240	11	16	1	14	4.0	—	—	25	0
Turkey													
16086	Turkey, avg, breast, w/skin, rstd	3 oz	85	161	24	0	0	6	1.8	2.1	1.5	63	0
51101	Turkey, avg, dark meat, w/o skin, rstd	3 oz	85	159	24	0	0	6	2.1	1.4	1.8	72	0
16028	Turkey, avg, dark meat, w/skin, rstd	3 oz	85	188	23	0	0	10	3.0	3.1	2.6	76	0
16158	Turkey, avg, light meat, w/o skin, rstd	3 oz	85	134	25	0	0	3	0.9	0.5	0.7	59	0
16027	Turkey, avg, light meat, w/skin, rstd	3 oz	85	168	24	0	0	7	2.0	2.4	1.7	65	0
16071	Turkey, avg, skin, rstd	1 ea	496	2192	98	0	0	197	51.3	83.8	45.0	560	0
16000	Turkey, avg, w/o skin, rstd	3 oz	85	145	25	0	0	4	1.4	0.9	1.2	65	0
16204	Turkey, ground, 10% fat, raw	3 oz	85	137	16	0	0	8	2.6	3.1	2.5	73	0
51133	Turkey, ground, 99% fat free, raw	4 oz	113	120	28	0	0	2	—	—	—	45	0
16351	Turkey, jerky, original, Original California	1 oz	28	80	14	3	0	1	0.0	—	—	30	60
Duck, Emu, Ostrich and Other													
15069	Cornish Game Hen, rstd	3 oz	85	221	19	0	0	15	4.3	6.8	3.1	111	27
16294	Duck, domesticated, whole, rstd, chpd	1 cup	140	472	27	0	0	40	13.5	18.1	5.1	118	88
16065	Goose, whole, w/o skin, raw	4 oz	113	183	26	0	0	8	3.2	2.1	1.0	95	14

Thia (mg)	Ribo (mg)	Niac (mg NE)	Vit B6 (mg)	Vit B12 (µg)	Fol (µg)	Vlt C (mg)	Vit D (IU)	Vit E (mg AT)	Cal (mg)	Iron (mg)	Magn (mg)	Phos (mg)	Pota (mg)	Sodi (mg)	Zinc (mg)	Wat (%)	Alco (g)	Caff (g)
0.02	0.07	2.25	0.25	0.00	75.8	0.4	—	8.4	22	1.22	41.3	370	272	131	1.7	1	0.00	0.00
0.02	0.07	2.25	0.25	0.00	75.8	0.4	—	8.4	22	1.22	41.3	370	272	1	1.7	1	0.00	0.00
0.43	0.37	5.57	1.07	0.00	315.9	1.5	—	49.0	117	5.78	171.4	1538	652	4	7.0	2	0.00	0.00
0.10	0.09	1.38	0.27	0.00	79.0	0.4	—	12.3	29	1.44	42.9	384	163	138	1.8	2	0.00	0.00
—	—	—	—	0.00	—	0.0	—	—	105	3.20	—	—	—	—	—	2	0.00	0.00
0.07	0.15	6.25	0.30	0.34	15.3	0.0	—	0.8	31	0.76	19.6	160	295	509	0.8	46	0.00	0.00
—	—	—	—	—	—	0.0	—	—	0	1.08	—	—	—	410	—	—	0.00	0.00
0.00	0.00	1.44	0.05	0.03	0.4	0.0	—	0.0	3	0.12	3.8	25	28	457	0.1	77	0.00	0.00
0.05	0.07	3.08	0.18	0.07	5.8	12.1	—	0.7	15	0.83	20.8	75	185	506	0.7	79	0.00	0.00
0.05	0.12	5.82	0.31	0.18	8.1	2.1	—	0.2	18	1.13	23.4	132	205	1118	1.3	67	0.56	0.00
0.07	0.10	12.56	0.54	0.31	3.4	0.0	—	0.4	14	0.97	26.4	209	235	67	0.9	60	0.00	0.00
0.05	0.10	11.65	0.50	0.28	3.4	0.0	—	0.2	13	0.87	24.7	194	218	63	0.9	65	0.00	0.00
0.03	0.10	7.19	0.28	0.20	2.6	0.0	—	0.2	11	0.75	20.4	140	159	54	0.8	68	0.00	0.00
0.10	0.11	8.94	0.37	0.25	12.8	0.0	—	0.9	17	1.05	20.4	157	171	234	0.8	52	0.00	0.00
0.07	0.10	11.68	0.49	0.28	5.1	0.0	—	0.5	14	1.00	25.5	198	220	65	0.9	57	0.00	0.00
0.05	0.10	10.81	0.47	0.27	3.4	0.0	—	0.2	12	0.91	23.0	182	208	60	0.9	62	0.00	0.00
0.10	0.18	4.76	0.20	0.23	15.3	0.0	—	1.0	18	1.22	17.0	123	157	251	1.8	49	0.00	0.00
0.07	0.20	5.82	0.27	0.25	9.4	0.0	—	0.7	14	1.27	20.4	150	196	76	2.2	51	0.00	0.00
0.05	0.18	5.40	0.25	0.25	6.0	0.0	—	0.5	13	1.15	18.7	143	187	74	2.1	59	0.00	0.00
0.00	0.01	1.02	0.07	0.03	0.5	0.0	1.9	0.1	2	0.20	3.0	24	29	13	0.3	53	0.00	0.00
0.07	0.25	4.13	0.18	0.47	14.5	0.0	—	0.8	20	0.92	21.3	138	256	434	1.9	49	0.00	0.00
—	—	—	—	—	—	0.0	—	—	0	0.00	—	—	—	65	—	—	0.00	0.00
0.07	0.10	4.90	0.23	0.21	8.0	0.3	8.8	1.4	12	0.91	14.6	146	180	388	0.8	49	0.00	0.00
0.07	0.10	5.03	0.23	0.23	8.2	0.3	9.0	1.5	12	0.93	15.0	150	184	399	0.8	49	0.00	0.00
0.07	0.20	6.67	0.36	0.38	10.2	0.0	—	0.2	10	1.29	23.8	202	257	108	1.9	75	0.00	0.00
0.07	0.10	11.59	0.62	0.43	4.5	0.0	—	0.2	12	1.00	28.4	253	286	58	0.7	74	0.00	0.00
—	—	—	—	—	—	0.0	—	—	0	0.72	—	—	—	480	—	—	0.00	0.00
—	—	—	—	—	—	0.0	—	—	20	0.72	—	—	—	450	—	—	0.00	0.00
0.05	0.10	5.40	0.40	0.31	5.1	0.0	—	0.2	18	1.19	23.0	179	245	54	1.7	63	0.00	0.00
0.05	0.20	3.09	0.31	0.31	7.7	0.0	—	0.5	27	1.98	20.4	174	247	67	3.8	63	0.00	0.00
0.05	0.20	3.00	0.27	0.31	7.7	0.0	—	0.5	28	1.92	19.6	167	233	65	3.5	60	0.00	0.00
0.05	0.10	5.82	0.46	0.31	5.1	0.0	—	0.1	16	1.14	23.8	186	259	54	1.7	66	0.00	0.00
0.05	0.10	5.34	0.40	0.30	5.1	0.0	—	0.1	18	1.20	22.1	177	242	54	1.7	63	0.00	0.00
0.10	0.72	13.17	0.40	1.19	19.8	0.0	—	2.6	174	8.88	79.4	680	794	263	10.3	40	0.00	0.00
0.05	0.15	4.63	0.38	0.31	6.0	0.0	—	0.3	21	1.50	22.1	181	253	60	2.6	65	0.00	0.00
—	—	—	—	—	—	0.0	—	—	22	1.28	22.9	140	207	109	2.5	71	0.00	0.00
—	—	—	—	—	—	0.0	—	—	0	1.44	—	—	—	65	—	—	0.00	0.00
—	—	—	—	—	—	0.0	—	—	20	1.08	—	—	—	550	—	31	0.00	0.00
0.05	0.17	5.01	0.25	0.23	1.7	0.4	10.2	0.2	11	0.76	15.3	124	208	54	1.3	59	0.00	0.00
0.23	0.37	6.75	0.25	0.41	8.4	0.0	—	1.0	15	3.77	22.4	218	286	83	2.6	52	0.00	0.00
0.15	0.43	4.84	0.73	0.56	35.2	8.2	—	1.3	15	2.91	27.2	354	476	99	2.7	68	0.00	0.00

PAGE KEY: A-108 Beverage and Beverage Mixes   A-110 Other Beverages   A-110 Beverages, Alcoholic   A-112 Candies and Confections, Gum   A-116 Cereals, Breakfast Type   A-120 Cheese and Cheese Substitutes   A-122 Dairy Products and Substitutes   A-124 Desserts   A-130 Dessert Toppings   A-130 Eggs, Substitutes, and Egg Dishes   A-132 Ethnic Foods   A-136 Fast Foods/Restaurants   A-150 Fats, Oils, Margarines, Shortenings, and Substitutes   A-150 Fish, Seafood, and Shellfish   A-152 Food Additives   A-152 Fruit, Vegetable, or Blended Juices   A-154 Grains, Flours, and Fractions   A-154 Grain Products, Prepared and Baked Goods

Code	Food Name	Unit/ Amt	Wt (g)	Energy (kcal)	Prot (g)	Carb (g)	Fiber (g)	Fat (g)	Sat (g)	Mono (g)	Poly (g)	Chol (mg)	Vit A (RE)
16064	Goose, whole, w/skin, raw	4 oz	113	421	18	0	0	38	11.1	20.2	4.3	91	19
81168	Ostrich, ground, brld	3 oz	85	149	22	0	0	6	1.5	1.8	0.6	71	0
51148	Pheasant, whole, ckd	3 oz	85	210	28	0	0	10	3.0	4.8	1.3	76	48
SALAD DRESSINGS, DIPS, MAYONNAISE, OR SPREADS													
Dips													
53685	Dip, bean	2 Tbs	35	40	2	6	0	1	0.5	—	—	5	0
27138	Dip, creamy ranch	2 Tbs	31	60	1	3	0	4	3.0	—	—	0	0
53554	Dip, French onion	2 Tbs	33	60	1	4	0	5	3.0	—	—	15	20
27136	Dip, green onion	2 Tbs	31	60	1	4	0	4	3.0	—	—	0	0
27132	Dip, guacamole	2 Tbs	32	60	1	4	0	4	3.0	—	—	0	0
90861	Dip, salsa con queso, medium	2 Tbs	32	42	1	5	1	2	0.5	—	—	5	19
44415	Dip, salsa, grande	2 Tbs	28	50	1	1	0	5	3.0	—	—	15	40
27143	Dip, spinach	2 Tbs	28	140	0	3	0	14	2.0	—	—	10	80
44414	Dip, Veggie	2 Tbs	28	50	1	2	0	5	3.0	—	—	15	60
44425	Guacamole, med	2 Tbs	28	57	1	3	2	5	1.0	—	—	0	10
Mayonnaise													
8069	Mayonnaise, fat free	1 Tbs	16	11	0	2	0	0	0.1	—	—	2	3
4070	Mayonnaise, light	1 Tbs	15	50	0	2		5	0.0	2.5	1.5	5	0
44719	Mayonnaise, rducd cal, cholest free	1 Tbs	15	49	0	1	0	5	0.7	1.1	2.8	0	0
8503	Mayonnaise, real	1 Tbs	14	100	0	0	0	11	1.5	—	—	5	0
Salad Dressings—Lower Calorie/Fat/Sodium/Cholest													
44731	Dip, hummus, low fat, dry mix	2 Tbs	15	75	3	8	2	3	0.0	—	—	0	0
44727	Salad Dressing, blue cheese, fat free	1 Tbs	17	20	0	4	1	0	0.0	0.0	0.1	1	1
44722	Salad Dressing, blue cheese, rducd cal	1 Tbs	16	14	0	2	0	0	0.1	0.2	0.1	2	11
44465	Salad Dressing, buttermilk, light	3.6 oz	100	225	1	16	1	17	1.3	5.4	4.3	21	19
8138	Salad Dressing, caesar, low cal	1 Tbs	15	16	0	3	0	1	0.1	0.2	0.4	0	0
44729	Salad Dressing, French, rducd cal	1 Tbs	16	32	0	4	0	2	0.3	0.5	1.2	0	3
44699	Salad Dressing, Italian	2 Tbs	31	70	0	0	0	8	1.0	—	—	0	0
44498	Salad Dressing, Italian, fat free	1 Tbs	14	7	0	1	0	0	0.0	0.0	0.0	0	1
44720	Salad Dressing, Italian, rducd cal	1 Tbs	14	28	0	1	0	3	0.4	0.7	1.6	0	0
44497	Salad Dressing, thousand island, fat free	1 Tbs	16	21	0	5	1	0	0.0	0.1	0.1	1	0
8545	Salad Dressing, vinaigrette, Italian, fat free	2 Tbs	35	35	0	8	0	0	0.0	0.0	0.0	0	0
8546	Salad Dressing, vinaigrette, raspberry, fat free	2 Tbs	35	35	0	8	0	0	0.0	0.0	0.0	0	0
Salad Dressings—Regular													
44705	Salad Dressing, caesar	2 Tbs	29	155	0	1	0	17	2.6	4.0	9.7	1	1
8015	Salad Dressing, French, cmrcl	2 Tbs	31	143	0	5	0	14	1.8	2.6	6.6	0	14
8569	Salad Dressing, French, creamy	2 Tbs	32	160	0	5	0	15	2.5	—	—	0	250
8579	Salad Dressing, honey dijon	2 Tbs	31	110	0	6	0	10	1.5	—	—	0	0
8612	Salad Dressing, Italian, zesty	2 Tbs	31	109	0	2	0	11	1.2	—	—	0	2
8479	Salad Dressing, Miracle Whip	1 Tbs	15	70	0	2	0	7	1.0	—	—	5	0
44590	Salad Dressing, ranch, cmrcl	1 oz	28	137	0	2	0	15	2.3	3.2	8.0	9	3
8024	Salad Dressing, thousand island, cmrcl	1 Tbs	16	58	0	2	0	5	0.8	1.2	2.8	4	4
SPREADS—CRACKER OR SANDWICH													
Salads													
57482	Cole Slaw, prep f/recipe	0.5 cup	60	41	1	7	1	2	0.2	0.4	0.8	5	39
56118	Salad, bean, three	0.5 cup	75	70	2	7	3	4	0.6	0.9	2.2	0	10

PAGE KEY: A-158 Granola Bars, Cereal Bars, Diet Bars, Scones, and Tarts   A-158 Meals and Dishes   A-162 Meats   A-168 Nuts, Seeds, and Products   A-170 Poultry   A-172 Salad Dressings, Dips, and Mayonnaise   A-172 Salads   A-174 Sandwiches   A-176 Sauces and Gravies   A-176 Snack Foods—Chips, Pretzels, Popcorn   A-178 Soups, Stews, and Chilis   A-180 Spices, Flavors, and Seasonings   A-182 Sports Bars and Drinks   A-182 Supplemental Foods and Formulas   A-184 Sweeteners and Sweet Substitutes   A-184 Vegetables and Legumes   A-198 Weight Loss Bars and Drinks   A-200 Miscellaneous

Thia (mg)	Ribo (mg)	Niac (mg NE)	Vit B6 (mg)	Vit B12 (µg)	Fol (µg)	Vit C (mg)	Vit D (IU)	Vit E (mg AT)	Cal (mg)	Iron (mg)	Magn (mg)	Phos (mg)	Pota (mg)	Sodi (mg)	Zinc (mg)	Wat (%)	Alco (g)	Caff (g)
0.10	0.28	4.09	0.43	0.38	4.5	4.8	—	2.0	14	2.83	20.4	265	349	83	2.0	50	0.00	0.00
0.18	0.23	5.57	0.43	4.88	11.9	0.0	—	0.2	7	2.92	19.6	191	275	68	3.7	67	0.00	0.00
0.05	0.15	6.40	0.63	0.61	4.3	2.0	—	0.2	14	1.22	18.7	206	230	37	1.2	54	0.00	0.00
—	—	—	—	—	—	0.0	—	—	0	0.36	—	—	—	140	—	70	0.00	0.00
—	—	—	—	—	—	0.0	—	—	0	0.00	—	—	20	210	—	—	0.00	0.00
—	—	—	—	—	—	0.0	—	—	0	0.00	—	—	—	230	—	—	0.00	0.00
—	—	—	—	—	—	0.0	—	—	0	0.00	—	0	20	190	—	—	0.00	0.00
—	—	—	—	—	—	0.0	—	—	0	0.00	—	0	25	240	—	—	0.00	0.00
—	—	—	—	—	—	0.0	—	—	19	0.00	—	—	—	254	—	—	0.00	0.00
—	—	—	—	—	—	1.2	—	—	20	0.00	—	—	—	130	—	—	0.00	0.00
—	—	—	—	—	—	0.0	—	—	0	0.36	—	—	—	200	—	—	0.00	0.00
—	—	—	—	—	—	0.0	—	—	20	0.00	—	—	—	125	—	—	0.00	0.00
—	—	—	—	—	—	1.8	—	—	10	0.18	—	—	—	147	—	66	0.00	0.00
—	—	—	—	—	—	0.0	—	0.5	1	0.01	—	4	8	120	—	82	0.00	0.00
—	—	—	—	—	—	—	—	0.6	—	—	—	—	—	125	—	51	0.00	0.00
0.00	0.00	0.00	0.00	0.00	0.0	0.0	—	0.9	0	0.00	0.0	0	10	107	0.0	56	0.00	0.00
—	—	—	—	—	—	0.0	—	0.4	0	0.00	—	0	0	75	—	20	0.00	0.00
—	—	—	—	—	—	0.0	—	—	0	0.54	—	—	—	240	—	—	0.00	0.00
0.00	0.01	0.00	0.00	0.03	1.0	0.0	—	0.0	12	0.00	1.5	18	33	136	0.0	68	0.00	0.00
0.00	0.00	0.00	0.00	0.01	4.5	0.0	—	0.1	11	0.01	0.6	8	8	258	0.0	78	0.00	0.00
0.01	0.02	0.00	0.02	0.00	4.0	0.7	4.9	1.6	125	0.87	6.0	193	132	932	0.6	62	0.00	0.00
0.00	0.00	0.00	0.00	0.00	0.3	0.0	—	0.1	4	0.02	0.3	3	4	162	0.0	73	0.00	0.00
0.00	0.00	0.00	0.00	0.00	0.3	0.0	—	0.5	2	0.05	0.0	2	13	160	0.0	59	0.00	0.00
—	—	—	—	—	—	0.0	—	—	0	0.00	—	—	—	350	—	71	0.00	0.00
0.00	0.00	0.01	0.00	0.03	1.7	0.1	—	0.1	4	0.05	0.7	15	14	158	0.1	80	0.00	0.00
0.00	0.00	0.00	0.00	0.00	0.4	0.1	—	0.1	1	0.01	0.3	1	5	199	0.0	70	0.00	0.00
0.03	0.00	0.03	0.00	0.00	1.9	0.0	—	0.1	2	0.03	0.6	0	20	117	0.0	66	0.00	0.00
—	—	—	—	—	—	0.0	—	—	0	0.00	—	—	—	280	—	—	0.00	0.00
—	—	—	—	—	—	0.0	—	—	0	0.00	—	—	—	35	—	—	0.00	0.00
0.00	0.00	0.00	0.00	0.00	0.9	0.0	—	1.5	7	0.05	0.6	6	9	317	0.0	34	0.00	0.00
0.00	0.01	0.05	0.00	0.03	0.0	0.0	—	1.6	7	0.25	1.6	6	21	261	0.1	37	0.00	0.00
—	—	—	—	—	—	0.0	—	—	0	0.00	—	0	20	270	—	35	0.00	0.00
—	—	—	—	—	—	0.0	—	—	0	0.00	—	0	35	210	—	—	0.00	0.00
—	—	—	—	—	—	0.2	—	—	1	0.05	—	4	9	505	—	53	0.00	0.00
—	—	—	—	—	—	0.0	—	0.0	0	0.00	—	0	0	95	—	—	0.00	0.00
0.02	0.01	0.00	0.00	0.09	1.1	1.0	0.8	1.3	9	0.18	1.4	46	18	231	0.1	38	0.00	0.00
0.23	0.00	0.07	0.00	0.00	0.0	0.0	—	0.6	3	0.18	1.2	4	17	135	0.0	47	0.00	0.00
0.03	0.03	0.15	0.07	0.00	16.2	19.6	—	0.1	27	0.34	6.0	19	109	14	0.1	82	0.00	0.00
0.03	0.05	0.21	0.01	0.00	28.0	2.0	—	0.9	18	0.74	13.7	38	123	260	0.3	81	0.00	0.00

PAGE KEY: A-108 Beverage and Beverage Mixes   A-110 Other Beverages   A-110 Beverages, Alcoholic   A-112 Candies and Confections, Gum   A-116 Cereals, Breakfast Type   A-120 Cheese and Cheese Substitutes   A-122 Dairy Products and Substitutes   A-124 Desserts   A-130 Dessert Toppings   A-130 Eggs, Substitutes, and Egg Dishes   A-132 Ethnic Foods   A-136 Fast Foods/Restaurants   A-150 Fats, Oils, Margarines, Shortenings, and Substitutes   A-150 Fish, Seafood, and Shellfish   A-152 Food Additives   A-152 Fruit, Vegetable, or Blended Juices   A-154 Grains, Flours, and Fractions   A-154 Grain Products, Prepared and Baked Goods

Code	Food Name	Unit/ Amt	Wt (g)	Energy (kcal)	Prot (g)	Carb (g)	Fiber (g)	Fat (g)	Sat (g)	Mono (g)	Poly (g)	Chol (mg)	Vit A (RE)
52061	Salad, chicken	0.5 cup	100	250	10	9	2	20	4.0	—	—	55	20
56253	Salad, crab	1 cup	208	282	27	11	1	14	2.0	3.5	7.1	142	37
56003	Salad, egg	1 cup	183	584	17	3	0	56	10.5	17.4	23.9	581	263
3312	Salad, fruit, w/citrus, fresh	1 cup	175	99	1	25	3	1	0.1	0.0	0.1	0	14
3311	Salad, fruit, w/o citrus, fresh	1 cup	175	101	1	26	4	1	0.1	0.1	0.2	0	34
69160	Salad, gelatin, fruity, prep f/recipe	1 ea	192	376	5	41	2	22	9.5	—	—	35	94
52029	Salad, macaroni, elbow, classic	0.5 cup	106	197	3	25	2	9	1.5	—	—	8	—
69196	Salad, Mediterranean Blend	2 cup	100	90	1	5	1	8	1.0	—	—	0	225
5637	Salad, mixed greens, raw	1 cup	55	9	1	2	1	0	0.0	0.0	0.1	0	150
4839	Salad, pasta, Greek, w/feta cheese	0.66 cup	140	200	6	27	3	8	2.0	—	—	5	—
56005	Salad, potato, prep f/recipe	0.5 cup	125	179	3	14	2	10	1.8	3.1	4.7	85	44
56257	Salad, seafood	0.5 cup	104	164	13	2	0	11	1.6	8.0	1.2	66	25
56256	Salad, shrimp	1 cup	182	282	27	6	1	17	2.6	4.5	8.4	206	42
5537	Salad, spinach, w/o dressing	1 cup	74	108	5	11	2	5	1.4	2.2	0.7	77	176
56643	Salad, taco	1.5 cup	198	279	13	24	—	15	6.8	5.2	1.7	44	93
52060	Salad, tuna	0.5 cup	100	260	12	9	2	19	3.0	—	—	30	20
SANDWICHES													
56647	Cheeseburger, reg, w/condiments	1 ea	113	295	16	27	—	14	6.3	5.3	1.1	37	97
66004	Hot Dog, plain, w/bun	1 ea	98	242	10	18	—	15	5.1	6.9	1.7	44	0
56667	Hot Dog, w/chili & bun	1 ea	114	296	14	31	—	13	4.9	6.6	1.2	51	7
56009	Sandwich, BLT, w/white	1 ea	124	318	10	29	2	18	4.1	—	—	20	49
56010	Sandwich, BLT, w/whole wheat	1 ea	137	339	12	29	5	20	4.9	—	—	23	56
56281	Sandwich, bologna	1 ea	83	256	7	26	1	13	4.1	6.3	2.1	16	37
56000	Sandwich, chicken, fillet, plain	1 ea	182	515	24	39	—	29	8.5	10.4	8.4	60	31
70755	Sandwich, egg cheese, medium	1 ea	119	350	12	30	1	20	8.0	—	—	110	0
56657	Sandwich, egg cheese, large	1 ea	146	340	16	26	—	19	6.6	8.3	2.6	291	201
66010	Sandwich, fish, w/tartar sauce	1 ea	158	431	17	41	0	23	5.2	7.7	8.2	55	33
56013	Sandwich, grilled cheese, w/white	1 ea	119	399	17	30	1	23	11.9	—	—	53	167
56014	Sandwich, grilled cheese, w/whole wheat	1 ea	132	431	20	30	4	27	13.8	—	—	60	192
56272	Sandwich, gyro	1 ea	105	170	12	21	1	4	1.5	1.4	0.4	34	11
56664	Sandwich, ham cheese	1 ea	146	352	21	33	—	15	6.4	6.7	1.4	58	96
56274	Sandwich, ham cheese, grilled	1 ea	141	381	21	30	1	20	7.9	7.9	2.4	54	106
56029	Sandwich, ham, w/white	1 ea	157	365	24	30	2	16	3.3	—	—	54	6
56030	Sandwich, ham, w/whole wheat	1 ea	169	379	27	29	4	18	3.9	—	—	59	7
56267	Sandwich, pastrami	1 ea	134	331	14	27	2	18	6.2	8.7	1.0	51	3
56040	Sandwich, peanut butter & jam, w/white	1 ea	101	348	11	47	3	14	2.7	—	—	1	0
56041	Sandwich, peanut butter & jam, w/whole wheat	1 ea	114	398	13	51	5	17	3.6	—	—	0	1
56277	Sandwich, pork	1 ea	136	324	26	32	1	9	2.9	4.1	1.0	62	1
56266	Sandwich, reuben	1 ea	181	464	21	30	3	29	9.9	9.7	6.7	82	94
66003	Sandwich, roast beef, plain	1 ea	139	346	22	33	—	14	3.6	6.8	1.7	51	22
56669	Sandwich, roast beef, w/cheese	1 ea	176	473	32	45	—	18	9.0	3.7	3.5	77	58
56286	Sandwich, salami	1 ea	82	234	8	25	1	11	3.4	5.2	1.9	19	35
56261	Sandwich, sloppy joe, w/bun	1 ea	186	358	18	36	2	15	5.0	6.6	1.4	46	73
56670	Sandwich, steak	1 ea	204	459	30	52	—	14	3.8	5.3	3.3	73	39
56048	Sandwich, tuna salad, w/white	1 ea	122	326	13	35	1	14	1.9	—	—	13	15
56052	Sandwich, turkey, w/white	1 ea	156	346	24	29	1	14	1.9	—	—	43	8
56053	Sandwich, turkey, w/whole wheat	1 ea	169	360	27	29	4	16	2.3	—	—	47	8

PAGE KEY: A-158 Granola Bars, Cereal Bars, Diet Bars, Scones, and Tarts   A-158 Meals and Dishes   A-162 Meats   A-168 Nuts, Seeds, and Products   A-170 Poultry   A-172 Salad Dressings, Dips, and Mayonnaise   A-172 Salads   A-174 Sandwiches   A-176 Sauces and Gravies   A-176 Snack Foods—Chips, Pretzels, Popcorn   A-178 Soups, Stews, and Chilis   A-180 Spices, Flavors, and Seasonings   A-182 Sports Bars and Drinks   A-182 Supplemental Foods and Formulas   A-184 Sweeteners and Sweet Substitutes   A-184 Vegetables and Legumes   A-198 Weight Loss Bars and Drinks   A-200 Miscellaneous

Thia (mg)	Ribo (mg)	Niac (mg NE)	Vit B6 (mg)	Vit B12 (µg)	Fol (µg)	Vit C (mg)	Vit D (IU)	Vit E (mg AT)	Cal (mg)	Iron (mg)	Magn (mg)	Phos (mg)	Pota (mg)	Sodi (mg)	Zinc (mg)	Wat (%)	Alco (g)	Caff (g)
—	—	—	—	—	—	1.2	—	—	40	0.36	—	—	—	600	—	—	0.00	0.00—
0.15	0.09	4.50	0.28	9.76	79.4	6.9	—	2.8	157	1.45	48.6	292	536	700	5.7	74	0.00	0.00
0.09	0.66	0.09	0.46	1.57	61.1	0.0	—	7.7	74	1.80	13.5	238	181	464	1.4	57	0.00	0.00
0.07	0.05	0.41	0.23	0.00	14.1	29.2	0.0	0.6	16	0.31	17.4	18	309	1	0.1	84	0.00	0.00
0.07	0.07	0.88	0.20	0.00	13.7	14.5	0.0	0.7	13	0.41	19.7	21	328	1	0.2	84	0.00	0.00
0.09	0.07	0.18	0.03	0.14	7.1	8.0	2.3	0.8	36	0.99	17.8	70	91	149	0.8	64	0.00	0.00
—	—	—	—	—	—	—	—	—	—	—	—	—	—	560	—	—	0.00	0.00
—	—	—	—	—	—	18.0	—	—	40	0.72	—	—	—	180	—	—	0.00	0.00
0.03	0.05	0.23	0.03	0.00	63.6	8.9	0.0	0.4	30	0.72	13.2	18	174	14	0.2	94	0.00	0.00
—	—	—	—	—	—	—	—	—	—	—	—	—	—	780	—	—	0.00	0.00
0.10	0.07	1.11	0.18	0.00	8.8	12.5	—	2.3	24	0.81	18.8	65	318	661	0.4	76	0.00	0.00
0.03	0.05	1.17	0.09	0.92	15.7	6.2	—	2.0	46	0.99	27.1	141	251	176	1.7	73	0.00	0.00
0.05	0.05	3.25	0.27	1.30	15.5	5.7	—	3.4	87	3.39	51.6	280	367	392	1.5	72	0.00	0.00
0.12	0.28	1.66	0.10	0.20	59.9	6.7	0.0	0.9	46	1.46	27.1	83	242	227	0.6	70	0.00	0.00
0.10	0.36	2.46	0.21	0.62	83.2	3.6	—	—	192	2.27	51.5	143	416	762	2.7	72	0.00	0.00
—	—	—	—	—	—	0.0	—	—	20	0.36	—	—	—	580	—	—	0.00	0.00
0.25	0.23	3.72	0.10	0.93	54.2	1.9	—	0.5	111	2.43	20.3	176	223	616	2.1	48	0.00	0.00
0.23	0.27	3.65	0.05	0.50	48.0	0.1	—	0.3	24	2.30	12.7	97	143	670	2.0	54	0.00	0.00
0.21	0.40	3.74	0.05	0.30	73.0	2.7	—	—	19	3.27	10.3	192	166	480	0.8	48	0.00	0.00
0.40	0.25	3.69	0.15	0.34	66.3	6.0	6.8	2.3	68	2.20	22.0	123	239	631	1.0	52	0.00	0.00
0.37	0.20	3.97	0.25	0.37	45.0	6.8	7.5	2.9	51	2.53	60.7	216	346	690	1.9	52	0.00	0.00
0.28	0.20	2.73	0.07	0.37	18.7	0.0	—	0.8	60	1.96	15.4	74	112	598	0.9	41	0.00	0.00
0.33	0.23	6.80	0.20	0.37	100.1	8.9	—	—	60	4.67	34.6	233	353	957	1.9	47	0.00	0.00
—	—	—	—	—	—	1.2	—	—	150	1.79	—	—	—	890	—	45	0.00	0.00
0.25	0.56	2.06	0.12	1.13	97.8	1.5	—	—	225	2.98	21.9	302	188	804	1.6	56	0.00	0.00
0.33	0.21	3.40	0.10	1.07	85.3	2.8	—	0.9	84	2.60	33.2	212	340	615	1.0	47	0.00	0.00
0.28	0.40	2.36	0.07	0.40	60.4	0.0	9.7	1.0	407	2.00	26.5	470	162	1155	2.0	37	0.00	0.00
0.23	0.36	2.46	0.15	0.46	36.6	0.0	10.8	1.4	439	2.31	68.2	619	264	1291	3.1	38	0.00	0.00
0.23	0.20	3.14	0.12	0.89	17.8	3.8	—	0.3	46	1.85	20.9	116	209	272	2.3	64	0.00	0.00
0.31	0.47	2.69	0.20	0.54	75.9	2.8	—	0.3	130	3.24	16.1	152	291	771	1.4	51	0.00	0.00
0.70	0.43	5.01	0.27	0.81	16.4	0.0	—	1.1	233	2.41	32.4	343	337	1465	2.5	47	0.00	0.00
0.89	0.43	6.82	0.38	0.61	59.8	0.1	25.1	2.5	76	3.09	32.1	270	384	1237	2.6	52	0.00	0.00
0.89	0.38	7.30	0.50	0.66	34.6	0.2	27.5	3.1	58	3.47	72.4	378	502	1339	3.7	53	0.00	0.00
0.28	0.27	4.76	0.12	0.97	21.2	2.0	—	0.3	68	2.64	23.1	135	243	1335	2.7	53	0.00	0.00
0.28	0.23	5.44	0.15	0.01	79.0	1.7	4.9	2.6	76	2.28	51.8	143	240	429	1.1	27	0.00	0.00
0.28	0.20	6.42	0.20	0.00	76.3	2.1	0.0	3.2	80	2.66	75.2	201	336	465	1.5	27	0.00	0.00
0.91	0.46	6.25	0.34	0.55	26.4	0.2	—	0.4	85	2.75	34.1	229	343	392	2.5	49	0.00	0.00
0.23	0.34	3.45	0.21	1.34	37.2	4.1	—	0.8	299	2.92	38.7	291	261	1348	4.0	53	0.00	0.00
0.37	0.31	5.86	0.25	1.22	57.0	2.1	—	0.2	54	4.23	30.6	239	316	792	3.4	49	0.00	0.00
0.38	0.46	5.90	0.33	2.05	63.4	0.0	—	—	183	5.05	40.5	401	345	1633	5.4	44	0.00	0.00
0.30	0.28	2.96	0.09	1.07	17.2	0.0	—	0.7	58	2.25	16.1	80	117	612	0.9	44	0.00	0.00
0.28	0.27	5.73	0.23	1.51	21.8	5.8	—	1.3	92	3.63	35.5	149	368	1008	3.2	61	0.00	0.00
0.40	0.37	7.30	0.37	1.57	89.8	5.5	—	—	92	5.15	49.0	298	524	798	4.5	51	0.00	0.00
0.30	0.23	5.88	0.12	0.66	62.5	1.1	72.0	2.8	76	2.40	24.5	152	168	588	0.7	46	0.00	0.00
0.31	0.28	9.27	0.41	1.74	60.3	0.0	15.0	3.3	72	2.18	30.9	250	306	1586	1.3	54	0.00	0.00
0.25	0.21	10.06	0.52	1.91	35.4	0.0	16.4	3.9	53	2.46	71.2	356	417	1734	2.2	54	0.00	0.00

PAGE KEY: A-108 Beverage and Beverage Mixes   A-110 Other Beverages   A-110 Beverages, Alcoholic   A-112 Candies and Confections, Gum   A-116 Cereals, Breakfast Type   A-120 Cheese and Cheese Substitutes   A-122 Dairy Products and Substitutes   A-124 Desserts   A-130 Dessert Toppings   A-130 Eggs, Substitutes, and Egg Dishes   A-132 Ethnic Foods   A-136 Fast Foods/Restaurants   A-150 Fats, Oils, Margarines, Shortenings, and Substitutes   A-150 Fish, Seafood, and Shellfish   A-152 Food Additives   A-152 Fruit, Vegetable, or Blended Juices   A-154 Grains, Flours, and Fractions   A-154 Grain Products, Prepared and Baked Goods

Code	Food Name	Unit/ Amt	Wt (g)	Energy (kcal)	Prot (g)	Carb (g)	Fiber (g)	Fat (g)	Sat (g)	Mono (g)	Poly (g)	Chol (mg)	Vit A (RE)
SAUCES AND GRAVIES													
Gravies													
53564	Gravy, beef, fat free	0.25 cup	60	20	0	5	0	0	0.0	0.0	0.0	5	0
53006	Gravy, beef, prep f/recipe	0.5 cup	135	107	3	7	1	8	1.9	3.4	2.0	3	150
53022	Gravy, chicken, can	0.25 cup	60	47	1	3	0	3	0.8	1.5	0.9	1	1
53565	Gravy, chicken, fat free	0.25 cup	60	15	1	3	0	0	0.0	0.0	0.0	5	20
53401	Gravy, country, dry mix	1 Tbs	6	22	1	4	0	1	0.1	0.4	0.0	0	0
53038	Gravy, mushroom, dry mix, svg	1 ea	21	70	2	14	1	1	0.5	0.3	0.0	1	0
53403	Gravy, onion, dry mix	1 Tbs	5	18	1	3	1	0	0.1	0.2	0.0	0	0
53044	Gravy, turkey, dry mix, svg	1 ea	7	26	1	5	—	1	0.1	0.2	0.2	1	1
Sauces													
53591	Marinade, cooking sauce, mesquite	1 Tbs	17	10	0	3	0	0	0.0	0.0	0.0	0	0
53587	Marinade, cooking sauce, teriyaki	1 Tbs	18	25	1	5	0	0	0.0	0.0	0.0	0	0
9559	Sauce, alfredo	0.25 cup	61	110	1	2	0	10	3.5	—	—	30	40
53000	Sauce, barbecue	1 cup	250	188	4	32	3	4	0.7	1.9	1.7	0	5
53320	Sauce, barbecue, sweet & sour	2 Tbs	34	45	0	10	0	0	0.0	0.0	0.0	0	0
53420	Sauce, barbecue, teriyaki	2 Tbs	36	60	0	12	0	0	0.0	0.0	0.0	0	0
9558	Sauce, cheese, cheddar, rts	0.25 cup	61	90	2	2	0	8	2.5	—	—	25	20
53523	Sauce, cheese, rts	0.25 cup	63	110	4	4	0	8	3.8	2.4	1.6	18	52
53474	Sauce, fish, rts	2 Tbs	36	13	2	1	0	0	0.0	0.0	0.0	0	1
53356	Sauce, Italian, rts	1 ea	1956	1917	33	362	27	37	5.1	23.3	5.3	0	1545
9425	Sauce, pasta, alfredo, classic	0.25 cup	61	110	1	3	0	10	3.5	—	—	25	100
53627	Sauce, pasta, garlic & herb, cnd	0.5 cup	126	50	2	10	2	0	0.0	0.0	0.0	0	40
53623	Sauce, pasta, garlic & onion, cnd	0.5 cup	125	40	2	9	2	0	0.0	0.0	0.0	0	30
53629	Sauce, pasta, traditional, cnd	0.5 cup	126	50	2	11	2	0	0.0	0.0	0.0	0	30
53540	Sauce, peanut	1 cup	240	749	31	29	8	63	12.8	30.0	17.1	0	1
7479	Sauce, picante, mild	2 Tbs	32	10	0	2	1	0	0.0	0.0	0.0	0	20
53284	Sauce, picante, med	2 Tbs	30	10	0	2	0	0	0.0	0.0	0.0	0	20
53221	Sauce, picante, hot	2 Tbs	30	10	0	2	0	0	0.0	0.0	0.0	0	0
53363	Sauce, pizza, deluxe, rts	0.25 cup	63	34	1	5	1	1	0.3	0.3	0.1	2	42
53425	Sauce, sloppy joe, cnd	0.25 cup	73	50	2	11	2	0	0.0	0.0	0.0	0	150
1709	Sauce, spaghetti, meatless, USDA, cnd	3.6 oz	100	48	1	9	—	1	0.2	0.2	0.5	0	34
51016	Sauce, spaghetti, traditional, cnd	0.5 cup	125	60	2	15	3	1	0.0	—	—	0	75
53011	Sauce, spaghetti, w/meat, cnd	1 cup	250	178	7	19	4	8	1.8	3.3	1.8	15	176
53524	Sauce, spaghetti/marinara, rts	0.5 cup	125	92	2	14	0	3	0.4	1.0	1.2	0	68
92310	Sauce, steak	1 Tbs	16	5	0	1	0	0	0.0	0.0	0.0	0	0
53352	Sauce, stir fry, all purpose, rts	1 Tbs	15	16	0	2	0	1	0.1	0.2	0.3	0	1
8983	Sauce, tartar	2 Tbs	28	139	0	1	0	15	2.7	0.7	2.3	11	6
90268	Sauce, white, dehyd, svg	1 ea	20	92	2	10	1	5	1.3	2.4	1.4	0	0
5181	Tomato Paste, unsalted, 6 oz can	1 ea	170	139	7	32	8	1	0.2	0.1	0.3	0	259
5180	Tomato Sauce, cnd	0.5 cup	122	39	2	9	2	0	0.0	0.0	0.1	0	42
SNACK FOODS—CHIPS, PRETZELS, POPCORN													
44061	Chips, bagel	5 pce	70	298	6	52	4	7	1.3	2.1	3.4	0	0
44256	Chips, corn, original	11 pce	28	140	2	19	2	6	0.5	—	—	0	0
44278	Chips, corn, original	32 pce	28	158	2	15	1	10	1.0	2.5	6.4	0	0
61236	Chips, potato, bkd	1 oz	28	133	1	20	1	5	0.7	2.8	1.2	0	0
43703	Chips, potato, classic	20 pce	28	150	2	15	1	10	3.0	—	—	0	0

PAGE KEY: A-158 Granola Bars, Cereal Bars, Diet Bars, Scones, and Tarts   A-158 Meals and Dishes   A-162 Meats   A-168 Nuts, Seeds, and Products   A-170 Poultry   A-172 Salad Dressings, Dips, and Mayonnaise   A-172 Salads   A-174 Sandwiches   A-176 Sauces and Gravies   A-176 Snack Foods—Chips, Pretzels, Popcorn   A-178 Soups, Stews, and Chilis   A-180 Spices, Flavors, and Seasonings   A-182 Sports Bars and Drinks   A-182 Supplemental Foods and Formulas   A-184 Sweeteners and Sweet Substitutes   A-184 Vegetables and Legumes   A-198 Weight Loss Bars and Drinks   A-200 Miscellaneous

Thia (mg)	Ribo (mg)	Niac (mg NE)	Vit B6 (mg)	Vit B12 (μg)	Fol (μg)	Vit C (mg)	Vit D (IU)	Vit E (mg AT)	Cal (mg)	Iron (mg)	Magn (mg)	Phos (mg)	Pota (mg)	Sodi (mg)	Zinc (mg)	Wat (%)	Alco (g)	Caff (g)
—	—	—	—	—	—	0.0	—	—	0	0.00	—	—	—	308	—	90	0.00	0.00
0.01	0.05	0.60	0.00	0.14	2.7	0.0	1.0	0.2	27	0.62	2.7	39	147	779	1.1	85	0.00	0.00
0.00	0.02	0.25	0.00	0.05	1.2	0.0	—	0.1	12	0.28	1.2	17	65	343	0.5	85	0.00	0.00
—	—	—	—	—	—	0.0	—	—	0	0.00	—	—	—	318	—	92	0.00	0.00
0.00	0.00	0.00	0.00	0.00	—	0.0	—	—	1	0.02	—	7	7	249	0.0	7	0.00	0.00
0.03	0.09	0.79	0.01	0.15	6.6	1.5	—	0.0	49	0.20	7.2	43	56	1402	0.3	3	0.00	0.00
0.02	0.01	0.00	0.01	0.00	—	0.0	—	—	1	0.10	—	10	25	229	—	8	0.00	0.00
0.00	0.02	0.18	0.00	0.03	5.7	0.0	—	0.0	10	0.23	3.1	18	30	307	0.1	5	0.00	0.00
—	—	—	—	—	—	1.8	—	—	0	0.00	—	—	25	400	—	—	0.00	0.00
—	—	—	—	—	—	3.0	—	—	0	0.00	—	—	40	480	—	64	0.00	0.00
—	—	—	—	—	—	0.0	—	—	40	0.00	—	—	—	390	—	76	0.00	0.00
0.07	0.05	2.25	0.18	0.00	10.0	17.5	—	0.0	48	2.25	45.0	50	435	2038	0.5	81	0.00	0.00
—	—	—	—	—	—	0.0	—	—	0	0.00	—	—	—	420	—	—	0.00	0.00
—	—	—	—	—	—	0.0	—	—	0	0.36	—	—	—	440	—	63	0.00	0.00
—	—	—	—	—	—	0.0	—	—	60	0.00	—	—	—	480	—	78	0.00	0.00
0.00	0.07	0.01	0.00	0.09	2.5	0.3	—	0.2	116	0.12	5.7	99	19	522	0.6	70	0.00	0.00
0.00	0.01	0.82	0.14	0.17	18.4	0.2	—	0.0	15	0.28	63.0	3	104	2779	0.1	71	0.00	0.00
2.41	1.42	35.63	5.40	0.00	508.6	131.1	—	37.8	1076	12.13	625.9	1350	11892	9584	8.2	76	0.00	0.00
—	—	—	—	—	—	0.0	—	—	40	—	—	—	—	340	—	75	0.00	0.00
—	—	—	—	—	—	6.0	—	—	40	1.08	—	—	—	390	—	88	0.00	0.00
—	—	—	—	—	—	6.0	—	—	40	1.08	—	—	—	390	—	89	0.00	0.00
—	—	—	—	—	—	6.0	—	—	40	1.08	—	—	—	390	—	87	0.00	0.00
0.11	0.14	16.63	0.58	0.00	99.2	27.1	—	12.4	52	2.29	200.9	460	901	580	3.7	47	0.00	0.00
—	—	—	—	—	—	0.0	—	—	0	0.00	—	—	—	230	—	92	0.00	0.00
—	—	—	—	—	—	0.0	—	—	0	0.00	—	—	—	230	—	91	0.00	0.00
—	—	—	—	—	—	19.8	—	—	0	0.00		—	—	260	—	91	0.00	0.00
0.03	0.02	0.89	0.09	0.00	6.3	7.1	—	1.6	34	0.56	13.2	32	223	117	0.2	87	0.00	0.00
—	—	—	—	—	—	0.0	—	—	0	0.72	—	—	—	420	—	—	0.00	0.00
0.02	0.11	0.73	0.05	0.00	—	3.9	—	—	20	0.89	13.0	25	292	590	0.2	87	0.00	0.00
—	—	—	—	—	—	9.0	—	—	40	1.44	—	—	—	590	—	84	0.00	0.00
0.12	0.11	3.47	0.31	0.49	25.0	18.8	1.2	3.0	54	2.09	43.2	104	742	982	1.3	85	0.00	0.00
0.02	0.07	4.90	0.21	0.00	13.8	3.9	—	2.5	34	1.05	26.2	45	470	601	0.7	82	0.00	0.00
—	—	—	—	—	—	0.0	—	—	0	0.00	—	—	—	200	—	90	0.00	0.00
0.00	0.00	0.14	0.00	0.00	0.6	0.7	—	0.0	2	0.10	1.5	4	8	233	0.0	74	0.00	0.00
—	—	—	—	—	—	0.7	—	—	6	0.14	—	—	38	153	—	39	0.00	0.00
0.03	0.07	0.14	0.01	0.15	6.7	0.6	—	0.1	133	0.10	7.7	49	73	675	0.2	2	0.00	0.00
0.10	0.25	5.23	0.37	0.00	20.4	37.3	—	7.3	61	5.07	71.4	141	1725	167	1.1	74	0.00	0.00
0.02	0.07	1.19	0.11	0.00	11.0	8.6	—	2.5	16	1.25	19.6	32	405	642	0.2	89	0.00	0.00
0.12	0.11	1.62	0.15	0.00	46.0	0.0	—	1.7	9	1.38	39.2	145	167	419	0.9	3	0.00	0.00
0.05	0.15	0.50	—	—	—	0.0	—	—	0	0.36	—	70	75	115	0.0	2	0.00	0.00
0.00	0.03	0.33	—	—	—	0.0	—	—	44	0.37	—	54	54	104	—	3	0.00	0.00
0.10	0.01	1.15	0.14	0.00	0.0	0.0	—	0.6	35	0.23	12.2	78	204	260	0.1	1	0.00	0.00
—	—	—	—	—	—	6.0	—	—	0	0.00	—	—	—	180	—	1	0.00	0.00

PAGE KEY: A-108 Beverage and Beverage Mixes   A-110 Other Beverages   A-110 Beverages, Alcoholic   A-112 Candies and Confections, Gum   A-116 Cereals, Breakfast Type   A-120 Cheese and Cheese Substitutes   A-122 Dairy Products and Substitutes   A-124 Desserts   A-130 Dessert Toppings   A-130 Eggs, Substitutes, and Egg Dishes   A-132 Ethnic Foods   A-136 Fast Foods/Restaurants   A-150 Fats, Oils, Margarines, Shortenings, and Substitutes   A-150 Fish, Seafood, and Shellfish   A-152 Food Additives   A-152 Fruit, Vegetable, or Blended Juices   A-154 Grains, Flours, and Fractions   A-154 Grain Products, Prepared and Baked Goods

Code	Food Name	Unit/ Amt	Wt (g)	Energy (kcal)	Prot (g)	Carb (g)	Fiber (g)	Fat (g)	Sat (g)	Mono (g)	Poly (g)	Chol (mg)	Vit A (RE)
61253	Chips, potato, fat free	100 g	100	379	10	84	8	1	0.2	0.0	0.3	0	2
44230	Chips, potato, original	18 pce	28	148	2	15	1	10	3.0	1.9	5.0	0	0
44241	Chips, potato, rducd fat	16 pce	28	128	2	18	1	7	1.0	1.6	4.1	0	0
44238	Chips, potato, unsalted	19 pce	28	158	2	16	1	10	3.0	—	—	0	0
44301	Chips, tortilla, blue corn	18 pce	28	110	3	22	2	2	0.0	—	—	0	0
44224	Chips, tortilla, cooler ranch	15 pce	28	138	2	18	1	7	1.5	1.9	2.2	0	0
61156	Chips, tortilla, light, bkd	10 ea	16	74	1	12	1	2	0.5	1.0	0.8	0	1
44225	Chips, tortilla, nacho cheesier	15 pce	28	138	2	17	1	7	1.5	1.9	2.2	0	0
4039	Chips, tortilla, salsa verde	12 pce	28	150	2	19	1	7	1.5	3.0	2.5	0	0
44223	Chips, tortilla, tstd corn	13 pce	28	138	2	18	1	7	1.5	—	—	0	0
44298	Chips, tortilla, yellow corn	18 pce	28	110	3	22	2	2	0.0	—	—	0	0
44087	Corn Cake, butter flvr	1 ea	9	34	1	7	0	0	0.1	0.1	0.1	0	4
44308	Corn Cake, caramel flvrd	1 ea	13	50	1	12	0	0	0.0	0.1	0.1	0	4
44031	Corn Nuts, plain	1 oz	28	126	2	20	2	4	0.7	2.7	0.9	0	0
44212	Fruit Leather, bar	1 ea	23	81	0	18	1	1	0.9	0.1	0.0	0	3
23404	Fruit Leather, roll, lrg	1 ea	21	78	0	18	1	1	0.1	0.3	0.1	0	3
44022	Popcorn Cake	1 ea	10	38	1	8	0	0	0.0	0.1	0.1	0	1
44014	Popcorn, caramel coated, w/o peanuts	1 oz	28	122	1	22	1	4	1.0	0.8	1.3	1	1
44038	Popcorn, cheese flvrd	1 cup	11	58	1	6	1	4	0.7	1.1	1.7	1	5
43701	Popcorn, Cracker Jacks, original	0.5 cup	28	120	2	23	1	2	0.0	—	—	0	0
44065	Popcorn, microwv	1 ea	87	435	8	50	9	24	4.3	7.1	11.7	0	13
44013	Popcorn, oil popped	1 cup	11	55	1	6	1	3	0.5	0.9	1.5	0	2
44072	Popcorn, white, air popped	1 cup	8	31	1	6	1	0	0.0	0.1	0.2	0	0
44015	Pretzels, hard	5 pce	30	114	3	24	1	1	0.2	0.4	0.4	0	0
44215	Pretzels, hard, chocolate coated	1 ea	11	50	1	8	0	2	0.8	0.6	0.2	0	0
61182	Pretzels, soft, med	1 ea	115	389	9	80	2	4	0.8	1.2	1.1	3	0
60899	Rice Cake, brown	1 ea	20	74	1	16	0	0	0.1	0.2	0.2	—	0
44017	Rice Cake, caramel corn, mini	1 ea	3	13	0	3	0	0	0.1	0.0	0.0	0	1
44016	Rice Cake, plain	1 ea	9	35	1	7	0	0	0.1	0.1	0.1	0	0
44032	Snack Mix, Chex	1 cup	42	181	5	28	2	7	2.4	3.9	1.1	0	6
57096	Snack, cheese n' crackers, pkg	1 ea	27	100	2	10	0	6	2.0	—	—	10	20
44248	Snack, cheese puffs, Cheetos	29 pce	28	158	2	15	1	10	2.5	2.7	3.1	0	0
44058	Trail Mix, regular	0.25 cup	38	173	5	17	2	11	2.1	4.7	3.6	0	1
44060	Trail Mix, tropical	1 cup	140	570	9	92	9	24	11.9	3.5	7.2	0	6
44059	Trail Mix, w/chocolate chips, salted nuts & seeds	0.25 cup	36	175	5	16	2	12	2.2	4.9	4.1	1	1
SOUPS, STEWS AND CHILIS													
Canned/Frozen/Prepared Soups, Stews and Chilis													
50595	Bouillon/Broth, beef, clear, cnd	1 cup	198	15	2	0	0	0	0.0	—	—	0	0
50596	Broth, chicken, clear, rts, cnd	1 cup	198	15	1	1	0	0	0.0	—	—	5	0
50312	Chili, con carne	1 cup	253	256	25	22	—	8	3.4	3.4	0.5	134	167
7760	Chili, vegetarian, cnd	1 cup	230	176	16	26	13	1	0.2	0.2	0.5	1	47
56001	Chili, w/beans, cnd	1 cup	256	287	15	30	11	14	6.0	6.0	0.9	44	87
50901	Chili, w/beef, rts, cnd	1 cup	245	190	16	34	8	2	0.5	—	—	5	100
28167	Chili, w/o beans, cnd	100 g	100	118	8	6	—	7	2.3	2.5	0.5	21	—
50406	Chowder, clam, New England, rts, cnd	1 cup	244	117	5	20	1	2	0.5	0.7	0.4	5	49

PAGE KEY: A-158 Granola Bars, Cereal Bars, Diet Bars, Scones, and Tarts   A-158 Meals and Dishes   A-162 Meats   A-168 Nuts, Seeds, and Products   A-170 Poultry   A-172 Salad Dressings, Dips, and Mayonnaise   A-172 Salads   A-174 Sandwiches   A-176 Sauces and Gravies   A-176 Snack Foods—Chips, Pretzels, Popcorn   A-178 Soups, Stews, and Chilis   A-180 Spices, Flavors, and Seasonings   A-182 Sports Bars and Drinks   A-182 Supplemental Foods and Formulas   A-184 Sweeteners and Sweet Substitutes   A-184 Vegetables and Legumes   A-198 Weight Loss Bars and Drinks   A-200 Miscellaneous

Thia (mg)	Ribo (mg)	Niac (mg NE)	Vit B6 (mg)	Vit B12 (µg)	Fol (µg)	Vit C (mg)	Vit D (IU)	Vit E (mg AT)	Cal (mg)	Iron (mg)	Magn (mg)	Phos (mg)	Pota (mg)	Sodi (mg)	Zinc (mg)	Wat (%)	Alco (g)	Caff (g)
1.08	0.11	6.44	0.80	0.00	45.0	9.3	—	0.0	35	3.56	70.0	167	1628	643	0.7	2	0.00	0.00
0.05	0.03	1.09	—	0.00	—	5.9	—	—	6	0.44	—	44	489	178	0.4	2	0.00	0.00
0.03	0.05	1.09	—	0.00	—	5.9	—	—	0	0.36	—	45	356	158	0.3	2	0.00	0.00
—	—	—	0.00	—	—	5.9	—	—	0	0.00	—	—	—	15	—	—	0.00	0.00
—	—	—	—	—	—	0.0	—	—	60	0.36	—	—	—	140	—	4	0.00	—
0.02	0.02	0.49	—	—	—	0.0	—	—	40	0.41	—	64	69	168	0.0	2	0.00	0.00
0.03	0.03	0.07	0.02	0.00	2.6	0.0	—	0.6	25	0.25	15.5	51	44	160	0.2	1	0.00	0.00
0.02	0.02	0.40	—	—	—	0.0	—	—	43	0.41	—	59	64	188	0.0	6	0.00	0.00
0.02	0.00	0.43	—	—	—	0.0	—	—	20	0.00	—	18	38	210	0.2	—	0.00	0.00
—	—	—	—	—	—	0.0	—	—	40	0.00	—	—	—	119	—	2	0.00	0.00
—	—	—	—	—	—	0.0	—	—	60	0.36	—	—	—	160	—	3	0.00	—
0.01	0.00	0.34	0.02	0.00	3.0	0.0	0.0	0.0	1	0.07	8.9	20	17	45	0.1	6	0.00	0.00
0.02	0.00	0.31	0.03	0.00	3.0	0.0	—	0.0	1	0.07	8.9	20	15	28	0.1	3	0.00	0.00
0.00	0.03	0.47	0.05	0.00	0.0	0.0	—	0.6	3	0.46	32.0	78	79	156	0.5	1	0.00	0.00
0.00	0.00	0.01	0.07	0.00	0.9	16.1	—	0.1	7	0.18	5.1	13	32	18	0.0	14	0.00	0.00
0.01	0.00	0.01	0.05	0.00	0.8	25.2	—	0.1	7	0.20	4.2	7	62	67	0.0	10	0.00	0.00
0.00	0.01	0.60	0.01	0.00	1.8	0.0	—	0.0	1	0.18	15.9	28	33	29	0.4	5	0.00	0.00
0.01	0.01	0.62	0.00	0.00	1.4	0.0	—	0.3	12	0.49	9.9	24	31	58	0.2	3	0.00	0.00
0.00	0.02	0.15	0.02	0.05	1.2	0.1	—	0.0	12	0.25	10.0	40	29	98	0.2	2	0.00	0.00
—	—	—	—	—	—	0.0	—	—	0	0.00	—	—	—	70	—	—	0.00	0.00
0.11	0.11	1.35	0.18	0.00	14.8	0.3	—	0.1	9	2.42	94.0	218	196	769	2.3	3	0.00	0.00
0.00	0.00	0.17	0.01	0.00	1.9	0.0	—	0.6	1	0.31	11.9	28	25	97	0.3	3	0.00	0.00
0.01	0.01	0.15	0.01	0.00	1.8	0.0	—	0.0	1	0.20	10.5	24	24	0	0.3	4	0.00	0.00
0.14	0.18	1.58	0.02	0.00	51.3	0.0	—	0.1	11	1.29	10.5	34	44	514	0.3	3	0.00	0.00
0.00	0.01	0.09	0.01	0.00	1.0	0.1	—	0.0	8	0.21	4.5	16	25	63	0.1	2	0.00	—
0.46	0.33	4.90	0.01	0.00	27.6	0.0	—	0.6	26	4.51	24.1	91	101	1615	1.1	15	0.00	0.00
—	—	—	—	—	—	0.0	—	—	5	0.15	—	—	67	57	—	5	0.00	0.00
0.00	0.00	0.10	0.00	0.00	0.6	0.0	0.0	0.0	1	0.02	2.6	6	6	14	0.0	2	0.00	0.00
0.03	0.00	0.58	0.05	0.00	1.8	0.0	0.0	0.0	1	0.12	14.2	33	25	14	2.0	3	0.00	0.00
0.66	0.20	7.15	0.66	5.26	21.2	20.2	—	0.1	15	10.50	26.8	79	114	432	0.9	4	0.00	0.00
—	—	—	—	—	—	0.0	—	—	60	0.36	—	—	—	331	—	—	0.00	0.00
0.10	0.05	0.72	—	—	—	0.0	—	—	22	0.58	—	15	20	365	0.0	2	0.00	0.00
0.17	0.07	1.76	0.10	0.00	26.6	0.5	—	1.3	29	1.13	59.2	129	257	86	1.2	9	0.00	0.00
0.62	0.15	2.06	0.46	0.00	58.8	10.6	—	3.1	80	3.70	134.4	260	993	14	1.6	9	0.00	0.00
0.15	0.07	1.60	0.09	0.00	23.6	0.5	—	3.9	40	1.23	58.4	140	235	44	1.1	7	0.00	2.18
—	—	—	—	—	—	0.0	—	—	0	0.00	—	—	—	890	—	98	0.00	0.00
—	—	—	—	—	—	0.0	—	—	0	0.00	—	—	—	960	—	—	0.00	0.00
0.12	1.13	2.48	0.33	1.13	45.5	1.5	—	1.6	68	5.19	45.5	197	691	1007	3.6	77	0.00	0.00
0.00	0.15	0.00	—	0.00	—	0.0	—	—	40	3.68	—	237	645	1144	0.6	79	0.00	0.00
0.11	0.27	0.92	0.34	0.00	58.9	4.4	—	1.5	120	8.77	115.2	394	934	1336	5.1	76	0.00	0.00
—	—	—	—	—	—	2.4	—	—	100	4.50	—	—	—	480	—	—	0.00	0.00
0.02	0.10	1.25	0.12	1.01	—	1.8	—	—	30	2.00	20.0	77	185	389	1.1	78	0.00	0.00
0.05	0.09	0.86	0.09	6.17	29.3	5.1	—	0.6	17	0.89	12.2	59	283	529	0.4	89	0.00	0.00

PAGE KEY: A-108 Beverage and Beverage Mixes A-110 Other Beverages A-110 Beverages, Alcoholic A-112 Candies and Confections, Gum A-116 Cereals, Breakfast Type
A-120 Cheese and Cheese Substitutes A-122 Dairy Products and Substitutes A-124 Desserts A-130 Dessert Toppings A-130 Eggs, Substitutes, and Egg Dishes A-132 Ethnic Foods
A-136 Fast Foods/Restaurants A-150 Fats, Oils, Margarines, Shortenings, and Substitutes A-150 Fish, Seafood, and Shellfish A-152 Food Additives
A-152 Fruit, Vegetable, or Blended Juices A-154 Grains, Flours, and Fractions A-154 Grain Products, Prepared and Baked Goods

Code	Food Name	Unit/Amt	Wt (g)	Energy (kcal)	Prot (g)	Carb (g)	Fiber (g)	Fat (g)	Sat (g)	Mono (g)	Poly (g)	Chol (mg)	Vit A (RE)
50907	Chowder, clam, New England, rts, cnd	1 cup	251	120	5	24	4	2	1.0	—	—	10	0
50647	Soup, bean & pork, cond, cnd, cmrcl	1 cup	269	347	16	46	16	12	3.1	4.4	3.7	5	180
50003	Soup, beef noodle, prep f/cnd w/water, cmrcl	1 cup	244	83	5	9	1	3	1.1	1.2	0.5	5	12
50399	Soup, beef vegetable, rts, cnd	1 cup	241	154	10	25	6	2	0.6	0.6	0.2	14	415
50686	Soup, chicken mushroom, cond, cnd, cmrcl	1 cup	251	274	9	19	1	18	4.8	8.1	4.6	20	25
50080	Soup, chicken mushroom, prep f/cnd w/water, cmrcl	1 cup	244	132	4	9	0	9	2.4	4.0	2.3	10	112
50982	Soup, chicken noodle, chunky, rts, cnd, svg	1 ea	243	114	8	14	—	3	0.8	1.2	0.6	24	262
50400	Soup, chicken noodle, rts, cnd	1 cup	237	76	6	9	1	2	0.4	0.6	0.4	19	182
50020	Soup, chicken rice, prep f/cnd w/water, cmrcl	1 cup	241	60	4	7	1	2	0.5	0.9	0.4	7	43
50091	Soup, chicken vegetable, prep f/cnd w/water, cmrcl	1 cup	241	75	4	9	1	3	0.8	1.3	0.6	10	193
50402	Soup, cream of broccoli, rts, cnd	1 cup	244	88	2	13	2	3	0.7	0.9	0.6	5	59
50654	Soup, cream of chicken, cond, cnd, cmrcl	1 cup	251	223	6	18	0	14	4.0	5.1	2.6	20	113
50666	Soup, cream of mushroom, cond, cnd, cmrcl	1 cup	251	213	4	17	0	15	3.4	2.8	3.6	0	20
50049	Soup, cream of mushroom, prep f/cnd w/water, cmrcl	1 cup	244	129	2	9	0	9	2.4	1.7	4.2	2	17
50197	Soup, cream of potato, prep f/cnd w/water, cmrcl	1 cup	244	73	2	11	0	2	1.2	0.6	0.4	5	76
50999	Soup, gumbo, zesty, rts, cnd	1 cup	244	100	6	15	3	2	1.0	—	—	10	40
50404	Soup, lentil, rts, cnd	1 cup	242	126	8	20	6	2	0.3	0.8	0.2	0	191
50405	Soup, minestrone, rts, cnd	1 cup	241	123	5	20	1	3	0.4	0.9	1.0	0	272
50486	Soup, onion, French, cond, cnd	0.5 cup	119	45	2	6	1	2	0.5	—	—	5	0
50403	Soup, pasta & garlic, rts, cnd	1 cup	243	100	4	20	3	1	0.3	0.4	0.5	5	311
50050	Soup, pea, green, prep f/cnd w/water, cmrcl	1 cup	250	165	9	26	3	3	1.4	1.0	0.4	0	20
50407	Soup, split pea, rts, cnd	1 cup	253	180	10	30	5	2	0.8	0.9	0.4	5	142
50504	Soup, tomato, cond, cnd	0.5 cup	122	90	2	20	1	0	0.0	0.0	0.0	0	100
50409	Soup, vegetable, rts, cnd	1 cup	238	81	4	13	1	1	0.3	0.4	0.3	5	640
57659	Stew, beef, cnd, svg	1 ea	232	218	11	16	3	12	5.2	5.5	0.5	37	385
7559	Stew, vegetarian	1 cup	247	304	42	17	3	7	1.2	1.8	3.8	0	232

Dry and Prepared Soups and Chilis

Code	Food Name	Unit/Amt	Wt (g)	Energy (kcal)	Prot (g)	Carb (g)	Fiber (g)	Fat (g)	Sat (g)	Mono (g)	Poly (g)	Chol (mg)	Vit A (RE)
90243	Broth, beef, dry cube, svg	1.33 ea	5	8	1	1	0	0	0.1	0.1	0.0	0	0
90247	Broth, chicken, cube, dry svg	1 ea	6	13	1	2	0	0	0.1	0.1	0.1	1	0
50037	Soup, chicken noodle, prep f/dehyd w/water	1 cup	252	58	2	9	0	1	0.3	0.5	0.4	10	5
50036	Soup, cream of chicken, prep f/dehyd w/water	1 cup	261	107	2	13	0	5	3.4	1.2	0.4	3	42
90346	Soup, minestrone, prep f/pkt w/water	1 ea	1142	354	20	54	—	8	3.7	3.3	0.5	11	137
50039	Soup, mushroom, prep f/dehyd w/water, pkt	1 ea	194	74	2	9	1	4	0.6	1.7	1.2	0	14
50040	Soup, onion, prep f/dehyd w/water, pkt	1 ea	184	20	1	4	1	0	0.1	0.2	0.1	0	0
92163	Soup, ramen noodle, any flvr, dry	3.6 oz	100	453	9	66	2	17	7.6	6.4	2.6	0	2
50042	Soup, tomato, prep f/dry w/water, pkt	1 ea	199	78	2	15	0	2	0.8	0.7	0.2	0	66
50044	Soup, vegetable beef, prep f/dry w/water	1 cup	253	53	3	8	1	1	0.6	0.5	0.1	0	25

Homemade/Generic Soups and Chilis

Code	Food Name	Unit/Amt	Wt (g)	Energy (kcal)	Prot (g)	Carb (g)	Fiber (g)	Fat (g)	Sat (g)	Mono (g)	Poly (g)	Chol (mg)	Vit A (RE)
50709	Broth, vegetable	1 cup	235	16	2	2	0	0	—	—	—	0	1
92757	Chili, con carne, w/beans & chicken	1 cup	254	217	17	27	7	5	1.2	1.9	1.5	33	124
50211	Chowder, fish	1 cup	244	194	24	12	1	5	2.4	1.9	0.6	56	63
50077	Soup, chicken gumbo, prep f/cnd w/water, cmrcl	1 cup	244	56	3	8	2	1	0.3	0.7	0.3	5	15

SPICES, FLAVORS, AND SEASONINGS

Code	Food Name	Unit/Amt	Wt (g)	Energy (kcal)	Prot (g)	Carb (g)	Fiber (g)	Fat (g)	Sat (g)	Mono (g)	Poly (g)	Chol (mg)	Vit A (RE)
90622	Salt Substitute, Mrs. Dash, original blend	0.25 tsp	1	0	0	0	0	0	0.0	0.0	0.0	0	0
26632	Salt Substitute, Nu-Salt, no sod, pkt	1 g	1	0	0	0	0	0	0.0	0.0	0.0	0	0
26014	Salt, table	0.25 tsp	2	0	0	0	0	0	0.0	0.0	0.0	0	0

PAGE KEY: A-158 Granola Bars, Cereal Bars, Diet Bars, Scones, and Tarts   A-158 Meals and Dishes   A-162 Meats   A-168 Nuts, Seeds, and Products   A-170 Poultry   A-172 Salad Dressings, Dips, and Mayonnaise   A-172 Salads   A-174 Sandwiches   A-176 Sauces and Gravies   A-176 Snack Foods—Chips, Pretzels, Popcorn   A-178 Soups, Stews, and Chilis   A-180 Spices, Flavors, and Seasonings   A-182 Sports Bars and Drinks   A-182 Supplemental Foods and Formulas   A-184 Sweeteners and Sweet Substitutes   A-184 Vegetables and Legumes   A-198 Weight Loss Bars and Drinks   A-200 Miscellaneous

Thia (mg)	Ribo (mg)	Niac (mg NE)	Vit B6 (mg)	Vit B12 (µg)	Fol (µg)	Vit C (mg)	Vit D (IU)	Vit E (mg AT)	Cal (mg)	Iron (mg)	Magn (mg)	Phos (mg)	Pota (mg)	Sodi (mg)	Zinc (mg)	Wat (%)	Alco (g)	Caff (g)
—	—	—	—	—	—	4.8	—	—	20	0.72	—	—	—	480	—	86	0.00	0.00
0.17	0.07	1.12	0.07	0.07	64.6	3.2	—	2.3	161	4.11	88.8	264	807	1907	2.1	70	0.00	0.00
0.07	0.05	1.07	0.03	0.20	19.5	0.2	—	0.7	15	1.10	4.9	46	100	952	1.5	92	0.00	0.00
0.10	0.11	2.80	0.25	0.31	24.1	4.6	—	0.5	14	1.77	31.3	99	605	405	1.3	85	0.00	0.00
0.05	0.23	3.25	0.10	0.12	5.0	0.0	—	1.6	58	1.75	17.6	55	316	1940	2.0	80	0.00	0.00
0.01	0.10	1.62	0.05	0.05	0.0	0.0	—	1.2	29	0.87	9.8	27	154	942	1.0	90	0.00	0.00
—	—	—	—	—	—	—	—	—	—	1.19	—	—	—	875	—	89	0.00	0.00
0.10	0.10	3.44	0.05	0.20	33.2	0.7	—	0.1	19	1.11	9.5	85	209	460	0.4	92	0.00	0.00
0.01	0.01	1.12	0.01	0.14	0.0	0.2	—	0.1	17	0.75	0.0	22	101	815	0.3	94	0.00	0.00
0.03	0.05	1.23	0.05	0.11	4.8	1.0	—	0.4	17	0.87	7.2	41	154	945	0.4	93	0.00	0.00
0.02	0.05	0.31	0.07	0.00	29.3	5.9	—	0.4	41	1.22	14.6	39	161	578	0.3	92	0.00	0.00
0.02	0.11	0.98	0.00	0.00	5.0	0.3	—	1.4	35	2.66	10.0	78	123	1644	0.7	83	0.00	0.00
0.10	0.10	1.05	0.00	0.00	5.0	0.0	—	2.0	30	2.78	10.0	65	156	1619	0.5	84	0.00	0.00
0.05	0.09	0.72	0.00	0.05	4.9	1.0	—	1.0	46	0.50	4.9	49	100	881	0.6	90	0.00	0.00
0.02	0.03	0.54	0.03	0.05	2.4	0.0	—	0.0	20	0.49	2.4	46	137	1000	0.6	92	0.00	0.00
—	—	—	—	—	—	3.6	—	—	40	0.72	—	—	—	480	—	88	0.00	0.00
0.10	0.09	0.69	0.15	0.00	101.6	1.0	—	0.6	41	2.66	41.1	128	336	443	1.0	88	0.00	0.00
0.15	0.07	1.02	0.14	0.00	60.3	0.7	—	0.7	39	1.69	31.3	87	306	470	0.7	87	0.00	0.00
—	—	—	—	—	—	0.0	—	—	20	0.00	—	—	—	900	—	90	0.00	0.00
0.23	0.12	2.03	0.10	0.00	63.2	0.0	—	0.5	51	0.87	34.0	87	299	450	0.6	88	0.00	0.00
0.10	0.07	1.24	0.05	0.00	2.5	1.8	—	0.4	28	1.95	40.0	125	190	918	1.7	83	0.00	0.00
0.18	0.07	1.15	0.18	0.02	50.6	0.0	—	0.5	43	1.95	35.4	137	463	420	1.0	82	0.00	0.00
—	—	—	—	—	—	6.0	—	—	0	0.72	—	—	—	710	—	80	0.00	0.00
0.07	0.07	1.83	0.07	0.07	28.6	1.4	—	0.1	31	1.51	21.4	74	290	466	0.4	91	0.00	0.00
0.17	0.14	2.85	0.30	0.86	25.5	10.2	—	0.2	28	1.64	32.5	128	404	947	1.9	82	0.00	0.00
1.73	1.48	29.63	2.72	5.42	254.4	0.0	—	1.2	77	3.21	313.7	543	296	988	2.7	70	0.00	0.00
0.00	0.00	0.15	0.00	0.05	1.5	0.0	—	0.0	3	0.10	2.4	11	19	1152	0.0	3	0.00	0.00
0.00	0.01	0.25	0.00	0.01	2.0	0.1	0.0	0.0	12	0.11	3.6	12	24	1536	0.0	2	0.00	0.00
0.20	0.07	1.09	0.02	0.05	17.7	0.0	—	0.1	5	0.50	7.6	30	33	578	0.2	94	0.00	0.00
0.10	0.20	2.60	0.05	0.25	5.2	0.5	—	0.6	76	0.25	5.2	97	214	1185	1.6	91	0.00	0.00
0.34	0.23	4.57	0.46	0.00	159.9	4.6	—	0.2	171	4.57	34.3	274	1531	4616	3.4	92	0.00	0.00
0.21	0.09	0.37	0.01	0.18	3.9	0.8	—	0.4	50	0.38	3.9	58	153	782	0.1	92	0.00	0.00
0.01	0.03	0.36	0.00	0.00	1.8	0.2	—	0.0	9	0.10	3.7	22	48	635	0.0	96	0.00	0.00
0.66	0.43	5.40	0.05	0.00	147.0	0.0	—	2.0	16	4.26	24.0	108	120	1160	0.6	5	0.00	0.00
0.05	0.03	0.58	0.07	0.05	6.0	3.4	—	0.4	40	0.31	9.9	50	221	708	0.2	90	0.00	0.00
0.02	0.03	0.46	0.05	0.25	7.6	1.3	—	0.2	13	0.86	22.8	35	76	1002	0.3	94	0.00	0.00
0.00	0.01	0.54	0.01	0.11	3.8	0.0	—	0.0	7	0.11	7.0	38	54	3114	0.0	95	0.00	0.00
0.21	0.23	5.17	0.36	0.11	58.0	21.4	—	1.7	58	2.68	53.1	195	682	874	1.5	79	0.00	0.00
0.17	0.25	2.88	0.36	1.25	16.3	7.3	—	0.4	148	0.70	49.1	298	711	180	1.1	83	0.00	0.00
0.01	0.05	0.66	0.05	0.01	4.9	4.9	—	0.4	24	0.89	4.9	24	76	954	0.4	94	0.00	0.00
—	—	—	—	0.00	—	0.0	—	—	0	0.00	—	—	—	0	—	—	0.00	0.00
—	—	—	—	—	—	0.0	—	0.0	0	—	0.0	—	530	0	—	—	0.00	0.00
0.00	0.00	0.00	0.00	0.00	0.0	0.0	—	0.0	0	0.00	0.0	0	0	581	0.0	0	0.00	0.00

PAGE KEY: A-108 Beverage and Beverage Mixes A-110 Other Beverages A-110 Beverages, Alcoholic A-112 Candies and Confections, Gum A-116 Cereals, Breakfast Type A-120 Cheese and Cheese Substitutes A-122 Dairy Products and Substitutes A-124 Desserts A-130 Dessert Toppings A-130 Eggs, Substitutes, and Egg Dishes A-132 Ethnic Foods A-136 Fast Foods/Restaurants A-150 Fats, Oils, Margarines, Shortenings, and Substitutes A-150 Fish, Seafood, and Shellfish A-152 Food Additives A-152 Fruit, Vegetable, or Blended Juices A-154 Grains, Flours, and Fractions A-154 Grain Products, Prepared and Baked Goods

Code	Food Name	Unit/Amt	Wt (g)	Energy (kcal)	Prot (g)	Carb (g)	Fiber (g)	Fat (g)	Sat (g)	Mono (g)	Poly (g)	Chol (mg)	Vit A (RE)
53439	Sea Salt	100 g	100	0	0	0	0	0	0.0	0.0	0.0	0	0
669	Seasoning, garlic salt	0.25 tsp	1	0	0	0	0	0	0.0	0.0	0.0	—	—
26604	Seasoning, lemon pepper	1 tsp	2	2	0	0	0	0	0.0	0.0	0.0	0	0
26028	Seasoning, poultry	1 tsp	2	5	0	1	0	0	0.0	0.0	0.0	0	4
26004	Spice Blend, curry, pwd	1 tsp	2	6	0	1	1	0	0.0	0.1	0.1	0	2
26001	Spice, basil, ground	1 tsp	1	4	0	1	1	0	0.0	0.0	0.0	0	13
26524	Spice, chili pepper, ground, domestic	1 tsp	2	6	0	1	1	0	—	—	—	—	42
26002	Spice, chili pepper, pwd	1 tsp	3	8	0	1	1	0	0.1	0.1	0.2	0	77
7395	Spice, cilantro, dehyd	100 g	100	265	31	34	11	8	0.2	3.7	0.5	0	3670
26003	Spice, cinnamon, ground	1 tsp	2	6	0	2	1	0	0.0	0.0	0.0	0	1
26019	Spice, clove, ground	1 tsp	2	7	0	1	1	0	0.1	0.0	0.1	0	1
26109	Spice, dill seed	1 tsp	2	6	0	1	0	0	0.0	0.2	0.0	0	0
26065	Spice, garlic powder	1 tsp	3	8	0	2	1	0	—	—	—	0	0
26008	Spice, onion, powder	1 tsp	2	7	0	2	0	0	0.0	0.0	0.0	0	0
26009	Spice, oregano, ground	1 tsp	2	5	0	1	1	0	0.0	0.0	0.1	0	10
26010	Spice, paprika	1 tsp	2	6	0	1	1	0	0.0	0.0	0.2	0	111
26522	Spice, pepper, black, ground	1 tsp	2	7	0	1	1	0	—	—	—	—	2
26628	Spice, peppermint, fresh	2 Tbs	3	2	0	0	0	0	0.0	0.0	0.0	0	14
26015	Spice, poppy seed	1 tsp	3	15	1	1	0	1	0.1	0.2	0.9	0	0
26631	Spice, spearmint, dried	1 Tbs	2	5	0	1	0	0	0.0	0.0	0.1	0	17
26033	Spice, thyme, ground	1 tsp	1	4	0	1	1	0	0.0	0.0	0.0	0	5
SPORTS BARS AND DRINKS													
62275	Bar, energy, apple cinnamon	1 ea	65	230	10	45	3	2	0.5	1.5	0.5	0	0
62714	Bar, energy, carrot cake	1 ea	68	234	10	41	5	4	1.8	—	—	0	884
62278	Bar, energy, chocolate	1 ea	65	230	10	45	3	2	0.5	0.5	1.0	0	0
62715	Bar, energy, chocolate almond fudge	1 ea	68	231	10	38	5	5	0.9	—	—	0	276
62709	Bar, energy, chocolate chip	1 ea	68	238	10	42	5	4	0.9	—	—	0	278
62831	Bar, energy, chocolate fudge brownie	1 ea	78	290	24	38	4	5	4.0	—	—	5	0
62561	Bar, energy, chocolate peanut butter	1 ea	65	230	10	45	3	3	0.5	1.5	1.0	0	0
62716	Bar, energy, cookies & cream	1 ea	68	225	10	39	5	4	1.5	—	—	0	277
62725	Bar, energy, honey peanut	1 ea	50	200	14	22	1	6	3.5	—	—	3	500
62710	Bar, energy, peanut butter	1 ea	68	240	12	38	5	5	0.8	—	—	0	277
62205	Bar, energy, peanut butter, Tiger's Milk	1 ea	35	140	6	18	1	5	1.0	—	—	0	150
62821	Bar, energy, vanilla crisp	1 ea	65	230	9	45	3	2	0.5	1.5	0.5	0	0
62833	Carbohydrate Gel, chocolate, pkt	1 ea	41	120	0	28	0	2	1.0	—	—	0	0
63031	Drink, protein, Max Whey, all flvrs, pwd, scoop	1 ea	27	88	20	3	0	1	—	—	—	25	0
62995	Formula, Myoplex Pro, vanilla, rtd	0.33 ea	250	110	15	8	2	2	0.5	—	—	13	168
20142	Sports Drink, btld	1 cup	241	60	0	15	0	0	0.0	0.0	0.0	0	0
20558	Sports Drink, grape, can/btl	1 cup	247	73	0	19	0	0	0.0	0.0	0.0	0	0
20559	Sports Drink, lemon lime, can/btl	1 cup	247	72	0	19	0	0	0.0	0.0	0.0	0	0
SUPPLEMENTAL FOODS AND FORMULAS—CHILD/ADULT													
Medical Nutritionals													
63162	Instant Breakfast, supplement, chocolate, rtu	1 ea	260	390	12	44	0	12	2.0	—	—	5	250
62761	Instant Breakfast, supplement, straw, liquid, rts	8 fl-oz	250	250	12	33	0	8	—	—	—	18	250
62760	Instant Breakfast, supplement, van, liquid, rts	8 fl-oz	250	250	12	33	0	8	—	—	—	18	250

PAGE KEY: A-158 Granola Bars, Cereal Bars, Diet Bars, Scones, and Tarts   A-158 Meals and Dishes   A-162 Meats   A-168 Nuts, Seeds, and Products   A-170 Poultry   A-172 Salad Dressings, Dips, and Mayonnaise   A-172 Salads   A-174 Sandwiches   A-176 Sauces and Gravies   A-176 Snack Foods—Chips, Pretzels, Popcorn   A-178 Soups, Stews, and Chilis   A-180 Spices, Flavors, and Seasonings   A-182 Sports Bars and Drinks   A-182 Supplemental Foods and Formulas   A-184 Sweeteners and Sweet Substitutes   A-184 Vegetables and Legumes   A-198 Weight Loss Bars and Drinks   A-200 Miscellaneous

Thia (mg)	Ribo (mg)	Niac (mg NE)	Vit B6 (mg)	Vit B12 (µg)	Fol (µg)	Vit C (mg)	Vit D (IU)	Vit E (mg AT)	Cal (mg)	Iron (mg)	Magn (mg)	Phos (mg)	Pota (mg)	Sodi (mg)	Zinc (mg)	Wat (%)	Alco (g)	Caff (g)
0.00	0.00	0.00	0.00	0.00	0.0	0.0	0.0	0.0	12	380.00	500.0	0	260	32000	870.0	7	0.00	0.00
—	—	—	—	0.00	—	—	—	—	—	—	—	—	—	240	—	11	0.00	0.00
0.00	0.00	0.00	0.00	0.00	0.0	0.0	0.0	0.0	3	0.10	0.8	1	6	461	0.0	2	0.00	0.00
0.00	0.00	0.03	0.01	0.00	2.1	0.2	0.0	0.0	15	0.52	3.4	3	10	0	0.0	9	0.00	0.00
0.00	0.00	0.07	0.01	0.00	3.1	0.2	0.0	0.4	10	0.58	5.1	7	31	1	0.1	10	0.00	0.00
0.00	0.00	0.10	0.02	0.00	3.8	0.9	0.0	0.1	30	0.58	5.9	7	48	0	0.1	6	0.00	0.00
—	—	—	—	0.00	—	0.7	—	—	4	0.23	—	—	—	3	—	14	0.00	0.00
0.00	0.01	0.20	0.10	0.00	2.6	1.7	0.0	0.8	7	0.37	4.4	8	50	26	0.1	8	0.00	0.00
0.93	1.59	9.68	1.46	0.00	137.0	139.0	—	—	1300	25.89	345.0	478	7189	371	6.0	4	0.00	0.00
0.00	0.00	0.02	0.00	0.00	0.7	0.7	0.0	0.0	28	0.87	1.3	1	12	1	0.0	10	0.00	0.00
0.00	0.00	0.02	0.00	0.00	2.0	1.7	0.0	0.2	14	0.18	5.5	2	23	5	0.0	7	0.00	0.00
0.00	0.00	0.05	0.00	0.00	0.2	0.4	0.0	0.0	32	0.34	5.4	6	25	0	0.1	8	0.00	0.00
0.00	0.00	0.01	—	0.00	—	0.1	—	—	3	0.01	—	—	38	1	—	6	0.00	0.00
0.00	0.00	0.00	0.02	0.00	3.5	0.3	0.0	0.0	8	0.05	2.6	7	20	1	0.0	5	0.00	0.00
0.00	0.00	0.09	0.01	0.00	4.1	0.8	0.0	0.3	24	0.66	4.0	3	25	0	0.1	7	0.00	0.00
0.00	0.03	0.31	0.07	0.00	2.2	1.5	0.0	0.6	4	0.50	3.9	7	49	1	0.1	10	0.00	0.00
—	—	—	—	0.00	—	0.0	—	—	8	0.15	—	—	—	0	—	12	0.00	0.00
0.00	0.00	0.05	0.00	0.00	3.6	1.0	—	0.0	8	0.15	2.6	2	18	1	0.0	79	0.00	0.00
0.01	0.00	0.02	0.00	0.00	1.6	0.1	0.0	0.0	41	0.25	9.3	24	20	1	0.3	7	0.00	0.00
0.00	0.01	0.10	0.03	0.00	8.5	0.0	—	0.0	24	1.39	9.6	4	31	6	0.0	11	0.00	0.00
0.00	0.00	0.07	0.00	0.00	3.8	0.7	0.0	0.1	26	1.73	3.1	3	11	1	0.1	8	0.00	0.00
1.50	1.70	20.00	2.00	6.00	400.0	60.0	—	18.4	300	6.30	140.0	350	110	90	5.2	—	0.00	0.00
0.37	0.28	3.54	0.41	0.98	87.0	67.1	—	20.2	275	5.32	103.2	298	246	170	3.2	17	0.00	0.00
1.50	1.70	20.00	2.00	6.00	400.0	60.0	—	18.4	300	6.30	140.0	350	145	90	5.2	—	0.00	15.00
0.38	0.31	3.63	0.43	0.98	84.6	65.7	—	20.8	278	5.73	128.3	304	232	139	3.7	19	0.00	0.00
0.34	0.28	3.49	0.38	0.98	85.6	66.1	—	20.3	265	5.21	95.5	286	206	76	3.5	15	0.00	—
1.50	1.70	20.00	2.00	6.00	400.0	60.0	—	18.3	300	6.30	140.0	350	—	150	5.2	—	0.00	—
1.50	1.70	20.00	2.00	6.00	400.0	60.0	—	18.3	300	6.30	140.0	350	140	95	5.2	—	0.00	—
0.34	0.27	3.45	0.43	0.98	85.1	66.2	—	20.3	279	5.23	102.6	266	212	179	3.2	20	0.00	0.00
0.60	0.50	9.00	0.60	1.20	80.0	60.0	80.0	13.6	100	3.59	40.0	100	115	220	3.0	—	0.00	—
0.40	0.30	6.25	0.41	0.98	96.2	65.8	—	20.4	268	5.30	113.7	305	301	289	3.6	15	0.00	—
1.26	0.60	3.00	0.60	1.50	—	6.0	60.0	—	300	2.70	100.0	100	—	75	—	—	0.00	0.00
1.50	1.70	20.00	2.00	6.00	400.0	60.0	—	18.3	300	6.30	140.0	350	110	90	5.2	—	0.00	0.00
—	—	—	—	—	—	9.0	—	2.8	0	0.00	—	—	40	50	—	—	0.00	25.00
—	—	—	—	—	—	0.0	—	—	0	0.00	—	—	—	35	—	10	0.00	—
0.25	0.33	3.32	0.33	1.33	120.0	15.0	66.7	4.5	116	—	59.3	141	167	177	2.5	—	0.00	0.00
0.00	0.00	0.00	0.00	0.00	0.0	0.0	0.0	0.0	0	0.11	2.4	22	26	96	0.0	94	0.00	0.00
—	—	—	—	—	—	0.0	—	—	0	0.00	—	—	—	32	28	—	0.00	0.00
—	—	—	—	—	—	0.0	—	—	0	0.00	—	—	—	32	28	—	0.00	0.00
0.37	0.43	5.00	0.50	1.50	100.0	15.0	—	—	250	4.50	100.0	250	430	120	3.8	—	0.00	—
0.37	0.43	5.00	0.50	1.50	1000.0	15.0	100.0	3.4	300	4.50	60.0	300	480	190	3.8	—	0.00	0.00
0.37	0.43	5.00	0.50	1.50	1000.0	15.0	100.0	3.4	300	4.50	60.0	300	480	190	3.8	—	0.00	0.00

PAGE KEY: A-108 Beverage and Beverage Mixes   A-110 Other Beverages   A-110 Beverages, Alcoholic   A-112 Candies and Confections, Gum   A-116 Cereals, Breakfast Type   A-120 Cheese and Cheese Substitutes   A-122 Dairy Products and Substitutes   A-124 Desserts   A-130 Dessert Toppings   A-130 Eggs, Substitutes, and Egg Dishes   A-132 Ethnic Foods   A-136 Fast Foods/Restaurants   A-150 Fats, Oils, Margarines, Shortenings, and Substitutes   A-150 Fish, Seafood, and Shellfish   A-152 Food Additives   A-152 Fruit, Vegetable, or Blended Juices   A-154 Grains, Flours, and Fractions   A-154 Grain Products, Prepared and Baked Goods

Code	Food Name	Unit/ Amt	Wt (g)	Energy (kcal)	Prot (g)	Carb (g)	Fiber (g)	Fat (g)	Sat (g)	Mono (g)	Poly (g)	Chol (mg)	Vit A (RE)
62136	Pudding, supplement, rtu, 5 oz can	1 ea	142	240	7	32	0	9	1.5	—	—	5	150
62795	Supplement Drink, Hi Protein, vanilla, rtu	1 cup	256	240	15	33	0	6	0.5	—	—	10	250
62796	Supplement Drink, Plus, vanilla, rtu	8 fl-oz	260	360	14	45	1	14	1.5	—	—	10	250
62162	Supplement Drink, vanilla, rtu	1 cup	256	240	10	41	0	4	0.5	—	—	5	250
Soy Nutritionals													
SWEETENERS AND SWEET SUBSTITUTES													
Jams and Jellies													
90974	Fruit Spread, apricot, 100% fruit	1 Tbs	19	40	0	10	0	0	0.0	0.0	0.0	0	0
90976	Fruit Spread, blueberry, 100% fruit	1 Tbs	19	40	0	10	0	0	0.0	0.0	0.0	0	0
90984	Fruit Spread, concord grape, 100% fruit	1 Tbs	19	40	0	10	0	0	0.0	0.0	0.0	0	0
90978	Fruit Spread, red raspberry, 100% fruit	1 Tbs	19	40	0	10	0	0	0.0	0.0	0.0	0	0
90979	Fruit Spread, strawberry, 100% fruit	1 Tbs	19	40	0	10	0	0	0.0	0.0	0.0	0	0
23054	Jam	1 Tbs	20	56	0	14	0	0	0.0	0.0	0.0	0	0
23205	Jam, apricot	1 Tbs	20	48	0	13	0	0	0.0	0.0	0.0	0	6
23288	Jam, concord grape	1 Tbs	20	50	0	13	0	0	0.0	0.0	0.0	0	0
92262	Jam, red raspberry	1 Tbs	20	50	0	13	0	0	0.0	0.0	0.0	0	0
23286	Jam, strawberry	1 Tbs	20	50	0	13	0	0	0.0	0.0	0.0	0	0
23003	Jelly	1 Tbs	19	51	0	13	0	0	0.0	0.0	0.0	0	0
23285	Jelly, apple	1 Tbs	20	50	0	13	0	0	0.0	0.0	0.0	0	0
23293	Jelly, concord grape	1 Tbs	20	50	0	13	0	0	0.0	0.0	0.0	0	0
90881	Jelly, mixed fruit	1 Tbs	20	50	0	13	0	0	0.0	0.0	0.0	0	0
23294	Jelly, strawberry	1 Tbs	20	50	0	13	0	0	0.0	0.0	0.0	0	0
23005	Marmalade, orange	1 Tbs	20	49	0	13	0	0	0.0	0.0	0.0	0	1
92229	Preserves	1 Tbs	20	56	0	14	0	0	0.0	0.0	0.0	0	0
92232	Preserves, apricot	1 Tbs	20	48	0	13	0	0	0.0	0.0	0.0	0	6
90891	Preserves, blueberry	1 Tbs	20	50	0	13	0	0	0.0	0.0	0.0	0	0
23297	Preserves, red raspberry	1 Tbs	20	50	0	13	0	0	0.0	0.0	0.0	0	0
23301	Preserves, strawberry	1 Tbs	20	50	0	13	0	0	0.0	0.0	0.0	0	0
Sugars, Sugar Substitutes, and Syrups													
25309	Honey, light	1 Tbs	21	64	0	17	0	0	0.0	0.0	0.0	0	0
25003	Molasses	1 Tbs	20	59	0	15	0	0	0.0	0.0	0.0	0	0
25201	Sugar, brown, unpacked	1 cup	145	547	0	141	0	0	0.0	0.0	0.0	0	0
63415	Sugar, powdered	0.25 cup	37	140	0	37	0	0	0.0	0.0	0.0	0	
25006	Sugar, white, granulated	1 tsp	4	16	0	4	0	0	0.0	0.0	0.0	0	0
25007	Sugar, white, granulated, pkt	1 ea	6	23	0	6	0	0	0.0	0.0	0.0	0	0
25010	Syrup, corn, dark	2 Tbs	41	117	0	32	0	0	0.0	0.0	0.0	0	0
25000	Syrup, corn, light	1 cup	328	961	0	261	0	0	0.0	0.0	0.0	0	0
63334	Syrup, dietetic	1 Tbs	15	6	0	7	0	0	0.0	0.0	0.0	0	0
23042	Syrup, pancake	1 Tbs	20	47	0	12	0	0	0.0	0.0	0.0	0	0
23090	Syrup, pancake, w/butter	1 cup	315	932	0	233	0	5	3.2	1.5	0.2	13	47
VEGETABLES AND LEGUMES													
VEGETABLES													
Fresh Vegetables													
5010	Alfalfa Sprouts, fresh	0.5 cup	16	5	1	1	0	0	0.0	0.0	0.1	0	3
7440	Artichokes, Calif, fresh	1 ea	340	85	7	20	10	0	0.0	0.0	0.0	0	0
5001	Asparagus, fresh	0.5 cup	67	13	1	3	1	0	0.0	0.0	0.1	0	51

PAGE KEY: A-158 Granola Bars, Cereal Bars, Diet Bars, Scones, and Tarts   A-158 Meals and Dishes   A-162 Meats   A-168 Nuts, Seeds, and Products   A-170 Poultry
A-172 Salad Dressings, Dips, and Mayonnaise   A-172 Salads   A-174 Sandwiches   A-176 Sauces and Gravies   A-176 Snack Foods—Chips, Pretzels, Popcorn
A-178 Soups, Stews, and Chilis   A-180 Spices, Flavors, and Seasonings   A-182 Sports Bars and Drinks   A-182 Supplemental Foods and Formulas
A-184 Sweeteners and Sweet Substitutes   A-184 Vegetables and Legumes   A-198 Weight Loss Bars and Drinks   A-200 Miscellaneous

Thia (mg)	Ribo (mg)	Niac (mg NE)	Vit B6 (mg)	Vit B12 (μg)	Fol (μg)	Vit C (mg)	Vit D (IU)	Vit E (mg AT)	Cal (mg)	Iron (mg)	Magn (mg)	Phos (mg)	Pota (mg)	Sodi (mg)	Zinc (mg)	Wat (%)	Alco (g)	Caff (g)
0.23	0.25	3.00	0.30	0.89	60.0	9.0	60.0	2.0	230	2.70	60.0	230	320	120	2.3	65	0.00	0.00
0.37	0.43	5.00	0.69	2.09	140.0	60.0	150.0	13.6	330	4.50	105.0	310	380	170	4.5	78	0.00	0.00
0.37	0.43	5.00	0.69	2.09	140.0	60.0	150.0	13.6	330	4.50	105.0	310	380	170	4.5	72	0.00	0.00
0.37	0.43	5.00	0.69	2.09	140.0	60.0	100.0	13.6	300	3.59	100.0	250	400	130	4.5	78	0.00	0.00
—	—	—	—	—	—	0.0	—	—	0	0.00	—	—	—	0	—	47	0.00	0.00
—	—	—	—	—	—	0.0	—	—	0	0.00	—	—	—	0	—	47	0.00	0.00
—	—	—	—	—	—	0.0	—	—	0	0.00	—	—	—	0	—	47	0.00	0.00
—	—	—	—	—	—	0.0	—	—	0	0.00	—	—	—	0	—	47	0.00	0.00
—	—	—	—	—	—	0.0	—	—	0	0.00	—	—	—	0	—	47	0.00	0.00
0.00	0.01	0.00	0.00	0.00	2.2	1.8	—	0.0	4	0.10	0.8	4	15	6	0.0	30	0.00	0.00
0.00	0.00	0.00	0.00	0.00	6.6	1.8	—	0.0	4	0.10	0.8	2	15	8	0.0	34	0.00	0.00
—	—	—	—	—	—	0.0	—	—	0	0.00	—	—	—	0	—	35	0.00	0.00
—	—	—	—	—	—	0.0	—	—	0	0.00	—	—	—	0	—	35	0.00	0.00
—	—	—	—	—	—	0.0	—	—	0	0.00	—	—	—	0	—	35	0.00	0.00
0.00	0.00	0.00	0.00	0.00	0.4	0.2	—	0.0	1	0.03	1.1	1	10	6	0.0	30	0.00	0.00
—	—	—	—	—	—	0.0	—	—	0	0.00	—	—	—	0	—	35	0.00	0.00
—	—	—	—	—	—	0.0	—	—	0	0.00	—	—	—	0	—	35	0.00	0.00
—	—	—	—	—	—	0.0	—	—	0	0.00	—	—	—	0	—	35	0.00	0.00
—	—	—	—	—	—	0.0	—	—	0	0.00	—	—	—	0	—	35	0.00	0.00
0.00	0.00	0.00	0.00	0.00	1.8	1.0	—	0.0	8	0.02	0.4	1	7	11	0.0	33	0.00	0.00
0.00	0.01	0.00	0.00	0.00	2.2	1.8	—	0.0	4	0.10	0.8	4	15	6	0.0	30	0.00	0.00
0.00	0.00	0.00	0.00	0.00	6.6	1.8	—	0.0	4	0.10	0.8	2	15	8	0.0	34	0.00	0.00
—	—	—	—	—	—	0.0	—	—	0	0.00	—	—	—	0	—	35	0.00	0.00
—	—	—	—	—	—	0.0	—	—	0	0.00	—	—	—	0	—	35	0.00	0.00
—	—	—	—	—	—	0.0	—	—	0	0.00	—	—	—	0	—	35	0.00	0.00
0.00	0.05	0.05	0.00	0.00	2.1	0.1	0.0	0.0	1	0.05	0.4	1	10	1	0.0	17	0.00	0.00
0.00	0.00	0.18	0.14	0.00	0.0	0.0	—	0.0	42	0.97	49.6	6	300	8	0.1	22	0.00	0.00
0.00	0.00	0.11	0.03	0.00	1.5	0.0	—	0.0	123	2.76	42.1	32	502	57	0.3	2	0.00	0.00
—	—	—	—	—	—	—	—	—	—	—	—	—	—	0	—	0	0.00	0.00
0.00	0.00	0.00	0.00	0.00	0.0	0.0	—	0.0	0	0.00	0.0	0	0	0	0.0	0	0.00	0.00
0.00	0.00	0.00	0.00	0.00	0.0	0.0	—	0.0	0	0.00	0.0	0	0	0	0.0	0	0.00	0.00
0.00	0.00	0.00	0.00	0.00	0.0	0.0	0.0	0.0	7	0.15	3.3	5	18	64	0.0	22	0.00	0.00
0.03	0.02	0.07	0.02	0.00	0.0	0.0	0.0	0.0	10	0.15	6.6	7	13	397	0.1	20	0.00	0.00
0.00	0.00	0.00	0.00	0.00	0.0	0.0	—	0.0	0	0.00	0.0	0	0	3	0.0	50	0.00	0.00
0.00	0.00	0.00	0.00	0.00	0.0	0.0	—	0.0	1	0.00	0.4	2	3	16	0.0	38	0.00	0.00
0.02	0.02	0.05	0.00	0.00	0.0	0.0	—	0.1	6	0.28	6.3	32	9	309	0.1	24	0.00	0.00
0.00	0.01	0.07	0.00	0.00	5.9	1.4	—	0.0	5	0.15	4.5	12	13	1	0.2	91	0.00	0.00
0.10	0.11	2.72	0.14	—	136.0	20.4	—	1.4	68	2.45	136.0	204	578	255	—	91	0.00	0.00
0.10	0.09	0.66	0.05	0.00	34.8	3.8	—	0.8	16	1.42	9.4	35	135	1	0.4	93	0.00	0.00

PAGE KEY: A-108 Beverage and Beverage Mixes   A-110 Other Beverages   A-110 Beverages, Alcoholic   A-112 Candies and Confections, Gum   A-116 Cereals, Breakfast Type   A-120 Cheese and Cheese Substitutes   A-122 Dairy Products and Substitutes   A-124 Desserts   A-130 Dessert Toppings   A-130 Eggs, Substitutes, and Egg Dishes   A-132 Ethnic Foods   A-136 Fast Foods/Restaurants   A-150 Fats, Oils, Margarines, Shortenings, and Substitutes   A-150 Fish, Seafood, and Shellfish   A-152 Food Additives   A-152 Fruit, Vegetable, or Blended Juices   A-154 Grains, Flours, and Fractions   A-154 Grain Products, Prepared and Baked Goods

Code	Food Name	Unit/ Amt	Wt (g)	Energy (kcal)	Prot (g)	Carb (g)	Fiber (g)	Fat (g)	Sat (g)	Mono (g)	Poly (g)	Chol (mg)	Vit A (RE)
5572	Beets, fresh, whole, 2"	1 ea	82	35	1	8	2	0	0.0	0.0	0.1	0	3
5678	Broccoflower, fresh	1 cup	100	32	3	6	3	0	0.0	0.0	0.1	0	7
6757	Broccoli, fresh	1 cup	71	24	2	5	2	0	0.0	0.0	0.0	0	47
5036	Cabbage, fresh, shredded	1 cup	70	17	1	4	2	0	0.0	0.0	0.0	0	13
5042	Cabbage, red, fresh, shredded	0.5 cup	35	11	1	3	1	0	0.0	0.0	0.0	0	39
9329	Carrots, baby, fresh	0.75 cup	85	40	1	9	2	0	0.0	0.0	0.0	0	1250
90429	Carrots, fresh, slices	1 pce	3	1	0	0	0	0	0.0	0.0	0.0	0	36
5049	Cauliflower, fresh	0.5 cup	50	12	1	3	1	0	0.0	0.0	0.0	0	1
90436	Celery, stalk, sml, 5" long, fresh	1 ea	17	2	0	1	0	0	0.0	0.0	0.0	0	7
7927	Chili Peppers, banana, fresh	1 cup	124	33	2	7	4	1	0.1	0.0	0.3	0	42
5359	Chives, fresh	1 Tbs	3	1	0	0	0	0	0.0	0.0	0.0	0	13
5560	Corn, white, sweet, kernels f/one ear, ckd, drained	1 ea	77	83	3	19	2	1	0.2	0.3	0.5	0	0
6015	Corn, white, sweet, kernels, fresh	1 cup	154	132	5	29	4	2	0.3	0.5	0.9	0	0
5379	Corn, yellow, sweet, kernels, ckd, drained	0.5 cup	82	89	3	21	2	1	0.2	0.3	0.5	0	21
5378	Corn, yellow, sweet, kernels, fresh	0.5 cup	77	66	2	15	2	1	0.1	0.3	0.4	0	15
7921	Cucumber, w/o skin, fresh, sliced	1 pce	7	1	0	0	0	0	0.0	0.0	0.0	0	1
5071	Cucumber, w/skin, fresh, slices	0.5 cup	52	8	0	2	0	0	0.0	0.0	0.0	0	5
5371	Eggplant, fresh, cubes	1 cup	82	20	1	5	3	0	0.0	0.0	0.1	0	2
26005	Garlic, cloves, fresh	4 ea	12	18	1	4	0	0	0.0	0.0	0.0	0	0
7081	Hummus, prep f/recipe	1 cup	246	435	12	49	10	21	2.8	12.1	5.1	0	1
5208	Kale, fresh, chpd	1 cup	67	34	2	7	1	0	0.1	0.0	0.2	0	1030
4851	Lettuce, crisphead, fresh, chpd	1 cup	55	8	0	2	1	0	0.0	0.0	0.0	0	28
5083	Lettuce, iceberg, fresh, chpd	1 cup	55	8	0	2	1	0	0.0	0.0	0.0	0	28
9316	Lettuce, iceberg, shredded	1.5 cup	100	15	1	3	1	0	0.0	0.0	0.0	0	20
5088	Lettuce, romaine, fresh, chpd	1 cup	56	10	1	2	1	0	0.0	0.0	0.1	0	325
5090	Mushrooms, fresh, pces/slices	0.5 cup	35	8	1	1	0	0	0.0	0.0	0.0	0	0
6494	Mushrooms, fresh, whole	1 cup	96	21	3	3	1	0	0.0	0.0	0.1	0	0
5099	Okra, ckd, drained, slices	0.5 cup	80	18	1	4	2	0	0.0	0.0	0.0	0	22
5775	Okra, fresh	0.5 cup	50	16	1	4	2	0	0.0	0.0	0.0	0	19
7498	Onion, red, fresh, chpd	1 cup	160	67	1	16	2	0	0.0	0.0	0.1	0	0
9548	Onion, sweet, fresh	100 g	100	32	1	8	1	0	—	—	—	0	0
5101	Onion, white, fresh, chpd	0.5 cup	80	34	1	8	1	0	0.0	0.0	0.1	0	0
7499	Onion, yellow, fresh, chpd	0.5 cup	80	34	1	8	1	0	0.0	0.0	0.0	0	0
26012	Parsley, fresh, chpd	0.5 cup	30	11	1	2	1	0	0.0	0.1	0.0	0	253
5124	Peppers, bell, green, sweet, fresh, chpd	0.5 cup	74	15	1	3	1	0	0.0	0.0	0.0	0	27
5128	Peppers, bell, red, sweet, fresh, chpd	0.5 cup	74	19	1	4	1	0	0.0	0.0	0.1	0	234
9242	Peppers, bell, yellow, sweet, fresh, chpd	0.5 cup	74	20	1	5	1	0	0.0	0.0	0.1	0	15
5143	Radishes, fresh, med, 3/4" to 1"	10 ea	45	7	0	2	1	0	0.0	0.0	0.0	0	0
7214	Rutabaga, fresh, cubes	0.5 cup	70	25	1	6	2	0	0.0	0.0	0.1	0	0
6861	Soybean Sprouts, mature, fresh	10 ea	10	12	1	1	0	1	0.1	0.2	0.4	0	0
5146	Spinach, fresh, chpd	1 cup	30	7	1	1	1	0	0.0	0.0	0.0	0	281
6863	Spinach, fresh, leaf	1 ea	10	2	0	0	0	0	0.0	0.0	0.0	0	94
7369	Squash, banana, fresh	0.75 cup	85	30	1	7	1	0	0.0	0.0	0.0	0	350
5801	Squash, butternut, fresh, cubes	0.5 cup	120	54	1	14	2	0	0.0	0.0	0.1	0	1277
90537	Squash, summer, all types, fresh, med	1 ea	196	31	2	7	2	0	0.1	0.0	0.2	0	39

PAGE KEY: A-158 Granola Bars, Cereal Bars, Diet Bars, Scones, and Tarts   A-158 Meals and Dishes   A-162 Meats   A-168 Nuts, Seeds, and Products   A-170 Poultry   A-172 Salad Dressings, Dips, and Mayonnaise   A-172 Salads   A-174 Sandwiches   A-176 Sauces and Gravies   A-176 Snack Foods—Chips, Pretzels, Popcorn   A-178 Soups, Stews, and Chilis   A-180 Spices, Flavors, and Seasonings   A-182 Sports Bars and Drinks   A-182 Supplemental Foods and Formulas   A-184 Sweeteners and Sweet Substitutes   A-184 Vegetables and Legumes   A-198 Weight Loss Bars and Drinks   A-200 Miscellaneous

Thia (mg)	Ribo (mg)	Niac (mg NE)	Vit B6 (mg)	Vit B12 (µg)	Fol (µg)	Vit C (mg)	Vit D (IU)	Vit E (mg AT)	Cal (mg)	Iron (mg)	Magn (mg)	Phos (mg)	Pota (mg)	Sodi (mg)	Zinc (mg)	Wat (%)	Alco (g)	Caff (g)
0.02	0.02	0.27	0.05	0.00	89.4	4.0	—	0.0	13	0.66	18.9	33	266	64	0.3	88	0.00	0.00
0.07	0.10	0.80	0.20	0.00	57.0	74.0	0.0	0.3	32	0.07	20.0	64	322	23	0.5	90	0.00	0.00
0.05	0.07	0.44	0.11	0.00	44.7	63.3	—	0.6	33	0.51	14.9	47	224	23	0.3	89	0.00	0.00
0.03	0.02	0.20	0.07	0.00	30.1	22.5	—	0.1	33	0.40	10.5	16	172	13	0.1	92	0.00	0.00
0.01	0.01	0.15	0.07	0.00	6.3	19.9	—	0.0	16	0.28	5.6	10	85	9	0.1	90	0.00	0.00
—	—	—	—	—	—	6.0	—	—	20	0.00	—	—	—	45	—	88	0.00	0.00
0.00	0.00	0.02	0.00	0.00	0.6	0.2	—	0.0	1	0.00	0.4	1	10	2	0.0	88	0.00	0.00
0.02	0.02	0.25	0.10	0.00	28.5	23.2	—	0.0	11	0.21	7.5	22	152	15	0.1	92	0.00	0.00
0.00	0.00	0.05	0.00	0.00	6.1	0.5	—	0.0	7	0.02	1.9	4	44	14	0.0	95	0.00	0.00
0.10	0.07	1.53	0.43	0.00	36.0	102.5	—	0.9	17	0.56	21.1	40	317	16	0.3	92	0.00	0.00
0.00	0.00	0.01	0.00	0.00	3.1	1.7	—	0.0	3	0.05	1.3	2	9	0	0.0	91	0.00	0.00
0.17	0.05	1.24	0.05	0.00	35.4	4.8	0.0	0.1	2	0.46	24.6	79	192	13	0.4	70	0.00	0.00
0.31	0.09	2.61	0.07	0.00	70.8	10.5	—	0.1	3	0.80	57.0	137	416	23	0.7	76	0.00	0.00
0.18	0.05	1.32	0.05	0.00	37.7	5.1	—	0.1	2	0.50	26.2	84	204	14	0.4	70	0.00	0.00
0.15	0.05	1.30	0.03	0.00	35.4	5.2	—	0.1	2	0.40	28.5	69	208	12	0.3	76	0.00	0.00
0.00	0.00	0.00	0.00	0.00	1.0	0.2	—	0.0	1	0.01	0.8	1	10	0	0.0	97	0.00	0.00
0.00	0.01	0.05	0.01	0.00	3.6	1.5	—	0.0	8	0.15	6.8	12	76	1	0.1	95	0.00	0.00
0.02	0.02	0.52	0.07	0.00	18.0	1.8	—	0.2	7	0.20	11.5	20	189	2	0.1	92	0.00	0.00
0.01	0.00	0.07	0.15	0.00	0.4	3.7	—	0.0	22	0.20	3.0	18	48	2	0.1	59	0.00	0.00
0.21	0.12	0.98	0.98	0.00	145.1	19.4	—	1.8	121	3.85	71.3	271	426	595	2.7	65	0.00	0.00
0.07	0.09	0.67	0.18	0.00	19.4	80.4	—	0.5	90	1.13	22.8	38	299	29	0.3	84	0.00	0.00
0.01	0.00	0.07	0.01	0.00	16.0	1.5	—	0.1	10	0.23	3.9	11	78	6	0.1	96	0.00	0.00
0.01	0.00	0.07	0.01	0.00	16.0	1.5	—	0.1	10	0.23	3.9	11	78	6	0.1	96	0.00	0.00
—	—	—	—	—	—	3.6	—	—	0	0.00	—	—	—	10	—	96	0.00	0.00
0.03	0.03	0.18	0.03	0.00	76.2	13.4	—	0.1	18	0.54	7.8	17	138	4	0.1	95	0.00	0.00
0.02	0.15	1.35	0.03	0.00	5.6	0.8	26.6	0.0	1	0.18	3.1	30	110	1	0.2	92	0.00	0.00
0.09	0.40	3.70	0.10	0.03	15.4	2.3	73.0	0.0	3	0.50	8.6	82	301	4	0.5	92	0.00	0.00
0.10	0.03	0.69	0.15	0.00	36.8	13.0	—	0.2	62	0.21	28.8	26	108	5	0.3	93	0.00	0.00
0.10	0.02	0.50	0.10	0.00	44.0	10.6	—	0.2	40	0.40	28.5	32	152	4	0.3	90	0.00	0.00
0.07	0.03	0.12	0.23	0.00	30.4	10.2	—	0.0	35	0.30	16.0	43	230	5	0.3	89	0.00	0.00
0.03	0.01	0.12	0.12	—	23.0	4.8	—	0.0	20	0.25	9.0	27	119	8	0.1	91	0.00	0.00
0.03	0.01	0.07	0.11	0.00	15.2	5.1	—	0.0	18	0.15	8.0	22	115	2	0.1	89	0.00	0.00
0.03	0.01	0.07	0.11	0.00	15.2	5.1	—	0.0	18	0.15	8.0	22	115	2	0.1	89	0.00	0.00
0.02	0.02	0.38	0.02	0.00	45.6	39.9	—	0.2	41	1.86	15.0	17	166	17	0.3	88	0.00	0.00
0.03	0.01	0.36	0.17	0.00	8.2	59.9	—	0.3	7	0.25	7.4	15	130	2	0.1	94	0.00	0.00
0.03	0.05	0.73	0.21	0.00	13.4	141.6	—	1.2	5	0.31	8.9	19	157	1	0.2	92	0.00	0.00
0.01	0.01	0.66	0.12	0.00	19.4	136.7	0.0	0.5	8	0.34	8.9	18	158	1	0.1	92	0.00	0.00
0.00	0.01	0.10	0.02	0.00	11.2	6.7	—	0.0	11	0.15	4.5	9	105	18	0.1	95	0.00	0.00
0.05	0.02	0.49	0.07	0.00	14.7	17.5	—	0.2	33	0.36	16.1	41	236	14	0.2	90	0.00	0.00
0.02	0.00	0.10	0.01	0.00	17.2	1.5	—	0.0	7	0.20	7.2	16	48	1	0.1	69	0.00	0.00
0.01	0.05	0.21	0.05	0.00	58.2	8.4	—	0.6	30	0.81	23.7	15	167	24	0.2	91	0.00	0.00
0.00	0.01	0.07	0.01	0.00	19.4	2.8	—	0.2	10	0.27	7.9	5	56	8	0.1	91	0.00	0.00
—	—	—	—	0.00	—	9.0	—	—	20	0.36	—	—	—	0	—	90	0.00	0.00
0.11	0.01	1.44	0.18	0.00	32.4	25.2	—	1.7	58	0.83	40.8	40	422	5	0.2	86	0.00	0.00
0.09	0.28	0.94	0.43	0.00	56.8	33.3	—	0.2	29	0.68	33.3	74	514	4	0.6	95	0.00	0.00

PAGE KEY: A-108 Beverage and Beverage Mixes   A-110 Other Beverages   A-110 Beverages, Alcoholic   A-112 Candies and Confections, Gum   A-116 Cereals, Breakfast Type
A-120 Cheese and Cheese Substitutes   A-122 Dairy Products and Substitutes   A-124 Desserts   A-130 Dessert Toppings   A-130 Eggs, Substitutes, and Egg Dishes   A-132 Ethnic Foods
A-136 Fast Foods/Restaurants   A-150 Fats, Oils, Margarines, Shortenings, and Substitutes   A-150 Fish, Seafood, and Shellfish   A-152 Food Additives
A-152 Fruit, Vegetable, or Blended Juices   A-154 Grains, Flours, and Fractions   A-154 Grain Products, Prepared and Baked Goods

Code	Food Name	Unit/ Amt	Wt (g)	Energy (kcal)	Prot (g)	Carb (g)	Fiber (g)	Fat (g)	Sat (g)	Mono (g)	Poly (g)	Chol (mg)	Vit A (RE)
90538	Squash, summer, all types, fresh, sml	1 ea	118	19	1	4	1	0	0.1	0.0	0.1	0	24
5833	Squash, winter, all types, fresh, cubes	0.5 cup	58	20	1	5	1	0	0.0	0.0	0.0	0	79
90604	Squash, zucchini, baby, med, fresh	1 ea	11	2	0	0	0	0	0.0	0.0	0.0	0	0
5519	Tomatoes, green, fresh, chpd	0.5 cup	90	21	1	5	1	0	0.0	0.0	0.1	0	58
3973	Tomatoes, orange, fresh	1 ea	111	18	1	4	1	0	0.0	0.0	0.1	0	166
90530	Tomatoes, red, cherry, fresh, year round avg	1 ea	17	3	0	1	0	0	0.0	0.0	0.0	0	14
5178	Tomatoes, red, ckd f/fresh w/o salt	0.5 cup	120	22	1	5	1	0	0.0	0.0	0.1	0	58
5177	Tomatoes, red, ckd f/fresh w/o salt, med	1 ea	123	22	1	5	1	0	0.0	0.0	0.1	0	59
5170	Tomatoes, red, fresh, year round avg, chpd/sliced	0.5 cup	90	16	1	4	1	0	0.0	0.0	0.1	0	76
6492	Tomatoes, roma, fresh, year round avg, fresh	1 ea	62	11	1	2	1	0	0.0	0.0	0.1	0	52
5547	Turnip Greens, chpd, fresh	1 cup	55	18	1	4	2	0	0.0	0.0	0.1	0	0
5183	Turnips, ckd, drained, cubes	0.5 cup	78	17	1	4	2	0	0.0	0.0	0.0	0	0
5306	Yams, fresh, cubes	0.5 cup	75	88	1	21	3	0	0.0	0.0	0.1	0	10
Cooked Vegetables													
4437	Artichokes, French, hearts, ckd, drained	0.5 cup	84	42	3	9	5	0	0.0	0.0	0.1	0	15
5000	Artichokes, globe, ckd, drained, med	1 ea	120	60	4	13	6	0	0.0	0.0	0.1	0	22
5003	Asparagus, ckd, drained	0.5 cup	90	20	2	4	2	0	0.1	0.0	0.1	0	90
5249	Bamboo Shoots, slices, ckd, drained	1 cup	120	14	2	2	1	0	0.1	0.0	0.1	0	0
5025	Beet Greens, ckd, drained	1 cup	144	39	4	8	4	0	0.0	0.1	0.1	0	1103
5022	Beets, ckd, drained, sliced	0.5 cup	85	37	1	8	2	0	0.0	0.0	0.1	0	3
5407	Borage, ckd, drained	100 g	100	25	2	4	1	1	0.2	0.2	0.1	0	438
5028	Broccoli, chpd, ckd, drained	0.5 cup	78	27	2	6	3	0	0.1	0.0	0.1	0	153
6092	Broccoli, spears, ckd f/fzn w/salt, drained	0.5 cup	92	26	3	5	3	0	0.0	0.0	0.1	0	103
5234	Broccoli, spears, ckd f/fzn, drained	0.5 cup	92	26	3	5	3	0	0.0	0.0	0.1	0	103
5653	Broccoli, stmd	1 cup	156	44	5	8	5	1	0.1	0.0	0.3	0	228
5033	Brussels Sprouts, ckd, drained, cup	0.5 cup	78	28	2	6	2	0	0.1	0.0	0.2	0	61
5038	Cabbage, ckd, drained, shredded	1 cup	150	33	2	7	3	1	0.1	0.0	0.3	0	21
5238	Cabbage, red, ckd, drained, shredded	0.5 cup	75	22	1	5	2	0	0.0	0.0	0.0	0	3
5358	Carrots, ckd f/fzn w/o salt, drained, slices	0.5 cup	73	27	0	6	2	0	0.1	0.0	0.2	0	1213
5889	Carrots, ckd f/fzn w/salt, drained, slices	0.5 cup	73	27	0	6	2	0	0.1	0.0	0.2	0	1213
5656	Carrots, stir fried	1 cup	156	67	2	16	5	0	0.0	0.0	0.1	0	3955
5655	Carrots, stmd	1 cup	156	67	2	16	5	0	0.0	Mono	0.1	0	3955
5052	Cauliflower, florets, ckd, drained	3 ea	54	12	1	2	1	0	0.0	0.0	0.1	0	1
7266	Cauliflower, green, ckd, head	0.2 ea	90	29	3	6	3	0	0.0	0.0	0.1	0	13
5894	Celery, ckd w/salt, drained, diced	0.5 cup	75	14	1	3	1	0	0.0	0.0	0.1	0	44
5056	Celery, ckd, drained, diced	1 cup	150	27	1	6	2	0	0.1	0.0	0.1	0	87
6093	Collards, chpd, ckd w/salt, drained	1 cup	190	49	4	9	5	1	0.1	0.0	0.3	0	1543
5061	Collards, chpd, ckd, drained	0.5 cup	80	21	2	4	2	0	0.0	0.0	0.1	0	650
6917	Corn, white, sweet, cob, ckd f/fzn w/salt, drained	1 ea	63	59	2	14	2	0	0.1	0.1	0.2	0	0
5567	Corn, white, sweet, cob, ckd f/fzn, drained	1 ea	63	59	2	14	1	0	0.1	0.1	0.2	0	0
6019	Corn, white, sweet, kernels, ckd f/fzn w/salt, drained	0.5 cup	82	66	2	16	2	0	0.1	0.1	0.2	0	0
5393	Corn, white, sweet, kernels, ckd f/fzn, drained	0.5 cup	82	66	2	16	2	0	0.1	0.1	0.2	0	0
6964	Corn, yellow, sweet, kernels, ckd f/fzn cob w/salt, drnd	0.5 cup	82	76	3	18	2	1	0.1	0.2	0.3	0	20
5365	Corn, yellow, sweet, kernels, ckd f/fzn cob, drained	0.5 cup	82	76	3	18	2	1	0.1	0.2	0.3	0	20
5639	Cucumber, ckd	1 cup	180	29	2	6	2	0	0.1	0.0	0.1	0	42
5456	Dish, broccoli, w/cheese sauce, ckd	0.5 cup	114	115	7	6	2	8	3.6	2.5	1.1	16	152

Thia (mg)	Ribo (mg)	Niac (mg NE)	Vit B6 (mg)	Vit B12 (µg)	Fol (µg)	Vit C (mg)	Vit D (IU)	Vit E (mg AT)	Cal (mg)	Iron (mg)	Magn (mg)	Phos (mg)	Pota (mg)	Sodi (mg)	Zinc (mg)	Wat (%)	Alco (g)	Caff (g)
0.05	0.17	0.56	0.25	0.00	34.2	20.1	—	0.1	18	0.40	20.1	45	309	2	0.3	95	0.00	0.00
0.01	0.03	0.28	0.09	0.00	13.9	7.1	—	0.1	16	0.34	8.1	13	203	2	0.1	90	0.00	0.00
0.00	0.00	0.07	0.01	0.00	2.2	3.8	0.0	0.0	2	0.09	3.6	10	50	0	0.1	93	0.00	0.00
0.05	0.03	0.44	0.07	0.00	8.1	21.1	—	0.3	12	0.46	9.0	25	184	12	0.1	93	0.00	0.00
0.05	0.03	0.66	0.07	0.00	32.2	17.8	—	—	6	0.51	8.9	32	235	47	0.2	95	0.00	0.00
0.00	0.00	0.10	0.00	0.00	2.5	2.2	—	0.1	2	0.05	1.9	4	40	1	0.0	94	0.00	0.00
0.03	0.02	0.63	0.09	0.00	15.6	27.4	—	0.7	13	0.81	10.8	34	262	13	0.2	94	0.00	0.00
0.03	0.02	0.64	0.10	0.00	16.0	28.0	—	0.7	14	0.83	11.1	34	268	14	0.2	94	0.00	0.00
0.02	0.01	0.52	0.07	0.00	13.5	11.4	—	0.5	9	0.23	9.9	22	213	4	0.2	94	0.00	0.00
0.01	0.00	0.37	0.05	0.00	9.3	7.9	—	0.3	6	0.17	6.8	15	147	3	0.1	94	0.00	0.00
0.03	0.05	0.33	0.14	0.00	106.7	33.0	—	1.6	104	0.61	17.1	23	163	22	0.1	90	0.00	0.00
0.01	0.01	0.23	0.05	0.00	7.0	9.0	—	0.0	26	0.14	7.0	20	138	12	0.1	94	0.00	0.00
0.07	0.01	0.40	0.21	0.00	17.2	12.8	—	0.3	13	0.40	15.8	41	612	7	0.2	70	0.00	0.00
0.05	0.05	0.83	0.09	0.00	42.8	8.4	—	0.2	38	1.08	50.4	72	297	80	0.4	84	0.00	0.00
0.07	0.07	1.20	0.12	0.00	61.2	12.0	—	0.2	54	1.54	72.0	103	425	114	0.6	84	0.00	0.00
0.15	0.12	0.98	0.07	0.00	134.1	6.9	—	1.3	21	0.81	12.6	49	202	13	0.5	93	0.00	0.00
0.01	0.05	0.36	0.11	0.00	2.4	0.0	—	0.8	14	0.28	3.6	24	640	5	0.6	96	0.00	0.00
0.17	0.41	0.72	0.18	0.00	20.2	35.9	—	2.6	164	2.74	97.9	59	1309	347	0.7	89	0.00	0.00
0.01	0.02	0.28	0.05	0.00	68.0	3.1	—	0.0	14	0.67	19.6	32	259	65	0.3	87	0.00	0.00
0.05	0.17	0.93	0.09	0.00	10.0	32.5	—	—	102	3.64	57.0	55	491	88	0.2	92	0.00	0.00
0.05	0.10	0.43	0.15	0.00	84.2	50.6	—	1.1	31	0.51	16.4	52	229	32	0.4	89	0.00	0.00
0.05	0.07	0.41	0.11	0.00	27.6	36.9	—	1.2	47	0.56	18.4	51	166	239	0.3	91	0.00	0.00
0.05	0.07	0.41	0.11	0.00	27.6	36.9	—	1.2	47	0.56	18.4	51	166	22	0.3	91	0.00	0.00
0.09	0.18	0.93	0.21	0.00	93.9	123.4	0.0	0.7	75	1.37	39.0	103	505	42	0.6	91	0.00	0.00
0.07	0.05	0.46	0.14	0.00	46.8	48.4	—	0.3	28	0.93	15.6	44	247	16	0.3	89	0.00	0.00
0.09	0.07	0.41	0.17	0.00	30.0	30.2	—	0.2	46	0.25	12.0	22	146	12	0.1	94	0.00	0.00
0.05	0.03	0.28	0.17	0.00	18.0	8.1	—	0.1	32	0.50	12.8	25	196	6	0.2	91	0.00	0.00
0.01	0.02	0.30	0.05	0.00	8.0	1.7	—	0.7	26	0.38	8.0	23	140	43	0.3	90	0.00	0.00
0.01	0.02	0.30	0.05	0.00	8.0	1.7	0.0	0.3	26	0.38	8.0	23	140	215	0.3	90	0.00	0.00
0.14	0.09	1.37	0.21	0.00	20.7	11.6	0.0	0.7	42	0.77	23.4	69	504	55	0.3	88	0.00	0.00
0.14	0.09	1.37	0.21	0.00	20.7	10.9	0.0	0.7	42	0.77	23.4	69	504	55	0.3	88	0.00	0.00
0.01	0.02	0.21	0.09	0.00	23.8	23.9	—	0.0	9	0.18	4.9	17	77	8	0.1	93	0.00	0.00
0.05	0.09	0.61	0.18	0.00	36.9	65.3	—	0.0	29	0.64	17.1	51	250	21	0.6	89	0.00	0.00
0.02	0.03	0.23	0.05	0.00	16.5	4.6	0.0	0.3	32	0.31	9.0	19	213	245	0.1	94	0.00	0.00
0.05	0.07	0.47	0.12	0.00	33.0	9.1	—	0.5	63	0.62	18.0	38	426	136	0.2	94	0.00	0.00
0.07	0.20	1.09	0.23	0.00	176.7	34.6	0.0	1.7	266	2.20	38.0	57	220	479	0.4	92	0.00	0.00
0.02	0.07	0.46	0.10	0.00	74.4	14.6	—	0.7	112	0.93	16.0	24	93	13	0.2	92	0.00	0.00
0.10	0.03	0.95	0.14	0.00	19.5	3.0	—	0.0	2	0.37	18.3	47	158	151	0.4	73	0.00	0.00
0.10	0.03	0.95	0.14	0.00	19.5	3.0	—	0.0	2	0.37	18.3	47	158	3	0.4	73	0.00	0.00
0.07	0.05	1.07	0.10	0.00	25.4	2.5	—	0.1	3	0.28	15.6	47	121	201	0.3	77	0.00	0.00
0.07	0.05	1.07	0.10	0.00	25.4	2.5	—	0.1	3	0.28	15.6	47	121	4	0.3	77	0.00	0.00
0.14	0.05	1.24	0.18	0.00	25.4	3.9	—	0.1	2	0.50	23.8	62	206	197	0.5	73	0.00	0.00
0.14	0.05	1.24	0.18	0.00	25.4	3.9	—	0.1	2	0.50	23.8	62	206	3	0.5	73	0.00	0.00
0.03	0.05	0.43	0.07	0.00	20.2	9.4	0.0	0.2	30	0.55	23.2	40	288	4	0.4	95	0.00	0.00
0.05	0.18	0.54	0.11	0.14	39.4	54.0	—	1.7	161	0.79	25.0	138	268	202	0.8	81	0.00	0.00

PAGE KEY: A-108 Beverage and Beverage Mixes   A-110 Other Beverages   A-110 Beverages, Alcoholic   A-112 Candies and Confections, Gum   A-116 Cereals, Breakfast Type   A-120 Cheese and Cheese Substitutes   A-122 Dairy Products and Substitutes   A-124 Desserts   A-130 Dessert Toppings   A-130 Eggs, Substitutes, and Egg Dishes   A-132 Ethnic Foods   A-136 Fast Foods/Restaurants   A-150 Fats, Oils, Margarines, Shortenings, and Substitutes   A-150 Fish, Seafood, and Shellfish   A-152 Food Additives   A-152 Fruit, Vegetable, or Blended Juices   A-154 Grains, Flours, and Fractions   A-154 Grain Products, Prepared and Baked Goods

Code	Food Name	Unit/ Amt	Wt (g)	Energy (kcal)	Prot (g)	Carb (g)	Fiber (g)	Fat (g)	Sat (g)	Mono (g)	Poly (g)	Chol (mg)	Vit A (RE)
5457	Dish, broccoli, w/cream sauce, ckd	0.5 cup	114	87	4	8	2	5	1.3	2.0	1.4	3	154
5989	Dish, succotash, ckd w/salt, drained	0.5 cup	96	110	5	23	5	1	0.1	0.1	0.4	0	29
5642	Eggplant, batter dipped, fried	1 pce	50	75	1	6	1	5	1.1	2.3	1.7	8	4
5072	Eggplant, ckd, drained, 1" cubes	0.5 cup	50	17	0	4	1	0	0.0	0.0	0.0	0	2
5673	Eggplant, stmd	1 cup	96	25	1	6	2	0	0.0	0.0	0.1	0	8
5640	Hominy, ckd	1 cup	165	119	2	24	4	1	0.2	0.4	0.7	0	0
7957	Hummus, cmrcl	1 cup	250	415	20	36	15	24	3.6	10.1	9.0	0	10
5075	Kale, ckd, drained	0.5 cup	65	18	1	4	1	0	0.0	0.0	0.1	0	885
5514	Mushrooms, batter dipped, fried	5 ea	70	156	2	11	1	12	1.5	3.6	6.0	2	6
5924	Mushrooms, ckd w/salt, drained, pieces	0.5 cup	78	22	2	4	2	0	0.0	0.0	0.1	0	0
5092	Mushrooms, ckd, drained	0.5 cup	78	22	2	4	2	0	0.0	0.0	0.1	0	0
5384	Mushrooms, shiitake, ckd, whole	4 ea	72	40	1	10	2	0	0.0	0.0	0.0	0	0
5657	Mushrooms, stmd	1 cup	156	39	3	7	2	1	0.1	0.0	0.3	0	0
5643	Mushrooms, stuffed	2 ea	48	138	5	13	1	7	2.2	3.1	1.6	6	50
5096	Mustard Greens, ckd, drained	1 cup	140	21	3	3	3	0	0.0	0.2	0.1	0	885
5644	Okra, batter dipped, fried	1 cup	92	175	2	14	2	13	1.7	3.1	7.1	2	39
5932	Okra, ckd f/fzn w/salt, drained, slices	0.5 cup	92	26	2	5	3	0	0.1	0.0	0.1	0	31
70623	Onion Rings	6 ea	88	222	3	27	—	12	1.9	4.1	5.1	0	9
6074	Onion, ckd w/salt, drained	0.5 cup	105	46	1	11	1	0	0.0	0.0	0.1	0	0
5529	Onion, pearl, ckd, whole	3 ea	45	20	1	5	1	0	0.0	0.0	0.0	0	0
7811	Onion, red, ckd, drained, chpd	0.5 cup	105	46	1	11	1	0	0.0	0.0	0.1	0	0
5650	Onion, stir fried	1 cup	210	80	2	18	4	0	0.1	0.0	0.1	0	0
5649	Onion, stmd	1 cup	210	80	2	18	4	0	0.1	0.0	0.1	0	0
5108	Onion, white, ckd, drained, chpd	0.5 cup	105	46	1	11	1	0	0.0	0.0	0.1	0	0
7812	Onion, yellow, ckd, drained, chpd	0.5 cup	105	46	1	11	1	0	0.0	0.0	0.1	0	0
5212	Parsnips, ckd, drained	1 cup	156	111	2	27	6	0	0.1	0.2	0.1	0	0
5662	Peppers, bell, green, sweet, chpd, stir fried	0.5 cup	68	18	1	4	1	0	0.0	0.0	0.1	0	39
5661	Peppers, bell, green, sweet, chpd, stmd	0.5 cup	68	18	1	4	1	0	0.0	0.0	0.1	0	41
9549	Peppers, bell, green, sweet, sauteed	100 g	100	127	1	4	2	12	1.6	2.3	5.9	0	28
5663	Peppers, bell, red, sweet, chpd, stmd	0.5 cup	68	18	1	4	1	0	0.0	0.0	0.1	0	368
5229	Poi	0.5 cup	120	134	0	33	0	0	0.0	0.0	0.1	0	7
9366	Potatoes, white, baby, ckd	0.5 cup	85	70	2	15	1	0	0.0	0.0	0.0	0	0
9368	Potatoes, yukon gold, ckd	0.5 cup	85	70	2	15	1	0	0.0	0.0	0.0	0	0
5426	Purslane, ckd, drained	0.5 cup	58	10	1	2	—	0	0.0	0.0	0.0	0	107
7226	Rutabaga, ckd, drained, mashed	0.5 cup	120	47	2	10	2	0	0.0	0.0	0.1	0	0
5459	Soybean Sprouts, mature, stmd	0.5 cup	47	38	4	3	0	2	0.3	0.5	1.2	0	2
6227	Spinach, chpd, fzn	0.33 cup	85	20	3	3	2	0	0.1	—	—	0	681
5972	Spinach, ckd w/salt, drained	0.5 cup	90	21	3	3	2	0	0.0	0.0	0.1	0	943
5147	Spinach, ckd, drained	0.5 cup	90	21	3	3	2	0	0.0	0.0	0.1	0	943
5670	Spinach, stmd	0.5 cup	95	21	3	3	3	0	0.1	0.0	0.1	0	607
5316	Squash, acorn, ckd, mashed	0.5 cup	122	42	1	11	3	0	0.0	0.0	0.0	0	100
5317	Squash, butternut, bkd, cubes	0.5 cup	102	41	1	11	3	0	0.0	0.0	0.0	0	1144
5455	Squash, spaghetti, bkd/ckd, drained	0.5 cup	78	21	1	5	1	0	0.0	0.0	0.1	0	9
6922	Squash, spaghetti, ckd w/salt, drained	0.5 cup	78	21	1	5	1	0	0.0	0.0	0.1	0	9
5975	Squash, summer, all types, ckd w/salt, drained	0.5 cup	90	18	1	4	1	0	0.1	0.0	0.1	0	20

PAGE KEY: A-158 Granola Bars, Cereal Bars, Diet Bars, Scones, and Tarts   A-158 Meals and Dishes   A-162 Meats   A-168 Nuts, Seeds, and Products   A-170 Poultry   A-172 Salad Dressings, Dips, and Mayonnaise   A-172 Salads   A-174 Sandwiches   A-176 Sauces and Gravies   A-176 Snack Foods—Chips, Pretzels, Popcorn   A-178 Soups, Stews, and Chilis   A-180 Spices, Flavors, and Seasonings   A-182 Sports Bars and Drinks   A-182 Supplemental Foods and Formulas   A-184 Sweeteners and Sweet Substitutes   A-184 Vegetables and Legumes   A-198 Weight Loss Bars and Drinks   A-200 Miscellaneous

Thia (mg)	Ribo (mg)	Niac (mg NE)	Vit B6 (mg)	Vit B12 (µg)	Fol (µg)	Vit C (mg)	Vit D (IU)	Vit E (mg AT)	Cal (mg)	Iron (mg)	Magn (mg)	Phos (mg)	Pota (mg)	Sodi (mg)	Zinc (mg)	Wat (%)	Alco (g)	Caff (g)
0.07	0.14	0.50	0.10	0.12	22.7	27.6	—	1.3	89	0.56	20.0	83	194	180	0.4	84	0.00	0.00
0.15	0.09	1.26	0.10	0.00	31.7	7.9	—	0.3	16	1.46	50.9	112	394	243	0.6	68	0.00	0.00
0.05	0.03	0.46	0.03	0.02	7.4	0.6	—	0.8	14	0.34	7.6	23	106	15	0.1	74	0.00	0.00
0.03	0.00	0.30	0.03	0.00	6.9	0.6	—	0.2	3	0.11	5.4	7	61	0	0.1	90	0.00	0.00
0.05	0.02	0.55	0.07	0.00	15.5	1.4	0.0	0.0	7	0.25	13.4	21	208	3	0.1	92	0.00	0.00
0.00	0.00	0.05	0.00	0.00	1.6	0.0	0.0	0.1	16	1.01	26.4	58	15	346	1.7	83	0.00	0.00
0.44	0.15	1.46	0.50	0.00	207.5	0.0	—	—	95	6.09	177.5	440	570	948	4.6	67	0.00	0.00
0.02	0.05	0.31	0.09	0.00	8.4	26.6	0.0	0.6	47	0.57	11.7	18	148	15	0.2	91	0.00	0.00
0.10	0.25	2.25	0.03	0.02	8.3	1.2	—	2.3	15	1.22	6.8	119	154	112	0.4	63	0.00	0.00
0.05	0.23	3.48	0.07	0.00	14.0	3.1	59.3	0.0	5	1.36	9.4	68	278	186	0.7	91	0.00	0.00
0.05	0.23	3.48	0.07	0.00	14.0	3.1	—	0.0	5	1.36	9.4	68	278	2	0.7	91	0.00	0.00
0.02	0.11	1.08	0.10	0.00	15.1	0.2	—	0.0	2	0.31	10.1	21	84	3	1.0	83	0.00	0.00
0.14	0.67	6.13	0.14	0.00	28.1	4.7	0.0	0.2	8	1.92	15.6	162	577	6	1.1	92	0.00	0.00
0.15	0.25	2.64	0.07	0.10	11.0	2.8	25.0	0.8	100	1.49	14.3	107	209	298	0.7	43	0.07	0.00
0.05	0.09	0.61	0.14	0.00	102.2	35.4	—	1.7	104	0.98	21.0	57	283	22	0.2	94	0.00	0.00
0.18	0.14	1.44	0.11	0.03	38.1	10.3	11.0	3.0	61	1.25	35.8	122	190	122	0.5	67	0.00	0.00
0.09	0.10	0.72	0.03	0.00	134.3	11.2	—	0.3	88	0.62	46.9	42	215	220	0.6	91	0.00	0.00
0.07	0.03	1.05	—	0.00	—	4.2	—	—	18	0.82	—	—	161	200	—	52	0.00	0.00
0.03	0.01	0.17	0.14	0.00	15.7	5.5	—	0.0	23	0.25	11.5	37	174	251	0.2	88	0.00	0.00
0.01	0.00	0.07	0.05	0.00	6.8	2.3	0.0	0.1	10	0.10	4.9	16	75	1	0.1	88	0.00	0.00
0.03	0.01	0.17	0.14	0.00	15.7	5.5	—	0.0	23	0.25	11.5	37	174	3	0.2	88	0.00	0.00
0.07	0.03	0.30	0.23	0.00	32.3	10.9	0.0	0.7	42	0.46	21.0	69	330	6	0.4	90	0.00	0.00
0.07	0.03	0.30	0.23	0.00	32.3	10.2	0.0	0.7	42	0.46	21.0	69	330	6	0.4	90	0.00	0.00
0.03	0.01	0.17	0.14	0.00	15.7	5.5	—	0.0	23	0.25	11.5	37	174	3	0.2	88	0.00	0.00
0.03	0.01	0.17	0.14	0.00	15.7	5.5	—	0.0	23	0.25	11.5	37	174	3	0.2	88	0.00	0.00
0.12	0.07	1.12	0.15	0.00	90.5	20.3	—	1.6	58	0.89	45.2	108	573	16	0.4	80	0.00	0.00
0.03	0.01	0.33	0.15	0.00	12.0	51.7	0.0	0.5	6	0.31	6.8	13	120	1	0.1	92	0.00	0.00
0.03	0.01	0.33	0.15	0.00	12.7	51.7	0.0	0.5	6	0.31	6.8	13	120	1	0.1	92	0.00	0.00
0.03	0.05	0.57	0.20	0.00	2.0	177.0	—	1.4	8	0.30	8.0	15	134	17	0.1	83	0.00	0.00
0.03	0.01	0.33	0.15	0.00	12.7	110.2	0.0	0.5	6	0.31	6.8	13	120	1	0.1	92	0.00	0.00
0.15	0.05	1.32	0.33	0.00	25.2	4.8	—	2.8	19	1.05	28.8	47	220	14	0.3	72	0.00	0.00
—	—	—	—	—	—	18.0	—	—	0	0.72	—	—	—	5	—	79	0.00	0.00
—	—	—	—	—	—	18.0	—	—	0	0.72	—	—	—	5	—	79	0.00	0.00
0.01	0.05	0.25	0.03	0.00	5.2	6.0	—	—	45	0.43	38.5	21	281	25	0.1	94	0.00	0.00
0.10	0.05	0.86	0.11	0.00	18.0	22.6	—	0.4	58	0.63	27.6	67	391	24	0.4	89	0.00	0.00
0.10	0.01	0.50	0.05	0.00	37.6	3.9	—	0.1	28	0.62	28.2	63	167	5	0.5	79	0.00	0.00
0.07	0.12	0.34	0.09	0.00	26.1	18.5	—	—	90	1.75	40.0	33	260	79	—	91	0.00	0.00
0.09	0.20	0.43	0.21	0.00	131.4	8.8	0.0	1.9	122	3.21	78.3	50	419	275	0.7	91	0.00	0.00
0.09	0.20	0.43	0.21	0.00	131.4	8.8	—	1.9	122	3.21	78.3	50	419	63	0.7	91	0.00	0.00
0.05	0.17	0.62	0.17	0.00	120.7	16.1	0.0	1.8	89	2.44	75.0	40	494	75	0.5	92	0.00	0.00
0.11	0.00	0.64	0.14	0.00	13.5	8.0	—	0.1	32	0.68	31.9	33	322	4	0.1	90	0.00	0.00
0.07	0.01	0.99	0.12	0.00	19.5	15.5	—	1.3	42	0.62	29.7	28	291	4	0.1	88	0.00	0.00
0.02	0.01	0.62	0.07	0.00	6.2	2.7	—	0.1	16	0.25	8.5	11	91	14	0.2	92	0.00	0.00
0.02	0.01	0.62	0.07	0.00	6.2	2.7	—	0.1	16	0.25	8.5	11	91	197	0.2	92	0.00	0.00
0.03	0.03	0.46	0.05	0.00	18.0	4.9	—	0.1	24	0.31	21.6	35	173	213	0.4	94	0.00	0.00

PAGE KEY: A-108 Beverage and Beverage Mixes   A-110 Other Beverages   A-110 Beverages, Alcoholic   A-112 Candies and Confections, Gum   A-116 Cereals, Breakfast Type
A-120 Cheese and Cheese Substitutes   A-122 Dairy Products and Substitutes   A-124 Desserts   A-130 Dessert Toppings   A-130 Eggs, Substitutes, and Egg Dishes   A-132 Ethnic Foods
A-136 Fast Foods/Restaurants   A-150 Fats, Oils, Margarines, Shortenings, and Substitutes   A-150 Fish, Seafood, and Shellfish   A-152 Food Additives
A-152 Fruit, Vegetable, or Blended Juices   A-154 Grains, Flours, and Fractions   A-154 Grain Products, Prepared and Baked Goods

Code	Food Name	Unit/ Amt	Wt (g)	Energy (kcal)	Prot (g)	Carb (g)	Fiber (g)	Fat (g)	Sat (g)	Mono (g)	Poly (g)	Chol (mg)	Vit A (RE)
5152	Squash, summer, all types, ckd, drained, slices	0.5 cup	90	18	1	4	1	0	0.1	0.0	0.1	0	20
5153	Squash, winter, ckd w/salt	1 cup	240	94	2	21	7	2	0.3	0.1	0.6	0	854
5667	Squash, zucchini, slices, stmd	0.5 cup	90	13	1	3	1	0	0.0	0.0	0.1	0	29
5327	Squash, zucchini, w/skin, ckd, drained, slices	0.5 cup	90	14	1	4	1	0	0.0	0.0	0.0	0	101
5059	Swiss Chard, ckd, drained, chpd	0.5 cup	88	18	2	4	2	0	0.0	0.0	0.0	0	536
5544	Taro, ckd, slices, Tahitian, Colocassia	0.5 cup	68	30	3	5	1	0	0.1	0.0	0.2	0	121
7277	Tempeh, ckd	3.6 oz	100	197	18	9	—	11	3.4	3.7	2.6	—	—
5536	Tomatoes, green, ckd/frd	1 ea	144	284	5	19	1	22	4.6	9.4	6.4	41	82
5628	Tomatoes, red, fried	1 ea	101	168	3	12	1	13	2.7	5.5	3.8	24	57
5185	Turnip Greens, chpd, ckd, drained	0.5 cup	72	14	1	3	3	0	0.0	0.0	0.1	0	549
6004	Turnip Greens, ckd w/salt, drained, chpd	0.5 cup	72	14	1	3	3	0	0.0	0.0	0.1	0	549
6233	Vegetables, mixed, broccoli cauliflower carrots, fzn	0.5 cup	92	25	2	5	2	0	0.0	—	—	0	500
6644	Vegetables, mixed, broccoli cauliflower, fzn	0.5 cup	91	22	2	4	—	0	0.1	—	—	0	41
5187	Vegetables, mixed, ckd f/fzn w/o salt, drnd, 10 oz pkg	1 cup	182	118	5	24	8	0	0.1	0.0	0.1	0	779
6007	Vegetables, mixed, ckd f/fzn w/salt, drained	0.5 cup	91	54	3	12	4	0	0.0	0.0	0.1	0	389
6224	Vegetables, mixed, fzn	0.33 cup	85	52	2	12	3	0	0.1	—	—	0	582
6010	Yams, ckd/bkd w/salt, cubes	0.5 cup	68	79	1	19	3	0	0.0	0.0	0.0	0	8
5168	Yams, ckd/bkd, cubes	0.5 cup	68	79	1	19	3	0	0.0	0.0	0.0	0	8

Frozen, Dehydrated, and Dried Vegetables

Code	Food Name	Unit/ Amt	Wt (g)	Energy (kcal)	Prot (g)	Carb (g)	Fiber (g)	Fat (g)	Sat (g)	Mono (g)	Poly (g)	Chol (mg)	Vit A (RE)
5361	Asparagus, spears, fzn	4 pce	58	14	2	2	1	0	0.0	0.0	0.1	0	55
6388	Broccoli, cuts, fzn	0.66 cup	90	25	2	4	2	0	0.0	0.0	0.0	0	40
6551	Broccoli, florets, select, fzn	1.33 cup	83	25	2	4	2	0	0.0	0.0	0.0	0	50
5740	Carrots, fzn, slices	0.5 cup	64	23	0	5	2	0	0.0	0.0	0.2	0	719
70617	Corn, cob, fzn	1 ea	174	212	6	45	—	6	1.1	0.2	0.3	0	59
6706	Corn, cob, Nibblers, fzn	1 ea	61	70	2	14	1	0	0.0	—	—	0	0
56958	Corn, cream style, fzn	0.5 cup	118	110	2	23	2	1	0.0	—	—	0	0
6392	Corn, niblets, fzn	0.66 cup	96	80	3	17	3	0	0.0	—	—	0	0
6018	Corn, white, sweet, kernels, fzn	0.5 cup	82	72	2	17	2	1	0.1	0.2	0.3	0	0
338	Dish, mixed vegetables, skillet, fzn	0.66 cup	82	25	2	4	2	0	0.0	0.0	0.0	0	200
6558	Mushrooms, dehyd	100 g	100	285	24	53	9	5	0.7	0.1	2.0	0	0
90491	Onion Rings, breaded, par fried, heated f/fzn	1 cup	48	195	3	18	1	13	4.1	5.2	2.5	0	11
5492	Onion, green, dehyd	100 g	100	295	20	66	10	2	0.3	0.3	0.6	0	5900
1830	Spinach, 80% ckd, fzn	3 oz	85	20	2	3	2	0	0.0	0.0	0.0	0	600
5446	Tomatoes, sun dried	0.5 cup	27	70	4	15	3	1	0.1	0.1	0.3	0	24
5821	Turnip Greens, fzn, chpd/dices, 10 oz pkg	0.5 cup	82	18	2	3	2	0	0.1	0.0	0.1	0	507
6395	Vegetables, stew style, fzn	0.5 cup	65	38	1	8	0	0	0.0	0.0	0.0	0	49

Canned Vegetables

Code	Food Name	Unit/ Amt	Wt (g)	Energy (kcal)	Prot (g)	Carb (g)	Fiber (g)	Fat (g)	Sat (g)	Mono (g)	Poly (g)	Chol (mg)	Vit A (RE)
7867	Artichokes, hearts, cnd, pieces	3 pce	80	30	2	5	0	0	0.0	0.0	0.0	0	10
6261	Asparagus, spears, cnd	128 g	128	20	2	3	1	0	0.0	0.0	0.0	0	40
6607	Beets, slices, cnd	0.5 cup	121	35	1	8	2	0	0.0	0.0	0.0	0	0
5199	Carrots, cnd, drained, slices	1 ea	3	1	0	0	0	0	0.0	0.0	0.0	0	31
7933	Chili Peppers, green, cnd	0.5 cup	70	15	1	3	1	0	0.0	0.0	0.1	0	8
6268	Corn, cnd	0.33 cup	77	70	2	15	2	0	0.0	0.0	0.0	0	0
6265	Corn, cream style, cnd	0.5 cup	127	100	2	22	1	0	0.0	—	—	0	20
51031	Corn, golden, cream style, cnd	0.5 cup	125	90	2	20	2	1	0.0	—	—	0	0

PAGE KEY: A-158 Granola Bars, Cereal Bars, Diet Bars, Scones, and Tarts   A-158 Meals and Dishes   A-162 Meats   A-168 Nuts, Seeds, and Products   A-170 Poultry
A-172 Salad Dressings, Dips, and Mayonnaise   A-172 Salads   A-174 Sandwiches   A-176 Sauces and Gravies   A-176 Snack Foods—Chips, Pretzels, Popcorn
A-178 Soups, Stews, and Chilis   A-180 Spices, Flavors, and Seasonings   A-182 Sports Bars and Drinks   A-182 Supplemental Foods and Formulas
A-184 Sweeteners and Sweet Substitutes   A-184 Vegetables and Legumes   A-198 Weight Loss Bars and Drinks   A-200 Miscellaneous

Thia (mg)	Ribo (mg)	Niac (mg NE)	Vit B6 (mg)	Vit B12 (µg)	Fol (µg)	Vit C (mg)	Vit D (IU)	Vit E (mg AT)	Cal (mg)	Iron (mg)	Magn (mg)	Phos (mg)	Pota (mg)	Sodi (mg)	Zinc (mg)	Wat (%)	Alco (g)	Caff (g)
0.03	0.03	0.46	0.05	0.00	18.0	4.9	—	0.1	24	0.31	21.6	35	173	1	0.4	94	0.00	0.00
0.20	0.05	1.67	0.17	0.00	67.2	23.0	—	0.3	34	0.79	19.2	48	1049	2	0.6	89	0.00	0.00
0.05	0.02	0.34	0.07	0.00	16.9	6.9	0.0	0.1	14	0.37	19.8	29	223	3	0.2	95	0.00	0.00
0.03	0.03	0.38	0.07	0.00	15.3	4.1	—	0.1	12	0.31	19.8	36	228	3	0.2	95	0.00	0.00
0.02	0.07	0.31	0.07	0.00	7.9	15.8	—	1.7	51	1.98	75.2	29	480	157	0.3	93	0.00	0.00
0.02	0.14	0.33	0.07	0.00	4.8	26.0	—	1.8	102	1.07	34.9	46	427	37	0.1	86	0.00	0.00
0.05	0.36	2.13	0.20	0.14	21.0	—	—	—	96	2.13	77.0	253	401	14	1.6	60	0.00	0.00
0.15	0.18	1.36	0.10	0.14	12.7	20.9	9.2	3.0	101	1.50	17.1	102	254	134	0.4	68	0.00	0.00
0.10	0.11	0.97	0.07	0.07	11.8	13.4	6.5	1.8	55	0.93	12.6	62	200	78	0.2	72	0.00	0.00
0.02	0.05	0.30	0.12	0.00	85.0	19.7	—	1.4	99	0.57	15.8	21	146	21	0.1	93	0.00	0.00
0.02	0.05	0.30	0.12	0.00	85.0	19.7	0.0	1.4	99	0.57	15.8	21	146	191	0.1	93	0.00	0.00
0.05	0.07	0.46	0.15	0.00	50.0	43.7	—	—	31	0.51	12.9	39	192	28	—	—	0.00	0.00
—	—	—	—	0.00	—	—	54.7	—	29	0.44	—	—	—	22	—	—	0.00	0.00
0.12	0.21	1.54	0.12	0.00	34.6	5.8	—	0.8	46	1.49	40.0	93	308	64	0.9	83	0.00	0.00
0.05	0.10	0.76	0.07	0.00	17.3	2.9	0.0	0.3	23	0.75	20.0	46	154	247	0.4	83	0.00	0.00
0.09	0.05	1.01	0.11	0.00	23.8	7.6	—	—	20	0.72	16.1	47	167	37	—	83	0.00	0.00
0.05	0.01	0.37	0.15	0.00	10.9	8.2	—	0.3	10	0.34	12.2	33	456	166	0.1	70	0.00	0.00
0.05	0.01	0.37	0.15	0.00	10.9	8.2	—	0.3	10	0.34	12.2	33	456	5	0.1	70	0.00	0.00
0.07	0.07	0.69	0.05	0.00	110.8	18.4	—	1.2	14	0.41	8.1	37	147	5	0.3	92	0.00	0.00
—	—	—	—	0.00	—	42.0	—	—	20	0.72	—	—	—	150	—	93	0.00	0.00
—	—	—	—	—	—	36.0	—	—	0	0.00	—	—	—	20	—	92	0.00	0.00
0.02	0.01	0.30	0.05	0.00	6.4	1.6	—	0.5	23	0.28	7.7	21	150	44	0.2	90	0.00	0.00
0.14	0.14	4.30	—	0.00	—	14.9	—	—	—	1.66	—	—	532	26	—	67	0.00	0.00
—	—	—	—	0.00	—	2.4	—	—	0	0.00	—	—	—	5	—	72	0.00	0.00
—	—	—	—	—	—	40.0	—	—	0	0.00	—	—	—	330	—	—	0.00	0.00
—	—	—	—	0.00	—	1.2	—	—	0	0.36	—	—	—	60	—	78	0.00	0.00
0.07	0.05	1.41	0.15	0.00	29.5	5.2	0.0	0.0	3	0.34	14.8	57	172	2	0.3	75	0.00	0.00
—	—	—	—	—	—	18.0	—	—	0	0.00	—	—	—	30	—	—	0.00	0.00
1.13	5.13	47.00	1.13	0.00	241.0	40.0	—	—	57	14.19	114.0	1187	4224	46	8.3	6	0.00	0.00
0.12	0.07	1.73	0.03	0.00	31.7	0.7	—	0.3	15	0.81	9.1	39	62	180	0.2	28	0.00	0.00
0.82	1.64	2.35	0.00	0.00	162.0	531.0	—	—	708	22.29	236.0	390	3034	47	5.2	4	0.00	0.00
—	—	—	—	—	—	6.0	—	—	60	0.36	—	—	—	115	—	93	0.00	0.00
0.14	0.12	2.44	0.09	0.00	18.4	10.6	—	0.0	30	2.45	52.4	96	925	566	0.5	15	0.00	0.00
0.03	0.07	0.31	0.07	0.00	60.7	22.0	—	1.9	97	1.24	22.1	22	151	10	0.1	93	0.00	0.00
0.05	0.01	1.05	—	0.00	—	2.3	—	—	0	0.00	—	—	152	38	—	85	0.00	0.00
—	—	—	—	0.00	—	3.6	—	—	0	1.08	—	—	0	200	—	91	0.00	0.00
—	—	—	—	—	—	12.0	—	—	0	0.36	—	—	—	450	—	95	0.00	0.00
—	—	—	—	—	—	0.0	—	—	0	1.08	—	—	—	260	—	92	0.00	0.00
0.00	0.00	0.01	0.00	0.00	0.3	0.1	—	0.0	1	0.01	0.2	1	5	7	0.0	93	0.00	0.00
0.00	0.01	0.43	0.07	0.00	37.5	23.8	—	—	25	0.92	2.8	8	79	276	0.1	93	0.00	0.00
—	—	—	—	—	—	2.4	—	—	0	0.00	—	—	—	230	—	77	0.00	0.00
—	—	—	—	—	—	2.4	—	—	0	0.00	—	—	—	430	—	80	0.00	0.00
—	—	—	—	—	—	2.4	—	—	0	0.36	—	—	—	360	—	81	0.00	0.00

PAGE KEY: A-108 Beverage and Beverage Mixes   A-110 Other Beverages   A-110 Beverages, Alcoholic   A-112 Candies and Confections, Gum   A-116 Cereals, Breakfast Type
A-120 Cheese and Cheese Substitutes   A-122 Dairy Products and Substitutes   A-124 Desserts   A-130 Dessert Toppings   A-130 Eggs, Substitutes, and Egg Dishes   A-132 Ethnic Foods
A-136 Fast Foods/Restaurants   A-150 Fats, Oils, Margarines, Shortenings, and Substitutes   A-150 Fish, Seafood, and Shellfish   A-152 Food Additives
A-152 Fruit, Vegetable, or Blended Juices   A-154 Grains, Flours, and Fractions   A-154 Grain Products, Prepared and Baked Goods

Code	Food Name	Unit/Amt	Wt (g)	Energy (kcal)	Prot (g)	Carb (g)	Fiber (g)	Fat (g)	Sat (g)	Mono (g)	Poly (g)	Chol (mg)	Vit A (RE)
51059	Corn, golden, whole kernel, cnd	0.5 cup	125	90	2	18	3	1	0.0	—	—	0	0
7855	Corn, whole kernel, cnd	0.5 cup	125	90	2	14	2	1	0.0	—	—	0	0
38077	Hominy, white, cnd	0.5 cup	82	59	1	12	2	1	0.1	0.2	0.3	0	0
5094	Mushrooms, cnd, drained, pces/slices	0.5 cup	78	20	1	4	2	0	0.0	0.0	0.1	0	0
5095	Mushrooms, cnd, drained, whole, med	1 ea	12	3	0	1	0	0	0.0	0.0	0.0	0	0
27169	Olives, black, jumbo, cnd	1 ea	8	7	0	0	0	1	0.1	0.4	0.0	0	3
9539	Olives, green, pickled, cnd	100 g	100	145	1	4	3	15	2.0	11.3	1.3	0	40
92209	Pickles, bread & butter	1 ea	8	6	0	1	0	0	0.0	0.0	0.0	0	1
90583	Pickles, dill, chpd/diced	1 cup	143	26	1	6	2	0	0.1	0.0	0.1	0	26
27028	Pickles, dill, low sod, med	1 ea	65	12	0	3	1	0	0.0	0.0	0.1	0	21
27039	Pickles, dill, rducd salt	1 ea	65	7	0	1	1	0	0.0	0.0	0.1	0	10
27013	Pickles, dill, slices	5 pce	35	6	0	1	0	0	0.0	0.0	0.0	0	6
27025	Pickles, sour	1 cup	155	17	1	4	2	0	0.1	0.0	0.1	0	22
90585	Pickles, sweet, slices	1 ea	7	8	0	2	0	0	0.0	0.0	0.0	0	1
5227	Pimentos, cnd	1 Tbs	12	3	0	1	0	0	0.0	0.0	0.0	0	32
5142	Pumpkin, cnd, unsalted	0.5 cup	122	42	1	10	4	0	0.2	0.0	0.0	0	1906
5964	Pumpkin, cnd, w/salt	0.5 cup	122	42	1	10	4	0	0.2	0.0	0.0	0	2702
27063	Relish, pickle, hotdog	1 Tbs	15	18	0	4	0	0	0.0	0.0	0.1	0	1
27052	Relish, pickle, sweet	1 cup	245	318	1	86	3	1	0.1	0.5	0.3	0	44
6393	Sauerkraut, crisp	30 g	30	5	0	1	1	0	0.0	0.0	0.0	0	0
5595	Spinach, cnd, not drained	0.5 cup	117	22	2	3	2	0	0.1	0.0	0.2	0	753
5599	Squash, zucchini, Italian style, cnd	0.5 cup	114	33	1	8	2	0	0.0	0.0	0.1	0	61
51000	Tomatoes, chunky, chili style, cnd	0.5 cup	128	30	1	8	2	0	0.0	0.0	0.0	0	50
51001	Tomatoes, chunky, pasta style, cnd	0.5 cup	128	45	1	11	2	0	0.0	0.0	0.0	0	50
6927	Tomatoes, crushed, cnd	0.5 cup	50	16	1	4	1	0	0.0	0.0	0.1	0	35
51005	Tomatoes, dices, cnd	0.5 cup	126	25	1	6	2	0	0.0	0.0	0.0	0	50
5630	Tomatoes, green, pickled	0.5 cup	71	26	1	6	1	0	0.0	0.1	0.1	0	59
6394	Tomatoes, pickled, halves	1 oz	28	5	0	1	1	0	0.0	0.0	0.0	0	0
6293	Tomatoes, puree, cnd	0.25 cup	63	20	1	4	0	0	0.0	0.0	0.0	0	50
9169	Tomatoes, stwd, cnd	0.5 cup	121	35	1	8	1	0	0.0	0.0	0.0	0	30
51020	Tomatoes, stwd, Italian recipe, cnd	0.5 cup	126	30	1	8	2	0	0.0	0.0	0.0	0	50
51022	Tomatoes, stwd, original recipe, cnd	0.5 cup	126	35	1	9	2	0	0.0	0.0	0.0	0	50
7885	Tomatoes, stwd, unsalted, cnd	0.5 cup	123	35	1	7	2	0	0.0	0.0	0.0	0	50
7896	Tomatoes, whole, peeled, cnd	0.5 cup	121	25	1	4	1	0	0.0	0.0	0.0	0	50
9520	Turnip Greens, cnd, unsalted	1 cup	144	27	2	4	2	0	0.1	0.0	0.2	0	858
51044	Vegetables, mixed, cnd	0.5 cup	124	40	2	8	2	0	0.0	0.0	0.0	0	225
5305	Vegetables, mixed, cnd, drained	0.5 cup	82	40	2	8	2	0	0.0	0.0	0.1	0	949
9522	Vegetables, mixed, cnd, unsalted	1 cup	182	67	3	13	6	0	0.1	0.0	0.2	0	2118
7873	Vegetables, peas & carrots, cnd	0.5 cup	123	50	4	10	3	0	0.0	0.0	0.0	0	500
Legumes													
7165	Beans, bbq	0.5 cup	100	160	6	32	6	2	0.5	—	—	—	—
7042	Beans, black turtle soup, mature, cnd	0.5 cup	120	109	7	20	8	0	0.1	0.0	0.2	0	0
7012	Beans, black, mature, ckd	1 cup	172	227	15	41	15	1	0.2	0.1	0.4	0	1
5213	Beans, blackeyed, immature, ckd, drained	0.5 cup	82	80	3	17	4	0	0.1	0.0	0.1	0	66
4450	Beans, blackeyed, mature, ckd	1 cup	172	200	13	36	11	1	0.2	0.1	0.4	0	3

PAGE KEY: A-158 Granola Bars, Cereal Bars, Diet Bars, Scones, and Tarts   A-158 Meals and Dishes   A-162 Meats   A-168 Nuts, Seeds, and Products   A-170 Poultry   A-172 Salad Dressings, Dips, and Mayonnaise   A-172 Salads   A-174 Sandwiches   A-176 Sauces and Gravies   A-176 Snack Foods—Chips, Pretzels, Popcorn   A-178 Soups, Stews, and Chilis   A-180 Spices, Flavors, and Seasonings   A-182 Sports Bars and Drinks   A-182 Supplemental Foods and Formulas   A-184 Sweeteners and Sweet Substitutes   A-184 Vegetables and Legumes   A-198 Weight Loss Bars and Drinks   A-200 Miscellaneous

Thia (mg)	Ribo (mg)	Niac (mg NE)	Vit B6 (mg)	Vit B12 (µg)	Fol (µg)	Vit C (mg)	Vit D (IU)	Vit E (mg AT)	Cal (mg)	Iron (mg)	Magn (mg)	Phos (mg)	Pota (mg)	Sodi (mg)	Zinc (mg)	Wat (%)	Alco (g)	Caff (g)
—	—	—	—	—	—	3.6	—	—	0	0.36	—	—	—	360	—	82	0.00	0.00
—	—	—	—	0.00	—	2.4	—	—	0	0.36	—	—	0	340	—	85	0.00	0.00
0.00	0.00	0.02	0.00	0.00	0.8	0.0	—	0.0	8	0.50	13.2	29	7	173	0.9	83	0.00	0.00
0.07	0.01	1.24	0.05	0.00	9.4	0.0	—	0.0	9	0.62	11.7	51	101	332	0.6	91	0.00	0.00
0.00	0.00	0.18	0.00	0.00	1.4	0.0	—	0.0	1	0.09	1.8	8	15	51	0.1	91	0.00	0.00
0.00	0.00	0.00	0.00	0.00	0.0	0.1	0.0	0.1	8	0.28	0.3	0	1	75	0.0	84	0.00	0.00
0.01	0.00	0.23	0.02	0.00	3.0	0.0	—	3.8	52	0.49	11.0	4	42	1556	0.0	75	0.00	0.00
0.00	0.00	0.00	0.00	0.00	0.3	0.7	—	0.0	3	0.02	0.2	2	16	54	0.0	79	0.00	0.00
0.01	0.03	0.09	0.01	0.00	1.4	2.7	—	0.1	13	0.75	15.7	30	166	1833	0.2	92	0.00	0.00
0.00	0.01	0.03	0.00	0.00	0.6	1.2	—	0.1	6	0.34	7.1	14	75	12	0.1	92	0.00	0.00
0.00	0.00	0.00	0.00	0.00	0.5	0.6	0.0	0.0	0	0.25	2.6	9	15	12	0.0	94	0.00	0.00
0.00	0.00	0.01	0.00	0.00	0.3	0.7	—	0.0	3	0.18	3.8	7	41	449	0.0	92	0.00	0.00
0.00	0.01	0.00	0.00	0.00	1.5	1.5	—	0.1	0	0.62	6.2	22	36	1872	0.0	94	0.00	0.00
0.00	0.00	0.00	0.00	0.00	0.1	0.1	—	0.0	0	0.03	0.3	1	2	66	0.0	65	0.00	0.00
0.00	0.00	0.07	0.02	0.00	0.7	10.2	—	0.1	1	0.20	0.7	2	19	2	0.0	93	0.00	0.00
0.02	0.07	0.44	0.07	0.00	14.7	5.1	—	1.3	32	1.70	28.2	43	252	6	0.2	90	0.00	0.00
0.02	0.07	0.44	0.07	0.00	14.7	5.1	—	1.2	32	1.70	28.2	43	252	295	0.2	90	0.00	0.00
0.00	0.00	0.00	0.00	0.00	0.8	0.9	0.0	0.0	4	0.20	3.2	3	31	81	0.0	69	0.00	0.00
0.00	0.07	0.56	0.03	0.00	2.5	2.5	—	0.2	7	2.13	12.2	34	61	1987	0.3	62	0.00	0.00
—	—	—	—	—	—	3.6	—	—	0	0.00	—	—	—	220	—	94	0.00	0.00
0.01	0.11	0.31	0.09	0.00	67.9	15.8	—	1.3	97	1.85	65.5	37	269	373	0.5	93	0.00	0.00
0.05	0.05	0.60	0.17	0.00	34.0	2.6	0.0	0.1	19	0.76	15.9	33	311	424	0.3	91	0.00	0.00
—	—	—	—	—	—	9.0	—	—	20	0.36	—	—	—	670	—	92	0.00	0.00
—	—	—	—	—	—	9.0	—	—	20	0.36	—	—	—	560	—	—	0.00	0.00
0.03	0.02	0.62	0.07	0.00	6.6	4.6	—	0.3	17	0.66	10.1	16	148	67	0.1	89	0.00	0.00
—	—	—	—	—	—	9.0	—	—	20	0.36	—	—	—	160	—	—	0.00	0.00
0.03	0.01	0.28	0.05	0.00	5.3	20.0	0.0	0.2	11	0.36	7.5	19	128	89	0.1	90	0.00	0.00
—	—	—	—	—	—	0.0	—	—	0	0.00	—	—	—	324	—	—	0.00	0.00
—	—	—	—	—	—	9.0	—	—	0	0.36	—	—	—	15	—	91	0.00	0.00
—	—	—	—	—	—	15.0	—	—	60	1.00	—	—	—	390	—	—	0.00	0.00
—	—	—	—	—	—	9.0	—	—	20	0.36	—	—	—	420	—	—	0.00	0.00
—	—	—	—	—	—	9.0	—	—	20	0.36	—	—	—	360	—	—	0.00	0.00
—	—	—	0.00	—	—	12.0	—	—	40	1.44	—	—	150	15	—	93	0.00	0.00
—	—	—	—	0.00	—	12.0	—	—	20	0.72	—	—	200	220	—	95	0.00	0.00
0.00	0.09	0.51	0.05	0.00	132.5	22.3	—	2.1	170	2.17	28.8	30	203	42	0.3	95	0.00	0.00
—	—	—	—	—	—	2.4	—	—	20	0.72	—	—	—	360	—	91	0.00	0.00
0.03	0.03	0.46	0.05	0.00	19.6	4.1	—	0.3	22	0.86	13.0	34	237	121	0.3	87	0.00	0.00
0.05	0.07	0.87	0.15	0.00	32.8	6.9	—	0.6	38	1.17	27.3	67	251	47	0.9	90	0.00	0.00
—	—	—	—	0.00	—	9.0	—	—	20	1.08	—	—	0	330	—	88	0.00	0.00
—	—	—	—	—	—	—	—	—	—	—	—	—	—	640	—	—	0.00	0.00
0.17	0.14	0.74	0.07	0.00	73.2	3.2	—	0.3	42	2.27	42.0	130	370	461	0.6	76	0.00	0.00
0.41	0.10	0.87	0.11	0.00	256.3	0.0	—	0.1	46	3.60	120.4	241	611	2	1.9	66	0.00	0.00
0.07	0.11	1.15	0.05	0.00	104.8	1.8	—	0.2	106	0.92	42.9	42	345	3	0.8	75	0.00	0.00
0.34	0.09	0.85	0.17	0.00	357.8	0.7	—	0.5	41	4.32	91.2	268	478	7	2.2	70	0.00	0.00

PAGE KEY: A-108 Beverage and Beverage Mixes   A-110 Other Beverages   A-110 Beverages, Alcoholic   A-112 Candies and Confections, Gum   A-116 Cereals, Breakfast Type   A-120 Cheese and Cheese Substitutes   A-122 Dairy Products and Substitutes   A-124 Desserts   A-130 Dessert Toppings   A-130 Eggs, Substitutes, and Egg Dishes   A-132 Ethnic Foods   A-136 Fast Foods/Restaurants   A-150 Fats, Oils, Margarines, Shortenings, and Substitutes   A-150 Fish, Seafood, and Shellfish   A-152 Food Additives   A-152 Fruit, Vegetable, or Blended Juices   A-154 Grains, Flours, and Fractions   A-154 Grain Products, Prepared and Baked Goods

Code	Food Name	Unit/ Amt	Wt (g)	Energy (kcal)	Prot (g)	Carb (g)	Fiber (g)	Fat (g)	Sat (g)	Mono (g)	Poly (g)	Chol (mg)	Vit A (RE)
7027	Beans, broad, mature, ckd	1 cup	170	187	13	33	9	1	0.1	0.1	0.3	0	3
7056	Beans, catjang cowpeas, ckd	1 cup	171	200	14	35	6	1	0.3	0.1	0.5	0	3
4441	Beans, chickpea, mature, ckd	0.5 cup	82	134	7	22	6	2	0.2	0.5	0.9	0	2
4465	Beans, cowpeas, immature, ckd, drained	1 cup	165	160	5	34	8	1	0.2	0.1	0.3	0	132
7018	Beans, cowpeas, mature, ckd	0.5 cup	86	100	7	18	6	0	0.1	0.0	0.2	0	2
4444	Beans, fava, mature, ckd	1 cup	170	187	13	33	9	1	0.1	0.1	0.3	0	3
7045	Beans, French, mature, ckd	1 cup	177	228	12	43	17	1	0.1	0.1	0.8	0	1
7175	Beans, garbanzo, cnd	0.5 cup	130	100	6	16	4	2	0.0	—	—	0	0
7001	Beans, garbanzo, mature, ckd	1 cup	164	269	15	45	12	4	0.4	1.0	1.9	0	3
7031	Beans, goa, mature, ckd	1 cup	172	253	18	26	4	10	1.4	3.7	2.7	0	0
7219	Beans, golden gram, mature, ckd	0.5 cup	101	106	7	19	8	0	0.1	0.1	0.1	0	2
7021	Beans, great northern, mature, ckd	1 cup	177	209	15	37	12	1	0.2	0.0	0.3	0	0
6219	Beans, green, cut, fzn	0.5 cup	83	25	1	6	2	0	0.0	—	—	0	44
6220	Beans, green, French cut, fzn	0.5 cup	83	25	1	6	2	0	0.0	—	—	0	38
5013	Beans, green, snap, ckd f/fzn, drained	1 cup	135	38	2	9	4	0	0.1	0.0	0.1	0	76
5856	Beans, green, snap, ckd w/salt, drained	1 cup	125	44	2	10	4	0	0.1	0.0	0.2	0	88
5009	Beans, green, snap, fresh	0.5 cup	55	17	1	4	2	0	0.0	0.0	0.0	0	38
6198	Beans, green, whole, deluxe, fzn	10 ea	40	11	1	2	1	0	0.0	—	—	0	27
6241	Beans, green, whole, fzn	21 ea	84	22	1	5	2	0	0.0	—	—	0	58
7008	Beans, kidney, all types, mature, ckd	1 cup	177	225	15	40	11	1	0.1	0.1	0.5	0	0
7047	Beans, kidney, red, mature, ckd	1 cup	177	225	15	40	13	1	0.1	0.1	0.5	0	0
7006	Beans, lentils, ckd f/dry w/o salt	0.5 cup	99	115	9	20	8	0	0.1	0.1	0.2	0	1
90019	Beans, lentils, mature, ckd w/salt	1 cup	198	230	18	40	16	1	0.1	0.1	0.3	0	2
6222	Beans, lima, baby, fzn	0.5 cup	94	126	7	24	6	0	0.1	—	—	0	22
7058	Beans, lima, baby, mature, ckd	0.5 cup	91	115	7	21	7	0	0.1	0.0	0.2	0	0
7010	Beans, lima, lrg, mature, ckd	1 cup	188	216	15	39	13	1	0.2	0.1	0.3	0	0
7059	Beans, mung, mature, ckd	0.5 cup	101	106	7	19	8	0	0.1	0.1	0.1	0	2
7022	Beans, navy, mature, ckd	1 cup	182	255	15	47	19	1	0.1	0.2	0.6	0	0
7050	Beans, pink, mature, ckd	1 cup	169	252	15	47	9	1	0.2	0.1	0.4	0	0
7013	Beans, pinto, mature, ckd	1 cup	171	245	15	45	15	1	0.2	0.2	0.3	0	0
7053	Beans, white, mature, ckd	1 cup	179	249	17	45	11	1	0.2	0.1	0.3	0	0
57290	Dish, green beans, French cut, w/toasted almonds, fzn	0.66 cup	81	51	2	6	2	3	0.3	—	—	0	33
5939	Peas, green, ckd f/fzn w/salt, drained	0.5 cup	80	62	4	11	4	0	0.0	0.0	0.1	0	53
5938	Peas, green, ckd w/salt, drained	0.5 cup	80	67	4	13	4	0	0.0	0.0	0.1	0	64
5116	Peas, green, fresh	1 cup	145	117	8	21	7	1	0.1	0.1	0.3	0	110
6226	Peas, green, fzn	0.5 cup	89	71	5	13	5	0	0.1	—	—	0	62
7020	Peas, split, ckd	1 cup	196	231	16	41	16	1	0.1	0.2	0.3	0	1
6364	Peas, sweet, fzn	0.66 cup	94	60	4	12	4	0	0.0	0.0	0.0	0	30
5971	Soybeans, green, ckd w/salt, drained	0.5 cup	90	127	11	10	4	6	0.7	1.1	2.7	0	14
7015	Soybeans, mature, ckd	1.25 cup	215	372	36	21	13	19	2.8	4.3	10.9	0	2
90028	Soybeans, mature, ckd w/salt	1.25 cup	215	372	36	21	13	19	2.8	4.3	10.9	0	2
5123	Vegetables, peas & carrots, ckd f/fzn, drnd	0.5 cup	80	38	2	8	2	0	0.1	0.0	0.2	0	749
Potatoes													
6179	Dish, baked potato & broccoli, w/cheese sauce	1 ea	339	403	14	47	—	21	8.5	7.7	4.2	20	315
5464	Dish, mashed potatoes, flakes, prep f/dry w/milk & butter	0.5 cup	105	102	2	11	1	5	2.9	1.2	0.1	15	46
5138	Dish, mashed potatoes, flakes, prep f/dry w/milk & margarine	0.5 cup	105	119	2	16	2	6	1.5	2.4	1.6	4	52

PAGE KEY: A-158 Granola Bars, Cereal Bars, Diet Bars, Scones, and Tarts   A-158 Meals and Dishes   A-162 Meats   A-168 Nuts, Seeds, and Products   A-170 Poultry   A-172 Salad Dressings, Dips, and Mayonnaise   A-172 Salads   A-174 Sandwiches   A-176 Sauces and Gravies   A-176 Snack Foods—Chips, Pretzels, Popcorn   A-178 Soups, Stews, and Chilis   A-180 Spices, Flavors, and Seasonings   A-182 Sports Bars and Drinks   A-182 Supplemental Foods and Formulas   A-184 Sweeteners and Sweet Substitutes   A-184 Vegetables and Legumes   A-198 Weight Loss Bars and Drinks   A-200 Miscellaneous

Thia (mg)	Ribo (mg)	Niac (mg NE)	Vit B6 (mg)	Vit B12 (µg)	Fol (µg)	Vit C (mg)	Vit D (IU)	Vit E (mg AT)	Cal (mg)	Iron (mg)	Magn (mg)	Phos (mg)	Pota (mg)	Sodi (mg)	Zinc (mg)	Wat (%)	Alco (g)	Caff (g)
0.15	0.15	1.21	0.11	0.00	176.8	0.5	—	0.0	61	2.54	73.1	212	456	8	1.7	72	0.00	0.00
0.28	0.07	1.22	0.15	0.00	242.8	0.7	—	0.6	44	5.21	164.2	243	641	32	3.2	70	0.00	0.00
0.10	0.05	0.43	0.10	0.00	141.0	1.1	—	0.3	40	2.36	39.4	138	239	6	1.3	60	0.00	0.00
0.17	0.23	2.30	0.10	0.00	209.6	3.6	—	0.4	211	1.85	85.8	84	690	7	1.7	75	0.00	0.00
0.17	0.05	0.43	0.09	0.00	178.9	0.3	—	0.2	21	2.16	45.6	134	239	3	1.1	70	0.00	0.00
0.15	0.15	1.21	0.11	0.00	176.8	0.5	—	0.0	61	2.54	73.1	212	456	8	1.7	72	0.00	0.00
0.23	0.10	0.97	0.18	0.00	132.8	2.1	—	0.2	112	1.90	99.1	181	655	11	1.1	67	0.00	0.00
—	—	—	—	—	—	0.0	—	—	40	1.44	—	—	—	340	—	—	0.00	0.00
0.18	0.10	0.86	0.23	0.00	282.1	2.1	—	0.6	80	4.73	78.7	276	477	11	2.5	60	0.00	0.00
0.50	0.21	1.42	0.07	0.00	17.2	0.0	—	0.2	244	7.44	92.9	263	482	22	2.5	67	0.00	0.00
0.17	0.05	0.57	0.07	0.00	160.6	1.0	—	0.2	27	1.40	48.5	100	269	2	0.8	73	0.00	0.00
0.28	0.10	1.21	0.20	0.00	180.5	2.3	—	0.5	120	3.76	88.5	292	692	4	1.6	69	0.00	0.00
0.03	0.07	0.02	0.03	0.00	10.8	8.9	—	—	35	0.70	16.6	22	128	3	—	—	0.00	0.00
0.05	0.07	0.25	0.03	0.00	11.1	7.6	—	—	38	0.79	18.3	21	141	3	—	—	0.00	0.00
0.05	0.11	0.51	0.07	0.00	31.1	5.5	—	0.5	66	1.19	32.4	42	170	12	0.6	91	0.00	0.00
0.09	0.11	0.76	0.07	0.00	41.2	12.1	—	0.6	58	1.60	31.2	49	374	299	0.5	89	0.00	0.00
0.05	0.05	0.40	0.03	0.00	20.4	9.0	—	0.2	20	0.56	13.8	21	115	3	0.1	90	0.00	0.00
0.01	0.03	0.11	0.01	0.00	4.7	4.3	—	—	15	0.31	8.0	10	71	1	—	—	0.00	0.00
0.05	0.07	0.25	0.03	0.00	9.8	9.1	—	—	32	0.64	16.8	21	149	2	—	—	0.00	0.00
0.28	0.10	1.01	0.20	0.00	230.1	2.1	—	0.1	62	3.93	74.3	244	717	2	1.8	67	0.00	0.00
0.28	0.10	1.01	0.20	0.00	230.1	2.1	—	1.5	50	5.19	79.7	251	713	4	1.9	67	0.00	0.00
0.17	0.07	1.04	0.18	0.00	179.2	1.5	—	0.1	19	3.29	35.6	178	365	2	1.3	70	0.00	0.00
0.33	0.14	2.09	0.34	0.00	358.4	3.0	—	0.2	38	6.59	71.3	356	731	471	2.5	70	0.00	0.00
0.09	0.07	1.12	0.15	0.00	83.2	18.0	—	—	32	1.85	45.1	96	471	114	0.9	65	0.00	0.00
0.15	0.05	0.60	0.07	0.00	136.5	0.0	—	0.2	26	2.18	48.2	116	365	3	0.9	67	0.00	0.00
0.30	0.10	0.79	0.30	0.00	156.0	0.0	—	0.3	32	4.48	80.8	209	955	4	1.8	70	0.00	0.00
0.17	0.05	0.57	0.07	0.00	160.6	1.0	—	0.2	27	1.40	48.5	100	269	2	0.8	73	0.00	0.00
0.43	0.11	1.17	0.25	0.00	254.8	1.6	—	0.0	126	4.30	96.5	262	708	0	1.9	64	0.00	0.00
0.43	0.10	0.95	0.30	0.00	283.9	0.0	—	1.7	88	3.89	109.9	279	859	3	1.6	61	0.00	0.00
0.33	0.10	0.54	0.38	0.00	294.1	1.4	—	1.6	79	3.56	85.5	251	746	2	1.7	63	0.00	0.00
0.20	0.07	0.25	0.17	0.00	145.0	0.0	—	1.7	161	6.61	112.8	202	1004	11	2.5	63	0.00	0.00
—	—	—	—	0.00	—	6.6	—	—	42	1.08	—	—	—	347	—	—	0.00	0.00
0.23	0.07	1.17	0.09	0.00	47.2	7.9	—	0.1	19	1.25	23.2	72	134	258	0.8	80	0.00	0.00
0.20	0.11	1.62	0.17	0.00	50.4	11.4	—	0.1	22	1.23	31.2	94	217	191	1.0	78	0.00	0.00
0.38	0.18	3.02	0.25	0.00	94.2	58.0	—	0.2	36	2.13	47.9	157	354	7	1.8	79	0.00	0.00
0.28	0.09	1.96	0.11	0.00	49.2	17.8	—	—	21	1.41	22.2	79	152	125	0.9	79	0.00	0.00
0.37	0.10	1.74	0.09	0.00	127.4	0.8	—	0.1	27	2.52	70.6	194	710	4	2.0	69	0.00	0.00
—	—	—	—	0.00	—	6.0	—	—	0	1.08	—	—	—	200	—	—	0.00	0.00
0.23	0.14	1.12	0.05	0.00	99.9	15.3	—	0.0	130	2.25	54.0	142	485	225	0.8	69	0.00	0.00
0.33	0.61	0.86	0.50	0.00	116.1	3.7	—	0.8	219	11.05	184.9	527	1107	2	2.5	63	0.00	0.00
0.33	0.61	0.86	0.50	0.00	116.1	3.7	—	0.8	219	11.05	184.9	527	1107	510	2.5	63	0.00	0.00
0.18	0.05	0.92	0.07	0.00	20.8	6.5	—	0.4	18	0.75	12.8	39	126	54	0.4	86	0.00	0.00
0.27	0.27	3.58	0.77	0.34	61.0	48.5	—	—	336	3.31	78.0	346	1441	485	2.0	70	0.00	0.00
0.14	0.05	0.80	0.10	0.11	6.3	10.6	12.9	0.1	30	0.17	11.5	41	170	172	0.2	81	0.00	0.00
0.11	0.05	0.69	0.00	0.00	7.3	10.2	—	0.7	51	0.23	18.9	59	245	349	0.2	76	0.00	0.00

PAGE KEY: A-108 Beverage and Beverage Mixes   A-110 Other Beverages   A-110 Beverages, Alcoholic   A-112 Candies and Confections, Gum   A-116 Cereals, Breakfast Type   A-120 Cheese and Cheese Substitutes   A-122 Dairy Products and Substitutes   A-124 Desserts   A-130 Dessert Toppings   A-130 Eggs, Substitutes, and Egg Dishes   A-132 Ethnic Foods   A-136 Fast Foods/Restaurants   A-150 Fats, Oils, Margarines, Shortenings, and Substitutes   A-150 Fish, Seafood, and Shellfish   A-152 Food Additives   A-152 Fruit, Vegetable, or Blended Juices   A-154 Grains, Flours, and Fractions   A-154 Grain Products, Prepared and Baked Goods

Code	Food Name	Unit/ Amt	Wt (g)	Energy (kcal)	Prot (g)	Carb (g)	Fiber (g)	Fat (g)	Sat (g)	Mono (g)	Poly (g)	Chol (mg)	Vit A (RE)
66107	Dish, mashed potatoes, real, premium, prep	0.5 cup	108	63	2	13	1	1	0.1	0.4	0.1	0	0
5137	Dish, mashed potatoes, w/whole milk	0.5 cup	105	87	2	18	2	1	0.3	0.1	0.1	2	4
5569	Dish, mashed potatoes, w/whole milk & butter	0.5 cup	105	119	2	18	2	4	1.8	1.3	0.2	12	38
5272	Dish, mashed potatoes, w/whole milk & margarine	0.5 cup	105	119	2	18	2	4	1.0	1.8	1.3	1	45
5786	Dish, potatoes au gratin, prep f/recipe w/butter	1 cup	245	323	12	28	4	19	11.6	5.3	0.7	56	164
5275	Dish, potatoes au gratin, prep f/recipe w/margarine	1 cup	245	323	12	28	4	19	8.6	6.3	2.6	37	167
70605	Dish, potatoes o'brien	0.5 cup	78	56	1	12	2	0	0.0	0.0	0.0	0	0
5787	Dish, potatoes o'brien, fzn	0.5 cup	97	74	2	17	2	0	0.0	0.0	0.1	—	14
5268	Dish, potatoes o'brien, prep f/recipe	1 cup	97	79	2	15	1	1	0.8	0.3	0.1	4	93
57362	Dish, potatoes, au gratin, prep f/dry	3 oz	85	90	3	14	—	2	—	—	—	—	—
70612	Dish, twice baked potatoes, w/butter	1 ea	143	204	4	27	4	9	3.1	3.1	0.5	0	86
5948	Potatoes, baked, peeled, salted	0.5 cup	61	57	1	13	1	0	0.0	0.0	0.0	0	0
5130	Potatoes, baked, peeled, unsalted	0.5 cup	61	57	1	13	1	0	0.0	0.0	0.0	0	0
6996	Potatoes, baked, salted	0.5 cup	61	57	2	13	1	0	0.0	0.0	0.0	0	1
5334	Potatoes, baked, unsalted, med, 2 1/4" to 3 1/4"	1 ea	173	161	4	37	4	0	0.1	0.0	0.1	0	3
7259	Potatoes, dehyd	100 g	100	367	8	81	3	1	—	—	—	—	0
5691	Potatoes, french fries, battered, shoestring, 80% ckd, fzn	3 oz	85	170	4	17	1	10	2.5	—	—	0	0
8900	Potatoes, french fries, crinkle, 1/2" x 1/2", 80% ckd, fzn	3 oz	85	170	3	24	2	7	2.0	—	—	0	0
5790	Potatoes, french fries, fzn	10 ea	65	101	2	16	2	4	0.6	2.4	0.4	0	0
5592	Potatoes, french fries, heated f/fzn w/o salt	10 ea	50	100	2	16	2	4	0.6	2.4	0.4	0	0
6413	Potatoes, french fries, waffle style	15 pce	84	140	2	22	2	5	1.5	2.0	0.0	0	0
6851	Potatoes, fresh, w/skin, med, 2 1/4" to 3 1/4"	1 ea	213	164	4	37	5	0	0.1	0.0	0.1	0	0
70611	Potatoes, hash browns, box, microwv	3.6 oz	100	193	2	23	1	10	2.6	3.5	0.0	0	0
70603	Potatoes, hash browns, shredded	0.5 cup	78	62	2	14	1	5	1.9	2.1	0.6	0	0
6402	Potatoes, patty, golden	1 ea	71	140	1	16	1	7	1.5	3.5	0.5	0	0
9250	Potatoes, red, w/skin, baked, med, 2 1/4" to 3 1/4"	1 ea	173	154	4	34	3	0	0.0	0.0	0.1	0	3
5512	Potatoes, rstd	1 ea	93	132	3	30	3	0	0.0	0.0	0.1	0	0
57368	Potatoes, scalloped, prep	3 oz	85	90	2	16	—	2	—	—	—	—	—
5339	Potatoes, skin, bkd	1 ea	58	115	2	27	5	0	0.0	0.0	0.0	0	1
70598	Potatoes, tater tots	0.5 cup	62	107	1	16	1	6	1.1	1.8	0.0	0	0
9247	Potatoes, w/skin, baked, med, 2 1/4"–3 1/4"	1 ea	173	163	4	36	4	0	0.0	0.0	0.1	0	3
7906	Potatoes, wedges, USDA, fzn	3 oz	85	105	2	22	2	2	0.5	1.2	0.1	0	0
5162	Sweetpotatoes, mashed f/cnd	1 cup	256	259	5	59	4	1	0.1	0.0	0.2	0	0
WEIGHT LOSS BARS & DRINKS													
Weight Loss Bars													
63408	Bar, diet, chocolate chip	1 ea	50	200	16	17	0	8	4.0	—	—	3	350
63370	Bar, diet, cranberry apple, granola	1 ea	56	220	8	35	1	5	3.5	—	—	5	150
8975	Bar, diet, hi prot & low carbohydrate, peanut butter	1 ea	50	190	22	2	0	5	2.5	—	—	0	0
62875	Bar, diet, hi prot, peanut butter	1 ea	70	250	30	11	2	6	3.5	—	—	0	0
62855	Bar, diet, oatmeal raisin	1 ea	56	220	8	36	2	5	3.5	—	—	3	350
62639	Bar, diet, peanut butter, breakfast & lunch	1 ea	34	150	5	19	2	6	2.5	—	—	5	250
63372	Bar, diet, peanut butter, granola	1 ea	56	220	8	35	1	6	3.5	—	—	5	150
Weight Loss Drinks													
62854	Drink, diet, cappuccino, milk base, rtd can	1 ea	345	220	10	42	5	1	0.5	0.5	0.0	5	350
62648	Drink, diet, choc fudge, milk base, rtd can	1 ea	345	220	10	42	5	3	1.0	1.5	0.5	5	350
63359	Drink, diet, chocolate, soy prot, rtd can	1 ea	345	230	12	39	5	3	1.0	1.5	0.5	0	350

Thia (mg)	Ribo (mg)	Niac (mg NE)	Vit B6 (mg)	Vit B12 (µg)	Fol (µg)	Vit C (mg)	Vit D (IU)	Vit E (mg AT)	Cal	Iron (mg)	Magn (mg)	Phos (mg)	Pota (mg)	Sodi (mg)	Zinc (mg)	Wat (%)	Alco (g)	Caff (g)
0.05	0.00	1.19	—	—	—	2.6	—	—	17	0.27	7.8	23	189	245	—	84	0.00	0.00
0.09	0.05	1.17	0.23	0.07	8.4	6.5	6.4	0.0	23	0.28	18.9	48	311	317	0.3	79	0.00	0.00
0.09	0.05	1.12	0.23	0.07	8.4	6.3	8.7	0.1	23	0.27	18.9	47	298	333	0.3	76	0.00	0.00
0.10	0.05	1.23	0.25	0.07	9.4	11.0	6.0	0.4	21	0.27	19.9	50	342	350	0.3	75	0.00	0.00
0.15	0.28	2.43	0.43	0.00	27.0	24.3	—	0.5	292	1.57	49.0	277	970	1061	1.7	74	0.00	0.00
0.15	0.28	2.43	0.43	0.00	27.0	24.3	—	1.3	292	1.57	49.0	277	970	1061	1.7	74	0.00	0.00
0.07	0.01	1.19	—	0.00	—	3.7	—	—	0	0.00	—	—	148	14	—	82	0.00	0.00
0.05	0.03	1.10	0.20		7.8	11.0	—	0.2	13	1.00	17.5	48	242	32	0.3	80	0.00	0.00
0.07	0.05	0.98	0.20	0.00	7.8	16.2	—	0.1	35	0.46	17.5	48	258	210	0.3	80	0.00	0.00
0.02	0.07	0.80	—	0.00	—	2.4	—	—	40	0.36	16.0	60	265	340	—	75	0.00	0.00
0.09	0.10	3.03	—	0.00	—	21.4	—	—	57	1.02	—	—	601	357	—	—	0.00	0.00
0.05	0.00	0.85	0.18	0.00	5.5	7.8	—	0.0	3	0.20	15.2	30	239	147	0.2	75	0.00	0.00
0.05	0.00	0.85	0.18	0.00	5.5	7.8	—	0.0	3	0.20	15.2	30	239	3	0.2	75	0.00	0.00
0.03	0.02	0.86	0.18	0.00	17.1	5.9	—	0.0	9	0.66	17.1	43	326	149	0.2	75	0.00	0.00
0.10	0.07	2.44	0.54	0.00	48.4	16.6	—	0.1	26	1.87	48.4	121	926	17	0.6	75	0.00	0.00
0.23	0.15	3.70	—	0.00	—	11.0	—	—	27	2.79	—	200	922	8	—	6	0.00	0.00
—	—	—	—	—	—	3.6	—	—	0	0.36	—	—	—	190	—	63	0.00	0.00
—	—	—	—	—	—	9.0	—	—	0	1.08	—	—	—	25	—	59	0.00	0.00
0.07	0.00	1.11	0.15	0.00	7.8	6.4	—	0.1	4	0.62	11.0	42	212	15	0.2	67	0.00	0.00
0.05	0.00	1.03	0.15	0.00	6.0	5.1	0.0	0.1	4	0.62	11.0	41	209	15	0.2	57	0.00	0.00
—	—	—	—	0.00	—	2.4	—	—	0	1.44	—	—	290	35	—	—	0.00	0.00
0.17	0.07	2.25	0.62	0.00	34.1	42.0	0.0	0.0	26	1.65	49.0	121	897	13	0.6	79	0.00	0.00
0.07	—	1.57	—	0.00	—	0.0	—	—	0	0.00	—	—	246	263	—	64	0.00	0.00
—	—	—	—	—	—	7.1	—	—	6	0.58	—	—	355	25	—	73	0.00	0.00
—	—	—	—	0.00	—	0.0	—	—	0	0.00	—	—	120	280	—	—	0.00	0.00
0.11	0.09	2.75	0.37	0.00	46.7	21.8	—	0.1	16	1.21	48.4	125	943	14	0.7	77	0.00	0.00
0.11	0.05	2.34	0.40	0.00	19.2	26.3	0.0	0.1	12	1.26	35.0	77	905	10	0.7	62	0.00	0.00
0.02	0.07	0.80	—	0.00	—	2.4	—	—	40	0.36	16.0	60	245	300	—	75	0.00	0.00
0.07	0.05	1.77	0.36	0.00	12.8	7.8	—	0.0	20	4.07	24.9	59	332	12	0.3	47	0.00	0.00
—	—	—	—	—	—	0.7	—	—	0	0.00	—	—	162	251	—	61	0.00	0.00
0.07	0.07	2.64	0.37	0.00	65.7	21.8	—	0.1	17	1.11	46.7	130	941	12	0.6	75	0.00	0.00
0.09	0.02	1.30	0.30	0.00	—	9.5	—	—	13	0.60	16.2	74	335	42	0.3	68	0.00	0.00
0.07	0.23	2.44	0.60	0.00	28.2	13.3	—	0.7	77	3.40	61.4	133	538	192	0.5	74	0.00	0.00
0.21	0.60	7.00	0.69	2.09	60.0	21.0	140.0	4.8	300	2.70	140.0	400	400	200	2.2	—	0.00	—
0.21	0.60	7.00	0.69	2.09	60.0	21.0	140.0	4.8	300	2.70	140.0	400	400	230	2.2	—	0.00	0.00
—	—	—	—	—	—	0.0	—	—	160	1.00	—	—	—	120	—	—	0.00	—
—	—	—	—	—	—	0.0	—	—	200	1.10	—	—	—	120	—	—	0.00	—
0.21	0.60	7.00	0.69	2.09	60.0	21.0	140.0	4.8	300	2.70	140.0	250	170	100	2.2	—	0.00	0.00
0.37	0.43	5.00	0.40	1.50	40.0	15.0	80.0	3.4	100	4.50	16.0	100	115	65	3.8	—	0.00	—
0.21	0.60	7.00	0.69	2.09	60.0	21.0	140.0	4.8	3000	2.70	140.0	400	400	320	2.2	—	0.00	—
0.51	0.60	7.00	0.69	2.09	120.0	60.0	140.0	13.6	400	2.70	140.0	400	600	220	2.2	—	0.00	—
0.51	0.60	7.00	0.69	2.09	120.0	60.0	140.0	13.6	400	2.70	140.0	400	600	220	2.2	—	0.00	—
0.44	0.50	6.00	0.60	2.09	160.0	30.0	120.0	3.4	400	4.50	100.0	300	700	420	3.8	—	0.00	—

PAGE KEY: A-108 Beverage and Beverage Mixes A-110 Other Beverages A-110 Beverages, Alcoholic A-112 Candies and Confections, Gum A-116 Cereals, Breakfast Type A-120 Cheese and Cheese Substitutes A-122 Dairy Products and Substitutes A-124 Desserts A-130 Dessert Toppings A-130 Eggs, Substitutes, and Egg Dishes A-132 Ethnic Foods A-136 Fast Foods/Restaurants A-150 Fats, Oils, Margarines, Shortenings, and Substitutes A-150 Fish, Seafood, and Shellfish A-152 Food Additives A-152 Fruit, Vegetable, or Blended Juices A-154 Grains, Flours, and Fractions A-154 Grain Products, Prepared and Baked Goods

Code	Food Name	Unit/ Amt	Wt (g)	Energy (kcal)	Prot (g)	Carb (g)	Fiber (g)	Fat (g)	Sat (g)	Mono (g)	Poly (g)	Chol (mg)	Vit A (RE)
62650	Drink, diet, milk choc, milk base, rtd can	1 ea	345	220	10	40	5	3	1.0	1.5	0.5	5	350
62646	Drink, diet, orange pineapple, rtd can	1 ea	360	220	7	46	5	1	0.0	0.0	0.0	5	500
62649	Drink, diet, straw cream, milk base, rtd can	1 ea	345	220	10	40	5	2	0.5	1.5	0.5	5	350
63374	Drink, diet, vanilla cream, low carb, rtd can	1 ea	350	190	20	7	5	9	1.5	6.0	1.5	15	350
63024	Shake, weight management, chocolate fudge, rtd	1 ea	250	100	15	5	—	2	0.0	—	—	15	150
63025	Shake, weight management, vanilla, rtd	1 ea	250	90	15	3	1	2	0.0	—	—	15	150
MISCELLANEOUS													
Baking Chips, Chocolates, Coatings, and Cocoas													
23519	Baking Chips, chocolate	31 pce	15	72	1	9	1	4	3.0	—	—	0	1
23012	Baking Chips, chocolate, semi sweet	10 pce	5	23	0	3	0	1	0.8	0.5	0.0	0	0
23200	Baking Chips, chocolate, semi sweet, w/butter	60 pce	28	135	1	18	2	8	5.0	2.8	0.3	5	2
23423	Baking Chips, M & M's, milk chocolate, mini bits	1 Tbs	14	71	1	10	0	3	2.1	1.1	0.1	2	6
23444	Baking Chips, milk chocolate, mini kisses	11 ea	15	80	1	9	0	4	3.0	—	—	5	0
4153	Baking Chips, Nestle Crunch, pieces	1.5 Tbs	15	80	1	10	0	4	2.0	—	—	0	0
23446	Baking Chips, Reese's peanut butter	1 Tbs	15	80	3	7	—	4	4.0	—	—	0	0
28299	Baking Chips, white chocolate, chunks	15 g	15	80	1	9	0	5	3.0	—	—	5	0
23401	Baking Chocolate, bar, semi sweet	0.5 oz	14	70	1	8	1	4	2.5	—	—	0	0
28063	Baking Chocolate, bar, unswtnd	0.5 oz	14	70	2	4	2	7	4.5	—	—	0	0
4355	Baking Chocolate, bar, white, premium	0.5 oz	14	80	1	8	0	4	3.0	—	—	5	0
28208	Baking Chocolate, unswntd, liquid	1 Tbs	15	71	2	5	3	7	3.8	1.4	1.6	0	0
28200	Cocoa Powder, unswntd	1 cup	86	197	17	47	29	12	6.9	3.9	0.4	0	0
Baking Ingredients													
28006	Baking Powder, low sod	1 tsp	5	5	0	2	0	0	0.0	0.0	0.0	0	0
28003	Baking Soda	1 tsp	5	0	0	0	0	0	0.0	0.0	0.0	0	0
51150	Candied Fruit	3.6 oz	100	321	0	83	2	0	0.0	0.0	0.0	0	2
26017	Cream of Tartar	1 tsp	3	8	0	2	0	0	0.0	0.0	0.0	0	0
3977	Pineapple, slices, natural glace	1 pce	63	180	0	46	0	0	0.0	0.0	0.0	0	0
28149	Yeast, active, dry	3.6 oz	100	333	39	43	24	5	1.2	2.6	0.8	0	0
28000	Yeast, baker's, dry active	1 tsp	4	12	2	2	1	0	0.0	0.1	0.0	0	0
Condiments													
9149	Catsup	1 Tbs	15	15	0	4	0	0	0.0	0.0	0.0	0	14
27032	Catsup, low sod	1 Tbs	15	16	0	4	0	0	0.0	0.0	0.0	0	16
90602	Catsup, low sod, pkt	1 ea	6	6	0	2	0	0	0.0	0.0	0.0	0	6
27004	Horseradish, prep	1 tsp	5	2	0	1	0	0	0.0	0.0	0.0	0	0
27000	Ketchup	1 Tbs	15	15	0	4	0	0	0.0	0.0	0.0	0	14
9151	Ketchup, low sod	1 Tbs	15	16	0	4	0	0	0.0	0.0	0.0	0	16
9152	Ketchup, low sod, pkt	1 ea	6	6	0	2	0	0	0.0	0.0	0.0	0	6
90931	Mustard, deli	100 g	100	113	5	10	6	7	0.3	—	—	0	4
27058	Mustard, dijon, Grey Poupon	0.5 cup	125	151	8	13	1	11	0.5	3.9	3.0	0	12
53254	Mustard, honey	1 ea	14	50	0	3	0	4	0.5	—	—	10	2
91801	Mustard, honey, fat free	1.5 Tbs	21	30	0	7	0	0	0.0	0.0	0.0	0	0
27070	Mustard, hot, pkt	1 ea	28	60	1	7	1	4	0.0	—	—	5	4
435	Mustard, yellow, prep	1 tsp	5	3	0	0	0	0	0.0	0.1	0.0	0	1
90211	Mustard, yellow, prep, pkt	1 ea	5	3	0	0	0	0	0.0	0.1	0.0	0	1
7523	Sauce, soy, dark	0.5 tsp	3	0	0	0	0	0	0.0	0.0	0.0	0	0

PAGE KEY: A-158 Granola Bars, Cereal Bars, Diet Bars, Scones, and Tarts   A-158 Meals and Dishes   A-162 Meats   A-168 Nuts, Seeds, and Products   A-170 Poultry
A-172 Salad Dressings, Dips, and Mayonnaise   A-172 Salads   A-174 Sandwiches   A-176 Sauces and Gravies   A-176 Snack Foods—Chips, Pretzels, Popcorn
A-178 Soups, Stews, and Chilis   A-180 Spices, Flavors, and Seasonings   A-182 Sports Bars and Drinks   A-182 Supplemental Foods and Formulas
A-184 Sweeteners and Sweet Substitutes   A-184 Vegetables and Legumes   A-198 Weight Loss Bars and Drinks   A-200 Miscellaneous

Thia (mg)	Ribo (mg)	Niac (mg NE)	Vit B6 (mg)	Vit B12 (µg)	Fol (µg)	Vit C (mg)	Vit D (IU)	Vit E (mg AT)	Cal (mg)	Iron (mg)	Magn (mg)	Phos (mg)	Pota (mg)	Sodi (mg)	Zinc (mg)	Wat (%)	Alco (g)	Caff (g)
0.51	0.60	7.00	0.69	2.09	120.0	60.0	140.0	13.6	400	2.70	140.0	400	600	220	2.2	—	0.00	—
0.51	0.60	7.00	0.69	2.09	120.0	60.0	140.0	13.6	350	2.70	140.0	400	500	180	2.2	—	0.00	0.00
0.51	0.60	7.00	0.69	2.09	120.0	60.0	140.0	13.6	400	2.70	140.0	400	600	220	2.2	—	0.00	0.00
0.51	0.60	2.00	0.20	0.60	120.0	60.0	140.0	13.6	400	2.70	140.0	400	400	200	2.2	—	0.00	0.00
0.30	0.34	0.40	—	1.50	120.0	15.0	—	4.1	100	0.00	80.0	150	280	170	3.0	—	0.00	—
0.30	0.34	—	0.40	1.50	120.0	—	—	4.1	100	0.00	80.0	150	170	170	3.0	—	0.00	0.00
—	—	—	—	—	—	0.0	—	—	5	2.00	—	—	—	31	—	4	0.00	—
0.00	0.00	0.01	0.00	0.00	0.1	0.0	—	0.0	2	0.15	5.4	6	17	1	0.1	1	0.00	2.93
0.01	0.02	0.11	0.00	0.00	0.9	0.0	—	0.3	9	0.88	32.6	37	103	3	0.5	1	0.00	17.57
0.00	0.02	0.02	0.00	0.03	0.7	0.1	—	0.1	16	0.17	6.5	24	42	10	0.2	2	0.00	2.50
—	—	—	—	—	—	0.0	—	—	20	0.00	—	—	—	15	—	2	0.00	—
—	—	—	—	—	—	0.0	—	—	0	0.00	—	—	—	25	—	2	0.00	—
—	—	—	—	—	—	0.0	—	—	0	0.00	—	—	—	35	—	—	0.00	0.00
—	—	—	—	—	—	0.0	—	—	20	0.00	—	—	—	15	—	0	0.00	—
—	—	—	—	—	—	0.0	—	—	0	0.72	—	—	—	0	—	3	0.00	—
—	—	—	—	—	—	0.0	—	—	0	1.44	—	—	—	0	—	4	0.00	—
—	—	—	—	—	—	0.0	—	—	20	0.00	—	—	—	15	—	3	0.00	—
0.00	0.03	0.31	0.00	0.00	2.9	0.0	—	0.9	8	0.62	39.8	51	175	2	0.6	1	0.00	7.05
0.07	0.20	1.87	0.10	0.00	27.5	0.0	—	0.1	110	11.92	429.1	631	1311	18	5.9	3	0.00	197.80
0.00	0.00	0.00	0.00	0.00	0.0	0.0	—	0.0	217	0.40	1.5	343	505	4	0.0	6	0.00	0.00
0.00	0.00	0.00	0.00	0.00	0.0	0.0	—	0.0	0	0.00	0.0	0	0	1259	0.0	0	0.00	0.00
0.00	0.00	0.00	0.00	0.00	0.0	0.0	—	0.0	18	0.17	4.0	5	57	98	0.1	17	0.00	0.00
0.00	0.00	0.00	0.00	0.00	0.0	0.0	—	0.0	0	0.10	0.1	0	495	2	0.0	2	0.00	0.00
—	—	—	—	—	0.00	—	0.0	—	0	0.00	—	—	5	40	—	27	0.00	0.00
10.00	5.00	41.00	—	—	—	6.0	—	—	73	6.00	—	898	1361	259	—	8	0.00	0.00
0.09	0.21	1.59	0.05	0.00	93.6	0.0	—	0.0	3	0.66	3.9	52	80	2	0.3	8	0.00	0.00
0.00	0.07	0.23	0.01	0.00	1.5	2.3	—	0.2	3	0.07	2.9	5	57	166	0.0	68	0.00	0.00
0.00	0.00	0.20	0.02	0.00	2.2	2.3	—	0.2	3	0.10	3.3	6	72	3	0.0	67	0.00	0.00
0.00	0.00	0.07	0.00	0.00	0.9	0.9	—	0.1	1	0.03	1.3	2	29	1	0.0	67	0.00	0.00
0.00	0.00	0.01	0.00	0.00	2.9	1.2	—	0.0	3	0.01	1.4	2	12	16	0.0	85	0.00	0.00
0.00	0.07	0.23	0.01	0.00	1.5	2.3	—	0.2	3	0.07	2.9	5	57	166	0.0	68	0.00	0.00
0.00	0.00	0.20	0.02	0.00	2.2	2.3	—	0.2	3	0.10	3.3	6	72	3	0.0	67	0.00	0.00
0.00	0.00	0.07	0.00	0.00	0.9	0.9	—	0.1	1	0.03	1.3	2	29	1	0.0	67	0.00	0.00
—	—	—	—	—	—	0.0	—	—	113	2.09	—	—	—	1553	—	74	0.00	0.00
0.17	0.11	2.55	0.10	0.00	0.0	1.0	—	—	170	3.25	—	273	222	3030	1.9	70	0.00	0.00
0.00	0.00	0.00	0.00	0.02	0.9	0.1	0.0	0.7	3	0.03	0.2	4	6	85	0.0	—	0.00	0.00
—	—	—	—	—	—	0.0	—	—	0	0.00	—	—	—	140	—	—	0.00	0.00
0.00	0.00	0.14	—	—	—	0.0	—	—	7	0.72	—	17	27	240	—	—	0.00	0.00
0.00	0.00	0.01	0.00	0.00	0.4	0.1	—	0.0	4	0.09	1.9	4	8	56	0.0	82	0.00	0.00
0.00	0.00	0.01	0.00	0.00	0.4	0.1	—	0.0	4	0.09	1.9	4	8	56	0.0	82	0.00	0.00
—	—	—	—	—	—	0.0	—	—	0	0.00	—	—	—	150	—	—	0.00	0.00

PAGE KEY: A-108 Beverage and Beverage Mixes A-110 Other Beverages A-110 Beverages, Alcoholic A-112 Candies and Confections, Gum A-116 Cereals, Breakfast Type A-120 Cheese and Cheese Substitutes A-122 Dairy Products and Substitutes A-124 Desserts A-130 Dessert Toppings A-130 Eggs, Substitutes, and Egg Dishes A-132 Ethnic Foods A-136 Fast Foods/Restaurants A-150 Fats, Oils, Margarines, Shortenings, and Substitutes A-150 Fish, Seafood, and Shellfish A-152 Food Additives A-152 Fruit, Vegetable, or Blended Juices A-154 Grains, Flours, and Fractions A-154 Grain Products, Prepared and Baked Goods

Code	Food Name	Unit/ Amt	Wt (g)	Energy (kcal)	Prot (g)	Carb (g)	Fiber (g)	Fat (g)	Sat (g)	Mono (g)	Poly (g)	Chol (mg)	Vit A (RE)
53614	Sauce, soy, light	1 Tbs	18	10	1	1	0	0	0.0	0.0	0.0	0	0
53530	Sauce, soy, low sod	1 Tbs	16	8	1	1	0	0	0.0	0.0	0.0	0	0
53471	Sauce, tabasco, rts	1 tsp	5	1	0	0	0	0	0.0	0.0	0.0	0	8
53099	Sauce, worcestershire	1 Tbs	17	11	0	3	0	0	0.0	0.0	0.0	0	2
53457	Vinegar, balsamic	1 Tbs	15	10	0	2	—	0	0.0	0.0	0.0	0	—
27007	Vinegar, cider	1 Tbs	15	2	0	1	0	0	0.0	0.0	0.0	0	0
92153	Vinegar, distilled	1 Tbs	17	2	0	1	0	0	0.0	0.0	0.0	0	0
27204	Vinegar, red wine	1 Tbs	16	0	0	0	0	0	0.0	0.0	0.0	0	0
Salsas													
92617	Salsa, lime & garlic	2 Tbs	32	15	0	3	1	0	0.0	0.0	0.0	0	40
92618	Salsa, rstd peppers & garlic	2 Tbs	32	10	0	2	1	0	0.0	0.0	0.0	0	40
53466	Salsa, rts	2 Tbs	32	9	0	2	1	0	0.0	0.0	0.0	0	10

Thia (mg)	Ribo (mg)	Niac (mg NE)	Vit B6 (mg)	Vit B12 (μg)	Fol (μg)	Vit C (mg)	Vit D (IU)	Vit E (mg AT)	Cal (mg)	Iron (mg)	Magn (mg)	Phos (mg)	Pota (mg)	Sodi (mg)	Zinc (mg)	Wat (%)	Alco (g)	Caff (g)
—	—	—	—	—	—	0.0	—	—	0	0.00	—	—	—	605	—	—	0.00	0.00
0.00	0.01	0.54	0.02	0.00	2.5	0.0	—	0.0	3	0.31	5.4	18	29	533	0.1	71	0.00	0.00
0.00	0.00	0.00	0.00	0.00	0.0	0.2	—	—	1	0.05	0.6	1	6	30	0.0	95	0.00	0.00
0.00	0.01	0.11	0.00	0.00	1.4	2.2	—	0.0	18	0.89	2.2	10	136	167	0.0	79	0.00	0.00
—	—	—	—	—	—	—	—	—	—	—	—	—	—	5	—	—	—	0.00
0.00	0.00	0.00	0.00	0.00	0.0	0.0	—	0.0	1	0.09	3.3	1	15	0	0.0	94	0.00	0.00
0.00	0.00	0.00	0.00	0.00	0.0	0.0	—	0.0	0	0.00	3.7	0	3	0	0.0	95	0.00	0.00
—	—	—	—	—	—	0.0	—	—	0	0.00	—	—	0	0	—	100	0.00	0.00
—	—	—	—	—	—	1.8	—	—	0	0.00	—	—	—	210	—	89	0.00	0.00
—	—	—	—	—	—	0.0	—	—	0	0.00	—	—	—	230	—	92	0.00	0.00
0.00	0.00	0.01	0.05	0.00	1.3	0.6	—	0.4	9	0.15	4.9	10	96	194	0.1	90	0.00	0.00

Glossary Terms

absorption The process by which nutrient molecules are absorbed by the GI tract and enter the bloodstream.

absorptive cells A class of cells, also called *enterocytes*, that cover the surface of the villi (fingerlike projections in the small intestine) and participate in nutrient absorption.

Acceptable Macronutrient Distribution Range (AMDR) Range of intake for a specific macronutrient that is associated with a reduced risk of chronic diseases while providing for recommended intakes of essential nutrients. AMDR are set for carbohydrate, protein, and fat (various forms); each is intended to provide guidance in dietary planning.

acesulfame K (ay-SUL-fame) An alternative sweetener that yields no energy to the body; it is 200 times sweeter than sucrose.

acetic acid (a-SEE-tic) A two-carbon fatty acid that is used in the synthesis of lipids.

$$CH_3-\overset{\overset{\textstyle O}{\|}}{C}-OH$$

acetylcholine (a-SEE-tul-coal-ene) A neurotransmitter released from nerve endings.

achlorhydria (ay-clor-HIGH-dre-ah) A decrease in stomach acid primarily due to age-associated loss of acid-producing gastric cells.

acidic pH A pH less than 7. Lemon juice has an acidic pH.

acquired immunodeficiency syndrome (AIDS) A disorder in which a virus (human immunodeficiency virus [HIV]) infects specific types of immune system cells. This leaves the person with reduced immune function and, in turn, defenseless against numerous infectious agents.

acrodermatitis enteropathica A rare inherited childhood disorder that results in the inability to absorb adequate amounts of zinc from the diet. Symptoms include skin lesions, hair loss, and diarrhea. If untreated, the condition can result in death during infancy or early childhood. Management of this condition is with zinc supplements.

actin (AK-tin) A protein in muscle fiber that, together with myosin, is responsible for contraction.

active absorption Absorption using a carrier and expending ATP energy. In this way the absorptive cell can absorb nutrients, such as glucose, against a concentration gradient.

active lifestyle A lifestyle that includes physical activity equivalent to walking more than 3 miles per day at 3 to 4 miles per hour in addition to the light physical activity associated with typical day-to-day life.

acute alcohol intoxication A temporary deterioration in mental function, accompanied by lack of coordination and partial paralysis arising from drinking alcoholic beverages too rapidly.

adenosine diphosphate (ADP) (ah-DEN-o-scene di-FOS-fate) A breakdown product of ATP. ADP is synthesized into ATP using energy from food-stuffs and a phosphate group (abbreviated P_1).

adenosine triphosphate (ATP) (ah-DEN-o-scene tri-FOS-fate) The main energy currency for cells. ATP energy is used to promote ion pumping, enzyme activity, and muscular contraction.

Adequate Intake (AI) Recommendations for nutrient intake when not enough information is available to establish an RDA. AIs are based on observed or experimentally determined estimates of the average nutrient intake that appears to maintain a defined nutritional state (e.g., bone health) in a specific population. Used when no RDA can be set.

adipose tissue (ad-i-POSE) A group of fat-storing cells.

ad libitum (ad-LIB-itum) At one's desire or pleasure.

ADP See *adenosine diphosphate.*

adrenergic (ADD-ren-er-gic) Relating to the actions of epinephrine and norepinephrine.

aerobic (air-ROW-bic) Requiring oxygen.

air displacement A method for estimating body composition that makes use of the volume of space taken up by a body inside a small chamber.

alcohol Ethyl alcohol or ethanol (CH_3CH_2OH).

alcohol abuse Alcohol consumption that results in severe physical, psychological, or social problems.

alcohol dehydrogenase (dee-high-DRO-jen-ase) The enzyme used in alcohol (ethanol) metabolism; the major enzyme used in the liver when alcohol is in low concentration.

alcohol dependence Repeated alcohol-related difficulties, such as a person's inability to control use, spending a great deal of time associated with alcohol use, continued use of alcohol despite physical or psychological consequences, persistent desire or unsuccessful efforts to cut down or control alcohol use, increased physical tolerance to alcohol's effects, and withdrawal symptoms.

aldosterone (al-DOS-ter-own) A hormone produced in the adrenal glands that acts on the kidneys, causing them to retain sodium and, therefore, water.

alkaline pH A pH greater than 7. Baking soda in water yields an alkaline pH.

allergen A foreign protein, or antigen, that induces excess production of certain immune system antibodies; subsequent exposure to the same protein leads to allergic symptoms. Whereas all allergens are antigens, not all antigens are allergens.

allergy A hypersensitive immune response that occurs when immune bodies produced by us react with a protein we sense as foreign (an antigen).

alpha (α) bond A type of chemical bond that can be broken by human intestinal enzymes in digestion; drawn as C—O—C.

alpha-linolenic acid (AL-fah-lin-oh-LE-nik) An essential omega-3 fatty acid with 18 carbons and 3 double bonds (C18:3, omega-3).

alpha-tocopherol (to-ca-FUR-all) The most potent form of vitamin E for antioxidant function in humans.

alveoli (al-VE-o-lye) Basic functional units of the lungs.

amenorrhea (A-men-or-ee-a) The absence of three or more consecutive menstrual cycles; the absence of menses in a female.

amines Can refer to hormones made of one or a few amino acids.

amino acid (ah-MEE-noh) The building block for proteins containing a central carbon atom with a nitrogen atom and other atoms attached.

amniotic fluid (am-nee-OTT-ik) Fluid contained in a sac within the uterus. This fluid surrounds and protects the fetus during development.

amphetamine (am-FET-ah-mean) A group of medications that stimulate the central nervous system and have other effects in the body. Abuse is linked to physical and psychological dependence.

amylase (AM-uh-lace) Starch-digesting enzyme from the salivary glands or pancreas.

amylopectin (AM-uh-low-pek-tin) A digestible branched-chain type of starch composed of multiple glucose units.

amylose (AM-uh-los) A digestible straight-chain type of starch made of multiple glucose units.

anabolic/anabolism (an-AH-bol-iz-um) Building compounds.

anaerobic (AN-ah-ROW-bic) Not requiring oxygen.

analog (AN-a-log) A chemical compound that differs slightly from another naturally occurring compound. Analogs generally contain extra or altered chemical groups and may have similar or opposite metabolic effects compared with the native compound. Also spelled *analogue.*

anal sphincters A group of two sphincters (inner and outer) that help control expulsion of feces from the body.

anaphylactic shock (an-ah-fih-LAK-tic) A severe allergic response that results in lowered blood pressure and respiratory and gastrointestinal distress. This reaction can be fatal.

androgenic (AN-dro-jenic) A general term for hormones that stimulate development in male sex organs—for example, testosterone.

android obesity (AN-droyd) The type of obesity in which fat is stored primarily in the abdominal area;

defined as a waist circumference greater than 40 inches (102 centimeters) in men and greater than 35 inches (89 centimeters) in women; closely associated with a high risk for cardiovascular disease, hypertension, and type 2 diabetes.

anemia (ah-NEM-ee-a) Generally refers to a decreased oxygen-carrying capacity of the blood. This can be caused by many factors, such as iron deficiency or blood loss.

anergy (AN-er-jee) Lack of an immune response to foreign compounds entering the body.

angiotensin I (an-jee-oh-TEN-sin) An intermediary compound produced during the body's attempt to conserve water and sodium; it is converted in the lungs to angiotensin II.

angiotensin II A compound produced from angiotensin I that increases blood vessel constriction and triggers production of the hormone aldosterone.

animal model Study of disease in laboratory animals that duplicates human disease. This can be used to understand more about human disease.

anorexia nervosa (an-oh-REX-ee-uh ner-VOH-sah) An eating disorder involving a psychological loss or denial of appetite followed by self-starvation; related in part to a distorted body image and to various social pressures commonly associated with puberty.

anthropometric assessment (an-throw-PO-met-rick) Pertaining to the measurement of body weight and the lengths, circumferences, and thicknesses of parts of the body.

antibody (AN-tih-bod-ee) Blood protein that inactivates foreign proteins found in the body. This helps prevent and control infections.

antibody-mediated immunity Specific immunity provided by B lymphocytes; also known as humoral immunity.

antidiuretic hormone (an-tie-dye-u-RET-ik) A hormone secreted by the pituitary gland that acts on the kidney to cause a decrease in water excretion. It is also called arginine vasopressin.

antigen (AN-ti-jen) Any foreign substance, generally large in size, that induces a state of sensitivity and/or resistance to microbes or toxic substances after a lag period; substance that stimulates a specific aspect of the immune system.

antioxidant (an-tie-OX-ih-dant) Generally a compound that stops the damaging effects of reactive substances seeking an electron (i.e., oxidizing agent). This compound prevents the breakdown of substances in food or the body, particularly lipids. An antioxidant is able to donate electrons to electron-seeking compounds. This in turn reduces electron capture and, thus, breakdown of unsaturated fatty acids and other cell (and food) components by oxidizing agents. Some compounds have antioxidant capabilities (i.e., stop oxidation) but are not electron donors per se.

anus (A-nus) Last portion of the GI tract; serves as an outlet for that organ.

aorta (a-ORT-ah) The major blood vessel of the body leaving from the left ventricle.

apoferritin (ape-oh-FERR-ih-tin) A protein in the intestinal cell that binds with the ferric form of iron (Fe^{3+}) to form ferritin.

apolipoprotein (ape-oh-LIP-oh-pro-teen) A protein attached to the surface of a lipoprotein or embedded in its outer shell. Apolipoproteins can help enzymes function, act as a lipid-transfer protein, or assist in the binding of a lipoprotein to a cell-surface receptor.

apoptosis (ah-pop-TOE-sis) A process that occurs over time in which enzymes in a cell sets off a series of events that disable numerous cell functions, eventually leading to cell death.

appetite The primarily psychological (external) influences that encourage us to find and eat food, often in the absence of obvious hunger.

arachidonic acid (ar-a-kih-DON-ik) An omega-6 fatty acid with 20 carbon atoms and 4 carbon-carbon double bonds (C20:4, omega-6); a precursor to some eicosanoids.

areola (ah-REE-oh-lah) The circular dark area of skin surrounding the nipple of the breast.

ariboflavinosis (ah-rih-bo-flay-vih-NOH-sis) A condition resulting from a lack of riboflavin. The *a* means "without," and the *osis* stands for "a condition of."

arithmetic ratio A series of numbers wherein the difference between each number is the same.

aromatherapy The use of the vapors of essential oils extracted from flowers, leaves, stalks, fruits, and roots for therapeutic purposes.

arrhythmias (ah-RITH-me-ahs) Abnormal heart rhythms that may be too slow, too early, too rapid, or irregular.

arteriole (ar-TEAR-e-ol) A tiny artery branch.

artery A blood vessel that carries blood away from the heart.

arthritis Inflammation at a point where bones join together. The disease has many possible causes.

ascites (a-SITE-ease) Fluid produced by the liver, accumulating in the abdomen, that is a sign of liver failure associated with cirrhosis.

aseptic processing (ah-SEP-tik) A method by which food and container are separately and simultaneously sterilized; it allows manufacturers to produce boxes of milk that can be stored at room temperature.

aspartame (AH-spar-tame) An alternative sweetener made of two amino acids and methanol; it is about 200 times sweeter than sucrose.

ataxia (a-TAX-ee-a) An inability to coordinate muscle activity during voluntary movement; incoordination.

atherosclerosis (ath-e-roh-scle-ROH-sis) A buildup of fatty material (plaque) in the arteries, including those surrounding the heart.

atom Smallest combining unit of an element. An atom contains protons, neutrons, and electrons.

ATP See *adenosine triphosphate.*

atria (A-tree-a) The two upper chambers of the heart, which receive venous blood.

atrophy (AT-row-fee) A wasting away of tissue or organs.

autodigestion Literally, "self-digestion." The stomach limits autodigestion by covering itself with a thick layer of mucus and producing enzymes and acid only when needed for digestion of foodstuff.

autoimmune Immune reactions against normal body cells; self against self.

avidin (AV-ih-din) A protein found in raw egg whites that can bind biotin and inhibit its absorption; cooking destroys avidin.

axon The part of a nerve cell that conducts impulses away from the main body of the cell.

bacteria Single-cell microorganisms; some produce poisonous substances that cause illness in humans. They contain only one chromosome and lack many of the organelles found in human cells. Some can live without oxygen and survive harsh conditions by means of spore formation.

basal metabolic rate (BMR) The rate of energy use (e.g., kcal/min) by the body when at rest and awake in a warm, quiet environment.

basal metabolism The minimal amount of energy the body uses to support itself in a fasting state when resting and awake in a warm, quiet environment. It amounts to roughly 1 kcal per kilogram per hour for men and 0.9 kcal per kilogram per hour for women.

benign Noncancerous; describes tumors that do not spread.

beriberi (BEAR-ee-BEAR-ee) The thiamin deficiency disorder characterized by muscle weakness, loss of appetite, nerve degeneration, and sometimes edema.

beta (β) bond A type of chemical bond that cannot be broken by human intestinal enzymes during digestion when it is part of a long chain of glucose molecules (e.g., cellulose); drawn as C⌒O⌣C.

betaine (bee-TAINE) A product of choline metabolism and a methyl ($—CH_3$) donor in methionine metabolism.

beta oxidation The breakdown of a fatty acid into numerous acetyl-CoA molecules.

BHA Butylated hydroxyanisole, a synthetic antioxidant added to food.

BHT Butylated hydroxytoluene, a synthetic antioxidant added to food.

bile A liver secretion that is stored in the gallbladder and released through the common bile duct into the duodenum. It is essential for the digestion and absorption of fat.

bile acids Emulsifiers synthesized by the liver and released by the gallbladder during digestion.

bilirubin (bi-li-RUBE-in) Bile pigment that is derived from hemoglobin during the destruction of red blood cells; excreted by the liver into the gallbladder.

binge-eating disorder An eating disorder characterized by recurrent binge eating and feelings of loss of control over eating that have lasted at least 6 months. Binge episodes can be triggered by frustration, anger, depression, anxiety, permission to eat forbidden foods, and excessive hunger.

bioavailability The degree to which the amount of an ingested nutrient is absorbed and is available to the body.

biochemical assessment An assessment focusing on biochemical functions (e.g., concentrations of nutrient by-products or enzyme activities in the blood or urine) related to a nutrient's function.

biochemical lesion An indication of reduced biochemical function (e.g., low concentrations of nutrient by-products or enzyme activities in the blood or urine) resulting from a nutritional deficiency.

bioelectrical impedance A method to estimate total body fat that uses a low-energy electrical current. The more fat storage a person has, the more impedance (resistance) to electrical flow will be exhibited.

biological value (BV) A measure of how efficiently food protein, once absorbed from the gastrointestinal tract, can be turned into body tissues.

biotechnology A collection of processes that involve the use of biological systems for altering and, ideally, improving characteristics of plants, animals, and other forms of life.

biotin (By-oh-tin) A water-soluble vitamin that, in coenzyme form, participates in reactions where carbon dioxide is added to a compound. It is an essential cofactor for enzymes involved in energy and amino acid metabolism and in fatty acid synthesis. Peanuts, liver, and egg are rich sources, but it can also be synthesized by intestinal bacteria.

bisphosphonates (bis-FOS-foh-nates) Compounds primarily composed of carbon and phosphorus that bind to bone mineral and in turn reduce bone breakdown.

bleaching process The process by which light depletes the rhodopsin concentration in the eye. This fall in rhodopsin concentration allows the eye to become adapted to bright light.

blood doping A technique by which an athlete's red blood cell count is increased. Blood is taken from the athlete, and the red blood cells are concentrated and then later reinjected into the athlete. Alternately, a hormone may be injected to increase red blood cell synthesis (erythropoetin [Epogen]).

B lymphocyte (LIM-fo-site) A type of white blood cell that recognizes antigens (e.g., bacteria) present in extracellular sites in the body and is responsible for antibody-mediated immunity. B lymphocytes originate and mature in the bone marrow and are released into the blood and lymph.

body mass index (BMI) Weight (in kilograms) divided by height (in meters) squared. A normal value is 18.5 to 24.9. A value of 25 or greater indicates a risk for body weight–related health disorders, such as type 2 diabetes and cardiovascular disease, especially when it is 30 or greater. 1 BMI unit equals 6–7 lb.

bolus (BOWL-us) A mass of food that is swallowed.

bomb calorimeter (kal-oh-RIM-eh-ter) An instrument used to determine the energy content of a food.

bond A sharing of electrons, charges, or attractions linking two atoms.

bone mass Total mineral substance (such as calcium or phosphorus) in a cross section of bone, generally expressed as grams per centimeter of length.

bone mineral density Total mineral content of bone at a specific bone site divided by the width of the bone at that site, generally expressed as grams per cubic centimeter.

bone remodeling A process by which bone is first resorbed by osteoclasts and then reformed by osteoblasts. This process allows the body to form bone where needed, such as in areas of high mechanical stress.

botulism A foodborne illness caused by the bacterium *Clostridium botulinum.*

bronchial tree (BRON-key-al) The bronchi and the branches that stem out to bronchioles.

bronchioles Smallest division of the bronchi.

brown adipose tissue (ADD-ih-pose) A specialized form of adipose tissue that produces large amounts of heat by metabolizing energy-yielding nutrients without synthesizing much useful energy for the body. The unused energy is released as heat.

buffers Compounds that cause a solution to resist changes in acid-base balance.

bulimia nervosa (boo-LEEM-ee-uh) An eating disorder in which large quantities of food are eaten at one time (binge eating) and then purged from the body by vomiting or by misuse of laxatives, diuretics, or enemas. Alternate means to counteract the excess energy intake are fasting and excessive exercise.

B-vitamins A group of several water-soluble vitamins that includes thiamin, riboflavin, niacin, pantothenic acid, biotin, vitamin B-6, vitamin B-12, and folate. All B-vitamins function as coenzymes.

cachexia (ka-KEX-ee-a) Widespread wasting of the body due to undernutrition.

calcitonin (kal-sih-TONE-in) A thyroid gland hormone that inhibits bone resorption.

calcitriol (kal-sih-TRIH-ol) The name sometimes given to the active hormone form of vitamin D [$1,25(OH)_2$ vitamin D] that contains a derivative of cholesterol as part of its structure.

calcium The major mineral component of bones and teeth; calcium also aids in nerve impulse transmission, blood clotting, muscle contractions, and other cell functions. Milk and milk products, leafy vegetables, and tofu are good sources.

calmodulin (kal-MOD-ju-lyn) A cell protein that binds calcium ions. The resulting calmodulin-Ca^{2+} complex influences the activity of some enzymes in the cell.

Campylobacter jejuni **(kam-PILE-o-bak-ter je-JUNE-ee)** A bacteria that produces a toxin that destroys the mucosal surfaces of the small and large intestines. *Campylobacter* is the leading cause of bacterial foodborne illness. The chief food sources are raw poultry and meat and unpasteurized milk. It is easily destroyed by cooking.

cancer A condition characterized by uncontrolled growth of abnormal body cells.

cancer initiation The stage in the process of cancer development that begins with alterations in DNA, the genetic material in a cell. These alterations may cause the cell to no longer respond to normal physiological controls.

cancer progression The final stage in the cancer process, during which the cancer cells proliferate, forming a mass large enough to significantly affect body functions.

cancer promotion The stage in the cancer process during which cell division increases, in turn decreasing the time available for repair enzymes to act on altered DNA, and encouraging cells with altered DNA to develop and grow.

capillary (KAP-ill-air-ee) A microscopic blood vessel that connects an arteriole and a venule; the functional unit of the circulatory system.

capillary bed Minute vessels one cell thick that create a junction between arterial and venous circulation. Gas and nutrient exchange occurs here between body cells and the bloodstream.

carbohydrate (kar-bow-HIGH-drate) A compound containing carbon, hydrogen, and oxygen atoms; most are known as *sugars, starches,* and *fibers;* supplies 4 kcal/gram.

carbohydrate counting Diet method that assigns a certain number of food exchanges or carbohydrate grams to each meal and snack. Insulin is matched to carbohydrate intake, and carbohydrate grams can come from several combinations of exchanges.

carbohydrate loading A process in which a very high carbohydrate intake is consumed for 6 days before an athletic event while tapering exercise duration in an attempt to increase muscle glycogen stores.

carbon skeleton What remains of an amino acid after the amino group ($-NH_2$) has been removed.

carcinogenic Describes a compound with the potential to cause cancer.

carcinoma Invasive malignant tumor derived from epithelial tissues that cover the body.

cardiac muscle Muscle that makes up the walls of the heart; produces rhythmical involuntary contractions.

cardiac output The amount of blood pumped by the heart.

cardiomyopathy Primary heart-muscle disease of unknown origin.

cardiovascular (heart) disease A general term that refers to any disease of the heart and circulatory system. This disease is characterized by the deposition of fatty material in the blood vessels (hardening of the arteries), which in turn can lead to organ damage and death; also termed coronary heart disease (CHD), because the vessels of the heart are the primary sites of the disease.

cardiovascular system The body system consisting of the heart, blood vessels, and blood. This system transports nutrients, waste products, gases, and hormones throughout the body and plays an important role in immune responses and regulation of body temperature.

cariogenic (CARE-ee-oh-jen-ik) Literally "caries producing"; a substance, often carbohydrate-rich (such as caramel), that promotes dental caries.

carnitine (CAR-nih-teen) A compound used to shuttle fatty acids from the cytosol of the cell into mitochondria.

carotenoids (kah-ROT-en-oyds) Pigment materials in fruits and vegetables that range in color from yellow to orange to red; three yield vitamin A activity in humans and thus are called provitamin A. Many have antioxidant properties as well. One example is beta-carotene.

carpal tunnel syndrome (CAR-pull) A disease in which nerves that travel to the wrist are pinched as they pass through a narrow opening in a bone in the wrist.

cartilage Connective tissue, usually part of the skeleton, that is composed of cells in a flexible network.

case-control study Studies in which individuals who have the condition in question, such as lung cancer, are compared with individuals who do not have the condition.

casein (KAY-seen) Protein found in milk that forms curds when exposed to acid and is difficult for infants to digest.

catabolic/catabolism (cat-ah-BOL-ik) Breaking down compounds.

catalase An enzyme that breaks down hydrogen peroxide (H_2O_2) to water.

catalase pathway An alternative enzyme pathway to alcohol metabolism; alcohol is broken down in conjunction with the breakdown of hydrogen peroxide (H_2O_2) by this enzyme.

catalyst (CAT-ul-ist) A compound that speeds reaction rates but is not altered by the reaction.

cecum (SEE-come) The first portion of the large intestine, which connects to the ileum.

celiac disease (SEE-lee-ak) An immunological or allergic reaction to the protein gluten in certain grains, such as wheat and rye. The effect is to destroy the intestinal enterocytes, resulting in a much reduced surface area due to flattening of the villi. Elimination of wheat, rye, and certain other grains from the diet restores the intestinal surface.

cell A minute structure; the living basis of plant and animal organization. In animals the cell is bounded by a cell membrane. Cells contain both genetic material and systems for synthesizing energy-yielding compounds. Cells have the ability to take up compounds from and excrete compounds into their surroundings.

cell differentiation The process of transforming an unspecialized cell into a specialized cell.

cell-mediated immunity A process in which T lymphocytes come in actual contact with the invading cells in order to destroy them.

cell nucleus An organelle bound by its own double membrane and containing chromosomes, the genetic information for cell protein synthesis.

cellulose (SELL-you-lows) A straight-chain polysaccharide of glucose molecules that is undigestible because of the presence of beta bonds; part of insoluble fiber.

Celsius A centigrade measure of temperature. For conversion: (degrees in Fahrenheit − 32) × 5/9 = °C; (degrees in Celsius × 9/5) + 32 = °F.

central nervous system (CNS) The brain and spinal cord portions of the nervous system.

cerebrovascular accident (CVA) (se-REE-bro-VAS-cue-lar) Death of part of the brain tissue due typically to a blood clot; also called *stroke*.

ceruloplasmin (se-RUE-low-PLAS-min) A blue, copper-containing protein in the blood that can remove an electron from Fe^{2+} (the ferrous form) to yield Fe^{3+} (the ferric form). The Fe^{3+} form of iron can then bind with iron transport and storage proteins, such as transferrin.

chain-breaking Breaking the link between two or more behaviors that encourage overeating, such as snacking while watching television.

chelates (KEY-lates) Complexes formed between metal ions and substances with polar groups, such as proteins. The polar groups form two or more attachments with the metal ions, forming a ringed structure. The metal ion is then firmly bound and sequestered.

chelation (key-LAY-shun) The use of medicinal compounds, such as ethylenediaminetetraacetic acid (EDTA), to bind metals and other constituents in the blood.

chemical reaction An interaction between two chemicals that changes both participants.

chemical score A ratio comparing the essential amino acid content of the protein in a food with the essential amino acid content in a reference protein. The lowest amino acid ratio calculated for any essential amino acid is the chemical score.

chief cell Gastric gland cell that secretes pepsinogen, precursor of pepsin.

chloride The major negative ion of extracellular fluid; aids in nerve impulse transmission and fluid balance in conjunction with sodium and potassium. It contributes to the function of white blood cells, aids in the transport of carbon dioxide from cells to the lungs, and is a component of hydrochloric acid production in the stomach. Salt supplies most of the chloride in the diet.

cholecystokinin (CCK) (ko-la-sis-toe-KY-nin) A hormone that stimulates enzyme release from the pancreas and bile release from the gallbladder.

cholera (KOL-er-a) See *Vibrio cholerae*.

cholesterol (ko-LES-te-rol) A waxy lipid found in all body cells, such as cell membranes. It has a structure containing multiple chemical rings. Cholesterol is found only in foods that contain animal products.

choline (COAL-ene) A water-soluble vitamin-like compound that functions as a precursor for acetylcholine, a neurotransmitter associated with attention, learning and memory, muscle control, and many other functions. Protein foods, especially eggs, are rich in choline.

cholinergic (coal-in-NER-jic) Relating to the actions of acetylcholine.

chromium A trace mineral that enhances the action of insulin. Egg yolks, whole grains, pork, nuts, and mushrooms are good sources.

chromosome A single large DNA molecule and its associated proteins containing many genes; stores and transmits genetic information.

chronic (KRON-ik) Long-standing, developing over time. When referring to disease, this term indicates that the disease progress, once developed, is slow and tends to remain; a good example is cardiovascular disease.

chylomicron (kye-lo-MY-kron) Lipoprotein made of dietary fats that are surrounded by a shell of cholesterol, phospholipids, and protein. Chylomicrons are formed in the absorptive cells (enterocytes) in the small intestine after fat absorption and travel through the lymphatic system to the bloodstream.

chyme (KIME) A mixture of stomach secretions and partially digested food.

cirrhosis (see-ROH-sis) A loss of functioning liver cells, which are replaced by nonfunctioning connective tissue. Any substance that poisons liver cells can lead to cirrhosis. The most common cause is chronic, excessive alcohol intake. Exposure to certain industrial chemicals can also lead to cirrhosis.

***cis* configuration** (sis) A form seen in compounds with double bonds, such as fatty acids, in which the hydrogens on both ends of the double bond lie on the same side of the plane of that bond.

citric acid cycle A pathway that breaks down acetyl-CoA, yielding carbon dioxide, $FADH_2$, $NADH + H^+$, and GTP. The pathway can also be used to synthesize compounds.

clinical assessment Physical evidence of diet-related disease. This type of assessment focuses on general appearance of skin, eyes, and tongue; evidence of rapid hair loss; loss of sense of touch; and loss of ability to cough and walk.

clinical lesion A sign seen on physical examination or a symptom perceived by the patient resulting from a nutritional deficiency.

clinical symptoms Generally, a change in health status noted by the individual (such as stomach pain) or noticed by a clinician during physical examination (the latter is technically called a clinical sign).

Clostridium botulinum (closs-TRID-ee-um bot-u-LYE-num) Bacteria that come from soil and may exist as bacteria themselves or in spore form in any food. As these bacteria multiply in food in the absence of air, they produce a deadly toxin. *C. botulinum* thrives primarily in canned food, especially improperly home-canned, low-acid foods such as string beans, corn, mushrooms, beets, asparagus, and garlic.

Clostridium perfringens (per-FRING-ens) Toxin-producing bacteria living throughout the environment, especially in soil, the intestinal tract of humans and animals, and sewage. *Clostridium* is called the "cafeteria germ" because most outbreaks of foodborne illness caused by it are associated with the food service industry or with events where large quantities of food are prepared and served. *Clostridium* thrives in an oxygen-free environment and forms heat-resistant spores.

coenzyme Compound that combines with an inactive protein, called an apoenzyme, to form a catalytically active enzyme called a holoenzyme. In this manner, coenzymes aid in enzyme function.

cofactor An organic or inorganic substance that binds to a specific region on an enzyme and is necessary for the enzyme's activity.

cognitive behavior therapy Psychological therapy in which the person's assumptions about dieting, body weight, and related issues are challenged. New ways of thinking are explored and then practiced by the person. In this way, the person can learn new ways to control disordered eating behaviors and related life stress.

cognitive restructuring Changing one's frame of mind regarding eating—for example, instead of using a difficult day as an excuse to overeat, substituting other pleasures or rewards, such as a relaxing walk with a friend.

colic (KOL-ik) Sharp abdominal pain that generally occurs in otherwise healthy infants and is associated with periodic spells of inconsolable crying.

colipase (co-LIE-pace) A protein secreted by the pancreas that changes the shape of pancreatic lipase, facilitating its action.

collagen (KOL-ah-jen) The major protein of the material that holds together the various structures of the body.

colostrum (ko-LAHS-trum) The first fluid secreted by the breast during late pregnancy and the first few days after birth. This thick fluid is rich in immune factors and protein.

comorbid A disease process that accompanies another disease. For example, if hypertension develops as obesity is established, hypertension is said to be a comorbid condition accompanying the obesity.

complement A series of blood proteins that participate in a complex reaction cascade following stimulation by an antigen-antibody complex on the surface of a bacterial cell. Various activated complement proteins can enhance phagocytosis, contribute to inflammation, and destroy bacteria.

complementary proteins Two food protein sources that make up for each other's inadequate supply of specific essential amino acids; together they yield a sufficient amount of all nine and so provide high-quality (complete) protein for the diet.

complete proteins Proteins that contain ample amounts of all nine essential amino acids.

compound A group of different types of atoms bonded together in definite proportion (see also *molecule*). Not all chemical compounds exist as molecules. Some compounds are made up of ions attracted to each other, such as Na$^+$Cl$^-$ (table salt).

compression of morbidity The delaying of the onset of disabilities caused by chronic disease.

concentration gradient Gradation in concentration that occurs between two regions having different concentrations.

conceptus (kon-SEP-tus) A generic term for any developmental stage derived from the fertilized ovum (zygote) until birth. The conceptus includes the extraembryonic membranes, as well as the embryo or fetus.

condensation reaction Chemical reaction in which a bond is formed between two molecules by the elimination of a small molecule, such as water.

congenital (con-JEN-i-tal) A term that means "present at birth." Thus, a congenital abnormality is a defect that has been present since birth. These defects may be inherited from the parents, may occur as a result of damage or infection while in the uterus, or may occur at the time of birth.

conjugase (KON-ju-gase) Enzyme systems in the intestine that enhance folate absorption; they remove glutamate molecules from polyglutamate forms of folate.

conjunctiva (kon-junk-TEA-vah) Mucous membrane covering the anterior surface of the eyeball and the posterior surface of the eyelids.

connective tissue Cells and their protein products that hold different structures in the body together. Some structures are made up of connective tissue—notably; tendons and cartilage. Connective tissue also forms part of bone and the nonmuscular structures of arteries and veins.

constipation A condition characterized by infrequent bowel movements.

contingency management Forming a plan of action to respond to a situation in which overeating is likely, such as when snacks are within arm's reach at a party.

control group Participants in an experiment who are not given the treatment being tested.

copper A trace mineral that aids in iron metabolism. It also functions in antioxidant enzyme systems and with enzymes involved in connective tissue metabolism and hormone synthesis. Liver, cocoa, beans, nuts, and whole grains are good sources.

cortical bone (KORT-ih-kal) Dense, compact, bone that constitutes the outer surface and shafts of bone; also called compact bone. Cortical bone makes up 75 to 80% of total bone mass.

corticosteroid (kor-ti-ko-STARE-oyd) A steroid produced by the adrenal gland, an example of which is cortisol.

cortisol (KORT-ih-sol) A hormone made by the adrenal glands that, among other functions, stimulates the production of glucose from amino acids and increases the desire to eat.

covalent bond (ko-VAY-lent) A union of two atoms formed by the sharing of electrons.

creatine (CREE-a-tin) An organic molecule in muscle cells that serves as a part of the high-energy compound creatine phosphate (or phosphocreatine).

creatinine (cree-A-tin-in) Nitrogenous waste product of the compound creatine found in muscles.

cretinism (KREET-in-ism) The stunting of body growth and mental development during fetal and later development that results from inadequate maternal intake of iodide during pregnancy.

Crohn's disease An inflammatory disease of the gastrointestinal tract, but generally more pronounced in the terminal ileum. A family history is a major risk factor. The disease limits the absorptive capacity of the small intestine.

crude fiber Outdated term for what remains of fiber after extended acid and alkaline treatment. Crude fiber consists primarily of cellulose and lignins.

cryptosporidiosis (krip-toe-spore-id-ee-O-sis) An intestinal disease, characterized by diarrhea, that originates from a protozoan parasite of the genus *Cryptosporidium.*

cyclamate (sigh-cla-MATE) An alternative sweetener that yields no energy to the body; it is 30 times sweeter than sucrose.

cyclooxygenase (sigh-clo-OXY-jen-ase) An enzyme used to synthesize prostaglandins, thromboxanes, and other eicosanoids. Abbreviated as COX.

cystic fibrosis (SIS-tik figh-BRO-sis) A disease that often leads to overproduction of mucus. Mucus can block the pancreatic duct, in turn decreasing enzyme output.

cytochrome (SITE-o-krome) Electron-transfer compound that participates in the electron transport chain.

cytochrome P450 A set of enzymes in cells that act on compounds foreign to the body. This action aids in their excretion, but also creates short-lived highly reactive forms.

cytokine (SITE-o-kine) A protein secreted by a cell that regulates the activity of neighboring cells.

cytoplasm (SITE-o-plas-um) The fluid and organelles (except the nucleus) in a cell.

cytosol The water-based phase of the cytoplasm; excludes organelles such as mitochondria.

cytotoxic T cell (cite-o-TOX-ik) Type of T cell that interacts with the infected host cell through special receptor sites on the T cell surface.

cytotoxic test An unreliable test to define food allergies that involves mixing white blood cells with food proteins.

Daily Reference Values (DRVs) Nutrient-intake standards established for protein, carbohydrate, and some dietary components lacking an RDA or a related nutrient standard, such as total fat intake. The DRVs for sodium and potassium are constant; those for the other nutrients increase as energy intake increases. The DRVs constitute part of the Daily Values used in food labeling.

Daily Values Standard nutrient-intake values developed by FDA and used as a reference for expressing nutrient content on nutrition labels. The Daily Values include two types of standards—RDIs and DRVs.

dark adaptation The process by which the rhodopsin concentration in the eye increases in dark conditions, allowing improved vision in the dark.

deamination (dee-am-ih-NA-shun) The removal of an amino group from an amino acid.

decarboxylation (dee-car-box-ih-LAY-shun) The action of removing one molecule of carbon dioxide from a compound.

decubitus ulcers (dee-CUBE-ih-tus) Chronic ulcers (also called bedsores) that appear in pressure areas of the skin over a body prominence. These sores develop when people are confined to bed or immobilized.

defecation Expulsion of feces from the rectum.

Delaney Clause A clause to the 1958 Food Additives Amendment of the Pure Food and Drug Act in the United States that prevents the intentional (direct) addition to foods of a compound that has been shown to cause cancer in laboratory animals or humans.

dementia (de-MEN-sha) General persistent loss or decrease in mental function.

denaturation (dee-NAY-ture-a-shun) Alteration of a protein's three-dimensional structure, usually because of treatment by heat, enzymes, acid or alkaline solutions, or agitation.

dendrite A relatively short, highly branched nerve cell process that carries electrical activity to the main body of the nerve cell.

dental caries (KARE-ees) Erosions in the surface of a tooth caused by acids made by bacteria as they metabolize sugars.

deoxyribonucleic acid (DNA) The site of hereditary information in cells; DNA directs the synthesis of cell proteins.

depolarization Reversal of membrane potential, which triggers generation of the nerve impulse in nerve cells.

dermatitis (dur-ma-TIE-tis) Inflammation of the skin.

dermis (DUR-miss) The second, or deep, layer of the skin under the epidermis.

DEXA See *dual energy X-ray absorptiometry.*

dextrin Partial breakdown product of starch that contains few to many glucose molecules. These appear when starch is being digested into many units of maltose by salivary and pancreatic amylase.

diabetes (DYE-uh-BEET-eez) A disease characterized by high blood glucose, resulting from either insufficient or no release of the hormone insulin by the pancreas or the general inability of insulin to act on certain body cells, such as muscle cells. The two major forms are type I (requires daily insulin therapy) and type 2 (may or may not require insulin therapy).

diastolic blood pressure (dye-ah-STOL-ik) The pressure in the arterial blood vessels when the heart is between beats.

dietary assessment An assessment that focuses on the typical food choices of the person, relying mostly on the recounting of one's usual intake or a record of one's intake of the previous day.

dietary fiber Fiber found in food.

Dietary Guidelines for Americans General goals for nutrient intakes and diet composition set by USDA and the Department of Health and Human Services.

Dietary Reference Intakes (DRIs) The term used to encompass the latest nutrient recommendations made by the Food and Nutrition Board, a part of the National Academy of Science. These include RDAs.

dietitian See *registered dietitian.*

diffusion The net movement of molecules or ions from regions of higher concentration to regions of lower concentration.

digestibility (dye-JES-tih-bil-i-tee) The proportion of food substances eaten that can be broken down into individual nutrients in the intestinal tract for absorption into the body.

digestion The process by which large ingested molecules are mechanically and chemically broken down to produce smaller molecules that can be absorbed across the wall of the GI tract.

digestive system The body system consisting of the gastrointestinal tract and accessory structures such as the liver, gallbladder, and pancreas. This system performs the mechanical and chemical processes of digestion, absorption of nutrients, and elimination of wastes.

diglyceride (dye-GLISS-er-ide) The breakdown product of a triglyceride consisting of two fatty acids bonded to a glycerol backbone.

dihomo-gamma-linolenic acid (dye-homo-gama-lin-oh-lenik) An omega-6 fatty acid with 20 carbons and three double bonds; the precursor to some eicosanoids.

direct calorimetry (kal-oh-RIM-eh-tree) A method of determining a body's energy use by measuring heat that is released from the body, usually using an insulated chamber.

disaccharides (dye-SACK-uh-rides) Class of sugars formed by the chemical bonding of two monosaccharides.

discretionary calories The amount of energy theoretically allowed in a diet after the person has met overall nutrition needs. This generally small amount of energy gives individuals the flexibility to consume some foods and beverages that may contain alcohol, added sugars, or added fats (e.g., many snack foods).

disordered eating Mild and short-term changes in eating patterns that occur in relation to a stressful event, an illness, or a desire to modify one's diet for a variety of health and personal appearance reasons.

distillation A physical method used to separate liquids based on their boiling points.

diuretic (dye-u-RET-ik) A substance that, when ingested, increases the flow of urine.

diverticula (DYE-ver-TIK-you-luh) Pouches that protrude through the exterior wall of the large intestine.

diverticulitis (DYE-ver-tik-you-LITE-us) An inflammation of the diverticula caused by acids produced by bacterial metabolism inside the diverticula.

diverticulosis (DYE-ver-tik-you-LOW-sus) The condition of having many diverticula in the large intestine.

DNA See *deoxyribonucleic acid.*

DNA transcription The process of forming messenger RNA (mRNA) from a portion of DNA.

docosahexaenoic acid (DHA) (DOE-co-sa-hex-ee-no-ik) An omega-3 fatty acid with 22 carbons and 6 carbon-carbon double bonds (C22:6, omega-3). It is present in large amounts in fatty fish and is slowly synthesized in the body from alpha-linolenic acid. DHA is especially present in the retina and brain.

dopamine (DOE-pah-mean) A type of neurotransmitter in the central nervous system that leads to feelings of euphoria, among other functions; it is also used to form norepinephrine, another neurotransmitter molecule.

double-blind study An experiment in which neither the participants nor the researchers are aware of each participant's assignment (test or placebo) or the outcome of the study until it is completed. An independent third party holds the code and the data until the study has been completed.

dual energy X-ray absorptiometry (DEXA) A highly accurate method of measuring body composition and bone mass and density using multiple low-energy X rays.

dual energy X-ray absorptiometry (DEXA) bone scan Method to measure bone density that uses small amounts of X-ray radiation. The ability of a bone to block the path of the radiation is used as a measure of bone density at that bone site.

duodenum (doo-oh-DEE-num, or doo-ODD-num) First portion of the small intestine; leads from the pyloric sphincter to the jejunum.

dyslipidemia (DIS-lip-ah-DEEM-E-ah) Generally refers to a state in which various blood lipids, such as LDL or triglycerides, are greatly elevated or in the case of HDL, very low.

early childhood caries Tooth decay that results from formula or juice (and even human milk) bathing the teeth as the child sleeps with a bottle in his or her mouth. The upper teeth are mostly affected because the lower teeth are protected by the tongue; formerly called *nursing bottle syndrome* and *baby bottle tooth decay.*

eating disorder Severe alterations in eating patterns linked to physiological changes. The alterations are associated with food restricting, binge eating, purging, and fluctuations in weight. They also involve a number of emotional and cognitive changes that affect the way a person perceives and experiences his or her body.

E. coli See *Escherichia coli.*

economic assessment An assessment that focuses on the ability of the person to purchase, transport, and cook food. The person's weekly budget for food purchases is also a key factor to consider.

ecosystem A "community" in nature that includes plants, animals, and the environment.

edema (uh-DEE-muh) The buildup of excess fluid in extracellular spaces.

eicosanoids (eye-KOH-san-oyds) Hormonelike compounds synthesized from polyunsaturated fatty acids, such as arachidonic acid. Within this class of compounds are prostacyclins, prostaglandins, thromboxanes, and leukotrienes.

eicosapentaenoic acid (EPA) (eye-KOH-sah-pen-tah-ee-NO-ik) An omega-3 fatty acid with 20 carbons and 5 carbon-carbon double bonds (C20:5, omega-3). It is present in large amounts in fatty fish and slowly synthesized in the body from alpha-linolenic acid. EPA is a precursor to some eicosanoids.

electrolytes (ih-LEK-tro-lites) Compounds that separate into ions in water and, in turn, are able to conduct an electrical current. These include sodium, chloride, and potassium.

electron A part of an atom that is negatively charged. Electrons orbit the nucleus.

electron transport chain A series of reactions using oxygen to convert NADH + H⁺ and FADH₂ molecules to free NAD⁺ and FDA molecules with the donation of electrons and hydrogen ions to oxygen, yielding water and ATP.

elements Substances that cannot be separated into simpler substances by chemical processes. Common elements in nutrition include carbon, oxygen, hydrogen, nitrogen, calcium, phosphorus, and iron.

elimination diet A restrictive diet that systematically tests foods that may cause an allergic response by first eliminating them for 1 to 2 weeks and then adding them back one at a time.

embryo (EM-bree-oh) In humans, the developing in utero offspring from about the beginning of the third week to the end of the eighth week after conception.

emulsifier (ee-MULL-sih-fire) A compound that can suspend fat in water by isolating individual fat droplets using a shell of water molecules or other substances to prevent the fat from coalescing.

endocrine gland (EN-doh-krin) A hormone-producing gland.

endocrine system The body system consisting of the various glands and the hormones these glands secrete. This system has major regulatory functions in the body, such as in reproduction and cell metabolism.

endocytosis (phagocytosis/pinocytosis) Forms of active absorption in which the absorptive cell forms an indentation in its membrane, and particles (phagocytosis) or fluids (pinocytosis) entering the indentation are then engulfed by the cell.

endometrium (en-doh-ME-tree-um) The membrane that lines the inside of the uterus. It increases in thickness during the menstrual cycle until ovulation occurs. The surface layers are shed during menstruation if conception does not take place.

endoplasmic reticulum (ER) (en-doh-PLAZ-mik re-TIK-u-lum) An organelle in the cytoplasm composed of a network of canals running through the cytoplasm. Rough ER contains ribosomes. Smooth ER contains no ribosomes.

endorphins (en-DOR-fins) Natural body tranquilizers that may be involved in the feeding response and function in pain reduction.

endothelial cells (en-doh-THEE-lee-al) A layer of flat cells lining the blood and lymphatic vessels and the chambers of the heart.

energy balance A state in which energy intake, in the form of food and beverages, matches energy expended, primarily through basal metabolism and physical activity.

energy density A comparison of the energy content of a food with the weight of the food. An energy-dense food is high in energy but weighs very little (e.g., many fried foods), whereas a food low in energy density such as an orange, weighs a lot but is low in energy content.

enriched A term generally meaning that the vitamins thiamin, niacin, riboflavin, and folate and the mineral iron have been added to a grain product to improve nutritional quality.

enterocytes (en-TER-oh-sites) Epithelial cells, which are highly specialized for digestion and absorption, that line the intestinal villi.

enterohepatic circulation (EN-ter-oh-heh-PAT-ik) A continual recycling of compounds between the small intestine and the liver; bile acids are one example of a recycled compound.

enzyme (EN-zime) A compound that speeds the rate of a chemical process but is not altered by the process. Almost all enzymes are proteins (some are made of nucleic acids).

epidemiology (ep-uh-dee-me-OLL-uh-gee) The distribution and determinants of diseases in human populations.

epidermis (ep-ih-DUR-miss) The outermost layer of the skin, composed of epithelial layers.

epigenetic carcinogens (promoters) (ep-ih-je-NET-ik car-SIN-oh-jens) Compounds that increase cell division and thereby increase the chance that a cell with altered DNA will develop into cancer.

epiglottis (ep-ih-GLOT-iss) Flap that folds down over the trachea during swallowing.

epinephrine (ep-ih-NEF-rin) A hormone produced by the adrenal gland in times of stress. It may also have neurotransmitter functions, such as in the brain.

epiphyseal line (ep-ih-FEES-ee-al) A line that replaces the epiphyseal plate when bone growth is complete.

epiphyseal plate A cartilage-like layer in the long bone. It functions in linear growth.

epiphyses (e-PIF-ih-seas) Ends of long bones. The epiphyseal plate—sometimes referred to as the growth plate—is made of cartilage and allows growth of the bone to occur. During childhood, the cartilage cells multiply and absorb calcium to develop into bone.

epithelial tissue (ep-ih-THEE-lee-ul) The surface cells that line the outside of the body and all passageways within it.

epithelium The covering of internal and external surfaces of the body, including the lining of vessels and other small cavities. It consists of epithelial cells joined by a small amount of cementing material.

equilibrium (ee-kwih-LIB-ree-um) In nutrition, a state in which nutrient intake equals nutrient losses. Thus, the body maintains a stable condition.

ergogenic (ur-go-JEN-ic) Work-producing. An ergogenic aid is a mechanical, nutritional, psychological, pharmacological, or physiological substance or treatment that is intended to directly improve exercise performance.

erythrocyte (eh-RITH-row-site) A mature red blood cell. It has no nucleus and a life span of about 120 days; contains hemoglobin, which transports oxygen and carbon dioxide.

erythropoietin (eh-REE-throw-POY-eh-tin) A hormone secreted mostly by the kidneys that enhances red blood cell synthesis and stimulates red blood cell release from bone marrow.

Escherichia coli Bacteria commonly found in the intestinal tract of humans and animals (commonly called *E. coli*). The especially virulent strains 0157:H7 and 0111:H8 have been found in undercooked beef, especially ground beef. Foods implicated in *E. coli* infection include unpasteurized milk, unpasteurized fresh apple cider, salad greens, cantaloupe, dry-cured salami, and many types of sprouts. Cooking destroys *E. coli*.

esophagus (eh-SOF-ah-gus) A tube in the GI tract that connects the pharynx with the stomach.

essential fatty acids Fatty acids that must be supplied by the diet to maintain health. Currently only linoleic acid and alpha-linolenic acid are classified as essential.

essential amino acids Amino acids that cannot be synthesized by humans in sufficient amounts or at all and therefore must be included in the diet; there are nine essential amino acids. These are also called *indispensable amino acids*.

essential nutrient In nutritional terms, a substance that, when left out of a diet, leads to signs of poor health. The body either can't produce this nutrient or can't produce enough of it to meet its needs. Then, if added back to a diet before permanent damage occurs, the affected aspects of health are restored.

esterification (e-ster-ih-fih-KAY-shun) The process of attaching fatty acids to a glycerol molecule, creating an ester bond and releasing water. Removing a fatty acid is called deesterification; reattaching a fatty acid is called reesterification.

Estimated Average Requirement (EAR) An amount of nutrient intake that is estimated to meet the needs of 50% of the individuals in a specific age and gender group.

Estimated Energy Requirement (EER) An estimate of the amount of energy intake that will balance energy needs of an average person within specific gender, age, and other considerations.

ethanol Chemical term for the form of alcohol found in alcoholic beverages.

eustachian tubes (you-STAY-shun) Thin tubes connected to the middle ear that open into the throat.

exchange The serving size of a food on a specific exchange list.

Exchange System A system for classifying foods into numerous lists based on the foods' macronutrient composition and establishing serving sizes, so that one serving of each food on a list contains the same amount of carbohydrate, protein, fat, and energy content.

exercise Physical activity that is done with the intent to provide a health benefit, such as improved muscle tone or stamina.

exocrine gland (EK-so-krin) A cluster of epithelial cells specialized for secretion. They have ducts that lead to an epithelial surface.

exocytosis (ek-so-sigh-TOE-sis) The process of cellular secretion in which the secretory products are contained within a membrane-enclosed vesicle. The vesicle fuses with the cell membrane and is open to the extracellular environment.

experiment A test made to examine the validity of a hypothesis.

extracellular fluid (ECF) Fluid present outside the cells; it includes intravascular and interstitial fluids; represents one-third of all body fluid.

extracellular space The space outside cells.

facilitated diffusion Absorption in which a carrier shuttles substances into the absorptive cell but no energy is expended. A concentration gradient higher in the intestinal contents than in the absorptive cell drives the absorption.

failure to thrive Inadequate gains in height and weight in infancy, often due to an inadequate food intake.

famine An extreme shortage of food that leads to massive starvation in a population; often associated with crop failures, war, and political unrest.

fasting hypoglycemia (HIGH-po-gligh-SEE-me-ah) Low blood glucose that follows about a day of fasting.

fat A general term that describes substances that dissolve in organic solvents such as benzene and ether. Fats are mostly composed of carbon and hydrogen, with relatively small amounts of oxygen and other elements.

fat-soluble vitamins Vitamins that dissolve in fat and such substances as ether and benzene, but not readily in water. These vitamins are A, D, E, and K.

fatty acid A chain of carbons chemically bonded together and surrounded by hydrogen molecules. These hydrocarbons are found in lipids and contain a carboxyl (acid

$$\overset{O}{\underset{\parallel}{}}$$

group $(-C-OH)$ at one end and a methyl group $(-CH_3)$ at the other.

feces (FEE-seas) Substances discharged from the bowel during defecation, including undigested food residue, dead GI tract cells, mucus, bacteria, and other waste material.

feeding center A group of cells in the hypothalamus that, when stimulated, causes hunger.

female athlete triad A condition characterized by disordered eating, lack of menstrual periods, and osteoporosis.

fermentation The metabolism, without the use of oxygen, of carbohydrates to alcohols, acids, and carbon dioxide.

ferritin A protein compound that serves as the storage form of iron in the blood and tissues.

fetal alcohol effect (FAE) (FEET-al) Hyperactivity, attention deficit disorder, poor judgment, sleep disorders, and delayed learning as a result of prenatal exposure to alcohol.

fetal alcohol syndrome (FAS) A group of irreversible physical and mental abnormalities in the infant that result from the mother's consuming alcohol during pregnancy.

fetus (FEET-us) The developing life form from about the beginning of the ninth week after conception until birth.

fiber Substances in plant foods that are not broken down by the digestive processes of the stomach or small intestine. These add bulk to feces. Fiber naturally found in foods is called dietary fiber.

flavin adenine dinucleotide (FAD) A compound that readily accepts and donates electrons and hydrogen ions; formed from the vitamin riboflavin.

fluoride A trace mineral that increases resistance of tooth enamel to dental caries. Typical sources are fluoridated water and toothpastes.

fluoroapatite (fleur-oh-APP-uh-tite) A fluoride-containing, acid-resistant crystalline substance that is produced during bone and tooth development. Its presence in teeth helps prevent dental caries.

folate A water-soluble vitamin that shares a close relationship with vitamin B-12. In its coenzyme form, folate is necessary for the synthesis of DNA and in the metabolism of various amino acids and their derivatives, such as homocysteine. It also functions in the formation of neurotransmitters in the brain. A maternal deficiency of folate can lead to neural tube defects in the very early development of the fetus. Asparagus, spinach, fortified grain products, and legumes are good sources.

folic acid The form of folate found in supplements and fortified foods.

folk medicine A medical treatment based on the beliefs, traditions, or customs of a particular society or ethnic/cultural group.

follicular hyperkeratosis (fo-LICK-you-lar high-per-ker-ah-TOE-sis) A condition in which keratin, a protein, accumulates around hair follicles.

foodborne illness Sickness caused by the ingestion of food containing toxic substances produced by microorganisms.

food diary A written record of sequential food intake for a period of time. Details associated with the food intake are often recorded as well.

food insecurity A condition of anxiety regarding running out of either food or money to buy more food.

food intolerance An adverse reaction to food that does not involve an allergic reaction.

food sensitivity A mild reaction to a substance in a food that might be expressed as light itching or redness of the skin.

fore milk The first breast milk delivered in the breastfeeding session.

fortified A term generally meaning that vitamins, minerals, or both have been added to a food product in excess of what was originally found in the product.

fraternal twins Offspring that develop from two separate ova and sperm and therefore have separate genetic identities, although they develop simultaneously in the mother.

free radicals Short-lived form of a compound that has an unpaired electron, causing it to seek an electron from another compound. Free radicals are strong oxidizing agents and can be very destructive to electron-dense cell components, such as the DNA and cell membranes.

free water The water not bound to the compounds in a food. This water is available for microbial use.

fructose (FROOK-tose) A monosaccharide with six carbons that/forms a five-membered or six-membered ring with oxygen in the ring; found in fruits and honey.

fruitarian (froot-AIR-ee-un) A person who eats primarily fruits, nuts, honey, and vegetable oils.

functional fiber Any fiber added to foods that has shown to provide health benefits.

functional foods Foods that provide health benefits beyond those supplied by the traditional nutrients they contain. For example, a tomato contains the phytochemical lycopene, so it can be called a functional food.

fungi Simple parasitic life forms, including molds, mildews, yeasts, and mushrooms. They live on dead or decaying organic matter. Fungi can grow as single cells, like yeast, or as multicellular colonies, as seen with molds.

galactose (gah-LAK-tos) A six-carbon monosaccharide that forms a six-membered ring with oxygen in the ring; an isomer of glucose.

galactosemia (gah-LAK-toh-SEE-mee-ah) A rare genetic disease characterized by the buildup of the single sugar galactose in the bloodstream, resulting from the inability of the liver to metabolize it. If present at birth and left untreated, this disease can cause severe mental retardation and cataracts in the infant.

gallbladder The organ attached to the underside of the liver and in which bile is stored and secreted.

gastric inhibitory peptide (GIP) (GAS-trik in-HIB-ih-tor-ee PEP-tide) A hormone that slows gastric motility and stimulates insulin release from the pancreas.

gastrin (GAS-trin) A hormone that stimulates enzyme and acid secretion by the stomach.

gastroesophageal reflux disease (GERD) (gas-troh-eh-SOF-ah-jee-al) Disease that results from stomach acid backing up into the esophagus. The acid irritates the lining of the esophagus, causing pain.

gastrointestinal distention (gas-troh-in-TEST-in-al) Expansion of the wall of the stomach or intestines due to pressure caused by the presence of gases, food, drink, or other factors. This expansion contributes to a feeling of satiety brought on by food intake.

gastrointestinal (GI) tract Comprises the main sites in the body used in digestion and absorption of nutrients. The GI tract consists of the mouth, esophagus, stomach, small intestine, large intestine, rectum, and anus.

gastroplasty (GAS-troh-plas-tee) Surgery performed on the stomach to limit its volume to approximately 30 milliliters.

gene expression (JEAN) The activation of a specific site on DNA, which results in either the activation or the inhibition of the gene.

generally recognized as safe (GRAS) A list of food additives that in 1958 were considered safe for consumption. Manufacturers were allowed to continue to use these additives, without special clearance, when needed for food products. FDA bears responsibility for proving they are not safe; it can remove unsafe products from the list.

genes (JEANs) The hereditary material on chromosomes that makes up DNA. Genes provide the blueprint for the production of cell proteins. The nucleus of the cell contains about 30,000 genes.

genetic engineering Manipulation of the genetic makeup of any organism with recombinant DNA technology.

genetically modified organism (GMO) Any organism created by genetic engineering.

genotoxic carcinogen (initiator) (JEH-no-TOK-sik car-SIN-oh-jen) A compound that directly alters DNA or is converted in cells to metabolites that alter DNA, thereby providing the potential for cancer to develop.

geometric ratio A series of numbers wherein the division of each number by the one to the left of it yields the same answer.

gestation (jes-TAY-shun) The period of intrauterine development of offspring, from conception to birth; in humans, gestation lasts for about 40 weeks after the woman's last menstrual period.

gestational diabetes (jes-TAY-shun-al) A high blood glucose concentration that develops during pregnancy and returns to normal after birth; one cause is the placental production of hormones that antagonize the regulation of blood glucose by insulin.

ghrelin A hormone made by the stomach that increases food intake.

glomerulus (glo-MER-you-lus) The capillaries in the kidney that filter waste products from the blood.

glucagon (GLOO-kuh-gon) A hormone made by the pancreas that stimulates the breakdown of glycogen in the liver into glucose; this breakdown increases blood glucose. Glucagon also performs other functions.

gluconeogenesis (gloo-ko-nee-oh-JEN-uh-sis) The production of new glucose by metabolic pathways in the cell. Amino acids derived from protein usually provide the carbons for this glucose.

glucose (GLOO-kos) A six-carbon carbohydrate found in blood as well as in table sugar bound to fructose; also known as *dextrose*, it is one of the simple sugars.

glucose polymer A carbohydrate source used in some sports drinks that consists of a few glucose molecules bonded together.

glutathione (gloo-tah-THIGH-on) A reducing agent. It can remove toxic peroxides that form in the cell during aerobic metabolism.

glutathione peroxidase (gloo-tah-THIGH-on per-OX-ih-dase) A selenium-containing enzyme that can destroy peroxides. It acts in conjunction with vitamin E to reduce free radical damage to cells.

glycemic index (GI) (gli-SEA-mik) The blood glucose response of a given food compared to a standard (typically, glucose or white bread).

glycemic load (GL) The amount of carbohydrate in a food multiplied by the glycemic index of that carbohydrate. The result is then divided by 100.

glycerol (GLIS-er-ol) A three-carbon alcohol that provides the backbone to form triglycerides.

glycocalyx (gli-ko-KAL-iks) Projections of proteins on the microvilli; they contain enzymes to digest protein and carbohydrate.

glycogen (GLI-ko-jen) A carbohydrate made of multiple units of glucose with a highly branched structure; sometimes known as *animal starch*. It is the storage form of glucose in humans and is synthesized (and stored) in the liver and muscles.

glycolipid (gli-ko-LIP-id) A lipid (fat) containing a carbohydrate group.

glycolysis (gli-KOL-ih-sis) The metabolic pathway that converts glucose into two molecules of pyruvic acid, with the net gain of two ATP and two NADH + 2H$^+$.

glycoprotein (gli-ko-PRO-teen) A protein containing a carbohydrate group.

glycosylation (gli-COS-ih-lay-shun) The process by which glucose attaches to (glycates) other compounds, such as proteins.

goiter (GOY-ter) An enlargement of the thyroid gland that can be caused by a lack of iodide in the diet.

goitrogens (GOY-troh-jens) Substances in food and water that interfere with thyroid gland metabolism and thus may cause goiter if consumed in large amounts.

Golgi complex (GOAL-jee) The cell organelle near the nucleus that processes newly synthesized protein for secretion or distribution to other organelles.

gout Joint inflammation caused by accumulation of a body compound called uric acid. Obesity is a risk factor for developing gout.

green revolution Increases in crop yields accompanying the introduction of new agricultural technologies in less developed countries, beginning in the 1960s. The key technologies were high-yielding, disease-resistant strains of rice, wheat, and corn; greater use of fertilizer and water; and improved cultivation practices.

growth hormone A pituitary hormone that stimulates body growth and release of fat from storage; it also has other effects.

gums Soluble fiber consisting of chains of galactose and other monosaccharides; characteristically found in exudates from plant stems.

gynecoid obesity (GI-nih-coyd) Obesity in which fat storage is located primarily in the buttocks and thigh area.

H₂ blockers Medications such as cimetidine (Tagamet) that block the increase of stomach acid production caused by histamine.

Harris-Benedict equation An equation that predicts resting metabolic rate based on a person's weight, height, and age.

heart attack Rapid fall in heart function caused by reduced blood flow through the heart's blood vessels. Often part of the heart dies in the process. It is technically called a *myocardial infarction*.

heartburn Pain caused by stomach acid backing up into the esophagus and irritating the tissue in that organ.

heart disease See *cardiovascular disease*.

heat cramps A frequent complication of heat exhaustion. They usually occur in individuals who have experienced large sweat losses from exercising for several hours in a hot climate and have consumed a large volume of water. The cramps occur in skeletal muscles and consist of contractions for 1 to 3 minutes at a time.

heat exhaustion The first stage of heat-related illness that occurs because of depletion of blood volume from fluid loss by the body. This depletion increases body temperature and can lead to headaches, dizziness, muscle weakness, and visual disturbances, among other effects.

heatstroke A condition in which the internal body temperature reaches 104°F. Sweating generally ceases if left untreated, and blood circulation is greatly reduced. Nervous system damage may ensue, and death is likely. Often the skin of individuals who suffer heatstroke is hot and dry.

helper T cell Type of T cell that interacts with macrophages and secretes substances to signal an invading pathogen; stimulates B lymphocytes to proliferate.

hematocrit (hee-MAT-oh-krit) The percentage of total blood volume occupied by red blood cells.

hematopoiesis (heem-oh-po-EE-sis) The production of blood cells.

heme iron (HEEM) Iron provided from animal tissues primarily as a component of hemoglobin and myoglobin. Approximately 40% of the iron in meat is heme iron; it is readily absorbed.

hemicellulose (hem-ih-SELL-you-los) A mostly insoluble fiber containing galactose, glucose, and other monosaccharides bonded together.

hemochromatosis (heem-oh-krom-ah-TOE-sis) A disorder of iron metabolism characterized by increased absorption of iron, saturation of iron-binding proteins, and deposition of hemosiderin in the liver tissue.

hemoglobin (HEEM-oh-glow-bin) The iron-containing protein in red blood cells that transports oxygen to the body tissues and some carbon dioxide away from the tissues. It is also responsible for the red color of blood.

hemolysis (hee-MOL-ih-sis) Destruction of red blood cells caused by the breakdown of the red blood cell membranes. This causes the cell contents to leak into the fluid portion (plasma) of the blood.

hemorrhage (hem-OR-ij) An escape of blood from blood vessels.

hemorrhagic stroke (hem-oh-RAJ-ik) Damage to part of the brain resulting from rupture of a blood vessel and subsequent bleeding within or over the internal surface of the brain.

hemorrhoid (HEM-or-oid) A pronounced swelling in a large vein, particularly veins found in the anal region.

hemosiderin (heem-oh-SID-er-in) An insoluble iron-protein compound found in the liver. Hemosiderin stores iron when the amount of iron in the body exceeds the storage capacity of ferritin.

hepatic portal system (vein) (he-PAT-ik) The vein in the GI tract that conveys blood from capillaries in the intestines and portions of the stomach to capillaries in the liver. Also simply referred to as portal vein.

hepatic vein (he-PAT-ik) The vein that drains the liver.

hepatitis A A virus found in the human intestinal tract and feces. It can contaminate many foods, especially shellfish and raw foods, and can endure significant heat, cold, and drying.

herbicide (ERB-ih-side) A compound that reduces the growth and reproduction of plants.

hexose (HEK-sos) A general term describing a carbohydrate containing 6 carbons.

high-density lipoprotein (HDL) The lipoprotein that picks up cholesterol from dying cells and other sources and transfers it to the other lipoproteins in the bloodstream as well as directly to the liver. A low blood HDL value increases the risk for cardiovascular disease.

high-fructose corn syrup A corn syrup that has been manufactured to contain between 40 and 90% fructose.

high-quality (complete) proteins Dietary proteins that contain ample amounts of all nine essential amino acids.

hind milk (HYND) The milk secreted at the end of a breastfeeding session; it is higher in fat than fore milk.

histamine (HISS-tuh-meen) A breakdown product of the amino acid histidine that stimulates acid secretion by the stomach and has other effects on the body, such as contraction of smooth muscles, increased nasal secretions, relaxation of blood vessels, and changes in constriction of airways.

homeostasis (home-ee-oh-STAY-sis) A series of adjustments that prevent change in the internal environment in the body.

homocysteine (homo-CYS-teen) An amino acid not used in protein synthesis, but instead arises during metabolism of the amino acid methionine. Homocysteine is likely toxic to many cells, such as those lining the blood vessels.

hormone A compound with a specific site of synthesis that, when secreted into the bloodstream, controls the function of cells in its target organ or organs. Hormones can be amino acidlike (epinephrine), proteinlike (insulin), or fatlike (estrogen).

hospice care (HAHS-pis) A facility offering care that emphasizes comfort and dignity in death.

human immunodeficiency virus (HIV) The virus that leads to acquired immunodeficiency syndrome (AIDS).

hunger The primarily physiological (internal) drive to find and eat food.

hydrogen peroxide Chemically, H_2O_2.

hydrogenation (high-dro-jen-AY-shun) The addition of hydrogen to a carbon-carbon double bond, producing a single carbon-carbon bond with two hydrogens attached to each carbon. Because hydrogenation of unsaturated fatty acids in a vegetable oil increases its hardness, this process is used to convert liquid oils into more solid fats, which are used in making margarine and shortening.

Trans fatty acids are a by-product of hydrogenation of vegetable oils.

hydrolysis (high-DROL-ih-sis) A chemical reaction in which a compound is broken down by the addition of water. One product receives a hydrogen ion (H^+), while the other product receives a hydroxyl ion (OH^-). Hydrolytic enzymes break down compounds using water in this manner.

hydrolysis reaction A chemical reaction in which a bond between two molecules is broken by the inclusion of a water molecule. The water donates a hydrogen to one reactant and a hydroxyl (–OH) group to the other reactant.

hydrophilic (high-dro-FILL-ik) Attracts water; literally means "water loving."

hydrophobic (high-dro-FO-bik) Repels water; literally means "water fearing."

hydroxyapatite (high-drox-ee-APP-uh-tite) A compound, composed primarily of calcium and phosphate, that is deposited into the bone protein matrix to give bone strength and rigidity ($Ca_{10}[PO_4]_6OH_2$).

hyperactivity A poorly defined term generally used to label inattention, irritability, and excessively active behavior in children. Technically referred to as attention deficit hyperactive disorder.

hypercalcemia (high-per-kal-SEE-mee-ah) A high concentration of calcium in the bloodstream. This condition can lead to loss of appetite, calcium deposits in organs, and other health problems.

hypercarotenemia (high-per-car-oh-teh-NEEM-ee-ah) Elevated amounts of carotenoids in the bloodstream, usually caused by consuming a diet high in carrots or squash or by taking beta-carotene supplements.

hyperglycemia (HIGH-per-gligh-SEE-me-uh) High blood glucose, above 125 mg/100 ml (dl) of blood.

hypergymnasia (high-per-jim-NAY-zee-ah) Exercising more than is required for good physical fitness or maximum performance in a sport; excessive exercise.

hyperlipidemia (high-per-lip-ih-DEE-me-ah) The presence of an abnormally large amount of lipids in the circulating blood.

hyperplasia (high-per-PLAY-zee-uh) An increase in cell number.

hypertension (high-per-TEN-shun) A condition in which blood pressure remains persistently elevated. Obesity, inactivity, alcohol intake, and excess salt intake all can contribute to the problem.

hypertrophy (high-PURR-tro-fee) An increase in tissue or organ size.

hypervitaminosis A (HIGH-per-vi-tah-mi-NO-sis) A condition resulting from intake of excessive amounts of vitamin A.

hypocalcemia (HIGH-po-kal-SEE-me-ah) Low blood calcium, typically arising from inadequate parathyroid hormone release or action.

hypochromic (high-po-KROM-ik) Describing pale red blood cells lacking sufficient hemoglobin as a result of iron deficiency. Hypochromic cells have a reduced oxygen-carrying ability.

hypoglycemia (HIGH-po-gligh-SEE-me-uh) Low blood glucose, below 40 to 50 mg/100 ml (dl) of blood.

hypothalamus (high-po-THALL-uh-mus) A region at the base of the brain that contains cells that play a role in the regulation of hunger, respiration, body temperature, and other body functions.

hypothesis (high-POTH-eh-sis) A tentative explanation by scientists to explain a phenomenon.

hysterectomy (hiss-te-RECK-toe-mee) Surgical removal of the uterus.

identical twins Two offspring that develop from a single ovum and sperm and, consequently, have the same genetic makeup.

ileocecal sphincter (ill-ee-oh-SEE-kal SFINK-ter) Ring of smooth muscle between the ileum of the small intestine and the colon.

ileum (ILL-ee-um) Terminal portion of the small intestine.

immune system The body system consisting of white blood cells, lymph glands and vessels, and various other body tissues. The immune system provides defense against foreign invaders, primarily because of the production of various types of white blood cells.

immunoglobulins (em-you-no-GLOB-you-lins) Proteins found in the blood that are responsible for antibody-mediated immunity and that bind specifically to antigen; also called *antibodies*. Immunoglobulins are produced by certain white blood cells in response to a foreign substance (antigen) in the bloodstream.

incidence The number of new cases of a disease in a defined population over a specific period of time, such as 1 year.

incidental food additives Additives that appear in food products indirectly, from environmental contamination of food ingredients or during the manufacturing process.

incomplete (lower-quality) protein Food protein that lacks ample amount of one or more of the essential amino acids needed to support human protein needs.

indirect calorimetry (kal-oh-RIM-eh-tree) A method to measure energy use by the body by measuring oxygen uptake. Formulas are then used to convert this gas exchange value into energy use.

infancy Earliest stage of childhood—from birth to 1 year of age.

infectious disease (in-FEK-shus) Any disease caused by an invasion of the body by microorganisms, such as bacteria, fungi, or viruses.

infrastructure The basic framework of a system or organization. For a society, this includes roads, bridges, telephones, and other basic technologies.

inorganic (in-or-GAN-ik) Any substance lacking carbon atoms bonded to hydrogen atoms in the chemical structure.

insensible water losses Water losses not readily perceived, such as water lost with each breath.

insoluble fibers Fibers that mostly do not dissolve in water and are not generally metabolized by bacteria in the large intestine. These include cellulose, some hemicelluloses, and lignins; more formally called *nonfermentable fibers.*

insulin (IN-su-lynn) A hormone produced by beta cells of the pancreas. Among other processes, insulin increases the synthesis of glycogen in the liver and the movement of glucose from the bloodstream into muscle and adipose cells.

integumentary system (in-teg-you-MEN-tah-ree) Having to do with the skin, hair, glands, and nails;

the largest organ in the body.

intentional food additive Additives knowingly (directly) incorporated into food products by manufacturers.

interferons (in-ter-FEAR-ons) A group of proteins released by virus-infected cells that bind to other cells, stimulating synthesis of antiviral proteins that in turn inhibit viral multiplication.

intermediate A chemical compound formed in one of many steps in a metabolic pathway.

international unit (IU) A crude measure of vitamin activity, often based on the growth rate of animals. Today these units have generally been replaced by precise measurement of actual quantities in milligrams or micrograms.

interstitial fluid (in-ter-STISH-al) Fluid between cells.

intracellular (in-tra-SELL-you-lar) Within a cell.

intracellular fluid Fluid contained within a cell; represents about two-thirds of all body fluid.

intravascular fluid (in-tra-VAS-kyu-lar) Fluid within the bloodstream (i.e., in the arteries, veins, capillaries, and lymph vessels); represents about 25% of all body fluids.

intrinsic factor (in-TRIN-zik) A substance present in gastric juice that enhances vitamin B-12 absorption.

in utero (in-YOU-ter-oh) "In the uterus," or during pregnancy.

in vitro (in-VEE-troh) Refers to experiments performed outside the body, such as in a test tube—literally, *in glass.*

in vivo (in-VEE-vo) Within the living body.

iodide A trace mineral that functions as a component of thyroid hormones. A deficiency can result in goiter. Iodized salt, saltwater fish, and iodide-fortified foods are good sources.

ion (EYE-on) An atom with an unequal number of electrons and protons. Negative ions have more electrons than protons; positive ions have more protons than electrons.

ionic bond (eye-ON-ik) A union between two atoms formed by an attraction of a positive ion to a negative ion, as seen in table salt (NA^+Cl^-).

iron A trace mineral that functions as a component of hemoglobin and other key compounds used in respiration; also important in immune function and cognitive development. Meats, seafood, molasses, and fortified foods are good sources.

irradiation (ir-RAY-dee-AY-shun) A process in which radiation energy is applied to foods, creating compounds (free radicals) within the food that destroy cell membranes, break down DNA, link proteins together, limit enzyme activity, and alter a variety of other proteins and cell functions of microorganisms that can lead to food spoilage. This process does not make the food radioactive.

ischemia (ih-SKI-mee-ah) Lack of blood flow due to mechanical obstruction of the blood supply, mainly from arterial narrowing.

ischemia stroke (ih-SKI-mik) A stroke caused by the absence of blood flow to a part of the brain.

isomers (EYE-so-mers) Different chemical structures for compounds that share the same chemical formula.

isotope (EYE-so-towp) An alternate form of a chemical element. It differs from other atoms of the same element in the number of neutrons in its nucleus.

jaundice (JOHN-diss) Yellowish staining of skin, sclerae of the eyes, and other tissues by bile pigments that build up in the blood.

jejunum (je-JOO-num) The first half of the small intestine (minus the first 12 in., which is the duodenum).

ketogenic (kee-toe-JEN-ik) A name often given to diets that lead to the abundant production of ketone bodies by the liver. This excess production can be caused by a low carbohydrate intake.

ketone bodies (KEE-tone) Incomplete breakdown products of fat, containing three or four carbons. Most contain a chemical group called a ketone, hence the name. An example is aceto acetic acid.

ketosis (kee-TOE-sis) The condition of having a high concentration of ketone bodies and related breakdown products in the bloodstream and tissues.

kidney nephrons (NEF-rons) The units of kidney cells that filter wastes from the bloodstream and deposit them into the urine.

kilocalorie (kill-oh-KAL-oh-ree) (kcal) The heat energy needed to raise the temperature of 1000 grams (1 L) of water 1 degree Celsius; also written as Calories, with a capital C.

kilojoule (KIL-oh-jool) (kJ) A measure of work. A mass of one kilogram moving at a velocity of 1 meter/sec possesses the energy of 1 kJ. One kcal equals 4.18 kJ.

kwashiorkor (kwash-ee-OR-core) A disease occurring primarily in young children who have an existing disease and who consume a marginal amount of energy and considerably insufficient amounts of protein in relation to needs. The child generally exhibits edema, poor growth, weakness, and an increased susceptibility to further illness.

lactase An enzyme made by absorptive cells of the small intestine; this enzyme digests lactose to glucose and galactose.

lactation The period of milk secretion following pregnancy; typically called *breastfeeding.*

lacteal (LACK-tee-al) A small lymphatic duct within a villus of the small intestine.

lactic acid (LAK-tik) A three-carbon acid formed during anaerobic cell metabolism; a partial breakdown product of glucose; also called *lactate.*

***lactobacillus bifidus* factor (lak-toe-bah-SIL-us BIFF-id-us)** A protective factor secreted in the colostrum that encourages growth of beneficial bacteria in the newborn's intestines.

lacto-ovo-pesco vegetarian (lak-toe-o-vo-pes-co-vej-eh-TEAR-ree-an) A person who consumes only plant products, dairy products, eggs, and fish.

lactoovovegetarian (lak-toe-o-vo-vej-eh-TEAR-ree-an) A person who consumes plant products, dairy products, and eggs.

lactose (LAK-tose) Glucose bonded to another sugar, galactose.

lactose intolerance A condition where noticeable symptoms such as abdominal gas and bloating appear as a result of severe lactose maldigestion.

lactose maldigestion (primary and secondary) Primary lactose maldigestion occurs when lactase production declines for no apparent reason. Secondary lactose maldigestion occurs when a specific cause, such as long-standing diarrhea, results in a decline in lactase production. The development of significant symptoms after lactose intake is called *lactose intolerance.*

lactovegetarian (lak-toe-vej-eh-TEAR-ree-an) A person who consumes plant products and dairy products.

lanugo (lah-NEW-go) Downlike hair that appears after a person has lost much body fat through semistarvation. The hair stands erect and traps air, acting as insulation for the body to compensate for the relative lack of body fat, which usually functions as insulation.

larva An early developmental stage in the life history of some organisms, such as parasites.

larynx (LAYR-ingks) The structure located between the pharynx and trachea that contains the vocal cords.

laxative A medication or other substance that stimulates evacuation of the intestinal tract.

lean body mass Body weight after subtracting fat storage weight. Lean body mass includes organs such as the brain, muscles, and liver as well as blood and other body fluids.

lecithins (LESS-uh-thins) A group of phospholipids containing two fatty acids, a phosphate group, and a choline molecule. Lecithins are a group of compounds, because they can differ based on the types of fatty acids found on each lecithin molecule.

leptin A hormone (167 amino acids) made by adipose tissue that influences long-term regulation of fat mass. Leptin also influences reproductive functions as well as other body processes such as insulin release.

let-down reflex A reflex stimulated by infant suckling that causes the release (ejection) of milk from milk ducts in the mother's breasts; also called *milk ejection reflex.*

leukemia (loo-KEY-mee-ah) A malignant neoplasm of blood-forming tissues, the bone marrow.

leukocyte (LOO-ko-site) A white blood cell.

leukotriene (LT) (loo-ko-TRY-een) An eicosanoid involved in inflammatory or hypersensitivity reactions, such as asthma.

life expectancy The average length of life for a given group of people (usually determined by the year of birth).

life span The potential oldest age a person can reach.

lignans A phytochemical class that acts as a phytoestrogen in the body. Food sources are whole grains and flax seeds.

lignins Insoluble fiber made up of a multiringed alcohol (noncarbohydrate) structure.

limiting amino acid The essential amino acid in the lowest concentration in a food or diet relative to body needs.

linoleic acid (lin-oh-LEE-ik) An essential omega-6 fatty acid with 18 carbon and 2 double bonds (C18:2, omega-6).

lipase (LYE-pase) Fat-digesting enzyme; lipase is produced by the stomach, salivary glands, and the pancreas.

lipid A compound composed of much carbon and hydrogen, little oxygen, and sometimes other elements. Lipids dissolve in ether or benzene, but not in water, and include fats, oils, and cholesterol.

lipid peroxidation (per-OX-ih-day-shun) A process initiated by an environmental component that induces the formation of an organic free radical, R•. In the formation of a fatty acid of this type, first a carbon-carbon double bond is broken. The resulting breakdown products react

with oxygen to form peroxides (a) or free radicals (b):

a.
$$\begin{array}{c} \quad H \quad H \\ \quad | \quad | \\ {-}C{-}C{-}O{-}O{-}H \\ \quad | \quad | \\ \quad H \quad H \end{array}$$

b.
$$\begin{array}{c} \quad H \quad H \\ \quad | \quad | \quad \bullet \\ {-}C{-}C{-}O{-}O \\ \quad | \quad | \\ \quad H \quad H \end{array}$$

lipogenesis (lye-poh-JEN-eh-sis) The building of fatty acids using derivatives of acetyl-CoA.

lipogenic (lye-poh-JEN-ik) The creation of lipid. The liver is the major organ with lipogenic potential in the human body.

lipolysis (lye-POL-ih-sis) The breakdown of triglycerides to glycerol and fatty acids.

lipoprotein (ly-poh-PRO-teen) A compound found in the bloodstream containing a core of lipids with a shell composed of protein, phospholipid, and cholesterol.

lipoprotein lipase (lye-poh-PRO-teen LYE-pase) An enzyme attached to the outside of endothelial cells that line the capillaries in the blood vessels; it breaks down triglycerides into free fatty acids and glycerol.

lipoxin (LX) (lih-POX-in) Eicosanoids made by white blood cells that are involved in the immune system and allergic responses.

lipoxygenase (lih-POX-ih-jen-ace) An enzyme used to synthesize leukotrienes and some other types of eicosanoids.

***Listeria monocytogenes* (lis-TEER-i-a mono-sy-TODGE-en-ees)** Bacteria widely distributed in the environment, often entering food from contamination with animal or human feces. Soft cheeses made with unpasteurized milk and unpasteurized milk itself are most often implicated. *Listeria* is very hardy, resisting heat, salt, cold, nitrate, and acidity much better than any other bacteria. Thorough cooking and pasteurization destroy *Listeria.*

liter (LEE-ter) (L) A measure of volume in the metric system. One liter equals 0.96 quarts.

liver Largest organ in the body, located in the abdominal cavity below the diaphragm; performs many vital functions that maintain balance in blood composition.

lobules (LOB-you-els) Saclike structures in the breast that store milk.

long-chain fatty acids Fatty acids that contain 12 or more carbons.

low birth weight (LBW) Referring to any infant weighing less than 5.5 pounds (2.5 kilograms) at birth; most commonly results from preterm birth.

low-density lipoprotein (LDL) The lipoprotein in the blood containing primarily cholesterol; elevated LDL-cholesterol is strongly linked to cardiovascular disease risk.

lower-body obesity The type of obesity in which fat storage is primarily located in the buttocks and thigh area.

lower esophageal sphincter (e-sof-ah-GEE-al SFINK-ter) A circular muscle that constricts the opening of the esophagus to the stomach.

lower-quality (incomplete) proteins Dietary proteins that are low in or lack one or more essential amino acids.

lumen (LOO-men) The inside of a tube, such as the inside cavity of the GI tract.

lymph (LIMF) A clear, plasmalike fluid that flows through lymph vessels.

lymphatic system (lim-FAT-ick) A system of vessels that can accept fluid surrounding cells and large particles, such as products of fat absorption. This lymph fluid eventually passes into the bloodstream via the lymphatic system.

lymphatic vessel (lim-FAT-ick) A vessel that carries lymph.

lymph duct A large lymphatic vessel that empties lymph into the circulatory system.

lymph node A small structure located along the course of the lymph vessels.

lymphocyte (LIM-fo-site) A class of white blood cells involved in the immune system, generally comprising about 25% of all white blood cells. There are several types of lymphocytes with diverse functions, including antibody production, allergic reactions, graft rejections, tumor control, and regulation of the immune system.

lymphoma (lim-FO-ma) A malignant tumor arising from lymph nodes or other lymph tissues.

lysosome (LYE-so-som) A cell organelle that contains digestive enzymes for use inside the cell for turnover of cell parts.

lysozyme (LYE-so-zime) A set of enzyme substances produced by a variety of cells; it can destroy bacteria by rupturing cell membranes.

macrocyte (MACK-ro-site) Literally "large cell," such as a large red blood cell.

macrocytic anemia (mack-ro-SIT-ik ah-NEM-ee-a) Anemia characterized by the presence of abnormally large red blood cells in the bloodstream.

macronutrient A nutrient needed in gram quantities in the diet. Fat, protein, and carbohydrates are macronutrients.

macrophage (MACK-ro-faj) Any large mononuclear phagocytic cell that is found in the tissues and is derived from a monocyte in the blood. Besides functioning as important phagocytes, macrophages secrete numerous cytokines and act as antigen-presenting cells.

macular degeneration A painless condition leading to disruption of the central part of the retina (in the eye) and, in turn, blurred vision.

magnesium (mag-NEE-zee-um) A major mineral essential to many biochemical and physiological processes, including calcium metabolism, active ATP formation, enzyme function, DNA and RNA synthesis, nerve and heart function, and insulin function. Spinach, squash, and wheat bran are good sources.

major mineral A mineral vital to health that is required in the diet in amounts greater than 100 mg/day; also called a *macromineral.*

malignant (ma-LIG-nant) Essentially, malicious. In reference to a tumor, the property of spreading locally and to distant sites.

malnutrition Failing health that results from long-standing dietary practices that do not meet nutritional needs.

malonyl-CoA (MAL-o-kneel) Building block in fatty acid synthesis:

$$\text{HO}{-}\overset{\displaystyle O}{\overset{\|}{C}}{-}CH_2{-}\overset{\displaystyle O}{\overset{\|}{C}}{-}\text{Coenzyme A}$$

maltase (MALL-tase) An enzyme made by absorptive cells of the small intestine; this enzyme digests maltose to two glucoses.

maltose (MALL-tos) Glucose bonded to glucose.

manganese A trace mineral that functions as a cofactor of some enzymes, such as those involved in carbohydrate metabolism and antioxidant protection. Nuts, oats, beans, and tea are good sources.

mannitol An alcohol derivative of fructose.

marasmus (ma-RAZ-mus) A disease that results from consuming a grossly insufficient amount of protein and energy; one of the diseases classed as protein-energy malnutrition. Victims have little or no fat stores, little muscle mass, and poor strength. Death from infections is common.

mass movement A peristaltic wave that simultaneously coordinates contraction over a large area of the large intestine. Mass movements propel material from one portion of the large intestine to another and from the large intestine into the rectum.

mast cell Tissue cell that releases histamine and other chemicals involved in inflammation.

meconium (me-KO-nee-um) The first thick, mucuslike stool passed by the infant after birth.

medium-chain fatty acid A fatty acid that contains 6 to 10 carbons.

megadose Intake of a nutrient far beyond estimates of needs to prevent a deficiency, or what would be found in a balanced diet; 2 to 10 times human needs is a starting point for such a dosage.

megaloblast (MEG-ah-low-blast) A large, nucleated, immature red blood cell in the bone marrow that results from the inability of a precursor cell to divide when it normally should.

megaloblastic anemia (MEG-ah-low-BLAST-ik) A form of anemia characterized by large, nucleated, immature red blood cells that result from the inability of precursor cells to divide normally.

memory cells B lymphocytes that remain after an infection to convey long-lasting or permanent immunity.

menaquinone A form of vitamin K found in fish oils and meats. It is also made by bacteria in the human intestine.

menarche (men-AR-kee) The onset of menstruation. Menarche usually occurs around age 13, 2 or 3 years after the first signs of puberty start to appear.

menopause (MEN-oh-paws) The cessation of menses in women, usually beginning at about age 50.

meta-analysis A summary of several scientific studies grouped together.

metabolic syndrome A condition in which the person has poor blood glucose regulation, hypertension, increased blood triglycerides, and other health problems. This condition is usually accompanied by obesity, lack of physical activity, and a diet high in refined carbohydrates. Also called *Syndrome X*.

metabolism (meh-TAB-oh-lizm) Chemical processes in the body that provide energy in useful forms and sustain vital activities.

metallothionein (meh-TAL-oh-THIGH-oh-neen) A protein that binds and regulates the release of zinc and copper in intestinal and liver cells.

metastasize (ma-TAS-tah-size) The spreading of disease from one part of the body to another, even to parts of the body that are remote from the site of the original tumor. Cancer cells can spread via blood vessels, the lymphatic system, or direct growth of the tumor.

meter A measure of length in the metric system. One meter equals 39.4 inches.

micelles (my-SELLS) Water-soluble spherical structures formed by lecithin and bile acids in which the hydrophobic parts of the molecules face inward and the hydrophilic parts face outward. Lipids enclosed within micelles do not separate out into an oily layer as they normally do when mixed with water.

microcytic (my-kro-SIT-ik) Describing red blood cells that are smaller than normal; literally, "small cell."

microcytic hypochromic anemia An anemia characterized by small, pale red blood cells that lack sufficient hemoglobin and thus have reduced oxygen-carrying ability. It is often also caused by an iron deficiency.

microfractures Small fractures, undetectable by X rays or other bone scans, that may develop constantly in bones.

micronutrient A nutrient needed in milligram or microgram quantities in a diet. Vitamins and minerals are micronutrients.

microsomal ethanol oxidizing system (my-kro-SO-mol) An alternative pathway for alcohol metabolism when alcohol is in high concentration in the liver; uses rather than yields energy for the body, in contrast to alcohol dehydrogenase activity.

microvilli (my-kro-VIL-eye) Microscopic, hairlike projections of cell membranes of certain epithelial cells.

minerals Elements used in the body to promote chemical reactions and to form body structures.

miscarriage Nonelective termination of pregnancy that occurs before the fetus can survive; typically called *spontaneous abortion*.

mitochondria (my-toe-KON-dree-ah) The main sites of energy production in a cell. They also contain the pathway for oxidizing fat for fuel, among other metabolic pathways.

modified food starch A product consisting of chemically linked starch molecules that is more stable than normal, unmodified starches.

molecule A group of atoms chemically linked together—that is, tightly connected by attractive forces (see also *compound*).

molybdenum (mo-LIB-den-um) A trace mineral that aids in the action of some enzymes in the body. Beans, whole grains, and nuts are good sources.

monoamine (MON-oh-ah-MEAN) A molecule containing one amide group.

monoglyceride (mon-oh-GLIS-er-ide) A breakdown product of a triglyceride consisting of one fatty acid bonded to a glycerol backbone.

monosaccharide (mon-oh-SACK-uh-ride) A simple sugar, such as glucose, that is not broken down further during digestion.

monounsaturated fatty acid (mon-oh-un-SAT-ur-ated) A fatty acid containing one carbon-carbon double bond.

morbidity A disease condition or state; illness.

mortality This represents a population's death rate. The term *morbidity* refers to the amount of sickness present.

motility Generally, the ability to move spontaneously. It also refers to movement of food through the GI tract.

mottling (MOT-ling) The discoloration or marking of the surface of teeth from exposure to excessive amounts of fluoride (also called *enamel fluorosis*).

mRNA translation The synthesis of polypeptide chains at the ribosome according to information contained in strands of messenger RNA (mRNA).

mucilages (MYOU-sih-laj) Soluble fiber consisting of chains of galactose and other monosaccharides; characteristically found in seaweed.

mucopolysaccharide (MYOO-ko-POL-ee-SAK-ah-ride) Substance containing protein and carbohydrate parts; found in bone and other organs.

mucosa (MYOO-co-sa) Mucous membrane consisting of cells and supporting connective tissue. In the digestive tract there is also a layer of smooth muscle supporting the mucosa. Mucosa lines cavities that open to the outside of the body, such as the stomach and intestine, and generally contains glands that secrete mucus.

mucous membranes (MYOO-cuss) Membranes that line passageways open to the exterior environment; also called *mucosae*.

mucus (MYOO-cuss) A thick fluid secreted by glands throughout the body. It contains a compound that has both a carbohydrate and a protein nature. It acts both as a lubricant and a means of protection for cells.

muscle fiber Essentially a single muscle cell. This is an elongated cell with contractile properties that forms the muscles of the body.

muscle tissue A type of tissue adapted for contraction.

muscular system The system consisting of smooth, cardiac, and skeletal muscle. This system produces body movement, maintains posture, and produces body heat.

mutagen (MYOO-tah-jen) Any agent that promotes a mutation (e.g., radioactive substances, X rays, or certain chemicals).

mutagenicity An agent that can induce or increase the frequency of mutation in an organism.

mutase (MYOO-tace) An enzyme that rearranges the functional groups on a molecule.

mutation (myoo-TAY-shun) A change in the chemistry of a gene that is perpetuated in subsequent divisions of the cell in which it occurred; a change in the sequence of the DNA.

mycotoxin (MY-ko-tok-sin) Toxic compounds produced by molds, such as aflatoxin B-1, found on moldy grains.

myelin sheath (MY-eh-lyn) A combined lipid and protein structure (lipoprotein) that covers nerve fibers.

myocardial depression Decreased activity of the heart muscle.

myocardial infarction (MY-oh-CARD-ee-ahl in-FARK-shun) Death of part of the heart muscle.

myofibrils (my-oh-FIB-rils) A bundle of contractile fibers within a muscle cell.

myoglobin (my-oh-GLOW-bin) The iron-containing protein that controls the rate of diffusion of oxygen (O_2) from red blood cells to muscle cells.

myosin (MY-oh-sin) A thick filament protein that connects with actin to cause a muscle contraction.

narcotic An agent that reduces sensations or consciousness.

negative energy balance The state in which energy intake is less than energy expended, resulting in weight loss.

negative nitrogen balance The state in which nitrogen losses from the body exceed intake, as in starvation.

neoplasm (NEE-oh-plaz-em) A new and abnormal growth of tissues, which may be benign or cancerous.

neotame A general purpose nonnutritive sweetener that is approximately 7000 to 13,000 times sweeter than table sugar. It has a chemical structure similar to aspartame. Neotame is heat stable and can be used as a tabletop sweetener as well as in cooking applications. It is not broken down to its amino acid components in the body after consumption.

nephron (NEF-ron) The functional unit of the kidney.

nerve A bundle of nerve cells outside the central nervous system.

nervous system The body system consisting of the brain, spinal cord, nerves, and sensory receptors. This system detects sensations and controls physiological and intellectual functions and movement.

nervous tissue Tissues composed of highly branched, elongated cells that transport nerve impulses from one part of the body to another.

neural tube defect A defect in the formation of the neural tube occurring during early fetal development. This type of defect results in various nervous system disorders, such as spina bifida. A very severe form is anencephaly. Folate deficiency in the pregnant woman increases the risk that the fetus will develop this disorder.

neuroendocrine (nyoo-row-EN-do-krin) Linked to the combined action of the endocrine glands and the nervous system. Examples include substances released from glands in response to nerve stimulation.

neuroglia (nyoo-row-GLEE-ah) (glial cells) Specialized support cells of the central nervous system.

neuromuscular junction (nyoo-row-MUS-kyo-lar) A chemical synapse between a motor neuron and a muscle fiber.

neuron (NYOUR-on) The structural and functional unit of the nervous system, consisting of cell body, dendrites, and axon.

neuropeptide Y (nyoo-row-PEP-tide) A small protein (36 amino acids) that increases food intake and reduces energy expenditure when injected into the brains of experimental animals.

neurotransmitter (nyoo-row-TRANS-mit-er) A compound made by a nerve cell that allows for communication between it and other cells.

neutron (NEW-tron) The part of an atom that has no charge.

neutrophil (NEW-tro-fil) A type of phagocytic white blood cell, normally constituting about 60 to 70% of the white blood cell count. Forms highly toxic compounds, which destroy bacteria.

neutrophil/activation (NEW-tro-fil) A type of white blood cell being prepared for immune response.

niacin A water-soluble vitamin that, in coenzyme form, participates in numerous oxidation-reduction reactions in cellular metabolic pathways, especially those used to produce ATP. Tuna, chicken, beef, peanuts, and salmon are good sources.

nicotinamide adenine dinucleotide (NAD) A compound that readily accepts and donates electrons and hydrogen ions; formed from the vitamin niacin.

night blindness A vitamin A deficiency condition in which the retina in the eye cannot adjust to low amounts of light.

nitrate A nitrogen-containing compound used to cure meats. Its use contributes a pink color to meats and confers some resistance to bacterial growth.

nitrosamine (ni-TROH-sa-mean) A carcinogen formed from nitrates and breakdown products of amino acids; can lead to stomach cancer.

nonessential amino acids Amino acids that can be synthesized by a healthy body in sufficient amounts; there are 11 nonessential amino acids. These are also called *dispensable amino acids.*

nonheme iron (non-HEEM) Iron provided from plant sources and elemental iron components of animal tissues. Nonheme iron is less efficiently absorbed than heme iron, and absorption is also more closely dependent on body needs.

nonpolar A neutral compound; no positive or negative poles present.

nonspecific immunity Defenses that stop the invasion of pathogens; requires no previous encounter with a pathogen.

no-observable-effect level (NOEL) The highest dose of an additive that produces no deleterious health effects in animals.

norepinephrine (nor-ep-ih-NEF-rin) A neurotransmitter released from nerve endings, and a hormone produced by the adrenal gland in times of stress.

norovirus A virus found in the human intestinal tract and feces. Food contamination by it occurs via direct hand-to-food contact, when sewage is used to enrich garden/farm soil, or when shellfish are harvested from waters contaminated by sewage. Cooking destroys the virus; shellfish and salads are the foods most often implicated. Noroviruses cause more cases of foodborne illness than any other microorganism. They can survive chlorination, and a relatively small amount can cause illness.

NSAIDs Nonsteroidal anti-inflammatory drugs; includes aspirin, ibuprofen, and naproxen.

nuclear receptor A site on the DNA in a cell where compounds (such as hormones) bind. Cells that contain DNA receptors for a specific compound are affected by that compound.

nucleolus (NEW-klee-o-less) Center for production of ribosomes within the cell nucleus.

nucleus (NEW-klee-us) In chemistry, the core of an atom; it contains protons and neutrons.

nutrient density The ratio derived by dividing a food's contribution to nutrient needs by its contribution to energy needs. When its contribution to nutrient needs exceeds its energy contribution, the food is considered to have a favorable nutrient density.

nutrient receptors Proposed sites in the small intestine that contribute signals to the brain that in turn elicit a feeling of satiety. These receptors are stimulated by nutrient exposure in the lumen of the small intestine.

nutrients Chemical substances in food that contribute to health, many of which are essential parts of a diet. Nutrients nourish us by providing energy, materials for building body parts, and factors to regulate necessary chemical processes in the body.

nutrition The science of food; the nutrients and the substances therein; their action, interaction, and balance in relation to health and disease; and the process by which the organism (i.e., body) ingests, digests, absorbs, transports, utilizes, and excretes food substances.

nutritional status The nutritional health of a person as determined by anthropometric measures (height, weight, circumferences, and so on), biochemical measurements of nutrients or their by-products in blood and urine, a clinical (physical) examination, a dietary analysis, and economic evaluation.

nutritionist A person who advises about nutrition and/or works in the field of food and nutrition. In many states in the United States, a person does not need formal training to use this title. Some states reserve this title for registered dietitians.

nutrition label A label containing "Nutrition Facts" that must be included on most foods. It depicts nutrient content in comparison to the Daily Values set by FDA. Canada has a separate set of nutrition labels.

obesity (oh-BEES-ih-tee) A condition characterized by excess body fat; typically defined in clinical settings as a body mass index (BMI) of 30 or above, but this cutoff is not always appropriate.

oleic acid (oh-LAY-ik) An omega-9 fatty acid with 18 carbons and one double bond (C18:1, omega-9).

olfactory (ol-FAK-toe-ree) Sense of smell.

olfactory cells Cells in the nasal region that discriminate numerous chemical molecules and transmit that information to the brain. This information represents one of the components of flavor.

oligosaccharides (ol-ih-go-SAK-ah-rides) From a nutritional standpoint, carbohydrates containing 3 to 10 single sugar units.

omega-3 (ω-3) fatty acid Unsaturated fatty acid with the first double bond on the third carbon from the methyl end ($-CH_3$).

omega-6 (ω-6) fatty acid Unsaturated fatty acid with the first double bond on the sixth carbon from the methyl end ($-CH_3$).

omnivore (AHM-nih-voor) A person who consumes foods from both plant and animal sources.

oncogene (AHN-ko-jeen) A protooncogene out of control.

oncotic force (ahn-KAH-tik) The osmotic potential exerted by blood proteins in the bloodstream.

opportunistic infection An infection that arises primarily in people who are already ill because of another disease.

organ A group of tissues designed to perform a specific function—for example, the heart. It contains muscle tissue, nerve tissue, and so on.

organelles (OAR-gan-ells) Compartments, particles, or filaments that perform specialized functions within a cell.

organic Any substance that contains carbon atoms bonded to hydrogen atoms in the chemical structure.

organism A living thing. The human body is an organism consisting of many organs that act in a coordinated manner to support life.

organ system A collection of organs that work together to perform an overall function.

osmolality (oz-mo-LAL-ih-tee) A measure of the total concentration of a solution; the number of particles of solute per kilogram of solvent.

osmosis (oz-MO-sis) The passage of a solvent such as water through a semipermeable membrane from a less concentrated compartment to a more concentrated compartment.

osmotic pressure The exerted pressure needed to keep particles in a solution from drawing liquid toward them across a semipermeable membrane.

osteoblast (OS-tee-oh-blast) Cells in bone that secrete mineral and bone matrix.

osteocalcin (OS-tee-oh-KAL-sin) A protein produced in bone that is thought to bind calcium; synthesis of osteocalcin is aided by vitamin K.

osteoclasts (OS-tee-oh-klasts) Bone cells that arise originally from a type of white blood cell. Osteoclasts secrete substances that lead to bone erosion. This erosion can set the stage for subsequent bone mineralization.

osteomalacia (OS-tee-oh-mal-AY-shuh) The weakening of the bones that occurs in adults as the result of poor bone mineralization linked to inadequate vitamin D status.

osteopenia (os-tee-oh-PEE-nee-ah) Decreased bone mass caused by cancer, hyperthyroidism, or other reasons.

osteoporosis (os-tee-oh-po-ROH-sis) Decreased bone mass where no obvious disease can be found. This bone loss is related to the effects of aging, genetic background, poor diet, and hormonal changes occurring in postmenopausal women.

ostomy (OS-toe-me) A surgically created short circuit in intestinal flow where the end point usually opens from the abdominal cavity rather than the anus, for example, a colostomy.

overnutrition A state in which nutritional intake greatly exceeds the body's needs.

ovum (OH-vum) The egg cell from which a fetus eventually develops if the egg is fertilized by a sperm cell.

oxalic acid (oxalate) An organic acid found in spinach, rhubarb, and other leafy green vegetables that can depress the absorption of certain minerals present in the food, such as calcium.

oxidation (ox-ih-DAY-shun) Loss of an electron by an atom or a molecule; in metabolism, often associated with a gain of oxygen or loss of hydrogen. Oxidation (loss of an electron) and reduction (gain of an electron) take place simultaneously in metabolism, because an electron that is lost by one atom is accepted by another.

oxidative phosphorylation The process by which energy derived from the oxidation of NADH + H$^+$ and FADH$_2$ is transferred to ADP + P$_i$ to form ATP.

oxidative stress The damage to lipids, proteins, and DNA produced by excessive production of free radicals.

oxidize (OX-ih-dize) In the most basic sense, either the loss of an electron or the gain of an oxygen in a chemical substance. This change typically alters the shape and/or function of the substance. An oxidizing agent is a substance capable of capturing an electron from another source. That source is then "oxidized" when it loses the electron.

oxidized LDL LDL that has been damaged by free radicals. Such damage is seen in both the lipids and proteins that make up this lipoprotein.

oxidizing agent In one sense, a substance capable of capturing an electron from another compound. A compound is "oxidized" when it loses an electron.

oxygenase (OK-si-jen-ace) Enzyme that incorporates oxygen directly into a molecule.

oxytocin (ok-si-TO-sin) A hormone secreted by the pituitary gland. It causes contraction of the musclelike cells surrounding the ducts of the breasts and the smooth muscle of the uterus.

p53 gene A tumor suppressant gene that can prevent inappropriate cell division.

palatable (PAL-it-ah-bull) Pleasing to taste.

pancreas (pan-KREE-us) Endocrine organ, located near the stomach, that secretes digestive enzymes into the small intestine and produces hormones, notably insulin.

pantothenic acid A water-soluble vitamin that functions as a component of coenzyme A (CoA), which itself plays a pivotal role in energy metabolism and fatty acid synthesis. Most foods are sources.

parasite An organism that lives in or on another organism and derives nourishment from it.

parasthesia (para-STEE-zya) An abnormal spontaneous sensation, such as of burning, prickling, and numbness.

parathyroid hormone (PTH) A hormone made by the parathyroid glands that increases synthesis of the vitamin D hormone and aids calcium release from bone and calcium uptake by the kidneys, among other functions.

parietal cell Gastric gland cell that secretes hydrochloric acid and intrinsic factor.

passive diffusion Absorption that requires permeability of the substance through the wall of the small intestine and a concentration gradient higher in the intestinal contents than in the absorptive cell.

pasteurizing (PAS-tur-i-zing) The process of heating food products to kill pathogenic microorganisms and reduce the total number of bacteria.

pathway A metabolic progression of individual steps from starting materials to ending products, such as $C_6H_{12}O_6$ (glucose) + O_2 eventually yielding CO_2 + H_2O.

pectin (PEK-tin) Soluble fiber containing chains of various monosaccharides; characteristically found between plant cell walls.

peer-reviewed journal A journal that publishes research only after two or three scientists who were not part of the study agree the study was well conducted and the results are fairly represented. Thus, the research has been approved by peers of the research team.

pellagra (peh-LAHG-rah) A disease characterized by inflammation of the skin, diarrhea, and eventual mental incapacity; results from an insufficient amount of the vitamin niacin in the diet.

pepsin (PEP-sin) A protein-digesting enzyme produced by the stomach.

peptide A few amino acids chemically bonded together; often two to four.

peptide bond A chemical bond formed between amino acids in a protein.

percentile Classification of a measurement of a unit into divisions of 100 units.

peripheral nervous system (PNS) (peh-RIF-er-al) The nerves of the nervous system that lie outside the brain and spinal cord.

peripheral neuropathy (peh-RIF-er-al nyoo-ROP-ah-thee) Impaired sensory, motor, and reflex actions affecting arms and legs and causing calf muscle tenderness and difficulty in rising from a squatting position.

peristalsis (per-ih-STALL-sis) A coordinated muscular contraction that propels food down the GI tract.

pernicious anemia The anemia that results from the inability to absorb sufficient vitamin B-12; it is associated with nerve degeneration, which can result in eventual paralysis and death.

peroxisome (per-OK-si-som) Cell organelle that uses oxygen to remove hydrogens from compounds. This produces hydrogen peroxide (H_2O_2), which breaks down into O_2 and H_2O.

peroxyl radical (per-OK-syl) A peroxide compound containing a free radical; designated ROO$^•$.

pesticide A general term for an agent that can destroy bacteria, fungi, insects, rodents, or other pests.

pH A measure of relative acidity or alkalinity of a solution. The pH scale is 0 to 14. A pH below 7 is acidic; a pH above 7 is alkaline.

phagocytic cells (fag-oh-SIT-ick) Cells that engulf substances; these cells include neutrophils and macrophages.

phagocytosis (FAG-oh-sigh-TOW-sis) A form of active absorption in which the absorptive cell forms an indentation, and particles or fluids entering the indentation are then engulfed by the cell.

pharynx (FAIR-ingks) The organ of the digestive tract and respiratory tract located at the back of the oral and nasal cavities.

phenylalanine (fen-ihl-AL-ah-neen) An essential (indispensable) amino acid.

phenylketonuria (PKU) (fen-ihl-kee-toh-NEW-ree-ah) A disease caused by a defect in the ability of the liver to metabolize the amino acid phenylalanine into the amino acid tyrosine. Toxic by-products of phenylalanine can then build up in the body and lead to mental retardation.

phosphocreatine (PCr) (fos-fo-CREE-a-tin) A high-energy compound that can be used to re-form ATP from ADP.

phospholipase (fos-fo-LY-pase) Enzyme that splits a fatty acid from a cell membrane phospholipid.

phospholipid Any of a class of fat-related substances that contain phosphorus, fatty acids, and a nitrogen-containing base. The phospholipids are an essential part of every cell.

phosphorus A major ion of intracellular fluid. It contributes to acid-base balance, bone and tooth strength, and various metabolic processes. Milk, milk products, and nuts are good sources.

photoisomerization (foto-eye-SOM-er-eye-zay-shun) Molecular isomerization of a compound by the energy of light.

photon (FO-ton) A unit of light intensity at the retina having the brightness of one candle.

photosynthesis (foto-SIN-tha-sis) The process by which plants use energy from the sun to produce energy-yielding compounds, such as glucose.

phylloquinone (fil-oh-KWIN-own) A form of vitamin K that comes from plants; also called *vitamin K₁*.

physical activity Any movement of the body caused by muscular contraction that results in the expenditure of energy.

physiological anemia The normal increase in blood volume in pregnancy that dilutes the concentration of red blood cells, resulting in anemia; also called *hemodilution*.

phytic acid (phytate) (FY-tick, FY-tate) A constituent of plant fibers that binds positive ions to its multiple phosphate groups.

phytobezoar (fy-tow-BEE-zor) A pellet of fiber characteristically found in the stomach.

phytochemical A chemical found in plants. Some phytochemicals may contribute to a reduced risk of cancer or cardiovascular disease in people who consume them regularly.

pica (PIE-kah) The practice of eating nonfood items, such as dirt, laundry starch, or clay.

pinocytosis (pee-no-sigh-TOE-sis) Formation of a vesicle that brings molecules into a cell; also called cell drinking.

placebo (plah-SEE-bo) A fake medicine used to disguise the roles of participants in an experiment; if fake surgery is performed, it is called a *sham operation*.

placenta (plah-SEN-tah) An organ that forms in the uterus in pregnant women. Through this organ, oxygen and nutrients from the mother's blood are transferred to the fetus and fetal wastes are removed. The placenta also releases hormones that maintain the state of pregnancy.

plaque (PLACK) A cholesterol-rich substance deposited in the blood vessels; it contains various white blood cells, smooth muscle cells, connective tissue (collagen), cholesterol and other lipids, and eventually calcium.

plasma The fluid, noncellular portion of the circulating blood. This includes the blood serum plus all blood-clotting factors. In contrast, serum is the fluid that results after the blood is first allowed to clot before being centrifuged; this does not contain the blood-clotting factors.

plasma cells A form of B lymphocytes that produce about 2000 antibodies per second.

polar A compound with distinct positive and negative charges (poles) on it. These charges act like poles on a magnet.

polyglutamate form of folate (POL-ee-GLOO-tah-mate) Folate with more than one glutamate molecule attached.

polyneuropathy (POL-ee-nyoo-ROP-ah-thee) A disease process involving a number of peripheral nerves.

polypeptide (POL-ee-PEP-tide) Fifty to 2000 or more amino acids bonded together.

polysaccharide (POL-ee-SACK-uh-ride) Large carbohydrates containing from 10 to 1000 or more glucose units; also known as *complex carbohydrates*.

polyunsaturated fatty acid A fatty acid containing two or more carbon-carbon double bonds.

pool The amount of a nutrient found within the body that can be easily mobilized when needed.

portal system A general term that describes veins in the GI tract that convey blood from capillaries in the intestines and portions of the stomach to the liver.

portal vein A large vein leaving from the intestine and stomach that connects to the liver.

positive energy balance State in which energy intake is greater than energy expended, generally resulting in weight gain.

positive nitrogen balance A state in which nitrogen intake exceeds related losses. This state causes a net gain of nitrogen in the body, such as when tissue protein is gained during growth.

post-translational processing Occurring or formed after protein synthesis is completed by the ribosomes.

potassium The major positive ion in intracellular fluid. It performs many of the same functions as sodium, such as fluid balance and nerve impulse transmission. Potassium also influences the contractility of smooth, skeletal, and cardiac muscle. Spinach, squash, and bananas are good sources.

power stroke Movement of the thick filament alongside the thin filament in a muscle cell, causing muscle contraction.

prebiotic A substance that stimulates bacterial growth in the large intestines.

precursor A compound that comes before; to precede.

preeclampsia (pre-ee-KLAMP-see-ah) Part of the disease called pregnancy-induced hypertension. This serious disorder can include high blood pressure, kidney failure, convulsions, and even death of the mother and fetus. Mild cases are known as preeclampsia; more severe cases are called eclampsia or, more correctly, toxemia.

pregnancy-induced hypertension A serious disorder that can include high blood pressure, kidney failure, convulsions, and even death of the mother and fetus. Although its exact cause is not known, an adequate diet (especially adequate calcium intake) and prenatal care may prevent this disorder or limit its severity. Mild cases are known as *preeclampsia;* more severe cases are called *eclampsia* (formerly called *toxemia*).

premenstrual syndrome (PMS) A disorder found in some women a few days before a menstrual period begins. It is characterized by depression, anxiety, headache, bloating, and mood swings. Severe cases are currently termed *premenstrual dysphoric disorder (PDD).*

preservatives Compounds that extend the shelf life of foods by inhibiting microbial growth or minimizing the destructive effect of oxygen and metals.

preterm An infant born before 37 weeks of gestation; such an infant is also referred to as *premature.*

prevalence The number of people at any one time who have a specific disease, such as obesity or cancer.

previtamin D$_3$ Precursor of one form of vitamin D, produced as a result of sunlight opening a ring on 7-dehydrocholesterol in the skin.

primary disease A disease process that is not simply caused by another disease process.

primary prevention The attempt to prevent a disease from developing in the first place—for example, following a diet low in saturated fat and cholesterol in an attempt to prevent cardiovascular disease.

primary structure of a protein The order of amino acids in the protein molecule.

prions (PRE-ons) Proteins involved in maintaining nerve cell function. Prions can turn infectious and lead to diseases such as bovine spongiform encephalopathy, also known as mad cow disease.

probiotic (PRO-bye-ah-tic) A product that contains specific types of bacteria. Use is intended to colonize the large intestine with the specific bacteria in the product. An example is yogurt.

progestins (pro-JES-tins) Hormones, including progesterone, that are necessary for maintaining pregnancy and lactation.

prognosis (prog-NO-sis) A forecast of the course and end of a disease.

prohormone Precursor of a hormone.

prolactin (pro-LACK-tin) A hormone secreted by the mother's pituitary gland. It stimulates the synthesis of milk in the breast.

prospective Research that follows individuals during a current course of treatment; contrast with retrospective research, which examines the past habits of individuals.

prostacyclin (PGI) (prost-tah-SIGH-klin) Eicosanoid made by the blood vessel walls that is a potent inhibitor of blood clotting.

prostaglandin (PG) (pros-tah-GLAN-din) One of several potent eicosanoid compounds made of polyunsaturated fatty acids that produce diverse effects in the body.

prostanoids (PROS-ta-noid) The group of prostaglandins, prostacyclins, and thromboxanes produced from 20 carbon (C:20) fatty acids; not as inclusive a term as *eicosanoids* because leukotrienes and lipoxins are not included.

prostate gland (PROS-tait) A solid, chestnut-shaped organ surrounding the first part of the urinary tract in the male. The prostate gland secretes substances into the semen.

protease (PRO-tea-ace) Protein-digesting enzyme.

protein Food and body components made of amino acids; proteins contain carbon, hydrogen, oxygen, nitrogen, and sometimes other atoms, in a specific configuration. Proteins contain the form of nitrogen most easily used by the human body. Supplies 4 kcal/gram.

protein-efficiency ratio (PER) A measure of protein quality in a food, determined by the ability of a protein to support the growth of a young animal.

protein-energy malnutrition (PEM) A condition resulting from regularly consuming insufficient amounts of energy and protein. The deficiency eventually results in body wasting, primarily of lean tissue, and an increased susceptibility to infections.

protein quality A measure of the ability of a food protein to support body growth and maintenance.

protein turnover The process by which a cell breaks down existing proteins and then synthesizes new proteins. Thus the cell can adapt to changing conditions: it will have the necessary proteins as the need for them arises.

prothrombin (pro-THROM-bin) One of the numerous proteins that participate in the formation of blood clots. Conversion of its precursor protein to the active blood-clotting factor in the liver requires vitamin K.

proton (PRO-ton) The part of an atom that is positively charged.

proton pump inhibitor A medication that inhibits the ability of gastric cells to secrete hydrogen ions. Examples are esomeprazole (Nexium) and lansoprazole (Prevacid). Low doses of this class of medications are also available without prescription (e.g., omeprazole (Prilosec)).

protooncogenes (pro-toe-ON-ko-jeans) Genes that cause a resting cell to divide.

provitamin Substance that can be made into a vitamin.

psyllium (SIL-ee-um) A mostly soluble type of dietary fiber found in the seeds of the plantago plant (native to India and Mediterranean countries).

pulmonary circulation (pulmonary circuit) The system of blood vessels from the right ventricle of the heart to the lungs and back to the left atrium of the heart.

pyloric sphincter (pi-LOR-ik SFINK-ter) Ring of smooth muscle between the stomach and the duodenum.

pyruvic acid A three-carbon compound formed during glucose metabolism; also called *pyruvate*.

racemase A group of enzymes that catalyzes reactions involving structural rearrangement of a molecule (e.g., conversion of D-alanine isomer to L-alanine isomer).

radiation Literally, energy that is emitted from a center in all directions. Various forms of radiation energy include X rays and ultraviolet rays from the sun.

raffinose (RAF-ih-nos) An indigestible oligosaccharide made of three monosaccharides (galactose-glucose-fructose).

rancid (RAN-sid) Containing products of decomposed fatty acids; they yield unpleasant flavors and odors.

reactive hypoglycemia (HIGH-po-gligh-SEE-mee-uh) Low blood glucose that may follow a meal high in simple sugars, with corresponding symptoms of irritability, headache, nervousness, sweating, and confusion; actually called *postprandial hypoglycemia*.

reactive oxygen species (ROS) Several oxygen derivatives produced during the formation of ATP. Formed constantly in the human body and shown to kill bacteria and inactivate proteins, they are also implicated in a number of diseases and inflammatory processes.

receptive framework for learning The process by which a person opens up to learning more about a problem; it usually involves seeking more information about the issue from books and people. In the case of seeking behavior changes, it involves examining background experience to evaluate whether a behavior change is feasible.

receptor (ri-SEP-ter) A site in a cell at which compounds (such as hormones) bind. Cells that contain receptors for a specific compound are partially controlled by that compound.

receptor pathway for cholesterol uptake A process by which LDL is bound by cell receptors and incorporated into the cell.

recombinant DNA (re-KOM-bih-nant) A molecule composed of the DNA of two different species spliced together, such as a combination of bacterial and human DNA used to produce unique bacteria that now can synthesize human proteins.

recombinant DNA technology A test tube technology that rearranges DNA sequences in an organism by cutting the DNA, adding or deleting a DNA sequence, and rejoining DNA molecules with a series of enzymes.

Recommended Dietary Allowances (RDAs) Recommended intakes of nutrients that are sufficient to meet the needs of almost all individuals (97%) of similar age and gender. These are established by the Food and Nutrition Board of the National Academy of Sciences.

Recommended Nutrient Intake (RNI) The Canadian version of RDA published in 1990.

rectum Terminal portion of the large intestine.

redox agents (RE-doks) Chemicals that can readily undergo both oxidation (loss of an electron) and reduction (gain of an electron).

reducing agent A compound capable of donating electrons (also hydrogen ions) to another compound.

reduction In chemical terms, the gain of an electron by an atom; takes place simultaneously with oxidation (loss of an electron by an atom) in metabolism because an electron that is lost by one atom is accepted by another. In metabolism, reduction is often associated with the gain of hydrogen.

Reference Daily Intakes (RDIs) Nutrient-intake standards set by FDA based on the 1968 RDAs for various vitamins and minerals. RDIs have been set for four categories of people: infants, toddlers, people over 4 years of age, and pregnant or lactating women. Generally the highest RDA value out of all categories is used as the RDI. The RDIs constitute part of the Daily Values used in food labeling.

registered dietitian (R.D.) A person who has completed a baccalaureate degree program approved by the American Dietetic Association, performed at least 900 hours of supervised professional practice, and passed a registration examination.

reinforcement A reaction by others in response to a person's behavior. Positive reinforcement entails encouragement; negative reinforcement entails criticism or penalty.

relapse prevention A series of strategies used to help prevent and cope with weight-control lapses, such as recognizing high-risk situations and deciding beforehand on appropriate responses.

remodeling The constant building and breakdown of bone throughout life.

renin (REN-in) An enzyme formed in the kidneys and released in response to low blood pressure; it acts on a blood protein called angiotensinogen to produce angiotensin I.

reproductive system The system consisting of the gonads, accessory structures, and genitals of males and females. This system performs the process of reproduction and influences sexual functions and behaviors.

requirement The amount of a nutrient required by one person to maintain health. This varies between individuals. We do not know our individual requirements for each nutrient.

reserve capacity The extent to which an organ can preserve essentially normal function despite decreasing cell number or cell activity.

resorption The loss of a substance by physiologic or pathologic means.

respiration The use of oxygen; in the human organism, the inhalation of oxygen and the exhalation of carbon dioxide; in cells, the oxidation (electron removal) of food molecules to obtain energy.

respiratory system The body system consisting of the lungs and various associated organs such as the nose and various conducting tubes. This system transports oxygen from outside air to the lungs and allows carbon dioxide to be expelled from the body. Oxygen and carbon dioxide are exchanged with the blood in the lungs. It also regulates acid-base balance in the body.

resting metabolism The amount of energy the body uses when the person has not eaten in 4 hours and is resting (e.g., 15 to 30 minutes) and awake in a warm, quiet environment. It is roughly 6% higher than basal metabolism because of the less strict criteria for the test. Often referred to as *resting metabolic rate (RMR)*.

retinoids (RET-ih-noyds) A collective term for the biologically active forms of vitamin A including retinol, retinal, and retinoic acid.

reverse transport of cholesterol The process by which cholesterol is picked up by HDL particles and transferred to the liver or to other lipoproteins that can dispose of it in the liver.

rhodopsin (row-DOP-sin) Photoreceptor in rod cells composed of 11-*cis*-retinal and opsin.

riboflavin (RYE-bo-fla-vin) A water-soluble vitamin that functions in coenzyme form in oxidation-reduction reactions, playing a key role in energy metabolism. Milk and milk products, liver, mushrooms, and green leafy vegetables are rich sources of riboflavin.

ribonucleic acid (RNA) (RI-bow-new-CLAY-ik) Single-stranded nucleic acid involved in the transcription of genetic information and translation of that information into protein structure.

ribose (RIGH-bos) A 5-carbon sugar found in genetic material—specifically, RNA.

ribosomes (RI-bow-soms) Cytoplasmic particles that mediate the linking together of amino acids to form proteins; attached to endoplasmic reticulum as bound ribosomes, or suspended in cytoplasm as free ribosomes.

rickets (RIK-its) A disease characterized by inadequate mineralization of the bones caused by poor calcium deposition during growth. This deficiency disease arises in infants and children with poor vitamin D status.

risk factor A term used frequently when discussing diseases and factors contributing to their development. A risk factor is an aspect of our lives—such as heredity, lifestyle choices (e.g., smoking), or nutritional habits—that make us more likely to develop a disease.

rough endoplasmic reticulum Portion of the endoplasmic reticulum that contains ribosomes. This is the site of protein synthesis in a cell.

R-protein A protein produced by the salivary glands that enhances absorption of vitamin B-12, possibly protecting the vitamin during its passage through the stomach.

RXR, RAR Abbreviations for retinoid X receptor and retinoic acid receptor. These two subfamilies of retinoid receptors in the nucleus interact with retinoic acid and bind with specific sites on DNA, allowing for gene expression.

saccharin (SACK-ah-rin) An alternative sweetener that yields no energy to the body; it is 300 times sweeter than sucrose.

saliva (sah-LIGH-vah) A watery fluid, produced by the salivary glands in the mouth, that contains lubricants, enzymes, and other substances.

salivary amylase (SAL-ih-var-ee AM-ih-lace) Starch-digesting enzyme produced by salivary glands.

salmonella (sal-mo-NELL-a) A large class of bacteria, many strains of which are toxic, commonly found in animal and human feces. Salmonella can multiply in raw meats, poultry, eggs, fish, sprouts, unpasteurized milk, and foods made with these products. Cooking destroys salmonella.

salt Generally refers to a compound of sodium and chloride in a 40:60 ratio.

sarcoma (sar-KO-mah) A malignant tumor arising from connective tissues.

sarcomere A portion of a muscle fiber that is considered the functional unit of a myofibril.

satiety (suh-TIE-uh-tee) A state in which there is no longer a desire to eat; a feeling of satisfaction.

saturated fatty acid A fatty acid containing no carbon-carbon double bonds.

scavenger pathway for cholesterol uptake A process by which LDL is taken up by scavenger cells embedded in the blood vessels.

scurvy (SKER-vee) The deficiency disease that results after a few weeks to months of consuming a diet that lacks vitamin C; pinpoint sites of bleeding on the skin are an early sign.

secondary deficiency A deficiency caused not by lack of the nutrient in question but by lack of a substance or process that is needed for that nutrient to function.

secondary disease A disease process that develops as a result of another disease.

secondary prevention Interventions to prevent further development of a disease so as to reduce the risk of further damage to health; for example, smoking cessation for a person who has already suffered a heart attack.

secretin (SEE-kreh-tin) A hormone that causes bicarbonate ion release from the pancreas.

secretory vesicles (see-KRE-tor-ee VES-ih-kels) Membrane-bound vesicles produced by the Golgi apparatus; contain proteins and other compounds to be secreted by the cell.

sedentary lifestyle A lifestyle that includes only the light physical activity associated with typical day-to-day life.

segmentation Contractions of the circular muscles in the intestines that lead to a dividing and mixing of the intestinal contents. This action aids digestion and absorption of nutrients.

selenium A trace mineral that functions as part of antioxidant enzyme systems and in thyroid hormone metabolism. Animal protein foods and whole grains are good sources.

self-monitoring A process of tracking a behavior and conditions affecting that behavior; actions are usually recorded in a diary, along with location, time, and state of mind. This can be a tool to help people understand more about their eating habits.

semiessential amino acids Amino acids that, when consumed, spare the need to use an essential amino acid for their synthesis. Tyrosine in the diet, for example, spares the need to use phenylalanine for tyrosine synthesis. Also called *conditionally essential amino acids.*

sensible water losses Water losses readily perceived, such as urine output and heavy perspiration.

sequestrants (see-KWES-trants) Compounds that bind free metal ions. By so doing, they reduce the ability of ions to cause rancidity in foods containing fat.

serotonin (ser-oh-TONE-in) A neurotransmitter synthesized from the amino acid tryptophan that affects mood (sense of calmness), behavior, and appetite and induces sleep.

serum (SEER-um) The portion of the blood fluid remaining after (1) the blood is allowed to clot and (2) the red and white blood cells and other solid matter are removed by centrifugation.

set point Often refers to the close regulation of body weight. It is not known what cells control this set point or how it actually functions in weight regulation. There is evidence, however, that mechanisms exist that help regulate weight.

sexually transmitted disease (STD) A contagious disease usually acquired by sexual intercourse or genital contact. Common examples include AIDS, gonorrhea, and syphilis. Also called *venereal disease.*

short-chain fatty acids Fatty acids that contain fewer than six carbon atoms.

sickle-cell disease (sickle-cell anemia) An illness that results from a malformation of the red blood cell because of an incorrect primary structure in part of its hemoglobin protein chains. The disease can lead to episodes of severe bone and joint pain, abdominal pain, headache, convulsions, paralysis, and even death.

sideroblastic anemia A form of anemia characterized by red blood cells containing an internal ring of iron granules. This anemia may respond to vitamin B-6 treatment.

sign A change in health status that is apparent on physical examination.

simple sugar Term used to describe the group of typical sugars in our diets: glucose, fructose, and sucrose.

skeletal fluorosis (flo-ROW-sis) A condition caused by a greatly excessive fluoride intake, characterized by weakened skeletal structure.

skeletal muscle Muscle tissue responsible for voluntary body movements.

skeletal system The system consisting of the bones, associated cartilage, and joints. This system supports the body, allows for body movement, produces blood cells, and stores minerals.

slough (SLUF) To shed or cast off.

small for gestational age (SGA) (jes-TAY-shun-al) Referring to infants who weigh less than the expected weight for their length of gestation. This corresponds to less than 5.5 pounds (2.5 kilograms) in a full-term newborn. A preterm infant who is also SGA will most likely develop some medical complications.

smooth endoplasmic reticulum Portion of the endoplasmic reticulum that does not contain ribosomes. This is the site of lipid synthesis in a cell.

smooth muscle Muscle tissue under involuntary control; found in the GI tract, artery walls, respiratory passages, the urinary tract, and the reproductive tract.

sodium The major positive ion in extracellular fluid. It is essential for maintaining fluid balance and conducting nerve impulses. Salt added to foods during their production supplies most of the sodium in the diet.

sodium bicarbonate (SO-dee-um bi-KAR-bow-nait) An alkaline substance made basically of sodium and carbon dioxide ($NaHCO_3$).

soft palate (PAL-it) The fleshy posterior portion of the roof of the mouth.

soluble fibers (SOL-you-bull) Fibers that either dissolve or swell in water and are metabolized (fermented) by bacteria in the large intestine. These include pectins, gums, and mucilages. More formally called *viscous fibers.*

solvent A liquid substance that other substances dissolve in.

sorbitol (SOR-bih-tol) An alcohol derivative of glucose that yields about 3 kcal/g but is slowly absorbed from the small intestine. It is used in some sugarless gums and dietetic foods.

specific heat The amount of heat required to raise the temperature of any substance 1°C compared with the heat required to raise the temperature of the same volume of water 1°C. Water has a high specific heat, meaning that a relatively large amount of heat is required to raise its temperature; therefore, it tends to resist large temperature fluctuations.

specific immunity The function of lymphocytes directed at specific antigens.

sphincter (SFINK-ter) A muscular valve that controls flow of foodstuff in the GI tract.

sphincter of Oddi Ring of smooth muscle between the common bile duct and the upper part of the small intestine (duodenum); also called the *hepatopancreatic sphincter.*

spontaneous abortion Cessation of pregnancy and expulsion of the embryo or nonviable fetus prior to 20 weeks gestation. This is the result of natural causes, such as a genetic defect or developmental problem; also called *miscarriage.*

spores Dormant reproductive cells capable of turning into adult organisms without the help of another cell. Various fungi and bacteria form spores.

sports anemia (ah-NEE-me-ah) A decrease in the blood's ability to carry oxygen, found in athletes, which may be caused by iron loss through perspiration and feces or increased blood volume.

stable isotope A specific, nonradioactive form of a chemical element. It differs from atoms of other forms (isotopes) of the same element in the number of neutrons in its nucleus. *Stable* means that the isotope is not radioactive, in contrast to some other types of isotopes.

stachyose (STACK-ee-os) An indigestible oligosaccharide made of four monosaccharides (galactose-galactose-glucose-fructose).

***Staphylococcus aureus* (staf-i-lo-COCK us OR-ee-us)** Bacteria found in nasal passages and in cuts on skin. The bacteria produce a toxin when contaminated food is left for an extended time at room temperature. Meats, poultry, fish, dairy products, and egg products pose the greatest risk. *Staphylococcus aureus* can withstand prolonged cooking.

starch A carbohydrate made of multiple units of glucose attached together in a form the body can digest; also known as *complex carbohydrate.*

stem cell Cell that, in an adult body, divides continuously and forms a supply of cells for differentiation.

stenosis (ste-NO-sis) Narrowing or stricture of a duct or canal.

steroids (STARE-oyds) A group of hormones and related compounds that are derivatives of cholesterol.

sterol (STARE-ol) A compound containing a multi-ring (steroid) structure and a hydroxyl group (–OH).

stimulus control Altering the environment to minimize the stimuli for eating—for example, removing foods from sight and storing them in kitchen cabinets.

stress fracture A fracture that occurs from repeated jarring of a bone. Common sites include bones of the foot.

striated muscle Muscles showing a striped pattern when viewed under the microscope. These stripes are due to presence and specific organization of the contractile proteins actin and myosin.

stroke The loss of body function that results from a blood clot or other change in arteries in the brain that affects blood flow. This in turn causes the death of brain tissue. Also called a *cerebrovascular accident*.

subclinical Disease or disorder that is present but not severe enough to produce signs and symptoms that can be detected or diagnosed.

submucosal layer (sub-myoo-KO-sal) A layer of blood and lymph vessels along with nerve fibers and connective tissue that stretch the whole length of the GI tract.

sucralose (SOO-kra-los) An alternative sweetener that has chlorines in place of three hydroxyl (–OH) groups on sucrose. It is 600 times sweeter than sucrose.

sucrase An enzyme made by the absorptive cells of the small intestine; this enzyme digests sucrose to glucose and galactose.

sucrose (SOO-kros) Fructose bonded to another sugar glucose; table sugar.

sugar Simple carbohydrate form with the chemical composition $(CH_2O)n$. Most sugars form ringed structures when in solution. Generally refers to monosaccharides and disaccharides.

sulfur A major mineral primarily functioning in the body in nonionic form as part of vitamins and amino acids. In ionic form, such as sulfate, it participates in the acid-base balance in the body. Protein-rich foods supply sulfur in the diet.

superoxide dismutase (soo-per-OX-ide DISS-myoo-tase) An enzyme that can quench (deactivate) a superoxide negative free radical ($O_2^{•-}$). This can contain the minerals manganese, copper, or zinc.

sympathetic nervous system Part of the nervous system that regulates involuntary vital functions, including the activity of the heart muscle, smooth muscle, and adrenal glands.

symptom A change in health status noted by the person with the problem, such as a stomach pain.

synapse (SIN-aps) The space between the end of one nerve cell and the beginning of another nerve cell.

system A collection of organs that work together to perform an overall function.

systemic circuit The part of the circulatory system concerned with the flow of blood from the left ventricle to the body and back to the right atrium.

systolic blood pressure (sis-TOL-lik) The pressure in the arterial blood vessels associated with the pumping of blood from the heart.

tagatose An isomer of fructose that is poorly absorbed and so yields only 1.5 kcal/g to the body. Tagatose is 90% as sweet as sucrose.

telomerase (teh-LO-mer-ace) Enzyme that maintains length and completeness of chromosomes.

telomeres (TELL-oh-meers) Caps at the end of chromosomes.

tendon Dense connective tissue that attaches a muscle to a bone.

teratogenic (ter-A-toe-jen-ic) Tending to produce physical defects in a developing fetus (literally means "monster producing").

tertiary structure of a protein (TER-she-air-ee) The three-dimensional structure of a protein formed by interactions of amino acids placed far apart in the primary structure.

tetany (TET-ah-nee) A body condition marked by sharp contraction of muscles and failure to relax afterward; usually caused by abnormal calcium metabolism.

theory An explanation for a phenomenon that has numerous lines of evidence to support it.

thermic effect of food (TEF) The increase in metabolism that occurs during the digestion, absorption, and metabolism of energy-yielding nutrients. TEF represents 5 to 10% of energy consumed.

thermogenesis The ability of humans to regulate body temperature within narrow limits (thermoregulation). Two visible examples of thermogenesis are fidgeting and shivering when cold. Other terms used to describe thermogenesis are adaptive thermogenesis and nonexercise activity thermogenesis (NEAT).

thiamin (THIGH-a-min) A water-soluble vitamin that functions in coenzyme form to play a key role in energy metabolism. Pork is a good source of thiamin.

thioredoxin (THIGH-o-re-dock-sin) A family of three selenium-dependent enzymes that have an antioxidant role and other roles in the body.

thrifty metabolism A metabolism that characteristically conserves more energy than normal, such that it increases risk of weight gain and obesity.

thromboxane (TX) (throm-BOK-sane) Eicosanoid made by blood platelets that is a stimulant of blood clotting.

thyroid hormone Hormone produced by the thyroid gland that increases the rate of overall metabolism in the body.

thyroid-stimulating hormone (TSH) The hormone that regulates the uptake of iodide by the thyroid gland and release of thyroid hormone. TSH is secreted in response to a low concentration of circulating thyroid hormone (thyroxine).

tissue (TISH-you) Collection of cells adapted to perform a specific function.

T lymphocyte (tee-LYMF-oh-site) A type of white blood cell that recognizes intracellular antigens (e.g., viral antigens in infected cells), fragments of which move to the cell surface. T lymphocytes originate in the bone marrow but must mature in the thymus gland.

tocopherols (tuh-KOFF-er-alls) A group of four structurally similar compounds that have vitamin E activity. The RRR ("d") isomer of alpha-tocopherol is the most active form.

tocotrienols (toe-co-TRY-en-ols) A group of four compounds with the same basic chemical structure as the tocopherols but containing slightly altered side chains. They exhibit much less vitamin E activity than the corresponding tocopherols.

Tolerable Upper Intake Level (UL) Maximum chronic daily intake of a nutrient that is unlikely to cause adverse health effects in almost all people in a population. This number applies to a chronic daily use.

total fiber Combination of dietary fiber and functional fiber in a food; also just called *fiber*.

total parenteral nutrition The intravenous provision of all necessary nutrients, including the most basic forms of protein, carbohydrates, lipids, vitamins, minerals, and electrolytes. This solution is generally infused for 12 to 24 hours a day in a volume of about 2 to 3 L.

toxic Poisonous; caused by a poison.

toxicity The capacity of a substance to produce injury or illness at some dosage.

toxin Poisonous compounds produced by an organism that can cause disease.

trabecular bone (trah-BEK-you-lar) The spongy, inner matrix of bone found primarily in the spine, pelvis, and ends of bones; also called cancellous bone. Trabecular bone makes up 20 to 25% of total bone mass.

trace mineral A mineral vital to health that is required in the diet in amounts less than 100 mg/day. Also called *micromineral*.

trachea (TRAY-key-ah) The airway leading from the larynx to the bronchi.

transamination (trans-am-ih-NAY-shun) The transfer of an amino group from an amino acid to a carbon skeleton to form a new amino acid.

***trans* configuration** Compound in which the hydrogens lie opposite each other across a carbon-carbon double bond.

***trans* fatty acids** A form of an unsaturated fatty acid, usually a monounsaturated one when found in food, in which the hydrogens on both carbons forming that double bond lie on opposite sides of that bond (*trans* configuration). Stick margarine, shortenings, and deep-fat fried foods in general are rich sources.

transferrin (trans-FER-in) A blood protein that transports iron in the blood.

transgenic Organism that contains genes originally present in another different organism.

transketolase (trans-KEY-toe-lace) An enzyme whose functional component is TPP (thiamin pyrophosphate); it converts glucose to various other sugars.

***Trichinella spiralis* (trik-i-NELL-a)** A parasitic nematode worm, found in wild game and pork, that causes the flulike disease trichinosis. It is easily destroyed by cooking. Modern sanitary feeding practices have drastically reduced *Trichinella* in commercial pork.

triglyceride (try-GLISS-uh-ride) The major form of lipid in the body and in food. It is composed of three fatty acids bonded to glycerol, an alcohol.

trimesters Three 13- to 14-week periods into which the normal pregnancy is somewhat arbitarily divided for purposes of discussion and analysis (the length of a normal pregnancy is about 40 weeks, measured from the first day of the woman's last menstrual period). Development of the offspring, however, is continuous throughout pregnancy, with no specific physiological characterizations demarcating the transition from one trimester to the next.

tropic hormone (TROW-pic) Hormone that stimulates the secretion of another secreting gland.

trypsin (TRIP-sin) A protein-digesting enzyme secreted by the pancreas to act in the small intestine.

tumor Mass of cells; may be cancerous (malignant) or noncancerous (benign).

tumor suppressor genes Genes that prevent cells from dividing.

type 1 diabetes A form of diabetes in which the person is prone to ketosis and requires insulin therapy.

type 2 diabetes A form of diabetes in which ketosis is not commonly seen. Insulin therapy can be used but often is not required. This form of the disease is often associated with obesity.

ulcer (UL-sir) Erosion of the tissue lining, usually in the stomach (gastric ulcer) or the upper small intestine (duodenal ulcer). These are generally referred to as *peptic ulcers.*

umami (you-MA-mee) A brothy, meaty, savory flavor in some foods. Monosodium glutamate enhances this flavor when added to foods.

undernutrition Failing health that results from a long-standing dietary intake that does not meet nutritional needs.

underwater weighing A method of estimating total body fat by weighing the individual on a standard scale and then weighing him or her again submerged in water. The difference between the two weights is used to estimate total body volume.

underweight A body mass index below 18.5. The cutoff is less precise than for obesity because this condition has been studied less.

unsaturated fatty acid A fatty acid with one or more carbon-carbon double bonds in its chemical structure.

upper-body obesity The type of obesity in which fat is stored primarily in the abdominal area; defined as a waist circumference more than 40 inches (102 centimeters) in men and more than 35 inches (88 centimeters) in women; closely associated with a high risk for cardiovascular disease, hypertension, and type 2 diabetes.

urea (yoo-REE-ah) Nitrogenous waste product of protein metabolism; major source of nitrogen in

$$\overset{O}{\underset{||}{}}$$

the urine, chemically NH_2-C-NH_2.

ureter (YOUR-ih-ter) Tube that transports urine from the kidney to the urinary bladder.

urethra (yoo-REE-thra) Tube that transports urine from the urinary bladder to the outside of the body.

urinary system The body system consisting of the kidneys, urinary bladder, and the ducts that carry urine. This system removes waste products from the circulatory system and regulates blood acid-base balance, overall chemical balance, and water balance in the body.

vagus nerves (VAY-guss) Nerves arising from the brain that branch off to other organs and are essential for control of speech, swallowing, and gastrointestinal function.

vegan (VEE-gun) A person who eats only plant foods.

vegetarian A person who avoids eating animal products to a varying degree, ranging from consuming no animal products to simply not consuming four-footed animal products.

vein A blood vessel that conveys blood to the heart.

ventricles (VEN-tri-kel) The two lower chambers of the heart, which contain blood to be pumped from the heart.

venule (VEN-yool) A tiny vessel that carries blood from the capillary to a vein.

very-low-calorie diet (VLCD) Diet that allows a person 400 to 800 kcal per day, often in liquid form. Of this, 120 to 480 kcals are carbohydrate; the rest is mostly high-quality protein. Also known as *protein-sparing modified fast (PSMF).*

very-low-density lipoprotein (VLDL) The lipoprotein created in the liver that carries both the cholesterol and the lipids taken up from the bloodstream by the liver and those that are newly synthesized by the liver.

Vibrio cholerae Bacteria found in human and animal feces; causes the severe illness known as cholera; most often transmitted via contaminated drinking water.

villi (VIL-eye) Fingerlike protrusions into the small intestine that participate in digestion and absorption of foodstuff.

virus The smallest known type of infectious agent, many of which cause disease in humans. Viruses do not metabolize, grow, or move by themselves. They reproduce by the aid of a living cellular host. A virus is essentially a piece of genetic material surrounded by a coat of protein.

visual cycle A chemical process in the eye that participates in vision. Forms of vitamin A participate in the process.

vitamin A A fat-soluble vitamin that exists in retinoid and carotenoid forms and is crucial to vision in dim light, color vision, cell differentiation, growth, and immunity. Significant food sources are beef liver, sweet potato, spinach, and mangoes.

vitamin B-6 A group of water-soluble vitamins that, in coenzyme form, play a role in more than 100 enzymatic reactions in the body, almost all of which involve nitrogen-containing compounds. These reactions include amino acid metabolism, heme synthesis, and homocysteine metabolism. Salmon, potatoes, and bananas are good sources.

vitamin B-12 A water-soluble vitamin that shares a close relationship with folate. In coenzyme form it participates in folate metabolism, in the citric acid cycle, and in the metabolism of fatty acids. Meats and shellfish are good sources; plants do not synthesize vitamin B-12.

vitamin C A water-soluble vitamin that is involved in many processes in the body, primarily as an electron donor; it is also known as ascorbic acid. Vitamin C contributes to collagen synthesis, iron absorption, and immune function. It also likely has in vivo antioxidant capability. Fruits and vegetables in general contain some vitamin C; citrus fruit, green vegetables, tomatoes, peppers, and potatoes are especially good sources.

vitamin D A fat-soluble vitamin that is crucial to maintenance of intracellular and extracellular calcium concentrations; it exists in cholecalciferol and ergocalciferol forms. Vitamin D is abundant in fatty fish such as herring, eel, salmon, and sardines. In North America, milk is generally fortified with 10 micrograms of vitamin D per quart.

vitamin E A fat-soluble vitamin that functions in the body as an antioxidant, preventing the propagation of free radicals; it exists as tocopherols or tocotrienols. Significant food sources are seeds, nuts, and plant oils.

vitamin K A fat-soluble vitamin that contributes to the synthesis by the liver of blood-clotting factors and the synthesis of bone proteins; it exists as phylloquinone or menaquinone. Green leafy vegetables such as brussels sprouts, kale, and lettuce are excellent sources.

vitamins Compounds needed in very small amounts in the diet to help regulate and support chemical reactions in the body.

VO_{2max} Maximum volume of oxygen that can be consumed per unit of time.

water The universal solvent of life; chemically, H_2O. The body is composed of about 60% water. Water (fluid) needs are about 13 8-oz cups per day for men and about 9 for women; needs are greater if one exercises heavily. Water serves as a solvent for many chemical compounds, provides a medium in which many chemical reactions occur, and actively participates as a reactant or becomes a product in some reactions. Without water, biological processes necessary to life would cease in a matter of days.

water-soluble vitamins Vitamins that dissolve in water. These vitamins are the B-vitamins and vitamin C.

Wernicke-Korsakoff syndrome Thiamin-deficiency disease caused by excessive alcohol consumption. Symptoms include eye problems, difficulty walking, and deranged mental functions.

whey (WAY) Proteins, such as lactalbumin, that are found in great amounts in human milk and are easy to digest.

white blood cells One of the formed elements of the circulating blood system; also called *leukocytes.* Five types of leukocytes are lymphocytes, monocytes, neutrophils, basophils, and eosinophils. White blood cells are able to squeeze through intracellular spaces and migrate. Leukocytes phagocytize bacteria, fungi, and viruses as well as detoxify proteins that may result from allergic reactions, cellular injury, and other immune system cells.

whole grains Grains containing the entire seed of the plant, including the bran, germ, and endosperm (starchy interior). Examples are whole wheat and brown rice.

xanthine dehydrogenase (ZAN-thin de-HY-droj-eh-nase) An enzyme containing molybdenum and iron that functions in the formation of uric acid and the mobilization of iron from liver ferritin stores.

xenobiotic (ZEE-no-bye-OT-ic) Compound that is foreign to the body. The principal classes are drugs, chemical carcinogens, and environmental substances such as pesticides.

xerophthalmia (zer-op-THAL-mee-uh) A condition marked by dryness of the cornea and eye membranes that results from vitamin A deficiency and can lead to blindness. The specific cause is a lack of mucus production by the eye, which then leaves it more vulnerable to surface dirt and bacterial infections.

xylitol (ZY-lih-tol) An alcohol derivative of the 5-carbon monosaccharide xylose.

Yersinia enterocolitica **(yer-SIN-ee-ya)** Bacteria found throughout the environment; present in feces; can contaminate food and water. It multiplies rapidly at room and refrigerator temperatures and is destroyed by thorough cooking.

zinc A trace mineral required for many enzymes, including those that participate in antioxidant enzyme systems. Zinc also stabilizes cell membranes and other body molecules. Seafood, meats, and whole grains are good sources.

zygote (ZY-goat) The fertilized ovum; the cell resulting from the union of an egg cell (ovum) and sperm until it divides.

zymogen (ZY-mow-gin) An inactive form of an enzyme that requires the removal of a minor part of the chemical structure for it to work. The zymogen is converted into an active enzyme at the appropriate time, such as when released into the stomach or small intestine.

Credits

© CORBIS website; **(bottom):** © PhotoDisc/Vol. 20; **p. 278 (top):** Ryan McVay/Getty Images; **(bottom):** © PhotoDisc Website; **p. 281(a,b):** Arthur Glauberman/Photo Researchers, Inc.; **p. 283:** © PhotoDisc/Vol. 25; **p. 284:** © CORBIS website; **p. 285:** McGraw-Hill Companies, Inc./Gary He, photographer; **p. 286:** © PhotoDisc Website; **p. 287:** Ryan McVay/Getty Images; **p. 288:** © PhotoDisc/Vol. 94

Chapter9

Opener: © PhotoDisc/Vol. 94; **p. 297:** Reproduced with permission. © Culinary Hearts Kitchen, 1982 © American Heart Association; **p. 304:** © Greg Kidd & Joanne Scott; **Fig 9-5 (both):** © PhotoDisc/Vol. 58; **Fig 9-6:** A Colour Atlas and Text of Nutritional Disorders by Dr. Donald D. McLaren/Mosby-Wolfe Europe Ltd.; **p. 310:** M. Freeman/PhotoLink/Getty Images; **Fig 9-10:** A Colour Atlas and Text of Nutritional Disorders by Dr. Donald D. McLaren/Mosby-Wolfe Europe Ltd.; **p. 315:** Hisham F. Ibrahim/Getty Images; **p. 316:** © Greg Kidd & Joanne Scott; **p. 321:** © Greg Kidd & Joanne Scott; **Fig 9-13:** © CORBIS/Vol. 83; **p. 324:** © CORBIS/Vol. 83; **p. 326:** © CORBIS website; **p. 328:** © PhotoDisc/Vol. 67

Chapter10

Opener: © PhotoDisc/Vol. 79; **p. 340:** Courtesy of National Pork Producers Council; **Fig 10-3:** A Colour Atlas and Text of Nutritional Disorders by Dr. Donald D. McLaren/Mosby-Wolfe Europe Ltd.; **p. 346:** CORBIS Modern Cuisine Vol. 43/MCU0062; **Fig 10-4:** A Colour Atlas and Text of Nutritional Disorders by Dr. Donald D. McLaren/Mosby-Wolfe Europe Ltd.; **p. 349:** © Mark Kempf; **p. 353:** CORBIS Food Perspectives Vol. 130/FPE0061; **p. 354:** © CORBIS/Vol. 202; **Fig 10-6 (top):** Michael Abbey/Photo Researchers, Inc.; **(bottom):** Biophoto Associates/SPL/Photo Researchers, Inc.; **p. 363:** CORBIS Vol. 30/FOD0028; **Fig 10-9:** A Colour Atlas and Text of Nutritional Disorders by Dr. Donald D. McLaren/Mosby-Wolfe Europe Ltd.;

p. 366: © Lex van Lieshout/imageshop/RF Alamy Images; **p. 368:** A Colour Atlas and Text of Nutritional Disorders by Dr. Donald D. McLaren/Mosby-Wolfe Europe Ltd.; **p. 369:** © Digital Vision; **p. 372:** Michael Matisse/Getty Images; **p. 379:** © Image Source/PunchStock; **p. 380:** Scott T. Baxter/Getty Images

Chapter 11

Opener: Ryan McVay/Getty Images; **p. 388:** © PhotoDisc; **p. 393, 394, 395:** MHHE Image Library; **p. 398 (top):** © CORBIS/Vol. 552; **(bottom):** © PhotoDisc; **p. 400:** Ryan McVay/Getty Images; **p. 401:** MHHE Image Library; **p. 402:** © PhotoDisc/Vol. 40; **p. 404 (top):** Rob Melnychuk/Getty Images; **(bottom):** MHHE Image Library; **p. 411:** The McGraw-Hill Companies, Inc./Andrew Resek, photographer; **p. 414:** © Yoav Levy/Phototake; **p. 416:** CORBIS Modern Cuisine/MCU0020; **p. 417:** CORBIS/CB012177; **p. 418:** © CORBIS website

Chapter 12

Opener: © PhotoDisc/Vol. 70; **p. 427:** Michael Lamotte/Cole Group/Getty Images; **p. 428:** Ohio State University Extension/Malcolm W. Emmons; **p. 429:** © PhotoDisc/Vol. 48; **Fig 12-3a:** SPL/Photo Researchers, Inc.; **Fig 12-3b:** Omikron/Photo Researchers, Inc.; **p. 433:** Ryan McVay/Getty Images; **p. 435:** Ohio State University Extension; **p. 437 (top):** © PhotoDisc/Vol. 59; **(bottom):** © CORBIS/Vol. #130; **Fig 12-4:** Dr. Amanda S. Prasad/American Journal of Medicine; **p. 439:** Courtesy Fishery Products Internationals, Danvers, MA; **p. 443:** © CORBIS/Vol. 43; **p. 444:** RF/CORBIS; **p. 446:** © Paul Casamassimo, DDS, MS; **p. 447:** © PhotoDisc/Vol. 02; **p. 448 (top):** CORBIS/CB035895; **(bottom):** Gordon Wardlaw; **p. 449:** MHHE Image Library; **p. 451:** Ryan McVay/Getty Images; **p. 452:** MHHE Image Library; **p. 458 (both):** © PhotoDisc/OS49; **p. 464:** The McGraw-Hill Companies, Inc./Andrew Resek, photographer

Chapter 13

Opener: Ryan McVay/Getty Images; **p. 469:** © CORBIS/Vol. 130; **p. 472:** The McGraw-Hill Companies, Inc./Gary He, photographer; **Fig 13-4:** © Samuel Ashfield/SPL/Photo Researchers, Inc.; **p. 481:** Pando Hall/Getty Images; **Fig 13-8:** © Rich O'Quihn University of Georgia; **Fig 13-9:** Courtesy of Life Measurement Instruments; **Fig 13-10 (all):** Diane Linsley/Linsley Photographics; **Fig 13-11:** © Gordon Wardlaw; **Fig 13-10:** DEXA; **p. 490:** © The Ohio State University Communications Photo Service, Jodi Miller; **p. 491:** © PhotoDisc/Vol. 82; **Fig 13-16 (1):** © Digital Vision; **Fig 13-16 (2):** JupiterImages; **Fig 13-16 (3):** Ryan McVay/Getty Images; **p. 495:** © PhotoDisc/Vol. 76; **p. 497:** © PhotoDisc/Vol. 20; **p. 498:** RF Getty Images; **p. 499:** © PhotoDisc/Vol. 20; **p. 503:** © PhotoDisc/Vol. 67

Chapter 14

Opener, p. 521 & 523: © PhotoDisc/EP040; **p. 524 (top):** © CORBIS/Vol. 223; **(bottom):** Karl Weatherly/Getty Images; **p. 525:** © PhotoDisc/Sports Metaphors; **p. 531:** © CORBIS/Vol. 20; **p. 532:** Ryan McVay/Getty Images; **p. 534 (top):** © James Mulligan; **(bottom):** RF/CORBIS; **p. 538 (top):** © Gordon Wardlaw; **(bottom):** PhotoLink/Getty Images; **p. 541:** © Royalty-Free/CORBIS; **p. 542:** © PhotoDisc/Vol. 51; **p. 543:** © CORBIS/Vol. 103; **p. 545:** © Getty Images/Vol. 1/Photolink; **p. 546:** McGraw-Hill Companies, Inc./Gary He, photographer; **p. 547:** Steve Cole/Getty Images

Chapter 15

Opener: © PhotoDisc/Vol. 67; **p. 560:** The McGraw-Hill Companies, Inc./Lars A. Niki, photographer; **p. 562 (top):** © PhotoDisc Website; **(bottom) & p. 563:** © Royalty-Free/CORBIS; **p. 564:** Ryan McVay/Getty Images; **p. 565:** Jim Arbogast/Getty Images; **p. 568 (top):** © PhotoDisc/Vol. 95; **(bottom):**

© Tom Steward Photography/CORBIS; **p. 570:** Royalty-Free/CORBIS; **p. 571:** © PhotoDisc/EP047; **p. 572 (top):** © PhotoDisc website; **Fig 15-3:** © Paul Casamassimo, DDS, MS; **p. 573:** © PhotoDisc/Vol. 83; **p. 574:** RF/CORBIS; **p. 575 (top):** © CORBIS/Vol. 552; **(bottom):** © PhotoDisc website; **p. 576:** © Royalty-Free/CORBIS; **p. 577:** The McGraw-Hill Companies, Inc./Gary He, photographer; **p. 579:** The McGraw-Hill Companies, Inc./Lars A. Niki, photographer

Chapter 16

Opener: © PhotoDisc/Vol. 46; **p. 589:** © CORBIS/Vol. 19; **p. 590:** Keith Brofsky/Getty Images; **p. 593:** Don Tremain/Getty Images; **p. 594:** Adam Crowley/Getty Images; **p. 596:** Getty Images; **p. 597:** Tracy Montana/PhotoLink/Getty Images; **p. 598:** RF/CORBIS; **p. 601:** USDA; **p. 602:** EyeWire Collection/Getty Images; **p. 603:** USDA; **p. 605:** © CORBIS/Vol. 83; **p. 607:** USDA; **p. 611:** © PhotoDisc/Vol. 192; **p. 612:** © Digital Vision/PunchStock; **p. 613:** © PhotoDisc/EP039; **p. 614:** © Royalty-Free/CORBIS

Chapter 17

Opener: © PhotoDisc/Vol. 61; **p. 623:** © PhotoDisc/EP077; **p. 626:** © PhotoDisc/Vol. 113; **p. 627:** © CORBIS/Vol. 135; **p. 631:** © CORBIS/Vol. 9; **p. 632 (top):** © PhotoDisc/Vol. 58; **(bottom):** © PhotoDisc/Vol. 113; **p. 634:** © CORBIS/Vol. 26; **p. 635:** © PhotoDisc/Vol. 113; **Fig 17-5:** © Paul Casamassimo, DDS,

MS; **p. 637:** Ryan McVay/Getty Images; **p. 638:** © CORBIS/Vol. 552; **p. 639:** Tim Hall/Getty Images; **p. 643:** © Greg Kidd and Joanne Scott; **p. 645:** © Joanne Scott; **p. 648:** USDA Photo by: Ken Hammond; **p. 649:** © Creatas/PunchStock; **p. 650:** © CORBIS/Vol. 124; **p. 651:** © CORBIS/Vol. 552; **p. 652 (top):** © CORBIS/Vol. 124; **(bottom):** © image100 Ltd; **p. 653:** RF/CORBIS; **p. 654:** Getty Images; **p. 656:** © CORBIS/Vol. 19; **p. 657 (top):** © PhotoDisc/Vol. 95; **(bottom):** © Stockbyte/PunchStock; **p. 658:** © PhotoDisc Website; **p. 662:** The McGraw-Hill Companies, Inc./Jill Braaten, photographer

Chapter 18

Opener: © PhotoDisc Website; **p. 667:** © RF/CORBIS; **p. 668:** Rim Light/PhotoLink/Getty Images; **p. 670 (both):** RF/CORBIS; **p. 672:** Mitch Hrdlicka/Getty Images; **p. 674:** Steve Mason/Getty Images; **p. 675:** © PhotoDisc website; **p. 676:** © CORBIS/Vol. 81; **p. 678 (both):** © RF/CORBIS; **p. 680:** © CORBIS/Vol. 81; **p. 681:** © Gordon Wardlaw; **p. 682:** Mitch Hrdlicka/Getty Images; **p. 686 (top):** © Gordon Wardlaw; **(bottom):** Keith Brofsky/Getty Images; **p. 687 (top):** Steve Mason/Getty Images; **(bottom):** © CORBIS/EP038; **p. 688:** © Getty Images/Digital Vision; **p. 689 & 690:** © PhotoDisc/Vol. 58; **p. 691:** © Royalty-Free/CORBIS; **p. 696:** © PhotoDisc/SS45

Chapter 19

Opener: © Digital Vision; **p. 701:**

© CORBIS/Vol. 12; **p. 707:** © Greg Wolff; **p. 712:** © The Ohio State University Communcations Photo Service; **p. 714:** Bob Montesclaros/Cole Group/Getty Images; **p. 716:** RF/CORBIS; **p. 717:** National Pork Producers Council; **p. 721:** © CORBIS/Vol. 83; **p. 722:** Jules Frazier/Getty Images; **p. 723:** © Object Series 36/PhotoDisc; **Fig 19-3a,b:** © Gordon Wardlaw; **p. 725:** © The Ohio State University Communications Photo Service; **p. 726:** RF/CORBIS; **p. 727:** © Royalty-Free/CORBIS; **p. 729:** Getty Images; **p. 731:** © The Ohio State University Communications Photo Service, Lloyd Lemmermann; **p. 732 (top):** © PhotoDisc/Vol. 49; **(bottom):** © PhotoDisc website; **p. 733:** © CORBIS/Vol. 552

Chapter 20

Opener: © PhotoDisc Website; **p. 744 (both):** © The Ohio State University Communications Photo Service; **Fig 20-1(reaching for food):** RF/CORBIS; **(others):** AP Wide World Photo; **p. 745:** RF/CORBIS; **p. 747:** USDA photo by Peter Manzelli; **p. 750:** © Royalty-Free/CORBIS; **p. 751:** © PhotoDisc/Vol. 25; **p. 753 & 754 (top):** © The McGraw-Hill Companies, Inc./Barry Barker, photographer; **(bottom):** © Getty Images/Digital Vision; **p. 756:** RF/CORBIS; **p. 758:** © CORBIS/Vol. 25; **p. 760:** PhotoLink/Getty Images; **p. 763:** Santokh Kochar/Getty Images; **p. 765 (top):** © CORBIS/Vol. 609; **(bottom):** © The Ohio State University Communications Photo Service, Jodi Miller

Index

Dietary Reference Intakes (DRIs): Recommended Intakes for Individuals, Electrolytes and Water

Food and Nutrition Board, Institute of Medicine, National Academies

Life Stage Group	Sodium (mg/d)	Potassium (mg/d)	Chloride (mg/d)	Water (L/d)
Infants				
0–6 mo	120*	400*	180*	0.7*
7–12 mo	370*	700*	570*	0.8*
Children				
1–3 y	1,000*	3,000*	1,500*	1.3*
4–8 y	1,200*	3,800*	1,900*	1.7*
Males				
9–13 y	1,500*	4,500*	2,300*	2.4*
14–18 y	1,500*	4,700*	2,300*	3.3*
19–30 y	1,500*	4,700*	2,300*	3.7*
31–50 y	1,500*	4,700*	2,300*	3.7*
51–70 y	1,300*	4,700*	2,000*	3.7*
> 70 y	1,200*	4,700*	1,800*	3.7*
Females				
9–13 y	1,500*	4,500*	2,300*	2.1*
14–18 y	1,500*	4,700*	2,300*	2.3*
19–30 y	1,500*	4,700*	2,300*	2.7*
31–50 y	1,500*	4,700*	2,300*	2.7*
51–70 y	1,300*	4,700*	2,000*	2.7*
> 70 y	1,200*	4,700*	1,800*	2.7*
Pregnancy				
14–18 y	1,500*	4,700*	2,300*	3.0*
19–50 y	1,500*	4,700*	2,300*	3.0*
Lactation				
14–18 y	1,500*	5,100*	2,300*	3.8*
19–50 y	1,500*	5,100*	2,300*	3.8*

NOTE: The table is adapted from the DRI reports. See www.nap.edu. Adequate Intakes (AIs) are followed by an asterisk(*). These may be used as a goal for individual intake. For healthy breastfed infants, the AI is the average intake. The AI for other life stage and gender groups is believed to cover the needs of all individuals in the group, but lack of data prevent being able to specify with confidence the percentage of individuals covered by this intake; therefore, no Recommended Dietary Allowance (RDA) was set.

SOURCE: *Dietary Reference Intakes for Water, Potassium, Sodium, Chloride, and Sulfate.* This report may be accessed via www.nap.edu.

Acceptable Macronutrient Distribution Ranges

Macronutrient	Range (percent of energy)		
	Children, 1–3 y	**Children, 4–18 y**	**Adults**
Fat	30–40	25–35	20–35
omega-6 polyunsaturated fats (linoleic acid)	5–10	5–10	5–10
omega-3 polyunsaturated fats[a] (α-linolenic acid)	0.6–1.2	0.6–1.2	0.6–1.2
Carbohydrate	45–65	45–65	45–65
Protein	5–20	10–30	10–35

[a]Approximately 10% of the total can come from longer-chain n-3 fatty acids.

SOURCE: *Dietary Reference Intakes for Energy, Carbohydrate, Fiber, Fat, Fatty Acids, Cholesterol, Protein, and Amino Acids* (2002). The report may be accessed via www.nar.edu.

Dietary Reference Intakes (DRIs): Tolerable Upper Intake Levels (UL[a]) , Vitamins

Food and Nutrition Board, Institute of Medicine, National Academies

Life Stage Group	Vitamin A (μg/d)[b]	Vitamin C (mg/d)	Vitamin D (μg/d)	Vitamin E (mg/d)[c,d]	Vitamin K	Thiamin	Riboflavin	Niacin (mg/d)[d]	Vitamin B-6 (mg/d)	Folate (μg/d)[d]	Vitamin B-12	Pantothenic Acid	Biotin	Choline (g/d)	Carotenoids[e]
Infants															
0–6 mo	600	ND[f]	25	ND	ND	ND	ND	ND	ND	ND	ND	ND	ND	ND	ND
7–12 mo	600	ND	25	ND	ND	ND	ND	ND	ND	ND	ND	ND	ND	ND	ND
Children															
1–3 y	600	400	50	200	ND	ND	ND	10	30	300	ND	ND	ND	1.0	ND
4–8 y	900	650	50	300	ND	ND	ND	15	40	400	ND	ND	ND	1.0	ND
Males, Females															
9–13 y	1,700	1,200	50	600	ND	ND	ND	20	60	600	ND	ND	ND	2.0	ND
14–18 y	2,800	1,800	50	800	ND	ND	ND	30	80	800	ND	ND	ND	3.0	ND
19–70 y	3,000	2,000	50	1,000	ND	ND	ND	35	100	1,000	ND	ND	ND	3.5	ND
>70 y	3,000	2,000	50	1,000	ND	ND	ND	35	100	1,000	ND	ND	ND	3.5	ND
Pregnancy															
≤18 y	2,800	1,800	50	800	ND	ND	ND	30	80	800	ND	ND	ND	3.0	ND
19–50 y	3,000	2,000	50	1,000	ND	ND	ND	35	100	1,000	ND	ND	ND	3.5	ND
Lactation															
≤18 y	2,800	1,800	50	800	ND	ND	ND	30	80	800	ND	ND	ND	3.0	ND
19–50 y	3,000	2,000	50	1,000	ND	ND	ND	35	100	1,000	ND	ND	ND	3.5	ND

[a]UL = The maximum level of daily nutrient intake that is likely to pose no risk of adverse effects. Unless otherwise specified, the UL represents total intake from food, water, and supplements. Due to lack of suitable data, ULs could not be established for vitamin K, thiamin, riboflavin, vitamin B-12, pantothenic acid, biotin, or carotenoids. In the absence of ULs, extra caution may be warranted in consuming levels above recommended intakes.

[b]As preformed vitamin A only.

[c]As α-tocopherol; applies to any form of supplemental α-tocopherol.

[d]The ULs for vitamin E, niacin, and folate apply to synthetic forms obtained from supplements, fortified foods, or a combination of the two.

[e]β-Carotene supplements are advised only to serve as a provitamin A source for individuals at risk of vitamin A deficiency.

[f]ND = Not determinable due to lack of data of adverse effects in this age group and concern with regard to lack of ability to handle excess amounts. Source of intake should be from food only to prevent high levels of intake.

SOURCES: Dietary Reference Intakes for Calcium, Phosphorus, Magnesium, Vitamin D, and Fluoride (1997); Dietary Reference Intakes for Thiamin, Riboflavin, Niacin, Vitamin B-6, Folate, Vitamin B-12, Pantothenic Acid, Biotin, and Choline (1998); Dietary Reference Intakes for Vitamin C, Vitamin E, Selenium, and Carotenoids (2000); and Dietary Reference Intakes for Vitamin A, Vitamin K, Arsenic, Boron, Chromium, Copper, Iodine, Iron, Manganese, Molybdenum, Nickel, Silicon, Vanadium, and Zinc (2001). These reports may be accessed via www.nap.edu.